THIRD EDITION

Community Health Nursing
Caring for the Public's Health

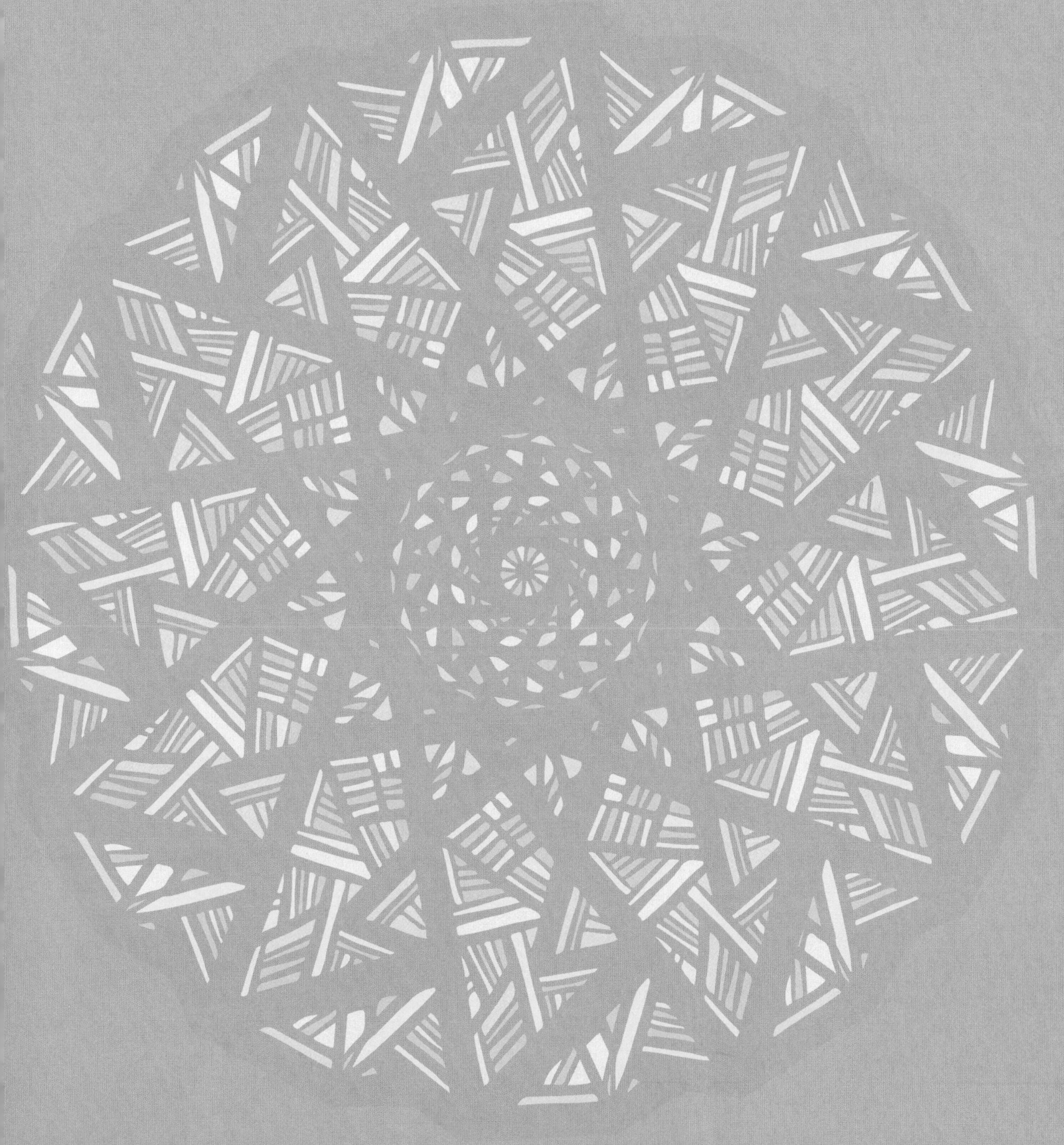

The Pedagogy

Community Health Nursing: Caring for the Public's Health, Third Edition, drives comprehension through various strategies that meet the learning needs of students, while also generating enthusiasm about the topic. This interactive approach addresses different learning styles, making this the ideal text to ensure mastery of key concepts. The pedagogical aids that appear in most chapters include the following:

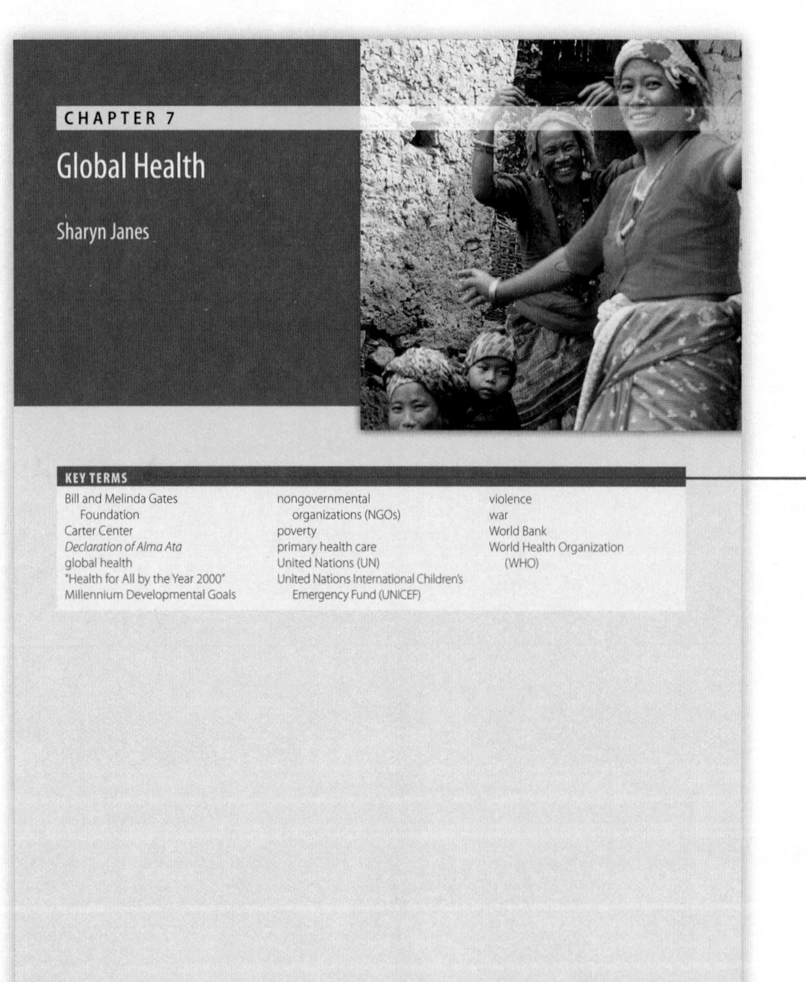

CHAPTER 7

Global Health

Sharyn Janes

KEY TERMS

Bill and Melinda Gates Foundation
Carter Center
Declaration of Alma Ata
global health
"Health for All by the Year 2000"
Millennium Developmental Goals
nongovernmental organizations (NGOs)
poverty
primary health care
United Nations (UN)
United Nations International Children's Emergency Fund (UNICEF)
violence
war
World Bank
World Health Organization (WHO)

Key Terms Found in a list at the beginning of each chapter, these terms will create an expanded vocabulary in community health nursing.

Questions to Consider These questions provide instructors and students with a snapshot of key information in each chapter. They serve as a checklist to help guide and focus study.

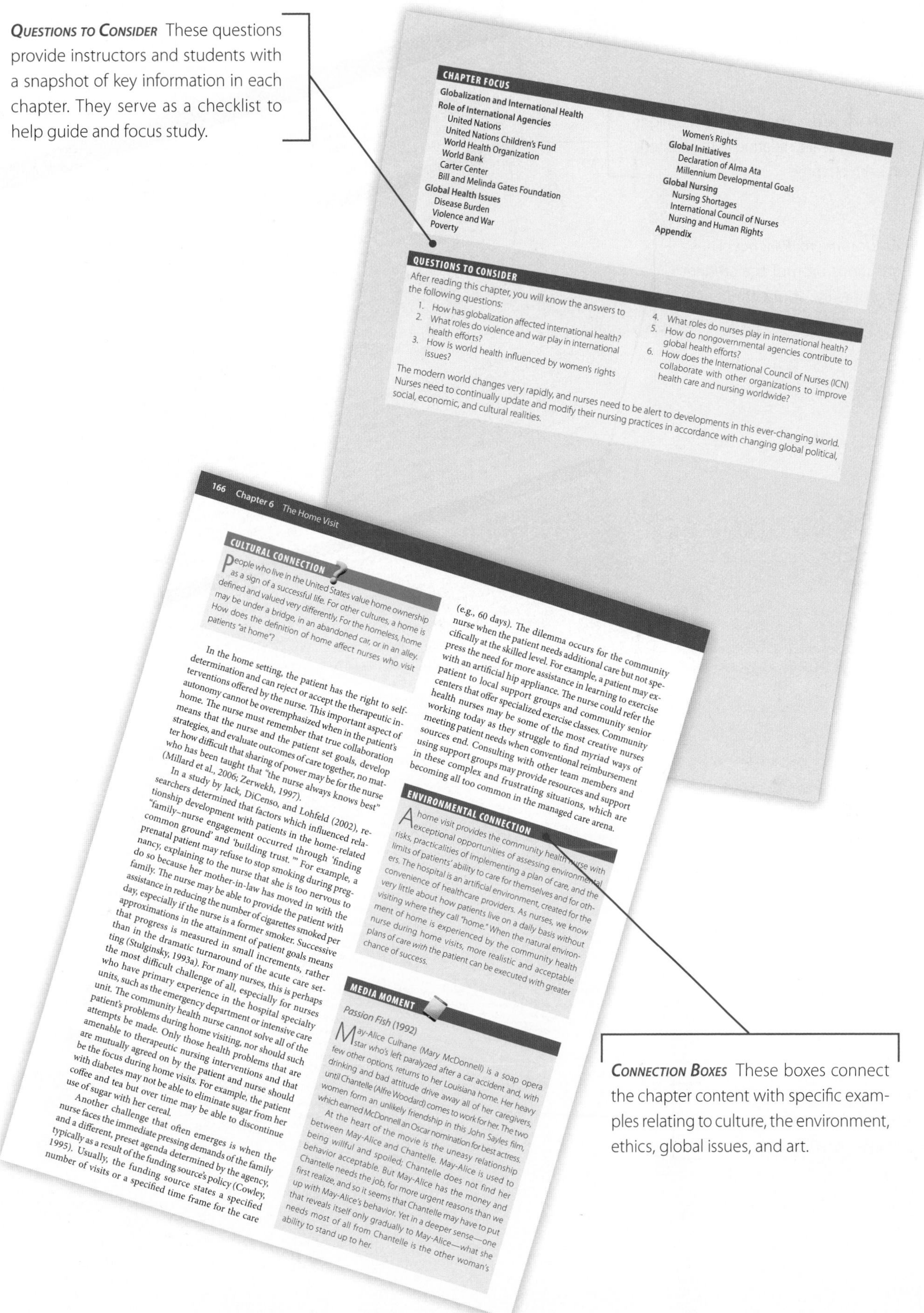

CHAPTER FOCUS

Globalization and International Health
Role of International Agencies
United Nations
United Nations Children's Fund
World Health Organization
World Bank
Carter Center
Bill and Melinda Gates Foundation
Global Health Issues
Disease Burden
Violence and War
Poverty
Women's Rights
Global Initiatives
Declaration of Alma Ata
Millennium Developmental Goals
Global Nursing
Nursing Shortages
International Council of Nurses
Nursing and Human Rights
Appendix

QUESTIONS TO CONSIDER

After reading this chapter, you will know the answers to the following questions:

1. How has globalization affected international health?
2. What roles do violence and war play in international health efforts?
3. How is world health influenced by women's rights issues?
4. What roles do nurses play in international health?
5. How do nongovernmental agencies contribute to global health efforts?
6. How does the International Council of Nurses (ICN) collaborate with other organizations to improve health care and nursing worldwide?

The modern world changes very rapidly, and nurses need to be alert to developments in this ever-changing world. Nurses need to continually update and modify their nursing practices in accordance with changing global political, social, economic, and cultural realities.

166 Chapter 6 The Home Visit

CULTURAL CONNECTION

People who live in the United States value home ownership as a sign of a successful life. For other cultures, a home is defined and valued very differently. For the homeless, home may be under a bridge, in an abandoned car, or in an alley. How does the definition of home affect nurses who visit patients "at home"?

In the home setting, the patient has the right to self-determination and can reject or accept the therapeutic interventions offered by the nurse. This important aspect of autonomy cannot be overemphasized when in the patient's home. The nurse must remember that true collaboration means that the nurse and the patient set goals, develop strategies, and evaluate outcomes of care together, no matter how difficult that sharing of power may be for the nurse who has been taught that "the nurse always knows best" (Millard et al., 2006; Zerwekh, 1997).

In a study by Jack, DiCenso, and Lohfeld (2002), researchers determined that factors which influenced relationship development with patients in the home-related "family–nurse engagement occurred through 'finding common ground' and 'building trust.'" For example, a prenatal patient may refuse to stop smoking during pregnancy, explaining to the nurse that she is too nervous to do so because her mother-in-law has moved in with the family. The nurse may be able to provide the patient with assistance in reducing the number of cigarettes smoked per day, especially if the nurse is a former smoker. Successive approximations in the attainment of patient goals means that progress is measured in small increments, rather than in the dramatic turnaround of the acute care setting (Stulginsky, 1993a). For many nurses, this is perhaps the most difficult challenge of all, especially for nurses who have primary experience in the hospital specialty units, such as the emergency department or intensive care unit. The community health nurse cannot solve all of the patient's problems during home visiting, nor should such attempts be made. Only those health problems that are amenable to therapeutic nursing interventions and that are mutually agreed on by the patient and nurse should be the focus during home visits. For example, the patient with diabetes may not be able to eliminate sugar from her coffee and tea but over time may be able to discontinue use of sugar with her cereal.

Another challenge that often emerges is when the nurse faces the immediate pressing demands of the family and a different, preset agenda determined by the agency, typically as a result of the funding source's policy (Cowley, 1995). Usually, the funding source states a specified number of visits or a specified time frame for the care (e.g., 60 days). The dilemma occurs for the community nurse when the patient needs additional care but not specifically at the skilled level. For example, a patient may express the need for more assistance in learning to exercise with an artificial hip appliance. The nurse could refer the patient to local support groups and community senior centers that offer specialized exercise classes. Community health nurses may be some of the most creative nurses working today as they struggle to find myriad ways of meeting patient needs when conventional reimbursement sources end. Consulting with other team members and using support groups may provide resources and support in these complex and frustrating situations, which are becoming all too common in the managed care arena.

ENVIRONMENTAL CONNECTION

A home visit provides the community health nurse with exceptional opportunities of assessing environmental risks, practicalities of implementing a plan of care, and the limits of patients' ability to care for themselves and for others. The hospital is an artificial environment, created for the convenience of healthcare providers. As nurses, we know very little about how patients live on a daily basis without visiting where they call "home." When the natural environment of home is experienced by the community health nurse during home visits, more realistic and acceptable plans of care with the patient can be executed with greater chance of success.

MEDIA MOMENT

Passion Fish (1992)

May-Alice Culhane (Mary McDonnell) is a soap opera star who's left paralyzed after a car accident and, with few other options, returns to her Louisiana home. Her heavy drinking and bad attitude drive away all of her caregivers, until Chantelle (Alfre Woodard) comes to work for her. The two women form an unlikely friendship in this John Sayles film, which earned McDonnell an Oscar nomination for best actress.

At the heart of the movie is the uneasy relationship between May-Alice and Chantelle. May-Alice is used to being willful and spoiled; Chantelle does not find her behavior acceptable. But May-Alice has the money and Chantelle needs the job, for more urgent reasons than we first realize, and so it seems that Chantelle may have to put up with May-Alice's behavior. Yet in a deeper sense—one that reveals itself only gradually to May-Alice—what she needs most of all from Chantelle is the other woman's ability to stand up to her.

Connection Boxes These boxes connect the chapter content with specific examples relating to culture, the environment, ethics, global issues, and art.

Research Alert These boxes highlight current research relating to the content in each chapter.

Application to Practice These questions prompt the student to critically apply their new knowledge to real-life situations.

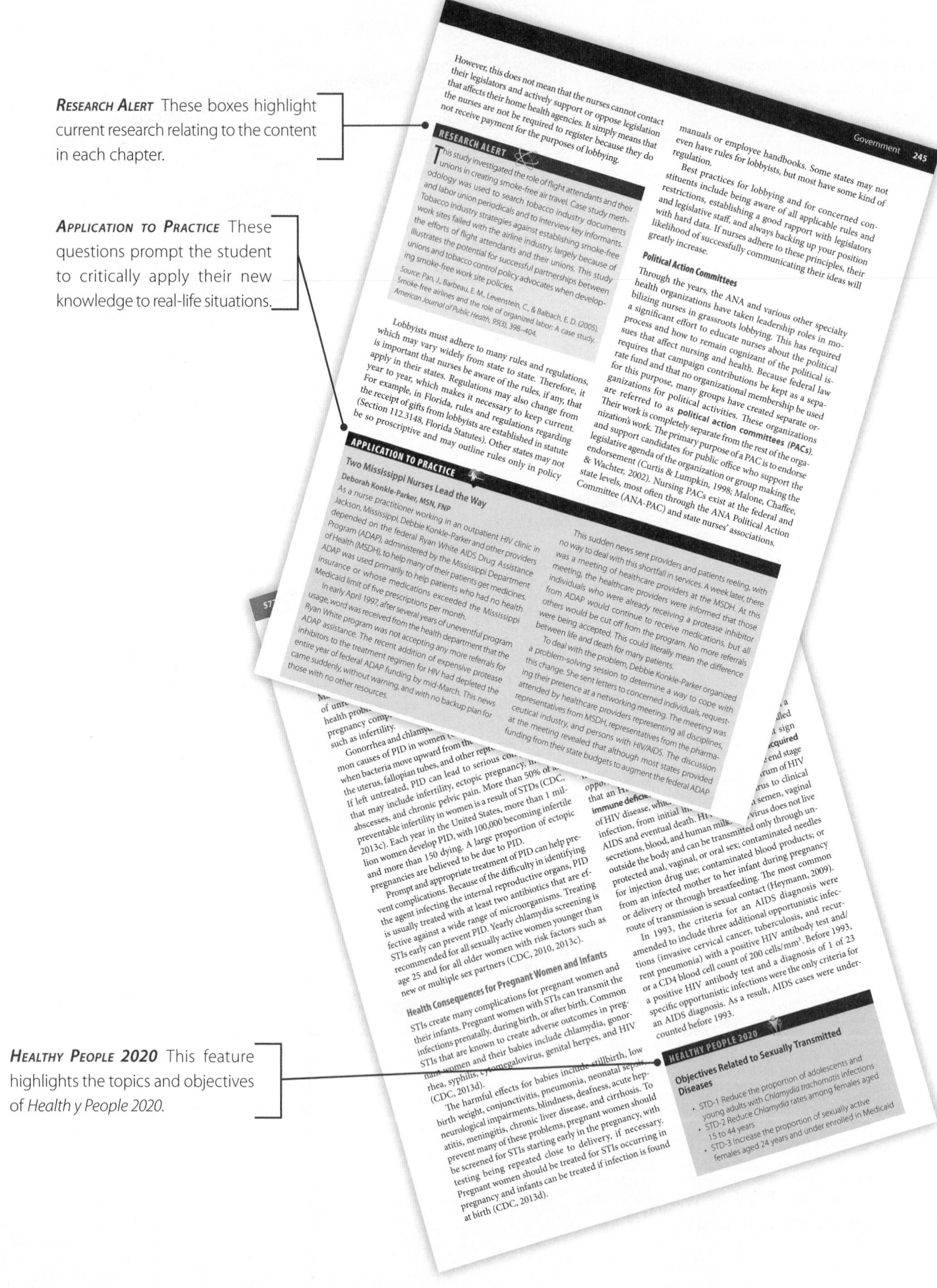

Healthy People 2020 This feature highlights the topics and objectives of *Health y People 2020.*

Affordable Care Act This feature highlights issues related to the Affordable Care Act.

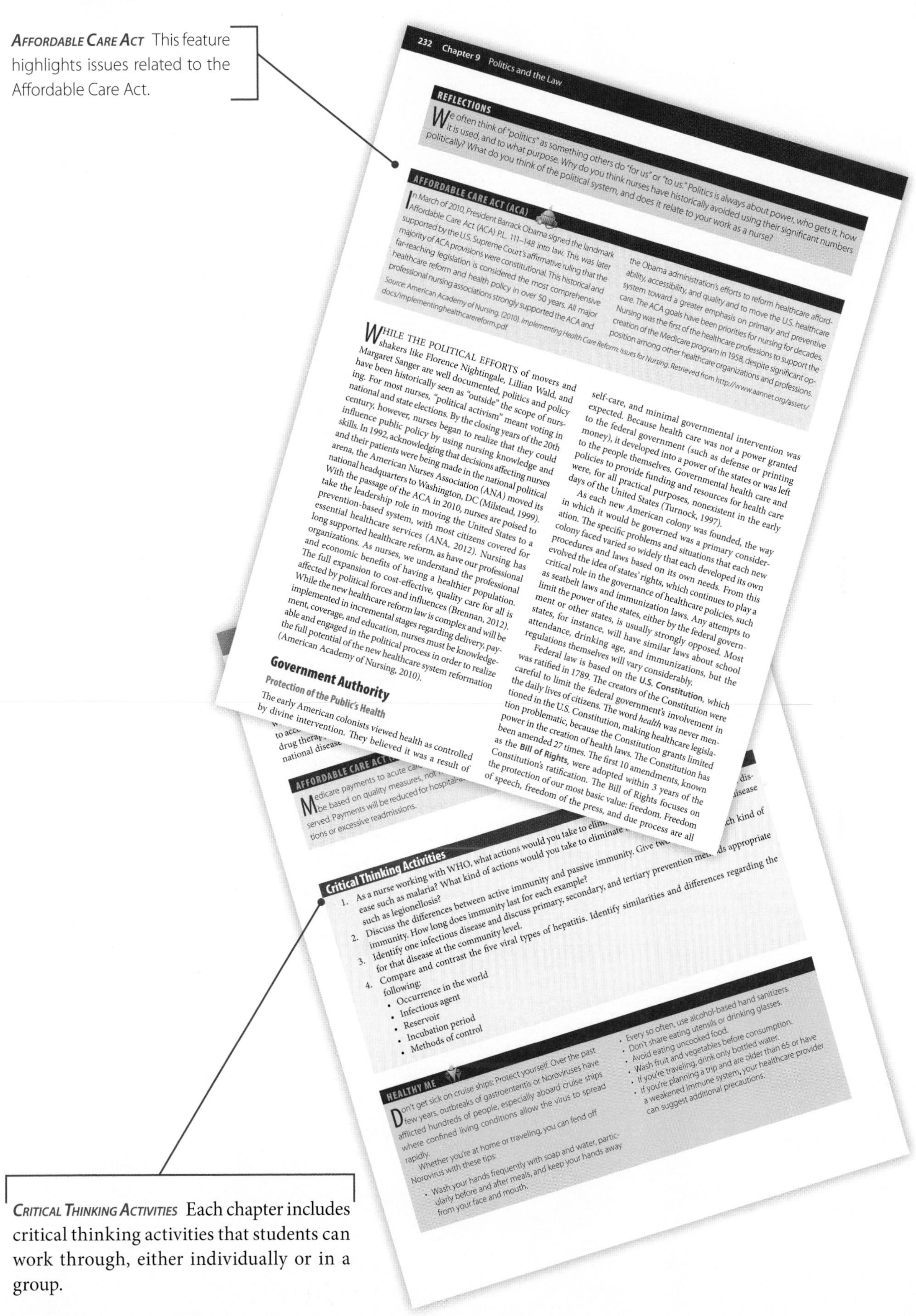

Critical Thinking Activities Each chapter includes critical thinking activities that students can work through, either individually or in a group.

THIRD EDITION

Community Health Nursing
Caring for the Public's Health

Edited by

KAREN SAUCIER LUNDY, PHD, RN, FAAN
Professor Emeritus
College of Nursing
The University of Southern Mississippi
Hattiesburg, Mississippi

SHARYN JANES, PHD, RN
Professor Emeritus
School of Nursing
Florida Agricultural and Mechanical University
Tallahassee, Florida

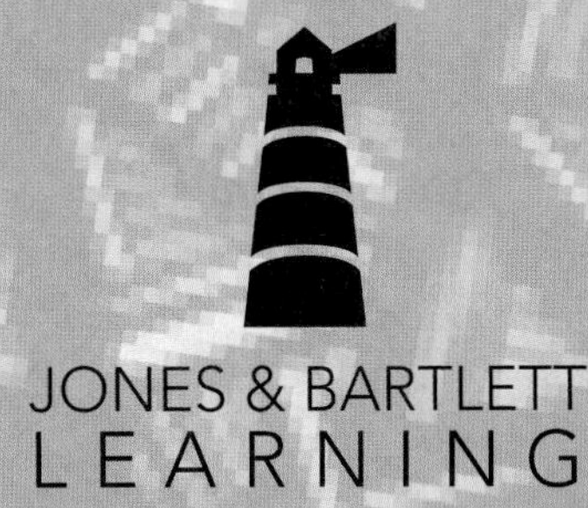

World Headquarters
Jones & Bartlett Learning
5 Wall Street
Burlington, MA 01803
978-443-5000
info@jblearning.com
www.jblearning.com

Jones & Bartlett Learning books and products are available through most bookstores and online booksellers. To contact Jones & Bartlett Learning directly, call 800-832-0034, fax 978-443-8000, or visit our website, www.jblearning.com.

Substantial discounts on bulk quantities of Jones & Bartlett Learning publications are available to corporations, professional associations, and other qualified organizations. For details and specific discount information, contact the special sales department at Jones & Bartlett Learning via the above contact information or send an email to specialsales@jblearning.com.

8715-1

Production Credits
VP, Executive Publisher: David Cella
Executive Editor: Amanda Martin
Associate Acquisitions Editor: Rebecca Myrick
Production Editor: Amanda Clerkin
Senior Marketing Manager: Jennifer Stiles
Art Development Editor: Joanna Lundeen
Art Development Assistant: Shannon Sheehan
VP, Manufacturing and Inventory Control: Therese Connell
Composition: Cenveo Publisher Services
Cover Design: Michael O'Donnell
Manager of Photo Research, Rights & Permissions: Lauren Miller
Cover Image: © Nataleana/Shutterstock, Inc.
Printing and Binding: Courier Companies
Cover Printing: Courier Companies

Library of Congress Cataloging-in-Publication Data
Community health nursing (Lundy)
Community health nursing : caring for the public's health / edited by Karen Saucier Lundy and Sharyn Janes. — Third edition.
p. ; cm.
Preceded by Community health nursing / Karen Saucier Lundy, Sharyn Janes. 2nd ed. c2009.
Includes bibliographical references and index.
ISBN 978-1-4496-9149-3
I. Lundy, Karen Saucier, editor. II. Janes, Sharyn, editor. III. Lundy, Karen Saucier. Community health nursing. Preceded by (work): IV. Title.
[DNLM: 1. Community Health Nursing. WY 106]
RT98
610.73'43—dc23

2014037459

6048

Printed in the United States of America
18 17 16 15 14 10 9 8 7 6 5 4 3 2 1

Contents

Unit 3
Care of Communities and Populations

Unit 4
Common Community and Population Health Problems and Issues

Preface

Community health nursing has historically responded to changes in healthcare needs of the population and met those needs in a variety of diverse roles and settings. In the 21st century, healthcare needs of the public can seem overwhelming to the beginning nurse. Since the publication of our first edition, the events of 9/11, Hurricane Katrina, the financial crisis of 2008, and the Affordable Patient Care and Protection Act (ACA) in 2010 have all changed the way we look at the public's health, security, inequity, social justice, and well being. The public's health has dominated the news in the past few years as a result of the passage of the federal ACA, which reforms a healthcare system in chaos, with a focus on prevention and health coverage for under and uninsured American citizens.

For those of us in community health, political, social, economic, cultural, and environmental issues have always been connected to population health outcomes. With recent national and global events, the public has become increasingly aware of the fragility of these interwoven influences on our existence within a global community. The healthcare system in the United States has produced technological advancements never thought possible at the beginning of the last century. Public health, along with scientific and technological progress, has resulted in an ever-increasing average life span for Americans, while other parts of the world struggle to meet basic healthcare needs. Greater life expectancy of individuals with chronic and acute conditions has continued to challenge the healthcare system's ability to provide efficient and quality care for its population.

As the population of the United States has become increasingly more diverse, the need for change in community health nursing is imperative; practice must now reflect an awareness of the diverse values and beliefs of populations from homeless veterans and the increasing number of older adults to children with chronic health conditions. Morbidity and mortality statistics reveal significant disparities among population groups, while socioeconomic and cultural factors contribute to persistent public health problems stemming from violence and substance abuse. Health care must be provided within a population's cultural context, whether influenced by culture, geographic location, age, gender, race, or ethnicity. In the *Third Edition* of this text, we have attempted to represent diversity among our authors, in the selection of chapter content, and in the general visual presentation of the text.

In spite of the overwhelming availability of health information via the Internet and other easily accessible sources to most of the U.S. population, we continue to be plagued with preventable illnesses that are largely a result of unhealthy life styles. In essence, despite advanced technology and unprecedented access to knowledge about health, our society remains unhealthy. We are faced with escalating childhood obesity and diabetes rates, family violence, alcohol and drug abuse, the reemergence of infectious diseases from last century, and chronic illnesses unknown in previous generations. Although the United States is the most advanced country in the world, it is far from being the healthiest. What can we do as nurses to promote healthy lifestyles, when all of our advanced diagnostics, therapies, surgeries, pharmacological agents, and an educated public present such great challenges? Public health has historically addressed these questions, with a focus on the health of populations, prevention, risk reduction, and the social and cultural environment. As student nurses in community health, sensitivity to one's own thoughts, feelings, and experiences are necessary for successful nurse interventions.

Through our unique pedagogical approach to learning, this text will offer the student a variety of ways to learn through self-reflection. Features such as poetry, art, music, films, literature, and narratives can help students move to a greater understanding of self through the shared experiences of others. This text will challenge the student to be fully engaged in the health of populations. The student will be confronted with one's own values and prejudices about poverty, racism, sexism, distribution of health resources, and personal and cultural beliefs. Personal beliefs affect one's ability to connect with and promote positive health changes in groups, families, and populations. Although text chapters can stand alone, students should become aware of the connections of all systems among the social, economic, historical, and political context that influence our effectiveness in connecting with patient populations in the promotion of our society's health.

By doing so, we hope to continue the tradition of a textbook that is more representative of what communities are in the United States—a unified society made up of many different populations and unique health perspectives.

This book is intended to serve as a primary text for undergraduate nursing students throughout the curriculum with an *emphasis on population-based nursing* directed toward health promotion and primary prevention in the community. It is both community-based and community-focused, reflecting the current dynamics of the healthcare system. The *Association of Community Health Nursing Educators Essentials of Baccalaureate Nursing Education for Entry Level Practice in Community/Public Health Nursing (C/PHN)* (2009) guided the conceptual development of chapter selection, structure, and content of the book.

Rising costs and an aging population have both contributed to the shift toward a population-based healthcare system. As the large cohort of Baby Boomers move into their aging years, their rising expectations for a healthy life span have resulted in a shift from episodic, acute care management to a more chronic focus on health and well being. Such a change has contributed to population-based outcomes and evidence-based practice. The community has largely become the setting for chronic illness management and prevention. All BSN nurses, to provide care for defined populations in all settings, must have the additional skills and knowledge in such areas as epidemiology and environmental sciences. Nurses will need to demonstrate skills in managed care at both the individual and group level, keeping an ever-vigilant eye on population influenced variables, such as age, gender, and cultural factors, whether in the acute/post acute setting or in community settings.

The cost and quality of health care in the United States continues to be the primary concern of its citizens. No longer just the interests of economists and policy makers, everyone has joined the debate about how to pay for the public's increasing expectations of quality health care at every life stage. More than 45 million U.S. citizens lack adequate health insurance while certain health indicators lag behind those of other comparable advanced countries who are spending far less for health care. The growing economic and health disparity between competing segments of the population has taken on national political significance, as all political parties struggle to find acceptable solutions. Health policy is no longer confined to nurses in leadership or government positions. Although nurses have historically remained uninvolved in the policy arena, this too is changing. The impact of federal and state policy on the delivery of community health services cannot be ignored if nurses in the community expect to influence the delivery of appropriate services to the population. This text provides chapters on economics, politics, and health policy by prominent nurse scholars who help beginning nurses understand how the knowledge of these often abstract forces that must be used in everyday clinical practice in all settings.

With the technological explosion of the 20th century, advances in digital technology have increased applications in telehealth, bringing together health providers and patients, without regard to geographical proximity. The community health nurse of the 21st century must use computer technology as the public health nurse of the 18th century used quill and ink. With faster and more current data access in community and acute care settings, new dimensions are emerging in patient assessment and intervention.

With rapid advances in *information technology* and *global travel*, global health issues create challenges for all nurses, not just those working in international settings. With the global community becoming smaller with every passing day, the spread of disease as well as health information occurs in hours rather than the years of the past. These dramatic risks have created the need for different approaches for the community health nurse. Travel nursing, both domestic and abroad, is one of the fastest growing areas in the nursing profession and challenges nurses to quickly adapt to changing physical and cultural environments. Vast opportunities now exist for nurses in global health, as formerly inaccessible populations throughout the world may now be reached through the advent of telehealth and telecommunications.

The passive health consumer of yesterday has given way to the well-informed, fully participating patient of today. With rapid and portable digital and media access to health information, which until recently has been available only to health professionals and scientists, individuals can participate as full partners in their care decisions and in the management of their health, which has raised expectations of care outcomes for patients and nurses. Through the phenomenal proliferation of the World Wide Web, most individuals can access unlimited information about health and health choices. This has greatly increased the power of consumer groups in health and has resulted in greater demands for services and access. The nurse in all settings will have even greater responsibilities in the educator role as community populations, patients, and families demand the most current information and become more assertive about securing services.

The increased interest in the *use of complementary and alternative, non-Western health practices* among Americans to enhance health, healing, and a more holistic sense of well being continues to influence the healthcare system. Nurses in the community are now confronted much more frequently with unfamiliar health practices that may or may not have a research basis for use. Attempts to legitimatize many unconventional approaches to health are occurring at research medical centers and through the federal government. A greater interest in the *spiritual aspects of health* is part of the movement among healthcare consumers for more emphasis on the subjective experience of health. With greater awareness of health information and greater participation in alternative health practices, community health nurses must be more prepared to understand these revolutionary changes. Nurses in the community are in an ideal position to help families and populations navigate through these uncharted and unfamiliar areas, making ethically sound and informed decisions. This text includes chapters on holistic health, health ministries, and spirituality to prepare the nurse for these challenges, breaking new ground for community health nursing textbooks.

With the extension of life through technology and improved living conditions, *end-of-life issues* have changed dramatically as well. The traditional approaches to caring for the dying are no longer as acceptable to patients accustomed to having more control in healthcare decisions. More patients and families are electing to die at home with hospice services and nurses as part of this team approach to a more dignified and humane end of life. In recognition of these needs, this text includes an extended section on hospice in the chapter on home health nursing. Recognizing the increased need for detailed information about home visiting, the *Third Edition* continues to offer a separate chapter on *home visiting.*

Nursing education is moving to integrate a more collaborative and interdisciplinary practice in the curriculum; therefore, this text features a unique *collaborative model of chapter authorship*. The BSN nurse will take the leadership role in such coordinated care in an increasingly complex healthcare system. Although most of our authors are community health nurse specialists, we also use other specialists in chapters that benefit from diverse perspectives. We believe that by securing well-known authors from nursing and other community health–related fields, we present a strong text and support our ideology of a more integrated approach to community health nursing. Further, *student nurses are included as authors of special features*, providing the reader with narrative accounts of the authenticity of student experiences in the community. The inclusion of clinical practitioners as authors further provides a clinical authenticity that is often missing from nursing textbooks.

A further strength of this text was in our review process. In addition to the traditional review process by community health nurse authors and faculty, we included nurses in other specialties; student nurses at all levels, including RN to BSN students; and beginning practicing nurses and experienced nurses in community health practice. These reviews were extremely enlightening, and we believe that through such an extensive and diverse group of reviewers, the *Third Edition* of this text is even more accessible for a broader section of nursing students.

Change has always been a certainty in the U.S. healthcare system. These changes present community health nurses with unlimited opportunities to influence the public's health. It is up to the student nurses of today to fully realize such possibilities. Nurses of the future must be in partnership with the healthcare system, which requires a broad understanding of community structure and process. The need for a commitment to lifelong learning and critical thinking skills emerge as vital for the nurse who will be successful in the challenging nursing roles of the future. We challenge faculty and students to use this text as the basis for their future professional practice, whatever the setting or role.

Dedication

I am honored to dedication this book to my family and friends who provide me with the love and commitment needed to see this new edition come to life. To bring a new edition of a text of this size and breadth to print consumes times, energy, and focus from so many. Special recognition to my husband, Dr. Joel Christopher Lundy, who acted as gentle critic and editor. For my son, Parker Lundy, who still believes that anything is possible. You are the joy of my existence and connection to the faculty of wonder. This edition is dedicated to the memory of my dearest friend and colleague, Dr. Sharyn Janes, who remained engaged, energized, and hopeful, despite the cancer through which she suffered during the development of this edition. Without her enduring light and positive energy, this book would not have happened. For your friendship and commitment to hope and all things good, I remain eternally grateful.

Introduction

The first edition of *Community Health Nursing: Caring for the Public's Health* broke new ground in our efforts to produce a readable, relevant, and interesting text, which reflected our passion for the fascinating and challenging field of public health. The *Third Edition* continues this tradition in our attempts to produce a book that both students and faculty should actually enjoy reading. Faculty are faced with a new generation of tech-savvy students who often eschew reading long, dry passages in traditional texts. We are committed to creating a text that is visually appealing, while presenting current information that transcends the traditional knowledge-based text in a variety of ways that students learn and experience the world of public and community health. Traditional texts that have virtually unchanged in format for decades no longer meet the needs of learners in the 21st century. Students are confronted with a myriad of information sources, from the Internet, social networks such as Twitter and Facebook, and media technology that appeals to all their senses. In order to meet the needs of students so that they will actually read texts, nursing educators must evolve with these ever-changing forms of communication, technology, and options for knowledge acquisition. This requires that we promote partnerships with students in their learning, rather than continue to perpetuate the authority hierarchy of teacher to student that has existed for centuries.

Both the National League for Nursing and the American Association of College of Nursing have called for new paradigm development and nursing education innovation to meet the demands of our future professional nurses. The shift to reflecting, learning, connecting, and thinking together *with* students drives the pedagogical changes in the *Third Edition* of our text. As a result of our commitment to create a text that addresses these critical changes in pedagogical approach, we have structured the text around reflective and connected learning thorough the inclusion of art, poetry, narratives, stories, media, and literature. We believe this approach can be a successful integration with traditional course content, either online or in the classroom, recognizing that students learn best using a variety of learning options. Chinn and Watson (1994, p. xv-xvi) advance that "Art allows us to locate ourselves in another space and place, to change our perception, our points of view." Although our text advances community health nursing to include diversity in knowing, learning, and caring, we are not breaking new ground.

In this text, we define art broadly, from photographs, film, and music to, poetry, literature, and personal narratives. We have included various personal narratives from nursing students and others in the text to capture interest and allow the student to place themselves in these personal stories. Further, through reading poetry or narratives, students can develop ethical knowledge and sensitivity, as well as promoting caring in a cultural context. Reading the chapter content for information and assuming a more active role through reflective reading and engagement of ideas will provide the student with opportunities to observe, experience, and analyze their own reactions to the broad field of public and community health. The depictions of illness, health, and healing through art, literature, and narratives can be powerful enhancements to student understanding of human experiences such as chronic illness, aging, and poverty. In short, they will have the opportunity of exploring art, literature, music, and narrative, connecting these with their own lives and interpreting the material according to their personal and professional life experiences.

Public and community nurses, perhaps more than other nursing specialties require that we enter the "other's world", not armed only with theoretical knowledge, but with a greater awareness of the human experiences of suffering, vulnerability, and life sustaining health practices. This greater awareness that human experiences are more than diagnoses or risk factors will further develop students' collaborative behaviors between the nurse and the populations we serve. This qualitative expression of the human experience in aesthetic knowing is "transformative and creative and promotes caring intention which can transform the learning experience of student nurses" (Purnell and Lynn, 2006, p. 9). Community health nursing is perhaps the oldest of all specialties; its historical roots lie in caring for people where they live, work and play, long before the development of hospital based "professional" care. As Jean Watson illuminates, "…Our Truths are co created through a process of values and meaning-making through language. When those values become human values of caring for self, others, and all living things, including planet Earth, and when the meaning-making of Truth involves humans and co creation of meaning via language, then another scenarios, different than the one we are used to, reveals the possibility of poeticizing as Truth…by inverting the paradigm and understanding human experiences from the inside out…". (Watson, 1994, p. 4, 15)

We hope that through the inclusion of these esthetic expressions of human experiences and health, our text can contribute to nurses' different ways of knowing and learning and thus, sensitize them to the development of holistic nursing practice in their selected fields, wherever they practice.

References

Purnell, J. J., & Lunn, C. E. (2006). Development of a model of nursing education grounded in caring and application to online nursing education. *International Journal for Nursing Caring, 10*(3), 8–16.

Chinn, P. L., & Watson, J. (1994). Art and aesthetics in nursing. New York, NY: National League for Nursing Press.

Watson, J. (1988). Nursing: Human science, human care. New York, NY: National League for Nursing.

Acknowledgments

Many people have contributed to the development and completion of all editions of this text. The chapter authors have honored us with their contributions to this text and have enriched our lives through our interactions with them. We thank them for helping this book come to life. The ideas and eventual structure of this text have evolved over countless conversations and interactions with faculty, colleagues, patients, and students over many years. We thank those who have inspired us and given us the hope and confidence that the unique format and presentation of this text meets the challenges of students and faculty in the 21st century. Our students continue to be the main inspiration for writing a text in community health nursing; as our future, they represent our best hope for a nurse-centered healthcare system for all. They have shared their stories, personal accounts, and daily reminders of what a textbook should be. We are honored to share many of their written narratives, poems, songs, and essays in the *Third Edition*. We remain in debt to the University of Southern Mississippi College of Nursing faculty and students for their encouragement and belief in seeing us through the *Third Edition* with their professional support. And for Jones & Bartlett Learning who believed in the continued importance of this project, especially Amanda Martin and Sara Bempkins. For those who participated in the critical review of this text, we thank them for their interest, enthusiasm, and courage to produce candid, detailed evaluations of this *Third Edition* throughout the many stages—and years—of development: Dr. Sherry Hartman, Dr. Kaye Bender; University of Southern Mississippi College of Nursing undergraduate and graduate students; Dr. Judith A. Barton; Dr. Ann Thedford Lanier, Dr. Cathy Hughes Dr. Joel Christopher Lundy, Marshall Parker Lundy, and Lilianna Kay Deveneau.

We would also like to acknowledge our colleagues in The *Association of Community Health Nursing Educators (ACHNE)* who provided valuable contributions through insightful and visionary input throughout the development of the *Third Edition*. Our best hope is that the *Third Edition* of the text in some small measure reflects the effort of so many who contributed to the final version of our *Third Edition*. Our names appear on the cover but the truest sense of authorship is shared with those named above and many unidentified friends, patients, family, and colleagues who are part of our life journey.

And lastly, we honor and acknowledge the work of our colleague and friend, Dr. Sherry Hartman, who contributed her energy and passion to all editions of this text. Her global insights, belief in humanity and justice for all, philosophical wisdom, and humor are woven throughout the text. We remain eternally grateful for her intellectual and personal presence in our lives.

Contributors

Joan H. Baldwin, DNSc, RN
Professor Emeritus
College of Nursing Brigham Young University
Provo, Utah

Judith A. Barton, PhD, RN
Associate Professor
School of Nursing
University of Colorado Health Sciences Center
Denver, Colorado

Kaye W. Bender, PhD, RN, FAAN
President and CEO
Public Health Accreditation Board
Alexandria, Virginia

Angela Chisum Blackburn PhD, ARNP, NNP-BC
Assistant Professor
Department of Nursing
University of West Florida
Pensacola, Florida

Ilene Purvis Bloxsom, RN, BSN, MSHA
Chief Nursing Officer
Dale Medical Center
Ozark, Alabama

Lucy Bradley-Springer, PhD, RN, ACRN, FAAN
Associate Professor and Director
Mountain Plains AIDS Education and Training enter
Associate Professor of Medicine
Adjunct Associate Professor of Nursing
Editor, *Journal of the Association of Nurses in AIDS Care*
University of Colorado Health Sciences Center
Denver, Colorado

Margaret A. Burkhardt, PhD, RN, CS, HNC
Associate Professor Emeritus
School of Nursing
West Virginia University
Director, Healing Matters
Morgantown, West Virginia

Angeline Bushy, PhD, RN, CS
Bert Fish Endowed Chair
Professor
School of Nursing
University of Central Florida-Daytona Beach
Daytona Beach, Florida

Patricia Butterfield, PhD, RN, FAAN
Professor and Dean
Washington State University
Intercollegiate College of Nursing
Spokane, Washington

Janie B. Butts, DSN, RN
Associate Professor School of Nursing
University of Southern Mississippi
Hattiesburg, Mississippi

Grace Coggio, PhD
Assistant Professor
Department of Communication Studies
University of Wisconsin, River Falls
River Falls, Wisconsin

Virginia Lee Cora, DSN, RN, CS
Adult/Geriatric Nurse Practitioner
Division of Geriatrics
School of Medicine
University of Mississippi Medical Center
Jackson, Misssissippi

Norma G. Cuellar, DSN, RN
Professor
The University of Alabama
Capstone College of Nursing
Tuscaloosa, Alabama

Lilianna K. Deveneau, BA, BS
St. Paul, Minnesota

Joseph E. Farmer, RN, MSN, ACRN, PhD(c)
Clinical Assistant Professor
Community and Mental Health Nursing
College of Nursing
The University of South Alabama
Mobile, Alabama

Sherry Hartman, DrPH, RN
Professor Emeritus
School of Nursing
University of Southern Mississippi
Hattiesburg, Mississippi

Jean Haspeslagh, DNS, RN
Professor Emeritus
School of Nursing
University of Southern Mississippi
Hattiesburg, Mississippi

Edith Hilton, PhD, DSN, MS, APRN, BC
Advanced Practice, Neurosciences
Northwestern Memorial Hospital
Chicago, Illinois

John Hodnett Jr., DNP, M.Ed., MSN, RN, LPC
Director of Clinical Operations
Sharkey-Issaquena Community Hospital
Instructor
The University of Mississippi Medical Center
School of Health Related Professions
Jackson, Mississippi

Cathy Hughes, DNP, MSN, RN
Assistant Professor, Clinical
College of Nursing
The University of Southern Mississippi
Hattiesburg, Mississippi

Loretta Sweet Jemmott, PhD, RN, FAAN
van Ameringen Professor
Psychiatric Mental Health Nursing
Director, Center for Health Disparities Research
School of Nursing
University of Pennsylvania
Philadelphia, Pennsylvania

Harriet J. Kitzman, PhD, RN, FAAN
Professor
Senior Associate Dean of Research
School of Nursing
University of Rochester
Rochester, New York

Pat Kurtz, PhD, RN
Professor Emeritus
School of Nursing
University of Southern Mississippi
Hattiesburg, Mississippi

Ann Thedford Lanier, PhD
Adjunct Professor
Department of Sociology
Texas Tech University
Lubbock, Texas
National Science Foundation (Ret.)
Washington, DC

Sarah Steen Lauterbach, MSPH, EdD, RN
Professor
College of Nursing
Valdosta State University
Valdosta, Georgia

Madeleine Leininger, PhD, RN, LHD, OS, CTN, FAAN, FRCNA, LL
Founder of Transcultural Nursing
Leader of Human Care Research
Adjunct Professor, University of Nebraska Medical Center (Omaha) College of Nursing
Professor Emerita, Wayne State University–Detroit
Omaha, Nebraska

Marshall Parker Lundy, BA
Active Psychiatric Treatment Technician
South Mississippi State Hospital
Purvis, Mississippi

Cynthia H. Luther, DSN, FNP, GNP
Assistant Professor
Director of Geriatric and Psychiatric Mental/Health Nurse Practitioner Tracks
The University of Mississippi Medical Center
Jackson, Mississippi

Frances Martin, PhD, FNP
School of Nursing
Medical College of Georgia
Athens, Georgia

Nancy Milio, PhD, MA, RN, FAPHA, FAAN
Professor Emeritus
Nursing and Health Policy and Administration
School of Public Health, Nursing
University of North Carolina at Chapel Hill
Chapel Hill, North Carolina

Cynthia O'Neill Morgan, PhD, RN
Pandemic Influenza Program Coordinator
Texas Department of State Health Services
Austin, Texas

Lindsay Lake Morgan, PhD, RN, GNP
Assistant Professor and Director
O'Connor Office of Rural Health Studies
Decker School of Nursing
Binghamton University
Binghamton, New York

Carol J. Nyman, CRN, FNP, MPH
Family Nurse Practitioner
U.S. Public Health Service
White Earth Indian Reservation
White Earth, Minnesota

Ruth A. O'Brien, PhD, RN, FAAN
Professor
School of Nursing
University of Colorado Health Sciences Center
Denver, Colorado

Bonita R. Reinert, PhD, RN, FAAN
Professor Emeritus
School of Nursing
University of Southern Mississippi
Hattiesburg, Mississippi

Bonnie Rogers, DrPH, COHN-S, FAAN
Associate Professor of Nursing and Public Health
Director, Occupational Health Nursing Program
Director/NC Education and Research Center
University of North Carolina at Chapel Hill
School of Public Health, Curriculum in Public Health Nursing
Chapel Hill, North Carolina

Marla E. Salmon, ScD, RN, FAAN
Robert G. and Jean A. Reid Endowed Dean and Professor
University of Washington
School of Nursing
Seattle, Washington

Betty Sylvest, DNS, RN, CNE
Associate Professor
Robert E. Smith School of Nursing
Delta State University
Cleveland, Mississippi

Heather Rakauskas Sherry, PhD
Director, Office of Articulation
Florida Department of Education
Former Legislative Analyst
Florida House of Representatives
Tallahassee, Florida

Gale A. Spencer, PhD, RN
Distinguished Teaching Professor
Decker Chair in Community Health Nursing
Decker School of Nursing
Binghamton University
Binghamton, New York

Linda Beth Tiedje, PhD, RN, MA, FAAN
Adjunct Associate Professor
College of Human Medicine
Department of Epidemiology
Michigan State University
East Lansing, Michigan

UNIT 1

The Context

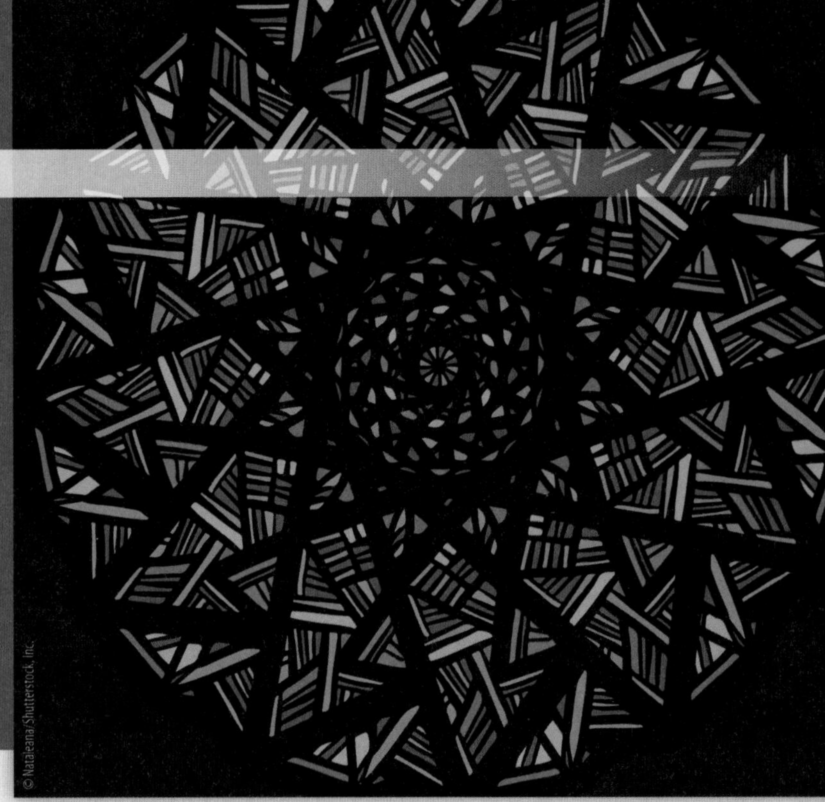

© Nataleana/Shutterstock, Inc.

COMMUNITY-FOCUSED NURSING

WHAT DOES IT MEAN to take care of a community? Community-focused nursing care is often difficult to define and even more difficult to practice. Baccalaureate nurses are educated to practice nursing in all healthcare settings. Community health nurses care for populations. Since the late 1800s, professional public health nurses have cared for communities. Those communities have changed over time, and the practice of community health nursing has changed as well. Community health nursing has evolved into a complex, multifaceted nursing specialty that is constantly challenged by rapidly changing delivery systems, including the passage of the Affordable Care Act (ACA, or "Obamacare") of 2010. While reading about the history of community and public health nursing, both similarities and differences in today's community health nursing practice will emerge. Community health nursing, which evolved from public health nursing and is accountable to the public for meeting the population's healthcare needs, has responded to changes in society to include the care of such diverse populations as schoolchildren, women with human immunodeficiency virus/acquired immune deficiency syndrome (HIV/AIDS), and the homeless. Unit 1 introduces the student to the world of the community health nurse: the focus, the settings, and the historical issues relevant to today's community health practice. As a broadly based specialty, community health nursing practice is more affected by structural changes in society than are other nursing specialties. The community health nurse must be aware of the healthcare system, social trends, economics, and culture to deliver effective care to the public. Unit 1 assists the student in understanding the uniqueness of community health nursing and the structural influences that must be considered when delivering effective care for an entire community.

CHAPTER FOCUS

A Closer Look at Health
- Historical Insights

Nursing in the 21st Century
- Educating Nurses for Community Health Nursing Practice

Community-Based, Population-Focused, Community Health Nursing: What's in a Name?
- Communities and Populations
- Acute Care Versus Community Health Nursing

Reform and the Reinvention of Systems of Care
- *Nursing's Agenda for Health Care Reform*
- Managed Care and the Future of Nursing

Back to the Future: From Hospital to Community, from Cure to Prevention
- Home Health Care
- Cure and Prevention: Can We Really Do It All?
- Benefits Versus Costs
- *Healthy People 2020:* Goals for the Nation
- Influences on a Community's Health: Culture, Environment, and Ethics

Epidemiology: The Science of Public Health

Measuring a Community's Health: How Do We Know When We Get There?

QUESTIONS TO CONSIDER

After reading this chapter, you will know the answers to the following questions:

1. How does the definition of health affect the way we care for populations?
2. How have settings and opportunities in the health-care system changed in recent decades?
3. What implications does the ACA have for nurses?
4. What is healthcare reform and prevention, and how do these changes influence health policy in the U.S. care system?
5. What is the significance of *Nursing's Agenda for Health Care Reform*?
6. What is *Healthy People 2020*, and how does it influence the healthcare system related to a policy of prevention?
7. What are the distinctions between the concepts of community health, population-focused care, and acute care?
8. What is a community, and what is a population?
9. What are the three major influences on community health?
10. What is epidemiology?
11. What is the relationship between the natural history of disease and the three levels of prevention?
12. How is a population's health measured?

CHAPTER 1

Opening the Door to Health Care in the Community

Karen Saucier Lundy, Sharyn Janes, and Sherry Hartman

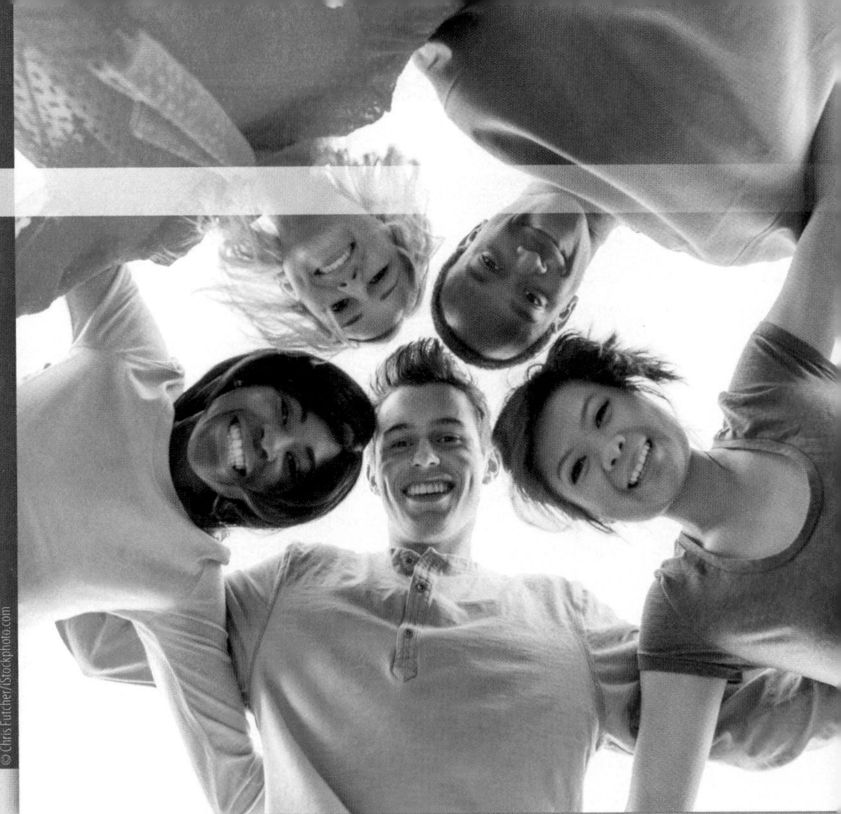

KEY TERMS

Affordable Care Act (ACA)
care management
community
community-based nursing
community health nursing
culture
environment
epidemiology
ethics
Florence Nightingale
health
healthcare reform
Healthy People 2020
home health care
managed care
Nursing's Agenda for Health Care Reform
Patient Protection and Affordable Care Act
population
population-focused care
populations of interest
primary prevention
public health nursing
secondary prevention
tertiary prevention
World Health Organization (WHO)

> We hear much of 'contagion and infection' in disease. May we not also come to make health contagious and infectious?
>
> —Florence Nightingale, 1890

> It is cheaper to promote health than to maintain people in sickness.
>
> —Florence Nightingale, 1894

REFLECTIONS

Firefighters Responding to 9/11 at Increased Cancer Risk
Coffee Linked to Lower Cancer Risks
Allergens Found High in Daycare Centers
Moderate Alcohol Consumption Appears to Slow Cognitive Decline in Older Women
States Wrestle with How to Accommodate Children Born in the U.S. to Illegal Immigrants
Dull, Low-Level Jobs Linked to Heart Problems
Teens Say Oral Sex Not Really Sex
Cosmetic Surgeons Focus More on Teen Set
Proximity to Power Lines at Birth May Increase Leukemia Risk
Middle-Age Obesity Predicts Old-Age Dementia
Obamacare Website Malfunctions Limit Access to Patient Enrollment in Insurance Marketplaces
The Robot Will See You Now: Is Your Doctor Becoming Obsolete?
Are Extended Work Hours for Nurses Worth the Health Risks?
Results from Harvard Nurses' Health Study Show That 70 Percent of Nurses Are Either Overweight or Obese
Cyberbullying Leads to Female Teen's Suicide
WHO Just Says No to Tanning Beds for Teens
Days Off in Fine Weather Linked to Melanoma-Courting Behavior
Energy Drinks and Adderall Use Results in Increase in Emergency Room Visits
TB Has Small Presence in America, But Remains Huge Worldwide
Is Your Desk Making You Sick? Computer Keyboards and Office Equipment Swarm with Germs
Cruise Ships May Be Hazardous to Your Health
Few Americans Following "Big Four" Healthy Lifestyle
Obesity in U.S. at Pandemic Level, May Decrease Life Expectancy for Younger Generations
Autism Linked to Allergic Disease During Pregnancy
Mental Disorders Strike Nearly Half of All Americans
Experts: AIDS Vaccine Years Away
Most Prescription Bottles Difficult for Elders to Read
Majority of Elders Do Not Take Drugs as Prescribed
Methamphetamine Now "Drug of Choice" in Rural U.S.
Drug Safety Fears Prompt Some Patients to Seek Alternative Pain Remedies
Aging in Brain Found to Hurt Sleep Needed for Memory
Antibiotics, Sex Hormones and Tranquilizers Found in Major U.S. Cities' Drinking Water
Women's Rights Linked with AIDS Epidemic in Africa
Security Concerns Hampering Polio Eradication Efforts in Pakistan

These headlines are all recent from media throughout the world. Sometimes it may seem that larger social issues are unrelated to nursing practice. As you will see in this text, however, community health nurses define health very broadly so that the connections between and among these headlines and our work in the community will become clearer. Almost every problem cited in the news can be linked to larger issues in public health.

After reading these headlines, think about the following questions:

- Why are illness and disease the focus of most health care in the U.S. healthcare system?
- Are you more interested in the "drama of trauma" in health care than community health nursing, such as educating people about prevention of disease and injury? If you are, you are not alone! Most student nurses and the public are more impressed with high-tech health care than with prevention.
- Think about why nurses might find self-care and prevention to be less interesting. Why do you?
- What do you know about the ACA (or "Obamacare") of 2010? Are you confused about how the new healthcare reform will affect you as a nurse?

THE WORLD OF NURSING and the nurse's role are always changing, but it is probably safe to say that those who choose nursing in the early decades of the 21st century are caught in unprecedented currents of change: revolutionary changes in healthcare delivery, changes in settings of care, and changes resulting from historical healthcare reform at the national level. Although bachelor of science in nursing (BSN)–prepared nurses have always been prepared and functioned to some degree within a community health framework, understanding the importance of population-focused and community health nursing practice knowledge and skills is critical to assuming a leadership role in the current healthcare system, regardless of setting. The passage of the **Patient Protection and Affordable Care Act**, also simply called the **Affordable Care Act** or ACA, on March 23, 2010—along with the confirmation of the Act's constitutionality by the U.S. Supreme Court on June 28, 2012—has been the most significant and sweeping healthcare reform legislation in the history of the U.S. healthcare system (American Academy of Nursing [AAN], 2010).

The ACA was created to increase access to affordable and accessible health care for millions of uninsured and underinsured Americans, with an emphasis on preventive health care, as well as protections for citizens from insurance companies denying coverage due to preexisting conditions and high-risk health conditions. The ACA's purpose is twofold: (1) to increase the number of Americans covered by health insurance and (2) to decrease the cost of health care. Prevention of illness and promotion of health are common threads throughout the ACA. The ACA most significantly reforms the way health insurance is purchased, requiring that all Americans purchase a private healthcare plan or pay a tax penalty. Americans who cannot afford private health insurance will either qualify for Medicare or Medicaid, or get assistance in the form of tax credits or tax breaks, among other types of financial support. The ACA has also resulted in one of the most debated and divisive pieces of federal legislation in recent years (Gable, 2011).

As student nurses, you will have varying opinions about the ACA, but as this text is published, ACA is the law, and it has already begun implementing dramatic and far-reaching changes within many facets of society. So, "What does that have to do with nursing?" you may be asking. Throughout the text, you will learn how the ACA will be implemented by the proposed timelines and the impact such reforms will have for all nurses.

The U.S. healthcare system has been challenged like never before to respond to bioterrorist threats unknown to nurses just a few years earlier. Following September 11, 2001, our world was forever changed. The loss of security in our communities remains a serious threat to our wellbeing. The unprecedented "disaster of disasters," Hurricane Katrina, forced us as a society to question our ability to respond to natural threats as well. Many of us watched in shock, and some of us experienced firsthand, the disintegration of an entire region along the Mississippi Gulf Coast and New Orleans. How could this happen in the United States? Even more importantly, how can we respond more efficiently and effectively to future disasters? The decade-long military conflict in the Middle East has resulted in thousands of disabling health conditions for veterans, increasing human and economic costs of a postwar society, and affecting veterans and their families.

These changes and other health crises have left us as a nation questioning our ability to respond to present and future public health needs. In this climate of disillusionment, Americans feel even more vulnerable than ever in terms of their safety, despite living in one of the most advanced nations in the world.

NOTE THIS!

Common Definitions in Community Health Nursing

Community health nursing is a systematic process of delivering nursing care to improve the health of an entire community (Nehls, Owen, Tipple, & Vandermause, 2001, p. 305).

Community-based nursing refers to the setting and the practice of the nursing role. The focus of community-based nursing care is primarily at the individual and family levels, which contribute to the health of the community. Community-based nursing often refers to nursing care provided outside of acute care settings.

Population-focused care refers to interventions aimed at health promotion and disease prevention that shape a community's overall health status.

Public health nursing is the practice of promoting and protecting the health of populations using knowledge from nursing, social, and public health sciences. The practice is population-focused, with the goals of promoting health and preventing disease and disability for all people through the creation of conditions in which people can be healthy (American Public Health Association, Public Health Nursing Section, 1996; American Nurses Association, 2013).

These forces for change have been developing for some time now, engulfing all healthcare professionals in the shifting sands of practice. In response to new demands, new opportunities, new possibilities, and a more complex healthcare environment, current nursing students pursue a curriculum that their predecessors would not recognize. The nurse's place in the healthcare system is at the patient's side, not just in the hospital, but in any setting and in a myriad of roles where people work, play, learn, worship, shop, explore the Internet, or call a hotline. The nurse has an opportunity to educate and promote health for people in broad and diverse communities. Further, travel nursing has emerged as a career choice that provides nurses with opportunities to work in different cultures, settings, and locales, not only in the United States, but throughout the world. In essence, every BSN nurse is a community health nurse: The degree to which this is true varies only in the specific demands of the nursing role and setting.

ART CONNECTION 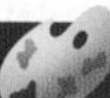

This feature will present a well-known art piece that contains a brief description of the significance of art to understanding the complexity of health, healing, and suffering. Select one of your favorite paintings and write a brief summary of how this art relates to health and healing.

As health care moves toward a more community-driven system, a change in focus becomes vital as we embrace a growing mindfulness to form partnerships with those served by community health nurses. New directions in health care are also occurring internationally, with community-based partnerships between healthcare providers and communities (Nehls & Vandermause, 2004). Even if the world around us appears to remain chaotic and complex, as some suggest, nursing ideals and commitments will fulfill the promise of the dreams that bring most nurses to the profession.

With the headlines often heralding hospital closures, insurance costs, patient access to ACA, mergers, and downsizing, where does that leave nurses? What is the story behind where we are today? What kind of job will there be for you after graduation? When you graduate from nursing school, you will join the more than 2.7 million registered nurses (RNs) in the United States? The good news is that the federal government predicts that RN will be one of the top careers with the most job openings in the future. Employment of RNs is expected to grow 26% from 2010 to 2020, faster than the average for all occupations (Bureau of Labor Statistics, 2012).

Rapid growth in this job market will be driven by technological and innovative advances in patient care and the ACA, which permit a greater number of health problems to be treated outside the traditional clinical/acute care setting. These changes, coupled with an increasing emphasis on preventive care as we learn more about what keeps people healthy, further expand the healthcare market (AAN, 2010).

A critical nursing shortage exists today in all areas of nursing and is projected to extend into the coming decades, especially for positions requiring a BSN. Travel nursing positions are in great demand in the United States and throughout the world. Nurses who can respond to different cultures and practice settings and adjust quickly to diverse care situations requiring community health and population-based skills will be in the greatest demand. In addition, the number of older people, who are much more likely than younger people to need nursing care, is projected to grow rapidly during the 21st century.

Although 61% of RNs still work in hospitals, that percentage has dropped more than five percentage points since 1992, and about 20% work part time, according to the Bureau of Labor Statistics (2012). The greatest changes have been an increase in the percentage of nurses who work in community-ambulatory care, home health, public health, and other community-based settings (U.S. Department of Health and Human Services [HHS], 2000). Dramatic changes in the way health care is delivered—and will be delivered in the future as the ACA continues to reshape the U.S. healthcare system—have led to the discharge of sicker patients to their homes. As managed care continues

BOX 1-1 Cornerstones of Public Health Nursing

Public health nursing practice:

- Focuses on entire populations
- Reflects the community's priorities and needs
- Establishes caring relationships with the community, families, individuals, and systems that comprise the populations public health nurses (PHNs) serve
- Is grounded in social justice, compassion, sensitivity to diversity, and respect for the worth of all people, especially the vulnerable
- Encompasses mental, physical, emotional, social, spiritual, and environmental aspects of health
- Promotes health through strategies driven by epidemiological evidence
- Collaborates with community resources to achieve those strategies, but can and will work alone if necessary
- Derives its authority for independent action from the Nurse Practice Acts

Source: Minnesota Department of Health Center for Public Health Nursing. (2004). *Cornerstones of public health nursing.* Retrieved from http://www.health.state.mn.us/divs/opi/cd/phn/docs/0710phn_cornerstones.pdf

A DAY IN THE LIFE

Working as a Nurse and Family Nurse Practitioner in Alaska: Just Another Day in a Frozen Paradise
Amanda Traver, FNP, MSN

The first word that comes to my mind after taking a job as a nurse in Alaska as a new BSN graduate is diversity—diversity in opportunities, diversity in the people I worked with, diversity in the type of injuries and illnesses, and diversity in my patients. I first came to Alaska as an Army nurse and functioned primarily in medical-surgical roles in military healthcare facilities. I saw more than my share of frostbite victims and all types of injuries related to living in this frigid environment. Once I completed my Army obligation, I realized just how even more diverse nursing could be. My options were numerous and diverse: working at the Army hospital as a civilian nurse, working in the local hospital, doing Medevac flights from rural villages in Alaska to regional medical centers such as Fairbanks or Anchorage, or working in the regional medical centers with Medevac flights from Fairbanks to Anchorage. What amazing choices! I eventually chose to work in the emergency room (ER) in the Fairbanks hospital.

As an ER nurse in Fairbanks, I was challenged with many diverse and complex patients. I will mention here only a few of my unique cases. There was the man who ran out to his outhouse "real quick" without his shoes at 30 degrees below zero and locked himself out of his house; he suffered severe frostbite on his feet. There was the man who was working for the forest service chopping down trees, when he turned around and looked straight into the eyes of a grizzly bear. He endured massive claw marks on his back and four deep teeth marks in his thigh before he could get his gun out of his pocket to shoot the bear. One of the highlights of my ER time was getting to know all the local alcoholics by name and their "drinks of choice." There were the usual gunshot wounds, car accidents, and domestic violence cases, but even with these typical ER cases, many were unique to Alaska's culture and environment, such as moose-versus-car accidents and harpoons impaled in patients' chests and limbs.

I returned to nursing school and successfully completed a family nurse practitioner (FNP) program. As I write this, I am in King Cove, Alaska, a small fishing village on the Aleutian chain, working as an FNP. Last night we had a tsunami warning. Recent patients included a man who had fallen, had a neck and head injury, and needed to be transported to a regional hospital. The wind was blowing at 35 miles per hour, with gusts up to 65 miles per hour, and snow squalls that made driving even more treacherous than usual. Only small, six-seater planes can land on the runway in King Cove, and that is in good weather. No planes can land on the runways at night. We had to request a Coast Guard helicopter to fly the patient across the bay to a town with a larger, lighted runway. A fishing boat was standing by to take the patient across the bay in case the helicopter could not get in. Fortunately, the Coast Guard helicopter was able to land. As we loaded the patient into the helicopter, the snow was blowing hard in our faces and the wind was howling. He was flown by helicopter to Fairbanks, where a plane picked him up and flew him to the larger medical center in Anchorage. Yes, I am a community health nurse, no matter where I practice. The community is my patient.

My next assignment will be in Nome, where I will work in the clinic and ER at the hospital for 5 months. My next assignment will be in Fairbanks for 6 months. Such is the life of a traveling FNP in Alaska—never a dull moment!

Even my time off in Alaska is diverse. I have learned to mountain bike and have been chased by a bear on a mountain biking trip. It was so close I could see the bear in my peripheral vision, feel her breath on my leg as I was pedaling, and feel the ground shaking as the bear ran. Fortunately, the bear left me alone.

I have learned to ice climb and mountain climb; I have backpacked in amazing, treacherous landscapes; and cross-country skiing is as close as my front yard. There are more pilots in Alaska per capita than anywhere else, and many places in Alaska are accessible only by plane. So I am now a licensed pilot and look forward to even more adventures in the remote, frozen wilderness. Who knows, perhaps one day I will be working as a nurse and a pilot transporting patients in the wild and beautiful state I now call home!

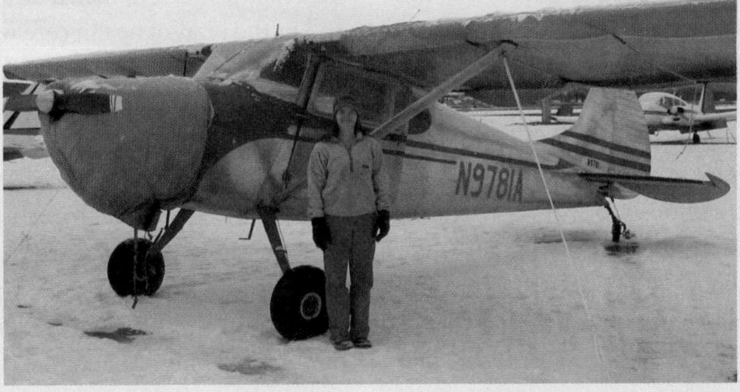

MEDIA MOMENT

View an episode of a current medical or health-related show on television, such as *Dr. Oz, Nurse Jackie, Grey's Anatomy*, or *Scrubs*. Can you identify a situation on the show where preventive interventions, such as patient or family education by a community health nurse, could have reduced or prevented the occurrence of a featured injury or disease? Why are these shows so popular with audiences when the worst-case scenario tends to occur?

A DAY IN THE LIFE

Martha Rogers, PhD, RN, FAAN, 1966

Nursing's story is a magnificent epic of service to mankind. It is about people: how they are born, and live and die; in health and in sickness; in joy and in sorrow. Its mission is the translation of knowledge into human service.

Nursing is compassionate concern for human beings. It is the heart that understands and the hand that soothes. It is the intellect that synthesizes many learnings into meaningful administrations.

For students of nursing, the future is a rich repository of far-flung opportunities around this planet and toward the further reaches of man's explorations of new worlds and new ideas. Theirs is the promise of deep satisfaction in a field long dedicated to serving the health needs of people.

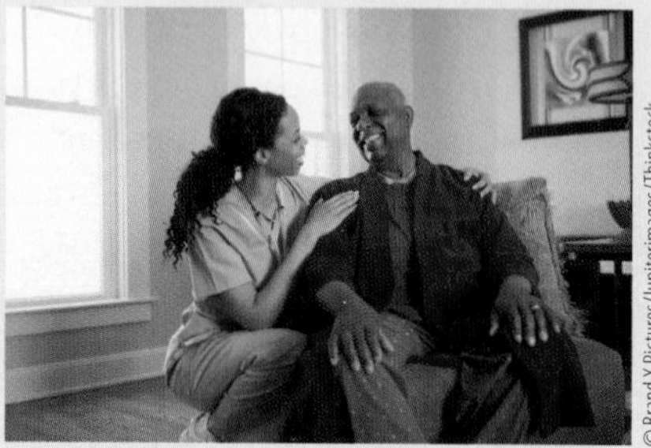

Home health nursing practice is the fastest-growing community health nursing role.

to result in fewer hospitalizations, nurses in acute care settings are facing assignments on a daily basis to different units and in diverse settings, including outpatient, home health, and other community-based agencies housed in or associated with their own facility (Gable, 2011).

As the patient census (the number of occupied beds in a hospital on a daily basis) fluctuates, nurses must be flexible, willing, and competent in multiple settings. So, no matter where you ultimately choose to work as a nurse, community health will be an influence on your choice of position, your role, and on your patients' lives. According to Gebbie (1996), the U.S. vision of public health is that of healthy people in healthy communities, because individual health can be fully realized only if the community itself is in good shape as well. (For a closer look at how much our health is influenced by public health measures, see the "Think About This" feature later in the chapter.)

Public health measures, such as immunizations, clean water, safe food, building working environments, sewage disposal, and disease surveillance and intervention, are virtually invisible and often of little interest to citizens and nurses alike *because of their success.* Florence Nightingale would be stunned at the accomplishments in society; during her lifetime, life expectancy was close to half what it is today in the United States. In the United States, we have experienced an extraordinary rise in life expectancy to 78.3 years in the second decade of the 21st century (U.S. Census Bureau, 2012). The gains in life expectancy have primarily come from public health interventions above, based on epidemiology, knowledge, and education of the population and research-based practices of health professionals and the public. The 1970s and 1980s saw a move toward an increase in population-focused research and practice, resulting in healthier communities. Examples of these interventions include anti-smoking campaigns to reduce tobacco use, hypertension and cardiac risk factor prevention and control, improved nutrition, auto and other transportation safety restraints for adults and children, and injury prevention. A reduction in childhood deaths of 40% and close to a 50% decline in cardiovascular-related deaths in adults have also contributed to the present health status and costs of our nation. Medical treatment alone can prevent only about 10% of "early" deaths (prior to expected life expectancy); however, population-based public health interventions (risk reduction of unhealthy lifestyle behaviors, such as sedentary lifestyle, diet, stress, occupational hazards, and substance abuse) have the potential to reduce approximately 70% of these early deaths (HealthyPeople.gov, 2013).

In this chapter, the history, context, and setting for nursing practice are discussed, as well as some of the current controversies and confusions specific to the new move to the patient's side in the community. So many things influence health: In this century we continue to find out through research how much in the environment, in our own behavior, and in the kind of health care we deliver affects whether we are healthy or ill. Why some people get sick and why some people do not have intrigued healthcare providers for centuries. This chapter introduces health as a concept, presents the historical insights we have learned, and reveals what we can expect nursing and health care to look like in the 21st century.

Sometimes the ways in which we use terms can confuse and obscure the focus of community and public health nursing. In this chapter the terms related to community, population, and nursing roles are discussed in the context of healthcare delivery. The ways in which a population's health is determined are introduced as are concepts related to disease and illness prevention and health promotion.

The term *community health nursing* will be used throughout this text to represent care directed toward improving the health of communities and population groups through prevention and risk reduction in all settings.

A Closer Look at Health

Before we can talk in more detail about the U.S. healthcare system and nursing roles in today's healthcare arena, we need an understanding of what health is. That seems simple; after all, everyone knows what health is. However, there are many definitions and descriptions of health depending on one's perspective and purpose.

The most well-known and widely cited description of health is the **World Health Organization's (WHO)** definition of **health** as a state of complete physical, mental, and social wellbeing, and not merely the absence of disease or infirmity (WHO, 1958). When this definition was first drafted in 1948, it began a trend that has persisted for more than 50 years to define health more broadly, including social terms in addition to medical terms.

In 1986, the WHO definition of health was expanded to include a community concept of health. WHO now defines health as the extent to which an individual or group is able, on the one hand, to realize aspirations and satisfy needs, and, on the other hand, to change or cope with the environment. Health is, therefore, seen as a resource for everyday life, not the objective of living; it is a positive concept emphasizing social and personal resources, in addition to physical capacities (WHO, 1986). An individual or community then must be able to attain and use resources effectively and exhibit resilience when facing change.

Although WHO's definition of health is the most widely accepted, many other definitions also imply a social or community focus. Health has been defined as a purposeful and integrated method of functioning within an environment (Hall & Weaver, 1977, p. 7), and as the common attainment of the highest level of physical, mental, and social wellbeing consistent with available knowledge and resources at a given time and place (Hanlon & Pickett, 1984). Even Florence Nightingale's definition of health as not only to be well, but also to use well every power that we have, can be used to describe health for both individuals and communities (Nightingale, 1860).

Many social issues surround the concept of health, making it difficult to limit it to only one definition and perspective. Health is defined by the society and culture in which we live. How individuals, families, and communities perceive what health means is often determined by social, cultural, and economic conditions that limit health choices (Kuss, Proulx-Girouard, Lovitt, Katz, & Kennelly, 1997). Put another way, health is highly dependent on where and how we live. A 20-year-old man may consider himself healthy only if he can run up the stairs at work. For an 80-year-old woman, retrieving her own mail at the mailbox may be her idea of health.

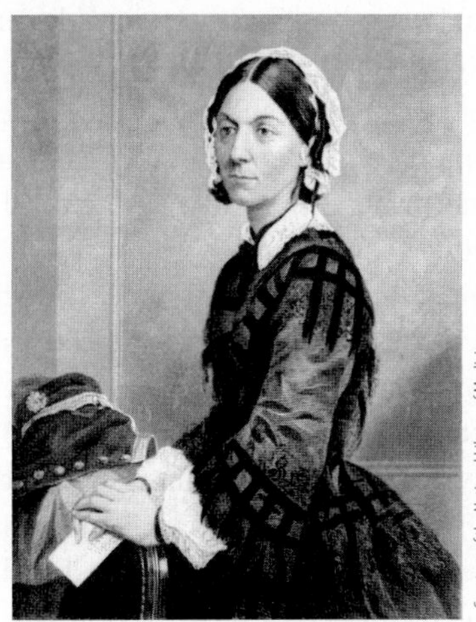
Courtesy of the National Library of Medicine

Young Florence Nightingale

Nurses differ in their perception of health and are influenced by their own background, age, and experiences. In a study that explored the perceptions of community health nurses about health, the nurses interviewed described health as an "interactive vision" between nurses and patients (Leipert, 1996). This vision of health varies with each nurse–patient relationship, depending on the values and characteristics of the nurse, the patient, and the setting where the interaction occurs. Some of the characteristics that can greatly affect the vision of health are age, culture, social environment, and economic status. Patients in this context include individuals, families, groups, and communities.

Historical Insights

Sickness and suffering have always been a part of human existence. As a result, from the beginning there have been men and women who served as caregivers to the sick and injured. Early on, most care was provided by family members. As human society evolved, moral consciousness became formalized into religious codes, and religious groups assumed more responsibility for the ill. Although their efforts were commendable, they were limited because so little was known about disease causation or prevention.

Florence Nightingale is recognized as the founder of modern professional nursing, and for developing the first school of nursing at London's St. Thomas Hospital in 1860. Although her initial efforts focused on preparing nurses to care for the sick in hospitals and infirmaries, she continued throughout her life to promote well nursing in the community. Nightingale's directive was to manipulate the patient's environment to allow nature to take its course in the healing process.

Through scientific inquiry during the 19th century, causes of the devastating communicable diseases of these earlier centuries began to emerge and professional intervention became possible. During the mid- to late 1800s, public health measures were established as the process of contagion between human hosts, and the environment became better understood.

Throughout the 20th century, medical science grew in leaps and bounds, and the manipulation of nature became the drive that resulted in significant medical discoveries and inventions. The United States experienced unprecedented growth in technology and medical science in this century. We learned more about the causes of diseases and generated a broad knowledge base about disease and injury detection, treatment, and prevention. The resulting healthcare system, which early on was divided into public and private sectors, focused on the diagnosis and treatment of disease in the highly specialized and centralized setting of the hospital. For most individuals, health care was synonymous with the local hospital.

During the 20th century, most nurses were employed in hospital settings as skilled caregivers for the acutely ill; nursing education was mostly focused on care of the sick. Nursing students gained experience almost exclusively in hospitals.

Nevertheless, even as the United States was credited worldwide with having the most advanced health technology for treating disease, and while healthcare spending vastly increased during the 1960s and 1970s, health professionals and the public increasingly expressed a growing concern that the healthcare needs of all citizens were not being met. As the 20th century came to a close, we came to realize that as a society our obligation is to provide an environment in which achievement of good health for all is not only possible but expected. Yet there are population groups—such as the homeless, the elderly, and the poor—whose illness and death rates exceed those of the general population and may require additional resources to achieve good health.

Healthcare costs in the United States already amount to more than 17% of the gross domestic product (GDP), more than twice that of other countries that can boast better health statistics. Americans would probably be willing to live with the high price tag of health care if it made us all healthier than people in other countries. However, that is not the case. In the United States, where the healthcare system is heralded as the most sophisticated in the world, when compared with similar countries such as the United Kingdom, Germany, or France, we are lagging behind in the following:

- The United States has high infant mortality rates relative to other highly developed industrialized nations.
- The United States ranks 25th in the world in life expectancy, behind Japan, Italy, France, and the Scandinavian countries.
- Prior to the passage of the ACA of 2010, at least one-third of the U.S. population had limited access to basic health services and one-third of the uninsured were children.
- Prior to the passage of the ACA of 2010, the United States was the only industrialized nation in the world without guaranteed access to basic healthcare services.

> It is from quiet places like this all over the world that the forces accumulate which presently will overbear any attempt to accomplish evil on a large scale. Like the rivulets gathering into the river, and the river into the seas, there come from communities like this streams that fertilize the consciences of men, and it is the conscience of the world that we are trying to place upon the throne which others would usurp.
>
> —*U.S. President Woodrow Wilson, address in Carlisle, England, December 29, 1918*

Much must be done in this country for many to achieve levels of health that are acceptable and equitable (AAN, 2010). Many deaths and disabilities could be reduced by environmental improvements and lifestyle changes. One hundred years ago, most deaths were caused by infectious diseases; today, the leading causes of death are related to societal influences, lifestyle, and behavioral choices. Progress in technology, while making our everyday lives easier and safer, has created and built environmental threats to our air, water, products, and food. Health problems such as addiction and violence have emerged as serious threats to our wellbeing and even survival. As Keck (1994) contends, "Good health cannot be achieved without a social concern for ethical, humane decision-making … a just and caring society does not withhold health care from its citizens; sickness, after all, is never something people deserve" (p. 4).

Beyond looking at our own country's struggle with internal decisions about healthcare delivery and connecting it with the broader determinants of health, there has been a concurrent recognition of the global connectedness and importance of concerns for health. The achievement of world health has increasingly become a global expectation. Although nurses are still needed as skilled caregivers who improve the health of individual patients, a broader perspective has evolved as population health interventions are realized to be at least equally, if not more, significant in the attainment of health for all. Solutions to the health problems of populations worldwide now exceed the resources and control of any one individual (Gostin, 2004; McKenzie & Pinger, 1997).

Nursing in the 21st Century

Hospitals in the early part of the new millennium are relinquishing their role as the recognized hub of care delivery, while delivery of healthcare services at home, at work, at play, in schools and churches, online, and on the telephone continues to increase. Who delivers health care, what is provided, and when and where patients are seen have changed. Trends related to cost containment, managed care systems, technology, societal expectations, and politics have all influenced these changes. Patients stay less often in the hospital, and when they do, they stay for fewer days. Patients are generally sicker both when they are admitted and when they are discharged than they have been in the past. There has not been a significant decrease in patient numbers, but rather the settings for care have changed; with this shift, population health issues have become more of a focus.

There are greater demands on the healthcare system now than ever before, including evidence-based practice, as health care becomes more focused on efficiency and quality in patient care (Ferguson & Day, 2007). Nurses, as the translators and caregivers for patients with more complex needs, are needed more than ever. Nurses, as always, continue to meet the needs of patients; we move to care for populations in whatever setting they are found.

> **GOT AN ALTERNATIVE?**
>
> Research indicates that at least 62% of the U.S. public uses some form of nontraditional or alternative medicine—yet few patients mention such measures when visiting their healthcare providers. Why do you think people are reluctant to share their use and interest in alternative health practices with nurses and physicians?
>
> *Source:* Barnes, P. M., Powell-Griner, E., McFann, K., & Nahin, R. L. (2004). Complementary and alternative medicine use among adults: United States, 2002. *Advance Data, 343*, 1–19.

In a study conducted by the American Nurses Association's (ANA) Department of Labor Relations and Workplace Advocacy, nurse executives from acute, home health, extended, and managed care settings reported on the skills seen as most important for the next generation of nurses. According to this study, nurses should possess skills of self-reliance, independence, flexibility, and decision making, as well as a systems-thinking approach to health care, patient education, critical thinking skills, and computer skills. The conclusion of the study was that nurses need to be prepared to provide the four "rights" of nursing practice: give the *right* care, in the *right* setting, at the *right* time, and at the *right* cost (Canavan, 1996).

Trossman (1998), in *American Nurse*, stated:

> Hospitals will still be a major place of employment for nurses. The type of work will slowly change, though, as these hospitals become the care zones for the nation's oldest and sickest individuals. At the same time, other settings, such as home health and community based care, will provide increased opportunities for RNs with a BSN degree. (p. 1)

Educating Nurses for Community Health Nursing Practice

The *Essentials of Baccalaureate Nursing Education for Entry Level Community/Public Health Nursing*, a document revised and endorsed by the Association of Community Health Nursing Educators (ACHNE) in 2009, provides recommendations regarding the baccalaureate educational content essential for entry level in community health nursing practice. ACHNE is the only organization that represents community health nurse educators throughout the United States and many other parts of the world. The original purpose of the *Essentials*, as put forth in the first edition in 1990, was to "delineate the essentials of education for entry level community health nursing practice." This remains a core purpose of the subsequent updates of the document. Changes in the healthcare system and the corresponding emergence of issues in community/public health nursing (C/PHN) education and practice necessitate an ongoing revision of entry-level C/PHN essentials. The objectives of the document are (1) to provide a framework for nursing educators in planning and implementing baccalaureate nursing curricula relevant to 21st century healthcare systems, and (2) to communicate to nursing, public health, and other communities the theoretical and clinical practice underpinnings necessary for C/PHN education and practice. For nursing to survive as a profession, ACHNE (2009) recognizes that nursing must evolve along with the changing healthcare system. Nurses of the future will practice in a more complex healthcare system that involves care of individuals outside of acute care and traditional hospital settings (community-based care) and care of populations (community-focused care). This text uses the ACHNE document as the basis for its content and organization (The full text of the ACHNE *Essentials of Baccalaureate Nursing Education for Entry Level Community/Public Health Nursing* can be accessed at http://www.achne.org/files/EssentialsOfBaccalaureate_Fall_2009.pdf).

One of the most intriguing and challenging aspects of the health problems that we face in the 21st century is that we already know about effective interventions for many diseases and conditions in our society. According to Salmon and Vanderbush (1990), never before have we known as much about health as we do now; what we don't know is how to put this knowledge into action (p. 192).

Community-Based, Population-Focused, Community Health Nursing: What's in a Name?

What does it mean that health care is moving to the community? Why are there so many terms to describe nurses who work with a community focus? Much of the confusion over the title of a nurse who focuses on prevention in nonacute populations reflects the diversity that has created new roles for nurses in the community. Both the terms *public health nursing* and *community health nursing* are used to describe a nurse who works with populations and toward goals associated with improving the health of communities, families, and individuals. The primary difference may mean little to you as a student nurse at this point. Community health nursing has been the accepted title for the past few decades. In recent years, public health nursing has reemerged as an accepted title for nurses who work with the entire public and populations with an emphasis on prevention, not just in an official public health agency, to improve the health of populations. Various groups representing all community and public health nurses in the United States through the Quad Council of Public Health Nursing Organizations continue to debate the appropriate title for the nurse who works with a community focus (ANA, 2013; American Public Health Association, 1996; ACHNE, 2009). The term *community health nursing* will be used throughout this text.

RESEARCH ALERT

Is aspirin a disease-preventing wonder drug for women? The answer to that question is a moving target. In 2005, a 10-year study of nearly 40,000 women, at the time the biggest and best such study yet undertaken, provided the first authoritative assessment of whether women could improve their long-term cardiovascular health by taking regular aspirin—a practice many had already begun based largely on data from studies of men.

The 2005 study, however, was disappointing to many women and their healthcare providers. It found that aspirin does not reduce the risk of a first heart attack for middle-aged women, as it does for men, but it does cut the risk of strokes, which is not the case for men. For women 65 and older, aspirin does lower the chances of having a heart attack, and its stroke-preventing benefits appear to be the greatest.

The findings suggested that the benefits of aspirin may not outweigh the risks for healthy women in their 40s and 50s, but once they hit their 60s, the balance shifts enough to make it worthwhile. Aspirin's major risk is of bleeding, which can cause serious problems including rare but deadly bleeding strokes. Women with high blood pressure and problems with stomach bleeding may be at particular risk.

As a result of that study and similar evidence, the U.S. Preventive Services Task Force issued a recommendation in 2009 that suggested that while preventive aspirin therapy was of benefit to men 45 and older, in women, it should not be initiated until age 55, and should only be considered if its potential benefits outweighed the risk of gastrointestinal bleeding. In other words, for women, the scenario was much more complicated.

Now a new set of data suggests that daily low-dose aspirin offers another potential benefit for women: a reduced risk of ovarian cancer. Researchers from the National Cancer Institute (NCI) reviewed data accrued between 1992 and 2007 from 12 population-based case–control studies of ovarian cancer, including 7,776 case patients and 11,843 control subjects. Their findings showed that aspirin use was associated with a reduced risk of ovarian cancer, especially among women who took low-dose aspirin daily. These findings suggest that the same aspirin regimen originally recommended to women for cardiovascular health could instead reduce the risk of ovarian cancer by 20% to 34%, depending on frequency of use and dose. Their findings were published February 4, 2014, in the *Journal of the National Cancer Institute*.

"Our study suggests that aspirin regimens, proven to protect against heart attack, may reduce the risk of ovarian cancer as well," said Britton Trabert of NCI's Division of Cancer Epidemiology and Genetics, one of the study's authors. However, she cautioned that the results, though "intriguing," were not enough to change the way clinicians advise women. "Additional studies are needed to explore the delicate balance of risk-benefit for this potential chemopreventive agent, as well as studies to identify the mechanism by which aspirin may reduce ovarian cancer risk," Trabert noted.

What can women take away from all this back and forth about whether they should or shouldn't take daily aspirin?

For one thing, they can recognize that there's now a strong body of data showing that men and women differ in fundamental ways on various aspects of health, and that research on men does not necessarily translate directly to women.

"This truly underscores the importance of studying medical therapies among women as well as men," said Julie Buring of the Brigham and Women's Hospital in Boston, who led the 2005 study. "We can't assume studies involving men apply to women."

It remains unclear why women respond differently, although some researchers have speculated that it may be due to hormonal differences or the fact that women tend to develop heart disease later in life.

"Age 50 in men is biologically about age 60 in women in terms of their risk of cardiovascular disease," Buring said.

Aspirin, an ancient medicine known for a century mainly as a way to alleviate headaches and fevers, became a key player in the fight against cardiovascular disease—the nation's leading killer—after doctors discovered its powers to prevent and help dissolve blood clots and reduce inflammation. These anti-inflammatory properties may be part of what enables it to stifle cancer, but the 2014 study suggests that there is more to aspirin's cancer-preventing capacity than that: Women who used other nonsteroidal anti-inflammatory drugs (NSAIDs) daily or weekly also saw a slight decline in ovarian cancer incidence, but it was considerably less than that seen with aspirin (about 10%) and was not statistically significant.

What these conflicting findings boil down to, in the end, is that prevention is not one-size-fits-all. "We know millions of people take aspirin thinking it will prevent them from having a heart attack," said Scott M. Grundy of the University of Texas Southwestern Medical Center in Dallas. "But there are risks, and there might be a huge number of women who might be taking aspirin who shouldn't be, because the risks may outweigh the benefit. We just hadn't had the data."

In the 2005 study, about half of a group of 39,876 women age 45 and older took 100 milligrams of aspirin every other day, while the other half took a placebo. After 10 years, the researchers found that aspirin did not reduce the overall risk of heart attacks. But aspirin did reduce by 17% the overall risk of strokes, which tend to strike women more than men, and cut the risk for the most common type of strokes by 24%. When the researchers did a separate analysis of women 65 and older, however, they found that those taking aspirin were 34% less likely to suffer heart attacks, and that the protection against strokes increased as well.

At the time that study was released, clinicians greeted the findings with relief. "This is the definitive trial that we've been waiting for," said Lori Mosca, a women's heart expert at Columbia University. "This answers a big question about whether healthy women have benefits from taking low-dose aspirin." Yet, with the newest evidence on the table, many healthcare providers will need to re-weigh the argument all over again—this time with patients' ovarian cancer risk in mind as well.

Sources: Ridker, P. M., Cook, N. R., Lee, I. M., Gordon, D., Gaziano, J. M., Manson, J. E., ... Buring, J. E. (2005). A randomized trial of low-dose aspirin in the primary prevention of cardiovascular disease in women. *New England Journal of Medicine, 552*(13), 1293–1304; Trabert, B., Ness, R. B., Lo-Ciganic, W. H., Murphy, M. A., Goode, E. L., Poole, E. M., ... Wentzensen, N. (2014). Aspirin, nonaspirin nonsteroidal anti-inflammatory drug, and acetaminophen use and risk of invasive epithelial ovarian cancer: A pooled analysis in the Ovarian Cancer Association Consortium. *Journal of the National Cancer Institute, 106*(2), djt431. doi: 10.1093/jnci/djt431; National Institutes of Health. (2014). Press release: NIH study finds regular aspirin use may reduce ovarian cancer risk. Retrieved from http://www.nih.gov/news/health/feb2014/nci-06.htm

Communities and Populations

When we think of the word "community," we may have many pictures in our mind, because the word has a variety of meanings. Andy Griffith lived in the community of Mayberry, and *Mr. Rogers' Neighborhood* is also a community. Most television situation comedies revolve around a community, such as the television shows *Seinfeld*, *Sesame Street*, or even *The Simpsons* and *South Park*. In this text, the word **community** is defined as a group of people who share something in common and interact with one another, who may exhibit a commitment with one another and may share a geographic boundary. A **population** is defined as a group of people who have at least one thing in common and who may or may not interact with one another. See **Box 1-2**.

BOX 1-2 Terms To Know

Community

A *community* is a group of people who share something in common and interact with one another, who may exhibit a commitment with one another, and who may share a geographic boundary.

Population

A *population* is a group of people who have at least one thing in common and who may or may not interact with one another.

Examples of communities include the following:

- Lesbians in a communal living setting
- The town of Golden, Colorado
- The faculty at Florida State University School of Nursing
- The Devil's Own neighborhood urban gang
- Sunshine Heights Retirement Village
- Elders with disabilities living in urban high-rise apartments

Examples of populations include the following:

- Teens who remain sexually abstinent
- Sexually active teenagers
- Nurses who work the night shift

- Female long-distance runners
- Teenagers with Down syndrome
- First-time mothers older than age 35
- People who text while driving

According to Schultz (1994), *interaction* is essential in a community, whereas members of a population may or may not interact with one another. To put it another way, communities are usually aware of their "communityness," which binds them into a collective entity and to which they give a name (Cottrell, 1976, pp. 114–115). Some populations evolve into communities over time. Elderly women who participate in a water aerobics class, for example, may develop into a cohesive interactive community that shares other common activities and interests.

> Small communities grow great through harmony, great ones fall to pieces through discord.
>
> —*Gaius Sallustius Crispus (c. 86–35/34* B.C.*), Roman historian*

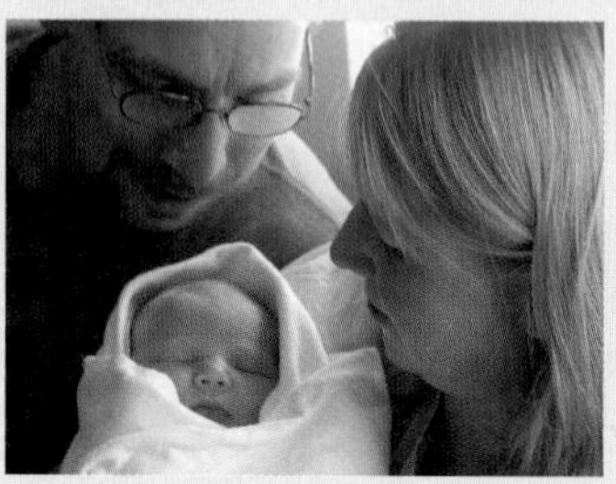
© Alan Heartfield/Shutterstock, Inc.

The average lifespan of Americans increased from 45 years to 75 years during the 20th century, but it is interesting to note that only five of those years are attributable to individual preventive or curative interventions such as cardiac surgery. Twenty-five of the additional years of life expectancy have resulted from public health efforts to provide for safe water, effective waste disposal, adequate housing, and other improvements in the overall health of communities (Bunker, Frazier, & Mosteller, 1994; Centers for Disease Control and Prevention [CDC], 2002).

There are many ways in which nurses are moving into new settings and expanding their application of community health nursing skills. Although these nurses are bringing expertise of acute care and technology to community settings, they are often lacking in their knowledge of community dynamics and public health concepts (Gebbie, 1996). If nurses are to continue to be a dynamic part of health care in the future, we must be able to understand the complex and community-focused nature of health promotion, illness prevention, recovery from illness and injury, and health restoration (Kurtzman, Ibgui, Pogrund, & Monin, 1980). We need to expand our knowledge and expertise in the care of individuals and our skills in hospital-based clinical management of illness and injury to include care of individuals in community settings (Hall & Stevens, 1995; Keller, Strohstein, Lia-Hoagberg, & Shaeffer, 2004). By using our expert knowledge and experience in medical–surgical, maternal–child, and psychiatric nursing, we can assist individuals, families, and groups to make choices that promote health and wellness (Smith, 1995).

Acute Care Versus Community Health Nursing

Let's compare acute care and community health nursing to more fully understand how these nursing roles differ both in setting and practice focus. In the acute care setting, there is the issue of provider control. Patients are well aware of who is in control in the hospital setting—the healthcare professional. The patient is in a subordinate position to the nurse, who remains the ultimate authority regarding when to go to sleep, what to wear, when and how much to urinate, what kind of diet to eat and when, and whether visitors are allowed. Treatments and interventions are done to the patient and scheduled at staff and hospital convenience. Patients, who are often identified by their condition (e.g., "the gallbladder in room 214"), are isolated from friends, family, and pets, who are excluded from the healthcare setting. Little individualized care that takes into consideration the patient's lifestyle and preferences is given. When a person changes into a hospital gown, the role of patient is assumed. Personal items such as medications, glasses, and false teeth are often relinquished, and self-care is limited, with permission often required from nurses for activities taken for granted at home. Many questions are asked, sometimes over and over by different health professionals, and most often these questions are of a very personal and intimate nature. Rarely does the patient receive any explanation for why information is needed, for to question is to risk being labeled a "difficult" patient—and we know what that means (Armentrout, 1998)! Refer to **Table 1-1** for differences in nursing interventions by setting.

The controlled environment of the acute care setting, however, has many benefits for the nurse:

- Predictable routine
- Maintenance of hospital policy
- Predictability of nursing and medical goals
- Resource availability, both human and material
- Collegial collaboration and consultation
- Controlled patient compliance with the plan of care: the patient takes correct medicine and treatment on time
- Standardization of care

The community setting is very different from acute care, especially in regard to the nurse–patient relationship. Nurses tend to be dependent on patients' willingness to share health information and to adhere to the plan of care, and patients

TABLE 1-1 Differences in Nursing Interventions by Setting

Health Problem	Acute Care Setting: Hospital	Community-Based Setting: Home Health
Osteoporosis resulting in degenerative hip disease	Treatment	Teach patient how to walk after surgery.
	Surgery and recovery (total hip replacement)	Involve family with encouraging activity and flexibility exercises.

on their own turf act very differently than they do in the acute care setting. A significant advantage is that the nurse is able to assess environmental conditions, food and other critical resources, lifestyle influences, and the social support system, such as friends, family, and pets. Transportation issues, which may affect the ability to adhere to medical and nursing goals, often become overriding concerns that are not even considered in the hospital setting.

In a community-based setting such as a school clinic, the nurse is dependent on the child's willingness to share information about his or her health concerns and on the teacher regarding any relevant learning issues that may affect the child's health. Educational goals are the primary concerns of the school, and the nurse must consider health in this total context.

The lack of colleagues to consult about problems and challenges encountered in community settings is often a cause of stress among new graduates and nurses who have never worked outside the controlled environment of the hospital and acute care settings (Armentrout, 1998).

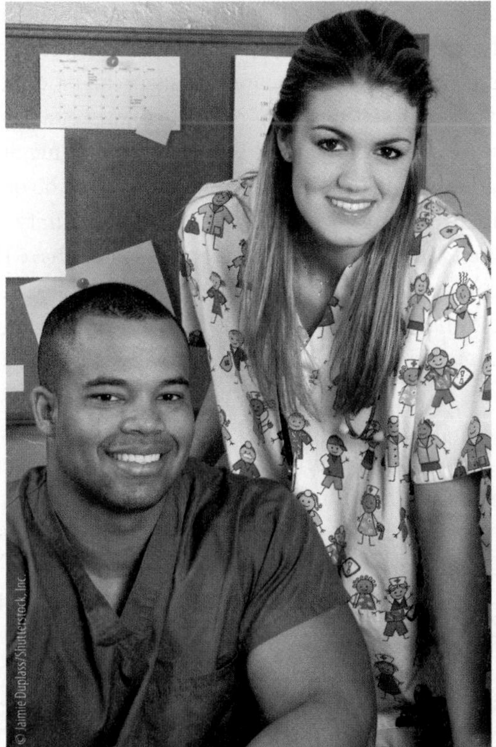

© Jaimie Duplass/Shutterstock, Inc.

Opening Doors. While the majority of RNs still work in hospitals, the number of them working in community-based settings continues to grow.

Benefits for the community-based patient include the following:

- Familiar and comfortable environment
- Routine that is less determined by the nurse or health professional
- Diverse resources, including friends, family, and pets, available for support and comfort
- Autonomy and choice in health decisions

Reform and the Reinvention of Systems of Care

Our healthcare system is but one of the many overlapping and interacting systems created by society. Societies create systems that reflect the commonly held values of that society. This is the realm of policy, politics, and power. For example, since the September 11, 2001 terrorist attacks on the United States, U.S. priorities have changed dramatically regarding safety and wellbeing. Bioterrorism and threats such as anthrax require public officials to use resources previously earmarked for other health priorities. Nurses have functioned in situations with increased stress, coping with the effects of national diseases themselves while still helping others deal with the ongoing trauma of a post-9/11 world (Davidhizar, Eshleman, & Wolff, 2003).

Healthcare reform initiatives have arisen in this realm of competing and conflicting values. Groups that advocate values related to protection, wellbeing, sustenance, quality of life, equity, fairness, and justice must often compete with other values related to economic self-interest. Even when values do not seem to be in conflict, the methods recommended to act on those values often cannot be agreed upon.

The capitalist values of the healthcare delivery system in the United States have also been questioned by healthcare leaders and policymakers in other countries (Moon, 1993; Morse, 2003). They often do not understand how the United States can consider itself a highly industrialized and civilized country and not provide basic, essential health care for all. A caring society would not allow individuals (especially children) to be deprived of health care. Many find our nonsystems approach to health care confusing. In a post-9/11 world, these chaotic times require even more thoughtful and prioritized planning to meet the critical population health needs of the most vulnerable groups in our society (Gostin, Boufford, & Martinez, 2004; Morse, 2003).

Indeed, few Americans would not argue that, although the health–illness system has changed with more vulnerable populations covered under the ACA, it still needs improvement. Many of the authors throughout this text make reference to **healthcare reform**. Enacted reforms, proposed reforms, and preferred reforms all have actual and possible effects on the populations for which nurses provide care and the conditions under which they provide it. Reform is not new, nor is it controlled; rather, it is episodic, responding to multiple forces for change. Reform implies some major change in the process of the delivery of health care. We often refer to reform as change that originates at the national level but is implemented by the states, by payers, or by provider systems. When change is not a "broad" and "sweeping" reform, it is considered an "incremental change," meaning smaller adjustments occur over time. This is the type of healthcare reform that occurred during the 1990s.

Historically, there have been numerous reform proposals. Major healthcare reform was attempted following World War II—in 1948, President Harry Truman proposed national health insurance. What many thought were the beginnings of broad health coverage were introduced in the 1960s as Medicaid and Medicare. In the 1970s, Senator Edward Kennedy (D-Massachusetts) was one of the major supporters of nationwide reform. The presidential campaigns of 2008 and 2012 were marked by passionate disagreements over health reform issues. Many such disagreements specifically focused on the ACA, which has been a key political issue since its passage in 2010 (even after the subsequent ruling by the Supreme Court in 2012 that the ACA is constitutional).

Nursing's Agenda for Health Care Reform

The failed effort of the 1990s to redesign the U.S. healthcare system had at least one positive consequence for nursing. In an unprecedented collaboration, more than 75 nursing associations endorsed the document jointly developed by the ANA and the National League for Nursing (NLN), ***Nursing's Agenda for Health Care Reform***. This document was significant in terms of its expression of nursing's values and in furthering an understanding of the profession itself. Values such as health services for all, illness prevention, and wellness were identified as prominent concerns. Many nurses played influential and visible roles during the healthcare reform attempts. Nursing supported the need for cost containment but wanted assurance of quality of care, reduced barriers to advanced practice nursing, and promotion of nursing care as the link between consumers and the healthcare system. According to the document, "the cornerstone of nursing's plan for reform is the delivery of primary healthcare services to households and individuals in convenient, familiar places" (ANA, 1991, p. 9).

Managed Care and the Future of Nursing

With the passage of the ACA, the controversial issues most debated are expanding federal coverage (access), controlling costs, and moving to evidence-based practice. Evidence-based practice directs care through verifiable research (Ferguson & Day, 2007). Many policy and regulation changes within the ACA, however, have had a significant impact on healthcare delivery systems and providers already. **Managed care** and a market approach based on "managed competition" have emerged as major strategies to control costs in the United States. These connected strategies have together transformed the organization and methods of care delivery.

Care management is a growing practice arena for nurses. Within the managed care environment, care management attempts to provide more timely and coordinated care for individuals. Individuals move among the following possible states: being well and promoting that state, having acute care needs, needing outpatient surgery, needing follow-up home care, and so on.

Healthcare organizations now see the economic and quality outcome benefits of caring for patients and managing patient care over a continuum of possible settings and needs. Traditional health care was episodic, with individuals moving with little connection from one episode of need to the next (often waiting until the need for care was acute) and one facility to another. When care is managed, the term *discharge planning* is now more accurately referred to as *transition planning* (Ferguson & Day, 2007). The patient does not leave the system, but merely requires another type of care, including wellness care or health promotion. Patients are followed much more closely both during illness care and with follow-up care when well. Care managers can practice from a base in many settings, including the offices of a payer. To more clearly conceptualize this change in thinking, instead of a patient being discharged from the hospital, he or she is described as being admitted *back* to the community.

When the healthcare providers in a system have the responsibility for all types of care for the plan's enrolled population, they have a financial incentive to coordinate or manage that care efficiently. The goal is to provide the best value in the most efficient way to be competitive in the healthcare market. A market economy with the addition of the ACA for healthcare delivery dramatically changes healthcare services and incentives. For nurses who are historically committed to doing whatever it takes for their patients, cost-consciousness is an unfamiliar and often resisted viewpoint.

Nurses in today's healthcare system must remain informed about the complexities of managed care if they are to sustain their professional identity and to assist patients in navigating this market system. The continued growth of managed care and the implementation of the ACA, as a system for health financing and delivery, provide unique challenges and opportunities for nurses, especially those prepared in community health. Nurses remain the only healthcare professionals who are specifically educated to assess health status and risks, unhealthy lifestyles, and health education needs for patients and families—who provide support and reassurance while caring for present and potential health problems and who act as advocates for primary and preventive care services. Managed care organizations, as well as all agencies that provide healthcare services in a managed care environment, have come to value quality and recognize the importance of prevention, wellness, and early intervention. The community health nurse is especially well prepared to provide managed care with the direction needed to focus on providing a full range of quality, cost-effective services in the promotion of a population's health.

> Money would be better spent in maintaining health in infancy and childhood than in building hospitals to cure diseases.
>
> —*Florence Nightingale, 1894*

Back to the Future: From Hospital to Community, from Cure to Prevention

As we have learned from the history of health care, early attempts to improve health, treat disease, and prevent disability occurred primarily in the home. The primary characteristic of the emerging system has been the move back to the community practice setting. Perhaps the major force behind much of the change has been economic, with efforts to contain what many see as the exploding costs of the U.S. healthcare system. The ACA came about primarily due to spiraling healthcare costs, which continue to delay economic recovery in the United States from the 2008 financial crisis. The stated purpose of the ACA is to "increase the number of Americans covered by health insurance and decrease the cost of health care." One cost-related factor encouraging a community focus has been the movement of patients out of expensive acute care facilities and into community settings, where many of their illness needs can be adequately met at a much lower cost. This movement has encouraged the growth of home care, hospice care, medical homes (coordinated and accessible care in a central home base for the patient through ACA legislative policies), nurse-managed clinics, outpatient treatment clinics, and outpatient surgeries. Another among the many results of cost-containment efforts has been the recognition of the connection between prevention and keeping populations healthy. Healthy populations have lower morbidity (disease rates) and mortality (death rates).

> My view, you know, is that the ultimate destination of all nursing is the nursing of the sick in their own homes. . . . I look to the abolition of all hospitals and workhouse infirmaries. But no use to talk about the year 2000.
>
> —*Florence Nightingale, 1867*

A DAY IN THE LIFE

Melanie C. Dreher, PhD, RN, FAAN

I am more convinced than ever that the major health problems in this and future decades—chronicity, aging, the personal and public health problems generated by social and economic dislocations, the prevention of illness, and the promotion of healthy communities—are all within the nursing genius to address and ameliorate. These are the very things that we are known for. They are the things we do best and we are the best to do them. . . . I truly believe that we are at a place in nursing that we will never see again. This is our big chance. . . . We cannot wait for anybody to let us do anything. . . . We have more capacity to play in the healthcare game, we have the obligation to take charge, to endorse professional values, and improve health outcomes.

Home Health Care

Home health care is the fastest growing community-based nursing role outside of the acute care setting. It is just one of many roles available in community health and is covered in depth in this text. Home health nursing is an example of an emerging role that has resulted from changes in the way health care is delivered and paid for.

One attempt at major healthcare cost containment in the early 1980s was the shift from cost reimbursement to prospective payment for hospital care, which means that payment is based on standard disease categories. Because of this change, hospitals could make money if they were efficient in taking care of patients' problems and could discharge them more quickly. Home health boomed as patients were discharged while still needing nursing care in their homes. Home health continues to grow and present new and challenging opportunities for nursing, with the implementation of the ACA and its emphasis on providing care in the most efficient environment to improve patient health outcomes and reduce hospitalizations.

Cure and Prevention: Can We Really Do It All?

Most people—even nurses—spend little time thinking about or planning for their own good health or the community's health. Research tells us that our health is influenced more by our social and biological environment, lifestyle choices, and self-care initiatives than by our inherited traits, yet we continue to pour money into newer and better treatments rather than into learning about what we can do to promote health and prevent illness from the beginning. We are discovering that we have overemphasized cure with a disease-based medical model for health care.

As early as 1977, the CDC reported an analysis of the proportional contributions to mortality in the United States of four health field elements: lifestyle, human biology, environment, and health care. Its conclusions were that approximately 50% of premature mortality in the United States is due to lifestyle, 20% to human biology, 20% to environment, and only 10% to inadequacies in health care. Seventy percent of the potential for reducing premature mortality lies in the areas of health promotion and disease prevention, but only about 3.5% of the healthcare dollar is spent in those areas. Therefore, although the health status of a population is related more to the determinants of health than it is to the causes of disease, we have developed a system that pays for illness care rather than a system designed to create the healthiest population possible.

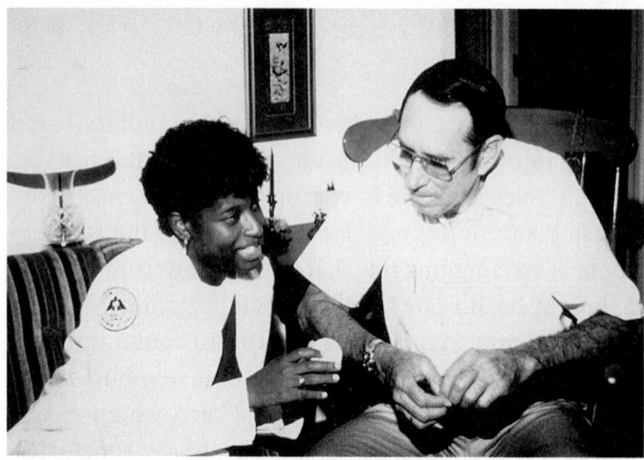

Home health nurses deliver care in the patient's home. A goal of home care is to teach self-care to patients and their families.

Certainly, access to competent and skilled health practitioners and technologies related to the diagnosis and treatment of disease is important, but no more so than having clean water to drink, safe food to eat, meaningful and safe employment with an adequate wage, adequate housing and child care, a good education, a life free of discrimination, and a safe environment. Such insights are leading to a "reinvention" of health services organizations at all levels—from single facilities organized to serve sick patients to complex networks organized to serve populations of mostly well people in the community (Friedman, 2013; Shortell & Gilles, 1995).

Prevention activities and population-focused care are often contrasted with the more immediately gratifying and exciting acute care. Community-focused care is long term, often behind the scenes, taken for granted, and largely unseen unless something goes amiss. Nurses have always promoted the welfare and health of those in their care. Wolf (1989) contends that nursing has difficulty being visible because much of the work of nursing goes unnoticed. Healthcare reform and the move to health promotion and illness prevention may provide the opportunity for nursing to shine as a profession. Public health's success literally makes it invisible to most of us.

Despite the excitement of acute care, many economic, social, and political factors suggest that the future focus of health care will be on health promotion and disease prevention in a health-based model with a community orientation (Friedman, 2013; Proenca, 1998). These areas and such networking have traditionally been the domain of the less visible and less financially supported practice of public health. Mechanic (1998) has pointed out that an alignment of public health with the growing managed care health plans would be a logical and potential benefit to the mission of the U.S. public health system. The vision of public health for more than a century has been one of health promotion and disease prevention that depends on a community perspective to activate identification of risks and protective and restorative interventions.

Healthcare providers in managed care plans are increasingly subject to competition and are evaluated on their successes in improving outcomes for their plan's enrollees. They have become more interested in the population activities and methods long carried out by public health. Acknowledging the economic value of population health promotion and disease prevention activities within the ACA and private healthcare marketplaces encourages the adoption of these approaches. Thus, for many nurses caring for individuals, the focus on community health nursing roles represents a transition to the community in practice setting.

Nurses have been optimistic about the trends in healthcare practice and reform. With the increasing impetus for health promotion, nurses seem well poised as a result of their long-standing commitment to and expertise in keeping people healthy. In the past, when nurses have made claims about the benefits of health promotion and disease prevention strategies, the thoughts have been on benefits to the individual, not on any financial benefit or loss. Now we as nurses are beginning to embrace the possibilities of teaming up with a market-driven business world to also realize financial benefits and improved health for populations.

Benefits Versus Costs

Anderson (1997) cautions against a naive understanding of what we take for granted. Indeed, she describes the case of smoking cessation programs, which have been proven to have economic benefits. However, a potential financial loss scenario is possible for preventing cardiopulmonary disease in middle-aged individuals. Prevention may actually increase managed care costs by prolonging a person's life and thus incurring greater costs for the complex medical problems of old age. Similarly, early detection of HIV in at-risk populations should permit early drug treatment to prevent costly AIDS-related illnesses. For a managed care organization, early detection would imply antiviral treatment costing thousands of dollars annually. Nondetection and an early death would actually save money for a private healthcare provider and increase its profits. Nurses are socialized to value life; healthcare companies are in business to make a profit first.

RESEARCH ALERT

Research has shown that children wearing Heelys sustain the same types of injuries as those wearing inline skates or riding skateboards or scooters. According to Vincent Iannelli, MD, two medical studies reported that children wearing Heelys had injuries ranging from "distal radius fractures and elbow injuries to a head injury that required surgery."

Although the manufacturer recommends wearing safety gear such as a helmet, wrist guards, and kneepads, very few children wear safety gear with Heelys. To prevent injuries, children should wear safety gear, remove the wheels when using Heelys in shoe mode, and avoid using the Heelys in skate mode in traffic, on stairs, or on uneven surfaces. Children should also avoid crowded areas and rolling faster than they can walk.

Many public places, including schools, ban the use of Heelys in skate mode and require children to take the wheels out of the Heelys before entering. Heelys should not be used in skate mode indoors. Falling into such indoor hazards as a table or display case can cause serious injury.

Parents should also know that W.A.T.C.H. (World Against Toys Causing Harm) included Heelys on their "10 worst toys" list.

With such dire warnings, nurses must realize the competing values often at work in the healthcare arena. Community-focused health promotion strategies also can face ideological, political, and religious differences that cause conflict. Much-needed sex education to prevent teenage pregnancy has long met with resistance from some groups. Strategies must be developed at the individual and societal levels to bring about change that aligns with all interested parties' goals and needs.

In the case of smoking cessation, for example, other community groups could be approached to encourage health promotion interventions and policies. Employers could be motivated to realize the financial gain of less employee illness and fewer workdays lost. They would then negotiate for managed care plans that cover health promotion activities (Friedman, 2013).

Healthy People 2020: Goals for the Nation

Even before the more recent reform efforts and regulations encouraged increased use of prevention practices, it became obvious in the 1970s, based on the CDC's study of premature deaths, that health promotion and disease prevention could save lives and perhaps reduce healthcare costs. In 1980, the federal government issued a set of national health objectives that were evaluated to measure the progress of U.S. health goals and healthcare services. The process proved valuable and was repeated with the issuing of a new set of objectives to guide the 1990s; that plan was titled *Healthy People 2000: National Health Promotion and Disease Prevention Objectives*.

The process was again repeated, culminating in the release of a *Healthy People 2010* document in October 2000. Two overarching goals—increase years of healthy life and eliminate health disparities—were proposed. Four enabling goals provided support; they were concerned with promoting healthful behaviors, protecting health, achieving access to quality health care, and strengthening community prevention. ***Healthy People 2020*** has been revised to focus on creating a society in which all citizens live long lives through an interactive website.

These objectives provide a tool that the creators envision for public health policymakers at the national, state, and local levels. Meeting these objectives requires that all healthcare providers move toward a community-based practice or focus. That is, providers must move from a focus on illness and cure to a focus on health promotion and illness prevention not only for populations at risk, but also for **populations of interest**—those people who are essentially healthy but whose health status could be improved or protected (Friedman, 2013; Keller et al., 2004).

> Preventable disease should be looked on as a social crime.
>
> —*Florence Nightingale, 1894*

HEALTHY PEOPLE 2020 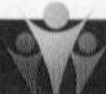

Introducing *Healthy People 2020*

Healthy People 2020 continues in this tradition with the launch on December 2, 2010 of its ambitious, yet achievable, 10-year agenda for improving the nation's health. *Healthy People 2020* is the result of a multiyear process that reflects input from a diverse group of individuals and organizations. For the first time, *Healthy People 2020* has an interactive website and database which provides statistical information about specific health issues and is searchable, making it accessible to citizens and health professionals, alike.

Vision

A society in which all people live long, healthy lives.

Mission

Healthy People 2020 strives to:

- Identify nationwide health improvement priorities.
- Increase public awareness and understanding of the determinants of health, disease, and disability and the opportunities for progress.
- Provide measurable objectives and goals that are applicable at the national, state, and local levels.
- Engage multiple sectors to take actions to strengthen policies and improve practices that are driven by the best available evidence and knowledge.
- Identify critical research, evaluation, and data-collection needs.

Overarching Goals

- Attain high-quality, longer lives free of preventable disease, disability, injury, and premature death.
- Achieve health equity, eliminate disparities, and improve the health of all groups.
- Create social and physical environments that promote good health for all.
- Promote quality of life, healthy development, and healthy behaviors across all life stages.

Four foundational health measures will serve as indicators of progress toward achieving these goals:

- General health status
- Health-related quality of life and wellbeing
- Determinants of health
- Disparities

Source: Healthy People 2020. Available at http://www.healthypeople.gov/2020/about/default.aspx
The topic areas and objectives of the *Healthy People 2020* agenda are available in interactive format online at http://www.healthypeople.gov/2020/topicsobjectives2020/.

Graphic Model of *Healthy People 2020*

The Federal Interagency Working Group developed a graphic model to visually depict the ecological and determinants approach that *Healthy People 2020* will take in framing the national health objectives. This particular graphic was designed to emphasize this new approach, and is not meant as a comprehensive representation of all public health issues and societal domains. The graphic framework attempts to illustrate the fundamental degree of overlap among the social determinants of health, and to emphasize their collective impact and influence on health outcomes and conditions. The framework also underscores a continued focus on population disparities, including those categorized by race/ethnicity, socioeconomic status, gender, age, disability status, sexual orientation, and geographic location.

Healthy People 2020

A society in which all people live long, healthy lives

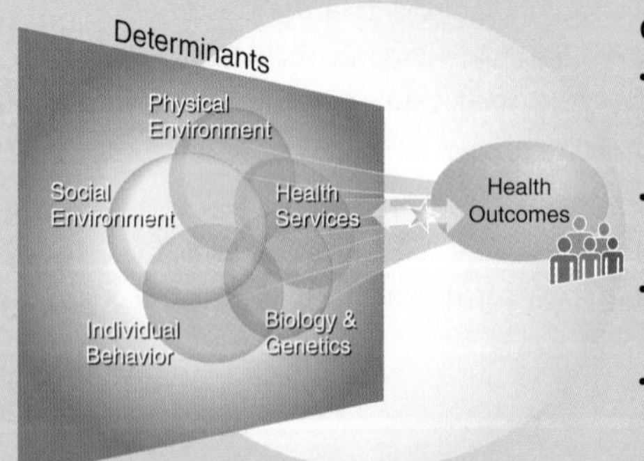
Determinants
Physical Environment
Social Environment
Health Services
Individual Behavior
Biology & Genetics
Health Outcomes
Overarching Goals:
• Attain high quality, longer lives free of preventable disease, disability, injury, and premature death.
• Achieve health equity, eliminate disparities, and improve the health of all groups.
• Create social and physical environments that promote good health for all.
• Promote quality of life, healthy development, and healthy behaviors across all life stages.

Figure 1-1 *Health People 2020 Graphic* Model

Reproduced from U.S. Public Health Service. Healthy People 2020. http://www.healthypeople.gov/2020/Consortium/HP2020Framework.pdf

Source: Healthy People 2020. Available at http://www.healthypeople.gov/2020/about/default.aspx

Influences on a Community's Health: Culture, Environment, and Ethics

Many different factors influence health care, making it difficult to decide which are the most important. For the nurse to isolate any one factor for assessment and intervention with both individuals and communities is like the captain of a ship seeing only the tip of the iceberg and not looking for the real threat to the ship's safety that lies underneath. However, three major components of health care are addressed in this chapter because they have a profound effect on all aspects of patient care: culture, environment, and ethics.

Culture

The numerous global, social, demographic, economic, and political changes in recent years have alerted health-care professionals to the need to provide attention to the increasing diversity in our society and the effect of that diversity on people's health (Meleis, 1996). International travel and advances in communication through the Internet, cell phones, and cable and satellite television make it essential for today's nurses to develop the skills needed to provide care that recognizes complexities and differences among patients (Janes & Hobson, 1998).

The United States is the most culturally diverse nation in the world. In fact, in 1994, *Time* magazine designated the United States the first universal nation (Grossman, 1994). In the 2010 U.S. Census, almost 30% of Americans were members of ethnic minority groups, including 13.1% African American, 16.9% Hispanic/Latino, 5.3% Asian/Pacific Islander, 1.2% American Indian and Alaska Native, and 2.4% identified themselves as two or more races.

Nurses must be sensitive to cultural differences to be able to provide the best possible care to individuals, families, and communities. But what, exactly, do we mean by the term *culture*? According to Leininger (1995), **culture** refers to the learned and shared beliefs, values, and lifeways of a designated or particular group that are generally transmitted intergenerationally and influence one's thinking and action modes. Giger and Davidhizar (1995) say that culture is a patterned behavioral response that develops over time as a result of imprinting the mind through social and religious structures and intellectual and artistic manifestations.

Purnell and Paulanka (2003) define culture as the totality of socially transmitted behavioral patterns, art, beliefs, values, customs, lifeways, and all other products of human work and thought characteristics of a population of people that guide their worldview and decision making. Obviously, culture is more than just ethnicity. Culture is language, religion, food, traditions, customs, clothing, and everything that makes one group of people unique and distinguishes it from other groups. Cultural values, beliefs, and behaviors can also be related to age, gender, sexual orientation, socioeconomic status, and profession. There is a culture of nursing that all nurses belong to, with its own language, values, and traditions that often clashes with patients whose cultural beliefs about health care differ from those of their nurses. Further, nursing as a profession struggles with a lack of cultural diversity itself, which presents yet another population that must be considered as we promote a holistic and representative profession.

When considering cultural issues, we need to look beyond the borders of our own country. Those who hold privileged and recognized positions in societies by virtue of specialized expertise, such as nursing, have an obligation to give back to those societies (Vilschick, 2003). To make such contributions, nurses should become "global citizens" holding a broad vision of international health. In today's connected world, no profession can be truly effective without interactions and viewpoints that include international perspectives. Community health nurses, especially, who by definition practice within a broad systems perspective, must incorporate understandings from international health efforts in their own interventions. Comparing and drawing insights from methods and successes of nurses in delivering care in other countries hold the promise of improving the care to U.S. patients. In addition, there is a need to understand and support collaborating agencies at the international level. Principles of pluralism, consultation, coherence, consensus, compassion, partnership, and cooperation are the hallmarks of nurses who practice and embrace global citizenship (Neufield, 1992). For example, control measures for effectively reducing HIV/AIDS have involved the active cooperation of most countries worldwide.

CULTURAL CONNECTION

After reviewing the section on culture in Chapter 1, why do you think nursing has had difficulty recruiting minorities and males into the profession?

Environment

The environment has been a concern for nursing since the days of Florence Nightingale. In *Notes on Nursing* (1860), Nightingale emphasizes the fact that recovery from illness can occur only in a bright, clean, well-ventilated environment. She states:

> The very first canon of nursing, the first and the last thing upon which a nurse's attention must be fixed, the first essential to a patient, without which all the rest you

can do for him is nothing, with which I had almost said you may leave all the rest alone, is this: TO KEEP THE AIR HE BREATHES AS PURE AS THE EXTERNAL AIR, WITHOUT CHILLING HIM.

When Nightingale spoke of the patient's environment, she meant the room in the hospital or home in which the patient stayed during the course of illness. In more recent years, the public health definition of **environment** has come to mean all the surroundings and conditions that affect the health of individuals, families, and communities, including the built environment. The environment has many different components, including social, cultural, political, economic, and ecological factors.

Environmental issues have been in the forefront of many political campaigns during the last several years and seem to be gaining momentum, with many governmental and private community groups supporting legislation to protect the environment (Graham, 1997). Most of this activity has been focused on the ecological component of environmental health—primarily clean air and water and a safe food supply. The created or built environment has only recently gained attention as another part of the environment, which affects a population's health. An example of the built environment is toxic workplaces with occupational hazards and homes with radon poisoning.

Nurses are beginning to take a more active role in promoting environmental health, reducing environmental health risks, and protecting Earth's resources. In fact, several nursing organizations, such as the American Holistic Nurses Association and the International Council of Nurses, have developed position statements to delineate the nurse's role in promoting environmental health. A specialty organization called Nurses for Environmental and Social Responsibility has been formed specifically to educate nurses and the public about environmental health hazards.

ENVIRONMENTAL CONNECTION

The work we are speaking of has nothing to do with nursing disease, but with maintaining health by removing the things which disturb it ... dirt, drink, diet, damp, draughts, and drains.

—Florence Nightingale, 1860

RESEARCH ALERT

How Safe Is Airline Drinking Water?

The Environmental Protection Agency (EPA) is the federal agency responsible for safe drinking water in communities, in public places, and on airplanes. In the summer and fall of 2004, the EPA tested drinking water aboard hundreds of randomly selected domestic and international passenger aircraft. The summer data showed that 13% of tested aircraft water failed to meet EPA standards; the fall 2004 testing showed that 17% failed the standards. Coliform bacteria, usually harmless, indicate that harmful organisms could be present and were found in unacceptable levels.

In response to these findings, the EPA embarked on a process to tailor the existing regulations for aircraft public water systems. In 2008, the EPA proposed the Aircraft Drinking Water Rule for public review and comment. The EPA will now have domestic airlines test themselves and submit results to the agency to see if the trend continues. Some self-sampling has begun, and airlines are adapting their routine disinfections to meet EPA guidance. Airlines now must disinfect water systems every 3 months and water carts and hoses leading to aircraft monthly.

Passengers with compromised immune systems should request canned or bottled beverages and avoid drinking coffee, tea, and other drinks prepared with tap water while on board airplanes. In the interim, to further protect the traveling public, the EPA placed 45 air carriers under Administrative Orders on Consent (AOCs), which will remain in effect until tailored aircraft drinking water regulations are final. These protocols will protect the public while existing regulations are being reviewed and data are being collected and analyzed from the aircraft drinking water. The air carrier AOCs combine sampling, best management practices, corrective action, public notification, and reporting and recordkeeping.

Source: Environmental Protection Agency (EPA). (2008). Airline water supplies. Retrieved August 28, 2008, from http://www.epa.gov/safewater/airlinewater

Ethics

Since the time of Florence Nightingale, the nursing profession has been addressing **ethics** concerns related to patient care issues. The ANA's (2008) *Code of Ethics for Nurses with Interpretive Statements* provides guidance for ethical decisions made by nurses in the clinical setting.

Ethical dilemmas have traditionally included such issues as informed consent and individual freedom of choice, autonomy, truth telling, protection of privacy and confidentiality, and discrimination. In addition, public

> Where justice is denied, where poverty is enforced, where ignorance prevails, and where any one class is made to feel that society is an organized conspiracy to oppress, rob and degrade them, neither persons nor property will be safe.
>
> *—Frederick Douglass (1818–1895), address on the 24th anniversary of emancipation, Washington, DC, 1886*

health nurses have had to make ethical decisions related to the dual obligation to protect the public's welfare while respecting the rights of individual patients (Folmar, Coughlin, Bessinger, & Sacknoff, 1997). According to Sorrell (2012), all nurses must consider healthcare reform and the public's health as a part of their ethical responsibility. Sorrell states that all health professionals should consider how "the implementation of the ACA relates to their role in understanding and trying to rectify conditions of injustice in health care. Changes in social attitudes and resources may require the combined efforts of different disciplines to identify the originating problem and find a way to remediate it."

BOX 1-3 About *Healthy People*

Healthy People provides science-based, 10-year national objectives for improving the health of all Americans. For more than 3 decades, *Healthy People* has established benchmarks and monitored progress over time in order to:

- Encourage collaborations across communities and sectors.
- Empower individuals toward making informed health decisions.
- Measure the impact of prevention activities.

Source: Reproduced from U.S. Public Health Service. Healthy People 2020. http://www.healthypeople.gov/2020/About-Healthy-People

ETHICAL CONNECTION

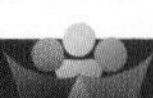

"Every community is an association of some kind and every community is established with a view to some good; for everyone always acts in order to obtain that which they think good. But, if all communities aim at some good, the state or political community, which is the highest of all, and which embraces all the rest, aims at good in a greater degree than any other, and at the highest good."

—Aristotle (384–323 B.C.)

Public health is concerned with ensuring the safety of the public's "good"—for example, through protection from hazards such as known infectious diseases where the administration of vaccinations ensures population and public protection. Such public interventions often inspire highly politicized legal debates, where the delicate balance between individual rights and freedom of choice is sacrificed for the sake of the community's right to good health. One such debate is over smoking bans in public places versus the right of individual tobacco users to exercise their rights to smoke in public places. How do you think Aristotle would respond to such a debate?

Today's changing healthcare delivery system brings with it additional ethical dilemmas for nurses. We are now concerned with problems related to equity in healthcare delivery, implementation of the ACA to improve

THINK ABOUT THIS

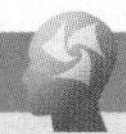

The first rays of sunlight peek through your bedroom curtains, accompanied by the fresh air of a new day. You breathe deeply and enjoy the clean air that public health protects by monitoring radiation levels and developing strategies to keep them low.

Rousing the children, you usher them into the bathroom for their showers. You brush your teeth, knowing the water won't make you sick because safe drinking water is the responsibility of public health.

You check your smile in the mirror. You can't remember your last cavity, thanks in part to the fluoride public health helps add to the water. Through similar programs, public health has always sought to promote good health by preventing disease altogether.

The family clambers to the table just as you finish pouring the milk, which is safe to drink because the State Department of Health checks and monitors it from the dairy to the grocery store.

After breakfast, you call your sister, who is pregnant with her first child, and find out her routine doctor's visit went perfectly. Even in the small town where she lives, your sister can visit a local doctor. Public health recognized the need for doctors in rural areas and helped place one there.

Your sister tells you her doctor suggested she visit the county health department and enroll in the Women, Infants, and Children (WIC) program, another public health service that ensures children get the proper nutrition to prevent sickness later in life.

You walk outside and guide the children into the car. You buckle their seatbelts without realizing it. Seatbelts have become a habit now, because public health has explained how proper seatbelt use has greatly reduced automobile-related deaths nationwide.

Playmates greet your children at the childcare center with yelps of youthful joy. As you watch the children run inside to play, you know they'll stay safe while you're away at work. Public health has licensed the center and made certain the staff knows the proper ways to avoid infectious disease outbreaks that can occur among young children.

And thanks to the immunizations your children have received, you know they'll be safe from life-threatening diseases like polio and whooping cough. In fact, public health has eliminated the deadly smallpox virus worldwide, so your children will never catch it. Maybe your children's children won't have to worry about polio or whooping cough.

You arrive at work and find a flyer for a new exercise program tacked to the bulletin board. You decide to sign up, remembering the public health studies that show you can reduce the risks of chronic disease by staying physically active.

The morning goes well, and you feel good because your company became a smoke-free workplace this month. Science shows that tobacco can cause cancer and other ailments in those who use tobacco and among those who breathe second-hand smoke. Public health encourages people and organizations to quit smoking so that all people can live more healthful lives.

Walking to a nearby fast-food restaurant for lunch, you pass a bike rider with a sleek, colorful helmet—another example of a public health message that can influence healthy behaviors. Inside, you order a hamburger and fries.

You notice the food service license signed by the State Health Officer on the wall, and you know the food is sanitary and free of disease-causing organisms. Still, a State Department of Health public service announcement from TV rings in your head, and you make a mental note to order something with a little less cholesterol next time.

You finish your day at work, pick up the kids, and head to the community park to let the children play. You watch the neighborhood children launch a toy sailboat into the park pond, knowing public health protects lakes and streams from dangerous sewage runoff.

At home, your spouse greets you at the door. You sort the mail and discover a letter from your uncle. He's doing fine after his surgery in the hospital and will head back to the nursing home in 2 days. You know he's getting quality care at both facilities because public health monitors and licenses them to ensure a commitment to quality standards. Even the ambulance that transported him to the hospital met public health standards for emergency medical services.

After dinner, you put the children to bed and sit to watch the evening news. The anchor details a new coalition dedicated to preventing breast and cervical cancer. A representative of the State Department of Health issues an open invitation for members from all walks of life. You jot down the telephone number and promise yourself you'll call first thing tomorrow.

As you settle into bed, you decide that public health is more than a point-in-time recognition. Without even realizing it, you'll rely on public health every day for an entire lifetime.

Source: Mississippi State Department of Health Annual Report (1997), pp. 2–3.

population health, environmental safety, politicization of healthcare interventions, euthanasia, elder abuse in nursing homes, provider–patient relationships, and community partnerships. Recent advancements in science and technology are presenting ethical dilemmas that Florence Nightingale could not have envisioned in even her wildest fantasies—for example, physician-assisted suicide, living wills, stem cell research, gene therapy, in vitro fertilization, and human cloning. All nurses would do well to follow Spicer's (1998) advice to nursing students in an editorial in *Imprint*: "As you prepare for your careers, remember your professional commitment to place your patient first in all decisions. Take time to establish your ethical boundaries. . . . Base your decisions from your head and your heart."

Epidemiology: The Science of Public Health

Epidemiology is the science that provides community and public health with a framework for addressing the primary, secondary, and tertiary health needs for a population and directs community health nursing practice. Whether a person is healthy or ill results from numerous constantly changing interacting forces. The actual occurrence of disease results from a triad of factors, referred to as the epidemiological model or triangle. This triad is composed of the host, the agent, and the environment. The *host* is the human body influenced by such variables as gender, age, race, and behavior. The *agent* is a physical, chemical, or biological element that can cause illness or injury. Examples might include tubercle bacilli or nicotine. The *environment* is perhaps the most complex component. As we learn more about health and its determinants, the environment holds more and more keys to explaining health risks to our human hosts. The environment not only includes the physical environment, such as climate and terrain, but also the sociocultural–political environment, such as poverty, racism, and other stressors that influence health.

Prevention strategies are made up of measures that protect people from disease and take the form of efforts that we use to protect ourselves and others from specific diseases and conditions and their resulting consequences. There are three levels of prevention: primary, secondary, and tertiary. Nurses in all settings use all three levels of prevention as a basis for practice. The nurse caring for patients in an acute care setting may primarily use secondary and tertiary interventions, whereas the occupational health nurse may use primary and secondary interventions in his or her role. These levels of prevention were originally conceptualized by Leavell and Clark in 1953 and were tied to what these authors described as the natural history of disease. Their assumption was that disease in humans is a process: The conditions that promote either health or disease are present in the human's biological, physical, emotional, and social environments as well as in the human host itself.

GLOBAL CONNECTION 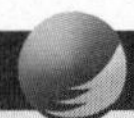

The Three Ps of Global Health:

Pollution
Population
Poverty

Source: Turnock, 1997.

The relationship between levels of prevention and the natural history of any given disease condition or health state is the basis for community health interventions. Disease occurs in two stages: prepathogenesis and pathogenesis. The intervention strategies or levels of prevention must coincide with predictable events within the stages of prepathogenesis (predisease) and pathogenesis (disease, condition, or injury). One can readily see that applying the levels of prevention requires that the nurse know the natural history of a given disease or condition. The less known about the disease or condition, the greater the likelihood of interventions occurring in secondary or tertiary prevention levels. In other words, the more we learn about disease, disability, and injury, the earlier we can intervene to prevent the illness from occurring. The goal of preventive health, then, is to intervene at the earliest possible stage in the natural history of disease to prevent complications, limit disability, and halt irreversible changes in health status (Leavell & Clark, 1979). The levels of prevention and examples are included as a boxed feature throughout the text (see Box 1-4).

BOX 1-4 Levels of Prevention

Primary Prevention

Health measures that focus on prevention of health problems *before* they occur.

Secondary Prevention

Health measures that begin when pathology is involved and is directed at early detection through diagnosis and treatment.

Tertiary Prevention

Health measures that are taken when an illness, injury, or disability is irreversible; interventions are focused on rehabilitation. The goal of these measures is to restore the person to the optimal level of health and function.

Primary prevention refers to those measures that focus on prevention of health problems before they occur. Primary prevention is not therapeutic, which means that it does not consist of symptom identification and use of the typical therapeutic skills of the nurse (Shamansky & Clausen, 1980). This level includes both generalized health promotion and specific protection against certain identified diseases or conditions. The purpose is to reduce the person's vulnerability to the illness by strengthening the human host's capacity to withstand physical, emotional, and environmental stressors. An example would be teaching a person about adequate nutrition, exercise, and hygiene. Specific protection includes numerous interventions associated with public health nursing: immunizations, bicycle helmets, automobile seatbelts, safety caps on electrical outlets, handrails on bathtubs, and drug education for children.

Secondary prevention begins when pathology is involved and is aimed at early detection through diagnosis and prompt treatment. This level of prevention is aimed at halting the pathological process, thereby shortening its duration and severity and getting the person back to a normal state of functioning. All screening tests, such as breast self-examinations, hypertensive assessments, and Pap smears, are included in this level of prevention. The goal of this level is to identify groups of individuals who have early symptoms of disease so that they may be treated as soon as possible in the natural history of the disease, condition, or injury. If the disease, condition, or injury cannot be cured, further complications and disability move the level of prevention to that of tertiary prevention.

Tertiary prevention consists of activities designed around rehabilitation of a person with a permanent, irreversible condition. The goal of tertiary prevention goes beyond halting the disease process to restoring the person to an optimal level of functioning within the constraints of the disability. Nursing strategies at this level might include teaching a stroke patient how to ambulate with assistance or teaching a child with cystic fibrosis how to reduce risks of respiratory infection while maintaining an active lifestyle.

The traditional epidemiological triad has focused on infectious disease as agent, human host, and physical environment. In most developed countries, in the past century there has been an epidemiological transition from infectious to chronic disease, such as cardiovascular disease, cancer, diabetes, asthma, and depression, and the environment has broadened to include the social and psychological environment, such as prejudice, racism, and stress.

The boundaries between secondary and tertiary prevention are often fuzzy and more difficult to identify as either one or the other. One feature that helps in this identification is that tertiary intervention takes place only if the condition results in a permanent disability (Shamansky & Clausen, 1980). This outcome may be influenced by the age or development of the patient rather than by the condition itself. For example, if a 15-year-old high school athlete suffers a simple broken femur during a soccer game, intervention would occur at the secondary prevention level. Although the athlete may require extensive physical rehabilitation after the cast is removed, unless there are serious complications, she should eventually be able to return to her normal state of health. Compare this situation with a 75-year-old man who falls from a roof and suffers the identical injury. Most likely, this patient would need both secondary and tertiary intervention strategies because of the aging process, recovery, and the likelihood of permanent disability resulting from this fall.

Shamansky and Clausen (1980) use the following example to illustrate how all levels of prevention are often used with the same patient and family:

> A nurse is conducting a group session with young parents and uses values clarification as a method to discuss issues of parental responsibility for providing a safe yet stimulating environment for the young, curious child. This is primary prevention: Health promotion occurs, because the discussion is general and directed toward nonspecific efforts to ensure the well-being of the young child.
>
> Later, on a home visit, the nurse encourages a mother to use screens on a second-story window, because she perceives the window is dangerously accessible to the active three-year-old. This, too, is primary prevention, an example of specific protection, because the nurse is attempting to remove a risk factor from the environment of a vulnerable child.
>
> If the screen is not used and the child falls out of the window onto a cement driveway below, the mother's and emergency personnel's use of appropriate emergency first aid would be secondary prevention through the use of prompt treatment. If the child sustained a severe head injury, was hospitalized (and secondary measures were used in the hospital), and later released to home care, teaching the mother to turn, feed, and give range-of-motion exercises would represent the disability limitation aspect of secondary prevention.
>
> Several months later, if the child is found to have some permanent brain damage, tertiary prevention would take the form of referrals to special education classes, or physical or speech therapy to increase the child's maximum potential level of functioning, although the damage itself is irreversible. (pp. 106–107)

NOTE THIS!

Why are American children getting heavier every year? Each day, most 8- to 18-year-olds spend an average of 4 hours watching television, videos, and DVDs; more than 1 hour on the computer; and about 50 minutes playing video games.

Measuring a Community's Health: How Do We Know When We Get There?

Outcomes and measurements of community health interventions take the form of health statistics such as birth rates, infant mortality rates, and incidence and prevalence rates for various diseases and age groups. Most threats to health do not occur at random (i.e., by chance). Natural forces influence health threats, but by no means do they dictate the outcome. In this century we have learned through epidemiological research that most threats or risks to our health and wellbeing are associated with patterns of human activity and behavior. It is those patterns that we use to evaluate health interventions and the multitude of influences on people's health (Cohen, 1989).

For example, breast cancer rates in the United States are high compared with other countries such as Japan and China. In other words, breast cancer is not universal among all females, nor is it randomly distributed in the global female population (Cohen, 1989).

We can see from epidemiological research that individual behavior has a significant effect on a person's chance of developing breast cancer. Breast cancer may be associated with a high-fat, high-protein, high-calorie diet, and with high levels of estrogen (either produced by the woman's own body or ingested in diet and medication). Women who do not have or nurse children or have them later in life also have higher rates of breast cancer. These lifestyle factors clearly influence a woman's chances of contracting breast cancer in her lifetime. The availability of cutting-edge technology, genomic research, and diagnostic interventions cannot prevent women from contracting breast cancer; these measures can improve chances of survival only after cancer is detected (Kolata, 1987; Marx, 1986; Winick, 1980).

In another example, maternal death risk in childbirth plummeted during the 20th century in developed countries as a result of application of prenatal care, use of antibiotics, and infectious disease control. In the United States, a woman has a 1 in 3,700 chance of dying in childbirth. By contrast, in Latin America, a woman's mortality risk is 1 in 130, and women in parts of Africa had an alarming 1 in 16 chance of dying as a result of childbearing (Whaley & Hashim, 1995).

Table 1-2 provides an illustration of the links among all levels of care. You will learn in this text how these group rates of disease, health, injury, and disability reflect more accurately the values of a society and how health professionals measure not only their interventions but the influences of many variables on health.

In a report by the Institute of Medicine (IOM, 2010), *The Future of Nursing: Leading Change, Advancing Health,*

TABLE 1-2 A Comparison of Individual, Family, Community, and Global Population-Focused Care

Individual Care	Family	Community	Global
Injuries suffered by women in violent spousal domestic relationship	Family dysfunctions, such as inability to provide appropriate behavioral roles and boundaries for conflict resolution	Children unable to function in school setting because of disruptive behavior in classroom	Women and children refugees in war-torn Pakistan and Afghanistan suffering from injuries as a result of acts of war violence
	Children exhibiting early and inappropriate use of firearms	Gang violence resulting in neighborhood isolation, decreased population, diminished economic base because of business closure, and decreased funds available for education and family assistance	

"nurses must be full partners, with physicians and other health professionals, in redesigning health care in the United States" (pp. 1–9). Public and community health nurses, because of their focus on prevention and health promotion, must lead the way in the evolving healthcare system of the United States in order to improve the public's health.

APPLICATION TO PRACTICE 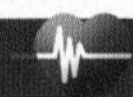

Community-Based Care: An Example from Practice

A 3-year-old child is brought to a public health department for her first set of immunizations. As the nurse assesses the child, she finds that the child has a generalized red rash all over her body. The mother complains that the child scratches and cries about the rash. She has been using a cortisone skin cream for 3 days, but the rash has worsened.

The nurse attends to the immediate concerns of the mother about home care, comfort measures, and possible causes. The nurse then delivers direct care to the child and to her family, while considering the following community implications:

- Does anyone else in the family exhibit those symptoms?
- Does the child go to day care?
- Have there been any other children in the clinic recently with similar symptoms? If so, how does this case compare with cases in recent months?
- What is the likely pathogen that is causing the rash?
- Are there any pregnant women in the clinic or in the home setting?

Consider the following questions:

1. What are possible conclusions that the nurse can make that have individual implications?
2. Are there community and public health issues that may be present that the nurse must address?

Conclusion

Community health and public health nursing care use a preventive focus with patients, communities, and populations, wherever they live, work, or reside. The focus of nurses' practice may be on the individual, but various influences on a community's health and the way in which the healthcare system has organized services around societal needs and expectations must also be considered. Nurses will play a critical role in the future of managed care, which is organized around prevention and a healthy population. Epidemiology is the science that provides community and public health with a framework for addressing the primary, secondary, and tertiary health needs for a population and directs community health nursing practice. The personal wellbeing of individuals is more than an individual matter. Humankind does not live in isolation, unaffected by others. Community health is a dynamic of the community and is influenced by the

LEVELS OF PREVENTION 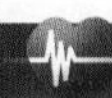

Primary: Teaching elementary school children how to avoid playground accidents.

Secondary: Assisting a class of children with how to know when to call parents or caregivers when they are injured

Tertiary: Providing education for parents when a child has experienced a serious injury, such as an amputated finger, about adaptation to schoolwork

AFFORDABLE CARE ACT (ACA)

The ACA was passed by Congress and signed into law by President Barrack Obama in March of 2010. The American Academy of Nursing strongly supported this major health-care reform, along with most of the professional nursing organizations in the United States. The new healthcare reform law was created to bring about major changes to the delivery of health care in the United States, particularly in regard to delivery and financing of health care to the uninsured and underinsured populations in the nation. Nursing plays a critical role in implementing the health reform changes that are often complex and vast in nature, providing wide access to essential healthcare services, preventive health care, improving quality of care, and controlling costs of health care.

context of where and how the population lives, works, and addresses healthcare needs. The ACA of 2010 is a challenge and opportunity for nurses to positively affect the health of the population.

HEALTHY ME

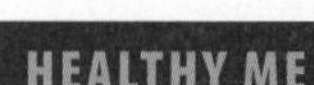

How do you cope with the stresses of nursing school using healthy practices?

Critical Thinking Activities

1. After reading "Think About This," respond to the following questions:
   - What are three risks described in the essay that were unknown a century ago?
   - What is the responsibility of the individual in creating a safe environment?
   - What are three public safety measures mentioned in the essay that do not exist in underdeveloped countries?
2. How can heart disease be both a personal health problem and a community health problem?
3. For several decades now, nurses have worked primarily in hospitals using a medical model approach to health and illness. Does nursing have a vision of the profession with community at the center, or has nursing become so institutionalized into hospital-based practice over the past decades that we will resist the tremendous opportunities to care for people in a myriad of settings and situations?
4. How has the ethic of caring for a patient's environment changed from Florence Nightingale's era?
5. How will the ACA of 2010 affect the delivery of nursing care services in all settings?

References

American Academy of Nursing (AAN). (2010). *Implementing health care reform: Issues for nursing.* Washington, DC: Author.

American Nurses Association (ANA). (1991). *Nursing's agenda for health care reform: Executive summary.* Washington, DC: Author.

American Nurses Association (ANA). (2008). *Code of ethics for nurses with interpretive statements.* Washington, DC: Author.

American Nurses Association (ANA). (2013). *Public health nursing: Scope and standards of practice.* Washington, DC: Author.

American Public Health Association, Public Health Nursing Section. (1996). *The definition and role of public health nursing: A statement of the APHA Public Health Nursing Section.* Washington, DC: Author.

Anderson, C. (1997). The economics of health promotion. *Nursing Outlook, 45*(3), 105–106.

Armentrout, G. (1998). *Community-based nursing: Foundation for practice.* Stamford, CT: Appleton & Lange.

Association of Community Health Nursing Educators (ACHNE). (2009). *Essentials of baccalaureate nursing education for entry level community/public health nursing.* Wheat Ridge, CO: Author. Retrieved from http://www.achne.org/files/EssentialsOfBaccalaureate_Fall_2009.pdf

Bunker, J. P., Frazier, H. S., & Mosteller, F. (1994). Improving health: Measuring effects of medical care. *Milbank Quarterly,* 72, 225–258.

Bureau of Labor Statistics. (2012). *Occupational outlook handbook,* 2012. U.S. Department of Labor. Retrieved from http://www.bls.gov/ooh/Healthcare/Registered-nurses.htm

Canavan, K. (1996). Nursing education on cusp of shift in focus: Faculty grapple with preparing students for changing health care delivery. *American Nurse, 28*(6), 1, 11.

Centers for Disease Control and Prevention (CDC). (2002). *Public health infrastructure: A status report.* Atlanta, GA: Author.

Cohen, M. (1989). *Health and the rise of civilization.* New Haven, CT: Yale University Press.

Cottrell, K. (1976). The competent community. In B. H. Kaplan, R. N. Wilson, & A. H. Leighton (Eds.), *Further explorations in social psychology.* New York, NY: Basic Books.

Davidhizar, R., Eshleman, J., & Wolff, L. (2003). Living with stress since 9/11. *Caring, 22*(4), 26–28, 30.

Ferguson, L. M., & Day, R. A. (2007). Challenges for new nurses in evidence-based practice. *Journal of Nursing Management, 15*(1), 107–113.

Folmar, J., Coughlin, S. S., Bessinger, R., & Sacknoff, D. (1997). Ethics in public health practice: A survey of public health nurses in southern Louisiana. *Public Health Nursing, 14*(3), 156–160.

Friedman, E. (June 2013). Which population: Whose health? *Hospitals and Health Networks.* Retrieved from http://www.hhnmag.com/hhnmag/HHNDaily/HHNDailyDisplay.dhtml?id=460002372

Gable, L. (2011). The Patient Protection and Affordable Care Act, public health, and the elusive target of human rights. *Journal of Law, Medicine and Ethics, 39*(3), 340–354.

Gebbie, K. M. (1996, November 18). *Preparing currently employed public health nurses for changes in the health care system: Meeting report and suggested action steps.* New York, NY: Columbia University School of Nursing Center for Health Policy and Health Sciences Research. (Report based on meeting in Atlanta, GA, July 11, 1996.)

Giger, J. N., & Davidhizar, R. E. (1995). *Transcultural nursing: Assessment and intervention* (2nd ed.). St. Louis, MO: Mosby.

Gostin, L. O. (2004). Health of the people: The highest law? *Journal of Law, Medicine and Ethics, 32*(3), 509–515.

Gostin, L. O., Boufford, J. I., & Martinez, R. M. (2004). The future of the public's health: Vision, values and strategies. *Health Affairs, 23,* 96–107.

Graham, K. Y. (1997). Ethics: Do we really care? *Public Health Nursing, 14*(1), 1–2.

Grossman, D. (1994). Enhancing your cultural competence. *American Journal of Nursing, 94*(7), 58–62.

Hall, J. E., & Weaver, B. R. (1977). *Distributive nursing practice: A systems approach to community health.* Philadelphia, PA: Lippincott.

Hall, J. M., & Stevens, P. E. (1995). The future of graduate education in nursing: Scholarship, the health communities, and health care reform. *Journal of Professional Nursing, 11*(6), 332–338.

Hanlon, J. J., & Pickett, G. E. (1984). *Public health: Administration and practice* (8th ed.). St. Louis, MO: Mosby.

HealthyPeople.gov. (2013). *Healthy People 2020.* Retrieved from http://www.healthypeople.gov/2020/default.aspx

Institute of Medicine (IOM). (2010). *The future of nursing: Leading change, advancing health.* Washington, DC: National Academies Press.

Janes, S., & Hobson, K. (1998). An innovative approach for affirming cultural diversity among baccalaureate nursing students and faculty. *Journal of Cultural Diversity, 5*(4), 132–137.

Keck, E. W. (1994). Community health: Our common challenge. *Family and Community Health, 17*(2), 1–9.

Keller, L. O., Strohstein, S., Lia-Hoagberg, B., & Shaeffer, M. A. (2004). Population-based public health interventions: Practice-based and evidence-supported. Part I. *Public Health Nursing, 21*(5), 453–468.

Kolata, G. B. (1987). Kung hunter-gathers Feminism, diet and birth control. *Science, 185,* 932–934.

Kurtzman, C., Ibgui, D., Pogrund, R., & Monin, S. (1980). Nursing process at the aggregate level. *Nursing Outlook, 28*(12), 737–739.

Kuss, T., Proulx-Girouard, L., Lovitt, S., Katz, C. B., & Kennelly, P. (1997). A public health nursing model. *Public Health Nursing, 14*(2), 81–91.

Leavell, H. R., & Clark, E. G. (1953). *Preventive medicine for the doctor in his community.* New York, NY: McGraw-Hill.

Leavell, H. R., & Clark, E. G. (1979). *Preventive medicine for the doctor in his community: An epidemiologic approach* (3rd ed.). Huntington, NY: RE Dreges.

Marx, J. (1986). Viruses and cancer briefing. *Science, 241,* 1039–1040.

Leininger, M. (1995). *Transcultural nursing: Concepts, theories, research, and practices* (2nd ed.). New York, NY: McGraw-Hill.

Leipert, B. D. (1996). The value of community health nursing: A phenomenological study of the perceptions of community health nurses. *Public Health Nursing, 13*(1), 50–57.

McKenzie, J. F., & Pinger, R. R. (1997). *An introduction to community health.* Boston, MA: Jones and Bartlett.

Mechanic, D. (1998). Topics of our times: Managed care and public health. *American Journal of Public Health, 88*(6), 84–85.

Meleis, A. L. (1996). Culturally competent scholarship: Substance and rigor. *Advances in Nursing Science, 19*(2), 1–16.

Moon, M. (1993). Health care reform. *Future of Children, 3*(2), 21–36.

Morse, S. S. (2003). Building academic-practice partnerships: The Center for Public Health Preparedness at the Columbia University Mailman School of Public Health, before and after 9/11. *Journal of Public Health Management & Practice, 9*(5), 427–432.

National Institutes of Health. (2014). Press release: NIH study finds regular aspirin use may reduce ovarian cancer risk. Retrieved from http://www.nih.gov/news/health/feb2014/nci-06.htm

Nehls, N., Owen, B., Tipple, S., & Vandermause, R. (2001). Lessons learned from developing, implementing and evaluating a model of community-driven nursing. *Nursing and Health Care Perspectives, 22*, 304–307.

Nehls, N., & Vandermause, R. (2004). Community driven nursing: Transforming nursing curricula and instruction. *Nursing Education Perspectives, 25*(2), 81–85.

Neufield, V. (1992). Training: A Canadian perspective. In Pan American Health Organization (Ed.), *International health: North-south debate.* (Human Resource Development Series, pp. 95, 193–203). Washington, DC: Pan American Health Organization.

Nightingale, F. (1860). *Notes on nursing: What it is and what it is not.* London, England: Harrison.

Proenca, E. J. (1998). Community orientation in health services organizations: The concept and its implementation. *Health Care Management Review, 23*(2), 28–38.

Purnell, L. D., & Paulanka, B. J. (2003). *Transcultural health care: A culturally competent approach* (2nd ed.). Philadelphia PA: F. A. Davis.

Salmon, M., & Vanderbush, P. (1990). Leadership and change in public and community health nursing today: The essential intervention. In J. C. McCloskey & H. K. Grace (Eds.), *Current issues in nursing* (3rd ed., pp. 187–193). St. Louis, MO: Mosby.

Schultz, P. R. (1994). On the matter of populations, aggregates, and communities. Unpublished manuscript, University of Washington, Seattle, WA.

Shamansky, S. L., & Clausen, C. L. (1980). Levels of prevention: Examination of the concept. *Nursing Outlook, 28*(2), 104–108.

Shortell, S. M., & Gilles, R. R. (1995). Reinventing the American hospital. *Milbank Quarterly, 73*(2), 131.

Smith, C. M. (1995). Responsibilities for care in community health nursing. In C. M. Smith & F. A. Maurer (Eds.), *Community health nursing: Principles and practice* (pp. 3–29). Philadelphia, PA: Saunders.

Sorrell, J. (2012). Ethics: The Patient Protection and Affordable Care Act: Ethical perspectives in 21st century health care. *OJIN: The Online Journal of Issues in Nursing, 18*(1). Retrieved from http://www.nursingworld.org/MainMenuCategories/ANAMarketplace/ANAPeriodicals/OJIN/Columns/Ethics/Patient-Protection-and-Affordable-Care-Act-Ethical-Perspectives.html

Spicer, G. (1998). Learning right from wrong. *Imprint, 45*(3), 4.

Trabert, B., Ness, R. B., Lo-Ciganic, W. H., Murphy, M. A., Goode, E. L., Poole, E. M., … Wentzensen, N. (2014). Aspirin, nonaspirin nonsteroidal anti-inflammatory drug, and acetaminophen use and risk of invasive epithelial ovarian cancer: A pooled analysis in the Ovarian Cancer Association Consortium. *Journal of the National Cancer Institute, 106*(2), djt431. doi: 10.1093/jnci/djt431

Trossman, S. (1998, March/April). Self-determination: The name of the game in the next century. *American Nurse*, 1.

Turnock, B. (1997). *Public health: What it is and how it works.* Germantown, MD: Aspen.

U.S. Census Bureau. (2012). *Statistical Abstract of the United States: 2012* (131st ed.). Retrieved from http://quickfacts.census.gov/qfd/states/00000.html

U.S. Department of Health and Human Services (HHS), Division of Nursing, Bureau of Health Professions, Health Resources and Services Administration. (2000). *National sample survey of registered nurses.* Washington, DC: U.S. Government Printing Office.

Vilschick, J. (2003, January/February). Lack of minority role models affects nursing shortage. Retrieved from http://minorityhealth.hhs.gov/assets/pdf/checked/Lack%20of%20Minority%20Role%20Models%20Affects%20Nursing%20Shortage.pdf

Whaley, R. F., & Hashim, T. J. (1995). *A textbook of world health: A practical guide to global health care.* Nashville, TN: Parthenon Publishing Group.

Winick, M. (1980). Nutrition in health and disease. New York, NY: John Wiley.

Wolf, Z. R. (1989). Uncovering the hidden work of nursing. *Nursing and Health Care, 10*(8), 462–467.

World Health Organization (WHO). (1958). *The first ten years of the World Health Organization.* New York, NY: Author.

World Health Organization (WHO). (1986). Health promotion: A discussion document on the concept and principles. *Public Health Reviews, 14*(3–4), 245–254.

CHAPTER FOCUS

Communities and Populations
- The Health of Communities and Populations
- Differences and Similarities Among Communities and Populations

Community Assessment Frameworks
- Community Empowerment
- Community Assessment Frameworks/Models

Using the Nursing Process for the Community
- Conducting a Community Assessment
- Community Diagnosis
- Planning and Prioritization Phase
- Implementation Phase
- Evaluation Phase

QUESTIONS TO CONSIDER

After reading this chapter, you will know the answers to the following questions:

1. What is a population-focused approach to health care and how will the Affordable Care Act (ACA) promote population health?
2. What is a community or population assessment?
3. How does the baccalaureate-prepared nurse use population assessment in healthcare and non-healthcare settings?
4. What is the "community as patient"?
5. What is the difference between a community and a population?
6. What do the terms *status, structure,* and *process* refer to?
7. What is the *Healthy Cities* initiative?
8. How are community assessment frameworks or models used in the assessment process?
9. What are examples of community assessment frameworks or models?
10. How does a community health nurse gain entry into the community?
11. What are the five methods of collecting community data?
12. What is a community diagnosis, and what is an example of one?
13. What occurs in the planning and prioritization phase of the community assessment process?
14. What occurs in the implementation phase of the community assessment process?
15. What are examples of strategies that the community health nurse can use to assist communities in healthy change?
16. What is media advocacy?

CHAPTER 2

Community and Population Health: Assessment and Intervention

Karen Saucier Lundy and
Judith A. Barton

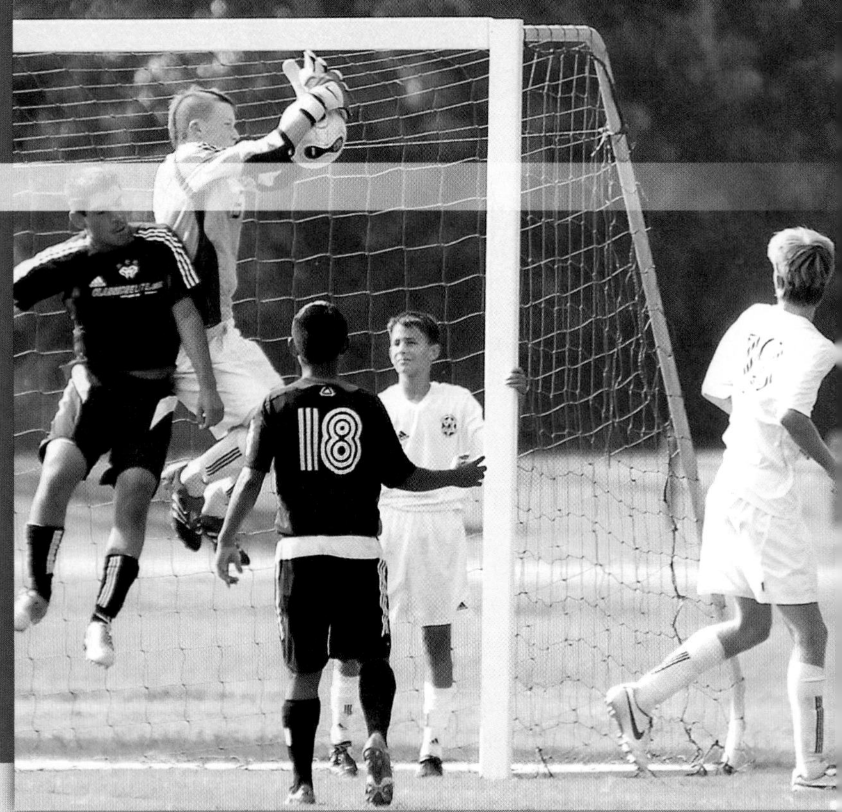

KEY TERMS

collaborative arrangement
community
community- and population-focused care
community as patient
community assessment
community assessment frameworks and models
community competency
community empowerment
community-focused intervention
community forums
community health diagnoses
constructed surveys
focus groups
healthy change
healthy communities
informant interviews
key informant
media advocacy
observation
planning phase
population
population assessment
population health
population-level interventions
primary informant
process
secondary analysis of existing data
secondary data
status
structure
windshield surveys

REFLECTIONS

Think about what living in a community means to you. How has it shaped your beliefs about health and what you do when you are sick? Did you spend your childhood and teen years in a small town, an urban area, or a suburb, or did you move around and spend time in many different types of communities? As a nursing student, think about the different communities where you feel most "at home" now. Describe these communities and indicate how they differ from those where you grew up in terms of health values.

COMMUNITY NURSES HAVE TRADITIONALLY conducted assessments of entire geopolitical communities and of vulnerable and diverse populations within communities, now commonly referred to as **population health**. The focus of the nursing assessment is on the community or population's health rather than on the individual's health status, and consequently the assessment takes on a different form and process (Nash, Reifsnyder, Fabius, & Pracillio, 2011). Perhaps the best and most dramatic example was the post–Hurricane Katrina public health disaster that occurred in New Orleans as a result of a lack of attention to planning for vulnerable population's health needs. Public health nurses, along with other disciplines, are challenged to balance these short-term crises with progress toward longer term goals, as we seek newer and better ways of solving health problems in our communities (Carney, 2006; Zandee, Bossenbroek, Slager, & Gordon, 2013).

Today more than ever, the community health nurse has the unique responsibility of defining problems and proposing solutions at the community/population level (Baldwin, Conger, Abegglen, & Hill, 1998; Gebbie, 1996; Keck, 1994; Williams & Highriter, 1978). Furthermore, baccalaureate-prepared nurses will be expected to practice population-based nursing in all settings as managed care of populations becomes the basis of organizational survival. In other words, community and population assessments are no longer confined to traditional community settings, but in all settings where health is the focus of research-based health interventions, including acute care, clinics, schools, the workplace, and hospitals.

The U.S. healthcare system is trending toward community- and population-focused care. The shift from location-based care (e.g., hospital, outpatient clinic care) to community-based care will demand a greater emphasis on nursing assessments of geopolitical communities and high-risk populations. In other words, to plan care, carry out interventions, and evaluate care outcomes when the patient is either a geopolitical community or a population, there is a need for all bachelor of science in nursing (BSN)–prepared nurses to have skills in community and population assessment. Although community and population assessment, planning, intervention, and evaluation are receiving greater attention in today's healthcare system, these skills have always been associated with community health nursing role expectations (Hegyvary, 1990). With the passage of the Patient Protection and Affordable Care Act (ACA) of 2010, community and population assessments will be required in several new provisions of the law, including hospitals, community organizations, and other health-related facilities in order to determine the community's health status and evaluation of unmet population health needs.

Historically, community/population assessment, the initial step in community-/population-focused care, was first seen as a nursing practice role by Florence Nightingale. Nightingale was concerned with assessing the physical and social environment as a possible cause of illness. Nightingale's own community assessments included an analysis of the 1861 census data of England, which served as the foundation of England's sanitary reform acts (Kopf, 1986). She also included community assessment as a nursing role for district nurses. These nurses were to assess both the physical and social environments of the community to determine which health teaching and social reform programs were needed by the community (Montero, 1985). From its earliest history, the nursing profession has viewed community and population assessment as an important role directed toward improving the health of entire communities.

Today, recommitment toward community and population assessment is a vital nursing practice role, as identified by all organizations that set standards for community health nursing (American Association of Colleges of Nursing [AACN], 2008; American Nurses Association, 2010; Association of Community Health Nursing Educators [ACHNE], 2009). This recommitment to seeing the community as patient has emerged as a critical function of the community health nurse as more and more research connects the important role that physical and social environments play in health and disease (Cassel, 1976; Gordon, 1990, 1993; Lalonde, 1974; Rodgers, 1984). Such findings also influence health policy formation, the establishment of priorities when financing health care, and the potential of the nursing community to establish itself as a leader in healthcare reform. Knowledge of community and population assessment is now considered essential for the baccalaureate nurse (Eide, Hahn, Bayne, Allen, & Swain, 2006; Ruth, Eliason, & Schultz, 1992). The diagnoses and interventions that result

BOX 2-1 Core Competencies for Public Health

Public health professionals should be able to do the following:

- Define a problem.
- Determine appropriate uses and limitations of quantitative and qualitative data.
- Select and define variables relevant to the defined public health problems.
- Identify relevant and appropriate data and information sources.
- Evaluate the integrity and comparability of data and identify gaps in data sources.
- Apply ethical principles to the collection, maintenance, use, and dissemination of data and information.
- Partner with communities to attach meaning to collected quantitative and qualitative data.
- Make relevant inferences from quantitative and qualitative data.
- Apply data-collection processes, information technology applications, and computer systems storage and retrieval strategies.
- Recognize how the data illuminate ethical, political, scientific, economic, and overall public health issues.

Source: Council on Linkages Between Academia and Public Health Practice: Core competencies for public health professionals, Washington, DC, 2010, USDHHS and Public Health Foundation. Available at http://www.phf.org/resourcestools/Documents/Core_Competencies_for_Public_Health_Professionals_2010May.pdf Accessed December 16 2013.

from the community and population assessment process are population-based, community-focused interventions (Pavlish & Pharris, 2012). Such interventions are directed at groups of persons within a community; activities are geared toward changes in community norms, greater consciousness about health issues and solutions, and healthy practices and behaviors, to name a few (Keller, Strohschein, Lia-Hoagberg, & Schaffer, 1998).

The core functions of public health nursing include assessment, policy development, and assurance. The basis for policy and assurance is the assessment of the community and population of interest for healthcare promotion. (See **Box 2-1** for specifics on the competencies for nurses and health professionals related to community and population assessment.)

This chapter introduces the concept of **community as patient**, explains how to get to know the community patient, and describes how to practice skills of community and population assessment in actual community assessment examples. The future of nursing depends to a large degree on our understanding of the "big picture" of healthcare delivery (Aiken & Salmon, 1994). We are becoming more and more dependent on outcomes and evidence-based measures, such as evaluation of morbidity and mortality statistics. In response, this chapter will help the beginning nurse use the community/population assessment process in all practice settings (Pavlish & Pharris, 2012; Reinhart, 1984; see **Box 2-2**).

This chapter also discusses how to interpret community- and population-level data and to plan interventions more appropriately and efficiently as we work within the limited resources of the present healthcare environment. Our healthcare system can no longer rely on quick fixes. For example, in developed countries the nature of fatal diseases has changed. In the course of recent human history, when people were fighting diseases such as smallpox, diphtheria, or polio, immunizations were an easy, quick, and sure prevention. As we have learned more about infectious disease and the contribution of human factors, such as lifestyle, heredity, and behavior, solutions have become more complex. Chronic disease and disabling conditions are continuing to grow as we extend the lifespan through technology and advancement of diagnosis and treatment. Today, many diseases and conditions require that we are much more attentive to the totality of variables that influence health and illness (Gebbie, 1996). Achieving prevention and control requires much more effort on the part of communities and changes in thinking about the impact of the structure of society (e.g., economics, culture, and politics) on the health of community (Community Health Advisor Network, 1999).

BOX 2-2 Ways in Which the Community Assessment/Population Assessment Can Be Used in the "Everyday Life" of a Practicing Nurse

- Applying for grants to provide health care for specific populations, such as pregnant adolescents
- Conducting a "mini" assessment during orientation to a new position in any setting to be better prepared for serving the agency's target population
- Avoiding burnout by going beyond personal care of patients, identifying better ways of delivering care, and using staff and material resources
- Justifying new projects by establishing the needs of a selected population
- Joining a community group such as the Parent Teacher Organization or American Cancer Society, volunteering to do an assessment and follow-through program planning
- Conducting an assessment of unfamiliar locales, both national and international, to determine possible relocation possibilities

Communities and Populations

The significance of the community/population nursing process becomes evident only when community health nurses define the community as patient. A nurse would not even consider omitting individual patient assessment and basing interventions only on intuition or a standard formula, but this is what happens when community health nurses fail to do a focused community/population assessment when planning and implementing health care for patients. For example, we would not examine just the arm of a patient and totally ignore the other systems of the body when we plan our nursing care. And yet by looking at only a few aspects of a selected community or population, such as the number and availability of hospitals, we are examining just the "arm" and ignoring the rest of the "body" of the community or population.

The first step in delivering **community- and population-focused care** is to define the boundaries of the group to be assessed. We often use the term **community** in various ways, so defining the boundaries of a community or population becomes critical in the early stages of **community-focused intervention.** Community is defined in this text as a group of people who share something in common, who interact with one another, and who may exhibit a commitment to one another. A **population** is defined as a group of people who have at least one thing in common and who may or may not interact with each other. From these definitions one can see that *interaction* is essential in a *community*, whereas members of a *population* may or may not interact with one another. To put it another way, community members are usually aware that they are part of a community and most often have an identified name. Populations may or may not have such self-awareness (**Box 2-3**). Some populations do evolve into communities. For example, adults who have disabilities and attend a day program in a certain community may develop into a cohesive, interactive group over time. Whether the population being assessed has self-awareness, the environment (e.g., the social, cultural, ecological environment of a particular community or the greater society) of the target population must be considered for effective health interventions to occur (Baldwin et al., 1998).

BOX 2-3 Examples of Communities and Populations

Examples of Communities

Retirement apartment community
Corvette Club of San Francisco
Town of Blackhawk, Colorado

Examples of Populations

Cross-country truck drivers
Elders with chronic asthma
College soccer players
Street musicians
Ice skaters

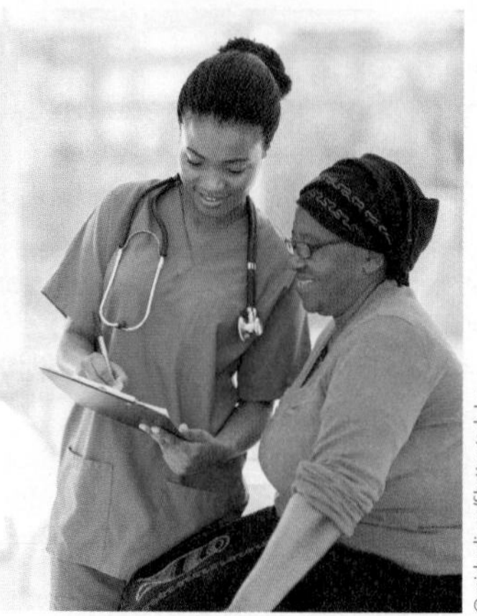

Nurse providing individual care.

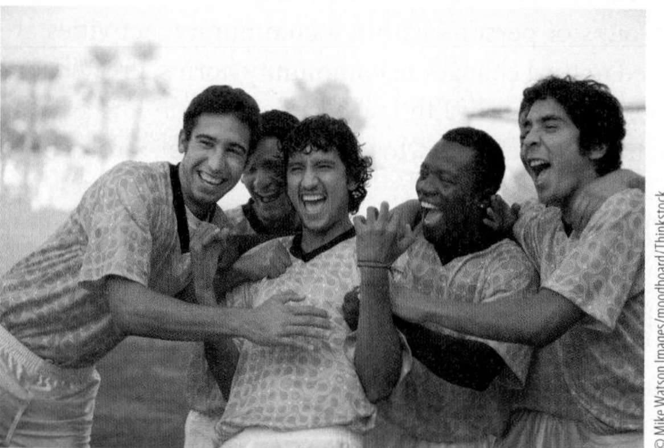

This college tennis team has formed a community after one year of common and meaningful interactions.

The Health of Communities and Populations

Public health professionals often describe **healthy communities** and populations in three different ways: status, structure, and process. See **Box 2-4** for a summary of these components.

Status is what we most commonly use to describe communities and populations and is the component you are most familiar with. When we talk about life expectancy rates and the morbidity (or illness) rates of a community or population, these are the "outcome" measures of *physical* or *biological* determinants of health. The *emotional aspects* of a community's or population's health status are often measured by such indices as specific mental health rates (e.g., suicide or drug addiction). The *social* determinants are reflected by such indices as crime rates and juvenile delinquency. As we have learned more about the health and the "ills" of modern society, we have discovered that most status outcome measures reflect the influences of all three

BOX 2-4 Basic Components of Community and Population Health with Example Indicators

Dimensions

Status

Vital statistics
Leading causes of death
Mental health statistics
Crime rates

Structure

Hospitals, community health clinics
Health professionals, government structures, and so on
Statistics related to use of health resources
Population characteristics (e.g., gender, age, socioeconomic status)

Process

Commitment of members
Self- and other awareness
Articulateness
Effective communication
Conflict resolution
Active participation by members
Management of social interactions with larger society/environment
Machinery for effective resource procurement and utilization

Source: This article was published in Community health nursing: Promoting health of aggregates, families, and individuals, M. Stanhope & J. Lancaster (Eds.), Community as patient: Using the nursing process to promote health by Schuster, G. F., & Goeppinger, J., pp. 289–314, Copyright Mosby 1996.

status components. For example, teen drug use is associated with risky behavior such as unprotected sex, which may result in high rates of teen pregnancy, sexually transmitted diseases, and associated higher infant mortality rates.

Structure refers to aspects of a community's or population's health such as health organizations, health professionals, utilization rates of health services and facilities, and characteristics of the community structure itself. How the community or population is structured is reflected in such measures as socioeconomic and educational levels; demographics of race, age, and gender; and the ways in which the members of a community access and use resources related to health. Research has linked education, socioeconomic status, and health outcomes, so these components are aspects that reflect the health status of a group to that end (Schuster & Goeppinger, 1996).

Process is a measure of community or population health that reflects how well a community/population functions to keep healthy. Just as the care of the individual patient commonly includes an assessment of personal competence to maintain health, so a community or population can be described in relation to **community competency**. This notion of community competency has been around for some time. George Herbert Mead (1934), the noted sociologist, linked our individual behaviors to what eventually emerges as collective behavior. These collective behaviors ultimately take the form of social institutions, such as a church, the Microsoft Corporation, or the American Red Cross. Mead contends that it is only this "organized self" and the resulting group response that makes communities possible and survival likely. For example, people exhibit varying degrees of competency at meeting social needs. Each individual who is intrinsically tied to the group through social interaction is changed by the interaction—each participant then not only becomes a part of the "other," but also learns his or her part as well as the part of the other (Mead, 1934). Cottrell (1976) defines community competence as a process in which the components of a community—families, organizations, and populations—"are able to collaborate effectively in identifying the problems and needs of the community; can achieve a working consensus on goals and priorities, can agree on ways and means to implement the agreed-on goals; and can collaborate effectively in the required action" (p. 197).

An important distinction must be made between individual competence and community competence: Although we often assume that a community made up of competent citizens and health professionals results in a competent community, these are not sufficient conditions. The complexity of community requires that we look not only beyond the individual parts of a community but also to the "whole" and the interactions between and among community constituents (Goeppinger, Lassiter, & Wilcox, 1982). Goeppinger, Lassiter, and Wilcox (1982) developed a nursing process–related model for community assessment designed to address the importance of community processes and community competence. To assess community competencies, the nurse examines the health capabilities and potential health actions of the community. The basic assumption of the community competency model is that health assessments need to include the community's strengths and abilities to improve their own health status. The model is based on research conducted by Goeppinger and Baglioni (1986) that was designed to discover indices of community competence. These competencies are not considered mutually exclusive, but are interrelated. **Table 2-1** summarizes essentials for community competency and includes examples from Goeppinger and Baglioni's research on indices of community competency.

TABLE 2-1 Essential Conditions for Community Competence

Commitment	Evidence that community members are attached to their community—people within the community demonstrate loyalty and pride
Self–other awareness	Evidence that community members are aware of how they fit into their community—as outsiders or insiders, as having power or not having power
Articulateness	Evidence that the community is able to clearly express its own issues, needs, and strengths as compared with other similar communities so as to effectively secure resources to meet needs
Effective communication	Evidence of good communication within a community—the people say that they feel they are always well informed about issues ahead of time so that good decisions can be made
Conflict containment and accommodation	Evidence that the community has been able to deal effectively with conflicts within the community such as growth policies or taxes for local school districts
Participation	Evidence that all populations (e.g., different age groups, ethnic groups) participate in community organizations and governmental decisions
Management of relations with larger society	Evidence that the community is able to secure resources from county, state, or federal governments as needed
Machinery for facilitating participant interaction and decision making	Evidence that a community's governmental structure has built-in processes that encourage participation by the members of the community for good decision making

Source: Adapted from Goeppinger, J., Lassiter, P. G., & Wilsoc, B. (1982). Community health is community competence. *Nursing Outlook*, 30(8), 464–467.

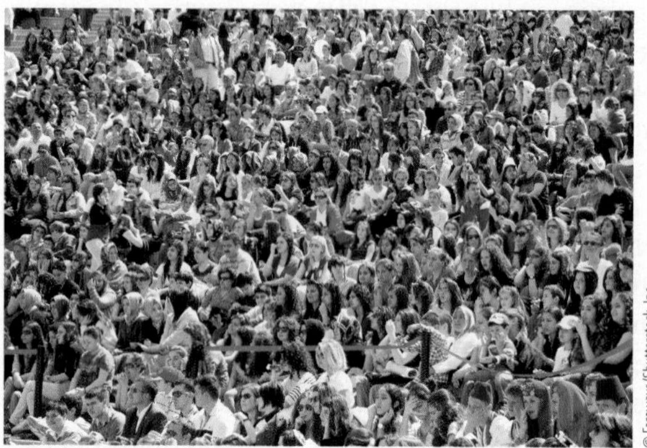

An example of a noninteracting population of young concertgoers.

Healthy Cities

The World Health Organization (WHO) developed the Healthy Cities initiative as a global approach to community-focused health promotion and preventive health. The Healthy Cities movement began in 1984 in Canada; in 1986, WHO initiated the project in Europe. The largest Healthy City in Europe in the WHO project is St. Petersburg, Russia, while Indiana and California have the longest history with Healthy Cities in the United States. Approximately half the world's population lives in urban areas, where health problems are the most complex. As an international movement, Healthy Cities (**Box 2-5**) now involves more than 1,000 cities throughout the world where public, private, and not-for-profit partnerships work together to address the complex health and environmental problems in urban areas (Flynn, Ray, & Rider, 1994). Based on the belief that the health of a community is largely influenced by the social and physical environments in which people live and work, Healthy Cities projects promote change in the complex web of city life (Flynn & Dennis, 1996). Community assessment is a critical and early step in the process of identifying the health needs of cities and working

BOX 2-5 What Does a Healthy City Look Like?

- Clean, safe, high-quality physical environment
- Stable and sustainable ecosystem
- Strong, mutually supportive, and nonexploitive community
- High degree of public participation in and control over decisions affecting citizens' lives, health, and wellbeing
- Meeting of basic needs (e.g., food, water, shelter, income, safe work) for the city's people
- Access to a wide variety of experiences and resources with diverse contacts, interaction, and communications
- Diverse, vital, and innovative city economy
- Connectedness with the city's past and heritage
- City structure that is compatible with and enhances the above qualities
- Optimal level of appropriate public health and illness care services accessible to all
- Good health status

Source: Healthy City Checklist. Copenhagen, WHO Regional Office for Europe, 2014, (http://www.euro.who.int/en/health-topics/environment-and-health/urban-health/activities/healthy-cities/who-european-healthy-cities-network/what-is-a-healthy-city/healthy-city-checklist, accessed July 4, 2008.

with residents to develop realistic and community-identified solutions (Hancock, 1993). The underlying philosophy of such an approach is based on the belief that when residents work out their own locally defined health issues, they will find sustainable solutions to those problems (Flynn, 1994; Lia-Hoagberg, Schaffer, & Strohschein, 1999).

Differences and Similarities Among Communities and Populations

Baccalaureate nurses are prepared to deliver population-focused care. The ACHNE has identified in its *Essentials of Baccalaureate Nursing Education for Entry Level Community/Public Health Nursing* (2009) community assessment, diagnosis, and community planning as essential skills for the BSN nurse.

For advanced-degree nurses specializing in community-based public health nursing, population-focused care becomes the primary focus of the role. For baccalaureate-prepared nurses not specializing in public health nursing, such care may be a secondary focus. However, baccalaureate-prepared nurses practicing in all settings (hospital settings and community settings) will need to have skills in population-focused care. Baccalaureate-prepared nurses will be expected to move beyond being able to just provide care for individual patients. They will be expected to move beyond incorporating only pathophysiological, psychological, pharmacological, and family factor knowledge into their nursing assessments of individual patients. They will need to incorporate population knowledge, including an understanding of the common needs of all patients who share one or more characteristics (Salmon, 1993).

These characteristics may include, for example, a common disease, gender, occupation, or age range. For example, an emergency department nurse noted that most of the patients she was caring for had some condition related to substance abuse. Perhaps they had been involved in an automobile accident caused by drunk driving, or perhaps they suffered a gunshot wound that occurred during a drug deal. Conducting a **population assessment** to better understand the demographic, political, economic, and health system factors affecting this population will eventually lead to **population-level interventions** such as an initiative to coordinate care of substance-abusing patients with mental health professionals. Such efforts may improve not only the health of the individuals within this population, but also the efficiency of the healthcare system (Keller, Strohschein, Lia-Hoagberg, & Schaffer, 2004; Keller, Strohschein, Schaffer, & Lia-Hoagberg, 2004).

Nurses also participate as team members in communitywide health assessments. **Community assessments** differ from population assessments only in that they are not focused on a specific group of individuals who share one or more common characteristics. City municipalities are an example of a community. The individuals in a city municipality interact to achieve goals of employment, the exchange of goods and services, law and order, and so on. A hospital is an example of a community. The individuals within the hospital environment interact to achieve the goals of the organization. You could think of community assessment as more expansive, more complex than a population assessment. In addition, the process of community assessment usually requires a team of researchers to complete a comprehensive analysis of the health of a community.

In the following section, four models for community assessment are presented. Please note that although these models use the language of community assessment and were developed for community assessment, they can be and are adapted for use in population assessments.

Community Assessment Frameworks

Just as there are models, theories, and organizing frameworks that guide nursing practice for individual and family care, there are theoretical perspectives for understanding community dynamics and assessing the needs and strengths or assets of communities. In addition to providing guidance on the criteria or systems to be assessed when the patient is a community, these theoretical perspectives provide guidance for the development of community diagnoses, program planning, and the process for data collection, analysis, and dissemination of the findings. All **community assessment frameworks and models** presented in this chapter are based on the underlying assumption that successful health programs are those that emerge from empowered communities that participate in all phases of program planning, implementation, and evaluation, with community assessment being the first phase of the empowerment process (Eisen, 1994).

EPIDEMIOLOGY AND THE COMMUNITY ASSESSMENT PROCESS

During the community assessment process, data can be organized by the epidemiological triad of host, agent, and environment. The interaction of these factors determines the health status of the community and can be used with any of the models described in this chapter. For example, the host is made up of the members of the community or population; the agent takes many forms, including influences such as stress, diet, racism, physical fitness, and access to health services; and the environment includes pollution, water quality, and weather conditions.

Community Empowerment

The WHO has provided leadership in the use of **community empowerment** as a means toward health for all. WHO's International Conference on Primary Health Care, held in 1978 at Alma-Ata, U.S.S.R., concluded that people throughout the world have little control over their own health care and that more positive health outcomes would occur if people had a greater sense of power over programs that address their needs (Glick, Hale, Kulbok, & Shettig, 1996). The term *community empowerment* means "a social-action process in which individuals and groups act to gain mastery over their lives in the context of changing their social and political environment" (Wallerstein & Bernstein, 1994). Based on the work of Brazilian educator Paulo Freire, community empowerment involves a participatory educational process in which people are not just the recipients of political, educational, or healthcare projects, but become active participants in naming their problems and proposing solutions. For example, empowerment projects should not begin with a nurse-conducted assessment of an at-risk population. Instead, participants from the identified population at risk are recruited by nurses to co-conduct the assessment. Of course, this recruitment process involves a level of trust that has developed between the nurses and the identified population at risk. For more information on building trust when the patient is a community, see "Gaining Entry into the Community" later in this chapter.

Community empowerment is also considered the prerequisite to health promotion. Indeed, the World Health Assembly observed, "the effective participation of the community is indispensable to guarantee the development of health activities and the prevention and control of disease" (WHO, 1985, p. 75). Just as individual patients cannot participate in health promotion until their basic needs are met and they feel some control over their lives, populations and communities must also feel empowered to participate in prevention and health-promoting projects.

Community assessment, viewed within the context of community empowerment, is just one part of the methodology that hopefully will lead to health for all. Community assessment is an essential component leading to effective, acceptable, affordable health care for our society and all other societies. It is one of the core competencies for nursing practice directed toward communities.

Keck (1994) believes that for community health to become a reality, all healthcare professionals will need to learn how to empower citizens to take responsibility for decision making related to the community's health, as well as their own. Empowering patients requires that health professionals give up some of their power and rely on true partnership and collaboration for the community good (Pavlish & Pharris, 2012). Such thinking brings resistance because to promote "power sharing" means to rely on community involvement, not just "lip service," for the advancement of a community's health status. An example of giving up power to the community is when the nurse facilitates the establishment of a board of directors for a community health center made up entirely of community members as the voting members with healthcare professionals as ad hoc members. Keck (1994) contends, "our common challenge [in community health] is the facilitation of that [empowering] process" (p. 8).

Community Assessment Frameworks/Models

Many community assessment frameworks and models have been designed to guide the process of community assessment. Two theoretical perspectives described here have either been developed by public health nurses or are often used by public health nurses when conducting a community assessment. Other important approaches to community assessment not included in this chapter are *Community Competence: A Positive Approach to Needs Assessment* by Goeppinger and Baglioni (1986) and *The Sunrise Model* by Leininger (1988).

Use of a framework or model to help guide a community assessment project is an essential step in the process. A framework/model provides a frame of reference for data collection. Concepts or elements within a theoretical framework or model can be transposed into categories for data collection, diagnosis, and planning. Examples of concepts or elements that can be transposed into categories for data collection include safety, community boundaries, lines of resistance, and government systems. The following sections of this chapter give examples of how theoretical concepts can be used as criteria for assessment, community diagnoses, and planning.

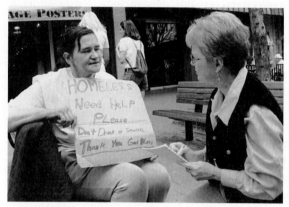

Chapter author Dr. Judith Barton conducting an interview, using the Lundy–Barton Systems Model as a theoretical guide to conduct a community health assessment with a community member who is homeless.

The *core* of any community is its people. Included in the core are the demographics of the population and their values, beliefs, and history. The core, in turn, affects and is affected by eight interacting subsystems. Those subsystems are physical environment, education, safety and transportation, politics

TABLE 2-2 Community-as-Partner Model: Concepts for Assessment

• **Community core**	• The people who reside in a geopolitical community or the population of a community. Criteria to evaluate when assessing the core include the community's history, current demographics, and the values and beliefs of community residents.
• **Interrelated subsystems:**	
Physical environment	• Observations of the climate, terrain, natural boundaries, commercial systems, neighborhoods, religious symbols, planning studies, and so on.
Health and social services	• Hospitals and clinics, home health care, extended care facilities, public health services, counseling and support services, clothing, food, shelter, and special needs services.
Economics	• Household median income, percentage of persons living in poverty, employment status, occupational categories, and union activity.
Safety and transportation	• Information about protection services (fire, police, water treatment, solid waste) and air quality. Information on public transportation.
Politics and government	• Type of city government, political action groups, and political party affiliation.
Communication	• Formal communication sources (e.g., newspapers) and informal communication sources (e.g., bulletin boards, posters).
Education	• Educational status of community members and educational sources.
Recreation	• Recreational facilities.
Stressors	• Tension-producing situations within the community, such as an increase in substance abuse among teens within the community.
Normal level of defense	• Health statistics for the community (e.g., mortality and morbidity).
Flexible line of defense	• Community responses to current stressors.
Lines of resistance	• Established strengths within the community (e.g., shelters, food banks).

Source: Data from Anderson, E. T., & McFarlane, J. (2003). *Community as partner: Theory and practice in nursing.* Philadelphia, PA: Lippincott.

and government, health and social services, communication, economics, and recreation. In addition to assessing the core people within a community and the eight interacting subsystems, the community-as-partner model directs the nurse to assess current stressors that are producing tension within the community, the normal level of defense or current level of health within the community, the flexible line of defense representing current temporary responses to stressors or threats to health within the community, and lines of resistance or established community strengths that weave through all the interacting subsystems. **Table 2-2** is a summary of all concepts or elements included in the community-as-partner model and their definitions.

After assessing *all* elements in the model, the researchers are directed to develop community diagnoses that include community responses to stressors (i.e., problem identification), causative factors leading to each problem, and a list of supporting data to validate each community diagnosis. In other words, the outcome of the community assessment using the community-as-partner model is a set of community diagnoses developed in the same format as nursing diagnoses. In turn, these community diagnoses lay the groundwork for health planning. For an example of a community diagnosis and plan see **Table 2-3**.

Although the community-as-partner model does not specifically direct the nurses to develop an interview guide based on the model's elements, an interview guide using an ethnographic, open-ended approach has been developed and can be found in **Box 2-6**.

RESEARCH ALERT

Teams of Community Health Workers and Nursing Students Effect Health Promotion of Underserved Urban Neighborhoods.

The purpose of this study was to explore the effectiveness of community health worker (CHW)/nursing student teams in promoting secondary protection and improving access to care for residents of three urban underserved neighborhoods. The research study also examined and measured CHW and resident satisfaction with such a program.

Quasi-experimental and nonexperimental designs were used with convenience samples consisting of residents who participated in the CHW program during 2005–2006, CHWs and residents who participated in the CHW program during 2005–2007, and a systematic random sample of residents across the three neighborhoods.

Continues

TABLE 2-3 Community Diagnosis for Health Planning Using the Community-as-Partner Model

Response (Problem)	Related to (Causes)	As Manifested by (Data)
Community disorganization and health/social services economic crisis	Increase in illegal immigrant workers from Mexico not eligible for government benefits Noncoordinated efforts between agencies within one community and among neighboring communities	Increase in nonreimbursed emergency department care at community hospital Increase in free school lunches at local school Increase in delayed prenatal care and lower birth weight infants
Goal	**Objective(s)**	**Evaluative Indicators**
Regional coordination of efforts to meet the needs of medical and social underserved population	Establish a task force made up of service providers and community leaders representing the medically and socially underserved populations to design appropriate and feasible solutions/programs to deal with current community disorganization and health/social services economic crises	Reduced nonreimbursed emergency department costs, free school lunches, and low birth weight rates Increase in first trimester prenatal care

Continued

Three quantitative measures were used in the study: a pre-/post-test with residents who participated in the program, a satisfaction survey of CHWs and participants, and a community assessment survey of the neighborhoods in which the program occurred.

CHW/nursing student teams were shown to increase awareness of community resources, increase access to dental care, decrease use of the ER, promote use of a medical home/regular source of care, and increase the percentage of people having their blood pressure screened in the last 2 years. Based on the results of this study, CHW/nursing student teams can positively impact the health of underserved populations.

Source: Zandee, G. L., Bossenbroek, D., Slager, D., & Gordon, B. (2013). Teams of community health workers and nursing students effect health promotion of underserved urban neighborhoods. *Public Health Nursing, 30*(5), 439–447.

Community-as-Partner Model

The *community-as-partner model* includes community assessment as the first phase of the nursing process to be used when the patient is a community. The model is based on nursing theorist Betty Neuman's (1989) total-person model for viewing individual patient problems. Nurse-authors Anderson and McFarlane (2003) developed the model to help guide public health nurses in their practice with communities. The authors explain that the title of the model is purposeful in that the underlying philosophy of the model is primary health care with an emphasis on community empowerment. The model is also intended to be a synthesis of public health and nursing.

The community-as-partner model is a systems perspective that gives direction to types of community systems (e.g., educational system and transportation system) that need to be assessed when conducting a community assessment. It also provides direction for the analysis of the data collected to illuminate community dynamics related to health. Concepts in the model include the *community core*, eight interacting community *subsystems*, community *stressors*, and boundaries titled *normal level of defense*, *flexible line of defense*, and *lines of resistance*.

ENVIRONMENTAL CONNECTION

Research has demonstrated a relationship between urban sprawl and greater risk of being overweight and obese. Urban sprawl is defined as a pattern of development across a metropolitan area where large percentages of the population live in lower density residential areas. Houses are on larger lots; cultural values reflect urban living and emphasize auto use. Consequences include a greater reliance on automobiles and decreased ability to walk to destinations, decreased neighborhood cohesion, and environmental degradation (e.g., greenhouse gas emissions and destruction of open spaces, decreased parks). The Centers for Disease Control and Prevention (CDC) has also released findings connecting urban sprawl with obesity, especially in the southern United States.

Source: Lopez, R. (2004). Urban sprawl and risk for being overweight or obese. *American Journal of Public Health, 94*(9), 1574–1579.

General Systems Model for Community Assessment

Lundy and Barton's (1995) *General Systems Model for Community and Population Assessment and Intervention*

BOX 2-6 Example of Key Informant Ethnographic Interview Guide Based on Community-as-Partner Model

Introduction by Interviewer

Explain the purpose of the interview (i.e., to better understand the culture and the customs of your community). In addition, confirm that you will be recording the interview so that you do not have to take notes the whole time. Tell the informant that he or she may ask you to stop the recording at any time. Finally, assure the informant that his or her identity will remain confidential in all reports.

Grand Tour Question: What is it like to live in your community?

Mini-Tour Questions (some of the following questions, which target community subsystems, may have been thoroughly covered in response to grand tour question):

- What do you do for fun?
- What would you tell someone new to your community about the natural resources (environment) in your community?
- What are the schools like? Where do people go if they want to further their education?
- How safe do you feel in your community? How do you get around (transportation) in your community?
- Who has the political power in the community (i.e., who is the most powerful figure[s] in your community)? Discuss your rationale (reasons).
- Describe your perceptions of the health of your community. Where do you personally go for your healthcare needs? How adequate are the services available to you?
- Please describe the formal and informal types of communication in your community.
- How would you describe the economic trends/future for your community? If I moved here, how easy would it be to make a living, buy groceries and clothes, and have a place to live?
- Can you tell me something about the cultural and spiritual/religious aspects of your community (e.g., family life, philosophy of community)?
- Is there anything else you would like to tell me about your community?

Source: Copyright 1996, The Regents of the University of Colorado. Used by permission.

is based on general systems theory as originally conceived by Von Bertalanffy (1968). A general systems approach is the basis for many nursing theories and has widespread usage in most all scientific disciplines. This approach to community assessment directs the research team to focus on the whole community, not on the parts of a community. Two broad concepts for assessment using this model include community structure and process.

The structure of any system can be defined as an arrangement of *interacting subsystems* or parts at a given point in time. The system as a whole has specified boundaries that determine what is inside the system and what is outside the system. In turn, each subsystem has boundaries that specify what is inside the subsystem and what is outside. Similar to the community-as-partner assessment model, subsystems within the community system include schools, churches, self-help groups, health systems, and so on. Systems also have a *suprasystem*, the larger construct of which the system is a part. For example, if the community system is identified as a municipality or a city, the county and state where the municipality is situated become suprasystems to the community system and have great relevance to the community system and the community assessment process.

Community health nurses using the general systems assessment approach to community assessment begin by identifying the target system and its boundaries. For example, if the assessment is to be carried out on a geopolitical community named Jonestown, the researchers must ask the following questions:

1. Do the boundaries for Jonestown stop at the city's geopolitical limits or does the community consider a neighboring smaller crossroads community as within its boundaries?
2. What are the critical subsystems within the target community system?
3. What are the critical suprasystems impacting the community?
4. What types of relationships exist among the subsystems and between the target community and its suprasystems?
5. Are the boundaries between subsystems, the system, and its suprasystems open and cooperative, or is there a lack of cooperation and support between these systems?
6. Does the target community system and its subsystems have a sense of integrity or are the boundaries too open?

In assessing *community process*, nurses need to determine how the community system works to meet its needs or goals. Questions to be asked include the following: How is the community system responding (termed *throughput*) to internal and external stimuli or *inputs*? What are the results or *outputs* of the community system's response?

(An example of a result or output to a stressor such as air pollution might be stricter auto emission policies.) Is the output successful (negative feedback) or does the Environmental Protection Agency fine the community for having too many poor air quality days per year (positive feedback). In other words, does the community return to a *steady state* or does it continue to experience *disequilibrium*? How can the community continue to grow from the ongoing processes of *input*, *response*, *output*, and *feedback*?

The Lundy–Barton Model also includes a process for the nurse to use as a follow-through to the community assessment. This process is a familiar one to both nursing and medicine. One assesses the patient (i.e., the community), arrives at several diagnoses, develops a plan of action, evaluates the outcomes, and revises the plan as needed. **Table 2-4** is a summary of all concepts found in the Lundy–Barton Model, their definitions, and examples of types of data to collect. A community assessment guide based on the Lundy–Barton Model can be found in the Appendix at the end of this chapter.

Using the Nursing Process for the Community

Conducting a Community Assessment

More often than not, a community assessment project will be guided by a blend of two or more theoretical perspectives. In addition, a community assessment model or blended model can be used to conduct a population assessment *in any practice setting*. For example, a nurse in a postpartum unit of a regional medical center noted that there had been an influx of Mexican immigrants. These immigrants were Spanish-speaking only, and no staff spoke Spanish, nor was patient education literature available in Spanish. The nurse in this case realized that she needed to provide the leadership role in conducting a population assessment. Her population assessment included an examination of population demographics in both the hospital and the general community. She then examined the hospital's human resources for language translation and available Spanish-language educational materials. She also interviewed personnel (key informants familiar with the population) on the unit and some of the inpatients as well (**primary informants**). The nurse, with the support of the nurse manager of the unit, raised the consciousness of the hospital administration that patient educational materials and translators should be available for Spanish-speaking patients. The nurse then developed a culturally sensitive child education program including written materials in Spanish. The program was implemented by nurses on the postpartum unit and was well accepted by the immigrant patients and nurses on the unit. Recommendations were made to the administration for the program's continuation with support from the Hispanic community. The nurse conducted key and primary informant interviews, gathered secondary data (e.g., community resources for the population and some census data on the population), and analyzed both sources of data to define the strengths and limitations of the population and recommendations for interventions at the population level. Clearly this nurse used her understanding of the connection between population health and individual care regardless of setting (Baldwin et al., 1998).

ETHICAL CONNECTION 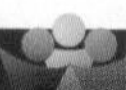

What about a population that chooses to ignore a critical health problem, as identified by the assessment? Considering the principle of autonomy, how would the community health nurse approach this challenge?

Once a theoretical perspective or a combination of theoretical perspectives has been chosen to guide the community assessment process, general tenets from the nursing process (i.e., assessment techniques, planning based on the assessment, interventions implemented at the community or population level, and evaluation) will apply. **Box 2-7** summarizes steps in the process of a community health assessment.

Gaining Entry into the Community

The collection of meaningful data about a community depends on the nurse's successfully gaining entry into the community. According to Goeppinger and Schuster, "gaining entry or acceptance into the community is perhaps the biggest challenge in assessment" (1988, p. 202).

Just as you would never just enter a patient's room in a hospital or knock on the door of a home health patient and say, "Turn over in bed, I am here to give you a 'shot,'" the population-focused nurse should not expect to just walk into a community and plan to conduct a community-focused intervention without going through some stages of getting to know the community as patient. As Kauffman (1994) explains in her study of the experience of white nurse researchers who conducted an ethnography of a senior citizen center in a poor, inner-city black ghetto, "getting in" a community is "a process of gaining, building, and maintaining trust with the group under study" (p. 179). Differences in characteristics such as social status, ethnicity, age, and class between the researchers, who are the *outsiders*, and the community being studied, the *insiders*, may create an environment of prejudicial and discriminatory responses that impede *getting in*. In other words, would the community be willing to share their issues with a community assessment team that just barged in and said they were here to study their health and healthcare needs? Would the results of an assessment set up in this manner produce valid results? Is it not possible that the outsiders could commit flagrant errors in their interpretations that might even promote prejudice and discrimination toward the very community that they intended to assist?

TABLE 2-4 Lundy–Barton Model: Concepts for Assessment with Example Questions

Community Structure	
• Target system	• *Observations*: Are the boundaries for the target community geopolitical or geographic? How would you describe the natural environment? Describe cultural symbols noted.
	• *Measurements*: Demographics, health and social service statistics.
	• *Interactions*: History of community, values and beliefs.
• Subsystems	• *Observations*: Windshield survey of public institutions such as schools, churches, businesses, recreational facilities, and so on.
	• *Measurements*: Literature on various subsystems within community.
	• *Interactions*: Interview key community leaders to find out how the community subsystems interact.
• Suprasystems	• *Observations*: Compare and contrast target community environment with suprasystems (e.g., in comparison to other cities within county).
	• *Measurements*: Demographic and health statistic data for most relevant suprasystem (e.g., state statistics) to compare target system with suprasystem.
	• *Interactions*: Interview key community leaders to find out how the target community interacts with state or county agencies.
Community Process	
• Goals	• *Observations*: Windshield survey may reveal new construction sites indicating growth direction.
	• *Measurements*: Seek community planning documents, interview key community leaders concerning goals of community.
	• *Interactions*: Does there seem to be agreement among key community leaders about community goals?
	• *Observations*: Attendance at community meetings to gain information about particular community stressors (inputs). Windshield survey to observe for environmental hazards.
• Inputs	• *Measurements*: Review of literature obtained from various community agencies to determine ongoing community initiatives (responses or throughputs). Interviews with key community members to learn more about final outcomes of initiatives and if the initiatives met their objectives (results or outputs and feedback).
• Responses/throughputs	
• Results/outputs	
• Feedback	• *Interactions*: Is the community experiencing a steady state or is it experiencing disequilibrium?

Source: This article was published in *Nursing process: Application of conceptual models*, 4th ed, P. J. Christensen & J. W. Kenney (Eds.),pp. 102–119, Lundy, K. S., & Barton, J. A. (1995). Assessment: Data collection of the community patient. Copyright Mosby 1995.

BOX 2-7 Steps in Community-Focused Intervention

Community defined; partnership established
Identification of the community
Promotion of the partnership of the community

Assessment

What are the characteristics of the population (age, gender, race)?
Which changes are occurring in the characteristics of the people in the community (births, deaths, migrations)?
Which health problems exist in the community (morbidity rates)?
Which health problems are causing deaths in the population (mortality rates)?
How do these health problems compare with other populations? Are they increasing or decreasing?

Nursing Diagnoses

Name the:

Risk of (a specific problem or health risk in the community)
Among (the specific group or population affected by the problem/risk)
Related to (strengths and weaknesses in the community that influence the specific health risk in the community)

Planning

Which factors that are changeable (environmental, behavioral) increase the risk of the health problem?
What can most effectively reduce risk among the population?
What can be done in the community to reduce risk?
How much change in the health problem is desired over what period of time in the population (goals and objectives)?
Who can most effectively affect the outcome of the plan?

Implementation

What is the role of the community health nurse in the action phase?
Which strategies can facilitate healthy change in the community?

Evaluation

Was the plan carried out?
Was it acceptable to the community or population?
Was the health problem changed as planned?
Was the program effective?
What would be done differently?
What are recommendations for future community health promotion?

Source: Community health nursing abstracts by SULLIVAN, JUDITH ANN, Reproduced with permission of BLACKWELL SCIENTIFIC PUBLICATIONS, in the format Republish in a book via Copyright Clearance Center.

Another strategy found to be helpful is to use a variety of communication channels to "reach" the target population. Using existing personal networks (e.g., clubs, social groups) and social institutions (e.g., voluntary health organizations, churches, schools) that the target population depends on for support and information can yield positive access results. If the target group has an established health network (e.g., a group of diabetic older adults), contacting those medical/health societies to seek support and approval can provide valuable entry. The nurse must be aware, however, that all members of a subgroup may not be reached through any one organization, thus necessitating the use of diverse means in attempts to initially establish contact with the target population (Keller, Strohschein, Lia-Hoagberg, & Schaffer, 2004). With the Internet, many new opportunities for developing contact and securing information about target groups are possible and hold great promise in this stage of community assessment. Another way to demonstrate the community team's commitment to reach the community is to participate in community activities. Community team members may stay in local motels, rather than chains, and patronize local eateries.

If the community assessment team is very different in social characteristics from the community under study, it would be easy for the outsiders to err by underestimating the effects of ethnicity, age, and class on insiders' responses (Richards et al., 2002). They may use inappropriate data-collection tools, or they may assume the insiders are just not knowledgeable enough or educated enough to be able to articulate their health beliefs and health issues. If the assessment team believes the community is not knowledgeable, they may patronize the group (i.e., treat the community with unseemly deference rather than as equals). Locals and important leaders in communities and target populations can function as valuable "cultural brokers," controlling entry into the group, especially to underserved populations. These brokers are often laypersons who might be called "natural helpers," people to whom the community turns for help in times of health concerns and other crises. Identifying these significant persons takes time because they may not be the formal leaders of a group. These brokers can impede "outside" projects or provide invaluable assistance in accessing the group. By serving as local "interpreters," these brokers can translate culture for both the health team and residents and promote collaboration for assessment activities.

Note that it is not detrimental to be an outsider when studying a community. The sociological concept of the "professional stranger" has taught us that being an outsider studying the group allows the researcher to avoid being caught up in the commitments of the group and therefore to be able to raise questions unlikely to be raised by insiders.

Kauffman (1994) proposes five phases of "getting in" to a community to build trust that will lead to a valid study of the community. These five phases are impressing, behaving, swapping, belonging, and "chillin' out." Kauffman points out that several phases may sometimes occur simultaneously. However, at all times the processes are mutual, interactive, and context specific.

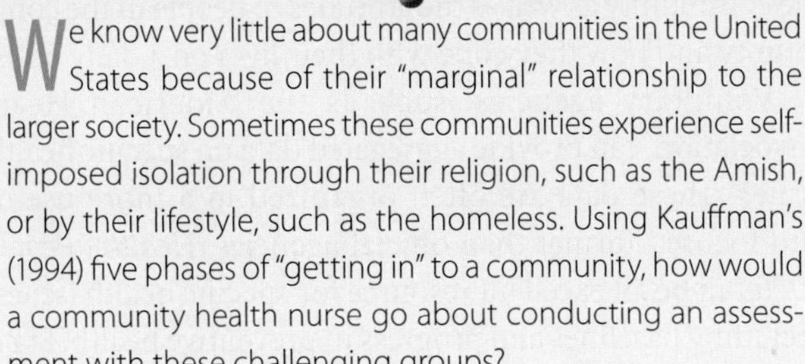

CULTURAL CONNECTION

We know very little about many communities in the United States because of their "marginal" relationship to the larger society. Sometimes these communities experience self-imposed isolation through their religion, such as the Amish, or by their lifestyle, such as the homeless. Using Kauffman's (1994) five phases of "getting in" to a community, how would a community health nurse go about conducting an assessment with these challenging groups?

Impressing is the initial and sometimes lengthy process of outsiders and insiders evaluating one another. Social myths are explored; stereotypes and traits of the other (e.g., skin color, clothes, social courtesies) are observed. Rejection is possible by either side. Strategies for the community assessment team to maintain include (1) maintaining political, institutional, and personal neutrality; (2) avoiding obligations to any sponsor or patron of the assessment project; (3) following the rules or customs of all the insiders, not just the leaders; (4) continuing to return to the community and clarifying the assessment process; (5) keeping abreast of local events; and (6) identifying key informants who represent all different groups within the community. An important aspect of a cultural system is its members' valued ideas—those notions about how things should be done. As is so often the case, community members and the community assessment team have different "valued ideas," and cultural clashes occur.

Behaving occurs when actions and interactions between outsiders and insiders begin to erode myths about each other, and each sees the other as fellow human beings, although each side may still guard against rejection. Strategies for continuing the trust-building process in this phase include (1) demonstrating nonjudgmental and unconditional regard, (2) being genuine and avoiding trying too hard to be accepted, (3) learning the language of the group (e.g., the meaning of cultural slang words, perhaps phrases of a foreign language), and (4) placing the insider as the esteemed teacher of community life and health. The gender and age of team members and community members can also play an important part in this phase. For example, using a very young community interviewer in an elderly population may be less effective than using a middle-aged person. Wax (1986) found that middle-aged or older women are more able than any other age or gender to collect data across ages and gender categories. Of course, generalizations must be avoided in any context; however, ignoring age and gender influences can often impede or distort data collection (Zandee et al., 2013).

Swapping involves reciprocal giving and sharing between the outsiders and insiders. Giving and sharing help break down the remaining barriers to mutual acceptance and trust between the outsiders and insiders. Strategies used in the swapping process include telling insiders more about the roles of the outsiders (e.g., health programs involved in, outcomes of previous community assessments). Going to community events is an important swapping activity that often allows for informal interviews.

Belonging is the culmination of the process. During this phase, outsiders and insiders are able to talk about issues that heretofore provoked discomfort. Issues such as racism, prejudice, and discrimination are open to discussion. Insider language no longer seems foreign to the outsider, who understands the meaning of the language. Greetings and good-byes include physical displays of affection such as hugging. Socially deviant acts such as drug use may no longer be hidden from the outsider.

Chillin' out begins as the outsiders near the end of their community assessment phase and begin (hopefully) a long-term partnership with the community for the improvement and maintenance of community health. Outsiders should give insiders an idea of what to expect in the future, such as the amount of help that will always be available from healthcare experts.

GLOBAL CONNECTION 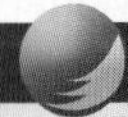

International travel nursing is rapidly becoming a growing field. How would knowing the community assessment process benefit a nurse who is traveling to a new city or country for the first time?

Collecting Data

What kinds of data do nurses look for when conducting a community assessment, and where do they find it?

The primary goal of data collection is to acquire meaningful and useful information about the community and its health. A systematic and informed nursing assessment in partnership with the community involves a variety of techniques and resources. The scope of a community or population assessment is determined by the purpose of the assessment and the complexity and nature of the identified community or population. For community assessments of large geopolitical communities, the process may take several months to a year or more and may require an interdisciplinary team.

Confidentiality regarding sensitive or controversial data is a critical issue for nurses conducting a community assessment (Goeppinger & Schuster, 1988). Just as a nurse must safeguard information obtained from the individual patient as an ethical and legal responsibility, the information derived from the community may involve a more concerted effort. Because there are often many team members collecting information from a variety of sources, it may be necessary to assign anonymous names to community members and even to other organizations within the community.

There are seven methods of collecting community data: **informant interviews**, **observation**, **secondary analysis of existing data**, **constructed surveys**, **focus groups**, **community forums**, and **windshield surveys**. The community health nurse should attempt to collect data using several different methods because no method is without bias. The process of using multiple complementary methods is termed *triangulation*.

Informant interviews involve directly questioning community residents. **Key informants** should be identified and interviewed early in the assessment process. These key informants are formal and informal leaders in the community who represent a cross section of age groups and ethnic groups. They include town officials, elected members, student and group leaders, and informal "spokespersons" such as barbers or postal carriers. The nurse uses appropriate communication techniques in directed conversations with selected members of a community. These interviews can be structured, with planned questions, or unstructured, in which the informants guide the interviews. Data gathered through informant interviews are considered subjective and can yield valuable information about the residents' perspectives on health values and health care; for example, how do the residents perceive their community healthcare services? Such data are recorded in the residents' own words and noted as direct quotations in the interaction column of the assessment tool. Both formal and informal leaders of groups and communities will yield important information about the community.

The nurse uses observation by purposefully looking and listening for significant events that are taking place in the community. Examples include city council meetings, high school basketball games, county fairs, barbershop conversations, and other similar social events. The nurse systematically records these observations. Relevant conversations of community residents are recorded in the interaction column of the assessment tool.

Secondary analysis is analysis of records, documents, and other previously collected data. The nurse may not have to collect new data when conducting the community assessment. Such data may already exist in the form of census data, historical accounts, diaries, previous studies of the community or aggregate, court records, minutes from community meetings, and research studies on population risks. The following Research Alert describes risks for cross-country truck drivers. The results of this research can be incorporated into a population assessment of cross-country truck drivers and is an example of the use of **secondary data** in a population health assessment. These are invaluable sources of information that can reveal the characteristics of the community as well as the attitudes of people in the community and how they cope with their lives on a daily basis.

Voluntary agencies, such as the American Heart Association, can provide aggregated data on specific health issues. These data are often organized in a more useful and focused format than official agencies. *Healthy People 2020* can be an excellent resource for specific health issues, including baselines and progress in preventive health. State health departments, the U.S. Public Health Service, the National Center for Health Statistics, and the U.S. Census Bureau provide a wide array of mortality and morbidity statistics and demographic profiles of populations. The CDC is an excellent source for information about national illness and health patterns as well as aggregated state health information.

RESEARCH ALERT

Long-haul truck drivers spend long hours on the road separated from family and other support systems, drive in hazardous conditions, and are often sleep deprived. Due to the demands of truck driving as an occupation, long-distance truck drivers are considered a population at risk for increased rates of drug use. Researchers and policymakers are especially interested in truck drivers' rates of drug use, the influence of drugs on truck accidents, and the link between drug use and fatigue. Studies have focused on identifying truck drivers at risk for abusing alcohol and drugs and investigating the drug use patterns of long-distance truck drivers.

Researchers interviewed 35 long-haul truck drivers at truck stops and loading facilities in cities and towns across Queensland, Australia. The majority of truck drivers interviewed reported high rates of over-the-counter, prescription, and illicit drug use. Reported use of amphetamines was particularly high.

In contrast to earlier studies that focused on fatigue as the motivating factor in drug use, the researchers found overlapping and changing motivations for drug use among the individual drivers. Using Becker's model of a drug use "career," they found that some of the drivers began using illicit drugs before they joined the truck driving occupation. They were motivated to use drugs by peer pressure, socialization, relaxation, wanting to fit their image of a truck driver, and addiction.

The results of this study indicate that social factors in addition to fatigue should be considered when developing drug prevention and treatment programs and policies for truck drivers.

Sources: Davey, J. J., Richards, N., & Freeman, J. (2007). Fatigue and beyond: Patterns of and motivations for illicit drug use among long-haul truck drivers. *Traffic Injury and Prevention, 8*(3), 7–18; Gay Anderson, D., & Riley, P. (2008). Determining standards of care for substance abuse and alcohol use in long-haul truck drivers. *Nursing Clinics of North America, 43*(3), 357–365.

In constructed surveys, community or aggregate members in a random sample of the population provide answers to written or oral questions. This technique is costly and time-consuming and is used only when other resources have been exhausted. Survey tools are available at the CDC website (http://www.cdc.gov) for a variety of attitude and opinion surveys with established reliability and validity for community data collection. For example, if a nurse is interested in abortion attitudes and if very little information is available through other techniques, a survey of community members may provide useful information about this issue.

A focus group can be used very effectively to derive information about health needs of specific groups in the community or population. The focus group is a qualitative approach to learning about subgroups within the population regarding sociocultural and other specific characteristics (Clark et al., 2003). Members of a focus group differ from other small groups in that the members are usually chosen to be fairly homogeneous in regard to specific characteristics, such as gender, age, or other social variables. By being highly selective about the membership of a focus group, the nurse can learn a great deal about that particular subpopulation's needs and perceptions about viable, acceptable solutions to health problems. The average group meeting lasts 2 to 3 hours and can be a very efficient way to determine group perceptions (Basch, 1987).

A community forum, which involves having an open meeting for all members of a community or population, can also be used to obtain information concerning the needs and perceptions of community members. In contrast to the focus group, a community forum is open to all; no attempt is made to structure a homogeneous group. A town hall meeting is a variation of the community forum that has gained popularity in recent decades; it was used by President Bill Clinton in 1994 and again, more than 2 decades later, by President Barack Obama in 2009 to bring their respective healthcare reform packages to the grassroots level. Even though community forums are not necessarily representative of the entire target population, they can be used effectively in a short period of time, with little cost, as one strategy for community members to voice their views.

The nurse can conduct a windshield survey of the geopolitical community as a technique for data collection. These observations through the window of an automobile are a way of collecting information about a community's environment. As an initial data-collection technique, a windshield survey often reveals common characteristics about how people live (e.g., transportation primarily by automobile, little pedestrian traffic), where they live, and the type of housing they live in.

Community Diagnosis

Conclusions about data collected on the community patient are a natural outcome of the assessment process. Eventually, these stated analyzed conclusions identify "labels" or names for the health problems in the community; these are called **community health diagnoses** (Higgs & Gustafson, 1985). The gathered data and generated data form a composite database. At this phase of the nursing process, as raw data are analyzed, themes begin to emerge and needs are noted, as are problems, strengths, and community resources. Community members continue to be involved in this process as both subjective and objective data are compiled (Keller, Strohschein, Lia-Hoagberg, & Schaffer, 2004; Keller, Strohschein, Schaffer, & Lia-Hoagberg, 2004).

Written community health diagnoses differ significantly from those written for the individual patient. Most systems of classification developed for nursing diagnoses have focused on the individual. Hamilton (1983) analyzed various theories and diagnostic classification schemata and concluded that research is needed in both the application of individual models of diagnoses and the clarification of the *target* of care, whether that be the community, individuals in the community, or individuals influenced by the community. Viewing the community as a patient who has varying degrees of ability to meet its own needs extends the focus to include response to illness and change, social problems, or any areas in which the community patient needs assistance in order to function optimally (Higgs & Gustafson, 1985). Data from the target community or population are compared with similar populations in other settings. Comparing data such as infant mortality rates or accident rates can reveal significant differences and point to specific disparate health risks in the target population. During this phase, the community health nurse compares conclusions about the community's health status with accepted standards of health, and judgments are made as to strengths and concerns of a community's functioning (Lundy & Barton, 1995).

Identified problems are now stated in the form of a community health diagnosis. Each diagnosis is documented, the recipient of care is identified (the community as opposed to the individual), and factors contributing to the problem are explicated.

A common nursing diagnosis format that has been modified for community use has been developed by Schuster and Goeppinger (1996) and Muecke (1984). Here the diagnosis takes the following form:

1. Risk of (a specific problem or health risk in the community)
2. Among (the specific group or population that is affected by the problem/risk)
3. Related to (strengths and weaknesses in the community that influence the specific problem or health risk in the community)

The following are some sample community/population diagnoses using the aforementioned format:

- Risk of lung infections among disaster workers related to debris from Hurricane Katrina recovery
- Risk of hearing loss among studio musicians related to constancy of loud music in occupational settings and nonuse of hearing protection
- Risk for increased incidence of pregnancy among teens at Rydell High School related to increased sexual activity and nonuse of contraceptive services or methods
- Risk for lung damage among migrant farm workers in the Louisiana delta related to presence of pesticide pulmonary irritants in the occupational environment
- Risk of eating disorders among professional ballet dancers related to occupational pressure to stay underweight for professional advancement
- Risk of sleep deprivation among nurses who are permanent night shift workers at Bayview Medical Center related to erratic and interrupted day sleep

MEDIA MOMENT

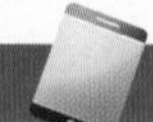

The Healing Heart: Communities Storytelling to Encourage Caring and Healthy Families (2003)

By A. Cox and D. Alperts, British Columbia, Canada: New Society Publishers

This book is a "basket of memories" that is meant to trigger memories for storytelling for use in personal and professional communities. The stories are for sharing among people of all ages, and many of the contributors preface their stories with work-related discussions about programs, projects, agencies, and the use of storytelling with their patients and its impact upon them. Communities include battered women, substance abuse and recovery patients, sex offenders, refugees, immigrants, and an adult prison group. The editors of the book maintain that the book is for people who work with communities so that they may learn to use storytelling in their work.

Planning and Prioritization Phase

During the **planning phase**, priorities are established, goals and objectives are identified based on those priorities, and community-focused interventions are developed. Unlike a clinical individual diagnosis, a community diagnosis requires more than simple establishment of the presence of a health problem. More than one health problem is always present in a community or population; consequently, diagnoses require prioritizing problems for community action. Criteria must be established to determine how resources and energies will be allocated toward addressing the identified needs (Watson, 1984).

The WHO has published criteria that may be used to prioritize health problems identified in communities. These criteria are listed in **Box 2-8**.

Goeppinger (1984) has also developed a set of criteria to guide the prioritization of community health problems. Those criteria are as follows:

- Community awareness of the problem
- Community motivation
- Nurse's or team's ability to influence problem solution
- Availability of expertise
- Severity of consequences to society if problems left unresolved
- Quickness with which the problem can be resolved

Reviewing the identified health problems using a set of criteria is a critical step in the process to address complex community health problems. In addition, community members representing multiple subpopulations within the community (e.g., different age groups, ethnic groups), community leaders, and assessment team members should be involved at this stage (Duiveman & Bonner, 2012).

Once the prioritized problem list emerges, goals, objectives, strategies, and plans are developed. *Goals* are broad and general statements of concern that are usually considered long range. *Objectives* are specific, measurable statements of desired outcomes and are often viewed as short term.

All planning group members, community representatives, and other experts within the appropriate areas are

BOX 2-8 Criteria for Selecting a Health Problem for Community Intervention

- Significance of the problem (in terms of numbers affected or consequences)
- Level of community awareness and priority
- Ability to reduce risk
- Cost of reducing risk (economic, social, ethical)
- Ability to identify the target population
- Availability of resources to intervene in the reduction of risk

Source: Adapted from World Health Organization (WHO). (1976, October 11–15). Criteria to be considered in selecting a preventive health action. In *Report of the first interdisciplinary workshop on psychosocial factors and health.* Stockholm, Sweden: Author.

involved in this process, especially those who will be most affected and who are in a position to influence the implementation of solutions. The importance of this involvement cannot be overemphasized. Many community interventions have failed and undermined future professional assistance because community teams excluded community members from participating in this process (Goodman et al., 1998). We know from research that when communities and populations develop a vested interest in the identification of health needs and proposed solutions, there is a greater likelihood of sustaining these intervention strategies over time. In other words, the community must be willing to "pay the price" of whatever objectives and goals are proposed (Watson, 1984).

Community health nurses are often members of teams who are conducting community- or population-level assessments, and as such the identified health problems and concerns are rarely limited to the use of nursing interventions (Robinson, 2005). The complexity of group-identified health concerns requires an interdisciplinary approach, and planning and intervention strategies usually reflect the involvement of other professionals (e.g., social workers, audiologists, physicians, and psychologists) and community resources' utilization (Duiveman & Bonner, 2012; Smith & Barton, 1992).

RESEARCH ALERT

Catholic Healthcare West (CHW) of San Francisco has developed a national Community Need Index (CNI) to identify and address barriers to healthcare access in communities. The CNI aggregates five socioeconomic indicators known to contribute to health disparity—income, culture/language, education, housing status, and insurance coverage—and applies them to every ZIP code in the United States. Each ZIP code is then given a score ranging from 1.0 (low need) to 5.0 (high need). Residents of communities with the highest CNI scores have been shown to be twice as likely to experience preventable hospitalization for manageable conditions—such as ear infections, pneumonia, or congestive heart failure—as residents of communities with the lowest CNI scores.

The CNI provides evidence for addressing socioeconomic barriers when considering health policy and local health planning. This tool links healthcare disparities between geographic regions and illustrates the acute needs of inner-city and rural areas. It may enable healthcare providers, policymakers, and others to allocate resources where they are most needed, using a standardized, quantitative tool.

Source: Roth, R. (2005). The "Community Need Index": A new tool pinpoints health care disparities in communities throughout the nation. *Health Progress, 86*(4), 32–38.

Implementation Phase

The implementation phase is the action phase. It translates the objectives and strategies into reality. Strategies should be selected based on not only currently available resources in the community but also the likelihood that the means will have some long-term availability. During implementation, lay leaders in the communities, professionals, and organizations must be included and their support acquired. In the long run, it is always better to educate others on how to implement these strategies than for the nurse and other team members to control the implementation (Barton, Smith, Brown, & Supples, 1993). The tendency toward paternalism is strong among health professionals and for many has been reinforced through acute care organizational structures and roles; one must safeguard against the problems of paternalism. In the implementation phase, those community leaders who have greatest probability of achieving success—those whom the community respects and looks to for guidance—are identified. In general, a pilot test should be planned if possible as a trial run of the implementation. In this way, using a few individuals from target groups for feedback, delivery, and design issues may be discovered before the major investments of time, energy, and resources (Clark, 1996). Pilot studies often reveal that more training is needed, along with more or different types of resources and more time. Minor flaws can be corrected; feedback can be collected from the pilot participants with ideas about how the implementation might be changed or improved; and fine-tuning can increase likelihood for success in the implementation (Schuster & Goeppinger,

1996). Box 2-8 and the following two Note This! boxes all provide examples of community-focused interventions implemented through a **collaborative arrangement** between health professionals and community leaders.

Role of the Community Health Nurse

The roles of the community health nurse (CHN) and other professionals depend on the nature of the health problem, the community's ability to make decisions, and professional and personal values and preferences. Also important is the history of the community's ability to solve its own problems. The nurse will play a different role in an established population where there is a history of successful health problem management, as opposed to one that is poorly organized and loosely connected to each other or that has vague community identity. In one case the nurse may serve only as advisor, whereas in another, the nurse must work with the community first to teach the community how to solve problems (Richards et al., 2002).

NOTE THIS!

Alaskans Race to Vaccinate: Children as a Population at Risk—A Community-Focused Intervention Implemented Through Collaboration Between Health Professionals and Target Population

A population assessment revealed that only 52.7% of the young children in Alaska were fully immunized. Through collaboration with several groups, including the University of Alaska Anchorage School of Nursing, the Iditarod Trail Committee, and the Indian Health Service, the Alaska Nurses Association established the I Did It By Two! Race to Vaccinate as a health project analogous to the Iditarod Sled Dog Race. The original Iditarod, in 1925, was an appropriate focus event because that relay, in which mushers and dogs carried antitoxin across 700 miles of Alaskan wilderness, halted a diphtheria epidemic. Alaska's "checkpoints" are 2, 4, and 6 months of age. The best possible "finishing time" is 12 to 15 months. Any child who reaches the long-distance goal by age 2 years wins an Iditarod certificate autographed by a musher. The Iditarod is the most famous sled dog race in the world, and the mushers who drive the sleds are influential spokespersons. The geographic outreach to connect with the target population was extensive, because the Iditarod Race runs from Anchorage to Nome, covering more than 1,049 miles. The immunization project has become the largest in the nation in conjunction with a sporting event. Outcome evaluation revealed first and second year immunization rates improved to more than 80% in targeted areas.

The Vaccinate Alaska Coalition (VAC), which cosponsors the Race to Vaccinate campaign, along with the Alaska State Health Department, received national recognition for their efforts to promote and provide immunization to people of all ages. Vaccinate Alaska Coalition (VAC) was a recipient of a 2003 Excellence in Immunization Award from the National Partnership for Immunization (NPI) in recognition of its sponsorship of the I Did It By Two! campaign and the Race to Vaccinate Campaign with the Iditarod Trail Sled Dog Race, which heightens public awareness of the critical need for timely immunization of children from birth through 2 years of age. For the campaign, children pass immunization "checkpoints" in order to cross the finish line and are declared "Winners in the Race to Vaccinate," just as mushers must pass checkpoints in the actual race. Since its inception, the Race to Vaccinate and the I Did It By Two! campaign participate in the Iditarod race by providing sled dogs and their mushers with race bibs, which display the Race to Vaccinate slogan. Four-time Iditarod champion Martin Buser and mushers Jon Little and Paul Gebhardt speak throughout Alaska about the crucial role of immunizations in lifelong good health.

Carolyn Keil, PhD, RN
Associate Professor, University of Alaska Anchorage
Project Director, Race to Vaccinate, 1992–1996

Sources: Adapted from Alaskans Race to Vaccinate. (1996). *Reflections* (4th Quarter); Roberts, K. (2003). Going the Distance: An itinerant nurse takes health care to the corners of Alaska. *American Journal of Nursing, 103*(12), 102–103; Alaska Department of Health and Social Services. (2005). *Strategic plan 2005–2007.* Juneau, AK: Division of Public Health.

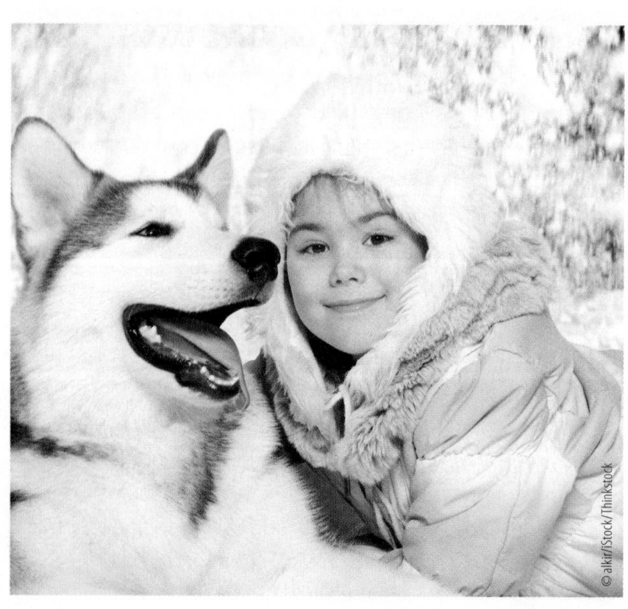

NOTE THIS!

Carter Center's Interfaith Health Program: Faith Population as Target Community, a Community-Focused Intervention Implemented Through a Collaborative Arrangement Between Health Professionals and Community Leaders

President Jimmy Carter and the Carter Center in Atlanta, Georgia, along with leaders from the Atlanta Interfaith Health Program, have developed a highly successful collaborative project to help faith communities nationwide prevent disease and promote wellness in their congregations. Through this program, Starting Point, religious groups and health professionals work together to identify risk factors, such as economics or age, and link resources to the church congregations. Dr. Fran Wenger of the Emory School of Nursing in Atlanta is one of the original organizers of this program and is responsible for training lay church leaders in identification of risk and the development of interventions. Religious groups across the country are building an impressive network of leaders, scholars, and community activists who share a common goal: to help people through their churches and religious groups lead more healthful lives. This effort uses a step-by-step training program in which lay volunteers in the church are prepared to be "health promoters." These volunteers then help identify group needs and then work to find appropriate resources, such as the American Cancer Society or the local Red Cross, to meet them. Jimmy Carter sums up the program in this way: "The key to empowering any community, be it religious or otherwise, is team work and a strong spirit of collaboration."

Source: Starting Point: Empowering Communities to Improve Health. A Manual for Training Health Promoters in Congregational Coalitions. Interfaith Health Program. (1997). Atlanta: The Carter Center.

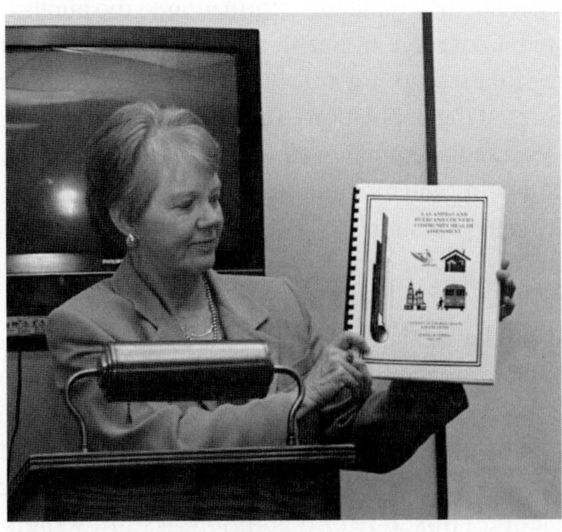

A community assessment report should be shared with target community. Dr. Judith Barton shares County Health Assessment with residents in rural Colorado.

Social Change and Community Action

The age-old question of how to "teach an old dog new tricks" leads us inevitably to the process of change. There are two types of change: unplanned or spontaneous change and planned change. There is considerable debate about the ultimate benefits of unplanned change, but the CHN is most interested in planned and directed change. Such community changes imply that the activities of the CHN are directed toward some goal or goals set in the planning stage of the nursing process (Richards et al., 2002). Intervention activities based on the concepts of planned change center on conscious, deliberate, and intentional actions directed toward **healthy change** in the community (Chin & Benne, 1989). Several forces influence the process of creating meaningful change.

The CHN intervenes in changing attitudes, values, knowledge, and skills of the community or population. Kurt Lewin (1951), in his force field theory, postulated that there are always two types of forces that affect the likelihood of change in any situation: driving forces and restraining forces. These two types of forces work in opposition to each other, and Lewin theorized that it is the relative strength of each force that determines whether change will occur. Force field theory postulates that when driving forces are stronger than restraining forces, change occurs.

Driving forces are those influences that favor change. Restraining forces, by contrast, impede change. For example, a group of restless teens, frustrated with the lack of unorganized recreational settings, may be a driving force that motivates a community to establish safe socialization sites for teens to gather. However, the same teen population might feel threatened by adults making the decisions about how these safe socialization sites operate and would, therefore, serve as a restraining force operating against change.

The role of the CHN in promoting healthy change involves manipulating the driving and restraining forces in ways that increase the likelihood of positive changes in the population. This occurs by increasing the driving forces while minimizing the restraining forces. The nurse in the change agent role can promote these changes through an understanding of the process. An underlying assumption of this process is that the community or population must participate in the planning of change (Tembreull & Schaffer, 2005). Some resistance to change can be assumed in most situations. To counter this resistance, the nurse engages the population members in planning the change. Such participation can result in decreased resistance to that change (Lippitt, Langseth, & Mossop, 1985).

Lay Advisors

Community members who hold more status and prestige in the community and are looked to by community members as the "movers and shakers" are the lay advisors who can make or break community intervention. By promoting new ideas and representing positive change, lay advisors provide the connection to the community while often displaying natural leadership abilities that can be encouraged and reinforced by the community health nurse (McKinley, 1973).

THINK ABOUT THIS 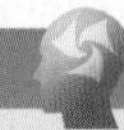

The virtual community assessment . . . try a community assessment board game!

Dr. Kathleen Masters has developed a board game based on the Lundy–Barton General Systems Tool for Community Assessment; it enables students to apply knowledge and practice skills necessary for performing a community assessment. Students are divided into teams who answer questions about their community by moving along spaces in "cars" through drawing "data" cards. Data include observations related to environment, demographic data, interviews with community residents, and observations of resident behavior. To advance, team members must answer correctly, move to interventions, and eventually reach the evaluation spaces on the board. Teams vote on correct diagnoses based on subjective and objective data presented.

This game helps students learn how to use the community assessment process in a fun way for a trial run before getting out in the real world!

Source: Masters, K. (2005). Development and use of an educator-developed community assessment board game. *Nurse Educator, 30*(5), 189–190.

Focus Groups

Small groups in the community are often the selected mechanism by which change is introduced and sustained. Existing community groups or new groups formed specifically around the community objectives are often successful in implementing healthy change. These groups link the individual to the community. Through formal groups such as church-related organizations or special interest groups, such as the Parent–Teacher Organization, nurses can provide the leadership both in initiating healthy change and promoting the group's efforts toward autonomy and self-care.

Policy and Legislation

To effect change at the governmental level, collective needs must be translated into a grassroots power base of influence. Nurses are often unfamiliar with this level of intervention and often need to build coalitions with other influential professional and organizational constituents to effect change. *Policy* refers to the principles and values that govern actions directed toward given ends; policy statements set forth a plan, direction, or goal for action. Because politics is often about scarce resources, the CHN involved in policy changes—whether at the local, state, national, or global level—effects healthy change in communities by influencing the distribution of resources, the amount of resources allocated, and the recipients of the allocated resources, that is, the target community (Chitty, 1997). Although different from politics, policy is shaped by politics (Mason, Talbott, & Leavitt, 1993).

Through the assessment process, the CHN identifies, along with the community or population, health needs or problems. Depending on the nature of the problem, the CHN can use his or her knowledge of the political process to influence the policy process, such as by drafting legislation, providing formal testimony as an advocate for the community, or lobbying governmental officials to make certain that those health issues are a priority for action. All activities are done with the community, by serving as both advocate and educator for the population in efforts to meet those identified goals (Chitty, 1997; Wallerstein, Duran, Minkler, & Foley, 2005).

Mass Media

The most common use of the mass media to promote healthy change in communities has been to communicate specific health information to larger audiences. Using a combination of media forms (e.g., television; radio; newspapers; newsletters; social networks, such as Twitter, Facebook, and LinkedIn; and magazines) provides a greater possibility for exposure and contact with the population. Some community members prefer oral delivery, contact, and consumption, whereas others are more visual, preferring to read (e.g., newsletters), watch television, or simply notice posters in selected community sites. Many population members might be more easily reached through the Internet. Internet and web-based instant communication, such as Facebook, Twitter, and other social networks/media, continue to be most successful in disseminating information to the public.

Media coverage of health issues and events can be a successful strategy for informing and motivating large numbers of the population (**Box 2-9**). A well-constructed, focused media campaign can be an excellent means for disseminating and modifying values about health. Such activities can be as simple as a well-timed letter to the editor, which can provide an excellent forum for airing of health concerns and eliciting feedback from the community. Securing the local newspaper's editorial support can be a major factor in soliciting legislators' and other policymakers' attention, particularly with controversial community issues. Press releases should also be considered standard fare for most community projects that serve a targeted population (**Box 2-10**). In addition, feature writers for local and state newspapers are always looking for stories of interest. Novel approaches to community programs, even the community or population assessment itself, should be

BOX 2-9 Steps in Using the Media for a Health Policy Intervention

1. Designate one member of the community team who has experience with media relations as spokesperson.
2. Identify health issues from goals that would be appropriately advanced in the media.
3. Work in conjunction with professional organizations and specialty groups to develop a media strategy.
4. Build coalitions with consumer groups and lay leaders in the community.
5. Go public through newspapers, television, radio spots, online social networks, and websites.
6. Evaluate effectiveness through community response: letters to the editor, phone calls, chat groups on the Internet, and online social networks, such as Facebook.

of interest to readers, particularly when the newspaper has a large readership. Other media tools include television and radio talk programs, beginning with local television stations and expanding to the networks. The coverage of community health issues not only helps inform the population about health issues but also is an excellent way of promoting positive, accurate public images of nursing in a health promotion role. Publicizing these nursing roles, goals, concerns, and accomplishments in the policy arena will serve to increase the likelihood of public support for nurse-initiated policy recommendations (Hanley, 1984).

BOX 2-10 Sample Press Release

For immediate release. October is Breast Cancer Awareness month. The focus on breast cancer targets all age groups of women and their partners in an effort to educate the public about the importance of early detection and treatment of breast cancer. The American Cancer Society sponsors the national campaign, and local health organizations, schools of nursing, and voluntary health groups working with the American Cancer Society provide speakers, materials, promotional media messages, and community-focused events. The Breast Cancer Awareness Committee of the greater Hattiesburg, Mississippi, area is a group of representatives from healthcare agencies, voluntary agencies, schools of nursing, and healthcare consumers who develop various projects in the community to enhance the public's awareness about breast cancer survival in the Pine Belt. BSN and RN students from the University of Southern Mississippi College of Nursing are involved in this collaborative effort as part of their community health educational experiences in their senior course, community health nursing. They have developed activities and projects that raise awareness on the college campus about the importance of breast self-examination (BSE). The students learn about the use of the media in community health education. Activities include sorority and fraternity presentations, newspaper press releases, television interviews, a website development focusing on men and breast cancer, and information booths at the student center and post office throughout the month of October.

Contact Persons:

Breast Cancer Awareness Team, Chairperson, Karen S. Lundy

Media Advocacy

Media advocacy is the strategic use of the mass media to advance healthy public policy by applying pressure to legislators and other policymakers (Wallack, Dorfman, & Woodruff, 1997). By focusing the attention of those who have the power to change policy, the media become a powerful tool for drawing attention to the actions of a specific group (e.g., the town council, a governing body, or a planning commission). This can also occur when the news story alerts people in the target population to an issue or an action and mobilizes community and population support. The goal in media advocacy is to have the news story told from a public health perspective. This means emphasizing the public policy dimensions of prevention and shifting the focus away from the individual health behavior to the cultural, social, economic, and political context of health issues. When the health issue is visible to large numbers of people, the issue becomes part of the public agenda. Thus, once a health issue is on the public agenda, media advocacy helps advance the goals of community policy by directing public attention to the actions of those responsible for enacting or opposing the policy. For example, one of the problems in the lack of initiatives concerning the acquired immune deficiency syndrome (AIDS) epidemic was the lack of media attention. The issue did not immediately make it to the national policy agenda as a result of complicated influences, primarily because the population initially at perceived risk was the male homosexual community, which had little success accessing the media. Without public attention on an issue or an event, the broader community remains in the dark, along with those who have the power to make the desired change (Wallack et al., 1997). According to Daniel Schorr, National Public Radio (now simply NPR) commentator, "If you don't exist in the media, for all practical purposes, you don't exist" (Communications Consortium Media Center, 1991, p. 7). By using the media to promote healthy change, Flynn (1998) advocates that nurses continue to think "upstream" and focus on fairness and equity in targeting those populations at risk.

Education

Educational strategies are perhaps the most common strategies used by CHNs in promoting health and preventing illness in individuals and communities. Educating the target population about available knowledge and community resources is common (Syme, 2004). The purpose of educating the target population about health issues and possible solutions is ultimately to create greater self-sufficiency and a community that is better prepared to make appropriate health-related decisions in the future (Magee, 2005). These include decisions about personal health behaviors, decisions about the use of available health resources, and decisions about societal health issues (Clark, 1996). Education strategies take many forms, including formal presentations, printed materials, community billboards, and other forms throughout the media and via the Internet. When current information and research are provided about health issues, people can become more involved in their own self-care and make informed decisions regarding personal behaviors that promote health; for example, should ear protection be used by persons in a rifle club, or should teens be held to a higher standard regarding alcohol use and driving automobiles? Health education can be viewed as a means of freeing people in populations from influences that lead them to unhealthy behaviors. Education is much more than merely imparting knowledge and skills; it includes helping people change their attitudes to those more conducive to healthful behavior. Teaching people to use resources—so that they learn not only what is available in the community but how to apply that knowledge in promoting healthy change—is an even more empowering strategy (Greenberg, 1989).

On a more global level, populations can be educated about decisions related to social health issues, such as AIDS or teen suicide risks. For example, educating the target population can assist people in determining whether they support legislation that requires motorcyclists to wear helmets or that bans smoking in public buildings. An informed population is better able to make decisions about major health issues that affect their lives (Clark, 1996).

ART CONNECTION 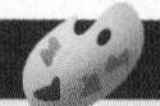

Explore the early paintings of Florence Nightingale, especially of those where she is working in the Crimean War. Do an environmental assessment of the painting, citing safety issues and health needs.

Evaluation Phase

To evaluate the effectiveness of implementations, the nurse evaluates the responses of the community to the interventions, the progress that has been made in affecting outcome measures (e.g., statistical changes), and how well the efforts have fared in comparison to the goals and objectives. Evaluation data are collected in various formats and should come from diverse viewpoints, both from the target population and from the team members (Anderson & McFarlane, 2003). Because the nursing process is cyclical instead of linear, evaluation as the final step in the process ultimately affects the next assessment. In community health interventions, there rarely is a true end point, but rather there is a dynamic interplay of the steps in a process. The effectiveness of community nursing interventions depends on continuous reassessment of the community's health and on appropriate revisions in the planning interventions. Essentially, evaluation boils down to this: What has been the intervention's impact on the health of the target population or community? Because the community is so complex and so many variables affect the outcome of health measures, it is often difficult to measure all the variables, including the interventions, that shaped the outcomes (Duiveman & Bonner, 2012). The nurse must be cautious about attributing changes to the interventions, or denying influence because of lack of concrete evidence that changes occurred. Was it worth the time and effort and resources? What would or could be done differently in the future? Equally important, the community must have an opportunity to shape the evaluation conclusions. Before a final analysis and evaluation report is finished, the team should seek input from the community and population members. Does the community deem the process a success? After all, the perceived results are most important in the final analysis and should be reported in the formal conclusions (Pavlish & Pharris, 2012).

The evaluation process entails both formative evaluation and summative evaluation. *Formative evaluation* measures focus on the process *during* the community interventions (Clark, 1996). For example, perhaps a strategy had been devised in which parents of young children would be offered a safety class on accident prevention at home. This class was initially offered on Saturday mornings. In the first two classes, only a few parents attended. It was discovered that Saturday mornings were often taken up with Little League sports and dancing lessons. The class was rescheduled for a weekday after work and attendance doubled within a week. In contrast, *summative evaluation* refers to the outcomes of the interventions, those measures that include end-of-intervention evaluations. Such measurements as satisfaction surveys, self-reports from parents of changes in their use of safety information in the home, or changes in the number of home accidents reported by the local hospital are all summative evaluation strategies (Benner & Meleis, 1978).

Putting the evaluation into lay terms in the final report to the community is expected of all community assessment team projects. The media (e.g., newsletters, local newspapers, television stations, and the Internet) and churches are appropriate resources for distributing the final report to the community. Whatever the outcome, because of the community assessment process, both the team members and the target population are changed (Magee, 2005). Closure in the form of a final report can have a critical impact on the future of the population's or community's response to health challenges and interventions.

Conclusion

Assessment of communities or populations is a critical nursing skill in the rapidly evolving U.S. healthcare system. The need for nurses to be able to assess communities and populations as the focus of nursing care has always been an integral skill for public health nurses working in official public health agencies. With an increasing focus on keeping participants of healthcare plans healthy, an emphasis on health promotion and prevention brings evidence-based, community-focused interventions to the forefront for professional nursing. In addition, healthcare agencies receiving federal funding to offset expenses incurred for treating the underinsured or noninsured are now required to assess the communities and populations they serve. In other words, there is a new emphasis on prevention rather than illness care pervading the U.S. healthcare system as outcome measures form the basis of reimbursement and service continuations. Preparation in community/population assessment is essential for nurses at the BSN level in all settings to promote the health of their patients.

AFFORDABLE CARE ACT (ACA) 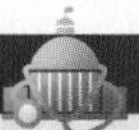

Community and population assessments will become more essential as the ACA extends to the community with greater emphasis on prevention and nonacute care settings.

LEVELS OF PREVENTION 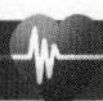

Primary: Conducting a population assessment for a group of healthy middle-aged adults in a church

Secondary: Assisting persons with hypertension with planning their diet and exercise to reduce the risks of their condition

Tertiary: Providing education for persons post-stroke to assist in safe mobility and self-care

Critical Thinking Activities

Population Assessment Guide for Community Health Nursing Students: An Introductory Field Experience for a Local Geopolitical Community

1. Before beginning your community assessment, identify the conceptual framework you would like to use in organizing your community assessment. Remember, a conceptual framework for community assessment will help you in knowing what data to collect, how you should collect the data, and how to interpret the analysis of data for community planning.
2. Go to the local library or to the Internet and access census data for your community before going out to the community so that you have a feel for the social status of your community. Necessary demographic data to collect include the following:
   - Total population for catchment area
   - Racial composition (%) for catchment area
   - Ethnic composition (%) for catchment area
   - Age distribution (% by category) for catchment area
   - Educational attainment (% by category) in catchment area
   - Percentage of all persons living below poverty level
   - Percentage of children younger than age of 5 years living below poverty level
   - Percentage of persons 65 years and older living below poverty level
   - Percentage of females 16 years and older who have children younger than 6 years of age and who work outside the home

Use census data to compare to your catchment area.

3. Meet with a key informant at the designated time. Ask the key informant to tell you what he or she knows about the immediate community in which the health center is located. What kind of people live in the community? What are some of the community's health issues (views of health are broad, including economic, political, cultural, education issues)? What does the key informant see as a primary strength of the community?

Ask your key informant about specific gathering places within the community where you might talk to community members, such as fire stations, housing offices, recreation centers, and so on.

Ask your key informant if it would be okay if you talked to a few of the patients waiting in the clinic area. Explain that you will introduce yourself as a student nurse who is conducting a community health needs assessment and you will then ask the waiting patients to just describe what it is like to live in this community.

4. Spend a little time in the clinic setting meeting some of the patients in the waiting rooms. Many of the clerks working in these clinics live in the neighborhood, and they may also be willing to talk to you. Be brave! Find out all you can about what it is like to live in the community. What is a strength of the community? What is a need? How has the community changed across time (history)? What is currently happening in the community? These are general "round the world" questions that can open up a full discussion. Write down the questions mentioned in this guide on an index card. When in doubt as to what to say next, just ask the person to more fully describe what they are talking about. For example, if the person is talking about gang crimes in the neighborhood, you can ask, "Can you tell me some more about this problem with gangs?"
5. Gather outside the clinic and take a windshield survey of your community (census tract boundaries). Pay attention to environmental characteristics such as range of housing, industry, recreation facilities, and so on.
6. Spend some time talking to members of the community who are located outside the clinic area. For example, you may venture into the recreation center and talk to a few people. Venture into a daycare center and ask to talk to the workers, children, and parents. Ask again about what it is like to live in the neighborhood.
7. Review any secondary data (e.g., health status reports) you were able to obtain from your key informant or others in the community.
8. Meet for lunch or an afternoon snack to analyze the findings from the secondary and primary sources. As a group, brainstorm about strengths and needs of the community assembled from observations, interviews, census data, and any previous reports you have been able to obtain. Develop two to three community diagnoses. Decide on an outline for a written report on your community assessment, and write a report on your community assessment as a group or divide up the outline for section writing.
9. Do an oral presentation of your community assessment. Share your findings with the "target" community and with your classmates.

Source: Adapted from Barton, J. (1997). "Undergraduate Mini Community Health Assessment." University of Colorado School of Nursing Health Sciences Center.

References

Aiken, L. H., & Salmon, M. E. (1994). Health care workforce priorities: What nursing should do now. *Inquiry, 31*, 318.

American Association of Colleges of Nursing (AACN). (2008). *The essentials of baccalaureate education for professional nursing practice*. Washington, DC: Author.

American Nurses Association (ANA). (2010). *Nursing: Scope and standards of practice* (2nd ed.). Silver Spring, MD: Author.

Anderson, E. T., & McFarlane, J. (2003). *Community as partner: Theory and practice in nursing* (4th ed.). Philadelphia, PA: Lippincott.

Association of Community Health Nursing Educators (ACHNE). (2009). *Essentials of baccalaureate nursing education for entry level community/public health nursing*. Wheat Ridge, CO: Author.

Baldwin, J. H., Conger, C. O., Abegglen, J. C., & Hill, E. M. (1998). Population-focused and community-based nursing—moving toward clarification of concepts. *Public Health Nursing, 15*(1), 12–18.

Barton, J. A., Smith, M., Brown, N. J., & Supples, J. M. (1993). Methodological issues in a team approach to community health needs assessment. *Nursing Outlook, 41*(6), 252–261.

Basch, C. (1987). Focus group interview: An underutilized research technique for improving theory and practice in health education. *Health Education Quarterly, 14*(Winter), 411–448.

Benner, P., & Meleis, A. (1978). Process or product evaluation? *Nursing Outlook, 23*, 302–307.

Carney, J. K. (2006). *Public health in action: Practicing in the real world*. Sudbury, MA: Jones and Bartlett.

Cassel, J. (1976). The contribution of the social environment to host resistance. *American Journal of Epidemiology, 104*(2), 107.

Chin, R., & Benne, K. D. (1989). General strategies for effecting changes in human systems. In W. L. French, C. H. Bell, & R. A. Zawacki (Eds.), *Organization development: Theory, practice and Research* (pp. 89–95). Homewood, IL: BPI Irwin.

Chitty, K. (1997). *Professional nursing: Concepts and challenges* (2nd ed.). Philadelphia, PA: Saunders.

Clark, M. J. (1996). *Nursing in the community* (2nd ed.). Stamford, CT: Appleton & Lange.

Clark, M. J., Cary, S., Diemart, G., Ceballos, R., Sifuentes, M., Atteberry, I., . . . Trieu, S. (2003). Involving communities in community assessment. *Public Health Nursing, 20*(6), 456–463.

Communications Consortium Media Center. (1991). *Strategic communication for non-profits: Strategic media—Designing a public interest campaign* (p. 7). Washington, DC: Benton Foundation and the Center for Strategic Communications.

Community Health Advisor Network. (1999). *Community facilitator implementation manual.* Jackson, MS: Freedom from Hunger.

Cottrell, L. S. (1976). The competent community. In B. H. Kaplan, R. N. Wilson, & A. H. Leighton (Eds.), *Further explorations in social psychology*. New York, NY: Basic Books.

Duiveman, T., & Bonner, A. (2012). Negotiating: Experiences of community nurses when contracting with clients. *Contemporary Nurse: A Journal for the Australian Nursing Profession, 41*(1), 120–125.

Eide, P. J., Hahn, L., Bayne, T., Allen, C. B., & Swain, D. (2006). The population-focused analysis project for teaching community health. *Nursing Education Perspectives, 27*(1), 22–27.

Eisen, A. (1994). Survey of neighborhood-based, comprehensive community empowerment initiatives. *Health Education Quarterly, 21*(2), 235–252.

Flynn, B. C. (1994). Partners for healthy cities. *Healthcare Forum Journal, 37*(3), 55–56.

Flynn, B. C. (1998). Communicating with the public: Community-based nursing research and practice. *Public Health Nursing, 15*(3), 165–170.

Flynn, B. C., & Dennis, L. I. (1996). Health promotion through healthy cities. In M. Stanhope & J. Lancaster (Eds.), *Community health nursing: Promoting health of aggregates, families and individuals*. St. Louis, MO: Mosby.

Flynn, B. C, Ray, D., & Rider, M. (1994). Empowering communities: Action research through healthy cities. *Health Education Quarterly, 21*(3), 395–405.

Gebbie, K. M. (1996, November 18). *Preparing currently employed public health nurses for changes in the health care system: Meeting report and suggested action steps*. New York, NY: Columbia University School of Nursing Center for Health Policy and Health Sciences Research. (Report based on meeting in Atlanta, July 11, 1996.)

Glick, D. F., Hale, P. J., Kulbok, P. A., & Shettig, J. (1996). Community development theory: Planning a community nursing center. *Journal of Nursing Administration, 26*(7/8), 44–50.

Goeppinger, J. (1984). Primary health care: An answer to the dilemmas of community health nursing? *Public Health Nursing, 3*, 129–140.

Goeppinger, J., & Baglioni, A. J. (1986). Community competence: A positive approach to needs assessment. *American Journal of Community Psychology, 13*, 507.

Goeppinger, J., Lassiter, P. G., & Wilcox, B. (1982). Community health is community competence. *Nursing Outlook, 30*(8), 464.

Goeppinger, J., & Schuster, G. (1988). Community as patient: Using the nursing process to promote health. In M. Stanhope & J. Lancaster (Eds.), *Community health nursing: Process and practice for promoting health*. St. Louis, MO: Mosby.

Goodman, R. M., Speers, M. A., McLeroy, K., Fawcett, S., Kegler, M., Parker, E., . . . Wallerstein, N. (1998). Identifying and defining the dimensions of community capacity to provide a basis for measurement. *Health Education Behavior, 2*(33), 258–278.

Gordon, L. J. (1990). Who will manage the environment? *American Journal of Public Health, 80*, 904–905.

Gordon, L. J. (1993). The future of environmental health and the need for public health leadership. *Journal of Environmental Health, 56*(5), 38–40.

Greenberg, J. S. (1989). *Health education: Learner-centered instructional strategies*. Dubuque, IA: W. C. Brown.

Hamilton, P. (1983). Community health diagnosis. *Advances in Nursing Science, 5*(3), 21–36.

Hancock, T. (1993). The evolution, impact and significance of the Healthy Cities/Healthy Communities movement. *Journal of Public Health Policy, 14*(1), 5–18.

Hanley, B. (1984). Legislation and policy. In J. A. Sullivan, *Directions in community health nursing*. Boston, MA: Blackwell.

Hegyvary, S. T. (1990). Education: Redefining community. *Journal of Professional Nursing, 6*(1), 7.

Higgs, Z. R., & Gustafson, D. D. (1985). *Community as patient: Assessment and diagnosis*. Philadelphia, PA: F. A. Davis.

Kauffman, K. S. (1994). The insider/outsider dilemma: Field experience of a white researcher "getting in" a poor black community. *Nursing Research, 43*(3), 179–183.

Keck, C. W. (1994). Community health: Our common challenge. *Family and Community Health, 17*(2), 1–9.

Keller, L. O., Strohschein, S., Lia-Hoagberg, B., & Schaffer, M. (1998). Population-based public health nursing interventions: A model from practice. *Public Health Nursing, 15*(3), 207–215.

Keller, L. O., Strohschein, S., Lia-Hoagberg, B., & Schaffer, M. A. (2004). Population-based public health interventions: Practice-based and evidence-supported (Part I). *Public Health Nursing, 21*(5), 453–468.

Keller, L. O., Strohschein, S., Schaffer, M. A., & Lia-Hoagberg, B. (2004). Population-based public health interventions: Innovations in practice, teaching, and management (Part II). *Public Health Nursing, 21*(5), 469–487.

Kopf, E. W. (1986). Florence Nightingale as statistician. In B. W. Spradley (Ed.), *Readings in community health nursing*. Boston, MA: Little, Brown.

Lalonde, M. (1974). *A new perspective on the health of Canadians—a working document*. Ottawa, Canada: Government of Canada.

Leininger, M. M. (1988). Leininger's theory of nursing: Cultural care diversity and universality. *Nursing Science Quarterly, 1*(4), 152–160.

Lewin, K. (1951). *Field theory in social science*. New York, NY: Harper.

Lia-Hoagberg, B., Schaffer, M., & Strohschein, S. (1999). Public health nursing practice guidelines: An evaluation of dissemination and use. *Public Health Nursing, 16*(6), 397–404.

Lippitt, G. L., Langseth, P., & Mossop, J. (1985). *Implementing organizational change*. San Francisco, CA: Jossey-Bass.

Lundy, K. S., & Barton, J. A. (1995). Assessment: Data collection of the community patient. In P. J. Christiansen & J. W. Kenney (Eds.), *Nursing process: Application of conceptual models* (4th ed.). St. Louis, MO: Mosby.

Magee, C. G. (2005). Public health consequences of imprisonment: Preventive care for women in prison: A qualitative community health assessment of the Papanicolaou test and follow-up treatment at a California state women's prison. *American Journal of Public Health, 95*, 10.

Mason, D., Talbott, S., & Leavitt, J. (Eds.). (1993). *Policy and politics for nurses: Action and change in the workplace, government, organization and community* (2nd ed.). Philadelphia, PA: Saunders.

McKinley, J. B. (1973). Social networks, lay consultation, and help-seeking behavior. *Social Forces, 53*(1), 275.

Mead, G. H. (1934). *Mind, self, and society*. Chicago, IL: University of Chicago Press.

Montero, L. A. (1985). Florence Nightingale on public health nursing. *American Journal of Public Health, 75*(2), 181.

Muecke, M. A. (1984). Community health diagnosis in nursing. *Public Health Nursing, 1*(1), 23–35.

Nash, D. B., Reifsnyder, J., Fabius, R. J., & Pracillio, V. P. (2011). *Population health: Creating a culture of wellness*. Sudbury, MA: Jones & Bartlett Learning.

Neuman, B. (1989). *The Neuman systems model: Application to nursing theory and practice*. Norwalk, CT: Appleton-Century-Crofts.

Pavlish, C. P., & Pharris, M. D. (2012). *Community-based collaborative action research: A nursing approach*. Burlington, MA: Jones & Bartlett Learning.

Reinhart, U. W. (1984). Rationing the health-care surplus: An American tragedy. *Nursing Economics, 1*(4), 210.

Richards, L., Kennedy, P. H., Krulewitch, C. J., Wingrove, B., Katz, K., Wesley, B., . . . Herman, A. (2002). Achieving success in poor urban minority community-based research: Strategies for implementing community-based research within an urban minority population. *Health Promotion Practice, 3*(3), 410–420.

Robinson, R. G. (2005). Community development model for public health applications: Overview of a model to eliminate population disparities. *Health Promotion Practice, 6*(3), 338–346.

Rodgers, S. (1984). Community as patient—a multivariate model for analysis of community and aggregate health risk. *Public Health Nursing, 1*(4), 210.

Ruth, J., Eliason, K., & Schultz, P. R. (1992). Community assessment: A process of learning. *Journal of Nursing Education, 31*(4), 181.

Salmon, M. E. (1993). Public health nursing—the opportunity of a century. *American Journal of Public Health, 83*, 1674–1675.

Schuster, G., & Goeppinger, J. (1996). Community as client: Using the nursing process to promote health. In M. Stanhope & J. Lancaster, *Community health nursing: Promoting health of aggregates, families and communities* (pp. 289–314). St. Louis, MO: Mosby.

Smith, M. C., & Barton, J. A. (1992). Technologic enrichment of a community needs assessment. *Nursing Outlook, 40*(1), 32–37.

Syme, S. L. (2004). Social determinants of health: The community as an empowered partner. *Preventing Chronic Disease*. Retrieved from http://www.cdc.gov/pcd/issues/2004/jan/03_0001.htm

Tembreull, C. L., & Schaffer, M. A. (2005). The intervention of outreach: Best practices. *Public Health Nursing, 22*(4), 347–353.

Von Bertalanffy, L. (1968). *General systems theory*. New York, NY: George Braziller.

Wallack, L., Dorfman, L., & Woodruff, K. (1997). Communications and public health. In F. D. Scutchfield & C. W. Keck (Eds.), *Principles of public health practice*. Albany, NY: Delmar.

Wallerstein, N., & Bernstein, E. (1994). Introduction to community empowerment, participatory education, and health. *Health Education Quarterly, 21*(2), 141–148.

Wallerstein, N., Duran, B., Minkler, M., & Foley, K. (2005). Developing and maintaining partnerships with communities. In B. A. Israel, E. Eng, A. J. Schulz, & E. A. Parker (Eds.), *Methods in community-based participatory research for health* (pp. 31–51). San Francisco, CA: Jossey-Bass.

Watson, N. M. (1984). Community as patient. In J. A. Sullivan (Ed.), *Directions in community health nursing*. Boston, MA: Blackwell.

Wax, R. H. (1986). Gender and age in fieldwork and field work education: "Not any good thing is done by one man alone." In T. L. Whitehead & M. E. Conaway (Eds.), *Self, sex and gender in cross-cultural fieldwork*. Urbana, IL: University of Illinois Press.

Williams, C. A., & Highriter, M. E. (1978). Community health nursing: Population focus and evaluation. *Public Health Reviews, 7*(2–4), 197.

World Health Organization (WHO). (1985). *Handbook of resolutions and decisions by the World Health Assembly and the Executive Board, 1972–1984* (Vol. 2[31], 42). Geneva, Switzerland: World Health Assembly.

Zandee, G., Bossenbroek, D., Slager, D., & Gordon, B. (2013). Teams of community health workers and nursing students effect health promotion of underserved urban neighborhoods. *Public Health Nursing, 30*(5), 439–447.

Appendix: The Lundy–Barton General Systems Model for Community and Population Assessment and Intervention

The unique responsibility of community health nursing practice is defining problems and proposing solutions at the population level. The process of making this connection from the individual to the community has proven to be an especially difficult task for the nurse conducting a community or population assessment. The community/population health assessment process is based on the understanding of the community as patient. This also includes populations within communities and society. Although nurses wouldn't consider the omission of individual patient assessment and base intervention on intuition, this is almost precisely what happens when we fail to do a thorough assessment when planning and delivering healthcare services to community populations. For example, we would not ever consider just examining the arm of a patient and totally ignoring the rest of the body when we plan nursing interventions. And yet by looking at only one aspect of the community/population, such as the physical parameters, we are just examining the "arm" and ignoring the "body" and "mind" of the community/population. One of the major difficulties in conducting a community/population assessment is that students and practicing nurses alike have often been limited to individualistic patient care. This focus on personal care sometimes presents difficulty in the transference of those skills to assessment and problem solving at the community and population levels.

The Lundy–Barton Model uses familiar systems theory and the nursing process to guide the collection and interpretation of data, development of problems and areas of need, and evaluation of nursing strategies to promote community health. The model includes a database, a needs list, assessment, and a plan to address each need with progress notes delineated for selected problems. Each of these components will be discussed in relation to community/population assessment with concurrent identification of the nursing process components.

Database (Assessment Phase: Nursing Process)

The collection of data corresponds to the assessment phase of the nursing process. The collection of data has one primary goal—to learn about the patient. The exploration of available data about the community can be general or quite specific, depending on the definition of the community or population and on the purpose of the project. An example of how the definition of community can affect the assessment of a community/population can be illustrated by the distinction of the community as a *place* or *nonplace*. A *place* community/population, according to Anderson and Carter (1974), refers to a specific geographic locality, one that can be defined by physical boundaries. This definition is the one most often used in health planning projects for specific urban or rural locales. A *nonplace* community/population is defined as one based on cooperation and commitment by its members to common goals and ideologies. A nonplace community/population is in a sense a "mind" community, such as the academic community, the virtual community of an Internet-based group within social networks (e.g., Facebook groups), or the nursing community. The distinction can also be made on the degree of attachment to a specific locale and the scope of activities, interest, and needs. Place communities have the greatest attachment to a specific locality, whereas nonplace communities usually have limited geographic ties. Nonplace communities generally are narrow in their scope of activities, interests, characteristics, and/or needs, whereas place communities have a wider scope of activities, interests, and needs. Defining the community/population as a place or nonplace will thus affect the direction and method of assessment (Anderson & Carter, 1974).

There are eight categories of data, which are presented in the following section and are considered necessary for the database of a community or population assessment.

Community/Population Profile

What makes the identified community different from any other community/population? The "community patient" is somewhat harder to get to know than the individual patient. Instead of using temperature, pulse, respiration, blood pressure, and so on, the indices of a community/population will take the form of *demographics* and *vital statistics*, such as morbidity/mortality rates, sex, age, ethnic and racial distributions, educational levels, occupation/employment patterns, and socioeconomic patterns. *Mortality rates* are important indices because they provide a picture of the health and living conditions of a community. The *infant mortality rate* is considered perhaps the most sensitive indicator of a community's health status; "such indices require a basic readjustment in thinking. A woman is either pregnant or not pregnant; a community is about 3% pregnant. A patient has or does not have heart disease; the community always has heart disease though the rate may go up or down" (Mattison, 1968).

Demographic data can be found in local and state health departments and on the Internet. U.S. census data are an excellent source for demographic data concerned with population density, population age distribution, occupational distribution, socioeconomic characteristics (income, education, employment), and marital status. Data concerning the kinds of family forms that are prevalent—young families with small children, percentage of women working, and so on—are also available from the U.S. Census Bureau and can provide useful information for the identification of family needs.

Information about how the population is distributed spatially is extremely important in considering the location, distribution, and delivery of health services. Whether a population is densely or sparsely populated has been shown to affect other aspects of people's lives such as norms, values, and types of health problems. Population density can also affect behavior and the emotional health of residents.

Information about the percentage of persons in each age category contributes to the assessment of health needs. Many times, when the age distribution is examined in a historical context, it becomes evident that there has been a population shift over time.

Morbidity and mortality statistics can help provide a statistical picture of the community or population in terms of the incidence and prevalence of specific diseases, health status, and deaths within a community. These statistics can be obtained through local and state health departments and the Centers for Disease Control and Prevention (for specific population groups such as teenagers); from special-interest groups, such as the American Cancer Society or the American Heart Association; or from the various population interest groups, such as women with HIV/AIDS. These data are most often obtained via the Internet.

Comparison of the Profile

Demographics and other statistics *should be compared* with adjoining communities or similar populations, the state, and/or the nation to ascertain the relative significance of the statistics. Not only can these comparisons provide clues as to what kinds of health problems and needs exist in a particular community, but they can also provide an evaluation of the effectiveness of existing health services and programs.

Psychological Climate

Just as an evaluation of an individual patient includes an examination of his or her psychological status, an assessment of the community/population is incomplete without evaluating the psychological aspects. There are three areas: (1) self-concept, (2) attitude toward health, and (3) history and changes over time. How the community/population views itself is usually based on history and traditions from the past. How does one find out what kind of *self-concept* the community or population has? Ask the members! Each community often thinks of itself in terms of descriptors such as "we are a friendly place," or "we just leave each other well enough alone," which can reflect whether the inhabitants see themselves as being connected to adjoining communities or separate from them. Listen to the people talking with one another—are the inhabitants proud of their community/population or are they somewhat distanced and seemingly apathetic? Does the population express powerlessness or worthlessness, such as women who have been abused by parents? Focus groups are an excellent means of listening to the voices of the often "hidden" community/population members: elderly, mothers of small children, people with disabilities, and so on (Clark et al., 2003).

In addition to evaluating the community/population's self-image as an indicator of the psychological climate, it is useful to determine the *community's attitude toward health in general.* Is health care a priority in the community/population? Indicators such as safety and public service media messages (e.g., radio, television, billboards) are evidence of the degree of voluntary efforts for the development of health programs and should aid in the assessment of where health fits into the community/population priority structure. What is the website of the community/population or group like? Is it current? Do members of the community interact with each other—either online on "blogs" or in person? Populations have a wide variety of attitudes and values about health. Teens may have very little interest in health because of their developmental level of self-awareness.

A third area to assess in terms of the psychological database is information concerning the *historical changes that a community/population has experienced* and its response to those changes. Understanding the history of the community or population—how and when it came to be, how it has responded to change (e.g., industrial growth, highway construction, rapid population growth or decline), and how it has dealt with health problems in the past—would all be helpful in planning realistically for health services. A community/population's experiences, its ability to mobilize resources, and dominant patterns of solutions to health problems all significantly affect how that community will respond to intervention. For example, the population of homosexual men has a long history of discrimination in the United States and may exhibit a distrust of the traditional healthcare system as a result. Knowledge about the community/population's past can give perspectives on its present and future. A community/population recovering from a catastrophic natural disaster, such as a major flood, may take years to recover. How a community has responded in the past to a disaster, such as Hurricane Katrina, can provide valuable information about the preparation of the community for any sudden changes or catastrophes.

Nutritional Evaluation

A history and evaluation of the community's nutritional status, as a part of the community/population assessment process, include identification of sources of food (e.g., homegrown, imported into community, processed foods, fast foods), ethnic or regional food prevalence, and food preparation customs (e.g., vegetarian, seafood availability, wild game). Morbidity/mortality statistics related to nutritional status and resources (e.g., goiter, cardiac disease, cancer) are also vital information to include in the nutritional assessment. A population of truck drivers, for example, may have nutritional patterns of consumption related to their erratic pattern of eating on the run.

Physical Fitness

In examining the community/population's "fitness," the presence or absence of exercise/fitness facilities available and/or used by the public, such as jogging and bicycling trails, are most certainly a reflection of its inhabitants' interest in physical fitness. Although most communities do not fall into a clear-cut category of either sedentary or active, one pattern usually tends to dominate and can provide important health status information. As a population, elders tend to be more sedentary than their younger counterparts.

Physical Examination

A physical examination of the community patient involves a hands-on type of approach. This obviously applies only to a geographic community. Shumway and Wisehart (1969) suggest using a walking tour to know a community at the resident level. They advise that getting "a feel for a community" involves a *systematic approach of observations* that can ultimately increase one's sensitivity to the surrounding ecological elements. If the community can be defined as a place community, the *geographic boundaries should be defined* and described as clearly as possible. Parameters can be defined in several ways: census tracts, natural boundaries (e.g., mountains, rivers), or roads and streets, specifically noting terrain, proximity to needed resources, and *isolation/proximity* to other communities. The *climate* has been demonstrated to have a significant effect on the health risks of a population. Whether the climate is desert or mountainous can affect the lives of the inhabitants in dramatic ways. Such factors as road conditions, animal vectors, housing conditions, and general appearances of the community should be noted in the physical assessment of the community.

Review of Systems

Once the "physical examination" has been done, it is important to conduct a review of systems within the community or population. This review should include an assessment of the services and facilities, human power, government (federal, state, county), and leadership (formal and informal) of health and nonhealth systems that affect the population or community.

The *health system* should include all organizations and services that provide health care. The private health services and public health services should be examined not only for availability and quality, but also for the degree of coordination between the services. The availability of homes for the elderly, services for the disabled (including accommodation in the community/population, such as access ramps), mental health services, and disaster preparedness for the community/population are examples of such services to be assessed. As community workers know all too well, it is often not a case of availability of needed services, but rather a lack of coordination within agencies, a lack of awareness of the services by the community members, an unwillingness by the members to use the facilities, or unacceptability of resources or services as a result of cultural differences. The source of health care is another important aspect of this assessment of healthcare systems specific to the community/population. Particularly in rural communities, the local pharmacist may be the primary source for health information and should be included in the assessment. Most members of a population seek health care and advisement on health issues from nonprofessionals daily. These sources should be identified in the assessment.

Nonhealth systems, such as the political system, the economic system, the educational system, and the religious system, should be assessed as critical influences on the health of a community/population. Health care does not exist in a vacuum apart from the other social structures within a community/population; it is influenced by and influences other systems within the community.

The *political system/atmosphere* of a community/population can be assessed through various sources: the local newspaper, community action groups, and/or previous history and political activities. The community/population should be assessed as liberal or conservative.

Klein (1965) identifies three important components of the political system that reflect interaction patterns of a community. This can also be applied to a population. *Authority* within a community often can be identified by the political leaders of a community—both elected, official leaders and nonofficial leaders (e.g., religious leaders). *Power* is often associated with authority but is not by any means limited to it. Power patterns in a community can often be identified by examining how formal decisions are made and who makes or vetoes them. *Prestige* is often based on social status, family class designation, and wealth. These three concepts—authority, power, and prestige—are closely linked.

The *social system* includes the prevalent norms and values as well as the dominant ethnic makeup of the community or population. Values influence norms and are often difficult to determine. Norms and values are intangible, so the community worker has to get a real feel for the group through direct involvement before they become apparent. Customs, specific town laws, and cultural patterns are reflective of that community/population's value system.

Communication patterns, both formal and informal, are an integral component of the social system. Communication as a necessary process by which people exchange information and interact with each other is basic to community living. *Informal* communication tends to occur wherever people collect—post offices, local cafes, recreation centers, barbershops, and so on. These informal relationships may occur online via social media, blogging, or other forms of virtual communication. How information is disseminated can be reflected in community bulletin boards, supermarket notice boards, Internet sources, and the like. Often, asking community/population residents where information is obtained will yield the most accurate information. The beauty shop or local bar might serve as the center for information dissemination. Without an understanding of who the key people and places are in terms of informal communication, meaningful, realistic programs can seldom be created.

Formal communication channels include all forms of media, including newspapers, television, and radio; the Internet via social networks such as Twitter, Facebook, and LinkedIn; and the postal system. These channels of communication can be used very effectively in the dissemination of health information, as well as in the identification of community/population ideas, attitudes, and health knowledge.

Information about *educational systems* includes public and private educational facilities, libraries, special educational services (pregnant teens, handicapped, adult education), and available resources. The *economic system* includes major businesses and industries as well as the census information previously mentioned—median family income, unemployment rates, major occupations, and percentage of families living below the poverty level.

The *religious system* is an important part of the community/population and can have a major influence on the political ideology and social norms and values of a community/population. Major denominations should be identified along with the major religious leaders of a community/population.

Services and community health programs sponsored by religious groups are an integral part of the community's healthcare delivery system.

Problem List (Nursing Diagnosis: Nursing Process)

The problem list corresponds to the nursing diagnosis component of the nursing process. As with individual nursing diagnoses, community/population diagnoses should specifically indicate that (1) *no* problems exist that demand intervention by the nursing discipline or by any other members of the health team or (2) needs exist as stated in terms of community problems that have evolved when basic human needs are either not being met or are being met inadequately.

Nursing diagnoses on the community/population level (as with the individual) use a humanitarian approach when specifying basic human needs. Examples of nursing diagnoses at the community level are as follows:

- Increased number of respiratory diseases related to air pollution
- Increased infant mortality rate related to increased teenage pregnancies
- Lack of neighborhood participation related to apathy

Problem Assessment and Plan Formulation (Planning: Nursing Process)

The integration of the two problem-solving methods of Problem-Oriented Medical Recording (POMR) and the nursing process requires that the nurse reassess each community diagnosis using the SOAP format. During this phase, each problem is individually described and evaluated with an intervention plan formulated for each problem. The specific components of the SOAP format follow:

- **Subjective data:** the community's point of view; how do persons in the community express the problem?
- **Objective data:** a summarization of vital statistics, health statistics, review of systems, environmental realities, and so on related to identified problem
- **Assessment:** an analysis of the identified needs or problem in terms of origination of the problem, overall impact, possible intervention points, and community/population parties that may have an interest in the problem and its solutions
- **Plan:** further diagnostic plans or an initial intervention plan developed for the identified problem in terms of short- and long-term goals/objectives with specific actions to be taken to accomplish each objective; health team members, community/population members, or organizations are designated to carry out specific actions

After each problem has been reassessed using the SOAP format, the problems are then prioritized. A committee of community/population members, experts, and community leaders should be involved in problem prioritization.

Progress Notes (Evaluation: Nursing Diagnosis)

The evaluation of the community/population assessment process should be documented in the form of progress notes. Progress notes are simply an appraisal of the effects of some predetermined plan to accomplish some measurable objective. During this phase of the POMR, new objectives and plans for each problem may be determined.

The Lundy–Barton General Systems Model for Community and Population Assessment and Intervention

I. Database (Assessment Phase)
  A. Definition of community or population
  B. Profile
    1. Demographics (census data)
    2. Morbidity (illness patterns)
    3. Birth rate
    4. Death rates by age
    5. Mortality rate (death rate)
    6. Socioeconomic characteristics
      a. Occupation/employment patterns
      b. Median income
      c. Percentage of families below poverty-level income
  C. Psychological climate
    1. Self-concept
    2. Attitude toward health
    3. Historical changes of community/population over time
  D. Nutritional evaluations
    1. Sources of food
    2. Statistics related to nutritional status
  E. Physical fitness
    1. Facilities
    2. Attitudes of residents
  F. Physical examination (for geographic communities)
    1. Systematic observation of community
    2. Defined parameters/boundaries
    3. Climate
    4. Location, topography, rural/urban
    5. Area in miles
    6. Environmental conditions
      a. General description
      b. Housing, quality and condition
      c. Sanitation, water supply, sewage, and trash disposal
      d. Degree of pollution (air, water)
      e. Presence of vectors
      f. Safety/protection
        (1) Police
        (2) Fire
        (3) Other
      g. Transportation
  G. Review of systems
    1. Health system
      a. Private, public services
        (1) Hospitals
        (2) Long-term care
        (3) Ambulatory service
          (a) Primary care
          (b) Mental health/substance abuse
          (c) Home health
          (d) Public health
      b. Resources for specific health needs (e.g., elderly, teen parents)
      c. Human power—need versus availability, type (health workers)
      d. Other healthcare or related resources
        (1) Occupational health service
        (2) School health
        (3) Voluntary agencies
        (4) Welfare agencies
        (5) Disaster preparedness services, usage and access
        (6) Other
    2. Nonhealth systems
      a. Political system/atmosphere
        (1) Dominant values
        (2) Authority; formal, nonformal leadership
        (3) Current political issues in community/population
      b. Social system
        (1) Prevalent norms
        (2) Cultural patterns/variables
        (3) Dominant values
        (4) Customs
        (5) Recreational/social facilities/activities
      c. Communication patterns
        (1) Informal and formal communication sources (e.g., newspapers, bulletin boards, Internet)
      d. Educational system
        (1) Public, private schools (number, type, student population, availability)
        (2) Values
        (3) Special educational services (e.g., pregnant teens, disabled, adult learners)
        (4) Libraries
      e. Economic system
        (1) Major businesses/industries
        (2) Marketing and shopping facilities
        (3) Leading occupations
        (4) Employment patterns
      f. Religious and belief systems
        (1) Major denominations and faith-based organizations
        (2) Religious and spiritual leadership

II. Problem List (Nursing Diagnosis)
   A. Identification of needs and assets from the assessment
III. Problem Assessment and Plan Formulation (Plan)
   A. Subjective data: community/population's point of view
   B. Objective data: nurse's point of view
   C. Assessment: interpretation of data
   D. Plan
      1. Short-term goals/objectives
      2. Long-term goals/objectives
      3. Specific actions for each objective/goal
   E. Prioritization of nursing diagnoses
IV. Progress Notes (Evaluation)
   A. Specification of any intervention implemented and evaluation of effectiveness
   B. Formulation of new objectives and plan

References

Anderson, R. E., & Carter, I. E. (1974). *Human behavior in the social environment: A social systems approach.* Chicago, IL: Aldine.

Clark, M. J., Cary, S., Diemart, G., Ceballos, R., Sifuentes, M., Atteberry, I., . . . Trieu, S. (2003). Involving communities in community assessment. *Public Health Nursing, 20*(6), 456–463.

Klein, D. C. (1965). Community and mental health: An attempt at a conceptual framework. *Community Health Journal, 1,* 301–308.

Lundy, K. S., & Barton, J. A. (1995). Assessment: Data collection of the community patient. In P. J. Christiansen & J. W. Kenney (Eds.), *Nursing process: Application of conceptual models* (4th ed.). St. Louis, MO: Mosby.

Mattison, B. (1968, June). Community health planning and the health professions. *Journal of Public Health, 58,* 1015–1021.

Shumway, S. M., & Wisehart, D. (1969). How to know a community. *Nursing Outlook, 17,* 63–64.

CHAPTER FOCUS

Classical Era

The Greeks and Health

Roman Era

Middle Ages

- Black Death
- The "Witch Craze" of the Early Middle Ages

The Renaissance

The Emergence of Home Visiting

The Reformation

The Advancement of Science and Health of the Public

The Dark Period of Nursing

Early Organized Health Care in the Americas: A Brave New World

- The Chadwick Report and the Shattuck Report

The Industrial Revolution

John Snow and the Science of Epidemiology

And Then There Was Nightingale . . .

- The Crimean Experience: "I Can Stand Out the War with Any Man"
- Florence Nightingale and Sanitation

Returning Home a Heroine: The Political Reformer

- Nightingale and Military Reforms
- The Nightingale School at St. Thomas: The Birth of Professional Nursing
- Taking Health Care to the Community: Nightingale and Wellness
- Nightingale's Legacy

Early Nursing Education and Organization in the United States

The Evolution of Nursing in the United States: The First Century of Professional Nursing

The Emergence of Community and Public Health Nursing

- Lillian Wald, Public Health Nursing, and Community Activism
- Dorothea Lynde Dix
- Clara Barton
- Birth of the Midwife in the United States
- The Nursing Profession Responds to the Great Depression and World War II
- Early Education and Standardization of Practice of Public Health Nursing
- Challenges of the 1930s
- Progressive Initiatives After the War Years
- Social and Political Influence of the 1960s and 1970s
- Public Health Nursing Services in the 1980s and 1990s

Science and Health Care, 1945–1960: Decades of Change

Years of Revolution, Protest, and the New Order, 1961–2000

Managed Care and Healthcare Reform: First Decades of the 21st Century

The Patient Protection and Affordable Care Act (ACA) of 2010

QUESTIONS TO CONSIDER

After reading this chapter, you will know the answers to the following questions:

1. When did humans first begin thinking about the causes of illness?
2. What were the contributions of the Greeks and Egyptians to our health practices today?
3. What are the origins of public health?
4. Who did the first home visits?
5. What were major health concerns of the Middle Ages?
6. What were Florence Nightingale's contributions to nursing as a profession?
7. What was the Chadwick Report, and why is it significant to community health nursing?
8. What role did William Rathbone play in the evolution of community health nursing?
9. Who is Lillian Wald, and why is she considered a prominent figure in the development of community health nursing in the United States?
10. What led to early standardization of public health nursing practice in the United States?
11. What are the major legislative events, discoveries, and inventions that have improved the health status of populations and communities?
12. What is the Patient Protection and Affordable Care Act of 2010 (ACA, or "Obamacare") and why is this healthcare reform legislation considered one of the most significant federal mandates for public and community health in the history of the United States?

CHAPTER 3

History of Community and Public Health Nursing

Karen Saucier Lundy and
Kaye W. Bender

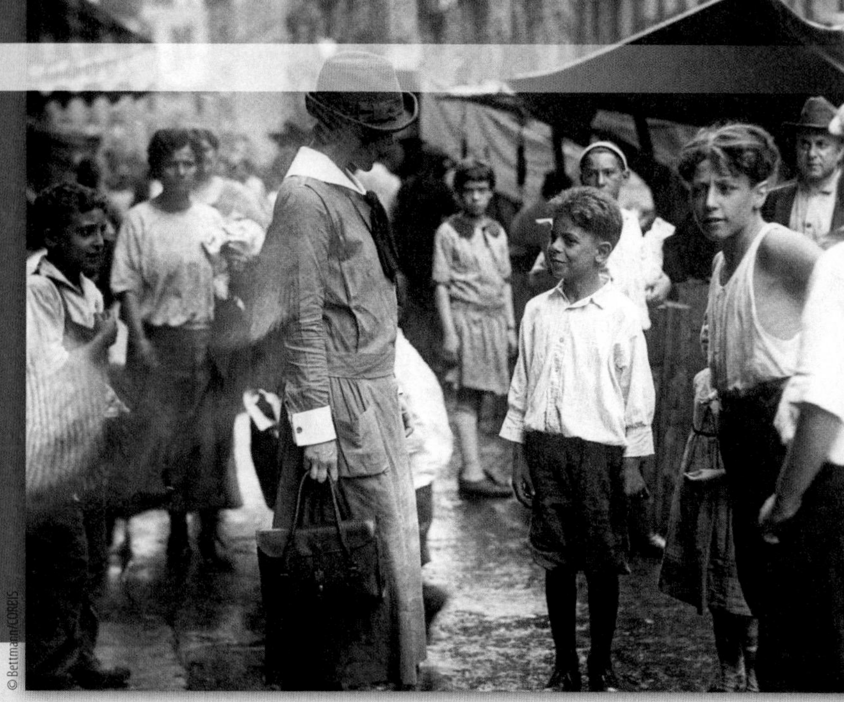

© Bettmann/CORBIS

KEY TERMS

American Journal of Nursing (AJN)
American Nurses Association (ANA)
Clara Barton
Black Death (bubonic plague)
Frances Payne Bolton
Mary Breckenridge
Mary Brewster
Cadet Nurse Corps
case management
deaconesses
Jane A. Delano
Dorothea Lynde Dix
Lavinia Lloyd Dock
Frontier Nursing Service
Goldmark Report
Annie Goodrich
Greek era
health visiting
Henry Street Settlement
Edward Jenner
Kaiserwerth Institute
Edwin Klebs
Robert Koch
Joseph Lister
managed care
Nightingale School of Nursing at St. Thomas
Nursing's Agenda for Health Care Reform
Louis Pasteur
Patient Protection and Affordable Care Act of 2010
William Rathbone
Reformation
Isabel Hampton Robb
Roman era
Margaret Sanger
Jessie Sleet Scales
Saint Vincent de Paul
Elizabeth Tyler
Lillian Wald

REFLECTIONS

What do you know about the history of health care and the role of nursing in health prevention and promotion? How do you define healing and healers as related to human history? How do you think Florence Nightingale would react if she were alive today regarding nursing, healing, and health care?

FOR AS LONG AS HUMANITY has existed, so have the nursing of the sick and community attempts to prevent illness. Health practices of early humans most likely evolved as a way for groups to survive. Many of these early causal links between humans and their environment were attributed to superstition and religion. Evidence from our earliest human ancestors suggests that techniques such as mind–body connections (e.g., voodoo, alchemy, and/or spells), isolation, migratory patterns, and/or societal estrangement of those community members who were defined by the group as sick were used to manage disease and protect the health of the community (Hanlon & Pickett, 1984).

Classical Era

More than 4,000 years ago, Egyptian physicians and nurses used an abundant pharmacological repertoire to cure the ill and injured. The Ebers Papyrus lists more than 700 remedies for ailments from snake bites to puerperal fever. The Kahun Papyrus (circa 1850 B.C.) identified suppositories (e.g., crocodile feces) that could be used for contraception (Kalisch & Kalisch, 1986).

Healing appeared in the Egyptian culture as the successful result of a contest between invisible beings of good and evil (Shryock, 1959). The physician was not a shaman; instead, there was specialization and separation of function, with physicians, priests, and sorcerers all practicing separately and independently. Some patients would consult the physician, some visited the shaman, and others sought healing from magical formulas. Many tried all three approaches. The Egyptians, quite notably, did not accept illness and death as inevitable but rather believed that life could be indefinitely prolonged.

Because Egyptians blended medicine and magic, the concoctions believed to be the most effective were often bizarre and repulsive by today's standards. For example, lizard's blood, swine's ears and teeth, putrid meat and fat, tortoise brains, the milk of a lactating woman, the urine of a chaste woman, and excreta of donkeys and lions were frequently used ingredients. At least some explanation for these odd ingredients can be found in the following:

> These pharmacological mixtures were intended to sicken and drive out the intruding demon, which was thought to cause the disease. Drugs containing fecal matter were in fact used until the end of the eighteenth century in Europe as common practice. (Kalisch & Kalisch, 1986)

As early as 3000 to 1400 B.C., the Minoans created ways to flush water and construct drainage systems. Circa 1000 B.C., the Egyptians constructed elaborate drainage systems, developed pharmaceutical herbs and preparations, and embalmed the dead. The Hebrews formulated an elaborate hygiene code that dealt with laws governing both personal and community hygiene, such as contagion, disinfection, and sanitation through the preparation of food and water. Hebrews, although few in number, exercised great influence in the development of religious and health doctrine. According to Bullough and Bullough (1978), most of their genus was religious, giving birth to both Christianity and Islam. The Jewish contribution to public health is greater in sanitation than in their concept of disease. Garbage and excreta were disposed of outside the city or camp, infectious diseases were quarantined, spitting was outlawed as unhygienic, and bodily cleanliness became a prerequisite for moral purity. Although many of the Hebrew ideas about hygiene were Egyptian in origin, Moses and the Hebrews were the first to codify them and link them with spiritual godliness. Their notion of disease was rooted in the "disease as God's punishment for sin" idea.

The civilization that grew up between the Tigris and Euphrates Rivers is known geographically as Mesopotamia (modem Iraq) and includes the Sumerians. Disease and disability in the Mesopotamian area, at least in the earlier period, was considered a great curse, a divine punishment for grievous acts against the gods. Having such a curse of illness resulting from sin did not exactly put the sick person in a valued status in the society. Experiencing illness as punishment for a sin linked the sick person to anything even remotely deviant: Such things as murder, perjury, adultery, or drunkenness could be the identified sins. Not only was the person suffering from the illness, but he or she was also branded by society as having deserved it. The illness made the sin apparent to all; the sick person was isolated and disgraced. Those who obeyed divine law lived in health and happiness. Those who transgressed the law were punished, with illness and suffering thought to be consequences. The sick person then had to make atonement for the sins, enlist a priest or other spiritual healer to lift the spell or curse, or live with the illness to its ultimate outcome. In simple terms, the person had to get right with the gods or live with the consequences (Bullough & Bullough, 1978). Nursing care by a family member or relative would be needed in any case, regardless of the outcome of the sin/curse/disease–atonement/recovery or death cycle. This logic became the basis for explanation of why some people get sick and some don't for many centuries, and it still persists to some degree in most cultures today (Achterberg, 1990).

> I have an almost complete disregard of precedent and a faith in the possibility of something better. It irritates me to be told how things always have been done . . . I defy the tyranny of precedent. I cannot afford the luxury of a closed mind. I go for anything new that might improve the past.
>
> You must never so much as think whether you like it or not, whether it is bearable or not; you must never think of anything except the need, and how to meet it.
>
> —*Clara Barton, Civil War nurse and founder of the American Red Cross*

The Greeks and Health

In Greek mythology, the god of medicine, Asclepius, cured disease. One of his daughters, Hygeia, from whose name we derive the word "hygiene," was the goddess of preventive health and protected humans from disease. Panacea, Asclepius's other daughter, was known as the all-healing "universal remedy"; today her name is used to describe any ultimate "cure-all" in medicine. Panacea was known as the "light" of the day, and her name was invoked and shrines built to her during times of epidemics (Brooke, 1997).

During the **Greek era**, Hippocrates emphasized the rational treatment of sickness as a natural, rather than god-inflicted, phenomenon. Hippocrates of Cos (460–370 B.C.) is considered the father of medicine because of his arrangements of the oral and written remedies and diseases, which had long been secrets held by priests and religious healers, into a textbook of medicine that was used for centuries (Bullough & Bullough, 1978). Hippocrates's contribution to the science of public health was his recognition that making accurate observations of and drawing general conclusions from actual phenomena formed the basis of sound medical reasoning (Shryock, 1959).

In Greek society, health was considered to result from a balance between mind and body. Hippocrates wrote a most important book, *Air, Water and Places*, which detailed the relationship between humans and the environment. It is considered a milestone in the eventual development of the science of epidemiology as the first such treatise on the connectedness of the web of life. This topic of the relationship between humans and their environment did not reoccur until the development of bacteriology in the late nineteenth century (Fromkin, 1998; Rosen, 1958).

Perhaps the idea that most damaged the practice and scientific theory of medicine and health for centuries was the doctrine of the four humors, first spoken of by Empedocles of Acragas (493–433 B.C.). Empedocles was a philosopher and a physician, and as a result, he synthesized his cosmological ideas into his medical theory. He believed that the same four elements (or "roots of things") made up the universe and were found in humans and in all animate beings (Bullough & Bullough, 1978). Empedocles believed that each human was a microcosm, a small world within the macrocosm, or external environment. The four humors of the body (blood, bile, phlegm, and black bile) corresponded to the four elements of the larger world (fire, air, water, and earth) (Kalisch & Kalisch, 1986). Depending on the prevailing humor, a person was sanguine, choleric, phlegmatic, or melancholic.

Because of this strongly held and persistent belief in the connection between the balance of the four humors and health status, treatment was aimed at restoring the appropriate balance of the four humors through the control of their corresponding elements. By manipulating the two sets of opposite qualities—hot and cold, wet and dry—balance was the goal of the intervention. Fire was hot and dry, air was hot and wet, water was cold and wet, and earth was cold and dry. For example, if a person had a fever, cold compresses would be prescribed for a chill and the person would be warmed. Such doctrine gave rise to faulty and ineffective treatment of disease that influenced medical education for many years (Taylor, 1922).

Plato, in *The Republic*, detailed the importance of recreation, a balanced mind and body, nutrition, and exercise. A distinction was made among gender, class, and health as early as the Greek era; that is, only males of the aristocracy could afford the luxury of maintaining a healthful lifestyle (Rosen, 1958).

In *The Iliad*, Homer's poem about the attempts to capture Troy and rescue Helen from her lover Paris, 140 different wounds are described. The mortality rate averaged 77.6%, with the highest mortality resulting from sword and spear thrusts and the lowest mortality resulting from superficial arrow wounds. There was considerable need for nursing care, and Achilles, Patroclus, and other princes often acted as nurses to the injured. The early stages of Greek medicine reflected the influences of Egyptian, Babylonian, and Hebrew medicine. Therefore, good medical and nursing techniques were used to treat these war wounds: The arrow was drawn or cut out, the wound washed, soothing herbs applied, and the wound bandaged. However, in sickness in which no wound occurred, an evil spirit was considered the cause. For example, the cause of the plague was unknown, so the question became how and why affected soldiers had angered the gods. According to *The Iliad*, the true healer of the plague was the prophet who prayed for Apollo to stop shooting the "plague arrows." The Greeks applied rational causes and cures to external injuries, while internal ailments continued to be linked to spiritual maladies (Bullough & Bullough, 1978).

Roman Era

During the rise and the fall of the **Roman era** (31 B.C.–A.D. 476), Greek culture continued to be a strong influence. The Romans easily adopted Greek culture and expanded the Greeks' accomplishments, especially in the fields of engineering, law, and government. The development of policy, law, and protection of the public's health was an important precursor to our modern public health systems (Fromkin, 1998; Rosen, 1958). For Romans, the government had an obligation to protect its citizens, not only from outside aggression such as warring neighbors, but also from inside the civilization in the form of health laws. According to Bullough and Bullough (1978), Rome was essentially a "Greek cultural colony" (p. 20).

During the 3rd century B.C., Rome began to dominate the Mediterranean, Egypt, the Tigris–Euphrates Valley, the Hebrews, and the Greeks (Boorstin, 1985). Greek science and Roman engineering then spread throughout the ancient world, providing a synthesized Greco-Roman foundation for eventual public health policies (Bullough & Bullough, 1978).

Galen of Pergamum (A.D. 129–199), often known as the greatest Greek physician after Hippocrates, left for Rome after studying medicine in Greece and Egypt and gained great fame as a medical practitioner, lecturer, and experimenter. In his lifetime, medicine evolved into a science; he submitted traditional healing practices to experimentation and was possibly the greatest medical researcher before the 17th century (Bullough & Bullough, 1978). Galen was considered the last of the great physicians of antiquity (Kalisch & Kalisch, 1986).

The Greek physicians and healers certainly made the most contributions to medicine, but the Romans surpassed the Greeks in promoting the evolution of nursing. Roman armies developed the notion of a mobile war nursing unit as their battles took them too far from home to be cared for by their wives and family. This portable hospital was a series of tents arranged in corridors; as battles wore on, these tents gave way to buildings that became permanent convalescent camps along the battle sites (Rosen, 1958). Many of these early military hospitals have been excavated by archaeologists along the banks of the Rhine and Danube Rivers. They had wards, recreation areas, baths, pharmacies, and even rooms for officers who needed a "rest cure" (Bullough & Bullough, 1978). Coexisting were the Greek dispensary forms of temples (*iatreia*), which started out as a type of physician waiting room. These eventually developed into a primitive type of hospital—that is, places for surgical patients to stay until they could be taken home by their families. Although nurses during the Roman era were usually family members, servants, or slaves, nursing had strengthened its position in medical care and emerged during the Roman era as a separate and distinct specialty (Minkowski, 1992).

During this era, the Romans developed massive aqueducts, bath houses, and sewer systems. Even though these engineering feats were remarkable at the time, poorer and less fortunate residents often did not benefit from the same level of public health amenities, such as sewer systems and latrines (Bullough & Bullough, 1978). However, the Romans did provide many of their citizens with what we would consider public health services.

NOTE THIS!

Did you know that engineers during the Roman era developed an aqueduct system capable of providing 40 gallons of water per person per day to Rome's 1 million residents, comparable to our consumption rates today?

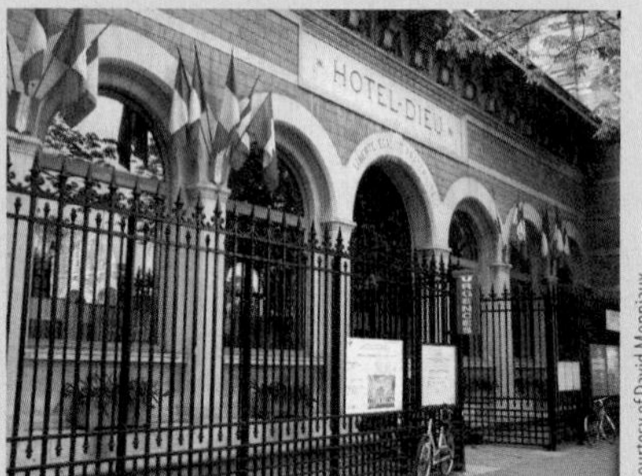

Courtesy of David Monniaux

As one of the oldest hospitals in existence, Hotel Dieu, in Paris, France, was founded in A.D. 650. The hospital is located adjacent to Notre Dame Cathedral on the Seine River and continues to provide state-of-the-art health care services. The motto of Hotel Dieu translates "Liberty, Equality, Brotherhood."

Middle Ages

The Middle Ages, or the medieval era, served as a transition between ancient and modern civilizations. The medical knowledge of the Greeks and Romans was preserved and expanded in the Islamic world, which underwent a "Golden Age" at this time but disappeared in Europe after the decline of the Roman Empire (476–1453 A.D.). While 9th- and 10th-century Muslim physicians such as Al-Razi, or Rhazes (841–926 A.D.), and Ibn-Sina, known as Avicenna (980–1037 A.D.), were developing the foundations of modern pharmacology in Persia, in Europe medicine was experiencing a reversal. Once again, myth, magic, and religion were explanations and cures for illness and health problems. For Europeans, the medieval world was the result of fusion among three streams of thought, actions, and ways of life—Greco-Roman, Germanic, and Christian—into one (Donahue, 1985).

CULTURAL CONNECTION

During the Early Middle Ages, Europeans seldom washed or changed their clothes more than once or twice a year. This lack of personal sanitation set up ideal conditions for the bubonic plague where one out of three faces disappeared from these human communities.

Source: Kelly, J. (2005). *The great mortality: An intimate history of the Black Death, the most devastating plague of all time.* New York, NY: HarperCollins.

Nursing was most influenced by Christianity with the beginning of **deaconesses**, or female servants, doing the work of God by ministering to the needs of others. Deacons in the early Christian churches were apparently available only to care for men; deaconesses cared only for the needs of the women. This role of the deaconess in the church was considered a forward step in the development of nursing, and in the 19th century it would strongly influence the young Florence Nightingale.

During this era, Roman military hospitals were replaced by civilian ones. In early Christianity, the *diakonia*, a kind of combination outpatient and welfare office, was managed by deacons and deaconesses and served as the equivalent of a hospital. Jesus served as the example of charity and compassion for the poor and marginal of society.

Communicable diseases were rampant during the Middle Ages, primarily because of the walled cities that emerged in response to the paranoia and isolation of the populations. Infection was next to impossible to control. Physicians had little to offer, deferring to the church for management of disease. Nursing roles were carried out primarily by religious orders. The oldest hospital (other than military hospitals in the Roman era) in Europe was most likely the Hôtel-Dieu in Lyons, France, founded in about 542 by Childbert I, king of France. The Hôtel-Dieu in Paris was founded in about 652 by St. Landry, bishop of Paris.

During the Middle Ages, charitable institutions, hospitals, and medical schools increased in number, with the religious leaders as caregivers. The word "hospital" which derives from the Latin *hospitalis*, meaning "service of guests," was most likely used for a shelter for travelers and other pilgrims as well as the occasional person who needed extra care (Kalisch & Kalisch, 1986). Early European hospitals were more like hospices or homes for the aged, sick pilgrims, or orphans. Nurses in these early hospitals were religious deaconesses who chose to care for others in a life of servitude and spiritual sacrifice (Minkowski, 1992).

Black Death

During the Middle Ages, a series of horrible epidemics, including the **Black Death (bubonic plague)**, ravaged the civilized world (Diamond, 1997; Fromkin, 1998). In the 14th century, Europe, Asia, and Africa saw nearly half their populations lost to the bubonic plague. According to Bullough and Bullough (1978), an interesting account of the arrival of the bubonic plague in 1347 claims that the disease had started in the Genoese colony of Kaffa in the Crimea. The story passed down through the ages was that the city was being besieged by a Mongol khan. When the disease broke out among the khan's men, he catapulted the bodies of its victims into Kaffa to infect and weaken his enemies. The soldiers and colonists of Kaffa then carried the disease back to Genoa.

THINK ABOUT THIS 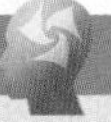

The Pima Indians of the American Southwest referred to the plague as *oimmeddam* or "wandering sickness." Below is an ancient Indian legend that describes the horror of their ancestors suffering from *oimmeddam.*

"Where do you come from?" an Indian asks a tall, black-haired stranger.

"I come from far way," the stranger replies, "from . . . across the Eastern Ocean."

"What do you bring?" the Indian asks.

"I bring death," the stranger answers. "My breath causes children to wither and die like young plants in the spring snow. I bring destruction. No matter how beautiful a woman, once she has looked at me, she becomes as ugly as death. And to men, I bring not death alone, but the destruction of their children and the blighting of their wives. . . . No people who look upon me are ever the same."

Worldwide, more than 60 million deaths were eventually attributed to this horrible plague. In some parts of Europe, only one-fourth of the population survived, with some places having too few people to bury the dead. Families abandoned sick children, and the sick were often left to die alone (Cartwright, 1972).

Nurses and physicians were powerless to avert the disease. Black spots and tumors on the skin appeared, and petechiae and hemorrhages gave the skin a darkened appearance. There was also acute inflammation of the lungs, burning sensations, unquenchable thirst, and inflammation of the entire body. Hardly anyone afflicted survived the third day of the attack. So great was the fear of contagion that ships were set to sail with bodies of infected persons without a crew, drifting through the North, Black, and Mediterranean seas from port to port with their dead passengers (Cohen, 1989). Bubonic plague is caused by the bacillus *Pasteurella pestis*, which is usually transmitted by the bite of a flea carried by an animal vector, typically a rat. After the initial flea bite, the infection spreads through the lymph nodes, and the nodes swell to enormous size; the inflamed nodes are called bubos, from which the bubonic plague derives its name. Medieval people knew that this disease was in some way communicable, but they were unsure of the mode of transmission (Diamond, 1997)—hence the avoidance of victims and a reliance on isolation techniques. The practice of quarantine in city ports was developed as a preventive measure and is still used today (Bullough & Bullough, 1978; Kalisch & Kalisch, 1986).

ETHICAL CONNECTION 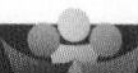

The Gallup Poll organization named nursing as the most "ethical" profession in the United States in 2013, according to a survey of American adults. More than 80% of respondents categorized nurses as having very high or high ethics. Nursing has been ranked the number one most ethical profession during the last 10 years, passed only in 2001 by fire fighters in the wake of the 9/11 terrorist attacks.

The plague had far-reaching social and religious consequences. The authority of the Catholic Church was weakened, due to the inability of priests to halt the disease and protect their parishioners from the Black Death, which was commonly assumed to be God's vengeance for the sins of humans. Although dreadful and terrifying, the plague brought about radical societal changes through the drop in value of land, due to a reduction in workers, thus raising the price of labor and ultimately ending Europe's feudal system (Fromkin, 1998).

The "Witch Craze" of the Early Middle Ages

As respected "wise women" through the centuries, during the Middle Ages midwives and women healers gradually transformed into members of a "demonized" avocation. As formal training in medicine gradually developed in Europe, leaders of the church and officials at the time restricted such education to men only, consequently creating a legal male monopoly of the practice of medicine and healing (Achterberg, 1990; Barstow, 1994; Briggs, 1996). As women found themselves "ineligible" to practice in their roles as healers, they faced an even greater threat as they were labeled as witches.

A revival of the Holy Inquisition, a body formed in France in 1022 and codified by the Catholic Church in the 1486 *Malleus maleficarum* (Hammer of Witches) by Pope Innocent VIII, allowed the persecutions to take form. By formalizing the legal punishment of witches and midwives, the Pope codified this "step-by-step, how-to manual" for dealing with the witch problem. Achterberg (1990) describes this significant endorsement in this way: "We are dealing here with an evil that surpasses rational understanding. Here was, indeed, the worst aberration of humanity and it trickled down the hierarchy of authority" (p. 86). The legal system throughout Europe became increasingly harsh with each new conviction, and as the distinction between sorcery and heresy was further blurred, those accused of witchcraft and heresy were found guilty of devil worship. With the support of both the church and civil authorities, as many as 250,000 women were accused, "tried," and tortured into making confessions and eventually burned at the stake simply for being women healers (Briggs, 1996). The accusers linked women's special healing "powers" to an alliance with Satan, and over three centuries they punished and eliminated women as perceived threats to their medical supremacy in society.

Our stereotype of a witch today reflects these ancient and deadly associations of women healers and evil magic: the elderly, unattractive woman dressed in black on a broomstick with a black cat at her side. Women in Europe who practiced as healers often used empirically sound herbal and alternative health practices (hence the caldron association), provided gynecological and obstetric care of women at all hours (hence the broom, because proper women did not go out at night and were presumed to "fly"), and relied on other women for advice and shared practices of healing (hence the "coven" association; Achterberg, 1990; Barstow, 1994). As described by Briggs (1996), "To this end they have allegedly flown by night to meetings where orgiastic, blasphemous or cannibalistic rituals symbolized their defection from social and personal virtue" (p. 4).

Briggs (1996) estimates that 100,000 trials of witches occurred in Europe between the years 1450 and 1750, with at least 50% of the accused being executed in brutal hangings and burnings. This "witch craze" reached its height during the 12th through 14th centuries in France, Germany, and other European countries (Achterberg, 1990; Barstow, 1994; Briggs, 1996). Religion, magic, healing, and witchcraft were inextricably linked throughout human history, but during this era dramatic changes in cultural values and paranoia about women's perceived powers resulted in a mass cultural movement to eliminate women as healers (Briggs, 1996; Minkowski, 1992).

The Renaissance

During the rebirth of Europe, great political, social, and economic advances occurred along with a tremendous revival of learning. Donahue (1985) contends that the Renaissance has been "viewed as both a blessing and a curse" (p. 188). There was a renewed interest in the arts and sciences, which helped advance medical science (Boorstin, 1985; Bullough & Bullough, 1978). Columbus and other explorers discovered new worlds, and belief in a sun-centered rather than earth-centered universe was promoted by Copernicus (1473–1543); Sir Isaac Newton's (1642–1727) theory of gravity changed the world forever. Gunpowder was introduced, and social and religious upheavals resulted in the American and French revolutions at the end of the 18th century (Weiner, 1993).

In the arts and sciences, Leonardo da Vinci, known as one of the greatest geniuses of all time, made a number of anatomical drawings based on dissection experiences. These drawings have become classics in the progression of knowledge about the human anatomy. Many artists of this time left an indelible mark and continue to exert influence today, including Michelangelo, Raphael, and Titian (Donahue, 1985; Minkowski, 1992; Weiner, 1993).

The Emergence of Home Visiting

In 1633, **Saint Vincent de Paul** founded the Sisters of Charity in France, an order of nuns who traveled from home to home visiting the sick. As the services of the sisters grew, St. Vincent appointed Mademoiselle Le Gras as supervisor of these visitors. These nurses functioned as the first organized visiting nurse service, making home visits and caring for the sick in their homes. De Paul believed that for family members to go to the hospital was disruptive to family life and that taking nursing services to the home enabled health to be restored more effectively and more efficiently (Weiner, 1993).

The Reformation

Religious changes during the Renaissance were to influence nursing perhaps more than any other aspect of society. Particularly important was the rise of Protestantism as a result of the reform movements of Martin Luther (1483–1546) in Germany and John Calvin (1509–1564) in France and Geneva, Switzerland. Although the various sects were numerous in the Protestant movement, the agreement among the leaders was almost unanimous on the abolition of the monastic or cloistered career. The effects on nursing were drastic: Monastic-affiliated institutions, including hospitals and schools, were closed, and orders of nuns, including nurses, were dissolved. Even in countries where Catholicism flourished, seizures of monasteries by royal leaders occurred frequently.

Religious leaders, such as Martin Luther in Germany, who led the **Reformation** in 1517, were well aware of the lack of adequate nursing care as a result of these sweeping changes. Luther advocated that each town establish something akin to a "community chest" to raise funds for hospitals and nurse visitors for the poor (Dietz & Lehozky, 1963; Fromkin, 1998). For example, in England, where there had been at least 450 charitable foundations before the Reformation, only a few survived the reign of Henry VIII, who closed most of the monastic hospitals (Donahue, 1985). Eventually, Henry VIII's son, Edward VI, who reigned from 1547 to 1553, was convinced and did endow some hospitals—namely St. Bartholomew's Hospital and St. Thomas's Hospital, which would eventually house the Nightingale School of Nursing in the 19th century (Bullough & Bullough, 1978).

GOT AN ALTERNATIVE?

Ehrenreich and English (1973), in their seminal work, *Witches, Midwives, and Nurses: A History of Women Healers*, note that in the Middle Ages it was the women who were testing new herbs and innovative ways of healing, leading to the adoption of humane, empirical paradigms of healing. All the while, they contend, their male counterparts clung to their ritualistic and outdated procedures, such as leeching, use of mercury, and purgation.

These authors contend that the witch craze, where thousands of women were tried and put to death, was a ruling-class campaign of terror against the female peasant healers who dared to introduce what is now considered holistic or complementary healing modalities. Given that God considered illness and suffering as payment for sin, anyone who offered healing interventions, such as boiling up herbs and potions in big pots, must be anti-God and, therefore, must be working for the "other side" or the Devil. It is hardly surprising, according to Ehrenreich and English, that nursing fell into disrepute by the 18th century, and that the only women who had any status for being involved in healing were those in holy orders. Yet for many poor people, their only remedies were these traditional healing "potions." As medicine grew with scientific models of illness management, these tried and tested remedies were held up as "old wives' tales."

Source: Ehrenreich, B., & English, D. (1973). *Witches, midwives, and nurses: A history of women healers.* Old Westbury, NY: Feminist Press.

The Advancement of Science and Health of the Public

It took the first 50 years of the 18th century for the new knowledge from the Enlightenment to be organized and digested, according to Donahue (1985). In Great Britain, **Edward Jenner** discovered an effective method of vaccination against the dreaded smallpox virus in 1798. Psychiatry developed as a separate branch of medicine, and instruments such as the pulse watch and the stethoscope were invented that measured and allowed for assessment of the body.

One of the greatest scientists of this period was **Louis Pasteur** (1822–1895). A French chemist, Pasteur first became interested in pathogenic organisms through his studies of the diseases of wine. His discovery, that heating wine to a temperature of 55° to 60°C killed the microorganisms that spoiled wine, was critical to the wine industry's success in France. This process of pasteurization led Pasteur to investigate many fields and save many lives from contaminated milk and food.

Joseph Lister (1827–1912) was a physician who set out to decrease the mortality resulting from infection after surgery. He used Pasteur's research to eventually arrive at a chemical antiseptic solution of carbolic acid for use in surgery. Widely regarded as the father of modern surgery, he practiced his antiseptic surgery with great results, and the Listerian principles of asepsis changed the way physicians and nurses practice to this day (Dietz & Lehozky, 1963).

Robert Koch (1843–1910), a physician known for his research in anthrax, is regarded as the father of microbiology. By identifying the organism that caused cholera, *Vibrio cholerae*, he also demonstrated its transmission by water, food, and clothing.

Edwin Klebs (1834–1913) proved the germ theory—that is, that germs are the causes of infectious diseases. This discovery of the bacterial origin of diseases may be considered the greatest achievement of the 19th century. Although the microscope had been around for two centuries, it remained for Lister, Pasteur, and Koch—and ultimately Klebs—to provide the missing link (Dietz & Lehozky, 1963; Fromkin, 1998; Rosen, 1958).

MEDIA MOMENT

***Troy* (2004)**

This movie starring Brad Pitt as Achilles is based on the epic poem *The Iliad* by Homer. The movie recounts the legend of the Trojan War, as the fortress city is attacked by a Greek army led by Menelaus of Sparta and Agamemnon of Mycenae.

Achilles, the mighty Greek warrior, had been dipped as an infant by his mother in the River Styx so that he would be invincible to iron weapons. Because his mother had held him by his heel, this was the only vulnerable part of his body. In the adaptation of Homer's *Iliad*, the Trojan warrior Paris (played by Orlando Bloom) shoots Achilles in the heel with a poison arrow and brings about his death. A simple superficial wound to the heel would not have been deadly; consequently, history provides us with an early account of biochemical warfare.

Source: Peterson, W. (Producer & Director). (2004). *Troy.* United States: Warner Bros.

NOTE THIS!

The Reformation had a devastating effect upon nursing. Imagine our situation in the United States if a decree went out that hospitals would be closed in 2 years. There would be no places available to care for the ill. Such were the conditions in England from 1538–1540 during the reign of Henry VIII. No provision was made for the sick and poor, there was no lay organization to replace those who had fled, and no one to develop or teach others to carry on.

Source: Dietz, D. D., & Lehozky, A. R. (1963). *History and modern nursing.* Philadelphia, PA: F. A. Davis.

The Dark Period of Nursing

The last half of the period between 1500 and 1860 is widely regarded as the "dark period of nursing" because nursing conditions were at their worst (Donahue, 1985). Education for girls, which had been provided by the nuns in religious schools, was lost. Because of the elimination of hospitals and schools, there was no one to pass on knowledge about caring for the sick. As a result, the hospitals were managed and staffed by municipal authorities; women entering nursing service often came from illiterate classes, and even then there were too few to serve (Dietz & Lehozky, 1963). The lay attendants who filled the nursing role were illiterate, rough, inconsiderate, and often immoral and alcoholic. Intelligent women and men could not be persuaded to accept such a degraded and low-status position in the offensive municipal hospitals of London. Nursing slipped back into a role of servitude as menial, low-status work. According to Donahue (1985), when a woman could no longer make it as a gambler, prostitute, or thief, she might become a nurse. Eventually, women serving jail sentences for crimes such as prostitution and stealing were ordered to care for the sick in the hospitals instead of serving their sentences in the city jail (Dietz & Lehozky, 1963). The nurses of this era took bribes from patients, became inappropriately involved with them, and survived the best way they could, often at the expense of their assigned patients.

During this era, nursing had virtually no social standing or organization. Even Catholic sisters of the religious orders throughout Europe "came to a complete standstill" professionally because of the intolerance of society (Donahue, 1985, p. 231).

MEDIA MOMENT

Martin Chuzzlewit **(1843–1844)**

By Charles Dickens

Charles Dickens created the immortal character of Sairey Gamp, who was a visiting nurse based on an actual hired attendant whom Dickens had met in a friend's home:

> She was a fat old woman, this Mrs. Gamp, with a husky voice and a moist eye, which she had a remarkable power of turning up and showing the white of it. Having very little neck, it cost her some trouble to look over herself, if one may say so, to those to whom she talked. She wore a very rusty black gown, rather the worse for snuff, and a shawl and bonnet to correspond. . . . The face of Mrs. Gamp—the nose in particular—was somewhat red and swollen, and it was difficult to enjoy her society without becoming conscious of the smell of spirits. Like most persons who have attained to great eminence in their profession, she took to hers very kindly; insomuch, that setting aside her natural predilections as a woman, she went to a lying-in [birth] or a laying-out [death] with equal zest and relish.

Sairey Gamp was hired to care for sick family members but was instead cruel to her patients, stole from them, and ate their rations; she was an alcoholic and has been immortalized forever as a reminder of the world in which Florence Nightingale came of age (Donahue, 1985; Minkowski, 1992).

Early Organized Health Care in the Americas: A Brave New World

In the New World, the first hospital in the Americas—the Hospital de la Purisima Concepcion—was founded some time before 1524 by Hernando Cones, the conqueror of Mexico. The first hospital in the continental United States was erected in Manhattan in 1658 for the care of sick soldiers and slaves. In 1717, a hospital for infectious diseases was built in Boston; the first hospital established by a private gift was the Charity Hospital in New Orleans. A sailor, Jean Louis, donated the endowment for the hospital's founding (Bullough & Bullough, 1978).

During the 17th and 18th centuries, colonial hospitals were often used to house the poor and downtrodden, though they bore little resemblance to modern hospitals. Hospitals called pesthouses were created to care for people with contagious diseases; their primary purpose was to protect the public at large, rather than to treat and care for the patients. Contagious diseases were rampant during the early years of the American colonies, often being spread by the large number of immigrants who brought these diseases with them on their long journeys to America. Medicine was not as developed as in Europe, and nursing remained in the hands of the uneducated. Average life expectancy at birth was only around 35 years by 1720. Plagues were a constant nightmare, with outbreaks of smallpox and yellow fever. In 1751, the first true hospital in the new colonies, Pennsylvania Hospital, was erected in Philadelphia on the recommendation of Benjamin Franklin (Kalisch & Kalisch, 1986).

By today's standards, hospitals in the 19th century were disgraceful, dirty, unventilated, and contaminated by infections; to be a patient in a hospital actually increased one's risk of dying. As in England, nursing was considered an inferior occupation. After the sweeping changes as a result of the Reformation, educated religious health workers were replaced with lay people who were "down and outers," in prison, or had no option left except to work with the sick (Kalisch & Kalisch, 1986).

The Chadwick Report and the Shattuck Report

Edwin Chadwick became a major figure in the development of the field of public health in Great Britain by drawing attention to the cost of the unsanitary conditions that shortened the lifespan of the laboring class and posed threats to the wealth of Britain. Although the first sanitation legislation, which established a National Vaccination Board, was passed in 1837, Chadwick found in his classic study, *Report on an Inquiry into the Sanitary Conditions of the Laboring Population of Great Britain*, that death rates were high in large industrial cities such as Liverpool. A more startling finding, from what is often referred to simply as the Chadwick Report, was that more than half the children of labor-class workers died by age 5, indicating poor living conditions that affected the health of the most vulnerable. Laborers lived only half as long as members of the upper classes.

One consequence of the report was the establishment of the first board of health, the General Board of Health for England, in 1848 (Richardson, 1887). More legislation followed that initiated social reform in the areas of child welfare, elder care, the sick, the mentally ill, factory health, and education. Soon sewers and fireplugs, based on an available water supply, appeared as indicators that the public health linkages from the Chadwick Report had an impact.

In the United States during the 19th century, waves of epidemics of yellow fever, smallpox, cholera, typhoid fever, and typhus continued to plague the population as in England and the rest of the world. As cities continued to grow in the industrialized young nation, poor workers crowded into larger cities and suffered from illnesses caused by the unsanitary living conditions (Hanlon & Pickett, 1984). Similar to what occurred with Chadwick's classic study in England, Lemuel Shattuck, a Boston bookseller and publisher who had an interest in public health, organized the American Statistical Society in 1839 and issued a census of Boston in 1845. Shattuck's census revealed high infant mortality rates and high overall population mortality rates. In his *Report of the Massachusetts Sanitary Commission* in 1850, Shattuck not only outlined his findings on the unsanitary conditions, but also made recommendations for public health reform that included the keeping of population statistics and development of a monitoring system that would provide information to the public about environmental, food, and drug safety as well as infectious disease control (Rosen, 1958). He also called for services such as well-child care, school-age children's health, immunizations, mental health, health education for all, and health planning. The Shattuck Report was revolutionary in its scope and vision for public health, but it was virtually ignored during Shattuck's lifetime. It would not be until 19 years later, in 1869, that the first state board of health was formed (Kalisch & Kalisch, 1986; Minkowski, 1992).

The Industrial Revolution

During the mid-18th century in England, capitalism emerged as an economic system based on profit. This emerging system resulted in mass production, as contrasted with the previous system of individual workers and craftsmen. In the simplest terms, the Industrial Revolution was the application of machine power to processes formerly done by hand. Machinery was invented during this era and ultimately standardized quality; individual craftsmen were forced to give up their crafts and lands and become factory laborers for the capitalist owners. All types of industries were affected; this newfound efficiency produced profits for owners of the means of production. As a result, the era of invention flourished, factories grew, and people moved in record numbers to work in the cities. Urban areas grew, tenement housing projects emerged, and overcrowded cities became serious threats to wellbeing (Donahue, 1985).

Workers were forced to go to the machines, rather than the other way around. Such relocations meant giving up not only farming, but also a way of life that had existed for centuries. The emphasis on profit over people led to child labor, frequent layoffs, and long workdays filled with stressful, tedious, unfamiliar work. Labor unions did not exist, nor was there any legal protection against exploitation of workers, including children (Donahue, 1985). All of these rapid changes and often threatening conditions were described in the work of Charles Dickens; in his book *Oliver Twist*, for example, children worked as adults without question.

According to Donahue (1985), urban life, trade, and industrialization contributed to these overwhelming health hazards, and the situation was confounded by the lack of an adequate means of social control. Reforms were desperately needed, and the social reform movement emerged in response to the unhealthy by-products of the Industrial Revolution. It was in this world of the 19th century that reformers such as John Stuart Mill (1806–1873) emerged. Although the Industrial Revolution began in England, it quickly spread to the rest of Europe and to the United States (Bullough & Bullough, 1978). The reform movement is critical to understanding the emerging health concerns that were later addressed by Florence Nightingale. Mill championed popular education, the emancipation of women, trade unions, and religious toleration. Other reform issues of the era included the abolition of slavery and, most important for nursing, more humane care of the sick, the poor, and the wounded (Bullough & Bullough, 1978). There was a renewed energy in the religious community with the reemergence of new religious orders in the Catholic church that provided service to the sick and disenfranchised.

Epidemics had ravaged Europe for centuries, but they became even more serious with urbanization. Industrialization had brought people to cities, where they worked in close quarters (as compared with the isolation of the farm) and contributed to the social decay of the second half of the 19th century. Sanitation was poor or nonexistent, sewage disposal from the growing population was lacking, cities were filthy, public laws were weak or nonexistent, and congestion of the cities inevitably brought pests in the form of rats, lice, and bedbugs, which transmitted many pathogens. Communicable diseases continued to plague the population, especially those who lived in these unsanitary environments. For example, during the mid-18th century typhus and typhoid fever claimed twice as many lives each year as did the Battle of Waterloo (Hanlon & Pickett, 1984). Through foreign trade and immigration, infectious diseases spread to all of Europe and eventually to the growing United States.

John Snow and the Science of Epidemiology

John Snow, a prominent physician, is credited with being the first epidemiologist. In 1854, he demonstrated that cholera rates were linked with water pump use in London (Cartwright, 1972; Johnson, 2006). Snow investigated the area around Golden Square in London and arrived at the conclusion that cholera was not carried by bad air, nor necessarily by direct contact. He formed the opinion that diarrhea, unwashed hands, and shared food somehow played a large part in spreading the disease.

People around Golden Square in London were not supplied with water by pipes, but rather drew their water from surface wells by means of hand-operated pumps. A severe outbreak of cholera occurred at the end of August 1853, resulting in at least 500 deaths in just 10 days in Golden Square. By identifying rates of cholera, Snow for the first time linked the sources of the drinking water at the Broad Street pump to the outbreaks of cholera, thereby proving that cholera was a waterborne disease. Snow's epidemiological investigation started a train of events that eventually would end the great epidemics of cholera, dysentery, and typhoid (Minkowski, 1992).

When Snow attended the now-famous community meeting of Golden Square and gave his evidence, government officials asked him what measures were necessary. His reply was, "Take the handle off the Broad Street pump." The handle was removed the next day, and no more cholera cases occurred (Snow, 1855). Although he did not discover the true cause of the cholera—the identification of the organism—he came very close to the truth (Johnson, 2006; Rosen, 1958).

And Then There Was Nightingale . . .

Florence Nightingale was named one of the 100 most influential persons of the last millennium by *Life* magazine (1997), one of only eight women so identified. Of those eight women, who included such luminaries as Joan of Arc, Helen Keller, and Elizabeth I, Nightingale was identified as a true "angel of mercy," having reformed military health care in the Crimean War and used her political savvy to forever change the way society views the health of the vulnerable, the poor, and the forgotten. She is probably one of the most written-about women in history (Bullough & Bullough, 1978). Florence Nightingale has become synonymous with modern nursing.

Florence Nightingale was the second child born to the wealthy English family of William and Frances Nightingale on May 12, 1820, in her namesake city, Florence, Italy. As a young child, Florence displayed incredible curiosity and intellectual abilities not common to female children of the Victorian age. She mastered the fundamentals of Greek and Latin, and she studied history, art, mathematics, and philosophy. To her family's dismay, she believed that God had called her to be a nurse (Bostridge, 2008). Nightingale was keenly aware of the suffering that industrialization created; she became obsessed with the plight of the miserable and suffering. Conditions of general starvation had accompanied the Industrial Revolution, along with overflowing prisons and workhouses, and displaced persons in all sections of British life. Nightingale wrote in the spring of 1842, "My mind is absorbed with the sufferings of man; it besets me behind and before. . . . All that the poets sing of the glories of this world seem to me untrue. All the people that I see are eaten up with care or poverty or disease" (Woodham-Smith, 1951, p. 31).

NOTE THIS!

Florence Nightingale never made a public appearance, never issued a public statement, and did not have the right to vote.

RESEARCH ALERT

As part of her work, Florence Nightingale collaborated with William Farr, the eminent medical statistician. Nightingale's epidemiological investigations, supported by Farr, illustrated that attention to environmental cleanliness was an important factor in preventing spread of disease (Bostridge, 2008). Nightingale channeled her investigations to support hospital reforms and the need for educated nurses who could provide better management of the hospital environment. Statistical support and solicited criticism allowed Nightingale to argue more forcefully for her reforms.

Source: Keeling, A. W. (2006). "Carrying ointments and even pills!" Medicines in the work of Henry Street Settlement visiting nurses, 1893–1944. *Nursing History Review, 14.*

For Nightingale, her entire life would be haunted by this conflict between the opulent life of gaiety that she enjoyed and the plight and misery of the world, which she was unable to alleviate. She was, in essence, an "alien spirit in the rich and aristocratic social sphere of Victorian England" (Palmer, 1977, p. 14). Nightingale remained unmarried, and at the age of 25, she expressed a desire to be trained as a nurse in an English hospital. Her parents emphatically denied her request, and for the next 7 years, she made repeated attempts to change their minds and allow her to enter nurse training. She wrote, "I crave for some regular occupation, for something worth doing instead of frittering my time away on useless trifles" (Woodham-Smith, 1951, p. 162).

During this time, Nightingale continued her education through the study of math and science, and she spent 5 years collecting data about public health and hospitals (Dietz & Lehozky, 1963). While in Egypt, Nightingale studied Egyptian, Platonic, and Hermetic philosophy; Christian scripture; and the works of poets, mystics, and missionaries in her efforts to understand the nature of God and her "calling" as it fit into the divine plan (Calabria, 1996; Dossey, 2000).

The next spring, Nightingale traveled unaccompanied to the **Kaiserwerth Institute** in Germany and stayed there for 2 weeks, vowing to return to train as a nurse. In June 1851, Nightingale took her future into her own hands and announced to her family that she planned to return to Kaiserwerth and study nursing. According to Dietz and Lehozky (1963, p. 42), her mother had "hysterics" and "scene followed scene." Her father "retreated into the shadows," and her sister, Parthe, expressed that the family name was forever disgraced (Cook, 1913).

In 1851, at the age of 31, Nightingale was finally permitted to go to Kaiserwerth. She studied there for 3 months with Pastor Fliedner. Her family insisted that she tell no one outside the family of her whereabouts, and her mother forbade her to write any letters from Kaiserwerth. While there, Nightingale learned about the care of the sick and the importance of discipline and commitment of oneself to God (Donahue, 1985). She returned to England and cared for her then-ailing father, from whom she finally gained some support for her intent to become a nurse—her lifelong dream (Bostridge, 2008).

In 1852, Nightingale wrote the essay "Cassandra," which stands today as a classic feminist treatise against the idleness of Victorian women. Through her voluminous journal writings, Nightingale reveals her inner struggle throughout her adulthood with what was expected of a woman and what she could accomplish with her life. The life expected of an aristocratic woman in her day was one she grew to loathe; throughout her writings, she poured out her detestation of the life of an idle woman (Nightingale, 1979, p. 5). In "Cassandra," Nightingale put her thoughts to paper, and many scholars believe that her eventual intent was to extend the essay to a novel. She wrote in "Cassandra," "Why have women passion, intellect, moral activity—these three—in a place in society where no one of the three can be exercised?" (Nightingale, 1979, p. 37). Although uncertain about the meaning of the name "Cassandra," many scholars believe that it came from the Greek goddess Cassandra, who was cursed by Apollo and doomed to see and speak the truth but never to be believed. Nightingale saw the conventional life of women as a waste of time and abilities. After receiving a generous yearly endowment from her father, Nightingale moved to London and worked briefly as the superintendent of the hospital Establishment for Gentlewomen During Illness, finally realizing her dream of working as a nurse (Bostridge, 2008; Cook, 1913).

The Crimean Experience: "I Can Stand Out the War with Any Man"

Nightingale's opportunity for greatness came when she was offered the position of female nursing establishment of the English General Hospitals in Turkey by the British Secretary of War, Sir Sidney Herbert. Soon after the outbreak of the Crimean War, stories of the inadequate care and lack of medical resources for the soldiers became widely known throughout England (Woodham-Smith, 1951). The country was appalled at the conditions so vividly portrayed in the *London Times*. Pressure increased on Sir Herbert to rectify the situation. He knew of one woman who was capable of bringing order out of the chaos and wrote the following now-famous letter to Nightingale on October 15, 1854, as a plea for her service:

> There is but one person in England that I know of who would be capable of organising and superintending such a scheme. . . . The difficulty of finding women equal to a task after all, full of horrors, and requiring besides knowledge and good will, great energy and great courage, will be great. Your own personal qualities, your knowledge and your power of administration and among greater things your rank and position in Society give you advantages in such a work which no other person possesses. (Woodham-Smith, 1951, pp. 87–89)

Nightingale took the challenge from Sir Herbert and set sail with 38 self-proclaimed nurses with varied training and experiences, of whom 24 were Catholic and Anglican nuns. Their journey to the Crimea took a month. On November 4, 1854, the brave nurses arrived at Istanbul and were taken to Scutari the same day. Faced with 3,000 to 4,000 wounded men in a hospital designed to accommodate 1,700 patients, the nurses went to work (Kalisch & Kalisch, 1986). This is the scene that the nurses faced: There were 4 miles of beds 18 inches apart. Most soldiers were lying naked with no bed or blanket. There were no kitchen or laundry facilities. The little light present took the form of candles in beer bottles. The hospital was literally floating on an open sewage lagoon filled with rats and other vermin (Donahue, 1985).

The barracks "hospital" was more of a death trap than a place for healing before Nightingale's arrival. In a letter to Sir Herbert, Nightingale, demonstrating her sense of humor, wrote, with tongue in cheek, that "the vermin might, if they had but unity of purpose, carry off the four miles of beds on their backs and march them into the War Office" (Stanmore, 1906, pp. 393–394).

By taking the newly arrived medical equipment and setting up kitchens, laundries, recreation rooms, reading rooms, and a canteen, Nightingale and her team of nurses proceeded to clean the barracks of lice and filth. Nightingale was in her element: She set out not only to provide humane health care for the soldiers, but also to essentially overhaul the administrative structure of the military health services (Williams, 1961). Nightingale and her nurses faced overwhelming odds and deplorable conditions. No accommodations had been made for their quarters, so they ended up in one of the hospital towers, 39 women crowded into six small rooms. In addition to having no furniture, one of the rooms even contained a long-neglected, forgotten corpse swarming with vermin! Ever the disciplinarian, Nightingale insisted on strict adherence to a standard nurse uniform: gray tweed dresses, gray worsted jackets, plain white caps, short woolen cloaks, and brown scarves embroidered in red with the words "Scutari Hospital" (Bullough & Bullough, 1978).

Florence Nightingale and Sanitation

Although Nightingale never accepted the germ theory, she demanded clean dressings; clean bedding; well-cooked, edible, and appealing food; proper sanitation; and fresh air. After the other nurses were asleep, Nightingale made her famous solitary rounds with a lamp or lantern to check on the soldiers. Nightingale had a lifelong pattern of sleeping few hours, spending many nights writing, developing elaborate plans, and evaluating implemented changes. She seldom believed in the "hopeless" soldier; instead, she saw only one that needed extra attention. Nightingale was convinced that most of the maladies that the soldiers suffered and died from were preventable (Williams, 1961).

Before Nightingale's arrival and her radical and well-documented interventions based on sound public health principles, mortality rates for the Crimea War were estimated to range from 42% to 73%. Nightingale is credited with reducing that rate to 2% within 6 months of her arrival at Scutari. She did so by conducting careful, scientific epidemiological research (Dietz & Lehozky, 1963). Upon arriving at Scutari, Nightingale's first act was to order 200 scrubbing brushes. The death rate fell dramatically once Nightingale discovered that the hospital was built literally over an open sewage lagoon. A dead horse was even retrieved from the sewer system under Scutari (Andrews, 2003).

> Bad sanitary, bad architectural, and bad administrative arraignments often make it impossible to nurse.
>
> —*Florence Nightingale*

GLOBAL CONNECTION 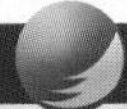

"I made up my mind that if the army wanted nurses, they would be glad of me, and with all the ardor of my nature, which ever carried me where inclination prompted, I decided that I would go to the Crimea; and go I did, as all the world knows."

—Mary Seacole

Mary Seacole, contemporary of Florence Nightingale, was named in 2004 the greatest black Briton of all time. Although few have heard of Seacole, she was an important figure in the establishment of nursing as a profession. The Royal College of Nursing President Sylvia Denton said of this honor: "Mary Seacole stood up against the discrimination and prejudices she encountered. Against all odds, Mary had an unshakeable belief in the power of nursing to make a difference."

Seacole was born in the early 1880s as Mary Grant, in Kingston, Jamaica, to a Scottish father and a free black Jamaican mother. Her mother taught her about Creole medicine and she grew up well educated. In 1838, she married Edward Seacole, who died shortly afterward. During their short marriage, they traveled around the Caribbean and Central America. After her husband's death, she returned to Kingston to help run the family boardinghouse. During two epidemics of cholera and one epidemic of yellow fever, she sharpened her skills as a nurse, even performing a postmortem autopsy of a baby who had died of cholera.

Seacole eventually traveled with her brother to other South American countries, establishing hotels and providing care for the sick. When she learned of the Crimean War, she traveled to England, at her own expense, and offered her services to the British Army. She was refused because of the color of her skin. The putdown did not deter Seacole, who funded her own 3,000-mile trip to Crimea, where she offered her services to Florence Nightingale. Nightingale refused her offer as a nurse, so Seacole set up a "hotel for invalids"—called the British Hotel—in nearby Baklava.

At her hotel, Seacole banned drunkenness and gambling, dispensed medicines, fed soldiers meals, and tended to the wounded on the battlefield under fire, making home visits to campsites in the area. Seacole's hotel was a financial disaster,

Continued

because she did not require payment for services and did not have the support of the British government. She used all of her savings to secure medicine and other needed supplies for the sick. When the Crimean War ended in 1856, Seacole was in severe debt and struggled in her lifetime residence in England. Her writings provided some financial support.

Through the years, historians have come to recognize Seacole's heroic and strong commitment to the development of war nursing. It is possible that Nightingale and Seacole never met. Historical evidence is inconclusive regarding the exact nature of their personal contact at Scutari. Nightingale's refusal to accept Seacole's offer to join her nurses at Sebastopol reflected the discrimination and prejudice of the day. Seacole received the Crimean Medal, the French Legion of Honor, and a Turkish Medal. She died in 1881 and is buried in London.

Selected References on the Life of Mary Seacole

Crawford, P. (1992). The other lady with the lamp: Nursing legacy of Mary Seacole. *Nursing Times, 88*(11), 56–58.

Gustafson, M. (1996). Mary Seacole, the Florence Nightingale of Jamaica. *Christian Nurse International, 12*(4), 9.

King, A. (1974). Mary Seacole, part I: A matter of life. *Essence, 4*(11), 32.

King, A. (1974). Mary Seacole, part II: The Crimea. *Essence, 4*(12), 68, 94.

Messmer, P. R., & Parchment, Y. (1998). Mary Grant Seacole: The first nurse practitioner. *Clinical Excellence for Nurse Practitioners, 2*(1), 47–51.

Payne, D. (1999). Face to face: Florence Nightingale and Mary Seacole battle it out face to face. *Nursing Times, 95*(19), 26–27.

According to Palmer (1982), Nightingale possessed the qualities of a good researcher: insatiable curiosity, command of her subject, familiarity with methods of inquiry, a good background of statistics, and the ability to discriminate and abstract. She used these skills to maintain detailed and copious notes and to codify observations. Nightingale relied on statistics and attention to detail to back up her conclusions about sanitation, management of care, and disease causation. Her now-famous "cox combs" are a hallmark of military health services management, through which she diagrammed deaths in the Army from wounds and from other diseases and compared them with deaths that occurred in similar populations in England (Palmer, 1977).

Nightingale was first and foremost an administrator: She believed in a hierarchical administrative structure with ultimate control lodged in one person to whom all subordinates and offices reported. Within a matter of weeks of her arrival in the Crimea, Nightingale was the acknowledged administrator and organizer of a mammoth humanitarian effort. From her Crimean experience on, Nightingale involved herself primarily in organizational activities and health planning administration. Palmer (1982) contends that Nightingale "perceived the Crimean venture, which was set up as an experiment, as a golden opportunity to demonstrate the efficacy of female nursing" (p. 4). Although Nightingale faced initial resistance from the unconvinced and oppositional medical officers and surgeons, she boldly defied convention and remained steadfastly focused on her mission to create a sanitary and highly structured environment for her "children"—the British soldiers who dedicated their lives to the defense of Great Britain. Proving her resilience and insistence on absolute authority regarding nursing and the hospital environment, Nightingale was known to send nurses home to England from the Crimea for suspicious alcohol use and character weakness.

It was her success at Scutari that enabled Nightingale to begin a long career of influence on the public's health through social activism and reform, health policy, and the reformation of career nursing. Using her well-publicized successful "experiment" and supportive evidence from the Crimean War, Nightingale effectively argued the case for the reform and creation of military health that would serve as the model for people in uniform to the present (D'Antonio, 2002). Nightingale's ideas about proper hospital architecture and administration influenced a generation of medical doctors and the entire world, in both military and civilian service. Her work in *Notes on Hospitals*, published in 1859, provided the template for the organization of military health care in the Union Army when the U.S. Civil War erupted in 1861. Her vision for health care of soldiers and the responsibility of the governments who send them to war continues today; her influence can be seen throughout the last century and into the 21st century, as health care for the women and men who serve their countries is a vital part of the wellbeing of not only the soldiers but also society in general (D'Antonio, 2002). See **Box 3-1**.

> Many soldiers wrote about their experiences of the Angel of Mercy, Florence Nightingale. One soldier wrote perhaps one of the most revealing tributes to this 'Lady with the Lamp':
>
> What a comfort it was to see her pass even. She would speak to one and nod and smile to as many more, but she could not do it all, you know. We lay there by hundreds, but we could kiss her shadow as it fell, and lay our heads on the pillow again content.
>
> —*Tyrell, 1856, p. 310*

BOX 3-1 Singing to Promote a Healthy Body and Soul: "The Nightingale's Song to the Sick Soldier"

Florence Nightingale set an example to all with her commitment and compassion to the weary and the sick. She had a special fondness for animals and birds and regularly showed compassion for them in correspondence. In one such letter to her cousin, she said, "There is nothing that makes my heart thrill like the voice of birds, much more than the human voice. It is the angels calling us with their songs." After her extraordinary acclaim resulting from her heroic actions during the Crimean War, numerous articles, songs, and poems of praise were written that linked Nightingale's compassion to the beautiful song of a nightingale. One such broadside that circulated after the war was published anonymously by *Punch* magazine entitled "The Nightingale's Song to the Sick Soldier." A broadside was a song or poem that was written to reflect the feelings and sentiment of the community.

The title of this poem is used as a metaphor for Nightingale's contribution to the war as a beautiful song. Last summer while preparing to enter nursing school, I volunteered at a hospital where my job was to help conduct recreational activities for the patients on the hospice ward. My favorite part of the day was when I got the chance to sing hymns to the patients. They would reach their hands out to me and smile. The nurses often remarked that many of these patients had not smiled in weeks. I was able to use singing as a way to touch the souls of the sick and bring comfort to those who were sad. After realizing how the singing touched my patients, I thought about how I could integrate singing, my other profession, into my nursing practice as a way to focus on the needs of the soul and the body. I believe that a nurse can communicate the joy that is inside us to the patient through the use of music as an act of compassion.

In this poem, Nightingale's legacy as a model, compassionate caregiver is conveyed through singing and the song of a nightingale. A song that was to keep a weary soldier alive and hopeful. It is this song that should be kept in the hearts of each nurse. It should radiate outwardly to "infect" all those around and emit a joyful spirit that is highly contagious.

Shandi Shiver, Senior BSN Nursing Student
Professional singer
The University of Southern Mississippi
School of Nursing

An African nurse from Jamaica, Mary Grant Seacole, offered her services to Nightingale after hearing of the need for nurses in Scutari. Although Nightingale rejected Seacole as a part of her nursing staff, Seacole persisted in her passion to provide care to the British military (Payne, 1999). Using her own money, she set up a type of inn that provided food and lodging for soldiers and their families near Scutari (Hine, 1989). Although Seacole is less well known than Nightingale, her contributions to nursing in wartime were significant in the history of minority nursing. Seacole is often referred to as "the other lady with the lamp" and "the Florence Nightingale of Jamaica." The School of Nursing in Kingston, Jamaica, is today named in her honor (Crawford, 1992).

Scores of books and articles have been written about Nightingale—she is an almost mythic figure in history. She truly was a beloved legend throughout Great Britain by the time she left the Crimea in July 1856, 4 months after the war ended. Longfellow immortalized this "Lady with the Lamp" in his poem of "Santa Filomena" (Longfellow, 1857).

Returning Home a Heroine: The Political Reformer

When Nightingale returned to London, she found that her efforts to provide comfort and health to the British soldier succeeded in making heroes of both Nightingale and the soldiers (Woodham-Smith, 1951). Both had suffered from negative stereotypes: The soldier was often portrayed as a drunken oaf with little ambition or honor; the nurse was perceived as a tipsy, self-serving, illiterate, promiscuous loser. After the Crimean War and the efforts of Nightingale and her nurses, both returned with honor and dignity, never more to be downtrodden and disrespected.

After her return from the Crimea, Florence Nightingale never made a public appearance, never attended a public function, and never issued a public statement (Bullough & Bullough, 1978). Even so, she single-handedly raised nursing from, as she put it, "the sink it was" into a respected and noble profession (Palmer, 1977). As an avid scholar and student of the Greek writer Plato, Nightingale believed that she had a moral obligation to work primarily for the good of the community. Because she believed that education formed character, she insisted that nursing must go beyond care for the sick; the mission of the trained nurse must include social reform to promote the good. This dual mission of nursing—caregiver and political reformer—has shaped the profession as we know it today, especially in the field of community health nursing. LeVasseur (1998) contends that Nightingale's insistence on nursing's involvement of a larger political ideal in the historical foundation of the field distinguishes us from other scientific disciplines, such as medicine.

How did Nightingale accomplish this transformation? You will learn throughout this text how nurses effect change through others. Florence Nightingale is the standard by which we measure our effectiveness. She effected change through her wide command of acquaintances: Queen Victoria was a significant admirer of her intellect and ability to effect change, and she used her position as national heroine to get the attention of elected officials in Parliament. She was tireless and had an amazing capacity for work. She used people (Bostridge, 2008). Everyone who could be of service to her was enlisted to help her meet her goals. Her brother-in-law, Sidney Herbert, was a member of Parliament and often delivered her "messages" in the form of legislation. When Nightingale wanted the public incited, she turned to the press, writing letters to the *London Times* and having others of influence write articles. She was not above threats to "go public" by certain dates if an elected official refused to establish a commission or appoint a committee. And when those commissions were formed, Nightingale was ready with her list of selected people for appointment (Palmer, 1982).

Nightingale and Military Reforms

The first real test of Nightingale's military reforms came in the United States during the "War Between the States"—the Civil War. Nightingale was asked by the Union to advise on the organization of hospitals and care of the sick and wounded. She sent recommendations back to the United States based on her experiences and analysis in the Crimean War, and her advisement and influence gained wide publicity. Following her recommendations, the Union Army set up a sanitary commission and provided for regular inspection of camps. Nightingale also expressed a desire to help with the Confederate military but, unfortunately, had no channel of communication with them (Bullough & Bullough, 1978).

The Nightingale School of Nursing at St. Thomas: The Birth of Professional Nursing

The British public honored Nightingale by endowing 50,000 pounds in her name upon her return to England from the Crimea. The money had been raised from the soldiers under her care and donations from the public. This Nightingale Fund eventually was used to create the **Nightingale School of Nursing at St. Thomas**, which was to be the beginning of professional nursing (Donahue, 1985).

Nightingale, at the age of 40, decided that St. Thomas's Hospital was the place for her training school for nurses. While the negotiations for the school went forward, she spent her time writing *Notes on Nursing: What It Is and What It Is Not*, which was published in 1859 (Bostridge, 2008). The small book of 77 pages, written for the British mother, was an instant success. An expanded library edition was written for nurses and used as the textbook for the students at St. Thomas. The book has since been translated into multiple languages, although it is believed that Nightingale refused all royalties earned from the publication of the book (Cook, 1913).

The nursing students chosen for the new training school were handpicked; they had to be of good moral character, sober, and honest. Nightingale believed that the strong emphasis on morals was critical to gaining respect for the new "Nightingale nurse," with no possible ties to the disgraceful association of past nurses. Nursing students were monitored throughout their 1-year program both on and off the hospital grounds; their activities were carefully watched for character weaknesses, and discipline was severe and swift for violators. Accounts from Nightingale's journals and notes revealed instant dismissal of nursing students for such behaviors as "flirtation, using the eyes unpleasantly and being in the company of unsavory persons." Nightingale contended that "the future of nursing depends on how these young women behave themselves" (Smith, 1934, p. 234). She knew that experiment at St. Thomas to educate nurses and raise nursing to a moral and professional calling represented a drastic departure from the past images of nurses and would take extraordinary women of high moral character and intelligence. Nightingale knew every nursing student (called a probationer), personally, often having the students at her house for weekend visits. She devised a system of daily journal keeping for the probationers; Nightingale herself read the journals monthly to evaluate their character and work habits. Every nursing student admitted to St. Thomas had to submit an acceptable "letter of good character," and Nightingale herself placed graduate nurses in approved nursing positions (Nightingale, 1915).

One of the most important features of the Nightingale School was its relative autonomy. Both the school and the hospital nursing service were organized under the head matron. This was especially significant because it meant that nursing service began independently of the medical staff in selecting, retaining, and disciplining students and nurses (Bullough & Bullough, 1978; Nightingale, 1915).

Nightingale was opposed to the use of a standardized government examination and the movement for licensure of trained nurses. She believed that schools of nursing would lose control of educational standards with the advent of national licensure, most notably those standards related to moral character. Nightingale led a staunch opposition to the movement by the British Nurses Association (BNA) for licensure of trained nurses, which the BNA believed critical to protecting the public's safety by ensuring the qualification of nurses by licensure exam. Nightingale was convinced that qualifying a nurse by examination tested only the acquisition of technical skills, not the equally important evaluation of character. She believed nursing involved "divergencies too great for a single standard to be applied" (Nutting & Dock, 1907; Woodham-Smith, 1951).

> I look to the day when there are no nurses to the sick but only nurses to the well.
>
> —*Florence Nightingale, 1893*

Taking Health Care to the Community: Nightingale and Wellness

Early efforts to distinguish hospital from community health nursing include Nightingale's views on "health nursing," which she distinguished from "sick nursing." She wrote two influential papers: "Sick-Nursing and Health-Nursing," which was read in the United States at the Chicago Exposition in 1893, and "Health Teaching in Towns and Villages" in 1894 (Monteiro, 1985). Both papers praised the success of prevention-based nursing practice. Winslow (1946) acknowledged Nightingale's influence in the United States by being one of the first in the field of public health to recognize the importance of taking responsibility for one's own health. As she wrote in 1891, "there are more people to pick us up and help us stand on our own two feet" (Attewell, 1996). According to Palmer (1982), Nightingale was a leader in the wellness movement long before the concept was identified. Nightingale saw the nurse as the key figure in establishing a healthy society, and she envisioned a logical extension of nursing in acute hospital settings to the broadest sense of community used in nursing today. Writing in *Notes on Nursing*, she visualized the nurse as "the nation's first bulwark in health maintenance, the promotion of wellness, and the prevention of disease" (Palmer, 1982, p. 6).

William Rathbone, a wealthy ship owner and philanthropist, is credited with the establishment of the first visiting nurse service, which eventually evolved into district nursing in the community. He was so impressed with the private-duty nursing care that his sick wife had received at home that he set out to develop a "district nursing service" in Liverpool, England. At his own expense, in 1859, he developed a corps of nurses who were trained to care for the sick poor in their homes (Bullough & Bullough, 1978; Howse, 2007; Minkowski, 1992). He divided the community into 16 districts; each was assigned a nurse and a social worker who provided nursing and health education. Rathbone's experiment in district nursing was so successful that he was unable to find enough nurses to work in the districts. Rathbone then contacted Nightingale for assistance. Her recommendation was to train more nurses, and she advised Rathbone to approach the Royal Liverpool Infirmary with a proposal for opening another training school for nurses (Rathbone, 1890). The infirmary agreed to Rathbone's proposal, and district nursing soon spread throughout England as successful "health nursing" in the community for the sick poor through voluntary agencies (Rosen, 1958).

Ever the visionary, Nightingale (1893) contended that "Hospitals are but an intermediate stage of civilization. The ultimate aim is to nurse the sick poor in their own homes" (Attewell, 1996). She also wrote in regard to visiting families at home (1894), "We must not talk to them or at them but with them" (Attewell, 1996). A service similar to that begun by Rathbone, **health visiting**, began in Manchester, England, in 1862 by the Manchester and Salford Sanitary Association. The purpose of placing "health visitors" in the home was to provide health information and instruction to families. Eventually, health visitors evolved to provide preventive health education and district nurses to care for the sick at home (Bullough & Bullough, 1978; Howse, 2007).

Nightingale's Legacy

When Nightingale returned to London after the Crimean War, she remained haunted by her experiences related to the soldiers dying of preventable diseases. She was troubled by nightmares and had difficulty sleeping in the years that followed. She wrote in her journal: "Oh my poor men; I am a bad mother to come home and leave you in your Crimean graves. . . . I can never forget. . . . I stand at the altar of the murdered men and while I live, I fight their cause" (Woodham-Smith, 1983, pp. 178, 193). Nightingale became a prolific writer and a staunch defender of the causes of the British soldier, sanitation in England and India, and trained nursing.

As a woman, Nightingale was not able to hold an official government post or to vote. Historians have had varied opinions about the exact nature of the disability that kept her homebound for the remainder of her life. Recent scholars have speculated that she experienced post-traumatic stress disorder from her experiences in the Crimea; there is also considerable evidence that she suffered from the painful disease brucellosis (Barker, 1989; Nightingale, 1915; Young, 1995). Nevertheless, Nightingale exerted incredible influence through friends and acquaintances, directing from her sickroom sanitation and poor law reform. Her mission to "cleanse" spread from the military to the British Empire; her fight for improved sanitation both at home and in India consumed her energies for the remainder of her life (Vicinus & Nergaard, 1990).

According to Monteiro (1985), two recurrent themes are found throughout Nightingale's writings about disease prevention and wellness outside the hospital. *The most persistent theme is that nurses must be trained differently and instructed specifically in district and instructive nursing.* Nightingale consistently wrote that the "health nurse" must be trained in the nature of poverty and its influence on health, something she referred to as the "pauperization" of the poor. She also believed that above all, health nurses must be good teachers about hygiene and helping families learn to better care for themselves (Nightingale, 1893). She insisted that untrained, "good intended women" could not substitute for nursing care in the home. Instead, Nightingale pushed for an extensive orientation and additional training, including prior hospital experience, before someone was hired as a district nurse. She outlined the qualifications in her paper "On Trained Nursing for the Sick Poor," in which she called for 1 month's "trial" in district nursing, 1 year's training in hospital nursing, and 3 to 6 months training in district nursing (Monteiro, 1985). According to Nightingale, "There is no such thing as amateur nursing."

The second theme that emerged from her writings was the focus on the role of the nurse. *Nightingale clearly distinguished the role of the health nurse in promoting what we today call self-care.* In the past, philanthropic visitors under the aegis of Christian charity would visit the homes of the poor and offer them relief (Monteiro, 1985). Nightingale believed that such activities did little to teach the poor to care for themselves and further "pauperized" them—keeping them dependent and vulnerable, unhealthy, prone to disease, and reliant on others to keep them healthy. The nurse had to help the families at home manage a healthy environment for themselves, and Nightingale saw a trained nurse as being the only person who could pull off such a feat. She stated, "Never think that you have done anything effectual in nursing in London, till you nurse not only the sick poor in workhouses, but those at home."

Although Nightingale is best known for her reform of hospitals and military health care, she was a great believer in the future of health care, which she anticipated should be preventive in nature and would more than likely take place in the home and community. Her accomplishments in the field of "sanitary nursing" extended beyond the walls of the hospital to include workhouse reform and community sanitation reform. In 1864, Nightingale and Rathbone once again worked together to lead the reform of the Liverpool Workhouse Infirmary, where more than 1,200 sick paupers were crowded into unsanitary and unsafe conditions (Bostridge, 2008). Under the British Poor Laws, the most desperately poor of the large cities were gathered into large workhouses. When they became sick, they were also sent to the workhouse. Trained nursing care in these venues was all but nonexistent. Through legislative pressure and a well-designed public campaign describing the horrors of the workhouse infirmary, reform of the workhouse system was accomplished by 1867. Although it was not as complete as Nightingale had wanted, nevertheless nurses were in place and being paid a salary (Nightingale, 1915; Seymer, 1954).

ETHICAL CONNECTION 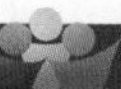

There are five essential points in securing the health of houses:

Pure air
Pure water
Efficient drainage
Cleanliness
Light

Sources: Nightingale, F. (1860). *Notes on nursing: What it is and what it is not.* London: Harrison; Cook, 1913, p. 133.

> To set these poor sick people going again, with a sound and clean house, as well as with a sound body and mind, is about as great a benefit as can be given them—worth acres of gifts and relief. This is depauperizing them."
>
> —*Florence Nightingale*

> My view you know is that the ultimate destination of all nursing is the nursing of the sick in their own homes. . . . I look to the abolition of all hospitals and workhouse infirmaries. But no use to talk about the year 2000.
>
> —*Florence Nightingale, letter to Henry Bonham Carter, 1867*

By 1901, Nightingale lived in a world without sight or sound, leaving her unable to write. Over the next 5 years, she lost her ability to communicate and most days existed in a state of unconsciousness. In November 1907, Nightingale was honored with the Order of Merit by King Edward VII, the first time the award was ever given to a woman. In May 1910, the Nightingale Training School of Nursing at St. Thomas celebrated its Jubilee. By that time, there were now more than 1,000 training schools for nurses in the United States alone (Cook, 1913).

Nightingale died in her sleep around noon on August 13, 1910, and was buried quietly and without pomp near the family's home at Embley, her coffin carried by six sergeants of the British Army (Bostridge, 2008).

Only a small cross marks her grave at her request: "FN. Born 1820. Died 1910." (Brown, 1988). The family refused a national funeral and burial at Westminster Abbey out of respect for Nightingale's last wishes. She had lived for 90 years and 3 months.

> Money would be better spent in maintaining health in infancy and childhood than in building hospitals to cure disease.
>
> —*Florence Nightingale, 1894*

> It is cheaper to promote health than to maintain people in sickness.
>
> —*Florence Nightingale, 1894*

A DAY IN THE LIFE

Barbara Dossey

Barbara Dossey is a noted Nightingale scholar and the author of the book *Florence Nightingale: Mystic, Visionary, Healer* (Philadelphia, PA: Lippincott Williams & Wilkins, 2000).

Was Nightingale a mystic? Mysticism is often defined as an individual's direct, unmediated experience of God. A mystic is a person who has such an experience, to a greater or lesser degree. Nightingale received her first call from God at age 16 and received three more direct calls from God in her life. She believed the messages of Christianity, but was tolerant and ecumenical in her attitude toward world religions. She wrote, "To know God we must study Him in the Pagan and Jewish dispensations as in the Christian."

Source: Creative Nursing by Creative Nursing Management, Inc. Reproduced with permission of Creative Nursing Management, Inc. in the format Book via Copyright Clearance Center.

Early Nursing Education and Organization in the United States

In the United States, the first training schools for nursing were modeled after the Nightingale School of Nursing at St. Thomas in London. Bellevue Training School for Nurses in New York City; Connecticut Training School for Nurses in New Haven, Connecticut; and the Boston Training School for Nurses at Massachusetts General Hospital in Boston were the earliest programs for trained nurses in the United States (Nutting & Dock, 1907). Based on the Victorian belief in the natural affinity for women to be sensitive, possess high morals, and be caregivers, early nursing training required that applicants be female. Sensitivity, high moral character, purity of character, subservience, and "ladylike" behavior became the associated traits of a "good nurse," thus setting the "feminization of nursing" as the ideal standard for a good nurse. These historical roots of gender- and race-based caregiving excluded males and minorities from the nursing profession, a trend that continued for many years and still influences career choices for men and women today. These early training schools provided a stable, subservient, white female workforce, as student nurses served as the primary nursing staff for these early hospitals.

A significant report, known simply as the **Goldmark Report** (more formally, *Nursing and Nursing Education in the United States*), was released in 1922; it advocated the establishment of university schools of nursing to train nursing leaders. The report, initiated by Nutting in 1918, was an exhaustive (500-page) and comprehensive investigation into the state of nursing education and training. Author Josephine Goldmark, a social worker and pioneer in research into nursing preparation in the United States, stated:

> From our field study of the nurse in public health nursing, in private duty, and as instructor and supervisor in hospitals, it is clear that there is need of a basic undergraduate training for all nurses alike, which should lead to a nursing diploma. (Goldmark, 1923, p. 35)

The first university school of nursing was established at the University of Minnesota in 1909. Although the new nurse training school was under the college of medicine and offered only a 3-year diploma, the Minnesota program nevertheless represented a significant leap forward in nursing education.

Nursing for the Future (the so-called Brown Report), authored by Esther Lucille Brown in 1948 and sponsored by the Russell Sage Foundation, was critical of the quality and structure of nursing schools in the United States. The Brown Report ultimately became the catalyst for the implementation of educational nursing program accreditation through the National League for Nursing (NLN; Brown, 1936, 1948).

Positive changes also occurred for minority and male nurses. As a result of the post–World War II nursing shortage, the associate degree in nursing (ADN) was established by Mildred Montag in 1952 as a 2-year program for registered nurses (Montag, 1959). In 1950, nursing became the first profession for which the same licensure exam, the State Board Test Pool, was used throughout the nation to license registered nurses (RNs). This increased mobility for the registered nurse resulted in a significant advantage for the relatively new profession of nursing (State Board Test Pool Examination, 1952).

THINK ABOUT THIS

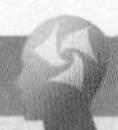

Some nurses believe that the legacy of Florence Nightingale is holding nursing back and represents the negative and backward elements of nursing. This view cites as evidence Nightingale's support for the subordination of nurses to physicians, opposition to registration of nurses, and failure to see mental health nurses as part of the profession. Wheeler has gone so far as to say, "The nursing profession needs to exorcise the myth of Nightingale, not necessarily because she was a bad person, but because the impact of her legacy has held the profession back too long." After reading this chapter, what do you think? Is Nightingale relevant in the 21st century to the nursing profession? Why or why not?

Source: Wheeler, W. (1999). Is Florence Nightingale holding us back? *Nursing 99, 29*(10), 82–23.

> Preventable disease should be looked upon as a social crime.
>
> —*Florence Nightingale, 1894*

The Evolution of Nursing in the United States: The First Century of Professional Nursing

Early nurse leaders of the century included **Isabel Hampton Robb**, who in 1896 founded the Nurses' Associated Alumnae. In 1911, this organization officially became known as the **American Nurses Association (ANA)**. **Lavinia Lloyd Dock** was a militant suffragist who linked women's roles as nurses to the emerging women's movement in the United States. By contrast, Isabel Hampton Robb—like Nightingale herself—opposed the women's suffragist movement, instead focusing on the need for women to own property in Great Britain. Her well-reasoned position was that property ownership was the link to women's voting power.

Mary Adelaide Nutting, Lavinia Lloyd Dock, Sophia Palmer, and Mary E. Davis were instrumental in developing the first nursing journal, ***American Journal of Nursing (AJN)***, in October 1900. Through the ANA and the *AJN*, nurses then had a professional organization and a national journal with which to communicate with one another (Kalisch & Kalisch, 1986).

State licensure of trained nurses began in 1903 with the enactment of North Carolina's licensure law for nursing. Shortly thereafter, New Jersey, New York, and Virginia passed similar licensure law for nursing. Professional nursing was well on its way to public recognition of practice and educational standards, as state after state passed similar legislation over the next several years.

Margaret Sanger worked as a nurse on the Lower East Side of New York City in 1912 with immigrant families. She was astonished to find widespread ignorance among these families about conception, pregnancy, and childbirth. After a horrifying experience with the death of a woman from a failed self-induced abortion, Sanger devoted her life to teaching women about birth control. A staunch activist in the early family planning movement, Sanger is credited with founding Planned Parenthood of America (Sanger, 1928).

THINK ABOUT THIS

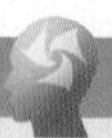

There have been many theories about the cause of Nightingale's chronic illness, which led to her being an invalid for most of her adult life. Many people have interpreted her condition as hypochondriacal, something of a melodrama of the Victorian times. Nightingale was rich and could take to her bed. Rumors have floated around among nursing students for years that she suffered from tertiary syphilis. She became ill during the Crimean War in May 1855 and was diagnosed with a severe case of Crimean fever. Today Crimean fever is recognized as Mediterranean fever and is categorized as brucellosis. Nightingale also developed ankylosing spondylitis, or inflammation of the spine.

For the next 34 years, Nightingale managed to continue her writing and advocacy, often predicting her imminent death. Some have claimed that she suffered from bipolar disorder, causing her to experience long periods of depression and remarkable bursts of productivity. Read about the various theories of her chronic disabling condition and reflect on your own conclusions about her mysterious illness.

Sources: Dossey, B. (2000). *Florence Nightingale: Mystic, visionary, healer* (Philadelphia, PA: Lippincott Williams & Wilkins); Nightingale suffered bipolar disorder. (2004). *Australian Nursing Journal, 12*, 2.

> As the modern nursing movement is emphatically an outcome of the original and general woman's movement . . . it would be a great pity for them [nurses] to allow one of the most remarkable movements of the day to go on under their eyes without comprehending it. . . . Unless we possess the ballot we shall not know when we may get up in the morning to find all that we had gained has been taken from us.
>
> —*Lavinia Lloyd Dock, 1907*

MEDIA MOMENT 

African American Nurses in History

Read more about the contributions of African American nurses . . .

Alexander, Z., & Dewjee, A. (1981). Mary Seacole. *History Today, 31*, 45.

Bell, P. L. (1993). "Making do" with the midwife: Arkansas's Mamie O. Hale in the 1940s. *Nursing History Review, 1*, 155–169.

Brewman, M. P. (1952). The Negro nurse. *Nation, 175*(8), 160.

Buhler-Wilkerson, K. (1992). Caring in its "proper place": Race and benevolence in Charleston, SC, 1813–1930. *Nursing Research, 41*(1), 14–20.

Campinha-Bacote, J. (1988). The Black nurses' struggle toward equality: An historical account of the National Association of Colored Graduate Nurses. *Journal of National Black Nurses Association, 2*(2), 15–25.

Carnegie, M. E. (1992). Black nurses in the United States: 1879–1992. *Journal of National Black Nurses Association, 6*(1), 13–18.

Chayer, M. E. (1954). Mary Eliza Mahoney. *American Journal of Nursing, 54*(4), 429–431.

Davis A. T. (1999). *Early black American leaders in nursing: Architects for integration and equality.* (National League for Nursing Series.) Sudbury, MA: Jones and Bartlett.

Doona, M. E. (1986). Glimpses of Mary Eliza Mahoney (7 May 1845–4 January 1929). *Journal of Nursing History, 1*(2), 20–34.

Elmore, J. A. (1976). Black nurses: Their service and their struggle. *American Journal of Nursing, 76*(3), 435–437.

George, V. D., Bradford, D. M., & Battle, A. (2000). Yesterday, today, and tomorrow: Transitioning through time with the Cleveland Council of Black Nurses. *Nursing & Health Care Perspectives, 21*(5), 219–227.

Goldstein, R. L. (1960). Negro nurses in hospitals. *American Journal of Nursing, 60*(2), 215–217.

Mabel Staupers, who led battle to end prejudice, dies at 99. (1990). *American Journal of Nursing, 9*(2), 121.

Mosley, M. O. P. (1995). Beginning at the beginning: A history of the professionalization of black nurses in America, 1908–1951. *Journal of Cultural Diversity, 2*(4), 101–109.

Mosley, M. O. P. (1995). Despite all odds: A three-part history of the professionalization of black nurses through two professional nursing organizations, 1908–1955. *Journal of National Black Nurses Association, 7*(2), 10–20.

Mosley, M. O. P. (1995). Mabel K. Staupers: A pioneer in professional nursing. *N & HC Perspectives on Community, 16*(1), 12–17.

Mosley, M. O. P. (1996). A new beginning: The story of the National Association of Colored Graduate Nurses, 1908–1951. *Journal of National Black Nurses Association, 8*(1), 20–32.

Smith, S. L. (1994). White nurses, black midwives, and public health in Mississippi, 1920–1950. *Nursing History Review, 2*, 29–49.

Staupers, M. K. (1937). The Negro nurse in America. *Opportunity, 15*(11), 339–341.

Staupers, M. K. (1961). *No time for prejudice: A story of the integration of Negroes in nursing in the United States.* New York, NY: MacMillan.

Tucker-Allen, S. (1997). The founding of the Association of Black Nursing Faculty: My memories of the first five years. *ABNF Journal, 8*(4), 73–80.

Washington, B. T. (1910). Looking through the years: 1910. Training colored nurses at Tuskegee. *American Journal of Nursing, 11*, 167–171. (Reprinted by permission in *Creative Nursing: A Journal of Values, Issues, Experience & Collaboration*, 3(1), 16, 1997.)

Wilkins, R. (1943). Black women in white. *Negro Digest, 1*(6), 61–63.

By 1917, the emerging nursing profession was driven by two significant events that dramatically increased the need for additional trained nurses in the United States: World War I and the influenza epidemic. Nightingale's work and the devastation of the Civil War had firmly established the need for nursing care in war. Mary Adelaide Nutting, who became a professor of nursing and health at Columbia University, chaired the newly established Committee on Nursing in response to the call for more nurses as the United States entered the war in Europe. U.S. nurses realized early on that World War I was unlike previous wars: It was a global conflict that involved coalitions of nations against nations, involving vast amounts of supplies and demanding the organization of all the nation's resources for military purposes (Kalisch & Kalisch, 1986). Along with **Lillian Wald** and **Jane A. Delano**, director of nursing in the American Red Cross, Nutting initiated a national publicity campaign to recruit young women to enter nurse training. The Army School of Nursing, headed by **Annie Goodrich** as dean, and the Vassar Training Camp for Nurses prepared nurses for the war and for home nursing and hygiene nursing through the Red Cross (Dock & Stewart, 1931). The Committee on Nursing estimated that there were at most 200,000 active "nurses" in the United States at the beginning of World War I, both trained and untrained, which was inadequate to support the military effort abroad (Kalisch & Kalisch, 1986). At home, the influenza epidemic of 1917–1919 led to increased public awareness of the need for public health nursing and public education about hygiene and disease prevention.

The successful campaign to attract nursing students focused heavily on patriotism, which ushered in the new era for nursing as a profession. By 1918, nursing school enrollments were up by 25%. In 1920, Congress passed a bill that provided nurses with military rank (Dock & Stewart, 1931). Following close behind, the passage of the 19th Amendment to the U.S. Constitution granted women the right to vote. According to Stewart (1921):

> Probably the greatest contribution of the war experience to nursing lies in the fact that the whole system of nursing education was shaken for a little while out of its well-worn ruts and brought out of its comparative seclusion into the light of public discussion and criticism. When so many lives hung on the supply of nurses, people were aroused to a new sense of their dependence on the products of nursing schools, and many of them learned for the first time of the hopelessly limited resources which nursing educators have had to work with in the training of these indispensable public servants. Whatever the future may bring, it is unlikely that nursing schools will willingly sink back again into their old isolation or that they will accept unquestionably the financial status which the older system imposed on them. (p. 6)

While nursing as a profession was emerging in the United States, it remained a "white, female only" career choice during these early years. Men and minorities were excluded from the field, and those who wanted to enter nursing school found themselves essentially "locked out." Eventually, quotas were established in select nursing programs to permit African Americans' and other minorities' admission. Even when these nurses graduated, they had very few employment opportunities owing to segregationist policies of hospitals and other health agencies. Males faced the same challenges, and eventually schools of nursing were developed specifically for male nurse training. Early roles for male nurses were limited to psychiatric facilities, where their strength and larger stature were considered advantages in dealing with these populations.

These early discriminatory policies reflected the era but were also patterned after Nightingale's belief that nursing was best suited for women and their nurturing instinct. Nightingale did not write specifically about the inclusion of minorities in the nursing profession. However, as indicated by her attitude toward Mary Seacole (as discussed earlier in this chapter), she seemed to have a preference for white female nurses as the face of the emerging profession of nursing.

The Emergence of Community and Public Health Nursing

The pattern for health visiting and district nursing practice outside the hospital was similar in the United States to that in England (Roberts, 1954). U.S. cities were besieged by overcrowding and epidemics after the Civil War. The need for trained nurses evolved as in England, and schools throughout the United States developed along the Nightingale model. Visiting nurses were first sent to philanthropic organizations in New York City (1877), Boston (1886), Buffalo (1885), and Philadelphia (1886) to care for the sick at home. By the end of the century, most large cities had some form of visiting nursing program, and some headway was being made even in smaller towns (Heinrich, 1983). Industrial or occupational health nursing was first started in Vermont in 1895 by a marble company interested in the health and welfare of its workers and their families. Tuberculosis (TB) was a leading cause of death in the 19th century; nurses visited patients bedridden from TB and instructed persons in all settings about prevention of the disease (Abel, 1997).

Lillian Wald, Public Health Nursing, and Community Activism

Lillian Wald, a wealthy young woman with a great social conscience, graduated from the New York Hospital School of Nursing in 1891 and is credited with creating the title "public health nurse." After a year working in a mental institution, Wald entered medical school at Woman's Medical College in New York. While in medical school, she was asked to visit immigrant mothers on New York's Lower East Side and instruct them on health matters (see **Box 3-2**). Wald was appalled by the conditions there. During one now famous home visit, a small child asked Wald to visit her sick mother.

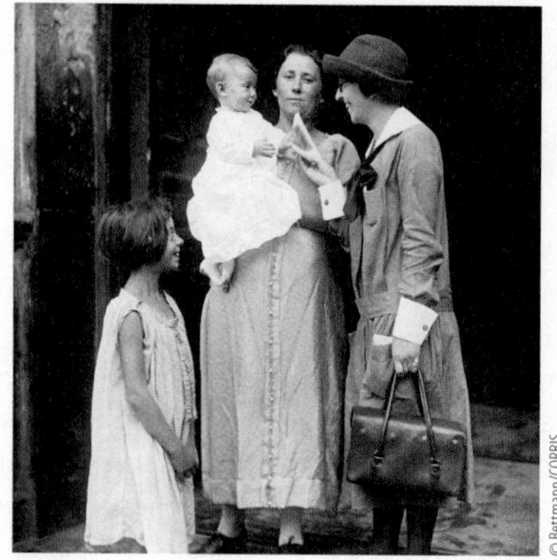

Nurse midwives in rural areas contributed to the decline in maternal and infant mortality during the 1950s.

And the rest, as they say, is history. According to Wald: "Nursing is love in action and there is no finer manifestation of it than the care of the poor and disabled in their own homes" (Wald, 1915, p. 14). What Wald found changed her life forever and secured a place for her in American nursing history. Wald said, "all the maladjustments of our social and economic relations seemed epitomized in this

BOX 3-2 Lillian Wald Takes a Walk

From the schoolroom where I had been giving a lesson in bed-making, a little girl led me one drizzling March morning. She had told me of her sick mother, and gathering from her incoherent account that a child had been born, I caught up the paraphernalia of the bed-making lesson and carried it with me.

The child led me over broken roadways . . . between tall, reeking houses whose laden fire-escapes, useless for their appointed purpose, bulged with household goods of every description. The rain added to the dismal appearance of the streets and to the discomfort of the crowds which thronged them, intensifying the odors which assailed me from every side. Through Hester and Division Streets we went to the end of Ludlow; past odorous fish-stands, for the streets were a market-place, unregulated, unsupervised, unclean, past evil-smelling, uncovered garbage cans . . .

All the maladjustments of our social and economic relations seemed epitomized in this brief journey and what was found at the end of it. The family to which the child led me was neither criminal nor vicious. Although the husband was a cripple, one of those who stand on street corners exhibiting deformities to enlist compassion, and masking the begging of alms by a pretense of selling, although the family of seven shared their two rooms with boarders—who were literally boarders, since a piece of timber was placed over the floor for them to sleep on—and although the sick woman lay on a wretched, unclean bed, soiled with a hemorrhage two days old, they were not degraded human beings, judged by any measure of moral values.

In fact, it was very plain that they were sensitive to their condition, and when, at the end of my ministrations, they kissed my hands (those who have undergone similar experiences will, I am sure, understand), it would have been some solace if by any conviction of the moral unworthiness of the family I could have defended myself as a part of a society which permitted such conditions to exist. Indeed, my subsequent acquaintance with them revealed the fact that miserable as their state was, they were not without ideals for the family life, and for society, of which they were so unloved and unlovely a part.

That morning's experience was a baptism of the fire. Deserted were the laboratory and the academic work of the college. I never returned to them. On my way from the sick-room to my comfortable student quarters my mind was intent on my own responsibility. To my inexperience it seemed certain that conditions such as these were allowed because people did not know, and for me there was a challenge to know and to tell. When early morning found me still awake, my naive conviction remained that, if people knew things—and "things" meant everything implied in the condition of this family—such horrors would cease to exist, and I rejoiced that I had a training in the care of the sick that in itself would give me an organic relationship to the neighborhood in which this awakening had come.

Source: Wald, L. D. (1915). *The House on Henry Street*. New York, NY: Henry Holt and Company.

brief journey" (p. 6). Wald was profoundly affected by her observations; she and her colleague, **Mary Brewster**, quickly established the **Henry Street Settlement** in this same neighborhood in 1893. She quit medical school and devoted the remainder of her life to "visions of a better world" for the public's health.

This effort later evolved into the Visiting Nurse Service of New York City, which laid the foundation for the establishment of public health nursing in the United States. The health needs of the population were met through addressing social, economic, and environmental determinants of health, in a pattern after Nightingale. The nurses helped educate families about disease transmission and stressed the importance of good hygiene. They provided preventive, acute, and long-term care. As such, the Henry Street Settlement went far beyond the care of the sick and the prevention of illness: It aimed at rectifying those causes that led to the poverty and misery.

Wald was a tireless social activist for legislative reforms that would provide a more just distribution for the marginal and disadvantaged in the United States (Donahue, 1985). She began her work with 10 nurses in 1893, which grew to 250 nurses serving 1,300 patients each day by 1916. During this same period, the budget for the service grew from nothing to more than $600,000 per year, all from private donations.

Wald hired African American nurse **Elizabeth Tyler** in 1906, which evidenced her commitment to cultural diversity. Although unable to visit white patients, Tyler made her own way by "finding" African American families who needed her service. In 3 months, Tyler had so many African American families in her caseload that Wald hired a second African American nurse, Edith Carter. Carter remained at Henry Street for 28 years until her retirement (Carnegie, 1991).

During her tenure at Henry Street, Wald demonstrated her commitment to racial and cultural diversity by employing 25 African American nurses over the years, and she paid them salaries equal to white nurses, and provided identical benefits and recognition to minority nurses (Carnegie, 1991). This practice was exceptional during the early part of the 20th century, a time when African American nurses were often denied admission to white schools of nursing and membership in professional organizations and were denied opportunities for employment in most settings. Because hospitals of this era often set quotas for African American patients, those nurses who managed to graduate from nursing schools found themselves with few patients who needed or could afford their services. African American nurses struggled for the right to take the registration examination available to white nurses.

Wald submitted a proposal to the city of New York after learning of a child's dismissal from a New York City school for a skin condition. Her proposal was for one of the Henry Street Settlement nurses to serve for free for 1 month in a New York school. The results of her experiment were so convincing that salaries were approved for 12 school nurses. From this beginning, school nursing was born in the United States and became one of many community specialties credited to Wald (Dietz & Lehozky, 1963).

In 1909, Wald proposed a program to the Metropolitan Life Insurance Company to provide nursing visits to its industrial policyholders. Statistics kept by the company documented the lowered mortality rates of policyholders attributed to the nurses' public health practice and clinical expertise. The program demonstrated savings for the company and was so successful that it lasted until 1953 (Hamilton, 1988).

RESEARCH ALERT

Three exceptional African American nurses—Jessie Sleet, Elizabeth Tyler, and Edith Carter—are considered pioneers in community health nursing. This research article details how these three African American community health nurses made significant contributions to the development of New York City's community health nursing by providing much-needed health care to unserved members of the African American community (1900–1937). They provided strong leadership in diverse roles such as supervisors, administrators, and educators in patients' homes, babies' health stations, settlement houses, and clinics. Their work occurred during a period of rapid industrialization, immigration, and great population growth in the midst of teeming slums, diseases, and death. In community health nursing history, it was a period of establishment, activism, expansion, and development. For these African American nurse pioneers, it was a time of significant challenges and growth. They faced educational, professional, and racial barriers and increased mortality among people of their own race. This research chronicles their brave and skilled efforts to transcend these barriers and improve the health of African American citizens during the early part of the 20th century.

Source: Mosley, M. O. (1996). Satisfied to carry the bag: Three black community health nurses' contributions to health care reform, 1900–1937. *Nursing History Review, 4,* 65–82.

Wald's other significant accomplishments include the establishment of the Children's Bureau, set up in 1912 as part of the U.S. Department of Labor. She was also an enthusiastic supporter of and participant in women's suffrage, lobbied for inspections of the workplace, and supported her employee, Margaret Sanger, in her efforts to give women the right to birth control. She was active in the American and International Red Cross and helped form the Women's Trade Union League to protect women from sweatshop conditions.

Wald first coined the phrase "public health nursing" and transformed the field of community health nursing from the narrow role of home visiting to the population focus of today's community health nurse (Robinson, 1946). According to Dock and Stewart (1931), the title of "public health nurse" was purposeful: The role designation was designed to link the public's health to governmental responsibility, not private funding. As state departments of health and local governments began to employ more and more public health nurses, their role increasingly focused on prevention of illness in the entire community. A distinction was made between the visiting nurse, who was employed by the voluntary agencies primarily to provide home care to the sick, and the public health nurse, who concentrated on preventive measures (Brainard, 1922). Early public health nurses came closer than hospital-based nurses to the autonomy and professionalism that Nightingale advocated. Their work was conducted in the unconfined setting of the home and community, they were independent, and they enjoyed recognition as specialists in preventive health (Buhler-Wilkerson, 1985). Public health nurses from the beginning were much more holistic in their practice than their hospital counterparts. They were involved with the health of industrial workers, immigrants, and their families, and were concerned about exploitation of women and children. These nurses also played a part in prison reform and care of the mentally ill (Heinrich, 1983).

Considered the first African American public health nurse, **Jessie Sleet Scales** was hired in 1902 by the Charity Organization Society, a philanthropic organization, to visit African American families infected by TB. Scales provided district nursing care to New York City's African American families and is credited with paving the way for African American nurses in the practice of community health (Mosley, 1996).

Dorothea Lynde Dix

Dorothea Lynde Dix, a Boston schoolteacher, became aware of the horrendous conditions in prisons and mental institutions when asked to conduct a Sunday school class in the House of Correction at Cambridge, Massachusetts.

She was appalled at what she saw and went about studying if the conditions were isolated or widespread; she took 2 years off to visit every jail and almshouse from Cape Cod to the Berkshire Mountains (Tiffany, 1890, p. 76). Her report was devastating. Boston was scandalized by the reality that the most progressive state in the union was now associated with such horrible conditions. The shocked legislature voted to allocate funds to build hospitals. For the rest of her life, Dorothea Dix stood out as a tireless zealot for the humane treatment of the insane and imprisoned. She had exceptional savvy in dealing with legislators: She acquainted herself with the legislators and their records and displayed the "spirit of a crusader." For her contributions, she is considered one of the pioneers of the reform movement in the United States, and her efforts are felt worldwide to the present day (Dietz & Lehozky, 1963).

Dix was also known for her work in the Civil War, having been appointed superintendent of the female nurses of the Army by the secretary of war in 1861. Her tireless efforts led to the recruitment of more than 2,000 women to serve in the Army during the Civil War. Officials had consulted Florence Nightingale concerning conditions in military hospitals and were determined not to make the same mistakes. Dix enjoyed far more sweeping powers than Nightingale, in that she had the authority to organize hospitals, to appoint nurses, and to manage supplies for the wounded (Brockett & Vaughan, 1867). Among her most well-known nurses during the Civil War were the poet Walt Whitman and the author Louisa May Alcott (Donahue, 1985).

Clara Barton

The idea for the International Red Cross was the brainchild of a Swiss banker, J. Henri Dunant, who proposed the formation of a neutral international relief society that could be activated in time of war. The International Red Cross was ratified by the Geneva Convention on August 22, 1864.

Clara Barton, through her work in the Civil War, had come to believe that such an organization was desperately needed in the United States. However, it was not until 1882 that Barton was able to convince Congress to ratify the Treaty of Geneva, thus becoming the founder of the American Red Cross (Kalisch & Kalisch, 1986). Barton also played a leadership role in the Spanish–American War in Cuba, where she led a group of nurses to provide care for both U.S. and Cuban soldiers and Cuban civilians. At the age of 76, Barton went to President McKinley and offered the help of the Red Cross in Cuba. McKinley agreed to allow Barton to go with Red Cross nurses, but only to care for the Cuban citizens. Once in Cuba, the U.S. military saw what Barton and her nurses were able to accomplish with the Cuban military, and American soldiers pressured military officials to allow Barton's help. Along with battling yellow fever, Barton was able to provide care to both Cuban and U.S. military personnel and eventually expanded that care to Cuban citizens in Santiago. One of Barton's most famous patients was young Colonel Teddy Roosevelt, who later became the president of the United States.

Barton became an instant heroine both in Cuba and in the United States for her bravery, tenaciousness, and organized services for the military and civilians torn apart by war. On August 13, 1898, the Spanish–American War came to an end. The grateful people of Santiago, Cuba, built a statue to honor Clara Barton in the town square, where it stands to this day. Tales of the work of Barton and her Red Cross nurses were spread through the newspapers of the United States and in the schools of nursing. A congressional committee investigating the work of Barton's Red Cross staff applauded the work of these nurses and recommended that the U.S. Medical Department create a permanent reserve corps of trained nurses. These reserve nurses became the Army Nurse Corps in 1901.

Barton also led the disaster recovery of the deadliest natural disaster in U.S. history, which surpassed even the recent Hurricane Katrina in its devastating death toll. On September 8, 1900, before hurricanes were even named, a vast storm with wind speeds exceeding 140 miles per hour blew into Galveston Bay. In 24 hours, wind and water had killed an estimated 6,000 people and destroyed an estimated 6,000 buildings. There was no federal help or resources, and the grieving survivors were faced with a federal government that "didn't do" relief for disasters. The only resources came from outside private donors, churches, and philanthropic organizations—and Clara Barton and her Red Cross nurses. One-sixth of the city's population was dead, and the sandbar of Galveston had no place to bury them. Clara Barton arrived on the scene quickly, and she organized efforts to comfort the survivors and provide healthcare services and community-based relief (Baker, 2006).

Clara Barton will always be remembered both as the founder of the American Red Cross and the driving force behind the creation of the Army Nurse Corps.

Birth of the Midwife in the United States

Women have always assisted other women in the birth of babies. These "lay midwives" were considered by communities to possess special skills and somewhat of a "calling." With the advent of professional nursing in England, registered nurses became associated with safer and more predictable childbirth practices. In England and in other countries where Nightingale-system nurses were prevalent, most registered nurses were also trained as midwives with a 6-month specialized training period. In the United States, the training of registered nurses in the practice of midwifery was prevented primarily by physicians. U.S. physicians saw midwives as a threat and an intrusion into medical practice. Such resistance indirectly led to the proliferation of "granny wives" who were ignorant of modern practices, were untrained, and were associated with high maternal morbidity (Donahue, 1985).

The first organized midwifery service in the United States was the **Frontier Nursing Service** founded in 1925 by **Mary Breckenridge.** Breckenridge graduated from St. Luke's Hospital Training School in New York in 1910 and received her midwifery certificate from the British Hospital for Mothers and Babies in London in 1925. She had extensive experience in the delivery of babies and midwifery systems in New Zealand and Australia. In rural Appalachia, babies had been delivered for decades by granny midwives, who relied mainly on tradition, myths, and superstition as the bases of their practice. For example, they might use ashes for medication and place a sharp axe, blade up, under the bed of a laboring woman to "cut" the pain. The people of Appalachia were isolated because of the terrain of the hollows and mountains, and roads were limited to most families. They also had one of the highest birth rates in the United States. Breckenridge believed that if a midwifery service could work under these conditions, it could work anywhere (Donahue, 1985).

Breckenridge had to use English midwives for many years and only began training her own midwives in 1939, when she started the Frontier Graduate School of Nurse Midwifery in Hyden, Kentucky, with the advent of World War II. The nurse midwives accessed many of their families on horseback. In 1935, a small 12-bed hospital was built at Hyden and provided delivery services. The nurse midwives under the direction of Breckenridge were successful in lowering the highest maternal mortality rate in the United States (in Leslie County, Kentucky) to substantially below the national average. These nurses, as at the Henry Street Settlement, provided health care for everyone in the district for a small annual fee. A delivery was assessed an additional small fee. Nurse midwives provided primary care, prenatal care, and postnatal care, with an emphasis on prevention (Wertz & Wertz, 1977).

The "Roaring Twenties" ushered American women—newly armed with the right to vote—into the new freedom of the "flapper era"—shrinking dress hemlines, shortened hairstyles, and the increased use of cosmetics. Hospitals were used by greater numbers of people, and the scientific basis of medicine became well established as most surgical procedures were done in hospitals. Penicillin was discovered in 1928, creating a revolution in the prevention of infectious disease deaths (Donahue, 1985; Kalisch & Kalisch, 1986). The previously mentioned Goldmark Report recommended the establishment of college- and university-based nursing programs.

Mary D. Osborne, who functioned as supervisor of public health nursing for the state of Mississippi from 1921 to 1946, had a vision for a collaboration with community nurses and granny midwives, who delivered 80% of the African American babies in Mississippi. The infant and maternal mortality rates were exceptionally high among African American families, and these granny midwives, who were also African American, were untrained and had little education.

Osborne took a creative approach to improving maternal and infant health among African American women. She developed a collaborative network of public health nurses and granny midwives in which the nurses implemented training programs for the midwives, and the midwives in turn assisted the nurses in providing a higher standard of safe maternal and infant health care. The public health nurses used Osborne's book, *Manual for Midwives*, which contained guidelines for care and was used in the state until the 1970s. They taught good hygiene, infection prevention, and compliance with state regulations. Osborne's innovative program is credited with reducing the maternal and infant mortality rates in Mississippi and in other states where her program structure was adopted (Sabin, 1998).

The Nursing Profession Responds to the Great Depression and World War II

With the stock market crash of 1929 came the Great Depression, which resulted in widespread unemployment of private-duty nurses and the closing of nursing schools, while simultaneously creating an increasing need for charity health services for the population. Nursing students, who had previously been the primary source of staff for hospitals, became scarcer. Unemployed graduate nurses were hired to replace them for minimal wages, a trend that was to influence the profession for years to come (MacEachern, 1932).

Other nurses found themselves accompanying troops to Europe as the United States entered World War II. Military nurses were a critical presence at the invasion of Normandy in 1938, as well as in North Africa, Italy, France, and the Philippines, where Navy nurses provided care aboard hospital ships. More than 100,000 nurses volunteered and were certified for military service in the Army and Navy Nurse Corps.

The resulting severe shortage of nurses on the home front resulted in the development of the **Cadet Nurse Corps. Frances Payne Bolton**, a Congresswoman from Ohio, is credited with the founding of the Cadet Nurse Corps through the Bolton Act of 1945. By the end of the war, more than 180,000 nursing students had been trained through this Act, while advanced practice graduate nurses in psychiatry and public health nursing had received graduate education to increase the numbers of nurse educators (Donahue, 1985; Kalisch & Kalisch, 1986).

Ernie Pyle, a famous correspondent in World War II, offered Americans a "front-seat view" of the war through his detailed journalistic accounts of daily life on the front. Pyle was the first journalist who put his own life in danger by reporting from the battlefront; he spent a great deal of time with soldiers during active combat and was killed during a sniper attack in Ie Shima, Japan, in 1942. Chaplin Nathan Baxter Saucier was assigned to retrieve his body, conduct his service, and assist the soldiers with building his coffin. The funeral service lasted only about 10 minutes. Pyle was buried with his helmet on, at Saucier's request. The Navy, Marine Corps, and Army were all represented at the service. Pyle was a highly regarded and humanistic voice for those serving America during World War II. Here is an example of his accounts of life for nurses in a field hospital in Europe:

> The officers and nurses live two in a tent on two sides of a company street—nurses on one side, officers on the other. . . . The nurses wear khaki overalls because of the mud and dust. Pink female panties fly from a line among the brown warlike tents. On the flagpole is a Red Cross flag made from a bed sheet and a French soldier's red sash. The American nurses—and there were lots of them—turned out just as you would expect: wonderfully. Army doctors and patients too were unanimous in their praise of them. . . . Doctors told me that in the first rush of casualties they were calmer than the men. For the first ten days they had to live like animals, even using open ditches for toilets but they never complained. One nurse was always on duty in each tentful of 20 men. She had medical orderlies to help her. The touch of femininity, the knowledge that a woman was around, gave the wounded man courage and confidence and a feeling of security. (Pyle, 1944)

During the midst of the Depression, many nurses found that the expansion and advances in aviation opened up a new field for nurses. In an effort to increase the public's confidence in the safety of transcontinental air travel, nurses were hired in the promising new role of "nurse-stewardess" (Kalisch & Kalisch, 1986). Congress created an additional relief program, the Civil Works Administration (CWA), in 1933 that provided jobs to the unemployed, including placing nurses in schools, public hospitals and clinics, public health departments, and public health education community surveys and campaigns.

The Social Security Act of 1935 was also passed by Congress to provide old-age benefits, rehabilitation services, unemployment compensation administration, aid to dependent and/or disabled children and adults, and monies to state and local health services. The Social Security Act included Title VI, which authorized the use of federal funds for the training of public health personnel. This led to the placement of public health nurses in state health departments and the expansion of public health nursing as a viable career path.

While nurses were forging new paths for themselves in various fields, Hollywood began featuring nurses in films during the 1930s. The only feature-length films to ever focus entirely on the nursing profession were released during this decade. *War Nurse* (1930), *Night Nurse* (1931), *Once to Every Woman* (1934), *The White Parade* (1934, Academy Award nominee for Best Picture), *Four Girls in White* (1939), *The White Angel* (1936), and *Doctor and Nurse* (1937) all used nurses as major characters. During the bleak years of the economic depression, young women found these nurse heroines who promoted idealism, self-sacrifice, and the profession of nursing over personal desires particularly appealing. No longer were nurses depicted as subservient handmaidens who worked as nurses only as a temporary pastime before marriage (Kalisch & Kalisch, 1986).

Early Education and Standardization of Practice of Public Health Nursing

After the turn of the century in the United States, infectious diseases such as smallpox, TB, malaria, cholera, and typhoid were practice priorities for public health nurses. The public health nurse often initially detected an infectious disease, then referred those patients to physicians for treatment, provided follow-up care to patients when indicated, and tried through education and demonstrations to family and caregivers to prevent the spread of disease. Progress for early education efforts was largely gained through experience. A 3-month orientation and observation process was established in the early 1920s for nurses new to the concepts and policies of public health nursing. The philosophy was simple: Public health nursing was about prevention of disease, the promotion of health, care of the sick, and rehabilitation to productive life (Erickson, 1996).

By 1927, the Rockefeller Foundation provided private funding for a training station for health workers in conjunction with several local county health departments. Nurses, physicians, and sanitarians from many states and foreign countries received public health orientation and training through this initiative before it was discontinued in 1932. In 1929, the Rockefeller Foundation provided grants through the Rosenwald Fund designated for programs to improve the health and lower the death rates of the African American population in the South. These funds, used to establish permanent public health nursing positions for African American nurses, targeted children in areas where nursing and sanitation would make a profound impact on health and health practices (Forbes, 1946).

Challenges of the 1930s

In 1933, President Roosevelt initiated the New Deal to relieve the economic hardship of the country. The Social Security Act in 1935 (Public Law No. 99-271) provided funding to increase public health programs, particularly to extend services and improve health care for mothers and children in rural areas suffering from economic stress. State boards of health secured funds in 1934 through the Children's Bureau of the U.S. Department of Labor for state supervisory nurses, regional supervisory nurses, and local county nurses. The goal of this special project was to place at least one public health nurse in each county in every state. The efforts to reach this goal were remarkable, but qualified public health nurses continued to be few in number (Association of State and Territorial Directors of Nursing [ASTDN], 1993).

The U.S. Public Health Service (USPHS), under the nursing consultation of Pearl Melver, provided leadership in the development of public health nursing services to the states. This effort was encouraged by the National Organization of Public Health Nursing and the Nursing Section of the American Public Health Association. Joint efforts of the federal public health nurses and those who were becoming organized in the states became the impetus for the growth of the specialty of public health nursing (ASTDN, 1993).

Another provision of the Social Security Act of 1935 was the establishment of Crippled Children's Services. Through this initiative, public health nurses were trained in rehabilitation nursing, primarily in orthopedics. These nurses visited crippled children in their homes, held conferences with parents, and assisted in field clinics (Roberts, 1985a).

Syphilis had also been recognized as a major source of morbidity and mortality for many years. In 1938, the USPHS and state boards of health cooperated in a major project to attempt to conquer the disease through case finding, treatment, follow-up contact, and education. Public health nursing was in the vanguard of this effort. Educational conferences were planned so that all public health nurses would have an opportunity to attend. Prenatal screening of patients for syphilis was being introduced as a standard nursing intervention at this time. These efforts were particularly successful in the South (Erickson, 1940; **Box 3-3**).

The country was gradually recovering from the Great Depression, and economic progress was accelerating. Farm production had broadened through diversification. New industries expanded the economy. The southern states, along with some of the eastern states, began to recognize the importance of nursing service in industrial hygiene programs. The U.S. Division of Industrial Hygiene asked for a public health nurse to plan and help institute nursing services. The prevention of disease, improvement of hazardous work conditions, promotion of health practices including nutrition, and first aid were the interventions to be provided through industrial nursing. As these nurses were employed, short-term educational and direct experience opportunities in areas with industrial nurses were

BOX 3-3 Public Health Milestones of the 1920s and 1930s

1920s	Frost established epidemiology as science basic to community health
1920s	National Organization for Public Health Nursing formed
1920s	Public Health Nursing Section of American Public Health Association formed
1921	First federal monies allocated for health and social welfare
1923	Health Organization of League of Nations founded
1925	Frontier Nursing founded
1930s	Association of State and Territorial Directors of Nursing formed
1930	Crippled Children's Programs established
1930	National Institutes of Health established
1935	Social Security Act passed
1938	American Public Health Association set standards for school health

Source: Data from Public Health Milestones in the 1920s and 1930s. APHA, 2006.

planned so that the nurses could receive the best preparation possible for the role (Morton, Roberts, & Bender, 1993; Roberts, 1985a, 1985b; Smith, 1934).

Progressive Initiatives After the War Years

By 1942, state boards of health and education began to enter operative agreements to strengthen public health nursing service to the school-age population. The role of the public health nurse in the school was generalized, but much emphasis was placed on health promotion, immunizations, nutrition, and correction of physical defects. Landmark legislation was passed by the U.S. Congress in March 1943, establishing the Emergency Maternity and Infant Care (EMIC) program for the care of the dependents of enlisted men of the U.S. armed services. The program was designed to provide for maternity care and acute illness care of the infants and was administered through the U.S. Children's Bureau. In less than a month, the program was initiated in almost all states. Training for public health nurses was once again funded by the federal government, and the role of the public health nurse expanded to include mothers and babies in a more formal way (ASTDN, 1935–1993).

The USPHS Division of Public Health Nursing conducted research during the mid-1940s to study public health nursing. The most significant recommendations included the designation of public health nursing in states as a major division of nursing, the recognition of public health nursing as a service delivery system to all public health divisions and programs, and the importance of educational and practice issues related to professional nursing. The studies cited a low educational level for public health nurses and strongly recommended upgrading educational qualifications. The studies critiqued the established expenditure of nursing time and activities, determining that many duties carried out by public health nurses could be delegated to clerical staff and health aides. Health aides were introduced to the public health team with high school graduates employed to support public health nursing. These individuals quickly became a valuable resource and support to public health nursing, performing both clerical and clinical support activities (ASTDN, 1935–1993).

In December 1947, senior cadet nurses had a 6-month general training in public health and polio care through the training center of the state boards of health. The purpose of the Cadet Nurse Corps Program, funded through the USPHS, was to encourage young women to study nursing and to augment the supply of nurses in all health services.

Nurses were returning to work following the close of World War II, although the overall demand for nurses continued to exceed the supply. Newly constructed hospitals, industry, and public health agencies were all clamoring and vying for the short supply of nurses. While more active professional nurses and more students in schools existed by the early 1950s than at any previous time, the increase in numbers and caliber of nurses had not kept pace with the need for service (ASTDN, 1935–1993).

Throughout the 1950s, the nursing home industry began to emerge, with licensure requirements for standards of operation developed to ensure quality of services and care. Communities were accommodating an increase in the number of elderly persons living with chronic and degenerative diseases. Public health nurses provided training courses for nurses' aides employed in nursing homes. Country public health nurses regularly visited the nursing homes within their communities, providing TB skin testing, administering flu vaccines, and providing technical assistance in nursing care. Nutritionists and physical therapists provided additional expertise to improve care processes and support public health nurses in the areas of rehabilitation and nutrition (Hanlon & Pickett, 1974a, 1974b; Morton et al., 1993).

A national trend began in the 1960s to release psychiatric patients from institutional care as improved psychotropic drugs and treatment modalities were available. Inadequate staffing at the state mental health institutions as a result of the nursing shortage was a complicating factor. The National Institute of Mental Health funded projects to study the impact that public health nurses might have on mental health care. A mental health nurse consultant was employed by many states to spearhead the research efforts of these projects. The projects' public health nursing activity was defined as "aftercare" and was designed to determine the effectiveness of integrating follow-up services to mental health patients and their families into general public health nursing service. Public health nursing services included case finding and referral, hospital discharge planning, home and family assessments before and after discharge to the home, and medication monitoring (Amendt & White, 1965; Cottrell, 1948). Mental health services remained an integral part of public health service delivery throughout this decade, with new activities enhancing the communities' focus (**Box 3-4**).

Great emphasis was placed on child health, growth, and development in the early 1960s. Communicable disease, intestinal parasites, and physical defects that had been so prevalent in the school-age population were greatly diminished. Evaluations of this population found the new concerns to be dental and oral defects, vision and hearing defects, mental and emotional disturbances, accidents,

BOX 3-4 Public Health Milestones of the 1940s and 1950s

1940s	Public health programs focused on health needs of the war period
1946	Centers for Disease Control and Prevention established by Congress
1946	Mahoney introduced use of penicillin for treatment of syphilis
1948	National Heart, Lung, and Blood Institute established
1948	World Health Organization established
1950s	Policy emphases on health and federal funds for states, environmental health issues, housing, behavior, medical care, and children's health
1950	Tuberculosis outpatient treatment becomes acceptable
1950	Introduction of the Salk vaccine
1950	White House Conference on Children and Youth

Source: Data from Public Health Milestones in the 1940s and 1950s. APHA, 2006.

and serious nutritional deficiencies. Continuing education was provided to enhance public health nurses' skills in observation, assessment, and nursing interventions in the care of children. Public health nurses began to be trained to assess developmental progress of children. Child health services provided by public health nurses included screening for physical defects, administration of immunizations, follow up to correct physical defects, referral for mental health evaluations, consultation with teachers, and health promotion in nutrition, accident prevention, and mental health (Roberts, 1985a).

An evaluation of the school health programs in the mid-1960s identified the need for additional nursing personnel to provide more direct preventive health services. Specialized federal funding through Title V grants was provided through the state departments of education to promote public health initiatives. Many schools recruited their nursing staff from the public health nursing workforce. Those public health nurses who went to schools took a broad view of child health and served as emissaries to school administrators and local boards' members. County public health nurses continued to serve as consultants to the schools in the areas of immunizations and communicable disease and as a referral source for Crippled Children's Services (Roberts, 1985a).

Immunizations administered by public health nurses were proving effective, yet surveys showed that many preschool and school-age children were not completely immunized. Boards of health, continuing their vigilance regarding children's health status, received federal grants under the Vaccination Assistance Act. In 1965, public health nurses administered an increased number of immunizations. The oral polio vaccine, known as the Sabin vaccine, became available in a sugar cube administration form. A measles vaccine became available in 1966 and rubella in 1969. Following mass initial immunization campaigns for both measles and rubella, the new vaccines were incorporated into routine immunization schedules for children (ASTDN, 1935–1993).

By the mid-1960s, federal funding for maternal/child health services required the incorporation of contraceptive information and general reproductive health into public health services. The objective was to reduce maternal and infant mortality and to generally improve the health and wellbeing of mothers and children. Some states had already identified the health problems associated with multiple unplanned and unwanted pregnancies and had been early leaders in efforts to repeal federal and state laws restricting birth control services. By 1944, these efforts had resulted in integrated family planning counseling and issuing of select supplies with maternity and postpartum services into many of the county health departments. Contraceptive supplies at that time included condoms and diaphragms. However, because of the wide divergence of public opinion, the development of the program was slow and unpublicized (ASTDN, 1935–1993: Morton et al., 1993).

Social and Political Influence of the 1960s and 1970s

By 1965, county health departments routinely provided contraceptive counseling and supplies. Oral contraceptives were also available by this time and gave women more convenient and accepted choices. Public health nurses promoted family planning and were key in identifying women at highest risk and need for such services. Family planning nursing visits increased across the country. Eventually, the federal government appropriated monies for additional education of public health nurses to function as family planning nurse practitioners (NPs).

Landmark legislation in 1965 amended the Social Security Act of 1935 by establishing Medicare, a health insurance plan for people 65 years of age and older and for those with long-term disabilities. The insurance plan included reimbursement for intermittent skilled nursing services provided to homebound persons. The purpose of home health services was twofold. Healthcare costs were beginning to skyrocket; home care would reduce costly hospitalization stays with the added benefit of patients being in familiar home settings, enhancing quality of life. The goal of the program was to rehabilitate patients to their maximum potential and to teach families to care for the physical and emotional needs of patients.

Public health nurses had been providing home nursing services on a limited basis since the inception of public health nursing, but this would be the first reimbursement established for direct nursing services. In addition, the reimbursable home health nursing services to be provided would require public health nurses to learn new assessment and rehabilitative technical skills. Federal regulations established for certification were monumental, however. Continuing education for the nurses and nurses' aides who were directly providing care was just one of the regulations that in itself would be an immense task once service delivery was fully implemented (Buhler-Wilkerson, 1993; Erickson, 1996; Institute of Medicine [IOM], 1988).

Federal grants through the USPHS were made available to support the implementation of home health. Nurse consultants, supervising nurses, and staff nurses attended university-supported educational offerings in rehabilitation care and techniques. Educational workshops were designed to upgrade nursing skills and techniques in rehabilitative care and on the conditions of participation of home health services. Additional workshop topics included documentation of skilled care and nursing care plans, medication administration and side effects, and the disease processes of many chronic health conditions.

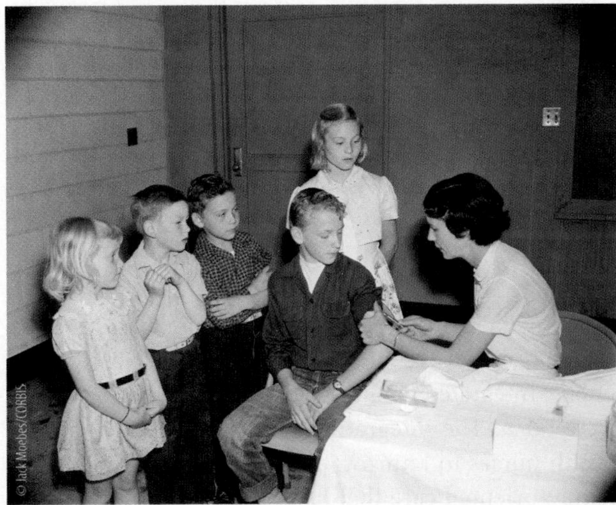

Public health nurses implemented the Salk vaccine beginning in 1955 in efforts to eradicate polio.

After federal costs studies were implemented by the public health nurses in home health care, it was demonstrated that additional auxiliary staff, including health aides and clerks, would allow public health nurses more time for nursing activities. Action was taken to create additional clerical and aide positions to support the nursing staff.

More liberal social values emerged, and the 1960s became known for having spawned a sexual revolution. These effects were recognized by the early 1970s. Communities were faced with tremendous increases in sexually transmitted diseases and teen pregnancy rates. Social programs in response to these increases were initiated in the 1960s and were formalized in public and community health efforts in all states. The establishment of Medicaid through the amendment to the Social Security Act, Title XIX, enhanced the delivery of healthcare services to a wider range of recipients. The quantity and variance of activities in public health nursing continued to increase.

All the while, the traditional programs of health protection and disease control moved forward, many with an accelerated pace. Collaboration with other agencies, institutions, and groups continued at a high level in an effort to coordinate resources to achieve the best possible public health service delivery. Medicaid programs enhanced the expansion of Crippled Children's Services as a payment mechanism for many previously uncovered services. Additional screening and specialty treatment clinics for neurology, heart, and orthopedics were established throughout the United States. Other initiatives also centered the delivery of child health services. Particularly in states with high infant mortality rates, state boards of health entered cooperative agreements in the 1970s to establish public health nursing positions in newborn intensive care units. The goal was to improve the communication, referral, and follow-up mechanisms for these high-risk infants after discharge from the hospital.

Title XIX of the Social Security Act (Medicaid) established Early and Periodic Screening, Diagnosis, and Treatment (EPSDT) in 1969 to improve the access to preventive and primary health care for low-income children. State boards of health used this opportunity to strengthen the delivery of well-child services. These physical screenings were made available primarily by public health nurses and were reimbursable nursing services, another recognition of the value of public health nursing service. The Denver Developmental Screening Test (DDST) was incorporated into the physical assessment, giving public health nurses a new tool to help find potential developmental delays and provide early intervention in the newborn to 6-year age groups. Workshops and in-service programs were conducted to teach the DDST standardized procedures.

BOX 3-5 Public Health Milestones of the 1960s and 1970s

1960s	Public health policy issues focused on inequality, integration, poverty, "the pill," housing environmental health, consumer protection, human rights, and peace
1960	Tuberculosis sanatoriums phased out and mainstream treatment begun
1961	First White House Conference on Aging
1961–1962	Sabin vaccine introduced
1962	National Institute of Child Health established
1964	*Surgeon General's Report on Smoking and Health* published
1965	Medicaid and Medicare programs enacted
1970	*Roe v. Wade*
1970	Occupational Safety and Health Administration established
1973	HMO Act passed
1976	National immunization program for "swine flu"
1978	Association of Community Health Nursing Educators formed
1979	Last outbreak of poliomyelitis in the United States
1979	First *Healthy People* report

Source: Data from Public Health Milestones in the 1960s and 1970s. APHA, 2006.

Medical technology continued to advance rapidly, including advances in genetic diagnostics and treatment. Routine screening for sickle-cell anemia was introduced and was integrated with EPSDT services. Other genetic technological advances determined that a contributing factor to the high incidence of mental retardation resulted from genetic disorders such as hypothyroidism and phenylketonuria (PKU). Medication and dietary treatments were developed for these genetic disorders that would improve the quality of life and life expectancy. Nursing interventions included a home assessment, treatment modalities ordered by the attending physician, provision of dietary supplements, and teaching basic child health care and special health care based on the genetic diagnosis derived from the screening (ASTDN, 1935–1993; Hanlon & Pickett, 1974b). Please refer to **Box 3-5** for milestones of the 1960s and 1970s.

A dramatic increase in home health nursing visits began at the close of the 1970s as a result of Medicare's implementation of diagnosis-related groups (DRGs), which were designed to lower costs through reduced institutionalization. Medicaid also reimbursed for home health services to eligible individuals not on Medicare and for some children with special healthcare needs. Private medical insurance plans and the Veteran's Administration were beginning to reimburse for home health services as well. Additional nursing positions were essential to meet the demand and to balance the quantity relationship with quality nursing care. As more acutely ill patients were cared for in the home and more advanced technological care was introduced into home health care, this specialty increased (ASTDN, 1935–1993).

Public Health Nursing Services in the 1980s and 1990s

As the 1980s began, the United States was experiencing an economic recession with skyrocketing interest rates and rising unemployment rates. National leadership was reducing funding for many of the social programs begun in the 1960s; the philosophy was that less governmental spending would enhance the national economy. The increased number of homeless persons became a national concern. Continuing concerns included illicit drug use, rising teen pregnancy rates, and alterations in family unit structures. Inadequate healthcare resources were also a continuing concern requiring cost containment, management of resources, and careful evaluation and incorporation of advancing technology. During this era, public health nursing services became varied throughout the country. In some states, basic services included both traditional preventive health services and family health services directed at high-risk mothers and babies and a reduction of unplanned pregnancies (ASTDN, 1935–1993).

Fortunately, public health nursing continued to grow and was a strong workforce in the country by the 1980s. Infant death rates declined significantly. Public health nurses participated in many research studies on public health problems such as congenital syphilis and TB preventive studies. Federal funding requirements changed from categorical grants to block grants. Categorical funding of the 1960s and 1970s had required that resources be restricted to the program that funded the resource; a nursing position funded by family planning, for example, was limited to family planning activities. Block funding allowed agencies more discretion on the use of these funds; therefore, services could be offered more efficiently to the public. Integrated public health nursing delivery systems were born. The integration of services allowed public health nurses to return to the more patient-oriented or family-oriented care that had been the traditional philosophy of public health nursing (ASTDN, 1993; Buhler-Wilkerson, 1993).

Genetics screening programs expanded as a result of advanced technology in the early 1980s. The first initiative was newborn screening for sickle-cell anemia. The goal was early detection of disease because early intervention could prevent common infections or premature deaths. State legislatures mandated hospitals to collect newborn screening specimens before infant discharge from the hospital. Screening included at least three genetic disorders: sickle-cell anemia, PKU, and hypothyroidism. Public health nurses were given the responsibility for following up with the newborns with a questionable or positive screen. Questionable screens for PKU and hypothyroidism require prompt attention because early treatment with diet and/or medication will prevent irreversible mental retardation and growth delay. The availability of public health nurses provided an effective means for timely follow up of screenings and for the implementation of medical and nursing care plans when indicated (ASTDN, 1993).

A crucial indicator of any state's quality of life is infant mortality. Public health nursing became a viable resource during the 1980s for delivering services (either personal or preventive) aimed at reducing infant mortality. The major cause of infant mortality was prematurity. Contributing factors included poor nutrition, smoking, teen pregnancy, and inadequate prenatal care. Socioeconomic factors such as inadequate housing, drug abuse, and lack of education were also contributing factors. Maternal risk scoring and documentation to ensure referrals to appropriate levels of care were standards of care. Tracking systems were intensified to ensure adequate levels of care.

Family planning services during the 1980s were also identified as a priority to reduce infant mortality. Risk factors included age and/or inadequate income to purchase contraceptive supplies. Public health nurses continued to promote family planning services, provide health promotion and education in their communities, and intensify tracking systems of teens and others at risk. The Special Supplemental Food Program for Women, Infants, and Children (WIC) continued to address infant mortality. WIC certification and nutrition education were integrated into maternal and child health nursing services' standards of care.

Congressional authorization gave states the option to expand their Medicaid programs in 1987. The services' expansion included case management of high-risk mothers and infants to ensure comprehensive care as a reimbursable service. Nutritionists, social workers, and public health nurses formed teams to establish care plans and assume case manager roles based on the patient's risk factors. Public health nursing activities included nursing assessments, home visits, health education, and communication with medical providers in an effort to improve the overall status of this high-risk population. Documentation of the care process was essential for continuity of care from the initial assessment and plan of care through implementation of services and ongoing evaluation.

Case management emerged during this decade as a new term, but the concept and the related activities of case management were the principles and foundations upon which public health nursing practice had been built. **Case management** is a program for intensive individual supervision, follow up, and referrals to appropriate levels of care. Public health nurses had been providing a form of case management through the years to many patients, such as those receiving TB treatment, those receiving home health services, and children with special healthcare needs.

School health nurses also became stronger in this era. School nurses strengthened the educational process of students by assisting them in improving or adapting to their health status. School nurses were available during school hours to serve as counselors and to provide case finding and referral to physicians, health departments, and other agencies as appropriate to meet the needs of school-age children. Activities included general health screening and referral, hearing and vision screening, identification of suspected abuse and neglect, substance abuse counseling, and appropriate decision making and support. In addition, school nurses provided classroom presentations on health issues and provided emergency care for injuries and illnesses at school.

Communicable disease had renewed public health interest in the nation throughout the 1980s. TB case rates were increasing. Measles cases were being reported among college-age students. New communicable disease concerns emerged in the 1980s, including increased incidence of hepatitis B, human immunodeficiency virus (HIV) infection, and acquired immune deficiency syndrome (AIDS). Case conferences with private medical consultants were established on a district level for initiation and ongoing review of treatment plans carried out by public health nurses. Drug resistance and failure to take medication were identified as major hindrances to individual cure and subsequent eradication of TB. In 1986, public health nurses initiated directly observed therapy (DOT) for TB cases. Rather than self-administration, patients would present to the health department or the public health nurse would visit the home for administration of medications. Later in the decade, public health officials recognized that the increase in TB cases was, in part, associated with the emerging HIV and AIDS cases. HIV screening became a standard of nursing care for all active TB cases.

Many states took an early stance to address measles among the college-age population in the mid-1980s as a result of the increased incidence of disease reported throughout the nation. The college-age population was at greatest risk for disease because they had been immunized with less-than-effective immunizations in the late 1960s or had not received the immunization. Collaboration with state college boards resulted in requirement of measles and rubella immunity for college admission. Public health nurses reviewed immunization records, provided screening tests when indicated, and administered immunizations to assist in the control of measles.

The first cases of AIDS were diagnosed in the early 1980s. Research soon unraveled part of the mystery of the disease. Risk factors for transmission of disease were identified, and a screening test for HIV, the virus that leads to AIDS, became available. Screening provided a means to detect HIV infection earlier and to provide appropriate counseling and education to alter risk behaviors and reduce transmission. Education of the public and high-risk individuals was the only effective weapon that public health had to address this disease. Public health nurses attended educational workshops to gain knowledge and skills for testing and counseling patients who requested testing. Health education materials were developed to support counseling and educational strategies. In addition, public health nurses implemented standards of care by integrating assessment of risk factors for patients receiving other public health services and by disseminating information through public presentations in schools and community organizations.

Progress continued for public health nurses during this era, yet dilemmas remain. A national nursing shortage was recognized, with all states feeling the effects. Public health felt the effects of the nursing shortage greatly, with the vacancy rates reaching 20% at times. A commission on nursing was organized by the Secretary of the U.S. Department of Health and Human Services (HHS) to examine and make recommendations regarding the nursing shortage. The commission's report, completed in 1989, cited the reality of the shortage and the impact on healthcare delivery. The shortage was determined to be the result of the increasing demand for nurses, and the report urged agencies to be attentive to using measures aimed at reducing the barriers to effective recruitment and retention (HHS, 1988).

One of the commission's recommendations was that nursing should have greater representation in the policy and decision-making activities of healthcare institutions. Acting on this recommendation, both public health nurses and their administrations developed mechanisms whereby public health nurses moved into broader policy-making roles. At the close of the decade, public health nursing continued as a strong force in the delivery of health care in many states and in health promotion and disease prevention in others. Public health nurses were instrumental in establishing and integrating new initiatives in public health to combat old public health problems and to address new public health concerns. The value of public health nursing activities continued to be recognized as reimbursement for selected activities and NP services were expanded.

The federal government's staggering budget deficits were the major national focus as the 1990s began. Healthcare costs were escalating, and governmental measures attempting to control increasing costs were not proving effective. The gloomy financial picture was exacerbated by Desert Storm, the U.S. military troops' assignment by President George H. W. Bush to protect Saudi Arabia and to retaliate for Iraq's invasion of Kuwait.

Current and emerging healthcare issues of the 1990s lay close to the heart of public health. The percentage of the population older than 65 continued to rise. Life expectancy in the United States had risen from 47 years in 1900 to 75 years in 1990. Infant mortality, although significantly declining through the years, required continued vigilance. The increased incidence of syphilis and other sexually transmitted diseases was of chief concern to public health. The number of persons infected with HIV and/or diagnosed with AIDS was increasing at alarming rates. Substance abuse continued to be a major problem, with studies identifying it as a contributing factor in 50% of all traffic accidents, in the transmission of HIV infection, and in infant morbidity and mortality.

Yet federal funding reductions were inevitable for public health as a result of the sluggish national economy as the United States entered the 1990s. Without significant infusions of money for additional staff, medications, vaccines, and health promotion/disease prevention activities, states faced increases in preventable diseases and deaths and a reversal of the recent favorable trends in lowering infant mortality and teen pregnancy. Difficult economic times resulted in the careful reviews of resources and the utilization of those resources. Focus was again directed toward enhancing nursing education and staff development, strengthening relationships with schools of nursing, and developing a quality assurance process for the integration of public health nursing services. Because of the large number of nurses employed, public health nurses were afforded greater access to approved continuing education opportunities specific to their area of practice. Select continuing education offerings, including TB updates, HIV testing and counseling courses, and community assessment, became required orientation for newly employed public health nurses (Gebbie, 1996).

The nation experienced a significant increase in the incidence of syphilis. Case rates were climbing and were

BOX 3-6 Public Health Milestones of the 1980s and 1990s

1980s	Public policy centered around AIDS, Medicare, Medicaid, tobacco control, international health, minority health, national healthcare reform, and national health objectives
1982	Warning labels on aspirin for Reye's syndrome prevention
1986	First anti-tobacco initiative by public health community
1988	*The Future of Public Health* published by the Institute of Medicine
1989	*Year 2000 Health Objectives* published
1990	*Healthy People 2000* report published
1991	*Healthy Communities 2000: Model Standards* published
1993	AZT sanctioned as able to reduce perinatal HIV
1996	*War and Public Health* published
1997	Plans underway for modern microbiological/biomedical laboratory capabilities
2000	*Healthy People 2010* published

Source: Data from Public Health Milestones in the 1980s and 1990s. APHA, 2000.

higher than they had been since the late 1940s. Much of the increased incidence was associated with drug abuse—the exchange of sex for drugs. Congenital syphilis was again an issue of public health concern for infant morbidity and mortality. Public health nursing protocols included standards of care for infected maternity patients and follow up for their newborn infants. Public health nurses increased their assessment for signs and symptoms of disease and for risk status of patients in their care, assisted disease intervention specialists with follow up of patients with positive laboratory results, and assisted with accessing medical treatment.

The incidence of another communicable disease, hepatitis B, was also increasing. With the advent of the hepatitis B vaccination, public health nurses implemented new protocols to screen maternity patients for hepatitis B and to provide follow up and immunization administration to the infants of infected mothers. Standing orders were written to effectively carry out the immunization and follow up of these infants. This was a major new public health initiative. See **Box 3-6** for a summary of activities during the 1980s and 1990s.

Federal monies increased for public health to address preventive intervention strategies for persons infected with HIV during the 1990s. States initiated programs to make select drugs available to patients. These programs required private physicians to submit medication orders for the patient. Public health nurses assisted patients with completing application forms, consulting private physicians regarding program guidelines, and adding medication.

Immunization administration had been a priority health effort for public health nurses since the early part of the century. A national emphasis reemerged in the early 1990s to meet a national objective to complete the immunization of 90% of all children by 2 years of age. The Centers for Disease Control and Prevention (CDC) identified barriers to children receiving their basic immunization series. The national discussion provided public health nurses with current knowledge on their assessment of simultaneous administration of several vaccines when indicated and on contraindications for immunization administration (HHS, 1992).

Science and Health Care, 1945–1960: Decades of Change

Dramatic technological and scientific changes characterized the decades following World War II, including the discovery of sulfa drugs, new cardiac drugs, surgeries, and treatment for ventricular fibrillation. The Hill-Burton Act, passed in 1946, provided funds to increase the construction of new hospitals. A significant change in the healthcare system was the expansion of private health insurance coverage and the dramatic increase in the birth rate, coined the "baby boom" generation. Clinical research, both in medicine and in nursing, became an expectation of health providers, and more nurses sought advanced degrees. The *Journal of Nursing Research* was first published, heralding the arrival of nursing scholarship in the United States.

Owing to increased numbers of hospital beds, additional financial resources for health care, and the post–World War II economic resurgence, an acute shortage of nurses occurred, and the existing staff faced increasingly stressful working conditions. Nurses began showing signs of the strain, engaging in debates about strikes and collective bargaining demands.

The composition of the nursing profession also changed. The ANA accepted African American nurses for membership, consequently ending racial discrimination in the dominant nursing organizations. The National Association of Colored Graduate Nurses was disbanded in 1951. Males entered nursing schools in record number, often as a result of previous military experience as medics. Prior to the 1950s and 1960s, male nurses had suffered minority status and were discouraged from nursing as a career. Seemingly forgotten by modern society, including Florence Nightingale and early U.S. nursing leaders, males made up more than one-half of the nursing care during medieval times. The Knights Hospitalers, Teutonic Knights, Franciscans, and many other male nursing orders had provided excellent nursing care for their societies. In fact, St. Vincent de Paul had first conceived of the idea of social service. Pastor Theodor Fliedner, teacher and mentor of Florence Nightingale at Kaiserwerth in Germany; Ben Franklin; and Walt Whitman (during the Civil War) all either served as nurses or were strong advocates for male nurses (Kalisch & Kalisch, 1986).

Years of Revolution, Protest, and the New Order, 1961–2000

During the social upheaval of the 1960s, nursing was influenced by many changes in society, such as the women's movement, the organized protest against the Vietnam War, the civil rights movement, President Lyndon Johnson's "Great Society" social reforms, and increased consumer involvement in health care. Specialization in nursing, such as cardiac intensive care unit (ICU), nurse anesthetist training, and the clinical specialist role for nursing emerged as a trend that affected both education and practice in the healthcare system. Medicare and Medicaid, enacted in 1965 under Title XVIII of the Social Security Act, provided access to health care for the elderly, the poor, and the disabled. The ANA took a courageous and controversial stand in that same year (1965) by approving its first position paper on nursing education, advocating for all nursing education for professional practice to take place in colleges and universities. Nurses returning from Vietnam faced emotional challenges through the recognition of post-traumatic stress disorder (PTSD), which affected some nurses' postwar lives.

With the increased specialization in medicine, the demand for primary care healthcare providers exceeded the supply. As a response to this need for general practitioners, Dr. Henry Silver (MD) and Dr. Loretta Ford (RN) collaborated to develop the first NP program in the United States at the University of Colorado (Silver, Ford, & Steady, 1967). NPs were initially prepared in pediatrics with advanced role preparation in common childhood illness management and well-child care. Silver and colleagues(1967) found that NPs could manage as much as 75% of the pediatric patients in community clinics, leading to the widespread use of NPs and growth of educational programs for NPs. The first state in 1971 to recognize diagnosis and treatment as part of the legal scope of practice for NPs was Idaho. Alaska and North Carolina were among the first states to expand the NP role to include prescriptive authority. By the new century, NP programs were offered at the MSN level in family nursing, gerontology, adult, neonatal, mental health, and maternal–child care; they have since expanded to include the acute care practitioner as well. Certification of NPs now occurs at the national level through the ANA and many specialty organizations, and NPs are licensed throughout the United States by state boards of nursing (Hagedorn & Quinn, 2004). The doctorate of nursing practice (DNP) has emerged in the past decade as the preferred educational preparation for all advanced practice nurses.

Managed Care and Healthcare Reform: First Decades of the 21st Century

Escalating healthcare costs resulting from the explosion of advanced technology and the increased lifespan of Americans led to the demand for healthcare reform in the late 1980s. The nursing profession heralded the way in healthcare reform when an unprecedented collaboration of more than 75 nursing associations, led by the ANA and NLN, published ***Nursing's Agenda for Health Care Reform.*** This document addressed the challenge of managed care in the context of cost containment and quality assurance of healthcare service for the nursing profession (ANA, 1991). **Managed care** is a market approach based on managed competition as a major strategy to contain healthcare costs; it remains a major system of care today, with expanded considerations as the ACA continues to influence the quality and costs of health care.

The IOM's (2008a) report *Assuring the Health of the Public in the 21st Century* builds upon its 1988 report and has major implications for public health policy development. The report contains several specific recommendations for strengthening the relationship between the vital sectors charged with protecting the public's health. The report proposes an ecological model upon which to base health professional education (including nursing education), clinical activities, and research with a population focus. Multiple determinants of health form the basis for an ecological model, which operates on the assumption that health is affected on several levels by these factors. Given that nurses make up the largest single workforce within the health system, the report's recommendations and the potential use of an ecological model as part of a population-focused practice have significant potential for creating new paths in nursing practice, education, and research.

A companion study by the IOM (2008b), *Who Will Keep the Public Healthy?*, builds on the ecological model and considers factors likely to affect public health in the 21st century, such as globalization, technological and scientific advances, and demographic shifts in the U.S. population. It defines a public health professional as a person educated in public health or a related discipline who is employed to improve health through a population focus. Eight new content areas for public health professionals to master are identified in this study: informatics, genomics, communication, cultural competence, community-based participatory research, policy and law, global health, and ethics.

Even as these studies were being conducted, public health history was being changed. Seasoned public health professionals, experiencing the erosion of the basic public health infrastructure created by state and local budget cuts, had predicted that the United States would be challenged significantly should any of the dilemmas of the past return. None of those predictions, however, accurately portrayed the impact that the events of September 11, 2001, and the subsequent anthrax threats would have on public health. Almost overnight, public health agencies and their partners became immersed in emergency preparedness activities that have now become routine. Public health professionals were challenged to place a high priority on such activities as syndromic surveillance, mass-casualty planning, handling of biological and chemical agents that would also be considered evidentiary material, and other similar work. New partners such as postal workers, law enforcement, and communication experts emerged. Public health nurses were also called upon to administer smallpox vaccine, something that had not been done in almost 2 decades. The beginning of the 21st century dawned with improved health status and a new public health threat: terrorism. Since September 11, 2001, terrorism has been a constant threat to the United States and to the global community.

ART CONNECTION 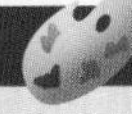

Research the web for early artwork where a nurse is featured from the 19th and 20th centuries. Describe how different these portrayals are from today's nurse.

The U.S. healthcare system continued to focus on federal coverage and spiraling costs during the first decade of the 21st century. The public and private sectors demonstrated increased dissatisfaction with healthcare access, quality, accessibility, and affordability. Healthcare organizations emerged in a managed care environment, involving public and private sectors of the healthcare industry. The economic and quality outcome benefits of caring for patients and managing their care over a continuum of possible settings and needs were seen as positive for many. Continuing into the second decade of the new century, patients are followed more closely within the system, during both illness and wellness. Hospital stays continue to be shorter, and more healthcare services are being provided in outpatient facilities and through community-based settings such as home health, occupational health, and school health. War, bioterrorism, an aging population, and emerging epidemics are just some of the challenges for today's nurses. Consensus regarding basic education and the entry level of registered nurses has not occurred. Relating to the global community as well as our own diverse population demands that nurses remain committed to cultural sensitivity in care delivery.

Because of professional nurses' engagement in healthcare reform—beginning with *Nursing's Agenda for Health Care Reform* (ANA, 1991) and in the years following—the profession was poised to take a leadership role in the passage of the **Patient Protection and Affordable Care Act (ACA) of 2010**. The purpose of the ACA is to provide affordable, quality health care to all Americans. The ACA was signed into law March 23, 2010 and upheld by the U.S. Supreme Court, which ruled it constitutional on June 28, 2012. The bill includes unprecedented preventive care and protections, including insurance companies no longer being able to deny individuals for preexisting conditions or to drop them from coverage when they get sick.

The history of health care and nursing provides us with ample examples of the wisdom of our forebears in the advocacy of nursing in these challenging settings and the unknown future. Nurses today, by considering the lessons of the past, become part of a profession that is well prepared to provide the full range of quality, cost-effective services needed in the promotion of health throughout the new century. See **Box 3-7**.

AFFORDABLE CARE ACT (ACA) 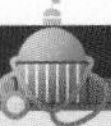

Nursing has been at the forefront of healthcare reform for many decades. The profession of nursing was the first of the health professions to support the creation of the Medicare program in 1958, in spite of critical opposition from the medical and hospital industries.

LEVELS OF PREVENTION 

Primary: Identify the primary healthcare interventions used by Florence Nightingale.

Secondary: What secondary interventions did Lillian Wald use?

Tertiary: How do tertiary interventions today differ from those in the past?

BOX 3-7 Public Health Milestones 2000–2013

2001	9/11 terrorist attacks (New York City and Washington, DC) and bioterrorist attacks lead to new initiatives in state and federal public health policies, organizational responses, and initiatives
	CDC investigates first anthrax case; the victim was a 63-year-old Florida man; patient first in a series of domestic terrorism victims of infection by anthrax sent through the mail
2003	Severe acute respiratory syndrome (SARS) coronavirus identified
2004	First state laws restricting access to over-the-counter medications used in methamphetamine production in Georgia
2005	Hurricane Katrina hits New Orleans and Mississippi Gulf Coast resulting in unprecedented public heath disaster and response at state and federal levels
	Rubella eliminated in the United States
2006	CDC recommends 15th and 16th routine immunizations for children and adolescents (rotavirus and human papillomavirus, respectively)
	CDC celebrates 60th anniversary.
2007	CDC issues federal order of isolation, the last such order being issued in 1963
2008	Large, multi-state foodborne illness outbreaks are detected and investigated, revealing gaps in food safety and the need to improve prevention efforts
2009	CDC identifies the novel H1N1 influenza virus
	H1N1 flu pandemic dominates CDC activities
2010	The Patient Protection and Affordable Care Act of 2010 (ACA) was signed into law, putting in place comprehensive U.S. health reform as the most significant federal mandate since the New Deal in the 1930s
	7.0 magnitude earthquake in Haiti; CDC response efforts help prevent 7,000 deaths from cholera
2011	Implementation of ACA: providing free preventive care for Medicare recipients; Community First Choice Option offers home- and community-based services to disabled individuals through Medicaid
	"Treatment as Prevention" as a means to reduce HIV transmission, after a research study showed that individuals who had started antiretroviral therapy immediately after diagnosis lowered the risk of HIV transmission to their uninfected sexual partners by as much as 96%
	Community resource programs enhanced to implement "test and treat" strategies for individuals and couples
	Increased treatment for HIV-positive mothers to prevent mother-to-child transmission
2012	Implementation of ACA: electronic health records, encouraging integrated health systems by providing incentives for healthcare providers to form Accountable Care Organizations (ACOs)
	U.S. Supreme Court decision upholds ACA against legal Constitutional challenges, with the exception of mandatory State expansion of Medicaid
	Greater investment in health information technology: privacy, accessibility and security of patient data, and social media educational efforts
2013-14	Implementation of ACA: Improved and expanded preventive health coverage for Medicaid recipients by providing new funding to state Medicaid programs and providers that chose to cover preventive services for patients at little or no cost

Critical Thinking Activities

1. Take a walk through your neighborhood and college campus. Identify public health measures that exist that can be traced to the Greek and Roman eras.
2. How do you think Lillian Wald would react to present-day public health departments?
3. How does the current interest in alternative and complementary health care relate to the Greeks' ideas about health?
4. How would you explain healthcare reforms of the 20th and 21st centuries in the United States to those from other comparable societies and countries?

References

Abel, E. K. (1997, November). Take the cure to the poor: Patients' responses to New York City's tuberculosis program, 1894–1918. *American Journal of Public Health, 87*, 11.

Achterberg, J. (1990). *Woman as healer: A panoramic survey of the healing activities of women from prehistoric times to the present.* Boston, MA: Shambhala.

Amendt, J. A., & White, R. P. (1965, July). Continued care services for mental patients. *Nursing Outlook*, pp. 57–60.

American Nurses Association. (1991). *Nursing's agenda for health care reform*. Washington, DC: Author.

American Public Health Association (APHA). (2006, November). *Public health milestones*. Unpublished paper. Washington, DC: Author.

Andrews, G. (2003). Nightingale's geography. *Nursing Inquiry*, *10*(4), 270–274.

Association of State and Territorial Directors of Nursing (ASTDN). (1993). *Historical summary of the Association of State and Territorial Directors of Nursing (1935–1993)*. Unpublished manuscript.

Association of State and Territorial Directors of Nursing (ASTDN). *Selected reports from annual meeting and correspondence, 1935–1993*.

Attewell, A. (1996). Florence Nightingale's health-at-home visitors. *Health Visitor*, *69*(10), 406.

Baker, K. (2006, April/May). The future of New Orleans: Can the disasters that befell other cities help save this one? *American Heritage*.

Barker, E. R. (1989). Care givers as casualties. *Western Journal of Nursing Research*, *11*(5), 628–631.

Barstow, A. L. (1994). *Witchcraze: A new history of the European witch hunt*. New York, NY: HarperCollins..

Boorstin, D. J. (1985). *The discoverers: A history of man's search to know his world and himself*. New York, NY: Vintage.

Bostridge, M. (2008). *Florence Nightingale: The making of an icon*. New York, NY: Farrar, Straus and Giroux.

Brainard, A. M. (1922). *The evolution of public health nursing*. Philadelphia, PA: Saunders.

Briggs, R. (1996). *Witches and neighbors: The social and cultural context of European witchcraft*. New York, NY: Penguin Books.

Brockett, L. P., & Vaughan, M. C. (1867). *Woman's work in the civil war: A record of heroism, patriotism and patience*. Philadelphia, PA: Zeigler, McCurdy.

Brooke, E. (1997). *Medicine women: A pictorial history of women healers*. Wheaton, IL: Quest Books.

Brown, E. L. (1936). *Nursing as a profession*. New York, NY: Russell Sage Foundation.

Brown, E. L. (1948). *Nursing for the future*. New York, NY: Russell Sage Foundation.

Brown, P. (1988). *Florence Nightingale*. Herts, UK: Exley Publications.

Buhler-Wilkerson, K. (1985). Public health nursing: In sickness or in health? *American Journal of Public Health*, *75*, 1155–1156.

Buhler-Wilkerson, K. (1993). Bringing care to the people: Lillian Wald's legacy of public health nursing. *American Journal of Public Health*, *83*(12), 1778–1786.

Bullough, V. L., & Bullough, B. (1978). *The care of the sick: The emergence of modern nursing*. New York, NY: Prodist.

Calabria, M. D. (1996). *Florence Nightingale in Egypt and Greece: Her diary and "visions."* Albany, NY: State University of New York Press.

Carnegie, M. E. (1991). *The path we tread: Blacks in nursing 1854–1990* (2nd ed.). New York, NY: National League for Nursing Press.

Cartwright, F. F. (1972). *Disease and history*. New York, NY: Dorset Press.

Cohen, M. N. (1989). *Health and the rise of civilization*. New Haven, CT: Yale University Press.

Cook, E. (1913). *The life of Florence Nightingale* (Vols. 1 and 2). London, UK: Macmillan.

Cottrell, H. (1948). *Mental health principles in the state and local health programs: A Commonwealth Fund demonstration* (Record Group 51, Vol. 36). Mississippi Department of Archives, Division of Public Health Nursing, Historical Files.

Crawford, P. (1992). "The other lady with the lamp": Nursing legacy of Mary Seacole. *Nursing Times*, *88*(11), 56–58.

D'Antonio, P. (2002). Nurses in war. *Lancet*, *360*(9350), 7–12.

Diamond, J. (1997). *Guns, germs, and steel: The fates of human societies*. New York, NY: W. W. Norton.

Dickens, C. (1844). *Martin Chuzzlewit*. New York, NY: Macmillan.

Dietz, D. D., & Lehozky, A. R. (1963). *History and modern nursing*. Philadelphia, PA: F. A. Davis.

Dock, L. N., & Stewart, I. M. (1931). *A short history of nursing* (3rd ed.). New York, NY: G. P. Putnam.

Donahue, M. P. (1985). *Nursing: The finest art*. St. Louis, MO: Mosby.

Dossey, B. M. (2000). *Florence Nightingale: Mystic, visionary, healer*. Springhouse, PA: Corporation.

Erickson, G. P. (1996, June). To pauperize or empower: Public health nursing at the turn of the 20th and 21st century. *Public Health Nursing*, *13*(3), 163–169.

Erickson, P. (1940). *The role of the public health nurse in the syphilis research project in Washington County*. Presented at the 1940 annual meeting of the Mississippi Nurses Association, Jackson, MS.

Forbes, M. D. (1946). *Report of a review of public health nursing in the Mississippi Board of Health* (Record Group 51, Vol. *36*). Mississippi Department of Archives, Division of Public Health Nursing, Historical Files.

Fromkin, D. (1998). *The way of the world: From the dawn of civilizations to the eve of the twenty-first century*. New York, NY: Random House.

Gebbie, K. M. (1996, November 18). *Preparing currently employed public health nurses for change in the health care system: Meeting report and suggested action steps*. New York, NY: Columbia University School of Nursing Center for Health Policy and Health Sciences Research. (Report based on meeting in Atlanta, GA, July 11, 1996.)

Goldmark, J. C. (1923). *Nursing and nursing education in the United States*. New York, NY: Macmillan.

Hagedorn, S., & Quinn, A. A. (2004). Theory-based nurse practitioner practice: Caring in action. *Topics in Advanced Practice Nursing eJournal*, *4*(4). Retrieved from http://www.medscape.com/viewarticle/496718_2

Hamilton, D. (1988). Clinical excellence, but too high a cost: The Metropolitan Life Insurance Company Visiting Nurse Service (1909–1953). *Public Health Nursing*, *5*, 235–240.

Hanlon, J. J., & Pickett, G. E. (1974a). Community nursing services. In J. J. Hanlon (Ed.), *Public health administration and practice* (pp. 533–547). St. Louis, MO: Mosby.

Hanlon, J. J., & Pickett, G. E. (1974b). Historical perspectives. In J. J. Hanlon (Ed.), *Public health administration and practice* (pp. 22–44). St. Louis, MO: Mosby.

Hanlon, J. J., & Pickett, G. E. (1984). *Public health administration and practice* (8th ed.). St. Louis, MO: Mosby.

Heinrich, J. (1983). Historical perspectives on public health nursing. *Nursing Outlook, 32*(6), 317–320.

Hine, D. C. (1989). *Black women in white: Racial conflict and cooperation in the nursing profession 1890–1950*. Bloomington, IN: Indiana University Press.

Howse, C. (2007). "The ultimate destination of all nursing": The development of district nursing in England, 1880–1925. *Nursing History Review, 15*, 65–94.

Institute of Medicine (IOM). (1988). *The future of public health*. Washington, DC: National Academies Press.

Institute of Medicine (IOM). (2008a). *Assuring the health of the public in the 21st century*. Retrieved from http://www.iom.edu/Activities/PublicHealth/PubHealth21stCen.aspx

Institute of Medicine (IOM). (2008b). *Who will keep the public healthy: Educating public health professionals for the 21st century*. Retrieved from http://www.iom.edu/CMS/3793/4723/4307.aspx

Johnson, S. (2006). *The ghost map: The story of London's most terrifying epidemic and how it changed science, cities and the modern world*. New York, NY: Penguin Books.

Kalisch, P. A., & Kalisch, B. J. (1986). *The advance of American nursing* (2nd ed.). Boston, MA: Little, Brown.

Le Vasseur, J. (1998). Plato, Nightingale, and contemporary nursing. *Image: Journal of Nursing Scholarship, 30*(3), 281–285.

Longfellow, H. W. (1857, November). Santa Filomena. *Atlantic Monthly, 1*, 22–23.

MacEachern, M. T. (1932). Which shall we choose: Graduate or student service? *Modern Hospital, 38*, 97–98, 102–104.

Minkowski, W. I. (1992). Women healers of the Middle Ages: Selected aspects of their history. *American Journal of Public Health, 82*(2), 288–295.

Montag, M. L. (1959). *Community college education for nursing: An experiment in technical education for nursing*. New York, NY: McGraw-Hill.

Monteiro, L. A. (1985). Florence Nightingale on public health nursing. *American Journal of Public Health, 75*(2), 181–185.

Morton, M., Roberts, E., & Bender, K. (1993). *Celebrating public health nursing: Caring for Mississippi's communities with courage and compassion, 1920–1993*. Jackson, MI: Mississippi State Department of Health.

Mosley, M. O. P. (1996). Satisfied to carry the bag: Three black community health nurses' contribution to health care reform, 1900–1937. *Nursing History Review, 4*, 65–82.

Nightingale, F. (1893). Sick-nursing and health-nursing. In *Women's mission* (pp. 184–205). (Arranged and ed. by Baroness Burdett-Coutts.) London, UK: Sampson, Law, Marston.

Nightingale, F. (1915). Florence Nightingale to her nurses: A selection from Miss Nightingale's addresses to probationers and nurses of the Nightingale school at St. Thomas's Hospital. London, UK: Macmillan.

Nightingale, F. (1979). Cassandra. In M. Stark (Ed.), *Florence Nightingale's Cassandra* (original work published in 1928). Old Westbury, NY: Feminist Press.

Nutting, M. A., & Dock, L. L. (1907). *A history of nursing* (Vol 1). New York, NY: G. P. Putnam.

The 100 people who made the millennium. (1997). *Life Magazine, 20*(10a).

Palmer, I. S. (1977, March/April). Florence Nightingale: Reformer, reactionary, researcher. *Nursing Research*, 13–18.

Palmer, I. S. (1982). *Through a glass darkly: From Nightingale to now*. Washington, DC: American Association of Colleges of Nursing.

Payne, D. (1999). Face to face: Florence Nightingale and Mary Seacole battle it out face to face. *Nursing Times, 95*(19), 26–27.

Pyle, E. (1944). *Here is your war: The story of G. I. Joe*. Cleveland, OH: World Publishing.

Rathbone, W. (1890). *A history of nursing in the homes of the poor*. Introduction by Florence Nightingale. London, UK: Macmillan.

Richardson, B. W. (1887). *The health of nations: A review of the works of Edwin Chadwick* (Vol. 2). London, UK: Longmans, Green.

Roberts, E. (1985a). *Highlights: Maternal and child health and crippled children's service, 1935–1985*. Jackson, MS: Mississippi Department of Health.

Roberts, E. (1985b, March). *The role of the southern nurse in public health*. Symposium on Southern Science and Medicine at the Education and Research Center, Jackson, MS.

Roberts, M. (1954). *American nursing: History and interpretation*. New York, NY: Macmillan.

Robinson, V. (1946). *White caps: The story of nursing*. Philadelphia, PA: Lippincott.

Rosen, G. (1958). *A history of public health*. New York, NY: M. D. Publications.

Sabin, L. (1998). *Struggles and triumphs: The story of Mississippi nurses 1800–1950*. Jackson: Mississippi Hospital Association Health, Research and Educational Foundation.

Sanger, M. (1928). *Motherhood in bondage*. New York, NY: Brentano's.

Seymer, L. (1954). *Selected writings of Florence Nightingale*. New York, NY: Macmillan.

Shryock, R. H. (1959). *The history of nursing: An interpretation of the social and medical factors involved*. Philadelphia, PA: Saunders.

Silver, H. K., Ford, L. C., and Steady, S. G. (1967). A program to increase health care for children: The pediatric nurse practitioner program. *Pediatrics, 39*(3).

Smith, E. (1934). *Mississippi special public health nursing project made possible by federal funds*. Paper presented at the 1934 annual Mississippi Nurses Association meeting, Jackson, MS.

Snow, (1855). *On the mode of communication of cholera*(2nd ed). London, England: Churchill Publishers.

Stanmore, A. H. G. (1906). *Sidney Herbert of Lea: A memoir*. New York, NY: E. P. Dutton.

The State Board Test Pool Examination. (1952). *American Journal of Nursing, 52*, 613.

Stewart, I. M. (1921). Developments in nursing education since 1918. *U. S. Bureau of Education Bulletin, 20*(6), 3–8.

Taylor, H. O. (1922). *Greek biology and medicine*. Boston, MA: Marshall Jones.

Tiffany, F. (1890). *The life of Dorothea Lynde Dix*. Boston, MA: Houghton Mifflin.

Tyrell, H. (1856). *Pictorial history of the war with Russia 1854–1856*. London, UK: W. and R. Chambers.

Vicinus, M., & Nergaard, B. (1990). *Ever yours, Florence Nightingale: Selected letters*. Boston, MA: Harvard University Press.

U.S. Department of Health and Human Services. (1988, December). *Final report of the Secretary's Commission on Nursing*. Washington, DC: Author.

U.S. Department of Health and Human Services, Public Health Services, Centers for Disease Control and Prevention. (1992, May). *Standards for pediatric immunization practice*. Atlanta, GA: Author.

Wald, L. D. (1915). *The house on Henry Street*. New York, NY: Henry Holt.

Weiner, D. B. (1993). The citizen patient in revolutionary and imperial Paris. Baltimore, MD: Johns Hopkins University Press.

Wertz, R. W., & Wertz, D. C. (1977). *Lying-In: A history of childbirth in America*. New Haven, CT: Yale University Press.

Williams, C. B. (1961, May). Stories from Scutari. *American Journal of Nursing, 61*, 88.

Winslow, C. E. A. (1946). Florence Nightingale and public health nursing. *Public Health Nursing, 38*, 330–332.

Woodham-Smith, C. (1951). *Florence Nightingale*. New York, NY: McGraw-Hill.

Woodham-Smith, C. (1983). *Florence Nightingale*. New York, NY: Atheneum.

Young, D. A. (1995). Florence Nightingale's fever. *British Medical Journal, 311*, 1697–1700.

CHAPTER FOCUS

Epidemiology Defined
Scope of Epidemiology
The Epidemiological, Research, and Nursing Processes
Natural History of Disease
Descriptive Epidemiology
- Use of Rates
- Sources of Data

Person, Place, and Time
- Person
- Place
- Time

Analytic Epidemiology

QUESTIONS TO CONSIDER

After reading this chapter, you will know the answers to the following questions:

1. What is the contribution of epidemiology to public health?
2. How do nurses use the principles of epidemiology?
3. How is the epidemiological process related to nursing and research?
4. What is the usefulness of rates in community health nursing?
5. What is the natural history of disease and what are the levels of prevention?
6. What are the *incidence* and *prevalence* rates?
7. What are the characteristics of a population by person, place, and time?
8. What are the characteristics of the four types of epidemiological research studies?
9. How can epidemiological research be used in community health nursing?

CHAPTER 4

Epidemiology of Health and Illness

Angeline Bushy and
Gail A. Harkness

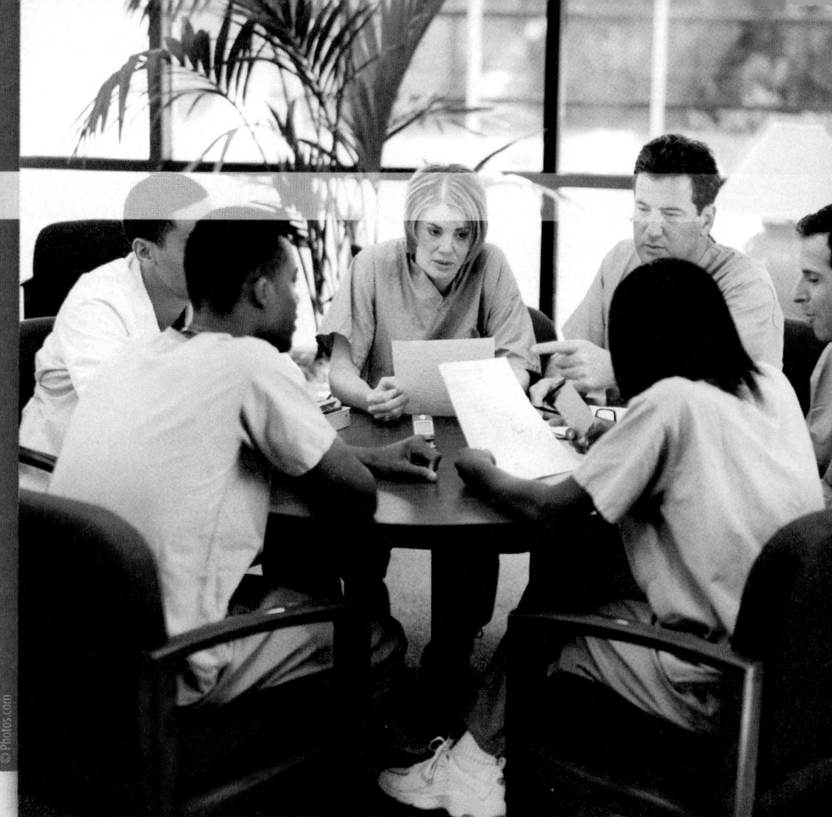

KEY TERMS

adjusted rates
case-control
cross-sectional
crude rates
ecological model
epidemic
epidemic curve
epidemiological triad
epidemiology
genomics
incidence
intervention
morbidity
mortality
period prevalence
point prevalence
prevalence
primary prevention
prospective
rate
retrospective
risk
risk factors
secondary prevention
specific rates
tertiary prevention
web of causation

"The work we are speaking of has nothing to do with nursing disease, but with maintaining health by removing the things which disturb it … dirt, drink, diet, damp, draughts, and drains."

—Florence Nightingale, 1860

REFLECTIONS

After reading the quote by Nightingale, think about this question: How are the "connections" in your life related to overall health and wellbeing? Think about your environment, your personal identity (e.g., gender and genetics), and the changing variables that can make you sick (e.g., stress) or keep you well (e.g., exercise, meditation).

DO YOU OFTEN WONDER HOW the human immunodeficiency virus (HIV) was discovered, or why we know that infant seats should be placed in the backseat of a car to reduce risks to babies? To understand the changes that can occur in the health of individuals or in various populations, it is necessary to identify the relationships between and among the various biological and psychosocial phenomena that underlie health and illness. Epidemiology, the basic science of preventive health, has provided a process for understanding these relationships by studying different populations of people in various situations. Through study of health problems as they occur in groups or populations, many characteristics of specific illness or disabilities can be identified that may not be evident in the study of individuals alone.

Health care for all individuals should be planned within the framework of family and personal friends, the immediate community culture where individuals live, and the larger world society (see **Figure 4-1**). Any individual's healthcare needs cannot be completely or correctly defined unless these broader factors are analyzed and appropriately incorporated into a plan of care. Just as information must be collected about individuals in assessing health problems, so data must be collected about groups, communities, and populations to assess the broader health needs of society. Epidemiological studies and results are increasingly important in the current U.S. healthcare system, because patient and population outcomes are increasingly tied to economic resources. Provisions of the Affordable Care Act (ACA) of 2010 that increase hospitals' financial accountability for preventable readmissions have heightened interest in identifying system-level interventions, such as epidemiology, to reduce readmissions. One study of readmissions due to complications in patients with congestive heart failure and acute myocardial infarction linked nurses' increased patient loads to an increase in readmission due to post-discharge complications (McHugh & Ma, 2013).

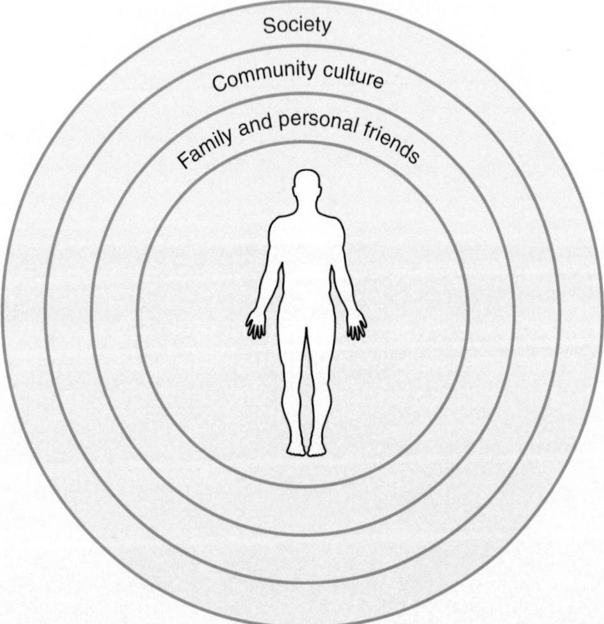

Figure 4-1 Individual within the framework of life.

For instance, the association between lung cancer and smoking might not have been ascertained by studying individual cases of lung cancer. Many smokers never develop lung cancer, and some nonsmokers do develop lung cancer. However, in 1950, Doll and Hill contrasted a group of lung cancer patients with a group of people who did not develop lung cancer. They clearly demonstrated that more people with lung cancer had smoked cigarettes than those people without the disease (Doll & Hill, 1950). This was substantiated by further research, and cigarette smoking is now considered a primary risk factor for lung and other cancers. This information has been the basis for national campaigns to decrease smoking among Americans. This example demonstrates the value of identifying certain characteristics or behaviors that increase risk of health problems even if the pathophysiology is not precisely known. Healthcare personnel can implement preventive health measures for both individuals and groups of people who are at high risk even if the causative factors are not known.

Epidemiology Defined

Epidemiology is the study of the distribution and the determinants of states of health and illness in human populations (Alanis, 1999; Gordis, 2004; Macha & McDonough, 2012). *Distribution* refers to the frequency of occurrence of states of health and illness; *determinants* refer to agents or factors that contribute to the cause of various states of health and illness. The word *epidemiology* is derived from Greek: *epi,* upon; *demos,* people; and *logos,* treatise. The ultimate goal of epidemiology is to use the information obtained from the study of the distribution and determinants of states of health and illness to prevent or limit the consequences of illness and disability in humans and maximize their state of health. Although the study of the influence of the environment on the occurrence of disease and the contagious nature of many diseases can be traced to Hippocrates, the techniques of modern epidemiological investigation were first developed in the mid-19th century.

William Farr, a physician from London, established the field of medical statistics. In 1839, he was appointed to the Office of the Registrar General for England and Wales. He set up a system for compilation of the numbers and causes of deaths and compared the deaths of workers in different occupations, the difference in mortality between men and women, and the effect of imprisonment on the frequency of death. He realized that studying the data from populations of people would provide much more information about human disease than studying individual cases (Humphreys, 1885).

During the mid-19th century, infectious diseases such as cholera and the plague were still killing much of the population of Europe. The primary goal then was to limit the spread of these devastating diseases and prevent their recurrence. John Snow, another British physician, investigated the **epidemic** of cholera that took place from 1848 to 1854. His classic investigation of the outbreak clearly established the rate as a fundamental tool of epidemiology. Snow investigated cholera outbreaks associated with water supplied from two different water companies. He demonstrated statistically that cholera was associated with the water company that obtained its water from an area of the Thames River that was heavily polluted with sewage, and not with the company that obtained its water farther upstream (Snow, 1855).

CULTURAL CONNECTION

African Americans as a group have a higher mean blood pressure than Caucasian Americans. Various hypotheses have been proposed to explain the differences between the races, such as genetic, social, economic, diet, and behavioral factors. To date, epidemiological studies have been inconclusive as to the exact causes for the differences.

Florence Nightingale was a contemporary of Farr and Snow and was significantly influenced by their statistical methods. Nightingale is probably best known for her work at the British military hospital in Scutari. British and French troops had invaded the Crimea on the north coast of the Black Sea, supporting Turkey in its dispute with Russia. Nightingale and her 38 nurses found the conditions appalling. Buildings were infested with rats and fleas,

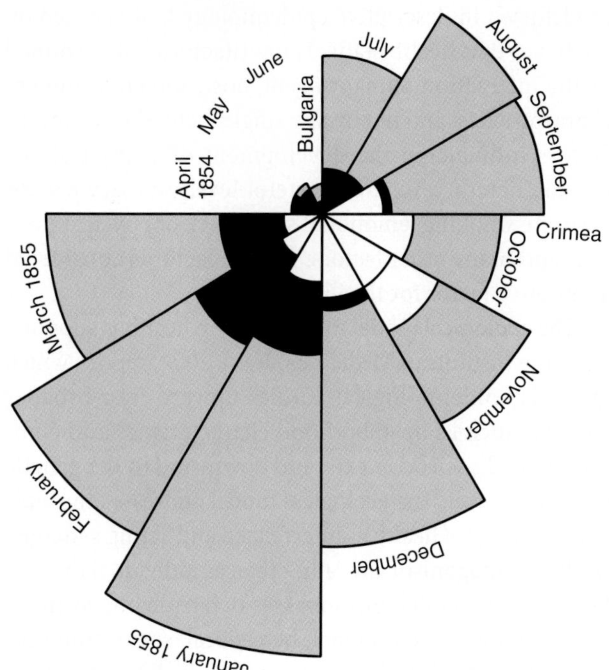

Figure 4-2 Nightingale's polar-area diagram.

streams of sewage flowed under the buildings, linens were filthy, and supplies were scarce. They initiated sanitary reforms, keeping records of illness and deaths. **Figure 4-2** shows a polar-area diagram designed by Nightingale to dramatize the needless deaths that occurred during the war and the effect of her reforms (Aiken, 1988; Bostridge, 2008; Cohen, 1984).

As a result of these early investigations, epidemiology traditionally has most often been associated with infectious diseases, with a focus on the **epidemiological triad**: agent, host, and environment (see **Figure 4-3**). That is to say one particular organism such as the measles virus (agent) infects the host (human) and, if the conditions are appropriate within the human (environment), morbidity (illness/symptoms) will occur. Essentially, the epidemiological triad remains a fundamental conceptual framework for the contemporary study of health problems.

Causal relations (one factor causing another particular event) are more complex than depicted in the epidemiological triangle. Therefore, the **web of causation** is another

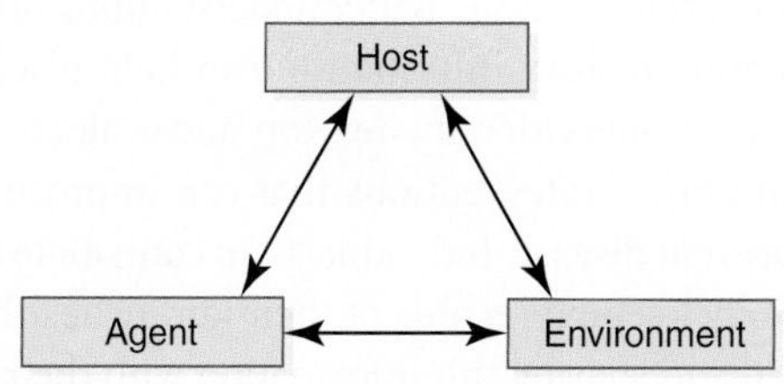

Figure 4-3 The epidemiological triad.

model used in descriptive epidemiology that is based on the belief that health status is multifactorial, determined by the interaction of many agent, host, and environment characteristics, and not by any single factor. For example, factors influencing the development of a heart attack include heredity, high cholesterol levels, dietary excess, cigarette smoking, emotional stress, lack of physical exercise, and many other factors. No one factor is considered a causative factor for the illness.

The **ecological model** for population health is supported by the Institute of Medicine's (IOM, 2002) report, which expands epidemiological studies upward into broader contexts such as neighborhood characteristics and community and social contexts, and downward to the genetic molecular level. The ecological model addresses multiple determinants of health as interrelated and acting synergistically or antagonistically rather than as individual discrete factors. This model encompasses determinants at many levels: biological, emotional, behavioral, socioeconomic, cultural, political, and environmental. The IOM's vision of healthy people in healthy communities requires a model that recognizes that healthy communities are more than a group of individuals who are healthy. But rather, contextual features of a community impact the health of the people who live there.

Risk is the probability that a particular event or outcome will occur within a specified time period. **Genomics** is the study of all the genes in a person, as well as the interactions of those genes with each other and a person's environment. All people are 99.9% identical in genetic makeup, but differences in the remaining 0.1% hold important clues about health and disease.

> Genomics plays a role in nine of the leading causes of death in the U.S. most notably cancer and heart disease. These diseases are partly the result of how genes interact with environmental and behavioral risk factors, such as diet and physical activity. Also, a large fraction of children's hospitalizations are due to diseases that have genetic components. By studying the relationship between genes, environment, and behaviors, researchers and practitioners can learn why some people get sick, while others do not. Family health history information can also help to identify people who may have a higher risk for certain diseases. Better understanding of genetic and family history information can help researchers and practitioners identify, develop, and evaluate screening and other interventions that can improve health and prevent disease. Individuals can contribute to their health by keeping records of their family health information and sharing this information with their doctor and with other family members. (CDC, n.d.)

Epidemiology can be considered as a *methodology* used to study health-related conditions and as a *body of knowledge* that results from research into a specific health-related condition (Alanis, 1999; Gordis, 2004). Using epidemiological research methodology to investigate health problems leads to the accumulation of a body of knowledge about that particular problem. (Epidemiological research methods are discussed later in the chapter.) Practitioners then can use this body of knowledge in their clinical decision making and in developing health services. For example, epidemiological research has associated hypertension, obesity, and smoking with increased incidence of heart disease. These are all potentially modifiable risk factors that often are associated with lifestyle and behavior choices. Nurses and other health professionals can use this information when assessing individual patients and helping them make choices about intervention techniques that may reduce their risk of heart disease. Also, community health nurses may initiate community-level programs to identify hypertension at an early stage, to stop smoking, or to decrease weight in an attempt to decrease the risk of heart disease for the population as a whole.

Scope of Epidemiology

The scope of epidemiology has been expanded and therefore changed in recent years. Not only are the distribution and determinants of illness and disease investigated, but variables that contribute to the maintenance of health are also studied. The evolving changes in demographic characteristics, the patterns of disease, methods of control and prevention of health problems, and the need for maintaining wellness have contributed to this shift in the scope of epidemiology. *Healthy People 2020* uses determinants of health to derive the objectives for the nation. The depth of topics covered by the objectives reflects the diversity of critical influences that determine the health of persons who live in communities. Improved public health services, increased life expectancy, increased frequency of noninfectious disease and chronic degenerative conditions, and advances in technology are continually changing the health needs of society. (See **Table 4-1** for a comparison of the leading causes of death in the United States over time.) Provision of present and future health care depends on (1) identifying health problems and needs, (2) collecting and analyzing data to identify factors that influence those health problems or needs, and (3) planning, implementing, and evaluating methods for prevention and control. These steps form the basis of the epidemiological process.

TABLE 4-1 Comparison of the Leading Causes of Death in the United States Between 1900 and 2010

1900	2000	2010
1. Major cardiovascular-renal diseases	1. Heart disease	1. Diseases of heart (heart disease)
2. Influenza and pneumonia	2. Cancer—malignant neoplasms	2. Malignant neoplasms (cancer)
3. Tuberculosis	3. Cardiovascular disease (strokes)	3. Chronic lower respiratory diseases
4. Gastritis, duodenitis, enteritis, colitis	4. Chronic lower respiratory disease	4. Cerebrovascular diseases (stroke)
5. Accidents	5. Unintentional injuries (accidents)	5. Accidents (unintentional injuries)
6. Malignant neoplasms	6. Diabetes mellitus	6. Alzheimer's disease
7. Diphtheria	7. Alzheimer's disease	7. Diabetes mellitus (diabetes)
8. Typhoid and paratyphoid fever	8. Influenza and pneumonia	8. Nephritis, nephrotic syndrome and nephrosis (kidney disease)
9. Measles	9. Kidney disease	9. Influenza and pneumonia
10. Cirrhosis of the liver	10. Septicemia	10. Intentional self-harm (suicide)

Sources: Reproduced from Kung, H. C., Hoyert, D. L., Xu, J., & Murphy, S. L. (2008). Deaths: Final data for 2005. *National Vital Statistics Report, 56*(10), 1–120.

The Epidemiological, Research, and Nursing Processes

The epidemiological process, the research process, and the nursing process have all evolved from steps in the problem-solving process. All three processes have similar basic components: defining the problem, gathering data, analyzing the data, and evaluating the results. The research process focuses on obtaining new knowledge about a health condition. The epidemiological process and the nursing process are more focused on planning for control, for prevention, or for intervention activities that will mediate a health condition (**Table 4-2**). The cyclical nature of the epidemiological process is illustrated in **Figure 4-4.**

TABLE 4-2 Similarities Between the Epidemiological Process, the Research Process, and the Nursing Process

Epidemiological Process	Research Process	Nursing Process
• Define Problem	• Define problem	• Assessment: Establish patient database
• Gather information from reliable sources	• Review literature	• Diagnosis: Interpret data Identify healthcare needs Select goals of care
• Describe problem by person, place, time	• Conceptualize problem	• Planning: Select process for achieving goals
• Formulate tentative hypothesis	• Define variables	• Implementation: Initiate and complete actions to achieve goals
• Analyze descriptive date to test hypothesis	• Identify methodology	• Evaluation: Determine extent of goal achievement
• Plan for control of the problem	• Collect data	
• Implement control plan	• Analyze data	
• Evaluate control plan	• Publish report	
• Prepare appropriate report	• Conduct further research	
• Conduct further research		

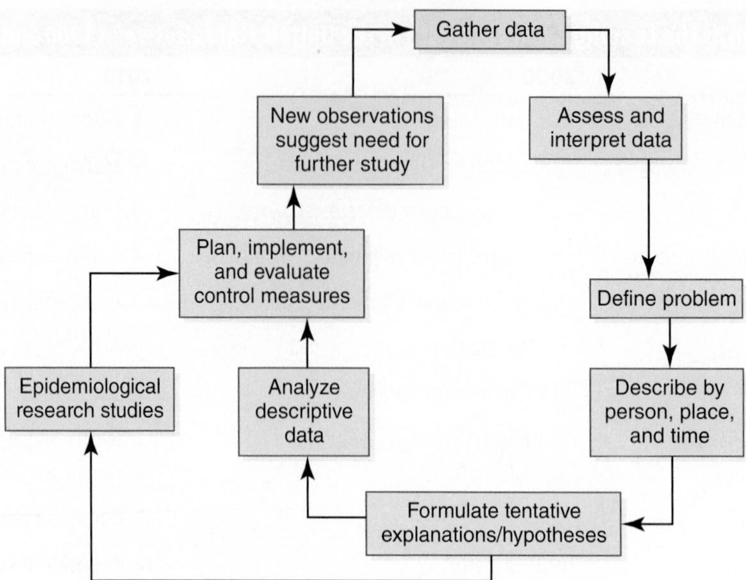

Figure 4-4 Model of epidemiological process.

RESEARCH ALERT

The purpose of this research study was to identify driving factors behind the incidence of macular edema (ME) in a population of insulin-dependent diabetics living in Wisconsin. Data were collected over the course of 25 years; participants included 955 individuals selected from 10,135 diabetic patients who received primary care in an 11-county area in southern Wisconsin from 1979 to 1980. This sample was composed of patients with type 1 diabetes diagnosed before age 30 years who participated in baseline examinations (1980–1982) and at least 1 of 4 follow-up (4-, 10-, 14-, and 25-year) examinations ($n = 891$) or died before the first follow-up examination ($n = 64$). Data collection at each follow-up exam included measuring weight, height, and blood pressure; dilating the pupils; taking stereoscopic color fundus photographs of seven standard fields (not done at 20-year follow up); performing a semiquantitative determination of protein levels in the urine; and determining blood glucose and glycosylated hemoglobin A1 levels from a capillary blood sample at the baseline, 4-, 10-, and 14-year follow ups and glycosylated hemoglobin A1c from venous blood at the 20- and 25-year follow ups. Cumulative 25-year incidence rates were calculated with a modification of the Kaplan-Meier approach to account for censored observations due to missed examinations and the competing risk of death. Although a number of factors, including patient sex, body mass index, smoking, elevated A1c, and hypertension were associated with the development of ME, the authors found that two factors—elevated systolic blood pressure and elevated A1c—were statistically significant in relation to ME, with proteinuria having marginal significance. In patients with diabetic retinopathy, elevated A1c had the strongest association with ME. Interestingly, hypertension was an inconsistent marker of ME; elevated diastolic blood pressure showed no significant correlation to ME, while systolic hypertension was correlated. These data suggest that improved glycemic control and blood pressure reduction may reduce incidence of ME in diabetic patients.

Sources: Klein, R., Knudtson, M. D., Lee, K. E., Gangnon, R., & Klein, B. E. (2008). The Wisconsin Epidemiologic Study of Diabetic Retinopathy XXIII: The twenty-five-year incidence of macular edema in persons with type 1 diabetes. *Ophthalmology, 116*(3), 497–503.

Natural History of Disease

In 1958, Leavell and Clark, two public health physicians, championed the cause of preventive medicine by emphasizing that prevention is required at every phase of the disease process among populations. They called the course of any disease process as it develops in humans the "natural history of the disease." For example, HIV disease progression, or the natural history of HIV disease, encompasses prevention of contracting HIV, HIV infection detection, asymptomatic HIV infection, period with symptoms, and finally acquired immune deficiency syndrome (AIDS) diagnosis (see **Figure 4-5**). During the *prepathogenesis* period, there are factors within individuals and their environments that may predispose or precipitate the disease. The initial interactions among agent, host, and environment occur during

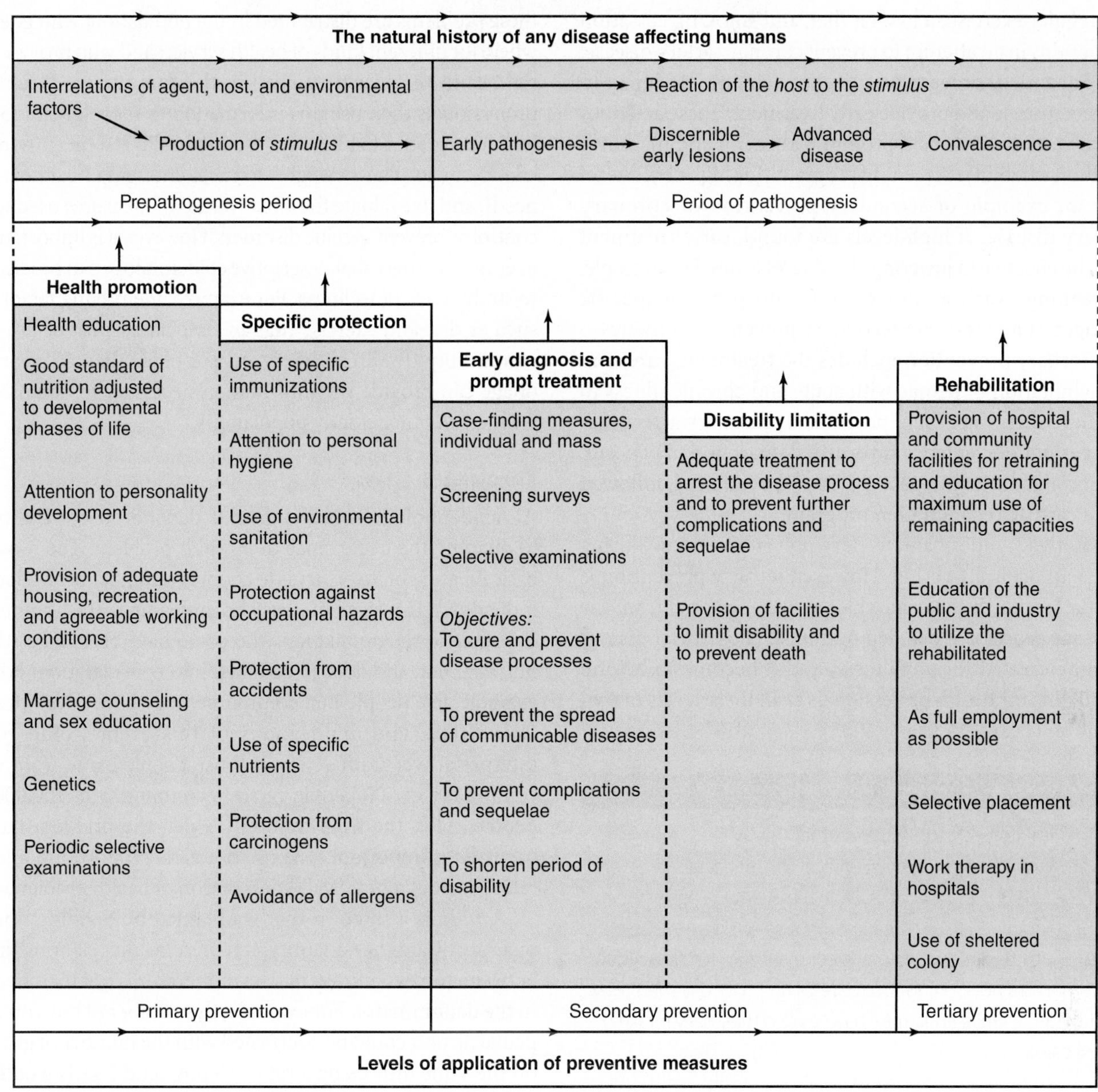

Figure 4-5 Levels of application of preventive measures in the natural history of disease.

Sources: Data from Leavell & Clark, 1965.

this period. For example, an individual may have an inherited predisposition to high cholesterol levels and may be obese, a smoker, and under excessive pressure at work in the prepathogenesis period. The period of *pathogenesis* begins when the host begins to respond with biological, psychological, or other changes. It is manifested by signs and symptoms that continue until the condition is resolved by recovery, disability, or death. If this individual is not able to modify the factors that predispose to disease, he or she is at high risk for a heart attack. As can be seen, this model applies to specific populations and the individuals who compose them.

Leavell and Clark (1958) identified *levels of prevention* for the prepathogenesis and pathogenesis periods as primary prevention, secondary prevention, and tertiary prevention.

Primary prevention includes activities that prevent a disease from becoming established and occurs during the prepathogenesis period. These activities include health promotion activities and specific protection activities such as immunizations and protection from hazards and hygiene. Because no symptoms of illness exist, primary prevention programs are directed toward either the general healthy population or toward a group of healthy people who are known to be at high risk for a particular disease, illness, or injury. For example, public health organizations and voluntary agencies have emphasized the importance of regular exercise, a low-fat diet, and smoking cessation programs in an attempt to prevent coronary artery disease.

Secondary prevention includes activities designed to detect disease and provide early treatment. These activities involve early diagnosis, prompt treatment, and measures to limit disability. Screening programs for high cholesterol are an example of secondary prevention of coronary artery disease. If high levels are found, early treatment can be effective in lowering cholesterol levels. For example, screenings such as monograms and prostate-specific antigen (PSA) tests are secondary prevention activities.

Tertiary prevention includes the treatment, care, and rehabilitation of people with acute and chronic illness to achieve their maximum potential. If coronary artery disease is not prevented, a myocardial infarction may occur. A coronary artery bypass graft may be required, followed by a cardiac rehabilitation program.

Both secondary and tertiary prevention occur during the pathogenesis period. However, tertiary prevention is initiated after irreversible changes have resulted from the disease process. A detailed outline of the natural history can be created for any illness, and it becomes a helpful guideline for health professionals at all three levels of prevention (Leavell & Clark, 1965).

ETHICAL CONNECTION 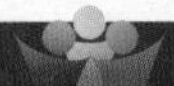

Epidemiological studies consistently show that Americans are getting fatter. The percentage of Americans who were obese in 1971 was 14.5%; in 2005, that percentage had climbed to a staggering 30.9%. The number of deaths per year associated with being overweight is estimated at 400,000. Adult women are now eating 335 more calories per day than they did in 1971, while adult men have upped their daily intake by 168 calories.

What ethical responsibilities do community health nurses have in the prevention of obesity versus the treatment of obesity-related diseases? Where are most of the resources spent in the healthcare system related to this serious, yet preventable health problem?

Descriptive Epidemiology

Descriptive epidemiology focuses on the frequency and distribution of states of health within a population. By describing characteristics of groups of people who have or do not have certain illnesses, factors that are associated primarily with the people who have the illness can be identified. These are called **risk factors**. Knowledge regarding risk factors provides supporting data to plan primary and secondary prevention activities. Generally, descriptive data can tell us what kind of people are at risk of developing certain health problems; what diseases, disabilities, or needs they have; how these problems are distributed in the population; who goes where for different kinds of health service; and who provides the health services they need in the community. Health professionals then use this information to set priorities for health programs, to find ways of using health resources more effectively, to plan strategies to meet emerging healthcare needs, and to evaluate the effectiveness of measures used to control or prevent specific disorders. However, it is important to emphasize here that descriptive epidemiology can be used to study states of wellness. For example, identifying factors such as diet and exercise that are associated with healthy, community-dwelling elderly people older than 85 years of age can provide the information necessary to enhance wellness in other elderly populations.

Use of Rates

All epidemiological investigations depend on the ability to quantify the occurrence of a health problem. The most basic measure of *frequency* is to count the number of affected individuals. However, this may be misleading. The number of people in the population who could have been affected, but were not, should also be taken into consideration. For example, five people in a community may have developed HIV/AIDS. The implications of this event would be interpreted very differently if those people came from a community of 500 people versus a community of 100,000 people. Also, the time frame in which the problem has occurred is important. The use of ratios, proportions, and rates provides a more valid description of health problems.

A *ratio* is a fraction that is obtained by dividing one quantity by another quantity; it represents the relationship between the two numbers. The numerator is not included in the denominator. For example, the number of boys on a pediatric unit could be contrasted with the number of girls on the same unit using a ratio: 10 boys and 5 girls would result in a 2:1 ratio of boys to girls.

A *proportion* is a type of ratio that includes the quantity in the numerator also as a part of the denominator. Therefore, it is the relationship of a part to the whole. Dividing the number of boys on the pediatric unit by the total number of boys and girls on the unit results in a proportion: 10 boys out of 15 boys and girls would result in a proportion of boys equal to 67%.

Two useful measures for comparing risks are relative risk (RR) and odds ratio. RR is the risk of an event (or of developing a disease) relative to exposure. RR is a ratio and probability of the event occurring in the exposed group versus a nonexposed group that can be found using the following equation:

$$RR = \frac{p \text{ event when exposed}}{p \text{ event when nonexposed}}$$

Suppose you are trying to find the RR of cancer associated with smoking, where a is the number of smokers with lung cancer, b is the number of smokers without lung cancer, c is the number of nonsmokers with lung cancer, and d is the number of nonsmokers without lung cancer. If $a = 20$, $b = 80$, $c = 1$, and $d = 99$, RR would be calculated as follows:

$$RR = \frac{a/(a+b)}{c/(c+d)} = \frac{20/100}{1/100} = 20.$$

Smokers would be 20 times as likely as nonsmokers to develop lung cancer. (Alternatively, RR can be calculated using MedCalc, an online calculator available for free at: http://www.medcalc.org/calc/relative_risk.php.) Another term for the RR is the risk ratio because it is the ratio of the risk in the exposed divided by the risk in the unexposed. RR is used frequently in the statistical analysis of binary outcomes where the outcome of interest has relatively low probability. It is thus often suited to clinical trial data, where it is used to compare the risk of developing a disease, in people not receiving the new medical treatment (or receiving a placebo) versus people who are receiving an established (standard of care) treatment. Alternatively, it is used to compare the risk of developing a side effect in people receiving a drug as compared to the people who are not receiving the treatment (or receiving a placebo; Macha & McDonough, 2012; Macintyre & Ellaway, 2000; Sheskin, 2004).

Rate is defined as a measure of frequency of an event or diagnosis in a defined population within a given time period. In other words, a rate is a proportion that includes the factor of time. Rates are the best indicators of the probability that a disease, condition, or event will occur; therefore, rates are the primary measurements used to describe occurrence. Rates take into consideration the population statistics and are frequently a more precise measure than is frequency. By using rates, it is possible to compare events that happen at different times and places and with different people. For example, rates make it possible to compare the occurrence of HIV/AIDS in two or more locations.

ENVIRONMENTAL CONNECTION

Many nursing students note that the environment gets little attention, compared to the person and agent parts of the epidemiological triangle in the nursing curriculum. What do you think?

A rate consists of two parts: a *numerator* and a *denominator*. The numerator is composed of the number of cases of the health problem being investigated within a given period. The denominator is the population at risk during the same period. If the period is long, the population at risk is often estimated at a midperiod, such as midyear. There are four basic principles that apply to the calculation of rates:

1. The numerator should include all events being measured; therefore, adequate information must be available.
2. Everyone in the denominator must be at risk for the event in the numerator.
3. A specific period must be indicated during which observations are made.
4. To make the rate a reasonable size to interpret and remove decimal points, the rate is multiplied by a base, usually a multiple of 10. Any base multiple of 10 may be chosen that results in a rate above the value of 1.

The formula for rate calculation follows:

$$Rate = \frac{\textit{Number of conditions or events occurring in a period of time}}{\textit{Population at risk during the same period of time}} \times \textit{Base multiple of 10}$$

Table 4-3 illustrates the calculation of rates that can be compared between cities.

An example of the difference between rates and ratios is shown in **Figure 4-6**. Legal abortion rates are defined as the number of legal abortions per 1,000 women age 15 to 44 years. Women experiencing legal abortions are in the numerator, and all women of childbearing age are in the

TABLE 4-3 Calculating and Comparing Rates Between Two Cities

City A	City B
• Number of hepatitis cases (conditions) = 45	• Number of hepatitis cases (conditions) = 341
• Population of City A = 153,000	• Population of City B = 1,326,000
• Hepatitis rate = 45/153,000 = 0.000294	• Hepatitis rate = 341/1,326,000 = 0.000257
• 0.000294 × 100,000 (base multiple of 10) = 29.4	• 0.000257 × 100,000 (base multiple of 10) = 25.7
• Hepatitis rate = 29.4 cases/100,000 people	• Hepatitis rate = 25.7 cases/100,000 people

Counting only cases, City B has a higher frequency of hepatitis. However, when the population at risk is included in the rate calculation, City A has more cases per population than City B.

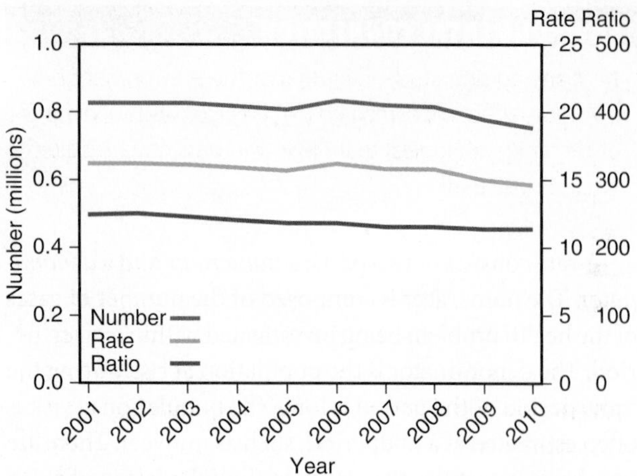

Figure 4-6 Number, rate, and ratio of abortions performed, by year—selected reporting areas,* United States, 1974–2010.

Source: Reproduced from CDC.

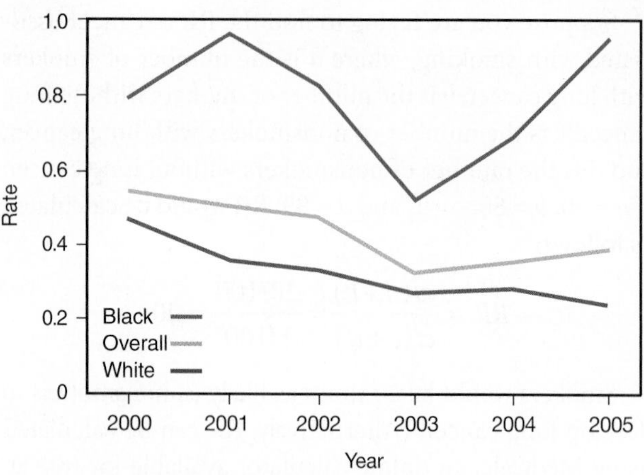

* Per 1,000 live births.
† Occurring in infants aged 0-6 days.
Rates for 2000-2005 correspond to surveillance areas participating since 2000, with the addition of Colorado in 2001. New Mexico, where surveillance began in 2004, is not included in comparison of incidence over time.

Figure 4-7 Rate of early onset group B streptococcal GBS disease by race and year.

Source: Reproduced from CDC.

denominator. The abortion ratio is the number of legal induced abortions per 1,000 live births. The numerator, the number of legal induced abortions, is not a part of the denominator, live births. Therefore, it is a ratio and not a rate. However, the number of legal induced abortions per 1,000 women of childbearing age is a rate, the abortion rate. Figure 4-6 shows the changes in the rates and ratio over a 10-year period (Centers for Disease Control and Prevention [CDC], 2013a).

Incidence Rates

Incidence is a form of rate that measures the *occurrence of new illnesses* in a previously disease-free group of people within a specific time frame, often 1 year. Therefore, it is a measure of the probability that people without a certain condition will develop the condition over a period of time. The numerator of incidence rates includes only the number of *new* conditions or events occurring within a period of time; therefore, the date of onset must be known. The general rules that apply to rates apply to incidence rates. Incidence rates and incidence ratios, especially **mortality** (death) rates, are often indices of the health of communities.

GLOBAL CONNECTION

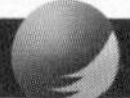

People living in Japan have from one-half to one-third the risk of dying from heart disease in comparison to people living in the United States, even when their mean cholesterol levels remain the same. When Japanese immigrants settle in the United States, within 5 years their risk for heart disease equals that of native U.S. citizens. How do you explain this difference?

Incidence rates can be used to determine trends over time. For example, **Figure 4-7** shows the rates of group B streptococcal (GBS) infection among infants in the United States (CDC, 2007b). This infection is the leading cause of bacterial disease and death among newborns in the United States and can cause illness and death in peripartum women and in adults with chronic medical conditions. Therefore, the incidence of this disease has been tracked in selected cities and their surrounding regions in different geographic locations. This incidence rate has been calculated as the number of infants infected per 1,000 live births. Figure 4-7 shows that while the incidence of GBS disease decreased among white infants after guidelines for preventing perinatal GBS disease were issued, it increased significantly among black infants. Continued surveillance is necessary to determine if this trend continues and to identify possible barriers to universal screening among black women (CDC, 2007b).

Prevalence Rates

Prevalence rates measure the number of people in a *given population who have an existing health problem within a specified time frame.* There are two types of prevalence rates. **Period prevalence** indicates the existence of a condition during an interval of time. **Point prevalence** refers to the existence of a condition at a specific point in time. **Prevalence** measures the amount of **morbidity** (illness) that exists in a community as a result of the health problem under investigation. Many healthcare workers believe that prevalence rates are more important than incidence rates

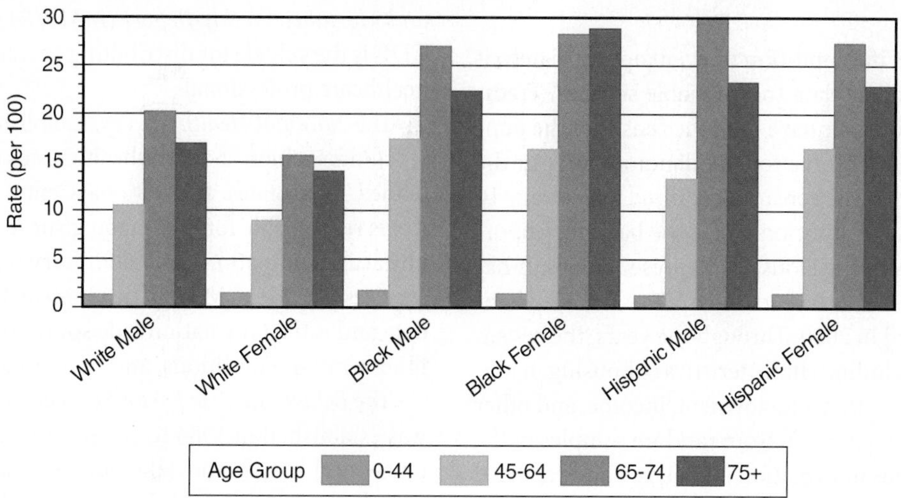

Figure 4-8 Age-specific prevalence of diagnosed diabetes by race/ethnicity and sex, United States, 2005.

Source: Reproduced from CDC.

in determining the total burden of the illness on the community. Community health nurses use prevalence data to plan for the allocation of resources in a community based on the amount of disease burden present. Knowledge of the prevalence of a condition such as diabetes mellitus within a population can lead to the prioritizing of facilities, services, and personnel to meet the special needs of diabetics in the community.

Prevalence is influenced by two factors: the number of people who have developed the condition in the past and the duration of their illness. A formula for prevalence is:

$$Prevalence = Incidence \times Duration\ of\ Illness$$

The longer the duration of a condition, the higher the prevalence rate in the community. This is best illustrated with chronic diseases. For example, there are many more cases of diabetes in a community than would be indicated by calculation of the incidence rate, which reflects new cases only. Although the incidence rate for diabetes is low, people live for many years with the illness, and the duration is high. Therefore, in calculating prevalence rates, the numerator consists of the number of *existing* cases of the condition or event that occur within a specified period. For example, the existing cases of diabetes mellitus include new cases that were recently diagnosed plus those cases diagnosed in the past who are currently living with the illness.

Crude, Specific, and Adjusted Rates

Other common rates include crude, specific, and adjusted rates. **Crude rates** measure the experience of health problems in populations of designated geographic areas. These broad descriptive statistics may obscure significant differences in the risk of developing various conditions. Factors such as age, gender, ethnicity, and other demographic factors are not taken into consideration. Therefore, **specific rates** for subgroups of the population may be calculated. These more detailed rates are commonly calculated to describe the distribution of health problems by age, gender, ethnicity, and other demographic characteristics. **Adjusted rates** have been standardized, removing the differences in composition of populations, such as age. **Figure 4-8** illustrates the prevalence of diabetes in four specific age groups. The rates are highest in the 65-to-74 and 75-plus categories. **Figure 4-9** illustrates age-adjusted rates of self-reported diabetes by race (CDC, 2007a). In this example, age adjustment removes age as a factor in the calculation of the rates. Therefore, the differences shown reflect a rather dramatic increase in diabetes mellitus in African American females. Knowledge of these factors can be helpful in assessing individual patients for their healthcare needs, as well as group needs for prevention and control programs.

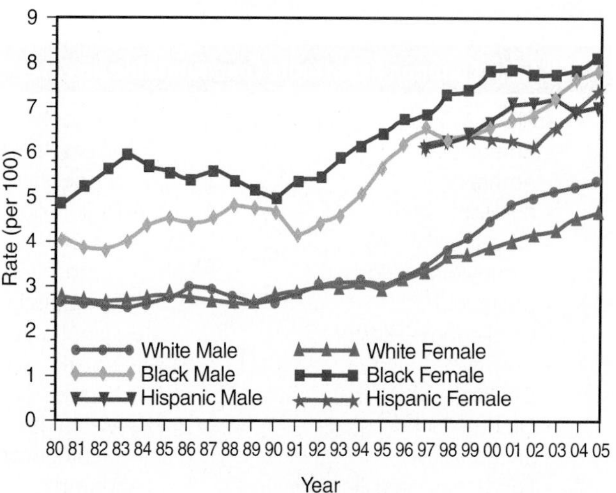

Figure 4-9 Age-adjusted prevalence of diagnosed diabetes by race/ethnicity and sex, United States, 1980-2005.

Source: Reproduced from CDC.

Sources of Data

To describe a specific condition or event appropriately, it is necessary to collect data from reliable sources. Traditionally, epidemiologists have used the census of the population as a reliable source for the denominators in the calculation of rates. The census is required once every 10 years by the U.S. Constitution and is the basis for apportionment of seats in the House of Representatives. It has been performed every 10 years since 1790. The 23rd census was completed in 2010. Through the years, the census has expanded, including characteristics of housing, nativity, migration, education, employment, income, and other information that is gathered from random samples of the population. Census information is analyzed and reported for the nation as a whole and in progressively smaller regions down to municipalities, census tracts, and blocks. Results are also reported in regions known as standard metropolitan statistical areas (SMSA). These regions are densely populated and are not necessarily bound by traditional state or county lines. The majority of the population of the United States lives within these areas.

Vital statistics are data collected from the continuous recording of events such as births, deaths, marriages, divorces, and adoptions, usually by state agencies. This information can be used to provide valid numerators and denominators for calculation of rates. CDC in Atlanta collects all information regarding reportable diseases from state health departments. A sample of common reportable communicable diseases is provided in **Box 4-1**. However, reportable diseases may vary somewhat from state to state and change as disease rates emerge and decline. The CDC also collects information about other infectious and noninfectious health problems through a series of more than 100 national surveillance programs. The *Morbidity and Mortality Weekly Report (MMWR)* published by the CDC is the vehicle for distributing current information to healthcare professionals.

The *National Health Survey*, established in 1956, provides information about the health needs of the population of the United States. The National Center for Health Statistics is responsible for the ongoing surveys of households, physical examinations and laboratory reports, and health services providers. Most of this information is prevalence data and is the only nationwide source of data on chronic illness, minor conditions, and functional problems.

The *Behavioral Risk Factor Surveillance System (BRFSS)* was established in 1984 to collect, analyze, and interpret behavioral risk factor data from all states. Information is gathered about health behaviors such as obesity, lack of physical activity, smoking, seatbelt use, and screening programs for breast cancer and elevated blood cholesterol. These BRFSS data were used in the formulation of national and state objectives for the years 2010 and 2020. Updated data are published regularly in the *MMWR*.

Any health-related information that has been collected about a group of people can be a source of data used to determine the distribution of states of health. Health-related information often is found in databases from healthcare institutions, disease registries, insurance companies, industries, accident and police records, private physicians' and health providers' offices, local surveys, and any other place where information is gathered. Community health nurses are likely to use these data when planning programs for groups of people with specific health needs and when information about the population is needed. These records reflect only those conditions or events that are characteristic of the people that sought the services of that agency or participated in the survey. These data are helpful in

BOX 4-1 Common Reportable Communicable Diseases

- AIDS
- Amebiasis
- Anthrax
- Botulism
- Brucellosis
- Campylobacteriosis
- Chancroid
- Chickenpox—Zoster
- Chlamydia
- Cholera
- Diphtheria
- Encephalitis
- Food-associated illnesses
- Giardiasis
- Gonorrhea
- Granuloma inguinale
- Hemophilus influenza
- Hepatitis A, B, non-A, non-B, unspecified
- Legionellosis
- Leprosy
- Leptospirosis
- Lyme disease
- Lymphogranuloma venereum
- Malaria
- Measles
- Meningitis
- Meningococcal infection
- Mumps
- Pertussis
- Plague
- Poliomyelitis
- Psittacosis
- Rabies
- Reye's syndrome
- Rocky Mountain spotted fever
- Rubella
- Salmonellosis
- Shigellosis
- Syphilis
- Tetanus
- Toxic shock syndrome
- Trichinosis
- Tuberculosis
- Tularemia
- Typhoid fever
- Typhus
- Yellow fever

establishing health services to meet their needs and in evaluating outcomes, but data must be interpreted carefully when applying the information to the community as a whole.

Person, Place, and Time

One of the first steps in investigating the distribution and determinants of a healthcare problem is to describe the problem *(what occurs)* in terms of person, place, and time. *Descriptive epidemiology* deals primarily with the study of the distribution of health problems. However, research studies that attempt to identify the determinants of a problem *(why it occurs)* depend on the accurate collection of descriptive data. Examining the information about person, place, and time can help identify the characteristics of people who develop a disease or illness and those who do not.

Person

Describing the person characterizes *who* develops the health problem. There are many variations among people based on genetic factors, biological characteristics, behavioral choices, lifestyle, and socioeconomic conditions. Because so many variations exist, incidence and prevalence rates should be calculated according to these factors. This can be done by examining individual case data and examining specific and adjusted rates. Age is the most important characteristic affecting health status, followed by sex. Therefore, age-specific rates and sex-specific rates are usually calculated when describing a problem. Age-specific rates are calculated using the number of people in a given age group who have the problem being investigated in the numerator, and the population at risk in the given age group in the denominator.

An example of age-specific rates follows. The study describes heat-related deaths in Maryland, Ohio, Virginia, and West Virginia when temperatures elevated for 2 weeks during June and July of 2012 (CDC, 2013b). **Figure 4-10** is a graph that shows that the average rate of heat-related deaths each year in males and females (CDC, 2012).

Using this knowledge, community health nurses could initiate multiple actions, either for individuals in their care or for groups. When a heat wave is forecast, primary prevention messages about how to avoid heat-related illness should be disseminated to the public. The elderly should be encouraged to maintain their fluid intake and assisted to increase their time in air-conditioned environments, making use of shopping malls and public libraries, even for part of the day. Alcohol consumption should be discouraged because it may cause dehydration and increase the risk for heat-related illnesses. Parents of young children should be educated about the increased heat sensitivity of young children and their need for adequate fluids. Daycare centers could be primary sites for dissemination of information.

Often, specific rates are presented in table or graph form, combining characteristics of persons and changes over time. **Figure 4-11** indicates the number of reported tuberculosis cases and the age characteristics of the cases by year, as well as the percentage change from 1993 to 2012 (CDC, 2003). More recent data are available on the Internet in the form of charts developed by the CDC; these may be downloaded from the CDC's website (http://www.cdc.gov/tb/statistics/surv/surv2012/default.htm). This information shows that people older than 65 are the most vulnerable to tuberculosis. Nurses use this knowledge in establishing primary prevention programs and in assessing their elderly patients for signs and symptoms that may be indicative of the infection.

Place

Where the rates of the health problem are the highest or the lowest can be determined by examining the characteristics of place. Understanding where illness occurs is a primary factor to be considered in planning prevention and control

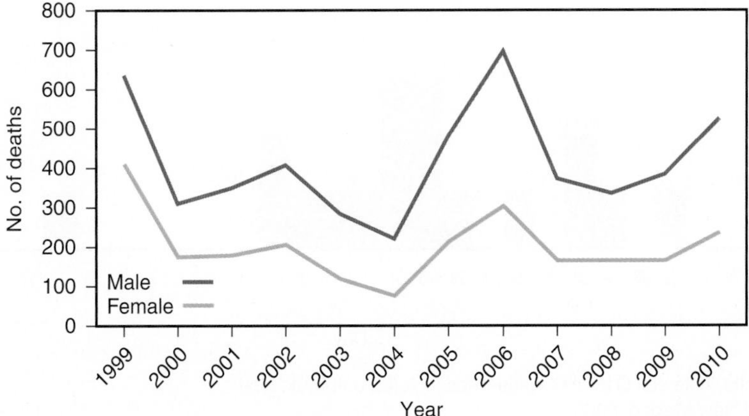

Figure 4-10 Number of heat-related deaths, by sex — National Vital Statistics System, United States, 1999–2010§.

Source: Reproduced from CDC.

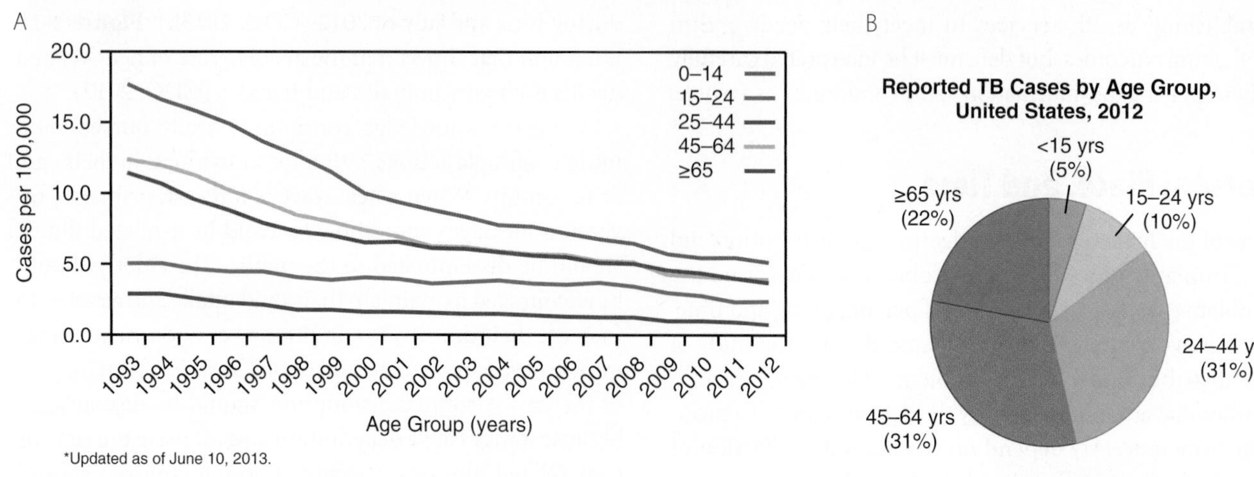

Figure 4-11 TB Case Rates* by Age Group United States, 1993–2012.

Source: Reproduced from CDC.

measures and making decisions about distribution of healthcare resources. Place can be a neighborhood, a healthcare facility, a town, a region, a nation, or any other natural or political boundary. The identification of health differences between urban and rural sectors or between similar localities is often helpful in investigating specific health needs of a community.

Place often is illustrated through the use of maps. For example, in an attempt to monitor progress to reduce the risk of severe adverse effects in children of mothers who consume alcohol, the CDC publishes the prevalence by state of reported frequent alcohol consumption among women of childbearing age. State health departments have used these data to determine priorities for their health objectives for 2020. For example, Wisconsin, Massachusetts, and Washington, DC have the highest prevalence rates (CDC, 2010) and should have targeted primary prevention programs toward this risk factor. Community health nurses would participate in the various efforts to reduce alcohol consumption in this age group.

Time

When health problems occur can be described by identifying short-term fluctuations measured in hours, days, weeks, or months; by periodic changes that are seasonal or cyclical; or by long-term changes over decades that reflect gradual changes. Describing the time of short-term outbreaks of infectious diseases is often performed by developing an **epidemic curve**. These graphs provide indications as to the mode of transmission and spread of the organism. **Figure 4-12** is an example of an epidemic curve. It depicts an outbreak of *Escherichia coli* O157:H7

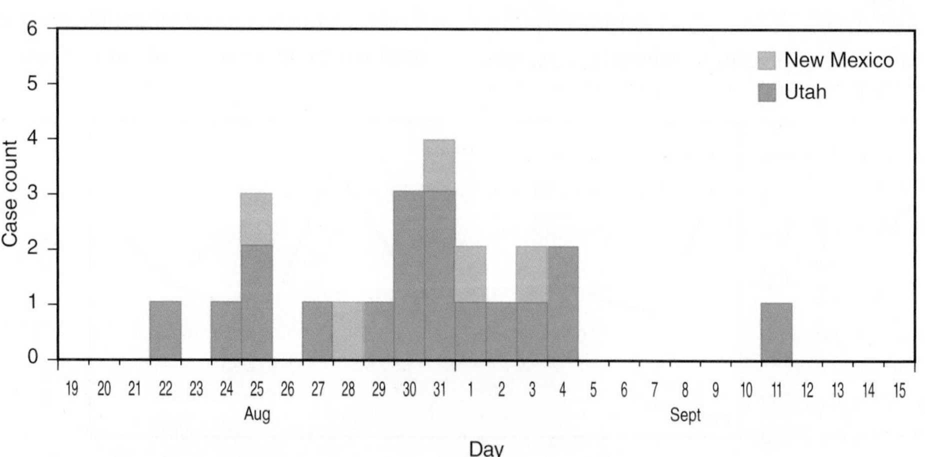

Figure 4-12 Epidemic curve by date of onset of confirmed cases.

Source: Reproduced from CDC.

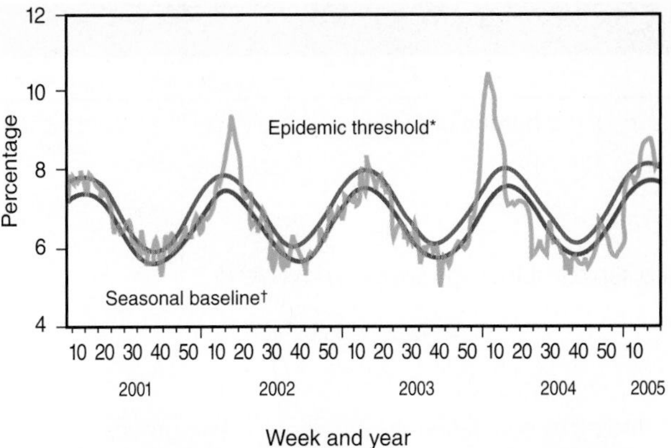

Figure 4-13

Source: Reproduced from CDC.

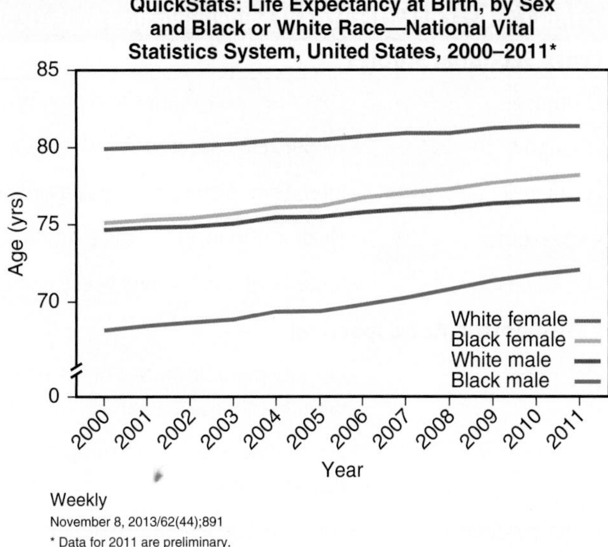

Figure 4-14 Life expectancy at birth, by sex and black or white race—National Vital Statistics System, United States, 2000–2011.*

Source: Reproduced from CDC.

associated with eating spinach in Utah and New Mexico in 2006 (Grant et al., 2008). Nationally, this outbreak involved 205 people. A multistate investigation was initiated, and the U.S. Food and Drug Administration (FDA) and the CDC advised the public not to eat bagged spinach. A case-control study and laboratory investigation conducted by the Utah and New Mexico Departments of Health confirmed 18 cases in Utah and 5 in New Mexico. Illness onset dates ranged from August 22 to September 11. *E. coli* O157:H7, which matched the national strain, was detected in three bags of spinach provided by case patients.

Periodic and *cyclical* changes also occur. For example, respiratory diseases are more common in the winter and spring (periodic), and hepatitis often increases in incidence every 7 to 9 years (cyclical). **Figure 4-13** reflects both periodic and cyclical changes in pneumonia and influenza mortality. A seasonal baseline is developed, and variations from this baseline determine whether an epidemic is occurring.

These types of data are the evidence base for many of the control, prevention, and surveillance activities that are initiated by public health departments and community agencies initiated to keep the public healthy.

Long-term changes or trends over time are shown in **Figure 4-14**. Significant changes in life expectancy at birth occurred between the years 2000 and 2011. The figure includes gender, a characteristic of persons to make the graph more meaningful.

Analytic Epidemiology

As discussed earlier in this chapter, *descriptive epidemiology* focuses on the distribution of health outcomes. Analytic epidemiology focuses on the determinants of health problems, or the *why*. When descriptive data are analyzed, the variations in person, place, and time often suggest tentative explanations or hypotheses. These hypotheses can then be tested through application of research methods in an attempt to find the reasons, or determinants, for these variations. This is a cyclical process because new knowledge may require further descriptive or analytic analysis.

Four types of studies are used in epidemiological analytic investigations: **cross-sectional**, **retrospective (case-control)**, **prospective**, and **intervention** (experimental) studies. The basic characteristics of these studies are outlined in **Table 4-4**. Ideally, the epidemiologist is seeking to establish a cause-and-effect relationship between the health problem or outcome that is being studied (dependent variable) and exposure factors (independent variables) that preceded it in time. Often, associations can be made between a condition and a specific factor, but a direct cause-and-effect relationship is weak or does not exist. More than one factor must be present for any illness to occur (multifactorial causation). Even in an infectious process, such as tuberculosis, presence of the organism alone is not sufficient to cause the disease. Characteristics of the agent, the host, and the environment all interact to determine the onset of the infection. For example, foodborne diseases are an important public health problem in the United States, and the nurse is well positioned to help prevent these infections through education about the handling and consumption of food. The highest risk group for hospitalization and death, as a result of foodborne diseases, includes persons 65 and older. These findings highlight the need

TABLE 4-4 Characteristics of Epidemiological Analytic Studies

Cross-Sectional Studies	
• Purpose	• Describe health states and provide a measure of the burden of a disease (prevalence) in a population
• Design	• All data are collected at the same time
• Data collection	• Interviews, observation, questionnaires
• Advantages	• Flexible, broad, economical, uncomplicated; rapid results, large samples possible
• Disadvantages	• Superficial, cannot infer cause and effect
Case-Control (Retrospective)	
• Purpose	• Identify possible causes or risk factors of a disease by comparing the difference in two groups: one with the disease (cases) and one without the disease (controls)
• Design	• Select case and control samples according to specific criteria. The dependent variable (case or not) has already occurred
• Data collection	• Trace past experience to determine relevant exposure factors (independent variables)
• Advantages	• First step in hypothesis testing, inexpensive, relatively small samples can be used, results obtained quickly
• Disadvantages	• Information about past exposure may not be available • Selection of appropriate control groups may be difficult • Temporal association between exposure and outcome may be difficult to determine • Potential selection, recall, and observation bias
Prospective, Cohort, or Longitudinal Studies	
• Purpose	• Determine the incidence of the health problem in a population at baseline, then follow the population over time to document the incidence of an outcome among exposed and nonexposed persons
• Design	• Samples chosen and observed forward in time
• Data collection	• Information on outcome variables obtained at specific intervals
• Advantages	• Incidence rates can be calculated directly • Time sequence easier to obtain • Effects of rare exposure can be investigated • Multiple outcomes may be studied
• Disadvantages	• May extend over a long period • Expensive • Case lost to follow up
Clinical, Experimental, or Intervention Studies	
• Purpose	• Determine whether a group with particular characteristics will benefit from interventions when compared with a group or groups who do not receive the intervention
• Design	• Randomly choose and assign groups to either a study group or control group • Introduce an intervention (independent variable) to the study group and compare with controls
• Data collection	• Collect data prospectively on a number of dependent variables
• Advantages	• Case and effect can be examined • Control over confounding variables
• Disadvantages	• Possible reactivity (Hawthorne effect) • Possible noncompliance with study protocols • Observation bias, placebo effect

for targeted population-focused action to address food safety gaps (CDC, 2013c). The more factors that can be identified as contributors to a disease process, the weaker the cause-and-effect relationship will be.

NOTE THIS! 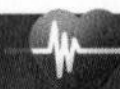

The Framingham Heart Study is a prospective study that has continued to follow the health characteristics of a community for more than 50 years. Much of the information about risk factors for coronary heart disease that underlies preventive programs was obtained from the results of this study.

APPLICATION TO PRACTICE

Using the Ethical Connection, identify primary and secondary interventions that would be feasible and appropriate for a group of elementary school children related to the risk of obesity. What additional information would you need regarding risk factors and interventions prior to designing health promotion programs for addressing them? How would you evaluate these interventions in terms of outcome effectiveness?

ART CONNECTION 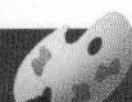

Select a favorite piece of art and identify the host, agent, and environment in the picture.

Conclusion

Promoting and preserving the health of populations are fundamental characteristics of community health nursing. Although nursing is a profession that focuses primarily on the individual, the person's healthcare needs cannot be completely or correctly defined unless family, personal friends, and the characteristics of the community and the society are considered. *Epidemiology,* the science of preventive medicine, provides a framework for studying and understanding these interactions. *Epidemiology* is the study of the distribution and the determinants of states of health and illness in human populations. The basic conceptual framework of epidemiology is the interaction among the agent, host, and environment—the epidemiological triad. Epidemiology is considered both as a methodology used to study health-related conditions and as an accumulated body of knowledge about a state of health. Nurses use the body of knowledge about health problems in their clinical decision making and may become involved in epidemiological research methods to gather new health-related information.

AFFORDABLE CARE ACT (ACA) 

Evidence-based programs that result from epidemiological studies will be used more and more as the mandatory basis for clinical practice in specific populations.

LEVELS OF PREVENTION 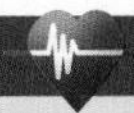

Primary: Educating persons about the necessity of recommended vaccines, such as the influenza vaccine.

Secondary: Providing a group education program for persons who have post-polio syndrome to reduce further complications.

Tertiary: Supporting the rehabilitation program of a person who has experienced severe and irreversible complications from West Nile disease.

Critical Thinking Activities

1. Using an example from your practice, identify two examples that illustrate how the epidemiological body of knowledge is used in clinical decision making.
2. Between January 1 and December 1, 2012, 25 new cases of tuberculosis were diagnosed in Big Valley, population 450,000. A prevalence survey taken the first week in January 2013 indicated that there were 250 cases on the list of active tuberculosis cases. There were 20 deaths due to tuberculosis recorded during this 1-year period. Using this information, calculate the following rates:
   a. What was the incidence rate per 100,000 population for tuberculosis during 2012?
   b. What was the prevalence rate per 100,000 population for tuberculosis during 2012?
   c. What was the cause-specific death rate per 100,000 for tuberculosis in 2012?
3. Discuss how nurses could use the case-control research methodology to answer questions in their practice.
4. A home health patient asks you if her husband should smoke cigarettes inside the house following the birth of their first child. How can you use epidemiological data to support your response to the family?

References

Aiken, L. (1988). *Assuring the delivery of quality patient care. State of the Science Invitational Conference: Nursing resources and the delivery of patient care* (NIH Publication No. 89-3008, pp. 3–10). Washington, DC: U.S. Department of Health and Human Services, Public Health Service.

Alanis, B. (1999). *Epidemiology in health care* (3rd ed.). Stamford, CT: Appleton & Lange.

Bostridge, M. (2008). *Florence Nightingale: The making of an icon.* New York, NY: Farrar, Straus and Giroux.

Centers for Disease Control and Prevention (CDC). (n.d.). Genomics and health. Retrieved from http://www.cdc.gov/genomics/public/index.htm

Centers for Disease Control and Prevention (CDC). (2003). Reported tuberculosis in the United States, 2002. *Surveillance Reports.*

Centers for Disease Control and Prevention (CDC). (2007a). Data and trends: National diabetes surveillance system. Retrieved from http://apps.nccd.cdc.gov/DDTSTRS/default.aspx

Centers for Disease Control and Prevention (CDC). (2007b). Perinatal group B streptococcal disease after universal screening recommendations—United States, 2003–2005. *Morbidity and Mortality Weekly Report, 56*(28), 701–705.

Centers for Disease Control and Prevention (CDC). (2010). State-specific weighted prevalence estimates of alcohol use among women 18–44 years of age, Behavioral Risk Factor Surveillance System, 2010. *Fetal Alcohol Spectrum Disorders–Data and Statistics.* Retrieved from http://www.cdc.gov/ncbddd/fasd/data.html

Centers for Disease Control and Prevention (CDC). (2012a). QuickStats: Number of heat-related deaths, by sex—National Vital Statistics System, United States, 1999–2010. *Morbidity and Mortality Weekly Report, 61*(36), 729.

Centers for Disease Control and Prevention (CDC). (2013a). Abortion surveillance—United States, 2010. *Morbidity and Mortality Weekly Report, 62*(8), 1–12.

Centers for Disease Control and Prevention (CDC). (2013b). Heat-related deaths after an extreme heat event—four states, 2012, and United States, 1999–2009. *Morbidity and Mortality Weekly Report, 62*(22), 433–436.

Centers for Disease Control and Prevention (CDC). (2013c). Incidence and trends of infection with pathogens transmitted commonly through food—foodborne diseases active surveillance network, 10 U.S. sites, 1996-2012. *Morbidity and Mortality Weekly Report, 62*(15), 283–287.

Cohen, B. (1984). Florence Nightingale. *Scientific American, 250*(3), 129.

Doll, R., & Hill, A. B. (1950). Smoking and carcinoma of the lung: Preliminary report. *British Medical Journal,* 2(4682), 739–748.

Gordis, L. (2004). *Epidemiology* (3rd ed.). Philadelphia, PA: Elsevier/Saunders.

Grant, J., Wendelboe, A., Wendel, A., Jepson, B., Torres, P., Smelser, C., & Rolfs, R. (2008). Spinach-associated *Escherichia coli* O157:H7 Outbreak, Utah and New Mexico, 2006. *Emerging Infectious Diseases, 14*(10), 1633–1636.

Humphreys, N. A. (1885). *Vital statistics: A memorial volume of selections from the reports and writings of William Farr.* London, UK: Sanitary Institute of Great Britain.

Institute of Medicine (IOM). (2002). *The future of public health in the 21st century.* Washington, DC: National Academies Press.

Kung, H. C., Hoyert, D. L., Xu, J., & Murphy, S. L. (2008). Deaths: Final data for 2005. *National Vital Statistics Report, 56*(10), 1–120.

Leavell, H. R., & Clark, E. G. (1958). *Preventive medicine for the doctor in his community: An epidemiologic approach* (2rd ed.). New York, NY: McGraw-Hill.

Leavell, H. R., & Clark, E. G. (1965). *Preventive medicine for the doctor in his community: An epidemiologic approach.* (3rd ed.) New York, NY: McGraw-Hill.

Macha J., & McDonough, K. (2012). *Epidemiology for advanced nursing practice.* Burlington, MA: Jones & Bartlett Learning.

Macintyre, S., & Ellaway, A. (2000). Ecological approaches: Rediscovering the role of physical and social environment. In L. Berkman & L. Kawachi (Eds.), *Social epidemiology* (pp. 332–348). New York, NY: Oxford University Press.

McHugh, M., & Ma, C. (2013). Hospital nursing and 30-day readmissions among Medicare patients with heart failure, acute myocardial infarction, and pneumonia. *Medical Care, 51*(1), 52–59.

MedCalc: Easy to Use Statistical Software. (2013). *Relative risk.* Retrieved from http://www.medcalc.org/calc/relative_risk.php

Murphy S. L., Xu, J. Q., & Kochanek K. D. (2013). Deaths: Final data for 2010. *National Vital Statistics Reports, 61*, 4. Hyattsville, MD: National Center for Health Statistics.

Sheskin, D. (2004). *Handbook of parametric and nonparametric statistical procedures* (3rd ed.). Boca Raton, FL: Chapman & Hall.

Snow, J. (1855). *On the mode of communication of cholera.* London, UK: Churchill. (Reproduced in *Snow on cholera.* [1965]. New York, NY: Hafner.)

CHAPTER FOCUS

The Evolving U.S. Healthcare Delivery System
- Private Healthcare Delivery
- Public Health Care
- Military Health Care
- Healthcare Reform

The Current U.S. Healthcare Delivery System
- Levels of Care
- Healthcare Providers
- Healthcare Settings
- Acute Care Facilities

Issues Affecting the Delivery of Healthcare Services
- Deregulation
- Emphasis on Secondary and Tertiary Healthcare Services
- Increasing Consumerism
- Technological Advances
- Increasing Longevity of Americans
- Defensive Health Care and Government Regulation

Managed Care

The Concept of Managed Care
- Managed Care Organizations
- Patient Care Outcomes

Health Politics and Policy
- Government Policy
- Public Opinion and Special-Interest Groups
- Nursing and Healthcare Policy

New Nursing Opportunities
- Advanced Practice Nurses
- Entrepreneurs
- Data Management
- Research

QUESTIONS TO CONSIDER

After reading this chapter, you will know the answers to the following questions:

1. How did the current U.S. healthcare system evolve to its present form?
2. What is the difference between private and public health care?
3. What are some of the current issues affecting health-care delivery in the United States, including the implementation of ACA?
4. How do politics and policy influence the healthcare delivery system?
5. What are some of the current and evolving health-care settings?
6. What impact is managed care having on healthcare delivery?
7. What are some potential roles for nurses within the changing healthcare system?

Health care is one of the largest industries in the United States, employing an estimated 16.4 million workers. The public's healthcare system in the United States includes the most technology-rich facilities and the most advanced practices in the world. The most well-educated physicians, nurses, and other healthcare workers use sophisticated treatments on a daily basis to prolong life and restore function. Less attention and resources have been focused on primary prevention and risk reduction.

CHAPTER 5

Transforming the Public's Healthcare Systems

Bonita R. Reinert and
Karen Saucier Lundy

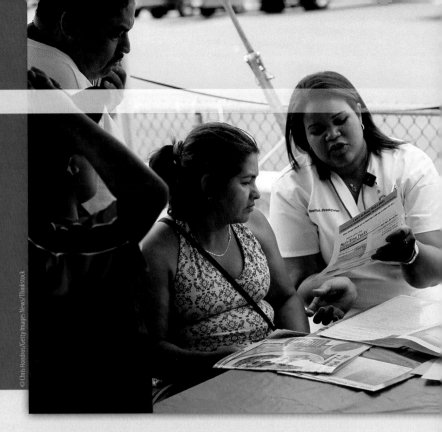

KEY TERMS

Affordable Care Act (ACA)
capitation
defensive health care
diagnosis-related groups (DRGs)
fee-for-service
healthcare delivery system
health maintenance organization (HMO)
integrated healthcare system
long-term care
managed care
managed care organization (MCO)
managed competition
point-of-service (POS) plan
preventive care
primary care
preferred provider organization (PPO)
prospective payment system (PPS)
secondary care
shelter nurse
tertiary care
third-party payer

REFLECTIONS

What has been your experience with health care in the United States as a nursing student and as a patient? What has it been like as an "insider" compared to your experience before you became a nursing student?

HEALTH CARE IS ONE of the largest industries in the United States, employing an estimated 16.4 million workers. This number is likely to grow significantly with the passage of the **Affordable Care Act (ACA)** in 2010, as millions more citizens gain access to health insurance and government-sponsored programs, such as Medicaid, beginning in 2014. The U.S. healthcare system is also unique in comparison with other developed countries around the globe. Almost all other comparable developed countries have universal healthcare coverage of some kind, in which the central government plays a central role in providing health care to all of its citizens. Passage of the ACA expands essential healthcare services via private and public reforms for all citizens by federal mandate. Expansion of health insurance and other public funding sources at an acceptable and affordable cost will remain a challenge for the next several years (see Box 5–1).

The U.S. healthcare system includes the most technology-rich facilities and the most advanced practices in the world. The best educated physicians, nurses, and other healthcare workers use sophisticated treatments on a daily basis to prolong life and restore function. As a result of the cutting-edge nature of this health care, the U.S. system is the most costly, in terms of resources, in the world. This chapter reviews components of the present healthcare system, with an emphasis on public and community health services, as prevention-oriented care becomes the economic incentive for major changes in the healthcare system (Shi & Singh, 2013).

The current patterns of healthcare delivery have resulted in an annual cost that exceeds $2 trillion, a figure that is significantly higher than the expenditures of any other industrialized nation. Costs continue to rise at an alarming rate. This figure represents 17.6% of the U.S. gross domestic product (GDP). Approximate expenditures for hospital care accounted for 30% of all national healthcare expenditures in 2011. Physician and clinical services accounted for 20%, prescription drugs for 10%, and nursing home care for 6%. With the extraordinary costs of health care in the United States, many residents have very limited access to even basic care. The Congressional Budget Office (CBO) estimates that 55 million U.S. citizens under the age of 65 are currently uninsured or underinsured (DeNavas-Walt, 2012). Those without access to health insurance are less likely to utilize primary, preventive services and less likely to seek care when hurt or ill until much later in the disease process—if they do at all.

Despite the advances in healthcare technology and high healthcare costs, clinical outcomes are not always significantly better in the United States when compared to other industrialized nations. In the 2011 National Scorecard on U.S. Health System Performance, which measures and monitors healthcare outcomes, quality, access, efficiency, and equity, the United States ranked 64 out of a possible 100. This score is a continuation of the steady decrease seen over 5 years, from the 67 received in 2006 to the 65 received in 2008. For one indicator, preventable mortality, the United States remained in last place among industrialized nations despite significant overall improvements—largely because other nations improved this metric even more (Commonwealth Fund Commission on a High Performance Health System, 2011). Access to health care is believed to be one of the determinants of the less than auspicious health indicators in the United States.

Lack of access to quality healthcare services can take several forms. For example, needed services may simply not be available in an accessible location or during hours when individuals are able to use them. The healthcare site may not be organized in a user-friendly manner so that individuals can obtain timely and acceptable services. For example, providers may not be as culturally sensitive or as multilingual as is needed in certain locations in the United States. Routine health care may also not be accessible because of a lack of personal funds and/or insurance coverage. Medications and special treatments may be beyond the financial resources of the individual despite a provider's carefully developed plan of care. Finally, individuals may not have a regular provider and thus may have to receive care from a variety of providers in a number of unconnected facilities. As a result, care may not be comprehensive or timely.

Although leaders in government, health care, and consumer groups continue to express concern over access issues, inequities in the current system are readily apparent. By most accounts, more than 47 million nonelderly Americans are uninsured (Kaiser Family Foundation, 2013). In addition, many more U.S. citizens are underinsured, and this figure is growing. Individuals working at part-time and minimum-wage jobs make up a large part of the uninsured and underinsured in this country.

A lack of insurance frequently results in a lack of prevention services and early interventions. Lack of adequate

BOX 5-1 Affordable Care Act (ACA) or "Obamacare": What Is It and Why Is It Necessary?

After decades of attempts to reform the U.S. health care system, in March 2010 President Barack Obama signed into law the Patient Protection and Affordable Care Act (P.L. 111–148) and the Health Care Education and Reconciliation Act of 2010 (P.L. 111–152). The two Acts are collectively known as the Affordable Care Act (ACA), or "Obamacare." The stated purpose of the ACA is to "increase the number of Americans covered by health insurance and decrease the cost of health care."

The American Public Health Association gives the following reasons for why the ACA was necessary:

1. Too many people lack healthcare coverage.
2. High healthcare costs threaten the country's economic stability, hindering our ability to reduce the federal deficit and to spend in other important areas, such as education, housing, and economic development. The United States spends 17.6% of its gross domestic product (GDP) on health care: approximately $2.6 trillion in 2012, which is one and a half times the amount spent by any other comparable country.
3. Despite high spending, our health outcomes are poor when compared with those of similar countries. The United States spends more on medical care than any other industrialized nation but ranks 26th among 36 countries in terms of life expectancy.
4. Our healthcare system emphasizes treatment instead of prevention. Seven in ten deaths in the United States are related to preventable conditions such as obesity, diabetes, high blood pressure, heart disease, and cancer, and three quarters of our healthcare dollars are spent treating such diseases. Only 3 cents per dollar spent (both public and private) on health care go toward prevention.
5. Health disparities exist among numerous vulnerable populations, including those related to income and access to coverage across demographics.

According to the U.S. Department of Health and Human Services, the ACA puts forth a new Patient's Bill of Rights and "gives Americans the stability and flexibility they need to make informed choices about their health." The features include:

1. Coverage
   - Ends pre-existing condition exclusions: Health plans can no longer limit or deny benefits due to a pre-existing condition.
   - Keeps young adults covered: If you are under 26, you may be eligible to be covered under your parent's health plan.
   - Ends arbitrary withdrawals of insurance coverage: Insurers can no longer cancel your coverage just because you made an honest mistake.
   - Guarantees your right to appeal: You now have the right to ask that your plan reconsider its denial of payment.
2. Costs
   - Ends lifetime limits on coverage: Lifetime limits on most benefits are banned for all new health insurance plans.
   - Reviews premium increases: Insurance companies must now publicly justify any unreasonable rate hikes.
   - Helps you get the most from your premium dollars: Your premium dollars must be spent primarily on health care—not administrative costs.
3. Care
   - Covers preventive care at no cost to you: You may be eligible for recommended preventive health services. No copayment for specific screening tests and pregnancy.
   - Protects your choice of doctors: Choose the primary care doctor you want from your plan's network.
   - Removes insurance company barriers to emergency services: You can seek emergency care at a hospital outside of your health plan's network.

Sources: Shi, L., & Singh, D. A. (2013). Essentials of the U.S. health care system (3rd ed.). Burlington, MA: Jones and Bartlett Learning; American Academy of Nursing, 2010, Healthcare.gov

prenatal care and infant immunizations, especially for the poor and minority populations, has sometimes led to illness and disability and, ultimately, increased financial demands on the public healthcare system. Statistically, African Americans fare worse in virtually every condition that affects health (Donatiello, Droese, & Kim, 2004). The rates of infectious disease such as tuberculosis, sexually transmitted diseases, and human immunodeficiency virus (HIV) continue to rise, especially within at-risk populations. A lack of accessible community mental health services has also resulted in a number of tragedies and untold stress for families.

Attempts to contain spiraling costs, deal with the dissatisfaction of consumers and providers, and address issues of uneven access and poor clinical outcomes have resulted in cost-containment legislation, new configurations of providers, and new ways of providing care. Because nursing care holds the answer to many of the current dilemmas, the nursing profession appears to be poised on the edge of an exciting and challenging future.

The Evolving U.S. Healthcare Delivery System

The term **healthcare delivery system** refers to a multilevel industry that transforms a variety of resources into essential services designed to meet the healthcare needs of a population. This transformation occurs through a complex set of interactions among consumers, providers, payers, employers, and the government. Resources include physical structures, personnel, technology, supplies, and financing, among other things. The system is both guided and, in some instances, undermined by competition, demands for profit, technological innovation, standards, and government regulations.

With growing concerns regarding out-of-control healthcare costs—a factor that further exacerbated the 2008 economic collapse—healthcare reform was once again a major political issue. President Obama signed into law, after a long and contentious legislative debate, the ACA of 2010. All major nursing organizations supported the ACA, including the American Nurses Association (ANA) and the American Academy of Nursing (AAN). Nursing organizations have long supported efforts to reform health care, recognizing their potential to expand access to cost-effective, quality care and to help shift the U.S. health system toward a greater emphasis on primary and preventive care—care that, in the long run, should lower healthcare costs for the population (AAN, 2010).

Many critics suggest that the U.S. healthcare system is not actually a system at all—that is, it is not a coordinated whole with interrelated parts. Instead, health care in this country often occurs as a series of fragmented episodes that may be isolated, unrelated, confusing, or even competing. Furthermore, in the United States there is no single source of oversight, policies, or goals, nor is there a set of shared values and concerns among the various entities in the delivery system.

Services in the United States may be provided in traditional settings, such as hospitals or physicians' offices, and in less traditional settings, such as shelters, specially equipped vans, or shopping malls. Patient care information may or may not be shared among the providers in the subsystems or even between providers at separate sites in a single subsystem. Furthermore, follow-up contact between providers and patients is rare.

CULTURAL CONNECTION

The healthcare system of a nation or society is influenced by the following factors:

- Political values and climate
- Level of economic development
- Technological progress
- Social and cultural values
- The physical environment
- Population characteristics
- Demographics
- Health trends

Source: Shi, L., & Singh, D. A. (2013). *Essentials of the U.S. health care system* (3rd ed.). Burlington, MA: Jones & Bartlett Learning.

Reimbursement may come from one or more of the following sources: private insurance companies, managed care organizations (MCOs), government agencies, foundations, and the patient. The patient is often the one who has to decide who to bill, what to do when reimbursement is denied, or who to talk to when the bill is only partially reimbursed.

Finally, services may need to be accessed in one or more of the following healthcare systems: private, public, and/or the military. Each system has a unique set of rules and requirements. Coverage may be overlapping, costs of care are different, and reimbursement occurs in different ways.

Private Healthcare Delivery

Our complicated private healthcare system has changed dramatically in the last 100 years. In the 19th century, family, servants, or close friends cared for patients in the home, with physicians making visits as needed. Treatment involved medicinal herbs and comfort measures. Medical knowledge was limited, and most medical practitioners in the United States lacked a standardized education. Medical treatments were based on common sense, and physicians often lacked acceptance as professionals. Care was purchased out of private funds or provided on a charity basis. The few hospitals that existed basically served indigent patients (i.e., without family or support) who found themselves at death's door. The medical treatments delivered in these early hospitals were often crude and seldom very effective.

After the middle of the 19th century, large leaps in medical knowledge occurred. These advances paved the way for significant gains in surgical interventions and the treatment of disease. The new, more sophisticated procedures required centralized facilities to house the new technology and train the personnel needed to provide patient care. This resulted in an era of extensive hospital construction, the institutionalization of health care, and the establishment of the hospital as the center of healthcare delivery (see **Box 5-2**).

BOX 5-2 Phases of Healthcare System Development

Development of the private healthcare delivery system occurred in several phases:

1. Prior to the 1850s: Illness and disability were handled at home. Few hospitals and clinics existed, and they provided mostly indigent care.
2. 1850–1930: Significant gains in medical knowledge occurred. Technology advances necessitated an increase in the number of hospitals and nurses.
3. 1930–1980: Health care became more organized. Insurance became available so people were more likely to go to hospitals for care.
4. 1980 to 2000: Soaring costs resulted in reorganization, restructuring, reallocation of scarce resources, and difficult ethical decisions.
5. 2000 to the present: Escalating healthcare costs and economic collapse led to healthcare reform, significantly the ACA, which was passed in 2010.

After World War I, the medical profession in this country grew in prestige and power. This transformation was based on several trends: movement to cities away from family and friends, advances in medical science and technology, organization of medicine and adoption of state licensing requirements, establishment of worker's compensation and growth of health insurance, and educational requirements for providers (Shi & Singh, 2013).

To ensure that hospital bills would be paid, insurance companies such as Blue Cross were formed. With the establishment of broader health insurance coverage, providers were at less financial risk, and insurance policies provided for the reimbursement of increasing numbers of patients. Patients selected the provider. Providers simply decided on the appropriate course of care for the patient, implemented that care, and then submitted bills at the end of the illness episode. This form of payment was known as fee-for-service.

Fee-for-service is a form of retrospective payment for health care in which a facility or provider submits a bill for services rendered at the completion of the healthcare episode. An advantage of this type of billing is that care is reimbursed according to the acuity of the patient's condition based on the services required. However, some healthcare experts now believe that paying a fee for each service performed encourages unnecessary services and frequent return visits, which in turn increases healthcare costs.

The Hill–Burton Act was passed in 1946 to help communities build hospitals. In the 1950s, the National Institutes of Health (NIH) became a major funding source for healthcare research. The Medicare Act was passed in 1965 to provide hospital insurance for the elderly. Each of these efforts increased the organizational strength of the U.S. healthcare system.

Two acts passed by Congress have significantly affected the methods by which hospitals are reimbursed for care. The Tax Equity and Fiscal Responsibility Act of 1982 (TEFRA) established a cost-per-case basis for Medicare-reimbursed inpatient services. The 1983 amendments to the Social Security Act established a prospective payment method of paying for inpatient services for Medicare patients based on a system of admitting diagnoses known as **diagnosis-related groups (DRGs)**.

Under the **prospective payment system (PPS)**, an annual fixed (prospective) rate was established for reimbursing providers for care based on 467 diagnoses or procedures. The prototype for the prospective payment system was developed at Yale University. Under the Yale program, reimbursement amounts bore "little or no relationship to length of stay, services rendered, or costs of care" (Williams & Torrens, 2008, p. 112). Rules stated that costs above the established amount for a given DRG would be absorbed by the hospital. If the care was delivered for less than the established amount, however, the hospital could keep the difference and make a profit.

Third-party payers are agencies or organizations such as insurance companies or health maintenance organizations (HMOs) that are responsible for all or part of an insured individual's healthcare costs. Third-party payers also adopted the DRG system as a part of their cost-saving measures. It has been suggested that prospective payment legislation introduced a new era of fiscal constraints, demands for accountability, and pressure to provide services in innovative ways. This new era involved the constant evaluation of practices, policies, and procedures to limit costs whenever possible and has resulted in concerns about access, equitable treatment decisions, and quality of care.

As a result of the need to control costs, provide quality care, and meet the needs of increasing numbers of individuals, a variety of creative and innovative healthcare organizations have developed. Often called alphabet health care, acronyms such as HMOs, preferred provider organizations (PPOs), point-of-service (POS) plans, and MCOs have become part of the new healthcare vocabulary (Feldstein, 2007). With these new healthcare models have come some difficult ethical questions. Is health care a right? If a treatment or procedure is available and you want it, should your insurance be required to pay for it? Who should decide on the appropriateness of medical treatment plans, the physician or the insurance company? These questions are probably going to be with us for a long time, because there are no easy answers.

Public Health Care

Public health can be defined as the health outcomes of a group of individuals, including the distribution of such outcomes within the group; the field of population health, which includes health outcomes, patterns of health determinants, and policies; and the interventions that link these two (Kindig & Stoddart, 2003). The U.S. public health system is made up of interwoven local, state, and national governmental agencies designed to look at broad community-based health issues and protect the general public from the hazards that result from living in populated urban areas.

Massachusetts was the first state to establish a state department of health modeled, in part, after the British General Board of Health. Lemuel Shattuck, from Massachusetts, produced a visionary report in 1850 entitled *Report of the Sanitary Commission of Massachusetts*. In that report, Shattuck outlined the health needs of the state and offered recommendations related to the need for sanitary engineers, accurate vital statistics, inspectors, food and drug regulations, public health education, and routine preventative health care for all citizens. Despite its carefully written and documented recommendations, however, this report was virtually ignored for almost 20 years.

In 1872, the Public Health Association was formed. Its membership focused on interdisciplinary efforts to improve health and developed a number of health promotion and illness prevention materials for the public. In the 1880s, based on work by Pasteur and Koch, public health moved from having a narrow emphasis on environmental sanitation to taking a broader view that included bacteriology and immunology.

ENVIRONMENTAL CONNECTION

While clean drinking water is taken for granted in the United States due to a long-standing commitment to public health and the availability of resources, 85% of the world's people live in the driest half of the planet, and therefore have more limited water access. The United Nations reported in 2013 that more than 780 million of the world's people lack clean drinking water and over 2.5 billion lack sanitation services (UN Water, 2013).

CULTURAL CONNECTION

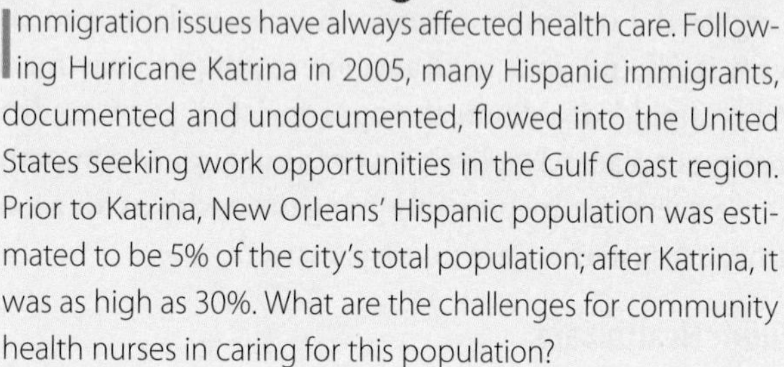
Immigration issues have always affected health care. Following Hurricane Katrina in 2005, many Hispanic immigrants, documented and undocumented, flowed into the United States seeking work opportunities in the Gulf Coast region. Prior to Katrina, New Orleans' Hispanic population was estimated to be 5% of the city's total population; after Katrina, it was as high as 30%. What are the challenges for community health nurses in caring for this population?

During the first decades of the 20th century, public health services began to expand in the United States. The Social Security Act of 1935 provided federal funding for support of local health departments and marked the first step toward the development of a nationwide network of public health agencies. Public health agencies were responsible for providing healthcare services to special populations such as urban poor, mothers, babies, and Native Americans, among others (Fairbanks & Wiese, 1998).

Today, public health agencies range in size and scope from local health departments to the Centers for Disease Control and Prevention (CDC) in Atlanta and focus on ensuring that the public health of the community is protected, promoted, and restored. To meet that overall goal, public health departments currently have a wide range of population-based goals (see **Box 5-3**). To meet the goal of healthy communities, public health agencies have expanded their core functions to include community assessment, policy development, limited medical services (e.g., immunizations, well-baby check-ups, sexually transmitted disease treatment, and surveillance), and program evaluation (Keck & Scutchfield, 1997).

BOX 5-3 Public Health Goals

The public health system is responsible for the following activities:

- Preventing epidemics and the spread of disease
- Reducing environmental hazards
- Preventing injuries
- Promoting healthy behaviors
- Providing disaster services
- Ensuring the quality and accessibility of health services

Source: Fairbanks, J., & Wiese, W. H. (1998). *The public health primer.* Thousand Oaks, CA: Sage.

RESEARCH ALERT

Many Native American nations, tribes, and bands are at an elevated risk for premature death from unintentional injury. The purpose of this study was to identify and characterize any association between prior injury and/or alcohol use contacts with the Indian Health Service (IHS) and subsequent alcohol-related injury death. Death certificates of Native Americans who died from injury in a rural IHS area over 6 consecutive years were linked to IHS acute care facility records and toxicology reports. Of the 526 injury deaths involving Native Americans in the IHS area studied, 411 (78%) were successfully linked to IHS records. Of these cases, 152 met the inclusion criteria, with an additional 98 cases identified as a comparison group.

No differences in alcohol use at time of death between groups with and without prior healthcare contact (for injury or alcohol) could be determined (81% versus 73%). A significant relationship was found between previous visits for acute or chronic alcohol use and subsequent alcohol-related fatalities ($p = .01$).

Based on these findings, injury-prevention activities in the population studied should be initiated at the time of any health system contact in which alcohol use is identified. Community health nursing interventions should be developed to educate patients and families about the risk of alcohol use and injury risk with any contact at point of service for this at-risk population.

Source: Sanddal, T. L., Upchurch, J., Sanddal, N. D., & Esposito, T. J. (2005). Analysis of prior health system contacts as a harbinger of subsequent fatal injury in American Indians. *Journal of Rural Health, 21*(1), 65–69.

Military Health Care

One of the most important fringe benefits of military life is a system of well-organized, comprehensive healthcare services provided at little or no extra cost (Williams &

Torrens, 2008). Military personnel are also covered for service-connected problems for life. Health care is always available when needed, although personnel may have little choice of provider. Finally, the military healthcare system emphasizes prevention in addition to illness care. The National Defense Authorization Act for fiscal year 2005 was designed to improve the comprehensiveness of the overall health benefits available to members of the National Guard, reservists, and their families.

Ambulatory care is provided in military base and regional clinics. Simple hospital services, including short-term stays, are available through base dispensaries or sick bays onboard ships. More advanced care is available in regional hospitals. Well-trained medics, nurses, and physicians, working in facilities owned by the U.S. government, provide most of the care. This system of care is well organized, integrated, and sophisticated.

Dependents and families of active-duty personnel are covered by an extensive health insurance plan known as TriCare. This program allows dependents and families to obtain health care from private clinics and practitioners, local hospitals, and HMOs when similar services are not available from a nearby military base.

A second program, the Veterans Administration (VA) healthcare system, is a hospital and long-term care system that exists to care for retired and disabled military personnel. Whereas a hospital clinic system is available for complicated ambulatory services, most simple ambulatory services are obtained through other systems of care. The VA healthcare system is probably the largest long-term care provider in the United States and is funded through an annual appropriation from Congress.

Healthcare Reform

The current U.S. healthcare delivery system is undergoing dramatic changes with the passage of the ACA. Advances in research and technology have resulted in the most sophisticated care in the world, and the most costly. At the same time, millions of Americans have limited or no access to healthcare services. When the uninsured do receive care, it is often in costly emergency departments and after the condition has become unnecessarily complex. Uncompensated care is on the rise, and many providers are limiting their numbers or refusing to care for uninsured or underinsured patients. Patients without a regular provider are often forced to seek care in emergency departments after their conditions have become serious and where care is often fragmented (Squires, 2012). Consequently, it is not surprising that healthcare reform has drawn the attention of many supporters.

Healthcare reform is not a new issue. The administrations of Franklin Roosevelt, Truman, Kennedy, Johnson, Nixon, Ford, Carter, George H. W. Bush, Clinton, and George W. Bush all attempted to design some type of healthcare reform. Only the Medicare Act, supported by President Kennedy before his death and passed by his successor, Lyndon Johnson, became law without undergoing major changes.

Each time, the need for healthcare reform was based on the need to control healthcare costs while providing access to quality healthcare services to increasing numbers of people. Prior to 1993, the prototypes for Clinton's healthcare reform bill had been debated through three elections and defeated by two legislatures because of concerns about increased costs and governmental control.

A massive reorganization attempt was started during the first year of President Clinton's administration under the direction of First Lady Hillary Rodham Clinton. This plan would have guaranteed all individuals access to a basic benefit package of selected primary and preventive services while ensuring cost containment and quality care.

The failure of the Clinton plan is generally attributed to a number of structural, strategic, and tactical mistakes. The opposition was well organized, the president had critics within his own party, the plan was too complex, the drafters of the plans were politically naive, and the president's political base of support was narrow. The arguments that were most often heard were that the plan was too expensive, it was too confusing, and taxpayers did not want to pay for health care for poor people. The failure of the plan left the United States and South Africa as the only major industrialized countries in the world without some form of universal insurance coverage. Although the reform package was never passed, healthcare changes did eventually occur. President Clinton's incremental initiatives, such as the Health Insurance Portability and Accountability Act of 1996, have succeeded.

In his health policy agenda, President George W. Bush focused less on broad, sweeping reform, and more on market-based, individualistic, incremental policies. Bush promoted health savings accounts, which allow people to create tax-free accounts to pay for out-of-pocket medical expenses, efforts to increase transparency in healthcare pricing and quality, and health information technology (Shi & Singh, 2013).

The Current U.S. Healthcare Delivery System

In response to a need for change, a number of new and innovative organizations are emerging, and many traditional components of the system are in transition because of the legal mandates set by the ACA. A single hospital operating independently or a physician/primary healthcare provider in an individual practice is becoming unusual. Hospitals, physicians, clinics, and other providers have been forced into a variety of interrelated systems. Growth and consolidation of smaller providers into larger organizations, horizontal and

ETHICAL CONNECTION 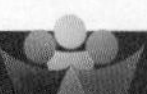

- According to the Institute of Medicine (IOM), uninsured Americans get about half the medical care of those with health insurance. As a result, they tend to be sicker and to die sooner.
- Approximately 45,000 unnecessary deaths occur each year because of lack of health insurance, according to a 2009 study in the *American Journal of Public Health*.
- When even one family member is uninsured, the entire family is at risk for the financial consequences of a catastrophic illness or injury.
- According to the American College of Emergency Physicians, healthcare costs for both the full-year and part-year uninsured have been estimated to total $176 billion dollars per year. The U.S. government's programs finance approximately 75% of this cost.
- The burden of uncompensated care has been a factor in the closure of some hospitals and the unavailability of services in others. Disruptions in service can affect all who are served by a facility, including those who have health insurance.
- The United States loses the equivalent of $65 billion to $130 billion annually as a result of the poor health and early deaths of uninsured adults, according to a 2004 IOM report.

"In light of the adverse consequences that uninsurance has for individuals, families, communities, and society as a whole, it should be painfully clear that our nation can no longer afford to ignore this problem," said IOM committee co-chair Arthur Kellermann, professor and chair of emergency medicine at Emory University School of Medicine in Atlanta. "We must find a way to cover the uninsured."

The committee's five guiding principles to judge proposed solutions are as follows:

1. Healthcare coverage should be universal.
2. Healthcare coverage should be continuous.
3. Healthcare coverage should be affordable to individuals and families.
4. The health insurance strategy should be affordable and sustainable to society.
5. Healthcare coverage should enhance health and wellbeing by promoting access to high-quality care that is effective, efficient, safe, timely, patient centered, and equitable.

Based on these facts and principles, what are our ethical responsibilities to providing basic health care to our citizens? Who is responsible? Who is most vulnerable?

Sources: Institute of Medicine, Committee on the Consequences of Uninsurance. (2004). *Insuring America's health: Principles and recommendations.* Washington, DC: National Academies Press; Wilper, A. P., Woolhandler, S., Lasser, K. E., McCormick, D., Bor, D. H., & Himmelstein, D. U. (2009). Health insurance and mortality in US adults. *American Journal of Public Health, 99*(12), 2289–2295; American College of Emergency Physicians. (2013). The uninsured: Access to medical care fact sheet. Retrieved from http://newsroom.acep.org/index.php?s=20301&item=30032

vertical integration of services within organizations, changes from government-owned facilities to private nonprofit and for-profit facilities, and diversification of traditional healthcare services are occurring at an amazingly rapid pace (Lee & Estes, 2003). Large purchasers of medical services are demanding wholesale prices for services and even dictating terms to providers. Insurance coverage is constantly changing, and patient choices have been reduced (Squires, 2012).

Levels of Care

The U.S. healthcare delivery system provides six basic levels of care: preventive, primary, secondary, tertiary, restorative, and continuing or long-term health care.

Preventive care includes education and screening programs. **Primary care** includes services directed at reducing the potential for a disease through continuous, coordinated, and comprehensive care. Preventive and primary care generally take place in the primary care provider's office.

Secondary care is concerned with early detection and treatment of acute illness and injury to prevent disability and mortality. This type of care usually occurs in the primary care provider's office or in a community hospital.

Tertiary care is concerned with slowing the progression of established disease, preventing further disability, and improving the individual's degree of functioning. It sometimes occurs in community hospitals and sometimes in large medical referral centers. Restorative care is part of tertiary care and includes hospice and chronic care and occurs in hospitals or special rehabilitation facilities. **Long-term care**, also usually a subset of tertiary care, occurs in long-term care facilities such as nursing homes and hospice facilities. Historically, the United States has focused most of its resources on tertiary care provided in large medical care institutions.

Healthcare Providers

Registered nurses (RNs) and physicians are the two largest groups of healthcare professionals. As health care has become more complex, however, the number and variety of providers has increased proportionately. The Commission on Accreditation of Allied Health Education Programs (CAAHEP) is the largest programmatic/specialized provider of accreditation in the health sciences field. In collaboration with its Committees on Accreditation, CAAHEP accredits more than 2,000 educational programs in 19 health sciences occupations across the United States and Canada (CAAHEP, 2008).

Physicians

Physicians are the second-largest group of healthcare professionals. A total of 921,904 physicians are currently practicing in the United States and its possessions (American Medical

Association [AMA], 2008). They diagnose and treat patients in an attempt to cure or improve the health of their patients. Physicians may be allopathic (MDs) or osteopathic (DOs).

In the past, most physicians were in solo practice. Today, many physicians are joining group practices or contracting with healthcare corporations. By joining groups, physicians are able to spread out both their workloads and their risks.

Nurses

Nurses are the largest group of healthcare providers. Approximately 3.1 million individuals hold nursing licenses in the United States (ANA, 2011). A nursing degree prepares an individual to work in many areas. For example, in 2011, approximately 57.3% of all registered nurses worked in hospitals; 8.7% worked in physician offices; 14% in home health care, nursing facilities, or outpatient care; and the rest in academic or civil service positions (Robert Wood Johnson Foundation, 2012). Nurses deliver and coordinate health care for patients within settings and across sites, collaborate with physicians, and carry out day-to-day treatments and care.

More than 250,000 registered nurses have the education and credentials to call themselves advanced practice nurses (ANA, 2011). The category of advanced practice nurse contains several different specialty areas, including clinical nurse specialists, nurse practitioners, nurse midwives, and nurse anesthetists. These advanced-level roles have grown over the years, usually in response to a physician shortage or a physician misdistribution. Each role has its own certification, rules and regulations, and state recognition process.

Nurses are currently at an important juncture in the development of the profession with the new healthcare reform of the ACA. They currently have the opportunity to show their value in providing quality care at a reasonable cost while obtaining positive patient outcomes (Buerhaus et al., 2012).

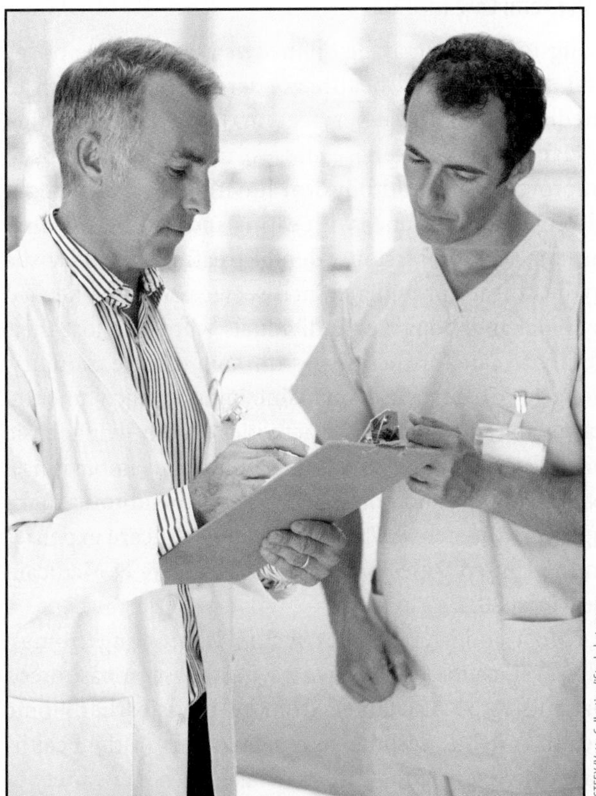

Physicians and nurses work in acute care settings in collaboration to improve health of patients.

NOTE THIS!

The American healthcare bill in 2009, according to the Commonwealth Fund's 2011 report, was approximately $7,960 per person.

Physician Assistants

Approximately 90,000 physician assistants (PAs) are currently practicing in the United States (American Academy of Physician Assistants [AAPA], n.d.b). The first training program for PAs was started at Duke University in 1965. As of 2011, the American Academy of Physician Assistants had accredited 156 PA programs in all 50 states (AAPA, n.d.a). The PA training program is typically the last 2 years of an undergraduate degree program and focuses on medical science and clinical skills. PAs work directly under the supervision and license of physicians, who are responsible for their performance. PAs can provide a variety of medical services as part of their role, such as history and physical examinations, minor medical diagnoses and care, follow-up care for acutely and chronically ill patients, hospital rounds, and surgical assistance, among other things.

Specialized Care Providers

Within the healthcare delivery system, certain groups of professionals provide focused care services. Examples are clinical psychologists, dentists, podiatrists, and optometrists. These professionals are licensed, although standards vary from state to state. They are usually addressed as "doctor," and in some areas they may have prescriptive authority and hospital privileges (i.e., they can admit and treat patients in a hospital setting). Their education is in depth in their specialty areas at a master's level or higher.

Technicians/Therapists

Many people who provide ancillary healthcare services are called technicians or technologists; examples include the medical laboratory technician or medical technologist, the medical record technician, the x-ray technician, and the dietary technician. Other ancillary healthcare professionals are called therapists; examples are respiratory, occupational, physical, mental health, and speech therapists. Each is educated and licensed to provide a specific service and is educated at a bachelor's level or higher.

MEDIA MOMENT 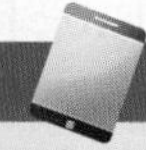

Daytime dramas ("soap operas") frequently use the hospital as a setting for plot lines. Millions of people watch these serials every day, which provide an artificial and often inaccurate portrayal of nurses, physicians, and the healthcare system. Rarely, if ever, is the issue of the cost of healthcare services mentioned. People in the series are often faced with near-death catastrophes, only to be saved at the last possible moment by some miraculous experimental treatment.

Other Providers

Other healthcare providers include professionals such as pharmacists and social workers. Pharmacists are specialists in the science of drugs and can make recommendations about drug therapy. Most programs preparing pharmacists are 5 years long and include an internship. Pharmacists are the third largest group of healthcare providers.

Social workers are assuming increasingly important roles in today's healthcare delivery system. These professionals counsel patients and families, often directing them to various healthcare resources. They may also be involved in discharge planning. Chaplains address the spiritual and emotional needs of patients and families from a nondenominational perspective.

Healthcare Settings

Services may be provided in traditional settings, such as hospitals, nursing homes, physicians' offices, ambulatory clinics, and homes. In addition, services may be provided in less traditional settings such as shelters, shopping malls, homeless shelters, pharmacies, schools, and job sites. Refer to the section "Community-Based Healthcare Settings" later in this chapter for more details.

Acute Care Facilities

Hospitals, or acute care facilities, make up the largest component of the U.S. healthcare delivery system and accounted for 31.6% of total U.S. health expenditures in 2012 (Centers for Medicare & Medicaid Services, 2012). Hospitals include federal, state, and local government facilities as well as those owned by private organizations. Privately owned hospitals include voluntary (not-for-profit) or proprietary (for-profit) hospitals. Religious and charitable groups operate voluntary hospitals and may be independent or represent HMOs or cooperatives. Individuals, partnerships, or corporations own proprietary hospitals. The early 2000s have seen an increase in investor-owned hospital corporations; the stock of these large corporations is traded on stock exchanges.

In the current healthcare market, many hospitals have established home health agencies to help patients as they transition from the hospital to the home environment. Community health nurses can provide a critical link between hospital care and home care.

Short-Term Specialized Care Facilities

Some facilities, such as mental health centers, substance abuse facilities, and rehabilitation centers, offer very specialized services. Patients are admitted to these facilities for a short-term stay to learn how to function with their disability. Another example of a short-term facility is a respite care facility that provides temporary inpatient services for individuals who usually are cared for at home. The purpose of respite care is to offer relief to the informal caregiver, usually a family member.

A short-term facility may be part of a network of coordinated services or a single independent entity. Centers may be staffed with a variety of healthcare providers, including physicians, nurses, and social workers. Short-term specialized care facilities discharge patients into the community after short stays. Community health nurses could provide family and home assessments to determine the patient's needs upon discharge and serve as a resource to patients once they are at home.

Long-Term Care Facilities

Long-term care may be defined as a wide range of social, personal, and healthcare services in addition to medical care. These services may include arranging social functions, exercise classes, and shopping trips to improve mental and physical function. Services might also include assistance with eating and bathing, arranging for therapy sessions, dental treatments, and visits by healthcare providers. Such services may be needed by older individuals or individuals who have lost their ability to care for themselves through disease or injury. Long-term care focuses on maintaining as much function as possible and emphasizes activities of daily living (basic needs such as eating, dressing, bathing, and ambulating). Nursing home and home healthcare expenditures make up approximately 8.2% of the total healthcare expenses in the United States (Centers for Medicare & Medicaid Services, 2012).

Most long-term care occurs in nursing homes. However, as the prospective payment system has forced patients to be discharged from hospitals earlier, home health care has become an essential part of the healthcare delivery system. Care may take place in a variety of other ways, such as through assisted living facilities and home healthcare agencies. Care is provided by registered nurses skilled in assessment and practical nurses and aides trained to provide safe patient care. Agencies receiving

Medicare reimbursement must be certified and must meet specified conditions and federal standards.

Technology previously found only in hospitals is now provided by home care agencies. These treatments may include intravenous feedings and medications, ventilators, portable dialysis machines, and cardiac monitoring, for example. Although home health care has changed dramatically, it is still the traditional practice area for community health nurses. In addition to skilled nursing care, home health care may include physical, occupational, or speech therapy; homemaker services; and home-delivered meals. Community health nurses must have excellent skills related to assessing community resources and individualized patient needs in each of these long-term care modalities.

Ambulatory Care Sites

Patients can receive care for conditions not requiring hospitalization at ambulatory care sites. Physician and clinical services account for 20.2% of the total healthcare expenses in the United States (Centers for Medicare & Medicaid Services, 2012). Many ambulatory care sites are affiliated with hospitals, whereas others operate independently. Traditional "walk-in" clinics have existed for many years and are often supported by government funding or charitable organizations. People often use these clinics in lieu of having a personal physician. Centers may operate on an appointment or drop-in basis. Some clinics are specialized, such as family-planning clinics or those offering only women's healthcare services, and nurse practitioners or PAs frequently provide the care. Community health nurses can provide essential services in assisting patients while they try to meet their healthcare needs and stay at home.

Rural health centers were developed as a result of federal funding and to meet the need for care in rural, impoverished areas with few or no local physicians. Teams of residents and physicians from medical centers, along with nurse practitioners and PAs, frequently provide much of the care in these centers. These providers may cover several clinics on a rotating basis. Community health nurses play an important role in providing continuity in the care of patients who are often seen by many different providers. See the "Ambulatory Care Center Nursing" section in the Research Alert later in this chapter for further discussion on ambulatory care in the community.

Daycare Centers

Daycare centers target specific patient populations. For instance, many daycare centers serve elderly persons who cannot be left alone for long periods of time but who can carry out activities of daily living. Other daycare centers serve patients who are physically or mentally challenged, such as those with cerebral palsy or Down syndrome or those with chemical dependencies. They care for individuals when family members are working and offer services such as meals, rehabilitation, and occupational therapy. Because the primary needs of these patients are in the area of personal care needs, nurses play an important role in these facilities.

The world's healthcare systems have more in common than you might think. For example, in Canada, which has a government-sponsored healthcare system, some 30% of health spending is privately financed. In our supposedly "free-market" U.S. healthcare system, more than 40% of health spending is taxpayer financed (Medicare, Medicaid, military), and the privately financed part is intensely regulated.

Nurse-Managed Health Clinics

Nurse-managed health clinics that provide direct care through professional nursing services are holistic and patient centered and are reimbursed at a reasonable cost. Accountability and responsibility for patient care and professional practice are those of the professional nurse. There are a variety of models that meet the needs of selected populations, such as free-standing clinics and school-based clinics, which may be affiliated with medical centers and schools of nursing. Nurse-managed health clinics are centers that have existed for many years, but with the passage of the ACA of 2010, expectations for growth and expansion of services in these types of community-based clinics are high. This may be especially beneficial for vulnerable populations that often lack access to traditional healthcare services (Hanson-Turton & Kinsey, 2001).

Hospices

A hospice, whether run by a public or private agency, is designed to care for terminally ill patients and their families by providing noncurative, supportive, and palliative services. Many patients receiving these services are suffering from cancer, although conditions such as acquired immune deficiency syndrome (AIDS), multiple sclerosis, or end-stage renal disease may also require hospice care. Although nurses play the major role in hospice care, a team approach including physicians, therapists, volunteers, and clergy is often used. Nursing activities focus on managing pain, treating symptoms, and preparing the patient and family for death and bereavement.

Hospice care has been the fastest-growing segment of Medicare-reimbursed care in recent years. The number of Medicare beneficiaries who used hospice for end-of-life care doubled between 2000 and 2010 (Medicare Payment Advisory Commission [MedPAC], 2012).

Retirement Communities

Since the 1990s, the number of retirement communities in the United States has increased significantly. These communities take many forms, such as entire small towns, retirement subdivisions, apartments or condominiums, and continuing-care communities. Although the services vary, retirement communities usually provide a number of levels of care.

In an arrangement known as assisted living, older people live independently with care nearby if needed. A convalescent center may be associated with the facility, and services such as physical and occupational therapy may be provided. Other healthcare services such as dental care may also be available. Residents are guaranteed access to various healthcare services, and the financial responsibilities are spread over the entire community. Some of the fees, such as entry fees, must be prepaid and may be very expensive. Entry fees and monthly maintenance fees are often high, thus limiting access to some of these facilities to the more affluent retirees.

Complementary/Alternative Health Care

Complementary and alternative health care involves nontraditional treatments such as acupressure, acupuncture, therapeutic touch, herbal treatments, hypnosis and imagery, and homeopathy. Complementary and alternative healthcare treatments are now being studied to see how they can be used to support more traditional medical plans of care.

Congress established the Office of Alternative Medicine in 1992 to sponsor research in this field to attempt to determine the value of nontraditional treatments on patient outcomes. Nurses have often been supportive of and practiced alternative health care. Current research has recently focused more attention on some of these modalities and made them more acceptable in mainstream health care.

GOT AN ALTERNATIVE?

The National Center for Complementary and Alternative Medicine (NCCAM) was established by Congress in 1992 to sponsor research into complementary and nontraditional treatments and their effects on patient health outcomes. The NCCAM is one of the 27 institutes and centers that make up the NIH. The NIH is one of eight agencies under the Public Health Service (PHS) in the U.S. Department of Health and Human Services (HHS).

NCCAM is dedicated to exploring complementary and alternative healing practices in the context of rigorous science, training complementary and alternative medicine (CAM) researchers, and disseminating authoritative information to the public and professionals.

Issues Affecting the Delivery of Healthcare Services

Many issues have contributed to the growth, complexity, and expense of the U.S. healthcare delivery system, such as deregulation, consumerism, technology, the graying of America, and our litigious society. (See **Box 5-4**.) Local, state, and federal governments have attempted to address these issues at one time or another. However, short-term fixes for any one factor have had little impact on the overall problem.

BOX 5-4 Key Concepts: Factors Affecting Healthcare Delivery

Failure of competition as a strategy following deregulation of health care
Emphasis on secondary and tertiary health care instead of prevention
Increasing consumerism
Escalating cost of technology
Aging of the population
Cost of defensive medicine
Government regulation and administrative costs

Deregulation

In the last few years, the United States has experienced deregulation of health care. The result has been a proliferation of facilities and technology (e.g., CAT scans and MRIs) in some urban areas, which has resulted in excess capacity and, in turn, increased competition. This expense is inevitably passed along to the patients. Also, the trend leads to misdistribution of essential services in underserved areas. Competition as a price control strategy has not helped to control healthcare costs. Americans still want the specialist, the newest technology, the cutting-edge treatment, and the hospital that looks like a four-star hotel: They simply hope their insurance will pay for it.

Emphasis on Secondary and Tertiary Healthcare Services

Historically, the U.S. healthcare system has allocated the majority of its resources to the care that occurs after the patient has become critically ill. Vast amounts of money have been spent on critical care units, technical procedures, and sophisticated surgical techniques, but little money has been devoted to preventing the illness in the first place. Education and screening services are often not reimbursed by third-party payers and are undervalued by busy providers. Although MCOs frequently say they value what these preventive services can accomplish, the cost is often more than they wish to pay. As a result, managed care often makes decisions about which preventive services are the most valuable and ignores the rest.

Increasing Consumerism

Healthcare consumerism encompasses the public's involvement in determining the type, quality, and cost of their health care. Today, consumers are reading, looking up information, subscribing to newsletters specializing in their healthcare problem, and attending support groups. They are better informed and asserting their right to have an active role in decisions related to their care.

In the past, the poor often either went without health care or had to be satisfied with a lesser quality of care. Values are changing, and equal access to health care is now viewed by many as a right.

Technological Advances

Advances made in technology have drastically changed health care and altered how physicians treat hospitalized patients. For example, the life expectancy of a person with diabetes has increased considerably in recent decades. New chemotherapy treatments have extended cancer patients' lives and, in some cases, greatly increased the quality of their lives. Heart, lung, and liver transplants—all of which were unheard of decades ago—have become commonplace. The latest antibiotic therapies ward off deadly diseases. Taken collectively, advances have reduced hospital stays and allowed people to live longer.

The new technology is expensive, and some advances have raised formidable ethical questions. If you can extend the life of an 80-year-old man for a short time by putting him on a ventilator, should you do it? If you can keep a premature baby alive on life support, but you know that the child has multiple irreparable problems that will result in incredible future costs, should you do it? For the cost of the care of one elderly man on a ventilator for several weeks, you could provide prenatal care to a large group of pregnant women.

RESEARCH ALERT

Public Not Taking Steps to Protect Their Health

Reeves and Rafferty found in their study of 153,000 Americans that only 3% of Americans follow the four basic healthy lifestyle habits that public health experts consider the cornerstones to a longer and better life: engaging in regular exercise, refraining from smoking, eating five or more fruits and vegetables daily, and maintaining a healthy weight. Many public health authorities believe that a person who follows the big four will have gone a long way toward reducing the risks of life-threatening chronic illnesses. The researchers noted:

> These data illustrate that a healthy lifestyle—defined as a combination of four healthy lifestyle characteristics—was undertaken by very few adults in the United States, and that no subgroup followed this combination to a level remotely consistent with clinical or public health recommendations.

The findings, they added, "support the need for comprehensive primary prevention activities to increase healthy lifestyles and to reduce the prevalence of chronic risk factors at the population level."

The researchers analyzed data from the 2000 Behavioral Risk Factor Surveillance System, which included 164,940 respondents aged 18 to 74 years. Participants were randomly telephoned and questioned about lifestyle habits, such as how often they drank fruit juice, ate green leafy vegetables, and the frequency and duration of physical activity.

Survey results showed the prevalence (95% confidence interval) of participants' four healthy lifestyle characteristics were as follows: nonsmoking, 76% (75.6%–76.4%); healthy weight, 40.1% (39.7%–40.5%); five fruits and vegetables a day, 23.3% (22.9%–23.7%); and regular exercise 22.2% (21.8%–22.6%). The overall prevalence of people engaging in all four healthy habits was a mere 3% (95% CI, 2.8%–3.2%) with little variation among subgroups (range, 0.8%–5.7%).

Researchers noted that one of the drawbacks to this study was its reliance on self-reported data. Still, it suggests healthcare providers have their work cut out for them.

"We believe that these findings serve to illustrate the health promotion crisis in the United States, characterized by excessive caloric intake, inadequate leisure time physical activity, increasing obesity, and high rates of cigarette use," the researchers wrote.

Currently, two-thirds of the entire U.S. population is overweight or obese. According to the Centers for Disease Control and Prevention, 22.5% of all U.S. adults (or 46 million people) smoke cigarettes. More men smoke than women—25.2% compared to 20%, respectively.

Source: Reeves, M. J., & Rafferty, A. P. (2000). Healthy lifestyle characteristics among adults in the United States. *Archives of Internal Medicine, 5*(165), 854–857.

Increasing Longevity of Americans

In the 2010 census, approximately 40.3 million individuals reported that they were 65 years of age or older. This represents 13.7% of the total U.S. population—and an increase of 1.3% from the 2000 census (U.S. Census Bureau, 2011). The fastest growing age group in the United States is people 85 and older. Because the heaviest users of health services are the elderly, more emphasis is being placed on their needs, the need for services has increased, and gerontology has become a significant branch of medicine and nursing. Topics such as living wills and power of attorney are becoming more widely discussed, as people become concerned about their ability to maintain life and the quality of that life.

Defensive Health Care and Government Regulation

Defensive health care is a practice of risk mitigation by physicians. It typically consists of avoiding risky procedures in patients who could potentially benefit from them and/or ordering medical tests, procedures, or further consultations that are not medically indicated in order to protect the physician from accusations of negligence (Sonal Sekhar & Vyas, 2013). Physicians are often forced to pay extremely high costs for malpractice insurance and attorneys' fees when they are sued. As a result, some physicians have simply stopped offering high-risk services such as obstetrics or have stopped providing care to indigent patients as a way to increase their profits.

The cost of defensive health care and government regulations has been a major factor affecting the delivery of health care in the United States. In addition, increased government regulation has caused many physicians to increase their office staff, reduce their patient load, or join healthcare systems where billing services are provided. As a result of these increased costs, the physician must become much more cost conscious, and health care has become a business rather than a service.

Managed Care

Total integration of services is expected to be the future economic structure of the U.S. healthcare delivery system. Networks are expected to compete for patients by becoming more efficient, charging lower prices, offering a wider range of services, and ensuring quality care for a fixed cost for the individual. They will maintain a central database to ensure that comprehensive care is delivered as the patient moves from provider to provider within the system. These networks are called managed care.

> I am interested in getting people to use the healthcare system at the right time, getting them to see the doctor early enough, before a small health problem turns serious.
>
> —*Donna Shalala, president of the University of Miami and former Secretary of Health and Human Services*

The Concept of Managed Care

The concept of managed care encompasses a wide variety of organizational structures and is quickly becoming the dominant management strategy in the U.S. healthcare delivery system. By definition, **managed care** refers to a system that, for a set fee, assumes responsibility and accountability for the health of a population through the use of effective, responsible, and cost-efficient care:

> Managed care integrates the financing and delivery of healthcare services to covered individuals, most often by arrangements with providers. These systems offer packages of healthcare benefits, explicit standards for the selection of healthcare providers, formal programs for ongoing quality assurance and utilization review, significant financial incentives for its members to use providers, and procedures associated with the plan. (ANA, 1998)

Managed care organizations (MCOs) first made their appearance in the 1970s and 1980s, when the insurance industry was faced with employers starting to self-insure and healthcare costs were soaring. The huge reserves of money that insurance companies had previously invested were being depleted. Strategically thinking insurance companies redefined their market and began developing MCOs.

The goals of managed care are achieved by keeping patients healthy and treating them in the lowest cost setting using providers that have also agreed to provide services at a reduced rate. Under this system, primary care replaces the hospital as the center of care. The goal is to keep people out of the hospital—not to keep the hospital beds full. More treatments and care are provided in clinics and physicians' offices. Ambulatory patients go home to recover from surgery rather than upstairs in the hospital for a leisurely recovery in a private room.

Managed care has transformed health care from a service industry into a competitive, market-driven business. The question now is whether healthcare decisions are made based on the patient's needs or on the need to show a profit for the organization and its stakeholders. Who is making the decisions about treatment options, and who is caring for the patient with complex, multisystem problems? Is the cheapest treatment always the best treatment? All of these questions are currently without answers.

> The care of human life and happiness, and not their destruction, is the first and only object of good government.
>
> —*Thomas Jefferson*

If managed care is considered the long-term answer to patient care questions, the answer lies in the premise that a healthy patient is cheaper to care for than an unhealthy one. Therefore, preventive care is the only answer. If managed care looks at the short-term answer, then cheaper is better.

Managed Care Organizations

The majority of MCOs can be categorized into three basic types: HMOs, PPOs, and POS plans. **Capitation** refers to the amount of money that is paid to an HMO to cover the cost of health care for a group of patients. An agency or organization representing a group of individuals seeking healthcare contracts with a group of providers and pays a predetermined fee periodically, usually quarterly.

Health Maintenance Organizations

Federally recognized **health maintenance organizations (HMOs)** are prepaid health management plans that offer an organized system for providing a predetermined set of healthcare services in a geographic area to a voluntarily enrolled group of people for an established fee. This system combines traditional insurance and healthcare delivery in one organization and provides a wide range of services, including inpatient and outpatient hospital care, infertility and mental health services, therapeutic x-ray treatments, alcohol and drug addiction treatment, and physical therapy.

HMOs were first established in 1973 under a federal program. The number of HMOs in existence grew dramatically over the next 30 years. Enrollment is voluntary; members have the option to select another plan. Because the fee paid by members is fixed annually, the organization tries to minimize costs. To do so, HMOs must place greater emphasis on health promotion and disease prevention. Some HMOs hire providers as employees, whereas others contract with providers for services.

Preferred Provider Organizations

A **preferred provider organization (PPO)** is a type of managed care plan composed of a group of physicians, and possibly one or more hospitals, which join forces to offer a prepaid healthcare plan to employers. In preferred provider arrangements, patients select their healthcare providers from the list of preferred providers and receive services at a discounted cost. If a consumer chooses to seek services from a provider who has not contracted with the plan, either a substantial deductible fee is assessed or the service is not covered. In the future, PPOs are likely to grow larger and include a wider range of providers.

Point-of-Service Plans

Point-of-service (POS) plans are also known as open-ended HMOs. POSs provide a set of services that are covered under the established fee, but members are also given the choice of going out of the network for services. Members share in costs with the HMO if they decide to go out of the network for care.

Multilevel Integrated Systems

The **integrated healthcare systems** of the future will consist of a mix of many types of healthcare facilities and providers connected through different types of contractual arrangements. These complex systems will be able to supply a broad range of services, from in-house care to outpatient care, from traditional to nontraditional care, within their own system (vertically integrated) or arrange for the services to be provided by other systems (horizontally integrated). Primary care providers, hospitals, retirement communities, wellness centers, pharmacies, health food outlets, rehabilitation centers, counseling centers, and many other types of providers from a large geographical area will be connected and accessible to members of these systems.

The process of changing traditional systems into new, multilevel integrated systems is often complicated and emotionally difficult. The literature is full of words designed to make the transformation process sound less cold and calculating. The first term to appear was "downsizing," which was immediately changed to "rightsizing." This term simply refers to cutting the number of funded positions to decrease costs. "Redesigning" was the next term to make an appearance; it referred to the process of examining all job descriptions to ensure equitable distribution of activities and reduce role overlap, excess specialization, and waste. The next term to appear was "restructuring," which refers to an assessment of the overall organizational structure in an attempt to improve productivity. Finally, "reengineering" refers to a comprehensive and often radical process to look at jobs and organizational structure as a way to form new relationships and new visions, and to improve functioning and productivity. As the evolution of these terms suggests, future integrated healthcare systems will be larger and more comprehensive.

Patient Care Outcomes

The term "patient care outcomes" refers to the consequences of care that the patient receives or does not receive. Outcome studies are becoming very popular in MCOs as a way to predict and provide effective patient care. These studies look for trends over time in patient status and adverse events. Adverse patient care outcomes are occurrences that are not expected as a result of the patient's disease process or treatment. Data obtained from patient care studies are then used as a basis for decisions, the development of policies and procedures, and changes in healthcare practice.

Efforts to improve patient care outcomes involve assessing individual patients' care and recovery and analyzing large data sets from across the country and world. Large national databases will be used in the future to provide predictive information on which to base treatments, types of care, lengths of care, and level of provider needed to achieve positive outcomes.

RESEARCH ALERT 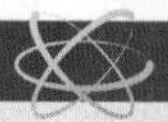

> Poor health was not just the result of random acts, bad luck, bad behavior or unfortunate genetics. Deliberate public policy decision about housing, education, parks and streets were the key drivers of racial differences in mortality.
>
> — David A. Ansell, County: *Life, Death and Politics at Chicago's Public Hospital (2011)*

Community-Based Healthcare Settings

Shelters in the Community

Another focus of community-based health nursing is that of the **shelter nurse**. Shelters are facilities established to assist people, who for one reason or another have found themselves to be homeless. While some shelters simply provide a place to get out of the weather, other shelters offer a wide range of services, often specializing in the concerns of specific populations such as the homeless, victims of abuse, or runaway youth.

Shelters are usually run by a combination of paid professionals and volunteer staff, including psychologists, nurses, attorneys, and others. Shelters may be sponsored by churches, community governments, and a variety of social agencies and are designed to provide a variety of services to people who often suffer from a variety of problems (Townsend, 2000). There is really no such thing as a typical shelter. The location of many shelters is kept confidential to protect the safety of the residents (Lundy, Sutton, & Foster, 2003).

Abuse Shelters Most cities in the United States now have shelters, or "safe houses," where women can go to obtain protection for themselves and their children. Most battered women who reside in shelters have experienced multiple traumatic events, with some even suffering from post-traumatic stress disorder (Humphreys, Lee, Neylan, & Marmar, 2001). Shelters not only provide a haven of safety to the abused and battered woman; they also provide health care, counseling, a milieu to express the intense emotions she may be experiencing, and a wealth of support including financial, social, and spiritual (Humphreys et al., 2001; Townsend, 2000).

Homeless Shelters In the United States, the homeless population is "among the poorest of the poor" (Zuvekas & Hill, 2000, p. 153) and consists not just of adult men and women, but also more than 1.6 million children (American Institutes for Research, National Center on Family Homelessness, 2010; Huang & Menke, 2001). A large segment of this population faces potential barriers to work, as many have serious mental and physical disabilities and others have single or multiple drug addictions (Hatton, 2001). In addition to meeting the medical and mental health needs of the homeless, shelters provide a safe, supportive environment for individuals who simply have no other place to go. While a small percentage of the homeless use the resources available to improve their lives, others become dependent on the provisions that the shelter offers (Lundy et al., 2003; Townsend, 2000).

Disaster Shelters When major flooding, tornadoes, landslides, and earthquakes strike, thousands of families are often displaced from their homes. For some families, displacement may be on a short-term basis. For others, their homes and all their belongings are gone. The greatest immediate need usually reported by most disaster victims is shelter (Daley, Karpati, & Sheik, 2001). This need is closely followed by food and hygiene requirements. Disaster victims include the young and the very old as well as those who are ill and those who are pregnant. Because of this, there is also a great demand in shelters for medications along with medical and nursing care (Daley et al., 2001).

The community health nurse, as a provider of care and manager of care in shelters, is in a unique position to help meet the needs of those people for whom shelters are their lifeline—the difference between life and death. It is essential that the shelter nurse exhibit the following competencies when working with all persons who enter a shelter in search of help and hope.

Professional behaviors essential to the shelter nurse include crisis intervention and counseling, health promotion and maintenance, screening and evaluation, provision of a therapeutic environment, assisting patients with self-care activities, administering and monitoring treatment regimens, health teaching, and outreach activities including home visits and community action (Townsend, 2000).

Shelter nurses must be able to accurately assess the needs of the population for whom they provide care. Depending on the type of shelter, nurses may care for patients with a multitude of physical needs, ranging from bruises and broken bones to pneumonia, sexually transmitted diseases (STDs), AIDS, substance abuse, tuberculosis, and dysentery.

Too often, however, it is the patient's spiritual and mental needs that are harder to assess. Shelter patients often suffer from mental illness, depression, anger, guilt, poor coping mechanisms, a multitude of stressors, and low self-esteem. Shelter nurses must be able to use therapeutic communication skills to develop a trusting relationship with their patients. It is the shelter nurse who is in the best position to let the shelter patient know that his or her feelings of anger and despair are normal and that others have experienced these same emotions in similar situations (Townsend, 2000). Through collaboration with the healthcare team, the nurse works with the patient in individual and group settings in an effort to develop coping skills that will serve as a stable base upon which the patient can begin to build a future.

One of the most important tasks of the shelter nurse is simply to care for the shelter patient. This starts with being nonjudgmental. It probably goes without saying that none of the shelter patients desire to be at the station in life in which they find themselves when they come to the shelter. Among the caring behaviors the shelter nurse must exhibit are listening, providing feedback, helping the patient to recognize available choices, and accepting and supporting the patient in whatever he or she chooses to do. One of the most important roles for nurses who work in shelters is that of educator, with emphasis on providing information about the availability of resources in the community (Townsend, 2000).

In addition to not having a place to live, shelter patients often lack the knowledge and skills that will help them to leave the shelter and function on their own. Patients may need assistance with completing paperwork to get federal or local assistance that will enable them to find a permanent home. They may need training or education to get a job, and many of the mentally ill lack the knowledge as to how to get the medications that will treat their mental illness. The shelter nurse may need to teach parenting skills, methods of building self-esteem, and alternative coping mechanisms to many of the shelter's patients. The mentally ill often need information about their medications to promote compliance. This includes when and how to take their medications as well as ways to reduce troublesome side effects. Some patients need assistance with hygiene and teaching about how to socially interact with others.

Nurses often serve as case managers for a selected group of patients who have been seen in shelters (Townsend, 2000). As case manager, the nurse coordinates services that are required to meet the needs of the patient. This is done in an effort to prevent avoidable episodes of illness—physical and mental—among these at-risk patients. Responsibilities include negotiating with many healthcare providers to obtain whatever services are needed by the patient. This coordination of services by the shelter nurse is done in an effort to optimize patient functioning and problem solving, improve work and socialization skills, promote leisure-time activities, and enhance the overall independence of the individual (Townsend, 2000).

The shelter nurse can participate in the research process at multiple levels. Areas of research involvement include identifying problem areas; collecting, analyzing, and interpreting data; applying findings; helping to evaluate, design, and conduct research; and using research available on the needs of shelter patients to formulate clinical pathways that will help to maximize outcomes for shelter patients (Hitchcock, Schubert, & Thomas, 1999). The shelter nurse can also keep abreast of current literature, share findings with other members of the healthcare team, and, when appropriate, apply findings to the care of shelter patients (Lundy et al., 2003).

Ambulatory Care Center Nursing Perhaps one of the most innovative and dramatic changes in community-based health care is in the diversity in care delivered in ambulatory care centers, from ambulatory surgical centers to ambulatory oncology care settings. These free-standing centers provide acute care to walk-in (ambulatory) patients without the custodial feel of traditional hospital care. These alternative sites for acute care have been very successful because of their efficiency, cost-effectiveness, and high degree of patient satisfaction. They can provide faster service with less paperwork and administrative time involvement. These ambulatory care centers are smaller in size than hospitals, employ fewer personnel, and have less technical equipment, which keeps costs down (Lundy et al., 2003).

Ambulatory Emergency/Trauma and Primary Care Centers These centers, often referred to as "urgent care," "urgicare," "minute clinics," or "walk-ins", do not perform major surgeries. Most are located in urban areas, shopping centers, and, most recently, retail stores. These community-based healthcare services have seen significant growth in the first part of the 21st century due to consumer demands for quick and inexpensive services. For example, when patients are unable to make an appointment with their primary caregiver, they can visit a CVS Minute Clinic or the Clinic at Wal-Mart to get a 5-minute strep test and fill any prescriptions at the same location. Influenza vaccinations are now available and administered at many pharmacies. Referrals can be made, based on diagnosis, to local full-service hospitals when patients need additional care.

As a relatively new resource for immediate and primary care, ambulatory centers are often staffed by family nurse practitioners, family practice physicians, registered nurses, licensed practical nurses, lab technicians, diagnostic technicians, and clerks. Ambulatory care centers try to enhance consumer satisfaction by being convenient, cost-effective, and caring. They do so by providing the four "A"s: They are affable, available, accessible, and affordable. These centers are often open 7 days a week, for 12 to 16 hours per day.

Minor illnesses, such as upper respiratory tract illnesses, impetigo, diarrhea, dehydration, urinary tract infections, asthma, and cellulitis can be easily diagnosed and treated at these clinics. Many also see more serious symptoms and illnesses such as chest pain, back pain, seizures, and anaphylaxis. Pregnancy tests are offered, along with suturing of lacerations, casting and splinting of fractures, and treatment of wounds, burns, and eye injuries. These centers offer limited diagnostic services, such as routine radiological services, complete blood cell counts, bacteriology, electrolytes, and toxicology tests.

The majority of patients are adults, although most centers see children as well. Return visits can be arranged but most customers are referred back to their family physician, nurse practitioner, or a specialist (Seidel, Henderson, & Lewis, 1991).

These relatively new healthcare services have been subjected to considerable criticism, especially from the medical community. Many critics view these "one-stop" services as inappropriate for children and others who need the comprehensive and continuous care delivered by a family healthcare provider (Lundy et al., 2003).

Ambulatory Surgery Centers Ambulatory surgery refers to a surgical process in which patients have surgery, recover, and are discharged home on the same day. Approximately 62% of all surgical procedures, whether performed in a hospital or a free-standing center, are now performed safely on an ambulatory basis without compromising the quality of care (Cullen, Hall, & Golosinsky, 2009). Surgical procedures generally do not exceed 90 minutes in length and require no more than 4 hours of recovery time.

Because of advances in anesthesia, surgical techniques, and a desire for convenience, free-standing, non-hospital surgical centers have grown significantly since the early 2000s. A 2006 CDC survey found that such centers perform roughly 43% of ambulatory procedures (Cullen et al., 2009). Cost containment is a major factor in the proliferation of same-day surgical centers. Each center has emergency equipment and trained personnel, including registered nurses. Pharmacy services are also available. Laboratory and radiological services may be performed on site or by referral to nearby facilities.

The American Academy of Ambulatory Care Nursing provides standards and guidelines for ambulatory centers in the community. Because of the brevity of patient contact in these centers, nurses must be focused and well educated as professionals in caring for persons who are frightened, stressed, and quickly discharged. The amount of time during which the ambulatory care center nurse stays with patients in these centers is short, so good communication skills are of special significance, to patients and their families and to other health professionals. Remaining focused and precise, nurses in these settings should communicate with deliberate and yet compassionate purpose due to the short length of time with the patients.

The ambulatory health center nurse conducts assessments, serves as an assistant to physicians as either a scrub or circulating nurse for surgical procedures, and takes histories during admission. Assessments after procedures are especially important at surgical centers because the collected data assist the physician in making the decision to discharge the patient.

The ambulatory center nurse makes quick decisions based on well thought-out clinical assessments and uses multiple interventions depending on the setting and diagnosis. Such a nurse analyzes data and integrates knowledge about the specific risks associated with the illness or procedure and takes appropriate action.

The nurse in the ambulatory care center must possess good interpersonal skills in which complex health and safety information can be conveyed in an understandable and concise manner to patients and their families, and in a respectful way to other workers and administration. Compassion for the patient and family is critical, because they are aware that they will be under medical supervision and care for only a short time. Nurses must promote self-care and confidence in the patient's ability to follow through with post-discharge instructions.

Much of the nurse role in an ambulatory care setting involves teaching of appropriate discharge measures. The nurse often follows up the following day to evaluate the health status of the patient after services have been delivered.

The nurse in the ambulatory care setting collaborates with other health professionals to share and manage critical information about the patient before, during, and after procedures. This team approach provides the patient with comprehensive care so that upon discharge, successful healing is more likely.

The ambulatory care center nurse manages a quick turnaround for patients with acute illnesses, which requires excellent organizational skills and a knowledge of critical information related to the specific illness or injury. Evaluation using outcome measurement can provide vital information about how to make the system work more efficiently while maintaining quality levels (Lundy et al., 2003; Williams, 1993).

Source: Lundy, K. S., Sutton, V., & Foster, B. (2003). The nurse's role in ambulatory health settings. In K. S. Lundy & S. Janes (Eds.), *Essentials of community-based nursing* (pp. 258–295). Sudbury, MA: Jones and Bartlett.

Health Politics and Policy

How did the U.S. healthcare delivery system become so expensive? Who should pay for the ever-increasing costs of health care and hospitalization? These questions have become the basis for untold numbers of legislative reports, articles, studies, and documentaries. The astronomical costs of some forms of treatment have made it impossible for the average patient to pay personally for needed medical, surgical, and nursing services. Single illness/episode bills well above $10,000 are no longer the exception. Many people rely on government interventions to help them deal with soaring costs and inaccessible services.

Government Policy

Health insurance provides protection against the high cost of medical care and hospitalization arising from illness or injury. Most Americans look to their jobs for health insurance, but increasingly insurance benefits are not available at work sites. The number of Americans who are uninsured or underinsured is increasing at an alarming rate. In response, Americans have appealed to their legislators for help.

Government policy focuses on health care on several levels. For example, federal legislation establishes boards to govern the practice of healthcare professionals and healthcare agencies, establishes commissions to examine healthcare delivery and make recommendations, and sets guidelines for the payment of Medicare benefits. State guidelines influence Medicaid benefits. Medicare and Medicaid guidelines affect the entire healthcare industry, because the government is the third-party payer for more than 40% of all U.S. expenditures for health care (Centers for Medicare & Medicaid Services, 2012).

The publication of *Healthy People 2020*, based on the progress made under *Healthy People 2000* and *2010* goals, again moved forward the U.S. agenda of disease prevention and health promotion for all citizens. The goals for the year 2020 retain three categories from the 2010 agenda—increasing the healthy lifespan, reducing health disparities, and increasing access to healthcare services—while adding the goal of creating social and physical environments that promote health for all (HHS, 2010). Prior to the publication of *Healthy People 2000*, these goals were not central in health legislation. However, in a time of increasing fiscal austerity, these goals make increasing economic sense: Keeping people well is much less costly than trying to cure or rehabilitate them.

Finally, there have been many debates about whether the United States should adopt a national health insurance plan or support market competition. Under a national plan, taxpayers would pay the government for the coverage, much like the way insurance companies currently collect funds from subscribers, and everyone would be covered at a predetermined basic level of services. The disadvantage is that government plans rarely operate very efficiently and many people feel that it is inappropriate for government to meddle in individuals' healthcare decisions. The ACA represented an attempt at a compromise between the two positions, requiring universal health coverage for all citizens but allowing private carriers to offer a range of policies for citizens to choose from and offering government support for the cost of policies to individuals who fell below a certain income level. Because certain aspects of implementation were left to states, the system is unevenly applied nationwide, and whether it will provide adequate coverage and cost reductions is an open question at the time of this writing.

Managed competition has been promoted as another way to keep healthcare costs at a reasonable level while ensuring quality care. Under this system, the government would allow a rivalry between healthcare providers for the purpose of attracting patients. However, an unequal distribution of the most ill patients might keep corporations from wanting to insure the very patients who need care the most.

Public Opinion and Special-Interest Groups

Public opinion expressed through special-interest groups is very influential in the development of public policy. Many special-interest groups, such as the American Hospital Association, the American Medical Association, and the American Insurance Association, spend huge amounts of time and money providing legislators with information on which to base healthcare decisions. Many legislators lack an in-depth understanding of healthcare issues. As a result, the information provided by special-interest groups often serves as a basis for healthcare decisions. When that happens, decisions may fail to reflect the best interests of the majority.

Nursing and Healthcare Policy

As the largest healthcare provider group, it is important for nurses to be both visible and vocal advocates for quality health care. To meet that important goal, the ANA has worked tirelessly over the years to develop an effective special-interest group infrastructure. In response to the healthcare reform issue, in 2007 the ANA formulated a position paper stating that the U.S. healthcare system needs restructuring, wellness promotion must become our emphasis, and universal access to healthcare services must be developed.

The ANA has been politically active in several other areas, including the area of healthcare rationing. When resources are limited, the question of healthcare rationing must be addressed. Of course, the well-insured individuals will worry about restrictions under such a system, and the uninsured or underinsured will worry that they will be excluded. Rationing can mean limiting access to care or limiting contact to the more expensive providers.

Through the years, ANA and state nurses organizations have continued to support legislation that aims to ensure basic healthcare services for everyone. To influence policy, nurses need to vote, be politically active in their states, and know which bills are being considered. To be politically active, you can work on someone's campaign, run for political office, support candidates financially, or simply stay in contact with elected state and federal officials and provide them with information when needed.

New Nursing Opportunities

As health care changes, the practice of nursing must also change. Nurses must stay knowledgeable about healthcare trends to make decisions about future careers. Those trends include things such as the growth in the healthcare workforce, the role of economics as a driving force, the changing U.S. demographics, the transformation of individual providers into multilevel corporations, the trend of physicians becoming employees, the philosophic move from "everything for a few" to "an adequate amount for many," and the increased importance of ambulatory care and home health care (Brennan, 2012; Huston & Fox, 1998). Some of the nursing roles related to these trends are discussed here. However, many future roles are yet to be created, as a result of dramatic changes in the healthcare system due to reform and the ACA (Robert Wood Johnson Foundation, 2012).

Advanced Practice Nurses

Advanced practice nursing is not a new category for nurses, but many of the traditional roles for nurses are changing. Nurse practitioners are moving into specialized areas such as geriatrics, acute care, and health care in correction facilities. Clinical nurse specialists are becoming experts in case management, genetics, and comprehensive cancer care. Nurse anesthetists and nurse midwives are managing patients with specialized needs. Advanced practice nurses are prepared to work with physicians, not for them. As specialties develop, nurses are finding ways to become experts in those areas. As more emphasis is placed on controlling healthcare costs, more providers will look to advanced practice nurses as providers of effective, quality, lower cost care. The doctorate of nursing practice (DNP) has emerged as the entry level for all advanced practice nurses. How this will impact the healthcare delivery system remains to be seen.

APPLICATION TO PRACTICE 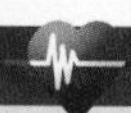

A pregnant woman with severe epilepsy has presented to the health department from a local obstetrical practice. She had been working part-time for a local grocer until her seizures became unmanageable, and she is no longer employed. The patient has been referred to the health department so that she can qualify for state funds for high-risk maternity care. The patient's husband works for a local manufacturing company and has HMO coverage for both himself and his wife through a company-sponsored managed care plan. The deductible and copayment are more than the couple can afford to pay, and they would like to find other resources to pay for the additional services needed to manage the epilepsy. The public health nurse checks with the state high-risk maternity care program and finds that the couple exceeds the income criteria and most likely will not qualify.

1. What are possible health and economic consequences if the patient's health is not managed appropriately during pregnancy?
2. Which system problems can you identify from the situation that result in ethical issues of treatment and care?
3. Who is responsible for seeing that this patient receives appropriate care at an affordable cost?

RESEARCH ALERT

The WIC (The Special Supplemental Nutrition Program for Women, Infants and Children) program provides food, education, and assistance with public health needs for women and children at nutritional risk. Close to 9.17 million persons participated in the WIC program in 2010. Over the decades, since its creation, WIC has produced many positive health outcomes, such as improved birth weights and childhood nutritional statuses. However, breastfeeding as the preferred method of infant nutrition has had less success in its promotion with the WIC program. WIC mothers are less likely to breastfeed their infants when compared to similar populations not on WIC. WIC prioritizes breastfeeding in its stated goals; however, only 0.6% of its budget is put toward breastfeeding initiatives, while infant formula accounts for 11.6% ($850 million) of WIC's budget. This inconsistency in the program's promotion of breastfeeding as the preferred choice for infant feeding in the first year of life is examined in this article and questions why WIC spends 25 times more on formula than on breastfeeding promotion.

Source: Baumgartel, K. L., Spatz, D. L., & American Academy of Nursing Expert Breastfeeding Panel. (2013). WIC (The Special Supplemental Nutrition Program for Women, Infants and Children): Policy Versus Practice Regarding Breastfeeding. *Nursing Outlook, 61,* 466–470.

Entrepreneurs

In the future, more nurses than ever before will own nursing businesses, such as independent nursing centers. In areas such as home health, healthcare management, insurance evaluation, environmental evaluation, workplace health care, caregiver support, program evaluation, and respite care, the opportunities are endless. Nurses will be in a position to contract with larger systems for consulting services and the application of specialized knowledge and skills. The emerging role of the nurse coach shows great promise in a reformed healthcare system.

Data Management

Public and private agencies are looking for nurses who are skilled at creating and managing large databases containing patient information, a field known as informatics. Every healthcare organization is struggling with the need to maintain information in a safe, yet easily accessible manner. Data must be available for evaluation and decision making. Nurses with an understanding of patient care data coupled with a working knowledge of computers, the workings of databases, and the use of evaluative statistics will be in the perfect position to fill these critical slots.

Research

We can no longer make decisions on the basis of what we have done before or what we think will work. Decisions must be based on data that can be seen, measured, and reproduced as needed, and then integrated with sound clinical practice experience based on research. We are moving into an age of evidence-based patient care. Consequently, patient-care research is more important today than at any time in the past. Nurse researchers try to develop an understanding of essential patient-care issues on which to base practice. They may be employees of an organization or working on a research project funded by the government or other organizations that fund research. Their work provides the structure for future practice that will identify efficient and effective healthcare practices that improve the lives of patients.

Conclusion

Some critics suggest that the U.S. healthcare system, which is supposed to guarantee access, innovation, and quality care, has instead become a system in crisis. A crisis exists in several areas: cost, availability, equity, efficiency, and responsiveness to public needs. This chapter discussed the history of the U.S. healthcare delivery system and described the changing components of that system. New roles for nursing are emerging as this healthcare system moves from one that was measured by the cost of its components to a system measured by the effectiveness of the care provided by its components.

ART CONNECTION 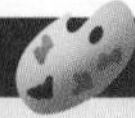

Look at paintings of Florence Nightingale. What are the differences in the depiction of her providing health care and that of the nurse today?

AFFORDABLE CARE ACT (ACA) 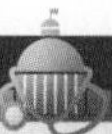

Healthcare spending in the United States since the 2010 passage of the ACA has risen by 1.3% a year, the lowest rate ever recorded, and healthcare inflation reached the lowest it has been in 50 years in 2013. How do you explain these changes in spending?

LEVELS OF PREVENTION 

Primary: Organize an influenza program for senior centers and offer the immunization at convenient times and places.

Secondary: Assist patients with self-help care practices once infected with the flu.

Tertiary: Consider vulnerable populations with chronic conditions such as asthma in the intervention of preventing further permanent damage from influenza infection.

HEALTHY ME 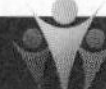

How do you utilize the healthcare system? Do you first seek advice from family and friends or from a healthcare provider? Think about how you stay well to avoid being a part of the acute care healthcare system.

Critical Thinking Activities

1. You are a 28-year-old single mother with three children. You are having pain in your stomach and trouble sleeping. You have no money and no insurance. How will you get someone to help you? What will you do if you need medication?
2. You are a 22-year-old single parent with two children ages 1 and 3 years. Your mother is unemployed and watches the children while you work. Your job does not provide you with insurance. Your state has refused to expand Medicaid to conform to the ACA, so although your pay is too high to allow you to be eligible for Medicaid and too low to allow you to afford insurance, you can't get a federal subsidy to purchase an insurance policy. Which types of services do you need from the Health Department?
3. In a world of limited resources, developing equitable health policies involves many difficult decisions. How would you answer the following questions?
   - Should an 85-year-old man with debilitating emphysema be placed on a respirator?
   - Should a 78-year-old woman with breast cancer be put on chemotherapy?
   - Should major health insurance plans reimburse for experimental treatments?
   - Should an insurance plan be required to pay for a liver transplant for an alcoholic?
   - Should a baby with multiple incurable birth defects be placed in a neonatal intensive care unit?

References

American Academy of Physician Assistants. (n.d.a). *Milestones in PA history.* Retrieved from http://www.aapa.org/WorkArea/DownloadAsset.aspx?id=789

American Academy of Physician Assistants. (n.d.b). *Quick facts: PAs and where they work.* Retrieved from http://www.aapa.org/the_pa_profession/quick_facts/resources/item.aspx?id=3848

American Academy of Nursing (AAN). (2010). *Implementing health care reform: Issues for nursing.* Washington, DC: Author.

American Institutes for Research, National Center on Family Homelessness. (2010). *What is family homelessness?: Children.* Retrieved from http://www.familyhomelessness.org/children.php?p=ts

American Medical Association (AMA). (2008). *Physician characteristics and distribution in the U.S.* Retrieved from http://www.ama-assn.org

American Nurses Association (ANA). (1998). *Managed care: Challenges and opportunities for nursing. Nursing facts.* Retrieved from http://www.nursingworld.org

American Nurses Association (ANA). (2011). *American Nurses Association fact sheet: Nursing by the numbers.* Retrieved from http://nursingworld.org

Brennan, A. M. (2012). The paradigm shift. *Nursing Clinics of North America, 47*(4), 455–462.

Buerhaus, P. I., DesRoches, C., Applebaum, S., Hess, R., Norman, L. D., & Donelan, K. (2012). Are nurses ready for health care reform? A decade of survey research. *Nursing Economics, 30*(6), 318–330.

Centers for Medicare & Medicaid Services. (2012). National health expenditure data tables. Retrieved from http://www.cms.gov/Research-Statistics-Data-and-Systems/Statistics-Trends-and-Reports/NationalHealthExpendData/downloads/tables.pdf

Commission on Accreditation of Allied Health Educational Programs (CAAHEP). (2008). *What is CAAHEP?* Retrieved from http://www.caahep.org/

Commonwealth Fund Commission on a High Performance Health System. (2011). *Why not the best? Results from the national scorecard on U.S. health system performance, 2011.* Retrieved from http://www.commonwealthfund.org/Publications/Fund-Reports/2011/Oct/Why-Not-the-Best-2011.aspx

Cullen, K. A., Hall, M. J., & Golosinsky, A. (2009). Ambulatory surgery in the United States, 2006 [Revised, 2009]. *National Health Statistics Reports No. 11,* Centers for Disease Control and Prevention. Retrieved from http://www.cdc.gov/nchs/data/nhsr/nhsr011.pdf

Daley, W. R., Karpati, A., & Sheik, M. (2001). Needs assessment of the displaced population following the August 1999 earthquake in Turkey. *Disasters, 25*(1), 67–75.

DeNavas-Walt, C. (2012). *Income, poverty and health insurance in the United States: 2011.* Washington, D.C.: U.S. Census Bureau.

Donatiello, J. E., Droese, P. W., & Kim, S. H. (2004). A selected, annotated list of materials that support the development of policies to reduce racial and ethnic health disparities. *Journal of the Medical Library Association, 92*(2), 257–265.

Fairbanks, J., & Wiese, W. H. (1998). *The public health primer.* Thousand Oaks, CA: Sage.

Feldstein, P. J. (2007). *Health policy issues: An economic perspective* (4th ed.). Chicago, IL: Health Administration Press.

Hanson-Turton, T., & Kinsey, K. (2001). The quest for self-sustainability nurse-managed health centers meeting the policy challenge. *Policy and Politics in Nursing Practice, 2,* 304–309.

Hatton, D. C. (2001). Homeless women and children's access to health care: A paradox. *Journal of Community Health Nursing, 18,* 25–35.

Hitchcock, J. E., Schubert, P. E., & Thomas, S. A. (1999). *Community health nursing: Caring in action.* Albany, NY: Delmar.

Huang, C. Y., & Menke, E. M. (2001). School-aged homeless sheltered children's stressors and coping behaviors. *Journal of Pediatric Nursing, 16,* 102–109.

Humphreys, J., Lee, K., Neylan, T., & Marmar, C. (2001). Psychological and physical distress of sheltered battered women. *Health Care Women International, 22,* 401–414.

Huston, C., & Fox, S. (1998). The changing healthcare market: Implications for nursing education in the coming decade. *Nursing Outlook, 46,* 109–114.

Kaiser Family Foundation. (2013). *Key facts about the uninsured population.* Retrieved from http://kff.org/uninsured/fact-sheet/key-facts-about-the-uninsured-population/

Keck, C. W., & Scutchfield, E. D. (1997). *Principles of public health practice.* Albany, NY: Delmar.

Kindig, D., & Stoddart, G. (2003). What is population health? *American Journal of Public Health, 93*(3), 380–383.

Lee, P. R., & Estes, C. L. (2003). *The nation's health* (7th ed.). Sudbury, MA: Jones and Bartlett.

Lundy, K. S., Sutton, V., & Foster, B. (2003). The nurse's role in ambulatory health settings. In K. S. Lundy & S. Janes (Eds.), *Essentials of community-based nursing* (pp. 258–295). Sudbury, MA: Jones and Bartlett.

Medicare Payment Advisory Commission. (2012). *Report to the Congress: Medicare payment policy (March 2012). Chapter 11: Hospice services.* Retrieved from http://www.medpac.gov/chapters/Mar12_Ch11.pdf

Robert Wood Johnson Foundation. (2012). *Nursing: Where the jobs are.* Retrieved from http://www.rwjf.org/en/about-rwjf/newsroom/newsroom-content/2012/03/nursing-where-the-jobs-are.html

Seidel, J. S., Henderson, D. P., & Lewis, J. B. (1991). Emergency medical services and the pediatric patient: Resources of ambulatory care centers. *Pediatrics, 88*(2), 230–235.

Shi, L., & Singh, D. A. (2013). *Essentials of the U.S. health care system* (3rd ed.). Burlington, MA: Jones & Bartlett Learning.

Shi, L., & Singh, D. A. (2014). *An update on health care reform in the United States.* Burlington, MA: Jones & Bartlett Learning.

Sonal Sekhar, M., & Vyas, N. (2013). Defensive medicine: A bane to healthcare. *Annals of Medical and Health Sciences Research, 3*(2), 295–296.

Squires, D.A., for The Commonwealth Fund. (2012). *Explaining high health care spending in the United States: An international comparison of supply, utilization, prices, and quality.* Retrieved from http://www.commonwealthfund.org/Publications/Issue-Briefs/2012/May/High-Health-Care-Spending.aspx

Towsend, M. C. (2000). *Psychiatric mental health nursing: Concepts of care* (3rd ed.). Philadelphia, PA: W.B. Saunders.

UN Water. (2013). Facts and figures. Retrieved from http://www.unwater.org/water-cooperation-2013/water-cooperation/facts-and-figures/en/

U.S. Census Bureau. (2011). *The older population: 2010, 2010 Census brief*. Retrieved from http://www.census.gov/prod/cen2010/briefs/c2010br-09.pdf

U.S. Department of Health and Human Services. (2010). *About Healthy People: Introducing Healthy People 2020*. Retrieved from http://www.healthypeople.gov/2020/about/default.aspx

Williams, S. J. (1993). Ambulatory health care services. In S. J. Williams & P. R. Torrens (Eds.), *Introduction to health services* (4th ed., pp. 108–133). Albany, NY: Delmar.

Williams, S., & Torrens, P. (2008). *Introduction to health services* (7th ed.). Clifton Park, NY: Cengage Delmar Learning.

Wilper, A. P., Woolhandler, S., Lasser, K. E., McCormick, D., Bor, D. H., & Himmelstein, D. U. (2009). Health insurance and mortality in US adults. *American Journal of Public Health, 99*(12), 2289–2295.

Zuvekas, S. H., & Hill, S. C. (2000). Income and employment among homeless people: The role of mental health, health and substance abuse. *Journal of Mental Health Policy Economics, 3*, 153–163.

CHAPTER FOCUS

The Home Visiting Process
Advantages of Home Visits
Effectiveness of Home Visits
Challenges of Home Visits
Distractions in the Home Environment

QUESTIONS TO CONSIDER

After reading this chapter, you will know the answers to the following questions:

1. What is a home health visit?
2. How is a home visit conducted?
3. What are the stages of a home visit?
4. What are the advantages and challenges of a home visit?
5. How effective are home visits in improving health for populations?

CHAPTER 6

The Home Visit

Karen Saucier Lundy

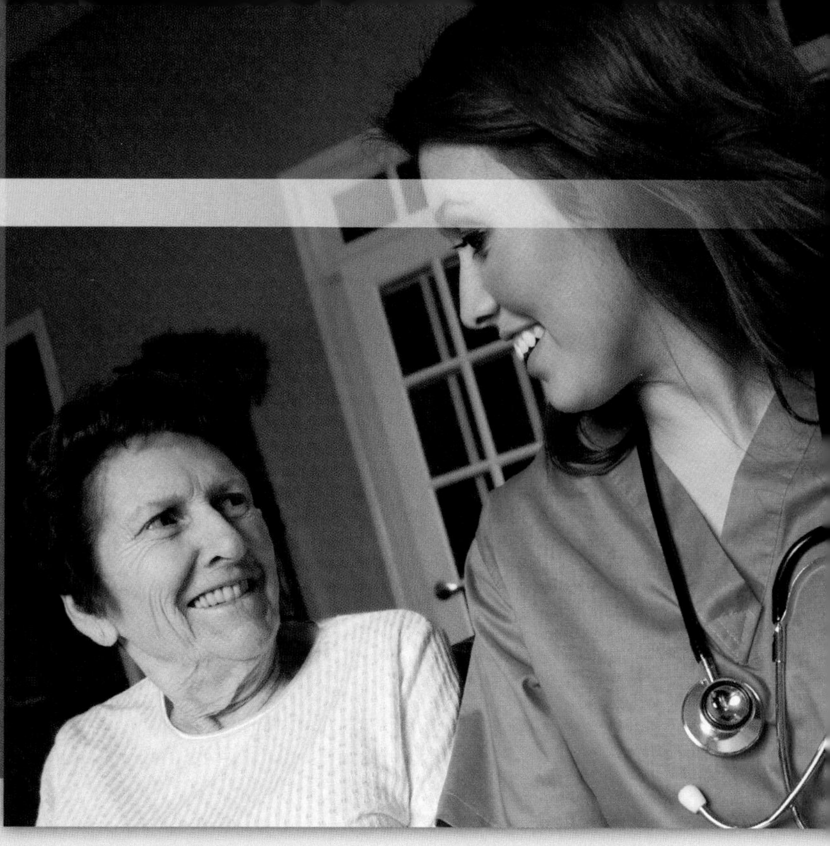

KEY TERMS

behavioral distractions
environmental distractions
nurse-initiated distractions
visiting nurse

Home is where the heart is.

—Pliny the Elder

Hospitals are an intermediate stage of civilization. While devoting my life to hospital work I have come to the conclusion that hospitals are not the best place for the poor sick except for surgical cases.

—Florence Nightingale, 1860

REFLECTIONS

The home was the earliest setting for nursing care. In today's society, most of us expect to go away from home to receive health care. What is your idea of home? Have you ever been on a home visit for providing health care? Think about how you might feel as a patient receiving a home visit from a nurse.

THANKS TO ADVANCES IN technology, nurses can now make "home visits" via the Internet using video through smartphones or computers. Many outpatient facilities consider a "home visit" to be calling a patient the day after treatment to assess the patient's condition. The Affordable Care Act (ACA) of 2010 included provisions that provide incentives to healthcare providers and organizations to keep patients at home as much as possible and out of institutional care settings. As technology evolves, should these types of "home visits" be considered appropriate substitutions for the actual in-home visit by a community health nurse? What are the ethical implications of changing our traditional concept of the home visit?

Since the beginning of time, humans have cared for their own at home, both in sickness and in health. Historically, homes were the earliest practice settings for nurses who worked in the community. Patients were seldom in hospitals, but rather recovered from illness at home and learned about disease prevention and treatment at home; as always, nurses reached out to them through the home visit. During the latter part of the 19th century and throughout the 20th century, community health nurses always had the home as a common setting for practice. As hospitals became more accessible and technology advanced, roles for nurses in the community became more specialized. One specialized role that emerged was that of the visiting nurse, organized by visiting nurse associations that were funded by philanthropic donations (Howse, 2007).

The evolution of home care in the United States resulted from social, economic, technological, demographic, and political forces that continue to shape our healthcare delivery system (National Association for Home Care [NAHC], 2010). By the end of World War II, the physician shortage and the continued explosion of medical technology in the hospital moved many physicians into hospitals, and physician home visiting became a thing of the past (Hafkenschiel, 1997). By the early 1960s, home care was primarily provided by public health and visiting nurses, who assessed patients, provided the necessary services, and managed the therapeutic plan of care. Public health nurses focused on prevention and education; visiting nurses provided sick care in the home. By 1963, according to the National Association for Home Care (2010), the number of home health agencies, primarily private philanthropic organizations, had grown to 1,100. The services they provided involved a variety of professional disciplines, including skilled nursing.

Nurses who make home visits today are employed by a variety of agencies, and their roles can encompass elements of both the **visiting nurse** (sickness care) and the public health nurse (health promotion, case finding, disease prevention, and education). However, in the current reimbursement-driven healthcare system, most nurses who visit patients at home tend to specialize in home health services, with an emphasis on illness care and post-hospital follow up, or public health services, which deliver care in the home and provide health education. With the increase in outpatient surgeries, prevention, chemotherapy, shorter hospital stays, and other services previously done on an inpatient basis, follow-up care at home will continue to be even more critical in a managed care environment. The role of the homecare nurse is increasingly more important as a specialty within community-based health care, especially with the goals of the ACA related to increased patient and population care outside of acute care and institutional settings.

Home health nurses may be employed by home health agencies, hospices, hospitals, public health departments, or clinics. Public health nurses may see patients at home through the auspices of the state health department, a local hospital, or a rural clinic. In this chapter, the home visit as a practice environment is described in the context of the emerging community-based healthcare system.

The Home Visiting Process

One simply has to look around any local hospital to see that it would seem to be much more efficient for patients to come to the nurse and other healthcare providers, where resources are plentiful. Certainly, one of the primary reasons that hospitals were first developed in the Middle Ages was so that caregivers could see more patients and observe them throughout the day and night. Yet there are very good reasons for seeing patients in their own homes. **Box 6-1** lists common purposes of home visiting; **Box 6-2** details the stages of the home visit, with information about the sequential steps in the home visiting process; **Box 6-3** provides information about differences between the home setting and the acute care setting; and **Box 6-4** provides hints on communicating effectively in the home setting.

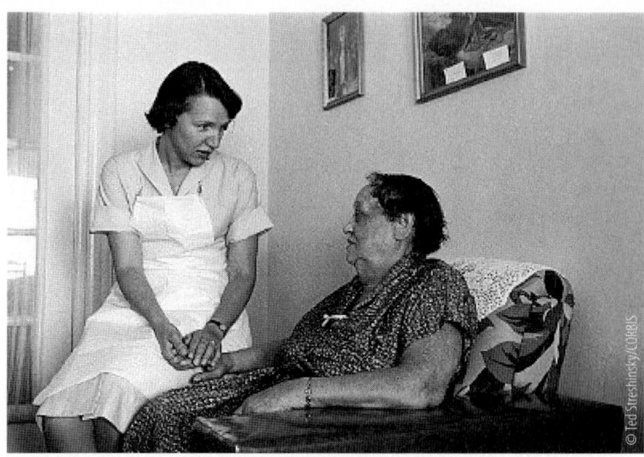

The acceleration of home health nursing came during the 1960s, when Medicare approved home health visits for reimbursement.

BOX 6-1 Purposes of Home Visits

Case Finding

- Public health and protection
- Abuse, neglect cases
- Communicable disease
- School-related health conditions

Illness Prevention and Health Promotion

- Prenatal and well-baby care
- Child development
- Elder care

Care of the Sick and Terminally Ill

- Home health
- Hospice

BOX 6-2 From Beginning to End ... Selecting a Successful Home Visit

Previsit/Planning Stage

- Determine which patients need to be seen.
- Prioritize the scheduled visits based on patient need, distance between visits, laboratory work, and coordination with other professionals and physician.
- Review the chart, orders, patient diagnosis, goals of care, and reasons for the home visit.
- Telephone the patient for validation of scheduled visit; ask patient about specific needs, such as supplies, and any special hazards, such as pets or environmental concerns; caregiver schedule.
- Secure directions to the home.
- Conduct inventory of bag, needed equipment and supplies for patients, and educational materials.
- Review safety considerations, such as timing of visit, environmental assessment.

Implementing the Visit

- Initiate the visit: introduction and identification of nurse to patient, brief social phase to establish rapport.
- Practice appropriate hygienic practices before patient assessment.
- Review plans for visit with patient.
- Determine expectations of patient regarding home visits.
- Conduct assessment: environment, patient, medication, nutrition, functional abilities and limitations, psychosocial issues, and evaluation of previous visit intervention effectiveness.
- Modify the plan of care based on patient need and situational dictates.
- Perform nursing interventions.
- Deal with distractions: environmental, behavioral, and nurse initiated.

Evaluating the Visit

- Evaluate effectiveness of interventions based on established short-term (response during visit) and long-term outcome criteria (effects of intervention at subsequent visits or other patient contact).
- Evaluate as to primary, secondary, tertiary interventions.
- Evaluate conduct of visit: availability of appropriate supplies, preparation of nurse for visit.

Documentation

- Document based on established outcome criteria and agency requirements.
- Validate diagnoses and additional health needs based on visit.
- Evaluate goals and objectives.
- Review actions taken, response of patient, and outcome of interventions (short and long term).
- Record both objective (nurse-based) and subjective (patient-based) data.
- As appropriate, use federal agency reimbursement guidelines, such as Medicare, for progress documentation and certification/recertification requirements.

Termination

- Termination begins with the first visit as nurse prepares the patient for time-limited nature of home visiting.
- Review goal attainment with patient/family and make recommendations and referrals as necessary for continued healthcare issues.
- Develop strategies for appropriate closure with patients who die, refuse visits, or are terminated because of nonreimbursable services.

BOX 6-3 Challenges in Home Settings

- *Control belongs to the patient* because care is being provided in his or her home.
- *A feeling of isolation and lack of support* often results from the nature of the home setting. There are no nurses or other team members in the next room to confirm an assessment or to distinguish an abnormal finding.
- *The home environment and family support system* are unpredictable and not always conducive to optimal care.
- *Dealing with multi-problem families* is difficult emotionally for the nurse, especially in the home setting where family dynamics and interactions are more intense and visible.
- *Difficulty in communicating with the various team members* can be a stressor.
- *The volume of documentation* required can be difficult as a result of the variety and demands of various funding sources and standards.
- *Frustrations with the system* are a common concern. There is often difficulty explaining Medicare or Medicaid's ever-changing requirements to patients and families, as well as to other providers.
- *Complex caseloads* that encompass all age groups with diverse problems are common in home care. The skills and knowledge required are broad, requiring the nurse to become a strong generalist.
- *Concern for personal safety* is an issue, because violence has increased in all delivery settings.

BOX 6-4 Secrets of Professional Conversation: The Home Visit

1. *Break the ice with a warm topic.* Try opening with a cliché such as the weather, pets, sports, children, yard flowers, garden, or any subject that interests *most* people. This often establishes a conversational bond that helps make the transition to other more sensitive topics easier. Example: "How has all this rain lately affected your garden?" Or, while pointing to pictures in home, ask, "Are these your children?"
2. *If you are extremely uncomfortable or have a sense of unidentified anxiety, explore possible source with the patient.* Often, nurses can sense nonverbal conflict in the home, with the patient, or with the family. By acknowledging this, valuable information can be elicited from the patient. Example: "Things seem a little unsettled today. Do you want to talk about anything before we get started with your assessment?"
3. *Pick up the pace by asking open-ended questions.* This forces discussion, because questions can't be answered with a simple yes or no. Answers will be longer so you will be able to notice other things that are being said to keep the conversation going. Example: "Why do you like living out in the country? What do you think about the new road going through town? What if . . .?"
4. *Show sincere interest.* Listening is a skill that must be practiced daily. This means making good eye contact. When the patient is speaking, our tendency is to spend that time planning what we will say next. This is not only discourteous and nontherapeutic, but also causes us to miss important information. Flatter your patient/family with sincere comments: All people crave appreciation. Make sure you *individualize* compliments with details, such as commenting on how much more energetic your patient is or noting that a young mother is attending to her new baby's cries very well. Listening is an excellent way to demonstrate your respect for your patient! Example: Instead of rehearsing your next line, focus on your *genuine* response to what he or she is saying. Challenge yourself to come up with questions about the points the person has raised.
5. *Develop a broad outlook.* Avoid using the word *I* too often. Watch the great conversationalists—Oprah Winfrey, Jane Pauley, Barbara Walters, Katie Couric, or Larry King—they seldom mention themselves, know a little bit about a lot of subjects, and demonstrate a curiosity about a broad range of topics. Example: Read the local newspaper daily and try to listen to at least one news show every other day. This ensures that you will expand your consciousness about community and national issues that concern your patients. Read a variety of opinions about a wide range of issues. Challenge yourself to think about things in new ways.
6. *Avoid judging others in advance (i.e., "prejudice").* Try to suspend judgment about your patient. Coming to conclusions about people before you have even entered their homes, based on what you have read in their chart or know about their income, shuts down your curiosity and prevents you from learning what you need to know about their health status. Example: In a home visit with a new mother who consistently misses clinic appointments, keep an open mind and ask her about other aspects of her life. Listen to her accounts of how her life has changed since giving birth.
7. *Quote your patient when possible.* A very flattering and confirming strategy to promote your patient's self-confidence is to use actual quotes from previous conversations (either from the same visit or previous visits, which means you have to really listen!) to illustrate health information. Example: "Since you mentioned last visit that you felt a 'bit better when I am able to cook my own breakfast,' I think that taking care of yourself as much as possible really makes a difference."

8. *End a conversation gracefully.* Breaking away from a conversation in the home can often be more difficult than starting one. After we "connect" with someone, most of us are hesitant to interrupt when we need to move on to other topics or to end the visit. The reality is that there will eventually come a point in any conversation when you will have to end it. Prepare when you enter the home to end the conversation. Example: Prepare an exit early on in a polite and friendly way. "I have so enjoyed our visit, but I must get going in order to see my other patients," or, "I see from the clock that it is near lunch and I know you must be hungry."

Source: Adapted from King, L. (1994). *How to talk to anyone, anytime, anywhere: The secrets of good conversation.* New York, NY: Crown.

Advantages of Home Visits

Community health nursing is holistic. Seeing patients in the artificial and controlled environment of a hospital reveals little to the nurse about the family's health influences and ability to carry out the plan of care (Persily, 2003). In the home, the nurse gets the complete picture, including environmental factors that affect health, social and psychological influences, relationships between and among family members, and the interaction of the patient with family and social networks. In a hospital, patients are separated from the context of their everyday lives: Healthcare providers control their every movement (including self-regulated body functions), they wear institutional clothes, and care is organized around physician and nurse schedules. Such separation of patients from the context of their lives makes it easier for nurses in the hospital to focus only on the biomedical aspects of disease (Liaschenko, 1994; Williams, 2004).

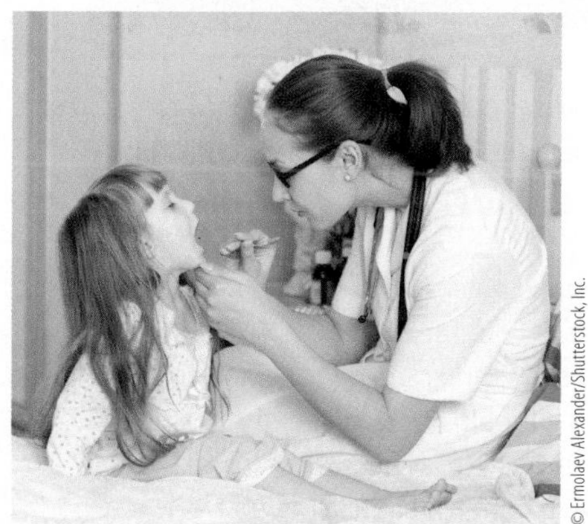

© Ermolaev Alexander/Shutterstock, Inc.

Home health visits take an average of 45 to 60 minutes to complete.

> Besides nursing the patient, she shows them in their own homes how they can call in official sanitary help to make their own poor room healthy, how they can improve appliances, how their homes may not be broken up.
>
> —*Florence Nightingale, 1890*

This is not the case in the home, where illness is but one aspect of the totality of the patient's living experience (Coffman, 1997; Williams, 2004). Hazards and resources are quickly evident and allow a more realistic plan of care to be established, which promotes the achievement of mutually set health strategies and goals. In addition, on a home visit, the nurse can see firsthand how well the patient can perform self-care and can make a more accurate evaluation of medical and nursing interventions. Such information can provide the nurse with valuable indicators in the evaluation of the effects of therapeutic interventions, as compared with the limited time and artificial constraints of the clinic or hospital environment (Liepert, 1996).

There are distinct advantages to the patient when care is provided in the home. For example, rather than having to obtain transportation to a healthcare facility, a home visit may be a more appropriate way to reach a patient. Transportation can be an obstacle for many patients, including those who do not have access to a private car or mass transit, are unable to drive, or are confined to their homes, especially those who live in rural areas. Another advantage is that patients are able to exercise more autonomy on their own turf, which allows the nurse to promote a sense of empowerment in the patient and family (Ruetter & Ford, 1996). The patient becomes part of the interdisciplinary team, rather than a dependent, passive recipient of care. As such, effective community health nurses can use the visit as a way to increase the patient's ability for self-care and enhance the sense of accomplishment in meeting health goals for self and family (Li, Liebel, & Friedman, 2013).

Home Call: Mother and Child

There's so little here: one table,
not laden, one blind
shut. One bulb
hung straight down. One woman,
not well (that look
of someone who won't talk
because they've been beaten
so the bruises don't show), and one

boy, dancing over, no
diaper, eager for the coin
of candy you lay in his
hand. He leans into your
yellow dress, reaching up,
a tendril attaching, lifting
out of the dark, unfurling
his last leaf. She watches him
watch you,
you with a house
she imagines half glass, where light
pours in, and everything
is already paid for: your
dress, the shine of health you wear
as though you own it, the look
of wealth, and (this too is
visible) the knowhow
to make the right phone calls,
calls to those, who, when you call,
will do what you say, pay
what you tell them, when
and to whom. You, she imagines,
who have at least two
of everything, you lift her son
to your yellow breast, that
well lighted place, where the air's
clean, and you don't
hate yourself, waiting in line
to pay for a sack of potatoes
you can't afford, She watches him
cling to you, she waits to see
what you will do; you who
have things, you who can
do things, you who can do
what you choose to, you
who can do something for them,
if you choose to, a little something
or nothing.

—*Marilyn Krysl*

Source: Krysl, M. (1989). *Midwife and other poems on caring*. New York, NY: National League for Nursing, pp. 11–12.

GLOBAL CONNECTION

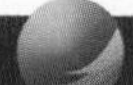

Home visiting in other countries may take the form of mandatory visits for mothers and babies, such as in Cuba and the United Kingdom. For remote villages, such as in the mountains of Nepal, how could home visiting be used as an efficient way of improving the health of community residents?

MEDIA MOMENT

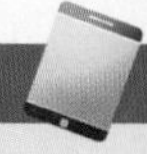

Marvin's Room (1996)

Bessie, played by Diane Keaton, is a straight-laced, devoted daughter providing total care for her ill father (Hume Cronyn) who must ask her estranged, bohemian sister, Lee (Meryl Streep), for help after Bessie suffers a health catastrophe. Bessie lives with her father and eccentric older aunt and has devoted her life to their care. Lee left the family years before and expresses little interest in the welfare of either her sister or her ailing father. She eventually makes the trip home to Florida with her two sons in tow. Leonardo DiCaprio effectively portrays the older, disturbed son who finds comfort with his newly found family. Old wounds are opened, and the movie provides an outstanding examination of life-choice consequences and the rewards of caring for others. Bessie has put her life on hold for years to care for her father, who "has been dying for 20 years—slowly, so that I won't miss anything." She doesn't see the years as wasted but rather says, "I've been so lucky to have been able to love someone so much."

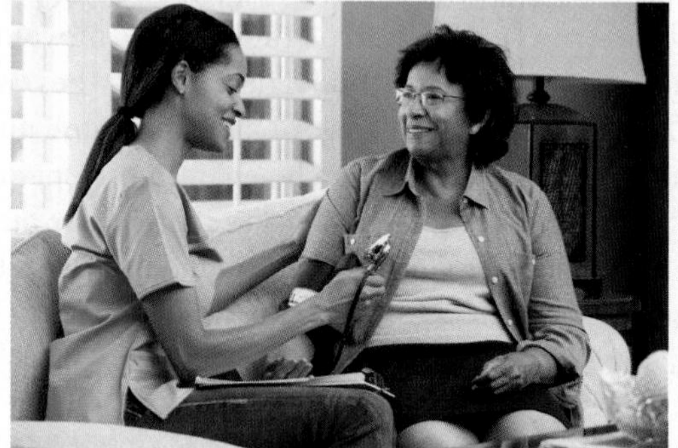

Home health nurses can assist elders to recover more quickly from acute episodes of age related conditions.

Knowing in Nursing (Art Connection)

I stepped outside of myself so that I could know
So that I could know the meaning of the earth
Its green springs and quiet winter nights.
So that I could know the depths
of the great, blue ocean
A place from which we all came.
I stepped outside of myself so that I could know
that there was more than the moon,
and the sun, and the stars ...
And that when I looked upon the earth
so that I could know the meaning of life and
appreciate its continuance in death.
I stepped outside of myself so that I could know
how to raise my arms in loving, caring ways
And say to those who would listen
Let me share myself with you and all that I know ...

—Robyn Rice, RN, MSN, PhD

RESEARCH ALERT 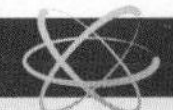

The Home Visit and the Nurse–Family Partnership: Evidence-Based Practice Research

The Nurse–Family Partnership (NFP), created by Dr. David Olds as an applied evidence-based practice home visiting model, is considered to be the most rigorously tested home visiting model in the United States. This Research Alert provides details of the actual research that supports the validity and successful outcomes of the NFP.

The cornerstone of the NFP model is the extensive research on the model conducted since the late 1970s. Randomized trials were conducted with three diverse populations beginning in Elmira, New York, in 1977; in Memphis, Tennessee, in 1987; and Denver, Colorado, in 1994. All three trials targeted first-time, low-income mothers. Follow-up research continues today, studying the long-term outcomes for mothers and children in the three trials.

The program effects that have the strongest evidentiary foundations are those that have been found in at least two of the three trials.

Consistent Program Effects[1]

- Improved prenatal health
- Fewer childhood injuries
- Fewer subsequent pregnancies
- Increased intervals between births
- Increased maternal employment
- Improved school readiness

Employing new and improved statistical analysis methods, Olds and his research team at the Prevention Research Center have been involved in an extensive reanalysis of certain outcomes from the 15-year follow up of the Elmira trial of NFP. An updated summary of the positive program effects is given here:

Benefits to Mothers

- 61% fewer arrests
- 72% fewer convictions
- 98% fewer days in jail[2]

Benefits to Children at Child Age 15

- 48% reduction in child abuse and neglect
- 59% reduction in arrests
- 90% reduction in adjudications as PINS (person in need of supervision) for incorrigible behavior[3]

Whereas the original analysis indicated that program effects were limited to the higher risk portions of the sample (where the mother was unmarried and from a low-income family at registration), the reanalysis indicates that the benefits of the program on the outcomes listed previously are present for the entire nurse-visited sample, irrespective of risk. Many of the program-control differences remain larger for the higher risk families, but the significance of the program effects now holds for the entire sample.

Earlier reported impacts of the Elmira program on "maternal behavioral problems due to substance abuse" and number of times the teens ran away were more accurately characterized as trends in initial follow-up reports. A 2010 analysis, however, found some encouraging results: Compared to individuals who did not participate in the nurse visitation program, girls who had been visited by nurses via the program were significantly less likely to be arrested and convicted of a crime, and they also had fewer children (11% versus 30% in controls) and less use of Medicaid services (18% versus 45%; Eckenrode et al., 2010).

Olds and his research team are committed to continually subjecting their work and earlier findings to the highest scientific standards and state-of-the-art statistical analysis.

About the Research Design

A randomized controlled trial is the most rigorous research method for measuring the effectiveness of an intervention. It is the type of study that the U.S. Food and Drug Administration (FDA) requires of new drugs or medical devices to determine their effectiveness and safety before they are made available to the public. Because of their cost and complexity, these kinds of trials are not often used to evaluate complex health and human services.

In addition, important data are continuously collected from NFP replication sites through the web-based Clinical Information System (CIS). These data are analyzed and returned to local NFP-implementing agencies to provide them with evidence of their progress toward NFP's three goals. For more details on the research, visit: http://www.nursefamilypartnership.org.

[1]Effects observed in at least two of three trials (Elmira, Memphis, and Denver).

[2]Impact on days in jail is highly significant, but the number of cases that involve jail time is small, so the magnitude of program effect is difficult to estimate with precision.

[3]Based on family court records of 116 children who remained in the study community for a 13-year period following the end of the program.

Sources: Eckenrode, J., Ganzel, B., Henderson, C. R., Smith, E., Olds, D. L., Powers, J., … Sidora, K. (2000). Preventing child abuse and neglect with a program of nurse home visitation: The limiting effects of domestic violence. *Journal of the American Medical Association, 284*(11), 1385–1391; Izzo, C., Eckenrode, J., Smith, E., Henderson, C. R., Cole, R., Kitzman, H., & Olds, D. L. (2005). Reducing the impact of uncontrollable stressful life events through a program of nurse home visitation for new parents. *Prevention Science, 6*(4), 269–274; Kitzman, H., Olds, D. L., Sidora, K., Henderson, C. R., Jr., Hanks, C., Cole, R., … Glazner, J. (2000). Enduring effects of nurse home visitation on maternal life course: A 3-year follow-up of a randomized trial. *Journal of the American Medical Association, 283*(15), 1983–1989; Olds, D. (2003). Reducing program attrition in home visiting: What do we need to know? *Child Abuse & Neglect, 27*(4), 359–361; Olds, D., Luckey, D., & Henderson, C. (2004). Can the results be believed? *Pediatrics, 115*(4), 1113–1114.

Home visits often take place over long periods, which affords the nurse ample opportunities for developing the authentic trust relationship necessary for a truly collaborative partnership to develop between nurse and patient. A result is that patients are often more willing to share sensitive and more intimate issues in the home setting, which allows the nurse to gain insight into complex interpersonal influences (Stulginsky, 1993a, 1993b; Williams 2004). Pregnant teens, for example, often need a different type of home visit, including a focus on the teen's developmental level and using narratives to assess the family (SmithBattle, Lorenz, & Leander, 2013).

MEDIA MOMENT 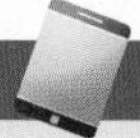

One True Thing (1998)

In this adaptation of Anna Quindlen's novel, when tough New Yorker Ellen Gulden (Renee Zellweger) discovers that her mother (Meryl Streep) has cancer, she quits her job, breaks up with her boyfriend, and moves back in with her parents to help out. Wanting nothing more than to ease her mother's suffering, she inadvertently uncovers several family secrets, including one about her philandering professor father (William Hurt). The movie's lesson is that we go through life telling ourselves a story about our childhood and our parents, but we are the authors of that story, and it is less fact than fiction.

Effectiveness of Home Visits

Research from a variety of studies indicates that successful home visiting programs have resulted in improved health outcomes. But how effective are home visits—such as those that are preventive in nature—in the long run?

In a landmark research study, prenatal and early childhood home visits by nurses reduced subsequent antisocial behavior and experimentation with drugs in adolescents born into high-risk families. The study, which evaluated the effects of home visits by nurses over the course of 15 years to low-income, unmarried women, found long-term benefits that included fewer episodes of children running away from home, fewer arrests and convictions, and decreased drug abuse when compared with similar groups of women who received prenatal and well-child care in a clinic. The adolescent children of these mothers also improved in terms of having fewer sexual partners, and they smoked and drank less than their peers who were not part of the home visiting programs (Izzo et al., 2005; Kitzman et al., 2000; Olds & Kitzman, 1993).

Zeanah, Larrieu, and Boris (2006) used the NFP program in Louisiana, focusing on the use of mental health professionals paired with visiting nurses, to successfully improve maternal and child health, especially in relation to social and developmental issues. In this and other settings where the NFP model has been used, the long-term preventive mental health impact has been impressive. Brown, McLaine, Dixon, and Simon (2006) found that focused home visits to children with elevated blood lead levels resulted in improved parent–child interaction and family housekeeping practices at the end of 1 year of visits, as well as a 47% decrease in blood lead levels in the children.

Other research has revealed that successful home visiting programs should be broad in focus (e.g., "improved pregnancy outcome" versus "hypertension management during pregnancy"), so as to contribute to the most lasting effects in health status. Also, home visits that occur over time and in greater frequency accomplish more in terms of improved health status for the patients than single visits (Barkauskas, 1983; Persily, 2003). Home visits to targeted high-risk groups who have complex and multiple needs have been linked with more significant changes in health status than visits to medium- or low-risk groups (Brown et al., 2006; Byrd, 1998 Deal, 1994; Dodge, Goodman, Murphy, O'Donnell, & Sato, 2013; Izzo et al., 2005; Olds & Kitzman, 1993; Persily, 2003; Roberts, Kramer, & Suissa, 1996; Zotti & Zahner, 1995). Numerous studies have demonstrated that home visiting by nurses to pregnant and postpartum women and their infants reduces risk factors that result in preterm births, abuse and neglect, and maternal health problems (Avellar & Supplee, 2013; Easterbrooks et al., 2013). In addition, home visits improve healthy behaviors and are cost-effective (Gomby, Larson, Lewit, & Behrman, 1993; Izzo et al., 2005; Olds, 1992; Olds, Henderson, Phelps, Kitzman, & Hanks, 1993).

Home health visits have been linked with fewer hospital readmissions, fewer emergency department visits, and cost savings when compared with acute care. A study of patients with congestive heart failure who were visited by home health nurses linked fewer hospital admissions—from 3.2 admissions per year to 1.2 admissions per year—with home health visits. The length of stay decreased from 26 days per year to 6 days per year (Kornowski, Zeeli, Averbuch, & Finkelstein, 1995).

Schoen and Anderson (1998), in their extensive review of the effectiveness of home visiting programs, found that the most successful programs have the following elements:

- A focus on families in greater need of services rather than universal programs
- Interventions that begin in pregnancy and continue through the second to fifth years of life

- Flexibility and family specificity regarding the duration and frequency of visits, according to the family's need and risk level
- Active promotion of positive health-related behaviors
- Use of a broad, multiproblem focus to address the full complement of family needs
- Assistance to the family with reduction of stress by improving the social and physical environment
- Use of nurses and professionals specifically prepared in home visiting

Challenges of Home Visits

Paradoxically, many of the aspects of home visiting that make it more advantageous for the nurse and patient than the hospital environment also contribute to the challenges of home visiting. Because the nurse is more independent and less tied to the physical constraints of the agency, professional isolation can be a problem, especially for a novice nurse. In the clinic or hospital, help or consultation with other professionals is only a few steps away. For the home visiting nurse, finding that help becomes more difficult and can be a source of considerable anxiety. With advanced technology, such as laptop computers and tablets, pagers, cell phones, mobile devices, and remote monitoring devices, the nurse must use different strategies for connecting with other professionals and their patients (Cipriano et al., 2014).

The intimacy of the home visit can create boundary issues for both the nurse and the patient. For example,

CULTURAL CONNECTION

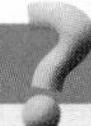

The NFP model has been utilized successfully in the remote swamps of southern Louisiana. This program was in place before Hurricane Katrina hit the area in August 2005.

Southern Louisiana is perhaps one of the most challenging locales for implementing the highly successful NFP project. Professional nurses, also referred to as "professional nurturers," visit poor and isolated mothers in the Cajun communities of Terrebonne and Lafourche parishes as part of the NFP program in Louisiana. Nurses visit mothers and babies up to the age of 2 to role-model good parenting practices and teach young families how to raise healthy children. This program is particularly challenging owing to the Cajun culture's resistance to government intervention programs and outsider intrusion. The area targeted by the NFP program was one of the poorest in the South before Hurricane Katrina struck, and it was hard hit by the hurricane. Yet due to the historically harsh living conditions of the swamps, few residents seemed to be concerned about the hurricane, according to one of the nurses in the program.

The Louisiana program focuses on an area an hour's drive southwest of New Orleans, along foggy, cypress tree–lined winding roads to the Gulf of Mexico. The Mississippi River sediment shaped this marshy delta, to which French Acadians migrated in the 18th century after being expelled by the British from Nova Scotia. Cajuns now live in one of the harshest environments in the United States and have built their lives for two centuries on one of the fastest-sinking lands on earth.

Louisiana has some of the lowest literacy and child poverty rates in the United States. Thirty percent of Louisiana's children grow up in poverty. Childrearing practices often reflect Cajun cultural beliefs, such as the notion that giving a baby a haircut before his first birthday will stunt his growth and damage his brain.

The NFP visiting nurse program has resulted in improved statistics, although the gains are modest when considered against most standards in public health. After 4 years, the Louisiana legislature doubled funding for the program, mainly through Medicaid. With more than 1,000 mothers and children who have finished the 2-year program, results are encouraging. By the time these children turned 2 years of age, almost 60% of the mothers who had started the program without a high school diploma or GED had one. Thirty percent of toddlers had scored in the top quartile of a national test for language development.

1. Why are the Cajuns of southern Louisiana seldom considered an ethnic group in the United States?
2. What are the political implications and possible blocks to implementing this type of program on a national basis?
3. Would these programs be in opposition to widely held American values of the sanctity of the family—for example, the idea that such programs intrude into a family's private life?
4. Does a program such as the NFP undermine other community efforts to fund public quality daycare centers, such as Head Start? Why or why not? What are possible compromises in funding these programs to promote better family outcomes and improve the community's overall health?

Sources: With kind permission from Springer Science & Business Media: Prevention Science, Reducing the impact of uncontrollable stressful life events through a program of nurse home visitation for new parents, 6(4), 2005, 269-274, Izzo CV et al.

RESEARCH ALERT

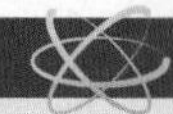

Recent advances in telecommunication technologies have enabled the direct provision of services to patients in the home using tools such as videophones and data transmission over phone lines. The present study compared nurse–patient interaction using two different video platforms designed for telehome care. One platform uses existing telephone lines (POTS video), and the other uses the Internet (IP video). The specific aims of this study were (1) to assess the degree of acceptance by nurses and patients of home video visits for nurse–patient interaction and (2) to compare preferences for delivery of home care between the two platforms, between video and live interaction, and between video and less frequent or no interaction.

The study used a quasi-experimental cross-over design. Nurse–patient pairs were assigned to conditions using a predetermined assignment procedure, alternating each new pair to start with one of the two platforms. Following that session, each participant pair then tested the second platform. Three simulated health problem scenarios, which focused on depression, anticoagulation therapy, and diabetes, were created for the study. A convenience sample of 26 practicing nurses and 18 volunteers serving as simulated patients participated in the study. Nurse case managers at the Iowa City Veterans Affairs Medical Center (VAMC) served as the nurse sample. Volunteer participants were recruited from the volunteer department at the same facility. Most of the volunteers (72%) were age 70 or older; 61% of the nurses were younger than 50 years old.

Most participants regularly wore corrective lenses (81% of nurses and 94% of volunteers); 11% of volunteers wore a hearing aid; and 17% reported having other hearing problems, while none of the nurses reported hearing problems. Forty percent of the volunteer patients reported that they were very or somewhat comfortable using a personal computer; 27% ($n = 4$) reported having a personal computer (PC) at home; and 20% ($n = 3$) had Internet access at home. All of the nurses regularly used computers at work, whereas most of the volunteers did not use the computer on a regular basis while at the medical center.

Description of POTS Video and IP Video Systems

The system selected for the plain old telephone service (POTS) video portion of the study was composed of a television monitor and a camera kit that combined a telephone, microphone, and video camera. To establish contact, the nurse activates the system using the remote control to enter the patient's telephone number. The patient at home responds by pushing the start button on the remote control device. During the visit, the nurse and the patient see and talk to each other, with all functions controlled by the nurse. At the end of the interaction, the patient presses the end-call button on the remote. The remote control device has one large green button to start the system and one large red end-call button to turn it off. This facilitates ease of use by older patients who may have limited dexterity or vision. In this study, the calls were placed on commercial telephone lines.

The Internet Protocol (IP)-based teleconferencing system consists of a small video camera with an integrated microphone that mounts on top of a PC monitor and connects to the PC via a USB port. To communicate using this platform, both the nurse and the patient need a PC, the video camera and software, and an Internet connection. To establish contact, the nurse activates the communication software, enters the patient's IP address, and clicks the dial button. When the patient has also activated the software on his or her PC and has established an Internet connection, the patient's software will recognize the incoming call and will emit an audible ring, much like a telephone call. The patient can then click a button to answer the call, and within a few seconds, the nurse and patient will be able to see and hear each other. To end the call, the nurse or patient clicks on the end-call button.

Each healthy adult volunteer played the role of a patient and was paired with a nurse. Seated in separate rooms, each patient–nurse pair conducted two simulated home visits on one of the video units being tested using a script prepared by the investigators. Scripts included typical patient problems addressed during a home care visit. Using the script, the nurse conducted a standard set of tasks or assessments that mimicked a home care visit. The nurse and patient each completed a short evaluation rating. The patient–nurse pair then conducted the same two simulated home visits using the same scripts on the second video unit, after which the nurse and patient again completed the same short evaluation rating. Following completion of the two simulated visits, the study coordinator conducted a brief open-ended interview with participants to discuss perceptions of the two platforms. These qualitative responses were recorded in notes taken by the study staff.

The three interaction scenarios simulated a nurse interacting with a patient with depression, a patient on anticoagulant therapy, and a patient with newly diagnosed diabetes. The scenarios were designed to maximize the features of the video component. The depression scenario required the nurse to observe the patient's facial expressions and body language. The anticoagulant scenario required the nurse to read the patient's medication bottle and to observe the patient's arms for signs of bruising. The diabetes scenario required the nurse to demonstrate the use of an insulin syringe to the patient. Each scenario was designed to be completed within 10 to 15 minutes.

Outcome Measures

An investigator-developed instrument was used that addressed patient–nurse communication using the video platforms. All items were scored using a 6-point Likert-type scale (1 = strongly disagree to 6 = strongly agree).

The first aim of the study was to assess the degree of acceptance of home video visits for nurse–patient interaction. For the first analysis, nurse and patient ratings were combined to compare POTS video to IP video. The IP video system was rated significantly higher ($p \leq 0.05$) in the following acceptance categories: trust that privacy is maintained; video visits as a replacement for nurse home visits; preference for the video visit compared to a nurse home visit; willingness to recommend the platform to others who need home care; willingness to use the platform if home care was needed; and recommending the platform to friends/patients. There were no significant differences between the POTS and IP system ratings for ease of use, visit taking too much time, and perceived expense of visit.

A separate analysis was conducted to compare patient and nurse ratings for each system. Patients rated the POTS video system significantly more favorably than did nurses, on the following criteria: acceptance of video visits as a replacement for nurse home visits, between the two platforms, and between video and live interaction.

Patients and nurses both preferred the IP video over the POTS system, citing superior visualization. Overall, patients ranked both platforms more favorably than did the nurses on acceptance of home video visits and preferences for more frequent visits relative to less frequent face-to-face visits.

Although the IP platform had higher overall ratings, a critical difference between the two platforms was ease of use. For example, some patients had a difficult time answering the call on the IP video system because they were not familiar or comfortable with using a computer. Although the study was initially designed to have both nurses and patients log on to the IP system, technical and end-user difficulties were so common in the first few sessions that the connection was instead established for the participants. Thus, ease of use is a critical consideration when selecting a home technology system.

Although participants preferred more frequent video visits compared to less frequent face-to-face visits, nurses emphasized the value of home visits. In the follow-up interviews, nurses often mentioned the importance of seeing a patient's surroundings and living conditions when conducting a home visit—a task that would be hampered by the narrow field of vision afforded by a video camera. Nurses expressed the need for personal contact with patients. However, they also acknowledged that video visits could be a good way to supplement face-to-face visits.

Home telehealth monitoring devices are quickly being adopted in practice settings. This study, by examining patient and nurse preferences for use, concluded that ease of use, clinical appropriateness, training, and support will affect the future growth of home telehealth.

Source: Wakefield, B. J., Holman, J. E., Ray, A., Morse, J., & Kienzle, M. G. (2004). Nurse and patient preferences for telehealth home care. *Geriatric Times, 5*(2), 27–30.

the boundary between professional distance and social intimacy because of the informality of the home is a constant challenge for the community health nurse. Certainly, there is a certain amount of socialization that occurs in all home visits as the nurse maintains therapeutic rapport and extends courtesy to her patient hosts. Nurses are always guests in the patient's home, and courtesies normally not extended in the hospital become critical in the home. Nurses also may find themselves disclosing more about themselves than they would in a hospital setting. Such self-disclosure must be monitored carefully so that the patient–nurse relationship remains therapeutic. For example, a nurse's concern about her own child's illness might be mentioned in casual comments and then become a significant source of anxiety for the elder patient who becomes overly worried about the child's wellbeing.

The nurse must also deal with the challenge that providing care may actually increase a person's feelings of vulnerability, simply by being seen at home by a nurse. The patient may perceive that by accepting the nurse's help, his or her own ability to give self-care is inadequate. In their ethnographic study, Magilvy, Brown, and Dydyn (1988) found that home health patients often expressed concerns about relying on a home health nurse as a sign of vulnerability. They expressed a need to maintain their independence and mobility and saw the nurse as a reminder of their dependency or reliance on outside help. Therefore, the nurse must constantly promote the collaborative nature of the patient–nurse relationship and frequently praise the patient for efforts to improve health, no matter how small or insignificant the changes might be. Nurses accustomed to using "take charge" skills such as are rewarded in the hospital often find that they may lead to failure in the home setting (Coffman, 1997; Liaschenko, 1994; Millard, Hallett, & Luker, 2006; Moser, Houtepen, & Widdershoven, 2007).

CULTURAL CONNECTION

People who live in the United States value home ownership as a sign of a successful life. For other cultures, a home is defined and valued very differently. For the homeless, home may be under a bridge, in an abandoned car, or in an alley. How does the definition of home affect nurses who visit patients "at home"?

In the home setting, the patient has the right to self-determination and can reject or accept the therapeutic interventions offered by the nurse. This important aspect of autonomy cannot be overemphasized when in the patient's home. The nurse must remember that true collaboration means that the nurse and the patient set goals, develop strategies, and evaluate outcomes of care together, no matter how difficult that sharing of power may be for the nurse who has been taught that "the nurse always knows best" (Millard et al., 2006; Zerwekh, 1997).

In a study by Jack, DiCenso, and Lohfeld (2002), researchers determined that factors which influenced relationship development with patients in the home-related "family–nurse engagement occurred through 'finding common ground' and 'building trust.'" For example, a prenatal patient may refuse to stop smoking during pregnancy, explaining to the nurse that she is too nervous to do so because her mother-in-law has moved in with the family. The nurse may be able to provide the patient with assistance in reducing the number of cigarettes smoked per day, especially if the nurse is a former smoker. Successive approximations in the attainment of patient goals means that progress is measured in small increments, rather than in the dramatic turnaround of the acute care setting (Stulginsky, 1993a). For many nurses, this is perhaps the most difficult challenge of all, especially for nurses who have primary experience in the hospital specialty units, such as the emergency department or intensive care unit. The community health nurse cannot solve all of the patient's problems during home visiting, nor should such attempts be made. Only those health problems that are amenable to therapeutic nursing interventions and that are mutually agreed on by the patient and nurse should be the focus during home visits. For example, the patient with diabetes may not be able to eliminate sugar from her coffee and tea but over time may be able to discontinue use of sugar with her cereal.

Another challenge that often emerges is when the nurse faces the immediate pressing demands of the family and a different, preset agenda determined by the agency, typically as a result of the funding source's policy (Cowley, 1995). Usually, the funding source states a specified number of visits or a specified time frame for the care (e.g., 60 days). The dilemma occurs for the community nurse when the patient needs additional care but not specifically at the skilled level. For example, a patient may express the need for more assistance in learning to exercise with an artificial hip appliance. The nurse could refer the patient to local support groups and community senior centers that offer specialized exercise classes. Community health nurses may be some of the most creative nurses working today as they struggle to find myriad ways of meeting patient needs when conventional reimbursement sources end. Consulting with other team members and using support groups may provide resources and support in these complex and frustrating situations, which are becoming all too common in the managed care arena.

ENVIRONMENTAL CONNECTION

A home visit provides the community health nurse with exceptional opportunities of assessing environmental risks, practicalities of implementing a plan of care, and the limits of patients' ability to care for themselves and for others. The hospital is an artificial environment, created for the convenience of healthcare providers. As nurses, we know very little about how patients live on a daily basis without visiting where they call "home." When the natural environment of home is experienced by the community health nurse during home visits, more realistic and acceptable plans of care *with* the patient can be executed with greater chance of success.

MEDIA MOMENT

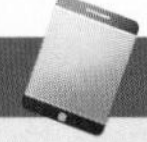

Passion Fish (1992)

May-Alice Culhane (Mary McDonnell) is a soap opera star who's left paralyzed after a car accident and, with few other options, returns to her Louisiana home. Her heavy drinking and bad attitude drive away all of her caregivers, until Chantelle (Alfre Woodard) comes to work for her. The two women form an unlikely friendship in this John Sayles film, which earned McDonnell an Oscar nomination for best actress.

At the heart of the movie is the uneasy relationship between May-Alice and Chantelle. May-Alice is used to being willful and spoiled; Chantelle does not find her behavior acceptable. But May-Alice has the money and Chantelle needs the job, for more urgent reasons than we first realize, and so it seems that Chantelle may have to put up with May-Alice's behavior. Yet in a deeper sense—one that reveals itself only gradually to May-Alice—what she needs most of all from Chantelle is the other woman's ability to stand up to her.

ETHICAL CONNECTION 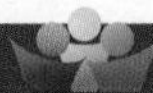

A nurse on a home visit is offered vegetables from the patient's garden. How would you respond to this situation? Is it always appropriate to refuse gifts from a patient? Why or why not?

Distractions in the Home Environment

Conducting a visit in the home, as compared with the nurse-controlled environment of the hospital, is unique in that the nurse must compete with many distractions. Although the distractions that nurses encounter on home visits may seem on the surface negative and interfere with the plan of care, Pruitt, Keller, and Hale (1987) contend that distractions can also provide valuable information about the patient's world. Distractions can generally be classified as environmental, behavioral, or nurse initiated.

Environmental distractions take the form of excessive stimuli, such as television and radio, children playing and making noise, phone calls, traffic, or construction noise. Other environmental sources of distraction may come from crowded or cluttered living conditions; the nurse almost always faces less than ideal living conditions on home visits. Nurses have their own picture of what an ideal living environment should look like, and such values influence the way distractions affect assessment and interventions. For example, the nurse may find a cluttered home a sign of a patient's depression or disinterest in a healthy environment. By remaining open to other explanations, the nurse may discover that the patient feels comforted by the various objects, furniture, and photos. How we "clutter" our homes has much to do with what is important to us—and to our patients—and thus can be a valuable way for us to learn about the patient's values. How we "use" our space, no matter how large or how small, reflects our values and lifestyles (Pruitt et al., 1987). Noticing how the furniture is arranged, the number and kinds of photographs around the home, and the kinds of objects displayed can help nurses understand a patient's family circle and ties as well as those things that bring the patient joy. The "doggie smell" and dog hair throughout the house may be what makes an elderly woman's house a home. Elders often have cluttered homes because they have accumulated the memories and possessions of a lifetime; they also may place furniture close together to make it easier to hear conversations.

The nurse can learn to minimize environmental distractions—for example, by asking to turn down or "mute" the television or avoiding visiting when the patient is most likely to be watching favorite television programs. Experienced home health nurses who visit patients over a long period of time are well aware of how important it is to avoid certain times of the day, such as when the patient's

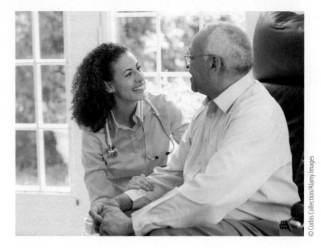

A nurse on a home visit.

favorite soap operas are on! If interruptions become a problem, observing how the patient reacts can provide the nurse with clues to how much of a threat the distraction is to the patient's health (Pruitt et al., 1987). One solution in visiting a pregnant woman with a 3-year-old child who may be distracting her is to have the child draw a picture for the nurse. Such a strategy can provide the nurse with ample time to perform assessment tasks with the mother. In a multiperson household where privacy is at a premium, retreating to a back room or even outside to a porch is often all that is necessary to obtain a few moments of distraction-free assessment time. Balancing courtesy with objectives for the visit becomes a skill that requires tact, humor, and creativity.

Another type of distraction is **behavioral distractions**. That is, the patient may exhibit behaviors that distract the nurse from the plan of care and goals of the home visit. Patients may avoid talking about health problems for a variety of reasons and may instead engage in social communication. Patients may have very real concerns that are not consistent with what the nurse sees as priority problems (Pruitt et al., 1987). By examining such avoidance, the nurse may find that these concerns should be addressed first. For example, a nurse who is seeing an older woman with diabetes may find that the patient refuses to discuss her daily blood sugars, but instead wants to talk about an auto accident that occurred the night before near the patient's home. Upon closer examination, the nurse finds that the accident has claimed the life of an elderly woman only casually known to the patient, and the patient then remarks, "It isn't too much longer that I will be able to drive, and then what will I do?" The patient was exposing her feelings of vulnerability about losing her mobility and independence. Other behaviors that may hinder the goals of the home visit include blocking or silence in response to inquiries related to health status. The nurse must use appropriate therapeutic communication techniques, such as refocusing, and exhibit patience to provide optimal comfort for the patient in the home environment.

GOT AN ALTERNATIVE?

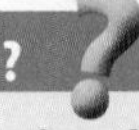

On a home visit, nurses often find out about folk remedies used by families for common health problems. In determining the appropriate response to these nontraditional or alternative health practices, the nurse should assess whether the practice is harmful, neutral, or beneficial. If the practice is neutral (such as keeping a good-luck charm in the baby's room), should the nurse take action with the family concerning the practice? How should the nurse intervene appropriately when the practice is determined to be harmful (such as pica eating), in contrast to being beneficial to the family's health (such as meditation and chanting)?

Nurse-initiated distractions can evolve from prejudices, fears, preoccupation with the tasks of home visiting, and reactions to lifestyles and living conditions different from the nurse's own. Homes of patients may be cluttered or appear unkempt, and these distractions can result in the nurse making judgments about the patient, even on an unconscious level. This "baggage" that all nurses carry with them on home visits should be carefully acknowledged and examined to prevent negative effects on nurse–patient interactions. Nurses may fear home visiting because of safety concerns, concerns over being alone without colleagues for support and consultation, and fears of being rejected by the patient. Practicing nursing in the uncontrolled environment of a patient's home can threaten even the most secure nurse in terms of autonomy and control. Other distractions that are common are talking on the phone with the home office or other healthcare professionals or making arrangements for other patients while in the patient's home. The nurse must be aware of how such distractions influence the nurse–patient relationship. While in the home, the patient should remain the focus as much as possible. By being preoccupied with staying on schedule, tasks, and documentation of the visit, the effectiveness of home visiting can be seriously threatened.

The nurse may also become frustrated with patients who are labeled as noncompliant or who seem to have contributed in some way to their health problems, such as emphysema in a smoker or liver cancer in an alcoholic. Understanding that these feelings are shared at one time or another by most nurses can be the first step to prevent them from affecting the care delivered. Talking with colleagues and having an open dialogue with other professionals in similar settings can help nurses understand not only the source of these distractions but also helpful ways that others have used to minimize their effects on patient care (Pruitt et al., 1987).

Conclusion

The origins of home visiting began with organized health care. Visiting families and patients in the home can provide the community health nurse with more realistic expectations of the family's needs and more appropriate interventions. Advantages and disadvantages of home visiting should be considered when choosing this setting for community-based nursing care.

APPLICATION TO PRACTICE

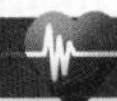

A community health nurse is following a child with high blood lead levels. During a follow-up visit to the clinic, the mother was distracted and kept looking at her watch while the nurse explained how important it was to keep the child from coming in contact with leaded paint. The child failed to keep an appointment with a university clinic for a chelation treatment. The community health nurse could not reach the mother because the phone had been disconnected.

On a home visit, the nurse found out that the father had been injured while working at his car repair service shop, located on the same lot as the family's mobile home. He had taken a temporary job while he recovered from the back injury, on an "as-needed" basis for a local garage, and used his own tow truck for jobs. He was on call 24 hours a day. Because of his business, many old cars were scattered all over the yard, explaining a potential source for the lead poisoning in the child. Also, the father's injury had kept him from repairing the family car, so the only transportation was the tow truck.

1. Identify three of the most serious health threats in this family.
2. Identify two nursing goals for this family.
3. What is the first action you would take on the first home visit?
4. What further information would be important to know about these family members?
5. Identify two strengths of this family.

AFFORDABLE CARE ACT (ACA)

The ACA Independence at Home Demonstration Program for chronically ill Medicare beneficiaries began in 2012. This program tests payment incentives and service delivery systems that utilize home-based, physician- and nurse practitioner–directed primary care teams to reduce expenditures and improve health outcomes. The program is seeking to reduce preventable hospitalizations, prevent hospital readmissions, reduce emergency department visits, improve health outcomes, improve the efficiency of care, reduce the cost of Medicare services, and achieve beneficiary and family caregiver satisfaction.

LEVELS OF PREVENTION 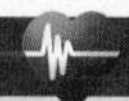

Primary: Home visit for a new healthy baby to assist the parents with basic health care and development milestones

Secondary: Home visit for a child with diabetes to assist parents with understanding the management of insulin administration

Tertiary: Home visit for an older woman to assist with post-leg amputation surgery (due to diabetes) care

HEALTHY ME 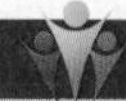

Have you ever been a patient in a hospital? If so, would you prefer to be taken care of at home for the same condition? Why or why not?

Critical Thinking Activities

1. Read the poem *Home Call: Mother and Child* by Marilyn Krysl earlier in this chapter.
   - How does the mother perceive the nurse in terms of power?
   - Do the status differences in the nurse and the mother affect the outcome of this home visit as intervention?
   - How could the nurse be culturally sensitive in this situation while educating the mother about appropriate child care?
   - How is power represented in this poem?
   - Identify one appropriate nursing intervention in the described home visit.
2. The following questions are common ones that student nurses ask about home visiting. As you read this chapter, reflect on your own responses to the questions.
   - What do patients in the home think of student nurses caring for them, especially if an instructor is not present?
   - What if the patient or family member asks me a question to which I don't know the answer?
   - What will I be expected to do as far as skills in the home setting?
   - What about safety issues?
   - What do I do if a patient "codes" while I am there?
   - Are there specific legal implications that I should be aware of in the home setting?

References

Avellar, S. A., & Supplee, L. H. (2013). Effectiveness of home visiting in improving child health and reducing child maltreatment. *Pediatrics, 132*(Suppl 2), S82–S89.

Barkauskas, V. H. (1983). Effectiveness of public health nurse home visits to primarous mothers and their infants. *American Journal of Public Health, 73*(5), 573–580.

Brown, M. J., McLaine, P., Dixon, S., & Simon, P. (2006). A randomized, community-based trial of home visiting to reduce lead levels in children. *Pediatrics, 117*(1), 147–153.

Byrd, M. E. (1998). Long-term maternal-child home visiting. *Public Health Nursing, 15*(4), 235–242.

Cipriano, P. F., Bowles, K., Dailey, M., Dykes, P., Lamb, G., & Naylor, M. (2013). The importance of health information technology in care and coordination and transitional care. *Nursing Outlook, 61*(6), 477–488.

Coffman, S. (1997). Home-care nurses as strangers in the family. *Western Journal of Nursing Research, 19*(1), 82–96.

Cowley, S. (1995). In health visiting: A routine visit is one that has passed. *Journal of Advanced Nursing, 22*, 276–284.

Deal, L. W. (1994). The effectiveness of community health nursing interventions: A literature review. *Public Health Nursing, 11*, 315–323.

Dodge, K. A., Goodman, W. B., Murphy, R. A., O'Donnell, K., & Sato, J. (2013). Randomized controlled trial of universal postnatal nurse home visiting: Impact on emergency care. *Pediatrics, 132*(Suppl 2), S140–S146.

Easterbrooks, M. A., Bartlett, J. D., Raskin, M., Goldberg, J., Contreras, M. M., Kotake, C., … Jacobs, F. H. (2013). Limiting home visiting effects: Maternal depression as a moderator of child maltreatment. *Pediatrics, 132*(Suppl 2), S126–S133.

Eckenrode, J., Campa, M., Luckey, D. W., Henderson, C. R., Jr., Cole, R., Kitzman, H., … Olds, D. (2010). Long-term effects of prenatal and infancy nurse home visitation on the life course of youths: 19-year follow-up of a randomized trial. *Archives of Pediatric & Adolescent Medicine, 164*(1), 9–15.

Gomby, D. S., Larson, J. D., Lewit, J., & Behrman, R. (1993). Home visiting analysis and recommendations. *The Future of Children, 3*, 6–22.

Hafkenschiel, J. (1997). Minding our business. Home health reimbursement and the 1997 Budget Act. *Home Care Provider, 2*(6), 279–281.

Howse, C. (2007). "The ultimate destination of all nursing": The development of district nursing in England, 1880–1925. *Nursing History Review, 15*, 65–94.

Izzo, C., Eckenrode, J., Smith, E., Henderson, C. R., Cole, R., Kitzman, H., & Olds, D. L. (2005). Reducing the impact of uncontrollable stressful life events through a program of nurse home visitation for new parents. *Prevention Science, 6*(4), 269–274.

Jack, S., DiCenso, A., & Lohfeld, L. (2002). Opening doors: Factors influencing the establishment of a working relationship between paraprofessional home visits and at-risk families. *Canadian Journal of Nursing Research, 34*(4), 59–69.

Kitzman, H., Olds, D. L., Sidora, K., Henderson, C. R., Jr., Hanks, C., Cole, R., ... Glazner, J. (2000). Enduring effects of nurse home visitation on maternal life course: A 3-year follow-up of a randomized trial. *Journal of the American Medical Association, 283*(15), 1983–1989.

Kornowski, R., Zeeli, D., Averbuch, M., & Finkelstein, A. (1995). Intensive home care surveillance prevents hospitalization and improved morbidity rates among elderly patients with congestive heart failure. *American Heart Journal, 4*, 762–766.

Li, Y., Liebel, D., & Friedman, B. (2013). An investigation into which individual instrumental activities of daily living are affected by a home visiting nurse intervention. *Age and Ageing, 42*(1), 27–33.

Liaschenko, J. (1994). The moral geography of home care. *Advances in Nursing Science, 17*, 16–26.

Liepert, B. D. (1996). The value of community health nursing: A phenomenological study of the perceptions of the community health nurses. *Public Health Nursing, 13*, 50–57.

Magilvy, J. K., Brown, N. J., & Dydyn, J. (1988). The experience of home health care: Perceptions of older adults. *Public Health Nursing, 5*(3), 140–145.

Millard, L., Hallett, C., & Luker, R. (2006). Nurse-patient interaction and decision-making in care. *Journal of Advanced Nursing, 55*(2), 142–150.

Moser, A., Houtepen, R., & Widdershoven, G. (2007). Patient autonomy in nurse-led shared care. *Journal of Advanced Nursing, 57*(4), 357–365.

National Association for Home Care (NAHC). (2010). *Basic statistics about home care: Updated 2010.* Washington, DC: Author. Retrieved from http://www.nahc.org/assets/1/7/10HC_Stats.pdf

Olds, D. L. (1992). Home visitation program for pregnant women and parents of young children. *American Journal of Diseases of Children, 146*, 704–708.

Olds, D. L., Henderson, C. R., Phelps, C., Kitzman, H., & Hanks, C. (1993). Effect of prenatal and infancy nurse home visitation on government spending. *Medical Care, 31*, 155–174.

Olds, D. L., & Kitzman, H. (1993). Review of research on home visiting for pregnant women and parents of young children. *The Future of Children, 3*(3), 53–92.

Persily, C. (2003). Lay home visiting may improve pregnancy outcomes. *Holistic Nursing Practice, 17*(5), 231–238.

Pruitt, R. H., Keller, L. S., & Hale, S. L. (1987). Mastering the distractions that mar home visits. *Nursing and Health Care, 8*, 344–347.

Roberts, I., Kramer, M. S., & Suissa, S. (1996). Does home visiting prevent childhood injury: A systematic review of randomized controlled trials. *British Medical Journal, 3122*(7022), 22–23.

Ruetter, L. I., & Ford, J. S. (1996). Perceptions of public health nursing: Views from the field. *Journal of Advanced Nursing, 24*, 7–15.

Schoen, S., & Anderson, S. (1998). The role of home visitation programs in improving health outcomes for children and families. *Pediatrics, 101*(3), 486–490.

SmithBattle, L., Lorenz, R., & Leander, S. (2013). Listening with care: Using narrative methods to cultivate nurses' responsive relationships in a home visiting intervention with teen mothers. *Nursing Inquiry, 20*(3), 188–198.

Stulginsky, M. M. (1993a). Nurses' home health experience. Part 1: The practice setting. *Nursing and Health Care, 14*, 402–407.

Stulginsky, M. M. (1993b). Nurses' home health experience. Part 2: The unique demands of home visits. *Nursing and Health Care, 14*, 476–485.

Williams, A. M. (2004). Shaping the practice of home care: Critical case studies of the significance of the meaning of home. *International Journal of Palliative Nursing, 10*(7), 333–342.

Zeanah, P. D., Larrieu, J. A., & Boris, N. W. (2006). Nurse home visiting: Perspectives from nurses. *Infant Mental Health Journal, 27*(1), 41–54.

Zerwekh, J. V. (1997). Making the connection during home visits: Narratives of expert nurses. *International Journal of Human Caring, 1*(1), 325–333.

Zotti, M. E., & Zahner, S. J. (1995). Evaluation of PHN home visits to pregnant women on WIC. *Public Health Nursing, 12*(5), 294–304.

CHAPTER FOCUS

Globalization and International Health

Role of International Agencies
- United Nations
- United Nations Children's Fund
- World Health Organization
- World Bank
- Carter Center
- Bill and Melinda Gates Foundation

Global Health Issues
- Disease Burden
- Violence and War
- Poverty
- Women's Rights

Global Initiatives
- Declaration of Alma Ata
- Millennium Developmental Goals

Global Nursing
- Nursing Shortages
- International Council of Nurses
- Nursing and Human Rights

Appendix

QUESTIONS TO CONSIDER

After reading this chapter, you will know the answers to the following questions:

1. How has globalization affected international health?
2. What roles do violence and war play in international health efforts?
3. How is world health influenced by women's rights issues?
4. What roles do nurses play in international health?
5. How do nongovernmental agencies contribute to global health efforts?
6. How does the International Council of Nurses (ICN) collaborate with other organizations to improve health care and nursing worldwide?

The modern world changes very rapidly, and nurses need to be alert to developments in this ever-changing world. Nurses need to continually update and modify their nursing practices in accordance with changing global political, social, economic, and cultural realities.

CHAPTER 7

Global Health

Sharyn Janes

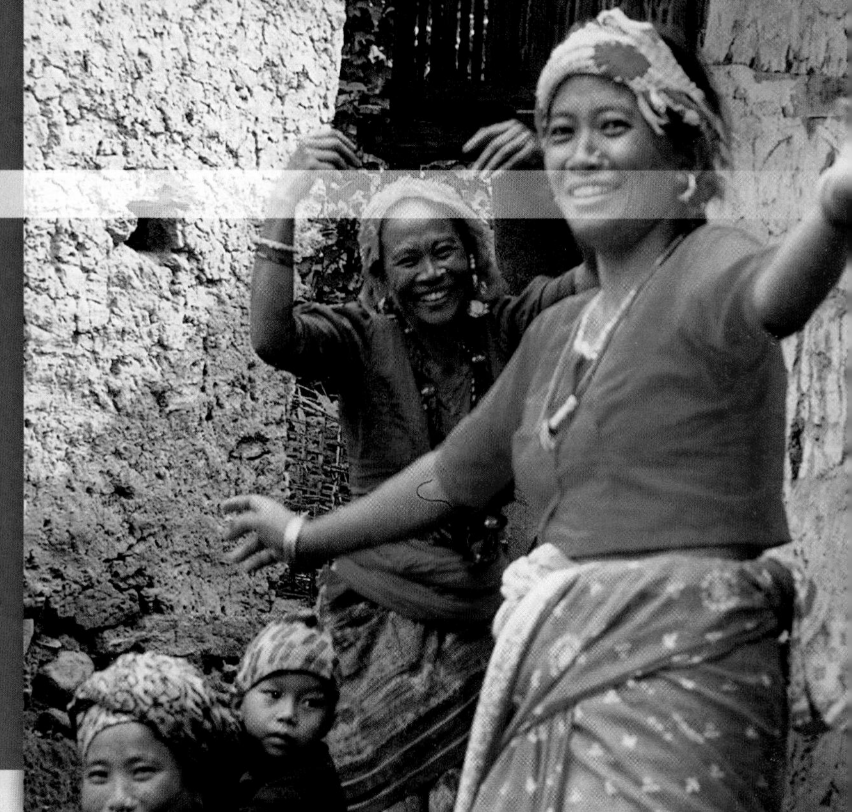

KEY TERMS

Bill and Melinda Gates Foundation
Carter Center
Declaration of Alma Ata
global health
"Health for All by the Year 2000"
Millennium Developmental Goals
nongovernmental organizations (NGOs)
poverty
primary health care
United Nations (UN)
United Nations International Children's Emergency Fund (UNICEF)
violence
war
World Bank
World Health Organization (WHO)

REFLECTIONS

As community health nurses, we are often overwhelmed with the problems facing the communities around us. How can we extend our care to the international community while still keeping our focus on the community in which we live and work? Is it possible to "think globally" and "act locally" without ever leaving our home communities? As one of the largest and most advanced countries in the world, what role should the United States play in helping global at-risk populations lead healthier lives?

AT THE BEGINNING of the 21st century, we are living in a global society. The Internet provides instant contact with people from many parts of the world. Through email and the Internet, there is immediate access to a wide variety of information in many different languages. Not only are we exposed to many cultures and ideologies, but, through rapid global transit, we are also exposed to many diseases and conditions only heard or read about in the past. Travel time has been reduced to hours to get to the other side of the world.

ART CONNECTION 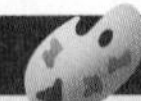

Locate an art example from a culture different from your own. Research the interpretation of the painting and the artist. How does art help broaden our understanding of diversity in a global community?

Globalization is not a new concept for nurses. "Travel nursing" dates back to the days of Florence Nightingale in the Crimea. Her influence was not only felt in her native England, but also throughout Europe, the Middle East, Australia, North America, and parts of Asia and Africa. Many of the healthcare challenges she faced in the mid-19th century are similar to the healthcare challenges faced by nurses in the 21st century. Nightingale's systematic approach to nursing became the basis for modern nursing. In 1899, the nursing profession, realizing the importance of a global approach to nursing, established the ICN, which was the first international organization for healthcare professionals. Today the ICN is a federation of 130 national nurses' associations, representing millions of nurses worldwide (ICN, 2013).

> Go to the people. Live with them. Learn from them. . . . Start with what they know; build with what they have. But with the best leaders, when the work is done, the task is accomplished, the people will say, 'We have done this ourselves'!
>
> —*Lao Tzu (700 B.C.)*

Globalization and International Health

Health professionals, particularly nurses, have a duty to influence global health care from preventive and restorative perspectives. Every nurse should consciously be involved with the business of **global health**, because health care is the business of nurses. The world is constantly changing, with poverty, epidemics, war, famine, rapid technological advances, environmental and natural disasters, and social injustice greatly influencing the health of the world's people (Basford, 2003).

Population demographics are shifting as the world's population expands. In 2012, the world population reached 7 billion, up from 6 billion in 1999, and it is expected to exceed 8 billion by 2025 (United Nations Department of Economic and Social Affairs [UNDESA], 2013). Ninety-nine percent of that growth is expected to occur in resource-poor countries. An estimated 4.3 people are born every second around the world (Population Reference Bureau [PRB], 2006). In many parts of the world, the population is aging, but in the countries affected by the human immunodeficiency virus (HIV) epidemic, life expectancy has dropped to 30–40 years. The current populations of these countries consist mostly of children and elders. The disappearance of the working-age population has greatly increased the levels of poverty for these regions in a world already overburdened by poverty.

CULTURAL CONNECTION 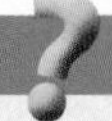

Do you consider poverty to be a cultural issue or an economic issue, especially as it relates to impoverished and underdeveloped countries?

As long as high birth rates and poverty continue to put pressure on populations, many people will see advantages in moving to countries believed to have more resources and greater opportunities. Each year, nearly 3 million migrants move from poor countries to wealthier ones. Increasingly, however, more of the migration is occurring between developing countries as the wealthier nations tighten immigration laws to protect themselves economically.

The population of the United States continues to diversify, with the number of foreign-born residents reaching

BOX 7-1 The World's 10 Largest Countries by Population, 2013 and 2050 (Projected)

2013		Projected 2050	
Country	**Population (millions)**	**Country**	**Population (millions)**
China	1,357	India	1,659
India	1,276	China	1,357
United States	316	Nigeria	432
Indonesia	248	United States	410
Brazil	195	Indonesia	372
Pakistan	190	Pakistan	361
Nigeria	173	Brazil	230
Bangladesh	156	Bangladesh	202
Russia	143	Democratic Republic of the Congo	184
Japan	117	Ethiopia	178

Source: Data from Population Reference Bureau, 2013.

an all-time high, even though the percentage of foreign-born individuals in the population is lower than it was in 1910. Even with this large number of immigrants, 60% of the U.S. population increase is attributable to natural increases (births minus deaths) in the native-born population. The United States is currently the world's third most populous country and is expected to remain so through at least 2050 (see **Box 7-1**).

Most European nations and some industrialized Asian nations such as Japan are dealing with population declines that may have negative economic consequences for these countries in the future. These countries are challenged with raising their extremely low birth rates and/or developing immigration policies and social programs that benefit their own citizens while encouraging people from other countries to migrate (PRB, 2006).

Role of International Agencies

United Nations

The **United Nations (UN)** was founded in 1945 when 51 nations came together after World War II to establish a commitment to world peace and security through international cooperation. Today, with a membership of 192 nations, the UN represents the interests of almost all countries of the world. When nations become members of the UN, they agree to accept the obligations of the UN Charter, which outlines the basic principles of international relations. However, the UN is not a form of world government. It does not make laws, but merely provides the means to help resolve global conflicts and formulate policies that affect all nations. All member nations, regardless of their size, wealth, or political system, have an equal vote in the decision-making process. While the UN cannot force any member nation to act on any recommendations made, its decisions reflect world opinion and represent the moral authority of the community of nations (UN, 2008).

The UN worked to combat all intolerance in all forms throughout the second half of the 20th century and continues to do so in the 21st century. In 1948, the Universal Declaration of Human Rights was drafted by the General Assembly of the UN to outline the basic rights and freedoms to which all peoples of the world are entitled. Two International Covenants were developed, which most UN member nations consider to be legally binding. One addresses economic, social, and cultural rights; the other addresses civil and political rights. These two covenants, along with the Universal Declaration of Human Rights, constitute the International Bill of Human Rights (UN, 2008).

Through the years, the UN has established special organizations, such as the United Nations Children's Fund, to address various social and economic issues. Several independent intergovernmental organizations are also related to the UN through special agreements but are not under UN authority. They have their own memberships, charters, budgets, and staffs (see **Box 7-2**). Also working closely with the UN are many independent **nongovernmental organizations (NGOs)**. The Carter Center and the Bill and Melinda Gates Foundation are just two of the many NGOs serving the vulnerable populations of the world.

A DAY IN THE LIFE

Now I want to pass on five lessons I have learned during 10 years as Secretary-General of the United Nations, lessons I believe the community of nations needs to learn as it confronts the challenges of the twenty-first century.

Lesson One: In today's world, we are all responsible for each other's security. Against such threats as nuclear proliferation, climate change, global pandemics, or terrorists operating from safe havens in failed nations, no state can make itself secure by seeking supremacy over all others. Only by working to make each other secure can we hope to achieve lasting security for ourselves.

Lesson Two: We are responsible for each other's welfare. Without a measure of solidarity, no society can be truly stable. It is not realistic to think that some people can go on deriving great benefits from globalization while billions of others are left out or thrown into abject poverty. We have to give all our fellow human beings at least a chance to share in our prosperity.

Lesson Three: Both security and prosperity depend on respect for human rights and the rule of law. Throughout history, human life has been enriched by diversity, and different communities have learned from each other. But if our communities are to live in peace, we must stress what unites us: our common humanity and the need for our human dignity and rights to be protected by law.

Lesson Four: Governments must be accountable for their actions, in the international as well as the domestic arena. Every state owes some account to other states on which its actions have a decisive impact.

Lesson Five: How can states hold each other accountable? Only through multilateral institutions. Those institutions must be organized in a fair and democratic way, giving the poor and the weak some influences over the rich and the strong. Developing countries should have a stronger voice in international financial institutions, whose decisions can mean life or death for their people.

More than ever, Americans, like the rest of humanity, need a functioning global system. Experience has shown, time and again, that the system works poorly when the United States remains aloof but functions much better when there is far-sighted U.S. leadership. That gives American leaders of today and tomorrow a great responsibility. The American people must see that they live up to it.

—Koffi A. Annan, United Nations Secretary General, 1997–2006, and 2001 Nobel Peace Prize recipient, excerpt from a speech at the Truman Presidential Museum and Library, Independence, Missouri, December 11, 2006

Every day the UN and its family of organizations, collectively known as the UN system, work to promote respect for human rights, protect the environment, fight disease, and reduce poverty. In addition, the UN system leads international efforts to stop drug trafficking and terrorism, assist refugees, clear landmines, and increase food production and distribution (UN, 2008).

United Nations Children's Fund

The **United Nations International Children's Emergency Fund (UNICEF)** was created in 1946 to assist millions of sick and hungry children in war-torn Europe and China.

ENVIRONMENTAL CONNECTION

You have noticed that everything an Indian does is in a circle, and that is because the Power of the World always works in circles, and everything tries to be round . . . . The Sky is round, and I have heard that the earth is round like a ball, and so are all the stars. The wind, in its greatest power, whirls. Birds make their nest in circles, for theirs is the same religion as ours . . . . Even the seasons form a great circle in their changing, and always come back again to where they were. The life of a man is a circle from childhood, and so it is in everything where power moves.

—Black Elk, Oglala Sioux holy man (1863–1950)

It soon became apparent that children all over the world needed help, so in 1950 its mandate was broadened to address the long-term needs of children and women in developing countries around the world. UNICEF became a permanent part of the UN system in 1953, when its name was shortened to the United Nations Children's Fund, though it retained UNICEF as its acronym (UNICEF, 2007).

Today, UNICEF's primary objective is to provide economic and humanitarian relief for the world's most disadvantaged children without discrimination. The children in the countries with the greatest need receive the highest priority. Special protection is ensured to children who are victims of war, disasters, extreme poverty, and all forms of violence and exploitation, and to those with disabilities (UNICEF, 2007).

UNICEF works to improve the lives of children in more than 190 countries around the world. Its programs and services are aimed at ending hunger and malnutrition, helping refugees, promoting the education of girls, controlling disease (primarily through immunization and HIV/acquired immune deficiency syndrome (AIDS) programs), saving the environment, and securing human rights (UNICEF, 2007).

World Health Organization

Organized efforts at providing a global health network date back to the 1830s, when an international alliance was formed to combat the cholera epidemic that was

BOX 7-2 Global Agencies: Autonomous Organizations Linked to the United Nations Through Special Agreements

Food and Agriculture Organization (FAO)	Works to improve agricultural productivity and food security, and to better the living standards of rural populations
International Atomic Energy Agency (IAEA)	Works for the safe and peaceful uses of atomic energy
International Civil Aviation Organization (ICAO)	Sets international standards for safety, security, and efficiency of air transport, and serves as the coordinator for international cooperation in all areas of civil aviation
International Fund for Agricultural Development (IFAD)	Mobilizes financial resources to raise food production and nutrition levels among the poor in developing countries
International Labour Organization (ILO)	Formulates policy and programs to improve working conditions and employment opportunities, and sets labor standards used by countries around the world
International Maritime Organization (IMO)	Works to improve international shipping procedures, raise standards in marine safety, and reduce marine pollution by ships
International Monetary Fund (IMF)	Facilitates international monetary cooperation and financial stability and provides a permanent forum for consultation, advice, and assistance on financial issues
International Telecommunication Union (ITU)	Fosters international cooperation to improve telecommunications of all kinds, coordinates usage of radio and TV frequencies, promotes safety measures, and conducts research
United Nations Educational, Scientific, and Cultural Organization (UNESCO)	Promotes education for all, cultural development, protection of the world's natural and cultural heritage, international cooperation in science, press freedom, and communication
United Nations Industrial Development Organization (UNIDO)	Promotes the industrial advancement of developing countries through technical assistance, advisory services, and training
Universal Postal Union (UPO)	Establishes international regulations for postal services, provides technical assistance, and promotes cooperation in postal matters
World Bank Group (WBG)	Provides loans and technical assistance to developing countries to reduce poverty and advance sustainable economic growth
World Health Organization (WHO)	Coordinates programs aimed at solving health problems and the attainment by all people of the highest possible level of health
	Works in such areas as immunization, health education, and the provision of essential drugs
World Intellectual Property Organization (WIPO)	Promotes international protection of intellectual property and fosters cooperation on copyrights, trademarks, industrial designs, and patents
World Meteorological Organization (WMO)	Promotes scientific research on the Earth's atmosphere and on climate change, and facilitates the global exchange of meteorological data
World Tourism Organization (WTO)	Serves as a global forum for tourism policy issues and a practical source of tourism know-how

Source: United Nations. (2008). *The UN in brief.* Retrieved from http://un.org/Overview/uninbrief/

sweeping Europe. Sporadic efforts continued throughout the next hundred years until the **World Health Organization (WHO)** was founded in 1948 through a special agreement with the UN. Today WHO, as a partner in the UN system, is responsible for directing and coordinating international health. The focus of WHO's work is producing and disseminating global health standards and guidelines, helping countries to address public health issues, and supporting health research (WHO, 2007). Its primary objective is for all

BOX 7-3 Notable Achievements of the World Health Organization

1948	The World Health Organization's Constitution was founded on April 7—a date now celebrated every year as World Health Day. The first World Health Assembly established its top priorities as malaria, women's and children's health, tuberculosis, venereal disease, nutrition, and environmental sanitation.
1952	Dr. Jonas Salk (United States) developed the first successful polio vaccine.
1952–1964	The global yaws-control program used long-acting penicillin with one single injection to control yaws, a crippling, disfiguring disease. By 1965, the prevalence of yaws was reduced by more than 95%.
1967	Dr. Christian Bernard (South Africa) conducted the first heart transplant surgery.
1974	The World Health Assembly adopted a resolution to create the Expanded Program on Immunization to bring basic vaccines to all children in the world.
1977	The first Essential Medicines List was developed, 2 years after the World Health Assembly introduced the concepts of "essential drugs" and "national drug policy."
1978	The International Conference on Primary Health Care, in Alma-Ata, Kazakhstan (former Soviet Union), set the historic goal of "Health for All."
1979	Smallpox—a disease that had maimed and killed millions—was eradicated. It was the first (and so far only) time that a major infectious disease has been eradicated and ranks as one of WHO's greatest achievements.
1983	Scientists at Pasteur Institute (France) identified HIV.
1988	The Global Polio Eradication Initiative was established.
2003	The first global public health treaty was adopted at the World Framework Convention on Tobacco Control. The treaty was designed to reduce tobacco-related deaths and diseases around the world.
2004	The Global Strategy on Diet, Physical Activity, and Health was adopted.
2005	The World Health Assembly revised the International Health Regulations.
2008	WHO introduced the safe surgery checklist to reduce surgical errors.
2009	An H1N1 pandemic response was initiated based on several years of preparations; a 5-year plan for prevention and control of noncommunicable diseases was launched.
2012	World health statistics found a 74% drop in mortality from measles due to global vaccination efforts.
2013	The Malaria Vaccine Technology Roadmap was launched with the goal of having a vaccine against *Plasmodium falciparum* available in 2015.

Sources: WHO, 2014a; WHO, 2013a, WHO, 2012a.

people to attain the highest possible level of health (see **Box 7-3**). WHO defines health as "a state of complete physical, mental, and social well-being and not merely the absence of disease or infirmity."

The WHO membership consists of 194 countries. Representatives from each of the member states meet every year at the World Health Assembly in Geneva, Switzerland, to set policy, approve the budget, and, every 5 years, to appoint a new Director-General. Their work is supported by the 34-member Executive Board, which is elected by the World Health Assembly (WHO, 2014a).

To better address the specific environmental, political, social, economic, and cultural needs associated with

> **I see the role of WHO as that of a global health guardian, a protector and defender of health, including the right to health. WHO is a custodian of technical expertise, but also of values, like social justice and equity, including gender equity. We must never forget our value system. Never forget the people. Public health is trained in compassion and driven by passion. This will always be our strength, our true comparative advantage.**
>
> *—Dr. Margaret Chan, WHO Director-General, Geneva, Switzerland, May 21, 2012*
>
> *Source:* Reproduced with permission of the publisher, from Dr. Margaret Chan, WHO Director-General. Geneva, World Health Organization, May 21, 2012.

BOX 7-4 World Health Organization Regional Offices

African Region: Brazzaville, Congo
Eastern Mediterranean Region: Cairo, Egypt
European Region: Copenhagen, Denmark
Region of the Americas: Washington, DC, United States
South-East Asia Region: New Delhi, India
Western Pacific Region: Manila, Philippines

Source: Data from World Health Organization. (2014). *About WHO.* Retrieved from http://www.who.int/about/en/

global healthcare issues in various parts of the world, WHO is divided into six major regions, each with its own regional office (see **Box 7-4**). More than 7,000 public health experts work in nearly 150 countries within these regions, as well as at the WHO headquarters in Geneva, Switzerland. In addition to medical doctors, professional nurses and midwives, public health specialists, researchers, and epidemiologists, WHO staff include administrative, financial, and information systems specialists, as well as experts in the fields of health statistics, economics, and emergency relief (WHO, 2014a).

World Bank

Since its creation in 1944 as an international financial institution associated with the UN, the **World Bank** has attempted to meet the needs of a changing world economy. The World Bank, which was originally called the International Bank for Reconstruction and Development, began its operations in Washington, DC, in 1946. Its primary function was to aid in the reconstruction of Europe after World War II. Now, the World Bank's priorities have evolved from rebuilding war-damaged European nations to alleviating poverty in developing countries. Since the 1970s, this organization has increasingly become more involved in health-related initiatives as a way to promote sustainable economic growth in its patient countries (Ruger, 2005); it even produces a blog on the topic of "healthy development," defined as investing for promotion of improved health (World Bank, 2014c).

Today the World Bank operates like a cooperative owned by 185 shareholder nations. The countries are represented by a board of governors, primarily consisting of ministers of finance or ministers of development from member nations, which meets once a year. The day-to-day work of the World Bank is conducted by 24 executive directors, who work at the World Bank headquarters. The five largest shareholder countries—France, Germany, Japan, the United Kingdom, and the United States—appoint an executive director from each, while other member countries are represented by 19 other executive directors. By tradition, the bank president is a citizen of the largest shareholder, the United States (World Bank, 2014c); its current president, Dr. Jim Yong Kim, holds doctoral degrees in both medicine and anthropology (World Bank, 2014b).

Over the past few decades, the World Bank has become increasingly instrumental in reducing poverty and raising the standard of living in many developing countries. Newly developed theories and evidence regarding successful economic development strategies have gradually changed the focus of the bank's lending policies.

MEDIA MOMENT 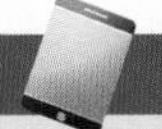

The Kite Runner (2007, film)

Based on the award-winning book by Khaled Hosseini, *The Kite Runner* film adaptation tells the story of Amir, who is haunted by the guilt of betraying his childhood friend Hassan. The story is set against a backdrop of tumultuous events, from the fall of the monarchy in Afghanistan through the Soviet invasion, the mass exodus of refugees to Pakistan and the United States, and the rise of the Taliban regime. The movie is about redemption for past grievances and serves as a metaphor about the dismal past of a struggling country and its hopeful future.

For example, in the 1950s and 1960s, promoting economic growth was viewed as the key to development. At that time, the World Bank focused primarily on large investments in physical capital and government infrastructures. However, during the 1970s and 1980s, while still providing funding for economic growth and infrastructure support for governments, the World Bank began to focus some of its efforts on meeting basic human needs such as health care and education, recognizing them as important factors in development. Investment in government power sectors was reduced from 21% in 1980 to about 7% in 2007. By comparison, direct funding for health, nutrition, education, pensions, and other social services increased from 5% to 22%. **Table 7-1** lists some of the recent core sector results reported by the World Bank.

While these successes are noteworthy, critics of the World Bank contend that more rapid progress is desperately needed. Major criticisms address the undemocratic governance and decision-making structures of the World Bank, which favor the elite interests within the wealthy nations. For example, the United States alone commands 16.4% of the World Bank's voting power. In its influential 1993 report *Investing in Health*, the World Bank stressed the importance of health to development while advocating for privatization of health services. In some situations, this approach has contributed to poor health outcomes

TABLE 7-1 World Bank Development Projects

Education
❑ More than 1 million additional teachers became qualified to teach at the primary level.
❑ More than 600,000 additional classrooms were constructed or rehabilitated.
Health
❑ More than 11 million people gained access to a basic package of health, nutrition, or population services.
❑ About 450,000 health personnel received training.
❑ More than 2,500 health facilities were constructed, renovated, and/or equipped.
❑ Almost 13 million children have been immunized, and close to 8 million received a dose of Vitamin A.
❑ About 28 million insecticide-treated malaria nets were purchased and/or distributed.
❑ More than 28,500 adults and children with HIV received antiretroviral combination therapy.
Road Transport
❑ About 3,790 km of rural roads and 1,900 km of nonrural roads were constructed or rehabilitated.
Water Supply
❑ Almost 6.8 million people in project areas were provided with access to Improved Water Sources.
❑ About 11,600 community water points were constructed or rehabilitated.
❑ About 334,000 new piped household water connections were established, and another 157,000 were rehabilitated.
❑ Close to 1,280 water utilities and water service providers are being supported.

Source: Data from World Bank, 2014c

by reducing access to health services for those who were unable to pay for such services. Many programs aimed at the poorest populations ignore structural deficiencies in social services (Birn & Dmitienko, 2005).

In 2003, the major international organizations representing nurses, teachers, and public-sector workers published serious criticisms of the World Bank's annual World Development Report (WDR). The ICN is the international federation for nurses' associations and unions, representing more than 12 million nurses in 129 countries; Education International (EI) is the global union federation for education unions, representing more than 26 million teachers in 155 countries; and Public Services International (PSI) is the global union federation for public-sector trade unions, representing more than 20 million workers in 149 countries (Communique, 2003). In a joint WHO communiqué, ICN, EI, and PSI expressed concerns that the latest WDR inaccurately placed the blame for the failure of health, education, water, and other utility services in developing countries on the poor performance of providers—nurses, teachers, utility workers, and other public employees. They argued that the World Bank has failed to recognize that nurses, teachers, and utility workers in developing countries are poor themselves. The ICN Executive Officer, Judith Outon, stated that there were many cases where nurses and other healthcare workers produced positive outcomes by working together with the people. She also pointed out that the current state of public services in developing countries was largely a result of reforms initiated by the World Bank (Communique, 2003). In the decade since then, the World Bank's leadership (and many of its priorities) have changed significantly; its eight millennium development goals include efforts to reduce child mortality, improve maternal health, and combat HIV/AIDS, malaria, and other diseases (World Bank, 2014b).

> We believe good health is a basic human right, especially among poor people afflicted with disease who are isolated, forgotten, ignored, and often without hope.
>
> —*Former U.S. President Jimmy Carter, founder and director of the Carter Center, Atlanta, Georgia*

Carter Center

The **Carter Center**, a nonprofit, NGO located in Atlanta, was founded by Jimmy and Rosalynn Carter in 1982. This private, nonpartisan organization is associated with Emory University and governed by an independent board of trustees, which is chaired by former U.S. President Carter. Its many projects are supported by donations from individuals, foundations, corporations, and countries. Activities directed by resident experts and scholars are designed and implemented in cooperation with Jimmy and Rosalynn Carter, networks of world

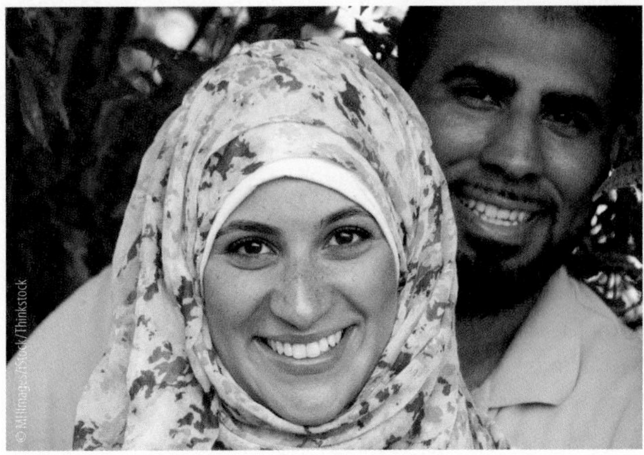

Muslim men and women vary considerably in their religious and cultural values. Community health nurses should avoid generalizations about this population regarding their health and religious practices.

leaders, other NGOs, and partners in the United States and the rest of the world (Carter Center, 2014).

The Carter Center has been instrumental in alleviating global health problems through its commitment to promoting peace and fighting disease. Its work is guided by a fundamental commitment to human rights and the alleviation of human suffering. The Carter Center has three main objectives: (1) prevent and resolve conflicts, (2) enhance freedom and democracy, and (3) improve health. The belief that all three of these objectives work together to affect the prosperity and stability of entire nations is central to the work of the Carter Center in serving the needs of millions of forgotten people around the world (Carter Center, 2014).

Bill and Melinda Gates Foundation

The **Bill and Melinda Gates Foundation** is a nonprofit NGO that was founded in 2000 by Bill Gates, cofounder and CEO of Microsoft, and his wife Melinda French Gates. In 2014, Bill Gates is the richest person in the world, with a net worth of more than $77 billion. Based in Seattle, Washington, the Gates Foundation is led by Chief Executive Officer Susan Desmond Hellman and co-chairs William H. Gates, Sr., Bill Gates, and Melinda French Gates. In developing countries, the foundation finances projects through its Global Development Programs and Global Health Programs that focus on reducing extreme poverty, improving health, and increasing access to public libraries. In the United States, programs are funded to ensure that all people have access to a good education and to technology in the public libraries. In its local region around Seattle, the foundation funds projects that focus on improving the lives of low-income families (Bill and Melinda Gates Foundation, 1999–2014).

A DAY IN THE LIFE 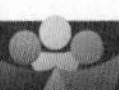

It is with a deep sense of gratitude that I accept this prize. I am grateful to my wife Rosalynn, to my colleagues at the Carter Center, and to many others who continue to seek an end to violence and suffering throughout the world. The scope and character of our Center's activities are perhaps unique, but in many other ways they are typical of the work being done by many hundreds of non-governmental organizations that strive for human rights and peace....

I am not here as a public official, but as a citizen of a troubled world who finds hope in a growing consensus that the generally accepted goals of society are peace, freedom, human rights, environmental quality, the alleviation of suffering, and the rule of law....

At the beginning of this millennium, I was asked to discuss, here in Oslo, the greatest challenge that the world faces. Among all the possible choices, I decided that the most serious and universal problem is the growing chasm between the richest and poorest people on earth ... and the separation is increasing every year, not only between nations but also within them. The results of this disparity are root causes of the world's unresolved problems, including starvation, illiteracy, environmental degradation, violent conflict, and unnecessary illnesses that range from Guinea worm to HIV/AIDS.

Most of the work of the Carter Center is in remote villages in the poorest nations of Africa, and there I have witnessed the capacity of destitute people to persevere under heartbreaking conditions. I have come to admire their judgment and wisdom, their courage and faith, and their awesome accomplishments when given a chance to use their innate abilities....

The bond of our common humanity is stronger than the divisiveness of our fears and prejudices. God gives us the capacity for choice. We can choose to alleviate suffering. We can choose to work together for peace. We can make these changes—and we must.

—Jimmy Carter, former U.S. President, Carter Center founder and director and 2002 Nobel Peace Prize recipient, excerpts from Nobel Peace Lecture, Oslo, Norway, December 10, 2002

Global Health Issues

Disease Burden

Infectious Diseases

Throughout history, infectious diseases were the leading causes of death throughout the world. By the end of the 20th century, however, medical science had developed successful prevention and treatment methods that greatly decreased the death rates from infectious diseases and raised the average life expectancy in middle- and higher income countries by decades. Nevertheless, infectious diseases continue to kill more than 13 million people every year and cause disability and suffering for millions of others. The organisms that cause these diseases continue to evolve, often requiring the development of new drugs and methods to prevent and/or treat them. New pathogens are emerging or evolving from infecting animals to infecting humans. Recent estimates show that infectious diseases are responsible for one-third of all global mortality. Most of these deaths occur in low- and middle-income countries, emphasizing the fact that infectious diseases present a very different experience for the poor and the wealthy (WHO, 2014b).

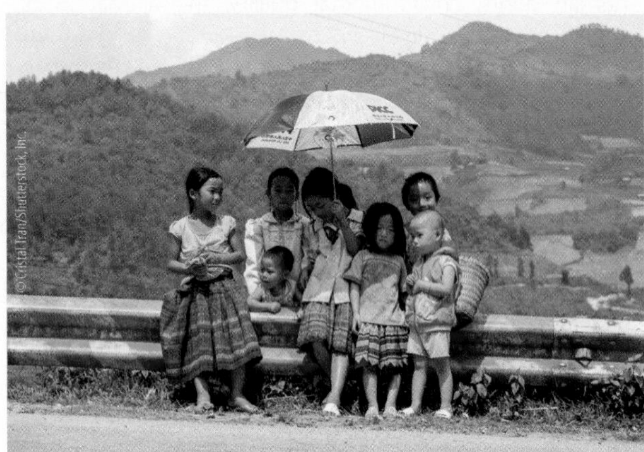

© Cristal Tran/Shutterstock, Inc.

Female children as young as 8 must take primary responsibility for younger children in many underdeveloped countries.

In low- and middle-income countries, three infectious diseases are among the top causes of death for adults ages 15 to 59: HIV/AIDS, tuberculosis (TB), and lower respiratory infections. HIV/AIDS causes 1.6 million deaths per year; the number has declined by almost a third since 2005 due to advances in prevention and treatment (UNAIDS, 2013). Similarly, the death rate from TB has declined by 45% since 1990; TB now causes approximately 1.3 million deaths per year (WHO, 2013a) and lower respiratory infections kill approximately 2.8 million people per year (Lozano et al., 2012), two-thirds of them children (Hustedt & Vazquez, 2010). In high-income countries, infectious diseases are not listed in the top 10 causes of death for adults. In low- and middle-income countries, 7 of the 10 leading causes of death for children younger than 14 years old are infectious diseases—many of them preventable—which kill about 6 million children each year (Black et al., 2008). The leading infectious diseases causing high mortality rates in children are lower respiratory infections, diarrheal diseases, and malaria (Disease Control Priorities Project, 2006a). One striking contrast is the steep decrease in deaths due to measles, which has declined 74% since 2000 due to global vaccination efforts (WHO, 2012b).

MEDIA MOMENT 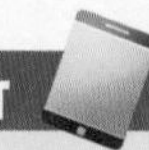

Rx for Survival: A Global Health Challenge (2006)

From vaccines to antibiotics, clean water to nutrition, bioterror threats to the HIV/AIDS pandemic, the six-part series *Rx for Survival* tells the tales of public health pioneers and captures the real-life drama of today's global struggle to overcome poor health and disease. Employing both historical dramatic sequences and current documentary stories, the series showcases milestones in public health history, such as the eradication of smallpox, alongside modern and future challenges, including severe acute respiratory syndrome (SARS), a potential global flu pandemic, and recovery from the Asian tsunami catastrophe. The series can be previewed and ordered at http://www.pbs.org/wgbh/rxforsurvival/series/about/index.html

Noncommunicable Diseases

In the 21st century, many developing countries are undergoing the same changes in the causes of morbidity and mortality that the developed countries experienced in the 20th century. Because of changes in diet and lifestyle and increases in life expectancy, many developing countries are seeing increases in the incidence of chronic diseases such as cardiovascular diseases, cancers, diabetes, and chronic respiratory diseases. These diseases, which until recently were largely confined to wealthy nations, have risen markedly in developing nations, and noncommunicable diseases now account for more than two-thirds of all deaths worldwide (Lozano et al., 2012).

Obesity is fast becoming one of the world's leading risk factors for premature death. One in four people in the world is too fat. One-third of total deaths worldwide are directly linked to excessive weight, lack of exercise, and tobacco use. Most distressing is the rapid spread of obesity beyond wealthy developed nations to some of the poorest countries in the world (MSNBC, 2004). Because infectious diseases, malnutrition, and maternal mortality are still responsible for 40% of deaths in these countries, the rapid rise in chronic diseases is creating a dual burden of disease that many of the healthcare systems in these poor countries are ill equipped to handle (Disease Control Priorities Project, 2006b).

Cardiovascular disease is now the number one cause of death worldwide. Eighty percent of the world's 13 million cardiovascular disease deaths occur in low- and middle-income countries. Conventional risk factors such as tobacco use, high blood pressure, high blood glucose, lipid abnormalities, obesity, and physical inactivity contribute to the vast majority of cardiovascular disease mortality and morbidity. Even in sub-Saharan Africa, high blood pressure, high cholesterol, extensive tobacco and alcohol use, and low

RESEARCH ALERT

To explore the state of reproductive health in Central and Eastern Europe since the dissolution of the Soviet Union, a study was conducted in two urban areas of the Ukraine. During a 19-month period between 1992 and 1994, 17,137 pregnancy outcomes were recorded. Sixty percent of the pregnancies were voluntarily terminated, generally before the 13th week. In pregnancies delivered after 20 weeks' gestation, fetal mortality was 29 per 1,000, nearly five times the rate among Caucasians in the United States. Perinatal mortality was estimated to be 35 per 1,000, about three times the U.S. rate. The data documented elevated reproductive risks in a former Soviet state. This study is believed to be the first to count and report pregnancy outcomes in the former Eastern bloc using World Health Organization definitions and research procedures.

Source: Little, R. E., Monaghan, S. S., Gladen, B. C., Shykryak-Nyzhnyk, Z., & Wilcox, A. J. (1999). Outcomes of 17,137 pregnancies in 2 urban areas of Ukraine. *American Journal of Public Health, 89*(12), 1832–1836.

vegetable and food consumption are among the top risk factors for disease. More 13- to 15-year-olds around the world are smoking than ever before, and obesity levels in children are increasing not only in the United States and Europe, but also in Brazil, China, India, and almost all island nations (Disease Control Priorities Project, 2006b).

Cancer is creating a quickly growing major global disease burden. The yearly incidence of cancer is projected to increase from 10 million to 15 million in 2020. Nine million cases are expected to occur in low- or middle-income countries. Cancer epidemiology differs between the developed and developing countries of the world, however. Developed countries have relatively high rates of lung, colorectal, breast, and prostate cancer; in these countries, there is a strong link between cancer and tobacco use, occupational carcinogens, diet, lifestyle, and obesity. By comparison, as many as 25% of cancers in developing countries are associated with chronic infections. Seven types of cancer account for 60% of all newly diagnosed cancer and cancer deaths in poorer countries: cervical, liver, stomach, esophageal, lung, colorectal, and breast (Disease Control Priorities Project, 2006b).

Diabetes is rapidly becoming a global pandemic, with 285 million adults affected worldwide (Shaw, Sicree, & Zimmet, 2010). The vast majority of affected persons have a diagnosis of type 2 diabetes, which until recently was an adult-onset disease, but is now being seen in more children, especially in the more-developed nations. This number is projected to grow 69% by 2030, a trend blamed on the epidemic increases in childhood obesity. In fact, today's youth are the first generation in history predicted to have a shorter life expectancy than their parents (Jain, 2004).

More than 141 million people with diabetes now live in low- and middle-income countries, which account for 72.5% of the world's total number of cases. These countries are spending between 2.5% and 15% of their annual health budgets on diabetic care. In 2025, it is predicted that more than 6% of the world's population will be diabetic, up 24% from 2003 levels (Disease Control Priorities Project, 2006b).

Chronic adult respiratory diseases, such as chronic obstructive pulmonary disease (COPD) and asthma, are major causes of the growing burden of chronic disease mortality and morbidity in the developing world. COPD, which includes emphysema, chronic bronchitis, and obstructive airway disease, is closely linked to cigarette smoking as well as to use of poorly vented, coal-burning cooking stoves. Asthma's prevalence worldwide is lower than the prevalence of other adult respiratory diseases, but studies done in some middle-income countries show that healthcare costs for asthma make up more than 1% of total healthcare costs (Disease Control Priorities Project, 2006b).

GLOBAL CONNECTION 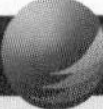

Bill Gates, founder of Microsoft, is the richest man in history, with an estimated fortune of $50–100 billion. Gates and his wife Melinda have also donated more money than anyone in history to projects designed to put computers in impoverished schools and have created a foundation that pours millions of dollars into global health problems, such as HIV/AIDS in Africa and other countries.

Violence and War

Levels of Violence

WHO (2002) defines **violence** as "the intentional use of force or power, threatened or actual, against oneself, another person, or against a group or community, that either results in or has a high likelihood of resulting in injury, death, psychological harm, maldevelopment, or deprivation" (p. 3). This definition includes all types of violence in all forms against individuals, families, and communities. *World Report on Violence and Health*, published by WHO in 2002, uses an ecological model to explore the biological, social, cultural, economic, and political factors that influence violent acts. The model categorizes violent behavior on four different levels—individual, relationship, community, and societal (WHO, 2002).

At the individual level, the model examines the biological and personal histories that influence whether an individual may become a perpetrator or victim of violence.

These factors may include not only demographic characteristics, such as age, education, and income, but also substance abuse, psychological or personality disorders, and a history of experiencing abuse or behaving aggressively. At the relationship level, the model looks at factors such as harsh physical punishment of children, lack of attention and bonding, family dysfunction, association with delinquent peers, and marital or parental conflict to determine how relationships with families, friends, intimate partners, and peers influence violent behavior. The community level examines schools, workplaces, and neighborhoods in an attempt to identify characteristics that may increase the risk for violence, such as poverty, high population density, low social capital, transient residents, and the existence of gangs or drug cultures. The fourth level looks at societal factors that create an environment that encourages or inhibits violence. Health, economic, educational, and social policies that maintain economic or social inequalities between groups in society are all factors that encourage violent acts (WHO, 2002).

Armed Conflict and War

Violent conflicts between nations and groups, acts of terrorism, rape as a weapon of war, the mass migration of people displaced from their homes, and gang warfare are occurring daily in many parts of the world. These acts of collective violence have devastating effects on physical and mental health, along with vast social, political, and economic consequences. During the last century, which was one of the most violent periods in human history, an estimated 191 million people lost their lives as a direct or indirect result of conflict. More than half of those fatalities were civilians. Besides the many thousands who are killed each year, there are huge numbers of people who are injured—including some who are mentally or physical disabled or physically mutilated. Torture and rape are used as methods to undermine communities, although exact numbers of people affected are not always known (WHO, 2002). **Box 7-5** outlines some of the causes of death for civilians during violent conflict or **war**.

BOX 7-5 The Consequences of Collective Violence

Increased civilian death rates during violent conflicts are usually due to the following causes:

- Injuries
- Decreased access to food
- Increased risk of communicable disease
- Decreased access to health services
- Decreased public health programs
- Poor environmental conditions
- Psychological distress

Source: Data from World Health Organization. (2002). *World report on violence and health* [abstract]. Geneva, Switzerland: WHO Press.

GOT AN ALTERNATIVE?

Herbal remedies are commonly used in many countries, such as Cuba and Jamaica, as an integral part of their healthcare system and are not considered "alternative."

Armed conflicts disrupt trade and other business activities, diverting resources from vital services and programs to pay for defense. Food production and distribution are slowed or stopped as thousands of people are displaced from their homes. Famine related to war, other armed conflicts, or genocide killed an estimated 40 million people in the 20th century (WHO, 2002).

Poverty

> There can be no peace as long as there is grinding poverty, social injustice, inequality, oppression, environmental degradation, and as long as the weak and small continue to be trodden by the mighty and powerful.
>
> —*Dalai Lama*

Poverty means powerlessness, lack of representation, and freedom. Almost half of the world's 7 billion people are poor. According to the World Bank, there are three levels of poverty: extreme, moderate, and relative. Extreme poverty, also known as absolute or abject poverty, is defined as living on less than $1 per day. At this income level, members of households are not able to meet basic needs for survival. They have chronic hunger, do not have access to health care, lack safe drinking water and sanitation, are uneducated and illiterate, and often do not have an adequate place to live or clothes to wear. Extreme poverty is the kind of poverty that kills. Moderate poverty is defined as living on less than $2 per day. At this income level, the basic survival needs of households are being met, but just barely. Relative poverty is defined as a household income below a given proportion of the national average. It means not having things that the middle class in countries take for granted (Sachs, 2005; World Bank, 2014c).

Extreme poverty now exists only in developing countries. In 2007, an estimated 1 billion people across the world lived in extreme poverty, down from 1.5 billion in 1981. While that decline indicates great global progress in poverty reduction, the progress has not been equal.

Rapid economic growth in East Asia, especially China, and the Pacific regions has greatly reduced levels of poverty in those regions, although rapid population growth has kept Asia in the lead with total numbers of poor people. South Asian countries have seen only moderate reductions in poverty levels, while poverty levels in the former Soviet Bloc countries in Eastern Europe and Central Asia increased in the last decade of the 20th century before declining slightly. However, sub-Saharan Africa has the largest proportion of poor people, with almost half of the population living in extreme poverty. The overall per capita income of African nations decreased by 14% between 1981 and 2001, and poverty levels in that region rose from 41% to 46% over the same period (Sachs, 2005; World Bank, 2014c). Much of that increase is related directly to HIV/AIDS, drought, isolation, and civil wars (Sachs, 2005).

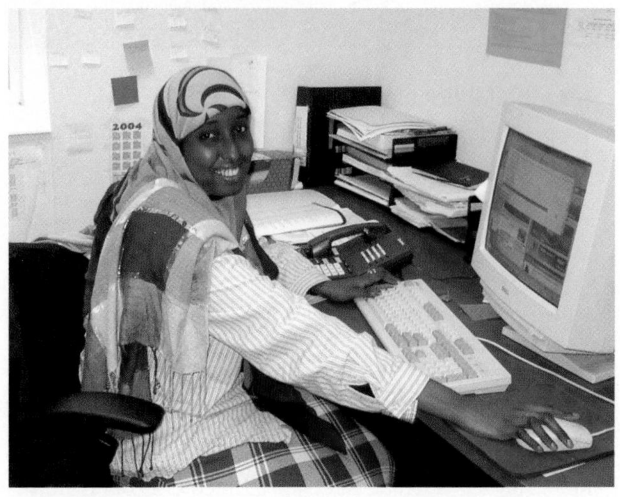

Women in many underdeveloped countries are making progress in careers previously restricted to men.

> The Millennium Declaration made clear, gender equality is not only a goal in its own right; it is critical to our ability to reach all the others.
>
> —*Kofi Annan, Secretary-General of the United Nations, 2004*

Women's Rights

Every day, all over the world, girls are kept out of school, beaten, ignored, forced to marry and have sex, sold as slaves, made to fight in wars, and asked to sit silently while others make decisions affecting their lives (UNICEF, 2014). In many countries of the world, women are not allowed to vote, own or inherit property, drive a car, get an education, or make any decisions about themselves or their children.

One woman dies from complications of pregnancy and childbirth every minute, accounting for more than half a million deaths worldwide each year. Ninety-nine percent of these deaths occur in the developing world, where the highest maternal mortality rates occur in sub-Saharan Africa, followed by South-Central Asia. According to WHO (2012a), a woman living in a developing country has a one in 416 chance of dying in pregnancy or childbirth during her lifetime, as compared with a one in 6,250 chance for a woman living in a developed country. Maternal mortality is both a human rights issue and an equity issue. Given that the vast majority of maternal deaths can be prevented with access to skilled prenatal, perinatal, and postnatal care, successful pregnancies and births should be a fundamental human right for all women (WHO, 2004).

Many women worldwide are victims of violence at all levels. Until recently, violence against women was considered to be a minor social problem by many governments and policymakers. This was especially true for women who were victims of violence perpetrated by their husbands or intimate partners. Beginning in the 1990s, however, the problem began to become more widely recognized as a serious human rights and public health issue. This rise in awareness was spurred on by the efforts of women's organizations and governments, which were committed to eliminating violence against women under international human rights laws. It is believed that the only way to effectively eliminate violence against women is through political will and by legal action in all sectors of society (WHO, 2005).

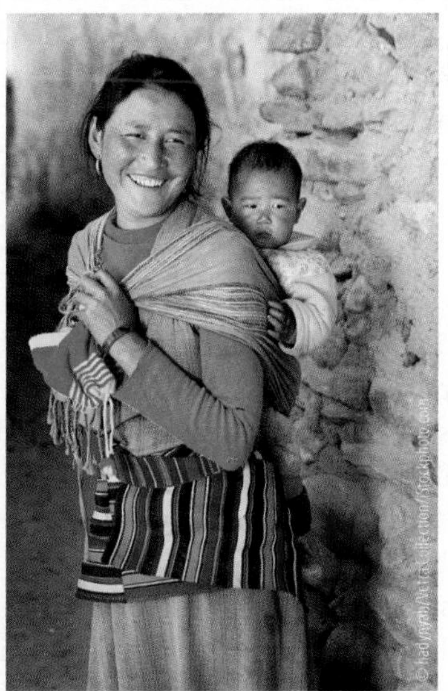

Although maternal mortality is still a significant problem for Nepalese women, it is being addressed by increases in postpartum care technology as Nepal struggles to improve the health status of women.

MEDIA MOMENT 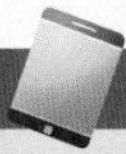

Slumdog Millionaire (2008)

This Academy Award winning movie is the story of Jamal Malik, an 18-year-old orphan from the slums of Mumbai, who has grown up on the streets. Malik is in the finals of a television quiz show, with 20 million rupees on the line as the final prize earnings. Prior to the last competition, he is arrested by the police who suspect Malik of cheating, due to his lack of formal education and a life lived as a homeless orphan. To prove his innocence, Jamal tells the story of his life in the slum where he and his brother grew up, of their adventures together on the road, of violent encounters with local gangs, and of Latika, the girl he cared for. Each chapter of his story reveals the key to the answer to one of the game show's questions. Jamal is released and returns to the game competition after explaining, through his experiences of life on the street, how he could know the correct answers. This story is one of street survival, created communities, and how we all learn through a diversity of experiences and circumstances.

> Women have an enhanced vulnerability to disease, especially if they are poor. Indeed, the health hazards of being female are widely underestimated. Economic and cultural factors can limit women's access to clinics and health workers. The World Health Organization reports that less is spent on health care for women and girls worldwide than for men and boys. As a result, women who become mothers and caretakers of children and husbands often do so at the expense of their own health. The leading causes of death among women are HIV/AIDS, malaria, complications of pregnancy and childbirth, and tuberculosis.
>
> —*Carol Bellamy, United Nations Children's Fund, New York, 2004*

In addition to violence, hunger, lack of education, and inferior legal status, HIV/AIDS and other infectious diseases disproportionately affect and further weaken the position of women in many of the world's poorest countries. Women typically have a more severe course of illness because of their lack of access to care, social inequalities, and restrictive cultural norms (Gerberding, 2004). In many cases the social, economic, and psychological effects of HIV are devastating. Fulfilling the traditional role of family caretaker means that women receive healthcare treatment only after the needs of their men and male children have been met. When their husbands or fathers die, the laws of many countries may allow women to lose their economic rights, which can leave them without property, without money, and without health care.

Global Initiatives

Declaration of Alma Ata

In 1978, 164 countries and 67 international organizations met in Alma Ata, Kazakhstan, for the International Conference on Primary Health Care. The nations of the world came together to recognize the concept of **primary health care** as a strategy to reach the goal of **"Health for All by the Year 2000."** The conference produced the document known as the ***Declaration of Alma Ata***, which was a major milestone for public health in the 20th century. The *Declaration* defined primary health care as:

> essential health care based on practical, scientifically sound, and socially acceptable methods and technology made universally accessible to individuals and families in the community through their full participation and at a cost that the community and country can afford to maintain at every stage of their development in the spirit of self-reliance and self determination. (Pan American Health Organization [PAHO], 2003)

The conference not only reaffirmed the WHO definition of health as a state of complete physical, mental, and social wellbeing and not merely the absence of disease or infirmity, but also declared health to be a fundamental human right. The attainment of the highest possible level of health was identified as an important global social goal that will require the action of all nations and the collaboration of many social and economic government agencies within and among governments.

The *Declaration of Alma Ata* promoted the concept that governments have a responsibility to promote the health of their citizens by providing adequate health and social services. Governments, international organizations, and the entire world community were challenged to work toward attaining a level of health for all peoples of the world that will permit them to lead socially and economically productive lives by 2000. Primary health care, as part of economic development and social justice, was designated as the key to attaining the goal. Countries were encouraged to work together, in recognition of the fact that the attainment of health by the people in any one country directly concerns and benefits every other country. All governments were encouraged to develop national policies, strategies, and plans of action to include primary health care as part of a comprehensive healthcare system (PAHO, 2003). The United States, while not creating policy to address the goal of Health for All by the Year 2000, developed the *Healthy People 2000* objectives, which was updated to *Healthy People 2010* in 2000, and *Healthy People 2020* in 2010.

At the Fifty-Sixth World Health Assembly meeting in 2003, 25 years after the *Declaration of Alma Ata*, WHO reviewed the health status of the world's citizens and the progress made toward the attainment of the Health for All by the Year 2000 goal. Evaluations identified a genuine commitment within countries to the principles of primary health care. In those countries where the development of primary health care has not been successful, failures were attributed to a lack of practical guidance for implementation, poor leadership, insufficient political commitment, inadequate resources, and unrealistic expectations (WHO, 2003).

MEDIA MOMENT

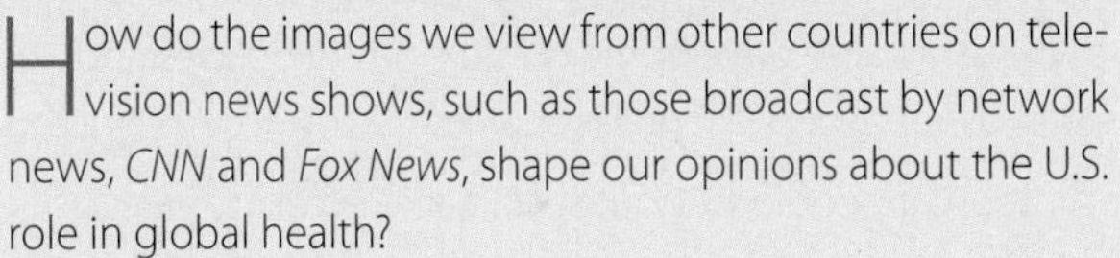

How do the images we view from other countries on television news shows, such as those broadcast by network news, *CNN* and *Fox News*, shape our opinions about the U.S. role in global health?

Millennium Developmental Goals

In 2000, the UN adopted the Millennium Declaration, which recognized that all governments not only have a responsibility to their own citizens, but also have a collective responsibility to uphold the principles of human dignity, equality, and equity for all of the world's people, especially the most vulnerable. Leaders from every country agreed on the importance of creating a world with less hunger, poverty, and disease; better survival rates for mothers and babies; better educated people; equal rights for women; and healthier environments (UN, 2000, 2006).

The UN **Millennium Developmental Goals** were developed to coordinate and strengthen unprecedented global efforts to meet the needs of the world's poorest people. A target date of 2015 for meeting these goals was agreed on by all of the world's governments and the leading global developmental institutions. **Box 7-6** lists the eight Millennium Developmental Goals.

Global Nursing

Nursing Shortages

WHO estimates it will take an additional 4.3 million healthcare workers (nurses, midwives, physicians, and support workers) to address the pandemic crisis of the shortage of global healthcare workers, which affects all countries of the world. Many developed nations are recruiting workers from less-developed nations to alleviate their staffing shortages. This practice has resulted in a global redistribution of healthcare workers and has left the countries with the greatest needs with the greatest shortages. African nations carry 25% of the world's disease burden but have only 3% of the world's healthcare workforce. There are many reasons why nurses and physicians migrate. While higher incomes are a major consideration, safer working conditions and better resources to provide quality care are equally important (Emory University, 2006).

International Council of Nurses

The ICN works to ensure quality nursing care for all, sound global health policies, the advancement of nursing knowledge, and the presence of a respected, competent, and satisfied global nursing workforce. Three goals and five core values guide all ICN programs and activities. The ICN's goals are to bring nurses together worldwide, to advance nurses and nursing worldwide, and to influence health policy. Its five core values are visionary leadership, inclusiveness, flexibility, partnership, and achievement. The ICN Code for Nurses is the foundation for ethical nursing practice throughout the world (ICN, 2013).

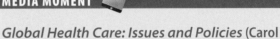

MEDIA MOMENT

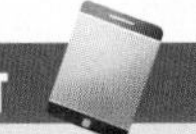

Global Health Care: Issues and Policies **(Carol Holtz, Jones & Bartlett Learning, 2013)**

This comprehensive book outlines the cultural, religious, economic, and political influences that impact global health care. Each chapter includes a summary of health policy issues in a specific global region, followed by an explanation of how these issues are affected by significant world events. Contributing authors are from various regions and countries of origin, which offer validity and authenticity to global perspectives of the current state of global health issues.

Nursing and Human Rights

Human rights are primarily concerned with the rights of individuals in relation to government. The goal of the global movement toward human rights is to ensure that all people have an opportunity to survive to achieve their full potential. Safe water and food, adequate nutrition, protection against slavery or torture, access to education, health care, and basic freedoms are the foundation for human rights. The Universal

BOX 7-6 United Nations Millennium Developmental Goals

Goals	Target
1. Eradicate extreme hunger and poverty.	Halve, between 1990 and 2015, the proportion of people whose income is less than $1 per day. Halve, between 1990 and 2015, the proportion of people who suffer from hunger.
2. Achieve universal primary education.	Ensure that, by 2015, children everywhere, boys and girls alike, will be able to complete a full course of primary schooling.
3. Promote gender equality and empower women.	Eliminate gender disparity in primary and secondary education, preferably by 2005, and in all levels of education no later than 2015.
4. Reduce child mortality.	Reduce by two-thirds, between 1990 and 2015, the under-5 mortality rate.
5. Improve maternal health.	Reduce by three-fourths, between 1990 and 2015, the maternal mortality ratio.
6. Combat HIV/AIDS, malaria, and other infectious diseases.	Have halted by 2015 and begun to reverse the spread of HIV/AIDS. Have halted by 2015 and begun to reverse the incidence of malaria and other major infectious diseases.
7. Ensure environmental sustainability.	Integrate the principles of sustainable development into country policies and programs and reverse the loss of environmental resources. Halve, by 2015, the proportion of people without sustainable access to safe drinking water and sanitation. By 2020, have achieved a significant improvement in the lives of at least 100 million slum dwellers.
8. Develop a global partnership for development.	Address the special needs of the least-developed, landlocked countries and small-island developing states. Develop further an open, rule-based, predictable, nondiscriminatory trading and financial system. Deal comprehensively with developing countries' debt. In cooperation with developing countries, develop and implement strategies for decent and productive work for youth. In cooperation with pharmaceutical companies, provide access to affordable essential drugs in developing countries. In cooperation with the private sector, make available the benefits of new technologies, especially information and communications.

Declaration of Human Rights, adopted by the UN in 1948, committed the international community to pursue a minimum standard of health care for all people (Williams, 2004).

Because the role and status of individuals in society strongly influence their health, human rights abuses contribute significantly to disease development. Nurses must care about human rights because their presence or absence affects a nurse's ability to practice nursing. The fundamentals of nursing are rooted in the act of

LEVELS OF PREVENTION 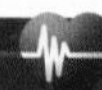

Primary: Develop educational programs for teens in Haiti on how to avoid risky behavior associated with HIV/AIDS.

Secondary: Screen Haitian teen population for HIV/AIDS.

Tertiary: Manage treatment protocols for those in Haiti infected with HIV/AIDS, with emphasis on prevention of spreading the disease and reducing complications from the disease.

A DAY IN THE LIFE

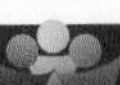

A Nursing Student's Story

Border issues affect everyone. During a clinical experience at a level 1 trauma center, another student and I were assigned to a room in the emergency department. A 16-year-old boy was brought in by the triage nurse. He was in obvious respiratory distress. He had renal failure, a Hickmann to right anterior chest wall, soiled dressings, bilateral rales, and +3 pitting edema. After assessment by the first-year resident, the chief resident was called and determined that this boy was not a candidate for emergency dialysis. An interpreter was called, and it was learned that the boy was from Honduras and had no medical coverage. He was admitted for observation. Following up on the patient's status the next day, we found the notation "illegal" recorded again and again in his medical record. Social Services could not help this young man. While we visited the patient, the chief nephrologist came to see him. He wanted us to translate for him as he gave discharge instructions. There would be no dialysis, and the Hickmann would not be removed. He said, "Marry a U.S. citizen or go back to your country. You will be discharged today."

We told the patient we were sorry and asked for his phone number. We told him we would try to do something. We knew that there is no hemodialysis in Honduras and that Social Services could have attempted to make referrals. We did some research and found a hospital willing to treat our patient and referred our patient there. In this cultural experience, we were able to integrate respect for human rights, patient advocacy, and ethics with critical care skills to assist this patient. We hope that we empowered this patient to use available community resources to care for himself despite cultural differences.

—Jamy Josey, BSN Nursing Student

1. What are the ethical issues this nurse faced?
2. What would you do for this patient if home health services were available after hospitalization?
3. How would this situation differ if a patient with the same condition were a U.S. citizen?

caring for other human beings. To provide the best nursing care, nurses must directly confront discrimination, poverty, and human rights abuses (Williams, 2004).

HEALTHY ME

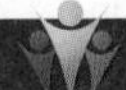

Have you visited another country? What was the first thing you experienced upon arrival? Did you experience "culture shock"? How did you react? Imagine how immigrants experience the United States for the first time. Consider the kind of support they need to succeed in a new culture.

Critical Thinking Activities

1. Which groups or organizations in your community are working locally to improve people's lives?
2. Are nurses actively involved with any of these groups? If so, in what capacity?

References

Basford, L. (2003). Global challenge: What if…? *Reflections on Nursing Leadership*, Fourth Quarter, 26–27.

Bill and Melinda Gates Foundation. (1999–2014). *Foundation fact sheet*. Retrieved from http://www.foundation.org/about/Pages/foundation-fact-sheet.aspx

Birn, A. E., & Dmitrienko, K. (2005). The World Bank: Global health or harm? *American Journal of Public Health, 95*(7), 1091–1092.

Black, R. E., Cousens, S., Johnson, H. L., Lawn, J. E., Rudan, I., Bassani, D. G., . . . Mathers, C. (2008). Global, regional, and national causes of child mortality in 2008: A systematic analysis. *Lancet, 375*(9730), 1969–1987.

Carter Center. (2014). *About the Center*. Retrieved from http://www.cartercenter.org/about/index.html

Communique. (2003, September 22). *World Bank report lets down 58 million public service employees*. Geneva, Switzerland: World Health Organization.

Disease Control Priorities Project. (2006a). *Infectious diseases*. Retrieved from http://www.dcp2.org/file/212/biovisio_breman.pdf

Disease Control Priorities Project. (2006b). *Noncommunicable diseases*. Retrieved from http://www.dcp2.org/file/58/dcpp-ncd.pdf

Emory University. (2006). Undelivered cures: 113 nations gather at Emory to tackle the global shortage of healthcare workers. *Emory and Global Health Magazine*.

Gerberding, J. L. (2004). Women and infectious disease. *Emerging Infectious Diseases, 10*(11). Retrieved from http://wwwnc.cdc.gov/eid/article/10/11/04-0800_article.htm

Hustedt, J. W., & Vazquez, M. (2010). The changing face of pediatric respiratory tract infections: How human metapneumovirus and human bocavirus fit into the overall etiology of respiratory tract infections in young children. *Yale Journal of Biology and Medicine, 83*(4), 193–200.

International Council of Nurses (ICN). (2013). *About ICN*. Retrieved from http://www.icn.ch/about-icn/about-icn/

Jain, A. (2004). Fighting obesity. *British Medical Journal, 328*, 1327–1328.

Lozano, R., Naghavi, M., Foreman, K., Lim, S., Shibuya, K., Aboyans, V., . . . Memish, Z. A. (2012). Global and regional mortality from 235 causes of death for 20 age groups in 1990 and 2010: A systematic analysis for the Global Burden of Disease Study 2010. *Lancet, 380*(9859), 2095–2128.

MSNBC. (2004). *"Globesity" gains ground as leading killer*. Retrieved from http://www.msnbc.msn.com/id/4900095/?GTI-3391

Pan American Health Organization (PAHO). (2003). *Primary health care: 25 years of the Alma Ata declaration*. Retrieved from http://www.paho.org/English/dd/pin/alma-ata._declaration.htm

Population Reference Bureau (PRB). (2006). *World population data sheet*. Retrieved from http://www.prb.org

Ruger, J. P. (2005). The changing role of the World Bank in global health. *American Journal of Public Health, 95*(1), 60–70.

Sachs, J. (2005, March 14). The end of poverty. *Time*, pp. 43–54.

Shaw, J. E., Sicree, R. A., & Zimmet, P. Z. (2010). Global estimates of the prevalence of diabetes for 2010 and 2030. *Diabetes Research & Clinical Practice, 87*(1), 4–14.

UNAIDS. (2013). *HIV/AIDS fact sheet*. Retrieved from http://www.unaids.org/en/resources/campaigns/globalreport2013/factsheet/

UNDP. (1998). *Human development report*. New York: Author.

UNICEF. (2007). *About UNICEF: Who we are*. Retrieved from http//www.unicef.org/about/who/index

UNICEF. (2014). *Voices of youth*. Retrieved from http://www.voicesofyouth.org/en

United Nations. (2000). *Resolution adopted by the General Assembly: United Nations Millennium Declaration*. New York, NY: Author.

United Nations. (2006). *The Millennium Development Goals report*. New York, NY: Author.

United Nations. (2008). *The UN in brief*. Retrieved from http://un.org/Overview/uninbrief/

United Nations Department of Economic and Social Affairs (UNDESA). (2013). *World Population Prospects: The 2012 revision*. Retrieved from http://www.unfpa.org/webdav/site/global/shared/documents/news/2013/KEY%20FINDINGS%20WPP2012_FINAL-2.pdf

Williams, A. B. (2004). Nursing, health, and human rights: A framework for international collaboration. *Journal of the Association of Nurses in AIDS Care, 15*(3), 75–77.

World Bank. (2014a). *Core sector indicators—Overview*. Retrieved from http://go.worldbank.org/M7RO39Y9D0

World Bank. (2014b). *Current president: Dr. Jim Yong Kim*. Retrieved from http://www.worldbank.org/en/about/president/about-the-office/bio

World Bank. (2014c). *What we do*. Retrieved from http://www.worldbank.org/en/about/what-we-do

World Health Organization (WHO). (2002). *World report on violence and health* [abstract]. Geneva, Switzerland: WHO Press.

World Health Organization (WHO). (2003). *International Conference on Primary Health Care, Alma-Ata: Twenty-fifth anniversary. Report by the Secretariat*. Geneva, Switzerland: WHO Press.

World Health Organization (WHO). (2004). *Press release: Making pregnancy safer*. Geneva, Switzerland: WHO Press.

World Health Organization (WHO). (2005). *Summary report: WHO multi-country study on women's health and domestic violence against women*. Geneva, Switzerland: WHO Press.

World Health Organization (WHO). (2007). *Working for health: An introduction to the World Health Organization*. Geneva, Switzerland: WHO Press.

World Health Organization (WHO). (2012a). *Fact sheet No. 348: Maternal mortality*. Retrieved from http://www.who.int/mediacentre/factsheets/fs348/en/

World Health Organization (WHO). (2012b). *World health statistics 2012*. Retrieved from http://who.int/gho/publications/world_health_statistics/2012/en/

World Health Organization (WHO). (2013a). *Fact sheet No. 104: Tuberculosis*. Retrieved from http://www.who.int/mediacentre/factsheets/fs104/en/

World Health Organization (WHO). (2013b). *Note for media: New malaria vaccines roadmap targets next generation products by 2030*. Retrieved from http://www.who.int/mediacentre/news/notes/2013/malaria-vaccines-20131114/en/

World Health Organization (WHO). (2014a). *About WHO*. Retrieved from http://www.who.int/about/en/

World Health Organization (WHO). (2014b). *Fact sheet: The Top 10 causes of death*. Retrieved from http://www.who.int/mediacentre/factsheets/fs310/en/index2.html

Appendix: Canada

Heather R. Sherry

Canada's healthcare system, commonly referred to as "Medicare," is designed to ensure reasonable access to healthcare services for all Canadian residents on a prepaid basis. It can be described as a series of 13 interlocking provincial and territorial health insurance plans and is funded predominantly through public tax dollars. Healthcare services are administered and delivered by the provincial and territorial governments, with funding assistance provided by the federal government. These services are provided to Canadian residents free of charge.

The *Canada Health Act (CHA)* is the federal legislation that governs the conditions under which provinces and territories may receive funding for the healthcare services they provide to Canadian residents. Provincial and territorial insurance plans must meet five specific criteria outlined in the CHA to be eligible for their full allocation of funding from the federal government:

- *Public administration*: The healthcare insurance plan of a province must be administered and operated on a nonprofit basis by a public authority appointed or designated by the government of the province. This public authority is accountable to the government and must be subject to audit.
- *Comprehensiveness*: The healthcare insurance plan of a province must insure all necessary health services including hospitals, physicians, and surgical dentists.
- *Universality*: All insured residents must be entitled to the same level of health care.
- *Portability*: Any resident who moves to a different province is guaranteed coverage from his or her home province during a minimum waiting period (also applies to residents who leave the country).
- *Accessibility*: All insured persons must have reasonable access to healthcare, and healthcare providers must receive reasonable compensation for their services.

As stated in the CHA, the primary objective of Canadian healthcare policy is "to protect, promote, and restore the physical and mental well-being of residents of Canada and to facilitate reasonable access to health services without financial or other barriers" (Canada Health Act 1985, c.6, s.3). In support of this objective, primary care doctors, specialists, hospitals, and dental surgery are all covered under provincial insurance policies. More than half of all doctors in Canada are primary care physicians, and the remaining doctors are specialists who provide services outside the scope of primary care physicians.

Although most basic healthcare services are provided under the provincial insurance plans, some services are not covered. For example, prescription medications, vision, and dental (nonsurgical) services are covered only through private insurance plans, which can be used to supplement primary health coverage. Private insurance plans are typically used by individuals with specific needs that are not covered by the primary plan and are often offered as part of employee benefits packages. In addition, many private clinics exist in Canada that offer specialized services. By law, they are not allowed to duplicate services provided by the CHA, but many still do. Residents often use these clinics to reduce the wait times that they can experience in the public healthcare system. This is controversial because there is a sense that the existence of these clinics creates an imbalance in the healthcare system that favors individuals with higher incomes.

Over the years, since public funding for health care began in Canada, the delivery of healthcare services has shifted away from hospitals and doctors and toward alternative care and public health interventions. Reforms have focused on primary healthcare delivery, which have included establishing 24-hour community healthcare centers, creating primary healthcare teams, emphasis on health promotion, prevention of illness and injury, management of chronic diseases, increased coordination and integration of comprehensive services, and improving the work environment of primary healthcare providers (Health Canada, 2009). Although there are some concerns about the efficiency of the Canadian healthcare system (which serves a population of more than 35 million people), Canadians as a whole continue to have a favorable health status. The average life expectancy in Canada is among the highest in the industrialized countries and the infant mortality rate is one of the lowest in the world.

References

Canada Health Act (R.S.C., 1985, c. C-6). Retrieved from http://laws-lois.justice.gc.ca/eng/acts/c-6/

Canadian Health Care, http://www.canadian-healthcare.org

Health Canada. (2009). Canada's Health Care System (Medicare). Retrieved from http://www.hc-sc.gc.ca/hcs-sss/medi-assur/index_e.html

Cuba

Juana Diasy Berdayes Martinez

Cuba, a Caribbean island nation with a population of more than 1 million, is located between the Caribbean Sea and the Atlantic Ocean, approximately 90 miles off the coast of the United States. After the Cuban Revolution in 1959, Cuba experienced many economic and social transformations, which led to the development of its current healthcare policy. The belief in the right to health care for all citizens and the duty of the state to guarantee it brought about the provision of free healthcare services for all Cuban citizens. A process of reorganization and expansion of the national healthcare system was initiated based on a primary care model. Several measures were taken to guarantee accessibility of healthcare services for all. For example, new hospitals were constructed in rural zones and mountain areas, greatly increasing the number of hospital beds nationwide. Health professionals no longer worked in private practices, but instead became a part of the government's primary care system (Jardnes, Ouvina, & Aneiro Riba, 1991).

From its beginnings, the Cuban public health system has included the participation of the community in its historic evolution. In 1964, the first polyclinic was created to deliver comprehensive health care to communities. Community participation in health care was reinforced in 1975 with the creation of health advisory committees. Health advisory committees consist of people in each community who participate in analyzing the health of the community and facilitating collaboration between the healthcare system and community residents. In 1984, the new Cuban primary care model was introduced with family physicians and nurses as essential components. Family practice physician offices, staffed by a physician and one or two nurses, began to spring up in every neighborhood. The principles of primary care proclaimed in Alma Ata in 1978 were applied in creative ways and adjusted to the economic and social conditions of Cuba. In this way, the truly humanistic dimensions of medicine and health care were applied to the care of people in their own communities. As a result, Cuba met the WHO's "Health for All by the Year 2000" objectives in 1985.

Since 1989, with the collapse of the Soviet Union (with which Cuba conducted 85% of its economic trade), the living conditions of the Cuban population have deteriorated. In addition, the longstanding economic embargo of Cuba by the United States has contributed significantly to the former country's economic depression. According to a 1997 study conducted by the American Association for World Health, the U.S. embargo has had a detrimental effect on the health and nutrition of large numbers of Cuban citizens. However, the negative impact has been offset by the commitment of the Cuban government to maintain a high level of budgetary support for the universal delivery of primary and preventive health care. The health services that have been affected most are organ transplant and other technology programs, surgical activity, the availability of medications, and the acquisition and maintenance of medical equipment. Despite these resource limitations, the goals of the Ministry of Public Health are focused on maintaining free and accessible health care for all citizens.

At present, Cuba has approximately 75,000 physicians and 103,000 nurses (World Bank, 2014a, 2014b). Many of these physicians and nurses work in family practice settings in the community, with an emphasis on health promotion and illness prevention. Nurses working in communities are in privileged situations to identify and satisfy the needs of families. By interacting with individuals and families in the community on a daily basis, nurses are able to develop a holistic view of the health status of the community and its members.

Despite the difficulties encountered during recent years, Cuba offers a healthcare system that is highly developed and effective. Because of the focus on primary care in the community, Cuba's main health indicators (such as average life expectancy and infant mortality) are comparable to those of industrialized nations, placing Cuba far ahead of the rest of Latin America and other developing countries around the world. Cuban collaboration on health is currently present in 66 countries in Latin America, the Caribbean, Asia, and Africa. With more than 23,000 Cuban health collaborators at work internationally, their contributions have been noteworthy in the face of serious health problems in many developing nations.

References

Jardnes, J. B., Ouviña, J., & Aneiro-Ribna, R. (1991). Education in the science of health in Cuba. *Public Health Cuban Magazine*, *25*(4), 387–407.

World Bank. (2014a). Data: Nurses and midwives (per 1,000 people). Retrieved from http://data.worldbank.org/indicator/SH.MED.NUMW.P3

World Bank. (2014b). Data: Physicians (per 1,000 people). Retrieved from http://data.worldbank.org/indicator/SH.MED.NUMW.P3

Jordan

Waddah Demeh

Jordan, a country with a population of 6.3 million, is located in the heart of the politically volatile Middle East, between Iraq, Saudi Arabia, Syria, West Bank, and Israel. The first Ministry of Health (MOH) was established in 1950 and the first health insurance system was implemented among Force Army members in 1963. Health services are provided through five major sectors:

- Ministry of Health: hospitals, clinics, and mother–child health centers
- Royal Medical Services (Force Army)
- Private sector: hospitals and clinics
- United Nation Relief and Work Agency (UNRWA): clinics and mother–child health centers
- Medical services at governmental universities: Jordan University Hospital and the Hospital of King Abed Allah Ibn al-Hussein

Jordan has limited financial resources and is still considered to be a developing country. Since King Abdullah II took the throne in 1999, health care, education, and technology have advanced quickly. Under his leadership, emphasis was placed on industry and the importance of Jordanian social and economic development. Jordan has approached development from a holistic perspective, realizing that poverty, illiteracy, and health form a triangle and must be addressed together. Advances in the struggle against poverty and illiteracy, in addition to the spread of sanitation, clean water, adequate nutrition, and housing, have resulted in a healthier Jordanian citizenry. The main goal of Jordan's health strategy has been to provide adequate health coverage to all. Jordan's public health system has concentrated on primary health care (e.g., childhood immunization and prenatal care) in all parts of the country, while leaving tertiary health care mostly to the private sector. Jordan's healthcare system has improved dramatically in the last few decades, placing it among the top 10 countries of the world in reducing infant mortality.

Jordan's health needs are met by a high ratio of medical personnel per capita, with the only personnel shortage being in trained local nurses. The government is establishing new nursing colleges and encouraging students to specialize in nursing by offering incentives for trained nurses and giving priority in employment for both male and female Jordanian nurses. Five of eight public universities have nursing colleges that offer both bachelor's and master's degrees in nursing, and two other private universities offer a degree in nursing as well.

Jordan is taking the lead in the Middle East region in recognizing nursing as an independent profession. In 2002, the Jordanian Nursing Council (JNC) was established to regulate the nursing profession through the development of bylaws and credentials policies as well as strategies to protect the health, safety, and welfare of the public. Some accomplishments of JNC to date include the following developments:

- Revising the current law and suggesting amendments
- Laying down the strategic planning of the JNC and the plan of action
- Forming committees to establish the clinical ladder
- Requesting institutions to participate in different committees that are defined in strategic planning (JNC, 2007)

Ninety-two percent of the population in Jordan is Muslim, and this plays a major role in individual and group perceptions about health. The purpose of Islam, as stated in the Qur'an, is to foster beneficial relations between individuals and groups to weld mankind into a true brotherhood. Families are considered the primary social unit in the community, and it is mainly women within families who care for and maintain essential family functions. They determine the nutritional status of the family; they manage and budget the household income; they teach, educate, and care for their children; and they provide health care to the household and community (Mahasneh, 2001).

Women in Jordan have many freedoms. The majority of young women attend universities, have voting rights, drive, and cover themselves only by choice. In fact, many young feminist women in Jordan today are returning to traditional Islamic values (including traditional dress) through the original interpretation of the Qur'an because they contend that the profit Muhammad defended the rights of women. These traditional religious beliefs influence their behavior on many levels, including teaching children to uphold the family honor in the name of God through maintaining virginity before marriage and not being seen alone with a man as a young girl. Shame brought on a family lasts generations and can influence family connections in the community. Men care for their families by protecting the women (Miller & Petro-Nustas, 2002).

References

Jordanian Nursing Council (JNC). (2007). *JNC home.* Retrieved from http://www.jnc.gov.jo/english/home.htm

Mahasneh, S. (2001). Health perceptions and health behaviors of poor urban Jordanian women. *Journal of Advanced Nursing, 36*(1), 58–68.

Miller, J., & Petro-Nustas, W. (2002). Context of care for Jordanian women. *Journal of Transcultural Nursing, 13*(3), 228–236.

UNIT 2

Influences on Community and Population Health

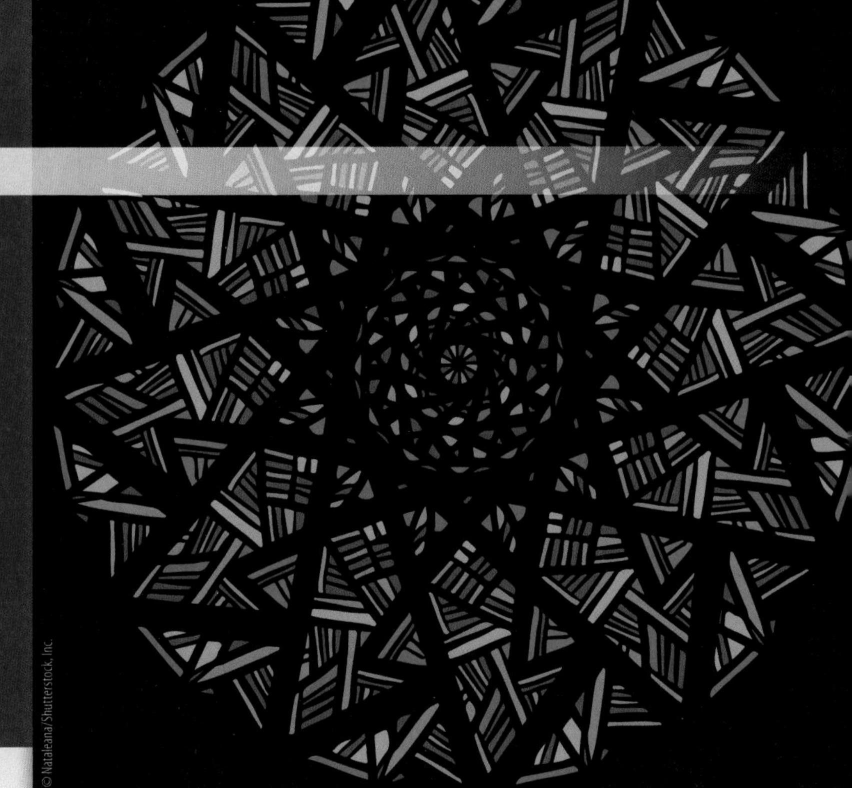

CHAPTER FOCUS

An Economic Approach to Health Care
- Markets and Competition
- Government Regulation and Involvement in Markets
- Market Failure in Health Care

History of U.S. Health Market
- Decreased Access: The Economic Barriers
- Influences on Costs and Access

Paying for Health Care
- Out-of-Pocket Payments and Charity
- Health Insurance
- Publicly Funded Insurance and Direct Care Programs

Cost Containment, Cost Analysis, and Quality

Public Health, Managed Care, and the Economics of Prevention
- Opportunities for Collaboration
- Counterforces to Collaboration
- Economics of Alternative Therapies

Significance of Economics for Community Health Nursing Practice

The Affordable Care Act (ACA)

Economics and Nightingale's Legacy

QUESTIONS TO CONSIDER

After reading this chapter, you will know the answers to the following questions:

1. Why is the U.S. healthcare market referred to as an "imperfect" market?
2. What are the major roles of government and private enterprise in the U.S. healthcare market?
3. What factors are contributing to high and rising healthcare costs?
4. What are the strategies used for cost containment of national health expenditures?
5. What are the financing, eligibility, and covered benefits of Medicare and Medicaid?
6. What other healthcare financing is covered by the government?
7. Why is it that, in spite of the availability of public and private health insurance programs, some U.S. citizens are without any coverage?
8. How and why might public health and managed care organizations collaborate?
9. How are community health nurses affected by the economic environment of their practice?
10. How will the Affordable Care Act of 2010 affect the future of healthcare financing?

CHAPTER 8

Economics of Health Care

Sherry Hartman and Dean Bauman

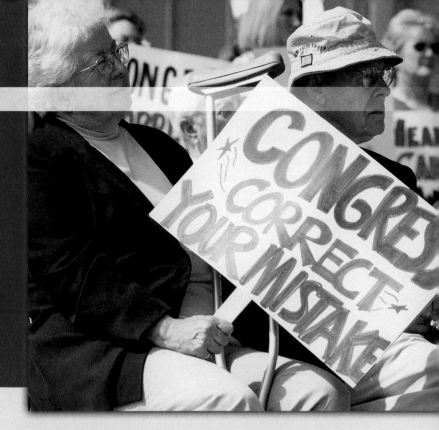

KEY TERMS

access to care
Affordable Care Act (ACA) of 2010
benefit period
categorical programs
categorically needy
Center for Medicare & Medicaid Innovation (CMMI)
community rating
competition
cost–benefit analysis
cost containment
cost-effectiveness analysis
cost-of-illness analysis
cost sharing
demand
entitlement
experience rating
free market competition
gross domestic product (GDP)
healthcare market
health insurance purchasing cooperative (HIPC)
imperfect market
inflation
managed care
marketplace
market failure
market justice
market
medically needy
Medigap insurance
opportunity cost
Patient-Centered Outcomes Research Institute (PCORI)
perfectly competitive market
price
relative value scale
resource utilization groups, version 3 (RUG-III)
self-insurance
social justice
standards of participation
supplier-influenced demand
supply
technology assessment
third-party payer
universal health care
welfare

REFLECTIONS

How much do you know about the real costs of health care and how nursing fits into the larger picture of economic markets? Why have nurses historically rejected the "irrelevant" knowledge about how the economic system of health care affects their practice and patient care?

Not so long ago, economic concerns were not considered an appropriate topic for basic nursing education, or perhaps even for advanced nursing. In-depth knowledge was essential only for nurse administrators who needed to deal with budgets and financial resources. In today's healthcare environment, however, nurses need to understand healthcare problems from many approaches and viewpoints. The science of economics is one of those approaches that has become increasingly important with the continued evolution of the U.S. health system. Even though "money concerns" have traditionally been resisted by general healthcare staff whose focus has been on meeting patient needs, most now acknowledge the impact of economics on healthcare problems and solutions. All levels of care providers need at least a rudimentary understanding of the economic workings of the system in which they practice at the institutional, national, and sometimes even global levels. Controlling costs, while maintaining quality and access, has become the major challenge of the 21st century. To do this, an understanding of economic descriptions and explanations of the healthcare market are necessary.

This text at times describes the context of and influences on healthcare practice, highlighting aspects of health problems from an economic point of view rather than strictly a biological or psychosocial perspective. Healthcare system analysts are concerned with the best structures for delivering the various needed healthcare services; health policymakers are concerned with deciding the best actions to take from among possible alternatives; health economists are concerned with the distribution of scarce resources among a defined population. These areas are interrelated: Economic analysis influences policy and budget decisions, which often drive the resulting healthcare delivery structures. The resultant structures, in turn, are analyzed in terms of how efficiently they distribute needed resources.

The goal of this chapter is to provide a basic knowledge of how economic theory is applied to the healthcare field, a brief history of how economics has been involved in healthcare legislation, and the current state of financing health care. The many sources of funding and reimbursement for health care are explained. Approaches to cost containment and methods of economic analysis are described, followed by a look at some of the relationships between private-sector health care and public health care. Finally, some of the implications of economics for community health nursing are summarized.

An Economic Approach to Health Care

Economics is the field of study that analyzes the production, distribution, and consumption of goods and services. Health economics, as a branch of economics, is concerned with issues relating to the production of goods and services in the healthcare sector of the economy, who gets access to the goods and services (distribution), and individual behavior in the consumption of health services. This is done by studying the structure of healthcare systems; individual behaviors that affect health, such as smoking and obesity; demographic shifts that affect the demand and supply of healthcare services; and the level of government involvement in the **healthcare market** and how this affects the behavior of individuals and firms (hospitals or insurance providers). **Figure 8-1** describes the areas that typify health economics.

A central focus of economics is the availability of resources. *Scarcity* describes a condition in which there are not enough resources to make the goods and services to fulfill all the wants and desires that individuals and households have (demand). This implies that constraints exist that limit the amount of goods that can be produced and consumed at a given time. In economics, this **opportunity cost** defines the true cost of a good or service in terms of other demands that money could have been spent on. This important concept makes explicit the fact that every decision involves tradeoffs, and these decisions affect how limited resources are used. Decision makers at every level face tradeoffs: For example Congress debates new healthcare legislation and hospital administrators decide on what new equipment to purchase (and thereby what will not be purchased). Opportunity cost is applied to both the production and consumption of goods and services.

Due to scarcity, it is necessary to achieve the greatest level of *efficiency* as possible in the production of a good or service so that more can be produced using those limited resources. It is also necessary to achieve the maximum degree of cost-effectiveness, which pertains to reaching preset healthcare goals at the least cost or maximizing

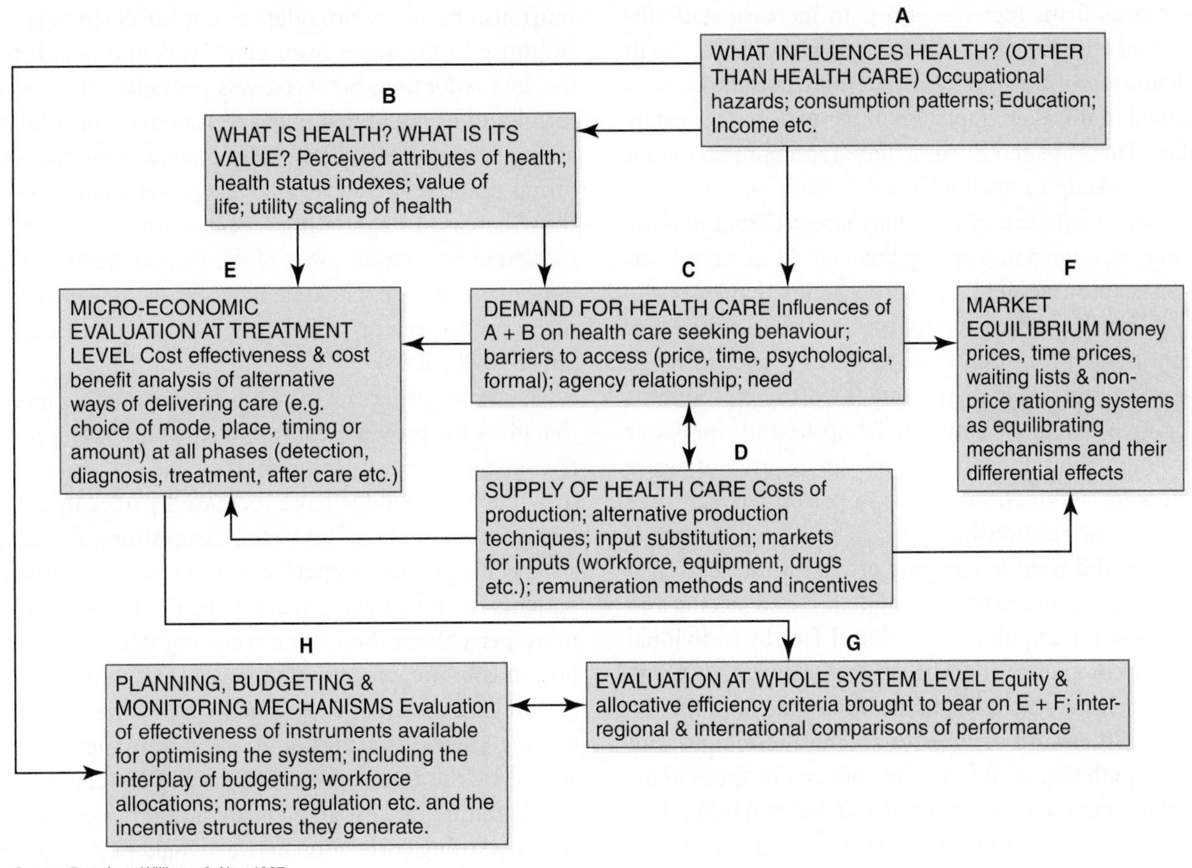

Figure 8-1 Plumbing diagram.

the health benefits of patients given a limited amount of resources or budget. A program is termed *inefficient* or not *cost-effective* if the same goals could be achieved at a lower cost and with fewer resources. These two terms historically lie at the center of the healthcare debate in the United States, between a purely privatized health system and a single-payer, **universal healthcare** system.

Markets and Competition

Like most sciences, economics is complex and broad in its scope. It frequently conceptualizes the processes and interactions around specific resources as a **marketplace**. In a marketplace, those who have something to sell and those who have needs or wants come together to make exchanges. There are various **markets** depending on the commodity being exchanged, such as the automobile market, the entertainment market, the housing market, and the healthcare market. In health care, the market includes all healthcare-related services that need to be distributed among the total U.S. population. Within that overall market are specific markets: the healthcare labor market, the homecare market, the hospital care market, the pharmaceuticals market, the personal health insurance market, the employer-paid health insurance market, and so on. A single hospital can also focus on its market: those potential users of its service and competing sellers in its service area. A market could also be defined geographically, such as the home healthcare market within a certain region.

The essence of a market is interaction between buyers and sellers. There is a particular amount of a product or service such as health care that buyers are willing and able to purchase and consume, which is referred to as the **demand** for the product. There is a certain amount that sellers or providers are willing to make available, which is referred to as the **supply** of the product. In both cases, the amount demanded or supplied is related to the **price** of the health product.

Competition in the market is the mechanism for setting price and quality. Suppliers compete for buyers of their products. Those who operate most efficiently (by satisfying buyers with the quality they want at the lowest possible cost) flourish; those who do not satisfy and retain consumers eventually close down. Price is most commonly the basis for competition, but competition can also be based on technical quality, amenities, access, or other factors. Efforts to operate efficiently increasingly impact the role of nurses as firms increase efforts to increase staff efficiency and eliminate over-staffing and redundancy. To fit the definition of a **perfectly competitive market**, such as described in this paragraph, a number of criteria must be fulfilled: These are described in the paragraphs that follow.

In a perfectly competitive market, consumers bear the financial consequences of their purchase decisions and are aware of price differences among products. Most Americans rely on reimbursement by third parties that bear the financial impact of decisions to receive care. This can cause patients to be price insensitive, to feel as if care is free, to believe they should get their money's worth for premiums paid, and to have no incentive to "shop around" for better prices. In general, most health consumers are not aware of prices for services, variations in prices between suppliers, and the relationship between price and quality. If consumers did want to compare prices for products, it is often hard to compare because of item-based pricing and negotiation for unpublished reduced fees by individual insurance companies or health plans (Deaton, 2006). Surgery, for example, includes charges for a surgeon, supplies, use of facilities, and services of an anesthesiologist and maybe a pathologist. Exact usage of each of these items sometimes cannot be anticipated and makes it difficult to determine a price prior to the service and compare it with a competitor's price. Even though health plans now negotiate fees for "packages" of services or benefits to overcome the pricing problems, these are not standardized and thus are still difficult to compare.

In a perfectly competitive market, there is unrestrained competition among providers. Unrestricted access to the market is blocked in several ways for some healthcare providers. An example is the case of advanced practice nurses, who often have not been free to set up primary care practices as they wish. Many states require medical oversight of nursing practice, such as permission for prescriptive privileges of nurse practitioners. Most **third-party payer** systems traditionally have not provided direct payment for nursing care. Instead, payment for most nursing care is included in hospital or clinic charges. If consumers must personally bear the cost for any nursing services they might receive directly, then services that could be offered by entrepreneurial nurses will have a limited demand in the market. Limits on entering the market for nurses and for some complementary or alternative healthcare practitioners are the same as giving physicians control over competitors. The results are lack of competition based on lower prices or on quality (Rambur & Mooney, 1998).

No single provider in a perfectly competitive market has monopoly power. Not only must providers be able to enter the market, but for competition to work, there must also be many providers vying for customers. One response to pressures from employers and health plans for cost reduction, however, was provider alliances and formation of integrated delivery systems. Consolidation among healthcare networks of hospitals and multispecialty group practices gives very large market shares to—and thus increased negotiating leverage for—these groups. In certain geographic areas of the United States, a single, large medical system has taken over as the sole provider of major health services, restricting competition (Rice, 1998; Shi & Singh, 2008).

Such mergers create local market negotiating leverage that gives the provider control over local services pricing (Berenson, 2005). In some markets, newly formed local provider monopolies have increased prices by 20% to 50%. For example, a 2011 study examining the cost of six specific procedures performed in hospitals found that patients in consolidated markets paid $4,561 to $13,690 more per patient than those receiving the procedures at hospitals in nonconcentrated markets (Robinson, 2011). Although consolidation probably is not the only factor driving such disparities, a 2013 white paper commissioned by the Robert Wood Johnson Foundation noted that literature on cost and consolidation has consistently shown a strong correlation between higher costs and consolidation (Balto & Kovacs, 2013).

In a perfectly competitive market, consumers have full information about the nature of the services they require, the results of their decisions, and the benefits they can obtain. In many instances, patient services are lifetime purchases with no opportunity to learn about quality differences through repeat purchases. In those cases, providers also have little reason to woo consumers by building a reputation for quality (Howell, 2006). The complexity of medical care itself and of the healthcare system makes informed choices difficult for patients. A consumer cannot know if a prescription or surgery is the better buy for his or her illness. There are so many choices of treatment—perhaps an acupuncturist would be a better buy. Treatment is sometimes urgently needed. Patients often do not have the time, skills, or resources to find needed information, and such information can be costly. In choice of health plan coverage, consumers do not know the differences between plan characteristics that indicate quality, convenience, flexibility, and extent of coverage. Even after a choice is made, consumers often cannot know if they made the right decision or what would have happened under other circumstances. Did the care cause the improvement or would it have happened anyway? What would have happened if another provider or treatment had been chosen?

In a perfectly competitive market, consumers and providers must act independently. Because of the "asymmetries of information" (Blumenthal, 1994, p. 252) in the healthcare market, patient consumers must depend on and accept the word of providers. Indeed, the words and advice of providers are as much the product being purchased as the examination or treatment. In a truly free market, the power lies with the consumer. However, physicians (suppliers) often are viewed as agents acting on behalf of patients. Thus, consumer demand is subject to artificial demand, commonly called **supplier-influenced demand** (Shi & Singh, 2008). In some cases, physicians own laboratories and invest in healthcare organizations, a relationship that may affect their ability to be impartial in recommending the use of these resources.

Providers of services in the free market seek to operate efficiently to maximize profits. Many providers of health care operate as nonprofit organizations. Their only constraint is to make their budgets balance such that expenditures equal revenues. Some may have goals beyond maximizing services, such as extending high salaries and benefits to administration, or improving organizational status with expensive equipment, regardless of whether the majority of patients need such technology. Conversely, workers in for-profit organizations may have adverse incentives owing to the firm's goal of profit. In the case of physicians, such conflicting goals can be seen when they focus on a specific patient and seek to exhaust every possibility for diagnosis and order many costly tests. Such conflict was a motivation for the capitated payment systems of early managed care, which encouraged less spending on care to realize higher retained profit. Concerns for quality have limited many such managed care restrictive methods, but perverse incentives still exist. Access and utilization barriers to managed care were the popular answer throughout the 1990s to market failure in health care.

The degree to which the markets in the healthcare industry fit these criteria is central to the policy and political arguments about which type of healthcare system the United States should adopt. If all of these criteria described the healthcare field as it truly is, then a privatized healthcare system would provide the most benefit at the lowest cost. For example, in many rural areas, the number of sellers (hospitals that provide the goods and services) is limited, and therefore the necessary requirement of many sellers does not exist. The 21st century has also seen a large amount of merger activity in the healthcare sector, from hospitals to insurance companies. Indeed, hospital consolidation "to create larger hospital systems with broader service reach and economies of scale to combat growing strategic, economic, and regulatory pressures" (Yanci, Wolford, & Young, 2013) is among the most significant trends in the industry. This results in fewer suppliers competing in a market. The requirement for complete information for all market participants is also difficult to meet. For example, individuals do not have access to all available information because they must take as truth the information a doctor provides regarding the goods and services that they require. That individual has no idea if various tests that a doctor orders them to get are relevant or cost effective.

If a market does not fit the criteria for a perfectly competitive market, it is subject to **market failure**. This means that the best possible results do not occur in a market "left on its own" and greater efficiency and cost-effectiveness could be acquired by the government intervening in the market. This has been the theoretical motivation for governments to regulate and participate in markets.

Government Regulation and Involvement in Markets

Rather than through markets, goods and services can also be distributed through the centralized decision making of the government. Through this system, buyers and sellers are directed to engage in exchanges based on a mandate rather than their own decision to buy based on the price mechanism. The stereotypical examples are the countries of the former Communist Bloc led by the Soviet Union. Most healthcare systems operate between these two extremes, using the market framework with government involvement in regulating the quality of services and providing financing to portions of the population. The United States has mainly a private system of financing and delivering health services. Sources of payment for U.S. health care are 55% from private sources and 45% from government sources at present; this is projected to shift to a 50-50 split by 2020 due to alterations in the market related to the 2010 Affordable Care Act (ACA) (Keehan et al., 2011). The majority of hospitals, physicians, and other healthcare providers are private businesses. From its earliest origins in a free market of direct exchange between individuals and their private physicians, the U.S. system moved slowly to more centralized decisions through government regulation. For example, federal and state governments determine public-sector expenditures, covered services, and reimbursement rates for Medicare and Medicaid services. They also regulate participants in the market by setting **standards of participation** for certification to provide services for Medicaid and Medicare patients. Such government regulations become the minimum standards of quality in other, private sectors of the health services market (Shi & Singh, 2008).

Over time, as the government role in the U.S. healthcare system has grown, there have been repeated attempts by both of the major political parties to control costs and government spending. The persistent high levels and rates of growth for healthcare expenditures remain dominant subjects of policy decisions in health care (Fuchs, 2005; Weinstein & Skinner, 2010). More private and public money being spent on health care means less money available to spend on other wants, needs, or investments in business activities. In the public sector, spending more on health care leaves less to spend on education, the military, the environment, and other needed public goods. As noted by Weinstein & Skinner (2010), there is concern over high U.S. spending because we may not be getting the value in improved health or patient satisfaction that other alternative policy and budget choices might provide. Some states have become frustrated with efforts at reform by the central government and have developed their own remedies. Massachusetts was the first state to require residents to carry health insurance, with employer contributions to employee coverage becoming mandatory. A few other states also considered legislation of some form of universal coverage, and at least 25 states considered employer mandates to increase coverage (Mantone, 2006).

Market Failure in Health Care

Those who believe in the superiority of competitive marketplaces base their preference on what would happen in an ideal perfect market that meets the criteria listed earlier. Although there may be success in applying free-market principles to the market where automobiles, condos, and refrigerators are exchanged for cash, these principles seem less appropriate for health care. The place where relief of pain, care of infections, and comfort of the spirit are exchanged for cash is thought to be very different (Berenson, 2005; Edwards, 2005; Rambur & Mooney, 1998).

History of U.S. Health Market

In the past, the patient or family expected to pay for their own health care. In 1940, 81.3% of health care was paid by the individual or the family, and 18.7% was financed by some intermediary third party. Of that 18.7%, 2.6% was from private insurance and 16.1% by public funding (Gibson & Waldo, 1982). Originally, the most powerful unions refused to support universal health care, because they feared government-provided health care would erode the need for the unions to exist (Altman & Shactman, 2011). However, this began to change during the Great Depression, beginning with the passage of the Social Security Act of 1935. The introduction of the first indemnity insurance plans, Blue Cross for hospital care and Blue Shield for physician care, diffused political demands for compulsory health insurance (Pulcini & Mahoney, 1998). A few short years after this, the U.S. government unintentionally initiated the creation of its very unique system of tying health care to employment. During World War II, the U.S. government enacted wage and price controls as it directed the war effort. Due to these controls on wages, firms had to find other means to attract workers, leading them to use benefit packages that included medical and dental insurance as incentives.

In 1959, with the Federal Employees Health Benefit Act, Blue Cross negotiated to provide health insurance coverage for federal employees and set the stage for its later involvement in Medicare and Medicaid. In the 1960s, with President Johnson's Great Society legislative efforts, a period of relative prosperity and a growing concern for poor and elderly populations, Medicaid (Title XIX) and Medicare (Title XVIII) programs were passed as amendments to the Social Security Act. At the same time, the federal government became more involved in health care with legislation establishing regional medical programs, comprehensive health planning, and extensive educational aid to medical and related health professions.

With the advent of the insurance system and government programs, by 2012, individual payout for health care was starkly different from that of 1940, with households paying directly for 29% of their care and 65% being paid by a third party—21% by private insurance sources (usually via an employer) and 44% from public funds (federal, 26%; state/local, 18%; Centers for Medicare & Medicaid Services, 2012).

It was soon evident that the costs of health care were escalating (see **Figure 8-2**). With the government and

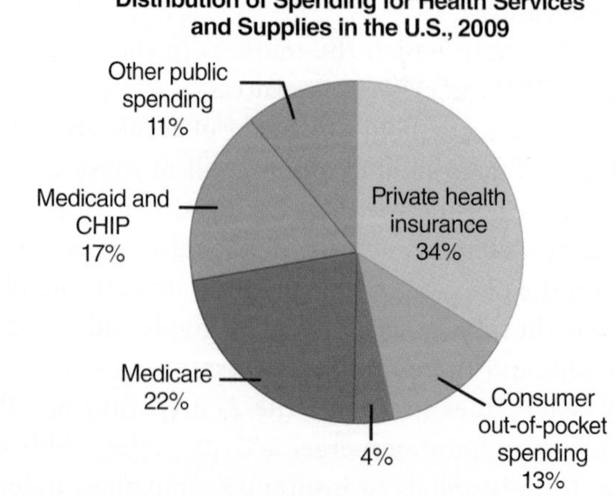

Figure 8-2 U.S. healthcare expenditures.

Source: Reproduced from CBO's 2011 Long-term budget outlook, Congressional Budget Office, June 2011.

third-party insurers paying so much for healthcare expenses, individuals did not have to bear the full cost of attaining healthcare services and products. The effect was as if individuals had more money to pay for care, increasing the amount of goods and services demanded. As economic theory predicts, increased sources of funds led to increased individual demand, and increasing revenues of the healthcare industry. Government intervention had contributed to rising costs (Finkler & Kovner, 1993, p. 80). This has resulted in a conflict in that voters do not want to pay more for health care but do not want limited access to goods and services. This has led to an apparent inability of society or government to limit the rising costs of health care and continues to be one of the roots of the present fiscal challenges in health care.

A commonly cited indicator of U.S. healthcare spending is related to the U.S. gross domestic product. **Gross domestic product (GDP)** is the monetary total of all finished goods and services (public and private) produced within a country in 1 year. Healthcare expenditures (which means all funds, private and public, spent on health care) as a percentage of the GDP are a standard measure for comparing and tracking changes in expenditure levels (Jacobs, 1997). In the United States, health care has had a long history of escalating costs, consuming an increasing share of the country's GDP. A graph of the rising expenditures from all sources shows a continuing amount being paid by private sources but a narrowing of the gap between government and private funding (see **Figure 8-3**). In 2004, private funding paid for 54.8% of U.S. health care ($1,030.3 billion), down from 59.5% in 1990. Currently, most people are still covered by employer-based health insurance.

Healthcare expenditures as a percentage of the GDP grew at an alarming rate for more than 30 years. In the early 1990s, policymakers predicted that, if left to grow unchecked, healthcare spending would reach 19% of the GDP by 2000 (White House Domestic Policy Council, 1993). This prediction proved to be high: In 2004, spending was 15.8% of the GDP and had not yet reached 18% as of 2012 (World Bank, 2014). **Figure 8-4** shows the continuing upward trend with some years of lower growth rates. In 1996, spending leveled off, with the growth rate of the overall economy exceeding the growth rate of healthcare expenditures. It had been predicted that the United States would top $1 trillion in healthcare spending by 1995 (Standard and Poor's Corporation, 1992), but with

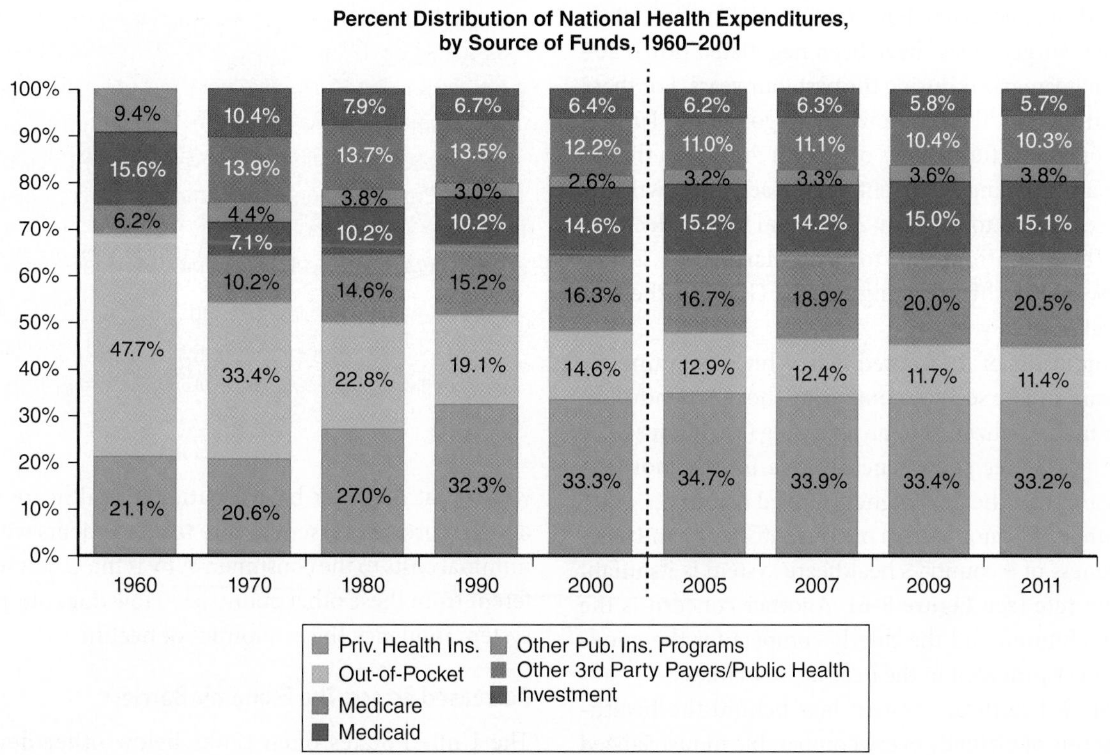

Figure 8-3 National health expenditures by source of funds, 1960 to 2011.

Source: Data from Kaiser Family Foundation calculations using NHE data from Centers for Medicare and Medicaid Services, Office of the Actuary, National Health Statistics Group, at http://www.cms.hhs.gov/NationalHealthExpendData/ (see Historical; National Health expenditures by type of service and source of funds, CY 1960–2011; file nhe2011.zip).

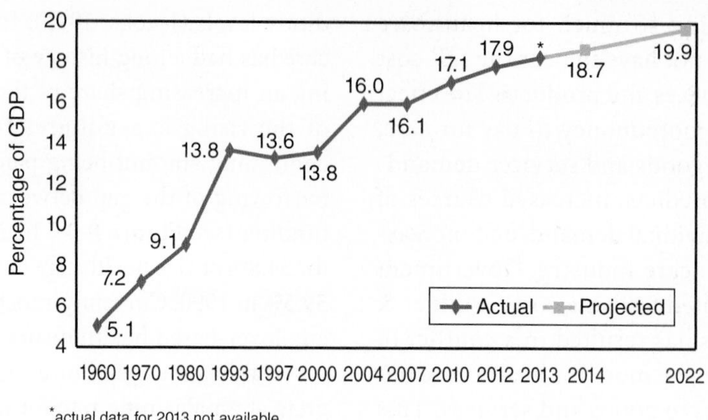

Figure 8-4 Actual and predicted national expenditures as a percentage of GDP, 1960 to 2010.
Source: Data from Centers for Medicare and Medicaid Services, Office of the Actuary, National Health Statistics Group, 2014.

the slower rate of growth, it was 1996 before the $1 trillion mark was passed.

The mid-1990s progress in reducing the rate of spending growth was unexpected. Analysts disagreed over the reasons for the slowed rate, but many believed the efficiencies introduced by increased **free market competition** and **managed care** were responsible. Economic analysts at the time did not view the lowered rates as a permanent trend. The limits of realizing improved efficiency without harming quality may have been reached as many factors continued to affect costs. For example, Halvorson (1999) noted that surgery fees "have been negotiated down 30–40% in many markets during the past four years. For these rock-bottom fees, there is nowhere to go but up" (p. 28). Projections show future rates of growth that are in the 7% to 7.5% annual range. Currently, the pace of growth has slowed compared to the early 2000s, and indeed declined slightly (by 0.2%) from 2009 to 2012 (Martin et al., 2014); at 17.2% in 2012, it is lagging behind GDP for the first time in almost 25 years.

An indicator of the United States' high spending for health care can be seen by comparing those expenditures to other industrialized nations' spending (see **Figure 8-5**). The United States spends nearly one-fourth more on health care than the next highest ranked country.

Another indicator used to measure efficiency and cost-effectiveness of a country's healthcare system is its infant mortality rate (see **Figure 8-6**). Another concern is the fact that children and the elderly compete for the goods and services provided in the healthcare market.

The U.S. healthcare system lags behind the healthcare systems of virtually every comparable industrialized nation in the world. The U.S. infant mortality rate is higher and life expectancy lower than in almost all countries who share similar populations and type of government. The United States is the only country in the industrialized world that does not have a national healthcare system, one that provides essential care to all residents with no or minimal costs to the consumer. Why is the U.S. system different from these other countries? How does our political system influence the economics of health?

A DAY IN THE LIFE

Health Policy and Ethics Analyst Emily Friedman

There is a new and growing class of uninsured people. Women aged 50 to 64 are disproportionally likely to be uninsured, often because they are not covered through spousal benefits that have ended because of loss of a job. . . . Older women . . . have been thrown into the individual health insurance market and can't afford coverage. I know a little about this first-hand. I am self-employed and buy my own health insurance. When I turned 50, my insurance sent me a birthday present of a 22% rate increase. That was followed this year with a 9% increase. There's a 14% rate increase on the way. When I am 55, I will be paying twice what I am paying now. I have a $500 deductible and have never filed a claim. I can afford it. But many cannot. I have friends who are working, yet who have sold belongings to pay for health care. The situation is very serious and it is happening to middle-class people.

—Emily Friedman, Health Policy and Ethics Analyst

Source: Brown, C. (1999). Ethics, policy, and practice: Interview with Emily Friedman. *Image: Journal of Nursing Scholarship, 31*, 259–262.

Decreased Access: The Economic Barriers

The United States often ranks below other developed countries in health status indicators. This problem can be described as follows: "The Americans who can afford health insurance, or who are well insured, can get the best care that medical technology can offer. Even so, the most

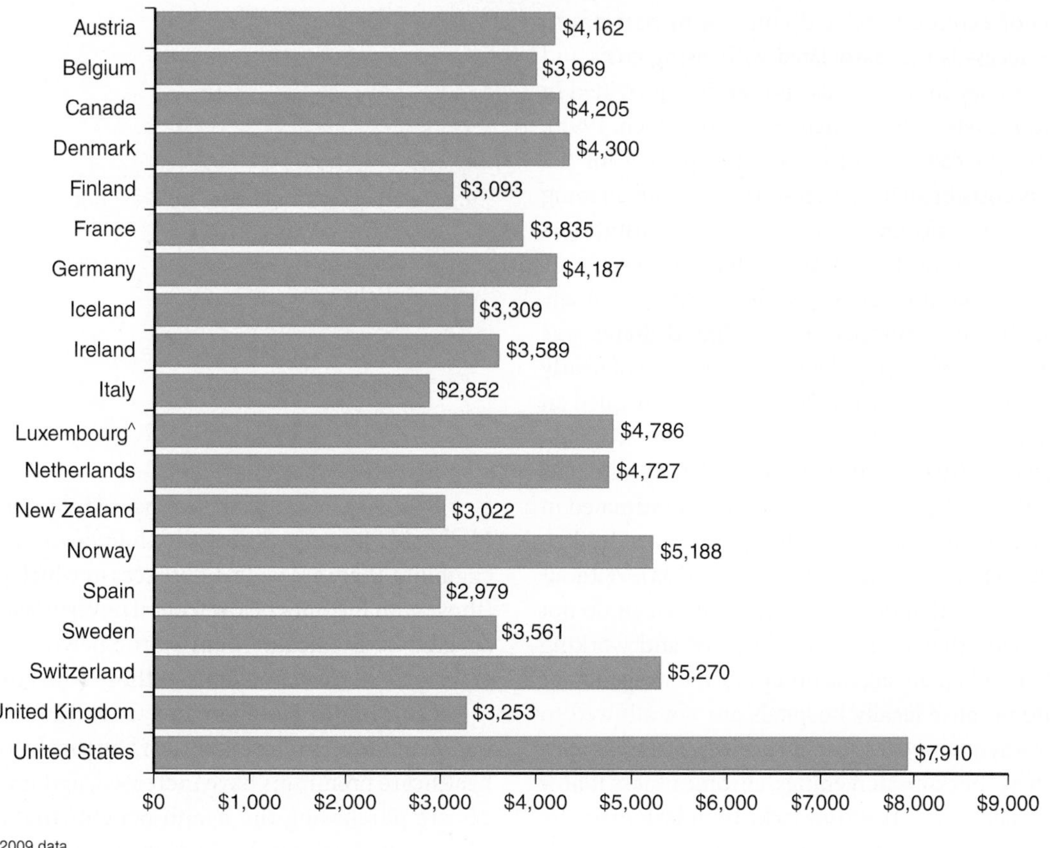

Figure 8-5 Total health expenditure in selected countries.

Note: Data for Japan, France, Germany, and Australia are for 2003.

Source: Data from http://kff.org/health-costs/slide/per-capita-total-current-health-care-expenditures-u-s-and-selected-countries-2010/

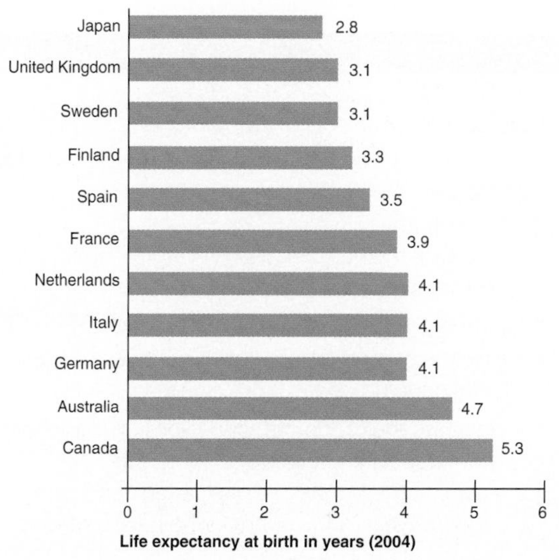

Figure 8-6 Infant mortality in selected countries.

Source: Data from OECD health date, 2006.

expensive care is often fragmented, or insufficient, and may not restore the patient to health or adequate functioning" (Kovner & Knickman, 2005, p. 4). Even though superior services are present, the dark side of the situation is that they are not accessible to all. **Access to care** means that people can get the health care they require when they need it. Inadequate access for millions of Americans is a core problem and has led to concern for how the healthcare system in the United States is structured.

The concept of access to health care has long been recognized as an issue and a responsibility for nurses (Stevens, 1992). Gulzar (1999) examined the concept of access to health care from a nursing perspective and delineated its many dimensions. She defined access to health care as "the fit among personal, socio-cultural, economic, and system-related factors that enable individuals, families, and communities to have timely, needed, necessary, continuous, and satisfactory health services" (p. 17). These include, for example, age, gender, ethnic, and cultural appropriateness; understandable language;

healthcare providers and facilities near where people live; available transportation; timeliness; and affordability.

The major economic-related concern to barriers to healthcare access is that associated with rising costs and an inability to pay for the goods and services provided in the healthcare system (Bodenheimer & Grumbach, 1995). Very few people can afford to pay out of pocket for the tremendous costs of an illness episode or for the ongoing expenses of a chronic illness, and long-term institutional care is far beyond most individuals' ability to pay. At its peak in 2010, the number of people younger than age 65 without health insurance in the United States was 49 million (15.9% of the population), an increase of nearly 10 million people (1.7%) from 2000, which continued an upward trend from the mid-1970s (Holahan & Cook, 2006). Between 2010 and 2014, however, that number has fallen slightly; the Kaiser Family Foundation estimated in 2012 that 47.3 million persons under age 65 lacked healthcare coverage (Kaiser Family Foundation, 2013a). Without coverage, people either do not seek needed care or do not pay for the care they do receive. The poor and working poor without adequate access do not lack emergency or urgent care because legally hospitals are not allowed to turn away anyone needing such services. It is primary care—such as checkups, screenings, chronic illness follow up, and prenatal care—that they lack. Their lack of access to primary care means that many of these individuals eventually need more costly and less timely treatment.

Although the number of people covered by Medicare and Medicaid has grown, there has been a drop in the number covered by private health insurance. Lack of insurance is not just a problem of the poor—the numbers of uninsured are growing among the middle class (see **Box 8-1**). Most of the uninsured do not qualify for Medicaid. Because states set their own standards for eligibility, there are wide differences in which poor people (those with incomes below federal poverty level [FPL]) are covered by Medicaid. Many of the newly uninsured are employed or are dependents of those who are employed.

According to Holahan and Cook (2006), the number of employers offering health benefits has declined as healthcare premiums have increased, and fewer employees are purchasing the health benefits that are offered. Changes in demographics and the workplace have played a role in the decline of employer-sponsored insurance. There has been a shift from employment in industries that historically provided high rates of health coverage to those that do not (from industrial manufacturing to services), as well as an increase in self-employment and small companies. Also, there has been a population

BOX 8-1 Influences on Rising Healthcare Costs

Increased government funding
Inflation
Imperfect market
Third-party payment
Rising drug costs
Increased use of technology for care
Increased wages for healthcare personnel
Population changes
Slow adoption of labor-saving technology
Administrative and medical excess
Medical practice styles
Emphasis on treatment versus prevention
Consumer expectations
Indigent care

HEALTHY PEOPLE 2020 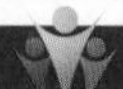

Objectives Related to Access to Quality Health Services

- Increase the proportion of persons with health insurance.
  - 1.1 Increase the proportion of persons with medical insurance.
  - 1.2 Increase the proportion of persons with dental insurance.
  - 1.3 Increase the proportion of persons with prescription drug insurance.
- Increase the proportion of insured persons with coverage for clinical preventive services.
- Increase the proportion of persons with a usual primary care provider.
- Increase the number of practicing primary care providers.
  - 4.1 Increase the number of practicing medical doctors.
  - 4.2 Increase the number of practicing doctors of osteopathy.
  - 4.3 Increase the number of practicing physician assistants.
  - 4.4 Increase the number of practicing nurse practitioners.
- Increase the proportion of persons who have a specific source of ongoing care.
  - 5.1 Increase the proportion of persons of all ages who have a specific source of ongoing care.
  - 5.2 Increase the proportion of children and youth aged 17 years and younger who have a specific source of ongoing care.
  - 5.3 Increase the proportion of adults aged 18 to 64 years who have a specific source of ongoing care.

Source: Reproduced from U.S. Department of Health and Human Services. (2010). Healthy People 2020. Retrieved from http://healthypeople.gov/2020/topicsobjectives2020/objectiveslist.aspx

5.4 Increase the proportion of adults aged 65 years and older who have a specific source of ongoing care.

- Reduce the proportion of persons who are unable to obtain or delay in obtaining necessary medical care, dental care, or prescription medicines.
  - 6.1 Reduce the proportion of persons who are unable to obtain or delay in obtaining necessary medical care, dental care, or prescription medicines.
  - 6.2 Reduce the proportion of persons who are unable to obtain or delay in obtaining necessary medical care.
  - 6.3 Reduce the proportion of persons who are unable to obtain or delay in obtaining necessary dental care.
  - 6.4 Reduce the proportion of persons who are unable to obtain or delay in obtaining necessary prescription medicines.
- Increase the proportion of persons who receive appropriate evidence-based clinical preventive services.
- Increase the proportion of persons who have access to rapidly responding prehospital emergency medical services.
  - 8.1 Increase the proportion of persons who are covered by basic life support.
  - 8.2 Increase the proportion of persons who are covered by advanced life support.
- Reduce the proportion of hospital emergency department visits in which the wait time to see an emergency department clinician exceeds the recommended timeframe.
  - 9.1 Reduce the proportion of all hospital emergency department visits in which the wait time to see an emergency department clinician exceeds the recommended timeframe.
  - 9.2 Reduce the proportion of Level 1–immediate hospital emergency department visits in which the wait time to see an emergency department clinician exceeds the recommended timeframe.
  - 9.3 Reduce the proportion of Level 2–emergent hospital emergency department visits in which the wait time to see an emergency department clinician exceeds the recommended timeframe.
  - 9.4 Reduce the proportion of Level 3–urgent hospital emergency department visits in which the wait time to see an emergency department clinician exceeds the recommended timeframe.
  - 9.5 Reduce the proportion of Level 4–semi-urgent hospital emergency department visits in which the wait time to see an emergency department clinician exceeds the recommended timeframe.
  - 9.6 Reduce the proportion of Level 5–nonurgent hospital emergency department visits in which the wait time to see an emergency department clinician exceeds the recommended timeframe.

Source: U.S. Department of Health and Human Services. (2010). *Healthy People 2020.* Retrieved from http://healthypeople.gov/2020/topicsobjectives2020/objectiveslist.aspx

movement from the northern and eastern regions of the United States to the south and west, which tend to have lower rates of employer-sponsored insurance and higher insurance rates. Employers who do offer health benefits are sharing more of the costs of rising premiums with their employees, often in the form of plans with high deductibles—$1,000 for single coverage and $2,000 for family coverage. Employee participation in high-deductible plans increased from 5% in 2007 to 8% in 2008 (Trapp, 2008).

Having private insurance does not guarantee financial access to care. Research based on data from the Commonwealth Fund Biennial Health Insurance Survey found that "the number of underinsured adults climbed to 25 million people in 2007, up from 16 million in 2003" (Collins, Kriss, Doty, & Rustgi, 2008). The study also found increases in the number of underinsured people reporting difficulty in paying their medical bills, from 34% of working-age adults in 2005 to 41% in 2007. The uninsured were twice as likely not to receive care, but three-fourths of those who went without were insured, and 46% had private insurance. Those who had Medicaid were as likely to go without care as the uninsured, because many physicians do not accept the coverage offered by Medicaid. Both the insured and the uninsured cited cost as the major barrier to seeking care (Collins et al., 2008).

Public programs are generally considered inadequate in terms of prenatal care (Hughes & Runyan, 2008) and mental health programs (Mechanic & Rochefort, 2008), and contractual arrangements for home health care can restrict needed visits in home healthcare services (Shaughnessy, Schlenker, & Hittle, 1995). By contrast, private coverage restricts access because of high out-of-pocket expenditures of copayments and deductibles, fixed indemnity (maximum payment allowed), and exclusions, such as for preexisting conditions. Exclusion may be for a set time after enrollment or may be permanent. Changing jobs can also trigger this restriction. Most Americans are underinsured for preventive services, catastrophic illness, and long-term care (Harrington & Estes, 2008). *The Healthy People 2020* objectives that address access issues are listed in the box feature, as does the ACA of 2010, described later on in the chapter.

Numerous negative outcomes for those who are uninsured or underinsured, lacking access to needed health care, have been documented.

Influences on Costs and Access

No single factor explains why health spending has grown at the rate it has over the past decades. Rather, several influences collectively contribute to the situation. As discussed earlier, there was an economic effect of increased demand as a result of *increased sources of funds from government and insurance coverage.* In addition, increases over the last few years have resulted from several sources.

Inflation, which is indicated by the rising consumer price index, has continued to affect all goods and services in the United States, but prices have increased at an even greater rate for healthcare services. Physicians and hospitals account for the greatest proportion of this increase. Expenditures for public health services account for only a little more than 3% of overall spending.

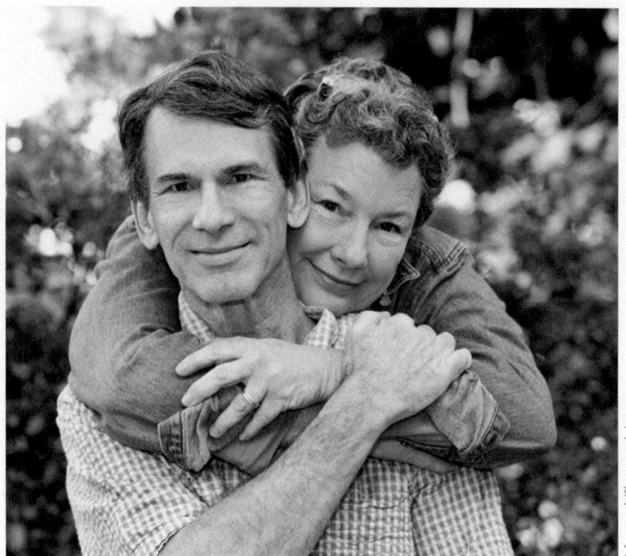

Many men and women are delaying retirement in order to maintain employer-sponsored health coverage.

Drug costs increased at nearly twice the annual rate of inflation between 2006 and 2010 (Government Accountability Office, 2011). Prices for generic drugs have decreased an average of 12.8% steadily since 2008, while prices of brand-name drugs increased an average of 21% (Express Scripts, 2012). Drug companies often market new, very expensive drugs directly to consumers, who then request them from their physicians. They also provide doctors with financial incentives to suggest these drugs to patients. In addition, companies raise the prices on older drugs that research shows to be most effective.

Most *advanced technology is expensive*. New and costly methods of care push prices up. One of the major contributors to healthcare services' inflation is increased use of technology, which often consists of newer and costlier treatments and methods of care. An excellent example is the availability of new treatments for women who are having difficulty conceiving. A single in vitro fertilization cycle costs $12,400 in the United States, and many women require two to three cycles of treatment to conceive (American Society for Reproductive Medicine, 2008). As newer technology is introduced, doctors and nurses become dependent on its use. More sophisticated technology requires more highly trained personnel to run it, and its complexity contributes to specialization among healthcare providers. This contributes to *higher personnel wages and benefit costs.* Consumers also become accustomed to having access to new technology and want the very latest in methods and equipment. Another obvious factor in rising costs is the *change in population demographics*. The overall U.S. population is growing partly as a result of immigration. Immigrants who enter the United States are often poorer and have more health problems. Providing healthcare access to these groups increases costs. Large populations alone can mean greater costs, but costs per capita (per person) in the United States have grown as well. In 1960, the healthcare costs per capita were $143; as of 2010, they were over $8,400 (Centers for Disease Control and Prevention [CDC], 2014) and are likely to continue rising. The higher costs per person can be partially explained by the changing demographics of an aging population. High-tech medicine and other factors have prolonged life. New terms, such as the "old old" and the "young old," have come into use as the population lives longer and "old" has new meaning. The over-85 group is growing at a rapid rate. Older persons require more health resources due to normal processes associated with aging as well as longstanding chronic illness. The need for more long-term care resources and personal health services is also increasing proportionately with the aging population.

Even though some are deprived of needed health care in the United States, there is also a factor of *excess* in the system. Excess comes in a variety of forms. High-tech equipment is expensive, as is the investment in space required to house it. Such technology often becomes used more frequently than necessary to justify its high cost. In a society where providers fear litigation, even when less expensive options may be equally effective, high-tech procedures may be overused in a type of *medical excess* that is referred to as "defensive medicine." Many argue that excessive and unwanted measures are used to prolong life past what is quality life for both terminally ill persons and the elderly.

Administrative excess contributing to increased costs includes both inefficiencies in systems of care and high administrative costs. Inefficient systems of care can be inferred from the patterns of differentiation in treatment and costs across geographic service areas, for example.

These differences, which are unexplained by other factors, are attributed to disagreement on "best practices" among direct care providers. Some practices are more expensive. For instance, the benefits of coronary artery bypass surgery over more conservative and less costly treatment are questioned. Greater numbers of hysterectomies and cesarean sections for women in some areas are explained by practice patterns that may not be cost-effective. Even with similar population attributes and illnesses, more days are spent in the hospital in some areas than in others. All of these discrepancies point to the need to look for more cost-effective clinical practices. Administrative costs, while accounting for a small proportion of the healthcare dollar, still come under criticism (Bodenheimer & Grumbach, 1995).

Closely associated with clinical practice patterns has been the *emphasis on cure over prevention of illness.* Practice is often guided by reimbursement patterns, and payment from most sources in the recent past has been made only when illness is present. Many economic analyses indicate that preventing illness is more cost-effective than waiting for a costly illness to be diagnosed, treated, and monitored. Managed care systems that focus on cost-effectiveness have begun to emphasize preventive care. The relationship of managed care and public health concerns for health promotion and disease prevention is addressed in detail later on.

Paying for Health Care

Access to health care is determined by financing. Thus, demand in the marketplace is directly related to the amount of financing. Services and treatments that are covered by a source of payment have greater demand than if those services were not covered. Financing of health care in the United States is complex. There are multiple sources of funds for health care. These funds, both public and private, are dispersed in a variety of programs and health plans through which resources are used to purchase services. **Figure 8-7** indicates the major sources of funds spent on personal health care.

Out-of-Pocket Payments and Charity

Those funds that are paid directly by individuals are sometimes called out-of-pocket payments. Some individuals or families assume all their own costs for healthcare services. This is possible when costs are low. A common example is the purchase of over-the-counter drugs. However, this is the least common method of paying for services. For most individuals, who are generally covered by either private or public insurance, the more common out-of-pocket expenses are in the form of **cost sharing**. These expenses include insurance premiums, insurance deductibles, copayment of a percentage of medical costs, costs above fixed payments, and noncovered services.

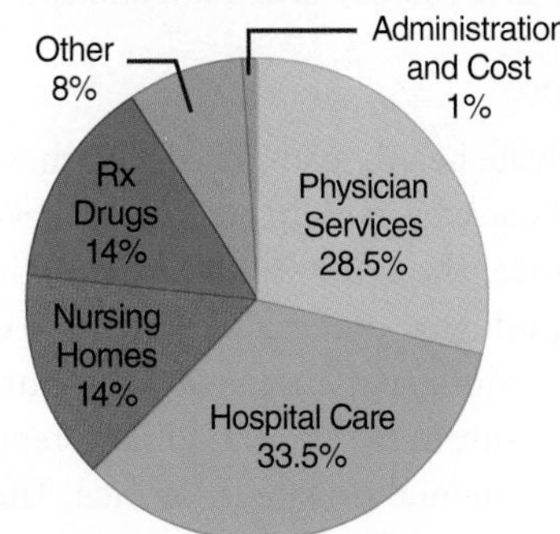

Figure 8-7 The nation's healthcare dollar: Where it went (2012.)
Source: Data from Center for Medicare & Medicaid Services (CMS). (2013). National Healthcare Expenditures. Retrieved from http://www.cms.gov/Research-Statistics-Data-and-Systems/Statistics-Trends-and-Reports/NationalHealthExpendData/downloads/tables.pdf

Because so many consumers are unable to meet the costs of services they need, and because providing health care to the suffering is seen by some as a moral imperative in modern societies, charity, insurance, and government sources provide funds in varying degrees (Wesson, 1999). Those who cannot afford to pay for needed care often turn to care financed by charity. Charity care has traditionally been seen as a religious duty or vocation, and various religious and secular organizations have offered care to the needy for little or no charge. Many physicians and other providers have also cared for the needy, either for free or based on a sliding scale. Philanthropic organizations financed by donors have established institutions to offer charitable care and special services. Another form of nongovernmental funds for health care is expenditures covering healthcare services provided for employees in industrial settings.

Health Insurance

Risk is central to the concept of insurance. Risk is the possibility of a substantial financial loss from costs of a health event that has a small probability of occurring. For a prepaid price (premium), companies offer specific benefits and protections from these risks. Health insurance is, therefore, a contractual agreement for payment of such healthcare costs and, therefore, protection from risk. This allows risk to be shifted from each specific individual to the group as a whole by pooling resources. The larger the group size, the more costs and risk can be shared among its members.

Health insurance is highly regulated by both federal and state governments. For example, significant federal reform was passed in 1996 with the Health Insurance Portability and Accountability Act (HIPAA). Key provisions of the act were portability of health insurance (if certain conditions of prior coverage are met), mental health parity as regards lifetime limits, mandatory minimum length of stay for obstetrics, the creation of tests of new funding methods (medical savings accounts), and fraud and abuse sanctions.

Private Insurance

Individual private health insurance is purchased by many Americans. Those who work in businesses that do not offer health insurance; the self-employed, including farmers; new college graduates; and early retirees are examples of those persons younger than age 65 who purchase their own private insurance. Many Medicare recipients also purchase supplemental private insurance. These types of policies do not spread risk as in group insurance, but base premiums on each individual's health risk.

Employment-Based Insurance

The most common kind of insurance is employer provided. That is, the employer pays all or most of the insurance premium as an employment benefit. In 2003, the average share of premiums paid by employers was 73%; the remaining 27% of premiums was paid by employees. By 2013, the employer's share had dropped by just 1%, but in the context of an almost 80% increase in overall premium costs, this meant that employees shouldered an additional 12% of the burden (Kaiser Family Foundation, 2013b). Health insurance as a fringe benefit became popular during World War II, when wages were frozen but benefits could be given to attract workers. It still is favored by tax policy, which does not apply income or Social Security tax to such benefits.

Premiums paid through employment are determined by group risks. An **experience rating** is based on a group's own health insurance claims experience. One group may be at greater risk due to occupational hazards and susceptibilities. Their premiums will be higher because they can be expected to have higher utilization of healthcare services. In contrast, **community ratings** base premiums on the utilization experience of a whole community so that rates are the same for everyone regardless of indicators of risk such as age or occupation.

As healthcare costs have risen, employers' insurance costs have risen as well. After salaries and raw materials, health care is the third highest cost category in U.S. corporations (Loubeau & Maher, 1996). Employers that compete in the global market are especially concerned because competitors in other countries with government-funded health care do not have the same costs and thus can set lower prices. In response, U.S. employers have initiated more and more cost-containment strategies, such as generic-only prescriptions, second opinions, preadmission testing, limiting procedures, and more outpatient surgery. For some employers (and individuals), **health insurance purchasing cooperatives (HIPCs)** help to lower costs. These organizations represent a number of employers, increasing the size of the group. By consolidating purchasing power and by realizing efficiencies in enrollment and premium collection, HIPCs can help small employers get lower rates than they could alone (Chollet, 1996). However, a main strategy has been to offer managed care plans as an exclusive or an alternative health plan. Managed care plans cover nearly 75% of employees with health insurance in both small and large firms (Shi & Singh, 2008).

Some employers with large workforces have begun to rely on **self-insurance**. Instead of paying premiums to an insurance plan, they assume healthcare cost risks by budgeting for medical claims from their employees. Government policy stimulated this option when it passed the Employee Retirement Income Security Act of 1974, which allowed for self-funded, nonprofit health plans by corporations. Such plans were exempted from taxes and certain mandatory benefits required of the regular plans (Health Insurance Association of America, 1991). For large employers, self-insurance was a better economic alternative. For employees, coverage can be less certain and they have less recourse for appealing claims that are not covered.

Some of the political debate over healthcare funding has centered on whether health insurance coverage should be mandated for all firms with workers. Proponents of such a policy believe it is sound business and will attract a stable, healthy workforce. Those opposed—mostly small business leaders—believe the expense would cause small businesses to become uncompetitive and fail, resulting in jobs lost.

Publicly Funded Insurance and Direct Care Programs

Public financing supports **categorical programs** that are developed to benefit a certain category of people. The largest of these are Medicare for the elderly and Medicaid for the indigent. The balance of government support goes to U.S. public health service hospitals, Veterans Affairs hospitals and health services, the Department of Defense for military personnel and dependents, the Indian Health Service (IHS), state and local support for inpatient psychiatric and other long-term care facilities, workers' compensation, public health activities, and other grants and initiatives. *In most cases the government provides the financing but obtains insurance and healthcare services through the private sector.* Payments are disbursed in programs of reimbursements, direct payment, grants, matching funds, and subsidies. Some programs combine federal and state funds. **Figure 8-8** shows the amounts of federal money spent on U.S. entitlement and welfare programs. The large impact of Medicaid, Medicare, and Social Security compared to other programs can be readily seen. Medicare and Medicaid are the primary subjects here, with other government health programs also being briefly explained to complete the picture of government financing.

MEDIA MOMENT

Fatal Care (1995)

This movie is based on the Robin Cook novel, which details the possible future of managed care. The main character has a child with cystic fibrosis and finds him in a hospital using a managed care system. Slowly, patients began to die mysteriously. Their deaths seem to follow a pattern of those who are the most costly in terms of health care and have the least chance of returning as healthy members of society. While this is a fictional mystery, it illuminates possible outcomes of a future managed healthcare system where costs determine patient outcomes.

John Q. (2002)

John Quincy Archibald's (Denzel Washington) son Michael collapses while playing baseball as a result of heart failure. John rushes Michael to a hospital emergency department, where he is informed that Michael's only hope is a transplant. Unfortunately, John's insurance will not cover his son's transplant. Out of options, John Q. takes the emergency department staff and patients hostage until hospital doctors agree to do the transplant. It offers an excellent examination and critical assessment of the "costs" of health care and determination of who has access to our latest technology.

Lorenzo's Oil (1992)

With this powerful 1992 drama, director–producer George Miller (*The Road Warrior*) proved that a movie about a disease does not have to be a typical disease-of-the-week movie. Based on the real-life case of the Odones family, the story concerns 5-year-old Lorenzo, suffering mightily from an apparently incurable and degenerative brain illness called A.L.D. His parents, an economist (Nick Nolte) and a linguist (Susan Sarandon), refuse to accept the received wisdom that there is no hope, and set about learning biochemistry to pursue a cure on their own. The film becomes an intriguing scientific mystery mixed with a story of pain, grief, and the strain on the two adults. Miller, a doctor himself, refuses to shrink from the chaos and horrors of a child's agony, and he and his wife spend their lives trying to find alternative cures, based on their knowledge of chemistry and diseases.

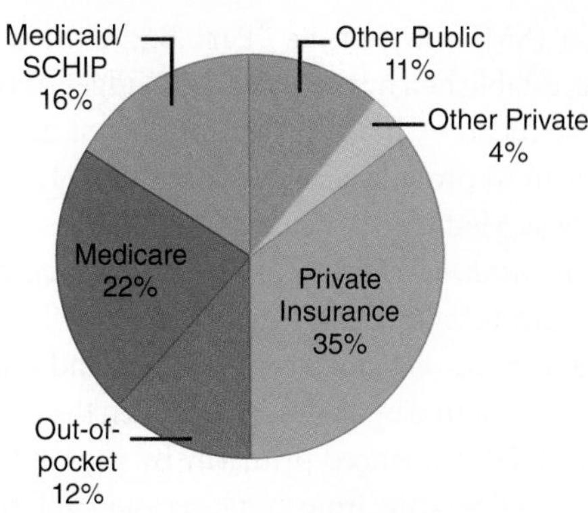

Figure 8-8 The nation's healthcare dollar: Where it came from (2012).

Source: Center for Medicare & Medicaid Services (CMS). (2013). National Healthcare Expenditures. Retrieved from http://www.cms.gov/Research-Statistics-Data-and-Systems/Statistics-Trends-and-Reports/NationalHealthExpendData/downloads/tables.pdf

Medicare

Title XVIII of the Social Security Act, entitled "Health Insurance for the Aged and Disabled," is commonly known as Medicare. Its beginning in 1966 was a historical benchmark. By giving health insurance to everyone older than 65 years of age who is covered by Social Security system entitlement, it signaled a giant step for government entry into personal healthcare financing. In 1973, other groups became eligible for benefits: persons entitled to Social Security or Railroad Retirement disability benefits for at least 24 months, persons with end-stage renal disease (ESRD) requiring continuing dialysis or kidney transplant, and certain otherwise noncovered persons who elect to buy into Medicare. The Health Care Financing Administration (HCFA) is responsible for overseeing the total program. Medicare covers approximately 50% of the medical expenses of the elderly (Lind/AARP, 2012).

Medicare consists of two parts, which differ in terms of their sources of funding and benefits: Hospital Insurance (HI), known as "Part A," and Supplementary Medical

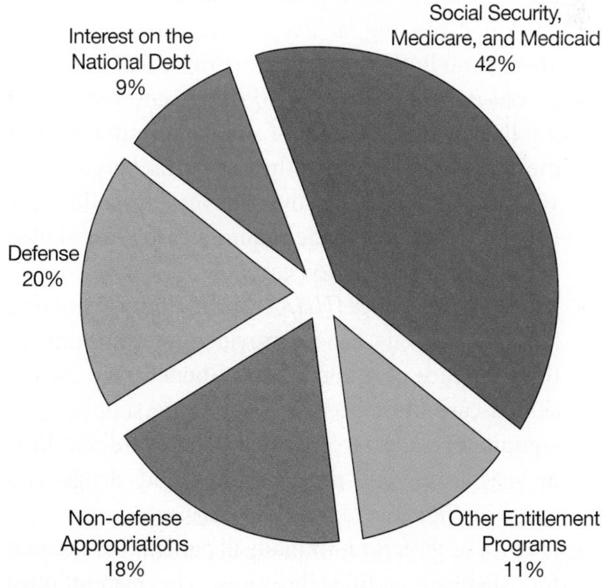

Figure 8-9

Source: Center on Budget and Policy Priorities.

Insurance (SMI), known as "Part B." A third part of Medicare, established by the Balanced Budget Act of 1997, was the Medicare+Choice program, known as "Part C," which began to provide services on January 1, 1998; it is now know as Medicare Advantage.

Hospital insurance, Part A, of Medicare is mandatory. It provides benefits for care provided in the hospital, outpatient diagnostic services, extended care facilities, and short-term care at home required by an illness for which the patient was hospitalized. HI is financed primarily by payroll taxes collected for Social Security from employees and self-employed workers. The tax is 1.45% of earnings paid by both employers and employees and 2.90% of earnings for self-employed persons. Prior to 1994, there was a ceiling on income taxed for Medicare, but the Omnibus Budget Reconciliation Act of 1993 (OBRA-93) made all earnings subject to Medicare tax. Part A HI has limits on care and requires deductibles and copayments based on the duration of services.

The following is an overview of the health benefits covered by Medicare's HI:

- *Inpatient hospital care* coverage includes a semi-private room, meals, regular nursing services, operating and recovery room, intensive care, inpatient prescription drugs, lab tests, x-rays, psychiatric hospital, inpatient rehabilitation, and long-term care hospitalization when medically necessary, as well as services and supplies used in the hospital. A maximum of 90 days is allowed per benefit period. Past the 90-days mark, there is a lifetime reserve of 60 inpatient days. A **benefit period** is an episode of illness starting with hospitalization and ending when the beneficiary has not been a patient in a hospital or skilled nursing facility for 60 consecutive days. There is no limit on the number of benefit periods.
- *Skilled nursing facility (SNF) care* is covered only if it follows within 30 days of a hospitalization of 3 or more days not including the day of discharge. Up to 100 days of care can be covered. Nursing facility care is not covered unless the required care is for skilled nursing or rehabilitation care.
- *Home health agency (HHA) care,* including care by a home health aide, can be provided intermittently in the residence of a home-bound beneficiary. Again, skilled care must be necessary. Some supplies and equipment may be provided. There are no time or visit limits. Full-time nursing, food, drugs, and blood are *not* covered as HHA services.
- *Hospice services* for terminally ill patients are covered for Medicare-certified hospices. The patient must have a life expectancy of less than 6 months and forgo benefits for traditional medical treatment for the terminal illness. Covered care includes pain relief, supportive medical and social services, physical therapy, nursing services, and symptom management.

Supplemental medical insurance, Part B, is available to almost all residents and certain aliens age 65 and older—even if not entitled to HI services; disabled persons who are eligible for HI are also covered by Part B. Coverage is voluntary and is financed by general tax revenues as well as a required monthly premium. Premiums are currently set at a level that covers 25% of the national expenditures for the aged beneficiaries. Although the majority of coverage goes to physician fees, SMI also covers many nonphysician services. To be covered, all services must either be medically necessary or be one of the prescribed preventive benefits (e.g., flu vaccinations). Special payment rules, including deductibles, maximum amounts payable, or higher cost sharing, apply to certain services and care. A yearly deductible and coinsurance of 20% of allowed charges are paid by the beneficiaries.

Medicare Advantage increases the managed care plans available to Medicare beneficiaries. Beneficiaries are given the option of a variety of risk-based plans, including coordinated care plans such as health maintenance organizations (HMOs), provider-sponsored organizations (PSOs), and preferred provider organizations (PPOs), as well as other approved alternatives to traditional Medicare. From the beginning of Medicare, alternative payment methodologies have existed for HMO-type providers. In 1995, less than 8% of the total Medicare population was enrolled in such plans. The goal has been to expand the number of managed care options and increase the number of contractors (Vladeck & King, 1997). Medicare Advantage offers beneficiaries a broad range of health plan options similar to those available in the private sector.

Market principles are evident in Medicare's performance as both a purchaser and a regulator of managed care. Beneficiaries are given information to allow them to compare their choices and make a selection based on individual preferences and market conditions. The Medicare Compare Database webpage, provided online by the Centers for Medicare & Medicaid Services (https://data.medicare.gov/), encourages Medicare consumers to "comparison shop" and offers beneficiaries the opportunity to check whether a provider is Medicare certified and what procedures and tests are covered under their plan.

Electing to participate in managed care plans may serve as an alternative to purchasing **Medigap insurance**, which is often desirable if the beneficiary has traditional fee-for-service coverage. Medicare can leave beneficiaries with substantial out-of-pocket costs. Because Part B excludes coverage for prescription drugs, glasses, dentures, hearing aids, yearly physical examinations, routine foot care, and dental care, many individuals supplement their Medicare benefits. Only 12% qualify for Medicaid to pick up these extra expenses, though some retirees have employer plans that cover extra expenses. The term "Medigap" is used to denote private health insurance that pays most of the healthcare service charges not covered by Parts A and B of Medicare. Such policies, which are offered by Blue Cross and Blue Shield and other commercial health insurance companies, must meet federal standards.

Methods of payment to providers of services for Medicare beneficiaries continue to change as cost-containment incentives are encouraged. Currently, hospitals are paid on a prospective payment system of fixed price per case for patients in diagnosis-related groups (DRGs).

Just as DRGs were implemented to contain hospital costs, **resource utilization groups, version 3** (RUG-III) were launched in July 1998 to contain costs in SNFs. They are designed to differentiate patients by their levels of resource use. Payment is made on a per diem rate that varies according to the RUG-III category. The goal is to relate pay to patient care requirements and to pay SNFs with different patient caseloads equitably (Shi & Singh, 2008). Likewise, HCFA has developed ambulatory patient groups (APGs) based on the same goals to be used in clinic settings. These have not been used in Medicare reimbursement yet, but some states have adopted the classification system for Medicaid programs (Shi & Singh, 2008).

Reimbursement for physicians prior to 1992 was for a "reasonable charge," which was the lowest of the actual charge, the customary charge, or the prevailing charge in the area. This has changed to payments based on lowest of submitted charges or a fee schedule based on a **relative value scale**. The relative values are based on the time, skill, and intensity it takes to perform a service. The scale places more value on care received through primary care physicians and emphasizes prevention and health promotion. Less value is placed on surgeries and high-technology use. Outpatient and home health services are currently reimbursed on a reasonable cost basis, but the 1997 Balanced Budget Act provided for implementing a prospective payment system for these services in the future. Claims for both HI and SMI are processed by nongovernment organizations that contract to serve as the fiscal agent between the federal government and providers. They function locally to apply coverage rules and are known as "intermediaries" and "carriers."

Medicaid

Because Americans contribute toward Medicare through taxes, it is considered an **entitlement** program due to them regardless of their wealth. Medicaid, however, is a **welfare** program, representing funds transferred from more economically affluent individuals to those in need.

Title XIX of the Social Security Act is a federal–state matching funds program with the intent to provide basic healthcare services to the economically indigent. The federal government provides matching funds based on the per capita income of each state. By law it cannot be more than 83% or less than 50% matching funds. There is no set limit on total federal outlays.

Within broad national guidelines that the federal government provides, each state: (1) establishes its own Medicaid eligibility standards; (2) determines the type, amount, duration, and scope of services; (3) sets the rate of payment for services; and (4) administers its own program. Policies vary greatly from state to state; thus a person who is eligible for Medicaid in one state may not be eligible in another state. In addition, eligibility and services in a state can change during a year.

The broad federal guidelines include certain mandated coverage as part of Medicaid. These include inpatient and outpatient hospital services, skilled nursing care, physician services, home health care, family planning services, and early and periodic screening, diagnosis, and treatment services for eligible children younger than age 26.

Recipients must establish their eligibility for Medicaid based on income and assets. In 2012, more than 72 million individuals were provided healthcare assistance, with a cost to the federal government of $435 billion. The Children's Health Improvement Program (CHIP) program (described in the next section) supported healthcare for 8.4 million children in 2012, costing an additional $12.2 billion (MACPAC, 2013).

The Medicaid program provides services to two broad groups of persons: the categorically needy and the medically needy. For the **categorically needy**, federal funds are matched for mandatory eligibility groups. These would include people receiving Supplemental Security Income (SSI) in some states; those who meet the requirements for the Aid to Families with Dependent Children (AFDC) that were in effect in their state prior to July 16, 1996; children younger than age 6 and pregnant women whose family income is below 133% of the FPL; and all children who are younger than age 19 in families with income at or below the FPL (the CHIP program also offers free or low-cost coverage for families with income in a range above the FPL based on family size). States also have the option of providing coverage to specified other categorically related groups and receive matching federal funds. One of these is the **medically needy**—persons who incur medical expenses beyond the scope of their income.

In 1996, the Personal Responsibility and Work Opportunity Act made sweeping welfare reforms that have had consequences for the Medicaid program. Changes in eligibility for SSI also had an impact. For aliens who lost SSI, Medicaid can continue only if they qualify under some other eligibility status. The new legislation ended the original foundation of the welfare system, Aid to Families with Dependent Children, and replaced it with Temporary Assistance for Needy Families (TANF). TANF is a block-grant program that limits lifetime cash welfare benefits to 5 years (or less at a state's option). Welfare funds are no longer unconditionally guaranteed to eligible poor families, but states are allowed to impose a wide range of other restrictions as well. For example, if recipients are not involved in work-related activities by the end of their second year on welfare, they must forfeit future benefits. Single mothers have an automatic 25% reduction in benefits if they refuse to help establish paternity of their children. Of significance for Medicaid was the delinkage of its benefits from welfare cash assistance. The law does not require persons covered by TANF to receive Medicaid. Because Medicaid eligibility is not linked to welfare, it is necessary to reach needy families and children who are outside of, as well as in, the welfare system to ensure as many children and families as possible obtain health insurance coverage.

Following the initiation of TANF, some states saw a drastic reduction in the number of children enrolled in Medicaid. Many believed that families were losing Medicaid as they transitioned off of welfare (Mississippi Health Advocacy Program, 1998). Guidelines for protecting and expanding health coverage in the post–welfare reform world have been developed by the Health Care Financing Administration (U.S. Department of Health and Human Services, 2008).

Other developments in Medicaid services are related to long-term nursing home care. Increasing numbers of elderly, in addition to the excessively high expense of long-term care institutions and home-based care, led to an increasing number of people becoming newly eligible for Medicaid coverage. Many with modest resources rapidly use them up in paying for nursing homes or home care. Nursing home expenses were just under $75,000 per year for a private room in 2007 (Genworth Financial, Inc., & National Eldercare Referral Systems, Inc., 2007). Middle-class individuals paying these costs quickly become medically needy and meet state guidelines for Medicaid. With Medicare coverage limited to only 3 months and little use of private insurance for nursing home coverage, Medicaid currently funds approximately half of annual nursing home care expenditures. Out-of-pocket payments make up the next largest percentage of funds. Very small shares of both institutional and home-bound long-term care services are paid by private insurance. Insurance for long-term care has been difficult to market. Younger, healthier groups whose enrollment would spread the risk and costs generally do not enroll. Therefore, long-term care insurance rates stay high and policies cover only a portion of expenses. Long-term care is expected to be an increasingly utilized provision of Medicaid, with efforts being focused on more community-based long-term care alternatives (Shi & Singh, 2008; Sultz & Young, 2014; Waid, 1998).

Reimbursement under Medicaid is made directly to providers. Rate-setting formulas, procedures, and policies vary widely among states. Fee-for-service systems of payment have dominated. However, federal waivers allow states to develop innovative delivery or reimbursement systems. The last few years have seen a growth in enrollment of Medicaid beneficiaries in managed care, from 56.72% of beneficiaries in 2000 to 65.4% in 2006. As with Medicare, public policymakers have been eager to realize the cost savings reported by private buyers of managed healthcare services. Competitive bidding strategies allow bids to be made by provider plans. Several states have converted their entire Medicaid programs into managed care.

Children's Health Insurance Program

One program initiated by the Balanced Budget Act of 1997 and reauthorized in 2009 is known as the Children's Health Insurance Program (CHIP). CHIP provided federal funds for states to expand Medicaid eligibility to include more uninsured children. These mostly low-income children could not qualify for Medicaid, yet their families could not afford private insurance.

Coverage could be provided by states through a Medicaid expansion, separate CHIP program, or a combination. Under a separate CHIP program, states could establish more flexible eligibility requirements. In some cases, states chose to implement coverage for low-income families—not just children—under CHIP. Also, eligibility for coverage could be expanded up to 200% of the poverty level. As with Medicare and Medicaid, managed care options were being offered.

CHAMPUS and Other Public Direct Care Programs

Another category of persons who have publicly funded healthcare insurance comprises military personnel and dependents. The Military Health Services System, funded under the Department of Defense, operates to provide medical services to active and retired members of the armed forces and their dependents. Care is provided through military facilities including hospitals and clinics and is supplemented by services purchased from civilian systems and paid for by the Civilian Health and Medical Program of the Uniformed Services (CHAMPUS). Services are free at military facilities; however, when care is received from civilian providers who are paid through CHAMPUS, there is cost sharing (deductibles and coinsurance) by the families. CHAMPUS does not cover active-duty service members (who receive all their care from the military facilities)—only retirees and dependents.

Linked to the military healthcare system is the Veterans Administration (VA) healthcare system. Through this system, the federal government acts as a direct supplier of services to veterans for war-related injuries and disabilities. For poor service personnel, care is also given for illness that is not related to military service.

The federal government is also involved in direct care to Native Americans living on reservations. The IHS provides inpatient and ambulatory clinic services through hospitals, health clinics, and ambulatory clinic facilities. These facilities operate at the local level to serve more than 1 million Native Americans. In 1976, tribal governments were granted authority to operate IHS facilities, which are often in remote areas and have low volume. The recent trend has been to refer and contract with private providers for specialty care and diagnostic services.

Other Public Sources of Healthcare Funding

The government funds numerous health programs for specific populations and specific health problems. Many of these have come about through amendments to the Public Health Service Act of 1994. The programs in place at most local health departments come from this funding and assist vulnerable at-risk groups. These programs cover immunizations, tuberculosis, venereal diseases, and family planning along with other services. Rural health clinics, migrant health clinics, and community health centers also are publicly funded. Community health centers operate with 28% of their funds authorized from the Public Health Service Act. These clinics, which pioneered the employment of nurse practitioners, serve as the primary safety net for the poor and underserved in both rural and inner-city settings (Shi & Singh, 2008).

Cost Containment, Cost Analysis, and Quality

Costs must be contained for the public to get maximum returns on prepaid private insurance, employer-sponsored insurance, and taxes paid toward healthcare programs. The maze of interconnecting factors related to the causes of high and rising healthcare costs, of course, guide the mechanisms chosen for controlling them. Mechanisms for **cost containment** include policy decisions at federal, state, local, and organizational levels. The forces influencing how these decisions are made are complex. Reform proposals show the policymakers' quandary in trying to rectify the cost and quality problems of the U.S. system. Proposals are for either total or incremental system changes or for changes in the financing of health care.

As has been pointed out earlier, economic trends related to costs in the last few years have so far shown results that encourage the strategy of market competition (although predictions of ability to sustain the trends vary). To quote a health services researcher, "The effects of what is now referred to as 'market driven' reform being played out through the proliferation and increasing gains by managed care in controlling costs are pervasively evident throughout virtually every component of the delivery system" (Sultz & Young, 2014). The managed care solution in relation to prevention and cost control is discussed later in the chapter.

Both regulatory and competitive strategies to control costs have been mentioned throughout the previous discussion in this chapter. **Box 8-2** summarizes some of the methods of these two strategies. One economic strategy that has become increasingly important for nurses and other providers is economic evaluation, which contributes to finding the most cost-effective ways of delivering care and treatments. At the level of practice guidelines and social policy, economic evaluation is essential. Economic evaluation can be used to help in resource allocation in

BOX 8-2 Cost-Containment Strategies

Controlling quantity of supply

- Incentives to decrease numbers of specialist physicians
- Certificate of need to limit technology duplication

Controlling price

- Reimbursement for lower cost providers such as nurse practitioners
- Reimbursement for:
  —DRGs: diagnosis-related groups
  —RBRVU: resource-based relative value units
  —APGs: ambulatory patient groups
  —RUGs: resource utilization groups

Controlling quantity of demand

- Patient cost sharing:
  —Increased proportion of premiums
  —Copayments
  —Deductibles
- Managed care to provide only necessary and appropriate services

Competition

- Insurers to shop for best benefit plans
- Managed care plans to shop for best provider contracts

Prioritizing through cost analysis

- Focus on prevention
- Reduced inefficiency of interventions

delivery of nursing care and to improve the overall quality of clinical care (Spetz, 2005; Stone, 1998).

Where once the focus of health decision making was only on the effectiveness of treatments and interventions, under competition providers are now competing for contracts with consumers. Consumers look around and make choices based on information about price, quality indicators, and levels of users' satisfaction. Insurers want to know which services to cover and how much to cover. Those who pay often make the treatment decisions. Policymakers want to know how to control public expenditures. Cost-evaluation assessments can be expensive, but, for stakeholders, competition provides the incentive to invest in the needed cost-effectiveness and quality outcomes data they provide. The data are used for internal decisions and now more and more often for letting potential buyers know about the "product" they are buying for "marketing" purposes.

To focus on quality and include cost in the analysis, a number of analytic techniques exist. These include cost-of-illness analysis, cost–benefit analysis, and cost-effectiveness analysis.

Cost-of-illness analysis estimates the total monetary effects of a specific disease or condition. It takes into account all the resources used to diagnose, treat, and cope with the illness (Max, 1997).

Cost–benefit analysis (CBA) uses such measures to compare benefits, in terms of disease prevention, with the costs of a program. In this technique, benefits are measured in monetary terms. CBA is the principal method used to evaluate decisions involving public expenditures. Decisions are based on alternatives providing the greatest net benefit, that is, the greatest level of economic efficiency (Moore, Laufer, & Conroy, 1998).

The Research Alert is an example of a cost–benefit study. The drawback of using this method to analyze health care is the difficulty of placing a dollar value on outcomes such as pain or grief or premature loss of life. The methods for determining such costs are developed in economics but are controversial (Thompson, 2003).

Cost-effectiveness analysis (CEA), sometimes considered a more acceptable healthcare valuation alternative, calculates a ratio in which health outcome is measured in health units, such as cases avoided or years of life saved. Cost of treatment or intervention is measured in dollars. Thus results are presented in terms of "cost per case prevented" or "cost per life saved." The purpose of CEA is to compare the relative value of different interventions in creating better health and/or longer life. Costs of alternative programs are compared based on a single nonmonetary outcome. CEA furnishes information that is useful in a variety of settings. In a managed care setting, an organization may wish to know the cost savings per low-birth-weight birth avoided as a consequence of a prenatal care outreach program. In addition, the organization could ask the cost of the program per year of life saved for its enrolled population. Analysis for a state health department might look at different strategies to control tuberculosis in the population. It could compare the cost-effectiveness of screening all community members versus screening only those at high risk based on history and exposure. In a larger context, the department might evaluate the costs per case of high blood lead level avoided as a result of an educational program aimed at housing repair to reduce dust and peeling paint.

RESEARCH ALERT

This study analyzed data to determine the cost-effectiveness of public nutrition education programs. Using program demographics and food-related dietary behaviors from participants in California's Expanded Food and Nutrition Education Program (EFNEP), researchers calculated benefit–cost ratios for the programs. EFNEP programs teach low-income families the basics of eating a balanced, nutritious diet, including how to shop for and prepare nutritious foods. The programs encourage increased consumption of fruits and vegetables, decreased consumption of fatty foods, and improved food safety and preparation. The long-term goal is to reduce the risk of chronic diseases and improve participants' health. To ensure continued funding, it is important to document the cost-effectiveness of EFNEP programs.

Researchers measured economic value "by comparing benefits (monetized in terms of decreased medical treatment costs) with costs (actual nutrition education expenses over a set time)." In addition to a list of program benefits and costs associated with EFNEP, the researchers assumed that there is a link between diet and chronic disease, they used a formula to quantify that relationship, and they calculated direct benefits as the money saved if treatment for a disease or condition could be prevented or delayed for 5 years. The initial benefit–cost ratio for California was 14.67 to 1.00, which means that for every $1.00 spent on EFNEP, $14.67 was saved in future medical costs. After performing sensitivity analyses to analyze the effects of changes in key variables, researchers found benefit–cost ratios ranging from 3.67 to 1.00, to 8.34 to 1.00, which means that for every $1.00 spent on nutrition education in California, $3.67 to $8.34 is saved.

Source: Joy, AB, Pradhan, V, Goldman, GE. 2006. Cost-benefit analysis conducted for nutrition education in California. Calif Agr 60:185-191. doi:10.3733/ca.v060n04p185

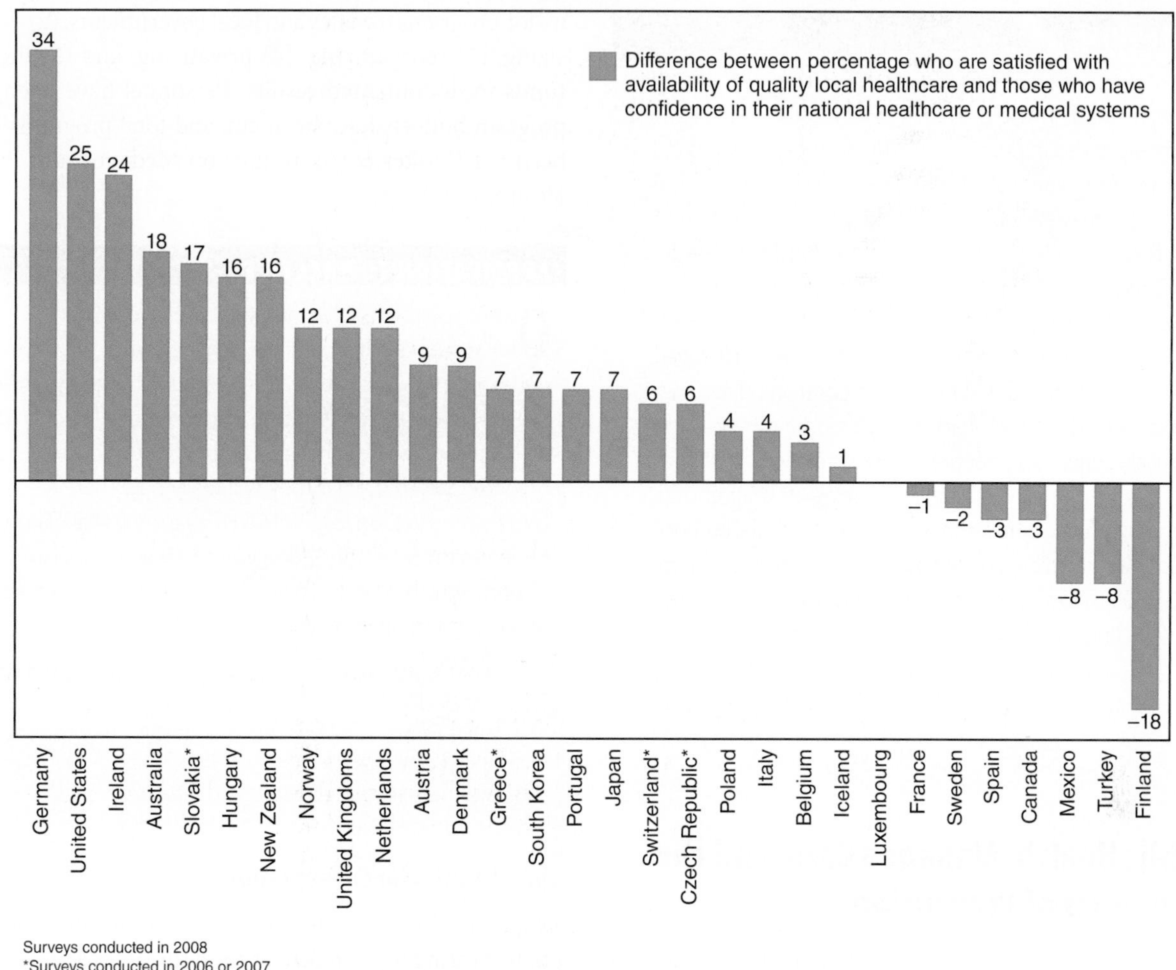

Figure 8-10 Differences in perceptions of local vs. national health care among OECD countries.

Source: http://www.gallup.com/poll/122393/oecd-countries-universal-healthcare-gets-high-marks.aspx

One other area in which cost–benefit and cost-effectiveness analyses are used is in the broader field of technology assessment. **Technology assessment**, a form of policy research, helps decision makers to deal with developing and using expensive healthcare practices and technologies. It is assessment that includes both cost–benefit analysis and outcome effectiveness analysis. In addition, it analyzes safety and social impact of technologies (Thompson, 2003).

CEA assists in setting priorities for the use of scarce resources. For instance, research was done on whether primary prevention by testing all individuals at age 30 for infection with *H. pylori*—a bacterial pathogen linked to gastric cancer—and treating those who tested positive was more cost effective than annual screening for individuals over the age of 50 who were considered high risk for gastric cancer (secondary prevention). While both methodologies produced cost savings in that they helped to reduce incidence of late-stage cancer diagnosis, which is generally considerably more expensive to treat and produces poorer outcomes, early eradication proved the more cost-effective method. However, once a patient reached the age of 45, the test-and-treat regimen did not seem any more effective, in terms either of cost or of preventive efficacy, than the surveillance method (Lee et al., 2007). Thus, while it may be worthwhile to channel resources into test-and-treat prevention for younger adults, annual screening based on risk factors is probably more beneficial, both in terms of cost and health, for reducing the costs of gastric cancer in individuals over 45.

Even though the influence of CEA on policy is not well documented, it is believed to have played a key role in some major decisions. Medicare's first preventive service—coverage of pneumococcal vaccine—was based on a CEA done by the Office of Technology Assessment. Cancer screening recommendations of the American Cancer Society are also based on CEA studies (Buerhaus, 1998; Gold, Siegel, Russell, & Weinstein, 1996).

NOTE THIS!

Contraceptives are cost-effective: For every $1 of public health funds invested in family planning, $4 to $14 of public funds are saved in pregnancy- and healthcare-related costs.

The vast majority of private insurers covers prescription drugs, but may exclude coverage for prescription contraceptives. Similarly, most policies cover outpatient medical services but often exclude outpatient contraceptive services for coverage.

Health insurance companies are more likely to cover sterilization or abortion services than contraceptives. This indicates the insurance community's tendency to pay for surgical services and not preventive care.

The Institute of Medicine Committee on Unintended Pregnancy recently recommended that "financial barriers to contraception be reduced by increasing the proportion of all health insurance policies that offer contraceptive services and supplies."

Source: American Public Health Association. (1998). Fact sheet: Prescription contraceptive equity. Retrieved from http://www.apha.org

Public Health, Managed Care, and the Economics of Prevention

The current economic environment has had consequences for the public health sector, which, following the attacks of September 11, 2001, and the ravages of Hurricane Katrina, has found "itself again at center stage, with the spotlights focused on its performance" (Beitsch, Brooks, Menachemi, & Libbey, 2006). Along with market forces playing a greater role in the total healthcare system, there has been a redefinition of government role. Even though government is a key instrument in community action, taxpayers appear unwilling to pay more money for publicly funded health programs (Appleby, 2006; Lasker & Committee on Medicine and Public Health, 1997). With costs rising, a tightening of public funds is the result. Although public health added new roles and responsibilities for responding to disasters, both human-made (September 11 attacks, bioterrorism) and natural (Hurricanes Katrina and Rita), and to emerging infectious diseases (avian flu and severe acute respiratory syndrome), funding for public health has not increased and is very limited in contrast to financial support for the private healthcare system (Beitsch et al., 2006). Tightening of funds threatens support for all of the health system's public goods: research, education of health professionals, population-based programs, and safety-net care for the uninsured and underinsured. Five mechanisms for federal cost cutting have been (1) moving authority and monetary responsibility for programs to states and local governments, (2) downsizing, (3) reorganizing, (4) privatizing, and (5) linking funds to documented results. Personnel have been cut, program budgets have been cut, and total programs have been cut (Lasker & Committee on Medicine and Public Health, 1997).

APPLICATION TO PRACTICE 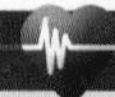

One of your patients at the clinic where you work comes in for a routine visit regarding her hypertension. In the midst of her visit, she tells you, "I am so confused. I have to make a decision about which Medicare plan to choose. I've only been on Medicare for 2 years and I've just begun to understand how it works and what they will really pay. There are gaps, but it is pretty good for me. Now they tell me I have a choice of changing plans. But I don't know what to do. How can I decide which is best for me? Surely you know more about these things than I do. What should I do?"

1. What is your role in such a situation? How would you respond?
2. What might you consider in educating this patient about care plans?
3. Are there resources you could refer her to?

Opportunities for Collaboration

In spite of the concerns about the cost-cutting effects on public health program delivery and threats of an **imperfect market** of privatized managed care, there are reasons for community health nurses to be encouraged by the rapid growth of managed care. One of the commonalities among all the payers of healthcare services has been cost-containment efforts through increased enrollment of their beneficiaries in managed care plans. The federal government has signed waivers to allow states to enroll Medicaid recipients in managed care plans; more than 74% of Medicaid beneficiaries receive healthcare services through managed care (Centers for Medicare & Medicaid Services, 2011). As of 2013, enrollment of Medicare beneficiaries in managed care was about 26% nationwide, although the percentage in each state varied considerably from one state to the next (Kaiser Family Foundation, 2013c); the effects of the 2010 ACA on both these figures have yet to be seen. Enrollment is encouraged and steadily increasing for employee-sponsored insurance as well. The positive element is the population orientation of managed care and the potential it has to strengthen public health efforts. Managed care links both the insurance and the delivery of services by paying care providers a set amount for all the services of their insured population. Thus, the care providers share the financial risk of the enrolled population's health status. The incentive is to keep the population healthy.

Managed care organizations providing health care become linked in two ways to public health efforts. First, they share the interest in using population-based methods of epidemiology to study, track, and understand their enrolled populations and to keep those populations healthy. Second, to keep their enrolled populations healthy, they are aware of the benefits of collaboration in the wider public health efforts that focus on preventing illness for the total population. Their enrolled populations are a part of the total population, of course. The total population achieves better outcomes with environmental protections, greater health awareness, early detection of disease, and improved health behavior. If the total population remains or becomes healthier, their enrolled populations do the same and the managed care organizations realize the benefits of decreased use of expensive services for preventable illnesses. Plans that can improve population health will control their costs and, therefore, will have a major advantage in a competitive market.

Prior to managed care, the influence and prestige of healthcare professionals outside of public health disciplines did not guide public opinion or government action toward prevention and health. The emphasis on cure of diseases over which there was more biological control left social and behavioral issues of health—such as drugs, alcohol, cigarettes, AIDS, and violence—with less attention and less funding. As noted earlier, a very small percentage of the U.S. national healthcare expenditures goes to public health activity (slightly more than 3%). The cost-effective methods of prevention and public health have not been recognized or valued by most individuals, groups, and governments in the United States. The more cost-effective prevention strategies are less dramatic. As Sultz and Young (2014) observe, "Unlike the recipients of heart transplants, … the media cannot show pictures of the hundreds of thousands of children who have *not* been crippled and have *not* died due to poliomyelitis since the successful programs have been initiated."

The shift in incentive from acute services as profitable to disease prevention as profitable is changing both who provides care and how care is provided (Shi & Singh, 2008). In contrast to most indemnity plans of insurance, managed care plans and providers are increasing preventive services such as screening, immunizations, and counseling for high-risk conditions. They encourage preventive services by increasing access to primary care providers. By making the providers accountable to the populations they care for and linking reimbursement for prevention to attaining certain goals, managed care methods could enhance the delivery of preventive services. If organized managed care plans, especially those enrolling public beneficiaries such as Medicaid, assume the services that have been offered by state and local health departments and publicly financed community health centers, these public services are affected. By losing Medicaid and other primary care patients to managed care plans, they must deal with shrinking budgets. Community health centers have reacted to competition by forming health plans of their own (Shi & Singh, 2008). Public health agencies are regrouping and devoting their resources to the core public health functions. If they are no longer competing for clinical patients and payments, they can focus on surveillance, community-wide interventions, and ensuring and enhancing access (Robbins & Freeman, 1999).

Some see these changes as encouraging and an imperative for collaboration and cooperation through partnerships between managed care organizations and public health agencies. The CDC has brought together members of the public health and managed care sectors at national conferences that focus on prevention (CDC, 1995). In addition, the CDC has formed partnerships with the American Association of Health Plans and The HMO Group, which have encouraged the managed care community to become involved in public health and preventive measures (Schauffler & Scutchfield, 1998).

The Committee on Medicine and Public Health reported on its mission and initiatives to join medical care and public health care (Lasker & Committee on Medicine and Public Health, 1997). Through this work, which was funded by both private and public funds, the committee examined 414 examples of collaborative efforts. They described the projects and indicated how the collaborative work was done. Benefits accrued to both health sectors: Public health agencies gained from the prevention efforts of managed care organizations, and the organizations benefited from the expertise of public health practitioners.

Managed care organizations are learning to conduct health assessments of the communities they serve and to identify areas where they can have a large influence on improving the communities' health (Shi & Singh, 2008). The collection and analysis of population-based data are the skills of public health that make collaboration welcome. Robbins and Freeman (1999), for example, have reported on a New England joint venture between the not-for-profit managed care organizations of the six states and those states' public health services. The goals these parties believe will be achieved are improved health and efficiency that reduce healthcare costs and, therefore, an increase in the political resolve to provide coverage for everyone.

Counterforces to Collaboration

The opportunities are not without problems, however, and the interface of public health with the new organized systems for delivering clinical care is evolving. One pressing issue is this: Who will care for the individuals who remain uninsured? Even with policy efforts to increase coverage for all, and especially for children, there still is not access for all. If health departments are expected to be the safety net, then they must be funded to do so. With Medicaid patients moving to managed care plans, public health can no longer cross-subsidize uninsured primary and preventive care with Medicaid funds.

Another issue for health departments is the "dumping" of services covered by private managed care plans. Plans may cover immunizations in their capitated fee, yet still send their enrollees to a health department for immunizations without reimbursing the department.

Coordination of state reporting for notifiable diseases, directly observed therapy, and sexually transmitted contact tracing may also be problematic, with managed care organizations seeing patients formerly seen by public health departments. Health departments must be able to obtain such patient enrollment and encounter information for surveillance and epidemiological studies. Clarification of these and other roles and responsibilities must be addressed in the midst of the new forces at work in the total system (Rosenbaum & Richards, 1996; Schauffler & Scutchfield, 1998).

Another barrier to collaboration is the nature of for-profit firms. Nonprofit providers are converting to for-profit organizations at an increasing rate. When accountability to their stockholders is their top priority, their motivation is naturally to seek short-term advantages that lead to a positive bottom line. An advantage could be realized in the short term by cutting preventive measures and increasing profits. Many know that their enrollees may change plans often and will not remain their financial responsibility if illness occurs in the future (Mechanic, 1998). Profit maximization can be socially undesirable when it leads to product quality effects. Clearly, withholding preventive services has an effect on individuals and on the larger public. The public has loudly criticized these and other business practices for decades: They want for-profit plans in health care to be accountable for the social responsiveness and social trust that any course in business ethics would encourage (Arrow, 1997; Porter, 2013).

RESEARCH ALERT

In recent decades, reductions in postpartum length of stay have been attempted in an effort to lower costly stays for newborns and their mothers. In spite of legislation and provider recommendations, many infants are discharged in less than 48 hours and do not have the recommended pediatrician-initiated reassessment within 48 hours of discharge. While such practices impact all newborns, they have a particularly significant impact on low-income families and are one factor in the United States' ranking as the industrialized nation with the highest infant mortality.

The Nurse–Family Partnership (NFP) began as a project seeking to identify whether adding nurse visits to postpartum mothers could improve outcomes in a cost-effective manner. It developed a program targeting low-income families with a focus on behavior modification to reduce or incentivize behaviors that affect infant mortality and morbidity, such as maternal or household smoking, parental substance abuse, immunizations, breastfeeding, and nutrition (Miller, 2012). Test projects in Elmira, NY; Memphis, TN; and Denver, CO proved successful and the program expanded.

In 2012, the Pew Charitable Trust commissioned a study to assess the effectiveness of the program from both a cost and efficacy perspective. This study analyzed costs, life status outcomes, functional outcomes, and return on investment in NFP services. It used those estimates to create an online, state-specific financial planning tool to allow states and communities to analyze the economics when deciding whether to invest in NFP activities.

The findings showed significant savings could be obtained by investing in nursing visits:

> NFP offers a mother lode of Medicaid savings. It reduces Medicaid spending on a first-born by 12%, yielding Medicaid savings of $20,003 per family served. If Medicaid fully funds the program, it recoups its costs before the child reaches age 5 and recoups 2.3 times its costs by the child's 18th birthday. NFP also reduces food stamp spending by 9% and TANF spending by 7%. Adding its reductions in special education, Child Protective Services, and criminal justice costs, total government savings are nearly $37,000 per family served. Thus, public NFP funding is a wise investment.
>
> NFP's cost-saving benefits are secondary to its effect on families. NFP lets first-borns with low-income parents get a safe and healthy start on life. It improves language development. It reduces crime, substance abuse, child maltreatment, preterm births, associated special needs, and infant mortality. Those life-changing benefits are the reason Medicaid, government, and society save money.

Source: Miller, T. R. (2012). *Executive Summary: Nurse-Family Partnership home visitation: Costs, outcomes, and return on investment.* Pew Charitable Trusts. Retrieved from http://www.pewstates.org/uploadedFiles/PCS_Assets/2013/Costs_and_ROI_executive_summary.pdf

Economics of Alternative Therapies

Among the many changes driven by economics that are important to community health nursing has been the increased acceptance of alternative therapies. Insurance plans and managed care organizations, driven by consumer demand and searching for lower cost services for their populations, have discovered alternative care methods. The economic impact of alternative care was realized with the publication of the landmark study by Eisenberg. Although this study included only 1,539 individuals, extrapolation of its results to the larger population indicated that more visits were made to alternative providers than to conventional primary care providers; $13.7 billion was spent, mostly out of pocket; and dollars spent exceeded out-of-pocket costs for hospitalization (Weeks, 1997). These numbers indicated a potential market for insurers and managed care.

In their quest to realize economic benefits, health plans have begun to include alternative therapy providers and treatment modalities in their plans. Alternative therapies most often are focused on holistic, wellness approaches that realize the benefits of prevention. Surveys of patients of alternative providers show that there are effects on use of conventional pharmaceuticals, necessity of conventional surgeries, development of self-care abilities, and reduced visits to conventional physicians after self-care education (Weeks, 1997). Providing a popular source of care in their plans may be a strategy by which managed care organizations can achieve multiple goals: increase market share by meeting a consumer demand, realize the cost savings of less technologically advanced treatments for illnesses, and use less services due to increased wellness. There are also possibilities for linkages and collaboration with public health in including alternative approaches to health. In Washington, for example, an integrated natural medicine/conventional medicine clinic is offered as a part of county services and it may be expanded. Other states are also interested in setting up such clinics (Weeks, 1997). Washington was also the first state to mandate health plan coverage of the full range of state-licensed providers such as naturopaths, acupuncturists, and chiropractors (Hamilton, 1996).

Plans that are beginning to create benefit packages for people interested in alternative care cover such alternatives as chiropractors, naturopaths, reflexology, rolfing, herbs, acupuncture, clinical nutritionists, massage, yoga, biofeedback, and chelation, among others (Hamilton, 1996; Weeks, 1997). For managed care organizations, these practices raise issues related to safety and efficacy documentation, which is not available in most cases.

Significance of Economics for Community Health Nursing Practice

Throughout this chapter, we have examined the implications of economics for the individuals, families, and communities for whom nurses care. It is easy to become immersed in the immediacy of individual nursing roles and remain unaware of the outside forces affecting practice. Today, economics—even more than social and political demands—drives our practice and the results for patients. Who gets seen? What treatment can they get? Who will treat them? What will the setting be? Who will you work with? Who will pay you? How will the ACA of 2010 affect the healthcare system? The answers to all these questions are influenced by economic considerations of financing of health and welfare services, reimbursement rates, insurance mechanisms, and means of delivery. In many ways, today's environment is favorable for community nurses as care continues to move into more cost-effective sites in the community, population-focused skills are needed, and disease prevention/health promotion is needed. Following are just some of the other implications for current practice in a rapidly changing environment.

Perhaps one of the most valuable interactions with patients is to address their needs as consumers in consumer-driven health care. As indicated earlier, informed consumers are vital for a market to work at its best. They need education, advocacy, and assistance. Beyond educating patients about their health or illness needs, nurses need to educate them for informed choices about their care. Even though Medicare covers screening mammograms, one in three women insured by Medicare did not receive a mammogram between 2004 and 2005 (Arvantes, 2008). Patients need assistance to increase their self-care knowledge, reinforce effective self-care, and partner with health providers. Nurses can reinforce the trend for consumers to be active and more informed about their healthcare options, including alternative therapies. As baby boomers enter the ranks of seniors, they are expected to use the Internet more than current seniors to access healthcare information (Gell, Rosenberg, Demiris, LaCroix, & Patel, 2013; Kaiser Family Foundation, 2005).

Importantly, in a consumer-driven health system, nurses can help consumers understand price, quality issues, and more. Educating and informing healthcare consumers about such things as discovering treatment options, reading quality reports, navigating complicated health plans, understanding payment systems, dealing with restrictions, and finding the service amenities they want will enable them to make market comparisons and choices. In addition to educating them to meet their own needs, consumers need "trusted partners to act as their agents" (Scandlen, 2005, p. 1557) in referrals to innovative providers, advocacy in appeals processes, and good documentation to ensure reimbursement.

When considering consumers in the marketplace, there are also opportunities as a nurse provider to inform health plan purchasers about the needs of their populations and how best to meet them. Employer health plans have tended to look only at cost and not consider quality in making plan decisions (Dentzer, 1998). Nurses have knowledge about quality and can purposefully encourage quality choices.

There are dynamic changes occurring in the nursing labor market. Reimbursement patterns and cost control have been the driving forces that moved jobs into the community setting, sought to replace or substitute nurses with cheaper labor sources, and are creating new roles. Demand management through telephone triage positions staffed by nurses eliminates unnecessary visits to clinics and emergency rooms (Larson-Dahn, 1998). In market settings, positions such as case manager, risk manager, provider liaison, benefits coordinator, utilization review coordinator, quality assurance coordinator, and positions utilizing population assessment skills are needed. There are new opportunities in prevention counseling services, and adding alternative therapies to practice options is encouraged by reimbursement trends.

Perhaps one of the most important labor market changes for nurses was gaining third-party reimbursement for advanced practice nurses (American Nurses Association, 1997). There had been reimbursement in specific rural areas, but the Balanced Budget Act of 1997 gave Medicare coverage to nurse practitioners and clinical nurse specialists for any service that would be covered under Medicare Part B when provided by a physician, regardless of geographic area. Nurses' reimbursement is capped at 80% of the physician rate. Direct reimbursement removed some of the barriers to entering the market, and the lower price for services made nurses more competitive. However, there are still significant labor market barriers including, for example, insurance companies that require billing under a physician's name or will credential only nurse practitioners employed by a physician and Medicare managed care organizations that will not allow nurse practitioners to be primary care providers. Free labor market competition for nurse providers still needs improvement (Ashby, 2006).

Community health nurses can optimize patient care by using economic information in coalition building, research, lobbying, negotiating with insurers, and influencing policy on healthcare allocation. In speaking the language of the marketplace, nurses can be more persuasive by having a broadly accepted reference point. In policy issues, nurses need to continually evaluate new or needed legislation that will affect patient care as well as themselves as consumers or providers. For example, mandatory overtime for nursing staff has become an unwelcome solution to the unmet labor market demand for nursing staff. The American Nurses Association has stated its support for legislation that limits mandatory overtime to 12 hours per 24-hour period and acknowledges that staffing concerns extend beyond acute care to community nursing as well (American Nurses Association, 2007).

Nurses can also participate in collecting, analyzing, and interpreting data for policy decisions. Spetz (2005) claims that the agenda for nursing research on cost-effectiveness is daunting. However, understanding economic evaluation methods such as CEA adds to nurses' ability to explain the value-added contribution of nursing services. As a necessary adjunct to evidence-based practice, CEA techniques have the potential to refine practice and lead to nursing interventions that utilize scarce resources for the best return in terms of health (Stone, Curran, & Bakken, 2002). Measures of effectiveness alone are not sufficient for ensuring the appropriateness or feasibility of interventions for specific settings or populations (Fielding & Briss, 2006; Siegel, 1998).

The Affordable Care Act

The goal of the **Affordable Care Act (ACA) of 2010** was not to remake the U.S. healthcare system (like the Clinton health reform bill proposed in the 1990s), but to build on top of the present system (Altman & Shactman, 2011). This process required frequent discussions with industry lobbyists and interest groups to get them to support the bill. The ACA continues to rely upon the existing employer-sponsored insurance system. Rather than mandating employers, the ACA instead charges a penalty fee to firms with more than 50 full-time employees who do not provide insurance, exempting those with less than 50 employees, and provides subsidies to those that choose to participate. The tax credits will be as high as 50% for firms that meet certain qualifications. Many fear that this will reduce the incentive for small businesses to expand, or result in the closure of firms over 50 full-time employees who are mandated to provide insurance but do not have the ability to pay the increased costs. Like the 2003 Medicare Prescription Drug, Improvement, and Modernization Act (MMA), the Affordable Care Act (2010) barely passed through Congress and created many fears of rising budget deficits.

As shown in **Figure 8-11**, the projections of the cost of the ACA's coverage provisions for those years have all been close to the original estimates on a year-by-year basis. Those amounts do not reflect the total budgetary impact of the ACA. That legislation includes many other provisions that, on net, will reduce budget deficits. Taking the coverage provisions and other provisions together, the Congressional Budget Office (CBO) and the Congressional Joint Committee on Taxation (JCT) have estimated that the ACA will reduce deficits over the next 10 years and in the subsequent decade.

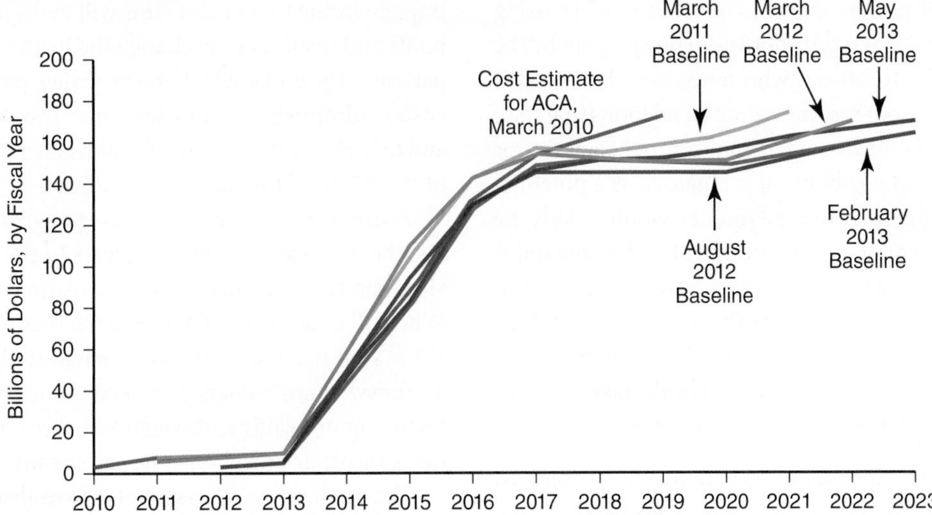

Figure 8-11 Comparison of CBO's estimates of the net budgetary impact of the coverage provisions contained in the ACA.
Source: http://www.gallup.com/poll/122393/oecd-countries-universal-healthcare-gets-high-marks.aspx

The CBO, in its July 2012 report to the House, noted the following expenditures during 2013 to 2022 for repealing the ACA, which if undertaken would lead to an increase in the deficit of $109 billion. This is due to the removal of penalties on the uninsured and taxes on premium "Cadillac" plans and an increase in spending due to a return to pre-ACA healthcare. CBO (2012) summarized the potential effects as follows: "About 30 million fewer nonelderly people would have health insurance in 2022 than under current law, leaving a total of about 60 million nonelderly people uninsured" (p. 9)

The ACA has three categories aimed at cost containment (Orszag, 2011). The first is simply reductions in Medicare reimbursements. This is accomplished by reducing growth rates of provider reimbursement rates and payments to hospitals for treating uninsured low-income patients. The second involves the private insurance market through a move toward uniform electronic standards for all insurance providers and taxes on "Cadillac" insurance plans. These are defined as plans that cost over $10,000 for individuals and over $27,500 for families, and will have a 40% tax on excess cost (Orszag, 2011). These create incentive for the plans to be redesigned so that they will not exceed these thresholds. The third category involves changing the structure of the health system so that payment is based on quality of service rather than quantity of services. This includes streamlining the number of treatment methods that are available (i.e., using the most effective treatment method rather than the one that reimburses the doctor or hospital the most). This is fundamentally a move from fee-for-service to fee-for-value. The move toward a system that uses electronic information will allow the type of data collection necessary to reveal the most effective treatment methods.

The ACA created a number of organizations to facilitate this change. One of these, the **Patient-Centered Outcomes Research Institute (PCORI)** describes its mission as follows: "The Patient-Centered Outcomes Research Institute (PCORI) helps people make informed healthcare decisions, and improves healthcare delivery and outcomes, by producing and promoting high integrity, evidence-based information that comes from research guided by patients, caregivers and the broader healthcare community" (PCORI, 2014). Another, the **Center for Medicare & Medicaid Innovation (CMMI)**, was created by Congress "for the purpose of testing 'innovative payment and service delivery models to reduce program expenditures ... while preserving or enhancing the quality of care' for those individuals who receive Medicare, Medicaid, or Children's Health Insurance Program (CHIP) benefits" (CMMI, 2014).

A third organization, the Independent Payment Advisory Board (IPAB), was established to maintain oversight of Medicare and Medicaid costs. This last organization has proven the most controversial; as described in a 2013 *New England Journal of Medicine* Perspective (Oberlander & Morrison, 2013), the board:

> is empowered to recommend changes to Medicare if projected per-beneficiary spending growth exceeds specified targets. Congress must consider Medicare reforms proposed by the board under special legislative rules, including limits on debate, which are designed to ensure speedy action. If Congress does not enact legislation containing those proposals or alternative policies that achieve the same savings, the IPAB's recommendations are to be implemented by the secretary of health and human services.

To some, these powers appear to be a means of bypassing congressional law-making authority—a power-grab by the executive branch. To others, who note that "the board is prohibited by law from making recommendations that raise revenues, increase cost sharing of Medicare beneficiaries, or restrict benefits and eligibility," it is regarded as a potential threat to providers, whose payments would likely be targeted in the event of cost overruns. A third complaint is the perennial distaste for yet another "layer of Washington bureaucracy" added to the healthcare system. In fact, as of March 1, 2014, the IPAB had yet to have members appointed, and little activity had been undertaken toward getting it operational. As noted in the Perspective article:

> Since Medicare spending is currently not projected to exceed the ACA's targets, there is no need for the administration to appoint members now. Yet the difficulties in launching the IPAB point to a more fundamental problem. The board's appeal lies largely in its aspiration to remove politics from Medicare—to create a policy-making process that is informed by experts and insulated from electoral pressures, interest-group demands, financial considerations, and partisan divisions. But given Congress's extreme partisan and ideological polarization … the IPAB's rough start should not be surprising. This is not the sort of political environment in which an independent board charged with making controversial decisions about one of America's most popular social programs is likely to thrive. These dynamics are unlikely to recede soon, which means that the IPAB is stuck in purgatory, neither operational nor canceled—an institution designed to be above politics that cannot escape the political binds holding it back. (Oberlander & Morrison, 2013)

Thus, the impact of the IPAB is presently nonexistent, and whether it can produce the results intended by Congress is unclear.

The ACA also established a hospital Value-Based Purchasing (VBP) program in Medicare. This will offer financial incentives to hospitals to improve the quality of care. Hospital performance is required to be reported publicly, beginning with measures relating to heart attacks, heart failure, pneumonia, surgical care, healthcare-associated infections, and patients' perception of care. This is also aimed at providing information to consumers so they can make the optimal decision on which hospital to use and create competition between hospitals for those consumers. The goal is to increase the information in the market, which is one of the conditions for a "free" competitive market.

To reduce administrative costs, the act will initiate changes meant to reduce reliance on paper records. This will be accomplished by standardizing billing and requiring the healthcare sector to begin adopting and implementing these rules. This will make it easier for hospitals and insurers to exchange the health information of patients. The end goal will be to reduce paperwork (labor costs), administrative burdens, and transcription errors, and to improve the quality of health care (U.S. Department of Health and Human Services, 2014).

Economics appears to be increasingly driving the U.S. healthcare system. Who gets access to the goods and services the sector provides? What treatment can they get? Who will treat them? Where will the treatment take place? What staff will see them? Where will staff pay originate? The answers are influenced by economic considerations of financing of health and welfare services, reimbursement rates, insurance mechanisms, and means of delivery.

The cost-cutting efforts may lead healthcare providers to move into more cost-effective sites in the community and to increase focus on disease prevention and health promotion.

Economics and Nightingale's Legacy

Even with the opportunities outlined previously, much in the current nursing literature reflects the uneasiness that nurses have with a healthcare system in which some are provided care and others, for lack of resources, go without. Historically, including during the failed Clinton administration attempt at comprehensive health reform, nurses have been advocates for access to quality, cost-effective healthcare services for all people. The gaps in access in the current system are obvious.

Nurses have also expressed misgivings about referring to those they care for as customers, buyers, or consumers. For some, the philosophy of health care as a business threatens the human interactions of nursing and creates an environment that restricts understanding of nursing's value and purpose (David, 1999; Heggen & Wellard, 2004). Nurses worry about the safety of vulnerable patients caught in cost-cutting efforts. Nurses have also questioned a system in which savings from cost cutting go into the pockets of high-salaried executives and stockholders (Gordon, 2008).

For community health nurses, a market system can seem at odds with the nation's public health goal to attain the highest levels of health and welfare for its citizens. Nurses appear to be struggling, as do other citizens, with the contrasting basic principles of justice underlying the production and distribution of healthcare resources. In broad contrast, these are market justice and social justice.

Approaching distribution by relying on capitalism and private for-profit enterprise is the **market justice** approach. Favoring the market is at the heart of the American traditions of individualism and limited government. The market solution is based on people's willingness and ability to pay. Those who cannot pay have individual accountability and do not receive services. People have the right to purchase the health goods they value. They purchase these goods with resources earned from their own efforts. The ideal results are economic efficiency. Market justice emphasizes individual rather than collective responsibility for health.

In contrast, a **social justice** approach holds health care to be a social good that should be collectively financed and available to all citizens regardless of ability to pay. Social justice favors societal responsibility for health care to be achieved through government initiative.

Elements of both market justice and social justice are present in the U.S. system (Shi & Singh, 2008). If the United States embraces the market system in health care, does this mean that collectively we believe only those who can pay should receive care or that people can only get the amount of care they can afford? As the only developed country in the world without some measure of universal healthcare coverage, it would seem so. Why we have adopted such a national stance has been the subject of much debate for decades. Our policies may be accurately reflecting the ethic of the U.S. citizenry (Rice, 1998). In a reported survey, it was found that only 23% of U.S. respondents agreed with the statement, "It is the responsibility of the government to take care of the very poor people who cannot take care of themselves" (Blendon et al., 1995). The U.S. response was considerably lower than the citizens of other countries (Blendon et al., 1995). Yet, in a more recent poll, 68% of respondents said that providing coverage for everyone is more important than keeping taxes down. This may be reflective of how the question is asked; however, approval for coverage for all dropped considerably when it might mean loss of any treatments currently covered by insurance, limits on doctor choice, or higher premiums (Appleby, 2006). This ethics quandary could explain the present inability of our policymakers to decide who, if anyone, is to provide health care to those who do not currently have economic access to such care.

Although the two differing ethics reflect values and beliefs about what is good or best, both beliefs seem to have flaws. Dowd (1999) has suggested that the question we really face is one of whether our problems are best solved by "imperfect government or imperfect markets" (p. 269). The United States is not alone in its struggle to deal with the economic challenges of health care. What is emerging internationally is discussion about a fundamentally different "third way" in health—a middle road between a centrally planned system and one based on market principles (Kritsotakis & Gamarnikow, 2004; LeGrand, 1999).

Nurses can better contribute to the ongoing dialogue if they understand the opportunities and the downfalls of the two economic approaches as they operate in our present system. Nurses can look back as far as Florence Nightingale and find the origins of our public involvement in what is good for society. LeVasseur (1998) describes the Nightingale legacy as a "guardian-like stamp on nursing" (p. 281). She says, "Nightingale showed a strong sense of responsibility to her society and a passion for reform. . . . It was not enough for Nightingale to have knowledge of the good, but it was important to put that knowledge into action as a guardian of the people" (p. 281). Nurses today need not and should not be passive participants in the broad marketplace of ideas about what our society values in health care.

HEALTHY ME 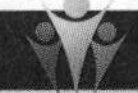

How much do you spend on health care per year? Include acute and preventive care expenses, such as medication, clinic visits, and exercise equipment and nutritional supplements.

AFFORDABLE CARE ACT (ACA)—WHY DO WE NEED IT?

- Too many people lack health coverage. Approximately 55 million Americans under the age of 65 are uninsured, representing 1 out of 5 in that population.
- U.S. healthcare spending is unsustainable, representing 17.9% of our GDP. Medicare alone represented 15% of our national budget in 2011, and this share is expected to grow as the baby boomer generation ages.
- Despite high spending, our health outcomes are poor. The United States spends significantly more on medical care than any other industrialized country but ranks 24th in life expectancy among these comparable countries.
- Our system emphasizes treatment instead of prevention. Seven out of 10 deaths in the United States are related to preventable diseases based on behavioral factors, such as obesity, diabetes, high blood pressure, heart disease, and cancer. Three-quarters of our healthcare dollar is spent treating such diseases. Only 3 cents of each (public and private) dollar is spent on preventive health care.
- Health disparities and inequities exist among numerous populations across demographic lines such as race, ethnicity, culture, income, and class. .
- Children and young adults under the age of 26 can be covered under their parents' health insurance.

Source: American Public Health Association. Fact Sheet "Why We Need the ACA", August, 2012. Retrieved from http://www.apha.org/NR/rdonlyres/19BEA341-A7C3-4920-B2BC-65BDC846B803/0/WhyWeNeedtheACA_Aug2012.pdf

Critical Thinking Activities

1. Explain how under imperfect market conditions, both prices and quantities of health care are higher than they would be in a highly competitive market.
2. Two emergency department nurses are debating the issue of access to health care. One is concerned about the stigma of those who are uninsured and claims that people without health insurance receive less health care and have poorer health than those with insurance. The other disagrees, claiming that hospitals, doctors, and public health clinics deliver large amounts of charity care, which allows uninsured people to have the services they need. Who has the stronger case? What does research tell us?
3. The following is a dialogue with former U.S. Department of Health and Human Services Secretary Donna Shalala and Princeton economist Uwe Reinhardt:

   Shalala: In fact, Medicare is the best payer in the system: It pays more quickly and better than most private systems do.

   Reinhardt: And it operates more cheaply. Medicare passes through much more money, about 97 cents of every premium dollar, because its administrative costs are so low. No private insurer can match that record. Most providers don't know this.

   Shalala: People just can't get the stereotype of big bureaucracy out of their heads. And the idea that Medicare's administrative expenses are 3% or 4% while the private sector spends 12% just doesn't register with many people particularly those who see health care as a business. (Shalala & Reinhardt, 1999)

4. Why might the difference exist between government and private spending? How might someone in a for-profit organization respond to this conversation?

References

Altman, S., & Shactman, D. (2011). *Power, politics, and universal health care: The inside story of a century-long battle.* Amherst, NY: Prometheus Books.

American Nurses Association. (1997). *Medicare reimbursement for NPs and CNSs.* Retrieved from http://www.nursingworld.org

American Nurses Association. (2007). *ANA position statement: Mandatory overtime.* Washington, DC: Author. Retrieved from http://www.nursingworld.org/MainMenuCategories/ThePracticeofProfessionalNursing/NurseStaffing/OvertimeIssues/Overtime.pdf

American Public Health Association (APHA). (1998). *Fact sheet: Prescription contraceptive equity.* Retrieved from http://www.apha.org/legislative/factsheets/fs2.htm

American Society for Reproductive Medicine (ASRM). (2008). *Frequently asked questions about infertility.* Retrieved from http://www.asrm.org/Patients/faqs.html

Appleby, J. (2006, October 16). Universal care appeals to USA: But what it would cost complicates the issue. *USA Today,* p. 4B.

Arrow, K. J. (1997). Social responsibility and economic efficiency. In T. Donaldson & T. W. Dunfee (Eds.), *Ethics in business and economics.* Brookfield, VT: Ashgate.

Arvantes, J. (2008). New study finds wide disparities in Medicare's quality of care. *AAFP News Now.* Retrieved from http://www.aafp.org

Ashby, M. (2006). Barriers to nurse practitioner reimbursement. *Pennsylvania Nurse, 61*(2), 19.

Balto, D. A., & Kovacs, J. (2013). Consolidation in health care markets: A review of the literature. White Paper submitted to the Robert Wood Johnson Foundation. Retrieved from http://www.dcantitrustlaw.com/assets/content/documents/2013/balto-kovacs_healthcareconsolidation_jan13.pdf

Beitsch, L. M., Brooks, R. G., Menachemi, N., & Libbey, P. M. (2006). Public health at center stage: New roles, old props. *Health Affairs, 25*(4), 911–922.

Berenson, R. A. (2005). Which way for competition? None of the above. *Health Affairs, 24*(6), 1536–1542.

Blendon, R. J., Benson, J., Donelan, K., Leitman, R., Taylor, H., Koeck, C., & Gitterman, D. (1995). Who has the best health care system? A second look. *Health Affairs, 14*(4), 220–230.

Blumenthal, D. (1994). The vital role of professionalism in health care reform. *Health Affairs, 13*(1), 252–256.

Bodenheimer, T. S., & Grumbach, K. (1995). *Understanding health policy: A clinical approach.* Stamford, CT: Appleton & Lange.

Brown, C. (1999). Ethics, policy, and practice: Interview with Emily Friedman. *Image: Journal of Nursing Scholarship, 31,* 259–262.

Buerhaus, P. I. (1998). Milton Weinstein's insights on the development, use and methodological problems in cost-effectiveness analysis. *Image: Journal of Nursing Scholarship, 30*(3), 223–227.

Center for Medicare & Medicaid Innovation. (2014). *About the CMS Innovation Center.* Retrieved from http://innovation.cms.gov/About/index.html

Centers for Disease Control and Prevention. (1995). Prevention and managed care: Opportunities for managed care, purchasers of health care, and public health agencies. *Morbidity and Mortality Weekly Report, 44,* 1–12.

Centers for Disease Control and Prevention. (2014). FastStats: Health expenditures. Retrieved from http://www.cdc.gov/nchs/fastats/hexpense.htm

Centers for Medicare & Medicaid Services. (2011). *2011 Medicaid managed care enrollment report: Summary statistics as of*

July 1, 2011. Retrieved from http://www.medicaid.gov/Medicaid-CHIP-Program-Information/By-Topics/Data-and-Systems/Downloads/2011-Medicaid-MC-Enrollment-Report.pdf

Centers for Medicare & Medicaid Services. (2012). *National health expenditures 2012 highlights.* Retrieved from http://www.cms.gov/Research-Statistics-Data-and-Systems/Statistics-Trends-and-Reports/NationalHealthExpendData/downloads/highlights.pdf

Centers for Medicare and Medicaid Services. (2014). *Table 1: National health expenditures aggregate.* Retrieved from http://www.cms.gov/Research-Statistics-Data-and-Systems/Statistics-Trends-and-Reports/NationalHealthExpendData/downloads/tables.pdf

Chollet, D. J. (1996). Redefining private insurance in a changing market structure. In S. H. Altman & U. E. Reinhardt (Eds.), *Strategic choices for a changing health care system.* Chicago, IL: Health Administration Press.

Collins, S. R., Kriss, J. L., Doty, M. M., & Rustgi, S. D. (2008). *Losing ground: How the loss of adequate health insurance is burdening working families.* Findings from the Commonwealth Fund Biennial Health Insurance Surveys, 2001–2007. Retrieved from http://www.commonwealthfund.org/Publications/Fund-Reports/2008/Aug/Losing-Ground--How-the-Loss-of-Adequate-Health-Insurance-Is-Burdening-Working-Families-8212-Finding.aspx

Congressional Budget Office (CBO). (2012). Effects on insurance coverage and their budgetary impact. Retrieved from http://www.cbo.gov/sites/default/files/cbofiles/attachments/43471-hr6079.pdf

Cowley, G., King, P., Hager, M., & Rosenberg, D. (1995, June 26). Going mainstream. *Newsweek,* pp. 56–57.

David, B. A. (1999). Nursing's conflicting values in competitively managed health care. *Image: Journal of Nursing Scholarship, 31*(2), 188.

Deaton, A. (2006, April). Letter from America: Trying to be a good hip op consumer. *Royal Economic Society Newsletter, 133,* 3–4.

Dentzer, S. (1998, January–February). A guide to managed care, part 2. *Modern Maturity,* 35–41, 43.

Dowd, B., (1999). An unusual view of health economics. *Health Affairs,* 18(1), 266–269.

Edwards, R. (2005). Blind faith and choice. *Health Affairs, 24*(6), 1624–1628.

Express Scripts. (2012). Drug trend quarterly spotlight. Retrieved from http://digital.turn-page.com/i/95262

Fielding, J. E., & Briss, P. A. (2006). Promoting evidence-based public health policy: Can we have better evidence and more action? *Health Affairs, 25*(4), 969–978.

Finkler, S. A., & Kovner, C. T. (1993). *Financial management for nurse managers and executives.* Philadelphia, PA: Saunders.

Fuchs, V. R. (2005). Health care expenditures reexamined. *Annals of Internal Medicine, 143*(1), 76–78.

Gell, N. M., Rosenberg, D. E., Demiris, G., LaCroix, A. Z., & Patel, K. V. (2013). Patterns of technology use among older adults with and without disabilities. *Gerontologist 54* (ePub ahead of print, December 2013). Retrieved from http://gerontologist.oxfordjournals.org/content/early/2013/12/29/geront.gnt166.abstract

Genworth Financial, Inc. & National Eldercare Referral Systems, Inc. (2007). *Genworth Financial 2007 cost of care survey.* Retrieved from https://longtermcare.genworth.com/comweb/consumer/pdfs/long_term_care/Cost_Of_Care_Survey.pdf

Gibson, R. M., & Waldo, D. R. (1982). National health expenditures, 1981. *Health Care Financing Review, 4*(1), 1–35.

Gold, M. R., Siegel, J. E., Russell, L. B., & Weinstein, M. C. (1996). *Cost-effectiveness in health and medicine.* New York, NY: Oxford University Press.

Gordon, S. (2008). Advocating for nursing. In C. Harrington & C. L. Estes (Eds.), *Health policy: Crisis and reform in the U.S. health care delivery system* (5th ed.). Sudbury, MA: Jones and Bartlett.

Government Accountability Office (GAO). (2011). *Prescription drugs: Trends in usual and customary prices for commonly used drugs.* Retrieved from http://www.gao.gov/products/GAO-11-306R

Gulzar, L. (1999). Access to health care. *Image: Journal of Nursing Scholarship, 31*(1), 13–19.

Halvorson, G. C. (1999). Health plans' strategic responses to a changing market place. *Health Affairs, 18*(2), 28–29.

Hamilton, J. (1996, May). Insurance for alternative treatments. *American Health,* 44.

Harrington, C., & Estes, C. L. (Eds.). (2008). *Health policy: Crisis and reform in the U.S. health care delivery system* (5th ed.). Sudbury, MA: Jones and Bartlett.

Health Insurance Association of America. (1991). *Source book of insurance data.* Washington, DC: Author.

Heggen, K., & Wellard, S. (2004). Increased unintended patient harm in nursing practice as a consequence of the dominance of economic discourses. *International Journal of Nursing Studies, 41,* 293–298.

Holahan, J., & Cook, A. (2006). *Why did the number of uninsured continue to increase in 2005?* Issue Paper Report #7571. Washington, DC: Kaiser Family Foundation. Retrieved from http://www.kff.org/uninsured/upload/7571.pdf

Howell, P. (2006). Market failure and public services. *Royal Economic Society Newsletter, 133,* 1.

Hughes, D., & Runyan, S. (2008). Prenatal care and public policy: Lessons for promoting women's health. In C. Harrington & C. L. Estes (Eds.), *Health policy: Crisis and reform in the U.S. health care delivery system* (5th ed.). Sudbury, MA: Jones and Bartlett.

Jacobs, P. (1997). *The economics of health care.* Gaithersburg, MD: Aspen.

Kaiser Family Foundation. (2005). *e-health and the elderly: How seniors use the Internet for health information.* Retrieved from http://kaiserfamilyfoundation.files.wordpress.com/2013/01/speaker-presentation.pdf

Kaiser Family Foundation. (2013a). Key facts about the uninsured population. Retrieved from http://kff.org/uninsured/fact-sheet/key-facts-about-the-uninsured-population/

Kaiser Family Foundation. (2013b). 2013 employer health benefits survey. Retrieved from http://kff.org/report-section/2013-summary-of-findings/

Kaiser Family Foundation. (2013c). Medicare Advantage fact sheet. Retrieved from http://kff.org/medicare/fact-sheet/medicare-advantage-fact-sheet/

Keehan, S. P., Sisko, A. M., Truffer, C. J., Poisal, J. A., Cuckler, G. A., Madison, A. J., . . . Smith, S. D. (2011). National health spending projections through 2020: Economic recovery and reform drive faster spending growth. *Health Affairs, 30*(8), 1594–1605.

Kovner, A. R., & Knickman, J. R. (2005). Overview: The state of healthcare delivery in the United States. In A. R. Kovner & J. R. Knickman (Eds.), *Jonas and Kovner's health care delivery in the United States* (8th ed., pp. 2–9). New York, NY: Springer.

Kritsotakis, G., & Gamarnikow, E. (2004). What is social capital and how does it relate to health? *International Journal of Nursing Studies, 41*(1), 43–50.

Larson-Dahn, M. (1998). An innovative approach to appropriate resource utilization. *Nursing Economics, 16*(6), 317–319.

Lasker, R. D., & the Committee on Medicine and Public Health. (1997). *Medical and public health: The power of collaboration.* New York, NY: The New York Academy of Medicine.

Lee, Y. C., Lin, J. T., Wu, H. M., Liu, T. Y., Yen, M. F., Chiu, H. M., . . . Chen, T. (2007). Cost-effectiveness analysis between primary and secondary preventive strategies for gastric cancer. *Cancer Epidemiology Biomarkers and Prevention, 16*(5), 875–885.

LeGrand, J. (1999). Competition, cooperation, or control? Tales from the British National Health Service. *Health Affairs, 18*(1), 27–39.

LeVasseur, J. (1998). Plato, Nightingale, and contemporary nursing. *Image: Journal of Nursing Scholarship, 30*(3), 281–285.

Lind, K. D., for the American Association of Retired Persons (AARP) Public Policy Institute. (2012). Setting the record straight about Medicare (Fact Sheet 249). Retrieved from http://www.aarp.org/content/dam/aarp/research/public_policy_institute/health/Setting-the-Record-Straight-about-Medicare-fact-sheet-AARP-ppi-health.pdf

Loubeau, P. R., & Maher, V. F. (1996). Any-willing provider laws: Point and counterpoint. *Medicine and Law, 15*(2), 219–226.

Mantone, J. (2006). Stating the case for coverage. *Modern Healthcare, 36*(18), 6–16.

Martin, A. B., Hartman, M., Whittle, L., Catlin, A., & National Health Expenditure Accounts Team. (2014). National health spending in 2012: Rate of health spending growth remained low for the fourth consecutive year. *Health Affairs, 33*(1), 67–77.

Max, W. (1997). Economic analysis in health care. In C. Harrington & C. L. Estes (Eds.), *Health policy and nursing: Crisis and reform in the U.S. health care delivery system* (2nd ed.). Sudbury, MA: Jones and Bartlett.

Mechanic, D. (1998). Topics for our times: Managed care and public health opportunities. *American Journal of Public Health, 88*, 874–875.

Mechanic, D., & Rochefort, D. (2008). A policy of inclusion for the mentally ill. In C. Harrington & C. L. Estes (Eds.), *Health policy: Crisis and reform in the U.S. health care delivery system* (5th ed.). Sudbury, MA: Jones and Bartlett.

Medicaid and CHIP Payment and Access Commission (MACPAC). (2013). Report to the Congress on Medicaid and CHIP: March 2013. Retrieved from http://cnsnews.com/sites/default/files/documents/MACPAC%20REPORT-2013.pdf

Miller, T. R. (2012). *Executive Summary: Nurse-Family Partnership home visitation: Costs, outcomes, and return on investment.* Pew Charitable Trusts. Retrieved from http://www.pewstates.org/uploadedFiles/PCS_Assets/2013/Costs_and_ROI_executive_summary.pdf

Mississippi Health Advocacy Program. (1998). *What welfare advocates need to know about low income families' eligibility for and entitlement to Medicaid: Action alert.* Jackson, MS: Author.

Moore, S., Laufer, F. L., & Conroy, M. B. (1998). The economics of health care. In D. J. Mason & J. K. Leavitt (Eds.), *Policy and politics in nursing and health care* (3rd ed.). Philadelphia, PA: Saunders.

Oberlander, J., & Morrison, M. (2013). Failure to launch? The Independent Payment Advisory Board's uncertain prospects. *New England Journal of Medicine, 369*(2), 105–107.

Orszag, P. (2011). How health care can save or sink America. *Foreign Affairs, 90*(4), 46–56.

Patient-Centered Outcomes Research Institute (PCORI). (2014). Mission and vision. Retrieved from http://www.pcori.org/about-us/mission-and-vision/

Porter, E. (2013, January 8). Health Care and Profits, a Poor Mix. *The New York Times.* Retrieved from http://www.nytimes.com/2013/01/09/business/health-care-and-pursuit-of-profit-make-a-poor-mix.html

Pulcini, J., & Mahoney, D. (1998). Health care financing. In D. J. Mason & J. K. Leavitt (Eds.), *Policy and politics in nursing and health care* (3rd ed.). Philadelphia, PA: Saunders.

Rambur, B., & Mooney, M. M. (1998). A point of view: Why point-of-care places are not free marketplaces. *Nursing Economics, 16*(3), 122–124, 146.

Rice, T. (1998). *The economics of health reconsidered.* Chicago, IL: Health Administration Press.

Robbins, A., & Freeman, P. (1999). How organized medical care can advance public health. *Public Health Reports, 114*, 120–125.

Robinson, J. (2011). Hospital market concentration, pricing, and profitability in orthopedic surgery and interventional cardiology. *American Journal of Managed Care, 17*(6), 241–248.

Rosenbaum, S., & Richards, T. B. (1996). Medicaid managed care and public health policy. *Journal of Public Health Management Practice, 2*(3), 76–82.

Scandlen, G. (2005). Consumer-driven health care: Just a tweak or a revolution? *Health Affairs, 24*(6), 1554–1558.

Schauffler, H. H., & Scutchfield, F. D. (1998). Managed care and public health. *American Journal of Preventive Medicine, 14*(3), 240–241.

Shalala, D. E., & Reinhardt, U. E. (1999). Viewing the U.S. health care system from within: Candid talk from HHS. *Health Affairs, 18*(3), 47–55.

Shaughnessy, P. W., Schenkler, R. E., & Hittle, D. F. (1995). Case mix of home health patients under capitated and fee-for-service payments. *Health Services Research, 30*(1), 1–8.

Shi, L., & Singh, D. A. (2008). *Delivering health care in America: A systems approach* (4th ed.). Sudbury, MA: Jones and Bartlett.

Siegel, J. E. (1998). Cost-effectiveness analysis and nursing research: Is there a fit? *Image: Journal of Nursing Scholarship, 30*(3), 221–222.

Spetz, J. (2005). The cost and cost-effectiveness of nursing services in health care. *Nursing Outlook, 53*(6), 305–309.

Standard and Poor's Corporation. (1992). *U.S. grapples with health care crisis.* Health care industry surveys, H15–H17.

Stevens, P. E. (1992). Who gets care? Access to health care as an arena for nursing. *Scholarly Inquiry for Nursing Practice*, *6*(3), 185–200.

Stone, P. W. (1998). Methods for conducting and reporting cost-effectiveness analysis in nursing. *Image: Journal of Nursing Scholarship*, *30*(3), 229–234.

Stone, P. W., Curran, C. R., & Bakken, S. (2002). Economic evidence for evidence based practice. *Journal of Nursing Scholarship*, *34*(3), 277–282.

Sultz, H. A., & Young, K. M. (2014). *Health care USA: Understanding its organization and delivery* (8th ed.). Burlington, MA: Jones & Bartlett Learning.

Thompson, K. M. (2003). Economic issues in health care. In L. A. Joel (Ed.), *Kelly's dimensions of professional nursing* (pp. 220–241). New York, NY: McGraw-Hill.

Trapp, D. (2008). Premiums for job-offered health insurance up 5% this year. *American Medical News.* Retrieved from http://www.ama-assn.org/amednews/2008/10/13/gvsb1013.htm

U.S. Department of Health and Human Services. (2014). *Read the law: The Affordable Care Act, section by section.* Retrieved from http://www.hhs.gov/healthcare/rights/law/index.html

Vladeck, B. C., & King, K. (1997). Medicare at 30: Preparing for the future. In C. Harrington & C. Estes (Eds.), *Health policy and nursing: Crisis and reform in the U.S. health care delivery system.* Sudbury, MA: Jones and Bartlett.

Waid, M. O. (1998). *Brief summaries of Medicare and Medicaid. Title XVII and Title XIX of the Social Security Act.* Report prepared for Health Care Financing Administration, U.S. Department of Health and Human Services.

Weeks, J. (1997). The emerging role of alternative medicine in managed care. *Drug Benefit Trends*, *9*(4), 14–16, 25–28.

Weinstein, M. C., & Skinner, J. A. (2010). Comparative effectiveness and health care spending—implications for reform. *New England Journal of Medicine*, *362*(5), 460–465.

Wesson, A. F. (1999). The comparative study of health reform. In F. D. Powell & A. F. Wesson (Eds.), *Health care systems in transition* (pp. 3–24). Thousand Oaks, CA: Sage.

White House Domestic Policy Council. (1993). *Health security: The President's report to the American people.* Washington, DC: Government Printing Office.

World Bank. (2014). *Data: Health expenditure, total (% of GDP).* Retrieved from http://data.worldbank.org/indicator/SH.XPD.TOTL.ZS

Yanci, J., Wolford, M., & Young, P. (2013). What hospital executives should be considering in hospital mergers and acquisitions. Retrieved from http://www.dhgllp.com/res_pubs/Hospital-Mergers-and-Acquisitions.pdf

CHAPTER FOCUS

Government Authority
- Protection of the Public's Health
- Power, Authority, and the Health of the Public
- Evolution of the Government's Role in Health Care

Government
- Federal Government
- State Government
- Local Government
- Different Types of Law
- How an Idea Becomes a Law
- How Nurses Can Get Involved

Regulation and Licensing of Nursing Practice
- The Regulatory Process
- Licensure

Nursing Practice and the Law
- Nursing Practice in Correctional Settings
- Forensic Nursing: An Emerging Nursing Role

QUESTIONS TO CONSIDER

After reading this chapter, you will know the answers to the following questions:

1. What is the role of the government in the health of its citizens?
2. How do the concepts of power and authority relate to public health regulation?
3. What is the history of governmental roles in health care?
4. What are the three branches of the federal government? What does each do in relation to health?
5. How is state government organized? How does it relate to health care?
6. What are the different kinds of laws?
7. What are the steps in the development of laws?
8. How can nurses be involved in the development of law and policy?
9. What are the primary issues related to regulation and licensure of nursing practice?
10. What settings are more likely to be influenced by legal issues in the practice of community health nursing and why?
11. What is the role of the nurse in correctional settings and in forensics?

CHAPTER 9

Politics and the Law

Karen Saucier Lundy, Sharyn Janes, and Heather Rakauskas Sherry

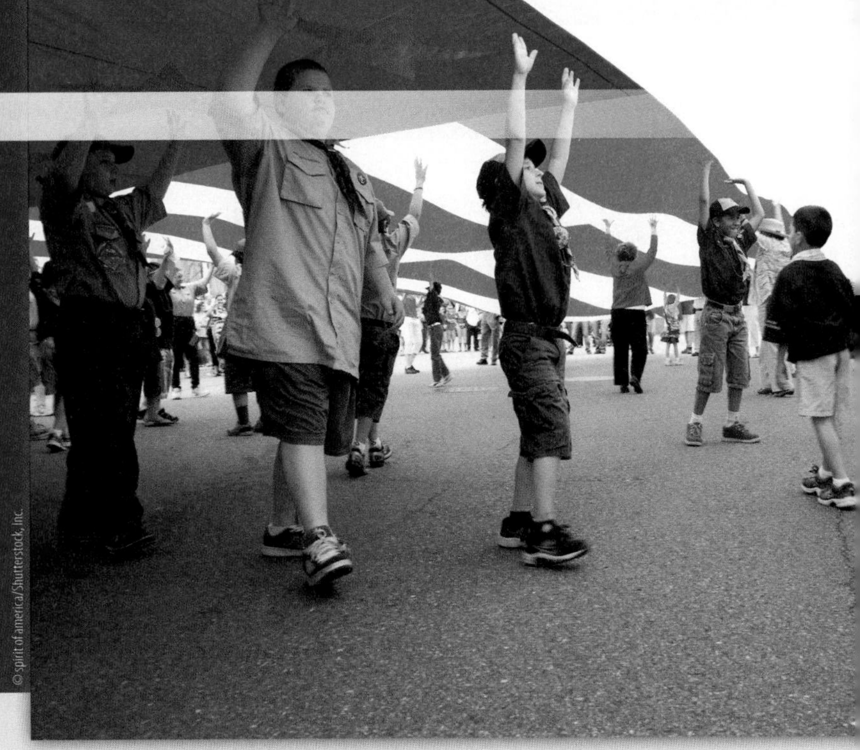

KEY TERMS

Bill of Rights
coercive power
connection power
constitutional law
correctional nursing
democracy
equality
executive branch
expert power
Federal Register
forensic nursing
freedom
information power
judicial branch
judicial or common law
legislative branch
legitimate power
liberty
licensure
lobbying
malpractice
negligence
Nurse Multistate Licensure Mutual Recognition Model
nurse practice act
police power
political action committees (PACs)
political power
power
Preamble of the U.S. Constitution
referent power
regulatory process
reward power
statutory law
U.S. Constitution

Never doubt that a small group of thoughtful, committed citizens can change the world; indeed, it's the only thing that ever does.

—Margaret Mead

The care of human life and happiness, and not their destruction, is the first and only object of good government.

—Thomas Jefferson

Abraham Lincoln did not go to Gettysburg having commissioned a poll to find out what would sell in Gettysburg. There were no people with percentages for him, cautioning him about this group or that group or what they found in exit polls a year earlier. When will we have the courage of Lincoln?

—Robert Coles

REFLECTIONS

We often think of "politics" as something others do "for us" or "to us." Politics is always about power, who gets it, how it is used, and to what purpose. Why do you think nurses have historically avoided using their significant numbers politically? What do you think of the political system, and does it relate to your work as a nurse?

AFFORDABLE CARE ACT (ACA) 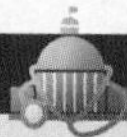

In March of 2010, President Barrack Obama signed the landmark Affordable Care Act (ACA) P.L. 111–148 into law. This was later supported by the U.S. Supreme Court's affirmative ruling that the majority of ACA provisions were constitutional. This historical and far-reaching legislation is considered the most comprehensive healthcare reform and health policy in over 50 years. All major professional nursing associations strongly supported the ACA and the Obama administration's efforts to reform healthcare affordability, accessibility, and quality and to move the U.S. healthcare system toward a greater emphasis on primary and preventive care. The ACA goals have been priorities for nursing for decades. Nursing was the first of the healthcare professions to support the creation of the Medicare program in 1958, despite significant opposition among other healthcare organizations and professions.

Source: American Academy of Nursing. (2010). *Implementing Health Care Reform: Issues for Nursing.* Retrieved from http://www.aannet.org/assets/docs/implementinghealthcarereform.pdf

WHILE THE POLITICAL EFFORTS of movers and shakers like Florence Nightingale, Lillian Wald, and Margaret Sanger are well documented, politics and policy have been historically seen as "outside" the scope of nursing. For most nurses, "political activism" meant voting in national and state elections. By the closing years of the 20th century, however, nurses began to realize that they could influence public policy by using nursing knowledge and skills. In 1992, acknowledging that decisions affecting nurses and their patients were being made in the national political arena, the American Nurses Association (ANA) moved its national headquarters to Washington, DC (Milstead, 1999). With the passage of the ACA in 2010, nurses are poised to take the leadership role in moving the United States to a prevention-based system, with most citizens covered for essential healthcare services (ANA, 2012). Nursing has long supported healthcare reform, as have our professional organizations. As nurses, we understand the professional and economic benefits of having a healthier population. The full expansion to cost-effective, quality care for all is affected by political forces and influences (Brennan, 2012). While the new healthcare reform law is complex and will be implemented in incremental stages regarding delivery, payment, coverage, and education, nurses must be knowledgeable and engaged in the political process in order to realize the full potential of the new healthcare system reformation (American Academy of Nursing, 2010).

Government Authority

Protection of the Public's Health

The early American colonists viewed health as controlled by divine intervention. They believed it was a result of self-care, and minimal governmental intervention was expected. Because health care was not a power granted to the federal government (such as defense or printing money), it developed into a power of the states or was left to the people themselves. Governmental health care and policies to provide funding and resources for health care were, for all practical purposes, nonexistent in the early days of the United States (Turnock, 1997).

As each new American colony was founded, the way in which it would be governed was a primary consideration. The specific problems and situations that each new colony faced varied so widely that each developed its own procedures and laws based on its own needs. From this evolved the idea of states' rights, which continues to play a critical role in the governance of healthcare policies, such as seatbelt laws and immunization laws. Any attempts to limit the power of the states, either by the federal government or other states, is usually strongly opposed. Most states, for instance, will have similar laws about school attendance, drinking age, and immunizations, but the regulations themselves will vary considerably.

Federal law is based on the **U.S. Constitution**, which was ratified in 1789. The creators of the Constitution were careful to limit the federal government's involvement in the daily lives of citizens. The word *health* was never mentioned in the U.S. Constitution, making healthcare legislation problematic, because the Constitution grants limited power in the creation of health laws. The Constitution has been amended 27 times. The first 10 amendments, known as the **Bill of Rights**, were adopted within 3 years of the Constitution's ratification. The Bill of Rights focuses on the protection of our most basic value: freedom. Freedom of speech, freedom of the press, and due process are all included. In recent years, the constitutional amendments have had relevance to healthcare issues. For example, the Fourteenth Amendment provides protection of personal liberty, such as a woman's right to choose to have an abortion. It is important to note, however, that neither the U.S. Constitution nor state constitutions guarantee access to health care. States retain whatever power the U.S. Constitution does not specifically define in federal law. State power concerning health care is termed **police power**. The state can use its power to protect the health, welfare, and safety of its citizens by establishing boards of nursing and medicine and passing immunization laws (Kelly & Joel, 1996).

Power, Authority, and the Health of the Public

Politics is always about **power**—who gets it, how it is obtained, how it is applied, and to what purposes it is used (Bacharach & Lawler, 1980). The German sociologist Max Weber defined power as the ability to control the behaviors of others, even in the absence of their consent (Weber, 1947). Power, then, is the capacity to participate effectively in a decision-making process. If citizens cannot or do not affect the process, they are powerless (Lenski, 1984).

Power can be classified as either legitimate or illegitimate. Power is considered legitimate if people recognize that those who apply it have the right to do so. This includes elected government officials, aristocracy, and those believed to be inspired by God. Weber referred to legitimate power as authority (Bacharach & Lawler, 1980). A simple illustration of this authority is that if the police stop you for speeding and levy a fine against you, you will recognize the law and the person carrying out the law as legitimate and you will probably obey. A political system can exist only if the people see the authority as legitimate. Most persons must see it as desirable, workable, and better than alternatives. We may complain about our legal system and its excesses or our Congress members and their self-serving interests, but most of us believe that the system works to our benefit most of the time. Once the bulk of citizens in any society no longer consider the political system legitimate, it is doomed, for its power can then rest only on coercion, which will eventually fail. Most revolutions, such as the French Revolution, the Iranian Revolution, and the American Revolution, were preceded by an erosion of the legitimacy of the existing political system (Robertson, 1981).

> Among the Indians there have been no written laws. Customs handed down from generation to generation have been the only laws to guide them. Every one might act different from what was considered right if he chose to do so, but such acts would bring upon him the censure of the Nation. . . . This fear of the Nation's censure acted as a mighty band, binding all in one social, honorable compact.
>
> —*George Copway (Kah-ge-ga-bowh), Ojibwa Chief, 1818–1863*

Concepts of Power

Political power is defined by Hewison (1994) as the "ability to influence or persuade an individual holding a governmental office to exert the power of that office to [effect] a desired change" (p. 1171). What allows some people to have more influence than others? Where does such power come from? Nurses can benefit from understanding these sources of power. French and Raven (1959) identify five power bases:

1. **Coercive power** is the use of force to gain compliance, often born out of real or perceived fear or threat to self. Police often use coercive power.
2. **Reward power** involves giving something of value for compliance. Compliance then results from the perceived potential for reward or favor of someone in power. A politician may help constituents obtain money for a new hospital in exchange for their political support.
3. **Expert power** results from expert knowledge or skills. Bill Gates has considerable expert power because of his expertise in computers and systems.
4. **Legitimate power** results from a title or position, such as an elected judge or the surgeon general.
5. **Referent power** results from being closely associated with someone who is powerful; for example, the aide or spouse of a senator. This can also be referred to as reflected power.

Hersey, Blanchard, and Natemeyer (1979) added two additional sources of power:

6. **Information power** results from the desire for information held by one person from one who does not have access to the information. This is commonly seen in the diplomatic corps of the United States.
7. **Connection power** results from the belief that a certain person has a special connection to a person or organization believed to be powerful. Lobbyists often use this kind of power when working with legislators' staff assistants (Helvie, 1998).

One primary way of gaining power as a nurse is through knowledge. Nurses can use their knowledge of politics, power, and the change process to introduce change favoring health in the legislative process. Nurses have historically had very little interest in achieving power. Others have too long been the "voice" of nursing, and nurses and their patients have suffered through lack of appropriate nurse advocacy (Huston, 1995).

Another way that nurses can achieve power is through affiliating with others who have similar interests in health. Through networking and using the power of numbers, nurses can facilitate communication and effect change through those in power positions (Anderson, 2006). Coalitions of people and organizations are most effective in bringing about change (Helvie, 1998).

> When nurses fully understand the impact of policy in the health care arena, when nurses fully understand the importance of tying outcomes research to public policy and when nurses fully understand the politics of health care, and mobilize their numbers and influence behind the political process, only then will the health system thrive and with nurses as key players.
>
> *—Betty Dickson, Lobbyist and Policy Consultant, Mississippi Nurses Association*

The idea of a nation-state is relatively new. The concept emerged in Europe only a few centuries ago, then spread to the Americas, and spread to most parts of Africa and Asia only during the 20th century. In the founding of the United States, a representative democracy was a new idea. **Democracy** comes from a Greek word meaning "rule of the people," and this is no doubt what Abraham Lincoln had in mind when he defined democracy as "government of the people, by the people, and for the people." Democracy in the United States requires that we recognize the powers of the government as being derived from the consent of the governed. We elect representatives who are responsible for making political decisions. According to Robertson (1981), "Representative democracy is historically recent, rare and fragile" (p. 488).

There are five basic conditions that must exist for a democracy to thrive:

1. Advanced economic development: This almost always involves an urbanized, literate, and sophisticated population that expects and demands participation in the political process.
2. Restraints on government power: This involves institutional checks on the power of the state (Robertson, 1981).
3. Consensus on basic values and a widely held commitment to existing political institutions.
4. Tolerance of dissent.
5. Access to information: A democracy depends on its citizens to make informed choices. There must be a free press.

Liberty Versus Equality

Freedom is defined in the United States as freedom "of"—freedom of speech, freedom of the press, and so on. In more socialist societies, freedom is defined as freedom "from"—freedom from hunger, freedom from unemployment, freedom from exploitation by people who want to make a fortune. In the United States, we equate freedom with **liberty**. Socialist societies equate freedom with **equality**. In general, the more liberty that exists in a society, the less equality. Your liberty to be richer than anyone else violates other people's right to be your equal; other people's right to be your equal violates your liberty to make a fortune. In the United States, we have chosen to emphasize liberty, which evolves from our value system. This emphasis can lead only to social inequality. Socialist societies emphasize equality, thus limiting personal liberty (Robertson, 1981).

In health care we often fail to understand why laws cannot be easily passed to impose penalties on persons who engage in risky behavior, such as requiring helmets for motorcyclists or tubal ligations for women who have injured their children through neglect or abuse. The answer lies in our emphasis on freedom in the United States and the limited power of the state. Recognizing and understanding these basic concepts about our government can help us use our skills and resources in the political process much more efficiently.

> Eternal vigilance is the price of liberty.
>
> *—Wendell Phillips, 1852*

Evolution of the Government's Role in Health Care

The **Preamble of the U.S. Constitution** states that one of the purposes of the federal government is to "promote the general welfare" of the people. This can be found in Article 1, Section 8. The federal government derives its power to become involved in healthcare activities from this simple declaration. Because of this very general statement, the degree of healthcare services provided by the federal government is often a source of conflict among the various constituents and political parties. As a capitalistic society, and lacking clear direction from the U.S. Constitution, the provision of health services for the general population has historically been the concern of private enterprise. Private physicians delivered services to patients, and patients in turn paid a fee for that service. This concept had been the foundation of medical care provision in the United States for nearly 200 years (Miller, 1992).

The first involvement of the federal government in health care was highly specialized for government employees. As early as 1796, the Marine Hospital Service was established to provide care for sick and disabled seamen. In 1852, St. Elizabeth Hospital in Washington, DC, was established to provide health care for federal employees. A landmark study, the Shattuck Report, written in 1850, recommended measures such as the creation of local and state boards of health; collection of vital statistics; and supervision of housing, factories, sanitation, and communicable disease control. Soon health departments in major cities became common. The Shattuck Report is considered the basis for the development of local and state health departments. Military personnel were soon cared for through the federal government, which eventually led to the Veterans Administration (VA). The VA is currently the largest healthcare system in the United States.

It was not until after World War II that the federal government ventured into health care and community health programs for the general population. In 1946, the Hill–Burton Act provided funds for building hospital facilities in many communities. Government funding for specific treatments for disease did not happen until the 1960s. Before the 1960s, the federal government primarily provided programs for the economically disadvantaged populations. The social welfare programs of the 1960s brought about the most dramatic changes in federal involvement in health care. The establishment of Medicare in 1965 was significant in that it became the first program to provide health services to citizens other than federal employees. The basic purpose of Medicare was to provide health care for the elderly. The Medicaid program was developed in 1965 and provided health care for low-income individuals. See **Box 9-1** for a list of the most significant health legislation acts passed during the "turning point decade" of the 1960s.

> If I were two-faced, would I be wearing this one?
>
> —*Abraham Lincoln*

The Civil Rights Act of 1964, although not directly related to health, provided fair access to health facilities for all races and genders. The Environmental Protection Agency (EPA), created through the National Environmental Policy Act, is historically one of the most significant pieces of U.S. environmental health policy. In recent years, significant legislation has been passed, including the Americans with Disabilities Act in 1990. This act increased the opportunities for Americans with disabilities to be integrated into mainstream society by removing physical barriers and improving public accommodation and services.

ETHICAL CONNECTION 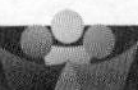

As a citizen of the United States, are we "free to be healthy" or to be "free from sickness"? What is the ethical responsibility of the government to safeguard such freedom?

Government

Federal Government

The federal government consists of three separate branches—executive (Office of the President), legislative (Congress), and judicial (federal court system). All three branches have a powerful impact on the healthcare delivery system and nursing practice (Shi & Singh, 2013). Nurses should be aware of how the different branches of the government affect healthcare policy and the ways that nurses can have a voice.

BOX 9-1 1965: What a Year for Health Law in the United States!

- Drug Abuse Control Amendments of 1965 (Public Law No. 89-74)
- Federal Cigarette Labeling and Advertising Act (Public Law No. 89-92)
- Construction Act Amendments of 1965 (Public Law No. 89-105)
- Community Health Services Extension Amendments of 1965 (Public Law No. 89-109)
- Health Research Facilities Amendments of 1965 (Public Law No. 89-115)
- Water Quality Act of 1965 (Public Law No. 89-234)
- Heart Disease, Cancer, and Stroke Amendments of 1965 (Public Law No. 89-239)
- The Clean Air Act Amendments and Solid Waste Disposal Act of 1965 (Public Law No. 89-272)
- Health Professions Educational Assistance Amendments of 1965 (Public Law No. 89-290)
- Medical Library Assistance Act (Public Law No. 89-291)
- Appalachian Regional Development Act of 1965 (Public Law No. 89-4)
- Older Americans Act (Public Law No. 89-73)
- Social Security Amendments of 1965 (Public Law No. 89-97)
- Vocational Rehabilitation Act Amendments of 1965 (Public Law No. 89-333)
- Housing and Urban Development Act of 1965 (Public Law No. 89-117)

Source: Data from Forgotson, E. H. (1967). 1965: The turning point in health law—1966 reflections. *American Journal of Public Health, 57*(6), 934–935.

Executive Branch

The **executive branch** consists of the president, the vice president, the Office of Management and Budget, and the administrative agencies, whose leadership is appointed by the president and approved by Congress. Presidential authority to exercise legislative leadership is clearly established by the Constitution and legislation, and accepted as a practical and political necessity (Anderson, 2006). The administrative agencies that have the greatest effect on healthcare policy and nursing education, research, and practice are the U.S. Department of Health and Human Services (HHS), the Department of Education, and the Department of Labor.

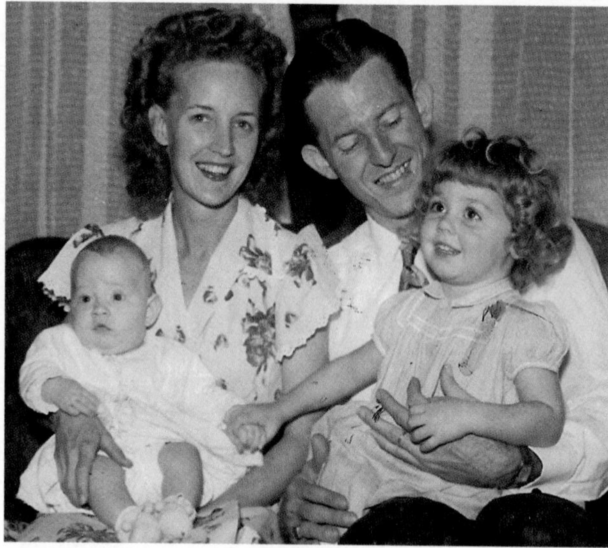

Families of the 1950s reflected a more traditional family form where mothers stayed home and fathers acted as the primary breadwinner. Children of these families make up the baby boomer generation and, as adults, now have very different values about gender roles within the family. Policies at all levels of government have been slow to respond to the dramatic changes in the diverse family forms of this century.

U.S. Department of Health and Human Services

The HHS is the federal agency most concerned with protecting the health of all Americans and providing essential human services, especially for those who are least able to help themselves. There are more than 300 programs under supervision, with a wide spectrum of activities and services. Some of these services include the following (HHS, 2014):

- Health and social science research
- Disease prevention, including immunization services
- Financial assistance and service for low-income families
- Child abuse and domestic violence prevention
- Medicare and Medicaid
- Food and drug safety
- Maternal and infant health improvement
- Services for older Americans
- Substance abuse treatment and prevention
- Health information technology
- Faith-based and community initiatives
- Comprehensive Native American health services
- Medical preparedness for emergencies, including potential terrorism

The HHS employs more than 60,000 people and administers more grant dollars than all other federal agencies combined. Its Medicare program is the nation's largest health insurer, handling more than 1 billion claims per year. Medicare and Medicaid together provide healthcare insurance for one in four Americans.

HHS funding for services is distributed primarily through federal, state, and local government agencies, although some services are provided through grants awarded to private-sector individuals or institutions. Programs, which are primarily located in Rockville, Maryland, are generally administered by 11 operating divisions, including eight agencies in the U.S. Public Health Service and three human services agencies. In addition, HHS programs provide for equitable treatment of beneficiaries nationwide and enable the collection of national health and other data. **Box 9-2** lists the health offices and services under the umbrella of HHS.

U.S. Public Health Agencies

National Institutes of Health The National Institutes of Health (NIH), located in Bethesda, Maryland, is the world's premier health research organization, supporting more than 38,000 research projects nationwide that

BOX 9-2 U.S. Department of Health and Human Services Agencies

U.S. Public Health Service Agencies

- National Institutes of Health
- Food and Drug Administration
- Centers for Disease Control and Prevention
- Indian Health Service
- Health Resources and Services Administration
- Substance Abuse and Mental Health Services Administration
- Agency for Healthcare Research and Quality
- U.S. Public Health Service Corps

Human Service Agencies

- Centers for Medicare & Medicaid Services
- Administration for Children and Families
- Administration on Aging

focus on diseases such as cancer, Alzheimer's disease, diabetes, arthritis, cardiovascular diseases, and human immunodeficiency virus (HIV)/acquired immune deficiency syndrome (AIDS). The NIH also includes the National Institute of Nursing Research (NINR). The research funded through NINR, which began as a center in 1986 and was elevated to institute status in 1993, focuses on health promotion and disease prevention, acute and chronic illness, and nursing systems (Bednash, Heylin, & Rhome, 1998).

Food and Drug Administration The Food and Drug Administration (FDA) is responsible for ensuring the safety of food and cosmetics and the safety and efficacy of pharmaceuticals, biological products, and medical devices.

Centers for Disease Control and Prevention Working with states and other partners, the Centers for Disease Control and Prevention (CDC)—established in 1946 and located in Atlanta, Georgia—provides a system of health surveillance to monitor and prevent disease outbreaks (including bioterrorism), implements disease prevention strategies, and maintains national health statistics.

The CDC director is also the administrator of the Agency for Toxic Substances and Disease Registry (ATSDR), which helps prevent exposure to hazardous substances from waste sites on the Environmental Protection Agency's National Priorities List.

The CDC's focus on the community allows nurses to make significant contributions in a variety of areas. Nurses are involved in the establishment of infection control guidelines; the prevention of substance abuse, HIV/AIDS, and other sexually transmitted infections; and in the areas of violence, adolescent and school health, women's health, children's health, and immunization (Bednash et al., 1998).

Health Resources and Services Administration The Health Resources and Services Administration (HRSA) provides access to essential healthcare services for people who are low income, are uninsured, or live in rural areas or urban neighborhoods where health care is scarce. HRSA-funded health centers provided medical care to almost 14 million patients at more than 3,700 sites in the United States in 2005. The agency, founded in 1982, helps prepare the U.S. healthcare system and providers to respond to bioterrorism and other public health emergencies, maintains the National Health Service Corps, and helps build the healthcare workforce through training and education programs.

Substance Abuse and Mental Health Services Administration Services to improve the quality and availability of substance abuse prevention, addiction treatment, and mental health care are provided by the Substance Abuse and Mental Health Services Administration (SAMHSA). Funding to support treatment for Americans with serious substance abuse or mental health problems is provided through block grants to states. Established in 1992, SAMHSA monitors the prevalence and incidence of substance abuse and identifies and disseminates information related to the best practices for prevention and treatment.

Agency for Healthcare Research and Quality The mission of the Agency for Healthcare Research and Quality (AHRQ), established in 1989, is to generate and distribute evidence-based information that improves healthcare delivery and outcomes.

U.S. Public Health Service Commissioned Corps The U.S. Public Health Service Commissioned Corps (PHS) is a uniformed service of more than 6,000 health professionals who serve in many HHS and other federal agencies. The PHS director is the Surgeon General of the United States, who is appointed by the president. PHS members, who are commissioned officers, include many nurses. The chief nurse holds the rank of rear admiral (HHS, 2014).

MEDIA MOMENT

A Civil Action (1998)

In this movie based on a true story, John Travolta stars as a personal-injury lawyer who sues a major corporation when the drinking water in Woburn, Massachusetts, is found to contain high levels of industrial solvents. Believing the contamination is responsible for the large number of leukemia deaths among the town's children, the citizens—led by a woman (Kathleen Quinlan) whose child has died—hire a lawyer to take on the corporate polluters. Beatrice and Grace are the real-life companies represented in the movie, and *A Civil Action* is based on Jonathan Harr's nonfiction bestseller, which won the National Book Award.

Thank You for Smoking (2005)

Big Tobacco spin-doctor Nick Naylor (Aaron Eckhart) is on a mission to make the country forget the dangers of his product. Rallying for the cause, he works to promote smoking in the movies and hush former employees who bad-mouth cigarettes, all the while trying to remain a good role model for his 12-year-old son. Maria Bello, Katie Holmes, Robert Duvall, and William H. Macy co-star in Jason Reitman's movie based on Christopher Buckley's novel. The movie provides thought-provoking satire on the continued debate between tobacco companies' right to advertise and the public health concerns related to tobacco use.

Infinitely Polar Bear (2014)

Cameron (Mark Ruffalo), who suffers from bipolar disorder, takes on care of his two daughters (Imogene Wolodarsky and Ashley Aufderheide) so his estranged wife (Zoe Saldana) can return to school to improve the family's financial prospects. The film touches upon the inherent conflicts of managing family life in the face of mental illness with edgy humor. Although his erratic and unpredictable mood changes make for some tension— a scene where Cameron's manic phase leads to binge drinking and being locked out by his daughters is at once laugh- and cringe-worthy—the film is a warm commentary on parenting's challenges at the best (and worst) of times, reminding us that people with mental illness have lives beyond the diagnosis.

Human Services Agencies

Centers for Medicare and Medicaid Services The Centers for Medicare and Medicaid Services (CMS), originally established as the Health Care Financing Administration in 1977, administers the Medicare and Medicaid programs, which provide health care to one in every four Americans. Medicare provides health insurance for more than 43 million elderly and disabled Americans. Medicaid, a joint federal–state program, provides health coverage for 51.6 million low-income people, including 25.1 million children, and nursing home coverage for low-income elders. CMS also administers the Children's Health Insurance Program (CHIP), which covers more than 8.9 million children (HHS, 2014).

Administration for Children and Families The Administration for Children and Families (ACF), established in 1991 by combining several existing programs, is responsible for 60 programs that promote the economic and social wellbeing of children, families, and communities. Some of the programs administered by the ACF are the state–federal welfare program called Temporary Assistance for Needy Families (TANF), which provides assistance to an estimated 4.4 million people, including 4 million children; the national child support enforcement system, which collects payments from noncustodial parents; and the Head Start program, which serves more than 900,000 preschool children. The ACF also funds programs to prevent child abuse and domestic violence and supports state programs to support foster care and provide adoption assistance (HHS, 2014).

GLOBAL CONNECTION 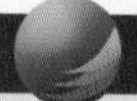

Other countries have different values concerning the obligation of government to fund basic and essential health care. Why is the United States different in this respect? Why has it rejected attempts in the past to "socialize" the U.S. healthcare system?

Administration on Aging Administration on Aging (AoA) programs provide services to older Americans living at home in the community through a nationwide aging services network. Services provided to elders include, but are not limited to, meals, transportation, caregiver support, personal care, information and assistance, nursing home ombudsman, elder rights protection, and health promotion. These services enable elders to remain healthy, secure, and independent (HHS, 2008).

Department of Education The U.S. Department of Education (DOE) provides billions of dollars each year for postsecondary education, including nursing education. Federal Family Education Loans (Stafford Loans), Pell Grants, and Federal Work Study programs are just a few of the sources of funding provided (Bednash et al., 1998; White, 2002).

Department of Labor The U.S. Department of Labor (DOL) is responsible for enforcing the Fair Labor Standards Act (minimum wage and overtime), the Employee Retirement Income Security Act (employee benefit and retirement plans), and the Occupational Safety and Health Act (OSHA) (job safety and health). All of these are important to nursing practice. The ANA has worked closely with the Department of Labor for over 20 years to ensure adequate funding for the health and safety of nurses in the workplace through enforcement of Occupational Safety and Health Act standards (Bednash et al., 1998; White, 2002).

Legislative Branch

The U.S. Congress is the **legislative branch** of the federal government. Congress has two houses with equal power: the Senate and the House of Representatives. The Senate has 100 members, two from each state. The House of Representatives membership varies according to the population. A representative is elected to represent a specific number of constituents, so states with larger populations have more representatives. The number of representatives a state has increases or decreases with corresponding changes in the state's population. The House of Representatives currently has more than 400 members. The sole legislative power of the federal government lies with the two houses of Congress (White, 2002). A partial list of the responsibilities of the U.S. Congress is outlined in **Box 9-3**.

Judicial Branch

The **judicial branch** of the federal government, known as the U.S. court system, consists of 94 federal district courts, 12 circuit courts of appeals, the U.S. Supreme Court, and several specialized courts to address customs, patents, military issues, and so on. A Supreme Court justice generally keeps his or her appointment until retirement or death. At that time, a replacement is

BOX 9-3 Responsibilities of the U.S. Congress

- Conduct hearings on issues that may generate federal legislation.
- Draft legislation.
- Estimate cost of proposed legislation.
- Enact legislation to create programs.
- Review legislated program operations.
- Determine the federal budget.
- Appropriate funds for federal operations.
- Decide entitlement policy (e.g., Medicare, Medicaid, Social Security).
- Confirm or reject presidential nominations for high-level federal positions (e.g., cabinet members, federal judges).

Source: Data from Bednash, G. P., Heylin, G. B., & Rhome, A. M. (1998). Federal government. In D. J. Mason & J. K. Leavitt (Eds.), *Policy and politics in nursing and health care* (3rd ed., pp. 436–457). Philadelphia, PA: Saunders.

appointed to the position by the president and approved by Congress (White, 2002).

Although the judicial branch of the government is not involved in making policy, the way in which the courts interpret the law may have a profound effect on health care, including nursing practice. The courts are often called upon to interpret and decide the meaning of statutory provisions that are ambiguous, unclear, and open to conflicting interpretation (Anderson, 2006). Nurses can affect the outcome of court cases by serving as expert witnesses or legal consultants (Bednash et al., 1998).

State Government

Although the role of the federal government is in the forefront of American politics, the truth is that most of the policies and laws related to nursing practice are created at the state level. The creation and enforcement of nurse practice acts and the regulation of nursing practice through licensing occurs at the state level. State governments consist of the same three branches as the federal government: executive, legislative, and judicial.

Executive Branch

The executive branch of all state governments consists of the governor and the attorney general. More than half of the states also have a lieutenant governor, who may or may not work closely with the governor, depending on the election politics of that state (Reinhard, 2002). Most governors are elected to 4-year terms and are eligible for reelection. The governor is responsible for presenting the state budget to the legislature and overseeing state spending. The governor's policy initiatives are often presented as part of the state budget proposal and may contain health-related programs. The lieutenant governor presides over state affairs in the absence of the governor and can influence health and social policies within the state. The attorney general represents the public's interests in legal cases coming before the court, not including the state supreme court. The attorney general's office is often called on to interpret the nurse practice act to clarify the intent of legislation or regulations (Gaffney, 1998).

GOT AN ALTERNATIVE?

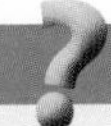

Vitamins and herbal supplements are not regulated by law in the United States. Do you think the FDA should regulate them as other "drugs"? Why or why not?

A DAY IN THE LIFE

In 1991, I received a telephone call from Geraldine Ferraro asking me to come to New York City to be interviewed for a leadership position on her campaign for a United States Senate seat representing the state of New York. How did Gerry find me and why did she want a nurse to work on a major national campaign?

My connection to Gerry followed one of the most important principles of political involvement and influence—"use your connections." I had spent a sabbatical year at the ANA working in the governmental affairs department. While there, I collaborated with one of the women who had been involved in Gerry's nomination for vice president of the United States in 1984. She knew Gerry was considering a run for the U.S. Senate, so she called her to recommend my political skills to her. Gerry indicated a strong interest in working with me because of my involvement with ANA, the first group to endorse her candidacy for vice president. Gerry called me and hired me a week later.

For a year and a half I worked as the upstate campaign coordinator. I was responsible for 54 of the 62 counties in the state, an area that covers over 40,000 square miles. I started with nothing except a great candidate. I had to organize an office, create a database of contacts, organize a grassroots network, raise thousands of dollars, and create fundraising and media events. Although I had been an active volunteer in numerous congressional and state legislative campaigns, I had never been a paid staff member. I did not have an appointed position in the political party, so I had to use all my communication skills, organizational skills, and nursing intuition to create a campaign presence in every one of the 54 counties under my leadership.

It helped to have a candidate with name recognition. When I called major democratic leaders and potential supporters, I didn't have to introduce my candidate. I used my connections and those of Gerry to build a grassroots structure. I focused on women's organizations, women leaders, nurses and their organizations, other health professionals, and any other men and women throughout the state who wanted to volunteer for Gerry. Gerry's candidacy energized and excited the electorate, as it had when she ran for vice president. It wasn't hard getting volunteers; it was only difficult organizing them to contribute in meaningful ways. Whether it was organizing events for fundraising, working with the media, conducting voter registration drives, or soliciting political endorsements, it took incredible planning and organizational skill and thousands of volunteer hours. I planned it all—over 200 events—supported by a grassroots structure of over 5,000 volunteers from every profession, occupation, and interest group who held campaign events, gave money, and worked for Gerry in their home communities.

The nurses came out in droves. Nurses who had never been involved politically suddenly wanted to help Gerry and listen to her message. Because I had been active in both the ANA-PAC and New York State political activities, I was able to help Gerry receive an early endorsement by the ANA-PAC and encourage the New York State Nurses Association to mobilize their members.

What was it like to work so closely for such a national and international "celebrity"? It was fun, grueling, exciting, challenging, and a once-in-a-lifetime experience. What made it easy was Gerry. She was personable, caring, and in many ways very much like her constituents. She had experienced poverty as well as success; she was a teacher and a lawyer; she was a mother, grandmother, and wife—so she knew about the issues and could relate to people throughout the country. She used me to draft her health platform and respected my expertise in teaching her about the issues. In addition, Gerry was able to bring the best political and media consultants to work with me and the campaign staff. Traveling with Gerry was the most fun of the entire year and a half. We would often spend two or three days alone traveling throughout the upstate counties, affording us an opportunity to become good friends. I was the oldest staff person, much closer in age to Gerry. That created a special bond that enabled me to have access to her and engendered mutual respect. At each event, I would sometimes look around as she was speaking and think how lucky I was to be able to have the opportunity to help elect someone whom I admired and believed could have been a fine senator. Unfortunately, that never happened. Gerry lost in the primary election by less than 10,000 votes out of 4 million cast. The country lost the chance to have a great senator. I gained a friend and stories for a lifetime.

—Judy Leavitt, MEd, RN, Campaign Manager for Geraldine Ferraro, Candidate for U.S. Senate in 1992

State Agencies

The power of state agencies to influence health and social policy varies across and within states (Reinhard, 2002). Typically, state agencies may be divided into five different categories:

1. Agencies led by elected officers such as secretaries of state, treasurers, and attorney generals
2. Agencies led by officers appointed by the governor or independent boards, such as secretaries of human services and commissioners of health
3. Professional licensing and regulatory boards, such as boards of nursing
4. Public authorities and corporations, such as higher education assistance authorities
5. Independent boards and commissions, such as councils of higher education and public utilities commissions

In many states, the Department of Health is a state organization whose primary purpose is to oversee and maintain the health of the community. The director of the state department of public health is appointed by the governor. In other states, the Department of Health may be a division within a larger government agency (Reinhard, 2002). There are many different functions of the department of public health, which may include data collection and surveillance, administration of Medicaid and other federally funded programs, public health programs, and hospital regulation (Gaffney, 1998).

Legislative Branch

State legislatures are the oldest part of the American government, existing long before the drafting of the U.S. Constitution. In fact, the Declaration of Independence was signed by representatives of the legislatures of the 13 colonies that became the original 13 states. State legislatures levy taxes, appropriate funding, and create and monitor agencies to carry out state business (Gaffney, 1998). Patterned after the federal legislature, all state legislatures (excluding Nebraska) consist of two houses: a Senate and a House of Representatives. In each state, the House of Representatives is larger than the Senate because senators represent larger districts within the state than members of the House. Therefore, each senator has a greater number of constituents.

Judicial Branch

State judicial systems are similar to that of the federal system. The state supreme courts serve to interpret the language of their state constitutions and apply it in the courtroom. In recent years, there have been many changes in state laws related to health care. Many more malpractice suits are being brought against physicians, nurses, and hospitals by people who believe that they have been injured as a result of negligence or inappropriate action (Gaffney, 1998).

Local Government

Local governments are the link between citizens and the state and federal governments. Local governments distribute billions of federal and state dollars to local community agencies to provide services. The quality of life in a community is determined by how local government officials make decisions about the delivery of services. Some of the services provided and monitored by local governments are public health, public education, drinking water, sewage disposal, police protection, and solid waste management (Majewski & O'Brien, 2006).

The number, size, and type of local government vary throughout the country depending on state and regional culture, economics, and geography. The U.S. Census Bureau has divided local governments into four categories: counties, municipalities, towns and townships, and special districts (Majewski & O'Brien, 2006). Local governments are divided into the same branches of government (with variations) as the federal and state governments.

> Let the strivings of Martin Luther King, Jr., to have been correct when he said that humanity can no longer be tragically bound to the starless midnight of racism and war.
>
> —*Nelson Mandela, Nobel Peace Prize acceptance speech, 1993*

Different Types of Law

According to *Webster's New World College Dictionary* (Agnus, 2004), a law is a rule of conduct established and enforced by the authority, legislation, or custom of a given community, state, or other group. There are three types of laws in the United States: constitutional law, legislation and regulation, and judicial or common law.

Constitutional law is derived from federal and state constitutions and is the supreme law of the land. The U.S. Constitution is the highest legal authority that exists, and no other law, state or federal, may overrule it. A state constitution is the highest state law authority, but any provisions that conflict with the federal constitution will be invalidated by the courts. It is not considered a conflict, however, if state constitutions provide more expansive individual rights than those guaranteed by the federal constitution (Kaplin & Lee, 2006).

Legislation and regulation, known as **statutory law**, are established through formal legislative processes. Each time the U.S. Congress or state legislatures pass legislation, the body of statutory law grows (Betts & Waddle, 2007). Statutes are enacted by federal and state governments. Local statutes, called *ordinances*, are enacted by local governing bodies, such as city and county councils (Kaplin & Lee, 2006).

Judicial or common law, known as case law, is derived from decisions made in the courtroom. Common law is based on the principles of justice, reason, and common sense rather than rules and regulations (Guido, 2001). Each time a judge or a jury makes a decision, the body of common law grows (Betts & Waddle, 2007). Decisions are made based on decisions from previous similar cases. Judges are bound by previous decisions (i.e., precedents) unless it can be shown that the previous rulings are no longer valid. Therefore, a decision made in a case with no predecessors is critical because it becomes a precedent-setting case.

Common law can be categorized as either civil or criminal. Civil law protects individuals and involves the enforcement of rights, duties, and other legal relations between private citizens (Betts & Waddle, 2007). For example, an individual can sue another individual or a company for not fulfilling the terms of a legal contract. Criminal law is a crime against the state and involves public concerns against unlawful behavior that threatens society (Betts & Waddle, 2007). Murder is an example of criminal law. Although the crime was committed against an individual, it threatens the security of society as a whole.

How an Idea Becomes a Law

In today's climate of healthcare reform, nurses must understand the legislative process to be able to influence the development of sound healthcare policy for their patients and for the profession of nursing (Abood & Mittelstadt, 2006; Santa Anna, 2006). Because the legislative process is similar at the state and federal levels, it is described at the state level in this chapter. Although the legislative pathway may differ slightly from state to state, the basic process is the same (Abood & Mittelstadt, 2006; Santa Anna, 2006). The state of Florida is used as the example.

A bill can be introduced only by a member of the legislature. Legislators introduce bills for many reasons, which may include pleasing a constituent or a special-interest group, declaring a position on an issue, getting publicity, or simply avoiding a political attack (Abood & Mittelstadt, 2006; Santa Anna, 2006). Companion bills (or twin bills) are sometimes introduced by legislators in the Senate and House of Representatives to increase the likelihood that the bill will pass and become law.

During a legislative session, the House and Senate meet separately and attempt to pass legislation that has previously been considered by a number of legislative committees. Committees are often referred to as the "heart of the legislative process" because they allow legislators to break down into smaller groups to discuss pertinent issues (Florida Senate, 2006). This enables members to have more in-depth discussions than would be possible if all issues were discussed by the entire legislature. Committees are established by authority of rules, which are adopted separately by the House and the Senate. The Speaker of the House and the President of the Senate, both of whom are elected by each body and represent the majority party, designate a chair and a vice-chair for each committee and appoint legislators to serve as committee members. Legislators usually serve on more than one committee.

There are three basic kinds of committees: standing, select, and conference committees. Standing committees are established by both the Senate and the House of Representatives to manage their business. They can be distinguished from each other by the kind of issues that they consider. For example, the Florida House of Representatives has a standing committee on healthcare regulation, which is responsible for considering bills relating to that particular area. The staff of this committee is responsible for doing the fact-finding groundwork for legislation that is referred to the committee for consideration. For example, if the committee were considering a bill proposing a change in the requirements for registered nurse (RN) licensure, it would study the current licensure requirements, find out why the sponsor of the bill (one or more of the representatives) believes the change is necessary, examine what the effects of the proposed change might be, and hear testimony from nurses, as well as the broader healthcare community, to gain insight about how they feel about the proposed change. Once all of these things are considered, the committee passes judgment on the proposed legislation. If the bill passes the committee, it travels either to the next committee of reference (if there is more than one) or to the floor of the House or Senate to be voted on by the respective body as a whole. If the committee does not pass the proposed legislation (reports unfavorably on the bill), the legislation will die unless two-thirds of the members vote to reconsider it. This is a very high percentage, and further consideration is unlikely to occur in this situation.

Committees wield significant power in the legislative process. The chair of each committee has a great deal of influence over legislation because he or she decides which bills will be heard by the committee. If a bill is not heard, it cannot be voted on and therefore cannot be passed. Committees also have the authority to amend proposed legislation, so the original bill may look very different by the time it reaches the floor of the House or Senate.

A second type of committee is the select committee. This type of committee is appointed to perform a particular task and goes out of existence when the purpose for which it was created has been accomplished (Florida House of Representatives, 2008). Also known as an "ad hoc" committee, a select committee may last anywhere from a few minutes to several years. For example, on the opening day of each legislative session, the Senate president will appoint a select committee to inform the House of Representatives that they are ready to begin conducting business. The Speaker of the House will appoint a similar committee that completes the ritual. These select committees complete their ceremonial function in a few minutes. By contrast, when an issue arises that merits special consideration, a select committee may be established to consider that particular issue in depth. For example, the 1999 Florida Legislature had to consider a comprehensive legislative package introduced by Governor Jeb Bush regarding education. Rather than refer the large number of bills to different standing committees, the Speaker of the House of Representatives appointed a Select Committee on Transforming Florida's Schools to consider the bills as a complete educational package. This committee consisted of members of the House of Representatives (from both political parties) and was chaired by the member who sponsored the legislation. It met for 2 weeks immediately before the legislative session, heard testimony from supporters and opponents, and was responsible for amending and voting on the bills in the package.

THINK ABOUT THIS 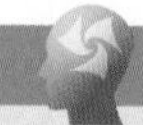

Nancy Pelosi, U.S. Representative from California, became the United States' first female Speaker of the U.S. House of Representatives in January 2007.

The third type of committee is a conference committee. Before the functions of this kind of committee can be described, it is necessary to further explain the process

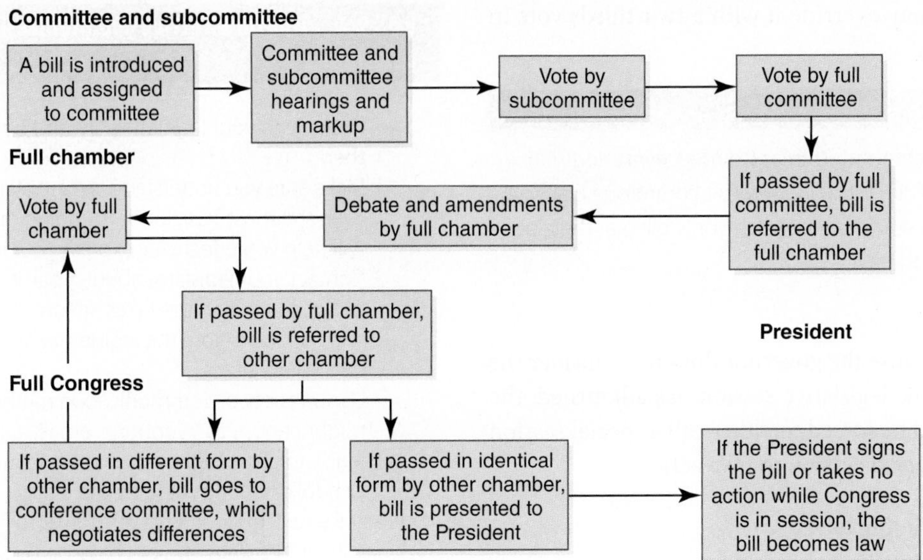

Figure 9-1 The legislative process.

of how a bill becomes a law. For a bill to be signed into law and become an act that is sent to the governor for consideration, it must pass both houses of the legislature in identical form. This is often more difficult than it sounds. First, the bill must have a sponsor in both the House and the Senate. These "companion" bills may be identical, similar, or very dissimilar. When a bill makes it through the committee process and is considered on the floor of the House or Senate, it goes through an amendatory process. Once amended, the bill requires a majority vote to pass.

Let's use RN licensure requirements as a hypothetical example. The House bill, after completing the committee process, increases both the level of education needed to obtain an RN license and the competencies required to pass the licensure exam. On the floor, House members amend the bill to add two more competencies. The bill, as amended, passes with a majority vote and is sent to the Senate for consideration. The Senate takes up the House bill and agrees with the increased educational requirements but decides to amend the bill because it does not agree with the competencies that the House has chosen. In the amendatory process, the Senate removes three of the competencies required in the House bill and adds two new competencies from the original Senate bill. The House bill, as amended by the Senate, then passes the Senate with a majority vote and is sent back to the House. If the House does not agree with the changes made by the Senate, they may reach an impasse. This often results in the bill's demise. However, if the proposed legislation is important to the leadership in each house, the presiding officers may appoint a conference committee in an attempt to reach a compromise agreement. If differences cannot be reconciled through the conference committee, the proposed legislation will fail. A conference committee is actually composed of two separate committees, one appointed by the president of the Senate and the other appointed by the speaker of the House. The two committees vote separately on all issues relating to the bill under consideration, and a majority of each committee must approve all changes (Florida Senate, 2008). If the conference committee can reach an agreement, the House and Senate must vote on the compromise on a "take it or leave it" basis and no amendments can be offered (Florida Senate, 2008). Usually, conference reports are submitted during the waning hours of a session, when time is short and legislators are unlikely to reject conference committee recommendations because it will most likely result in the failure of the bill (Florida House of Representatives, 2008).

It is important to realize that many bills make it through the committee process but never get heard on the floor of the House or Senate. The presiding officers of each house, through the standing committees on rules and calendar, have control over which bills will be considered by the full House or Senate. Just as in committee, if a bill is not heard on the floor, it cannot be voted on and therefore cannot pass.

If a bill makes it through the committee process and passes both houses in identical form, it is called an *act*. Each act is sent to the governor for consideration, and he or she may either sign it into law, allow it to become law without his or her signature, or veto it. If an act is vetoed, the legislature may override it with a two-thirds vote in both houses.

NOTE THIS!

A conference committee is appointed every legislative session to consider the budget. This committee is always important because the budget is the only bill that the legislature is *required* to pass.

However, because the governor does not consider the acts until after the legislative session has adjourned, the legislature would be forced to either call a special session or wait until the next session to take action.

How Nurses Can Get Involved

Nurses can become involved in the political process at various levels. The first and most important thing is to be an informed voter. Nurses should watch the news, read the newspaper, surf the Internet, and be aware of what the candidates stand for on the national, state, and local levels regarding health issues and policy. Listen and read diverse opinions about issues related to health and nursing, whether via blogs, social networks (such as Facebook or LinkedIn), or health-related websites in order to be a well-informed professional who advocates for the public's health. Nurses should also find out where candidates stand on the issues that are important to them as nurses. This can be accomplished with just a minimal amount of investigation. Nurses should also become members of their professional organizations, because organized lobbying via political action committees (PACs) influences state and national health policy directly related to nursing and the public's health (Brennan, 2012). Nurses can contact the professional organizations to which they belong to find out which candidates they support. If a candidate is an incumbent, his or her voting record on issues of importance should be checked. Nurses must make phone calls, write letters, and ask questions!

Once legislators are in office, nurses should get to know them and make themselves and their views known to them. **Box 9-4** provides some tips for effectively communicating ideas to legislators.

BOX 9-4 Tips for Effective Communication with Legislators

- Know who your legislators are and how to contact them.
- Make sure you understand the legislative process. Even the most basic understanding of the process will help you effectively express your ideas.
- Contact your legislator about a particular issue before the legislature takes action on it. Most matters coming before the legislature are well publicized before session.
- Use a variety of communication methods. You might choose to telephone, email, fax, or visit your legislator. You might also choose to give testimony at public hearings held by the legislature.
- Tell your legislator what effect you think a particular bill, if it becomes law, will have on you, your children, business, or community. Be concise, but specific.
- Be polite, even if you disagree strongly with the legislator you are addressing. Lawmakers cannot please everyone. Your communication will be more effective if you are reasonable in your approach.
- Suggest a course of action and offer assistance. Don't make promises or threats.

Source: Florida Senate. (2006). Effective communication with a legislator. Retrieved from http://www.flsenate.gov

To have one of your ideas introduced as a bill, you must first find a sponsor in both the House and the Senate. The best scenario would be to approach a potential sponsor who is influential among legislators and who has a record of sponsoring successful legislation in your area of interest. This person will be likely to have more success in building coalitions among members than a less experienced legislator. It is also helpful if the legislator feels strongly about the issue, because he or she will be more likely to fight for the proposed legislation.

Some legislative bodies place limits on the number of bills that can be filed by a particular member. It is necessary to investigate whether limitations exist and, if so, approach potential sponsors early. Timing can be crucial, especially if the issue of concern is a highly publicized one. Be aware of media coverage and strategically plan your moves.

Lobbying

Lobbying is defined as "influencing or attempting to influence legislative action or non-action through oral or written communication or attempting to obtain the goodwill of a member or employee of the Legislature" (Section 11.045 Florida Statutes). A lobbyist is a person who is employed and receives payment for the primary purpose of lobbying on behalf of another person, group, or governmental entity. Most states, if not all, require lobbyists to be registered as such. This registration allows citizens to be informed about activities that are aimed at influencing government decision making. For example, when major legislation relating to health care is being considered, it may be beneficial to know which groups have hired lobbyists to promote their interests and monitor their activities and expenditures.

For example, home health agencies may hire lobbyists whose principal responsibilities are to represent the organization's interests to the legislature and other government agencies. Nurses employed by a home health agency would not be considered lobbyists unless their most significant work responsibility dealt with governmental affairs.

However, this does not mean that the nurses cannot contact their legislators and actively support or oppose legislation that affects their home health agencies. It simply means that the nurses are not be required to register because they do not receive payment for the purposes of lobbying.

RESEARCH ALERT 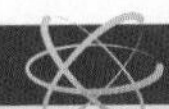

This study investigated the role of flight attendants and their unions in creating smoke-free air travel. Case study methodology was used to search tobacco industry documents and labor union periodicals and to interview key informants. Tobacco industry strategies against establishing smoke-free work sites failed with the airline industry, largely because of the efforts of flight attendants and their unions. This study illustrates the potential for successful partnerships between unions and tobacco control policy advocates when developing smoke-free work site policies.

Source: Pan, J., Barbeau, E. M., Levenstein, C., & Balbach, E. D. (2005). Smoke-free airlines and the role of organized labor: A case study. *American Journal of Public Health, 95*(3), 398–404.

Lobbyists must adhere to many rules and regulations, which may vary widely from state to state. Therefore, it is important that nurses be aware of the rules, if any, that apply in their states. Regulations may also change from year to year, which makes it necessary to keep current. For example, in Florida, rules and regulations regarding the receipt of gifts from lobbyists are established in statute (Section 112.3148, Florida Statutes). Other states may not be so proscriptive and may outline rules only in policy manuals or employee handbooks. Some states may not even have rules for lobbyists, but most have some kind of regulation.

Best practices for lobbying and for concerned constituents include being aware of all applicable rules and restrictions, establishing a good rapport with legislators and legislative staff, and always backing up your position with hard data. If nurses adhere to these principles, their likelihood of successfully communicating their ideas will greatly increase.

Political Action Committees

Through the years, the ANA and various other specialty health organizations have taken leadership roles in mobilizing nurses in grassroots lobbying. This has required a significant effort to educate nurses about the political process and how to remain cognizant of the political issues that affect nursing and health. Because federal law requires that campaign contributions be kept as a separate fund and that no organizational membership be used for this purpose, many groups have created separate organizations for political activities. These organizations are referred to as **political action committees (PACs)**. Their work is completely separate from the rest of the organization's work. The primary purpose of a PAC is to endorse and support candidates for public office who support the legislative agenda of the organization or group making the endorsement (Curtis & Lumpkin, 1998; Malone, Chaffee, & Wachter, 2002). Nursing PACs exist at the federal and state levels, most often through the ANA Political Action Committee (ANA-PAC) and state nurses' associations.

APPLICATION TO PRACTICE 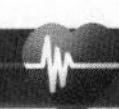

Two Mississippi Nurses Lead the Way

Deborah Konkle-Parker, MSN, FNP

As a nurse practitioner working in an outpatient HIV clinic in Jackson, Mississippi, Debbie Konkle-Parker and other providers depended on the federal Ryan White AIDS Drug Assistance Program (ADAP), administered by the Mississippi Department of Health (MSDH), to help many of their patients get medicines. ADAP was used primarily to help patients who had no health insurance or whose medications exceeded the Mississippi Medicaid limit of five prescriptions per month.

In early April 1997, after several years of uneventful program usage, word was received from the health department that the Ryan White program was not accepting any more referrals for ADAP assistance. The recent addition of expensive protease inhibitors to the treatment regimen for HIV had depleted the entire year of federal ADAP funding by mid-March. This news came suddenly, without warning, and with no backup plan for those with no other resources.

This sudden news sent providers and patients reeling, with no way to deal with this shortfall in services. A week later, there was a meeting of healthcare providers at the MSDH. At this meeting, the healthcare providers were informed that those individuals who were already receiving a protease inhibitor from ADAP would continue to receive medications, but all others would be cut off from the program. No more referrals were being accepted. This could literally mean the difference between life and death for many patients.

To deal with the problem, Debbie Konkle-Parker organized a problem-solving session to determine a way to cope with this change. She sent letters to concerned individuals, requesting their presence at a networking meeting. The meeting was attended by healthcare providers representing all disciplines, representatives from MSDH, representatives from the pharmaceutical industry, and persons with HIV/AIDS. The discussion at the meeting revealed that although most states provided funding from their state budgets to augment the federal ADAP dollars, Mississippi did not. It was decided that to change this policy, it was important to become an organized body to influence the legislators. The Mississippi HIV/AIDS Assembly was formed, with Debbie Konkle-Parker as its chair. The Mississippi HIV/AIDS Assembly consisted of two committees: (1) the AIDS Aware committee for mobilizing grassroots lobbying efforts around the state and (2) the Health Provider Network of interdisciplinary healthcare providers who could mobilize organizational lobbying efforts. Shortly after this meeting, the MSDH found a way to temporarily redirect some of the money from other parts of the Ryan White program to re-enroll some patients who had been dropped from the program. But that effort was only putting a "Band-Aid" on the problem until further funding could be obtained.

The Health Provider Network set about the task of determining the direction of the work of the assembly, and the AIDS Aware committee gathered grassroots support for their efforts. The highest priority goal was supporting the Health Department's request for $500,000 from the state budget for ADAP. Although this amount was much less than what was actually needed, it was determined that politically this was an amount that reasonably could be requested by the Health Department. The Mississippi AIDS Assembly requested $2 million from the legislature, which was the estimate of how much money was actually needed to meet the extent of the problem in Mississippi.

Through these two committees, several different actions were taken, including providing speakers to bring attention to the issue for the public; maintaining a "silent" presence, including media coverage at a key budget hearing meeting; attending a meeting of the legislature's public health committee where bills were decided on before being brought to the floor; and applying consistent pressure on legislators to consider this issue. Multiple mailings went out to individuals throughout the state, encouraging personal communication with their legislators and a "spreading of the word."

The result of this yearlong work was the first-ever state dedication of $750,000 to the Mississippi Ryan White AIDS Drug Assistance Program, with more to follow each year. This funding allowed a return of new referrals to the program and an immediate lessening of the waiting list of individuals needing medications.

Connie Thompson, BSN, RN

As the infection control coordinator of a medical center in Jackson, Mississippi, Connie Thompson played a big role in the efforts of the Mississippi HIV/AIDS Assembly and eagerly joined in the excitement surrounding its legislative victory. But after the excitement faded away, Thompson realized that this was only the beginning. More funding and services were needed, not only for persons living with HIV/AIDS, but for persons living with any chronic, disabling disease.

In August 1998, under the leadership of Thompson, a variety of Mississippi organizations and agencies joined forces in an effort to influence legislative healthcare issues for disabled persons. Eventually this group formed a coalition of more than 50 organizations and agencies known as the Coalition for Uninsured Mississippians, representing thousands of Mississippians with disabilities or chronic illnesses who are denied access to health insurance each year. These individuals—persons with cancer, heart disease, HIV, diabetes, asthma, lupus, arthritis, and other diseases—earn a little more money, either from disability payments or job income, than the maximum allowed to qualify for Medicaid. However, they don't make enough money to be able to afford expensive private health insurance.

As a result, these men, women, and children are forced to make frequent visits to hospital emergency departments for basic health care. Or worse, they do not seek care at all until a crisis occurs that requires inpatient hospitalization. Proper disease management with regular clinic visits for appropriate follow up and networking for patient care and services would maintain optimal health standards for these individuals. Quality of life for these persons would greatly improve and health care would be more cost-effective if they had access to health insurance.

The Coalition for Uninsured Mississippians sought support from Mississippi's citizens for a legislative bill that would allow disabled persons with incomes below 250% of the federal poverty level to buy in to Medicaid coverage. The purchase of this coverage would be based on a sliding scale fee. Both the Balanced Budget Act of 1997 and encouragement from the HHS were used to support the coalition's action.

Within 2 months of the coalition's initial meeting, a petition supported by thousands of Mississippians had been sent to the co-chairs of the joint subcommittees of health and welfare of the state legislature. A statewide Forum for Effective Advocacy of Chronic Illnesses and Disabilities was held to discuss the issues, and a task force was formed to meet with the director of the division of Medicaid to look for solutions. Connie Thompson, as the facilitator of the Coalition for Uninsured Mississippians, was invited to serve on the attorney general's Partners for a Healthy Mississippi task force.

As a result of the coalition's efforts, a bill to expand Medicaid coverage by authorizing a buy-in opportunity to workers who are disabled and earning less than 250% of the federal poverty level was drafted and signed into law by the Mississippi legislature and the governor during the 1999 legislative session.

In both of these scenarios, nurse-led public policy strategies, starting with simple problem-solving meetings, have achieved the goal of improving health care for some of Mississippi's poor and vulnerable citizens.

Deborah Konkle-Parker, MSN, FNP

Regulation and Licensing of Nursing Practice

The Regulatory Process

Although it is important for nurses to be involved in the legislative process, it is equally important for nurses to understand the **regulatory process**. According to *Webster's New World College Dictionary* (Agnus, 2004), *regulation* is the act of controlling, directing, or governing according to a rule, principle, or system. Once bills are passed into law by the legislative branch of government, they must be implemented by the administrative agencies of the executive branch (Abood & Mittelstadt, 1998; Loquist, 1999; White, 2002). Legislation is purposely expressed in broad terms to provide flexibility and adaptability of laws over time. Regulation is expressed in very specific terms describing how the administrative agency with jurisdictional authority will implement the law (Loquist, 1999; Santa Anna, 2002). The legislative process is used to create policy and laws to address a particular issue when none exist. Regulation is used to clarify and interpret existing policy and laws and decide what methods will be used to enforce them (Loquist, 1999; Santa Anna, 2002).

Regulations frame the way health policy is transposed into services and programs. Although regulations are a direct result of passed legislation, they are shaped into their final forms by the ongoing involvement of healthcare professionals and their professional organizations, third-party payers, consumers, and other special-interest groups. Before a federal agency can implement a law, it must publish the proposed regulation or set of regulations in the **Federal Register**. The publication of the proposed regulations affords anyone with any interest in the regulations the ability to react to them before they become finalized. Commenting on proposed regulations before they are finalized is one of the most important, but often neglected, parts of the legislative process (Abood & Mittelstadt, 1998).

The U.S. Constitution dictates that the government has a duty to protect its citizens. The Tenth Amendment to the U.S. Constitution provides the states with all the powers not specifically reserved for the federal government. Regulation of healthcare professions is one way that each state exercises its responsibility to protect the health, safety, and welfare of its residents.

Nursing practice in each state is governed by a **nurse practice act**, which includes the laws and regulations that control the requirements for entry into practice, the standards for acceptable practice, the standards for continuing competence, and the disciplinary actions taken for misconduct (Betts & Keepnews, 2002; Loquist, 1999; National Council of State Boards of Nursing [NCSBN], 2009). The state nurse practice act is the most important piece of legislature for nurses because it governs every facet of nursing practice (Guido, 2001).

Each state legislature designates a board of nursing to administer the nurse practice act. There are boards of nursing in all 50 states, the District of Columbia, and four U.S. territories (NCSBN, 2006; NCSBN, 2009). The most critical role of the board of nursing is to ensure the safety of the public by monitoring the competency of practicing nurses through licensure (Loquist, 1999).

Licensure

A license is a formal permission authorized by law to do something (Agnus, 2004). Nurses must be licensed in a state in order to work as an RN, licensed practical nurse (LPN), or licensed vocational nurse (LVN). **Licensure** provides the public with the greatest level of protection, because it protects the title of RN or LPN and delineates the scope of nursing practice (Loquist, 1999; NCSBN, 2006). Requirements for licensure include proof of graduation from an approved academic program, a passing score on the licensing examination, and personal qualifications such as citizenship or visa permits, good physical and mental health, and good moral character (Barnum, 1997; Guido, 2001; Loquist, 1999).

All states administer licensing examinations using a standardized national test developed and administered by the NCSBN. Licensing examinations are called the National Council Licensing Examination for Registered Nurses (NCLEX-RN) and the National Council Licensing Examination for Practical Nurses (NCLEX-PN). Traditionally, nurses have been required to be licensed in the state in which they practice. If a nurse moves to a different state, he or she must obtain a license from the new state. A national examination makes seeking reciprocity (recognition of licensure from one state to another) an easy process if the nurse has a valid license in one state (Betts & Waddle, 1993; Guido, 2001).

In recent years, the use of telecommunication technology has transformed the healthcare delivery system and challenged the individual state licensing system. Mergers of healthcare systems have produced giant corporations that operate across state lines. Nurses serve as case managers for patients living in many different states and staff regional or national telephone advice and consultation hotlines (Hutcherson & Williamson, 1999; Loquist, 1999; Wakefield, 1999; Reinhard, 2002). As nurses began practicing in several states at the same time, separate licenses had to be obtained from each state. This policy is impractical and expensive.

In response to the licensing dilemma, the NCSBN adopted a new model for nursing regulation in 1997 called the **Nurse Multistate Licensure Mutual Recognition Model**. According to the ANA, multistate licensure allows a nurse to practice in several states while holding a license in only one state. States enter into interstate compact agreements to coordinate activities associated with licensure. This mutual recognition model, now called the Nurse Licensure Compact (NLC), allows nurses to practice in states that have adopted an interstate compact with each other. The nurses are held accountable for compliance with the laws and regulations of each state's nurse practice act. Twenty four states are presently participating in the NLC and more states are considering or have passed legislation to join the NLC (NCSBN, 2014).

State boards of nursing are responsible not only for ensuring the competency of nurses entering into practice, but also for monitoring the competence of those nurses already in practice. Most nurse practice acts have provisions that require employers to report any violations. Procedures for reporting misconduct, conducting investigations, and issuing sanctions are outlined in the regulations of each state's or territory's nurse practice act. Licensed nurses are responsible for knowing the laws and regulations that govern nursing practice in their states (Loquist, 1999; NCSBN, 2006; NCSBN, 2009).

Nursing Practice and the Law

The most common lawsuits filed against healthcare professionals involve the principles of **negligence** and **malpractice**, which fall under the classification of tort law. Torts are legal wrongs committed against another person or against the property of another person. The wrongdoing may be intentional or unintentional and must result in physical, emotional, or economic harm (Betts & Waddle, 1993; Guido, 2001; Pozgar, 2004).

Although the terms *negligence* and *malpractice* are often used interchangeably, there is a fine distinction between them. *Negligence* is a general term that describes the failure to act as any prudent or reasonable person would act in a specific circumstance. *Malpractice* is a more specific term that considers a professional standard of care as well as the professional status of the healthcare provider. To be liable for malpractice, the person committing the misconduct must be a professional acting in a professional role. Professional misconduct includes either doing something that should not be done (commission) or not doing something that should be done (omission) (Betts & Waddle, 1993; Guido, 2001; Pozgar, 2004).

For a nurse to be found guilty of malpractice in a court of law, the following must have existed:

- A duty was owed to the patient.
- There was a breach of the duty owed to the patient.
- Harm was caused to the patient.
- The harm was foreseeable.
- The action or inaction of the nurse caused the harm (Guido, 2001; Pozgar, 2004).

Nursing Practice in Correctional Settings

The role of the community health nurse in correctional settings is relatively new. Health care for this population has unique challenges for the nurse in this specialized legal setting (see the Levels of Prevention box at the end of the chapter). The basis of correctional health care is providing primary care for inmates from the time of entry into the system, through transfers to other facilities, and to final release from custody back to the community (Earley, 1999). Nurses in correctional facilities provide health care to populations incarcerated in jails, prisons, juvenile detention facilities, and similar settings. Ages range from youths to aged adults. Women, although representing only 10% to 12% of the incarcerated population, make up a growing number of persons in correctional facilities (Freudenberg, Daniels, Crum, Perkins, & Richie, 2005; Hufft & Kite, 2003).

Although often not fully realized by the general population, the existence of health care in correctional facilities is based on the Eighth Amendment of the U.S. Constitution, which prohibits "cruel and unusual punishment" of those convicted of crimes. Furthermore, as a public health concern, correctional institutions are reservoirs of physical and mental illness, which constantly spill back into the community. Appropriate treatment must be provided, with a focus on prevention of transmission of communicable disease. The health of the general community is affected as the inmate population continues to increase.

The consequences of untreated illness in the system are not just for the inmate or even just to the correctional system. These are public health problems that require effective management and close collaboration between correctional health and the public health system (Conklin, Lincoln, & Flanigan, 1998; Freudenberg et al., 2005).

Incarcerated populations have greater health risks than the general population for communicable disease, especially HIV and tuberculosis; violence-associated risks; decreased educational levels; substance abuse; and poverty. Not only do inmates have higher risks for many of these health problems upon admission, but environmental conditions within the correctional facility and behaviors associated with incarceration lend themselves to the spread of communicable disease. The nurse in the correctional setting can provide interventions aimed at interrupting the chain of contagion and can educate the inmates about self-care and protection from these risks. Inmate education is an essential function of **correctional nursing**. The goals are for inmates to remain healthy while incarcerated and to return to the community properly educated about remaining free of communicable disease, as well as to prevent others from becoming infected. Peer education groups have been an effective strategy in the correctional system (Conklin et al., 1998; Heines, 2005).

Forensic Nursing: An Emerging Nursing Role

Forensic nursing, one of the fastest growing specialties in the field of nursing, is the necessary link between health care and law enforcement. In 1992, 70 sexual assault nurses met in Minneapolis, Minnesota, and founded what would become the International Association of Forensic Nurses (IAFN). The ANA recognized forensic nursing as a nursing practice specialty in 1996. Forensic nurses can be found working in rape crisis centers, emergency departments, and nursing homes, among other places. In some parts of the United States, forensic nurses serve as coroners and death investigators to assist law enforcement officers in the investigation of homicides or other unexplained deaths.

The practice roles for forensic nurses encompass several different areas of expertise, including sexual assault nurse examiners, forensic correctional nurses, forensic pediatric nurses, and forensic psychiatric nurses. In addition to providing essential nursing services such as appropriate physical care and emotional support to victims of crime, the duties of forensic nurses include collecting and handling police evidence and providing expert testimony in court (Yost & Burke, 2006). While still a relatively new nursing specialty, forensic nurses have successfully bridged the gap between health care and law enforcement, resulting in a high demand for this valuable area of nursing expertise.

LEVELS OF PREVENTION 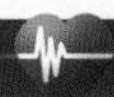

Activities in Correctional Facilities

Primary:
- Stress reduction education
- Prenatal care
- Immunizations
- Violence prevention

Secondary:
- Treatment of infections
- Trauma care for injuries
- Screening for suicide risk
- Disaster and emergency care

Tertiary:
- Injury rehabilitation
- Diabetes foot care
- Stroke rehabilitation

Conclusion

Nurses in the community must remain current and informed about politics and law as related to public health nursing practice (Buerhaus et al., 2012). The political system is ultimately about the distribution of power through formalized and complex systems of law, policy, and regulatory control mechanisms. Settings within the community have legal implications for the nurse, and there are emerging opportunities for nurses within the political/legal community, such as correctional and forensic nursing. Furthermore, for nurses to maintain control of professional nursing practice, understanding and applying political knowledge helps secure our future in the healthcare delivery system. New opportunities exist for community health nurses to influence the healthcare delivery system at the local, state, and national levels with the passage of the ACA of 2010.

HEALTHY ME 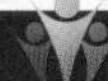

How much do you think about politics affecting your health? Give examples of ways that you use the healthcare system (prescriptions, services, etc.) and how the political system plays a role in each.

Critical Thinking Activities

1. Do all three types of law apply to professional nursing practice? In what ways?
2. In what ways can nurses influence legislation that affects nursing practice?
3. What types of nursing situations may lend themselves to malpractice suits?
4. What steps can you take to avoid a lawsuit?
5. Is there a particular "type" of patient who will sue? What makes you think so?

References

Abood, S., & Mittelstadt, P. (1998). Legislative and regulatory processes. In D. J. Mason and J. K. Leavitt (Eds.), *Policy and politics in nursing and health care* (3rd ed, pp 384–396). Philadelphia, PA: W.B. Saunders.

Abood, S., & Mittelstadt, P. (2006). Legislative and regulatory processes. In D. J. Mason, J. K. Leavitt, & M. W. Chaffee (Eds.), *Policy and politics in nursing and health care* (5th ed.). Philadelphia, PA: Saunders.

Agnus, M. E. (2004). *Webster's new world college dictionary* (4th ed.). New York, NY: MacMillan.

American Academy of Nursing (AAN). (2010). *Implementing health care reform: Issues for nursing.* Washington, DC: Author.

American Nurses Association (ANA). (2012). Affordable Care Act is still the law. *American Nurse, 44*(4), 1–13.

Anderson, J. E. (2006). *Public policymaking* (6th ed.). Boston, MA: Houghton Mifflin.

Bacharach, S. B., & Lawler, E. J. (1980). *Power and politics in organizations.* San Francisco, CA: Jossey-Bass.

Barnum, B. S. (1997, August 13). Licensure, certification, and accreditation. *Online Journal of Issues in Nursing.* Retrieved from http://www.nursingworld.org/MainMenuCategories/ANAMarketplace/ANAPeriodicals/OJIN/TableofContents/Vol21997/No3Aug97/LicensureCertificationandAccreditation.html

Betts, V. T., & Waddle, F. I. (1993). Legal aspects of nursing. In K.K. Chitty (Ed.), *Professional nursing: Concepts and challenges.* Philadelphia, PA: W.B. Saunders.

Bednash, G. P., Heylin, G. B., & Rhome, A. M. (1998). Federal government. In D. J. Mason & J. K. Leavitt (Eds.), *Policy and politics in nursing and health care* (3rd ed., pp. 436–457). Philadelphia, PA: Saunders.

Betts, V. T., & Keepnews, D. (2002). Nursing and the courts. In D. J. Mason, J. K. Leavitt, & M. W. Chaffee (Eds.), *Policy and politics in nursing and health care* (4th ed., pp. 471–478). St. Louis, MO: Saunders.

Betts, V. T., & Waddle, F. I. (2007). Legal aspects of nursing. In K. K. Chitty & B. P. Black (Eds.), *Professional nursing. Concepts and challenges* (5th ed.). Philadelphia, PA: Saunders.

Brennan, A. M. (2012). The paradigm shift. *Nursing Clinics of North America, 47*(4), 455–462.

Buerhaus, P. I., DesRoches, C., Applebaum, S., Hess, R., Norman, L. D., & Donelan, K. (2012). Are nurses ready for health care reform? A decade of survey research. *Nursing Economics, 30*(6), 319–330.

Conklin, T., Lincoln, T., & Flanigan, T. (1998). A public health model to connect correctional health care with communities. *American Journal of Public Health, 88*(8), 1249–1251.

Curtis, B. T., & Lumpkin, B. (1998). Political action committees. In D. J. Mason & J. K. Leavitt (Eds.), *Policy and politics in nursing and health care* (3rd ed., pp. 546–554). Philadelphia, PA: Saunders.

Earley, J. (1999, Spring/Summer). Nursing behind bars. *Minority Nurse*, pp. 22–25.

Florida House of Representatives. (2008). *The council-committee process.* Retrieved from http://www.myfloridahouse.gov/contentViewer.aspx?category=PublicGuide&file=About_The_Legislative_Process_The_Committee_Process.html

Florida Senate. (2006). Effective communication with a legislator. Retrieved from http://www.flsenate.gov/About/EffectiveCommunication

Florida Senate. (2008). Committees. Retrieved from http://www.flsenate.gov/Committees

Forgotson, E. H. (1967). 1965: The turning point in health law—1966 reflections. *American Journal of Public Health, 57*(6), 934–935.

French, J. R., & Raven, B. (1959). The basis for social power. In D. Cartwright (Ed.), *Studies in social power.* Ann Arbor, MI: University of Michigan Press.

Freudenberg, N., Daniels, J., Crum, M., Perkins, T., & Richie, B. E. (2005). Coming home from jail: The social and health consequences of community reentry for women, male adolescents, and their families and communities. *American Journal of Public Health, 95*(10), 1725–1736.

Gaffney, T. (1998). State government. In D. J. Mason & J. K. Leavitt (Eds.), *Policy and politics in nursing and health care* (3rd ed., pp. 417–427). Philadelphia, PA: Saunders.

Guido, G. W. (2001). *Legal issues in nursing* (3rd ed.). Upper Saddle River, NJ: Prentice Hall.

Heines, V. (2005). Speaking out to improve the health of inmates. *American Journal of Public Health, 95*(10), 1685–1688.

Helvie, C. O. (1998). *Advanced practice nursing in the community.* Thousand Oaks, CA: Sage.

Hersey, P., Blanchard, K., & Natemeyer, W. (1979). Situational leadership: Perception and impact of power. *Group Organizational Studies, 4*, 418–428.

Hewison, A. (1994). The politics of nursing: A framework for analysis. *Journal of Advanced Nursing, 20*, 1170–1175.

Hufft, A., & Kite, M. M. (2003). Vulnerable and cultural perspectives for nursing care in correctional systems. *Journal of Multicultural Nursing & Health, 9*(1), 18.

Huston, C. J. (1995, Fall). Nursing and political action in the twentieth century: From separation to fusion. *Revolution: The Journal of Nurse Empowerment*, 50–53.

Hutcherson, C., & Williamson, S. H. (1999). Nursing regulation for the new millennium: The mutual recognition model. *Online Journal of Issues in Nursing.* Retrieved from http://www.nursingworld.org/MainMenuCategories/ANAMarketplace/ANAPeriodicals/OJIN/TableofContents/Volume41999/No1May1999/MutualRecognitionModel.html

Kaplin, W. A., & Lee, B. A. (2006). *The law of higher education* (4th ed.). San Francisco, CA: Jossey-Bass.

Kelly, L. Y., & Joel, L. A. (1996). *The nursing experience* (3rd ed.). New York, NY: McGraw-Hill.

Lenski, G. E. (1984). *Power and privilege.* Chapel Hill, NC: University of North Carolina Press.

Loquist, R. S. (1999). Regulation: Parallel and powerful. In J. A. Milstead (Ed.), *Health policy and politics: A nurse's guide* (pp. 105–146). Gaithersburg, MD: Aspen.

Majewski, J. V., & O'Brien, M. C. (2006). Local government. In D. J. Mason, J. K. Leavitt, & M. W. Chaffee (Eds.), *Policy and politics in nursing and health care* (5th ed.). Philadelphia, PA: Saunders.

Malone, P. S., Chaffee, M. W., & Wachter, M. B. (2002). The power and influence of special interest groups in health care. In D. J. Mason, J. K. Leavitt, & M. W. Chaffee (Eds.), *Policy and politics in nursing and health care* (4th ed. pp. 627–638). St. Louis, MO: Saunders.

Miller, D. F. (1992). *Dimensions of community health.* Dubuque, IA: W.C. Brown.

Milstead, J. A. (1999). Advanced practice nurses and public policy, naturally. In J. A. Milstead (Ed.), *Health policy and politics: A nurse's guide* (pp. 1–41). Gaithersburg, MD: Aspen.

National Council of State Boards of Nursing (NCSBN). (2006). *What boards do.* Retrieved from https://www.ncsbn.org/521.htm

National Council of State Boards of Nursing (NCSBN). (2009). Changes in Healthcare Professions' Scope of Practice: Legislative Considerations. Retrieved from https://www.ncsbn.org/ScopeofPractice_09.pdf

National Council of State Boards of Nursing (NCSBN). (2014). Nurse license compact. Retrieved from https://www.ncsbn.org/nlc.htm

Pozgar, G. D. (2004). *Legal aspects of health care administration* (9th ed.). Sudbury, MA: Jones and Bartlett.

Reinhard, S. C. (2002). State government: 50 paths to policy. In D. J. Mason, J. K. Leavitt, & M. W. Chaffee (Eds.), *Policy and politics in nursing and health care* (4th ed., pp. 491–497). St. Louis, MO: Saunders.

Robertson, I. (1981). *Sociology* (2nd ed.). New York, NY: Worth.

Santa Anna, Y. (2006). Legislative and regulatory processes. In D. J. Mason, J. K. Leavitt, & M. W. Chaffee (Eds.), *Policy and politics in nursing and health care* (5th ed.). Philadelphia, PA: Saunders.

Shi, L., & Singh, D. A. (2013). *Essentials of the U.S. health care system.* (3rd ed.). Burlington, MA: Jones & Bartlett Learning.

Turnock, B. J. (1997). *Public health: What it is and how it works.* Gaithersburg, MD: Aspen.

U.S. Department of Health and Human Services (HHS). (2010). *Healthy People 2020: Topics and objectives.* Retrieved from http://www.healthypeople.gov/2020/TopicsObjectives2020/

U.S. Department of Health and Human Services (HHS). (2014). *HHS: What we do.* Retrieved from http://www.hhs.gov/ocio/about/whatwedo/what.html

Wakefield, M. K. (1999). Have license, will travel. *Nursing Economics, 17*(2), 114–116.

Weber, M. (1947). *The theory of social and economic organization* (Ed. and Trans. A. M. Henderson & T. Parsons). New York, NY: Oxford University Press.

White, K. M. (2002). The federal government. In D. J. Mason, J. K. Leavitt, & M. W. Chaffee (Eds.), *Policy and politics in nursing and health care* (4th ed., pp. 515–533). St. Louis, MO: Saunders.

Yost, J. R., & Burke, T. L. (2006). Forensic nursing: An aid to law enforcement. *FBI Law Enforcement Bulletin, 75*(2), 7–12.

CHAPTER FOCUS

Health Policy and Public Policy
- Goals Versus Policies
- Purpose of Public Policy
- Choosing Policies
- History of Health Policy in the United States
- Present Need for Public Health Policy

Public Health and Public Policy

Policy Development
- Policy Environment
- Public Health Advocacy and Action
- Policy Shape and Setting
- Policy Goals, Tools, and Resources
- The Players as Stakeholders
- Player Connections

Information for Action

Policy Development Strategies
- Bargaining
- Information Through the Mass Media
- Health Information
- Mass Media and the Case of Healthcare Reform: A Cautionary Tale

Implementation
- Evaluation

Nurses in Communities, Public Health Policy, and Primary Prevention
- Advocacy Tools of the Future

QUESTIONS TO CONSIDER

After reading this chapter, you will know the answers to the following questions:

1. What is health policy and how is it related to the healthcare system?
2. What are the purposes of health policy?
3. How have health policies been developed from a historical perspective in the United States?
4. Why is health policy needed in the United States?
5. What is the policymaking process?
6. How can the tobacco control health issue be used to illustrate successful public health policymaking?
7. How are policies developed and by whom?
8. How are policies evaluated in the United States?
9. Who are stakeholders and how do they influence policy development?
10. What is the role of community health nurses in the health policymaking process?

CHAPTER 10

Health Policy

Nancy Milio, Marti Jordan, and Karen Saucier Lundy

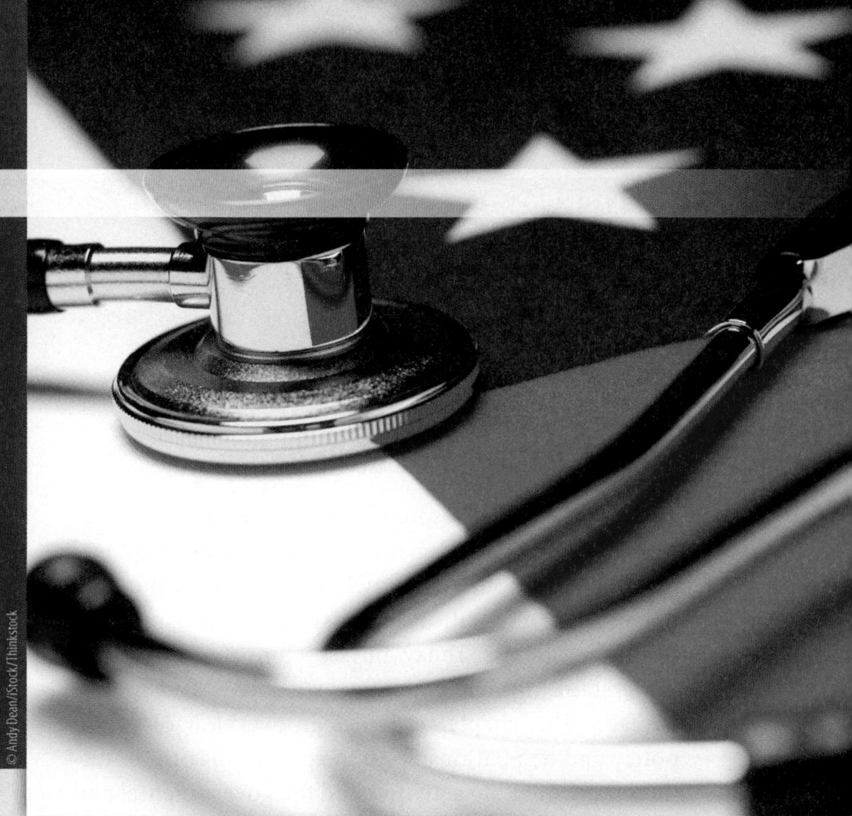

KEY TERMS

appropriations
authorization
bargaining
collaboration
cooperation
fiscal policy
health policy
impacts
organization policy
outcomes
outputs
policy environment
policy instruments
public health prevention policies
public policy
rule making
stakeholders
strategic information

> Policy is like a play in many acts, which unfolds inevitably once the curtain is raised. To declare then that the performance will not take place is an absurdity. The play will go on, either by means of the actors or by means of the spectators who mount the stage.
>
> —Klemens von Metternich, 1880

> Manner of living, wages, the condition of industry and commerce, public administration, years of abundance and those of famine—everything that contributes to affluence and civilization—produce great variations in death rate. Affluence and wealth . . . is in truth the most important of all hygienic factors, namely that which best assures the very preservation of life.
>
> —Rene Villerme, mid-19th century

REFLECTIONS

Nurses have been slow as a profession to view health policy as a priority in our practice. Why do you think knowledge about policy and health care is rarely considered? Do you often think of "politics" as something essential in the practice of community health nursing? In this chapter you will learn about not only the process of healthcare policy development but also the critical nature of such knowledge to the promotion of nursing care of populations.

Health Policy and Public Policy

To meet the social responsibility of the health professions to promote and maintain health in all segments of the population, our knowledge and skills must go beyond the biomedical and psychosocial aspects of health and illness. Today, nurses' competence requires understanding health policy—what it is and how it is made. This chapter provides an overview of health policy and its relationship to the public's health. It outlines policymaking activities and the governmental and other "players" (or stakeholders) that influence those processes. It is important for nursing as a profession and for those in practice to understand policy development in local, state, and national contexts to recognize when community health might be affected and to find ways to influence policies to promote and protect health. This awareness can guide nursing's contribution to policy action on behalf of people's health.

Health policy is public (governmental) policy that affects health and health care in national, state, and local arenas. It covers a broad range, including economic, housing, environmental, budgetary, and health services policy. Typically, the public, politicians, press, and professionals see health policy as including mainly those laws and practices affecting the agencies (public and private) that finance and organize the delivery of personal health services. Considerable policy *is* concentrated on finance, because almost 18% of the U.S. gross domestic product—about $2.8 trillion per year—is devoted to health-related expenditures. However, much more than health services policy affects people's health (Lasker, 1997). Health is significantly related to income and other measures of socioeconomic status such as educational opportunities, affordable housing, investments in children's welfare, improvements in working conditions and benefits, and community support (Hatcher, 2003; Sultz & Young, 2014; Syme, Lefkowitz, & Krimgold, 2004).

Like all **public policy**, health policy is a guide to government action to alter what would otherwise occur, seeking more desirable or acceptable prospects. It points the way and enables effective action to coherent activity by public and private institutional systems. It is a decision about amounts and allocations (or distribution) of resources in organizations and governments.

The overall amount (i.e., the budget of governments or institutions) is a statement of commitment to a certain area of social or community or organizational relevance or concern, like health services or education. The distribution of that amount within the budget is a statement of the true priorities of the policymakers, regardless of their statements about goals or mission. Together, the total amount and its allocation are called **fiscal policy**.

Goals Versus Policies

Goals, by themselves, are not policies. Although policies have goals, they are much more than that. For example, the goals of *Healthy People 2000*, *Healthy People 2010*, and *Healthy People 2020* were not policies because they had no instruments or resources specifically allocated to carry them out, other than having national health agencies monitor national progress toward the goals. The documents did not carry the force of law, which derives from one of the three constitutional sources of policy: Congress (legislation), the executive branch (the president's executive orders, which remain in force throughout his or her term of office and apply only to the executive branch), or independent regulatory agencies, created by Congress, having a specific jurisdiction, such as the U.S. Food and Drug Administration and the Environmental Protection Agency. None of these institutions is absolute; all are subject to constitutional checks and balances. The job of the courts is to interpret—not create—policy; however, in doing so, they inevitably influence policy, as do myriad organizations and groups in and outside government.

None of these three types of policy bodies at the national level, nor their counterparts in states and localities, is required to follow statements about national goals. Goals are useful as a framework and a source for policy ideas but are not in themselves sufficient for effective policy. They must first be fully formulated and adopted in legislation, executive order, or regulation, which are accompanied by the broad methods (or legal instruments discussed in the following paragraphs) and authorized funds to carry them out. Otherwise, they remain at a voluntary level of action, dependent on the willingness of relevant groups to invest their own resources to follow them (Fairman and D'Antonio, 2013).

For example, by the late 1990s, states had adopted only some of the *Healthy People 2000* goals and were either unwilling or unable to track more than 40% of them, quite apart from authorizing funds to achieve them. In some states this monitoring capacity actually declined as a result of funding cutbacks. In addition, monies allocated to use the data often did not have high priority: Just 6 in 10 states included some environmental health objectives in their public health planning and fewer than 10 states provided air-quality data, taking more than 2 years to distribute it; fewer than half the states provided childhood poverty data and took more than 4 years to give it to local health departments; and fewer than 25 states collected data on injuries (Krieger, Chen, & Ebel, 1997; National Association of County and City Health Officials [NACCHO], 1998; Public Health Foundation, 1998).

Although *Healthy People 2020*, the most recent set of objectives, outlines 571 objectives in 41 focus areas, it has only four overarching goals: (1) to attain high-quality, longer lives free of preventable disease, disability, injury, and premature death; (2) to achieve health equity, eliminate disparities, and improve the health of all groups; (3) to create social and physical environments that promote good health for all; and (4) to promote quality of life, healthy development, and healthy behaviors across all life stages. These represent an expansion of the 2010 goals, which were simply to increase years of healthy life in the population as a whole and to eliminate disparities among groups.

Healthy People 2020, often called a road map for U.S. public health, is not supported by an effective or efficient public health infrastructure. The current public health system in the United States relies on a fragmented assortment of individual agencies, states, and communities to develop strategies for meeting the *Healthy People 2020* goals and to identify and provide the resources needed to accomplish them (Lurie, 2004). Some of the provisions of the Affordable Care Act (ACA) of 2010 were included as an effort to address this fragmentation—for example, the initiative to promote adoption of electronic health records. Even so, the reforms enacted in this law are far from comprehensive in terms of unifying public health.

The clearest and most accurate sign or indicator to determine whether actual policy change has occurred in any governmental body or other organization—health center, school, home care agency—is a change in the size and/or allocation of its resources: money, the authority and responsibilities vested in certain positions (e.g., staff nurses), and other resources. When organizations, as a result of policy changes, conduct their services differently, as staff do things differently, consumers can also behave differently: Patterns change. **Organization policy** is that of a single organization or a type of organization (e.g., public schools), either public (e.g., health department) or private (e.g., churches or childcare centers or corporations), and it is closely tied to governmental policy changes.

Purpose of Public Policy

The purpose of policymaking is to shape the direction and pace of change in a preferred direction by modifying current patterns of action. It is not to change the behavior of every individual, each of whom is free to follow a policy or not, perhaps with possible personal consequences, such as refusing a vaccine or driving faster than the speed limit at the risk of injury or fine.

Rather, the aim of policymaking is to change the decisions of organizations about their use of resources. This, in turn, changes the activities of managers and staff, clients, and customers from former patterns toward new patterns in governmental agencies, nonprofit organizations, and commercial organizations, whether construction firms, restaurants, regulatory agencies, schools, or clinics. A school board policy requiring the availability of healthy foods in cafeterias will change the types of foods that schools buy, the menus and methods of preparation used by kitchen staff, and the pattern of foods that students and teachers will eat, thereby promoting health.

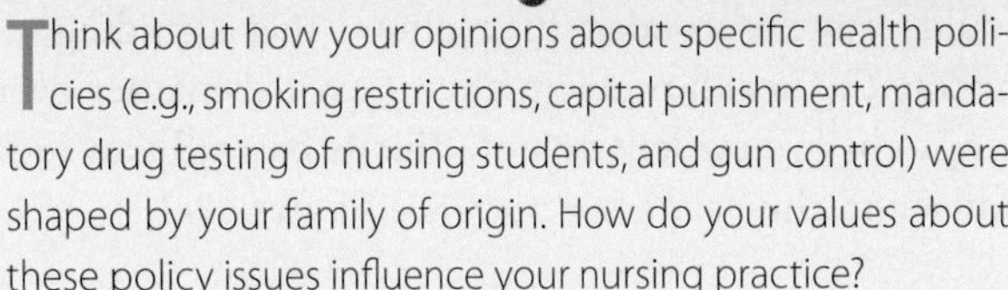

CULTURAL CONNECTION

Think about how your opinions about specific health policies (e.g., smoking restrictions, capital punishment, mandatory drug testing of nursing students, and gun control) were shaped by your family of origin. How do your values about these policy issues influence your nursing practice?

Choosing Policies

To address any health problem, there are always several choices (including doing nothing). We know, for example, that about 310,000 mostly low-income children aged 1–5 years in the United States have health-damaging blood levels of lead, mainly from exposure to lead-based paint in old houses and environmental contamination. The problem is three times worse in African American children, even when they are not living in old housing and are not in the lowest income bracket, indicating discrimination in the choice of neighborhoods available to some African American families (Centers for Disease Control and Prevention [CDC], 2013; Government Accountability Office, 1998). Here are the policy choices:

- Healthcare systems can conduct outreach, screening, and treatment.
- Community coalitions can form to conduct outreach, screening, and treatment.
- State Medicaid agencies can require Medicaid contractors to provide and report on these services for their enrollees.

Intervention Strategy	Focus
Individual-directed, information-mediated change	• Homes and communities (e.g., computers, TV campaigns, health fairs) • Organization settings (e.g., counseling; computers; small-group training of patients, clients, customers, health care practitioners, librarians, teachers, clergy)
Organization-directed change	• Policy bodies: – Congress, legislatures – Independent regulatory agencies – Government administration (e.g., executive orders, rule making) • Specific organizations: – Government organizations (e.g., health departments, housing, schools) – Nongovernment organizations (e.g., managed care organizations, community health centers, companies, retailers)

Figure 10-1 Strategies for prevention and health promotion basically aim at either (1) changing individuals' behavior or physical condition through information/education or clinical means (or changing individual practitioners) or (2) changing the decisions of organizations about their use of resources through policy efforts. This, in turn, changes the activities of managers, staff, clients, and customers in policy and service organizations in the public and private sectors.

These policy changes—with their goals, means, and accompanying shift in budget and program resources—would result in secondary prevention—that is, finding and treating the health problem after it exists, whether overt symptoms are evident or not. This is basically an individual and clinical perspective. See **Figure 10-1**.

> We all declare for liberty; but in using the same word, we do not all mean the same thing. With some the word 'liberty' may mean for each man to do as he pleases with himself, and the product of his labor; while with others the same may mean for some men to do as they please with other men, and the product of other men's labor. Here are two, not only different, but incompatible things, called by the same name—liberty.
>
> —*Abraham Lincoln*

ENVIRONMENTAL CONNECTION

How has the American with Disabilities Act changed the work environment for people with disabilities? How has it changed the work environment for people without disabilities?

To adopt a public health, population-oriented, primary preventive policy approach—to prevent the problem before it begins—additional choices are possible:

- Require lead paint removal and environmental code enforcement after providing information to landlords, polluting organizations, tenants, and homeowners
- Develop safe, affordable housing
- Provide for safe and effective schools and schooling, including job training and jobs development
- Work for pro-community/antidiscrimination changes

All this effort would require entry by health proponents into the complex and long-term processes that result in organizational and public policy change. Policy does not just happen. It is determined by organized groups in and outside government and, therefore, can be observed, analyzed, and understood well enough to promote health-supporting development. Policymaking processes shape policy content as groups that are affected by them (stakeholders) attempt to influence policy development to favor their own needs and priorities (Fairman and D'Antonio, 2013). See **Box 10-1** for a partial list of stakeholders in healthcare policy decisions.

The results often have indirect or direct impact on population health. Indirect effects include access to the conditions for healthful living, such as housing, jobs, information and education, health care, protective environments, tax equity, and civil rights (Hatcher, 2003; Milio, 1997; Syme et al., 2004). The coalition of environmental health organizations, for example, worked to influence Congress in the 1970s to pass historic laws protecting air, water, and habitats. The laws have been effective in directly improving the health of millions of Americans and indirectly affecting health by preserving the viability of agricultural land needed for sustaining food and nutrition for future generations.

BOX 10-1 Major Stakeholders in U.S. Health Policy

- The public (health consumers—which include patients, families, and consumer organizations such as the American Association of Retired Persons, the American Cancer Society, the American Heart Association, labor organizations, etc.)
- Employers (public and private employers and employer organizations representing small and large businesses)
- Providers (physicians, dentists, nurses, nurse practitioners, physician assistants, pharmacists, podiatrists, chiropractors, and allied health professionals)
- Hospitals (general, specialty, teaching, rural, profit or nonprofit, independent, or multifacility systems)
- Alternative therapy organizations (providers of alternative health interventions such as rolfing, yoga, spiritual healing, relaxation techniques, herbal remedies, energy healing, megavitamin therapy, acupuncture, acupressure, and massage therapy)
- Insurance industry (managed care organizations, Blue Cross/Blue Shield, and other private insurance companies)
- Long-term care (nursing homes, home health agencies, rehabilitation facilities, etc.)
- Mental health (psychiatric hospitals, community mental health facilities, and many community-based ambulatory care services)
- Voluntary facilities and agencies (HIV/AIDS support groups; addiction support groups such as Alcoholics Anonymous, Narcotics Anonymous, Overeaters Anonymous; and public education and lobbying groups such as Mothers Against Drunk Driving)
- Health professions education and training institutions (schools of public health, medicine, nursing, dentistry, allied health, pharmacy, optometry, etc.)
- Professional associations (national, state, and regional organizations representing healthcare professionals or institutions such as the American Nurses Association, the American Medical Association, the American Public Health Association, and the American Hospital Association)
- Other health industry organizations (pharmaceutical companies, medical supply and equipment companies, and information and management system suppliers)
- Research communities (educational institutions, government agencies such as the National Institutes of Health or the Agency for Healthcare Research, and not-for-profit foundations such as the Pew Charitable Trusts, the Robert Wood Johnson Foundation, and the Bill and Melinda Gates Foundation)

Source: Sultz, H. A., & Young, K. M. (2014). *Health care USA: Understanding its organization and delivery* (8th ed). Burlington, MA: Jones & Bartlett Learning.

> There is nothing more difficult to plan, more doubtful of success, nor more dangerous to manage than the creation of a new system.
>
> —*Machiavelli, The Prince, 1512*

History of Health Policy in the United States

Historically, the United States has enacted broader health policies than those in recent years. During much of the 1990s, health policy had been viewed narrowly, focusing on health services delivery and the economics of it, while weakening environmental health, healthful living conditions, and primary public health prevention legislation (Center for the Future of Children, 1997; Fairman & D-Antonio, 2013; U.S. Department of Health and Human Services [HHS], 1995; Wakefield, Gardner, & Guillett, 2002).

> The master of every ship of the United States arriving from a foreign port . . . shall pay . . . twenty cents per month for every seaman employed . . . to provide for . . . the sick or disabled seamen in [government] hospitals . . . now established in the several ports.
>
> —*The U.S. Fifth Congress, July 16, 1798*

Some of the major steps in health policy since the start of the nation include the first national health service and national health insurance program set up before the end of the 18th century. This was, and in modified form continues to be, a system of government health care paid by private employer insurance for the U.S. Merchant Marine. A larger and fully tax-supported national health service is the one provided to Congress and the president, the only fully socialized medical system in the United States today. These are national governmental healthcare systems that are available to everyone in special groups. Most advanced countries have national systems available to their entire population, including immigrants.

Constitutional provisions in our national and state governments to protect the health, safety, and welfare of people authorize, but do not require, governments to use legal tools to realize these purposes. For example, if health were part of the Bill of Rights, governments would be legally required—would be liable—to protect health.

Other early national health policies include the Pure Food and Drug Act (1906); the Social Security Act and its income support for the poor, blind, disabled, and elders and health services for mothers and children (1935); and the first environmental law, the Water Pollution Control Act of 1948. The Economic Opportunity Act was to

BOX 10-2 Selected History of Important Federal Health Legislation

Pure Food and Drug Act, 1906
Maternity and Infancy Act, 1921
Social Security Act, 1935
Nurse Training Act, 1941
Public Health Services Act, 1944
Hospital Survey and Construction Act (Hill–Burton Act), 1946
Federal Employee Health Benefits Act, 1959
Health Professions Educational Assistance Act, 1963
Older Americans Act, 1965
Highway Safety Act, 1966
Child Nutrition Act, 1966
National Environmental Policy Act, 1969
Comprehensive Drug Abuse Prevention and Control Act, 1970
Occupational Health and Safety Act, 1970
Consumer Product Safety Act, 1972
Toxic Substances Control Act, 1976
Rural Health Clinics Act, 1977
Comprehensive Smoking Education Act, 1984
Emergency Medical Treatment and Active Labor Act, 1986
Omnibus Health Act (Medicaid expansions), 1986
Americans with Disabilities Act, 1990
Preventive Health Amendments Act, 1992
Health Center Consolidation Act, 1996
Health Insurance Portability and Accountability Act, 1996
Child Abuse Prevention and Treatment Act, 2003
Medicare Prescription Drug Improvement and Modernization Act, 2003
Combating Autism Act, 2006
Traumatic Brain Injury Act, 2008
Patient Protection and Affordable Care Act, 2010

develop poor communities and end poverty (1964); the National School Lunch and Child Nutrition Amendments included the Special Supplemental Nutrition Program for Women, Infants, and Children (WIC; 1972) (Weissert & Weissert, 1996). See **Box 10-2** for a partial list of health legislation that has been passed.

RESEARCH ALERT 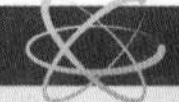

This study analyzed the ethical, public policy, and educational issues that arise in the United States and United Kingdom when genomic information acquired as a result of genetic testing is introduced into healthcare services. The research findings concluded that individual, family, and societal issues may conflict with current healthcare practices and policies when genetic testing is done, but current health policies do not fully address these concerns. In addition, healthcare providers, including nurses, are not fully prepared to incorporate genetic testing into their practice.

Source: Williams, J., Skirton, H., & Masny, A. (2006). Ethics, policy, and educational issues in genetic testing. *Journal of Nursing Scholarship, 38*(2), 119–125.

Present Need for Public Health Policy

Although overall U.S. death rates are declining, continuing gaps in health between disadvantaged and other populations are increasing in many respects. In addition, disability from chronic illness is widespread (Cutler & Sheiner, 1999; Klijs, Nusselder, Looman, & Mackenbach, 2011; Wakefield et al., 2002). Health inequalities in morbidity, mortality, and disability are strongly related to poverty and income inequality. Gaps in health between low- and high-income groups are expected to increase further as wealth inequalities continue to grow (Hatcher, 2003; Kaplan, 1996; Montgomery, Kiely, & Pappas, 1996).

Widening health gaps are not accounted for by biomedical and behavioral risk factors alone. Rather, they are affected by a complex web of linked living standards as experienced in jobs and workplaces, homes, and communities (Karlsson, Nilsson, Lyttkens, & Leeson, 2010). In turn, these are related to how supportive public policies are in these sectors (Hatcher, 2003; Syme et al., 2004). Virtually all measures of health and illness are worse among poor people compared with their better-off counterparts, regardless of ethnicity, gender, or age. Because of the breadth of the determinants of health, much has been written about the need for broad social and economic policies to promote health.

Evidence shows that public health–oriented public policies make a difference. For example, Social Security retirement income has been the single most important policy to reduce poverty in the United States, especially among elders, thereby contributing to healthful living standards for millions of people. A special tax credit for full-time working parents was supposed to be an important policy to prevent several million children from living in poverty (National Center for Children in Poverty [NCCP], 1998). The federal child and dependent care tax credit reduces the amount of taxes working families with childcare expenses must pay. All families at all income levels are eligible for the tax credit (NCCP, 2007).

Despite this, the tax credit was not enough to prevent an overall increase in child poverty since the 1980s because of low-wage jobs and national and state policies that cut back resources available to poor families. In addition, the credit is nonrefundable, limiting its value to low-income families. The credit cannot exceed the taxes that a family owes, and no benefit is provided for families who do not pay taxes because their income is too low. A single-parent family with two children is not required to pay taxes if their income is below $15,000 per year. To be eligible for the tax credit, a family must be responsible for paying expenses related to the care of children under the age of 13 (or older dependents who are not able to care for themselves) that occur while the parents or legal guardians are working or looking for work. In 2014, taxpaying families with two or more children could claim up to $6,000 in annual childcare expenses, and families with one child could claim up to $3,000. The credit equals 20% to 35% of the amount claimed, which provided a maximum tax credit of $2,100 for families with two or more children (NCCP, 2014).

The fact remains that 32.3 million children in the United States are growing up in low-income families. More than 80% of these children have at least one working parent whose income is not sufficient to support the family. In most cases, it is not until a family of four reaches an income level of $35,000–$70,000 per year (150%–300% of the federal poverty level) that parents are able to provide their children with the basic necessities, such as food, housing, and health care (NCCP, 2014).

Public Health and Public Policy

Public health is a governmental (public) responsibility embodied in federal and state agencies, including the CDC, the Environmental Protection Agency, and state and local health departments. They are, in principle, accountable for the health of all the people, extending beyond the health of particular individuals, as is done in personal health services.

Public health policy involves promoting and protecting health, preventing disease, and preserving life through policies that ensure the determinants of health for all segments of the population (Rose, 1985, 1990). When it is effective, it makes healthy choices equitably available to all groups—about where to live, work, learn, obtain needed services and information, and participate in public life in safe, supportive, and sustainable environments (Fairman and D'Antonio, 2013).

According to the Institute of Medicine (1988), the mission of public health is:

> fulfilling society's interest in assuring conditions in which people can be healthy . . . to generate organized community efforts to address the public interest in health by applying scientific and technical knowledge to prevent disease and promote health. . . . [It] is addressed by private organizations, but the governmental public health agency has a unique function: to see to it that vital elements are in place and that the mission is adequately addressed.

This echoes the historic understanding of the public health mission:

> Public health is the science and art of preventing disease, prolonging life and promoting health . . . through organizing community efforts for sanitation of the environment, the control of communicable infections, the education of the individual in personal hygiene, the organization of medical and nursing services for the early diagnosis and preventive treatment of disease, and the development of the social machinery to ensure everyone a standard of living adequate for the maintenance of health, so organizing these benefits as to enable every citizen to realize his birthright of health and longevity. (Winslow, 1920)

This public health enterprise, undertaken by government agencies and other allied groups, ranging from local health centers to national voluntary organizations like the American Public Health Association and public-interest groups such as the Brady Campaign to Prevent Gun Violence, requires organizational and organized action directed toward all types of entities, including policy bodies and the public. This historic approach of public health during most of its first century resulted in major successes, such as regulating sewage, water supplies, and housing conditions, decades before vaccines were discovered (Institute of Medicine, 1988).

ENVIRONMENTAL CONNECTION

The banning of trans fats from New York City restaurants became effective in 2006. Do you support such a policy? Why or why not? How far can government policies go before the infringement of individual freedom of choice conflicts with our basic political values?

As illustrated earlier, policies change organizations (and their resource allocations and programs) so that populations can have more healthful choices about where and how to live. Examples of **public health prevention policies** include tobacco control—for example, higher cigarette taxes of 50 cents in Oregon reduced smoking by 18% in youth; communicable disease prevention, such as when public and private provider subsidies produced large increases in immunization rates, especially among poor and minority children; abortion funding for poor women, which resulted in an increase in early prenatal care, fewer teen births, and lower rates of low-birth-weight babies and infant death; and containment of alcohol liberalization, handgun controls, and motorcycle safety measures, all of which achieved widespread long-term health benefits (Center for Health Economics Research, 1993; Kraus, Peek, & Williams, 1995; National Cancer Institute, 1991; Office of Disease Prevention and Health Promotion, 1994; Pentz et al., 1989; Teh-Wei, Hai-Yen, & Keeler, 1995).

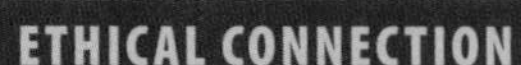

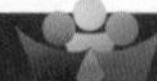

"There are two levers to set a man in motion, fear and self-interest."

—Napoleon Bonaparte, 1769–1821,
French general and emperor

How does this quotation relate to health policy? Is the fear of sickness and/or death related to national health policies on organ donation or cloning? How?

Policy Development

What follows is first an overview of the policymaking process and then an illustration of each step in policy development.

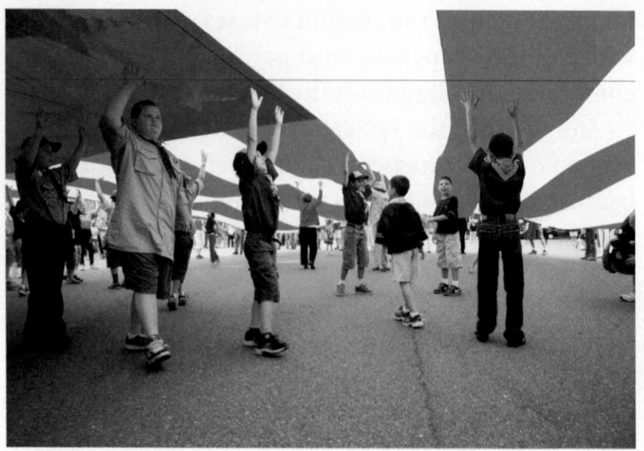

Policy Environment

Policy development does not occur on a clean slate. It always has precursors in earlier eras, deriving from experience with similar issues and societal assumptions about the role of government (Laumann & Knoke, 1987). Most importantly, it is formed in a context of near-term limiting and enabling circumstances. These are important to be aware of to plan effective strategies to influence policymaking.

Figure 10-2 depicts the connections between policymaking and health (Milio, 1976, 1986, 2000). It shows how policy works through organizational action, which shapes community environments, living patterns, and ultimately population health. This occurs in a **policy environment** or context that encompasses circumstances affecting whether and how policymaking proceeds, regardless of the type of policy in question. Important factors include the demographic and epidemiological nature of the population (e.g., an aging population, high rates of smoking), the economy and technology (e.g., inflation,

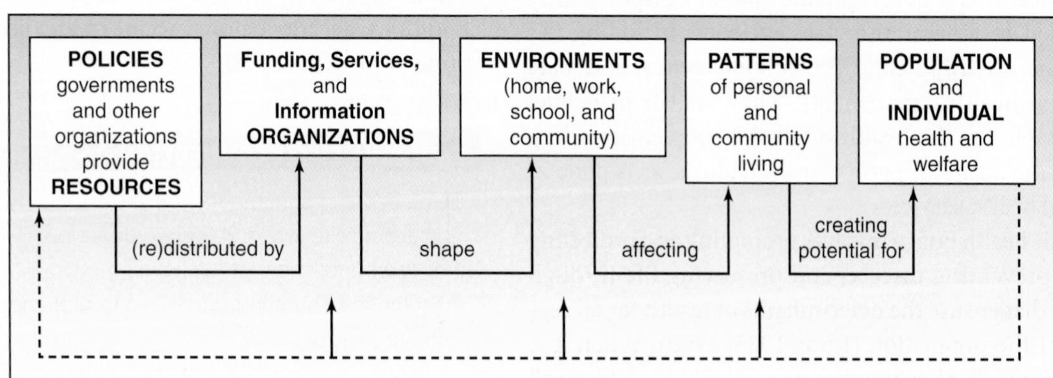

Figure 10-2 Depiction of the connections between policymaking and health. Policy works through organizational action, which shapes community environments, affecting living patterns and ultimately population health. The changes that result in all these areas then feed back (dotted lines) and are taken into account in ongoing efforts to find acceptable and effective ways to deal with public health problems.

unemployment, extent of information technology), the socioeconomic and ethnic makeup of communities (e.g., poverty and discrimination), the distribution of resources (e.g., homelessness and extremes in wealth), political party agendas, organizational hierarchies (e.g., dominant interest groups), and even sudden disasters—national emergencies from weather or war, for example, can stop all policy development as policymakers attend to (costly) emergency measures. All these things must be considered to some extent by policy participants. All this information is available and needed for effective policy work by interested nurses and is best done on an organized and thought-out basis.

Yet, however rapidly changing and uncertain the environment is, the policymaking time clock is ticking, and the electoral calendar moves on. To be effective, policy action and influence must be exerted in time and be timely, in tune with the environment.

The media are in a unique position among organizations (see **Figure 10-3**). They are not only channels for information, but they also create and shape issues (Horton, 2006; Mason, Dodd, & Glickstein, 2007; Minkler, 2004), such as portraying teen violence as a parental problem rather than a public health problem that could be alternatively addressed by, among other things, handgun control. For example, Japan, where handguns are banned, had 11 handgun killings in 2007, whereas the United States had 9,146 and Canada had 173 (Krause & Berman, 2007). Media portrayals set up ideas and expectations about the kinds of solutions needed to address problems (Amundson, Lichter, & Lichter, 2005; Bomlitz & Brezis, 2008; Mason et al., 2007).

As members of global, profit-making corporations, the media seek to attract audiences and advertisers and often shape programming with this aim. For example, news and weather have become "infotainment" rather than accurate and sometimes unpleasant depictions of complex realities (Cappella & Jamieson, 1996). Other players in the policy arena actively attempt to use the media for strategic purposes. Organized interest groups can indirectly reach policymakers and the public through the mass media (Columbia Institute, 1995; Mason, Dodd, & Glickstein, 2007).

The public in this framework consists of several populations that are affected by policymakers' decisions, such as audiences, voters, taxpayers, consumers, and donors to parties and interest groups. Policy choices set the parameters for health in the form of access to services, products, processes, prices, taxes, and information. Most of the public are not active members of interest groups. Through these complex processes, then, ongoing outcomes of policymaking create the conditions for the health of populations, especially of disadvantaged subgroups.

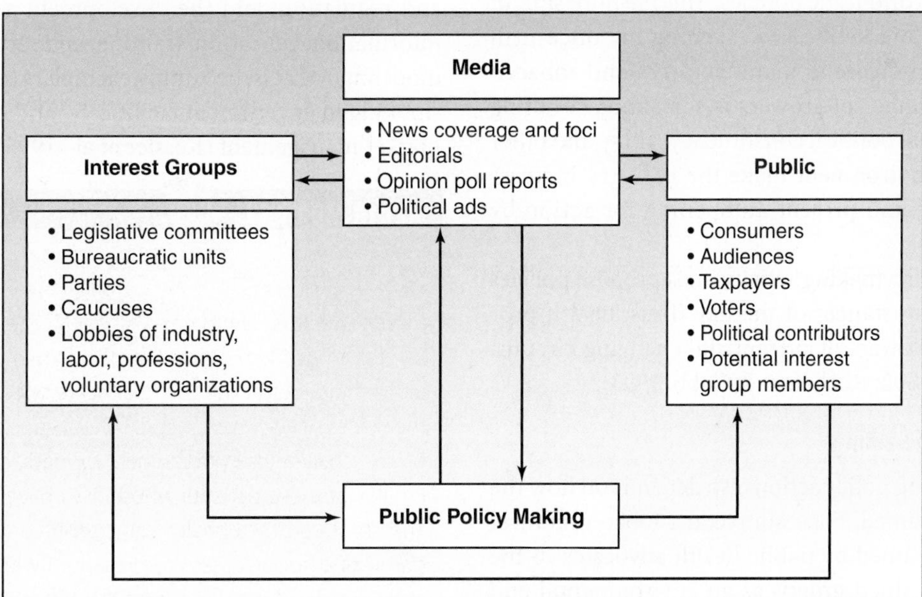

Figure 10-3 The media are not only channels for information; they also create and shape issues. Media portrayals set up ideas and expectations about the kinds of solutions needed to address problems. Other players in the policy arena actively attempt to use the media for strategic purposes. Organized interest groups within and outside government can indirectly reach policymakers and the public through the mass media. The "public" is actually several populations that are affected by policymakers' decisions, such as audiences, voters, taxpayers, consumers, and donors to parties and interest groups.

ETHICAL CONNECTION 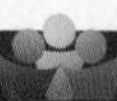

"Price is what you pay. Value is what you get."

—Warren Buffet, American investment entrepreneur

What are the ethical implications of this quotation in relation to healthcare policy in the United States? Is health care a good "value" in the United States as compared to other commodities? Why or why not?

Public Health Advocacy and Action

The Case of Tobacco Control: A Success Story

Antismoking policy development in the United States in the 1980s and 1990s offers many lessons in public health policymaking (Heiser & Begay, 1997; Jacobson, Wasserman, & Raube, 1993). Some states passed strong laws (e.g., widespread bans on smoking in public places and private worksites and large penalties), whereas others enacted weaker legislation (e.g., narrow restrictions, smokers' rights clauses, minor penalties). More effective policymaking involved legislative leadership, strong coalitions, and support by top public health and government officials.

Environmental Context

In the anti-tobacco case, the policy environment includes the shrinking of the U.S. tobacco market and costly legal challenges facing the tobacco industry. This impelled cigarette manufacturers to seek overseas markets, facilitated by liberal world trade policies. This offshore shift of production and marketing is weakening the once-firm alliance between cigarette manufacturers and tobacco farmers. The number of growers is shrinking, resulting in a less influential political constituency. These and other aspects of the environment make the industry increasingly vulnerable and present an opening for action by health advocates.

Successful policymaking activity must propose policies that fit the circumstances of the day. Thus, health proponents must be aware of current and changing circumstances (Milio, 2002; Rochefort & Cobb, 1993).

Policy Shape and Setting

Health-supporting policy action also depends on how the policy issue is framed. For example, the tobacco-control issue could be framed by public health advocates in the health field and allied groups as an environmental and child health issue, or by pro-tobacco groups as one of smokers' right to take personal risks in using a legal product. The policy outcome could be very different depending on who defines the problem (Milio, 2002).

The policy arena—that is, where the action takes place—in local, state, or national jurisdictions, is another consideration. Successful tobacco control advocates used the open arenas of legislatures or the public referendum process and sought news media coverage to amplify their position in contrast to the highly paid, behind-the-scenes activities and television advertising of the industry.

For example, for some anti-tobacco campaigns, local ordinances may be more readily enacted rather than state law, despite the narrower public health impact at local levels. Sufficient community-level action can be a learning laboratory and can create political conditions for stronger statewide policies. Nurses, as members of health or other groups, have been and can continue to be part of any or all such efforts.

Policy Goals, Tools, and Resources

The design of an effective policy includes goals and the means to reach those goals. The goals should eventually be specified as measurable objectives to help focus activity and track progress. The strength (or absence) of means is important for the forward movement and implementation of a policy. Without measurable objectives, progress toward health goals becomes contentious; without sound means and resources, little program action is likely to occur.

Policy effectiveness depends on adequate financing and the choice of legislative tools used. The means to achieve policy goals involve a limited list of **policy instruments** (legal tools) that are used by most governments. These tools include economic incentives (e.g., tax breaks, subsidies) to businesses, governments, and taxpayers; mandates and regulation; and the development and provision of information, education, training, and services. Others are modeling—that is, becoming exemplars (e.g., not allowing smoking in government facilities)—and market power or market management (Kessler et al., 1996).

MEDIA MOMENT 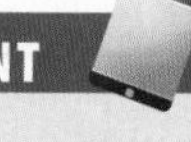

Sicko (2007)

Documentary filmmaker Michael Moore was nominated for an Academy Award for this film in 2008. It is a raw, unflinching look at the U.S. healthcare system, told through the voices of everyday people faced with extraordinary and bizarre challenges in their quest for basic health coverage. Profiles of these patients whose lives have been disrupted and shattered by a health catastrophe and resulting economic and social losses are presented with sensitivity and even humor. Moore does a comprehensive job of reviewing the historical evolution of the U.S. healthcare system. Moore quickly moves to the healthcare systems of Canada, Cuba, Great Britain, and France, examining these systems as compared to the United States. The film ends with an emotional gathering of rescue workers who responded to the

September 11, 2001 terrorist attacks who have since been denied medical treatment and yet remain hopeful in their unusual acts of diplomacy and compassion. This is a movie that everyone who works in the healthcare system should see and discuss!

Tools, such as market management or market power, are used when, for example, governments buy public employee health insurance plans that cover only smoking-cessation programs and collaborate with public health organizations in passing clean indoor air laws (Sofaer, Woolley, & Mauery, 1997). When governments buy only recycled paper or healthy foods, the market price is often lowered for everyone.

Some of these tools are clearly more powerful than others in their potential effectiveness. For example, economic and regulatory instruments are more effective than information and education to ensure healthful changes in organizations and individuals: Smoking rates drop faster with a high tobacco tax and no-public-smoking rules than with sharing of information on health effects alone, especially among teens. However, the more effective means are the most difficult to get adopted, because they have a higher political cost—that is, it is riskier to offend commercial groups by using economic instruments such as a tobacco tax increase than to simply inform the public of health risks through warning labels on cigarettes. This was clear in tobacco-control cases.

The Players as Stakeholders

Policies develop through the actions of the players and their relationships as they try to shape decisions about who pays and who gets what of the determinants of health. The players are the organized groups—**stakeholders**—whose interests are affected by current and prospective policies. They include political parties, the media, bureaucracies, voluntary and commercial organizations, public-interest groups, and professional associations.

A policy issue draws the attention of public and private stakeholders who view a policy change as important to their interests. These stakeholders perceive themselves to be importantly affected by a change in policy. Their interests are the things they need to survive, including finances (from grants, contracts, dues, or sales), facilities, staff, authority, control, status, legitimacy, and image.

GLOBAL CONNECTION 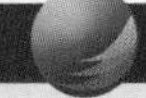

How do U.S. health policies—for example, policies about smoking restrictions—affect global health?

In turn, these resources affect a group's bargaining power. Stakeholders include elected or other officials, legislative committees, parties, and bureaus; commercial, scientific, and medical groups; and voluntary nonprofit organizations, including public interest groups (Daniels, Glickstein, & Mason, 2012; DiMaggio & Anheier, 1990; Feldstein, 1996; Jasanoff, 1993; Nathanson, 2005; Rice, 2002; Warner, 1991).

The underlying interest of political and other governmental leaders is to retain power and authority. For businesses, increased profits and market share are important. Professionals want to acquire grants, higher career status, and control over their practice. Voluntary organizations must please their boards and donors; advocacy groups must satisfy their supporters (e.g., governing board, funders, membership), both existing and potential. Each group attempts to engage in political activity in ways that will shape any particular policy to favor its own interests (Benjamin, Perfetto, & Greene, 1995; Nathanson, 2005; Rice, 2002).

In the case of tobacco policy, the involvement of major health-related organizations illustrates these self-regarding calculations and accounts for their sometimes sideline roles in the policymaking process. State health departments, public health associations, medical societies, and large voluntary organizations did no more than lend their names to the anti-tobacco coalitions that were fighting for strong tobacco-control legislation. Each of these mainline organizations had competing priorities, such as fears of budget cuts from opposition lawmakers, lack of staff, or legal restrictions in some local health departments. The medical societies chose to use their political capital to seek better clinical payment rates, and the large nonprofit groups feared a backlash from some donors. These organizational decisions about public health advocacy were strategic choices made by each organization that took into account the tradeoffs in resources for the group and its purposes. In one state, "risk protection" was required before a state chapter of the American Cancer Society publicly agreed to lead a tobacco taxation campaign (Heiser & Begay, 1997).

> Each of us must choose whether to live our lives narrowly, selfishly and complacently or to act with courage and faith. We are not governed by fate or mysterious forces of history. It is the sum of our choices that will determine the kind of America and the kind of world in which we live.
>
> —*Madeleine Albright, U.S. Secretary of State, George Washington University Commencement, May 21, 2000*

Player Connections

Alliances are more reliable and long-lasting when they are based on written agreements, agreed rules, or intense resource exchange. **Collaboration** differs from **cooperation** by the exchange of tangible assets (e.g., part-time staff or use of printing equipment in the former, as contrasted with the verbal support and good will in cooperative ties). For example, the California Nurses Association gained much more public support than it could have otherwise in a recent referendum on state healthcare reform by allying with labor unions and others and sharing staff.

To influence policymakers in the face of competition by well financed, large-scale commercial interests, as in tobacco control, requires strategic planning, continuous management, and joint efforts, despite the difficulties of coalition formation (Heiser & Begay, 1997; Kegler, 1995; Nathanson, 2005; Rice, 2002).

Information for Action

Information is basic to policymaking. It is used to monitor, analyze, evaluate, report, and critique an issue. It becomes action-oriented when used for informing, educating, persuading, mediating, activating, or mobilizing others to act (Lindblom & Cohen, 1979; Ray & Roberts, 2002).

The strategic problem for proponents of health-supporting policy is to use selected types of information to convince target groups that their policy position is economically feasible (to its supporters and users), politically acceptable (to the more powerful groups affected by it), socially approved within the milieu in which it is to operate, and administratively and technologically possible (Milio, 2000; Ray & Roberts, 2002). To do this, a wide range of **strategic information** is needed—about the policy environment and the problem; the purposes, interests, and tactics of the players; and the degree of support among constituencies, as gauged by polls and endorsements. This must be sought and developed by policy proponents; thus the need for an organized and sustained effort.

Studies can stimulate new ways to conceive policy problems and solutions and occasionally are directly incorporated into policy development, such as the knowledge that high tobacco taxes are the most effective way of reducing smoking in young people (Beyer & Trice, 1982; Brewer & De Leon, 1983; Brint, 1990; Webber, 1987). "Research that demonstrates that a course of action being contemplated by policymakers may (or may not) lead to undesirable or unexpected consequences can contribute significantly to policymaking" (Shi & Singh, 2008, pp. 554–555).

This wide array of information goes far beyond typical health status data and includes a variety of material available from all the social–political–economic disciplines and policy think tanks (institutes and centers). This information is often available on the Internet. The task, then, is to effectively use that information to influence policymaking in language, formats, and amounts that are suited to each target group, including the press and the public.

GOT AN ALTERNATIVE? 

Should regulation of herbal therapies be the responsibility of the U.S. Food and Drug Administration? What are advantages and possible negative consequences of regulating this type of nontraditional treatment?

Policy Development Strategies

The most effective policymaking activities, demanding the most resources, include lobbying legislative or bureaucratic policymakers directly or through their constituents; ensuring the election or appointment of supportive political leaders; and engaging in litigation. Less effective means, often used by small groups, involve developing publicity through the media and organizing demonstrations, conferences, and public education programs (Nathanson, 2005; Walker, 1991). All such activities have long been on the agendas of national, state, and, to some extent, local nursing organizations. Their voice is always stronger when allied with other groups, as occurred in the national healthcare reform effort of 1993–1994.

Bargaining

The central strategic activity to influence policies and move them through the phases of policymaking is negotiation. This process always involves compromise. Effective **bargaining** requires taking account of the interests of governments and other target groups and being willing to

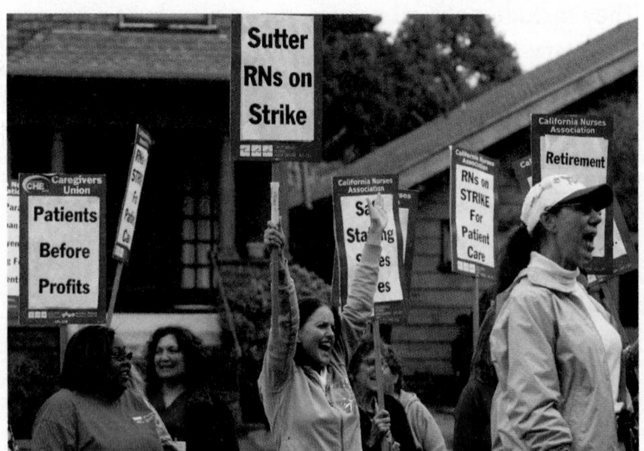
Sutter RNs on Strike
Caregivers Union
Patients Before Profits
California Nurses Association
Retirement
RNs on STRIKE For Patient Care

Nurses and other lobbying groups work to influence health policy through legislation.

trade away some less valued interests to gain others in the foreseeable future, such as agreeing to a 50-cent tobacco tax instead of a dollar so that political support for adoption is easier to gain.

Public distortion of facts by opponents requires prompt public rebuttal by health proponents, such as when tobacco proponents maintained that there is no scientific proof of the health effects of smoking (Heiser & Begay, 1997). By contrast, to obtain political and organizational endorsement, proponents must demonstrate the political support needed by elected and bureaucratic officials—for example, by providing credible evidence of support from opinion polls and sponsorship by local groups and agencies. This involves developing information on group support for proponents' policy preferences or offering a promise by coalition members of future support for the policymaker's agenda.

Information Through the Mass Media

People's information is obtained directly from experience or through various interpersonal and technological channels. All such conduits select and shape the information they pass on according to their own priorities (Minkler, 1997). The media mix includes storage tools (DVDs, Blu-ray, CDs, SD cards, etc.) and transmission channels (TV networks, cable, satellite, radio, print media, etc.), all of which are merging on the Internet. This rapidly expanding web of information sources has implications for both policy development activities and health information/education.

Mass media affect policymaking in many ways. They convey information and messages that influence perspectives and actions, depending on when, how, and in what social and information contexts they are received.

The media set the agenda, telling people which issues are important to think and talk about. They also frame or focus on certain aspects of issues, helping shape how people and policymakers understand them. This is especially true for the formation of short-term public opinion about public health issues, such as environmental pollution and poverty.

As commercial organizations, the media depend on advertisers. They select content and target audiences to attract viewers for their sponsors. Larger audiences mean higher prices for advertising and higher revenues. Prime-time news media focus on mainstream issues. For example, 4 years passed before the prime-time new media began covering human immunodeficiency virus/acquired immune deficiency syndrome, after the disease became widespread in the United States, believing that it was a minor problem of interest only to homosexuals and intravenous drug users but not to the population at large (Edgar, Fitzpatrick, & Freimuth, 1992).

The media in this way reinforce mainstream views and set expectations about reality, including racial and gender stereotypes. For example, heavy viewers—those who watch more television (or videos) daily than others (more than 4 hours)—are more likely to overestimate the prevalence of divorce, illegitimacy, abortions, sexually transmitted diseases, and crime (Edgar et al., 1992). This perception clearly has implications for the kinds of demands the public makes (or indicates in polls) for public policy action.

Health Information

Education and information are part of the package of useful policy tools and are longer lasting when accompanied by other stronger tools. Public health media campaigns are usually limited to attempts to influence *individual* behavior rather than to mold public opinion about policy issues. As costly as they are, however, these health education campaigns by themselves mainly affect knowledge or awareness, and only occasionally do they influence short-term behavior (Public Health Service, Office of Technology Assessment, 1991; Rice & Atkin, 1994).

Several conditions must be in place to translate awareness of a health problem into changes in personal behavior, especially for the long term. The message must have the following characteristics:

- Targeted and attractive for specific groups
- Conveyed over multiple channels long enough for "saturation" of the target groups
- Integrated with local interpersonal communication
- Supported by environmental, organizational, and policy changes to ensure long-term behavior change, such as increases in tobacco taxes and laws against smoking in public places

A new and important aspect of health information campaigns is the need to identify the most appropriate channels for dissemination. Where traditional print or television media were the primary means of communication for most of the 20th century, in 2014 information is disseminated through multiple means: print, television, online articles (which can be in type, video, or slide format), social media campaigns, webinars, chats, texts, or any combination of these. Moreover, which channel is used depends on who the intended audience is. A newspaper article on the impact of a new strain of flu that hits young adults hardest is not likely to reach that target audience unless it is published online as well as in print, and disseminated via social media (Facebook, Twitter, YouTube, etc.). At the same time, however, older adults who may not be as knowledgeable or interested in online communication may not respond to a campaign that uses such channels to the exclusion of more traditional media.

So, for example, outreach attempting to raise awareness of osteoporosis screening in older adults that is exclusively available online may fail to reach many members of its target audience who lack the skills, interest, or access to Internet-based literature.

Mass Media and the Case of Healthcare Reform: A Cautionary Tale

Policy issues raised in the mass media can have adverse public health policy effects. Issues are often defined too simply, solutions described too superficially, and legitimacy conferred on only selected groups because of what "sells" to audiences and advertisers. In the Internet era, information travels extraordinarily quickly, which means that "bad" information can become entrenched in the public mindset before updated or more accurate data emerge. Particularly with respect to online and social media news, the information being disseminated is frequently inaccurate or overstated and, according to one study, slanted toward negative information ("Learn of this new threat to your health!") as opposed to positive health promotion (Miller, 2013). This in itself suggests the need for greater attention to the electronic world by the public health community as the experience of healthcare reform portrays.

A series of studies covering the introduction and failure of the Clinton healthcare plan from September 1993 to July 1994 demonstrates how mass media are woven into policymaking processes and shows how important it is to take the media into account in health policy development (Braun, 1995; Cappella & Jamieson, 1994, 1996; Columbia Institute, 1995). Findings show the following:

- Although the media devoted much time and space to healthcare reform, two-thirds of all coverage was on political strategy, not content; the pros and cons of each major proposal or areas of agreement.
- Coverage was not balanced, giving more attention to the president's plan while others, like the single-payer bill, had no real public airing. Without public knowledge about options, there was little likelihood of support for a compromise bill.
- The tone of the stories was that politicians act out of self-interest rather than commitment to the public good. Randomized viewer studies showed that strategy-based (versus issue-centered) stories created perceptions of policymakers as posturing, deceptive, self-interested, and unconcerned with the welfare of citizens. Groups viewing only issue-centered stories were less cynical.
- News coverage of political advertising, by emphasizing the attack and controversial nature of the ads, dramatically enlarged the ads' audiences and collectively aired an additional 15 minutes of free nationwide television exposure. The ads' sponsors then had incentive to prepare ever more extreme ads, costing more than $50 million. These ads succeeded in reaching legislators on key committees and their media market viewers.
- The public was found to be generally poorly informed (e.g., 75% did not know the administration was the main proponent of an employer mandate requiring them to offer insurance to workers [favored by a majority of people]), fewer than half had heard of the single-payer bill, and they wanted much more information and blamed the media for not providing it.
- Reporting of opinion polls was uncritical; it magnified the impact of uninformed opinion, creating "news" out of uninformed opinion (failing to qualify the results according to people's depth of knowledge) and influencing the actions of leading members of Congress and perhaps also of undecided viewers.
- The advertising, polls, and media coverage of them ultimately had an impact on Congress's rejection of major reform. Leaders said that public opinion was as influential in the debate as the administration itself, that interest-group advertising (mainly by health insurance and business interests) was persuasive, that the public was not well informed on the issues, and that the media had done a poor job of helping people understand the issues. Despite this, leading members and staff of the House and Senate said their main sources of information about public opinion were the polls (mainly reported in the media), the trade group lobbies, and the media (Columbia Institute, 1995).

In large part, most of the media-based issues within healthcare reform reflected a failure of policy experts ("wonks") to translate their intentions into language easily understood by people who were not involved with the details, and to offer a story equally as dramatic and interesting as the tales—sometimes invented—told by opponents of the reforms. Most of these failings were repeated during the passage of the ACA in 2010. One essay chronicling the mistakes of the ACA's passage and implementation noted that "the Obama plan, like . . . the Clintons' plan before it . . . [put] wonks . . . in charge and there seems to have been little checking to see if real people could handle it" (Drew, 2013). Policy fights and failures represent a much more dramatic story than consensus and successes; as the essay points out, "anecdotes about people losing their policies . . . make for more dramatic news stories than the advances already achieved under the law; there's been little attention to the already slowing rate of growth in the cost of health care—one of the law's major goals" (Drew, 2013). Particularly given the speed at which news and opinions "go viral" in the Internet age, and the negative slant of such stories with respect to health (Miller, 2013), failure to manage mass media communications can be a death knell for even the best crafted policy.

RESEARCH ALERT 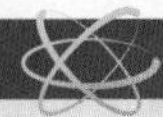

This study examined the effects of policy variables on enrollment in the Special Supplemental Nutrition Program for Women, Infants, and Children (WIC) using Aday and Anderson's framework for the study of access. Secondary analysis of data from public documents and agencies for the 50 states was done. Independent variables were the ratio of the federal WIC grant to the eligible population, state supplementation of WIC, administrative and food dollars per person, WIC population per clinic, and WIC priority categories served. The dependent variable was the eligible WIC population enrolled. State supplementation of the WIC budget, administrative and food dollars per person, cost of living, population density and distribution, and ratio of the federal WIC grant to the eligible population accounted for 85% of the variance in WIC enrollment. Recommendations included reorienting the federal funding formula toward enrollment incentives, state supplementation of WIC, and examination of administrative and food costs.

Source: Wimmer, M. (2003). The effects of policy on enrollment in the Special Supplemental Nutrition Program for Women, Infants, and Children. *Policy, Politics, & Nursing Practice, 4*(3), 210–220.

Implementation

Congressional adoption of policies, known as **authorization**, only begins the next major phase of policymaking: making a policy effective in the real world. Policies require **appropriations**, approved amounts of funds to be available over 1 year or more, to put the policy into effect. To complete the task, the monies must be allocated (i.e., distributed by an authorized agency, usually a government bureau, in the form of grants, contracts, or other payments).

Prior to this dispersal of funds, the policy must be interpreted in specific terms, known as **rule making**; opened to public comment for 30 to 60 days (always published in the weekly *Federal Register*); finalized; and then publicized to eligible recipient organizations, such as state agencies and community groups, including health centers and home health agencies. These potential users must apply for the funds by proposing what programs they will conduct with the monies. The awardees then implement programs, such as community or employee tobacco education, smoking-cessation programs, or payment for the costs of setting up smoke-free workplaces.

Finally, the authorized agencies must monitor and enforce the rules that guide application of the policy and eventually feed this information back into the final phase of policymaking: evaluation. At any point in implementation, groups may contest the process in court if they think it is proceeding too slowly or too quickly, fairly or unfairly.

> In this and like communities, public sentiment is everything. With public sentiment, nothing can fail; without it, nothing can succeed.
>
> —*Abraham Lincoln, 1858*

The complexity of policy implementation processes, as federal and state funds are dispersed into programs across communities, means that there are infinite ways for opponents to change the pace and direction of a policy. For example, in Massachusetts and California, where tobacco-control coalitions succeeded in passing tobacco tax referenda against strong industry lobbying, the actual use of the millions of new dollars became another source of contention. Rather than the intended use of the funds for anti-tobacco programs, policymakers attempted to use the monies for other, sometimes political, purposes such as financing hospital care in response to the hospital lobby (Begay & Glantz, 1997).

In one state, the anti-tobacco coalition sued the state in court and won, requiring authorization and allocation of the funds for the stated smoking prevention and control purposes. In the other state, the coalition negotiated a compromise on the use of the funds, but this resulted in a decline in appropriations for tobacco control over the next several years. Analysis of such experiences can help inform future public health policy efforts.

Evaluation

Research findings (i.e., science-based information)—in contrast to opinions and impressions—are often not available or are not used much by policymakers. Studies must be translated first into the organizational or political priorities of policymakers. The timing of findings makes a difference too in whether they are used, for instance, before interest groups have developed around a policy issue, or much later, when social acceptance improves (Brint, 1990; Brooten, Brown, Miovech, & Youngblut, 2006). Most evaluation consists of the impressions of user groups and program reports on **outputs**, such as numbers of people served, numbers reached by public education campaigns, new smoke-free workplaces, the decline of cigarette sales, and financial reports. Policy **impacts** include the indirect effects of a policy, sometimes unintended or unwanted. For example, when strict local no-smoking laws were passed in New York, bars and restaurants did not lose business as the tobacco industry had warned (Engelen, Farrelly, & Hyland, 2006). When the WIC program was implemented, it created new local food retail jobs and improved local economies (National Farmers Association, 1996).

Outcomes—that is, changes in people's health—are more rare, sometimes because they can be seen only after a longer period of time than policymakers are willing to wait (such as a decline in lung cancer), and sometimes because health indicators often require additional spending for evaluation research—monies that are often not available. Evaluation is thus both a political and scientific process, and its results determine whether a policy will be revised, cut back, or repealed (Hanley, 2006; Zervigon-Hakes, 1995).

The lesson is clear: Policymaking for health continues long after adoption and requires that proponents continue to monitor the processes and to take action to preserve the health effectiveness of any specific policy. This kind of "watchdog" activity is often done by public interest groups, such as the Coalition on Smoking and Health, the Brady Campaign to Prevent Gun Violence, and the Center for Public Environmental Oversight in Washington, DC. Governments also have monitoring agencies, including the Government Accountability Office of Congress to oversee legislative results and the Office of Management and Budget, which oversees the effectiveness of most executive branch agencies for the White House.

Nurses in Communities, Public Health Policy, and Primary Prevention

The tobacco coalitions all succeeded to some degree in obtaining public resources to prevent the biggest single cause of death in populations. Yet the largest risk factor threatening health and life, one not often discussed or addressed by the health sector, is the gross and growing disparity in social and economic determinants of health between the nation's disadvantaged communities and others (Krieger, 1994; Link & Phelan, 1995; Wexler & Copeland, 2003). It is possible for the public health community to initiate and work with coalitions in local, state, and national strategies to improve the conditions in which people live. This includes nurses, who see the effects of poverty and discrimination based on ethnicity, age, and other factors. They have been and, to fulfill their professional duty, should continue to be involved at every level, either through their practice settings, nurse groups, or by joining allied groups. To promote primary prevention policies, it is necessary to involve a wide range of organizations that affect living conditions and to focus on priority public, institutional, or corporate policies.

> Americans will always do the right thing . . . after they have exhausted all the other possibilities.
>
> —*Winston Churchill*

Among the many community conditions needed to support population health are housing, child welfare, and access to comprehensive primary care (Federman et al., 1996; Montgomery et al., 1996; NCCP, 2007). With the kind of policy groundwork outlined previously, these issues can become priorities for health departments and other parts of the health community. Policy proposals can then be developed to ensure more healthful living conditions. A few examples follow.

Neighborhoods with high rates of unemployment, poverty, high rent, and crowded housing are associated with a high incidence of low-birth-weight babies. Adverse living situations predispose people to toxicities, infections, contagions, accidents, strains on eyesight, unhealthy food storage and use, and mental health stresses from lack of privacy, the inability to work at home, and lack of recreation opportunities (Martin, 1977; Roberts, 1997; Sherman & Redlener, 2003).

The availability and adequacy of housing significantly affect health through the following strategies:

- The siting of housing—whether near polluting industries or near transportation routes to access job opportunities, education and health services, and stores
- Local environmental controls and maintenance, such as water supply and waste management
- Housing structure involving overcrowding, ventilation, lighting, and temperature control

Thus, legitimate public health activities include improved zoning, environmental regulations, and building codes; the development of adequate low-rent housing and transportation systems; support for tenant organizations and citizen grievance processes; and open hearings on housing issues. Although not under the direct control of health departments, community health organizations and agencies can form coalitions and raise these issues by defining the type and scope of health issues and the policy changes needed to support health, as well as through work with local and state organizations in housing, economic development, land use, and the environment to advise on and advocate changes (Hardy & Satterthwaite, 1987; Rice, 2002; Slater & Carlton, 1985).

On a smaller scale, taking account of commercial establishments' interest in safe and expanding markets, local governments and community organizations, led by health departments or other health advocacy groups, can use their market power to influence the proportion of healthy foods in the local food supply and to limit access to tobacco (CDC, 1999). For instance, they could require that cafeterias in their facilities offer healthier food choices. This would encourage food suppliers to change their supplier contracts to retain their own contracts, with ripple effects on food-processing corporations. The new options in these facilities would result in changes in eating habits for clients and employees while at the same time suggesting an exemplary "healthful practices" model for the public and the media. Nurses, for example, could propose healthy food options in their worksite cafeterias in state and local health agencies, schools, hospitals, health maintenance organizations, prisons, military installations, vending machines, and so on.

With rising child impoverishment and lack of health care, child health and welfare are at risk (Cohen, 2002). Specific, focused policies proposed by nurses allied with child welfare proponents (Deal & Shiono, 1998) that are worthy of advocacy efforts include the following:

> The new technologies hold promise for a greatly enhanced system that can meet the changing needs of an information-based society. At the same time, these technologies will generate a number of significant social problems. How these technologies evolve, as well as who will be affected positively or negatively, will depend on decisions now being made in both the public and private sectors . . . making choices about universal service is essentially making choices about equality of opportunity. Defining universal service is, in effect, making choices about the nature of society itself.
>
> —*Office of Technology Assessment, U.S. Congress, Critical Connections, 1990*

- An increase in cigarette excise taxes
- Strong indoor and outdoor air quality control and enforcement
- An above-poverty-level minimum wage
- Handgun control
- Repair of the welfare and prevention safety net
- Comprehensive maternal–child care and child day care

Advocacy Tools of the Future

Electronic networks are a new set of tools to extend the sources of support and strengthen the advocacy efforts for the public's health. Community-based groups, allied with the public health community, raise and amplify issues, propose solutions, establish their legitimacy, and join larger coalitions. These advocacy networks, linked to national and local watchdog groups, supply timely and accurate information not only about problems, but also about program and policy solutions and sources of technical assistance. Perhaps most importantly, these electronic links coordinate joint advocacy efforts and alert local groups to timely actions in local, state, and national policy arenas, including coordination of email, fax, phone, social media, or letter-writing campaigns to pass, for example, a tobacco tax or handgun registration.

The case has been made in public health forums and studies for electronic networks to link public health and other community organizations to improve community health, especially in poor areas. This collaboration supports core public health functions through strengthening services delivery, education, environmental health, community mobilization, and policy advocacy (Lasker, Humphreys, & Braithwaite, 1995; Jennings, Thompson, & Roberts, 2002; Milio, 1995, 1996). Nurses are in a position to point out the importance of electronic linkages with community organizations to develop and reinforce health and community partnerships.

Conclusion

An understanding of health policymaking and the mission of public health is not merely an academic exercise. It is essential to the health professions and their institutions because practitioners in nursing and other health fields are in applied—not academic—disciplines. Our privileges are derived from our social responsibility to ensure the health of all populations. An awareness of the health effects of a wide range of public and corporate policies, the public reporting of these effects, and efforts to promote health-supporting policies fall within the scope of the health community and in our activities within other groups. Participation in any aspect of these complex and ongoing policy processes can engage us as individuals. But more often, policy work requires action through organizations to sustain the necessary long-term effort to ensure effective health-supporting policies.

The leaders in nursing of the 19th and 20th centuries were great women with broad vision and understanding of the issues of their day. They engaged political, social, and healthcare groups in improving both the healthcare system and the health of all the people, especially the rural and urban poor, immigrants, and other vulnerable groups. The 21st century is at least as challenging and requires comparable vision, commitment, and energy.

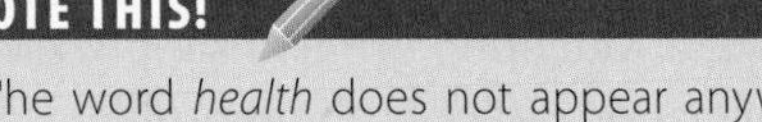

NOTE THIS!

The word *health* does not appear anywhere in the U.S. Constitution or Bill of Rights.

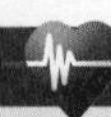

LEVELS OF PREVENTION

Primary: Education about the dangers of smoking for teens

Secondary: Promoting programs for those who are attempting to quit smoking

Tertiary: Providing care and education for populations with chronic obstructive pulmonary disease due to long-term smoking

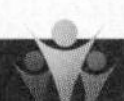

HEALTHY ME

Identify a health policy that affects your life and health, such as no smoking in buildings, no cell phone use while in a moving vehicle, or wearing seatbelts in cars. How does this affect your attitude about mandatory laws and policies in terms of personal compliance?

Critical Thinking Activities

1. Select a community health problem, such as teen suicide or school violence. Chapter author Dr. Milio contends, "Media are not only channels for information . . . they also create and shape issues." Think of several examples from the media in which your selected health issue is presented as a problem or a solution. Who is blamed for the problem? Are solutions identified? Who are the stakeholders in any policymaking related to your identified problem?
2. If you could design a website that influences health policy for children with learning disabilities, what components would you include? How would you include the public in its development and implementation? Who would you include as experts on your website? Decide how you could link your website to other advocacy groups. Design an evaluation of this project as related to effectiveness in policymaking.

References

Amundson, D. R., Lichter, L. S., & Lichter, S. R. (2005). *What's the matter with kids today? Television coverage of adolescents in America.* Prepared for the Frameworks Institute. Retrieved from http://www.frameworksinstitute.org/assets/files/PDF/Youth_Whats_the_Matter.pdf

Begay, M., & Glantz, S. (1997). Question 1 tobacco education expenditures in Massachusetts, USA. *Tobacco Control, 6*, 213–218.

Benjamin, K., Perfetto, E., & Greene, R. (1995). Public policy and the application of outcomes assessments: Paradigms vs politics. *Medical Care, 33*(4), AS299–AS306 suppl.

Beyer, J., & Trice, H. (1982). The utilization process: A conceptual framework and synthesis of empirical findings. *Administrative Science Quarterly, 24*(4), 591–622.

Bomlitz, L. J., & Brezis, M. (2008). Misrepresentation of health risks by mass media. *Journal of Public Health, 30*(2), 202–204.

Braun, S. (1995, March/April). Media coverage of health care reform. A content analysis. *Columbia Journalism Review*, supplement, 1–8.

Brewer, G., & De Leon, P. (1983). *Foundations of policy analysis.* Homewood, IL: Dorsey.

Brint, S. (1990). Rethinking the policy influence of experts: From general characterizations to analysis of variation. *Sociological Forum, 5*(3), 361–385.

Brooten, D., Brown, L. P., Miovech, S. M., & Youngblut, J. M. (2006). Politics of nursing research. In D. J. Mason, J. K. Leavitt, & M. K. Chaffee (Eds.), *Policy and politics in nursing and health care* (5th ed.). Philadelphia, PA: Saunders.

Cappella, J., & Jamieson, K. (1994). *Public cynicism and news coverage in campaigns and policy debates: 3 field experiments.* Research report. Philadelphia, PA: Annenberg School for Communication.

Cappella, J., & Jamieson, K. (1996). *Media in the middle: Coverage of the health care reform debate of 1994.* Research report. Philadelphia, PA: Annenberg School of Mass Communications.

Center for the Future of Children. (1997, Spring). Welfare to work. *Future of Children, 7*, 1.

Center for Health Economics Research. (1993). *Access to health care: Indicators for policy.* Princeton, NJ: Robert Wood Johnson Foundation.

Centers for Disease Control and Prevention (CDC). (1999). *Physical activity and good nutrition.* Atlanta, GA: Author.

Centers for Disease Control and Prevention (CDC). (2013). *Lead.* Retrieved from http://www.cdc.gov/nceh/lead/

Cohen, S. S. (2002). Child care policy making. In D. J. Mason, J. K. Leavitt, & M. K. Chaffee (Eds.), *Policy and politics in nursing and health care* (4th ed., pp. 669–675). St. Louis, MO: Saunders.

Columbia Institute. (1995, May). *What shapes lawmakers' views? A survey of members of Congress and key staff on health care reform.* Washington, DC: Author.

Cutler, D., & Sheiner, L. (1999). *Demographics and medical care spending: Standard and non-standard effects.* Unpublished paper. Boston, MA: Harvard School of Public Health.

Deal, L., & Shiono, P. (1998). Medicaid managed care and children: An overview. *Future of Children, 8*(2), 93–104.

DiMaggio, P., & Anheier, H. (1990). The sociology of non-profit organizations and sectors. *Annual Review of Sociology, 16*, 137–159.

Drew, E. (2013). Obama: The first term did it. *The New York Review of Books.* Retrieved from http://www.nybooks.com/blogs/nyrblog/2013/nov/23/obama-first-term/

Edgar, T., Fitzpatrick, M. A., & Freimuth, V. S. (1992). *AIDS: A communication perspective.* Hillsdale, NJ: Lawrence Erlbaum.

Engelen, M., Farrelly, M., & Hyland, A. (2006, July). *The health and economic impact of New York's clean indoor air act.* Albany, NY: New York State Department of Health.

Fairman, J., & D'Antonio, P. (2013). History counts: How history can shape our understanding of health policy. *Nursing Outlook, 61*(5), 346–352.

Federman, M., Garner, T. I., Short, K., Cutter, W. N., 4th, Kiely, J., Levine, D., . . . McMillen, M. (1996, May). What does it mean to be poor in America? *Monthly Labor Review, 119*(5), 3–17.

Feldstein, P. J. (1996). *The politics of health legislation. An economic perspective.* Chico, CA: Health Administration Press.

Government Accountability Office (GAO). (1998). *Elevated blood lead levels in children.* Washington, DC: U.S. Congress.

Hanley, B. E. (2006). Policy development and analysis. In D. J. Mason, J. K. Leavitt, & M. K. Chaffee (Eds.), *Policy and politics in nursing and health care* (5th ed.). Philadelphia, PA: Saunders.

Hardy, J., & Satterthwaite, D. (1987). Housing and health. *Cities, 4*, 221–235.

Hatcher, B. J. (2003). The Maternal and Child Health Community Leadership Institute: Putting the Health for All Framework into action. In H. M. Wallace, G. Green, & K. J. Jaros (Eds.), *Health and welfare for families in the 21st century* (2nd ed., pp. 41–51). Sudbury, MA: Jones and Bartlett.

Heiser, P., & Begay, M. (1997). Campaign to raise the tobacco tax in Massachusetts. *American Journal of Public Health, 87*, 968–973.

Horton, K. B. (2006). Lobbying: An inside view. In D. J. Mason, J. K. Leavitt, & M. K. Chaffee (Eds.), *Policy and politics in nursing and health care* (5th ed.). Philadelphia, PA: Saunders.

Institute of Medicine. (1988). *The future of public health.* Washington, DC: National Academies Press.

Jacobson, P., Wasserman, J., & Raube, K. (1993). Politics of antismoking legislation. *Journal of Health Policy, Policy & Law, 18*, 787–818.

Jasanoff, S. (1993). *The fifth branch: Science advisors as policymakers.* Cambridge, MA: Harvard University Press.

Jennings, C. P., Thompson, L., & Roberts, D. (2002). Achieving health literacy. In D. J. Mason, J. K. Leavitt, & M. K. Chaffee (Eds.), *Policy and politics in nursing and health care* (4th ed., pp. 107–111). St. Louis, MO: Saunders.

Kaplan, H. (1996). Inequality in income and mortality in the US: Analysis of mortality and potential pathways. *British Medical Journal, 312*, 999–1003.

Karlsson, M., Nilsson, T., Lyttkens, C. H., & Leeson, G. (2010). Income inequality and health: Importance of a cross-country perspective. *Social Science & Medicine, 70*(6), 875–885.

Kegler, M. (1995). *Community coalitions for tobacco control: Factors influencing implementation.* PhD dissertation. Chapel Hill, NC: University of North Carolina School of Public Health.

Kessler, D. A., Witt, A. M., Barnett, P. S., Zeller, M. R., Natanblut, S. L., Wilkenfeld, J. P., . . . Schultz, W. B. (1996). The Food and Drug Administration's regulation of tobacco products. *New England Journal of Medicine, 335*(13), 988–994.

Klijs, B., Nusselder, W. J., Looman, C. W., & Mackenbach, J. P. (2011). Contribution of chronic disease to the burden of disability. *PLoS ONE, 6*(9), e25325. doi:10.1371/journal.pone.0025325

Kraus, J., Peek, A., & Williams, S. (1995). Compliance with the 1992 California motorcycle helmet use law. *American Journal of Public Health, 85*(3), 96–99.

Krause, K., & Berman, E. G. (Eds). (2007). *Small Arms Survey 2007: Guns and the city.* Geneva, Switzerland: Small Arms Survey Project.

Krieger, N. (1994). Epidemiology and the web of causation. *Social Science & Medicine, 39*, 887–903.

Krieger, N., Chen, J. T., & Ebel, G. (1997). Can we monitor socioeconomic inequalities in health? A survey of US health departments' data collection and reporting practices. *Public Health Report, 112*(6), 481–491.

Lasker, R. (1997). *Medicine and public health.* New York, NY: New York Academy of Medicine.

Lasker, R., Humphreys, B., & Braithwaite, W. (1995, July). *Making a powerful connection: The health of the public and the national information infrastructure. Report of the Public Health Data Policy Coordinating Committee, U.S. Public Health Service.* Washington, DC: U.S. Government Printing Office.

Laumann, E., & Knoke, D. (1987). *The organizational state.* Madison, WI: University of Wisconsin Press.

Lindblom, C., & Cohen, D. (1979). *Useable knowledge.* New Haven, CT: Yale University Press.

Link, B., & Phelan, J. (1995). Social conditions as fundamental causes of disease. *Journal of Health & Social Behavior, 2*(special issue), 80–94.

Lurie, N. (2004). The public health infrastructure: Rebuild or redesign? In C. Harrington & C. L. Estes (Eds.), *Health policy: Crisis and reform in the U.S. health care delivery system* (4th ed., pp. 184–187). Sudbury, MA: Jones and Bartlett.

Martin, A. (1977). *Health aspects of human settlements: A review.* Geneva, Switzerland: World Health Organization.

Mason, D. J., Dodd, C. J., & Glickstein, B. (2007). Role of the media in influencing policy: Getting the message across. In D. J. Mason, J. K. Leavitt, & M. K. Chaffee (Eds.), *Policy and politics in nursing and health care* (5th ed.). Philadelphia, PA: Saunders.

Milio, N. (1976, March). A framework for prevention: Changing health damaging to health generating life patterns. *American Journal of Public Health, 66*, 35–38.

Milio, N. (1986). *Promoting health through public policy*. Ottawa, Canada: Canadian Public Health Association.

Milio, N. (1995). Beyond informatics: Community electronic networks and public health. *Journal of Public Health Management & Practice, 2*(3), 6–11.

Milio, N. (1996). *Engines of empowerment: Using information technology to create healthy communities and challenge public policy*. Chico, CA: Health Administration Press.

Milio, N. (1997). Case studies in nutrition policymaking: How process shapes product. In B. Garza (Ed.), *Beyond nutrition information*. Ithaca, NY: Cornell University Press.

Milio, N. (2000). Evaluating health promotion policies: Tracking a moving target. In I. Rootman, M. Goodstadt, L. Potvin, & J. Springett (Eds.), *Evaluation of health promotion: Principles and perspectives*. Copenhagen, Denmark: World Health Organization.

Milio, N. (2002). Where policy hits the pavement: Contemporary issues in communities. In D. J. Mason, J. K. Leavitt, & M. K. Chaffee (Eds.), *Policy and politics in nursing and health care* (4th ed., pp. 659–668). St. Louis, MO: Saunders.

Miller, A. S. (2013). The zombie apocalypse: The viral impact of social media marketing on health. *Journal of Consumer Health on the Internet, 17*(4), 362–368.

Minkler, M. (Ed.). (1997). *Community organizing and community building for health*. New Brunswick, NJ: Rutgers University Press.

Minkler, M. (Ed.). (2004). *Community organizing and community building for health* (2nd ed.). New Brunswick, NJ: Rutgers University Press.

Montgomery, L., Kiely, J., & Pappas, G. (1996). Effects of poverty, race, and family structure of US children's health: Data from the National Health Interview Survey, 1978 through 1980 and 1989 through 1991. *American Journal of Public Health, 86*(10), 1401–1405.

Nathanson, M. D. (2005). *Health care providers' government relations handbook*. Sudbury, MA: Jones and Bartlett.

National Association of County and City Health Officials (NACCHO). (1998). *NACCHO study of electronic communication capacity of local health departments*. Washington, DC: Author.

National Cancer Institute. (1991). *Strategies to control tobacco use in the United States: A blueprint for public health action in the 1990s*. Smoking and Tobacco Control Monographs 1. Bethesda, MD: Author.

National Center for Children in Poverty (NCCP). (1998). *Young children in poverty*. New York, NY: Columbia University School of Public Health.

National Center for Children in Poverty (NCCP). (2007). *Federal child and dependent care tax credit*. New York, NY: Columbia University School of Public Health.

National Center for Children in Poverty (NCCP). (2014). *Basic facts about low-income children: Children under 18 years, 2012*. Retrieved from http://www.nccp.org/publications/pub_1089.html

National Farmers Association Market Nutrition Programs. (1996). *Program impact report*. Washington, DC: Author.

Office of Disease Prevention and Health Promotion. (1994). *For a healthy nation: Returns on investment in public health*. Atlanta, GA: U.S. Department of Health and Human Services.

Pentz, M., Brannon, B. R., Charlin, V. R., Barrett, E. J., MacKinnon, D. P., & Flay, B. P. (1989). The power of policy: The relationship of smoking policy to adolescent smoking. *American Journal of Public Health, 79*(7), 857–862.

Public Health Foundation. (1998). *Measuring health objectives and indicators: 1997 state and local capacity survey*. Washington, DC: Author.

Public Health Service, Office of Technology Assessment. (1991). *Adolescent health* (vol. 1). Washington, DC: U.S. Congress.

Ray, M. M., & Roberts, S. (2002). Lobbying policymakers: Individual and collective strategies. In D. J. Mason, J. K. Leavitt, & M. K. Chaffee (Eds.), *Policy and politics in nursing and health care* (4th ed., pp. 551–561). St. Louis, MO: Saunders.

Rice, R. (2002). Coalitions: A powerful political strategy. In D. J. Mason, J. K. Leavitt, & M. K. Chaffee (Eds.), *Policy and politics in nursing and health care* (4th ed., pp. 121–129). St. Louis, MO: Saunders.

Rice, R., & Atkin, C. (1994). Principles of successful public communication campaigns. In J. Bryant & D. Zillman (Eds.), *Media effects: Advances in theory and research* (pp. 365–387). Hillsdale, NJ: Lawrence Erlbaum.

Roberts, E. (1997). Neighborhood social environments and the distribution of low birth weights in Chicago. *American Journal of Public Health, 87*, 597–603.

Rochefort, D., & Cobb, R. (1993). Problem definition, agenda access, and policy choice. *Policy Studies Journal, 21*(1), 56–71.

Rose, G. (1985). Sick individual and sick populations. *International Journal of Epidemiology, 14*, 32–38.

Rose, G. (1990). Future of disease prevention: British perspectives on the US Preventive Services Task for Guidelines. *Journal of General Internal Medicine, 5*, S128–S132.

Sherman, P., & Redlener, I. (2003). Homeless women and their children in the 21st century. In H. M. Wallace, G. Green, & K. J. Jaros (Eds.), *Health and welfare for families in the 21st century* (2nd ed., pp. 469–480). Sudbury, MA: Jones and Bartlett.

Shi, L., & Singh, D. A. (2008). *Delivering health care in America: A systems approach* (3rd ed.). Sudbury, MA: Jones and Bartlett.

Slater, C., & Carlton, B. (1985). Behavior, lifestyle, and socioeconomic variables as determinants of health status: Implications for health policy development. *American Journal of Preventive Medicine, 1*, 25–33.

Sofaer, S., Woolley, S. F., & Mauery, D. R. (1997). *Models for assessing the impact of changes in health care delivery and financing on community tuberculosis prevention and control programs*. Research report. Washington, DC: George Washington University Center for Health Outcomes Improvement Research.

Sultz, H. A., & Young, K. M. (2014). *Health care USA: Understanding its organization and delivery* (8th ed). Burlington, MA: Jones & Bartlett Learning.

Syme, S. L., Lefkowitz, B., & Krimgold, B. K. (2004). Incorporating socioeconomic factors into U.S. health policy: Addressing the barriers. In C. Harrington & C. L. Estes (Eds.), *Health policy: Crisis and reform in the U.S. health care delivery system* (4th ed., pp. 78–82). Sudbury, MA: Jones and Bartlett.

Teh-Wei, H., Hai-Yen, S., & Keeler, T. (1995). Reducing cigarette consumption in California: Tobacco taxes vs an anti-smoking media campaign. *American Journal of Public Health, 85*, 1218–1222.

U.S. Department of Health and Human Services (HHS). (1995, April). *Personal Responsibility Act of 1995: Preliminary impacts.* Washington, DC: Author.

Wakefield, M.K., Gardner, D. B., & Guillett, S. E. (2002). Contemporary issues in government. In D. J. Mason, J. K. Leavitt, & M. K. Chaffee (Eds.), *Policy and politics in nursing and health care* (4th ed., pp. 421–437). St. Louis, MO: Saunders.

Walker, J. (1991). *Mobilizing interest groups in America: Patrons, professions, and social movements.* Ann Arbor, MI: University of Michigan Press.

Warner, K. (1991). Tobacco industry scientific advisors: Serving society or selling cigarettes? *American Journal of Public Health, 81*(7), 839–842.

Webber, D. J. (1987). Factors influencing legislators' use of policy information and implications for promoting greater use. *Policy Studies Review, 6*(4), 64–80.

Weissert, C., & Weissert, W. (1996). *Governing health: The politics of health policy.* Baltimore, MD: Johns Hopkins University Press.

Wexler, S., & Copeland, V. C. (2003). Combating family poverty: A review of the American welfare system. In H. M. Wallace, G. Green, & K. J. Jaros (Eds.), *Health and welfare for families in the 21st century* (2nd ed., pp. 119–137). Sudbury, MA: Jones and Bartlett.

Winslow, C. E. A. (1920, March). The untilled field of public health. *Modern Medicine*, 183.

Zervigon-Hakes, A. (1995). Translating research into public programs and policies. *Future of Children, 5*(3), 175–191.

CHAPTER FOCUS

Community-Based Transcultural Nursing
Scope of Transcultural Nursing Cultures
Transcultural Nursing Principles
Transcultural Concepts
Leininger's Theory of Culture Care Diversity and Universality

Development of the Theory
Goal of the Theory
Assumptions of the Theory
The Sunrise Model: A Visual Guide for the Theory
Application of the Theory and Model

QUESTIONS TO CONSIDER

After reading this chapter, you will know the answers to the following questions:

1. What is community-based transcultural nursing?
2. What are the principles of transcultural nursing?
3. What is culturally competent nursing care?
4. What is the theory of culture care diversity and universality?
5. How did the theory of culture care diversity and universality develop?
6. How is the sunrise model used as a guide for the theory?
7. How are the theory of culture care diversity and university and the sunrise model used to provide culturally competent nursing care?

Establishing new knowledge and practice pathways is always a major challenge, for new pathways may create fears and uncertainty; yet these pathways are essential to meet community, societal, and global human needs.

CHAPTER 11

Transcultural Nursing Care in the Community

Madeleine Leininger and Sharyn Janes

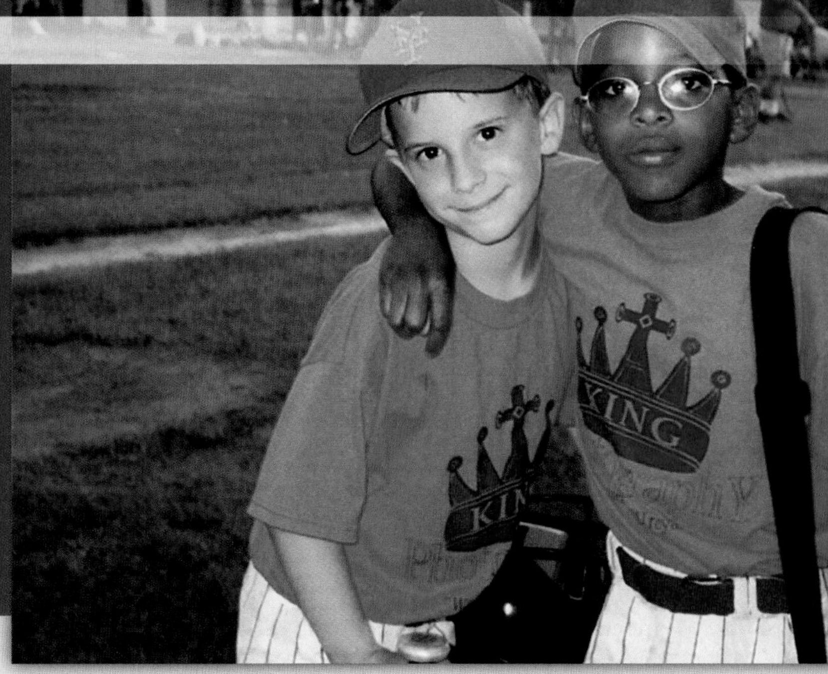

KEY TERMS

caring
cultural backlash
cultural barriers
cultural bias
cultural blindness
cultural clashes
cultural ignorance
cultural imposition
cultural lifeways
cultural pain
cultural shock
cultural values
cultural variation
culturally competent care
culture
culture bound
emic view
ethnocentrism
etic view
generic care
immigrants
nursing
professional care
refugees
stereotyping

> Keep, ancient lands, your storied pomp!" cries she
> With silent lips. "Give me your tired, your poor,
> Your huddled masses yearning to breathe free,
> The wretched refuse of your teeming shore.
> Send these, the homeless, tempest-tossed, to me;
> I lift my lamp beside the golden door.
>
> —*Emma Lazarus (1849–1887), U.S. poet, Written for inscription on the Statue of Liberty*

REFLECTIONS

Children are not born "cultured." Humans are not hard-wired genetically to their culture. Each generation transmits culture to its children through a "cultural blueprint." Our primary cultural influences come from our family and the community of our childhood. As we grow older, our blueprint also grows culturally, as we move from our family of origin to school, church, and peers. In today's media-saturated world, our cultural identity is reinforced through all forms of media. We often associate culture with the "other," those unlike ourselves. Just as a fish is unaware that he or she is "wet," so culture is largely unconscious. That which is considered "normal" exerts a powerful effect on our ideas about health and illness, even from whom and where we seek health care.

As a student nurse, how have your cultural "imprints" affected your care of "others," especially those from widely diverse cultures and populations? Have you been in a situation where your own cultural beliefs have been challenged? What did this feel like, and how is it related to your role as a nurse?

NURSING IS PROGRESSING THROUGH the second decade of the 21st century with many new challenges, pathways, and opportunities. In the 21st century, nurses are and will continue to be involved with many immigrants, refugees, travelers, and strangers coming from many different places. Many nurses will live in a variety of different geographic locations and practice nursing in largely unfamiliar cultural and physical environments.

Today's nurses are learning to use transcultural nursing concepts, principles, and practices to help them function in different community and cultural contexts. Transcultural nursing has become one of the most essential and relevant pathways to meet the holistic and special needs of people from diverse and similar cultures. As nurses learn about the essential and desired care expectations of different cultures, they become aware of different ways to provide culturally competent and sensitive care. Transcultural nursing focuses on holistic and comprehensive ways to know and serve people of diverse cultures throughout the life cycle. The primary goals of *transcultural community-based nursing* are to help people of different and similar cultures maintain their health, prevent illnesses or disabilities, and die in culturally congruent and meaningful ways. Nurses in the 21st century are challenged to adopt this perspective to become better professional nurses.

Transcultural community-based nursing is essential for the future of the profession. Along with transcultural definitions, concepts, principles, and practices, a brief history of transcultural nursing is provided in this chapter to describe the growth of the field since the 1950s. The theory of culture care diversity and universality is presented in the final section of this chapter as an important perspective from which transcultural nursing can be studied and assessed. The theory can be used to assist nurses in providing culturally safe, effective, and congruent nursing care. Throughout this chapter, some reflective questions and examples are posed to help nurses reflect on the cultural beliefs, values, and lifeways that exist in different cultures.

Because transcultural community-based nursing is the goal for the 21st century, it is important to understand some definitions of common terms related to the field of transcultural nursing; these are outlined in **Box 11-1** (Leininger, 1995, 2006).

Community-Based Transcultural Nursing

Community-based transcultural nursing refers to the creative use of transcultural nursing concepts, principles, research, knowledge, and practices that focus on large overall designated communities or geographic contexts to provide culturally competent nursing care. Most communities have many diverse cultural groups with some similar and some sharply diverse cultural lifeways.

The following fundamentals describe the nature, characteristics, and power of cultures; the concept of care; and transcultural nursing:

- Cultures tend to be stable, yet they may change over time in beliefs, values, and cultural lifeways.
- Cultural patterns, norms (rules), and practices are powerful influences on human care and transcultural community practices.
- Cultural values and beliefs vary between and within cultures and must be understood to develop culturally congruent care practices.
- Cultural rituals, symbols, taboos, and practices are important to identify and understand for transcultural nursing.
- Transcultural nursing necessitates studying the total lifeways of people, including influences on care related to religion or spirituality, politics, economics, technologies, kinship ties, environment, and specific values and practices.
- Different modes of communication; use of space, land, and property; and use of home remedies are all part of discovering the transcultural nursing care needs of people.

BOX 11-1 Definitions

- **Culture**: The learned, shared, and transmitted values, beliefs, norms, and lifeways of a particular group that guide their thinking, decisions, and actions in patterned ways
- **Cultural values**: The powerful directive forces that give order and meaning to people's thinking, decisions, and actions
- **Cultural variations**: The subtle or obvious variables among and between cultures that make them unique with respect to traditional or nontraditional ways of living
- **Cultural lifeways**: The patterned ways of living of a particular individual or group
- **Cultural imposition**: The tendency to impose one's beliefs, values, and lifeways on another individual or culture, due largely to ignorance about a culture
- **Ethnocentrism**: The belief that one's own ways of living or doing are the best, most preferred, or superior to others
- **Stereotyping**: The undesirable tendency to pre-judge and fix cultures into rigid and biased ways, due largely to ethnocentrism and racism
- **Cultural blindness**: The inability to recognize one's own values and lifeways or those of another culture, making culture invisible
- **Cultural clashes**: Major conflicts in valuing and understanding differences between cultures and variability among or within cultures
- **Caring**: Actions and activities directed toward assisting, supporting, or enabling another individual or group with evident or anticipated needs to improve a human condition or lifeway, or to face death
- **Nursing**: A learned humanistic and scientific profession and discipline focused on human caring
- **Emic view**: The insider's or local perspective about cultures, families, lifeways, and health care
- **Etic view**: The outsider's or external perspective about cultures, families, lifeways, and health care
- **Culturally competent care**: The deliberate and creative use of transcultural nursing knowledge and skills to assist or facilitate individuals or groups to maintain their wellbeing, recover from illness, or face a disability or death

- Different cultures in a community have different lifeways that must be considered by nurses.
- Different cultures have different caregivers to heal, cure, or assist their people.
- Cultural gatekeepers are found in communities that protect, defend, and uphold cultural values, beliefs, and desired lifeways.
- Transcultural care needs and expectations vary among communities and cannot be assumed to be alike.
- In every community there will be subcultures that are slightly different from the dominant culture and that require attention from the transcultural nurse. These subcultures include the homeless, homosexuals, gangs, drug users, individuals from poor and affluent social classes, and others.

Although nurses have traditionally worked with people in communities, providing care in homes, schools, industrial plants, clinics, and other settings, the major missing dimension has been knowledge of the cultural background of the people and how to care for them in that context. Cultural factors have been taken for granted and often viewed as less important or not even recognized. With the advent of transcultural nursing came a new and heightened awareness of the importance of culturally based knowledge. It was soon discovered that nurses prepared in transcultural community-based nursing were able to demonstrate the use of their knowledge with specific cultures in beneficial ways. Nurses working in community or public health settings found that transcultural nursing concepts were important in providing effective care. In fact, nurses who were skilled and prepared to work with different cultures realized the unique care needs of patients and became confident with individuals, groups, families, and communities (Leininger, 1981, 1988, 1995, 2006).

Beginning in the mid-1970s, community health nurses encountered many new cultural strangers, such as immigrants, refugees, migrant workers, and others, and felt helpless in knowing how to understand and help them. That is when many community nurses began to enroll in transcultural nursing courses. The need for transcultural community-based care was clearly evident as they told their stories about trying to help cultural strangers who seemed to suddenly come into their nursing world. Some nurses did not understand why some patients wanted their children to be cared for before any adults. Other nurses were baffled by strange terms such as *susto*, *evil eye*, and *sacred objects to heal* because they were terms specific to cultures and to cultural healthcare practices. Without understanding these terms and many others, nurses were disadvantaged. Many nurses said they had to almost completely relearn nursing from a different perspective, because many of their previous nursing ideas did not fit with specific cultures. Indeed, some nursing knowledge learned earlier was counter to what some cultures needed

(Leininger, 1988, 1995, 2006). Some nurses became excited and developed creative ways to use transcultural nursing knowledge and skills in community contexts. They became firm advocates of transcultural nursing and encouraged other nurses to learn how to care for diverse cultures in their community experiences.

NOTE THIS!

Foreign-born residents comprise nearly 13% of the U.S. population. As of 2011, 24% of all children in the United States lived with at least one immigrant parents. With their American-born children, foreign-born persons account for more than half of the U.S. population growth.

Migration Policy Institute. (2013). Frequently requested statistics on immigrants and immigration in the United States. Retrieved from http://www.migrationpolicy.org/article/frequently-requested-statistics-immigrants-and-immigration-united-states

RESEARCH ALERT

This research investigated the nature, relationships, and implications of metaphor in the expressions of good and evil in Chinese, Vietnamese, Ethiopian, Somali, French, and English. A grounded theory research method was used in the collection of metaphoric expressions of good and evil from study participants who were fluent in both their native languages and English. The researcher, by means of dialogue and open-ended interviews with the study participants, examined both the literal and idiomatic meanings of these expressions.

From this examination, the expressions were categorized based on the underlying conceptual metaphor. The parts of the underlying metaphor were compared and contrasted with selected examples in each language group. Following this analysis, the researcher discussed the implications for moral, cognitive, and curriculum theories, which were justified based on the study results.

The results support a theory of universal moral conceptualization, with human wellbeing as the guiding principle for metaphoric representation of good and evil. The results also suggest a paired structure to human mental operations, which link the imagination and the reason as an interdependent dynamic of cognition. From the cognitive theory flows a curriculum theory, which makes inclusion of both the imagination and the reason imperative to moral teaching that is neither trivial nor arbitrary.

Source: Dunlap, R. K. (2005). *Common minds: A study of metaphors of good and evil across selected languages*. Unpublished dissertation, Belmont College.

What are some of the major reasons why transcultural nursing is important today? Which transcultural nursing concepts, principles, and research findings can help community nurses? First, any human community has people who are born, live, become ill or maintain health, and die within a community perspective (Leininger, 1981, 1988, 1995, 2006). Humans are culturally rooted, acting and making decisions daily that are based on largely unspoken values, beliefs, and cultural community lifeways (Leininger, 1970, 1978). Moreover, most cultures have beliefs about the way they prefer caregivers to care for them. They have ideas that certain decisions and actions can lead to their health and wellbeing or help them face illnesses, disabilities, and death. Such community beliefs and expectations are extremely important to families and individuals. Although individuals or families may not always be willing to talk openly or directly with their nurses, their expectations still exist.

As a nurse enters the home of an individual or a family, the people remain alert to see whether he or she will be responsive to their cultural beliefs, values, mannerisms, dress, language, and symbols. For example, a community nurse who was knowledgeable about Vietnamese culture allowed a young Vietnamese mother to demonstrate how she cared for her infant's upper respiratory infection. The nurse was readily accepted by the mother, the family, and the community because she understood and respected traditional Vietnamese infant care.

People do not always consciously make known their cultural values, beliefs, and lifeways to others in daily conversations. However, if important cultural practices are violated or neglected, they will often speak out. They often go back to their cultural history to support their actions and beliefs and may say things like, "Well, it has always been this way," or, "This is how we have always believed and lived and my grandparents have lived that way, too." Sometimes, a nurse may not like to be told how to do things by nonprofessionals and may view the family as uncooperative, resistant, or difficult to work with when they fail to respond to the nurse's expectations. When resistance is met, the nurse should stop, listen, and learn from the people who understand cultural care decisions and actions. There are many examples of why families of specific cultural backgrounds are not willing to yield to an outsider's views. Transcultural nursing gives active and serious attention to the people's views, while the professional's views are secondary.

Integrating transcultural knowledge and skills into community nursing is related to the principle that cultures have a right to have their cultural values known, respected, and appropriately used in nursing and related healthcare services (Leininger, 1970, 1988, 1995, 2006). Humans have a right to physical and psychological health care, and their cultural care needs should be treated with equal importance because cultural factors greatly influence how people act, feel, and perceive their environment. However, the physical and mental needs of patients are generally emphasized more in nursing education and practice than the cultural needs. A person's culture often receives limited attention or is avoided by nurses because they do not understand it. Community nurses who have been oriented to transcultural nursing are alert to cultural care factors and use specific strategies and principles to help those of different cultural backgrounds living in a community. Cultural care needs are emphasized, and physical and emotional needs are met within a cultural perspective (Leininger, 1978, 1996).

Culturally congruent care provides culture-specific care decisions and actions for therapeutic benefits that fit with the cultural needs and expectations of patients. Transcultural nursing knowledge can assist nurses in providing culturally congruent care for individuals and families in different communities. Nurses must remain cognizant of culture-specific care that is compatible with the values and beliefs of individual cultures. This can be accomplished by being attentive to subtle differences and similarities among cultures and recognizing care differences and similarities among patients in various living or working contexts. Maintaining a comparative perspective and not assuming all cultures are alike is important. There often is a tendency to label and lump all members of a particular culture together when considering healthcare needs. However, there is great variability between and within cultures and among individuals and families, and these differences must be considered when providing culture-specific and culturally congruent care. To assume that all people in a particular culture are the same is stereotyping and leads to negative outcomes. For example, to avoid stereotyping, one should not assume that all Chinese men are stoic and fit clearly into one particular behavior style. Instead, it is recommended that one observe the actual behaviors and subtle impressions that do not place the Chinese man in a rigid position at all times.

Providing culturally based community caring is directly related to the nurse's intent or desire to heal patients, prevent unnecessary illnesses, and support people in achieving their daily living goals and needs. It is impossible to achieve such important goals unless the nurse knows and practices holistic culturally based care. Holistic culturally based care includes assessing the influences of religion, politics, technology, education, kinship (family), and specific cultural values and beliefs within the patient's own environment. All these factors can and do influence the patient's way of living and responding to nursing care. The theory of culture care diversity and universality provides this holistic, yet specific, care perspective to heal and help people in congruent or meaningful ways. Patients have a right to have these diverse factors influencing their wellbeing understood and respected by healthcare providers. For example, if a nurse fails to explore the social and religious concerns of a Mexican American patient's family, the patient might report that he or she received no nursing care at all.

NOTE THIS!

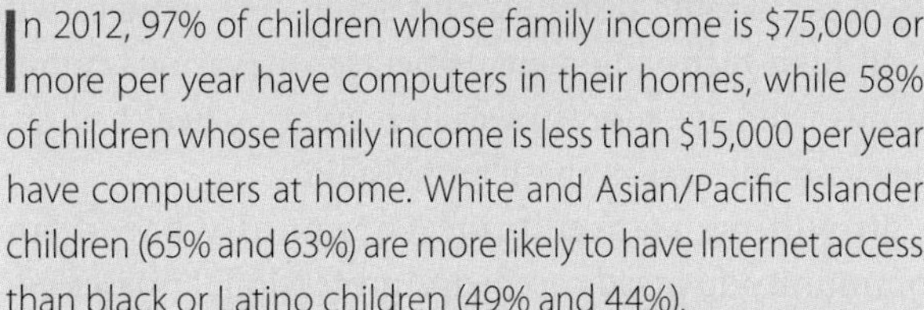

In 2012, 97% of children whose family income is $75,000 or more per year have computers in their homes, while 58% of children whose family income is less than $15,000 per year have computers at home. White and Asian/Pacific Islander children (65% and 63%) are more likely to have Internet access than black or Latino children (49% and 44%).

Source: Child Trends Databank. (2013). Home computer access and Internet use. Retrieved from http://www.childtrends.org/?indicators=home-computer-access

APPLICATION TO PRACTICE

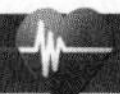

As a community health nurse you are making home visits twice a week to Mrs. Mendoza, who lives in a rural community. Mrs. Mendoza is an 82-year-old Mexican American woman with a below-the-knee amputation of her left leg related to her diabetes mellitus. She lives with her 50-year-old son and two teenage grandsons. It is difficult to communicate with Mrs. Mendoza or to do any diabetic teaching because you do not speak Spanish and no one in the Mendoza household speaks English. During your first five visits, the neighbor who lives down the road was willing to come to Mrs. Mendoza's house during your visits to serve as your interpreter. However, on your sixth visit, you discover that the neighbor is not at home. Because you are unable to communicate with Mrs. Mendoza, you go to each of her neighbors' houses looking for someone who can speak English but find none of them at home. Frustrated and behind schedule, you return to Mrs. Mendoza's house to learn that her son, who has been at home during all of your visits, is able to speak English fluently.

- How do you feel when you learn that Mrs. Mendoza's son can speak English?
- Why do you think he did not tell you he could speak English earlier?
- What could you have done to make the situation different?

Health care in the future will become more community focused and will emphasize maintaining health and preventing, in addition to treating, illnesses. As the largest group of healthcare providers, nurses will be extremely important in providing care to various cultural groups. The ways in which different cultures prevent illnesses and maintain health will be a major focus of community health nursing in the 21st century and beyond. The community will be recognized as the natural and familiar context for all human caring and health services, becoming the dominant mode over hospital care as the paradigm shifts related to the 2010 Affordable Care Act (ACA) become entrenched (Leininger, 1995, 1997b, 2006). Hospital services will decrease and will largely focus on treating special diseases, chronic illnesses, and acute emergencies with costly high-tech equipment. Patients from various cultural groups will have more power in regulating health care as they gain cultural strength and visibility.

Providing transcultural community-based and community-focused care helps professional nurses gain satisfaction and rewards from their important nursing contributions to society. As community nurses incorporate transcultural nursing into their work roles, the public will more easily recognize their significant and unique contributions. Traditional community and public health principles blended with transcultural nursing principles will take on new meaning and relevance in growing multicultural communities (DeSantis, 1997; Horn, 1979; Leininger, 1988; Luna, 1998; Shapiro, Miller, & White, 2006).

Macrocultures

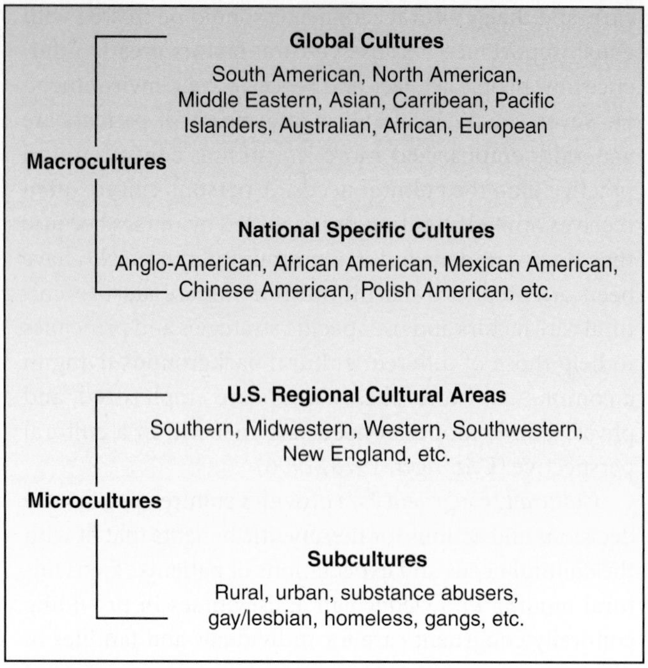

Global Cultures
South American, North American, Middle Eastern, Asian, Carribean, Pacific Islanders, Australian, African, European

National Specific Cultures
Anglo-American, African American, Mexican American, Chinese American, Polish American, etc.

Microcultures

U.S. Regional Cultural Areas
Southern, Midwestern, Western, Southwestern, New England, etc.

Subcultures
Rural, urban, substance abusers, gay/lesbian, homeless, gangs, etc.

Figure 11-1 Scope of transcultural nursing cultures.

Scope of Transcultural Nursing Cultures

There are various types and sizes of community cultures. Some communities are very large (macrocultures) and others are considerably smaller (microcultures; see **Figure 11-1**). Nurses should make an effort to grasp the nature and scope of the communities in which they are working and be aware of the different microcultures and macrocultures that exist within a particular environment.

Transcultural Nursing Principles

One of the most important goals of transcultural nursing is to enter the patient's world and assist in therapeutic and beneficial ways. Providing culturally congruent care to people in a community first necessitates a careful assessment of the cultural needs of the people. After analyzing the cultural assessment data, the nurse should use transcultural principles, concepts, and research to develop and implement a culturally congruent plan of care. Working with different cultures requires that the nurse have "holding" (prelearned) knowledge about specific cultures. It is important that the nurse be able to carefully blend his or her *etic* (or professional knowledge) with the patient's *emic* (or traditional and folk knowledge). These two categories of knowledge sometimes come together, but great discrepancies can exist and need to be resolved for the safety and health of the patient. Rather than focus on medical treatments that may not fit the cultural needs of patients and may be useless or even detrimental, transcultural nursing focuses more on the information, beliefs, and practices of those being treated. Patients expect that their traditional beliefs and practices will be respected and that appropriate rituals will be used to assist them in recovery or death within their cultural environment. Therefore, when possible, culturally appropriate interventions should be the preferred treatment, which may create a challenge for healthcare professionals. Understanding general transcultural nursing principles can help nurses bridge the gap between emic and etic points of view (**Box 11-2**).

ENVIRONMENTAL CONNECTION

Where we live shapes our culture in ways that are seldom noticed. For example, people who live in tropical climates often express their culture through colorful clothing, art, and architecture that reflects warmth and promotes cooling.

Transcultural Concepts

To understand transcultural nursing as used within community nursing contexts, knowledge of several major concepts is essential. Some of these concepts come from anthropology, but others have been developed as basic

BOX 11-2 Transcultural Nursing Principles

1. All human cultures have diverse living, caring, and healing modes that nurses need to study and understand to work effectively with people of different cultures.
2. Care is a basic human need, and it is the essence and dominant focus of the nursing profession.
3. Understanding one's own culture is the first essential expectation to understand other cultures or subcultures.
4. People have the right to have their cultural values known, respected, understood, and used appropriately in nursing and healthcare services.
5. Transcultural nursing is concerned with the comparative values, beliefs, and practices of specific cultures to provide meaningful, safe, and specific healthcare practices.
6. Nurses use humanistic and scientific cultural care knowledge as they provide care to different cultures. Humanistic care aspects make people remain human, and scientific research findings about cultures and care guide nurses' decisions and actions.
7. Understanding culture care differences and similarities enables the nurse to respect patients and assist them to grow, function, maintain their wellbeing or health, and prevent illnesses and premature death.
8. Willingness to enter the patient's world and become an active and interested participant is essential in maintaining effective nurse–patient or nurse–family relationships.
9. Listening, respecting, and being attentive to what patients of different cultures say or do are essential to understanding them and providing meaningful and beneficial nursing services.
10. A nurse's ability to speak the patient's cultural language opens the door to understanding what the patient is seeking or experiencing.
11. If the patient's cultural lifeways, values, and caring expressions do not immediately "make sense," the nurse must continue to make an effort to understand them.
12. In every culture, care, healing, and health practices are greatly influenced by patients' worldviews, environmental context, and social structure features (including the religious or spiritual beliefs, kinship ties, political–legal views, economic aspects, technologies, and specific cultural historical values).
13. Every culture usually has two major types of healthcare systems: generic (indigenous, traditional, folk) and professional (learned in schools). Nurses need to understand both to provide culturally congruent care.
14. Cultures have their own culturally defined ways to promote and maintain health, face death, and deal with unfavorable sociocultural conditions and crises.
15. Healthcare practices in Western and non-Western cultures have major differences that need to be understood when planning and providing care to patients.

Source: Leininger, 1995, 2006.

transcultural nursing concepts. Although a few basic definitions were presented at the beginning of this chapter, there are some that merit further clarification with clinical examples to illustrate them.

Because an important goal of transcultural nursing is to provide culturally competent care, it needs to be considered at the outset. *Culturally competent care* refers to the use of culturally based knowledge in creative, congruent, and meaningful ways to provide beneficial and satisfying health care to diverse cultures. As nurses work with other cultures, they combine their patients' traditional knowledge with their own professional nursing knowledge to provide meaningful, safe, and responsible care. The nursing interventions must fit or be reasonably tailored to incorporate cultural values, beliefs, and practices to be effective and acceptable to the people. Nurses should encourage all members of the healthcare team to consider the cultural values of their patients when making decisions related to their health care.

The concept of cultural values is critical in health care because all cultures want their values and beliefs respected and upheld. *Cultural values* are the powerful directive forces that give order and meaning to why people think, act, and

MEDIA MOMENT

Selected Films About Culture

Film	Culture
The Milagro Beanfield War	Mexican
Passion Fish	Louisiana Cajun
Belizaire the Cajun	Louisiana Cajun
Sherman's March	Southern United States
To Kill a Mockingbird	Southern United States
Crimes of the Heart	Southern United States
Do the Right Thing	African American

Continues

MEDIA MOMENT (*CONTINUED*)

The Color Purple	African American
The Brothers McMullen	Irish American
Witness	Amish
Divine Secrets of the Ya Ya Sisterhood	Southern United States
Spanglish	Mexican American
A Love Song for Bobby Long	Southern United States
Barbershop	African American
Woman, Thou Art Loosed	African American
The Untold Story of Emmett Louis Till	African American
The Human Stain	African American

make decisions. For example, the extended family of an African American pregnant woman living in the rural South told the visiting nurse about their culture and what they valued. Several of the women said, "We value our greens, soul food, peas, pork, and special pregnancy foods." These mothers made clear the cultural values that needed to be considered by the nurse for the family's general nutrition and for the mother during pregnancy. The foods were viewed as essential for their health care, so the nurse included as many of these foods as possible in the nutritional plan for the pregnant mother, making modifications only where necessary.

Two concepts that are extremely helpful to nurses are emic and etic views. *Emic view* refers to what the local people or the "insiders" hold as important to know and believe. For example, a Philippine elderly mother and family believe that when the grandmother gets old, she should not live in a nursing home. Instead, they hold the emic view that the sons, daughters, and grandchildren should care for their elders. This emic or local Philippine view is different from Anglo-American families, who often believe that their elders will probably go to a nursing home for care and protection.

Etic view refers to an external or outsider's view of a culture. For example, many Anglo-American nurses believe that when elders reach about 80 years old, they should consider being placed in a nursing home so that they will not be a burden to other family members. This etic or outsider's view is very different from what the Philippine families value, wanting their elders to be cared for by family members in their homes and not in institutions such as nursing homes. The Philippine emic view and the Anglo-American nurses' etic view are very different and can often be a source of cultural conflicts and stresses.

ETHICAL CONNECTION 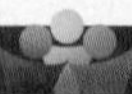

Gay children, especially teenage males, are committing suicide in unprecedented numbers. When you think of culture, does your idea about being a "culture" include people who have different sexual orientations, such as lesbianism, homosexuality, and bisexuality? Why or why not? What are the ethical implications of our ideas about what is and what is *not* a culture? How do these ideas affect our ability to provide care for all?

Generic and professional care are related to emic and etic views. **Generic care** is the folk, naturalistic, or traditional health practices that cultures have known and used over time. In contrast, **professional care** is what is learned from nursing, medicine, and other healthcare education programs. Generic and professional care practices often have many differences that must be recognized and addressed. For example, several Mexican American families visited by a community health nurse wanted the nurse to know and integrate their generic (folk or naturalistic) care with the professional nursing care. They also wanted the community nurse to acknowledge that Mexican fathers are the ones responsible for major family decisions, such as signing treatment consent forms for family members. Respecting these important generic or folk family considerations was essential for the nurse to provide culturally congruent care.

Another set of closely related concepts is ethnocentrism and cultural imposition. *Ethnocentrism* refers to the belief that one's own ways are the best, most superior, or preferred ways of acting, believing, or valuing something. An example of this concept is Anglo-American nurses who contend that managed care is the best way to provide health services. Nursing students may also be ethnocentric, believing that faculty lectures are the best way to help students learn about nursing and, therefore, rejecting other methods of teaching. Ethnocentrism takes a strong position that there is only one "right" way to do things.

Cultural imposition refers to one group of people forcing their cultural beliefs, values, and patterns of behavior on others as a result of ethnocentrism, cultural biases, ignorance, or various other reasons. An example is an Anglo-American nurse who imposes her beliefs that women should be equal partners with their husbands in making healthcare decisions for the family on a Mexican American mother. This can create conflict within the family, causing difficulty for the woman and possibly leading to the family's total rejection of the nurse's care. Cultural imposition practices are one of the most common nursing care problems encountered with patients from different cultures.

Cultural ignorance refers to insufficient knowledge about a specific culture to provide safe and meaningful care. This chapter includes many examples of cultural ignorance as a major problem in nursing practices. Lack of knowledge often leads to destructive care practices and nontherapeutic outcomes for patients.

Cultural bias refers to a strong position that all decisions must be based on one's own values and beliefs. For example, nurses who firmly value nursing homes at the end of life, with no other alternative plan, can be considered culturally biased. It is a largely one-sided, rigid, and persistent stance. If nurses are not able to recognize and understand their cultural biases, these biases can greatly interfere with patients' choices, interests, and even therapeutic care practices. Both nurses and patients may have biases that should be recognized and discussed so that acceptable compromises can be reached.

GLOBAL CONNECTION 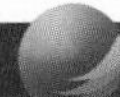

No event can be beyond expectations,
Fear, contradiction, or compel surprise, for Zeus,
Father of Olympians, has made night at full noon,
darkness mid the brilliance of the sun—
and pale fear has seized men.
Henceforth, nothing for them is certain:
One may expect everything,
And none among you should be astonished to see,
One day, the deer, preferring the sonorous tides
Of the sea to the land,
Borrow from the dolphins their sea pasture,
While the latter plunge into the mountains.

—Archilochus, 700 B.C.

How do you interpret this poem from ancient Greece regarding the need for humans to connect culturally to one another? Can we ever be completely open to all cultures as nurses?

MEDIA MOMENT 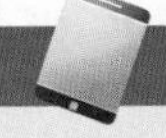

As the world continues to "shrink" as a result of the reach of television and the Internet to even the most remote parts of the world making information available instantly, we truly are becoming a global community of consciousness.

Cultural shock refers to a state of being disoriented or unable to respond appropriately to a situation or person because of complete strangeness or unfamiliarity with what was seen or experienced. This concept is often seen between nurses and patients from different cultures. For example, a community nurse entered the home of a very poor Native American family and found there were six children (ages 3 to 10 years) sleeping on the floor with dirty blankets. The nurse also discovered that the children ate only bread and beans each day and that the house was very dirty. The nurse was shocked by the conditions and did not know what to say or do, so she left the home. She reported that she found an "unbelievable home situation" and became helpless and confused. Because of her cultural shock, she was not able to assess the overall health of the children or work with the family to meet their healthcare needs.

Cultural pain refers to the considerable discomfort, suffering, or unfavorable response experienced by an individual or group belonging to a particular culture when insulting and offensive comments are made by an outsider. Cultural pain is more common than realized among health personnel (Leininger, 1997a). For example, an African American family experienced cultural pain when an Asian American community health nurse showed facial disgust when she saw the family eating "chitlins" (choice intestinal animal products). The nurse emphatically said, "That food is not good for you and you should not be eating such food." She also referred to the family as a "Negro" family, which was most offensive to them. As a consequence, the African American family experienced cultural pain from the nurse's gestures and comments.

Cultural variation refers to the slight or marked variability among or between cultures that makes them unique or different. This variability is often due to differences between traditional and nontraditional lifeways over time. For example, Mexicans, Puerto Ricans, and Cubans show slight or major cultural variability in beliefs and lifeways because of different historical and cultural backgrounds, yet some similarities in language, values, and beliefs have been identified that result in them being known collectively as Hispanics or Latinos. Likewise, many Native Americans show cultural variability among the nearly 540 Native American nations in the United States. Nurses need to learn about variations between and among cultures and if there are changes in these cultures over time.

Cultural barriers refer to obstacles that interfere with cultures accessing or achieving their desired goals or opportunities. This concept was evident when an Anglo-American community nurse always made an appointment to care for an Arab-Muslim family at noon, which was their prayer time. The nurse insisted that the family members see her at noon, when it was convenient for her to give a special medication and check the father's blood pressure. Coming at noon was a cultural barrier to the Arab-Muslim family, because it interrupted their prayer time, so they refused the community nurse's services.

Stereotyping refers to putting a label on members of a culture or subculture that reflects fixed characteristics perceived as belonging to that particular group without considering individual or group differences or cultural variability. For example, a nurse may stereotype Native Americans as "lazy and unreliable alcoholics" or label Vietnamese as "passive, unwilling to learn English, and too difficult to understand and help." Anglo-American patients may be labeled as "pushy, selfish, and materialistic." Such rigid stereotyping statements are imprecise and crude labels that cause cultural pain and inaccurate assessments. Stereotypes are usually negative, but positive generalizations may also be harmful. For example, some nurses may assume that all Asian Americans are high achievers or that all Jewish people are wealthy. All professional nurses should be keenly aware of stereotyping to avoid its potentially negative consequences.

GLOBAL CONNECTION

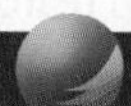

The concept of transcultural nursing was developed by Dr. Madeline Leininger to prepare nurses for working with various cultures throughout the world. She has had extensive experience with many cultures around the globe, conducting research on cultural beliefs, values, and health practices.

Culture bound refers to specific care, health, and illness conditions that are unique or particular to a culture and often exist within a specific geographic area. For example, *kuru* is a condition observed in the Eastern Highlands of New Guinea. It is culture bound and unique to the geographic area and female gender (Leininger, 1995). Some New Guinea women who are pregnant become weak and anorexic and die within 9 to 10 months. Other examples of cultural-bound conditions, such as Arctic hysteria, running amok, *susto*, and mushroom madness, are found with specific cultures in certain geographic areas. Often, there may be no medical cure, but nursing care is essential.

Cultural backlash is a phenomenon that occurs when a culture has been "bought" or encouraged to use another culture's values, material goods, beliefs, and lifeways. This often proves to be unsuitable and leads to serious unfavorable outcomes. Taking on another culture's values or material goods leads to anger and disappointment because the other ideas or things do not fit the culture. For example, using self-care theory and practices in a non-Western culture may contradict cultural beliefs and lifeways. Western nursing faculty or practitioners may impose their practices on a non-Western culture, but the ideas and practices are not congruent with the cultural lifeways. As a consequence, non-Western nurses or patients may turn against the Western nurses as a cultural backlash for imposing their ideas or values on them. Cultural ignorance, cultural imposition, and culturally imperialistic behavior are often the factors contributing to cultural backlash. This is a serious and growing problem in cultural education as well as in nursing practice and exchange.

Immigrants and **refugees** are two different groups of people who are often confused with each other. An immigrant is a person who voluntarily chooses to come to another country for various reasons, which may include seeking new opportunities for employment. For example, Europeans immigrated to America in the early colonial days and started life anew. Today thousands of immigrants continue to come to the United States each year. In contrast, refugees are people who have been suddenly forced to leave their homeland and come to another country for survival because of political oppression, social injustices, destructive war conditions, or other threatening circumstances. For example, in the 1970s and 1980s, many Vietnamese, Laotians, Cambodians, and Filipinos left their homelands to escape oppressive war forces and/or because they were suddenly driven out of their country (Leininger, 1995). Nurses need to understand the historical shifts of different immigrants and refugees because their care and health needs are different. The community nurse is expected to understand and care for these strangers almost overnight as newcomers to the community.

Basic transcultural nursing ideas should be used to guide community nurses in their assessment and understanding of families and individuals from diverse cultures. All nurses should understand these fundamental concepts before beginning to work in the community so that they can avoid cultural clashes, cultural imposition, and other potentially negative outcomes with patients. It is a nurse's ethical and moral responsibility to study transcultural nursing principles before working with patients of diverse cultures and not to assume one can "wing it" (Leininger, 1990). Self-awareness, along with the use of transcultural knowledge, can lead to successful and effective culturally congruent nursing care.

MEDIA MOMENT

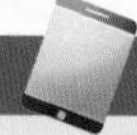

***The Culture of Fear: Why Americans Are Afraid of the Wrong Things* (2000)**

—By Barry Glasner, New York, NY: Basic Books

Americans are afraid of many things in our culture that shouldn't frighten us, according to Barry Glasner. In this book, which is devoted to challenging conventional wisdom, Glasner critically examines such issues as violence in schools, breast cancer, environmental threats, and the influence of popular media on what we "think is true."

NOTE THIS!

In Japan, bowing is part of a typical greeting. The depth of the bow is determined by how much respect the person bowing wishes to convey.

Leininger's Theory of Culture Care Diversity and Universality

Development of the Theory

The development of the theory of culture care diversity and universality began in the mid-1950s in the search for a body of transcultural nursing knowledge to guide nursing decisions and actions in the care of the culturally different (Leininger, 1991, 1995, 2006). As in any discipline or profession, theories are used to discover, explain, predict, and generate new knowledge or reaffirm existing knowledge. Without theories, nursing would have no scientific way to explain or interpret what happens and why. Nursing theories and clinical practices are interdependent because clinical practices need theories, and theories use clinical data to examine outcomes. These ideas led to the development of the theory of culture care diversity and universality as the scientific base for the substantive body of knowledge known as transcultural nursing (Leininger, 1970, 1991, 1995, 2006).

Interestingly, in the 1950s, there were virtually no nursing theories, and none that were focused on culture and caring phenomena. In that era nurses were preoccupied with meeting the post–World War II medical disease symptoms and treatment regimes prescribed by physicians. Very few nurses were interested in developing nursing theories to advance nursing knowledge. There were nurses interested in research, borrowing research methods from other disciplines, but few were thinking about nursing theories and nursing research methods that would focus on specific culture care phenomena. There was a need to focus on care as the essence of nursing with a transcultural nursing perspective and to develop a theory that (1) focused on culture and caring, (2) was a holistic theory that would include the total human being in a cultural context, (3) would generate practical knowledge to guide nursing care decisions and practices related to specific cultures, and (4) would provide a new kind of comparative nursing care that would be meaningful to different cultures and have healing or beneficial outcomes (Leininger, 1991, 1995, 2006).

GOT AN ALTERNATIVE?

A Mexican American woman ties a good-luck talisman around her newborn baby's neck to protect her from "mal ojo," or bad eye. How would you assess this cultural practice?

The theory of culture care diversity and universality was the first nursing theory to focus on culture and care in different cultures with multiple holistic factors influencing care (Leininger, 1991). The theory helps nurses discover and use culture care findings in community-based practices in primary, secondary, or tertiary care settings. It is useful in community nursing because it is practical and comprehensive regarding culture and care aspects. It is a theory that can be used with individual cultures or with several cultures, depending on the nurse's practice or research interests. In using the theory, nurses search for care meanings that can be used to provide culturally congruent care.

In developing the theory, it was assumed that there were cultural differences (diversities) as well as some universals (commonalities) that could be found in different cultures in which nurses were expected to provide care. It was further assumed that factors such as worldview and social structure features (e.g., religion and spirituality, kinship, philosophy of life, economics, politics, education, technology, and specific cultural values, beliefs, and lifeways) would significantly influence culture and care in different environmental contexts. In addition, transcultural nursing care would be influenced by both generic (folk or local) and professional care practices. Finally, there would be three major modes to guide cultural care decisions and actions: (1) culture care preservation or maintenance, (2) culture care accommodation or negotiation, and (3) culture care structuring or repatterning (Leininger, 1991; Leininger & McFarland, 2002, p. 84):

- "Culture care preservation or maintenance refers to those assistive, supportive, facilitative, or enabling professional actions and decisions that help people of a particular culture to retain and/or maintain meaningful care values and lifeways for their well-being, to recover from illness, or to deal with handicaps or dying."
- "Culture care accommodation or negotiation refers to those assistive, supportive, facilitative, or enabling creative professional actions and decisions that help people of a certain culture (or subculture) to adapt to or to negotiate with others for meaningful, beneficial, and congruent health outcomes."
- "Culture care structuring or repatterning refers to the assistive, supportive, facilitative, or enabling professional actions and decisions that help clients reorder, change, or modify their lifeways for new, different, and beneficial healthcare outcomes."

Goal of the Theory

The goal of the theory is to discover ways to provide culturally congruent and responsible transcultural nursing care (Leininger, 1991, 1995, 2006). The purpose of the theory is to discover, document, explain, and interpret culturally congruent care with individuals or groups under study (Leininger, 1991). The theory provides research findings that are tailored to meet the patients' holistic cultural needs and expectations. As a new theory, it brought together synthesized research knowledge of culture care that had not been previously discovered and had been neglected in nursing practice. Many cultures are pleased to learn that their cultural values and beliefs are used in transcultural nursing.

Assumptions of the Theory

To fully understand the theory and its relationship to transcultural community-based nursing, the following assumptions and premises that guide nurses in the use of the theory must be examined. They are specifically focused on community-based transcultural nursing care to help community nurses use the assumptions in meaningful ways (Leininger, 1991). The theory assumes:

1. Care is the essence and the central dominant, distinct, and unifying focus of nursing.
2. Humanistic and scientific care are essential for human growth, wellbeing, health, survival, and the ability to face death and disabilities.
3. Care (caring) is essential to curing or healing, for there can be no curing without caring. (This assumption was held to have profound relevance worldwide.)
4. Culture care is the synthesis of two major constructs that guide the researcher to discover, explain, and account for health, wellbeing, care expressions, and other human conditions.
5. Culture care expressions, meanings, patterns, processes, and structural forms are diverse, but some commonalities (universalities) exist among and between cultures.
6. Culture care values, beliefs, and practices are influenced by and embedded in the worldview, social structure factors (e.g., religion, philosophy of life, kinship, politics, economics, education, technology, and cultural values), and the ethnohistorical and environmental contexts.
7. Every culture has generic (lay, folk, naturalistic; mainly emic) and usually some professional (etic) care to be discovered and used for culturally congruent care practices.
8. Culturally congruent and therapeutic care occurs when culture care values, beliefs, expressions, and patterns are explicitly known and used appropriately, sensitively, and meaningfully with people of diverse or similar cultures.
9. Leininger's three theoretical modes of care offer new, creative, and different therapeutic ways to help people of diverse cultures.
10. Qualitative research paradigmatic methods offer important means to discover largely embedded, covert, epistemic, and ontological culture care knowledge and practices.
11. Transcultural nursing is a discipline with a body of knowledge and practices to attain and maintain the goal of culturally congruent care for health and wellbeing.

The Sunrise Model: A Visual Guide for the Theory

The sunrise model was developed to visualize the different dimensions of the theory as nurses study different cultures (see **Figure 11-2**; Leininger, 1991, 1995, 2006). Nurses can use this conceptual model to see the different areas that need to be examined in assessing and planning care for patients of different cultures. Although the model is *not* the theory, it is a valuable guide to grasp the holistic aspects of humans living in a particular culture. This model can be used by community nurses to assess the cultural care factors of patients (individuals and groups, especially families) to get a holistic or complete picture of the patient's cultural world. By using this model, nurses avoid partial or incomplete assessments that fail to know the patients and their total reality in a cultural context. Patients who have had nurses who used this model often say, "At last, nurses are looking at my total life and not just my body, diseases, emotional symptoms, or other pieces of me." Patients want nurses to know what guides their daily living along with their cultural values, beliefs, and practices.

By using the sunrise model, nurses remain focused on the theory to identify differences and similarities of care dimensions as expressed and practiced in the culture. Whether working with individuals, families, or groups, nurses should be aware that the traditional physical,

THINK ABOUT THIS 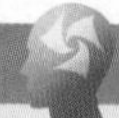

Recently celebrities such as Mel Gibson and Michael Richards ("Kramer" from the *Seinfeld* television series) have been thrust into the spotlight for being insensitive and even bigoted. Do well-known celebrities represent values that many of us share, or are these simply isolated incidents that would not receive any attention if the persons involved were not famous? Do you see the public's reaction to such celebrity comments or behavior as exceptions to most of our cultural values, or should we seriously consider these exhibitions as evidence that racial and ethnic bias exist in the United States to a greater degree than is commonly believed?

psychological, and social components of care are not specifically identified in the sunrise model because these factors are embedded within the social structure and worldview and are included in both the generic and professional aspects of care. Moreover, gender, class, sexual orientation, and other factors are likewise an integral part of the areas identified in the model, but they are not specifically labeled. The environmental, historical, and language contextual aspects are given attention in the model as they provide holistic ideas relative to community-based transcultural nursing and health practices.

Community nurses generally use this model to assess patients' needs. Nurses can start anywhere in the model with what patients want to talk about. It is the patients or families who take the lead to tell their health or illness story. The nurse is expected to follow their lead. In so doing, the nurse gets access to emic patient information and does not push for etic data or professional information alone. As the nurse assesses the patient, the goal is to enter the world of the patient rather than the world of the nurse. This allows the patient to tell his or her story and explain how health, illness, and care are known to him

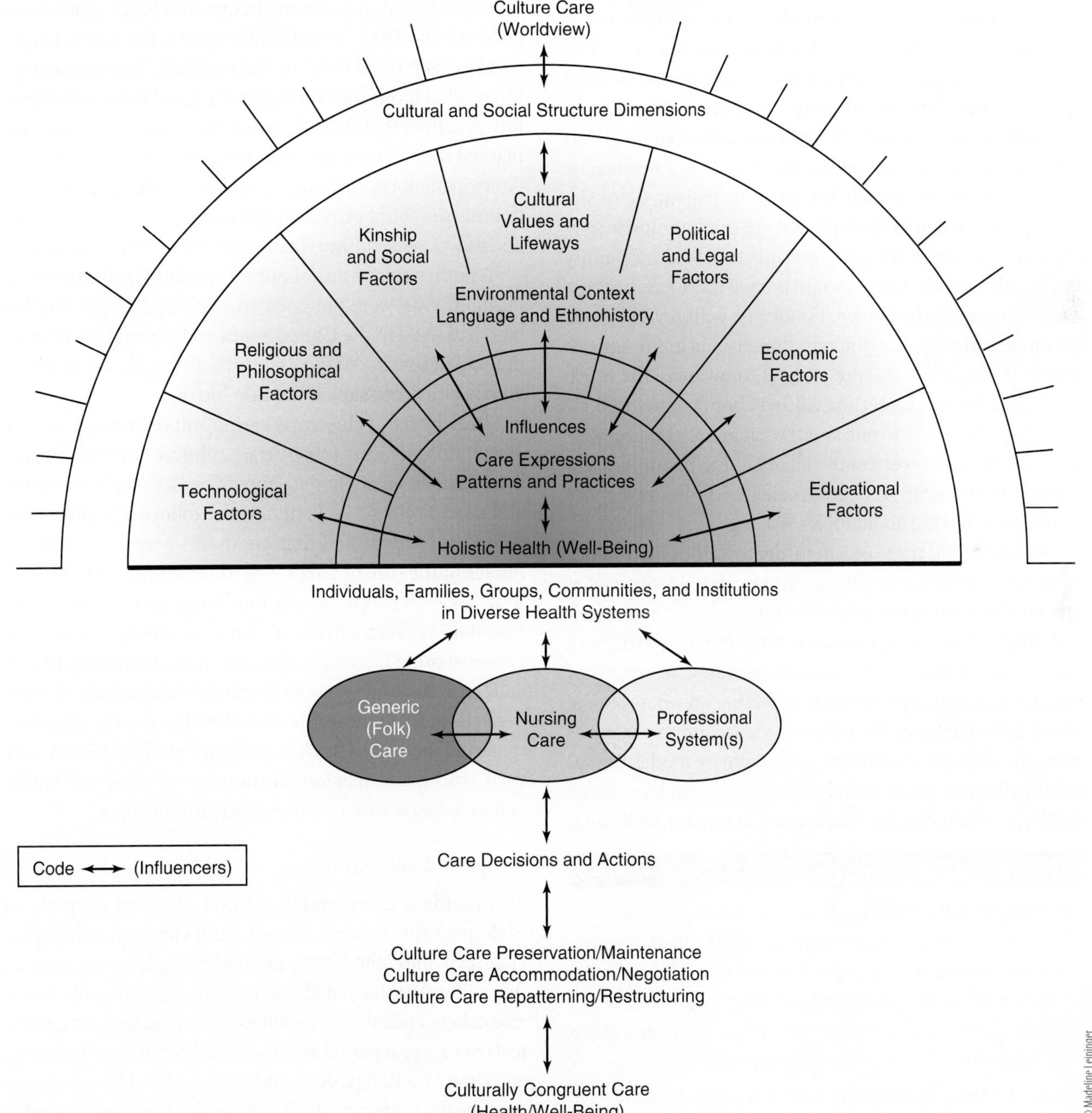

Figure 11-2 Leininger's sunrise model.

or her. This ethnonursing, people-centered approach has been developed to characterize transcultural nursing as an approach truly interested in discovering the person's worldview and other aspects influencing one's wellbeing (Leininger, 1985, 1991, 1995, 2006). It allows the nurse to discover the meaning and experiences of care and health and identify which factors are cultural facilitators or barriers to good health.

The ethno (people) nursing approach to health assessment requires that the nurse understand his or her own culture before trying to discover another culture. If the nurse is not first aware of his or her own culture, then cultural clashes, cultural imposition, and other problems may occur. With this people (ethno) approach, the nurse strives to get the emic or the patient's worldview. The nurse is an active observer of the patients or families in their homes or local environments. This natural context provides rich and accurate data that are usually different from data obtained in an unnatural or unfamiliar environment such as a hospital or clinic. As the nurse actively listens to the patient, he or she becomes attuned to the patient's ways of thinking and knowing. For example, if the patient wants to talk about family and health care, the nurse should pursue this focus because it is of interest to the patient. Gradually, with several visits, the nurse addresses the different dimensions in the sunrise model. If the patient did not address some areas, the nurse carefully asks the patient to "tell me about" these aspects. Initially, patients like to talk about what interests them most or what they are most comfortable talking about. Once a trusting relationship develops, patients will become more comfortable talking about topics that are more sensitive.

Nurses should try to obtain in-depth, rather than superficial, knowledge about patients and work to identify what care factors seem to have the most influence on their health and illness status. This process is done in a co-participant (nurse with patient) way to arrive at accurate assessments or research findings. By constantly reflecting on what is being stated and clarifying the patients' views and experiences using the different dimensions of the sunrise model, nurses usually discover some entirely new or different knowledge that has not been taught or addressed in nursing textbooks.

RESEARCH ALERT

Immigrants in the United States lose their native language in just three generations. Latino children by the third generation are overwhelmingly English only in their language skills. Only 17% with three or four foreign-born grandparents speak Spanish fluently. If the child has only one parent or grandparent who is foreign born, this rate drops to 5%.

Source: Rumbaut, R., Massey, D., & Bean, F. (2006). Linguistic life expectancies: Immigrant language retention in Southern California. *Population and Development Review, 32*(3), 447–460.

Application of the Theory and Model

Greek American Families

A Greek American family was very pleased when visited by a nurse in their home, because they could share many ideas about their generic herbs (folk practices) and how herbs were used to treat "little or big illnesses." They showed the nurse where the herbs grew in their home environment (backyard) and how and why they used herbs to "keep well." The Greek American family members talked about caring practices at home (emic) and how different they were from hospital (etic) care. The family said, "We do not like to go to the hospital unless desperately ill because the hospital is a sick place and they use medicines and foods that are not good for us. They do not understand what Greek people need to keep them well." In their kitchen, they showed the nurse what foods they thought were good to eat and shared folk practices that they use when they become ill. They explained to the nurse how they would like to be cared for as Greek patients in the hospital and stated that they believed that nurses could provide quality care for them if they understood Greek culture (Leininger, 1991, 1995, 1996, 2006).

As other transcultural nurses studied Greek American families, data were obtained from several Greek families who had lived in the United States and Canada for 20 years but had never shared their culture and healthcare practices with health professionals because "no one seemed interested in Greek beliefs, values, and caring" modalities (Leininger, 1991). Rosenbaum's (1990) transcultural nursing research has provided in-depth data about Greek Canadian widows and care. From several studies, the following culture care values were identified that are used today as a guide for nurses in the care of Greek American families: (1) Prevent illnesses with proper Greek foods and exercise and avoid hospitals, (2) keep active with family and religious services, (3) assist other Greek families with herbal remedies to prevent illnesses, and (4) show hospitality to strangers as a caring action. In all these Greek studies, the dominant factors that influenced the Greek families in the United States were their worldview, religion, kinship, specific cultural family values, generic care practices, and ethnohistory.

Philippine American Families

To provide a comparative cultural view, an example of Philippine Americans is offered. Both Greek and Philippine cultures in the United States are good examples to teach nurses that cultural values and lifeways do not change readily. Nurse researchers studied several Philippine families in an urban context over a 2-year period and discovered culture care meanings and desired actions that should be considered by nurses and other health professionals. The Philippine families had lived in Midwestern, urban America for approximately 20 years, but their traditional cultural values, beliefs, and lifeways were still more apparent than Anglo-American values and lifeways. It was determined that the provision of culturally congruent care for Philippine families should include (1) maintaining smooth relationships with the family (*Pakikisama*), (2) remaining alert to "saving face" by avoiding shame and being demeaning in public talk, (3) showing respect for and deference to authority (especially elders), (4) showing mutual reciprocity by sharing between people (*Utang Na Loob*), (5) knowing how to provide holistic caring practices, (6) demonstrating gentle and tender ways of caring, and (7) remaining pleasant when caring for others, especially family members (Leininger, 1991).

These care meanings fit well with the dominant Philippine cultural values of (1) family unity and closeness, (2) respect for authority and elders, (3) leaving oneself to God (*Behala Na*), (4) use of hot/cold theory in care and health practices, (5) folk foods and care practices, (6) the importance of religion in caring practices (the majority are Roman Catholics), and (7) nurses showing an obligation to family members when caring for them.

Using the sunrise model as a guide, kinship (family and social) ties, religion, cultural values, environment, generic herbs and treatment, and historical factors all need to be considered to get a holistic care perspective. Although the research with the Greek American and Philippine American families identified distinct differences between the two cultures, there were many commonalities, such as an emphasis on religion, family ties, historical factors, generic care, and use of their home environment resources. In working with these two cultures, professional nursing and medical practices were not relied on entirely, but rather the inclusion of generic family care with folk care practices was important to maintain and preserve the families' wellbeing.

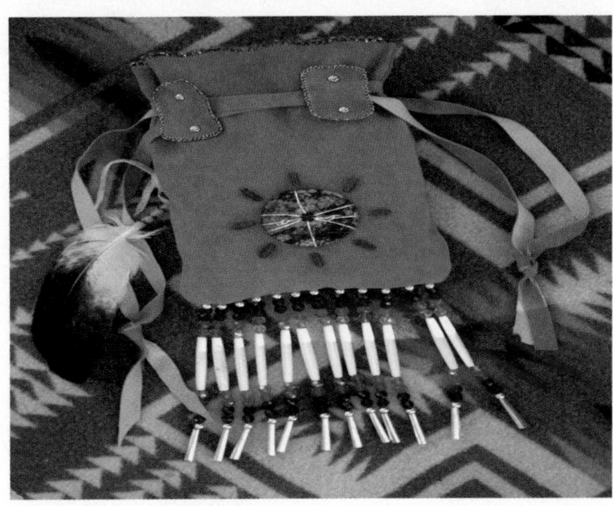

This is a traditional Navajo medicine bag used to promote healing and well-being. Each bag is created specifically for the individual and often contains medicinal herbs, semiprecious stones, beading, and animal fetishes.

CULTURAL CONNECTION

> I feel as if getting my skin painted gave me an identity; it was about fitting into my own skin. In our caring profession of nursing, will nursing accept me and my tattoos?
>
> —*Serena Williamson, student nurse*

Tattoos are simply symbols. They are along the same lines as stretch marks in childbirth, as reminders of a battle faced, an idea in time, and an immortalized piece of the past.

Barely 2 months into nursing school, I was warned by the main nurse recruiter of the bigger hospital in town that I would "never work in their facility." Next, a nursing faculty member told me that with my visible tattoos, I would never have a job as a professional nurse. Ironically enough, I interviewed with the same recruiter and received a position in the "banned" facility the summer between my junior and senior years of nursing school.

So, I guess you could say I am used to the negative reaction that tattoos elicit. Nurses are not any different from the public; they just have the "professional image" hammer to use.

My professionalism is questioned and denied with one glance at my uncovered, tattooed arm. So I do what many people with tattoos do in these settings: I cover up. Asking people who are not tattooed about tattoos has elicited many interesting responses: "What are you going to do when your skin sags?" "What will your grandchildren think?" Then there are the gender-specific questions: "How do you handle the pain?", "What does your mother/father/boyfriend/aunt think?", and my favorite, "Tattoos on women—well, they are just loose women."

Social stigmas placed on tattoos are simply that—socially created and change as society changes. As we all know, we are taught certain things about certain "groups" and we can accept them without reservation or question, have experiences that confirm or refute the teachings, or never buy into them in the first place.

By the way, my tattoo artist told me he rarely tattoos a biker.

During my obstetrics clinical rotation, I observed in the antepartum clinic that, of the 15 patients we saw that day, 9 had visible tattoos. Maybe this was an atypical clinic, maybe not. Or just maybe, many, if not most, of our hospital patients of the future will have tattoos.

My tattoo symbolizes and is a metaphor of the many parts of my personal struggles and instrumental components of who I am today. The swan is how I see myself now, the ugly duckling who morphed into a "swan"—as a viable and productive member of society: The swan is black to represent my place in my family—forever the black sheep. Tiger lilies are the backdrop of the design: They represent my beloved deceased grandmother,

Continues

CULTURAL CONNECTION (*CONTINUED*)

who shaped my whole reality. I remember her yard being a gorgeous field of tiger lilies in the summer.

The most unexpected aspect of my tattoo experience was how it has changed the way I feel about my body. I met with my tattoo artist, Jeremy Justice, and gave him a brief idea of what I had in mind. He drew the tattoo especially for my body and told me that it would not look good on someone without curves. Now every time I look at my back and see how my waist curves in its natural state, I experience contentment. Using my skin as a canvas for the art of my life made me feel like I fit into it.

—Serena Williamson, senior nursing student,
University of Southern Mississippi School of Nursing,
Hattiesburg, Mississippi

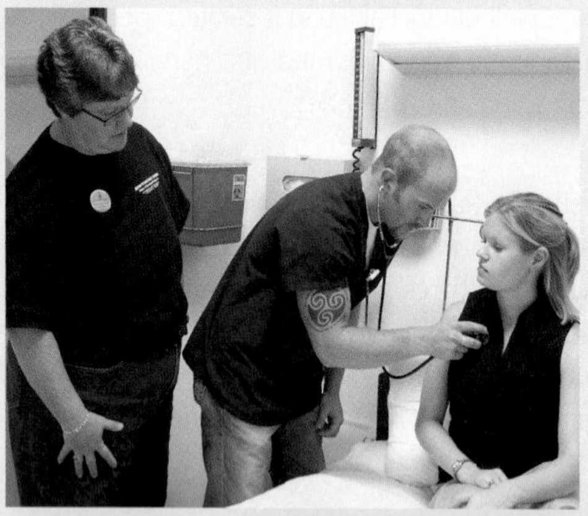

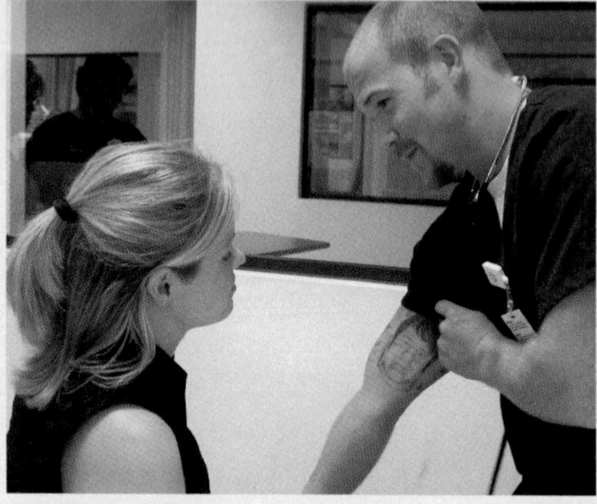

My older brother, Bhron, was 8 years older than me. He died on March 7, 2004, at the age of 29 from a toxic combination of Soma [carisoprodol] and alcohol, after a night on the town with me. I found him on the kitchen floor around 8:00 the next morning at my parents' house in Meridian, Mississippi.

I was asleep on the couch, and my father awakened me, saying to "come in the kitchen—something is wrong." I walked into the kitchen to find my brother lying on the floor with one leg propped up and his hands over his chest as if he was asleep. My first thoughts were to laugh, because I thought he had just fallen asleep on the floor. However, within a few seconds, I realized something was really wrong. His color was pale and his throat looked swollen and engorged. I quickly dropped to my knees and felt for a pulse. As I touched him, he seemed so cold and stiff . . . I knew then he had passed some hours before we found him. At this point, I knew there was nothing to do . . . I struggled with the idea of beginning CPR, but knew there was no point. I looked at my father as he stood next to the refrigerator showing a blank stare and said, "He's gone, Dad" . . . then I asked him to call an ambulance. He didn't respond, so I yelled it again . . . this time he ran to the phone and called 911. As my father dialed the number, he said to me "I've got to tell your mother. . . ."

I asked him not to, not yet . . . but he insisted, dropped the phone, and walked to my mother's bedroom. . . . I grabbed the phone, told the dispatcher the address and what had happened. She asked if I would like to perform CPR as she could instruct and help me to do so. . . . I explained to her that I knew how to perform CPR and that my brother had been dead for a while and that there was no point.

As I was on the phone, I could hear my mother come running up the hallway screaming frantically, "What's going on?" As she turned the corner to the kitchen and saw my brother, I heard the most blood-curdling scream in my life . . . I didn't know what to do. I found myself in a position in which I had to control the situation. My father didn't seem to know what to do; he just stood there with a blank stare. My mother was frantically crying and screaming.

I met the paramedics outside and informed them of the situation as they rushed into the house. Once they got inside to my brother and assessed him, I remember seeing one of the paramedics who had a disappointed and sad look on his face, as he made contact with the others. He shook his head. Soon the police showed up and had to conduct their work.

As all this was going on, I went to sit in another room just to try to calm myself . . . much of this event was a blur . . . family members began showing up . . . after a few hours of blur and so much emotion and crying, I had to leave . . . and so I did . . . I got in my car and left for Hattiesburg to get away from everything and just sit alone at my apartment. . . .

I got the tattoo of my brother not only in memory, but also as a way for him to "live" through me . . . it has become a way for me to deal with it. I'm often approached about my tattoo and I am automatically inclined to tell the story of how he passed. Rather than carry a picture of my brother in my wallet or put one in my car or room, I have a permanent picture of my brother that is always with me and in a place I can always see.

Along with the portrait of my brother, I decided to expand the ideal of our brotherhood. Bhron and I had a favorite movie that we watched together many times, called the *Boondock Saints*. The movie is about two brothers with matching tattoos (which my brother and I have on our backs), who believe they are divinely obligated to rid their city and the world of sinners and evil.

With this movie in mind and my heritage of Scotch–Irish, I decided to use the first and last sentences of a prayer the two brothers would say to themselves often, after purging the sinners... "And shepherds we shall be, for thee my lord for thee... in nomine Patris, et Filii, et Spiritus Sancti," which translates to "in the name of the Father, the Son, and the Holy Spirit."

I also found a Celtic trinity symbol, which I thought was perfect with the quote, the movie, my heritage, and my brother. This symbol correlates with many other ancient symbols, including triskeles and mandalas, in which one continuous line forms the symbol and there are no closings to the design.... I drew the design with a few personal adjustments and added the quote around the symbol.... I also decided to put my brother's name on the back of my arm and add clouds around everything to "finish" the painting around my arm.

My tattoos have brought me praise as well as disapproval. I cannot think of a day that goes by that at least one person has not approached me or commented on my tattoo. Most of the people who make comments are younger and closer to my age. They ask me where I got it, what it means, and they usually compliment my tattoo. In contrast, I get strange or disappointing looks from members of the older generation. I sometimes feel like an outcast or someone that isn't to be trusted, based on these "disgusted looks."

In the hospital, I have received disapproving looks and comments from coworkers, physicians, and patients. I usually brush their disapproval off, but sometimes find myself taking them

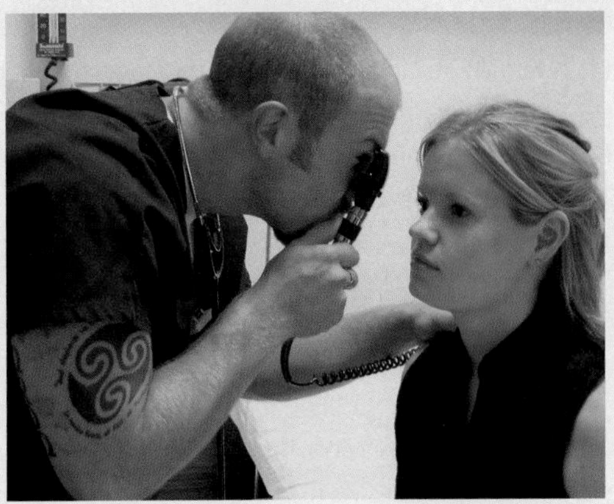

as direct and personal attacks. Maybe tattoos aren't what most people would do to commemorate a deceased relative, but to me it seems very appropriate. I try to cover my tattoos while at work or in clinicals for nursing school, because I do not want my ideals to affect the persona of my professionalism in a clinical setting. My tattoos are a direct reflection of my life experiences; they are not a reflection of my abilities as a professional nurse. I am very proud of my tattoos—I would never go back and change a thing.

—Noah Seth Jordan, student nurse, University of Southern Mississippi School of Nursing

APPLICATION TO PRACTICE 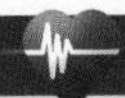

Read the following statements about cultural values and use them to perform a "self-check" of your own cultural identity and attitudes about caring for diverse populations:

- You are different from me because you are

  ______________________________.

- We are different from each other and this makes me feel

  ______________________________.

- The difference between us makes you

  ______________________________.

- You threaten my traditions, my core values, my sense of entitlement, my power. I must protect myself from you if your

- ____________________ shows enough to remind me just how dangerous you can be. I want you to be more like me because

  ______________________________.

- You make me feel vulnerable, out of control, and powerless, and your culture seems wrong because of

  ______________________________.

- If you get too close, I will

  ______________________________.

- I will protect myself and teach my children to protect themselves from people like you, different from us, because of

  ______________________________.

- I will teach my children with whom they must not play or walk to school with because of

  ______________________________.

- I want you to speak my language; I do not want to learn yours because of

  ______________________________.

Source: Davanaugh, G. F. (1991). *Psychiatric mental health nursing*. Philadelphia, PA: Lippincott.

DAY IN THE LIFE

Nursing students and others frequently ask me: How did transcultural nursing get started? In the 1950s I envisioned the field of transcultural nursing as an important and neglected area of study and practice. I was working as a child psychiatric clinical nurse specialist in a child guidance agency and discovered that children and families who come from different cultures could not be cared for or treated in the same way. I observed that children of African, Appalachian, German, Jewish, and other cultures clearly revealed differences in their eating, sleeping, playing, interaction, and sociocultural patterns. Because nurses were the major direct and continuous healthcare providers, they needed to understand these differences. I realized that my basic nursing program failed to prepare me to effectively deal with different cultures and types of care. I was culturally ignorant of the values, beliefs, and lifestyle practices of people. I had no idea how cultures could exert such a powerful force on people's health and wellbeing. I soon realized that nursing and other healthcare providers tended to treat all people alike, treating people as if they were mainly biophysical and psychological beings who were devoid of culture. Healthcare providers acted with limited knowledge and cultural influences on healing and wellbeing.

These realities led me to pursue graduate study in anthropology so that I could learn from scholars who had been studying cultures around the world for over 100 years. After learning from the experts in anthropology, I faced the challenge of how to develop the new field of transcultural nursing. One of the first tasks was to establish courses and programs in transcultural nursing, which entailed preparing faculty and practitioners to become transcultural nurse generalists and specialists in a field unknown to nurses. It also involved stimulating nursing leaders and organizations, as well as nursing students, to become interested in transcultural nursing knowledge and practices.

Almost 5 decades later, transcultural nursing knowledge is recognized as essential for teaching, research, practice, and consultation worldwide. Nursing students have been the strongest and most persistent promoters of transcultural nursing, along with patients who recognize that they have a right to have their cultures respected and given attention in health services. Schools of nursing, as well as many hospitals, clinics, and community agencies, are giving attention to diverse cultures in education and clinical services. This attention is necessary to meet accreditation requirements. Community health nurses continue to see the urgent need for transcultural nursing as they care for many families of different cultures. Because patients are increasingly dismissed from hospitals early, it is the role of community health nurses to maintain care services and relationships with cultural groups, including many new immigrants, refugees, and other newcomers to their communities.

In the early years there were nurses who were resistant to transcultural nursing. They were afraid to deal with cultural factors and wanted to protect themselves by not getting involved in areas they did not understand. Transcultural nursing education has helped many nurses face their fears and move forward to become more competent practitioners.

Transcultural nursing concepts, principles, theories, and research findings are guiding nurses to provide transcultural nursing services in the community, hospitals, clinics, hospices, and many other settings where nurses work. The *Journal of Transcultural Nursing* was established in 1988 and provides a rich source of transcultural nursing research findings and other information. In addition, many books, articles, and other publications focus on transcultural nursing to guide nurses in their practices.

The Transcultural Nursing Society, established in 1974, offers regional, national, and global conferences where nurses can meet with other transcultural nurses to share ideas and experiences and expand their worldview. In 1988, the Transcultural Nursing Society began to certify nurses to ensure that they could provide safe, competent, and effective care to people of diverse cultures. Today, there are more than 100 certified transcultural nurses (CTN), but many more are preparing themselves to meet the certification requirements. The Transcultural Nursing Society became the first organization to provide certification of nurses worldwide, which is a hallmark for future nursing directions.

—Madeleine Leininger

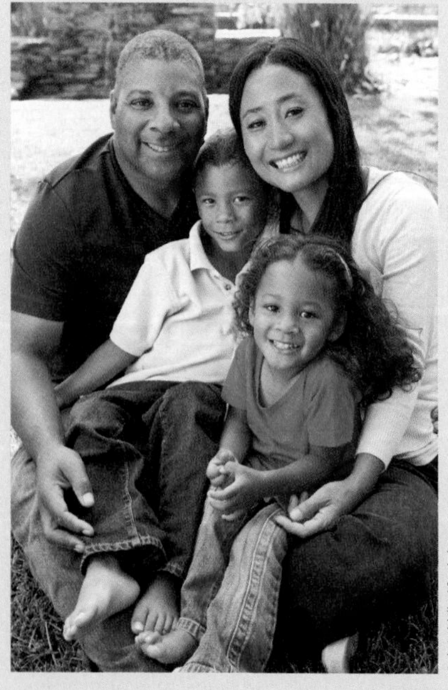

Conclusion

As we enter the 21st century, the theory of culture care diversity and universality has become a major theory to guide nurses in arriving at community-based transcultural nursing. It is the only theory that has an explicit nursing research method designed to tease out relevant and appropriate culture care data. All too often, borrowed theories and methods from other disciplines fail to tap into nursing care phenomena, and the methods often prove to miss the cultural, environmental, and historical factors that hold special meaning and are stated in the people's language modes (Leininger, 1985, 1991, 1995, 2006). Moreover, since the 1970s, transcultural nursing researchers have found that qualitative research methods, such as ethnonursing, provide a wealth of rich culture and care data that are meaningful, specific, and appropriate in providing transcultural nursing care. It should be noted that research studies done in hospitals and clinics tend to reveal less opportunity for cultural informants to be heard or to get care that is culture specific and culturally congruent, unless the nurse is prepared in transcultural nursing and is a strong leader to support patients.

HEALTHY ME 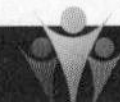

What was it like growing up and learning cultural values about health in your family? How do those values affect you as an adult with specific health and illness concerns?

LEVELS OF PREVENTION 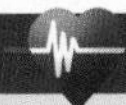

Primary: Teaching a class for college students about cultural sensitivity

Secondary: Utilizing transcultural nursing principles to assist the group with resolution after a culturally insensitive comment has been made

Tertiary: A family from a different country is living in the United States and experiences a hate crime. Refer family to appropriate supportive resources in the community and contact legal authority.

Critical Thinking Activities

1. How many different cultural groups are there in your community? Who are they?
2. What are some of their traditions and values?
3. How are they different from you?
4. How are they like you?

References

DeSantis, L. (1997). Building healthy communities with immigrants and refugees. *Journal of Transcultural Nursing, 9*(1), 20–31.

Horn, B. M. (1979). Transcultural nursing and child-rearing of the Muckleshoot people. In M. M. Leininger (Ed.), *Transcultural nursing: Proceedings from four transcultural nursing conferences* (pp. 57–69). New York, NY: Masson.

Leininger, M. (1970). *Nursing and anthropology: Two worlds to blend.* New York, NY: Wiley. (Reprinted in 1994 by Greyden Press, Columbus, OH).

Leininger, M. (1978). *Transcultural nursing*. Columbus, OH: Greyden Press.

Leininger, M. (1981). *Care: An essential human need.* Thorofare, NJ: Charles B. Slack.

Leininger, M. (1985). *Qualitative research methods in nursing.* New York, NY: Grune & Stratton.

Leininger, M. (1988). *Care: Discovery and uses in clinical and community nursing.* Detroit, MI: Wayne State University Press.

Leininger, M. (1990). *Ethical and moral dimensions of care*. Detroit, MI: Wayne State University Press.

Leininger, M. (1991). *Cultural care diversity and universality: A theory of nursing.* New York, NY: National League for Nursing Press.

Leininger, M. (1995). *Transcultural nursing: Concepts, theories, research, and practice.* Columbus, OH: McGraw-Hill.

Leininger, M. (1996). Quality of life from a transcultural nursing perspective. *Nursing Science Quarterly, 9*(2), 71–78.

Leininger, M. (1997a). Cultural pain. *Images of Nursing* (Summer Edition), 19–20.

Leininger, M. (1997b). Future directions in transcultural nursing in the 21st century. *International Nursing Review, 44*(1), 19–23.

Leininger, M. (2006). Culture care diversity and universality theory and evolution of the ethnonursing method. In M. M. Leininger and M. R. McFarland (Eds.), *Culture care diversity and universality: A worldwide nursing theory* (2nd ed., pp. 1–41). Sudbury, MA: Jones and Bartlett.

Leininger, M., & McFarland, M. R. (2002). *Transcultural nursing: Concepts theories, research and practice* (3rd ed.). New York, NY: McGraw-Hill.

Luna, L. (1998). Culturally competent health care: A challenge for nurses in Saudi Arabia. *Journal of Transcultural Nursing, 9*(2), 8–15.

Rosenbaum, J. (1990). Culture care of older Greek-Canadian widows within Leininger's theory of culture care. *Journal of Transcultural Nursing, 2*(1), 3–9.

Shapiro, M. L., Miller, J., & White, K. (2006). Community transformation through culturally competent nursing leadership: Application of theory of culture care diversity and universality and tri-dimensional leader effectiveness model. *Journal of Transcultural Nursing, 17*(2), 113–118.

CHAPTER FOCUS

Virtue or Character Ethics

Principle-Based Ethics: Developing Moral Rules

Utilitarian Theories: Doing the Most Good for the Most People

Deontological Theories: Balancing Rights and Obligations

Justice in Health Care

Communitarian Ethics

Values and Health Policy

Ethic of Care

Ethical Problems Faced by Community Nurses: The Research

Ethical Decision Making

Service-Learning: Discovering the Self and Developing Community Values

QUESTIONS TO CONSIDER

After reading this chapter, you will know the answers to the following questions:

1. What is bioethics, and how is it important to the community nurse?
2. What is the ethics of virtue, and what part do virtues play in the practice of nursing?
3. What is meant by principle-based ethics?
4. How does Kant's deontological approach differ from Mill's utilitarian approach?
5. What role does each of the four major ethical concepts—beneficence, nonmaleficence, autonomy, and justice—play in community nursing practice?
6. How can healthcare resources be distributed in a fair manner?
7. How does the ethical theory of care differ from or agree with other theories?
8. What information does the nurse need to make ethically based decisions?
9. What is service-learning, and how does it apply to community health?

A different way of thinking about right and wrong actions may be needed in working with aggregate populations in the community. The situation becomes more complex when we attempt to weigh individual rights and privileges against what is best for the larger group.

CHAPTER 12

Ethics and Health

Pat Kurtz and Janie B. Butts

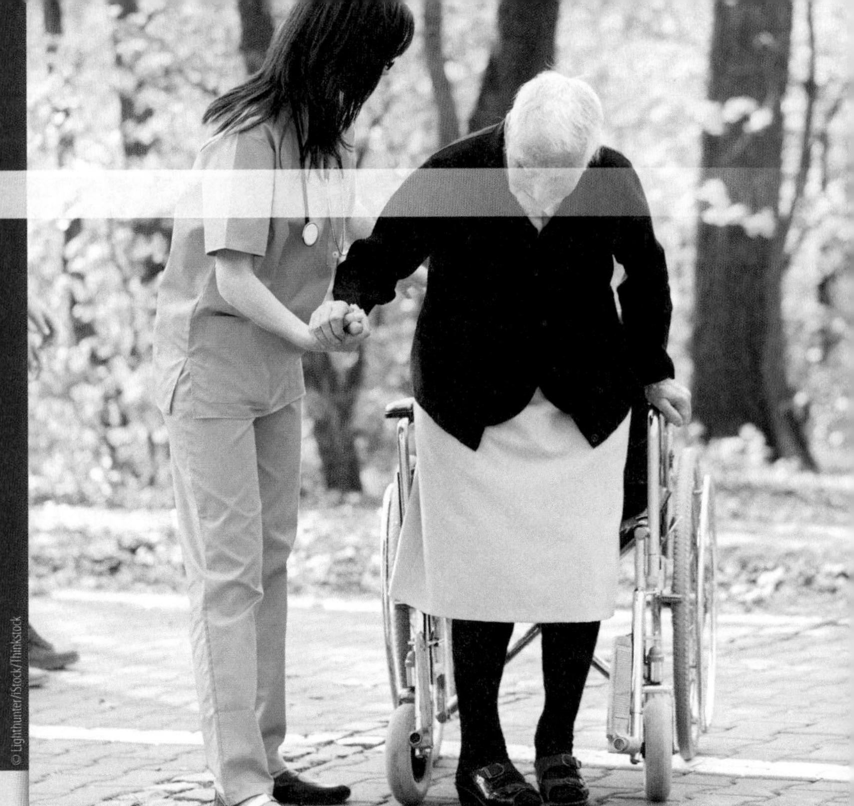

© Lighthunter/iStock/Thinkstock

KEY TERMS

autonomy
beneficence
bioethics
casuistry
compassion
conscientiousness
consequentialism
deontological
discernment
ethic of care
ethical decision making
ethical dilemma
ethics
integrity
justice
nonmaleficence
service-learning
trustworthiness
utilitarianism
virtue ethics

REFLECTIONS

A state legislature allotted its state health department $750,000 to match federal funding for medication sufficient to treat 20 patients with acquired immune deficiency syndrome (AIDS). However, there were 100 patients who needed the help. Public health nurses in each district were asked to select patients for the medication program.

A terminally ill cancer patient who is in great pain begs the nurse for more medication than the physician has ordered. What should the nurse do?

A man was diagnosed and treated for a venereal infection by his family nurse practitioner. He agreed that his wife should also be treated, but he did not want her to know that he acquired the disease from a prostitute and infected her. He asked the nurse practitioner if there was any way to avoid sharing this information.

When faced with situations like these, it sometimes feels like there are no "right" actions. What are your reactions to the three ethical dilemmas? What other information would be helpful to know about these situations to make a decision?

THE SITUATIONS WE encounter as healthcare professionals may be complex and puzzling dealing with serious issues of wellbeing, life, and death. Our early experiences are usually of little help in guiding our actions in such complex situations. The philosophical discipline of **ethics** is the study of how we should behave, or how to determine the right thing to do in our interactions with others. **Bioethics** is the common name for the study of ethics as it relates to health and the moral problems that arise as a result of advances in health technologies and our increasing ability to do more to treat illness and prolong life. Ethical theories provide a guide to examining ethical situations and to articulating preferred ways of living and behaving as healthcare practitioners. We must, however, remain aware that differences of opinion exist among those well versed in ethics and bioethics regarding which theories best fit which cases, as well as what role character development plays in preparation for acting ethically in the community.

As our understanding of the universe, the nature of human behavior, and societal relationships have increased or changed, theories about ethical behavior have been modified and new theories developed. One essential difference in the various approaches to ethical decision making has to do with the target of the action. For whom or for what are we interested in doing the right thing—ourselves, a coworker, an individual patient, a family, an organization, a community, a nation, or the world? Unfortunately, what may seem to be the ethical thing to do for one person or group may not be the ethical thing for another. A situation characterized by conflicting actions or obligations is known as an **ethical dilemma**.

Because of the variety of settings in which nurses practice and the philosophical assumption of the nursing community that nurses care for the whole person, nurses are often involved in all aspects of the patient's life as they relate to health. In 1990, Bishop and Scudder pointed out that a major characteristic of nursing is that nurses practice "in-between." Decades later, this statement still holds. By in-between care, they mean that in addition to giving direct care to the patient, nurses must manage and coordinate other aspects of the patient's care. This management includes advocating for the patient with the physician and other healthcare providers, interpreting the patient's needs to the agency, and interpreting agency policy and other constraints to patients and families. For a community health nurse, it may also mean advocating for agencies and policies in the political arena.

For the nurse practicing in the community, the community itself is another interested party in the patient's health care. Community health nurses are accountable for all individual patients and populations in the community. Rich (2013b) emphasizes that nurses are "collectively committed to the common good of alleviating patients' suffering and promoting patients' wellbeing." A different way of thinking about ethical actions may be needed in working with aggregate populations. One or more ethical theories or approaches will guide nurses' actions (Rich, 2013a).

Ethical issues or dilemmas become more complex when we attempt to weigh individual rights and privileges against assessments of what is best for a larger group. Ethical decisions are often made from an array of competing "oughts" and choices that include justice in distribution, the patient's comfort level or happiness, the patient's wishes, the expense of services, the patient's responsibility in acquiring a condition, and the social role of the patient. Oughts refer to normative inquiry of ethical behavior, or how people ought to behave if making a choice in certain situations. Choices refer to the recognition that competing goods exist but that valid justification exists for one choice over another.

One approach to increasing competence in dealing with ethical matters is to begin with clarification of our own values and identifying and understanding the values by which other people live. The cultural competence required for expert nursing care is a specific ethical demand on members of the profession to know and respect the values of others. Steele and Harmon (1983) and Uustal (1993) have developed strategies to aid in values clarification. The steps in the clarification process help people discover which values they hold and how strongly they hold them in relation to others. Values are often the result of years of consciously seeking information and weighing the importance of one point of view against another. However, they are also simply adopted from family tradition, religious teaching, or modeling people whom we admire without much reflection. These acquired values of individuals play a role in their moral behavior.

Over the millennia, philosophers, ethicists, theologians, and others have attempted to formulate principles and rules that will guide us in ethical behavior. This chapter presents some of the basic principles of classical ethical theories (virtue ethics, deontology or formalism, and utilitarianism or consequentialism), as well as more recent formulations of biomedical ethics and care ethics. It includes a special focus on the justice issue of distribution of care and on the value systems that influence our national agendas for health care. Finally, research findings related to ethical dilemmas identified by community health nurses are reviewed and frameworks for **ethical decision making** are presented.

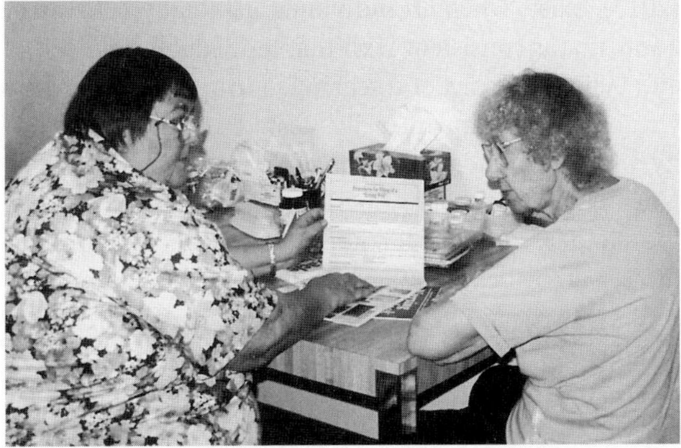

Pat Kurtz , chapter author, counseling an elderly patient about a living will.

Virtue or Character Ethics

One of the earliest philosophical approaches to correct behavior was that of **virtue ethics**. According to this approach, if a person has a "good" character, that person will behave ethically as a matter of course. Virtue ethics is based on the writings of the Greek philosopher Aristotle (384–382 BCE). Aristotle (Apostle, 1975) believed that there was general agreement that everyone has a "life goal" and that ultimate life goal is "happiness." Although each person has a different definition of happiness, Aristotle believed that happiness is achieved by what he called "excellence in performing rational activities" (thinking), which includes "excellence in choosing."

Behavioral choices lie on a continuum between ultimate extremes. Gluttony or self-denial might be the two extremes of a continuum representing eating or any other behavior relating to psychological or physiological needs. Rashness and cowardice might be the extremes of a risk-taking continuum. Aristotle argued that the best choices lie between the two extremes, preferably somewhere in the middle, which he called the *golden mean*. The person who selects and acts on these middle-ground choices is virtuous. However, the mean for each virtue is unique for each type of virtue and situation; in other words, the mean is not a mathematical average that is consistent for all virtues (Rich, 2013a). A person who acts in a pattern of consistency born of practice is thought to have good character.

Aristotle believed that becoming a virtuous person was a matter of habit and could be learned over time. The more one acts virtuously, the stronger the character trait becomes. In the throes of a crisis, character traits come to the fore and are more likely than relying on sudden decision making to result in good outcomes. From this standpoint, part of becoming a "good" nurse would require that students should practice a life of moderate choices that consistently lead to the most right professional actions in given circumstances. That is, the virtuous nurse would simply be disposed to do the ethically virtuous thing, rather than having to reason to an ethical solution by some procedure. The word *ethics* actually stems from the Greek word *ethos*, which means "well-developed habits."

Like many other experiences in life, a given behavior may or may not be considered virtuous, depending on the culture of the individual. Honesty is often considered a virtue. However, if you belong to a criminal community or to a poverty-stricken family or community, honesty may not be valued in the same way it is in a community of middle-class property owners. Likewise, not all virtues are ethical in nature. Cheerfulness may be considered a virtuous social trait, but it is ethical only when displayed within an ethical situation. Even a right action is not ethical by itself, according to Aristotle, unless the action comes from ethical motivation. In other words, to be considered virtuous, not only must the behavior be the right action, purposefully done, but it must also come from an ethically appropriate inner urge to do the right thing. **Box 12-1** describes characteristics of virtue ethics.

Characteristic of certain roles, occupations, and professions are expectations that their practitioners will have

BOX 12-1 Virtue Ethics: Aristotle

- The ultimate goal of life is to achieve happiness, which comes from excellence of thinking.
- An important aspect of excellence of thinking is excellence of choosing virtuous action—the golden mean.
- A virtuous action is moral only when it is done from a motivation to do the right thing.
- Virtue, for those of good character, is learned over time by the practice of acting in virtuous ways.
- Virtues are partly discerned from observing instances of sustained exemplary behavior by role models.

character and virtues beyond those of other people. In the case of nursing, it is expected that nurses will be (possess the virtue of) caring and will express that caring in all aspects of patient–nurse interaction. As a virtue, caring may be considered a mean between extremes on a continuum of attention to and feeling for others. At the one extreme would be rejection and callousness; at the other extreme would be over-involvement and indulgence. From a patient's point of view, caring includes or implies other virtues. For example, if nurses are caring, they are also trustworthy and can be relied upon to give fitting priority to the patient's welfare.

The Florence Nightingale Pledge identifies some virtues that were expected of nurses in the past. These virtues include purity, obedience, loyalty, and willingness to assume the handmaiden role to the physician (Davis & Aroskar, 1991). Changes in the societal expectations of the role of women in general and expectations from within nursing have devalued some of these historical virtues and replaced them with virtues of assertiveness, loyalty to and advocacy for the patient, and willingness to take appropriate risks.

It is not uncommon for nurse educators and other nurses to question the virtuousness of today's nursing students and novice nurses. They complain that some nurses are joining the profession for its high salaries and security and do not show the ethical character traits of caring and the strict honesty that they believe are required of nurses.

Beauchamp and Childress (2013) identified five virtues that they consider primary to the ethics of health professionals: compassion, discernment, trustworthiness, integrity, and conscientiousness

Compassion, a notion related to caring, includes an active and decisive concern for others and an awareness of their pain or suffering. The compassionate person is disposed to respond with appropriate feelings of sympathy and mercy, as well as a desire to help decrease pain and other suffering. Ethically, being disposed to show these feelings also may be a critical factor in a patient's perception of being cared for.

While compassion has a strong emotional component, **discernment** is an intellectual trait that involves "the ability to make fitting judgments and reach decisions without being unduly influenced by extraneous considerations, fears, personal attachments, and the like" (Beauchamp & Childress, 2013, p. 39). The discerning person is able to take decisive action based on insight resulting from a history of clear judgment and understanding. The person is able to make ethical judgments without being unduly influenced by other personal or political factors. The person sees to the heart of the matter without the bias of personal involvement or personal feelings, without the common ethical flaw known as "conflict of interest." The discerning person is able to see what needs to be done, when, and in what way in situations involving ethical considerations.

Trustworthiness is a character trait that gives other people confidence that an individual consistently acts in moral character to make ethical decisions. Beauchamp and Childress believe that the presence or lack of trustworthiness may be the most influential factor in whether a relationship continues between a patient and a caregiver. For sure, trustworthiness is one of the most essential virtues that one can practice in medical and health care. For many years in national Gallup polls, nurses have been consistently rated by the public as being the most trustworthy group among professionals.

Integrity, according to Beauchamp and Childress (2013), exists when an individual habitually behaves in a way that is consistent with that individual's core values and beliefs. Persons of integrity, so to speak, "walk their virtuous talk." Moral integrity means "soundness, reliability, wholeness, and integration of moral character" (p. 40). Nurses maintain professional integrity when they practice the standards of ethical conduct of their profession. For nurses, ethical conduct is outlined with nine provisions in the American Nurses Association (ANA; 2001) *Code of Ethics for Nurses with Interpretive Statements*. Sometimes integrity can be disturbed when the individual faces conflicts that lead to the need to compromise beliefs and values. *Moral distress* is a term connected to the tension people experience as a result of compromising their ethical principles.

When people are motivated by their mental faculty to do what is ethical just because the action is the right thing to do, they are acting conscientiously. Beauchamp and Childress (2013) characterize this behavior as the virtue of **conscientiousness** that comes about as a result of long-standing self-reflection on one's beliefs and feelings about "obligatory or prohibitive, right or wrong, good or bad, and virtuous or vicious behavior" (pp. 42–43). Acting conscientiously requires a balancing act. If an individual or a group makes a decision based on a conscientious objection, the decision could adversely affect or compromise patient interests. The same could be true for a group of people who conscientiously object to a public health policy that serves the communal good over individual interests. Balancing guides nurses and other professionals to protect both the individual interests and the communal good.

Principle-Based Ethics: Developing Moral Rules

In principle-based approaches to ethics, the right or ethical action is determined not by the virtues (or habits) of individuals or authoritative tradition, but rather by the support of a set of beliefs developed by careful reasoning. Such beliefs include ideas about who has what kinds of rights and which rights or obligations have priority over other rights and obligations. For example, who has the right to make decisions about a patient's health care, and in what ways are healthcare providers obligated to support a decision with which they disagree? The two major principle-based approaches are utilitarianism and deontology.

Utilitarian Theories: Doing the Most Good for the Most People

The primary belief of people who have adopted the utilitarian position is that the most ethical action is the one that results in the greatest good (happiness) for the greatest number. A corollary to this notion would be that the best action is the one that causes the least harm to the fewest people. The philosopher cited most frequently as a proponent of **utilitarianism** is John Stuart Mill (1806–1873).

To a utilitarian, the important thing is not so much your good will toward others, but rather the consequences that result from your action. (Utilitarianism is also known as **consequentialism**.) Determining which action to take requires that all possible actions in the situation and the potential outcomes of each be examined for every person or group who may be involved. After the different outcomes are weighed and balanced, the action that leads to the best outcome for the most people is selected.

The utilitarian approach has obvious limitations. The first that may come to mind is the problem of how we can know what the outcomes will be for all the persons involved, because many factors beyond our control—or even beyond our knowledge—influence outcomes. Another problem arises when the preferred action and/or outcome is itself unethical. An example would be falsifying records in a home health agency so that the insurers will continue to pay for visits to otherwise ineligible patients. If the purpose of the falsification was to continue needed services to patients who would otherwise not receive them, the consequence is positive for the patient; however, the means are still unethical (and illegal). Recognizing this possible misuse of the theory as a rationalization for unethical behavior, Mill (1859/1871/1993) acknowledged that some behaviors were inherently unethical and could not be condoned, no matter what the favorable outcome. He specifically cited slavery as an example.

A more relevant issue in our time might be the use of migrant labor at pay rates below minimum wage and without decent provisions for living to produce cheaper food for the larger U.S. population. To avoid the misuse of this ethical approach, commonly expressed as "the ends justify the means," there must be general agreement about the ethical appropriateness of the proposed action and possible outcomes.

Another common criticism of the utilitarian approach is that it may not be practical for the average person. The principle of maximizing benefit for the greatest number may place the individuals making the decision in a position of always having to sacrifice their own preferences for the greater good. This self-sacrifice may be too difficult for the average person and raises questions about what the limits of our obligation to maximize benefit in that way are and whether it is even possible to make fair decisions in situations in which we may either be benefited or harmed. For example, suppose you are asked to support legislation that would provide increased health benefits for you and your family. After examining the proposed legislation, you realize that it will exclude many needy people who are benefiting from current legislation. In this instance, opposition to the proposed legislation would benefit more people, but at your expense.

The utilitarian approach is also criticized because it appears to give undue advantage to the majority population. For example, legislation that mandates increased health benefits (e.g., mammography) for participants in a health maintenance organization (HMO), Medicaid recipients, or those who have other private insurance will benefit a large number of people. At the same time, it excludes a minority who have no insurance and who may have more need for the services but lack the ability to pay for them. The criterion of justice (discussed in detail later)—so important in other approaches—may be missing from the utilitarian approach. **Box 12-2** lists the major descriptors of utilitarianism/consequentialism.

A major area in which utilitarianism aids decision making is in public policy development, wherein it is often referred to as *cost–benefit analysis*. It is the presumed goal of policymakers that whatever money is appropriated or whatever regulations are adopted will further the general good of society. Developing public policy requires the careful examination of all possible options and the

BOX 12-2 Utilitarianism/Consequentialism

- The major determinant of ethical behavior is that it provides the most benefit to the most people or the least harm to the fewest people.
- The decision to act must be based on a careful examination of all possible actions in the situation and the possible consequences of each action.
- Regardless of consequences, actions themselves must be deemed to be ethical.

probable consequences of each. It is not uncommon that legislation is passed with good intentions, only to find later that a group of people has been left out, that the new legislation conflicts with other important practices, or that it encourages poor or fraudulent practices. It is important that nurses be at the decision-making table to provide data about these options and consequences from their perspectives as caregivers and advocates.

ETHICAL CONNECTION 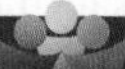

Stason and Weinstein studied the cost-effectiveness of screening for and treating hypertension using data from the Framingham longitudinal study and results of other hypertension studies. They projected various models of cost from initial screening to long-term treatment, considering such factors as dropout rates; nonadherence to medication; side effects; probability of more expensive events, such as stroke and myocardial infarction; and age. They found that it is more cost-effective to fund programs designed to increase adherence to the treatment regimen for those already in treatment than to institute screening for new cases. They also found that it is more cost-effective if hypertensive men start treatment when they are young, but women begin when they are older. The recommendation was that *if* screening is instituted, the focus should be on young men and older women.

What are the disadvantages to this utilitarian approach? Do you agree or disagree with this approach?

Source: Stason, W. B., & Weinstein, M. C. (1977). Public health rounds at the Harvard School of Public Health: Allocation of resources to manage hypertension. *New England Journal of Medicine, 296*(3), 732–739.

Deontological Theories: Balancing Rights and Obligations

Ethical theories categorized as **deontological** uphold the position that whether an action is ethical depends on the action itself—principally the motivational basis for the action. The word "deontological" was originally meant to differentiate an ethic of duty from the more utilitarian ethic of consequences.

Immanuel Kant (1724–1804) is the philosopher who proposed the basis for our major theory of deontological ethics in his attempt to elaborate a rationale for ethical behavior based on pure reason, rather than tradition or authoritative pronouncement. Kant (1785/1997) proposed two foundational principles, or rules, that he called "categorical imperatives" or unconditional "ethical laws." "Law" here means the generalized reason for an action, which would hold universally and which everyone must follow. If a rule meets that criterion, then it will always be true for every similar instance, and the individual is therefore obligated to follow the rule in every instance.

For example, you might want to determine whether it is ethical to lie to a patient about a diagnosis or prognosis. Is lying ethical? Based on Kant's procedures to determine the imperative, you would first determine whether lying could be an acceptable ethical behavior for every person in every circumstance. Rationally, you would have to conclude that it could not; otherwise, no relationships that required trust could be developed. Therefore, lying is not ethical and is not acceptable in any situation. "Never lie" would be a categorical imperative. It could be argued, however, that some healthcare patients are special cases and that telling them the truth might cause psychological harm. Therefore, it is more ethical to lie than to risk causing harm. The imperative that one should never lie would have to be rejected or, at least restated, if this is thought to be true.

GOT AN ALTERNATIVE? 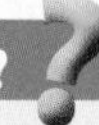

As more people seek out alternative health practices, nurses face a challenge. Nurses are often less familiar with these nontraditional treatments, so how can they practice in an ethical manner when their values are based on traditional medical treatment?

Kant's second principle is that everyone should be treated as ends and not means to an end. Modern versions of deontological theory all include this second imperative in rules related to respect for individuals (the principle of autonomy). **Box 12-3** describes deontological ethics according to Kant.

We have many examples of other approaches to this rule-based ethics. Of specific interest are theories of justice, notably those of Rawls and Nozick, which are discussed later. The Roman Catholic tradition, which originated from the Judeo-Christian ethic, has influenced the issue of assurance of social justice, both globally and in Western ethics (Butts, 2013). Another illustration of Roman Catholic influence is the Ten Commandments,

BOX 12-3 Deontological Ethics: Immanuel Kant

- Individuals establish their own moral rules based on the criterion that the generalized intention of their action could apply to everyone—that is, could become a "law."
- The rules apply to every similar situation.
- People must be treated as ends and not means (given respect as autonomous persons).

which are universal rules proposed for adherents of those religions. In addition, Butts (2013) stated that the Roman Catholic tradition has heavily influenced the landmark right-to-life/right-to-die court decisions, such as the Karen Ann Quinlan case (1975) and the Terri Schiavo case (1990/2005). Codes of ethics for professional groups are also examples of approach.

Nurses rely to a large extent on guidance in ethical matters from the ANA (2001) *Code of Ethics* and accompanying interpretive comments. This code, which is a non-negotiable guide for ethical behavior, focuses on professional responsibilities and on obligations of the nurse toward all patients. It clearly includes the community as a type of patient and the role of the nurse in the community. It does not go into detail about ethics with populations but is clearly consistent with the recently published code of ethics for public health team members. The "Principles of the Ethical Practice of Public Health" are listed in the Cultural Connection feature. Modern bioethics is another form of the deontological approach to ethics. Two events have influenced the development of modern bioethical theory: the medical experiments of German physicians during World War II (Davis & Aroskar, 1991) and the increasing development and use of technology in medicine (Beauchamp & Childress, 2013). In the first instance, interest in gaining new knowledge that would be helpful in the Nazi war effort, together with a disrespect for certain groups of people (e.g., Jews, Gypsies, mentally challenged), motivated Nazi doctors to perform experiments that were excruciatingly painful, degrading, and murderous. Revelation of these experiments at the Nuremberg trials following the war shocked the world community and increased awareness of humankind's capacity for inflicting harm. Further awareness and shock came with the revelation of inhumane research being conducted in the United States. Some, like the Tuskegee syphilis study being conducted on Southern African American men (in which researchers knowingly failed to treat study participants with the penicillin that would have cured their syphilis), were even supported by the U.S. Public Health Service. The results of these and other revelations were a series of national and international codes of ethics for the conduct of research.

The introduction of increasingly more sophisticated technology over the last several decades has enabled healthcare providers to perform complicated surgical procedures, such as heart bypass and organ transplants; to keep premature infants alive; to identify genetic abnormalities in a fetus; and to maintain nutrition, hydration, and respiration in patients in irreversible coma. In the struggle to find the right actions in these and other situations, solutions for many ethical dilemmas were eventually sought from the courts.

ETHICAL CONNECTION 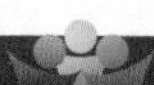

In 1932, the U.S. Public Health Service funded research to study the natural course of syphilis, a disease that at the time had no known, reliable treatment. Subjects for that study consisted of a group of 200 African American men who were infected with the disease and 100 African American men who were uninfected from the small area of Tuskegee, Alabama. The study continued for 40 years, during which time the infected population became more ill and had a much higher mortality rate than the uninfected control group. By the 1940s, it was found that penicillin was an effective treatment; however, none of the men were given the antibiotic. Many of the men did not know that they were subjects of a research study, were not told that penicillin would help them, and faithfully continued to appear for the periodic exams, believing that they were being treated. Articles reporting on the study were published in medical journals and, in addition to the nurse and physicians involved, many physicians from the Tuskegee medical center and around the state knew about the work. It was not until the project was exposed in 1972 in a Washington newspaper that the public became aware and expressed outrage about it. At this point the study was finally discontinued.

Source: Brandt, A. M. (1978). Racism and research: The case of the Tuskegee syphilis study. *Hastings Center Report, 8*(6), 21–29.

CULTURAL CONNECTION 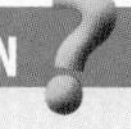

Principles of the Ethical Practice of Public Health, Version 2.2

1. Public health should address principally the fundamental causes of disease and requirements for health, aiming to prevent adverse health outcomes.
2. Public health should achieve community health in a way that respects the rights of individuals in the community.
3. Public health policies, programs, and priorities should be developed and evaluated through processes that ensure an opportunity for input from community members.

Continues

4. Public health should advocate and work for the empowerment of disenfranchised community members, aiming to ensure that the basic resources and conditions necessary for health are accessible to all.
5. Public health should seek the information needed to implement effective policies and programs that protect and promote health.
6. Public health institutions should provide communities with the information they have that is needed for decisions on policies or programs and should obtain the community's consent for their implementation.
7. Public health institutions should act in a timely manner on the information they have within the resources and the mandate given to them by the public.
8. Public health programs and policies should incorporate a variety of approaches that anticipate and respect diverse values, beliefs, and cultures in the community.
9. Public health programs and policies should be implemented in a manner that most enhances the physical and social environment.
10. Public health institutions should protect the confidentiality of information that can bring harm to an individual or community if made public. Exceptions must be justified on the basis of the high likelihood of significant harm to the individual or others.
11. Public health institutions should ensure the professional competence of their employees.
12. Public health institutions and their employees should engage in collaborations and affiliations in ways that build the public's trust and the institution's effectiveness.

The development and dissemination of the "Principles of the Ethical Practice of Public Health" is funded primarily by the Centers for Disease Control and Prevention (CDC) through the Public Health Leadership Society (PHLS). The Center for Health Leadership and Practice, Public Health Institute, is acknowledged for its role in the initial development of the principles. PHLS also acknowledges the work of the members of the original PHLS Ethics Work Group (responsible for drafting the code) and the current members of the PHLS Standing Committee on Ethics.

ENVIRONMENTAL CONNECTION

Toxic waste dumps and other contaminants that affect people's health are often located near impoverished and vulnerable populations. What are the ethical implications of this practice, and how does it reflect government accountability for safeguarding the health of all its citizens?

> Be kind, for everyone you meet is fighting a hard battle.
>
> —*Plato*

Beginning in 1977, Beauchamp and Childress (2013) identified four bioethical principles that are now recognized globally as essential to a theory of modern bioethics: **autonomy** (respect for human dignity of all persons), **nonmaleficence** (refraining from harm), **beneficence** (promoting good), and **justice** (fair distribution of burdens and benefits). Other principles, such as sanctity of life, truthfulness, confidentiality, and gratitude, are sometimes added to this list by other writers on ethics (Burkhardt & Nathaniel, 1988; Butts & Rich, 2013; Uustal, 1993). Some ethicists prioritize these principles by saying, for example, that when there is a conflict between principles, the principle of autonomy will take precedence. Others believe that none of the obligations that arise in the course of relationships is primary. Each principle may be overridden in a situation of conflict with another ethical obligation.

Respect for the Autonomy of the Individual

Beauchamp and Childress (2013) defined respect for autonomy as the self-determination of moral decisions that are free from controlling interferences by others and from any personal limitations that prevent meaningful choice, such as lack of understanding. Having respect for an individual's autonomy means understanding and acting on the belief that people have the right to make decisions and take actions based on their own beliefs and value systems.

The concept of autonomy is further elaborated by arguing that respect for autonomy is not just the negative action of not interfering, but also includes the obligation to take positive actions to promote the individual's capacity to be autonomous. An example of a positive action might be to provide care that will restore an individual's capacity to think clearly after a period of confusion. Working with family members to limit their pressure on the patient for a particular decision and providing

> The Buddhist Avatamsaka Sutra contains a story about how all perceiving, thinking beings are connected in a way that is similar to a universal community. The story is about the heavenly net of the god Indra. 'In the heaven of Indra, there is said to be a network of pearls, so arranged that if you look at one you see all the others reflected in it. In the same way each object in the world is not merely itself but involves every other object and in fact is everything else. In every particle of dust there is present Buddhas without number.'
>
> —*Sir Charles Eliot, as cited in F. Capra,* The Tao of Physics *(1999, p. 296)*

information to an individual or community group that needs to make a good decision regarding health care are other examples. Principles of privacy and confidentiality both are derived from respect for autonomy, as is the principle of informed consent, which refers to the patient's agreement to undergo a medical or nursing treatment or be a research subject.

Nonmaleficence

"First, do no harm" has been part of the Hippocratic Oath taken by physicians for centuries and has been a cornerstone of ethical practice in medicine and nursing. For many experts, the principles of nonmaleficence and beneficence are the ends of a continuum relating to harm and obligations to help (Beauchamp & Childress, 2013. In this context, the principle with the highest priority of obligation is that of inflicting no harm. The second priority is that a person should prevent harm. The third priority is that of removing harm. The fourth priority is that of doing or promoting good. Rules that may be said to emerge from the nonmaleficence principle include not killing, not causing pain or suffering, not incapacitating others, not offending others, and not depriving others of the "goods of life." Major ethical issues related to nonmaleficence deal with treatments used to prolong life, such as intubation and artificial feeding.

Justice

Justice may be defined generally as "fair, equitable, and appropriate treatment in light of what is due or owed to persons" (Burkhardt & Nathaniel, 1998, p. 57). The major focus of ethical theories of justice in relation to health care is the concept of "right to health care," often meaning the right to government-subsidized health care for everyone. The arguments for or against the existence of such a right are consistent with the debaters' philosophical and political belief systems regarding the role of government in the lives of individuals.

> Although we can distinguish between ethics and politics, they are inseparable. For we cannot understand ethics without thinking through our political commitments and responsibilities. And there is no understanding of politics that does not bring us back to ethics. Ethics and politics as disciplines concerned with praxis are aspects of a unified, practical philosophy.
>
> —R. J. Bernstein. (1998). *The new constellation: The ethical–political horizons of modernity–postmodernity*. Cambridge, MA: MIT Press.

In addition to being a major concept in the principlist approach to ethics, there are theories of distributive justice that articulate, order, and justify principles that specify just distributions of benefits and burdens (Beauchamp & Childress, 2013). Buchanan (1992) identifies four major theories of justice: utilitarianism, Rawls' justice as fairness, rights-based egalitarianism, and Marxist egalitarianism.

Beneficence

The principle of beneficence has to do with obligations to act in ways that would benefit or provide some good to others. Beauchamp and Childress (2013) focus on two aspects of beneficence: positive beneficence and utility. Positive beneficence provides the rationale for a number of specific moral rules generally accepted by our society (**Box 12-4**).

BOX 12-4 Rules of Positive Beneficence

- Protect and defend the rights of others.
- Prevent harm from occurring to others.
- Help persons with disabilities.
- Rescue persons in danger.

Source: Bauchamp, T., & Childress, J. (1994). *Principles of Biomedical Ethics* (4th ed.). New York, NY: Oxford University Press.

Theoretical arguments about beneficence have to do with the extent to which we are obligated to people who are not in a special relationship with us, the way in which children, parents, and friends are. Are we obligated to everyone, or only to special people? Formalized relationships between healthcare providers and patients have been identified as special relationships that do obligate the provider.

MEDIA MOMENT 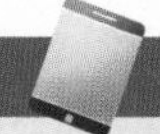

Ethics for the New Millennium (2001)

By the Dalai Lama, New York, NY: Penguin Putnam.

In a modern society characterized by insensitivity to violence, ambivalence to the suffering of others, and a high value placed on the profit motive, is talk of ethics anything more than a temporary salve for our collective conscience? The Dalai Lama thinks so. In his *Ethics for the New Millennium,* the exiled leader of the Tibetan people shows how the basic concerns of all people—happiness based in contentment, appeasement of suffering, forging meaningful relationships—can act as the foundation for a universal ethics.

According to Donaldson (1992), the philosopher David Hume (1711–1776) is credited with first identifying the circumstances under which justice is necessary:

- *Dependence*. Individuals are not self-sufficient. They require the cooperation of nature and of other humans to "achieve certain critical goods."
- *Moderate scarcity*. Some scarcity is required because if there is an overabundance, justice is not required; if there is severe scarcity, a decent life is impossible to achieve.
- *Restrained benevolence*. Humans are generous, but only to a point. They may frequently sacrifice at all levels (family–country), but over the long term, they show a deep-seated resilience to self-interest.
- *Individual vulnerability*. No matter what one's status, anyone can be subject to attack from others.

Utilitarianism and its criticisms were discussed earlier in this chapter. Rawls' "justice as fairness" theory was developed partly as a response to the shortcomings of utilitarianism. Rawls (1999) asks that we imagine an ideal situation in which the principles of justice for a democratic and free society are developed from an "original position" by a group of representative people who are unbiased, in a situation of equality. This "original position" is one where the framers work from a "veil of ignorance," where they do not know who they may be or what position they may hold within the society. Rawls believes that the group members would want to maximize their own positions, whatever those may turn out to be and so, through deliberative rationality, would agree to accept his two principles of justice. **Box 12-5** presents these principles.

The "just savings principle" refers to Rawls' belief that every generation has an obligation to "save" for future generations. Thus, each generation should pass on to the next generation an amount of capital (e.g., factories, infrastructure, and other resources) and those institutions that would ensure their liberty and wellbeing; these assets include ideas and culture. Although it is expected that a given generation will pass on the opportunity for a better life, it is not expected that the generation will unduly deprive itself to do so. Each generation receives from the previous one and gives to the next. What seems to be a reasonable savings depends on the circumstances of each generation.

The general rules are those that would be worked out from the "original position" in which the group members, working behind the "veil of ignorance," do not know which will be their generation. Current generational issues include our Social Security system, natural resource usage, transportation infrastructure, and educational systems.

BOX 12-5 Rawls' Principles of Justice

First Principle

Each person is to have an equal right to the most extensive total system of basic liberties possible in the society. These liberties can be restricted only for the sake of overall liberty. Liberty may be restricted in only two cases: (1) A less extensive than possible liberty must strengthen the total system of liberties for everyone, and (2) a less than equal liberty must be accepted by those affected.

Second Principle

Social and economic inequalities are to be to the most benefit of the least advantaged, and offices and positions must be open to all under conditions of fairness of opportunity. Justice takes priority over efficiency and maximizing the sum of advantages. There are two exceptions: (1) Any inequality of opportunity must be to the advantage of those with lesser opportunity, and (2) an excessive rate of savings must generally decrease the burden of those who bear the hardship.

Critics of Rawls say that his theory demands too much from those who are better off, even when those who are worse off would not suffer or their conditions could not be improved. He is also accused of being too optimistic about the general acceptance of the ideal situation. If too many of the citizens are alienated from the culture, consensus may not be attainable.

Adherents to the philosophy of radical libertarianism take the position that the role of the state is to enforce property rights—not to redistribute wealth, except to rectify past violations of individual property rights. Nozick (1974) responded to Rawls' theory by asserting that enforced redistribution of goods violates individual rights requiring interference with individuals' lives, causing unacceptable disruption. In addition, the redistribution is intuitively unjust. According to Buchanan (1992), Nozick's critics respond that current tax laws provide redistribution with only minimal disruption, and we cannot assume that injustice doesn't arise after an accumulation of individual transactions that, by themselves, appear to be fair.

The original Marxist theories proposed that the need for redistribution would disappear after a class leveling occurred and a common control of the means of production was implemented. Clearly, that has not happened in communist systems, and more moderate Marxists now believe that there will always be a need for a principle of enforced distributive justice. They focus now on Marx's vision of a more rational and humane, post-capitalist society.

MEDIA MOMENT 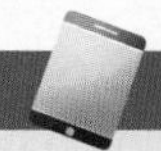

Our Endangered Values: America's Moral Crisis (2006)

By Jimmy Carter, New York, NY: Simon & Schuster.

President Jimmy Carter, Nobel Peace Prize Winner, is one of the most respected voices in the United States today in the areas of human rights, diplomacy, and good government. In his book, *Our Endangered Values: America's Moral Crisis,* Carter presents a series of essays that outline his views about the key ethical and moral issues looming in the 21st century. Topics such as war, environmental negligence, the death penalty, civil liberties, moral responsibilities to the poor, and the separation of church and state are critically debated in the context of Carter's worldview and spiritual philosophy about our role as world citizens.

Justice in Health Care

Although Rawls' theory does not specify health care as a social good, Daniels (1985) believes that a theory of "just health care" was compatible as an extension of Rawls' general theory of justice and developed his theory based on assumptions of "rights to health care" in relation to individual needs. Daniels' composite list of rights is presented here:

- Society has the duty to its members to allocate an adequate share of its total resources to health-related needs, such as the protection of the environment and the provision of medical services.
- Society has the duty to provide a just allocation of different types of health services, taking into account the competing claims of different types of health needs.
- Each person is entitled to a fair share of such services, where "fair share" includes an answer to the question, "Who should pay for the services?" (p. 8)

For Daniels (1985), needs are defined as being "necessary to achieve or maintain species-typical functioning" (p. 26). If there is impairment of this functioning through either disease or disability, individuals are restricted in the expression of the normal range of opportunity their own talents and skills would otherwise allow them. Daniels proposed that the greater the impairment, the more important it is to prevent, cure, or compensate for the disease conditions.

In Daniels' (1985) theory, "normal range of opportunity" is defined for individuals as the reasonable life plans available to them in their particular society if they were healthy. This definition implies that there will still be differences among individuals (e.g., normal genetic endowment and cultural expectations and limitations). The emphasis is on fairness, meaning that society must refrain from imposing barriers to equal opportunity and must correct for interferences to equal opportunity. The assumption of the Rawlsian "veil of ignorance" should be applied here in regard to decisions about needs.

Allocation of societal resources among all social needs and among the various levels of healthcare needs (prevention, cure, restoration, and extended support) requires both moral judgment and extensive empirical knowledge about allocation consequences. Daniels (1985) also points out that protection of opportunity must not undermine a society's productive capacity.

In his analysis, Daniels (1985) deals with two related issues in the application of his theory: equitable access to health care and paternalism. Three general approaches may be taken in dealing with the issue of access. The first is utilization rates, by which differences and similarities in usage among groups are identified. For example, if a service is utilized equally between upper- and lower-class subgroups, equality of access is thought to exist. The second is the process approach, in which process variables are examined to determine whether some variable, such as geographic distance or waiting time, makes the process more burdensome for some. The third approach, the market approach, determines that access is equitable if there are no information, supply, or financial barriers that prevent access to what is referred to as a "reasonable" or "decent basic minimum" of service. Daniels asserts that the "decent minimum" in health care should reflect our ideas of "tolerable life prospects."

Daniels (1985) also proposed a "theory of justifiable paternalism," which relates to issues of equitable risk prevention in the prevention of disease. Reduction of disease risk may include general measures, such as mandatory water and waste treatment from which everyone benefits equally; alternatively, it may be specific, targeting workplace risks where only some individuals are affected. Regulating workplace risk by imposing standards and rules is said by some to be in conflict with an individual's freedom in lifestyle choices and the right to take risks voluntarily.

What needs to be considered is whether the workers (1) are truly informed of all risks to health, (2) are truly able to make a choice without depriving themselves of a reasonable living, and (3) are not subject to overt or covert coercion. Daniels (1985) states:

> In general we ought to preserve autonomy. . . . But we are not bound to preserve the illusion of autonomy. If unregulated worker "choices" about risk-taking must fail, or generally do fail, to be informed, competent, or truly voluntary, then we are not compromising autonomy by intervening. (p. 159)

Communitarian Ethics*

Because of the relationships involved, a community has a "moral nature" as compared to the nature of a population. *Communitarian ethics* is based on the position that all foundational ethics derives from communal values, the common good, societal good, traditional practices, and virtuous actions (Beauchamp & Childress, 2013). Communitarian ethics is applicable to moral relationships within any type of community, both large and small. As an ethical approach, it is distinguished because the epicenter of communitarian ethics is the community rather than beginning from the point of any one individual (Wildes, 2000). Populations in general, and moral communities in particular, are also the starting points for community nursing.

Some ethicists have tried to draw a strong distinction between ethical approaches that emphasize individualism and autonomy as differentiated from communitarian ethics, which emphasizes a common good. However, it is reasonable to assume that people can be interested in both their own wellbeing and the common good of the communities to which they belong. The value of considering communitarian ethics lies in the benefit that can be gained from illuminating and appreciating the relationships and interconnections between people who are often overlooked in everyday life. Although personal moral goals are significant, the importance of forming strong communities and identifying the moral goals of those communities must be appreciated for both individuals and communities to flourish.

An important point that distinguishes communitarian ethics from other ethical approaches, such as deontology or utilitarianism, is communitarians' acceptance that humans naturally favor the people with whom they live and have frequent interactions. Deontologists, for example, base their ethics upon the existence of a more impartial stance toward the persons who are the receivers of their morally related actions.

Communitarians accept partiality as a way of relating to others but also believe that it is realistic to develop empathy and compassion toward people who are personally unknown to them. Nussbaum (2004) suggested that people often develop an "us versus them" mentality, especially when they are separated by significant cultural differences. People are able to generate sympathy when they hear about epidemics and disasters occurring on continents that are far away, but it is usually difficult for people to sustain that level of sympathy for more than a short period of time. People tend to stop and notice others' needs but soon turn back to their own personal lives. According to Nussbaum, humanity will "achieve no lasting moral progress unless and until the daily unremarkable lives of people distant from us become real in the fabric of our own daily lives" (p. 958) and until people include others that they do not know personally within the important sphere of their lives. Nurses must broaden their scope of concern to include people affected by healthcare disparities, diseases, and epidemics all over the world.

> A human being is a part of the whole, called by us the 'universe,' a part limited in time and space. He experiences himself, his thoughts and feelings, as something separated from the rest, a kind of optical delusion of his consciousness. This delusion is a kind of prison for us, restricting us to our personal desires and to affection for a few persons nearest to us. Our task must be to free ourselves from this prison by widening our circle of compassion to embrace all living creatures and the whole of nature in its beauty.
>
> —*Albert Einstein*

All communities have an organizing core vision about the meaning of life and how one ought to live. Community nurses have an important role in bringing populations and communities together to work toward a common humanitarian good. Transforming communities from a "them versus us" mentality to one that seeks a common good is possible through education (Nussbaum, 2004). "Children [and people] at all ages must learn to recognize people in other countries as their fellows, and to sympathize with their plights. Not just their dramatic plights, in a cyclone or war, but their daily plights" (p. 959). This need for empathetic understanding also is important within one's own country, state, town, and neighborhood. Many people are suffering within the United States because they lack adequate health care, food, environmental sanitation, and housing.

The education of communities often occurs through role modeling. Members of communities learn about what is and is not accepted as moral through personal and group interactions and dialogue within their communities. Narratives are told about the lives of exemplars, such as Florence Nightingale in nursing, to illustrate moral living. In Nightingale's efforts to improve social justice and health protection through environmental measures and her efforts to elevate the good character of nurses, she

* This section was adapted from the following source: Rich, K. L. (2013). Public health nursing ethics. In J. B. Butts & K. L. Rich (Eds.), *Nursing ethics: Across the curriculum and into practice* (pp. 321–369). Burlington, MA: Jones & Bartlett Learning.

exhibited moral concern for her local society, the nursing profession, and people remote from her local community, such as people affected by the Crimean War. In learning from Nightingale's example, communitarian-minded nurses are in an excellent position to educate the public and other healthcare professionals about why they in many ways should assume the role of being their "brother's and sister's keeper."

Values and Health Policy

As Schlesinger (2002) explains, historically a market-based model for health care has had a variable level of support in the United States. Support has markedly increased since the beginning of the Reagan administration in the early 1990s. The market-based model views health care as a commodity similar to material goods, subject to the laws of supply and demand in relation to availability and cost. It has competed with two alternative models: the medical professionalism model and the societal rights model.

THINK ABOUT THIS 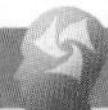

Where, after all, do universal human rights begin? In small places, close to home—so close and so small that they cannot be seen on any map of the world. Yet they are the world of the individual person: the neighborhood he lives in; the school or college he attends; the factory, farm, or office where he works. Such are the places where every man, woman, and child seeks equal justice, equal opportunity, equal dignity without discrimination. Unless these rights have meaning there, they have little meaning anywhere. Without concerted citizen action to uphold them close to home, we shall look in vain for progress in the larger world.

—Eleanor Roosevelt (1884–1962), U.S. author, diplomat, and First Lady, statements at presentation of "In Your Hands: A Guide for Community Action for the Tenth Anniversary of the Universal Declaration of Human Rights," March 27, 1958

How has the United States changed since 1958 in regard to justice, as related to health care?

The medical professionalism model rejects the idea that consumers are competent to make good medical choices, arguing that medical care is too complex and still under development. Proponents of this model believe that medical providers should make healthcare decisions. The Great Depression of the 1930s saw the emergence of the "societal rights" framework. In the early 1940s, President Franklin Roosevelt called for the rights for all to medical care and the opportunity to achieve and enjoy good health.

The role of the government within the medical professional model is to promote scientific knowledge and the training of professionals. By contrast, in the social rights model, the role of government is to ensure a standard of equality and equal access to services. The then-dominant "rights" model during the 1960s and 1970s saw increases in the role of the government with the establishment and expansion of programs such as Medicare, Medicaid, and other health and social programs. The swing toward the market model was driven primarily by the marked increases in the costs of these healthcare programs. In the market model, the role of government is to support fair competition among providers.

Political conservatives have been among the entities most interested in cost reduction and in reduction of the role of government in health services. However, liberals were also supportive of "managed competition," believing it would transform medical care by breaking up the entrenched interests of the medical profession and make it more responsive to consumers—hence the support from the Clinton administration for expansion of managed care.

In spite of the support from both conservatives and liberals, there had been little real progress toward healthcare reform prior to the passage of the Affordable Care Act (ACA) in 2010. Many proposals had been attempted, but until recently, at least, the reform had been limited. In an effort to understand these failures, Schlesinger (2002) carried out a series of research studies examining the values held by liberals and conservatives of both the "Washington elite" (congressional staff who had designated responsibility for health issues) and the general public. Respondents were supportive of a market model, yet they held very different views about issues of responsibility and equity in health care.

Schlesinger found that while 58% of congressional health staff supported the market model for healthcare reform, only 41% of the general public did so. When he compared the congressional staff with the general public on the responsibility measures, he found that market advocates among the elite were almost twice as likely as nonadvocates to agree that individuals should be responsible for their own health care. By comparison, market advocates of the public were slightly less likely than nonadvocates to support the personal responsibility statements. The differences between the groups were even more pronounced when Schlesinger considered the norms of fairness items. He concluded that these differences between the general public and the congressional elite may account for the problems that have emerged in trying to implement a market approach to healthcare reform.

Ethic of Care

The previously discussed theories have in common the use of moral principles to guide behavior. These theories are concerned with the rights of individuals within a society and the obligations of individuals to others and to society. A more recently developed theory, known as the **ethic of care**, takes a different position—namely, that relationships and responsibilities are more important than rights and obligations or outcomes. In this approach, the primary focus is on the wellbeing of the whole person. This means that the nurse is concerned with all aspects of the patient's wellbeing, not merely the disease process. Care is designed for needs in all realms—physical, psychological, social, and spiritual—with the understanding that each affects the others and the totality of health. The broader social environment that affects the patient, such as the family, is also of concern. Nursing actions are deemed ethical when they take into consideration this whole person, who is labeled "the patient". They are unethical when they focus on the disease process or disability.

There is also a component of compassion, which is a precursor to caring. The nurse who practices from this care approach will be concerned with developing personal characteristics and taking actions that will show caring. This ethical approach is still developing within nursing, where care has always been central. There are many barriers within the present healthcare system that interfere with care for the whole person, such as a technology focus, managed care, and specialization (Purtillo, 1999).

The ethic of care rings true for many nurses who believe it describes the context of and their feelings about their work. It is the connectedness and responsibility for having met the needs of individuals under their care that give satisfaction. Benner (1984) provides many examples from her interviews that support this view.

The person living a caring ethic bases his or her actions on the needs of those for whom the individual cares, either naturally or in a formal caring relationship. For the community health nurse, the focus changes from the individual to the population, but responding to needs at all levels remains the same (see **Box 12-6**).

BOX 12-6 The Ethic of Care

- The focus is on the whole individual.
- The caregiver has a responsibility to meet the needs of those for whom the person is caring.
- There is an affective element of compassion in the relationship.

Ethical Problems Faced by Community Health Nurses: The Research

Several studies identifying the ethical problems related to community health nursing have been conducted by nurse researchers in both the United States and other countries. In one study, Aroskar (1989) sent questionnaires to more than 1,000 staff nurses who worked in community health and public health agencies in Minnesota. More than 300 nurses responded, listing the problems they had encountered. Aroskar categorized the problems according to the type of ethical conflict they represented. These categories and some examples are shown in **Box 12-7**.

BOX 12-7 Community Health Nursing Problems Categorized by Ethical Conflict

Conflict Between Autonomy and Beneficence

- Getting patients to be responsible for their own care and wellbeing
- Wishes and rights of patients about living, dying, and refusing treatment
- Unnecessary treatment (use of narcotics)
- Apparent negligence of a child without evidence to report
- Refusal of treatment when the patient's condition is deteriorating

Conflict Between Truth-Telling and Nonmaleficence

- Stretching the truth or game-playing to satisfy criteria for treatment
- Withholding information or lying to the patient about diagnosis or treatment
- Nonbetrayal of colleagues to the patient and/or family about quality of care

Distributive Justice

- Unnecessary government subsidization for low-income families
- Lack of funds for medical care
- Struggle for equal care, regardless of race or finances

Source: This article was published in Nursing Clinics of North America, 24(4), Aroskar, M., Community health nurses: Their most significant ethical decision-making problems, pp. 967–975, Copyright Elsevier 1989.

In a survey of 40 public health nurses in southern Louisiana, Folmar, Coughlin, Bessinger, and Sackoff (1997) found similar results to those uncovered by Aroskar.

In another study, using a list of 39 ethical problems, 745 hospital and community nurses were asked to indicate each one they had encountered in the last 12 months.

The researchers (Wagner & Ronen, 1996) reported the 10 most frequently encountered dilemmas. Again, the major issues were similar to those found in previous studies. The community health nurses reported similar issues to those faced by the hospital nurses, but generally encountered them less frequently.

Gremmen (1999), using a grounded study method, interviewed 33 Dutch visiting (district) nurses, asking them about what they considered to be central to their work. This researcher was interested in the nurses' moral reasoning about their work. The theoretical focus of her study was on the apparent conflict between an ethic of care and an ethic of justice. The nurses described how they handled situations in which patients were resistant to treatment. Analysis of the interview data showed three parts to the process the nurses described, which Gremmen labeled "tuning in to the patients' lives," "convincing or even pushing patients while not forcing them," and "not withdrawing from patients while disagreeing with them." It was her conclusion that care and justice are both crucial to the work of public health nurses and can be complementary.

As part of a study of 30 community health nurses in British Columbia, Canada, Duncan (1992) asked them to report the clinical situations that created ethical dilemmas. One condition involved "patients' rights," specifically related to high-risk families, adults with mental health concerns, and adolescents who were at risk but didn't want their families involved. A second condition was described as "system interaction"—that is, problematic situations between nurses and consumers and problems with inadequate resources. "Allocation of resources" included problems about limiting resources for resistant patients, allocating visits, and effectiveness. "Nurses' rights" was the final condition. Employment contracts, high caseloads, and limited resources jeopardized the nurses' rights to act according to their own values.

> It is not unusual that moral uncertainty is first experienced and escalates to moral distress as patients' rights are not respected or as institutional constraints are applied and nurses feel unable to act on their moral choices and judgments.
>
> —A. Hamrick. (2000). Moral distress in everyday ethics. *Nursing Outlook, 48,* 199.

Oberle and Tenova (2000) asked 22 Canadian public health nurses the following: "Please describe a frequently recurring ethical problem (or problems) that you have experienced in practice—something that has been a common problem for you." Follow-up questions related to support and how they resolved the problems. The researchers identified the following five themes based on their analysis of the transcribed interviews:

- *Relationships with healthcare professionals.* Relationships were ethical problems when they prevented the nurse from delivering optimal care—for example, the physician denigrating the nurses' advice, one-way communication only, and observing inferior care.
- *Systems issues.* Systems issues included resource distribution, such as performance of quality care with inadequate resources; choices about offering programs, including how much and to whom; and too few resources.
- *Patient relationships.* This theme encompassed issues such as the context and nature of the relationships, empowerment versus dependency, and boundary setting. The fact that the patient controlled the continued existence of the relationship challenged the nurses to find ways to establish working and trusting relationships. They had to decide between not intervening in some events to maintain the relationship and taking action to stop risky behavior (e.g., poor parenting). Professional versus personal relationship issues were more problematic in rural settings, when patients were encountered in social settings.
- *Respect for persons.* Respecting autonomy was interlaced with all the themes and was seen as foundational to public health nursing. The issues in regard to autonomy were the questioning of whose rights (among family members) should be supported, deciding when someone was unable to make their own decisions, and learning how to be a confidante and still maintain confidentiality when the information was something that would be helpful to other providers.
- *Putting self at risk.* Situations involving risks to the nurse's personal integrity and physical danger were the issues in this theme.

Ethical Decision Making

Dozens of institutes and centers, most of which are associated with universities, focus on the study of bioethics. Some universities offer degree programs in ethics and in clinical ethics. More and more often, healthcare agencies use qualified ethicists on ethics committees as consultants to help them with ethical problems. In larger agencies, nurses are able to consult ethicists to help them with ethical decision making.

Often, however, nurses themselves must reason through the ethical problems they encounter. Several authors have presented decision-making models, most of which are based on a problem-solving format. The common steps in the process include the following:

1. Determine how these problems affect the autonomy and quality of life of the individual. For example, is the person mentally competent? Is the health problem life-threatening? Is the individual able to communicate and relate to others? To what extent can the individual care for himself or herself? Is the problem likely to get worse? What kinds of treatments are available, proposed, and usual? Are the treatments likely to have positive outcomes? How painful or intrusive are they? What information does the person have about the problem?
2. Separate the ethical issues from those of a strictly medical nature and determine which individuals and groups will be affected by the decision. For example, what is important for the patient? Which principles are involved: respecting the person, preventing harm, doing good, providing justice, maximizing outcomes for the greater number? Who are the stakeholders in this situation: family, hospital or agency administration, physicians, nurses, the community?
3. Identify and understand the values of those who will be affected, including those of the nurse. What do the individuals involved think about relevant issues, such as quality of life, prolonging life at all costs, autonomy in the face of increased risks, suffering, and the responsibilities of caring?
4. Develop alternative options and weigh them in the light of the rights and obligations of all concerned. What harms and benefits accrue to each of the stakeholders in relation to each option? If a patient refuses chemotherapy, for example, does this decision conflict with the physician's belief that such treatment will be beneficial? Will a family member feel guilty because "everything possible" wasn't done? Are there financial savings for third-party payers?
5. Decide on a course of action and later evaluate the outcome. Part of the decision includes determining who should make the decision.

This framework was designed primarily for use in situations involving individual or family care. Kass (2001) has developed a six-step framework for public health and aggregate populations that poses questions to be asked of program developers:

1. *What are the public health goals of the proposed program?* The goals should be related to reduction of morbidity or mortality. The goal may be an intermediary one, but there should be awareness of the relationship to the ultimate goal.
2. *How effective is the program in achieving its stated goals?* This step requires that assumptions about the effects of the program be identified and documented to the extent possible from previous research or program results.
3. *What are the known or potential burdens of the program?* There are usually three major burdens associated with public health programs: risks to privacy and confidentiality, risks to liberty, and risks to justice. Disease surveillance and vital statistics, communicable disease reporting, and contact tracing all have the risk of loss of confidentiality. The burdens of these programs are borne by the target groups for the benefit of all others, and there is a risk of biased reporting. Health education programs include the possibility that they may not work, may involve manipulation or coercion, and are potentially paternalistic. If findings from research studies are never implemented, there is potential harm to participants who have been misled about the goals of the project. Regulation and legislation constrain freedom of choice and often target some groups for the benefit of others (immunization, motorcycle helmets, smoking).
4. *Can burdens be minimized? Are there alternative approaches?* Programs must be modified to impose the least burden possible without decreasing effectiveness.
5. *Is the program implemented fairly?* Burdens and benefits must be distributed fairly and not solely to specific targeted populations without adequate justification.
6. *How can the benefits and burdens of a program be fairly balanced?* Health officials and professionals have a responsibility to promote programs that increase health benefits and to prevent programs that are unethical. Minority opinions must be taken into account; however, dissent is not a reason not to implement a program. The greater the burden imposed by a program, the greater must be its benefits.

One time-honored approach to ethical decision making entails comparing the present case to those in the past. This process, known as **casuistry**, starts with identifying the relevant points and finding how this case is the same or different and which principles then apply. This approach has been foundational for developing church and judicial precedents.

Service-Learning: Discovering the Self and Developing Community Values*

One skill needed for developing ethical responses is what is called a *moral imagination*. In Kohlberg's terms, the imagination develops with moral growth (Kohlberg, 1981). This imagination gives one the ability to see the moral dimensions of more situations and to empathize with more issues, sides, and sentiments. Such an active imagination is developed with experience and contact with events, situations, and others' ideas. What are your beliefs about the importance and effects of your own personal decisions and actions in the world of nursing and society? How might you find out? What are your values, positions, and beliefs about those people beyond your familiar community? How have you learned those values? Might they change? Do you really know your community? Who do you want to include or exclude from your personal community and why? What are the experiences of people who are different from you? The more these questions are asked and reflected on, the greater the moral imagination.

Even though learning by experience has always been a part of nursing through clinicals, practicums, and laboratory assignments, a new interest has grown in a different form of experiential learning called **service-learning**. Service-learning emphasizes needs and benefits to an actual group of persons or community rather than solely focusing on student academic and career learning. It is also distinguished by having an overt goal of developing a social consciousness, values, and skills regarding civic responsibility. In addition, to truly be service-learning, it must include a strong emphasis on personal insight with planned methods and scheduled time for self-reflection and self-discovery.

The focus with this approach is on the lessons learned and insights gained from performing service work, not just clinical or professional intervention. The learner in performing a service is a "servant" to others. Many in nursing believe that service-learning can help nursing develop and strengthen the legacy of values believed to underlie both nursing and public health. Service-learning lets students face situations in which they foster intangible qualities and values such as empathy, self-awareness, self-confidence, a caring activism to advocate for health, a sense of democratic civic responsibility, a global ecological awareness, cultural competence, and social justice. These are learned in such a way as to become part of a student's life experiences; in turn, these experiences develop the moral imagination.

Even if your university does not have a service-learning program, you can apply some of the methods yourself. When working in community centers, such as daycare centers, Meals on Wheels, senior centers, youth services, soup kitchens, drug education programs, and so on, think beyond the patients' immediate health concerns. Think also about what it feels like to see you "serving" them. Is "serving" a positive image for nurses? How can a group or community best be "served"? What is in their best interest? What gets in the way of meeting their needs? How can members of the group be empowered to help themselves? Which organizational, local, state, or federal policies need to be changed to assist them? How do you feel about the needy? What did you or anyone else do to contribute to their situation? What are your beliefs about them and their situations? Are justice and care present in their lives? How much are you influenced by the beliefs of your friends, family, church, and the dominant society? Do you have any obligations to the members of the group beyond their physical health concerns? Would your personal beliefs and values ever make a difference?

Conclusion

Because of the special relationship nurses have as care providers to their patients, they are frequent participants in ethical decision making related to patients, families, and the community. Expectations of the community and the profession require that nurses possess certain virtues that will promote trust in all their professional relationships. Ethical decision making is based on the particular values individuals have acquired both as children and as thinking adults.

This chapter has presented the major thinking of philosophers, theologians, and other ethicists over the centuries. It should be clear that there is disagreement on generalities and on specifics. It is characteristic of the United States that there is wide variation in cultural, religious, educational, and ethnic backgrounds, and it is inevitable that values will also differ. We do, however, have many values in common. More recent philosophical approaches (post-modernism) present the view that there are no certainties and no foundational beliefs: We must each make our own way.

The value of understanding the principles of ethical theories is that it provides us with starting points for thinking through and developing our own set of beliefs, and our own frame of reference for the practice of nursing. For whether we like it or not, we are involved in situations that demand an ethical response almost daily in our work.

* This section was written by Dr. Sherry Hartman, Associate Professor Emeritus, University of Southern Mississippi, College of Nursing.

APPLICATION TO PRACTICE 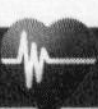

The Need for Home Care

Lila S., age 68, was referred to a home health agency after her discharge from an acute care agency, where she had been hospitalized for pneumonia and stabilization of her diabetes with insulin regulation. She lived with her 6-year-old granddaughter in a small, grimy, cluttered trailer. The whereabouts of the girl's father were unknown, and her mother was in and out of drug treatment units.

Lila's poor eyesight from cataracts made it difficult for her to test her blood glucose or measure her insulin. Painful leg ulcers and arthritis made it difficult for her to walk.

Medicaid allowed four home visits by the nurse. This nurse had made home visits to Lila in the past and saw that her ability to care for herself had decreased and that she would need more help in the future. Lila S. has always been quite independent and does not agree that she is not taking care of herself well. She believes it is important that she maintain a home for her granddaughter.

Medical Issues

- It is important that Lila's glucose be monitored and that her insulin dosage be adjusted accordingly. Her diabetes is fairly stable but needs careful monitoring because of the severe episode of hyperglycemia that accompanied the pneumonia.
- Lila's poor eyesight increases the probability that she will make errors in her diabetes regimen.
- Lila's leg ulcers require care and should be monitored by a knowledgeable person.
- Lila's diminished mobility decreases her ability to go to sources of help.

Based on her assessment, the nurse decides that Lila S. needs a nurse to visit several times a week to monitor the glucose readings and help her adjust dosage and inject her insulin. Ideally, these visits should be done every day. An appeal made to the Medicaid reviewer for additional visits was denied, and the home health agency closed the case.

Ethical Issues

The nurse understood that the agency must have reimbursement for the services it provides; however, she believed that she and the agency had an obligation to continue care that they had begun for this patient, who was obviously in need and whose lack of care might be life-threatening. Legally, no such obligation exists. Various possibilities were discussed with the patient, including trying to find someone she could live with or who could live with her, or going to a nursing home. Lila S. was insistent that she remain at home and care for her granddaughter. The ethical issues involved in this situation are as follows:

- The right of the patient to decide how she wants to live (autonomy)
- The responsibility of the nurse to do no harm or to prevent harm by not abandoning the patient (nonmaleficence) or causing harm to the granddaughter
- The responsibility of the nurse to provide competent care, directly or indirectly, to the patient (beneficence)
- The justice of a healthcare system that will not pay for needed health care that would be less expensive and likely prevent the otherwise high probability that the patient will need more expensive care later

Utilitarian Approach

Utilitarians would start with the question, "Who would be affected by decisions in this instance?" The person most affected is the patient herself; the next most affected is her granddaughter. The nurse and the home health agency also have some stake. Finally, society in general may be affected. In determining what would accomplish the most good for the most people, the effect of the decision on society would have the highest priority. Continuing home care to this patient might be expensive at the time, but the long-range projection is that without the immediate care, the patient will probably need much more expensive treatment and additional hospitalizations later. Based on concrete information about costs, utilitarians would most likely decide in favor of continuing visits. They may also attempt to change the laws or regulations that tend to prohibit the more cost-effective solution.

Deontological Approach

The deontological, rule-based approach would examine the rights and obligations of the participants and determine which had higher priority. The foremost right is the right of the patient to make her own decisions based on her own values. The providers are obligated to determine whether the patient is competent to make rational decisions.

There is no reason to believe that Lila S. is incompetent, except for her unawareness that she is less able to care for herself. She values her independence and should be allowed to remain in her home. The providers are then obligated to allow and, preferably, support that choice by providing services to help her remain at home.

Another right of the individual is that of not being harmed by others. The healthcare providers must examine the medical and social information to determine whether the actions they take will be harmful in any way. Given the current situation, two alternatives present themselves. First, Lila S. remains in her home. It is probable that her diabetes will again go out of control. She will need hospitalization and may possibly need amputations. In this instance, she remains autonomous but incurs harm in the progression of her health problems. A second alternative is that Lila S. is persuaded to enter a nursing home, where she can get daily help with her medical and physical needs. The harm in this scenario is that her sense of self as an independent person may be damaged, and she may feel guilty for not taking care of her granddaughter. Whether the deontologist values autonomy or nonmaleficence most, the preferred solution for Lila S. would be continuing home visits.

Additional harm may be incurred by separating the granddaughter from her grandmother, who has provided a stable home and, presumably, love. If the granddaughter were older, she might be enlisted to help with the insulin injections, and perhaps the grandmother will not suffer any serious problems until the granddaughter is of an age to help.

The justice consideration is readily evident in this case: What would seem to be a decent minimum of care cannot be provided because the woman is poor. It is not clear that Lila S. was born disadvantaged, except that diabetes has a large genetic component. Being poor does mean you may not get the early health care you need and may suffer more negative consequences than others.

Caring Approach

The major focus of the caring approach to this ethics problem will be the responsibilities of the nurse to the patient with whom she has a formal caring relationship. The legal contract for the relationship stipulates a certain number of visits, but the emotional contract has a broader scope. The patient will expect that the nurse will do everything possible to help her achieve her health goals. These expectations may include not abandoning the patient while she still needs help.

The nurse will respond to these expectations and try various avenues to enlist the help Lila S. needs to remain at home. If all else fails and the agency cannot continue visits; the Medicaid administration will not change the ruling; and no relatives, friends, or neighbors can be found to help, there is one last solution. The nurse may decide to utilize personal time, such as lunch hours to provide the needed nursing care. This kind of devotion is above and beyond what is expected legally or ethically, but the feeling of responsibility for some patients may generate that kind of behavior.

In all of the approaches described for this case, the issue of financial support is important. If finances were not a barrier, Lila would get all the help she needed to maintain herself and her granddaughter at home and satisfactorily manage her health needs. It is impossible to consider health care for individuals or groups without considering the benefits and cost to society. Even though a person may take a deontological or a caring approach to ethical decision making, most of the time the ultimate financial outcome must be considered.

ART CONNECTION

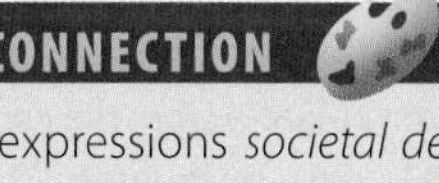

The expressions *societal decline, decay or decadence,* and *indulgent behavior* are generally referred to as a decline or decay of ethics, morals, and social norms in the abstraction. This concept is often portrayed in history and in art as people acting in a self-indulgent manner in a celebratory setting. Common usage of these conditions generally accepts the idea that such declines inevitably precede the destruction of the select culture or society. Social generation is related to ethics in the chaos of such rapid change in normative ethics and rules. In the late 19th century, Henryk Siemiradzki, a Russian painter, portrayed the imminent fall of the Roman Empire through his painting *Roman Orgy in the Time of Caesars* (1872). Find an image of the painting on the Internet and describe how the painting reflects the mood of decadence, moral conflict, and self-indulgence. Discuss how this painting reflects the contents of this chapter.

LEVELS OF PREVENTION

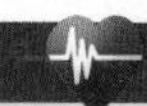

Primary: Using the ANA's *Code of Ethics for Nurses* as a guide to practice

Secondary: Acknowledging that principles of ethics may result in an ethical dilemma and conflict, such as mandatory reporting of a patient with a sexually transmitted infection to the state department of health.

Tertiary: If an ethical violation has occurred as a result of mandatory reporting of an infectious disease, explain to the patient why the violation occurred.

AFFORDABLE CARE ACT (ACA)

The nursing profession was the first of all health professions and professional health groups to support the creation of the Medicare federal program in 1958. How does this reflect our ethical values about health care?

Source: American Academy of Nursing. (2010). *Implementing Health Care Reform: Issues for Nursing.* Retrieved from http://www.aannet.org/assets/docs/implementinghealthcarereform.pdf

Critical Thinking Activities

1. Some nursing students cheat on examinations. This implies an absence of virtue, and many believe that those individuals cannot then be trusted to be honest about the care they give to patients, because they may endanger patients by lying to protect themselves about errors or omissions of treatment. Should dishonest students be denied a license to practice nursing? What is the responsibility of other students who know about the cheating?
2. As a patient or as a family member of a patient, what virtues would you expect of a nurse? Is it reasonable to expect these virtues?
3. A 14-year-old girl revealed to the school nurse that she was sexually active and wanted contraceptive medications. She had seen many of her peers become pregnant, and she stated that she was not ready for a child, but planned to continue her sexual activity. What are the ethical considerations for the nurse in this situation?
4. John, age 32, is known to the public health clinic staff from his visits for intramuscular haloperidol injections. He has spent time in the state hospital, where he was diagnosed with paranoid schizophrenia. John was stabilized on medication and discharged to live with his sister, who is married and has four children. He stayed with her only 2 weeks; he now lives under a bridge. He eats irregularly and has poor hygiene. The original plan was for John to be seen at the mental health clinic, but he refuses to go there. Most of the time his sister is able to persuade him to obtain his medication at the public health clinic. Recently, his sister reported that John is thin and appears ill. He refuses to return to her home and, when pressed, becomes angry and shouts that he wants to be left alone. The sister has appealed to the clinic staff to do something. What are the ethical considerations in this situation?
5. Select a local public health program you know about, or develop one you believe your community needs. Show how this program does or does not meet the ethical criteria proposed by Kass (2001).
6. In a large general hospital, many nurses and auxiliary personnel complain to the clinic staff about chronic back pain related to their jobs. The hospital administration has not been responsive to their complaints. Is this an instance in which regulation of ergonomic devices by the Occupational Safety and Health Administration should be required, or would this be unnecessary paternalism?
7. Develop a healthcare plan for your state that follows Daniels' justice theory. Start by identifying your values and goals.

HEALTHY ME

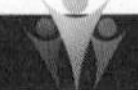

Develop your own written ethical code of conduct and values about caring for populations in terms of working with scarce resources, such as time, resources, and energy.

References

American Nurses Association (ANA). (2001). *Code of ethics for nurses with interpretive statements.* Silver Spring, MD: Author.

Aristotle. (1975). *Aristotle's Nichomachean ethics* (trans. and ed. by H. Apostle). Grinnell, IA: Peripatetic Press.

Aroskar, M. (1989). Community health nurses: Their most significant ethical decision-making problems. *Nursing Clinics of North America, 24*(4), 967–975.

Beauchamp, T., & Childress, J. (2013). *Principles of biomedical ethics* (7th ed.). New York, NY: Oxford University Press.

Benner, P. (1984). *From novice to expert: Excellence and power in clinical nursing practice.* Menlo Park, CA: Addison-Wesley.

Bernstein, R. J. (1998). *The new constellation: The ethical–political horizons of modernity–postmodernity.* Cambridge, MA: MIT Press.

Bishop, A. H., & Scudder, J. (1990). *The practical, moral, and personal sense of nursing: A phenomenological philosophy of practice.* Albany, NY: State University of New York Press.

Buchanan, A. (1992). Distributive justice. In L. Becker & C. Becker (Eds.), *Encyclopedia of ethics* (Vol. I, pp. 655–661). New York, NY: Garland.

Burkhardt, M., & Nathaniel, A. (1998). *Ethics and issues in contemporary nursing.* Albany, NY: Delmar.

Butts, J. B. (2013). Ethical issues in end-of-life nursing care. In J. B. Butts & K. L. Rich (Eds.), *Nursing ethics: Across the curriculum and into practice* (3rd ed., pp 243–286). Burlington, MA: Jones & Bartlett Learning.

Butts, J. B., & Rich, K. L. (Eds.). (2013). *Nursing ethics: Across the curriculum and into practice* (3rd ed.). Burlington, MA: Jones & Bartlett Learning.

Daniels, N. (1985). *Just health care.* New York, NY: Cambridge University Press.

Davis, A., & Aroskar, M. (1991). *Ethical dilemmas and nursing practice.* Norwalk, CT: Appleton & Lange.

Donaldson, T. (1992). Circumstances of justice. In L. Becker & C. Becker (Eds.), *Encyclopedia of ethics* (Vol. I, pp. 653–655). New York, NY: Garland.

Duncan, S. (1992). Ethical challenges in community health nursing. *Journal of Advanced Nursing, 17*, 1035–1041.

Folmar, J., Coughlin, S., Bessinger, R., & Sackoff, D. (1997). Ethics in public health practice: A survey of public health nurses in southern Louisiana. *Public Health Nursing, 14*(3), 156–160.

Gremmen, I. (1999). Visiting nurses' situated ethics: Beyond care versus justice. *Nursing Ethics*, 6(6), 515–528.

Kant, I. (1997). *Groundwork of the metaphysics of morals* (original work published 1785; trans. and ed. by M. Gregor). Cambridge, UK: Cambridge University Press.

Kass, N. (2001). An ethics framework for public health. *American Journal of Public Health*, *9*(11), 1776–1782.

Kohlberg, L. (1981). *The philosophy of moral development: Moral stages and the idea of justice (essays on moral development, volume 1).* New York, NY: Harper & Row.

Mill, J. (1993). *On liberty and utilitarianism*. New York, NY: Bantam Books. (Original work published 1859/1871)

Nozick, R. (1974). *Anarchy, state, and utopia*. New York, NY: Basic Books.

Nussbaum, M. (2004). Compassion and terror. In L. P. Pojman (Ed), *The moral life: An introductory reader in ethics an literature* (2nd ed., pp 937–961).

Oberle, K., & Tenora, S. (2000). Ethical issues in public health nursing. *Nursing Ethics*, *7*(5), 425–439.

Purtillo, R. (1999). *Ethical dimensions in the health professions* (3rd ed.). Philadelphia, PA: Saunders.

Rawls, J. (1999). *A theory of justice* (rev. ed.). Cambridge, MA: Belknap Press.

Rich, K. L. (2013a). Ethical theories and approaches. In J. B. Butts & K. L. Rich (Eds.), *Nursing ethics: Across the curriculum and into practice* (3rd ed., pp. 3–30). Burlington, MA: Jones & Bartlett Learning.

Rich, K. L. (2013b). Public health nursing ethics. In J. B. Butts & K L. Rich (Eds.), *Nursing ethics: Across the curriculum and into practice* (3rd ed., pp. 321–369). Burlington, MA: Jones & Bartlett Learning.

Schlesinger, M. (2002). On values and democratic policy making: The deceptively fragile consensus around market-oriented medical care. *Journal of Health Politics, Policy, and Law*, *27*(6), 889–925.

Steele, S., & Harmon, V. (1983). *Values clarification in nursing* (2nd ed.). Norwalk, CT: Appleton-Century-Crofts.

Uustal, D. (1993). *Clinical and ethical values: Issues and insights*. East Greenwich, RI: Educational Resources in Health Care.

Wagner, N., & Ronen, I. (1996). Ethical dilemmas experienced by hospital and community nurses: An Israeli survey. *Nursing Ethics: An International Journal for Health Care Professionals*, *3*(4), 294–304.

Wildes, K. (2000). *Moral acquaintances: Methodology in bioethics.* Notre Dame, IN: University of Notre Dame Press.

CHAPTER FOCUS

Upstream Thinking: Making Connections Between Environmental and Human Health

Trends in Exposure and Disease

A World View

The Environment and Health

- Environmental Health Policy: Historical Perspectives
- Recent Environmental Health Issues
- Historical Perspectives on Environment and Health
- Origins of Environmental Health Policy
- Environmental Policy: Government and Public Roles

Nursing and the Environment

Roles of the Community Health Nurse

- Identifying Risks
- Assessing Exposures
- Communicating Risks
- Assessing and Referring Patients

Ethical Principles Addressing Environmental Health Nursing

QUESTIONS TO CONSIDER

After reading this chapter, you will know the answers to the following questions:

1. Which specific global environmental threats affect public health?
2. What are current trends in disease and exposure in the environment?
3. What is the history of environmental health in the United States?
4. What is environmental health policy?
5. How does environmental health policy evolve?
6. What is the government's role in environmental health policy?
7. What are the specific roles of the community health nurse in promoting a healthy environment?
8. What is an exposure assessment, and how is it conducted?
9. What is the role of effective communication in the education of community residents?
10. What is upstream thinking, and how is it related to environmental health?
11. What are the key ethical principles related to the environment?
12. How does a community health nurse develop a clinical practice in environmental health?

CHAPTER 13

Environmental Health

Carole J. Nyman,
Patricia Butterfield,
and Karen Saucier Lundy

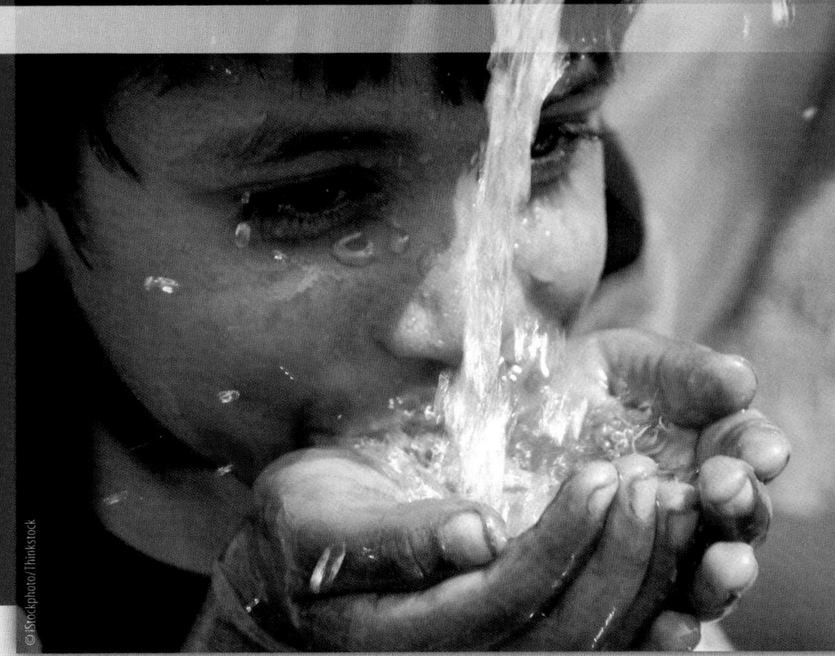
© iStockphoto/Thinkstock

KEY TERMS

environmental health
environmental justice
risk assessment
risk management
social justice
toxicology
toxins
upstream thinking

> Only after the last tree has been cut down,
>
> Only after the last river has been poisoned,
>
> Only after the last fish has been caught,
>
> Only then will you find that money cannot be eaten.
>
> —Cree Indian Philosophy

> There are five essential points in securing the health of houses:
>
> 1. Pure air
> 2. Pure water
> 3. Efficient drainage
> 4. Cleanliness
> 5. Light
>
> —Florence Nightingale, 1860

REFLECTIONS

As you reflect on your personal relationship with the environment, how do these quotes reflect changes through the past century of humans and their environment? As nurses, do we consider environmental influences as we care for our patients?

WHEREVER A POPULATION EXISTS, THE IMPACT of environmental agents on human health is obvious when exposures are high and health effects are immediate. Nurses are most likely to see this type of situation in emergency departments or poison control centers. Frantic parents might call to report that their 3-year-old daughter was found playing with a bag of fertilizer in the garage. A young father, stripping woodwork in a spare basement room, may be brought into the emergency departments by his wife after being overcome by fumes from paint stripper. An elderly woman may be found unconscious in her home after using her gas stove burners to heat her small apartment. In each situation, nurses and other professionals organize a collective response to an immediate health crisis precipitated by an environmental agent. Detoxification procedures begin, and emergency efforts focus on protecting a person's target organ systems. In these scenarios, the link between an environmental exposure and human health is clear. It is easy to see that harmful consequences can result from a single exposure to a toxic agent.

However, acute exposures represent only the tip of the iceberg in the domain of environmental health. In most situations, associations between exposures and disease are not easily traced; years or decades may have elapsed between exposure to the agent of concern and subsequent health effects. In addition, exposures may have occurred in small doses over time or may involve contact with a variety of compounds that interact with each other to cause small changes that ultimately lead to disease. An additional complicating factor is that, for many environmental factors, inconclusive science characterizes associations between exposure and the development of disease. Climate change (or "global warming") remains a constant concern throughout the world, and the 21st century continues to see the results of these changes in extreme weather patterns and effects on the global population.

Because of these and other considerations, environmental health is one of the most challenging and rapidly developing aspects of community health nursing. Fortunately, for many nurses, it is also one of the most rewarding areas of practice. Florence Nightingale is considered the first to recognize the role of the nurse in addressing environmental issues in the hospital, at home, in the workplace, and in the community. In 2010, the American Nurses Association added environmental health principles to its Standards of Professional Practice, which further recognizes the critical expectations of the professional nurse's role in knowing environmental risks and implementing risk-mitigation strategies. Nurses have a unique place in the promotion of a healthy environment and prevention of environmental hazards for all populations. The American Nurses Association's Principles of Environmental Health for Nursing Practice are provided in **Box 13-1**.

BOX 13-1 American Nurses Association's Principles of Environmental Health for Nursing Practice

1. Knowledge of environmental health concepts is essential to nursing practice.
2. The Precautionary Principle guides nurses in their practice to use products and practices that do not harm human health or the environment and to take preventive action in the face of uncertainty.
3. Nurses have a right to work in an environment that is safe and healthy.
4. Healthy environments are sustained through multidisciplinary collaboration.
5. Choices of materials, products, technology, and practices in the environment that impact nursing practice are based on the best evidence available.
6. Approaches to promoting a healthy environment respect the diverse values, beliefs, cultures, and circumstances of patients and their families.
7. Nurses participate in assessing the quality of the environment in which they practice and live.
8. Nurses, other healthcare workers, patients, and communities have the right to know relevant and timely information about the potentially harmful products, chemicals, pollutants, and hazards to which they are exposed.
9. Nurses participate in research of best practices that promote a safe and healthy environment.
10. Nurses must be supported in advocating for and implementing environmental health principles in nursing practice.

Source: American Nurses Association. (2007). *Principles of Environmental Health for Nursing Practice*. Silver Spring, MD: Author.

Upstream Thinking: Making Connections Between Environmental and Human Health

One of the most challenging areas in environmental health is linking a past exposure from 10 to 20 years ago with the development of a current health problem. Even though we are intellectually aware that some agents have health consequences that may not be seen for years or decades, it can be difficult to take such a distant and uncertain threat seriously.

One conceptual approach that has been used in interdisciplinary public health efforts, referred to as **upstream thinking**, uses the analogy of a river to demonstrate connections between preceding exposures and later health consequences. This approach is based on an article by McKinlay (1979), who tells the story of a physician friend and his struggle to keep from feeling overwhelmed by the enormity of health problems that he encounters in clinical practice. The friend notes that he feels as if he is so caught up in rescuing individuals from the river that he has no time to look upstream to see who is pushing them in. In this analogy, the river represents illness and health providers' efforts to rescue people from illness. However, in this portrayal no one receives care until they are downstream in the river of illness, which precludes efforts to intervene before illness develops.

McKinlay (1979) challenges providers to look upstream, where the real problems lie. The river analogy includes many concepts in community health nursing, including epidemiology, the natural history of disease and levels of prevention. The power of the upstream conceptualization of health lies in its simplicity and the ease with which one can connect the correlates and causes of disease with their consequences.

Upstream thinking lends itself well to health problems of environmental origin and can be helpful in guiding practice decisions that have long- and short-term consequences for our patients. Examples of environmental upstream nursing actions include the following:

- Instructing a patient to wear a respirator when stripping paint from an old home
- Encouraging farmers who work with pesticides to refrain from wearing their work boots into the house
- Developing a school policy to establish waiting periods for children to be off playgrounds and recreational areas, such as sports fields, following applications of fertilizers and herbicides
- Educating new parents about the need for safe materials, nontoxic furniture and decorations in a newborn nursery

In each situation, the nurse is acting from a primary prevention viewpoint to prevent or minimize the occurrence of an exposure. It is not necessary to know the toxicology of all of the agents involved. Nurses can initiate an action and then seek guidance from experts in toxicology or other disciplines. The goal is to minimize the opportunity for harm by linking an understanding of nursing actions at the present time with the prevention of harmful health effects in the future (Butterfield, 1990; Butterfield & Postma, 2009).

Trends in Exposure and Disease

Health professionals and citizens are generally aware of the delicate balance that exists between the environment and global health. A goal of policymakers, both in the United States and elsewhere, has been to increase technology without compromising public health and safety. With increasing technological advancements, also come known and unknown environmental toxins. Unfortunately, despite our knowledge of the links between environmental contaminants and health problems, our society continues to manufacture, use, and dispose of many potentially hazardous chemicals. In 2012, U.S. industry reported the release of 3.63 billion pounds of potentially toxic chemicals into the air, water, and soil (U.S. Environmental Protection Agency [EPA], 2012). The widespread use of chemicals with toxic effects (**toxins**) highlights the importance of educating nurses who can work to reduce exposures to those substances in homes, workplaces, and public areas. Many cases of environmentally induced illness can be prevented, but it requires actions that have not traditionally been a central part of community health nursing (Butterfield, 2002; Butterfield & Postma, 2009; Kleffel, 1996). As can be understood from Box 13-1, nurses play a critical role in maintaining knowledge about known and possible toxins and promoting healthy environmental conditions for populations, especially those who are vulnerable, such as children, those with compromised immune systems and chronic conditions, and the elderly.

A World View

Despite efforts to reduce industrial pollution and automobile emissions, increasing numbers of citizens the world over are facing health risks from environmental toxicants. Because of the rapid increase in the world's population, small changes in urbanization and agricultural production can have large consequences on global public health (Briggs, 2003). The health consequences of increased industrial globalization and planetary climate change are problems for the world that no single nation can hope to address alone (Kirk, 2002). The relationships of industrialization and deforestation to the emergence of new diseases and the reemergence of diseases previously thought to be under control (e.g., tuberculosis) are of special concern. Recent ecological changes associated with human health problems include the following:

- Population movements and the intrusion of humans into new habitats, particularly tropical forests
- Deforestation, with new forest–farmland margins that expose farmers to new vectors of disease (Daszak, Tabor, Kilpatrick, Epstein, & Plowright, 2004)

- Irrigation, especially primitive systems that serve as breeding areas of arthropods
- Rapidly expanding urbanization, with vector populations finding urban breeding grounds in standing water and sewage (Patz et al., 2004)
- Changes in agricultural practices, such as the use of antimicrobial-supplemented animal feeds and the crowding of animals in confined spaces
- The growth in large corporate farms, including farmed fish and seafood, and corporations that produce massive amounts of toxins that are released into the environment, often with insufficient and inconsistent regulatory compliance or government oversight
- Climate change resulting in massive numbers of persons who are affected by typhoons, earthquakes, droughts, and other extreme weather conditions, resulting in mass relocation to unfamiliar and potentially toxic terrains
- Increasing number of political refugees crossing national boundaries and living in crowded, unhealthy conditions resulting from numerous wars and military/national conflicts
- Nuclear accidents, such as the Fukushima disaster in Japan in March 2011, in which a major earthquake touched off a 15-meter high tsunami, disabling the power supply that cooled three Fukushima Daiichi reactors (All three cores largely melted in the first 3 days. Nuclear hazardous materials continue to be monitored worldwide after the catastrophe.)

These problems require a perspective that goes beyond national boundaries and mobilizes global concern and cooperation. Import policies in developed nations need to address the transfer of natural resources from developing countries, such as mineral wealth, oil, and exotic lumber. Environmentally sound practices in the mining, agriculture, and forestry industries need to be enhanced through cooperative efforts between industry and citizen groups. Several disease surveillance organizations have requested additional funding for the development of a system that could coordinate global reporting of disease surveillance and control efforts. Better diagnostic techniques, prevention strategies, and risk factor analysis must be taught to healthcare professionals worldwide. More funding for basic and applied research related to the environment and infectious diseases can yield significant improvements in public health. Education for a global perspective is needed to address the issue of infectious disease within the context of shared environmental responsibility. As our planet moves from a national to an international perspective on health problems, it is easy to see that environmentally destructive practices in one country can lead to health problems in many other parts of the world.

The Centers for Disease Control and Prevention (CDC)(2013a) continues to analyze the public health consequences from global heat waves and extreme weather conditions—increasingly common events that are setting alarming new records for low and high temperatures as well as producing greater intensity of storms, floods, and droughts. Many scientists have hypothesized that global changes in weather patterns will lead to critical changes in disease occurrence over the next few decades.

The Environment and Health

A healthy environment is one in which people—whether at home, in schools, at workplaces, or in their communities—have access to safe food and water, have adequate sanitation, and are protected from risks associated with chemical pollution, environmental degradation, and disasters (World Health Organization, 2005). The term **environmental health** refers to freedom from illness or injury related to toxic agents and other environmental conditions that are potentially detrimental to human health (Pope, Snyder, & Mood, 1995). Healthcare providers' roles in environmental health are expanding to include caring for people with exposures to hazards in their homes, workplaces, and communities through contaminated air, water, and soil.

Because "environment" is such a universal concept, it can be difficult to define the boundaries of environmental health. The application of environmental health in clinical practice ranges from descriptions of hospital rooms to international and global perspectives on the health of the planet. Although a hospital room differs from a global ecology perspective in complexity and other dimensions, both views can provide insights into opportunities for health at the individual and collective levels. Just as the scope of clinical practice varies from individual emergencies to situations in which a healthcare provider is charged with the health assessment of populations, so too must the scope of environmental health assessment vary across situations.

Because of the rapid increase in chemical production and use since World War II, synthetically derived chemicals are often considered inherently dangerous. However, each environmental agent must be studied and understood; it is a big mistake to overgeneralize and say that all synthetic products are dangerous and that all natural products are inherently safe. Some of the biggest threats to human health throughout human history have come from "natural" substances such as lead, mercury, and arsenic. Furthermore, chemicals are often considered the only source of environmental health threats; however, physical agents (e.g., noise, vibration, ionizing radiation) and biological agents (e.g., bacterial contamination, fungal spores, viruses) also play significant roles in health problems of environmental etiology.

CULTURAL CONNECTION

Some cultural and religious groups do not believe in the use of added minerals, such as fluoride, to drinking water. With current research providing evidence that fluoridated drinking water dramatically reduces tooth decay in children, how can these belief systems be respected while still preserving the health of the population?

Environmental Health Policy: Historical Perspectives

In Europe and North America, early environmental health regulations focused exclusively on sanitation, water quality, and housing. The public health implications of these regulations cannot be overemphasized; mortality rates dropped significantly following the institutionalization of quality standards for drinking water and sewage disposal (Kotchian, 1997). Following the publication of Rachel Carson's *Silent Spring* in 1962, citizen groups mobilized in support of more comprehensive legislation to protect the environment and endangered species. Examples of legislation passed during the 1960s and 1970s include clean air and water acts, occupational health and safety acts, toxic substances controls acts, and the Poison Prevention Packaging Act. During these two decades, the EPA, Occupational Safety and Health Administration (OSHA), and Nuclear Regulatory Commission were also established (Stevens & Hall, 1997).

Public and governmental actions addressing environmental health continue to this day, although some observers believe that responses have not been sufficient to reduce the health risks in the environment. Community right-to-know federal legislation, enacted in 1987, authorizes citizens' access to information addressing the presence, management, and release of hazardous chemicals in their community. Information addressing the storage and use of more than 300 chemicals was collected by the EPA, assembled into databases called the Toxic Release Inventory, and made available to the public. The Pollution Prevention Act of 1990 authorized data-collection activities addressing toxic chemicals that leave a community facility. These recent governmental efforts have greatly enhanced the ability of citizens to gain access to environmental data from their neighborhood. Such data can empower citizens to advocate on behalf of their community and hold government and private officials accountable for policy decisions.

Despite recent advances in environmental information through Internet access, some environmental advocates point out that, although some environmental risks have been minimized or eliminated, new risks have been identified but not addressed. Citizen advocacy groups have observed that many health and safety regulations have not been uniformly implemented or enforced; loopholes exist in others. In addition, some policymakers and legislators believe that environmental initiatives and laws are not in the best interests of the economy; thus, laws, standards, or initiatives have been canceled, weakened, or not given the funds they need to be effective.

In regard to the built environment, many scientists are beginning to view cities and towns almost as ecosystems and to critically examine the placement of roads, sidewalks, and buildings. Using mapping (e.g., with global positioning system [GPS] technology) and other research techniques, they can compare differences in obesity levels between neighborhoods with and without sidewalks (Booth, Pinkston, & Poston, 2005). Other scientists are examining the complex relationships among neighborhood factors such as walkability, grocery store access, and the availability of bike paths. Their studies are beginning to quantify what we already know intuitively: Depending on their attributes, "places" can promote or inhibit health in the same way that a poor diet can. In fact, the more we learn about built environment, the more scientists are beginning to see links between physical and mental health and automobile use (or overuse; Pohanka & Fitzgerald, 2004).

Since the early 2000s, children's environmental health issues have also become the focus of greater scientific scrutiny. An increasing recognition that children absorb chemicals in different ways than adults has led to studies examining children's exposure to substances such as pesticides, mercury, and tobacco smoke (Hill & Butterfield, 2006; Reddy, Reddy, & Reddy, 2004). One big concern is the cumulative effect of exposure to multiple chemicals over a child's life. Historically, cancer studies have been conducted to examine links between a single agent (e.g., benzene) and a single type of cancer. Now, however, scientists are beginning to recognize the limitations of looking at just one agent at a time and are beginning to look at exposure to multiple chemicals in human milk, in drinking water, and in school settings (Shendell, Barnett, & Boese, 2004). Close to 30 million U.S. citizens drink water that exceeds one or more of the EPA's safe drinking water standards, and 50% of the population of the United States lives in areas that exceed national air quality standards.

Recent Environmental Health Issues

In the second half of the 20th century, awareness of the damage to the environment and its resulting effect on health grew dramatically. Population growth (see **Figures 13-1** and **13-2**), urban spread, advanced

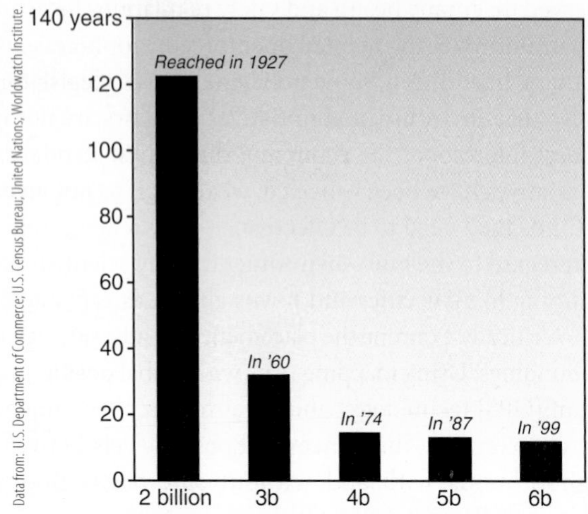

Figure 13-1 Years taken to reach one billion markers.

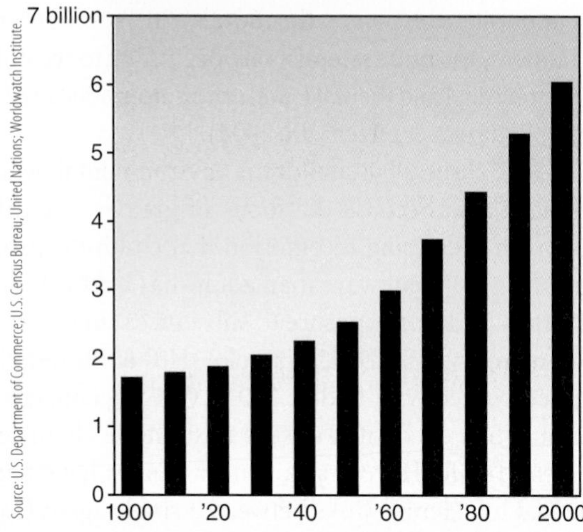

Figure 13-2 Estimates of world population.

technology, industrialization, and modern agricultural methods were the source of great progress, but they also led to the creation of environmental hazards that may not have been observed previously. It seems as if news outlets feature stories on new threats almost daily, leaving citizens to sort out the difference between hype and reality. Three trends that seem here to stay include: (1) the focus on the built environment, (2) an emphasis on children's environmental health, and (3) the environmental justice movement.

The environmental justice movement has played a critical role in changing government policies addressing the placement and operation of factories and other industrial facilities in the United States. When citizens began to protest the placement of factories in minority neighborhoods, state and local policymakers began to examine historical (and current) business and zoning regulations. What they found was a pattern of putting "dirty" businesses in poorer or minority communities, while higher income neighborhoods remained free of such facilities (Frumkin, 2005). From these beginnings came the environmental justice movement, which sowed the seeds of activism across the nation. Today, environmental justice has come to be known as the fair treatment and meaningful involvement of all people, regardless of race, color, national origin, or income, with respect to the development, implementation, and enforcement of environmental laws, regulations, and policies (EPA, 2014).

Historical Perspectives on Environment and Health

The science of epidemiology has been closely linked to environmental health since the original work done by John Snow in 1854. The same deductive processes in inquiry that Snow used to link cholera deaths to contaminated Thames River water have been used countless times over the past century to link environmental agents with disease occurrence. Because the basic tenets of descriptive epidemiology (i.e., time, person, and place) have been such a powerful tool in establishing links between environmental agents and disease, this approach to scientific inquiry has stood the test of time for investigations of environmentally induced diseases at both local and global levels.

Some argue that epidemiological methods have been more effective in addressing infectious and acute diseases than chronic conditions. There may be some validity to this position, because links between exposure and disease are most easily made when the induction period is relatively brief. However, in recent years, chronic disease epidemiology has played an important role in furthering an understanding of relationships between environmental exposures and several types of cancer, neurological impairment, and autoimmune conditions. Examples in this area include associations between the following:

- Asbestos exposure and mesothelioma
- Prenatal exposure to diethylstilbestrol (DES, a form of estrogen given to pregnant women in the 1950s and 1960s to prevent miscarriage) and a rare form of cervical cancer
- Occupational exposure to vinyl chloride (used in the manufacture of polyvinyl chloride plastic pipe) and the development of liver cancer
- Various toxins linked to Alzheimer's disease

One of the biggest challenges in the area of chronic disease epidemiology is to establish evidence of exposure dose for agents without biomarkers (i.e., physiological fingerprint of exposure). In these cases, exposure has most often been "estimated" using a questionnaire or interview guide. This method of estimating exposure can be problematic for exposures that may (or may not) have happened years or decades ago. More recently, the CDC began to test citizens for body burden levels of a variety of environmental chemicals. In 2003, the CDC released findings that included citizens' blood and urine levels for 116 chemicals, including selected insecticides and herbicides, dioxins, phytoestrogens, and lead. Preliminary findings revealed that only 2.2% of children (ages 1–5 years) were found to have elevated blood lead levels—an improvement from the 4.4% rate seen in the 1990s.

The *Fourth National Report on Human Exposure to Environmental Chemicals, Updated Tables, September 2013* (2013a) provides new CDC data since the release of the *Fourth Report, 2009*. Since the publication of the Fourth Report, 201 chemicals have been updated and data on 49 chemicals have been added. This update also includes new data for 91 chemicals measured in serum-pooled samples. Readers are advised to review this publication for the most recent and complete biomonitoring data on the CDC website (http://www.cdc.gov/exposurereport/).

The authors of this report noted that is it important to remember that there has been no baseline information available for most of these chemicals; therefore, one cannot say whether the levels found are safe or unsafe. The important gap that this study fills is in providing baseline information so that we can begin to understand what are "normal" ranges for these chemicals. There is good news on the horizon. The CDC is releasing new reports via their website on a more frequent basis, so that scientists can begin to understand trends in chemical exposures. Understanding these exposures will provide a scientifically accurate foundation for the development of U.S. chemical reduction policies For the most up-to-date information, go to their website (http://www.cdc.gov/exposurereport/).

Origins of Environmental Health Policy

Although concerns for environmental risks to health and safety have existed to some extent for centuries, the current widespread awareness and concern about these risks among public and private sectors are relatively recent phenomena. With the Industrial Revolution in the 1800s, the developed world, including the United States, focused on modernization and rapid production of goods and services. Concerns about depletion of natural resources or damage and hazards resulting from the products and wastes of industrialization were not yet realized or acted on. During this time, however, there was growing concern for working conditions and safety of workers, as reflected in the movement to organize and unionize the workforce to demand safe work environments, among other improvements.

In the early decades of the 1900s, concerns about environmental health and safety were demonstrated by governments with the passage of laws to protect the public from hazardous goods in the marketplace. In the United States, for example, the Pure Food and Drug Law was passed in 1906 and the Food and Drug Administration was established in 1931 (Henson, Robinson, & Schmele, 1996).

In the next several decades of the 1900s, war efforts and postwar industrial rebuilding consumed the energies of governments and the public. Again, the international production of war and postwar goods and services took precedence, and the lay public held a belief that their governments would protect them from environmental risks and hazards.

The birth of the consumer-driven environmental movement that continues today can be traced to the 1960s and 1970s. Multiple trends and events served to

APPLICATION TO PRACTICE 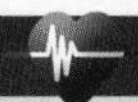

Health Policy Actions Result from Community Involvement

Pam and Steven are registered nurses practicing at a mobile clinic that provides health care for migrant farm workers and their families in a Midwestern state. They discuss the numerous children with skin and respiratory complaints that they have recently seen at the clinic. A review of clinic records reveals that more than twice the expected number of children had been seen in the clinic presenting with skin irritations, headaches, or abdominal cramping. The nurses begin to gather more detailed interview data from mothers who bring their children to the clinic with these symptoms. They learn that mothers are bringing their infants to the fields because there is no affordable day care available in this area. Older children work with their parents picking vegetables. They discuss their observations with the clinic's medical director and a toxicology consultant from the Migrant Council. They learn that the symptoms they have observed are common in pesticide exposure or poisoning.

A team from the clinic and Migrant Council visits the local vegetable fields and finds multiple exposure risks for children. Some mothers carry infants into the fields in cloth carriers as they pick crops. Other infants are left at the edges of the crop rows in child carriers and strollers. Children as young as 4 years old pick vegetables next to their parents. Rubber gloves and other protective coverings are not available in sizes small enough for child

(Continued)

APPLICATION TO PRACTICE (*CONTINUED*)

workers. Some children are observed picking pesticide-dusted vegetable and eating them unwashed for lunch. On review of applicable federal and state laws, they find that while regulations protecting children from pesticides in foods are strict and clear, they are much less clear regarding protection of adults or children who harvest that food. Laws regulating or providing for safety for agricultural child workers are also not clear.

The team meets to examine the data collected and formulate an approach. They decide that an immediate priority is to reduce the potential pesticide exposures in this local area. They plan to work with farm owners to provide low-cost or no-cost day care and child-sized protective equipment. They also plan educational programs for migrant parents, offered after hours in their housing areas, focused on reducing exposures. Because migrant workers travel after harvest to other agricultural areas, reducing the problem in this area alone will not protect the children as they move to other areas. The team identifies informal leaders in the group of migrant workers and provides them with training in community development so that they will be better able to advocate for safe working conditions on behalf of their group wherever they work. The team also contacts legislators and policymakers to advocate for improved regulations to protect migrant workers and their families from pesticide exposures.

Source: Adapted from Crenson, M. (1997, December 28). Kids at work in fields of unseen danger. *Missoulian*, p. A4.

raise international consciousness that some aspects of the environment had become a growing risk to public health and safety. Disenchantment with postwar living conditions and the realization of the environmental effects of nuclear proliferation and war occurred after World War II. Public cynicism toward the government and other institutions occurred in the United States during and after the Vietnam War era. Several widely read exposés of environmental hazards also were published during this time. One influential publication, *Silent Spring* (Carson, 1962), predicted the poisoning and destruction of the natural environment in the name of progress with the use of pesticides. Rachel Carson's book was history making in its effect on thought and policymaking following its publication. Consumerism gained momentum during this time as a result of the efforts of national leaders and consumer advocate groups. All of these trends and events resulted in public concern and activism followed by governmental responses to citizens' growing environmental awareness.

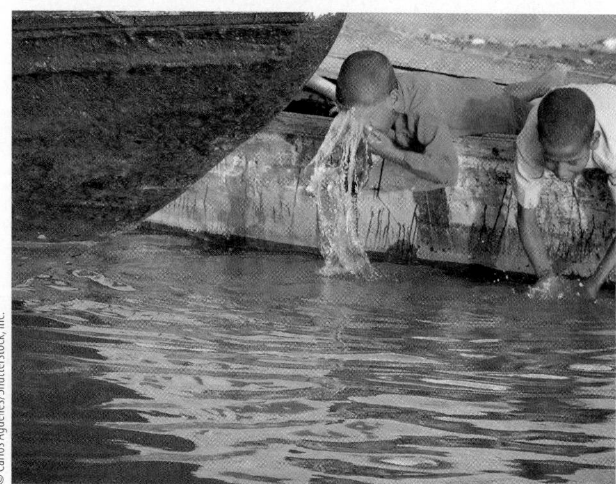

> The nation that destroys its soil destroys itself.
>
> —*Franklin D. Roosevelt*

Environmental Policy: Governmental and Public Roles

One of the primary purposes of government in a democratic society is to protect and safeguard the governed or the public. To fulfill this purpose, the government passes laws and enacts rules and regulations to prevent and reduce risks to the public. Government agencies and offices have been created to identify and monitor risks and hazards, monitor compliance with rules, and gather data to inform policymakers. Government initiatives have been implemented because of priorities of elected or appointed officials as well as in response to pressures from an environmentally conscious public.

Despite all of this governmental activity, our environment still poses hazards to the safety and health of the public. In many cases, the dangers are more complicated now than ever before. Reasons for that increased risk include the following:

- Environmental health has been addressed in a piecemeal fashion instead of in a potentially more effective comprehensive plan.
- Proposed policies and laws that improve the health of the environment are often perceived to be in conflict with what is in the best interest of business and the economy.
- Laws and policies cannot solve all environmental problems and risks without voluntary actions by individuals, groups, and organizations.
- Science has not been able to keep pace with potential environmental hazards and pollutants.
- In a world of finite resources, the costs of cleaning and protecting the environment are in competition with the costs of other desired and needed social programs.

At the local and national levels, policymakers set national and state priorities among competing social programs, establish standards for environmental hazards and risks, take action against those who violate standards, and allocate billions of federal and state funds according to these established priorities. A broad set of population health goals to be achieved by the year 2000 was established by the U.S. Public Health Service in 1990 and was reaffirmed with the publication of *Healthy People 2010*, and now the *Healthy People 2020* objectives, which include environmental health as a priority area; these objectives serve as the basis for federal and state policy formulation and action (U.S. Department of Health and Human Services, 2014). Selected objectives related to the environment are listed in the *Healthy People 2020* feature that follows.

The public plays an important role in setting the stage for policy decisions by expressing its values and in the actions it takes as an electorate. Policymakers are also influenced by organized interest groups and elected and appointed officials who represent these interests. In the environmental health arena, these groups have traditionally been organized into two factions: (1) businesses and industries that depend on the environment for raw materials and/or disposal of waste and (2) citizen groups and voluntary organizations that have an interest in preventing or limiting the extraction of raw materials or disposal of waste. Nurses can work to foster health communication between groups and direct the dialogue to areas of common ground. In addition to participation of citizens, nurses can enlarge their role in environmental health policymaking by increasing their political expertise and activity as professionals.

In the United States, policymakers and the public alike trust the nursing profession to be advocates for patients and to speak and act on behalf of the health of the population. Nurses are considered reliable and trustworthy sources of information about threats to health and also represent the largest group of healthcare professionals among the voting age population. By staying informed of current and accurate information on environmental risks, organizing and becoming actively involved with groups of nurses and others around environmental issues, and actively communicating with and lobbying policymakers and organized interest groups, nurses can effectively influence public policy. In the practice arena, nurses can also inform and mobilize citizen groups and other professionals to become actively involved in communicating with and lobbying policymakers about environmental issues of concern to themselves and their communities.

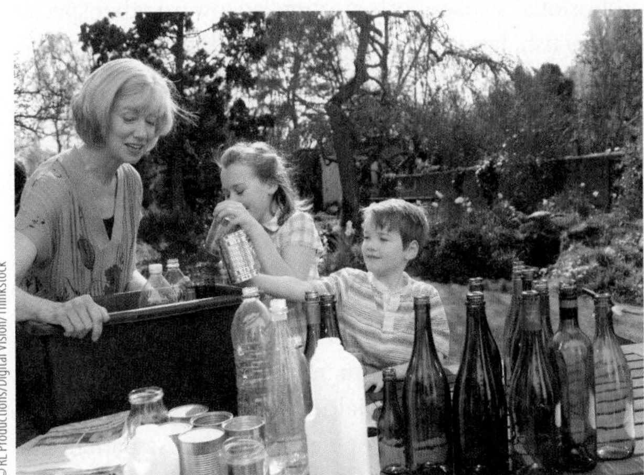

© RL Productions/Digital Vision/Thinkstock

Recycling efforts have increased with significant environmental benefits.

HEALTHY PEOPLE 

Selected Objectives Related to Environmental Health

EH-8.1: Eliminate elevated blood lead levels in children.

EH-9: Minimize the risks to human health and the environment and hazardous sites.

EH-10: Reduce pesticide exposures that result in visits to the health facility.

EH-11: Reduce the amount of toxic pollutants released into the environment.

EH-13: Reduce indoor allergen levels.

EH-18: Decrease the number of U.S. homes that are found to have lead-based paint or related hazards.

Source: U.S. Department of Health and Human Services. (2014). Environmental health objectives. Retrieved from http://healthypeople.gov/2020/topicsobjectives2020/objectiveslist.aspx?topicId=12

> Within the last few years, a large part of London was in the daily habit of using water polluted by the drainage of its sewers and water closets. This has happily been remedied. But, in many parts of the country, well water of a very impure kind is used for domestic purposes. And when epidemic disease shows itself, persons using such water are almost sure to suffer.
>
> —*Florence Nightingale, 1860*

Nursing and the Environment

Nursing's efforts to promote health by influencing environmental conditions predate the modern environmental movement by more than a century. Florence Nightingale, the founder of modern nursing, developed her theory of nursing with a strong emphasis on the individual's environment. Although the term "environment" did not appear in her published works, she addressed health using five environmental dimensions: (1) pure, fresh air; (2) pure water; (3) efficient drainage; (4) cleanliness; and (5) light—that is, direct sunlight (Nightingale, 1969/1860). To Nightingale, the environment was the surrounding context in which the individual lived: a person's health or illness was a direct result of environmental influences. Deficiencies in any of the five factors produced a health deficit. Nightingale also stressed the importance of a comfortably warm, noise-free environment and a good diet. Although originally intended to address a hospital environment, her concepts were broad enough to serve as a basis for public health nursing, and they remain integral parts of nursing and health care.

Nursing has long noted the influence of the environment on health and has assumed the role of managing the interaction between patients and their environments. Often, nursing's approach has been to assist the patient to adapt to the environment; thus, the focus for intervention was changing the individual or community patient to facilitate a better match with the environment. An emerging role for nursing today is to intervene directly in environmental factors in an attempt to change unhealthy conditions and mobilize individuals or communities to do the same. Nurse scientists are conducting studies in environmental factors directly, such as water and air quality, policies, laws that influence the health of the population, and conditions in workers' environments to improve understanding of healthful and unhealthful environmental conditions and the interventions that can improve them.

ETHICAL CONNECTION 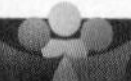

Attempts to ban smoking in bars have resulted in community divisiveness over public health and individual right to freedom of expression, especially in small, western U.S. towns. As a community health nurse, how can you provide advocacy for the entire population in this environmental health issue?

GOT AN ALTERNATIVE? 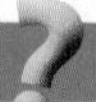

Using organic or nontoxic household products in the home is safer for the environment and for the residents of both the home and the community. One common concern is the high cost of these products. What can the community health nurse do in regard to educating families about reducing environmental toxins when the costs of these products limit their use among disadvantaged families?

Just as it is a challenge to draw a circle around the concept of environmental health, so, too, is it difficult to delineate the unique role of nursing in addressing environmental health issues. Many professional disciplines—from wildlife biologists to microbiologists to engineers—consider environmental health problems within their domain of expertise. Environmental health is an area in which many different professionals are needed to prevent, minimize, and improve environmental problems. Both basic and applied research efforts are required to understand all of the implications of environmental health problems. Professional nurses are well suited to participate in collaborative efforts because they have historically functioned at the center of the healthcare team. However, nursing efforts are focused exclusively on human health, in contrast to some professions, whose efforts are directed toward other species such as fish, large mammals, and plant life. Nursing interventions are directed toward preventing and minimizing the effects of environmental health problems on persons of all ages. This focus does not mean, however, that concerns about animal and plant life are dismissed or that health connections between species are not recognized.

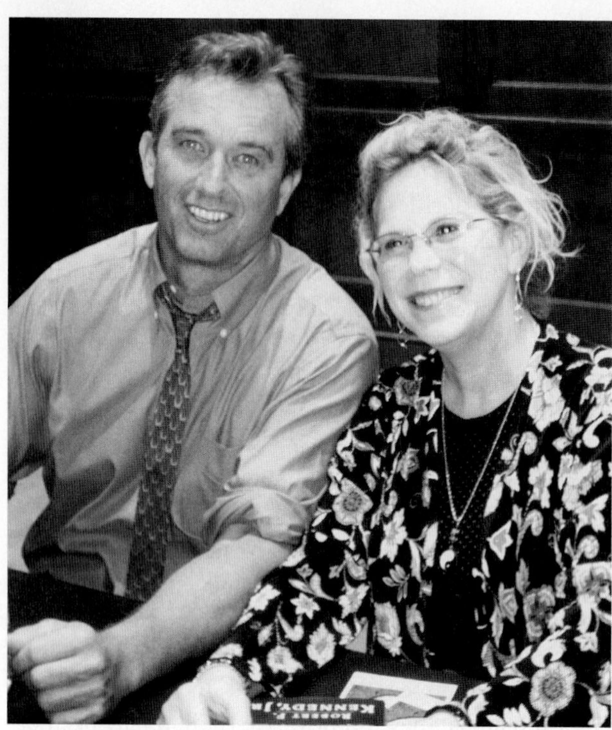

Robert Kennedy, Jr., environmental activist, attorney, and author of *Crimes Against Nature*, with text author Dr. Karen Saucier Lundy.

Community health and occupational health are the nursing practice specialties often associated with health hazards in the physical environment. In view of the universal presence of environmental hazards, it is critical that nurses in all practice specialties have an understanding of environmental health (Pope et al., 1995). As patient advocates, all nurses need to be concerned about the health of the environment because it is a major determinant of their patients' health.

Roles of the Community Health Nurse

Nursing has a long history of identifying health risks and intervening directly on behalf of patient health. The role of the nurse in providing pure water, a restful setting, and a hygienic hospital environment was among the early environmental concerns of the nursing profession. By the late 1800s and early 1900s, nursing became concerned with identifying and resolving communicable disease outbreaks, improper food handling, inadequate disposal of wastes, and unsafe water supplies (Tiedje & Wood, 1995). During the growing environmental awareness of the 1960s and 1970s, nursing expanded its environmental concerns to include identification and interventions related to exposures to toxins and chemicals from the home and community environments. More recently, nursing has acknowledged that the environment relevant to our patients' health is larger and more multifaceted than was appreciated previously. Accordingly, nursing's concerns have expanded to regional, national, and global physical environmental hazards as well as influences arising from the social, economic, psychological, and political environments.

RESEARCH ALERT 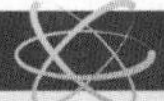

Amaya and colleagues have documented high rates of exposure to lead, trace elements, and pesticides in Hispanic persons residing in United States–Mexico border communities. As one part of a larger study examining the serum lead levels in pregnant Hispanic women, a case investigation of a family with two children with elevated lead levels was conducted. Dust samples were collected both inside and outside the residence; additional samples were taken from water, paint, and cookware in the home. The evidence supported a hypothesis that primary exposure occurred from battery recycling and burning of electrical wire conducted on the premises by the father and grandfather of the children. Steps to ameliorate exposure pathways were undertaken by community health nurses working with the family. Monthly lead levels taken on both children declined over the next 4 months. Unfortunately, the family moved away without notice and was lost to follow up 9 months after the initial event.

Such investigations capitalize on the risk communication skills of nurses working in border communities. Nurses' abilities to locate and intervene effectively with disenfranchised families are unsurpassed among health professions. Case-series and case-control studies by nurse scientists can yield important findings at the local and national levels, while furthering the role of nursing and the environmental health sciences. Elevated blood lead levels have been reported in approximately 8% of low-income children in El Paso County, Texas. Nursing research addressing the areas of risk communication, healthcare access, and intervention strategies with families at risk for lead exposure can lead to a significant reduction of persons affected by this serious health problem.

Source: Amaya, M. A., Ackall, G., Pingitore, N., Quiroga, M., & Ternazas-Ponce, B. (1997). Childhood lead poisoning on the US–Mexico border. A case study in environmental health nursing lead poisoning. *Public Health Nursing, 14*, 353–360.

Identifying Risks

Community health nurses often emphasize primary prevention activities that address environmental health because many environmentally induced illnesses are preventable through risk management activities. In concert with other professionals, community health nurses often conduct a systematic review of risks known as a quantitative **risk assessment**. Risk is the probability of injury, disease, or death for individuals or populations exposed to hazardous substances; it may be expressed numerically (e.g., "one in 1 million"), but this rate is often impossible to estimate. In such situations, risk may be expressed using terms such as high, medium, or low. The steps involved in a risk assessment are outlined in **Box 13-2**. **Risk management** involves developing and evaluating possible regulatory actions guided by the risk assessment plus other ethical, political, social, economic, and technological factors (U.S. Congress, Office of Technology Assessment, 1990).

It is important to consider the depth of inquiry when addressing the role of nursing in environmental health. Which areas of inquiry contain the dimensions of environment that fall within the scope of nursing? Surely, given enough time and paper, one could generate a seemingly endless list of questions that relate human health to the environment. The challenge then lies in the ability to focus nursing assessment activities into areas that are most obvious to the clinical or research area of interest. One would expect to see overlapping areas of focus between environmental health, as it relates to professional nursing, and other professions such as **toxicology**, pharmacology, and the behavioral sciences. The goal in such a case is not to stake out a new specialty area for nursing practice,

BOX 13-2 Steps in an Environmental Risk Assessment

1. *Hazard identification:* Does the agent cause the adverse effect?
2. *Exposure assessment:* Which exposures are currently experienced or anticipated?
3. *Dose–response assessment:* What is the relationship between the dose and incidence?
4. *Risk characterization:* What is the estimated incidence of the adverse effect in a given population?

but rather to integrate knowledge from nursing and other disciplines and apply this knowledge to the patients' needs for health promotion or restoration.

Looking at the environment from a broad view, environmental factors are involved in almost all disease risks and include areas such as housing, nutrition, socioeconomic status, and lifestyle. Even the health of persons with genetic disorders can often be enhanced through nursing actions addressing personal and societal aspects of the environment. Environmental health includes a concern for not only the physical environment, but also the interrelated social, economic, psychological, and political environments. Such conditions as poverty, powerlessness, social injustice, and racism that arise from diverse environmental factors can reduce opportunities for health and contribute to illness just as certainly as do chemical or physical agents. A central goal of this chapter is to provide information that allows for a richer understanding of the connectedness among many features of the environment.

THINK ABOUT THIS

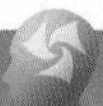

After the damage inflicted by Hurricane Katrina and the resulting levee break in New Orleans in August 2005, the area's unprecedented environmental debris and hazards created the nation's greatest recycling challenge. The sheer volume of debris created by Katrina was staggering—including about 25 million cubic yards of "green waste" (tree limbs, trunks, leaves, dead bushes), enough to fill up the Louisiana Superdome nearly twice. Some had to be incinerated, some was used as cover in landfills due to the time factor, and much is now being used as lawn and garden mulch and composting material. Flooded vehicles and hundreds of thousands of destroyed refrigerators, washing machines, and other appliances have yielded about 280,000 tons of steel, according to Louisiana state officials. Many builders, restoration experts, artists, and grassroots organizations have recycled much of the debris into jewelry and for use in the restoration of homes.

Although information addressing physical agents predominates this chapter, it is important to understand that aspects of the social and economic environment are also centrally linked to opportunities for health in civilizations throughout the world.

Assessing Exposures

Community health nurses often participate in exposure assessments following the development of a case or suspected cluster of disease. Because of their methodical skills in home assessment, nurses are often called on to conduct comprehensive exposure assessments in homes or occupational settings. Strong interview, observation, and family assessment skills are needed by nurses to collect these data in a clear and systematic manner. Clues to potential solutions to environmental risks may occur during the course of community or home assessments, although the resolution of some risks may require the expertise of nonnursing professionals. Home visits often require follow-up conversations with toxicologists, industrial hygienists, or other scientists who have expertise with the exposures of interest.

Exposure assessments are much simpler when patients present with an acute illness, such as acute pesticide poisoning or inhalation fever. Assessments become much more complex when the specific types of agents have not been considered a priori or when the induction period between exposure and disease occurrence is unknown. The greatest challenges occur in persons with chronic disease or disease of unknown cause or when exposure to small doses of multiple agents has occurred over years or decades. In these types of clinical situations, it is very unusual to make a link between disease and a specific type of exposure with a high degree of confidence. Unusual conditions and rarer forms of cancer, such as the association between asbestos and development of mesothelioma, are the exception and can often be narrowed down to a specific place and time in one's life. **Box 13-3** includes

BOX 13-3 Conducting a Home Assessment and Environmental Exposure History

A public health nurse has been assigned to a home that may be hazardous for the family to live in. A reference has been made to the public health nurse by a home health nurse who has been visiting the family, which includes one elder over 65, two parents, and two children under the age of 6. The nurse uses the following guide to make his assessment and determine any risks that may be threatening to the family's health and wellbeing.

Areas of Visual Inspection

Examine areas in the immediate vicinity of the home for the presence of the following:

- Water hazards
- Automobiles, farms, or other large equipment
- Garbage/waste storage containers
- Garages, sheds, or other outbuildings for safety hazards
- Chemical storage areas
- Pets or livestock

- Areas where rats or mice could live around home or outbuildings
- General age and condition of home (e.g., presence of peeling paint, metal edges from siding)

Consider whether any of the aforementioned items constitute a health threat to any family members or to the community in general.

Questions to Consider in Assessing Environmental Agents in the Home

Ask family members about the following:

- Hobbies or crafts involving potential for lead exposure (e.g., stained glass, ceramic glazing)
- Potential for significant exposure to gasoline or diesel exhaust from car repair activities or from nearby traffic
- Safe storage of food (stored where vermin cannot contaminate food) and proper cooking and refrigeration facilities
- Storage and use of insecticides, lawn care products, fertilizers
- Use of deodorizers and candles with additives for aroma
- Home heating—type of furnace, use of wood stoves
- Use of cleaning products that are strong irritants
- Fumigants or other products used for tick or flea control in the home
- Storage of food in copper or brass containers (can contaminate food with copper or lead)
- Exposure to wood preservatives (e.g., pentachlorophenol) in log homes
- Potential for lead exposure through lead-based plumbing
- Source of water (municipal or private well)
- Any seasonal changes in water sources during the year (e.g., private well during the winter and water delivered to a cistern during the summer months)
- Recent home renovation activities such as sanding or stripping of old paint that could result in lead exposure to family members

Questions Addressing Symptoms Related to Environmental Agents in the Home

Do any members of the family have symptoms that they attribute to an environmental exposure? If so, elicit the nature of symptoms, duration, fluctuations in symptoms over the day and from week to week, seasonal changes, and related symptoms in other family members or others who spend extended time in the home.

Ascertaining Agent-Specific Data from Individuals

Exposures

- Concurrent and past exposures to metal, dust, fibers, fumes, chemicals, biological hazards, radiation, noise, vibration
- Typical workday (job tasks, location, materials, agents used)
- Changes in routines or processes
- Other employees or household members similarly affected

Health and Safety Practices at Worksite

- Ventilation
- Medical and industrial hygiene surveillance
- Employment examinations
- Personal protective equipment (e.g., respirators, gloves, coveralls)
- Lockout devices, alarms, training, drills
- Personal habits (smoking, eating in the work area, handwashing with solvents)

Work History

- Description of all prior jobs, including short-term, seasonal, or part-time employment and military service
- Description of present job(s)

Environmental History

- Present and prior home locations
- Jobs of household members
- Home insulating, heating, and cooling system
- Home cleaning agents
- Pesticide exposure (e.g., pet flea treatments, roach and ant sprays)
- Water supply
- Recent renovation/remodeling
- Air pollution, indoor and outdoor
- Hobbies: painting, sculpting, welding, woodworking, piloting, autos, firearms, stained glass, ceramics, gardening
- Hazardous wastes/spills exposure
- Presence of pets and animals
- Use of protective devices when using any known toxins at home, in the workplace, and in the community

Medical History

- Past and present medical problems
- Medications

Source: Adapted from Agency for Toxic Substances and Disease Registry, U.S. Department of Health and Human Services. (2000). *Case studies in environmental medicine: Taking an exposure history.* Retrieved from http://www.atsdr.cdc.gov/csem/csem.asp?csem=17&po=0

basic information addressing the components of a home assessment and environmental exposure history. As one would expect, data collection is customized to address the unique aspects of the exposures, setting, and persons involved in the situation.

Communicating Risks

Often, the most successful strategies for responding to environmental risks affecting a community involve empowering citizens to address the problem. If successful, these strategies result not only in the resolution of the immediate problem but also in the creation of a group able to address future threats. Nurses should be encouraged to become familiar with the principles of environmental risk communication. An increased availability of information to the public increases the possibility that the community health nurse will be sought for advice and further information. Nurses are trusted in a community, and the public values their opinions. It is professionally responsible to share science-based information with persons most affected by that information. Nurses should understand the influence of the environment and environmental agents on human health based on knowledge of relevant epidemiological, toxicological, and exposure factors.

Basic principles of risk communication can be used in many environmental health situations, ranging from a toxic spill incident to a neighborhood meeting to discuss groundwater contamination. Overall, risk communication focuses on telling citizens what is known about a risk situation in a clear and forthright manner. In addition, it is important to directly explain what information is not currently known and the process by which additional information will be communicated to all parties. Basic guidelines addressing the principles of risk communication are listed in **Box 13-4**. Infants and children have a unique vulnerability to being exposed to chemical agents.

Communicating a balanced view of these risks to parents is a challenge for nurses in the community. An example of this challenge involves the practice of breastfeeding. For many years, nurses have played a significant role in policies and clinical actions that support breastfeeding practices in new mothers. This advocacy role has been based on scientific findings that human milk is the ideal infant food, because of the easy digestibility of milk proteins, the presence of maternal antibodies, and safety from contamination through the use of improperly sanitized bottles, among other health benefits.

- Since the 1990s, scientists have become increasingly aware that human milk also carries a host of potentially serious risks to infant health. The greatest concern has been physiological evidence that many chemicals to which the mother has been exposed are transferred into breast milk. Of special interest are the findings from studies that examine the metabolism and fate of chemicals that have extremely long half-lives (i.e., years and decades) within human populations. Such agents include polychlorinated organic pollutants, such as organochlorine pesticides, polychlorinated biphenyls (PCBs), and polychlorinated dibenzodioxins and dibenzofurans, (PCDDs/PCDFs), as well as some forms of metals such as methylmercury. In most cases, persons ingest these agents in their diets, usually from contaminated fish and animal products such as meats, fats, cheese, and eggs. In large doses, many pesticide products and mercury compounds have

BOX 13-4 Basic Guidelines for Risk Communication

Don't confuse people's understanding a risk with their acceptance of it—anger and resentment are often expressed when people are unwittingly exposed to an environmental hazard and feel that they have no control over the situation.

Avoid trivializing the risk or minimizing people's concerns. Frustration needs to be heard and acknowledged, not suppressed. It is important to listen attentively and respectfully to all concerns and respond in a clear manner with whatever information is currently available. Say what is known, and also say what is not known. Gaining trust from the audience in a public meeting will not usually occur if people perceive that they are being patronized or placated. It is best to say what is currently known about the situation of concern and what is not known.

Often, health providers do not have all the information at hand or are waiting for additional information to come in (e.g., laboratory values or diagnostic tests from exposed persons). State clearly what information is not currently available and when that information will be available. Respond to the different needs of different audiences. In an incident that involves a pesticide spill at a local school, the parents of schoolchildren will probably have different concerns than the janitor and physical facilities staff at the school. Think about your audience in advance—try to anticipate what questions you would have if you were in the audience and direct the discussion from that perspective.

Recognize that input from the public can help your agency make better decisions. Holding private meetings or trying to avoid public input is likely to fuel distrust in community members. By building in opportunities for affected persons to help remedy an environmental hazard situation, those persons gain a sense of control over the situation and feel like they are helping themselves and others. Think broadly about how to use citizens' help to get mailings out, set up phone trees, and form advocacy groups. If you do not allow citizens to work with you and your agency, they may begin to work against you.

Source: Adapted from Hance, B. J., Chess, C., & P. M. Sandman, P. M. (1990). *Improving dialogue with communities: A risk communication manual for government.* Trenton, NJ: New Jersey Department of Environmental Protection. Used by permission.

> affected neurobehavioral, neuromotor, and speech development. Unfortunately, much less is known about the long-term effects of low-dose exposure in human milk. For a variety of feasibility and methodological reasons, scientific studies of low-dose and early-life exposures are extremely difficult to conduct. Such studies often help in the incremental advancement of scientific understanding but are not able to yield clear-cut answers to clinical questions (Gladen et al., 1999; Hooper, 1999; Landrigan, 2002). According to the CDC, although some women may have detectable levels of chemical agents in their breast milk, no established "normal" or "abnormal" levels exist to aid in clinical interpretation. As a result, breast milk is not routinely tested for environmental pollutants.
>
> Breastfeeding is still recommended despite the presence of chemical toxins. For the vast majority of women, the benefits of breastfeeding appear to far outweigh the risks. To date, effects on the nursing infant have been seen only where the mother herself was clinically ill from a toxic exposure.

Infants and children are particularly susceptible to the toxic effects of chemical exposure for a number of reasons. Pound for pound of body weight, a child eats much more food than an adult. Youngsters between the ages of 1 and 5 years eat and drink three to four times more food and water than do adults. In addition to this increased food intake, there is evidence that compared with adult bodies, the metabolic pathways of children have a diminished ability to metabolize or detoxify chemical agents effectively. Children's daily activity patterns, such as playing on the ground and hand-to-mouth behavior, can also increase their exposure to some environmental toxicants. Because of incomplete scientific evidence about the long-term consequences of exposure to chemical agents, primary prevention activities that reduce the opportunity of exposure provide the first and most important line of defense on behalf of children's health (Schmidt, 1999).

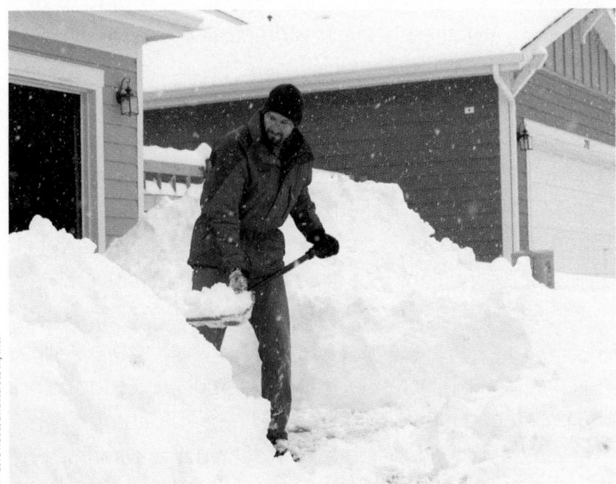

The physical environment in which we live, such as the Colorado winter above, greatly affects a population's health.

Assessing and Referring Patients

A critical piece of comprehensive nursing practice is the identification of high-risk patients so that these individuals can be referred for further evaluation and follow up. To provide such care for these patients, nurses must have a good understanding of the environmental health resources located within their geographic area. In many communities, professionals with environmental health expertise, such as industrial hygienists, physicians, and toxicologists, are located in the state health department. Other experts may be located in occupational health clinics in both hospital and community settings. For nurses working in agricultural communities, expertise in environmental health may often be found through contacts with county extension agents, pest management specialists, migrant and seasonal farm worker clinics, or agricultural medicine programs (Shreffler, 1996). It is essential that patients be referred to resources that are culturally and socioeconomically appropriate (Pope & Rall, 1995).

There is some evidence from applied research studies that both pediatric and adult patients are falling through the cracks of the health system when they are in need of specialized environmental health services. In a review of children residing in New York City, Markowitz, Rosen, and Clemente (1999) estimated that only 60% of high-risk children were being screened for lead poisoning; of those children who were found to have elevated lead levels, nearly 60% were not receiving timely follow up by healthcare providers. In a more recent study that specifically looked at immigrant children in New York, researchers found risk of lead poisoning was five times higher in foreign-born children than in U.S.–born children, suggesting environmental exposures prior to arrival might compound the problem (Tehranifar et al., 2008). In another study examining the health consequences of lead exposure, elevated values were associated with an increased risk for hypertension later in life (Korrick, Hunter, Rotnitzky, Hu, & Speizer, 1999). According to the CDC, primary prevention is a strategy that emphasizes the prevention of lead exposure, rather than a response to exposure after it has taken place. Primary prevention is necessary because the effects of any lead appear to be irreversible (CDC, 2005, 2013a).

A third environmental health study focused on persons at increased risk of developing lung cancer caused by both household radon exposure and cigarette smoking. Researchers developed statistical models of risk and determined that the most effective strategy to reduce the risk

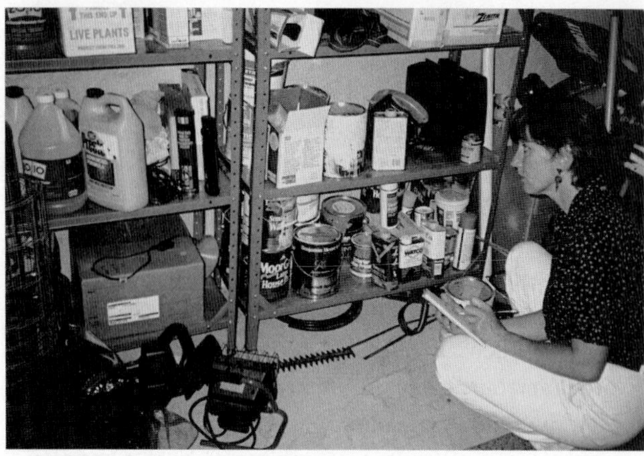

Chapter author Dr. Patricia Butterfield conducting a home environmental exposure assessment.

of radon-related cancer was smoking cessation. Stopping smoking was more effective in reducing cancer risk than directly reducing the levels of radon in the home (Mendez, Warner, & Courant, 1998). Although it is always optimal to reduce disease risk through all possible means (e.g., smoking cessation plus radon-reduction interventions), this study demonstrates the importance of addressing both environmental and behavioral means to minimize disease risk in exposed persons.

Community health nurses are the health providers most familiar with their patients' home setting, lifestyle, work habits, and environmental exposures. Because of their unique presence in a variety of patient settings, nurses may become aware of patients' environmental health risks and work toward directing them to an appropriate source of evaluation and treatment. See the Application to Practice feature addressing household environmental assessment and interventions for children with asthma.

APPLICATION TO PRACTICE

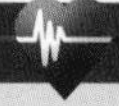

Asthma Management in a Young Girl

A public health nurse working in an urban area has been coordinating services with the school nurse practitioner at Northside Elementary, a primary school located in a low-income neighborhood. The nurse practitioner calls to request a home assessment for 7-year-old Lateesha. Lateesha is in the second grade, and the teacher notes that she has performed poorly in the classroom compared with her skill level during the previous year. In a phone interview, the mother states that she thinks the child's inattentiveness in the classroom results primarily from several recent colds that required Lateesha to miss school. The mother notes that Lateesha has missed 8 days of school so far this year and has had some difficulty with the make-up work following these absences.

When the nurse visits the home, she notes that Lateesha's mother, brother, sister, and grandmother live in a three-bedroom apartment near the school. When entering the home, the nurse notes that the room is very warm and sees an older model space heater in the kitchen area. The mother explains she wants to keep it warm for Lateesha's 4-year-old sister, who has complained that the apartment is too cool during winter. The nurse also notes several ashtrays in the living room and the presence of Tigger, the family cat. The mother informs the nurse that Lateesha has had four severe colds since October and that the last physician they saw at the clinic suggested that Lateesha has asthma. The mother received two types of inhalers for Lateesha following this clinic visit but notes that no one explained whether Lateesha is to use the inhalers every day or only after she develops a cold or breathing difficulties.

What should be the focus of the interventions of the community health nurse with this family?

NOTE THIS!

A remarkable decrease in the incidence of many childhood communicable diseases has occurred during this and the last century in U.S. populations; these conditions include diphtheria, pertussis, and polio. Unfortunately, this progress against many communicable diseases has been offset by an equally remarkable increase in asthma occurrence in both pediatric and adult populations in industrialized nations throughout the world. Overall asthma prevalence has increased by 58% since 1980; the mortality rate has increased by 78%. Children from urban areas and racial/ethnic communities have experienced the greatest increases in both prevalence and mortality. Hospitalization and morbidity rates for nonwhite children are almost twice those for white children. Asthma symptoms are caused by hyperresponsiveness of the airways to a number of common environmental allergens, including dust mites, animal dander, cockroaches, fungal spores, and pollens. Exacerbation of asthma has also been associated with air quality problems such as increased levels of sulfur dioxide, nitrogen dioxide, and ozone. Cigarette smoking and exposure to secondhand smoke also contribute to exacerbation of several childhood conditions such as otitis media, pneumonia, bronchitis, and asthma. Currently, approximately 30% of American preschoolers are exposed to residential tobacco smoke. Just as the precipitating factors for asthma are multiple, so too must be prevention efforts by nurses and other health providers. These efforts need to address household and community-based patterns of exposure as well as continuity of care and ongoing management for affected persons.

Sources: Clark, N. M., Brown, R. W., Parker, E., Robins, T. G., Remick, D. G. Jr, Philbert, M. A., . . . Israel, B. A. (1999). Childhood asthma. *Environmental Health Perspective, 107*(Suppl. 3), 421–429; Eggleston, P. A., Buckley, T. J., Breysse, P. N., Wills-Karp, M., Kleeberger, S. R., & Jaakkola, J. J. (1999). The environment and asthma in U.S. inner cities. *Environmental Health Perspectives, 107*(Suppl. 3), 439–450, CDC, 2013b).

Ethical Principles Addressing Environmental Health Nursing

Nurses have a duty to safeguard patients from environmental hazards and risks regardless of patients' income, insurance status, or lack of access to care. The nurses' *Code of Ethics* addresses responsibilities to collaborate with other health professionals and citizens in promoting community and national efforts to meet the health needs of the public (American Nurses Association, 2001).

Justice is a highly valued ethical principle in most societies today and is one of the beliefs that guide the practice of nursing. The concept of fairness of opportunity is a value in the United States that is supported in laws that forbid discriminatory treatment that limits one's opportunities on the basis of unchangeable characteristics such as gender, race, or socioeconomic status. **Social justice** means fairness or equality in the distribution of the benefits and burdens of society. According to the principles of social justice, no one person or group should have a disproportionate share of the benefits available to a society nor of the burdens that are present.

When applied to environmental health, principles of social justice suggest that the ability to live in a healthy environment as part of the process for attaining or maintaining health should be available to all. Because health is of fundamental importance to having opportunities for life, liberty, and the pursuit of happiness, environmental risks that take place or are allowed to persist differentially that are based on gender, race, or socioeconomic status would not be consistent with justice or fairness of opportunity (Daniels, 1985). **Environmental justice** is not served when some persons or groups have disproportionate shares of the benefits of healthy environments and others have disproportionate shares of the burdens of contaminated ones.

Most environmental hazards do not pose uniform or equal risks to the health of an entire population. Some widespread hazards, such as global warming, acid rain, and air or water pollution, involve an entire region or country, but most environmental health concerns involve different exposures within the same population. Some exposures occur because of behaviors or practices that could be considered changeable as a result of choices the individual makes. The decision to not wear protective gear when applying pesticides is an example of a choice that could easily be changed from health damaging to health protecting. Some exposures occur, however, because of unchangeable characteristics or circumstances of some individuals in the population, such as socioeconomic status, race, powerlessness, age, or gender. Lead exposure, for example, is most common in children who live in low-income housing. The disposal of toxic waste into sites located near low-income neighborhoods whose residents lack the financial resources and power to prevent it is another example of disproportionate exposure to environmental hazards (Bullard, 1990, 1993).

The distinction between changeable and unchangeable courses of action may not always be clear. For example, the training one receives about pesticide safety and the availability of safety equipment may affect the use of safety measures more than personal choice. Many environmental risks occur from exposures to toxic substances on the job. Some individuals may have the ability to change

MEDIA MOMENT 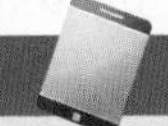

Last Child in the Woods: Saving our Children from Nature-Deficit Disorder (2008)

By Richard Louv. New York, NY: Algonquin Books

Richard Louv brings together critical research that links direct exposure to nature as essential for a child's healthy physical and emotional development. There is a growing body of evidence linking the lack of nature in children's lives and the rise in obesity, diabetes, attention disorders, and depression. Louv provides guidance to readers on how to reverse this trend and encourage children (and parents) to experience the healing and essential aspects of nature.

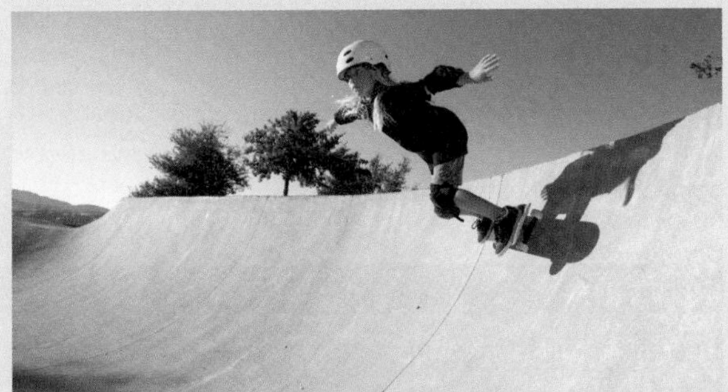

Children are more vulnerable to environmental risks than adults due to greater time outdoors, immaturity of their immune systems, and other developmental differences.

occupations to reduce risks, but many others cannot reasonably entertain such an option. It also may be possible to alter some risks such as living in low-income housing with lead-based paint. In this example, although residents' incomes and ability to relocate may be unchangeable, they can work to improve the safety in their current housing and influence landlords to correct or reduce environmental hazards such as lead-based paint.

Nurses play a role in promoting environmental justice in several ways. Educating individuals on ways to reduce exposure to toxic substances is important. Giving information about contacts in health departments or work safety committees is helpful to individuals and groups. Helping groups organize and present a united voice to industries and politicians is important to people who may otherwise have been powerless to protest. Community health nurses know the strengths of their communities and are able to identify the people who provide leadership to the group. Community health nurses are also already sensitive to their community's cultural or ethnic attributes, which may affect the process of seeking environmental justice.

MEDIA MOMENT

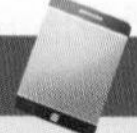

Erin Brockovich **(2000)**

In this film based on a true story, Julia Roberts stars as an unemployed single mother who becomes a legal assistant instrumental in bringing a case against a giant California energy company for releasing a cancer-causing chemical into the drinking water supply for the small town of Hinkley. Despite having little formal legal training, Brockovich successfully initiates one of the biggest class-action environmental lawsuits in American history, winning a settlement of over $300 million from the company.

Activists concerned about environmental hazards and social justice have also begun to work with and for disadvantaged groups to increase their awareness of unequal environmental risks and possible strategies to improve them. Disadvantaged, at-risk groups in a particular area may not be organized into a functioning community or have community or neighborhood organizations that can be readily mobilized for action. In this case, activists work with whatever organizations exist or form an informal group of concerned residents who may get others involved over time. An environmental hazard close to where people live is an issue that can be effective in organizing and mobilizing citizens to work together as a group (Butterfield & Postma, 2009).

Conclusion

The role of community health nurses in environmental health is evolving in several ways:

- From illness treatment to illness recognition and prevention
- Toward a multidisciplinary foundation of basic and applied science
- Toward an emphasis on activities in which nursing excels, such as risk communication, community-based investigations, and patient advocacy strategies
- Toward an integration of environmental health principles into all domains of nursing practice and research

Knowledge of pollutants—whether physical, chemical, or biological—is characterized by incomplete science. The field is constantly changing, with the discovery of new hazards, but also innovative ways of minimizing hazard use and exposure. Nurses can participate in advancing environmental health science by participating in applied research activities on behalf of vulnerable groups or those disproportionately exposed to agents of concern. A list of websites that provide scientifically sound environmental health information is provided in **Table 13-1**.

Nurses have functioned at the fringe of power and politics, which has often been detrimental to the nursing profession, perhaps even to health care. In the field of environmental health, nurses are capable of making great contributions to the social, political, and economic forces that presently guide environmental healthcare policy. By broadening nurses' understanding of the environment, new horizons in environmental health can be developed and expanded on behalf of the health of our patients, our nation, and our planet.

GLOBAL CONNECTION

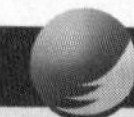

Home to only 4.4% of the world's population, the United States accounts for about 19% of the Earth's greenhouse gas emissions.

Source: U.S. Environmental Protection Agency. (2008). Global greenhouse gas emissions data. Retrieved from http://www.epa.gov/climatechange/ghgemissions/global.html

NOTE THIS!

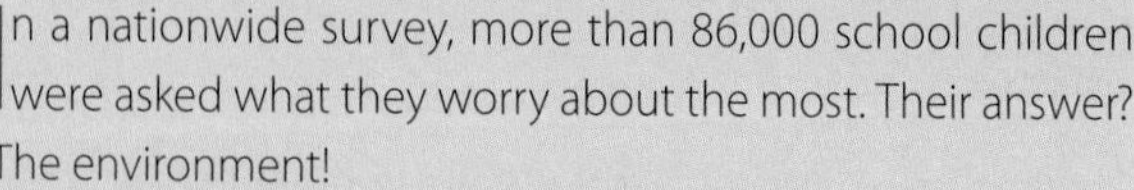

In a nationwide survey, more than 86,000 school children were asked what they worry about the most. Their answer? The environment!

Source: Environmental and Occupational Sciences Institute, Public Health and Risk Communication Division.

TABLE 13-1 Resources for Environmental Health Information

Agency or Organization	Purpose	URL
Agency for Toxic Substances and Disease Registry (ATSDR)	Part of the U.S. Department of Health and Human Services. Conducts public health assessments of waste sites, health consultations concerning specific hazardous substances, and applied research in support of public health assessments. Supports an environmental health nursing initiative. Also provides an exceptional list of fact sheets for specific toxics and a comprehensive group of case studies addressing specific exposures.	http://www.atsdr.cdc.gov/
American Association of Occupational Health Nurses (AAOHN)	Professional organization for occupational and environmental health nurses. Provides information resources about nursing and environmental health.	http://www.aaohn.org/practice/standards.html
Association of Occupational and Environmental Clinics	Conducts information sharing, education, and research through a network of clinics. Provides professional training, community education, exposure and risk assessment, clinical evaluations, and consultation services.	http://www.aoec.org/
Environmental Protection Agency (EPA)	Employs 18,000 people across the United States, including in its headquarters offices in Washington, DC; 10 regional offices; and more than a dozen labs. Develops and enforces regulations addressing environmental protection, performs research, and provides educational support throughout the country.	http://www.epa.gov/
EnviRN	An information resource site operated by the University of Maryland School of Nursing.	http://envirn.umaryland.edu
National Center for Environmental Health (NCEH)	Part of the Centers for Disease Control and Prevention. Works to prevent illness from interactions between people and the environment. Especially committed to safeguarding the health of vulnerable populations.	http://www.cdc.gov/nceh/
National Environmental Education and Training Foundation	An environmental education site with links to nursing and health education materials.	http://www.neetf.org/
National Institute of Environmental Health Sciences (NIEHS)	Part of the National Institutes of Health. Works to reduce the burden of human illness from environmental causes by understanding each of these elements and how they interrelate.	http://www.niehs.nih.gov/
RN No Harm	An American Nurses Association program focusing on the prevention of pollution and medical waste from hospitals and clinics.	http://www.nursingworld.org/rnnoharm/

APPLICATION TO PRACTICE 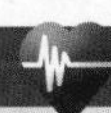

Broadening Nurses' Expertise in Environmental Health Clinical Practice: Thinking Upstream

Over the course of several years, a public health nurse was asked about water quality issues by patients attending the well-child clinic. These questions most commonly addressed parents' concerns about potable water contamination, and the nurse believed she was unqualified to answer these types of questions. After spending a few hours at home reviewing water quality information on the EPA's website, the nurse decided to seek some advice from the health department director about the lack of preparation to respond to patients' questions regarding environmental health. The director suggested that the nurse

(Continued)

APPLICATION TO PRACTICE (*CONTINUED*)

spend some time with a water quality specialist, who was located within another department, and authorized time for the nurse to work 1 week in that department. During her week with environmental health personnel, the nurse worked in the field when the environmental engineer inspected the installation of a private well west of town. She made a special effort to talk with all of the people in the environmental health department so that she had a better understanding of the full range of expertise within the department. After working in the field, she visited the laboratory to observe testing procedures for water quality and to learn about the different water tests available to the public.

When she returned to the well-child clinic the following week, the nurse decided to allocate at least half an hour per day to developing a resource library on water quality issues in the clinic. She obtained educational brochures from the environmental health department; in addition, she established a system where nurses could give interested patients a plastic bottle for water sampling and have them send it directly to the laboratory for analysis. The nurse also asked the environmental engineer to make his phone number available to respond to any questions from patients about their water and septic systems.

Over the next year, the nurse provided continuing education for the nursing staff until they became more comfortable providing patients with specific information about water quality and differentiating between questions they could answer and those that were best referred to the engineers and scientists in the other department. Nurses came to understand that the prevention of problems held the key to long-term sustainability of water quality in their community and ecosystem. Many of the same principles of prevention that were so familiar to them in public health nursing could be applied equally well to actions to reduce opportunities for water pollution.

During the next few months, the nursing staff reached beyond their original contacts with the environmental health department and extended further into partnerships with other environmental information and advocacy groups in the area. They worked with the local university's pollution prevention program to display and educate patients about the safe disposal of household products and solvents, to reduce solid waste, and to increase participation in recycling of paint and motor oil. Nurses found that they could often incorporate several minutes of "pollution prevention" instruction into many well-child visits and that parents were often appreciative of this information. The nurses worked to make other health departments aware of their efforts and presented a summary of their program at their annual public health association conference. As a culmination of their work, the nurses developed a website to educate professional colleagues throughout the nation on their growing expertise in water quality and pollution prevention.

Daffodils

I gathered in the first of the daffodils this morning
And built a fire.
We always have one more cold day before the Easter
Out the window beyond the streaks of slow soft rain I see
The green netting of spring—high in the trees.
I remember how—on days like this— when I was very young
I fought to keep from running away
Such promises the yellow flowers made.

—Ann Thedford Lanier

HEALTHY ME

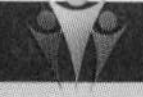

How often do you get outside? We spend more and more time inside than anytime in history, much having to do with advances in technology. Spend time outside almost each day, just to walk and benefit from the healing elements of nature.

ART CONNECTION

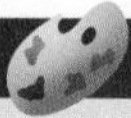

Peruse the Internet for art of the environment which is of interest to you. This can be of nature, from flowers to people outside their homes. How does the art affect you? Does it calm you? What is your overall sense of how art represents one aspect of how the environment affects our lives on a daily basis?

LEVELS OF PREVENTION

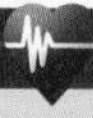

Primary: Educating families about the risk of radon in homes

Secondary: Assisting a family in seeking appropriate resources to help them remove the radon from the house and screening all members for radon poisoning

Tertiary: Taking appropriate action and seeking assistance from professionals to support the family should there be radon damage to any of the family members

Critical Thinking Activities

1. Take a walk or a drive around your own neighborhood and identify any potential environmental health risks. What kind of prevention interventions can be done to minimize exposure to these hazards? As a nursing student, what role can you play?

References

Agency for Toxic Substances and Disease Registry, U.S. Department of Health and Human Services. (2000). *Case studies in environmental medicine: Taking an exposure history*. Retrieved from http://www.atsdr.cdc.gov/CSEM/exphistory/ehcover_page.html

American Nurses Association (ANA). (2001). *Code of ethics for nurses with interpretive statements*. Silver Spring, MD: Author.

American Nurses Association (ANA). (2010). *Nursing: Scope and standards of practice* (2nd ed.). Silver Spring, MD: Author.

Booth, K. M., Pinkston, M. M., & Poston, W. S. C. (2005). Obesity and the built environment. *Journal of the American Dietetic Association, 105*(Suppl. 5), 110–117.

Briggs, D. (2003). Environmental pollution and the global burden of disease. *British Medical Bulletin, 68*, 1–24.

Bullard, R. D. (1990). *Dumping in Dixie: Race, class, and environmental quality*. Boulder, CO: Westview Press.

Bullard, R. D. (1993). *Confronting environmental racism: Voices from the grassroots*. Boston, MA: South End Press.

Butterfield, P. G. (1990). Thinking upstream: Nurturing a conceptual understanding of the societal context of health behavior. *ANS: Advances in Nursing Science, 12*(2), 1–8.

Butterfield, P. G. (2002). Upstream reflections on environmental health: An abbreviated history and framework for action. *ANS: Advances in Nursing Science, 25*(1), 32–50.

Butterfield, P. G., & Postma, J. (2009). ERRNIE research team: The TERRA framework: Conceptualizing rural environmental health inequities through an environmental justice lens. Upstream reflections on environmental health: An abbreviated history and framework for action. *ANS: Advances in Nursing Science, 32*(2), 107–117.

Carson, R. (1962). *Silent spring*. Boston, MA: Houghton Mifflin.

Centers for Disease Control and Prevention, National Center for Environmental Health. (2013a). *Fourth national report on human exposure to environmental chemicals* (NCEH Pub No. 03-0022). Retrieved from http://www.cdc.gov/exposurereport/pdf/FourthReport.pdf

Centers for Disease Control and Prevention. (2005). *Preventing lead poisoning in young children*. Atlanta, GA: Author.

Centers for Disease Control and Prevention. (2013b). *Low level lead exposure harms children: A renewed call for primary prevention report of the advisory committee on childhood lead poisoning prevention*. Atlanta, GA: Author. Retrieved from http://www.cdc.gov/nceh/lead/acclpp/final_document_030712.pdf

Clark, N. M., Brown, R. W., Parker, E., Robins, T. G., Remick, D. G. Jr, Philbert, M. A., . . . Israel, B. A. (1999). Childhood asthma. *Environmental Health Perspective, 107*(Suppl. 3), 421–429.

Crenson, M. (1997, December 28). Kids at work in fields of unseen danger. *Missoulian*, p. A4.

Daniels, N. (1985). *Just health care*. Cambridge, UK: Cambridge University Press.

Daszak, P., Tabor, G. M., Kilpatrick, A. M., Epstein, J., & Plowright, R. (2004). Conservation medicine and a new agenda for emerging disease. *Annals of the NY Academy of Science, 1026*, 1–11.

Eggleston, P. A., Buckley, T. J., Breysse, P. N., Wills-Karp, M., Kleeberger, S. R., & Jaakkola, J. J. (1999). The environment and asthma in U.S. inner cities. *Environmental Health Perspectives, 107*(Suppl. 3), 439–450.

Frumkin, H. (2005). Health, equity, and the built environment (editorial). *Environmental Health Perspectives, 113*(5), A290–A291.

Gladen, B. C., Monaghan, S. C., Lukyanova, E. M., Hulchiy, O. P., Shkyryak-Nyzhnyk, Z. A., Sericano, J. L., & Little, R. E. (1999). Organochlorines in breast milk from two cities in Ukraine. *Environmental Health Perspectives, 107*(6), 459–462.

Henson, R. H., Robinson, W. L., & Schmele, J. A. (1996). Consumerism and quality management. In J. A. Schmele (Ed.), *Quality management in nursing and healthcare*. Albany, NY: Delmar.

Hill, W. G., & Butterfield, P. G. (2006). Environmental risk reduction for rural children. In H. J. Lee & C. A. Winters (Eds.), *Rural nursing: Concerns, theory and practice* (2nd ed.). New York, NY: Springer.

Hooper, K. (1999). Breast milk monitoring programs (BMMPs): World-wide early warning systems for polyhalogenated POPs and for targeting studies in children's environmental health. *Environmental Health Perspectives, 107*(6), 429–430.

Kirk, M. (2002). The impact of globalization and climate change on health: Challenges for nursing education. *Nurse Education Today, 22*(1), 60–71.

Kleffel, D. (1996). Environmental paradigms: Moving toward an eccentric perspective. *ANS: Advances in Nursing Science, 18*(4), 1–10.

Korrick, S. A., Hunter, D. J., Rotnitzky, A., Hu, H., & Speizer, F. E. (1999). Lead and hypertension in a sample of middle-aged women. *American Journal of Public Health, 89*(3), 330–335.

Kotchian, S. (1997). Perspectives on the place of environmental health and protection in public health and public health agencies. *Annual Review of Public Health, 18*, 245–259.

Landrigan, P. J. (ed.) (2002). Chemical contaminants in breast milk. *Environmental Health Perspectives, 110*(6), A313–A315.

Louv, R. (2008). *Last child in the woods: Saving our children from nature-deficit disorder*. Chapel Hill, NC: Algonquin Books.

Markowitz, M., Rosen, J. F., & Clemente, I. (1999). Clinician follow-up of children screened for lead poisoning. *American Journal of Public Health, 89*(7), 1088–1089.

McKinlay, J. B. (1979). A case for refocusing upstream: The political economy of illness. In E. G. Jaco (Ed.), *Patients, physicians, and illness* (3rd ed., pp. 9–25). New York, NY: Free Press.

Mendez, D., Warner, K. E., & Courant, P. N. (1998). Effects of radon mitigation vs. smoking cessation in reducing radon-related risk of lung cancer. *American Journal of Public Health, 88*(5), 811–812.

New Jersey Department of Environmental Protection. (1990). *Improving dialogue with communities: A risk communication manual for government*. New Brunswick, NJ: Author.

Nightingale, F. (1969). *Notes on nursing*. New York, NY: Dover. (Originally published by D. Appleton and Company, 1860)

Patz, J. A., Daszak, P., Tabor, G. M., Aguirre, A. A., Pearl, M., Epstein, J., . . . Bradley, D. J. (2004). Unhealthy landscapes: Policy recommendations on land use change and infectious disease emergence. *Environmental Health Perspectives, 112*(10), 1092–1098.

Pohanka, M., & Fitzgerald, S. (2004). Urban sprawl and you: How sprawl adversely affects worker health. *AAOHN Journal, 52*(6), 242–246.

Pope, A. M., & Rall, D. P. (Eds.). (1995). *Environmental medicine: Integrating a missing element into medical education*. Washington, DC: National Academies Press.

Pope, A. M., Snyder, M. A., & Mood, L. H. (Eds.). (1995). *Nursing, health and the environment: Strengthening the relationship to improve the public's health*. Washington, DC: National Academies Press.

Reddy, M. M., Reddy, M. B., & Reddy, C. F. (2004). Scientific advances provide opportunities to improve pediatric environmental health. *Journal of Pediatrics, 145*(2), 153–156.

Schmidt, C. W. (1999). Poisoning young minds. *Environmental Health Perspectives, 107*(6), A302–307.

Shendell, D. G., Barnett, C., & Boese, S. (2004). Science-based recommendations to prevent or reduce potential exposure to biological, chemical, and physical agents in schools. *Journal of the School of Health, 74*(10), 390–396.

Shreffler, M. J. (1996). An ecological view of the rural environment: Levels of influence on access to health care. *Advanced Nursing Science, 18*(4), 48–59.

Stevens, P. E., & Hall, J. M. (1997). Environmental health. In J. M. Swanson & M. A. Nies (Eds.), *Community health nursing: Protecting the health of aggregates* (2nd ed., pp. 736–765). Philadelphia, PA: Saunders.

Tehranifar, P., Leighton, J., Auchincloss, A. H., Faciano, A., Alper, H., Paykin, A., & Wu, S. (2008). Immigration and risk of childhood lead poisoning: Findings from a case–control study of New York City children. *American Journal of Public Health, 98*(1), 92–97.

Tiedje, L. B., & Wood, J. (1995). Sensitizing nurses for a changing environmental health role. *Public Health Nursing, 12*(6), 356–365.

U.S. Congress, Office of Technology Assessment. (1990, April). *Neurotoxicity: Identifying and controlling poisons of the nervous system* (Publication No. OTA-BA-436). Washington, DC: U.S. Government Printing Office.

U.S. Department of Health and Human Services (HHS). (2014). *History and development of Healthy People*. Retrieved from http://healthypeople.gov/2020/about/history.aspx

U.S. Environmental Protection Agency. (2012). *2012 TRI national analysis*. Retrieved from http://www2.epa.gov/toxics-release-inventory-tri-program/2012-tri-national-analysis

U.S. Environmental Protection Agency. (2014). *Environmental justice*. Retrieved from http://www.epa.gov/compliance/environmentaljustice/

World Health Organization, Regional Office for South-East Asia. (2005). *Sustainable development and healthy environments*. Retrieved from http://www.searo.who.int/en/section23.htm

Appendix
Environmental Agents and Their Adverse Health Effects

Note: This table is not meant to be comprehensive, but to provide examples of several types of agents.

Agent	Exposure	Route of Entry	System(s) Affected	Primary Manifestations	Aids in Diagnosis	Remarks
Metals and Metallic Compounds						
ARSENIC	Alloyed with lead and copper for hardness; manufacturing of pigments, glass, pharmaceuticals; byproduct in copper smelting; insecticides; fungicides; rodenticides; tanning	Inhalation and ingestion of dust and fumes	Neuromuscular Gastrointestinal Skin Pulmonary	Peripheral neuropathy, sensory–motor Nausea and vomiting, diarrhea, constipation Dermatitis, finger and toenail striations, skin cancer, nasal septum perforation Lung cancer	Arsenic in urine	
ARSINE	Accidental byproduct of reaction of arsenic with acid; used in semiconductor industry	Inhalation of gas	Hematopoietic	Intravascular hemolysis; hemoglobinuria, jaundice, oliguria or anuria	Arsenic in urine	
BERYLLIUM	Hardening agent in metal alloys; special use in nuclear energy production; metal refining or recovery	Inhalation of fumes or dust	Pulmonary (and other systems)	Granulomatosis and fibrosis	Beryllium in urine (acute); beryllium in tissue (chronic); chest x-ray; immunological tests (such as lymphocyte transformation) may also be useful	Pulmonary changes virtually indistinguishable from sarcoid on chest x-ray.
CADMIUM	Electroplating; solder for aluminum; metal alloys, process engraving; nickel–cadmium batteries	Inhalation or ingestion of fumes or dust	Pulmonary Renal	Pulmonary edema (acute); emphysema (chronic) Nephrosis	Urinary protein	Also a respiratory tract carcinogen.
CHROMIUM	In stainless and heat-resistant steel and alloy steel; metal plating; chemical and pigment manufacturing; photography	Percutaneous absorption, inhalation, ingestion	Pulmonary Skin	Lung cancer Dermatitis, skin ulcers, nasal septum perforation	Urinary chromate (questionable value)	

(Continued)

Agent	Exposure	Route of Entry	System(s) Affected	Primary Manifestations	Aids in Diagnosis	Remarks
Metals and Metallic Compounds *(continued)*						
LEAD	Storage batteries; manufacturing of paint, enamel, ink, glass, rubber, ceramics, chemical industry	Ingestion of dust, inhalation of dust or fumes	Hematological Renal Gastrointestinal Neuromuscular Central nervous system (CNS) Reproductive	Anemia Nephrotoxicity Abdominal pain ("colic") Palsy ("wrist drop") Encephalopathy, behavioral abnormalities Spontaneous abortion	Blood lead Urinary ALA Zinc protoporphyrin; free erythrocyte protoporphyrin	Lead toxicity, unlike that of mercury, is believed to be reversible, with the exception of late renal and some CNS effects.
MERCURY Elemental	Electronic equipment; paint; metal and textile production; catalyst in chemical manufacturing; pharmaceutical production	Inhalation of vapor; slight percutaneous absorption	Pulmonary CNS	Acute pneumonitis Neuropsychiatric changes (erethism); tremor	Urinary mercury	Mercury illustrates several principles. The chemical form has a profound effect on its toxicology, as is the case for many metals. Effects of mercury are highly variable. Though inorganic mercury poisoning is primarily renal, elemental and organic poisoning are primarily neurological.
MERCURY Inorganic Organic	Agricultural and industrial poisons	Some inhalation and gastrointestinal (GI) and percutaneous absorption Efficient GI absorption, percutaneous absorption, and inhalation	Pulmonary Renal CNS Skin CNS	Acute pneumonitis Proteinuria Variable Dermatitis Sensorimotor changes, visual field constriction, tremor	Urinary mercury Blood and urine mercury	The responses are difficult to quantify, so dose-response data are generally unavailable. Classic tetrad of gingivitis, sialorrhea, irritability, and tremor is associated with both elemental and inorganic mercury poisoning; the four signs are not generally seen together. Many effects of mercury toxicity, especially those in CNS, are irreversible.
NICKEL	Corrosion-resistant alloys; electroplating; catalyst production; nickel–cadmium batteries	Inhalation of dust or fumes	Skin Pulmonary	Sensitization dermatitis ("nickel itch") Lung and paranasal sinus cancer		

ZINC OXIDE	Welding byproduct; rubber manufacturing	Inhalation of dust or fumes that are freshly generated		"Metal fume fever" (fever, chills, and other symptoms)	Urinary zinc (useful as an indicator of exposure, not for acute diagnosis)	A self-limiting syndrome of 24–48 hours with apparently no sequelae.
HYDROCARBONS						
BENZENE	Manufacturing of organic chemicals, detergents, pesticides, solvents, paint removers; used as a solvent	Inhalation of vapor; slight percutaneous absorption	CNS Hematopoietic Skin	Acute CNS depression Leukemia, aplastic anemia Dermatitis	Urinary phenol	Note that benzene, as with toluene and other solvents, can be monitored via its principal metabolite.
TOLUENE	Organic chemical manufacturing; solvent; fuel component	Inhalation of vapor, percutaneous absorption of liquid	CNS Skin	Acute CNS depression Chronic CNS problems such as memory loss Irritation dermatitis	Urinary hippuric acid	
XYLENE	A wide variety of uses as a solvent; an ingredient of paints, lacquers, varnishes, inks, dyes, adhesives, cements; an intermediate in chemical manufacturing	Inhalation of vapor; slight percutaneous absorption of liquid	Pulmonary Eye, nose, throat CNS	Irritation, pneumonitis, acute pulmonary edema (at high doses) Irritation Acute CNS depression	Methylhippuric acid in urine, xylene in expired air, xylene in blood	
KETONES Acetone (methyl ethyl ketone—MEK, methyl *N*-propyl ketone—MPK, methyl *N*-butyl ketone—MBK, methyl iso-butyl ketone—MIBK)	A wide variety of uses as solvents and intermediates in chemical manufacturing	Inhalation of vapor, percutaneous absorption of liquid	CNS Peripheral nervous system (PNS) Skin	Acute CNS depression MBK has been linked with peripheral neuropathy Dermatitis	Acetone in blood, urine, expired air (used as an index for exposure, not for diagnosis)	The ketone family demonstrates how a pattern of toxic responses (i.e., CNS narcosis) may feature exceptions (i.e., MBK peripheral neuropathy).
FORMALDEHYDE	Widely used as a germicide and a disinfectant in embalming and histopathology, for example, and in the manufacture of textiles, resins, and other products	Inhalation	Skin Eye Pulmonary	Irritant and contact dermatitis Eye irritant Respiratory tract irritation, asthma	Patch testing may be useful for dermatitis	Recent animal tests have shown it to be a respiratory carcinogen. Confirmatory epidemiological studies are in progress.

(*Continued*)

Agent	Exposure	Route of Entry	System(s) Affected	Primary Manifestations	Aids in Diagnosis	Remarks
HYDROCARBONS *(continued)*						
TRICHLOROETHYLENE (TCE)			Nervous Skin Cardiovascular	Acute CNS depression Peripheral and cranial neuropathy Irritation, dermatitis Dysrhythmias	Breath analysis for TCE	TCE is involved in an important pharmacological interaction. Within hours of ingesting alcoholic beverages, TCE workers experience flushing of the face, neck, shoulders, and back. Alcohol may also potentiate the CNS effects of TCE. The probable mechanism is competition for metabolic enzyme.
CARBON TETRACHLORIDE	Solvent for oils, fats, lacquers, resins, varnishes, other materials; used as a degreasing and cleaning agent	Inhalation of vapor	Hepatic Renal CNS Skin	Toxic hepatitis Oliguria or anuria Acute CNS depression Dermatitis	Expired air and blood levels	Carbon tetrachloride is the prototype for a wide variety of solvents that cause hepatitis and renal damage. This solvent, like trichloroethylene, acts synergistically with ethanol.
CARBON DISULFIDE	Solvent for lipids, sulfur, halogens, rubber, phosphorus, oils, waxes, and resins; manufacturing of organic chemicals, paints, fuels, explosives, viscose rayon	Inhalation of vapor, percutaneous absorption of liquid or vapor	Nervous Renal Cardiovascular Skin Reproductive	Parkinsonism, psychosis, suicide Peripheral neuropathies Chronic nephritic and nephrotic syndromes Acceleration or worsening of atherosclerosis; hypertension Irritation; dermatitis Menorrhagia and metrorrhagia	Iodine azide reaction with urine (nonspecific since other bivalent sulfur compounds give a positive test); CS_2 in expired air, blood, and urine	A solvent with unusual multisystem effects, especially noted for cardiovascular, renal, and nervous system actions.
STODDARD SOLVENT	Degreasing, paint thinning	Inhalation of vapor, percutaneous absorption of liquid	Skin CNS	Dryness and scaling from defatting; dermatitis Dizziness, coma, collapse (at high levels)	A mixture of primarily aliphatic hydrocarbons, with some benzene derivatives and naphthalenes	

ETHYLENE GLYCOL ETHERS Ethylene glycol monoethyl ether—Cellosolve, ethylene glycol monoethyl acetate—Cellosolve acetate, methyl- and butyl-substituted compounds such as ethylene glycol mono-methyl ether-methyl Cellosolve	The ethers are used as solvents for resins, paints, lacquers, varnishes, gum, perfume, dyes, and inks; the acetate derivatives are widely used as solvents and ingredients of lacquers, enamels, and adhesives. Exposure occurs in dry cleaning, plastic, ink, and lacquer manufacturing, and textile dying, among other processes	Inhalation of vapor, percutaneous absorption of liquid	Reproductive CNS Renal Liver		Ethylene glycol ethers, as a class of chemicals, have been shown in animals to have adverse effects including reduced sperm count and spontaneous abortion, as well as CNS, renal, and liver effects	
ETHYLENE OXIDE	Used in the sterilization of medical equipment, in the fumigation of spices and other foodstuffs, as a chemical intermediate	Inhalation	Skin Eye Respiratory tract Nervous system	Dermatitis and frostbite Severe irritation; possibly cataracts with prolonged exposure Irritation Peripheral neuropathy		Recent animal tests have shown it to be carcinogenic and to cause reproductive abnormalities. Epidemiological studies indicate that it may cause leukemia in exposed workers.
DIOXANE	Used as a solvent for a variety of materials, including cellulose acetate, dyes, fats, greases, resins, polyvinyl polymers, varnishes, and waxes	Inhalation of vapor, percutaneous absorption of liquid	CNS Renal Liver	Drowsiness, dizziness, anorexia, headaches, nausea, vomiting, coma Nephritis Chemical hepatitis		Dioxane has caused a variety of neoplasms in animals.
POLYCHLORINATED BIPHENYLS (PCBs)	Formerly used as dielectric fluid in electrical equipment and as a fire-retardant coating on tiles and other products. New uses were banned in 1976, but much of the electrical equipment currently used still contains PCBs	Inhalation, ingestion, skin absorption	Skin Eye Liver	Chloracne Irritation Toxic hepatitis	Serum PCB level for chronic exposure	Animal studies have demonstrated that PCBs are carcinogenic. Epidemiological studies of exposed workers are inconclusive.

(Continued)

Agent	Exposure	Route of Entry	System(s) Affected	Primary Manifestations	Aids in Diagnosis	Remarks
IRRITANT GASES						
AMMONIA	Refrigeration; petroleum refining; manufacturing of nitrogen-containing chemicals, synthetic fibers, dyes, and optics	Inhalation of gas	Upper respiratory tract Eye Moist skin	Upper respiratory irritation Irritation Irritation		
HYDROCHLORIC ACID	Chemical manufacturing; electroplating; tanning; metal pickling; petroleum extraction; rubber, photographic, and textile industries	Inhalation of gas or mist	Upper respiratory tract Eye Mucous membrane, skin	Upper respiratory irritation Strong irritant Strong irritant		
HYDROFLUORIC ACID	Chemical and plastic manufacturing; catalyst in petroleum refining; aqueous solution for frosting, etching, and polishing glass	Inhalation of gas or mist	Upper respiratory tract	Upper respiratory irritation		In solution, causes severe and painful burns of skin and can be fatal.
SULFUR DIOXIDE	Manufacturing of sulfur-containing chemicals; food and textile bleach; tanning; metal casting	Inhalation of gas, direct contact of gas or liquid phase on skin or mucosa	Middle respiratory tract	Bronchospasm (pulmonary edema or chemical pneumonitis in high dose)	Chest x-ray, pulmonary function tests	Strong irritant of eye, mucous membranes, and skin.
CHLORINE	Paper and textile bleaching; water disinfection; chemical manufacturing, metal fluxing; detinning and dezincing iron	Inhalation of gas	Middle respiratory tract	Tracheobronchitis, pulmonary edema, pneumonitis	Chest x-ray, pulmonary function tests	Chlorine combines with body moisture to form acids, which irritate tissues from nose to alveoli.
OZONE	Inert gas-shielded arc welding; food, water, and air purification; food and textile bleaching; emitted around high-voltage electrical equipment	Inhalation of gas	Lower respiratory tract	Delayed pulmonary edema (generally 6–8 hours following exposure)	Chest x-ray, pulmonary function tests	Ozone has a free-radical structure and can produce experimental chromosome aberrations; it may thus have carcinogenic potential.

NITROGEN OXIDES	Manufacturing of acids, nitrogen-containing chemicals, explosives, and more; by-product of many industrial processes	Inhalation of gas	Lower respiratory tract	Pulmonary irritation, bronchiolitis fibrosa obliterations ("silo filler's disease"), mixed obstructive–restrictive changes	Chest x-ray, pulmonary function tests	
PHOSGENE Isocyanates TDI (toluene diisocyanate) MDI (methylene diphenyl diisocyanate) Hexamethylene diisocyanate and others	Manufacturing and burning of isocyanates, and manufacturing of dyes and other organic chemicals; in metallurgy for one separation; burning or heat source near trichloroethylene Polyurethane manufacture; resin-binding systems in foundries; coating materials for wires; used in certain types of paint	Inhalation of gas Inhalation of vapor	Lower respiratory tract Predominantly lower respiratory tract	Delayed pulmonary edema (delay seldom longer than 12 hours) Asthmatic reaction and accelerated loss of pulmonary function	Chest x-ray, pulmonary function tests Chest x-ray, pulmonary function tests	Isocyanates are both respiratory tract "sensitizers" and irritants in the conventional sense.
ASPHYXIANT GASES (simple asphyxiants: nitrogen, hydrogen, methane, and others)	Enclosed spaces in a variety of industrial settings	Inhalation of gas	CNS	Anoxia	O_2 in environment	No specific toxic effect; act by displacing O_2.
CHEMICAL ASPHYXIANTS						
CARBON MONOXIDE	Incomplete combustion in foundries, coke ovens, refineries, furnaces, and more	Inhalation of gas	Blood (hemoglobin)	Headache, dizziness, double vision	Carboxyhemoglobin	
HYDROGEN SULFIDE	Used in manufacturing of sulfur-containing chemicals; produced in petroleum product use; decay of organic matter	Inhalation of gas	CNS Pulmonary	Respiratory center paralysis, hypoventilation Respiratory tract irritation	PaO_2	
CYANIDE	Metallurgy, electroplating	Inhalation of vapor, percutaneous absorption, ingestion	Cellular metabolic enzymes (especially cytochrome oxidase)	Enzyme inhibition with metabolic asphyxia and death	SCN in urine	

(Continued)

Agent	Exposure	Route of Entry	System(s) Affected	Primary Manifestations	Aids in Diagnosis	Remarks
PESTICIDES						
ORGANOPHOSPHATES (malathion, parathion, and others)		Inhalation, ingestion, percutaneous absorption	Neuromuscular	Cholinesterase inhibition, cholinergic symptoms: nausea and vomiting, salivation, diarrhea, headache, sweating, meiosis, muscle fasciculations, seizures, unconsciousness, death	Refractoriness to atropine; plasma or red cell cholinesterase	As with many acute toxins, rapid treatment of organophosphate toxicity is imperative. Thus diagnosis is often based on history and a high index of suspicion rather than biochemical tests. Treatment is atropine to block cholinergic effects and 2-pyridine aldoxime methyl chloride (2-PAM) to reactivate cholinesterase.
CARBAMATES (carbaryl [Sevin] and others)		Inhalation, ingestion, percutaneous absorption	Neuromuscular	Cholinesterase inhibition, cholinergic symptoms: nausea and vomiting, salivation, diarrhea, headache, sweating, meiosis, muscle fasciculations, seizures, unconsciousness, death	Plasma cholinesterase; urinary 1-naphthol (index of exposure)	Treatment of carbamate poisoning is the same as that of organophosphate poisoning except that 2-PAM is contraindicated.
CHLORINATED HYDROCARBONS Chlordane DDT Heptachlor Chlordecone (Kepone) Aldrin Dieldrin Uridine		Inhalation, ingestion, percutaneous absorption	CNS	Stimulation or depression	Urinary organic chlorine, or *p*-chlorophenol acetic acid	The chlorinated hydrocarbons may accumulate in body lipid stores in large amounts.
BIPYRIDYLS Paraquat Diquat		Inhalation, ingestion, percutaneous absorption	Pulmonary	Rapid massive fibrosis, only following Paraquat ingestion		An interesting toxin in that the major toxicity, pulmonary fibrosis, apparently occurs only after ingestion.

Source: Tarcher, A. B. (Ed.). (1992). *Principles and practice of environmental medicine.* New York, NY: Plenum Press.

UNIT 3

Care of Communities and Populations

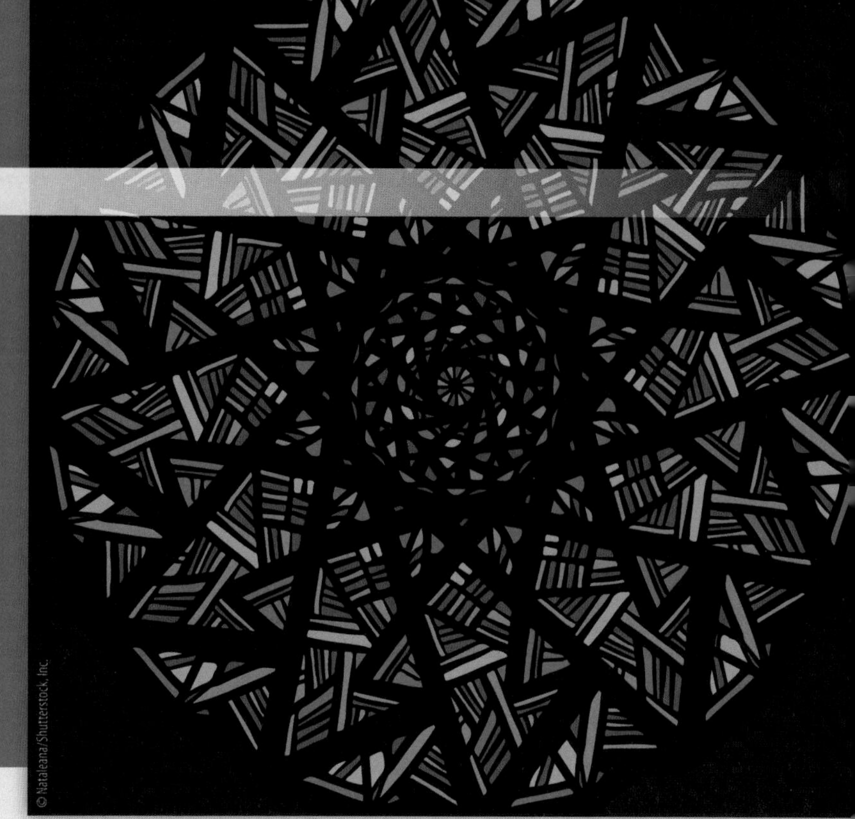
© Nataleana/Shutterstock, Inc.

CHAPTER FOCUS

Basic Concepts of Health and Health Promotion
- Selected Definitions of Health Promotion and Wellness
- Community Health Promotion and Wellness

Factors Influencing Health Promotion and Wellness
- Changes in Societal Expectations
- Shifting Sands of the Healthcare Delivery System
- U.S. Government Initiatives
- Affordable Care Act
- Public–Private Partnerships
- Growing Consumerism and Emphasis on Self-Care

Models of Health Promotion and Wellness
- Holistic Wellness: Self-Inventory of Personal Wellness
- Using the Medicine Wheel
- The 4+ Model of Wellness
- How to Use the 4+ Model of Wellness with Individuals, Families, Populations, and Communities
- The Pender Health Promotion Model
- Life Stages Conceptual Framework

QUESTIONS TO CONSIDER

After reading this chapter, you will know the answers to the following questions:

1. What is the difference between health promotion and wellness?
2. What are levels of prevention?
3. What do health promotion and wellness look like?
4. Which factors influence health promotion and wellness?
5. What are the different models for health promotion?
6. How can community health nurses use these models in the promotion of health in their patients?
7. How can a nurse use these concepts to promote self-health?

CHAPTER 14

Health Promotion and Wellness

Joan H. Baldwin,
Cynthia Conger,
and Betty Sylvest

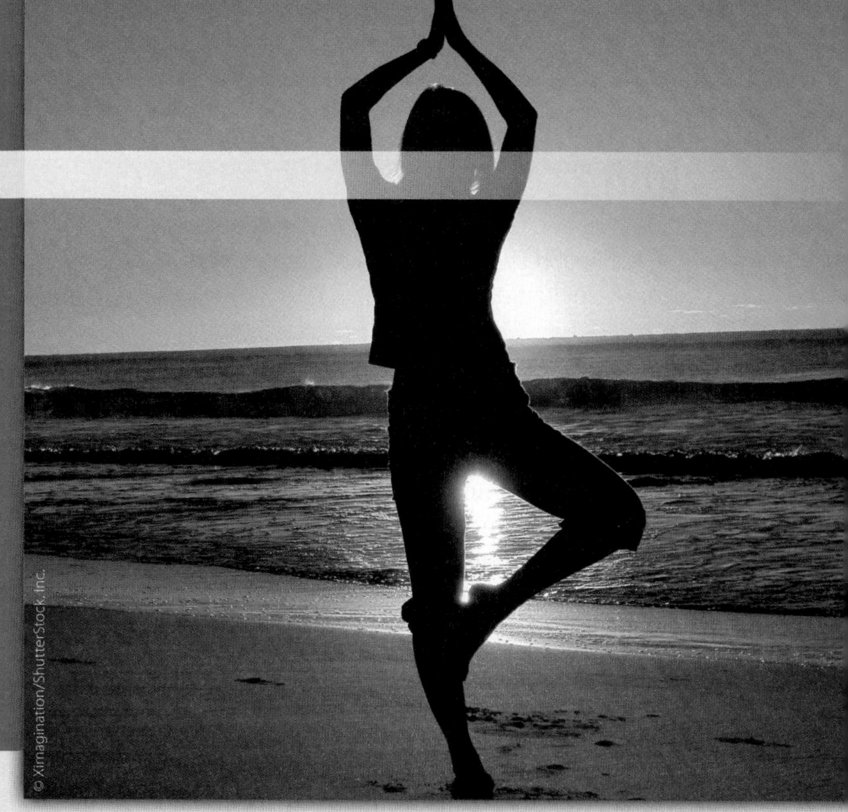

KEY TERMS

chronic diseases and health promotion
health-promoting behaviors
health promotion
high-level wellness
levels of prevention
personal health promotion
professional health promotion
wellness

> It is not stress that kills us, it is our reaction to it.
>
> —Hans Selye

REFLECTIONS

At the end of the day, what do you do to remain healthy? What does being healthy mean to you? Has the meaning of health changed since you entered nursing school? Why do you think nursing is among the least healthy of all the helping professions?

HEALTH PROMOTION AND WELLNESS are important concepts throughout nursing education and practice in all settings. Nurses promote good health and wellness for themselves, their loved ones, and patients. Generally, the major steps to health and wellness include healthy eating, proper exercise, adequate sleep, and time to unwind and manage stress. Health promotion in this respect has always been a nursing focus. As the healthcare delivery system moves further into managed care, however, **health promotion** and **wellness** become still more important. Health promotion and disease prevention are the keys to managing healthcare costs. Promoting the health of individuals, families, populations, and communities is essential in nursing practice not only because it is the humane and ethical thing to do, but also because it has practical and economic benefits.

It may be surprising to learn that there are several different definitions for the terms *health promotion* and *wellness*. There are definitions of health promotion and wellness for self, for other individuals, and even for populations and communities.

What do nurses really mean when they say they promote good health and wellness? There are many aspects of health promotion and wellness that will be important to know as a professional nurse. In this chapter, we (1) briefly discuss basic concepts of health and health promotion as related to the concept of disease prevention, including definitions of *health promotion* and *wellness* as the terms are used in this chapter; (2) delineate factors influencing health promotion and wellness; (3) demonstrate some ways of looking at health promotion and wellness by discussing some models of health promotion, risk evaluation, and analysis tools, plus wellness guides that might be useful to know about to promote health and wellness; and (4) introduce three models of wellness.

Basic Concepts of Health and Health Promotion

How people generally define health may influence how they define health promotion (Baldwin, 1995; Bryer, Cherkis, & Raman, 2014; Green & Raeburn, 1990; Raphael, 2000). For instance, if health is considered the absence of disease, the definition of health promotion would necessarily include the idea of disease prevention. However, if health is defined as a concept that expresses the positiveness of a full and joyful life, disease prevention is not a part of the definition. Edelman and Fain (1998) speak of this second characterization of health as "expanding consciousness, pattern or meaning recognition, personal transformation, and tentatively, self-actualization" (p. 9). One example is a woman living with a chronic disease such as diabetes, who still considers herself a healthy person; she may see herself being as far along toward self-actualization as she can be.

In 1983, Brubaker conducted a linguistic analysis of the term *health promotion* in nursing literature and found that it was rarely defined specifically and often used as though it had the same meaning as disease prevention. There continues to be debate about the definition of health promotion and whether the definition must necessarily include disease prevention.

Historically, health promotion as a concept has been linked with disease prevention. Clark and Leavell (1965) depicted three **levels of prevention**—primary, secondary, and tertiary—in a model. Primary prevention includes health promotion as part of the model. When primary prevention methods are used, the basic premise of the model is that health-promotion activities "serve to further general health and well-being" (Clark & Leavell, p. 20). Because this is a model describing disease-prevention factors, it leads one to connect health promotion with disease prevention. In this particular model, primary prevention methods include **health-promoting behaviors** that are designed to improve general health and wellbeing, with the emphasis being on preventing a disease in the first place. For instance, brushing teeth after meals is one step in preventing tooth decay, which would also be good for general health.

As early as 1965, Clark and Leavell noted, "health promotion is not applied for specific disease and as yet is not widely utilized" (p. 24). Identifying health-promoting strategies for secondary and tertiary prevention still seems to be a bit difficult today, but health-promoting activities are important in these levels as well. *Secondary prevention* refers to the early detection of disease and prevention of disease sequelae—defined as "an aftereffect of disease, condition, or injury; a secondary result" (*Webster's Collegiate Dictionary*, 2004). A health-promoting action for a woman who has a diagnosis of fibrocystic breast disease would be to avoid caffeine. Poe and O'Neill (1997) determined that caffeine slows the process of the body's natural defenses, which normally results in the elimination of precancerous cells. Therefore, the potential for proliferation of abnormal cells is increased with caffeine ingestion. Tertiary prevention focuses on the minimization of loss of function as a result of disease. Health-promoting activities in tertiary prevention might include training for a competition by a diabetic skier who has only one leg. Good and reasonable physical fitness promotes health.

Today there are also reasons for using health-promotion strategies, behaviors, or actions without necessarily having to consider prevention of disease. Someone may choose certain health-promoting actions just because the actions make the person feel good or healthy. For example, many people like to walk or run several times a week and comment that if they don't walk or run, they don't have as much energy during the day. In this example, these people are not specifically concerned about preventing disease; they just want to feel as good as they can.

GLOBAL CONNECTION

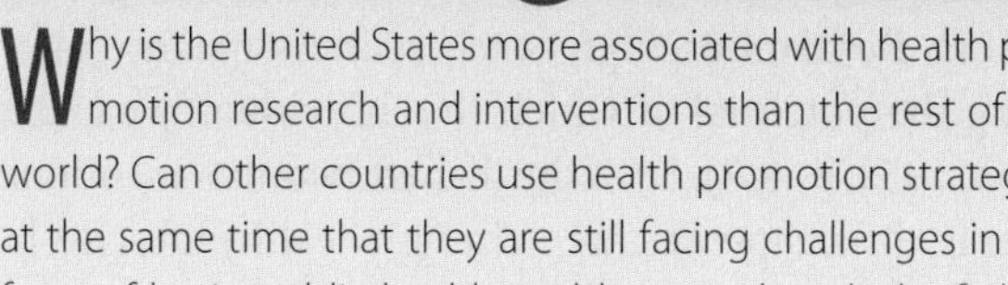

Why is the United States more associated with health promotion research and interventions than the rest of the world? Can other countries use health promotion strategies at the same time that they are still facing challenges in the form of basic public health problems such as lack of clean drinking water and infectious diseases?

The World Health Organization (WHO) has a number of subagencies related to worldwide health promotion. One of these, the International Union for Health Promotion and Education, has an official publication called *Global Health Promotion* that it uses to disseminate practical information for professionals around the world. The goal of the Chronic Diseases and Health Promotion program is "to provide leadership and direction of global, regional, and national efforts to promote health and to prevent and control major chronic diseases and their risk factors" (WHO, 2013a).

Selected Definitions of Health Promotion and Wellness

For the purposes of this chapter, health promotion has two definitions depending on if the nurse is applying health-promotion strategies to other people or if the nurse is promoting his or her own health. The definition of **professional health promotion** on behalf of others reflects the "organized actions or efforts that enhance, support, or promote the well-being or health of individuals, families, groups, communities, or societies" (Kulbok, Baldwin, Cox, & Duffy., 1997, p. 17). An example of this definition is a school nurse teaching elementary school children the importance of washing hands to eliminate germs and dirt. The nurse first coats the children's hands with an invisible product that can be washed away with soap and water. After handwashing, a special light is shined on the children's hands; areas not carefully washed clean of the product glow green, demonstrating to the children that if hands are not carefully washed, "germs" may remain, much like the green, glowing product. Health education programs and physical education activities, to name two possibilities, are also examples of professional health promotion on behalf of others.

Personal health promotion reflects more emphasis on self-actualization and taking care of oneself. This definition identifies what motivates people "to attain and maintain their highest state of wellness, overall fitness, and self-actualization" (Baldwin, 1992, p. 10). For instance, the school nurse may recognize that walking daily for 30 minutes after work maintains physical fitness, dissipates work stress, and provides a sense of renewal and joy as he or she appreciates the spring flowers blooming.

GOT AN ALTERNATIVE?

Back injuries are the most common occupational injury reported by nurses during their careers. Avoiding back injuries is more than proper body mechanics: New lifting technology in healthcare facilities and self-care exercise, such as yoga, tai-chi, and weight-bearing and strengthening exercises, are all important prevention strategies that nurses should use to avoid this chronic, often disabling condition. Mitchell, O'Sullivan, Burnett, Straker, and Rudd (2008) researched the occurrence of low back pain in nursing students and through their careers and found that although many facilities have programs to prevent back injuries, these programs are not used on a regular basis by students or nurses. Many studies have assessed the likelihood of nurses developing back injuries at some point in their career (Dent, 2010.)

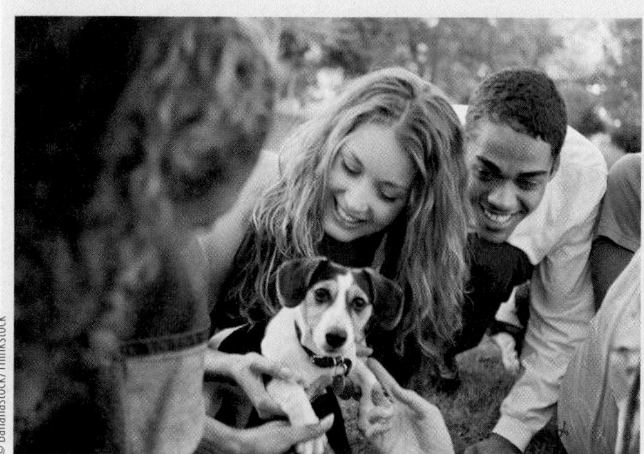

Positive and nurturing relationships with friends and pets are associated with good health.

BOX 14-1 Key Concepts: Definitions of Health Promotion

Health promotion by professionals on behalf of others is "organized actions or efforts that enhance, support, or promote the wellbeing or health of individuals, families, groups, communities, or societies" (Kulbok et al., 1997, p. 17).

Personal health promotion is identification of what motivates people "to attain and maintain their highest state of wellness, overall fitness, and self-actualization" (Baldwin, 1992, p. 10).

What is the relationship between health promotion and wellness? As defined in this chapter, health promotion relates to behaviors or activities that result in wellness. Dunn (1959, 1980) describes **high-level wellness** as "an integrated method of functioning which is oriented toward maximizing the potential of which the individual is capable" (p. 447). The concept of high-level wellness is based on the assumption that every individual, regardless of personal challenges, has a potential for wellness within the limits placed by the challenge. In other words, high-level wellness is the highest level of wellbeing that a person can reach. To attain high-level wellness, there must be harmony in all aspects of a person's life. **Box 14-1** lists two definitions of health promotion.

Health promotion and wellness, particularly when defined for one's own use, are closely related or even interrelated. In this chapter, *wellness* is a state of being; *health promotion* is how one gets there (**Box 14-2**). How one attains and maintains wellness is accomplished through various health-promoting behaviors. In 2013, the U.S. Department of Health and Human Services published a list of healthy behaviors leading to prevention of major diseases. Health prevention behaviors include: (1) exercise and fitness; (2) diet, nutrition and eating right; (3) healthy lifestyle (i.e., weight loss if obesity present, smoking and tobacco cessation, limited drinking of alcohol, prevention of injury or accidents); (4) vaccination/immunization; (5) health screenings; (6) healthy environmental factors.

WHO (2013a) presented the Chronic Diseases and Health Promotion (CHP) whose mission was to provide direction and leadership on the global, regional, and national fronts. This direction was designed to promote health, helping to control chronic diseases and risk factors. The objectives for the CHP were to provide advocacy for health promotion and chronic disease control by providing guidelines for chronic disease prevention. The CHP was charged with promoting health especially for the poor and disadvantaged populations. The CHP was charged with the prevention of early deaths and avoidance of unnecessary disabilities related to the affects of chronic major diseases, hoping to prevent blindness and deafness.

BOX 14-2 Definitions of Wellness, Health-Promoting Behaviors, and the Interrelationship Between Health Promotion and Wellness

High-level wellness is "an integrated method of functioning which is oriented toward maximizing the potential of which the individual is capable" (Dunn, 1959, p. 447).

Health-promoting behaviors are "any actions or behaviors taken by individuals to improve or promote well-being or health" (Kulbok et al., 1997, p. 17). These "behaviors [are those] that enhance, support, encourage and/or promote a healthy state" (Kulbok, Carter, Baldwin, Gilmartin, & Kirkwood, 1999).

The *interrelationship of health promotion and wellness* can be represented by the idea that wellness is a state of being, and health promotion is how one gets there.

A person can be sick and be moving toward wellness using health-promoting actions or behaviors or can have a chronic disease and actually be experiencing high-level wellness. Remember, high-level wellness means "maximizing the potential of which the individual is capable" (Dunn, 1959, p. 447). So, if the diabetic woman mentioned earlier in this chapter is maintaining a healthy lifestyle, has no difficulty managing her diabetes, is happy, and feels well balanced in her life, it could be said that the woman is likely to be experiencing high-level wellness. The woman is maximizing the potential of which she is capable.

The woman with diabetes is the one most likely to know what her maximum potential can be and how close she is to reaching it in her life. What high-level wellness is, using Dunn's (1959) definition, for any particular person is defined by that person and may change over time.

How can a 22-year-old student nurse who is in a car accident and becomes a paraplegic reach high-level wellness? According to the aforementioned definitions, the student nurse has the potential to be more or less well within the boundaries of the limits set by the condition. "Wellness is a bridge that takes people into realms far beyond treatment or therapy—into a domain of self-responsibility and self-empowerment" (Ryan & Travis, 1991, p. 3). The student nurse has choices. Relating to personal life, the student nurse has the choice to (1) do nothing about overcoming the physical, emotional, mental, and spiritual challenges of being a paraplegic; (2) learn to use a wheelchair to go to classes and elsewhere; or (3) perhaps even go so far as to become a gold medalist in the Paralympics. Professionally, the student nurse can bend to the pressure of the barriers and drop out of the nursing program or fight the system to remain, making adjustments as necessary. There is no reason that a full, satisfying, professional nursing career should be out of reach for this student.

It is important to note that nurses do not define high-level wellness for patients, but rather they assist patients in identifying what they are capable of reaching to maximize their potential for high-level wellness. Remember what was noted earlier in the chapter: High-level wellness is the highest level of wellbeing *that patients can reach*. An overweight, heavy-smoking, heavy-drinking person may think, and even state, the belief that he or she is healthy, but given Dunn's definition, it is unlikely that the person is experiencing high-level wellness and maximizing his or her potential to the best of his or her abilities. It is relatively easy to apply this concept to individuals, but how does high-level wellness translate to communities?

According to WHO (2013b), "Health promotion is the process of enabling people to increase control over, and to improve, their health. It moves beyond a focus on individual behavior towards a wide range of social and environmental interventions" (para 1)

Models of Health Promotion

While the definition of health promotion has been universally adopted, there have been a number of different approaches to promoting health. Since the 1960s, three key models of health have influenced health promotion. The *biomedical model of health* (pre-1970s):

- Focuses on risk behaviors and healthy lifestyles
- Emphasizes health education—changing knowledge, attitudes, and skills
- Focuses on individual responsibility
- Treats people in isolation of their environments

The *social model of health* (from the 1970s onward):

- Addresses the broader determinants of health
- Involves intersectoral collaboration
- Acts to reduce social inequities
- Empowers individuals and communities
- Acts to enable access to health care

The *ecological model of health* (from the late 1970s onward):

- Acknowledges the reciprocal relationship between health-related behaviors and the environments in which people live, work, and play (behavior does not occur in a vacuum)
- Considers the environment is made up of different subsystems—micro, meso, exo, and macro
- Emphasizes the relationships and dependencies between these subsystems
- Is comprehensive and multifaceted, using a shared framework for change at individual and environmental levels (Victorian Health Promotion Foundation, 2013)

The future role of nursing in health promotion will be in education, practice, and research settings where nurses will participate in the advancement of health promotion not only to the mainstream but to the forefront of nursing practice. The future must focus on teaching people how to remain healthy using evidence-based practice, which will affect health promotion (Chiverton, Votava, & Tortoretti, 2003).

Community Health Promotion and Wellness

Communities have potential for high-level wellness, too. Communities can be defined within geographic boundaries or as population groups with special needs or interests (Baldwin, Conger, Abegglen, & Hill, 1998). Communities usually have systems in place, such as planning commissions or committees, to identify what is high-level wellness for that group. For example, one element of wellness identified in the motto for Sandy City, Utah, is support for family values. One way the community supports family values is by promoting healthy family activities. Toward this end, the community master plan establishes a network of neighborhood parks that will be developed as neighborhoods expand. This process maximizes the potential of the community to reach what it has defined as high-level wellness.

The Role of the Nurse in Health Promotion

According to Hartford (2009), nurses are high-level thinkers with exceptional skills and considerable ability to communicate, negotiate, coordinate, and collaborate in the delivery of health care in the community. Each interaction with people of the community gives the nurse an opportunity to provide education related to health promotion. The nurse listens to the people and gains insight into what level of wellness the person exists in. The nurse can assist the person in developing a personal goal of working toward wellness (as perceived by the person).

> Life is short, the art long, opportunity fleeting, experience treacherous, judgment difficult.
>
> —*Hippocrates (460–377 B.C.)*

Some community interventions that support wellness are relatively easy to identify by community members. Others, especially related to population wellness, are more difficult for communities to pinpoint. Nurses often collaborate with community groups to identify these strengths, assets, problems, and needs.

People with chronic and even terminal diseases may live their lives in such a healthy and balanced manner that high-level wellness might be attained, at least for a time. A person can use health-promotion behaviors and activities even if ill or diseased "to become an active participant in the healing process instead of a passive recipient" (Ryan & Travis, 1991, p. 3).

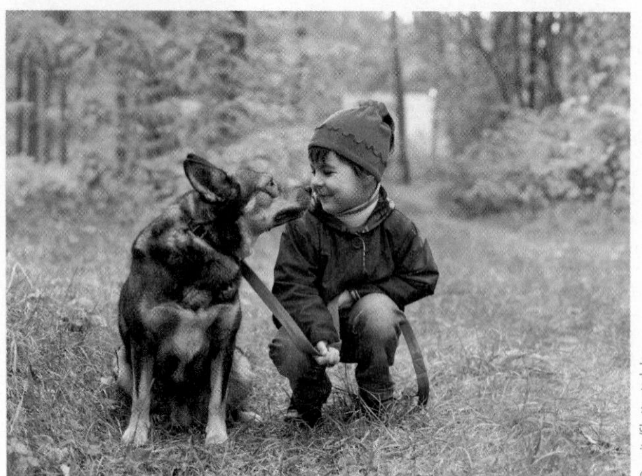
© vvvita/Shutterstock, Inc.

Learning to care for pets can promote health through teaching compassion and caring to children.

CULTURAL CONNECTION

You have noticed that everything an Indian does is in a circle, and that is because the Power of the World always works in circles, and everything tries to be round. . . . The Sky is round, and I have heard that the earth is round like a ball, and so are all the stars. The wind, in its greatest power, whirls. Birds make their nests in circles, for theirs is the same religion as ours. . . . Even the seasons form a great circle in their changing, and always come back again to where they were. The life of a man is a circle from childhood, and so it is in everything where power moves.

—Black Elk, Oglala Sioux holy man, 1863

Factors Influencing Health Promotion and Wellness

Health care in the United States is finally experiencing a shift in focus from a rather one-sided emphasis on present and potential disease to a more balanced focus that includes an equal emphasis on health promotion, wellness, risk reduction, and disease prevention (Baldwin et al., 1998). Educating patients, defined as individuals, families, populations, or communities, regarding their health requires information about health-promotion activities that the patients consider relevant to them. It is because of this shift in focus that we now are more strongly accentuating the importance of understanding the "whys" and "how-to's" of health promotion and wellness. Some of the factors influencing health promotion and wellness are the changes in societal expectations, shifting sands of the healthcare delivery system, U.S. government initiatives, public–private partnerships, and growing consumerism and emphasis on self-care.

Changes in Societal Expectations

Over the years, people in the United States have vacillated as to what good health and wellness are all about. Some cultures had lifestyles that encompassed running and athletic feats, such as hunting, that sustained life; other groups were much more sedentary. Types of foods eaten varied, and little attention was paid to which foods were healthy and which foods were not; the important thing was being able to eat. Prior to the 1960s, the social system was such that the majority of people spent more time worrying about food, shelter, and safety (lower levels of Maslow's hierarchy) than self-actualization (Maslow, 1970). The relationship of lifestyle and health had not been established scientifically. Health was primarily defined as the absence of disease, and healthcare delivery and research focused on controlling and trying to cure communicable diseases. The media played little or no role in sharing health-related information with the public other than reporting morbidity and mortality information.

Since the 1960s, societal expectations have changed. Increasing affluence has allowed the majority of society to move beyond a primary concern with food, shelter, and safety toward achieving self-esteem and self-actualization (Maslow, 1970). High-level wellness is a state of self-actualization, "maximizing the potential of which the individual is capable" (Dunn, 1959, p. 447). During the 1950s and 1960s, the leading causes of morbidity and mortality moved from communicable disease to chronic disease. With this shift, the healthcare profession had less success in controlling the causes of disease or in curing some of the diseases. Instead of cure, the focus became symptom management. It became more obvious that the method of control for chronic disease begins with health promotion and specific preventive measures.

MEDIA MOMENT 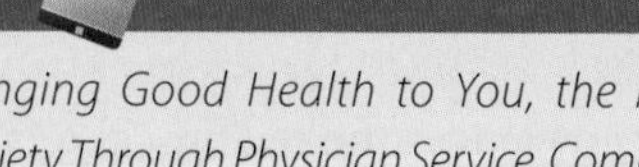

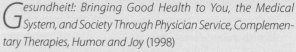

Gesundheit!: Bringing Good Health to You, the Medical System, and Society Through Physician Service, Complementary Therapies, Humor and Joy (1998)

By Patch Adams and Maureen Mylander, Rochester, VT: Inner Traditions International.

All those who loved the movie *Patch Adams* will want to read this enjoyable book to learn more about the revolutionary ideas of this fascinating physician and his successful practice at the Gesundheit Institute in Northern Virginia.

Dr. Adams is a social revolutionary who presents his unique approach to "free medicine" through a collection of essays. Adams believes that today's high-tech medicine is too costly, impersonal, and boring. He demonstrates how healing can be a loving, creative, and humorous human-to-human experience between practitioner and patient, rather than a for-profit business. Through the efforts of Adams and his colleagues, the Gesundheit Institute was operated as a free healthcare service, without payment, malpractice insurance, or formal facilities.

Adams's book is an excellent example of the possibilities of how complementary and conventional medicine can be combined to deliver services to patients in a partnership based on mutual respect and a commitment to a vision of what good health can be.

Since the mid-1960s, there has been a proliferation of research relating health promotion and wellness to lifestyle practices. This information has become so popular that the media have developed an interest in reporting health-promotion strategies. Today, experts on morning television programs regularly report the latest in health-related research and health-promotion strategies. With these societal changes in perception and the increasing costs of health care, pressure came to bear to look for the most cost-effective methods to deliver health care.

Shifting Sands of the Healthcare Delivery System

The healthcare delivery system, as a fee-for-service system, focused on the treatment of illness rather than on health promotion and prevention of disease (Butterfield, 1993). However, research has demonstrated that the causes of most chronic illness are the practice of health-depleting behaviors *and* social and environmental barriers that limit the choices individuals, families, populations, and communities have relating to health-promoting activities. In addition, in a seminal article by McGinnis and Foege (1993), the chief preventable causes of death are translated to lifestyle choices and social influences. These causes include tobacco use; poor diet and activity patterns; alcohol consumption; exposure to environmental microbial or toxic agents; inappropriate use of firearms; promiscuous, unprotected sexual behaviors; motor vehicle accidents; illicit drug use; and socioeconomic barriers.

There are many social barriers that limit the choices patients have in relationship to health-promoting activities. Prime examples are those who live in inner cities or who live in rural or frontier areas. Food choices are limited by distance to full-service grocery stores and availability of transportation. The stores that are available tend to be small, family-owned markets or gas station mini-marts. Both provide limited choice of foods at prices higher than full-service chain stores. In addition, gas station mini-marts may not sell produce, but do sell high-fat, high-calorie, and high-sugar convenience foods.

With the move to managed care and other community-based services for individuals and families and the realization that chronic illness and even death are grounded, for the most part, in lifestyle choices and social barriers, the focus of health care is changing. The principles of managed care require that health-promotion and disease-prevention activities be included in practice at both individual and population levels to prevent the costly occurrence of chronic disease and disability. For managed care organizations to realize a profit, risk groups must be managed at the individual and the aggregate levels (Baldwin et al., 1998). Also, managed care organizations are becoming more involved in community activities such as community-based health centers, health fairs, Healthy Communities programs, and school-based clinics. Many managed care systems and other insurance companies encourage health-promotion education, activities, and behaviors for their members. In addition, industries have included wellness programs for employees, which may offer various types of reimbursement incentives, from lowering insurance premiums to giving bonuses to those members and employees who demonstrate health-promoting behaviors.

Social media is being used across the generations. According to a study by Kaiser Permanente, half of internet users are noted to be between the ages of 50 and 63 and about one in three users are aged 64 and older (Benner, 2013). Social media is playing a major role in the health literacy of patients. Patients can find information related to any illness via the internet. Social media contacts via avenues such as "tweeter", "Facebook", "Yahoo messenger" as well as many other websites provide information related to healthcare and health in general. This could also be a hindrance to healthy lifestyles (Holiday, 2013).

HEALTHY PEOPLE 2020 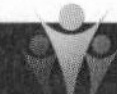

Health Determinants and Health Outcomes by Life Stages Conceptual Framework

Healthy People 2020 provides a set of 10-year national goals and objectives for improving Americans' health. This proposal contains 42 areas and nearly 600 objectives in which there are 1,200 measures. The Leading Health Indicators are those general areas that are labeled as high priority":

- Access to health services
- Clinical preventive services
- Environmental quality
- Injury and violence
- Maternal, infant, and child health
- Mental health
- Nutrition, physical activity, and obesity

(Continued)

HEALTHY PEOPLE 2020 (*CONTINUED*)

- Oral health
- Reproductive and sexual health
- Social determinants
- Substance abuse
- Tobacco

Source: Healthy People 2020. (2011). Leading health indicators: Development and framework. Retrieved from http://www.healthypeople.gov/2020/LHI/development.aspx

U.S. Government Initiatives

In the late 1970s, the Surgeon General of the United States, in a document entitled *Healthy People*, reported to the nation about the expectations at that time regarding health promotion and disease prevention in this country (Baldwin, 1992, 1995; Kulbok & Baldwin, 1992; U.S. Public Health Service [USPHS], 1979). The Surgeon General stated, "Let us make no mistake about the significance of this document, it represents an emerging consensus among scientists and the health community that the Nation's health strategy must be dramatically recast to emphasize the prevention of disease" (USPHS, 1979, p. vii).

In 1980, target outcomes, in the form of objectives for the year 1990, were given relating to the reduction of premature mortality in four age groups (Maiese & Fox, 1998). At that time, prevention of disease was the main thrust, with health-protection factors addressed and health promotion mentioned. Revised and updated objectives, written in 1990 for the year 2000 (*Healthy People 2000: National Health Promotion and Disease Prevention Objectives*), changed the order of health priorities. Health promotion became the first consideration in the list of three important factors: health promotion, health protection, and preventive services (Baldwin, 1992; Kulbok & Baldwin, 1992). The HHS published the document *Healthy People 2010 Objectives: Draft for Public Comment* (1998b) to elicit public and professional input into the developed national objectives for the year 2010. In November 2000, the second edition of *Healthy People 2010: Understanding and Improving Health* was published. These objectives were again updated in 2011 with the release of *Healthy People 2020*, which includes an assessment of progress toward health goals and the description of additional goals that 10 years of change and experience have brought to the forefront.

Nurses must be involved at all levels of policy development. They have been members of task forces developing the components of each *Healthy People* document, and via the Internet, nurses have had opportunity to give input and feedback on the *Healthy People 2020* development. An interactive database system, *DATA 2020*, has been developed and contains the most recent national and state data related to all of the objectives and subgroups of *Healthy People 2020*. These data are updated quarterly (Centers for Disease Control and Prevention [CDC], 2014). Health behaviors are also tracked by state with the Behavioral Risk Factor Surveillance System (BRFSS), which can be found on the CDC website (http://www.cdc.gov/brfss/). The *Healthy People 2020* document provides a wonderful opportunity for nursing students to assess populations within their local regions related to progress toward one or more of the objectives.

Through the years, the Institute of Medicine of the National Academies and the Secretary's Advisory Committee on National Health Promotion and Disease Prevention set out to provide several recommendations for the HHS as the leading health indicators. These indicators were developed and released as part of the *Healthy People 2020* initiative (HHS, 2011).

Affordable Care Act

On March 23, 2010, President Obama signed the Affordable Care Act (ACA). The law put in place comprehensive health insurance reforms that were to roll out over four years and beyond. The following is an overview of the healthcare law as it was proposed to roll out from 2010 to 2015.

2010: A new Patient's Bill of Rights goes into effect, protecting consumers from the worst abuses of the insurance industry. Cost-free preventive services begin for many Americans.
2011: People with Medicare can get key preventive services for free and also receive a 50% discount on brand-name drugs in the Medicare "donut hole."
2012: Accountable Care Organizations and other programs help doctors and healthcare providers work together to deliver better care.
2013: Open enrollment in the Health Insurance Marketplace begins on October 1st.
2014: All Americans will have access to affordable health insurance options. The Marketplace allows individuals and small businesses to compare health plans on a level playing field. Middle and low-income families will get tax credits that cover a significant portion of the cost of coverage. The Medicaid program will be expanded to cover more low-income Americans. All together, these reforms mean that millions of people who were previously uninsured will gain coverage, thanks to the ACA.

New Consumer Protections

- **Putting Information for Consumers Online.** The law provides for where consumers can compare health insurance coverage options and pick the coverage that works for them. *Effective July 1, 2010.*
- **Prohibiting Denying Coverage of Children Based on Pre-Existing Conditions.** The healthcare law includes new rules to prevent insurance companies from denying coverage to children under the age of 19 due to a pre-existing condition. *Effective for health plan years beginning on or after September 23, 2010 for new plans and existing group plans.*
- **Prohibiting Insurance Companies from Rescinding Coverage.** In the past, insurance companies could search for an error, or other technical mistake, on a customer's application and use this error to deny payment for services when he or she got sick. The healthcare law makes this illegal. After media reports cited incidents of breast cancer patients losing coverage, insurance companies agreed to end this practice immediately. *Effective for health plan years beginning on or after September 23, 2010.*
- **Eliminating Lifetime Limits on Insurance Coverage.** Under the law, insurance companies will be prohibited from imposing lifetime dollar limits on essential benefits, like hospital stays. *Effective for health plan years beginning on or after September 23, 2010.*
- **Regulating Annual Limits on Insurance Coverage.** Under the law, insurance companies' use of annual dollar limits on the amount of insurance coverage a patient may receive will be restricted for new plans in the individual market and all group plans. In 2014, the use of annual dollar limits on essential benefits like hospital stays will be banned for new plans in the individual market and all group plans. *Effective for health plan years beginning on or after September 23, 2010.*
- **Appealing Insurance Company Decisions.** The law provides consumers with a way to appeal coverage determinations or claims to their insurance company, and establishes an external review process. *Effective for new plans beginning on or after September 23, 2010.*
- **Establishing Consumer Assistance Programs in the States.** Under the law, states that apply receive federal grants to help set up or expand independent offices to help consumers navigate the private health insurance system. These programs help consumers file complaints and appeals; enroll in health coverage; and get educated about their rights and responsibilities in group health plans or individual health insurance policies. The programs will also collect data on the types of problems consumers have and file reports with the HHS to identify trouble spots that need further oversight. *Grants Awarded October 2010.*

Improving Quality and Lowering Costs

- **Providing Small Business Health Insurance Tax Credits.** Up to 4 million small businesses are eligible for tax credits to help them provide insurance benefits to their workers. The first phase of this provision provides a credit worth up to 35% of the employer's contribution to the employees' health insurance. Small nonprofit organizations may receive up to a 25% credit. *Effective now.*
- **Offering Relief for 4 Million Seniors Who Hit the Medicare Prescription Drug "Donut Hole."** An estimated four million seniors will reach the gap in Medicare prescription drug coverage known as the "donut hole" this year. Each eligible senior will receive a one-time, tax free $250 rebate check. *First checks mailed in June 2010 and will continue monthly throughout 2010 as seniors hit the coverage gap.*
- **Providing Free Preventive Care.** All new plans must cover certain preventive services such as mammograms and colonoscopies without charging a deductible, co-pay, or coinsurance. *Effective for health plan years beginning on or after September 23, 2010.*
- **Preventing Disease and Illness.** A new $15 billion Prevention and Public Health Fund will invest in proven prevention and public health programs that can help keep Americans healthy—from smoking cessation to combating obesity. *Funding begins in 2010.*
- **Cracking Down on Health Care Fraud.** Current efforts to fight fraud have returned more than $2.5 billion to the Medicare Trust Fund in fiscal year 2009 alone. The new law invests new resources and requires new screening procedures for health care providers to boost these efforts and reduce fraud and waste in Medicare, Medicaid, and the Children's Health Improvement Program (CHIP). *Many provisions effective now.*

Increasing Access to Affordable Care

- **Providing Access to Insurance for Uninsured Americans with Pre-Existing Conditions.** The Pre-Existing Condition Insurance Plan provides new coverage options to individuals who have been uninsured for at least six months because of a pre-existing condition. States have the option of running this program in their state. If a state chooses not to do so, a plan will be established by the Department of Health and Human Services in that state. *National program effective July 1, 2010.*

- **Extending Coverage for Young Adults.**Under the law, young adults will be allowed to stay on their parents' plan until they turn 26 years old (in the case of existing group health plans, this right does not apply if the young adult is offered insurance at work). Check with your insurance company or employer to see if you qualify. *Effective for health plan years beginning on or after September 23.*
- **Expanding Coverage for Early Retirees.** Too often, Americans who retire without employer-sponsored insurance and before they are eligible for Medicare see their life savings disappear because of high rates in the individual market. To preserve employer coverage for early retirees until more affordable coverage is available through the new exchanges by 2014, the new law creates a $5 billion program to provide needed financial help for employment-based plans to continue to provide valuable coverage to people who retire between the ages of 55 and 65, as well as their spouses and dependents. *Applications for employers to participate in the program available June 1, 2010.* For more information on the Early Retiree Reinsurance Program, visit www.ERRP.gov.
- **Rebuilding the Primary Care Workforce.** To strengthen the availability of primary care, there are new incentives in the law to expand the number of primary care doctors, nurses, and physician assistants. These include funding for scholarships and loan repayments for primary care doctors and nurses working in underserved areas. Doctors and nurses receiving payments made under any state loan repayment or loan forgiveness program intended to increase the availability of healthcare services in underserved or health professional shortage areas will not have to pay taxes on those payments. *Effective 2010.*
- **Holding Insurance Companies Accountable for Unreasonable Rate Hikes**. The law allows states that have, or plan to implement, measures that require insurance companies to justify their premium increases will be eligible for $250 million in new grants. Insurance companies with excessive or unjustified premium exchanges may not be able to participate in the new health insurance exchanges in 2014. *Grants awarded beginning in 2010.*
- **Allowing States to Cover More People on Medicaid.** States will be able to receive federal matching funds for covering some additional low-income individuals and families under Medicaid for whom federal funds were not previously available. This will make it easier for states that choose to do so to cover more of their residents. *Effective April 1, 2010.*
- **Increasing Payments for Rural Health Care Providers.** Today, 68% of medically underserved communities across the nation are in rural areas. These communities often have trouble attracting and retaining medical professionals. The law provides increased payment to rural health care providers to help them continue to serve their communities. *Effective 2010.*
- **Strengthening Community Health Centers.** The law includes new funding to support the construction of and expand services at community health centers, allowing these centers to serve some 20 million new patients across the country. *Effective 2010.*

Improving Quality and Lowering Costs

- **Offering Prescription Drug Discounts.** Seniors who reach the coverage gap will receive a 50% discount when buying Medicare Part D covered brand name prescription drugs. Over the next 10 years, seniors will receive additional savings on brand name and generic drugs until the coverage gap is closed in 2020. *Effective January 1, 2011.*
- **Providing Free Preventive Care for Seniors.** The law provides certain free preventive services, such as annual wellness visits and personalized prevention plans for seniors on Medicare. *Effective January 1, 2011.* Learn more about preventive services under Medicare.
- **Improving Health Care Quality and Efficiency.** The law establishes a new Center for Medicare & Medicaid Innovation that will begin testing new ways of delivering care to patients. These methods are expected to improve the quality of care and reduce the rate of growth in healthcare costs for Medicare, Medicaid, and CHIP. Additionally, by January 1, 2011, HHS will submit a national strategy for quality improvement in health care, including by these programs. *Effective no later than January 1, 2011.*
- **Improving Care for Seniors After They Leave the Hospital.** The Community Care Transitions Program will help high-risk Medicare beneficiaries who are hospitalized avoid unnecessary

readmissions by coordinating care and connecting patients to services in their communities. *Effective January 1, 2011.*

- **Introducing New Innovations to Bring Down Costs.** The Independent Payment Advisory Board will begin operations to develop and submit proposals to Congress and the President aimed at extending the life of the Medicare Trust Fund. The Board is expected to focus on ways to target waste in the system and recommend ways to reduce costs, improve health outcomes for patients, and expand access to high-quality care. *Administrative funding becomes available October 1, 2011.* Learn more about strengthening Medicare.

Increasing Access to Affordable Care

- **Increasing Access to Services at Home and in the Community.** The Community First Choice Option allows states to offer home- and community-based services to disabled individuals through Medicaid rather than institutional care in nursing homes. *Effective beginning October 1, 2011.*

Holding Insurance Companies Accountable

- **Bringing Down Healthcare Premiums.** To ensure premium dollars are spent primarily on healthcare, the law generally requires that at least 85% of all premium dollars collected by insurance companies for large employer plans are spent on healthcare services and healthcare quality improvement. For plans sold to individuals and small employers, at least 80% of the premium must be spent on benefits and quality improvement. If insurance companies do not meet these goals, because their administrative costs or profits are too high, they must provide rebates to consumers. *Effective January 1, 2011.*
- **Addressing Overpayments to Big Insurance Companies and Strengthening Medicare Advantage.** Today, Medicare pays Medicare Advantage insurance companies over $1,000 more per person on average than is spent per person in Traditional Medicare. This results in increased premiums for all Medicare beneficiaries, including the 77% of beneficiaries who are not currently enrolled in a Medicare Advantage plan. The law levels the playing field by gradually eliminating this discrepancy. People enrolled in a Medicare Advantage plan will still receive all guaranteed Medicare benefits, and the law provides bonus payments to Medicare Advantage plans that provide high quality care. *Effective January 1, 2011.*

Improving Quality and Lowering Costs

- **Linking Payment to Quality Outcomes.** The law establishes a hospital Value-Based Purchasing program (VBP) in Traditional Medicare. This program offers financial incentives to hospitals to improve the quality of care. Hospital performance is required to be publicly reported, beginning with measures relating to heart attacks, heart failure, pneumonia, surgical care, healthcare associated infections, and patients' perception of care. *Effective for payments for discharges occurring on or after October 1, 2012.*
- **Encouraging Integrated Health Systems.** The new law provides incentives for physicians to join together to form "Accountable Care Organizations." These groups allow doctors to better coordinate patient care and improve the quality, help prevent disease and illness and reduce unnecessary hospital admissions. If Accountable Care Organizations provide high quality care and reduce costs to the health care system, they can keep some of the money that they have helped save. *Effective January 1, 2012.*
- **Reducing Paperwork and Administrative Costs.** Health care remains one of the few industries that relies on paper records. The new law will institute a series of changes to standardize billing and requires health plans to begin adopting and implementing rules for the secure, confidential, electronic exchange of health information. Using electronic health records will reduce paperwork and administrative burdens, cut costs, reduce medical errors and most importantly, improve the quality of care. *First regulation effective October 1, 2012.*
- **Understanding and Fighting Health Disparities.** To help understand and reduce persistent health disparities, the law requires any ongoing or new federal health program to collect and report racial, ethnic, and language data. The Secretary of Health and Human Services will use this data to help identify and reduce disparities. *Effective March 2012.*

Increasing Access to Affordable Care

- **Providing New, Voluntary Options for Long-Term Care Insurance.** The law creates a voluntary long-term care insurance program—called CLASS—to provide cash benefits to adults who become disabled. Note: On October 14, 2011, Secretary Sebelius transmitted a report and letter to Congress stating that the Department does not see a viable path forward for CLASS implementation at this time.

Improving Quality and Lowering Costs

- ***Improving Preventive Health Coverage.*** To expand the number of Americans receiving preventive care, the law provides new funding to state Medicaid programs that choose to cover preventive services for patients at little or no cost. *Effective January 1, 2013.*
- **Expanding Authority to Bundle Payments.** The law establishes a national pilot program to encourage hospitals, doctors, and other providers to work together to improve the coordination and quality of patient care. Under payment "bundling," hospitals, doctors, and providers are paid a flat rate for an episode of care rather than the current fragmented system where each service or test or bundles of items or services are billed separately to Medicare. For example, instead of a surgical procedure generating multiple claims from multiple providers, the entire team is compensated with a "bundled" payment that provides incentives to deliver healthcare services more efficiently while maintaining or improving quality of care. It aligns the incentives of those delivering care, and savings are shared between providers and the Medicare program. *Effective no later than January 1, 2013.*

Increasing Access to Affordable Care

- **Increasing Medicaid Payments for Primary Care Doctors.** As Medicaid programs and providers prepare to cover more patients in 2014, the Act requires states to pay primary care physicians no less than 100% of Medicare payment rates in 2013 and 2014 for primary care services. The increase is fully funded by the federal government. *Effective January 1, 2013.*
- **Open Enrollment in the Health Insurance Marketplace Begins.** Individuals and small businesses can buy affordable and qualified health benefit plans in this new transparent and competitive insurance marketplace. *Effective October 1, 2013.*

New Consumer Protections

- **Prohibiting Discrimination Due to Pre-Existing Conditions or Gender.** The law implements strong reforms that prohibit insurance companies from refusing to sell coverage or renew policies because of an individual's pre-existing conditions. Also, in the individual and small group market, the law eliminates the ability of insurance companies to charge higher rates due to gender or health status. *Effective January 1, 2014.*
- **Eliminating Annual Limits on Insurance Coverage.** The law prohibits new plans and existing group plans from imposing annual dollar limits on the amount of coverage an individual may receive. *Effective January 1, 2014.*
- **Ensuring Coverage for Individuals Participating in Clinical Trials.** Insurers will be prohibited from dropping or limiting coverage because an individual chooses to participate in a clinical trial. Applies to all clinical trials that treat cancer or other life-threatening diseases. *Effective January 1, 2014.*

Improving Quality and Lowering Costs

- **Making Care More Affordable.** Tax credits to make it easier for the middle class to afford insurance will become available for people with income between 100% and 400% of the poverty line who are not eligible for other affordable coverage. (In 2010, 400% of the poverty line comes out to about $43,000 for an individual or $88,000 for a family of four.) The tax credit can be advanced, so it can lower your premium payments each month, rather than making you wait for tax time. It's also refundable, so even moderate-income families can receive the full benefit of the credit. These individuals may also qualify for reduced cost-sharing (copayments, co-insurance, and deductibles). *Effective January 1, 2014.*
- **Establishing the Health Insurance Marketplace.** Starting in 2014 if your employer doesn't offer insurance, you will be able to buy it directly in the Health Insurance Marketplace. Individuals and small businesses can buy affordable and qualified health benefit plans in this new transparent and competitive insurance marketplace. The Marketplace will offer you a choice of health plans that meet certain benefits and cost standards. Starting in 2014, Members of Congress will be getting their healthcare insurance through the Marketplace, and you will be able buy your insurance through the Marketplace too.
- **Increasing the Small Business Tax Credit.** The law implements the second phase of the small business tax credit for qualified small businesses and small nonprofit organizations. In this phase, the credit is up to 50% of the employer's contribution to provide health insurance for employees. There is also up to a 35% credit for small nonprofit organizations. *Effective January 1, 2014.* Learn more about the small business tax credit.

Increasing Access to Affordable Care

- **Increasing Access to Medicaid.** Americans who earn less than 133% of the poverty level (approximately $14,000 for an individual and $29,000 for a family of four) will be eligible to enroll in Medicaid. States will receive 100% federal funding for the first three years to support this expanded coverage, phasing to 90% federal funding in subsequent years. *Effective January 1, 2014.*
- **Promoting Individual Responsibility.** Under the law, most individuals who can afford it will be required to obtain basic health insurance coverage or pay a fee to help offset the costs of caring for uninsured Americans. If affordable coverage is not available to an individual, he or she will be eligible for an exemption. *Effective January 1, 2014.*

Improving Quality and Lowering Costs

- **Paying Physicians Based on Value Not Volume.** A new provision will tie physician payments to the quality of care they provide. Physicians will see their payments modified so that those who provide higher value care will receive higher payments than those who provide lower quality care. *Effective January 1, 2015.*

The ACA provides 10 essential health benefits:

1. Ambulatory patient services
2. Prescription drugs
3. Emergency care
4. Mental health services
5. Hospitalization
6. Rehabilitative and habilitative services
7. Preventive and wellness services
8. Laboratory services
9. Pediatric care
10. Maternity and newborn care (Lalli, 2013, pp. 23–24)

Public–Private Partnerships

Through a cooperative agreement between the American Public Health Association (APHA) and the CDC, a major collaborative process resulted in another document, *Healthy Communities 2000: Model Standards: Guidelines for Community Attainment of the Year 2000 National Health Objectives* (APHA, 1991). The approach and document are considered valuable resources for communities wanting to explore and develop local health-promotion standards. The APHA built on the *Healthy People 2000* objectives, developing step-by-step criteria for each objective. Each objective had a measurable "goal" attached to it. For instance, the objective to reduce coronary heart disease deaths might have a measurable goal to reduce *x* amount of these deaths per 100,000 people by some specific date. These guidelines for attaching measurable criteria to the national objectives have been adapted and used by leaders, including nurses and other healthcare professionals in many states, counties, regions, cities, and even some neighborhoods, who wish to facilitate more healthful lifestyles for the populations they serve. At present, the Healthy Communities program offers a number of tools and training processes, including grants and evaluation services, via the CDC's website.

The Healthy Cities program originated in 1985 with a presentation at an international meeting in Canada. The theme of the presentation was that health is the result of much more than medical care; people are healthy when they live in nurturing environments and are involved in the life of their community (Duhl, 1986). A publication developed as part of this initiative, *Healthy People in Healthy Communities: A Guide for Community Leaders* (HHS, 1998a), links healthy cities with healthy people to create a healthy community in a guide to how other cities and communities developed and implemented their healthy community initiatives.

ENVIRONMENTAL CONNECTION

Tobacco companies have mounted extensive media campaigns targeting ethnic, lower income urban areas while promoting their products. What are the possible environmental and ethical outcomes of these free-market-economy activities in regard to public health?

There have been numerous partnerships and group efforts in which nurses have collaborated with Healthy Cities and Communities projects throughout the country. Flynn and other community health nurses began "Healthy Indiana," which was an early forerunner of ensuing Healthy Cities and Communities programs (Kellogg Foundation, 1988). Other examples include work with homeless populations (Moore, Neff, Smith, & Weber, 1999) and nurse managed care centers (Drapo & Woods, 1992). The growth of community nursing organizations demonstrates how nurses believe our focus should be on partnering and collaborating with communities and special populations in health-promoting efforts. Nurse educators and local public health nursing directors continue to forge collaborative bonds with cities, communities, and target population groups in developing community/population health-promotion needs and assets assessments (Baldwin, 1995; Raphael & Bryant, 2002).

The following is an example of nursing student involvement with community-level health promotion interventions. The Brigham Young University College of Nursing in Provo, Utah, offers a community/population assessment elective course to nursing undergraduate students and university honor students. Various city and county health departments and local communities have requested assistance in assessing the needs of key population groups. For example, the members of the Healthy Taylorsville Project requested the class's help in assessing the needs and viewpoints of the youth of the community. The college students collaborated with the school superintendent, principals, teachers, counselors, and junior and senior high school students. They produced a document outlining the needs of the youth and their suggestions and ideas about health-promotion strategies for the city of Taylorsville (Browning, Huls, Rather, & Stout, 1997). One example of the Taylorsville youths' suggestions was to place stoplights at two of the busiest streets in the growing city so that students could safely cross those streets to get to and from school. The document will be a major guide toward anticipated changes for many of the needs stated by the youth (J. I. Morgan, Director of Administrative Services, personal communication, Taylorsville, Utah, March 1998).

Growing Consumerism and Emphasis on Self-Care

Since the late 1960s, consumers of health care have increasingly demanded information relating to their health care and to items that promote health. In the past, consumers almost complacently accepted what physicians and others in control of healthcare systems told them regarding their health care. Over the last few decades, consumers have become better educated and more proactive in demanding their rights and insisting that healthcare professionals be accountable for their actions. Evidence can be seen in the proliferation of satisfaction surveys, opinion polls, and litigation, as well as in the nature of advertising, and exercise activities that claim to be health promoting are seen throughout the media. People are requesting more information on labels so that they can discern whether the item contains anything that might be non-health promoting, especially something that might trigger an allergy or be too high in calories. The health-promotion aspects of education have become a major focus for all age and ethnic groups. The Mississippi Public Broadcasting (MPB) organization posted in the publication "Southern Remedy: Teaching other to use Southern Remedy's adult healthy eating plate designed to help Mississippians make more informed choices about the food they consume. A tool recommended by MPB is a "healthy eating plate". They also propose specific points such as: (1) calories are fuel; (2) everything in moderation; (3) variety is the spice of life; (4) go natural; (5) limit empty calories; and (6) don't be too hard on yourself (Southern Remedy, 2014).

Who is responsible for health? There is an expanding awareness that consumers must bear the responsibility for their own health. How can consumers do this? Self-care is the answer. Self-care is defined as those "activities initiated or performed by an individual, family, or community to achieve, maintain, or promote maximum health" (Steiger & Lipson, 1985, p. 12). Orem (1985) defines self-care as "the production of actions directed to self or to the environment in order to regulate one's functioning in the interest of one's life, integrated functioning, and well-being" (p. 31).

> Let us rise up and be thankful, for if we didn't learn a lot today, at least we learned a little; and if we didn't learn a little, at least we didn't get sick; and if we got sick, at least we didn't die; so let us all be thankful.
>
> —*Buddha (563–483 BC)*

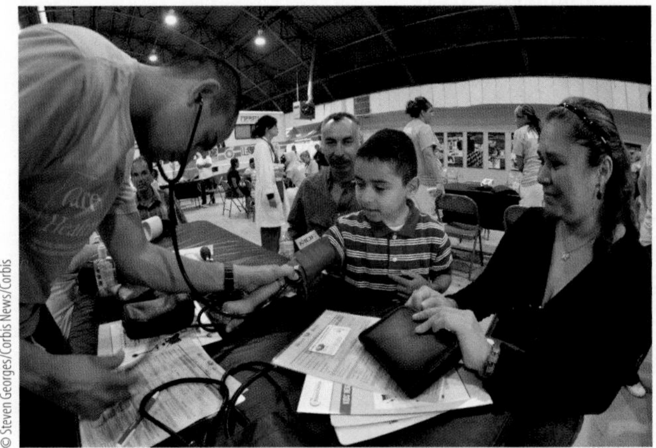

© Steven Georges/Corbis News/Corbis

Health fairs are effective ways to reach specific populations for health promotion in communities.

The impetus for the current interest in self-care began anew in the late 1970s and early 1980s. The HHS (1982) published a document titled *Forward Plan for Health 1977–1981*. It seems remarkable to consider today, that for the first time ever, the authors of this report boldly suggested that lifestyle and psychosocial factors had a great impact on morbidity and mortality. A number of health-promotion elements such as nutrition, exercise, and fitness were mentioned.

DAY IN THE LIFE

Janet Quinn

A healing environment is one that facilitates the emergence of the Haelan effect, the synergistic, organismic, multidimensional response of whole persons in the direction of healing and wholeness. Healing, the emergence of right relationship at, between, and among all the levels of human being, is always accomplished by the one healing. No one and no thing can heal another human being. All healing is creative emergence, new birth, the manifestation of the powerful inner longing, at every level, to be whole. . . . We can remove barriers to the healing process. We can participate in creating environments that will support healing. We can become midwives to this process of healing, creating, and being a safe, sacred space into which the healing might emerge. We can literally become the healing environment.

—Janet F. Quinn, 1992, in Holding Sacred Space: The Nurse as Healing Environment. *Holistic Nursing Practice, 6*(4), 26–36.

RESEARCH ALERT 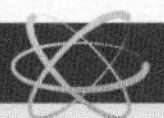

The authors of a randomized controlled trial compared the outcomes of individuals chosen to participate in the 8-week People with Arthritis Can Exercise (PACE) program with those who did not receive the PACE intervention. The mean age of the 347 participants was 70, 90% were women, and all reported limitations due to arthritis. Patients completed a Health Assessment questionnaire and tests of physical function and physical activity. Researchers measured outcomes at baseline and 8 weeks, and the intervention group completed self-assessments at 3 and 6 months. Researchers adjusted the outcomes for possible confounding variables.

One-hour PACE program classes were conducted twice a week for 8 weeks. The mean number of classes attended by the intervention group was 9.4. After 8 weeks, patients in the intervention group had reduced pain and fatigue, and improved arthritis management. Program participants who continued the program for 6 months had better outcomes in pain, fatigue, and stiffness versus those in the control group.

Source: Barclay, L., & Vega, C. (2008). Eight-week exercise program may benefit elderly patients with arthritis. *Medscape Medical News.* Retrieved from http://www.medscape.org/viewarticle/568653

In addition to the emphasis placed by government documents at that time, the popular press also supported the notion. In his book *Megatrends*, Naisbitt (1982, p. 131) forecast that self-care emphasizing health-promotion strategies would move health care out of the medical-institutional illness model into an era of self-responsibility for health and wellness. In 1999, the USPHS published a well-received book, *Promoting Physical Activity: A Guide for Community Action*. Shortly thereafter, several other exercise-motivation books appeared on the scene (Marcus & Forsyth, 2002).

The demand for self-care is currently coming from people themselves, private insurance carriers, managed care organizations, employers, and communities. In the past, individuals would never consider questioning the diagnoses or orders of their physicians. Insurance carriers now insist that there be at least two healthcare professionals' opinions before major surgery.

In addition, consumers are demanding information about complementary treatment options in addition to allopathic treatments suggested by physicians. Insurance and managed care companies are providing self-care books that assist subscribers to self-diagnose and self-treat simple illnesses and injuries, as well as offer tips on health-promoting activities for all members of the family. Incentives include managed care organizations paying bonuses to members for smoking cessation, weight loss, and other health-promoting activities that move the members toward high-level wellness. At the workplace, large companies implement organizational wellness programs that assist employees to maximize personal wellness. Research has shown that an employee experiencing high-level wellness uses fewer sick days and is more productive on the job (HHS, 1998b; National Institute for Occupational Safety and Health, 1996). At home or from a local library or other community establishment, patients can access numerous websites on any subject relating to self-care.

Self-care and consumerism are processes that assist people to know about health-promoting items and activities. At the population and community levels, the Healthy Cities and Communities program depends heavily on people within communities to identify problems and assets and engage in problem solving and self-care to correct problems and promote maximal community wellness. The success of the *Healthy People 2020* objectives for the nation is equally dependent on patient education in health-promotion and self-care strategies as well as policy changes to improve social conditions allowing for the context within which personal choices about health are made. To make informed health-promoting decisions, appropriate and correct health-promotion information must be available to patients, as well as to legislators who make the policies.

NOTE THIS!

The percentage of Americans who walk to work dropped from 5.6% in 1980 to 3.9% in 1990 and 2.9% in 2000. Walking has been replaced by the automobile or mass transit. The change in residence for most Americans, from the city to the suburbs, has created the necessity for people to drive cars to their places of employment and has reduced the time that most people have at home. Urban sprawl has created fewer opportunities for employment in one's community, therefore increasing commute time and providing fewer chances for walking to work. Commute times are getting longer. The percentage of workers who reach their jobs in less than 20 minutes dropped to 47% in 2000 after hovering around 50% for decades.

—Alan Pisarski, *Commuting in America. III.* Transportation Research Board, National Research Council, October 16, 2006.

Kylatra (2014) reported that the average American may commute up to 25.5 minutes to and from work each day. That equates to approximately 204 hours of commuting each year. The time spent during commuting alters your body's responses. Body functions that may be altered with commuting are:

1. Elevated blood sugar
2. Higher cholesterol levels
3. Increased risk of depression
4. Increased risk of anxiety
5. Decline in happiness and life satisfaction
6. Spikes in blood pressure
7. Long-term elevation of blood pressure
8. Drops in cardiovascular fitness
9. Alterations in sleep patterns
10. Increases in back pain and discomfort.

Models of Health Promotion and Wellness

Numerous models of health promotion and wellness might be useful guides to assessing and promoting health and wellness in communities, populations, families, and individuals. Many models have been constructed to explain, assess, plan, or evaluate health-promotion education programs; states of health, wellness, and illness; and preventive measures.

As early as 1952, researchers expressed the need for a model to help explain and predict why certain at-risk populations took preventive actions and others did not, even when there was very little or nothing being charged for the preventive services (Rosenstock, 1974). The first popular model developed was the health belief model (Becker, 1974; Hochbaum, 1958; Padilla & Bulcavage, 1991; Rosenstock, 1974). In this model, "the individual's weighing of the positive and negative valences of the threats of illness was emphasized" (Baldwin, 1992, p. 27). How the individual perceived his or her susceptibility to an illness and what might be the perceived benefits and barriers to doing something about preventing the illness were important factors in the health belief model. Even when the individual decided it was in his or her best interest to take some action to prevent the illness, there needed to be a trigger or cue to action to motivate the person to carry out the action (Baldwin, 1992; Rosenstock, 1974).

Several other models have been developed that might be useful to the nurse of today. As researchers continue the quest to predict and explain which factors contributed to health-promoting and health-protecting behaviors, the multidimensionality of the process became clearer. Further developments of the predictors of preventive health behavior originating in the health belief model were instigated in later models. Cognitive factors such as patients' definitions of health and perceptions about health behaviors, including benefits, barriers, and control, were seen as important to patients' health-promoting behaviors. Modifying factors, ranging from demographic, biological, behavioral, and interpersonal factors to environmental issues, including access to care, as well as factors that might influence the initiation of health-promoting and health-protective behaviors, were explored. Many of these multidimensional factors can be seen in the health-promotion models constructed in the 1980s and early 1990s (Palank, 1991; Pender, 1987; Simmons, 1990) and in health-hazard risk evaluation and appraisal tools and wellness guides, which began appearing in the early 1970s and 1980s.

Health-hazard risk evaluation and appraisal tools are commonly designed in survey questionnaire form to provide quantitative data elicited from patients' responses regarding lifestyle and health habits. Questions regarding activities of daily living ranging from personal health habits, such as "How often do you brush your teeth?", "In what way and how often do you exercise?", and "Are you sexually active?" to questions about seatbelt use and consumption of caffeine products, are often asked. Often, information is required regarding family and personal medical histories and various demographic data. The information from these questionnaires can then be compared with known national and local health statistics to make predictions and health-promotion recommendations regarding morbidity and mortality risks for the patients. Wellness guides are generally in a question-and-answer form, designed to appeal to consumers who may have a common health or wellness question or concern.

In the late 1980s, the *Guide to Clinical Preventive Services* (U.S. Preventive Services Task Force, 1989) was developed. In 1995, a second edition was published to help guide primary care health professionals providing preventive services. These tools and guides are used by physicians' and nurse practitioners' offices, hospitals, health departments, managed care systems, and other agencies to assist healthcare professionals in counseling patients about reducing potential risks and increasing health-promoting behaviors. Models, tools, and guides continue to be designed to help explore factors involved in health promotion and wellness decision making for individuals, families, populations, and communities.

Three recent models are described to demonstrate how these techniques might be used to assess and facilitate wellness interventions: (1) holistic wellness: self-inventory of personal wellness using the medicine wheel (McDonald, 1997), (2) the 4+ model of wellness (Baldwin & Baldwin, 1998), and (3) the Pender health promotion model (Pender, 2011). These models are similar in some respects to earlier models and tools in the assessment of multidimensional variables affecting health and wellness, but they differ somewhat in their approaches. Both of these models may be used with any ethnic population, as may several of the earlier models. The holistic wellness model allows patients to identify aspects that determine wellness and to define what well and unhealthy states are for them. The 4+ model of wellness also encourages patient participation in the assessment of wellness and adds two other dimensions: the consideration of what might be the sources of nurture and depletion for a patient and ways that the nurse might facilitate interventions with the patient, focusing on those sources of nurture and depletion to promote health and wellness.

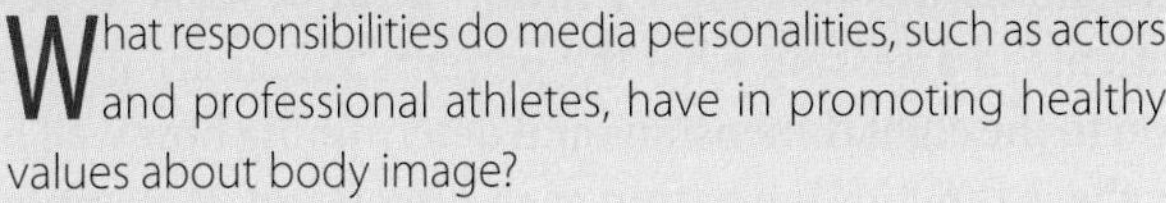

ETHICAL CONNECTION

What responsibilities do media personalities, such as actors and professional athletes, have in promoting healthy values about body image?

Holistic Wellness: Self-Inventory of Personal Wellness Using the Medicine Wheel

The medicine wheel is a sacred symbol that is common to almost all Native American tribes. Ivan McDonald, a member of the Blackfeet tribe and health educator for Indian Health Services in Browning, Montana, developed

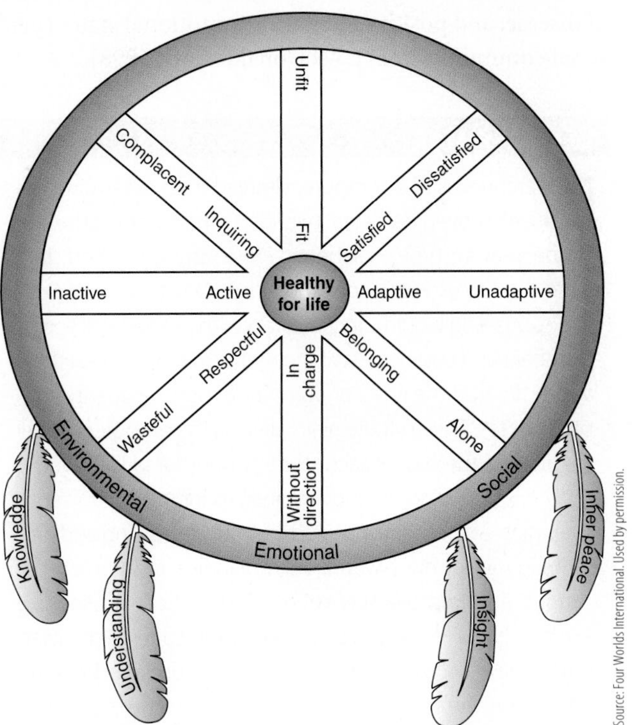

Source: Four Worlds International. Used by permission.

Figure 14-1 Holistic wellness: Self-inventory of personal wellness using the medicine wheel.

the holistic wellness model using the medicine wheel as a basis (see **Figure 14-1**). Although the descriptors for this model are specific to the values and beliefs of the Blackfeet culture of Native Americans, the wheel can be used to assess wellness for any person of any culture. The descriptors of "healthy" states and "unhealthy" states for the spokes of the wheel should reflect the individuality of the person.

The holistic wellness model is grounded in the Native American understanding of existence. The medicine wheel, as a representation of this understanding, is depicted as a circle that comprises the four sacred directions. Each direction represents not only one of the basic elements necessary for survival, but also a human element.

The East is symbolic of the sun and fire and of one's own creative spirit. The South represents water and one's emotions. The West is the place of Mother Earth and one's intuition—the place of magic and dreams. The North represents air and minds filled with wisdom as one learns about the mystery of life.

Holistic wellness defines health in terms of the whole person, not only in terms of physical illness. The model represents how Native American people understand health as a balance within the person and between the person and everything around him or her—physical, vocational, psychological, social, emotional, environmental, spiritual, and intellectual. It focuses on optimal health, prevention of disease, and positive mental and emotional states (personal communication, I. McDonald, April 1998).

RESEARCH ALERT 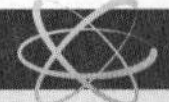

Researchers used a computer simulation to determine the cost-effectiveness of lifestyle intervention or metformin for preventing type 2 diabetes. Previously published data were used to estimate how and at what cost diet and exercise counseling would affect patients with prediabetes versus the effect and cost of prescribing metformin. The researchers also estimated the costs of doing nothing for patients with prediabetes. They put the estimates into a computer model to calculate the cost of each strategy per year of life saved.

The results of the computer analysis indicated that both strategies—prescribing diet and exercise counseling and prescribing metformin—would delay diabetes, reduce complications, and improve survival rates. The effect of diet and exercise, however, was favorable for all adult ages, while metformin was not cost effective after age 65. Compared with no prevention, the cost estimate for diet and exercise counseling was about $8,800 and the cost estimate for metformin was about $29,000 per quality-adjusted life-year saved.

Source: Herman, W. H., Hoerger, T. J., Brandle, M., Hicks, K., Sorensen, S., Zhang, P.,...Ratner, R. E. (2005). The cost-effectiveness of lifestyle modification or metformin in preventing type 2 diabetes in adults with impaired glucose tolerance. *Annals of Internal Medicine* (pp. 323–332). Diabetes Prevention Program Research Group.

The spokes of the medicine wheel radiate from a center circle that represents wellness or "Healthy for Life." The spokes contain dimensions of the specific wellness (e.g., the physical wellness spoke has the dimensions of unfit and fit), with the more positive part of the dimension being closest to the center "Healthy for Life" circle in the figure. The spokes are defined as follows:

- *Physical wellness*: maintenance of your body in good condition by eating right, exercising regularly, avoiding harmful habits, and making informed, responsible decisions about your health
- *Vocational wellness*: enjoyment of what you are doing to earn a living and/or to contribute to society
- *Psychological wellness*: maintenance of mental health or the ability to think reasonably clearly and to avoid wildly distorting reality
- *Social wellness*: ability to perform the expectations of social roles effectively, comfortably, and without harming others
- *Emotional wellness*: understanding emotions and knowing how to cope with problems that arise in everyday life; ability to endure stress
- *Environmental wellness*: minimizing personal and global risks to health, socioeconomic status, education, and various other environmental factors that affect health, such as noise pollution, radiation, air pollution, and water pollution
- *Spiritual wellness*: a state of balance and harmony with yourself and others; includes trust, integrity, principles, ethics, the purpose or drive in life, basic survival instincts, feelings of selflessness, degree of pleasure-seeking qualities, commitment to some higher process or being, and the ability to believe in concepts that are not subject to a "state of the art" explanation
- *Intellectual wellness*: having a mind open to new ideas; covers such activities as speaking, writing, analyzing, critical thinking, and judgment

The eagle feathers at the bottom of the wheel represent the progression of personal development: knowledge, understanding, insight, and inner peace. Each element is a higher level than the one before. However, the element before must occur before one can aspire to the next level. The progression of the feathers is similar to the progression for each dimension reflected in the spokes of the wheel. As the patient develops inwardly toward Healthy for Life, there is progress from knowledge to inner peace.

The holistic wellness model includes social and environmental aspects as they relate to a person's wellness. From the perspectives of many cultures, a person's wellness depends on social relationships and harmony with the environment. For example, for some societies in Australia and Mexico, physical illness can be caused by breaches of social norm. Although this is not necessarily a common idea in many Western societies, from the worldview of most cultures, personal illness or wellness may be a result of social and environmental interactions.

How to Use the Holistic Wellness Model

The nurse could use the holistic wellness model as a visual depiction of a patient's self-defined wellness state. The model can be used by health professionals to help patients in assessing what the patient's values are in relation to the eight dimensions and determining how well he or she is functioning within each dimension. It is important to note, though, that if one dimension becomes the focus of changing behaviors, other dimensions may suffer from lack of attention. Therefore, facilitating interventions through the use of this model requires that the nurse and the patient together consider how to strengthen all of the dimensions as equally as possible. In addition, the holistic wellness model is handy for quick evaluations of progress. It is also important to understand that the balance may shift depending on circumstances and that, as symbolized by the medicine wheel, there is constant motion.

Several examples of how to intervene and facilitate the patient's consideration of a more healthful lifestyle using health-promoting behaviors include the following: (1) If the patient considers himself or herself to be on the unfit dimension of the "Physical" spoke, discuss ways for the patient to become more fit. What does the patient like to do for exercise, and what can the patient physically and realistically do? If walking is difficult for an elderly person, perhaps suggest starting with moving every possible body joint two or three times during a television or radio commercial or for a rest while reading. (2) If the patient believes he or she is inactive on the Spiritual spoke, review what spirituality means to the patient and see if he or she can discover ways to become more active in that realm. (3) If the patient sees that he or she is without direction on the Emotional spoke, address things that might be done by the patient to make him or her feel more in charge of life. The major issue here is what the patient believes he or she can realistically do to develop health-promoting behaviors that will lead to the patient being more healthy for life.

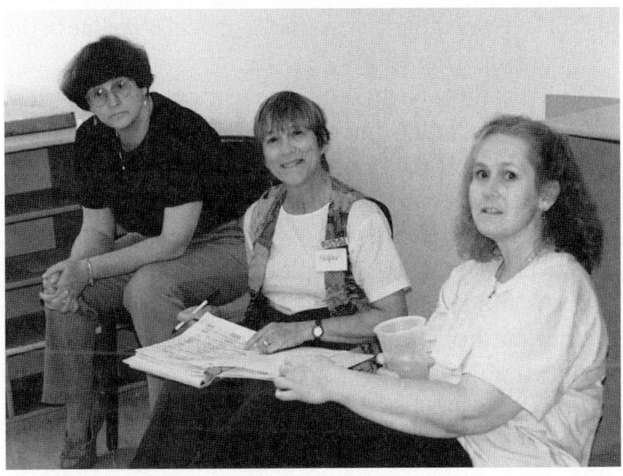

Chapter author, Dr. Joan Baldwin, discusses a health promotion project with nursing students.

At a community level, the model could be applied by changing the names on the outer ring of the medicine wheel. For example, things such as public transportation, community pride, healthcare services, and so on could substitute for the physical, spiritual, and psychological elements. The spokes would translate similarly. For instance, public transportation might be present (meaning all possible modes of transportation are available) to absent (meaning there is no public transportation in the community). The feather could be redefined as knowledge to data, understanding to information, insight to creative solutions, and inner peace to harmony of factors.

The 4+ Model of Wellness

The 4+ model of wellness (Baldwin & Baldwin, 1998) is designed to assist with critical thinking about things that might negatively deplete or positively nurture wellness in a patient. There are two layers, much like transparent plastic overlays, to this model: (1) the four domains of inner self and (2) the outer systems. When layer 2 is placed over layer 1, the total 4+ model of wellness appears.

The 4+ model of wellness begins with the inner self layer, depicting a sphere containing the four domains of inner self (see **Figure 14-2**) of the patient. The patient might be oneself, another individual, a family, a population, or a community. The four domains of inner self are intellectual, physical, emotional, and spiritual (or spirit).

This portion of the 4+ model of wellness appears simple but is really quite complex. The intellectual component of the inner self relates to how the patient thinks. The physical is how the patient moves and senses things and includes all of the patient's physiological (or inner workings, as in the case of a community as patient) aspects. How a patient feels anger, excitement, and so on is reflected in the emotional aspect, and the spiritual denotes the fire that drives the engine that connects one to others and to a higher power. The spiritual domain also includes the capacity to give love. Thus, the spiritual domain within each of us seems to have more than one role. This domain is likely to be the most complex and sometimes difficult to understand, although it is one of the most important to consider.

Achieving a holistic and harmonious state within the inner self is one part of the model. For example, think of the four domains of inner self as a tire. When all four of the

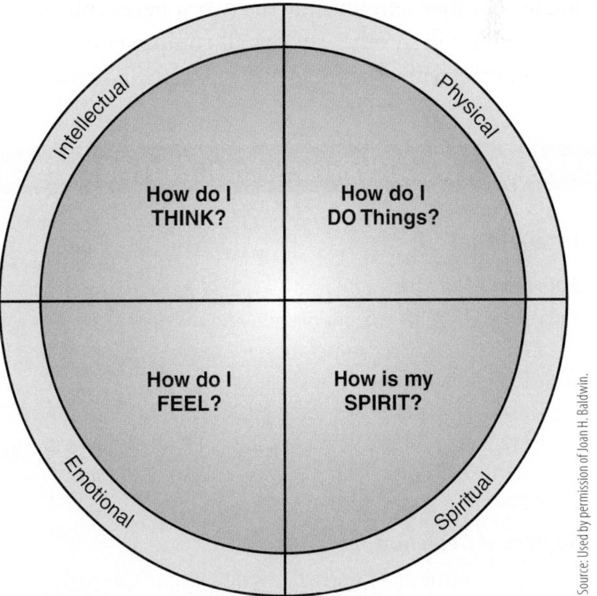

Figure 14-2 The 4+ model of wellness: The four domains of inner self.

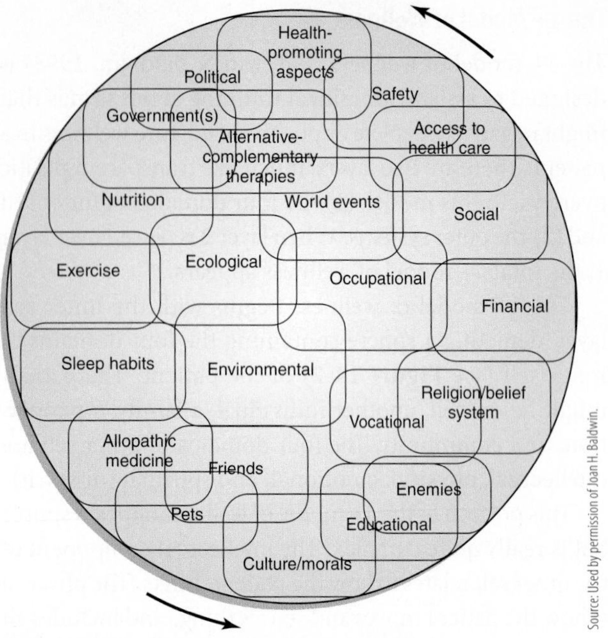

Figure 14-3 The 4+ model of wellness: The outer systems.

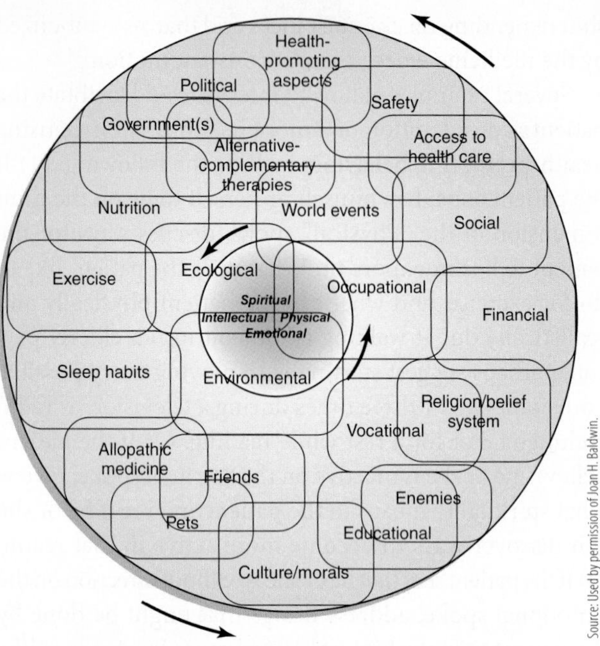

Figure 14-4 The 4+ model of wellness: The four domains of inner self plus the outer systems.

domains—intellectual, physical, emotional, and spiritual—are "pumped up," the tire is rounded and rolls along evenly. This is what is meant by a holistic and harmonious state. This healthy state of harmony is further affected by interconnectedness and interaction with systems outside the inner self, which are depicted in the second overlay—the outer systems (see **Figure 14-3**)—as facets of another sphere surrounding the sphere of the four domains of inner self.

All of the elements of the outer systems sphere interact and interconnect with one another and with all the four domains of inner self. Imagine the two spheres constantly rotating about each other so that all components of each sphere interact with other elements within their own sphere and with one another at some time. **Figure 14-4** depicts the idea of layering the spheres—the 4+ model of wellness: the four domains of inner self plus the outer systems.

Think of the total model as a patient system, one system with many moving components. Using the 4+ model of wellness, the nurse can look for things that might be depleting the elements of the inner self rather than nurturing the elements toward harmony. By working with the patient to consider things that might deplete any one or all of the four domains and thinking of ways to strengthen those things that nurture the patient, the nurse and patient may be able to identify health-promoting actions for the patient. Selected sources of nurture and depletion are listed in **Box 14-3**.

BOX 14-3 The 4+ Model of Wellness: Selected Sources of Nurture and Depletion

Intellectual

Sources of Nurture

- Books/intellectual media activities
- Observation/contemplation
- Experience/critical thinking
- Knowledge building more knowledge
- Practicing "brain work"—that is, children's play and games; children learn this way and so do adults
- Planning for the future

Sources of Depletion

- Brainwashing—imposed conditioned responses
- Mind-numbing repetition
- Boredom
- Noise
- Interruption
- Stresses/stressors
- Codependent behavior encouraged by a perpetrator—can lead to post-traumatic stress syndrome

Emotional

Sources of Nurture

- Relief from stress
- Accomplishments
- Winning
- Physical wellbeing, exercise, diet

- Rest/relaxation
- Meditation/biofeedback, etc.
- Ability to "vent" appropriately

Sources of Depletion

- Physical illness
- Weak intelligence (inability to solve a problem)
- Isolation/noise/threats

Physical

Sources of Nurture

- Appropriate nutrition
- Outdoor/indoor activities/exercise
- Rest/relaxation
- Physical "work"
- Biofeedback/complementary health therapies, and so on
- Appropriate physiological working
- Physical therapy

Sources of Depletion

- Disease/illness/prepathogenesis
- Toxins/environmental hazards
- Drug/substance abuse
- Poor nutrition/diet
- Lack of sleep
- Noise
- Stress/stressors/allergies
- Excessive exercise/exertion
- Trauma

Spiritual

Sources of Nurture

- Giving love/connecting with others
- Being of service/loving animals
- Beauty/music/art
- Quiet/peace, meditation/prayer
- Physical exercise/cheering
- Being loved/hugs and pat-pats
- Intellectual stimulus/creating

Sources of Depletion

- Too much demand for support of others
- Failure to experience connectedness, love, belonging

Source: Baldwin & Baldwin, 1998. Used by permission of Joan H. Baldwin.

General Observations

Strength in any domain, if not in excess, can nurture the other three domains. Also, depletion of any domain weakens and drains the other three domains.

Spiritual Domain

On first consideration, the emotional and spiritual domains may appear similar, but in this model, these areas are quite different from each other. In this model, *spiritual* means the spirit or fire one has within. Excessive emotional highs may deplete the spirit. Of importance in this model is that *spiritual* does not mean religion or religious. Religion is actually a piece of the outer system that affects the inner self. Parts of a religion may, indeed, nurture the spirit, but sometimes, as in the case of overzealousness, depletion of the spirit may occur.

Observations About Excesses

Excessive striving in any area can be destructive in all four domains. An illustration would be someone who exercises to an extreme, to the detriment of personal relationships with others.

Excessive pain can be a depleting factor. For example, it is hard to think when you are suffering severe pain. One kind of severe pain is depression. Severely depressed people become so immobilized in several of the domains that they cannot move themselves toward strength in any of the areas through simple exercise or nutrition or even interaction with loving people. Serious disease or weakness (which can cause excessive physiological and other problems) can deplete several domains and can be a major factor in the patient suffering a downward spiral to total collapse and death.

Any excesses or "lacks" within any of the four domains throw the inner self sphere extremely "off balance or out of harmony." Think of the inner self sphere as being a tire; the difference in pressure on any portion of the tire will throw the tire off balance. People in various cultures speak of the tremendous importance of balance or harmony in a person's life.

Contemporary researchers and authors are proposing that changing and growing systems do not necessarily seek total equilibrium, that constant change alters the state of harmony or balance constantly (Coveney & Highfield, 1990; Prigogine & Stengers, 1984; Wheatley, 1994). This might explain how the assessment of a patient on one day may be far different from a similar assessment another day or even later in the same day. This is why it is important to observe the patient over time—to get a broader picture of what might be occurring within that patient's system. There does not have to be "equilibrium" to have balance or harmony; in fact, a well-functioning system is always in a state of nonequilibrium because it constantly and inevitably changes focus. A system that is flexible and open can constantly move, changing and adjusting to regain harmony or a state as close to harmony as possible (Wheatley, 1994).

How to Use the 4+ Model of Wellness with Individuals, Families, Populations, and Communities

The nurse should begin by assessing the four domains of inner self for oneself or a patient. Then, the components of the outer systems, which encircle and move around the four domains of the inner self sphere, must be considered. By using the total 4+ model of wellness to assess the interactions and interconnectedness of the elements in the outer systems to all aspects of the inner self, the nurse will be able to critically assess and analyze much about himself or herself or others. The nurse and the patient may be able to determine which factors to work on strengthening or nurturing and which factors might be diminished or deleted to "pump up" the patient system's wellness. Remember that the patient can be a family, group, population, or community, as well as an individual.

Individuals

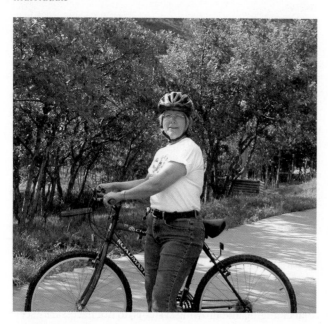

Staying active as we age is an important way to improve the health of the population.

Consider a significantly overweight, older man as an individual patient. The patient has been prescribed a diet that is nutritionally sound and, if followed, should help him lose weight. The patient could be thinking he is trying to follow his prescribed diet, and he is perplexed about not being successful in losing weight. The nurse could explore with the patient as many aspects as possible of his four domains of inner self, as well as the outer system components, to begin to figure out what interventions might facilitate health-promoting behaviors for this patient. After working with the patient to assess what might be sources of nurture and depletion for each of his four domains, the nurse (and, in some difficult cases, a team of healthcare professionals), along with the patient, would develop a wellness plan. Ideally, finding ways to nurture the patient's four domains and considering how the depleting sources could be diminished would constitute the initial part of the plan. For example, there might be work environment stressors (sources of depletion), such as the fact that doughnuts and other high-sugar, high-fat, and high-calorie foods are encouraged at break time at the workplace, which makes adhering to the prescribed diet difficult. Brainstorming with the patient about how he might discuss his need to be on the prescribed diet with his supervisor and how difficult it has been not to eat the doughnuts when they are in full view could be one step in the process.

There will be some sources of nurture that the patient could also strengthen. A source of nurture might be that the man has a dog as a pet. Possibly the man and his dog could work with children in a daycare center for developmentally disabled children. There have been many research articles relating the health-promoting aspects of the human–animal bond (Edney, 1992; McConnell, Brown, Shoda, Stayton, & Martin, 2011; National Institutes of Health, 1987). In addition, the process of connecting older people with younger people has many nurturing benefits (Piper, 1999). A service opportunity such as this could possibly nurture all four of the patient's domains, and certainly would nurture the individuals who are the recipients of this service.

RESEARCH ALERT 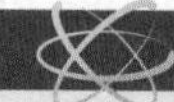

An exploration of the research in several disciplines related to the use of animals for therapy in health care demonstrated applicability of the findings to enhance health-promoting nursing interventions for patients. A selective historical tour of the literature regarding the human–animal bond and its therapeutic effect in health care is a segue to more recent research on the subject. Considerations about the pros and cons of having animals interact with hospitalized patients are developed. The link between the benefits of stress reduction and positive psychoneuroimmunology changes in patients as a result of human–animal bonding therapies emerges as the strongest health-promotion possibility for the use of this animal-assisted therapy.

Source: Jorgenson, J. (1997). Therapeutic use of companion animals in health care. *Image: The Journal of Nursing Scholarship, 29*(3), 249–254.

Another important factor to remember when working with any patient is that the patient's goals or priorities in life may not be the same as what you might consider his, her, or its (in the case of a family, population, or community) goals or priorities "should" be. This is equally important to remember when establishing things that nurture or deplete a patient. These also are factors in why patients do not always do what a healthcare professional tells them to do. Too often, if patients choose not to do what the healthcare professional says, or cannot do something for some valid reason, healthcare professionals indicate that the patients are "noncompliant" or cannot figure out why patients do not do what is "good" for them. These episodes sometimes create ethical concerns, especially concerning whose needs are not being met. Building trust, rapport, and respect with patients often encourages the patients, in due time, to follow healthcare professionals' suggestions for health-promoting behaviors.

Families

Using the 4+ model of wellness when assessing more than one individual becomes more complex than assessing an individual. Consider a family as a large patient system consisting of several smaller systems, or individual family members. Look for sources of nurture for the family. These sources might include things such as being broad-minded, being creative, having good problem-solving skills, being flexible, having family members who are interconnected with each other and the outer systems of the family, sharing spirituality, and being appropriately nurturing of the family's spirit and the spirits of others. A family that has developed these characteristics and continues to derive nurture from them among others demonstrates a fair amount of harmony, health, and wellness. In the family Application to Practice, look for potential sources of nurture and depletion in the various family patients.

APPLICATION TO PRACTICE

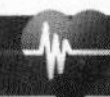

How Everything Affects Everything: A Saga of One Man's Life and the Negative Influences on Him and the Families Involved

Sam had a difficult childhood. His mother left the family when Sam was about 3 or 4 years old. His father probably was devastated, but Sam was too young to understand all that had happened. Sam's paternal grandparents raised Sam because Sam's father had to work long hours to even begin to make enough money to sustain himself, much less Sam. Sam's grandfather was strict and was sometimes abusive to Sam's grandmother. No one in the family seemed to recognize that Sam believed that he was responsible in some way for his mother's leaving.

As Sam grew older, he became angry that his mother had left him although he seemed to appreciate the fact that his grandparents took some amount of care of him. He was certain his father had no real love for him. Sam was a fairly bright young boy and did well in school. Sometime in his teens, Sam began experimenting with marijuana. He managed to graduate from high school and began doing manual labor and odd jobs. He still lived with his grandparents.

Sam had several girlfriends over the next few years. The girls and many of his friends were younger than he was by several years. Sam was always the leader of the group. He and his friends abused alcohol and began taking many other kinds of "street drugs." Sam verbally abused his friends and girlfriends by telling them they were stupid and so on. Eventually he married one of the young women. After a time he was not only abusing her verbally, but also forcing her to start taking some of the drugs that he was taking.

Sam and his wife had a child. Amazingly, the child was healthy. As the child grew, Sam insisted on having the child by his side when Sam wanted the child to be there. Otherwise, Sam ignored the child. Sam said he "loved" the child, yet burdened the young child (then about 3 or 4 years of age) with Sam's concerns about money and Sam's belief that the child's mother was no good. Sam also continued to have sexual liaisons with other women. Sam's wife made several attempts to leave Sam, especially after some fairly severe beatings. The child often observed these situations. After several years of abuse, Sam's wife left him and took the child with her to live elsewhere. Sam threatened to find her and kill her if the child was not returned. After almost 2 years of legal interventions, Sam's wife won a divorce and legal physical custody of the child (meaning that the child would live with her, but that Sam might have some input into the raising of the child). Sam tolerated this process for a short time before he began verbally harassing and threatening his ex-wife on the phone.

There were several more months of harassment, which led to the involvement of police and other legal interventions. When Sam was finally arrested for selling drugs and being intoxicated, among other things, the court agreed that Sam would be denied contact with his son.

1. Using the 4+ model of wellness of Sam's four domains, how many were affected by his early life? By his high school adventures? By his adult life?
2. What additional information is needed in the scenario to assess Sam's wellness in the time before he went to jail? Consider what effect the outer systems components (e.g., social, vocational, environmental) may have had on Sam.

3. Which sources of nurture and/or depletion are recognizable? Which of Sam's domains may have been affected, given the sources of nurture and/or depletion noted?
4. Which health-promoting behaviors of Sam's family might have helped Sam during his early development? List Sam's family's possible sources of nurture and depletion.
5. While considering the 4+ model of wellness, which sources of nurture and/or depletion did the family of the ex-wife and child have? How might a nurse assist them to assess their own four quadrants individually and as a single-parent family?
6. How might a nurse help the ex-wife and child develop the health-promoting behaviors they might need individually and as a single-parent family?
7. Think about Sam's abuse of and involvement with substances. Consider his desire for drugs, his early life, and the life he was living as an adult. What view/attitudes might a nurse take as a logical and ethical approach toward Sam?

Populations and Communities

Now think about how the 4+ model of wellness might be used to examine a population or a community. If a family is a patient system, then a population or a community can also be a patient system; individuals within the population and individuals and target (or at-risk) populations within a community are the smaller systems within the larger patient system of population or community. Remember that your own goals, values, and priorities are not necessarily those of populations or communities. These patient systems also have their own goals, values, and priorities that can create ethical dilemmas for the nurse.

MEDIA MOMENT 

Life Is Beautiful (1997)

This film is about the endurance of the human spirit and a sense of humor even in the worst of human conditions: a Nazi concentration camp. A Jewish Italian waiter named Guido (Roberto Benigni) is sent to a Nazi concentration camp during World War II, along with his wife (Nicoletta Braschi) and their young son (Giorgio Cantarini). Refusing to give up hope, Guido tries to protect his son's innocence by pretending that their imprisonment is an elaborate game and that everything is bearable with a great sense of humor, with the grand prize being a tank. Benigni also directed. Italian with English subtitles.

Patch Adams (1998)

After committing himself to a mental institution, Hunter "Patch" Adams (Robin Williams) realizes that introducing his fellow patients to humor significantly improves their quality of life. Upon leaving the institution, he decides to become a physician who cures people using laughter rather than cold, analytical processes. Although jeopardizing his future in medicine, Patch continues his unconventional, yet promising healing methods.

Amélie (2001)

Amélie (Audrey Tautou) lives alone and works in a café. When she finds a box of toys hidden for 40 years behind a baseboard in her apartment, she is inspired to return the items to their entire rightful owner—no small or easy task. This journey and acts of anonymous generosity spark more benevolent acts. A celebration of life, *Amélie* reminds us of the small wonders that are all around us—if only we pause to look.

French with English subtitles. Nominated for multiple Academy Awards.

Sources of nurture for populations and communities may be similar to those for a family. As the patient system becomes larger (as with more than one individual), the sources of nurture also become broader in many cases. Freedom from harassment, threats, or violence could be added to any level of patient system sources of nurture but often seems to be pertinent to an at-risk or target population or community. Sources of depletion for a population could be the reverse of the sources of nurture. For instance, an at-risk population of unwed pregnant teenagers might be depleted by harassment, ridicule, or shunning by others with extreme moral views against unmarried young women being sexually active. The target population and community Application to Practice describes some of the things a nurse needs to consider when using the 4+ model of wellness.

APPLICATION TO PRACTICE 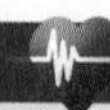

A Target Population Within a Community

The Teen Mothers' High School Program, which was located in one of the local high schools in the town of Urbansville, was used by more than 100 young single women each year for 5 years. The City Council decided to participate in the formation of a community health-promotion program called "Healthy Urbansville." The council members wanted to improve the health-promoting aspects of their city. They called on leaders in the educational facilities in town, police/sheriff and fire departments, local business people, ecclesiastical representatives (e.g., of churches, temples, synagogues), and other local interested citizens, including representatives of the youth groups and senior citizens' centers, to be part of this community effort.

The city was fairly large and contained many community resource agencies and emergency funding processes to assist those in need. The city was located in an urban area of the western region of the country, with many parks and recreation areas. The city prided itself on the good relationships between its diverse populations, the cleanliness of the city, and the efforts toward appropriate city growth that had been in place for several years. There were several excellent libraries, theater and other media options, art and history museums, and restaurants of all kinds. Biomedical and complementary integrative health therapies co-existed. There were churches of many different denominations readily accessible by most of the populations. Transportation opportunities were well distributed throughout the city, although there were continuing construction projects at various times throughout the dry seasons. There were, as in any large city, varying socioeconomic groups, including many homeless. Illicit drug dealing was being combatted daily by the police and others, but it was not out of hand. Violence was occasional, with robberies and burglaries being highest during the hotter months. Overall, the city considered itself a city with a future.

One of the major concerns of the Healthy Urbansville group that came forth after an in-depth community/population assessment process, which included the use of several surveys (plus the 4+ model of wellness), was that the rising numbers of teen pregnancies had a depleting effect on the community as a whole; families and resources within the community were hard hit. The age ranges of the teenage mothers was between 14 and 17; there were presently 1,000 young women in this age group, according to the most recent statistics. Statistically, teen pregnancies resulted in higher mortality rates than other age groupings. This concern became the main priority of the Healthy Urbansville group.

1. Using the 4+ model of wellness and given what this case study indicated, which assets (or sources of nurture) and which problems (sources of depletion) might exist in the Urbansville community?
2. What might be the sources of nurture in the intellectual domain of the community? In the physical, emotional, and spiritual domains of the community?
3. Think of the teenage mothers in this community. What questions might you have regarding this target (at-risk) population? What are some of the sources of nurture (or assets) that might affect young women in the age group between 14 and 17 years of age? What are some of the potential sources of depletion (or problem areas) that might affect young women in this age group?
4. Given the sources of nurture (or assets) identified, which interventions might be made to strengthen these in the young women? What might be done to diminish or delete the depleting sources (or problems)?
5. List several interventions for both the community and target population that could facilitate health-promoting behaviors, either individually or by working to diminish a source of community depletion.

The Pender Health Promotion Model

The Pender Health Promotion Model (Pender, 1987, 2011) was developed by University of Michigan nursing professor Dr. Nola Pender over the course of several decades to complement models of health protection. It takes the position that three specific areas are crucial to health promotion: an individual's experiences and characteristics, behavior-specific cognition and affect, and the actual or intended behavioral outcomes. In terms of its focus, it takes a clear position that health promotion requires a conscious, intentional alteration of patients' behaviors toward health and healing; the role of the nurse is to offer guidance on the steps or techniques that can best assist the patient in this endeavor.

The basic assumptions of this model, as described in Pender's manual (2011), are as follows:

1. Persons seek to create conditions of living through which they can express their unique human health potential.
2. Persons have the capacity for reflective self-awareness, including assessment of their own competencies.
3. Persons value growth in directions viewed as positive and attempt to achieve a personally acceptable balance between change and stability.
4. Individuals seek to actively regulate their own behavior.
5. Individuals in all their biopsychosocial complexity interact with the environment, progressively transforming the environment and being transformed over time.
6. Health professionals constitute a part of the interpersonal environment, which exerts influence on persons throughout their lifespan.
7. Self-initiated reconfiguration of person–environment interactive patterns is essential to behavior change.

In this model, the nurse takes on a multifaceted role as educator, sounding board, and guidance counselor, using knowledge of health promotion and of the patient's personal character and environment to assist the patient in directing his or her efforts to alter behavior in a health-supporting direction.

Life Stages Conceptual Framework

During the huge undertaking by a 50-member multiple federal interagency workgroup, the birth of the Healthy People 2020 Leading Health Indicators (LHIs) came to fruition. The leading party was the HHS. The *Healthy People 2020* LHIs were selected and organized using a Health Determinants and Health Outcomes by Life Stages Conceptual Framework that was intended to place attention on both the individual determinants as well as societal determinants affecting the public's health and contributing to health disparities across the lifespan, thereby bringing to the forefront strategic opportunities to promote health and improve the quality of life for the American people (HHS, 2014).

Determinants of Health and Health Disparities Biological, social, economic, and environmental factors—and their interrelationships—influence the ability of individuals and communities to make progress on these indicators. Addressing these determinants is key to improving population health, eliminating health disparities, and meeting the overarching goals of Healthy People 2020.

Health Across the Life Stages The LHIs will be examined using a life stages perspective. This approach recognizes that specific risk factors and determinants of health vary across the lifespan. Health and disease result from the accumulation (over time) of the effects of risk factors and determinants. Intervening at specific points in the life course can help reduce risk factors and promote health. The life stages perspective addresses one of the four overarching goals of Healthy People 2020.

AFFORDABLE CARE ACT (ACA)

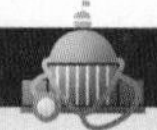

One of the main reasons the ACA was critical as healthcare reform legislation in the United States is that 7 in 10 deaths in the United States are related to preventable diseases such as obesity, diabetes, high blood pressure, heart disease, and cancer, and three-quarters of our healthcare dollars are spent treating such diseases. However, only 3 cents of each dollar spent on health care in the United States (public and private) go toward prevention and wellness.

Source: American Public Health Association. (2012). Why do we need the Affordable Care Act? Retrieved from http://www.apha.org/NR/rdonlyres/19BEA341-A7C3-4920-B2BC-65BDC846B803/0/WhyWeNeedtheACA_Aug2012.pdf.

Conclusion

This chapter discusses basic concepts of health and health promotion as related to disease prevention, including definitions of *health promotion* and *wellness* as the terms are used in this chapter; delineation of factors influencing health promotion and wellness; a brief summary of some ways of looking at health promotion and wellness by describing some models, guides, and tools involved in health protection, health promotion, wellness and risk evaluation, analysis, and reduction; and introduction of three models of wellness. Key concepts, case studies, research alerts, and critical thinking activities are presented to reinforce concepts and assist in "pushing the envelope" and expanding ideas for health-promotion interventions.

LEVELS OF PREVENTION

Primary: Exercising on a regular basis, including aerobic work, stretching, and weight training

Secondary: Getting mammogram or prostate screenings, depending on appropriate schedule according to age and family history

Tertiary: Assisting a diabetic who has lost a toe and must learn through physical therapy how to maintain balance

HEALTHY ME

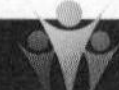

What do you do *each* day to create a "healthy you"? List those activities that you purposely do in order to promote your health while a nursing student.

Critical Thinking Activities

1. Can a person who has been diagnosed with bipolar disorder and who is appropriately and successfully being managed with medications achieve high-level wellness?
2. Can a community experiencing a severe gang problem achieve high-level wellness? If so, how might this be done?
3. How might the Jedi Women (a community action group consisting of single low-income mothers) define high-level wellness for their group? What activities might stimulate the group toward self-actualization?

4. Which social barriers might keep patients from exploring health-promoting activities, including healthy eating, exercising, and so forth?
5. Why is it that lifestyle choices and social limitations and barriers exist? Which situations might be lending themselves to building social barriers for patients?
6. Some population and community patients have noticeable limitations to their lifestyle choices, as noted in this chapter. Consider the populations that lived in major cities, as well as in rural and/or frontier areas, in the United States 50 years ago. Compare the positives and negatives of their lifestyle choices at that time to similar populations of today.
7. Discuss things a community or society could do to support an individual's self-care activities.
8. Describe how consumerism and self-care activities might encourage health-promotion and wellness behaviors.
9. Make a table with two columns. In the first, list self-care activities you engage in to nurture your wellness. In the second, list self-care activities you have not been doing but should. Plan interventions to include at least two new health-promoting behaviors in your daily life.
10. Identify two populations to which you belong. List five self-care practices these populations engage in for the benefit and nurture of their members.
11. How can communities engage in self-care?
12. Redefine the descriptors "unhealthy" and "well" for each of the spokes of the holistic wellness model as they fit into your or your patient's cultural perspective.
13. Discuss the meaning of knowledge, understanding, insight, and inner peace, which are found on the eagle feathers on the bottom of the holistic wellness model (Figure 14-1), as they might fit your or your patient's culture.
14. With the patient, evaluate the patient's health at each spoke (see Figure 14-1). Consider each spoke as having a weak or more negative dimension (e.g., on the Physical spoke, unfit would be the weak dimension and fit would be the healthy dimension). Have the patient place a dot on the spoke where the patient thinks he or she is at the time on that spoke's dimension. The closer the patient places the dot to the center of the wheel on any given spoke/dimension, the healthier the person considers himself or herself in regard to that dimension. Once a dot is placed on each spoke, the dots are connected to form a circle. The nurse and the patient can visually evaluate whether the circle is balanced and where the weak dimensions are.
15. Discuss potential interventions and/or changes the patient might decide to make to move himself or herself more toward the center of the holistic wellness wheel (Figure 14-1) toward being "healthy for life."
16. For your own community, identify the system dimensions that would be important to assessing wellness.
17. Refer to Box 14-3. Which other items could be added to the box to describe sources of nurture and sources of depletion for each of the four domains for an individual, a family, a population, or a community?
18. From Box 14-3, choose a source of nurture in one of the domains and describe how that source of nurture might affect another domain in a patient.
19. How might an excess of any factor affect any (or all) of a patient's domains?
20. If a person has a physical injury, which of the other domains besides the physical one might be affected? In what way(s)?
21. Consider a woman who is the sole support of several children and must also be the caregiver for an elderly, ill parent. Which domains(s) in that person might be affected? How?
22. If that woman becomes totally depleted in several of her domains, how will the domains of the family she is caring for be affected? Describe.

References

American Public Health Association (APHA). (1991). *Healthy communities 2000: Model standards: Guidelines for community attainment of the year 2000 national health objectives* (3rd ed.). Washington, DC: Author.

Baldwin, E. M., & Baldwin, J. H. (1998). *4+ model of wellness*. Unpublished manuscript.

Baldwin, J. H. (1992). Moving towards harmony: Types and meanings of cues that prompt health-promoting decisions in women in the middle years. Doctoral dissertation, Catholic University of America, Washington, DC. *UMI Dissertation Abstracts*, Order No. 9220772.

Baldwin, J. H. (1995). Are we implementing community health promotion in nursing? *Public Health Nursing, 12*(3), 159–164.

Baldwin, J. H., Conger, C. O., Abegglen, J. C., & Hill, E. M. (1998). Population-focused and community-based nursing—moving toward clarification of concepts. *Public Health Nursing, 15*(1), 12–18.

Becker, M. H. (Ed.). (1974). *The health belief model and personal health behavior*. Thorofare, NJ: Charles B. Slack.

Benner, D. M. (2013). The demographics of social media users—2012. Pew Research Center's internet & American Life Project. Kaiser Permanente Foundation.

Browning, B., Huls, J., Rather, R., & Stout, L. (1997). *Taylorsville youth assessment*. Unpublished manuscript. Provo, UT: Brigham Young University College of Nursing.

Brubaker, B. H. (1983, April). Health promotion: A linguistic analysis. *Advances in Nursing Science, 5*, 1–14.

Butterfield, P. G. (1993). Thinking upstream: Conceptualizing health from a population perspective. In J. M. Swanson & M. Albrecht (Eds.), *Community health nursing: Promoting the health of aggregates* (pp. 68–80). Philadelphia, PA: Saunders.

Centers for Disease Control and Prevention (CDC). (2014). *Healthy People 2020*. Retrieved from http://www.cdc.gov/nchs/healthy_people/hp2020.htm

Chiverton, P. A., Votava, K. M., & Tortoretti, D. M. (2003). The future role of nursing in health promotion. *American Journal of Health Promotion, 18*(2), 192–194.

Clark, E. G., & Leavell, H. R. (1953/1965). Levels of application of preventive medicine. In H. R. Leavell & E. G. Clark (Eds.), *Preventive medicine for the doctor in his community: An epidemiologic approach* (3rd ed., pp. 14–38). New York, NY: McGraw-Hill.

Coveney, P., & Highfield, R. (1990). *The arrow of time: A voyage through science to solve time's greatest mystery*. New York, NY: Fawcett Columbine.

Dent, S. (2010). The Nurse's Guide to Preventing Back Pain. Retrieved from http://nursinglink.monster.com/nurse-supervisor-jobs/articles/12074-the-nurses-guide-to-preventing-back-pain

Drapo, P. J., & Woods, E. (1992). Preparing community health nurses for the real world: Power, politics, and poverty. In *1991 Papers: State of the art in community health nursing education, research, and practice* (pp. 47–51). Lexington, KY: ACHNE.

Duhl, L. J. (1986). *Health planning and social change*. New York, NY: Human Sciences Press.

Dunn, H. L. (1959). High-level wellness for man and society. *American Journal of Public Health, 49*, 789.

Dunn, H. L. (1980). *High level wellness*. Thorofare, NJ: Charles B. Slack.

Edelman, C. L., & Fain, J. A. (1998). Health defined: Objective for promotion and prevention. In C. L. Edelman & C. L. Mandle (Eds.), *Health promotion throughout the lifespan* (4th ed., pp. 3–24). St. Louis, MO: Mosby.

Edney, A. T. B. (1992). Companion animals and human health. *Veterinary Record, 130*(4), 285–287.

Green, L. W., & Raeburn, J. (1990). Contemporary developments in health promotion: Definitions and challenges. In N. Bracht (Ed.), *Health promotion at the community level* (pp. 19–44). Newbury Park, CA: Sage.

Hartford, J. (2009). The role of the nurse in health promotion. *Hospital News*. Retrieved from http://www.hospitalnews.com/the-role-of-the-nurse-in-health-promotion/

Hochbaum, G. M. (1958). *Public participation in medical screening programs: A socio-psychological study*. (Publication No. 572). Bethesda, MD: Public Health Service.

Holiday, R. (2013). e-Patient Engagement. Mississippi Health Care Symposium on Health Literacy. Mississippi Education Consortium for the Doctorate of Nursing Practice. HRSA Grant Number D09HP22638.

Kellogg Foundation funds 3-year "Healthy Cities Indiana" project. (1988). *American Journal of Public Health, 78*(12), 5.

Kulbok, P. A., & Baldwin, J. H. (1992). From preventive health behavior to health promotion: Advancing a positive construct of health. *Advances in Nursing Science, 14*(4), 50–64.

Kulbok, P. A., Baldwin, J. H., Cox, C. L., & Duffy, R. (1997). Advancing discourse on health promotion: Beyond mainstream thinking. *Advances in Nursing Science, 20*(1), 13–21.

Kulbok, P. A., Carter, K. F., Baldwin, J. H., Gilmartin, M. J., & Kirkwood, B. (1999). The multidimensional health behavior inventory. *Journal of Nursing Measurement, 7*(2), 177–195.

Kylatra, C. (2014). 10 things your commute does to your body. Retrieved from 10%20Things%20Your%20Commute%20Does%20to%20Your%20Body

Lalli, F. (2013). The affordable care act & you: The new health law ensures you have access to these 10 essential health benefits. *AARP: The magazine*. Mattoon, IL: RR Donnelley.

Maiese, D. R., & Fox, C. E. (1998). Laying the foundation for Healthy People 2010—The first year of consultation. *Public Health Reports, 113*, 92–95.

Marcus, B., & Forsyth, L. (2002, December). *Motivating people to be physically active*. Washington, DC: Human Kinetics.

Maslow, A. W. (1970). *Motivation and personality*. New York, NY: Harper & Row.

McConnell, A. R., Brown, C. M., Shoda, T. M., Stayton, L. E., & Martin, C. E. (2011). Friends with benefits: On the positive consequences of pet ownership. *Journal of Personality and Social Psychology, 101*(6), 1239–1252.

McDonald, I. (1997). *Holistic wellness: Self inventory of personal wellness utilizing the medicine wheel*. Unpublished manuscript.

McGinnis, J. M., & Foege, W. H. (1993). Actual causes of death in the United States. *Journal of the American Medical Association, 270*(18).

Moore, V., Neff, D., Smith, G., & Weber, J. (1999). *The homeless in Utah County: Food & Care Coalition*. Unpublished manuscript. Provo, UT: Brigham Young University College of Nursing.

Naisbitt, J. (1982). *Megatrends*. New York, NY: Warner Books.

National Institute for Occupational Safety and Health. (1996). *National Occupational Research Agenda*. (DHHS [NIOSH] Publication No. 96-115). Washington, DC: U.S. Government Printing Office.

National Institutes of Health. (1987). *The health benefits of pets*. (Publication No. 1998-216-107). Washington, DC: U.S. Government Printing Office.

Orem, D. E. (1985). *Nursing: Concepts of practice* (3rd ed.). New York, NY: McGraw-Hill.

Padilla, G. V., & Bulcavage, L. M. (1991). Theories used in patient/health education. *Seminars in Oncological Nursing, 7*(2), 87–96.

Palank, C. L. (1991). Determinants of health-promotive behavior: A review of current research. *Nursing Clinics of North America, 26*(4), 815–832.

Pender, N. (1987). *Health promotion in nursing practice* (2nd ed.). East Norwalk, CT: Appleton & Lange.

Pender, N. (2011). *The health promotion model manual.* Retrieved from http://deepblue.lib.umich.edu/bitstream/handle/2027.42/85350/HEALTH_PROMOTION_MANUAL_Rev_5-2011.pdf

Piper, M. (1999). *Another country: Navigating the emotional terrain of our elders.* Los Angeles, CA: Riverhead Books.

Poe, B. S., & O'Neill, K. O. (1997). Caffeine modulates heat shock induced apoptosis in the human promyelocytic leukemia cell line HL-60. *Cancer Letters, 121*, 1–6.

Prigogine, I., & Stengers, I. (1984). *Order out of chaos.* New York, NY: Bantam Books.

Raphael, D. (2000, December). The question of evidence in health promotion. *Health Promotion International, 15*(4), 355–367.

Raphael, D., & Bryant, T. (2002). The limitations of population health as a model for a new public health. *Health Promotion International, 17*(2), 189–199.

Rosenstock, I. M. (1974). Historical origins of the health belief model. In M. H. Becker (Ed.), *The health belief model and personal health behavior* (pp. 1–8). Thorofare, NJ: Charles B. Slack.

Ryan, R. S., & Travis, J. W. (1991). Introduction. In R. S. Ryan & J. W. Travis (Eds.), *Wellness: Small changes you can use to make a big difference* (p. 3). Berkeley, CA: Ten Speed Press.

Simmons, S. J. (1990). The health-promoting self-care system model: Directions for nursing research and practice. *Journal of Advances in Nursing, 15*(10), 1162–1166.

Southern Remedy. (2014). Teaching others to use Southern Remedy's adult healthy eating plate. Mississippi Public Broadcasting.

Steiger, N. J., & Lipson, J. C. (1985). *Self-care nursing: Theory and practice.* Bowie, MD: Brady Communications.

U.S. Department of Health and Human Services (HHS). (1982). *Forward plan for health 1977–1981.* Washington, DC: U.S. Government Printing Office.

U.S. Department of Health and Human Services (HHS). (1998a). *Healthy people in healthy communities: A guide for community leaders.* Washington, DC: Office of Disease Prevention and Health Promotion.

U.S. Department of Health and Human Services (HHS). (1998b). *Healthy People 2010 objectives: Draft for public comment.* Washington, DC: U.S. Government Printing Office.

U.S. Department of Health and Human Services (2000). *Healthy People 2010: Understanding and improving health* (2nd ed.). Washington, DC: U.S. Government Printing Office.

U.S. Department of Health and Human Services. (2011). *Healthy People 2020: Leading health indicators development and framework.* Retrieved from http://www.healthypeople.gov/2020/LHI/development.aspx

U.S. Preventive Services Task Force. (1989). *A guide to clinical preventive services: An assessment of the effectiveness of 169 interventions.* Baltimore, MD: Williams & Wilkins.

U.S. Public Health Service (USPHS). (1979). *Healthy people: The surgeon general's report on health promotion and disease prevention* (DHEW Publication No. 79-55071). Washington, DC: U.S. Department of Health, Education, and Welfare.

U.S. Public Health Service (USPHS). (1999). *Promoting physical activity: A guide for community action.* Washington, DC: Human Kinetics.

Victorian Health Promotion Foundation (VHPF). (2013). *Defining health promotion.* Retrieved from http://www.vichealth.vic.gov.au/Publications/VCE/Defining-health-promotion.aspx

Webster's Collegiate Dictionary (11th ed.). (2004). Springfield, MA: Merriam-Webster, Inc.

Wheatley, J. (1994). *Leadership and the new science: Learning about organization from an orderly universe.* San Francisco, CA: Berrett-Koehler.

World Health Organization. (2013a). *Chronic diseases and health promotion.* Retrieved from http://www.who.int/chp/about/en/index.html

World Health Organization. (2013b). *Health promotion.* Retrieved from: http://www.who.int/topics/health_promotion/en

CHAPTER FOCUS

Development of Health Ministries
- History of Ministering: Hospitals, Hospitality, and Religious Communities
- Nightingale's Legacy: Relationship of Nursing to Early Models
- Philosophical Underpinnings

Health Ministry in Action

Relationship Between Community Health Nursing and Faith Communities
- Faith Community Nursing

Missionary Nursing
- Roles and Practice of Missionary Nurses

Spirituality Versus Religion in Health Care
- Providing Spiritual Care
- Barriers to Providing Spiritual Health Care
- Morals, Ethics, and Spirituality in Health Care
- HIPAA and Spirituality
- Praying with Patients
- Rituals

QUESTIONS TO CONSIDER

After reading this chapter, you will know the answers to the following questions:

1. What are health ministries?
2. How did health ministries begin?
3. How does spirituality relate to health?
4. How is the faith community an ideal setting for the role of the community health nurse?
5. What are examples of models of health ministries?
6. What is faith community nursing?
7. How can nurses function to promote health in health ministry programs?
8. What are some of the unique challenges faced by nurses practicing in a faith community?
9. What are some of the attributes needed to succeed in faith community nursing?

Wouldn't it be wonderful if faith groups adopted one small area and made sure that every single child was immunized, that every person had a basic medical exam, and that every woman who became pregnant would get prenatal care? Are these goals possible? We believe the answer is yes.

CHAPTER 15

Health Ministries: Health and Faith Communities

Lilianna K. Deveneau and
Karen Saucier Lundy

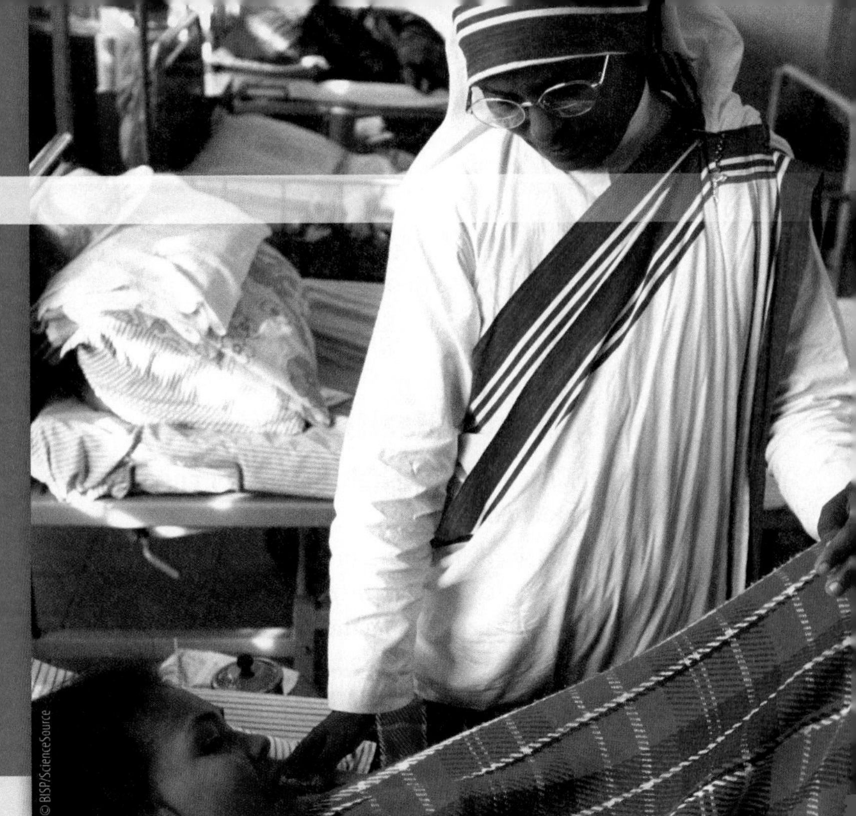

KEY TERMS

extrinsic religiosity
faith community
health ministry
holistic care
intrinsic religiosity
missionary nursing
religion
rituals
spirituality

> Prayer does not use up artificial energy, doesn't burn up any fossil fuel, doesn't pollute. Neither does song, neither does love, neither does the dance.
>
> —Margaret Mead

> Never worry about numbers. Help one person at a time, and always start with the person nearest you.
>
> —Mother Teresa

> Blessed are those who have not seen and yet believe.
>
> —Jesus, John 20:29

> Every human being is the author of his own health and disease.
>
> —Buddha

> If the only prayer you say in your whole life is 'Thank you,' that would suffice.
>
> —Meister Eckhart, 4th century theologian and mystic

REFLECTIONS

These quotations represent many different expressions of spirituality. How do you define spirituality? What are common themes in the quotes? Are religion and spirituality the same? As you read this chapter, consider the ways in which community health nurses should include the spiritual aspect of health in caring for populations.

Development of Health Ministries

History of Ministering: Hospitals, Hospitality, and Religious Communities

Health ministry refers to the practice of incorporating spirituality into patient care, thereby caring for the individual as a whole—addressing the mind, body, and spirit. Caring for a patient's physical and spiritual wellbeing dates back to the first models of the nursing profession (Watson, 2005; Young & Koopsen, 2011 and is an important factor in one's overall health. In fact, the words "health," "holy," and "whole" are derived from the Saxon word *hal* and the Greek word *holos*, meaning whole (Dossey and Keegan, 2013; Young & Koopsen, 2011).

The history of "ministering" comes from the earliest accounts of efforts to help and to care for the unfortunate, often those who were unable to afford private care in their homes. "Hospitality" was offered by religious communities who saw it as their responsibility to provide comfort and care. Hospitals originated as places where this ministering to (care of) the sick took place. Religious communities, lay and formal, have a history of providing advocacy for and access to care. Concern for the underserved focused on the disadvantaged, the elderly, women and children, the disabled, and the chronically ill (Wall & Nelson, 2003) and sought to overcome barriers of suffering and injustice with faith communities as the focus of interventions. The work of the Carter Center at Emory University (**Box 15-1**)

BOX 15-1 The Carter Center's Interfaith Health Program: Realigning Community Assets Through Collaboration of Faith Communities and Health Organizations in Building Healthier Communities

The Carter Center's interest in the role of faith communities in improving community health began in the 1980s. A national symposium, "Closing the Gap," signaled the beginning of concerted efforts to bring together the most significant health science and the most relevant knowledge and experience from theology for both the faith community and health science and health service institutions. At that time, the Carter Center identified faith communities as the most underused resource group, with potential to help in closing the gap for improving America's health.

In 1989, a conference on *Striving for Fullness of Life: The Church's Challenge in Health* was sponsored by the Carter Center and the Wheat Ridge Foundation. This conference focused on building healthy lives through public health measures such as preventing disease, disability, and premature death. This proved to be an important step forward, but it did not address the need for shifts in how congregations viewed their roles in the larger community and how health institutions and organizations perceived the assets of congregations.

The Interfaith Health Program was formed in 1992 to respond to the challenge of helping to build healthier communities by engaging leaders from the health sciences and theology along with community representatives from health services and congregations to find ways to realign faith and health assets for the good of the community.

The Five Gap Model was used to ask the right questions when searching for strategies. The gaps include the following:

- The gap between what is already known and what is applied
- The gap between what every faith group affirms as their concern for social justice and what they do
- The gap between successful working models and general application in other communities
- The gap perpetuated by faith groups working in isolation from each other and health agencies
- The gap between present wants and future needs

Using the Five Gap Model, we focused on promotion of congregational health ministries, one of the key strategies of the Interfaith Health Program. The Atlanta Health Ministry Model was developed and then used in two African American communities and one multicultural community in Atlanta. This health ministry model was based on the participatory approach proposed by Paulo Freire, the Brazilian grassroots educator and author of *Pedagogy of the Oppressed* (1970). Some of the core principles of the Atlanta Health Ministry Model (Droege & Wenger, 1997, p. 14) are as follows:

- Education is never neutral; it is either liberating or domesticating.
- People will act on issues that evoke strong feelings.
- People are creative and intelligent with the capacity for action.
- Genuine dialogue is needed if communities are to share, listen, and learn.

Several key action steps characterized the approach used in Atlanta. First, a working group of 15 religious leaders participated in a 6-month planning process to determine the most effective way to enlist faith communities to increase engagement in health-promotion activities. This process served to nurture a network of potential collaborators.

Second, in each neighborhood, local pastors (or priests, rabbi, and imam) were invited to join a network of congregations, with each network governed by a Health Ministry Council. This council was formed by the participating congregations and staffed by a network coordinator. Third, the training of Congregational Health Promoters was at the heart of the program. The training program was coordinated by the Neil Hodgson Woodruff School of Nursing at Emory University, with nursing instructors who understood the participatory teaching-learning process leading the training sessions.

The goal of this approach was to build on the capacities of the congregations and communities rather than to fix problems or to predetermine what needs to be learned.

Each participating congregation designated two natural leaders from within the congregation to join the training program, which consisted of 20 to 24 hours of 2- to 3-hour sessions. Although the emphasis was on lay health leadership, some professionals such as nurses and social workers participated in the training. As the need was expressed by the participants, local health resource persons came to discuss specific health services in the community. When the trainees recognized the need to learn more about a resource, such as nutritional information or heart health resources, the nursing instructor would make the connections for them, always emphasizing how they can assume that role in the future.

So, what has happened in these neighborhoods since the initial training period? In a largely African American community, Atlanta Health Ministries, a nonprofit organization with 501(c)3 status, was established. It has several active committees, with one of them being Congregational Health Promoters. In a very multiethnic community, there is a Congregational Health Ministry program as part of the Chamblee–Doraville Ministry Center. A Congregational Health Ministry Coordinator, who is a parish nurse employed by St. Joseph's Mercy Care System, conducts training sessions in Spanish and English and serves as a mentor for all of the congregational health promoters in the neighborhood, which includes Korean, Vietnamese, African American, Hispanic, and dominant-culture American congregations.

A commitment to cultural openness is inherent in all of the initiatives of the Interfaith Health Program: "Cultural openness refers to a life-long stance that promotes cultural self awareness and continuing development of transcultural skills" (Wenger, 1998, p. 164). As boundaries are spanned among

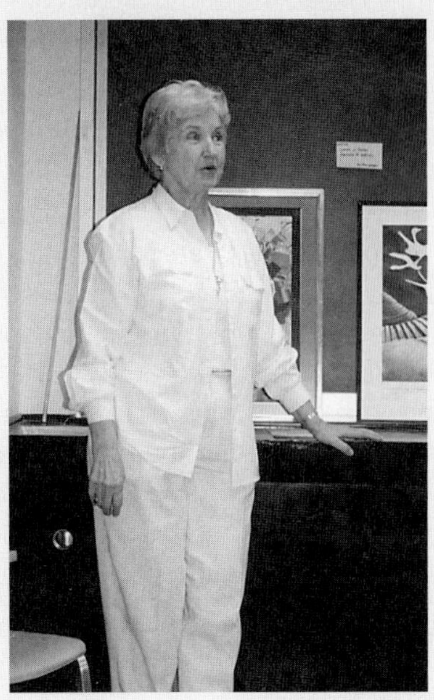

Anna Frances Wenger, PhD, RN, FAAN, the Carter Center

disciplines and within communities, the persons engaged in faith and health ministries need to constantly renew their commitment to learn about the meaning of faith and health within the worldviews of the people. Respect for differences, although important, is not enough (Wenger, 1998). Transcultural knowledge and skills are essential components when engaging in health ministries and building partnerships.

Two other initiatives of the Interfaith Health Program are directed toward moving the faith and health movement forward. Whole Communities Collaborative is a network of faith and health leaders from five specific communities within the United States where local working groups exchange ideas and develop local activities that bring faith-based communities and health organizations together for the good of the larger community or neighborhood. The other initiative is referred to as the Faith and Health Consortium. This network focuses on academic/community partnerships. There are five sites in the United States and one in South Africa where at least a school of theology or seminary and a school of public health have formed an agreement to promote disciplinary and interdisciplinary courses, research studies, and service projects that involve the integration of faith and health concepts. Schools of nursing, medicine, social work, and allied health are included whenever possible. The Faith and Health Consortium working groups always include community partners because of the underlying premise that the education of professionals, in addition to research and service projects, needs ongoing involvement with representatives from the community to keep the academic endeavors grounded within socio-cultural contexts. Both of these networks have developed collaborative

(Continued)

BOX 15-1 (*continued*)

relationships through regular monthly conference calls and periodic meetings attended by representatives from the local site working groups.

Building partnerships between health institutions and faith communities requires an appreciation of assets or strengths that are already present within the community. Most of the work of the Interfaith Health Program focuses on alignment of assets for improvement of community health. Faith-based congregations are one of the most enduring assets within a community. Gary Gunderson (1997, 1998), director of the Interfaith Health Program, has outlined the following eight key strengths of congregations that highlight congregations as strategic partners in building healthier communities:

1. The power to accompany, to be physically present
2. The power to convene in small and large groups across interest lines
3. The power to connect, to form human networks across which resources flow
4. The power to frame, to story, and to set events and data in a meaningful context
5. The power to give sanctuary to people, programs, ideas, and dialogue
6. The power to bless, forgive, and nurture hope amid its opposite
7. The power to pray and to mark the boundary between holy and human
8. The power to endure and to maintain the sense of time and development

The challenge for health professionals and congregational leaders is to intentionally search for ways that the assets of health and faith structures can be aligned for the benefit of the community at large. Our aspiration is that the most relevant health science and the most mature faith will guide the alignment of assets that will build strong partnerships for healthier communities.

Source: Anna Frances Z. Wenger, PhD, RN, FAAN, Affiliate Faculty, Neil Hodgson Woodruff School of Nursing; Faith and Health Consortium Coordinator, Interfaith Health Program, Rollins School of Public Health, Emory University, Atlanta, Georgia.

and the Park Ridge Center for the Study of Health, Faith, and Ethics are two examples of current health ministries.

Health ministries have experienced a resurgence in recent healthcare theory and practice because of numerous trends in society. The aging U.S. population is not only increasing in number, but also raising issues of values, quality of life, and caring for those who now are living longer. Moreover, recently studies have begun to focus on the health benefits of spirituality and religion; this trend has already led to changes in nursing theory and practice as a way to improve patients' quality of life.

The link between caregiving and spirituality is present throughout history. For over 100,000 years, shamans, medicine men and women, or healers were believed to have powers that enabled them to connect to one's spirit to promote healing. These beliefs and practices can still be seen today in as much as 70–90% of the world's population (Young & Koopsen, 2011).

Nursing care, in its modern sense, can be traced back before the beginning of Christianity. In Babylonia, for example, the ancient Code of Hammurabi suggests personal care was given to patients between visits with the physician (O'Brien, 2014). The first medical textbook, known as the *Ebers Papyrus*, was created in ancient Egypt around 1500 BCE, although it is believed to have been copied from texts almost 2,000 years older (Frank, 1953; O'Brien, 2014). Ancient Rome is also credited with medical advances. Cato the Elder discovered treatments for gout, colic, constipation, side aches, and indigestion (Bullough & Bullough, 1969; O'Brien, 2014). In China, herbs were used for their curative properties and adapted by nursing therapy practices (Sellew & Nuesse, 1946; O'Brien, 2014). Finally, in ancient Israel, a religious practice of giving a percentage of one's possessions, known as tithing, allowed for the creation of "houses for strangers," later known as hospitality houses or charity houses (O'Brien, 2014). These discoveries paved the way for the advancement of care.

The Old and New Testaments of the Christian Bible refer to nurses, the nurse–patient relationship, and caring for others. Biblical references are still used to describe nurses, including the title "angels of mercy" and nurses "answering the call" to be a caregiver or "answering God's call" (Young & Koopsen, 2011). Monasteries, originally founded to provide a site for poverty, chastity, and obedience, became centers for nursing the sick and wounded by the 5th century (Donahue, 1985; O'Brien, 2014), and continued these services through the time of Florence Nightingale and beyond.

MEDIA MOMENT

Popular medical television programs, such as *House, Scrubs, Nurse Jackie,* and *Grey's Anatomy,* seldom address religious or spiritual aspects of care. Why do you think these aspects of health are avoided?

Nightingale's Legacy: Relationship of Nursing to Early Models

> For what is Mysticism? Is it not the attempt to draw near to God, not by rites or ceremonies, but by inward disposition? Is it not merely a hard word for "The Kingdom of Heaven is within"? Heaven is neither a place nor a time.
>
> —*Florence Nightingale, 1873*

> Religion is meant to be light, sign, watermark, path. Religion becomes a map to a place no one has ever been. But the going on is up to me. And the way I go is my spirituality.
>
> —*Joan Chittister, OSB*

Early models of health ministry can be traced to Florence Nightingale and her own preparation for nursing. Believing that her purpose was to care for the sick, the underserved, and the disadvantaged, Nightingale sought nursing training, but the only formal education in caring for the sick available to her was a 3-month experience at the Institution of Deaconesses at Kaiserworth, Dusseldorf, Germany. The institution had 100 beds, and there were 116 deaconesses (so-called Protestant nurses) in training to provide care. It has been argued that Nightingale's primary purpose was not necessarily religious, but spiritual (Dossey, 1998). Historically, Nightingale followed a long line of healers—shamans, witches, midwives, and deaconesses. She wanted to answer what she believed to be her vocation—her call. Her primary commitment was to actualize her spiritual convictions in acts of social justice.

Organized religion has many icons and symbols that represent values related to good and evil, the sacred and profane, and the expected actions of believers. Think of your own experiences with these symbols and your reaction to them. Now consider your reaction to religious symbols unfamiliar to your own values. How difficult is it to accommodate your patients' religious beliefs and values associated with their symbols in healthcare settings?

Read the "Day in the Life" feature by Donna Doherty and consider how one nurse dealt with this conflict. Was she accepting or did she simply tolerate her patients' religious values? Why or why not?

Dossey, through her extensive research of Nightingale's writings, casts her as a genuine 19th-century mystic: "I plotted her life as such and found it to be similar to recognized mystics, such as St. Catherine of Siena, St. Catherine of Genoa, and St. Teresa of Avila" (Dossey,

DAY IN THE LIFE

Working with Patients of Different Faiths

By Donna Doherty, MSN, RN

The following story about spirituality and my experience in a home health setting will challenge your approach to religious and faith belief systems. Nursing is more than science. It is a true healing art that touches the soul when practiced with love.

Allen M. was an 84-year-old man who was dying. He had lived a full life and had personal photos on the walls with presidents, mayors, governors, and movie stars. He was comfortable with himself and his surroundings. He always had a smile. His walls were covered with hundreds of books—books on every subject. His paintings and drawings mirrored a love of life and people that I rarely have seen.

Allen practiced a healing modality called Reiki. He would constantly send energy and prayers for other people even though he was very ill. He would say, "In healing others, I heal myself." His favorite reply to good conversation was, "That's beautiful."

Every day that I visited as his home health nurse was an eye-opening experience. Most days Allen would be in prayerful meditation. He would be kneeling in front of an altar on his sun porch—soft music playing, incense burning, a Chinese gong standing on the altar, a laughing Buddha in position, and an artificial waterfall in place. This made the area an optimal healing environment for him.

I would assess his health status, answer questions, and teach him information about his illness. In the course of evaluating issues that were of concern to him, the conversation turned to the terminal part of his illness. He openly discussed funeral plans. I had assumed that he would have a Buddhist service. I was surprised to learn that he had been a lifelong Episcopalian. His church had been planning an elaborate service. He was very pleased with this but he wanted to honor the Buddhist part of his life. He asked me to help him plan the service. It would be a memorial ceremony.

The conflicts in me arose. Would I be dishonoring my beliefs in honoring his? Was it really my place to help Allen with this task? Nurses are placed in unusual circumstances sometimes. I prayed about this and in doing so realized that the greatest gift that we have been given is free will. Right or wrong, good or bad, we can choose who we are. The freedom that Allen demonstrated in his personal worship was dear to him. He had lived a full life in service to others. He never forced his views on others.

I carry these special memories with me always. Honoring the spiritual beliefs of my patients comes naturally to me.

(Continued)

DAY IN THE LIFE *(CONTINUED)*

If I had constructed a boundary between the spiritual beliefs, it would not have served any purpose but to create a stagnation in the healing process. I allow the spiritual interaction to flow like water, always moving, cleansing, and ending at its natural conclusion.

The memorial service was, in Allen's words, "beautiful."

as quoted in Manthey, 1999, p. 3). Nightingale heard the voice of God for the first time on February 7, 1837, at the age of 16. She wrote, "God spoke and called me to his service" (Dossey, 1998). Although many have compared Nightingale's experience to Joan of Arc's experience, for Nightingale, there were no further "instructions" from God for another 16 years. From that point on, her life was a journey of spiritual enlightenment, through her writings, research, and obsession with the creation of the professional nurse.

Recent attention to Nightingale's philosophical leanings shows how committed she was to the integration of spirituality in nursing, clearly differentiating between spirituality and religion, which she saw as only one possible expression of spiritual life. Nightingale distinctly articulated a concept of spirituality that was broader than religion. Spirituality was, for her, a connection between an inner self and a higher reality through creative energy. Such energy was the most powerful resource for healing (Anderson, 1996; Macrae, 1995).

Nightingale, it seems, was as ahead of her time in health ministry and spirituality in nursing as she was in epidemiology and community health nursing. Today, the growing commitment to **holistic care** is pushing nursing and medicine, as well as other disciplines, to reexamine the place of spirit in relationship to body and mind. Differences between spirituality and religion, and **extrinsic** and **intrinsic religiosity** are poorly understood and often badly articulated (Couture, 2003; Dossey, 1998; Zinnbauer et al., 1997).

> If grace is so wonderful, why do we have such difficulty recognizing and accepting it? Maybe it's because grace is not gentle or made-to-order. It often comes disguised as loss, or failure, or unwelcome change.
>
> —*Kathleen Norris*

Philosophical Underpinnings

The philosophical underpinnings of faith communities remain essentially unchanged. At their best, communities of faith seek ways to continue a tradition of service, often to those who need it most.

The commitment is to health and wholeness for self and others. Participation in advocacy, health education, promotion, and illness prevention are intrinsically linked to spiritual health. Such a health ministry functions within a self-understanding of compassion and care that encompasses faith, lived out in the concept of care; hope, actualized within a context of care; and love, which becomes the blueprint for the conduct of care.

Nightingale was raised in a Unitarian and Anglican home. Although she came to disdain organized religion, she was an intensely spiritual person. She wrote in 1852 of her dissatisfaction with the Church of England and the Catholic Church:

> The wound is too deep for the Church of England to heal. I belong as little to the Church of England as to that of Rome—or rather my heart belongs as much to the Catholic Church as to that of England—oh, how much more. The only difference is that the former insists peremptorily upon my believing what I cannot believe, while the latter is too careless and indifferent to know whether I believe it or not. (Dossey, 1998)

While Nightingale believed in the messages of Christianity, she demonstrated an unconventional tolerance and acceptance of other world religions. She wrote, "To know God we must study Him in the Pagan and Jewish dispensations as in the Christian" (Dossey, 1998, p. 48). This thread of unity to the whole continued throughout her life's writings. Dossey noted that Nightingale studied the St. James version of the Bible with great intensity, providing written annotations on almost every page. She wrote her own ideas, meanings, and interpretations in English, French, Greek, and Italian, with a blank page between most every printed page of the Bible (Dossey, 1998).

> A religion that takes no account of practical affairs and does not help to solve them is no religion.
>
> —*Mahatma Gandhi*

> God inspires people to help other people who have been hurt by life, and by helping them, they protect them from the danger of feeling alone, abandoned or judged.
>
> —*Rabbi Harold Kushner, Author of When Bad Things Happen to Good People*

Though Florence Nightingale proclaimed spirituality as elemental to nursing, declaring it the most potent resource for healing, the roots of modern Western medicine can be traced to the French philosopher, scientist, and mathematician Rene Descartes (1596–1650). His belief that the church should cultivate the spirit and allow science to heal the body is known as the Cartesian split. This dichotomous outlook asserted medicine should consist only of the rational and observable. Consequently, religion and spirituality became dismissed in the scientific realm. The Cartesian model provided a basis for medicine, and its practices are still seen today (Messikomer & DeCraemer, 2002; Young & Koopsen, 2011). The ancient foundations of spirituality within nursing and the Western model of medicine through rationality and observation create tension within both practitioners and patients.

Faith Community Nursing Within the United States

Despite the questions concerning the role of spirituality in health, caretakers continued to practice faith-based care. In fact, the first organized group of nurses in the United States was the Sisters of Charity in Emmitsburg, Maryland, established in 1803 (Koenig, 2008; Young & Koopsen, 2011). Throughout the next two centuries, demands for healthcare providers, coupled with the rapid development of technology, created a more complex nursing field in which science reigned while spirituality practices were de-emphasized (Koenig, 2008; McSherry & Draper, 1998; Young & Koopsen, 2011). Though this trend continued, in the late 1970s and 1980s, Reverend Dr. Granger Westberg originated the concept of congregational or parish nurses (O'Brien, 2014; Young & Koopsen, 2011). In 2005, the term *parish nursing* was changed to *faith community nursing* in the American Nurses Association's (ANA's) *Scope and Standards of Practice* to include health ministry nurse, parish nurse, congregation nurse, crescent nurse, and health and wellness nurse (ANA & Health Ministries Association [HMA], 2005; O'Brien, 2014).

The philosophy of faith community nursing continues today, placing spirituality central to healthcare practices (O'Brien, 2014). The faith community combines a love for humanity, a willingness to serve, and a belief in a higher power, God, creator, or connectedness with all things with the education of a nurse. Spirituality is essential to health care (Watson, 2005; Taylor, 2007; Young & Koopsen, 2011), and yet the only formal education most nurses receive on this topic is basic and is covered only during one's training period (Koenig, 2008). One choice nurses have to avoid this is to become a faith community nurse (FCN). This often includes an association with a specific congregation, church, mosque, temple, or other religious center. FCNs are experienced registered nurses (RNs) with specialized training in holistic health and spiritual care (Tuck, Wallace, & Pullen, 2001), which can include classes such as philosophy, health assessment, psychosocial issues, community resources, and relevant professional, legal, and ethical issues common to their specific roles and locations Young & Koopsen, 2011). FCNs perform all independent functions of a professional nurse while promoting health and healing as a member of a specific **faith community**. Moreover, FCNs work with their congregations to promote health and healing and to prevent disease. Finally, they serve as the following (O'Brien, 2014; Young & Koopsen, 2011):

- Personal health counselors
- Advocates and community liaisons
- Support group facilitators
- Referral agents
- Integrators of faith and health
- Participants in quality assessments, community collaboration, performance appraisal, and research

Health education in the church community takes the form of classes, literature, newsletters, and web-based information. Support groups, especially those that are age focused, such as daycare for preschool children or for elderly community members, make a substantial contribution to a community's wellbeing, as do focused issue groups that provide a forum for shared experiences such as separation or bereavement.

Community service initiatives like care teams, providing housing with Habitat for Humanity, literacy programs such as Operation Read, and one-on-one caring outreach programs are all examples of health ministries. Giving space and time to support groups, such as Alzheimer's caregivers and self-help groups including Alcoholics Anonymous (AA) and Celebrate Recovery (CR), fills a larger community health need.

There are currently thousands of FCNs in each state, and they are increasing in number around the globe (Young & Koopsen, 2011). FCN has been declared a specialty in community nursing by the ANA and HMA, and is therefore expected to continue to gain popularity among nurses.

RESEARCH ALERT

Nothing is so firmly believed as what is least known.

—*Montaigne, 1588*

A study of 1,931 older residents of Marin County, California, analyzed the association between attending religious services and all-cause mortality over a 5-year period looking at six confounding factors: demographics, health status, physical functioning, health habits, social functioning, and support and psychological state. Persons who attended religious services had lower mortality rates than those who did not, and religious attendance tended to be slightly more protective when coupled with high social support. This study lends

(*Continued*)

RESEARCH ALERT (*CONTINUED*)

credence to the existence of a "protective effect" of religious attendance on health; a broad implication is the potential benefit of partnerships between religious organizations and health-promotion efforts.

Source: Oman, D., & Reed, D. (1998). Religion and mortality among the community-dwelling elderly. *American Journal of Public Health, 88*(10), 1469–1475.

Health Ministry in Action

THINK ABOUT THIS 

"I have an almost complete disregard of precedent and a faith in the possibility of something better. It irritates me to be told how things always have been done. I defy the tyranny of precedent. I cannot afford the luxury of a closed mind. I go for anything new that might improve the past."

—Clara Barton, *A Chosen Faith*

What do you think Clara Barton means in her last statement, "I go for anything new that might improve the past"?

DAY IN THE LIFE

An FCN Speaks

When we began this program, I asked that it be called Health Ministry and that I'd be called the Health Ministry Coordinator, not parish nurse. I certainly wanted to attract the help of nurses in the congregation, but by inviting anyone who was interested, we ended up with a dynamite Wellness Cabinet. We had a variety of health-related professionals volunteer but I was most amazed that we attracted business people whose services and savvy could benefit the elderly, and a group of stay-at-home moms who organized themselves into a subgroup they wanted to call the Postal Ministry (sending cards to the homebound, sick, and grieving).

> I confused things with their names: that is belief.
>
> —*Jean-Paul Sartre*

> What keeps us alive, what allows us to endure? I think it is the hope of loving, or being loved.
>
> —*Meister Eckhart*

THINK ABOUT THIS 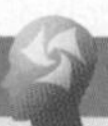

Our common threads: How world religions express "The Golden Rule"

Christian: Do unto others as you would have them do unto you.

Bahai: Blessed are those who prefer others to themselves.

Buddhism: Hurt not others in ways that you yourself would find hurtful.

Judaism: What is hateful to you, do not do to your neighbor. That is the entire Torah. The rest is commentary. Go and learn.

Islam: No one is a believer until you desire for another that which you desire for yourself.

Sikhism: Be not estranged from one another for God swells in every heart.

Jainism: In happiness and suffering in joy and grief, regard all creatures as you would yourself.

MEDIA MOMENT 

Byock, I. (2004). *The Four Things That Matter Most, A Book about Living.* New York, NY: Atria Books

A review by Maryfran Stulginsky, RN, MS, FCN

It is a fallacy to assume that the receivers of care in any faith community are typically staunch believers. Church communities are like any other … heterogeneous … some folks are traditionalists, some liberal, some lax, some affiliating to keep peace, some just showing up out of obligation or image, the list can go on and on. But, when crisis occurs, the belief that the faith community is a good place to start looking for help is pretty consistent. Most of what FCNs do comes second nature, but the most challenging piece of this practice, both for the novice and the experienced, is providing spiritual care.

It can be absolutely frightening, especially when you are aware that the person you are trying to help is on a completely different wave length from you spiritually. You are a believer; they are not. You see God as a loving presence ready to forgive; they see God as a harsh judge anxious to punish wrongs. You believe in hope; they have none left. Although I always pray for wisdom before every visit and feel generally prepared, I have recently found a resource that's been extremely helpful and given me greater confidence in what I do.

I use *The Four Things That Matter Most, A Book About Living,* by Ira Byock, MD to guide my discussions with patients and families. Ira Byock is a palliative care physician; his suggestions come from his practice. He proposes that four simple statements—"Please forgive me," "I forgive you," "thank you," and "I love you"—provide a clear path to emotional wellness. Being able to say and act on these statements can provide the tools for living a meaningful life, improving relationships, and healing what may appear hopeless.

For me, the book's message is simple: Healing and wholeness are always possible. The pages contain actual dialogues with patients, giving the reader ideas about what words to use, how to sequence specific discussions, and how to bring up difficult topics. The four statements are a useful framework for spiritual assessment, intervention, and evaluation: "Is there a need for forgiveness, do you need to forgive a situation or someone in your life, is there someone you need to thank or hear 'thank you' from, is there someone whose 'I love you' you hope to hear, is there someone you need to say 'I love you' to?"

Although the book quotes lines from famous religious and secular figures and states that its ideas reflect the teachings of most of the world's religions, it is not particularly theological. Nurses versed in their faith's sacred writings can easily call forth passages that frame and add weight to the discussion. For persons with no faith orientation, it is secular enough. Its ideas are universal. And, for those haunted by religious messages from their past, which cause them to reject formal religion, the four simple statements enable grace to be at work through the presence of the nurse.

For One More Day (2006)

By Mitch Albom, New York, NY: Hyperion.

What would we do if we had just 24 more hours to spend with our deceased loved ones? Author Mitch Albom gives us a glimpse into one suicidal man's experience of 24 hours with his mother, who died 12 years before.

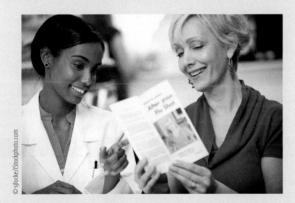

Pharmacist counseling church members at health fair about prescription drug therapy.

RESEARCH ALERT 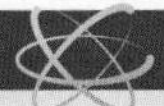

Research Call to Action

Despite the growth of faith community nursing, very few (usually only two to three studies yearly) formal research studies specific to the practice are found in the Cumulative Index to Nursing and Allied Health Literature database. Most of what exists to date are studies looking at the FCN curriculum, congregational needs assessments, typical FCN interventions, and perceptions of FCN. In recognition of this issues, the International Parish Nurse Resource Center (IPNRC) organized a research meeting with its educational affiliates in 2006 to address the dearth of FCN research. Several of those affiliates responded with ideas and projects that are now ongoing. The IPNRC encourages individual parish nurse research and especially welcomes projects focused on programs and interventions carried out on a routine basis that would enable analytical evaluation so as to report outcomes (IPNRC 2008).

Faith-Based AIDS Care and Support

In a recent study, researchers sought to examine the role of religious organizations in the provision of HIV/AIDS-related assistance in Africa. Data were collected from Christian religious organizations in southern Mozambique. Bivariate comparisons and logistic regression analysis of survey data were performed, and an analysis of the qualitative data complemented the quantitative data.

The analysis revealed little involvement of religious organizations in provision of assistance. Instead, most assistance was decentralized and consisted of psychological support and some personal care and household help. Material or financial help was rare. Assistance to nonmembers of congregations was reported more often than to members. Members of larger and better secularly connected congregations were more likely to report assistance than were members of smaller and less secularly engaged ones. Assistance was reported more in cities than in rural areas. Women were more likely to report assisting congregation members than men were, but the reverse was true for assistance provided to nonmembers. The cooperation of religious organizations in provision of assistance was hindered by financial constraints and institutional rivalry. The conclusion and implications for policy were to involve religious organizations in provision of HIV/AIDS-related assistance by taking into account that organization's resources, institutional goals, and social characteristics.

Source: Agadjianian, V., & Sen, S. (2007). Promises and challenges of faith-based AIDS care and support in Mozambique. *American Journal of Public Health, 97*(2), 362–366.

MEDIA MOMENT 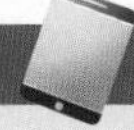

Carson, V., & Koenig (2008). *Spiritual Dimensions of Nursing Practice*. West Conshohocken, PA: Templeton Press

This book is considered a classic in guiding nursing's role in spiritual health. This seminal work on spirituality and

(*Continued*)

MEDIA MOMENT (*CONTINUED*)

health has been revised and updated since the original 1989 edition. The new edition is coauthored by Harold Koenig, a psychiatrist and director of Duke University's Center for Spirituality, Theology and Health. It builds on the original foundations laid in the first, provides perspectives on new research in the spiritual dimensions of nursing care, applies nursing theory to spiritual care, and addresses the spiritual needs of nurses and patients. It also looks at ethical issues in nursing and legal decisions that impact healthcare issues. Populations across the entire lifespan are considered as are the spiritual implications of chronic illness and death. A variety of faith backgrounds is addressed, along with religious practices of both theistic and pantheistic believers. This book is essential for nurses looking to prepare to meet the needs of patients from a variety of religious traditions.

CULTURAL CONNECTION 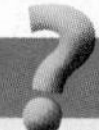

Caring for People of the Muslim Faith

Those who practice the religion of Islam are called Muslims; there are approximately 1.1 billion Muslims worldwide. Some 10–26% of Muslims are Arab; the majority of Muslims worldwide are Asian or African. Islam is one of the largest and fastest growing religions in North America, yet nurses in the United States are often unfamiliar with the cultural needs of this faith.

Islamic beliefs include the revealed word of God to the Prophet, Muhammad, and are based on the belief in one God, Allah. *Islam* means surrender or obedience to the will of God. Its scripture is called the Quran and is considered God's revelation to the Prophet Muhammad through the Angel Gabriel, which began in about the year AD 610.

Muslims strive to live their lives in surrender to Allah through the five basic pillars or requirements of the faith: the affirmation that "there is no god but God, and Muhammad is the Messenger of God; the five daily ritual prayers; the giving of alms to the poor; the observance of Ramadan (fasting from dawn to sunset during the month of Ramadan); and the religious pilgrimage to Mecca. Muslims see Muhammad as the continuation of a lineage of prophets including Adam, Noah, Abraham, Moses, David, and Jesus, so they seek a sense of community with the People of the Book, including Jews and Christians. Jihad is a duty to God and is to be both individual and communal.

Health is very much a part of Muslims' everyday life, from food practices, exercise, and the seeking of outside medical treatment for illness. Modesty through dress customs is often the most unfamiliar practice to U.S. nurses when interacting with Muslim families. There is considerable diversity in dress according to individual and cultural identities. Both men and women are modest and uncomfortable with unnecessary body exposure. Women may wear a body covering called a *hijaab*, a *burka'a*, and the *khumar*. The specific wearing of these garments is cultural rather than religious. Diet restrictions include consumption of only kosher or halal-prepared meat, as well as prohibition of pork and alcohol. Muslims should be well informed and provided alternatives in the use of medications that contain alcohol.

Islamic teachings regulate relationships between men and women. It is preferred to have healthcare providers who are of the same sex as the patient and Muslim if possible.

When a patient is dying, in either the home or the hospital, the nurse can respect the Muslim faith by turning the patient on his or her right side to face Mecca and allowing visitors to recite the prayer of allegiance to Allah. When death occurs, the body must be covered at all times. Muslims prefer that only health professionals of the same sex as the patient touch the body. Preparations are extensive and include washing and perfuming the body and then wrapping it in a white sheet by family members of the same sex. Autopsies are usually not performed and the body is buried with a simple prayer. The body is buried directly into the ground without a coffin, again facing Mecca. All of this takes place within a very short period of time, often within hours after death. The bereavement period is confined to 3 days, and children are not exposed to death or death rituals.

Nurses in the community should ask the patients and families of the Muslim faith which practices are comforting for them. One suggestion is to ask, "Do you have spiritual or religious beliefs that are important for your health care?" and respond in kind.

Source: Ott, B. B., Al-Khadhuri, B., & Al-Junaibi, S. (2003). Preventing ethical dilemmas: Understanding Islamic health care practices. *Pediatric Nursing, 29*(3), 227–230.

DAY IN THE LIFE

A New Faith Community Nurse

By Maryfran Stulginsky, RN, MS, FCN

Father asked me to speak at all the Masses about our new Health Ministry Program. His goal was for the congregation to visually see and hear me, to be able to associate the service with a face, and to get a sense of what Health Ministry was about. My goals were certainly similar, but I wanted to use this opportunity to impart another message. I wanted the congregation to understand that this new offering was a ministry, a living out of the gospel message, not just a social program. And, that the new parish nurse saw herself as a minister, part of the pastoral team called to serve the congregation.

That Sunday I introduced myself and the new Health Ministry Program. I outlined what was initially going to be offered: home visits, an emergency meal program, and an invitation to anyone in the congregation to share their health-related, social outreach skills with the community by joining our Wellness Committee. I pointed out that this new program was a way to respond to many of our faith's directives: Visit the sick, comfort the sorrowful, love one another. Then I used scripture to paint the picture:

"I believe that two scriptural stories can describe even better than I can what health ministry is about. The first is the story about the Agony in the Garden; the second is the story about the Good Samaritan.

The Agony in the Garden story has Jesus in incredible pain over what his suffering will be. He's anticipating his suffering and death by crucifixion. Around him are his friends ... all asleep, oblivious to the anguish he is experiencing alone. Health ministry calls us to stay awake and be present to the hurting among us. Often we cannot change outcomes of suffering people, but we can stay alert and walk with them as they stagger painful roads.

The second story is about the Good Samaritan. Everybody knows it, but you may not have ever thought about it in this manner. The Good Samaritan found the hurting man, he assessed his injuries, he thought about how he might help, he sought the intervention of the innkeeper and negotiated care in the immediate community, and he departed the scene and then returned to evaluate what happened in his absence. Health ministry includes all these steps. As a pastoral team, with information you share with us confidentially, we will be taking those same Good Samaritan Steps. Health ministry cares about people—body, mind, and soul—and these two stories demonstrate how we will be showing that care here at St. Francis of Assisi."

DAY IN THE LIFE

Elisabeth Kübler-Ross

It's only when we truly know and understand that we have a limited time on earth—and that we have no way of knowing when our time is up—we will then begin to live each day to the fullest, as if it was the only one we had.

There is no joy without hardship. If not for death, would we appreciate life? If not for hate, would we know the ultimate goal is love? At these moments, you can either hold on to negativity and look for blame, or you can choose to heal and keep on loving.

The most beautiful people we have known are those who have known defeat, known suffering, known struggle, known loss, and have found their way out of the depths. These persons have an appreciation, a sensitivity, and an understanding of life that fills them with compassion.

Elisabeth Kübler-Ross was a pioneer in research of death experiences in children and adults.

HEALTHY PEOPLE 2020

Implications for Faith Communities

- Organize/prioritize programming around those issues identified in the congregational assessment and common to the *Healthy People* list.
- Identify and focus on the pre-existing social determinants impacting health that are present in the congregation.
- Investigate resources and plan programming in order to improve health equity.
- Develop methods to impart health and wellness information via the Internet.
- Investigate sites and guide the faith community's use of reliable, evidence-based web resources.
- Educate the ministry staff on ways faith community endeavors can respond to nationwide health guidelines.

Relationship Between Community Health Nursing and Faith Communities

Faith Community Nursing

An appropriate and challenging intervention for the community health nurse is putting the theological foundations of health ministries into action. Given that the professional discipline of nursing incorporates the physical, emotional, cultural, and spiritual domains of practice, and because professional nursing partners with professionals from a variety of disciplines and community members with varying life experiences, health ministry activities are a natural arena for nurses working in community-based and population-focused practice. See **Box 15-2**.

> Nurses have long observed that when illness or brokenness occurs, patients—whether individually or with their family or friends—may turn to their source of spiritual strength for reassurance, support, and healing.
>
> —*Faith Community Nursing: Scope and Standards of Practice (ANA & HMA, 2005)*

BOX 15-2 Fast Facts About FCN

- Faith Community Nursing (FCN) nursing is an ANA-recognized specialty.
- FCN partners health issues with the faith of the client.
- FCNs are licensed RNs governed by their state's nurse practice act, the *Code of Ethics for Nurses with Interpretative Statements* (ANA, 2001), and *Faith Community Nursing: Scope and Standards of Practice* (ANA & HMA, 2005).
- A specialized (30-hour continuing education units) curriculum best enables nurses to practice as FCNs.
- The curriculum addresses prayer, self-care, ethical issues, documentation, health promotion, life issues of violence, suffering and grief, assessment, and care coordination.
- FCNs can be found in all 50 states and around the world.
- FCNs can be called parish nurse, church nurse, faith community nurse, crescent nurse, health minister, or congregational nurse (depending upon the congregation).
- FCNs often serve geographic neighbors of a congregation.
- There are approximately 15,000 parish nurses in the United States.
- Thirty-five percent of U.S. FCNs have paid positions; the rest are volunteers.
- The IPNRC and the HMA are the professional organizations of FCN.

BOX 15-3 Assumptions of Faith Community Nursing

- Health and illness are human experiences.
- Health is the integration of the spiritual, physical, psychological, and social aspects of the patient.
- Health promotes a sense of harmony with self, others in the environment, and a higher power.
- Health may be experienced in the presence of disease or injury.
- The presence of illness does not preclude health nor does optimal health preclude illness.
- Healing is the process that integrates the body, mind, and spirit to create wholeness.
- Health is a sense of wellbeing, even when the patient's illness is not cured.

Source: American Nurses Association & Health Ministries Association. (2005). *Faith Community Nursing: Scope and Standards of Practice.* Silver Spring MD: American Nurses Publishing.

BOX 15-4 Resources for New Faith Communities

Bennett, R., & Hale, W. D. (2009). *Building Healthy Communities Through Medical-Religious Partnerships.* Baltimore, MD: Johns Hopkins University Press.

This text offers guidance to medical practitioners seeking to incorporate the healing benefits of faith and belief into their practice by means of developing partnerships with religious leaders and communities.

Patterson, D. L. (2008). *Health Ministries: A Primer for Clergy and Congregations.* Cleveland, OH: Pilgrim Press.

This text is a comprehensive primer on developing and managing health ministries.

ETHICAL CONNECTION 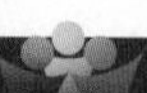

Health ministry programs are often associated with specific religious denominations (e.g., Catholic, Protestant). How can community health nurses implement healthy lifestyles in the role of a parish or missionary nurse when the specific religious doctrine contradicts the nurse's values about health and disease intervention?

APPLICATION TO PRACTICE 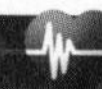

Hilda left a message on my voicemail asking for a nursing visit. She stated she had "heart and breathing trouble" and another personal problem that she had to talk over. Upon entering her home later that day, I met Hilda's son, who looked about 40, and appeared to be an adult with developmental disabilities; his language was simple, his movements somewhat uncoordinated, and his behavior child-like. During the entire visit, Hilda's son never left her side.

Hilda was in her recliner using oxygen, which she reported to use "most of the time." A physical assessment, a med review, and her medical history verified a fragile cardio-respiratory condition. I clearly determined she was a parishioner who needed to be followed in order to observe changes and prevent hospitalizations. But, I've learned that often what I perceive to be someone's issue is not always why I am invited into the home. For this reason, my standard line always is, "What would you like me to do for you?" Good thing I asked.

Hilda's concern was not about herself. Hilda told me that her son had recently become active at a center for disabled adults where he met a younger woman and "the two of them are in love, and all over each other!" I found out that both adult children were being cared for by aging parents who talked about the situation and who shared similar concerns: the future care of their disabled children after they were gone and the potential arrival of an unplanned grandchild. Hilda spoke to her son's doctor about her fears, and he suggested sterilization. The doctor then spoke to Hilda's son, and presumably informed consent existed because Hilda's son told me, "I don't want to make a baby, I can't take care of a baby, and neither can my girlfriend." The issue of concern was that sterilization was not sanctioned by Hilda's faith, and she was too embarrassed to talk out her concerns with a clergyman. She feared that she was sinning simply in considering this option and that if in fact she encouraged her son to accept the procedure, she was dooming them both to hell. Her son told me, "I don't want to do anything my mother thinks is wrong."

The challenge in practicing nursing in a faith setting is that even when nurses may believe that the greater good is served by supporting specific health-related decisions, they cannot endorse what is forbidden by the tenets of the religious denomination they represent. In addition, for some churchgoers, discussions about situational reasoning or prayerful decision making fall on deaf ears, especially when considering a deviation from the law as they understand it. "Permission" can only come from the Father or Reverend or the Rabbi or Imam. Such was the case with Hilda. With her consent, my intervention was to seek out an understanding clergyman, whom I knew would be sympathetic to their situation. I explained the issues and asked him to go see mother and son. Whatever was said during that visit gave comfort enough for Hilda to make arrangements for her son to have the medical procedure they both felt he should have.

MEDIA MOMENT

What Dreams May Come (1998)

This movie features Robin Williams and his search for heaven after losing his own life, and the lives of his children and his wife. Cuba Gooding, Jr. is the angel who guides his journey into the afterlife and search for his family, which is his "heaven." The movie does not venture into specific religious doctrine, which allows for people of all faiths to appreciate the experience of good and evil in a beautifully filmed story.

Schindler's List (1993)

Steven Spielberg's Best Picture–winning film about Holocaust-era Germany is based upon the true story and carries the tagline: "Whoever saves one life, saves the world entire."

Amadeus (1984)

This is the story of an institutionalized composer, Antonio Salieri, who is driven insane by envy because he compares his modest musical talents to the genius of his rival, Mozart, yet he cannot comprehend why God would give so great a musical gift to such a vulgar and sinful person.

Arts and Faith, an online discussion group comprised of film critics and other movie buffs, compiles its list of the top 100 spiritually significant films ever made. The list is continually updated. For more information go to http://www.filmsite.org/top100spiritual.html

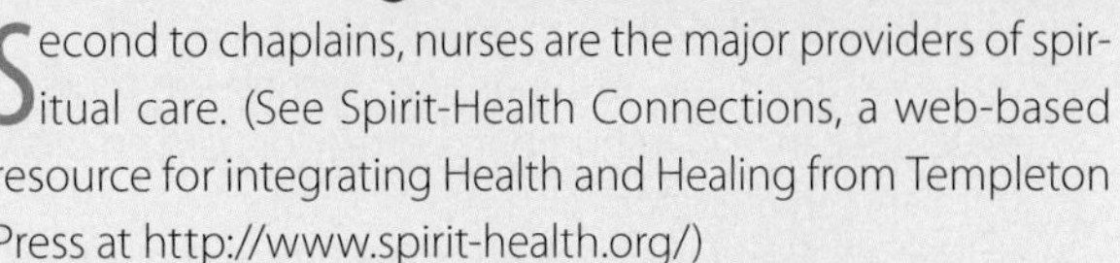

DID YOU KNOW?

Second to chaplains, nurses are the major providers of spiritual care. (See Spirit-Health Connections, a web-based resource for integrating Health and Healing from Templeton Press at http://www.spirit-health.org/)

MEDIA MOMENT

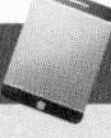

Bridge Over Troubled Water

Lyrics and music by Paul Simon (1970)

The 2011 documentary, *The Harmony Game: The Making of Bridge Over Troubled Water,* tells the story behind Simon and Garfunkel's award-winning song, which has been recorded by many of the world's greatest vocalists. In this film, Paul Simon spoke about writing this song as "a little hymn." The song was written by Simon about providing comfort to a person in need.

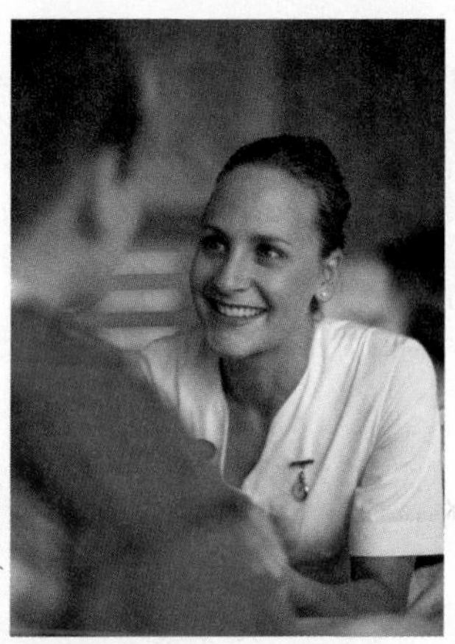

© Stockbyte/Thinkstock

Health fair at church provides opportunities for the nurse to discuss drug use with children.

THINK ABOUT THIS

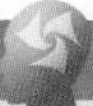

Where do I start? How do health ministries really "get off the ground"?

1. Start small. Focus on a minimum of time, money, and people. Start with blood pressure screening; involve the congregation in the planning and involvement of the activity.
2. Be visible at all times. This can be done easily with a monthly bulletin board in the religious structure, which features new information about healthy lifestyles each month.
3. Don't waste time. Avoid meetings if possible; do not get bogged down in structure, policy, and committees, which can lead to unnecessary work and time.

(Continued)

THINK ABOUT THIS (*CONTINUED*)

Most health ministries are made up of volunteers; requiring too many meetings and creating too much structure can lead to burnout and lack of participation from church members.

4. Ask others for what you need. Many health projects can be very inexpensive if you ask local businesses to provide services or goods in exchange for public recognition of their donation. Health fairs are excellent ways to involve the religious community.
5. Play it safe. Avoid hands-on care: Make home visits, use referrals and consultation as primary interventions, and focus on education. Avoid any medical treatments, and always make sure you are covered through the religious organization's insurance.
6. Know your congregation. Do assessments of members' needs often, and plan health projects *with* them, not *for* them.
7. Document all health-related activities associated with health ministry, no matter how small. This practice provides the nurse and the ministry with outcome data that serve as evidence of effectiveness and promote continuation of health services.
8. Think broadly. Include health professionals in the community and congregation, as well as those who are interested in health. Keep your "arms open" for health ministry involvement.
9. Don't give up. Ministers and congregations come and go, priorities change, and some programs are successful while some are not. Keep your eye on the long-term goal of keeping spirituality and health as an expected part of ministries.

Source: Adapted from Klammer, L. M. (2006, January). Starting a church health ministry. *Clergy Journal*.

DAY IN THE LIFE

FCNs Address the Question: "What attributes do you see as vital for the success of your practice as a Faith Community Nurse?"

Flexibility

Flexibility is so incredibly important. No two days are ever the same. Most days driving to work I have a plan that includes visits scheduled, meetings to attend, and projects to address. Then I check my voicemail and everything can go out the window. One of those days I'll never forget was when the religious education coordinator called to say an 8-year-old student who had just missed last week's Sunday school class due to what was presumed to be flu was now on a respirator and expected to die of viral meningitis. Family was gathered at the hospital and the pastor was in attendance. Of course, the day's plan was scratched so I could begin to consider grief support for the family, write up a notice to go out to parents explaining viral meningitis and their children's possible exposure, connect with the child's school nurse so we could coordinate a joint effort for coping with panicked parents, and make contact with a grief-support crisis team to see about coming to Sunday School 5 days later.

Trust

Sometimes people call the church based on a very simple belief: trust. People believe that they can count on a faith community to help them. After all, aren't churches in the business to help? And then sometimes a "church nurse" is seen as less threatening than clergy, because once upon a time they had a bad experience and the baggage still weighs them down.

Ability to Respect Confidentiality

My greatest challenge when I first started was confidentiality. I had been a church member for a long time, and now all of a sudden I was ministering to friends and acquaintances. I needed to reassure people over and over again that what I knew and what they shared with me as their nurse was confidential. There was a lot of skepticism. And there were a lot of hurt feelings too, when I refused to talk about parishioners' conditions and share what I knew with friends the client and I both had in common.

Spiritual Maturity

Sometimes we meet people who want no part of God, or the church for that matter. But they want help so they invite you in. And by presence, consistency, and nonjudgmental outreach, we try to model God. But if you are spiritually mature, you know that you are not there to use your position to evangelize. Sometimes a good experience helps some people find a new or renewed sensitivity to their spiritual dimension, but it doesn't always happen, and you need to be okay with that. It doesn't mean you've failed. We are not supposed to be in this to convert! I like Mother Teresa's line, "O God, let your light shine through me."

Good Communication Skills

More than anything else, I listen and clarify what I've heard people say. It's amazing how many people just ache to have someone listen to them. I've learned that my body language, the tone of voice I use, and having a sense of humor are all so very important.

Ability to be Present

I recently heard Anne Lamott speak. She told us that she believes that Jesus tells us in prayer, "I hear it, I get it, me too." Those words really resonated with me. They actually echoed words of wisdom from the Rabbi who taught one of my parish nurse classes years ago. He constantly reminded us that being present to people was "what God does."

Willingness to Learn New Skills

There's so much on-the-job training in this role. There are clinical situations you've never dealt with before, and you need to be willing to research answers, look for resources, spend time, network, and be humble enough to ask others for help.

Ability to Go It Alone

This practice is so solitary, and because of that, you have to generate your own community. Not many of us work with partners. Sure, we are part of a pastoral staff, but no one else on staff does what we do. None of them can do our job in our absence. Essentially, we have a private nursing practice out of a church. No nurse supervisor is guiding or evaluating us. No continuing education is provided in house, and there are no nursing team meetings to help you unpack a difficult situation. It's you alone in your office dealing with issues, you alone in your car working in the community, you alone in the home and at the bedside. So, you have make sure you connect with other nurses doing the same thing, like we do here—to share resources, share stories, lift each other up.

Source: Voices of the Main Line Philadelphia Faith Community Nurse Support Group

MEDIA MOMENT

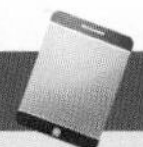

A Faith Like Mine: A Celebration of the World's Religions Through the Eyes of Children (2005)

By Laura Buller, New York, NY: DK Publishing.

This book provides an illuminating and comprehensive look at the world's many and diverse religions through the eyes of children. It gives parents and caregivers a theological tour of faith as seen through the perspectives of children growing up in each of the religious traditions. From Buddhism, Islam, Judaism, Christianity, and Sikhism to lesser known religions, such a Zoroastrianism and Shintoism, few religions are left out. Having a clearer view of what it means to be people of "faith" can provide nurses and others with an introduction to the world's faiths and an appreciation of how much they all have in common. Respect for life, beauty, tradition, and a reassuring faith emerge as common patterns that can promote understanding and acceptance for all faiths, even as we embrace our differences.

The document entitled *Scope and Standards of Parish Nursing*, prepared by the HMA, was adopted by the ANA in 1998 and updated in 2005 as *Faith Community Nursing: Scope and Standards of Practice*. The HMA is a professional interfaith organization that encourages faith communities to work with professionals, lay individuals, and agencies to promote health and wellness. Both nurses and others interested in health ministries make up its membership. The document describes to the profession and to the public this evolving "specialty practice of nursing and of health ministry" (ANA/HMA, 2005, p. 3). Further, the document describes the independent practice of nursing, as defined by the jurisdiction's nursing practice act, in health promotion within the context of the patient's values, beliefs, and faith practices. The patient focus of a parish nurse is the faith community, including its family and individual members and the community it serves.

Basic preparation courses recommended for the FCN and endorsed by the IPNRC consist of at least 30 hours of coursework in parish nursing. Information can be obtained from this center, which advocates, develops, and promotes quality programs and current resources. The center provides consultation and is on the cutting edge of research in parish nursing. The annual Westberg Symposium provides the valued benefits of education and networking. Spiritual maturity, professional practice experience, competent communication and negotiation skills, and a commitment to assessment of personal holistic health are necessary to achieve success in parish nursing.

Parish nursing's philosophy first of all maintains that the spiritual dimension is central to the practice (Patterson, 2006; Solari-Twadell & McDermott, 1999); see **Box 15-5**. The intentional and compassionate caring of nursing evolves from the spiritual dimension inherent in all humankind.

ETHICAL CONNECTION

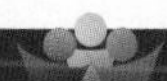

The 2005 *Faith Community Nursing: Scope and Standards of Practice* cited difficulty finding all-inclusive terminology to describe the beliefs and practices of the many dissimilar traditions now embracing the practice of FCN in rural areas, towns, and cities (ANA & HMA, 2005).

BOX 15-5 Components of Parish Nursing

- Intentional and compassionate caring
- Focus on faith community and ministry
- Strengths of congregation are paramount
- Partnership with church community
- Attention to relationship between health, spiritual health, and healing

Source: Solari-Twadell, P. A., & McDermott, M. A. (Eds.). (1999). *Parish nursing: Promoting whole person health within faith communities.* Thousand Oaks, CA: Sage.

CULTURAL CONNECTION

Prayers from the World's Religions

"When you arise in the morning, give thanks for the morning light, for your life and strength, give thanks for your food and the joy of living. If you see no reason for giving thanks, the fault is in yourself."

—Tecumseh, Native American

"Mystery of Life, Source of All Being, we are thankful for the gifts of life and being, of love and connection. We are thankful for all the wonders of the world around us. We are thankful for each other and for all the members of our global family. As we make our Family Pledge, may we have eyes that see, hearts that love, and hands that are ready to serve in love and in kindness, with caring and with courage. Blessed Be."

—Unitarian Universalist Prayer

"Even as a mother at the risk of her life watches over and protects her only child, so with a boundless mind should one cherish all living things. Let none by anger or hatred wish harm to another. May all beings be happy. May they live in safety, free from fear and distress."

—Buddhist Prayer

"O Thou kind Lord! These lovely children are the handiwork of the fingers of Thy might and the wondrous signs of Thy greatness. O God, protect these children. Graciously assist them to be educated and enable them to render service to the world of humanity. O God, these children are pearls. Cause them to be nurtured within the shell of Thy loving kindness. Thou are the Bountiful, the All-Loving."

—Baha'I Prayer

"All praise is due to You, our Lord, Guardian, and Cherisher of the Universe, who has sent the prophets to teach us how to live as full human beings. Make us among those who can truly say, 'We hear and obey.' Awaken in our hearts those attributes you love the best, and help us to be Merciful, Compassionate, Forgiving, Truthful, Just, and Patient with each other and with all those around us. Make us worthy to be counted in the community of Your Beloved, who said, 'The best of you are those who are the best to their families.'"

—Islamic Prayer

"Loving God, you sent Jesus to show us how to live in peace and love for one another. Jesus, you are our rock and our salvation. You showed us to love as you have loved us and to care for those who are less fortunate. You forgave those who hurt you. Your heart went out to people no one else cared about. Jesus, send us your Spirit to help each of us be truthful whenever we speak, loving whenever we act, and courageous whenever we find violence or injustice around us. We ask this in your holy name and that of the Father, the Son, and the Holy Ghost."

—Christian Prayer

"O God, God of my brothers and sisters, relations and friends, God of my ancestors, God of all connections with all things; You, through all obstacles; You, in our emptiness and in our abundance; You, in our search for peace, You. We have given ourselves to sacred collation with You in the Repair of the world, *Tikkun*. As You make peace there, let there be peace among us, among all peoples, changing the world one person at a time, one family at a time, one community at a time, one world. Amen."

—Jewish Prayer

This feature graciously contributed by Jean A. Haspeslagh, DNS, RN.

GOT AN ALTERNATIVE?

Research has associated stained glass with inducing relaxation and a sense of peaceful self-consciousness and promoting meditation. How can our knowledge of the influence of color be used in creating a therapeutic environment for our patients, either in a healthcare facility, in a church, at home or in our built environment?

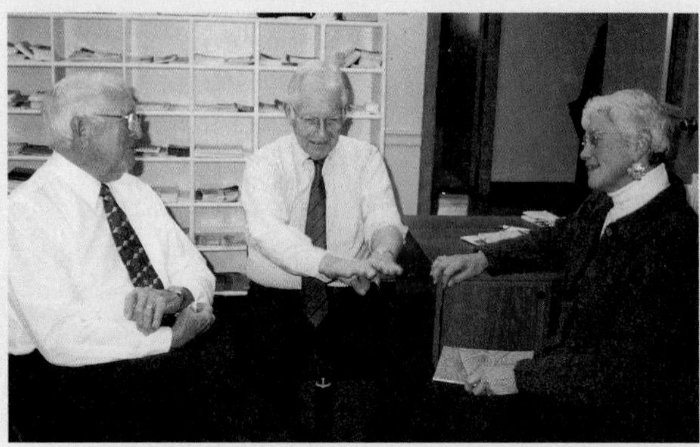

Ruth Berry (right) counseling church members between church services.

ENVIRONMENTAL CONNECTION

Expand your definition of environment to include the physical and symbolic aspect of a church or religious gathering place. How does the religious or faith-related physical environment affect the health and wellbeing of the population?

DAY IN THE LIFE

Maryfran Stulginsky, RN, MS, FCN

From the moment I began my work at the parish, handicapped accessibility in the church and its buildings was an issue for me and for members of the community. The church was over 100 years old. There was a first-floor side entrance that enabled worship access, but as for the rest of the campus, stairs were everywhere. Meetings were held in the parish office, and attending them required climbing steps (up and down). If you had to use the bathroom once you got to the first floor meeting, you needed to renegotiate steps again because the bathroom was actually on ground level. In the school where the seniors first met, they had to climb an incredibly steep set of stairs to get to their space. Off the meeting room was a tiny, antiquated, makeshift bathroom. Although it was on the same level, it was awkward for people using walkers. When the meeting room changed to a ground-level space elsewhere in the school, the bathroom access became a challenge again. More steps, luckily not that many and not that steep but there was "No room for a ramp," I was told, due to architectural issues. Money was always the issue cited. And it was! Conversion of old buildings is costly, and major renovations were required. Theoretically, I could understand, but it was always hard justifying the choice "not to spend money on costly renovations" to the increasing older population who told me they felt excluded from meetings and activities because of poor access.

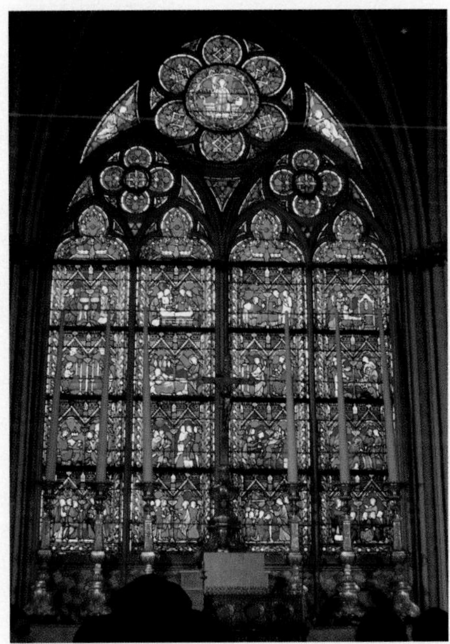

The stained glass of the windows at Notre Dame Cathedral in Paris, France depicts spiritual connectedness to the Creator, light, warmth, comfort, conscience, hope, and continuity. Stained glass has long been part of organized religion.

ENVIRONMENTAL CONNECTION

Expand your definition of environment to include the physical and symbolic aspects of a church or religious gathering place. How does the religious "environment" affect the health and wellbeing of the church population?

Missionary Nursing*

A discussion of health ministries and faith community nursing would be incomplete without reviewing the role of missionary nurses. In the United States, the number of nurses who serve/work as missionary nurses continues to increase yearly. Exact figures are unavailable because these nurses serve/work at private, local, state, national, and international levels. Another reason that exact numbers are unavailable is to protect the safety of missionary nurses, some of whom work in countries where their faith is at risk due to unstable political environments.

Many of the major denominations in the United States have nurses who serve/work as missionary nurses. Examples include the International Mission Board of the Southern Baptist Convention, the Presbyterian Church in America, the General Board of Global Ministries, and the United Methodist Church.

Some missionary nurses may serve/work on a short-term or part-time basis, for a period of weeks or months. Many work full-time in other nursing roles and participate in focused mission projects on their vacation days or take temporary leave time to do so. These short-term or part-time missionary nurses routinely participate in mission trips to areas of the United States or to areas abroad (e.g., Mexico, Honduras, Ukraine) where underprivileged and underserved populations are in dire need of food, clothes, medicine, and health care. The missionary teams that travel to these areas to meet the specific needs of patients and communities include various combinations of nursing, medical, surgical, dental, and lay volunteers. Each mission trip is as unique as the patients and communities to which it ministers. Interpreters are used, as needed, to overcome language and cultural barriers. Often, makeshift healthcare clinics are set up in churches, in schools, or outside under canopies. Many of these clinics are primitive;

*The section on missionary nursing is authored by Barbara Foster, RN, MSN, Instructor, Division of Associate Degree Nursing, Copiah–Lincoln Community College, Wesson, Mississippi, and adapted from Lundy, K. S., Sutton, V., & Foster, B. (2003). The nurse's role in ambulatory health settings. In K. S. Lundy & S. Janes (Eds.), *Essentials of community-based nursing* (pp. 259–291). Sudbury, MA: Jones and Bartlett Publishers.

others may be equipped with some modern technology, if electricity is available. Frequently, missionary teams not only provide health care, but also assist with the building of churches, houses, and schools.

Other missionary nurses are career missionary nurses, working for years or even a lifetime in this capacity. Missionary nurses work as a "home missionary" in the United States or as a "foreign missionary" in other countries. Career (i.e., full-time) missionary nurses who work abroad become totally immersed in the culture of the people whom they serve and learn to speak the native language fluently. Many of the foreign countries in which they reside are impoverished, war-torn, and desperate for physical, nursing, medical, and spiritual attention. Missionary nurses who work full-time often find themselves in unsafe conditions owing to governments that are resistant to outside interventions.

Roles and Practice of Missionary Nurses

Missionary nurses focus on meeting the physical, spiritual, and emotional needs of their patients. They often report that serving in this role provides almost indescribable personal fulfillment and job satisfaction and consider missionary nursing to be a "calling." These nurses often refer to **missionary nursing** as "pure nursing," unencumbered by the demands of paperwork, documentation, and other system restraints. Nursing schools are seeing an increase in the number of students who seek to become missionary nurses or who begin mission work as nursing students during school vacations; many nursing students receive credit for clinical hours by participating in mission trips. Missionary nursing is based on the principles and philosophy of community health nursing.

The needs of patients and communities vary greatly, depending on the location, culture, economy, type of

GLOBAL CONNECTION 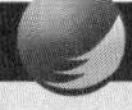

Missionary nursing is a specialty within health ministries. How can nurses provide care in other cultures and faiths than their own without experiencing ethical and professional conflicts?

APPLICATION TO PRACTICE 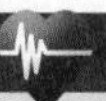

A Health Fair: Medicines and More

"Medicines and More" was the result of interest expressed on the part of members of the Wellness Committee of the Second Presbyterian Church in Lexington, Kentucky. A retired health professional and an older adult caregiver commented that they were concerned about numerous conversations and observations regarding confusion with medications. Quickly, the committee's discussion included stories of inquiries regarding multiple names for medicines, complex over-the-counter preparations, duplicate medicines for the same ailment, values and dangers of herbal preparations, problems eating or not eating food with medicines, medication errors indicating the need for reinforcement of emergency assistance, and others.

Members decided a fair would reach many people quickly. Although a major target was the older population, the committee believed that the information was valuable for members of all ages, for families, and for individuals who were living alone. Because members already gathered on Sunday mornings for educational and worship services and because many elderly persons regularly participated in the monthly "Retirees Lunch," the committee decided to plan the event to coincide with established habits. The committee members further decided that because they wanted to provide information applicable for all ages and for the total congregation, they would schedule the fair during and following the Retirees Lunch in a room adjacent to the dining room. Families and those members not participating in the lunch were guided directly to the fair location following worship service. Retirees would be the special fair participants after lunch.

After agreeing upon a number of objectives, the members listed tasks and eagerly offered to take responsibility for the many jobs. These jobs included marketing and publicity, obtaining resources, volunteering for hosting the various exhibits, taking blood pressure readings, greeting community presenters, and monitoring flow on the day of the fair.

The parish nurse contacted the local health department nutritionist and the university's college of pharmacy. A pharmacy brown-bag event was very popular, and the nutritionist provided helpful information regarding food–medicine interaction, supplements, and herbal preparations. Committee members contacted a local hospital's homecare agency for information on lifeline emergency calling. The senior nursing student contacted the local police department for 9-1-1 guidelines, supplied various phones for demonstration and practice, and obtained literature and posters at the State Pamphlet Library. In collaboration with the parish nurse, a County Cooperative Extension "lookalikes" display was updated. Children and adults were able to view models and a brochure depicting potentially dangerous and confusing foods, medicines, and household products.

To encourage participation at all exhibits and to obtain evaluation data, members who completed surveys were eligible to win loaves of whole-wheat variety breads. The committee reviewed the evaluations within 2 weeks, reported the results and extended thanks to planners and attendees in the congregation's newsletter, and gained information for planning future programs regarding nutrition and exercise.

Effective and enjoyable health fairs can be simpler or more elaborate than the one described. The community presenters gained a new resource for their information. Both the pharmacists and the nutritionist expressed that they had never envisioned the benefits of providing health information in a faith community setting, and the county's extension agency appreciated help in renewing their display and obtaining feedback for additional outreach options. Collaborating with these professionals and their agencies created new partnerships with mutual benefits.

APPLICATION TO PRACTICE 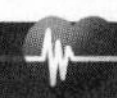

Creating Personal Medical and Health Profiles

Personal medical profiles were used by the FCN at Our Mother of Good Counsel Church, Bryn Mawr, Pennsylvania as one way to introduce her practice to its senior community. The FCN attended the monthly senior meeting where she offered blood pressure screening, but she was seeing only a small percentage of the total group and picking up referrals on an even smaller number. There had to be a way for her to reach more people and place herself front and center as a resource for the seniors.

The FCN was already writing a weekly wellness tip in the parish bulletin. Each week she addressed a health-related topic, offering current information and local/web-based resources connected to it. The wellness tips covered a wide variety of holistic health issues. Numerous people shared how useful the information was (sometimes telling the nurse it was their favorite thing to read during dull sermons!). For this reason, it was a perfect venue to introduce the medical profile service.

One week's tip painted a picture of a typical senior visit to the emergency department (ED) or a new doctor's office—the sites, the sounds, the tension, the fidgeting, then the barrage of questions typically asked about current medicines and past medical history. The nurse then described the client's possible emotional state: anxious, in pain, frightened. Wasn't trying to call up pertinent information on demand difficult? Often, memory did not serve. Or, suppose someone else was speaking on your behalf and they just did not know your story? What if the senior had a short, typed medical profile in his or her wallet that could be handed over to the questioning person?

The nurse suggested anyone interested in creating such a document contact her for a home visit. The medical profiles created were typed on the FCN's computer (password protected), could be updated as needed, and multiple hard copies were left in the home. Profiles included such information as date of birth, all current medications, allergies, past medical and surgical history, the client's current doctors and their contact information, dates of last screening procedures, the existence of a living will and medical power of attorney, and so forth. The service was a success and proved to be an ongoing request during the FCN's tenure at the parish. What was especially gratifying was the feedback from the ED staff at the nearby hospital and many local physicians' practices. Parishioners would report that they were often asked, "Do you by chance go to that church where their nurse does medical profiles? Do you have one?" One doctor in the congregation who saw many of the parish seniors in his office called it a "Godsend."

MEDIA MOMENT 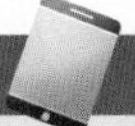

Lessons from the *Lotus Sutra*

Karen Rich, PhD, RN

The *Lotus Sutra,* one of the Buddha's last teachings, is sometimes referred to as the "King of Sutras" (Thich Nhat Hanh, 2003). In the *Lotus Sutra,* the Buddha introduced many bodhisattvas to his followers. A bodhisattva is an enlightened being who vows, through compassion, to help all other beings attain enlightenment. Bodhisattvas realize the teachings of the Buddha "to look and listen with the eyes of compassion" and understand that "compassionate listening brings about healing" (Thich Nhat Hanh, 1998, p. 86).

In caring for elderly patients and populations, nurses can be compared to compassionate bodhisattvas who facilitate elders' wellbeing. Elders suffer from many losses in their lives, both large and small. Loss of loved ones, health, mobility, beauty, and status are only a few of these losses. Although their patients' losses may go unnoticed by nurses, the events can have intense effects on elderly patients. Simmons (2000) has called "the work of learning to live richly in the face of loss learning to fall" (p. xi). Letting go can be terrifying for elders. Living can be terrifying, too, because one must learn to let go to live.

The ubiquitous losses and changes that occur with old age can result in anxiety about life's unpredictability. Elderly patients must depend on and trust in the moral goodness of healthcare professionals even when they are confronted with attitudes of ageism and when their care is not given serious consideration because no cure can be achieved. When an elder reacts to these insults by developing a hardened resistance toward life's fluctuations, impermanence, and loss, the outcome may be anger and depression.

(Continued)

MEDIA MOMENT (*CONTINUED*)

Compassion is the desire to separate others from suffering and the desire for others to experience wellbeing. Like the bodhisattvas described in the *Lotus Sutra,* compassionate nurses can dedicate themselves to helping patients overcome suffering and its causes. Nurses who exhibit the virtue of compassion can help elders learn to relax in the face of life's changes rather than tightening into an unhealthy resistance. All people suffer, yet all people desire wellbeing regardless of their age. "Compassion is not a relationship between the healer and the wounded. It is a relationship between equals" (Chodron, 2001, p. 50).

Compassion requires communicating with patients from one's heart. For many elders, the world is a lonely place with no one to listen to their feelings or understand their lives. Nurses who have a sincere desire to take action to alleviate the suffering of this vulnerable group are widening the circle of compassion in the world. Research has shown that elders have a higher response to placebo treatment than is normally expected (Soloman, 2001). This higher response has been attributed to the attention that elderly persons receive because of their participation in research studies. Elders must be very lonely indeed for this slight attention to be so important to them.

Unpredictability is inherent in the daily life of elders, and impermanence and loss have a glaring presence that is difficult for the aged to ignore. Nurses might do well to remember the teachings of the *Lotus Sutra* when caring for elderly individuals and populations—to look and listen with the eyes of compassion and that compassionate listening brings about healing.

Karen Rich, PhD, RN, Associate Professor,
The University of Southern Mississippi College
of Nursing, Hattiesburg, Mississippi

government, and access to affordable health care. Missionary nurses must be committed to serving and ministering to the differing needs of patients and communities with diverse cultures and populations. The primary purpose of missionary nursing is to meet the spiritual, physical, and emotional needs of persons in need throughout the world.

Communication skills and therapeutic communication are essential to the role of missionary nurses. Often, different languages and cultures represent barriers to communication. Missionary nurses must exhibit flexibility, patience, and a willingness to work within different health systems. Patients' values regarding health and nursing roles are often dramatically different from the values of the nurse. Missionary nurses tend to focus on basic professional values, such as compassion and nonjudgmental attitudes, rather than the proscribed roles typical in U.S. health care, so as to provide culturally appropriate care.

Missionary nurses utilize population-based skills of the community health nurse, such as community assessment, to provide culturally relevant care as defined by the community. Specific needs are then prioritized by the community and the mission healthcare team. Collaboration among fellow members of the missionary team and community members enables missionary nurses to plan ways to meet specific needs, often in a very short time span. Goals may be set to meet the needs of these communities on a short-term basis and then provide direction for subsequent mission trips.

> They must be true Nurses to be true Missionaries.
>
> —*Florence Nightingale, 1892*

Missionary nurses utilize and apply nursing research and outcomes management in various ways. For example, the specific needs of various populations and diverse cultures may be compared on private, local, state, national, and international levels. Data may be analyzed and used in different ways to meet the unique needs of each culture and population group. Various caring interventions and missionary nursing activities then focus on these findings to provide needed services.

Missionary nurses should learn all they can about the cultures of the populations and communities they serve, both prior to leaving their home country and after comparing this information upon arrival. Teaching is also an important component of missionary nursing. For example, in some countries cholera is a constant threat to the health of a community, so missionary nurses may teach ways to prevent cholera. Language and cultural barriers are frequently encountered and must be overcome to enable nurses to establish helping, trusting relationships.

Missionary nurses may formally or informally manage the care of patients and communities from diverse cultures. Managing care requires spiritual maturity, therapeutic communication, negotiation skills, and a personal commitment to the overall health and wellbeing of patients and communities. Missionary nurses pay particular attention to the spiritual needs of patients. Whenever possible, basic needs, such as food, water, clothing, and housing, are provided.

Spirituality Versus Religion in Health Care

While FCNs are affiliated with a specific church, mosque, temple, or congregation, each nurse can implement aspects of spirituality into his or her practice methods. In fact, because nurses spend the most time with patients of all healthcare workers, they are in a unique position to establish trust and provide spiritual care (Young & Koopsen, 2011). Hospitals and other patient care facilities are beginning to integrate spiritual models into their practices, and some are even requiring spiritual assessments of their clients. For example, the Joint Commission requires healthcare management teams to consider a client's spiritual values, beliefs, and needs when delivering care (Young & Koopsen, 2011). This has led to many healthcare organizations adopting statements to support the "dignity, culture, beliefs, practices, and spiritual needs of all patients, their caregivers, and hospital personnel" (Young & Koopsen, 2011). But what does spirituality mean, and is that different from religion?

Spirituality is derived from the Latin word *spiritus*, meaning breath and spirit or soul (Young & Koopsen, 2011). Defining this abstract concept is difficult, due to the highly subjective, personal, and individualistic nature of the concept (Coyle, 2002). It has been described as a belief in a universal power working in one's life (Young & Koopsen, 2011), an interconnectedness with all things and an awareness of the purpose and meaning of life (Walton, 1996), or any act that nourishes the soul or spirit (Watson, 2005). **Religion**, on the other hand, is formed from the Latin word *religare* which means to reconnect or retie (Burkhardt & Nagai-Jacobson, 2002) and usually refers to a system of shared beliefs and values.

Several conceptual differences include the following (Eliopoulos, 2014; Young & Koopsen, 2011):

- Religion is more authoritative and systematic, using a set of rules or guidelines for beliefs and behaviors, which is usually written.
- Religion separates one group from another, while spirituality is universal and emphasizes unity and focuses on the commonalities between all belief systems, such as love, peace, and forgiveness.
- Spirituality attempts to connect the mind, body, and spirit.
- Spirituality focuses on one's emotions and inner experience, while religion seeks to create a community.
- The language used in religion describes belief systems and guidelines for worship, whereas words used to explain spirituality are more ethereal, abstract, and focused on interconnectivity.

Therefore, a person can be spiritual, religious, both, or neither.

By including one's spirituality into a patient's health care, practitioners can provide comfort and ease suffering, create more meaningful interactions, gain a better understanding of the patient and his or her needs, and become more familiar and confident in one's own beliefs, all of which lead to better overall care. Koenig (2007) asserts, "This area of care is vitally important to a patient's psychological, social, and physical health, and thus should be addressed." (p. 78)

There are many benefits to a holistic care approach. Treating the mind, body, and spirit not only creates a deeper relationship between caregiver and patient, but can contribute to long-term mental and physical health benefits and overall wellness. These include lower mortality and less disease (Young & Koopsen, 2011) and provision of hope, strength, and emotional support (Skokan & Bader, 2000), which can influence a person's will to live and therefore one's potential to heal. Burkhardt and Nagai-Jacobson (2002) declare, "Healing and spirituality are intimately connected. Grounded in the understanding that spirituality is the essence of who we are as human beings, we believe that healing is essentially a spiritual process that attends to the wholeness of a person." (p. 10) Research has demonstrated many positive links between spirituality/religion and health.

It is important to watch for these negative health risks and provide counsel or make referrals as needed.

Providing Spiritual Care

Now that we understand how crucial spiritual care is to one's overall health, how can we integrate this type of care into daily practice?

Recently, nurse scholars have begun to reintegrate spiritual care into practice, resulting in the rediscovery of holistic care (O'Brien, 2014). Watson (2013) believes, "A values-based, theory-guided approach to human caring and health care change illuminate the need for a major shift to occur. This is essential to achieve the authentic changes needed for nursing and human caring to survive in the coming era." This includes acknowledging the following (Watson, 2005):

- Human caring is not to be bought and sold as if it were a commodity.
- Caring and economics can coexist to achieve cost-effectiveness and cost-benefits.
- Nurses have a covenant with the public to provide human caring.
- Providing care should not be based upon a consumerist customer model.

- Both patients and healthcare providers require a caring and healing environment.
- The transition of health care to include human caring must begin from inside the healthcare system.

These beliefs have been incorporated into an ethical practice model known as Jean Watson's Theory of Human Caring. This model includes the following elements (Watson Caring Science Institute, 2013):

- Transpersonal caring relationship—moves beyond one's self to connect with or embrace the spirit or soul of the other through the process of caring and healing
- Caring moment/caring occasion—focuses on the uniqueness of the self, the other, and the moment, and being open to new possibilities
- Expanded views of self and other persons (transpersonal mind-body-spirit unity of being)
- Caring-healing consciousness and intentionality to care and promote healing—interconnectedness between caregiver and patient
- Unbroken wholeness and connectedness of all
- Advanced caring-healing modalities/nursing arts as a future model for advanced practice of nursing
- Care-supporting factors (also known as "Clinical Caritas Processes" or "The Ten Caritas" from the Greek word meaning "to cherish"):
    - Formation of a humanistic-altruistic system of values
    - Installation of faith-hope
    - Cultivation of one's sensitivity to one's self and to others
    - Development of a helping-trusting, human caring relationship
    - Promotion and acceptance of the expression of positive and negative feelings
    - Systematic use of a creative, problem-solving, caring process
    - Promotion of transpersonal teaching-learning
    - Provision for a supportive, protective, and/or corrective mental, physical, societal, and spiritual environment
    - Assistance with gratification of human needs
    - Allowance for existential-phenomenological-spiritual forces

This theory or approach to caring is centered upon intentional relationship building, connecting, and caring to promote a healing environment (Watson, 2005) and can therefore be implemented in all healthcare situations, regardless of one's religious or spiritual beliefs. By focusing on human dignity and respect, practitioners can care for patients in a humanistic way, touching the lives of their patients while promoting health and healing.

Whereas Watson focuses on transpersonal care, Leininger's Transcultural Nursing Theory, also known as Culture Care Theory, compares various cultures in an attempt to understand similarities (culture universal) and differences (culture specific) across human groups (Leininger, 2002). Important concepts within the theory include the following beliefs (Leininger, 2002):

- Cultural competence is an important component of nursing.
- Perceptions of illness and wellness are shaped by one's culture, as well as individual factors such as perception, coping, skills, and social ability.
- Healthcare providers should supply programs, policies, and services to meet the needs of each culturally diverse population encountered, which requires creativity and flexibility.

Incorporating these models into practice can allow us to care for each patient on individual, cultural, physical, and emotional levels. "Consistent with the wisdom and vision of Florence Nightingale, nursing is a lifetime journey of caring and healing, seeking to understand and preserve the wholeness of human existence and to offer compassionate, informed, knowledgeable human caring to society and humankind" (Watson, 2005).

Barriers to Providing Spiritual Health Care

"At its most basic level, nursing is a human-caring, relational profession. It exists by virtue of an ethical-moral ideal, and commitment to provide care for others" (Watson, 2005). While caring for one's spiritual state is an integral part of treating the person as a whole, many nurses are hesitant to approach the subject. One reason for this may be that nurses have fought to ensure their profession is as "medical," objective, and research-based as physician practices, and spirituality is a difficult factor to measure and therefore prescribe or address (Young & Koopsen, 2011). Other reasons include a lack of spiritual training or awareness, embarrassment, confusion regarding policies, the lack of time with each patient, a lack of privacy with the patient, beliefs that spirituality/religion should not be discussed by anyone other than a spiritual/religious provider, and a fear of embarrassing, angering, or offending the patient (Burkhardt & Nagai-Jacobson, 2002; Koenig, 2007; Young & Koopsen, 2011).

Patients can also be apprehensive to discuss spiritual needs. This may be due to a fear of being misjudged, a lack of knowledge about spirituality and/or its influences on health, fear of embarrassment, or an inability to communicate due to physical or emotional barriers or prejudices about their healthcare providers (Keonig, 2008; McSherry & Cash, 2000; Young & Koopsen, 2011).

Multiple solutions exist to provide spiritual care to patients. First, it is important to remember the distinctions between religion and spirituality. By providing spiritual care, one is nourishing the spirit, or the most human elements of a person. One can provide spiritual care simply by having a deep conversation concerning the patient's fears, hopes, anxieties, and wishes. By separating religious practices such as reciting scripture, praying, or chanting from spiritual exercises such as meditation or guided imagery, addressing the patient holistically becomes much more comfortable. It is also important to keep the potential benefits of holistic care in mind when assessing each patient. Finally, by helping to create rituals for a patient, a nurse or other healthcare provider can allow a space for each patient to address his or her own spiritual needs while simultaneously experiencing other health benefits that accompany positive habitual behaviors.

Morals, Ethics, and Spirituality in Health Care

Though healthcare providers have a responsibility to assess a patient's spiritual needs (Koenig, 2007), this should be done in a respectful manner. Further, the practitioner should take care to avoid imposing one's own beliefs or values on the patient (Young & Koopsen, 2011). Healthcare providers are allowed to conduct a simple spiritual assessment, but anything beyond this requires a patient's permission (Koenig, 2007). This would include praying with a patient, contacting a religious or spiritual provider for the patient such as a pastor or chaplain, recommending religious or spiritual resources, or reciting Biblical or other religious verses or texts. When in doubt, it is best to err on the side of caution; always ask the patient's permission if you are unsure or believe your actions may be beyond the scope of a simple spiritual assessment.

Some points to keep in mind include the following:

- Patients may be self-sufficient in their spirituality and may not have spiritual needs all the time or wish to inform healthcare providers about those needs (Young & Koopsen, 2011).
- Nonbelievers can experience distress when exposed to religious beliefs (Koenig, 2007)
- Those who are confident in their own spiritual beliefs appreciate their own traditions while attempting to understand other people's views on spirituality (Burkhardt & Nagai-Jacobson, 2002)
- Religious beliefs and spirituality become more prominent and essential to patients during times of stress, loss, illness, or the possibility of surgery or rehab (Young & Koopsen, 2011). Involvement in religion and spirituality also increase with age (Young & Koopsen, 2011).
- Practitioners should set aside their own beliefs and help clients search for their own belief system that will give them strength, joy, and wellness (Young & Koopsen, 2011).
- While nurses may not feel comfortable providing spiritual care, they should always be sensitive to the spiritual needs of the patient (O'Brien, 2014).

HIPAA and Spirituality

There are many concerns and misconceptions regarding what kinds of information can be released to the public, particularly in matters of religion and spirituality. The Health Insurance Portability and Accountability Act of 1996 (HIPAA) and the Standards for Privacy of Individually Identifiable Health Information, or "Privacy Rule," ensure that individual health information is protected, while allowing the flow of healthcare information needed to provide quality care and to protect the public's wellbeing (U.S. Department of Health and Human Services [HHS], 2003). The HIPAA Privacy Rule *does* allow hospitals and other covered healthcare providers to inform the clergy about parishioners in the hospital if the patient has agreed to the request (HHS, 2003). Moreover, clergy do not need to ask for a patient by name and can request information regarding patients of a particular religion. However, hospitals are not required to collect such information, nor are patients required to provide an answer (www.aha.org). When a patient is unable to provide or objects to religious preferences due to incapacity or emergency, healthcare providers can still disclose the patient's information to the clergy or other religious officials if the disclosure is consistent with any known or prior expressed preferences and is within the patient's best interests as determined by that healthcare provider (HHS, 2003).

Though clergy are allowed to request lists of patients with specific religious and/or spiritual beliefs, the Privacy Rule states that health care "does not include methods of healing that are solely spiritual. Therefore, clergy or other religious practitioners that provide solely religious healing services are not healthcare providers within this rule, and consequently are not covered entities for the purposes of this rule" (HHS, 2003, Part 160 Subpart A, General Provisions, Section 160.103). As a result, some pastoral care providers or clergy persons may be limited in providing care based on the role description of their position and in accordance with HIPAA regulations (O'Brien, 2014). This adds to the importance of collecting a patient's religious and/or spiritual preferences during patient intake and regular checkups. Therefore, if a patient would like clergy, chaplain, pastoral, or other religious/spiritual care, he or she can request it at any time and should be provided the opportunity to do so.

Praying with Patients

Research is beginning to look at the positive health effects of praying, which have only recently been acknowledged by the medical community (Carson & Koenig, 2008; Young & Koopsen, 2011). However, although prayer can be healing, comforting, and calming, healthcare providers must understand that praying with patients is not always appropriate. It is important to gain the patient's permission before attempting to pray, create a private environment, compose a personal prayer specific to that patient's needs, and monitor the patient's verbal and nonverbal responses (Taylor, 2002; Young & Koopsen, 2011).

Just as patients have the right to privacy and prayer and may choose whether or not to partake in religious and spiritual exercises, these freedoms also apply to practitioners. Therefore, while nurses should always be sensitive to the spiritual needs of the patient (O'Brien, 2014), if a patient asks a healthcare provider to partake in any religious or spiritual practice that makes the caregiver uncomfortable, such as prayer, he or she also has a right to respectfully decline. Instead, healthcare workers can ask the patient's permission to contact a religious or spiritual care provider on the patient's behalf.

Winslow and Winslow (2003) state that although prayer may be beneficial to patient care, this process must be "guided by ethical reflection." Finally, nurses should keep in mind that praying with patients is a privilege and should be approached with the utmost respect, dignity, and care. It is therefore imperative to use ethics, reasoning, and good judgment surrounding this type of care.

Rituals

Creating rituals to suit patients' physical and mental needs is an innovative way to incorporate spirituality without imposing religion or invading patient privacy, because rituals allow patients to develop their own sense of spirituality.

Rituals are repeated practices that involve completing tasks, hobbies, or pastimes with mindfulness. They allow individuals to reconnect with their sense of self and can therefore greatly improve spiritual health. Various rituals are seen throughout many cultures and religions and contain specific steps for recovery while reducing fear, anxiety, depression, and feelings of helplessness (Dossey & Keegan (2013). These practices can be secular or spiritual and allow for sacred time and space in our lives (Burkhardt & Nagai-Jacobson, 2002). Examples can include:

- Daily walks
- Time spent in nature, such as in trails or gardens
- Meditation
- Writing or journaling
- Creating art or music
- Prayer
- Family picnics or celebrations
- Cooking
- Guided imagery
- Yoga
- Sunday meals with friends

Creating personalized rituals is an important aspect of healing (Young & Koopsen, 2011). Healthcare providers can help patients discover a ritual to fit their individual physical, mental, and spiritual abilities and needs.

Rituals can be healing practices in many ways:

- They help individuals to connect to resources deep within themselves, loved ones, community, and a higher power (Burkhardt & Nagai-Jacobson, 2002).
- They provide highly structured practices that can provide rules for behavior (Achterberg, Dossey, & Kolkmeier, 1994).
- Focusing on the present relieves the mind of anxiety, fear, judgments, and pressing concerns (Reynolds, 2001).
- Calming images such as waterfalls, flowers, mountains, or the ocean produce positive changes in the body physiologically, biochemically, and immunologically (Freeman, 2008).
- Many religions consider nature to be the handiwork of a higher power and therefore being in nature has a calming effect that allows people to feel connected with a greater force or creator (Taylor, 2002).
- Rituals involving physical activity have added physiological and biochemical health benefits because of the body's release of serotonin and dopamine during exercise, which promote feelings of happiness.

Rituals can be done every day, no matter how much or how little time one has—from a 1-hour walk to a 5-minute journey to a waterfall in one's mind—and is a minimalist way to promote spirituality, healing, and wellness.

Conclusion

Whether one is an FCN, missionary nurse, or general care practitioner, human caring can be implemented in one's routine to create meaningful relationships with patients; encourage mind, body, and spirit wellness; and promote preventative care. Spirituality and religion have been found to have beneficial effects on patient health and can be integrated into the healthcare system through faith care nursing, clergy/pastoral/spiritual visits, human caring techniques, or through daily rituals. By caring for patients on a human level, we can promote lasting care and be changed as nurses while influencing the lives of our patients and our communities.

LEVELS OF PREVENTION

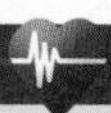

Primary: Conducting nutrition classes for preteens on healthy snacks

Secondary: Identifying preteens at risk for obesity-related health issues

Tertiary: Working with youth leaders in faith organizations to develop exercise and nutritional programs for preteens with diabetes

HEALTHY ME

How do you define spirituality? What role does it play in promoting and maintaining good health and a balanced life?

Critical Thinking Activities

1. Identify a health issue in your home community that could potentially be addressed by building a partnership with a local faith community.
   a. In what ways could a faith community address the problem to enhance public sector efforts?
   b. What kind of partnerships could be forged with the faith community to enhance their contribution?
   c. What are the steps that need to be taken to initiate a plan?
   d. How will your own faith experience influence your participation?

References

Achterberg, J., Dossey, B., and Kolkmeier, L. (1994). *Rituals of healing: Using imagery for health and wellness.* New York, NY: Bantam Books.

American Nurses Association (ANA). (2001). *Code of ethics for nurses with interpretive statements.* Silver Spring, MD: Author.

American Nurses Association & Health Ministries Association (2005). *Faith community nursing: Scope and standards of practice.* Silver Spring, MD: American Nurses Publishing.

Anderson, A. A. (1996). Florence Nightingale: Construction of a profession. *Anglican Theology and Review, 78*(3), 404–420.

Bennet, R., & Hale, W. (2009). *Building healthy medical-religious partnerships.* Baltimore, MD: Johns Hopkins University Press.

Bullough, V. O., & Bullough, B. (1969). *The emergence of modern nursing* (2nd ed.). New York, NY: Macmillan.

Burkhardt, M.A., & Nagai-Jacobson, M.G. (2002). Spirituality: Living our connectedness. New York, NY: Delmar Thomson Learning.

Carson, V., & Koenig, H. (2008). *Spiritual dimension of nursing practice.* West Conshohocken, PA: Templeton Press.

Chodron, P. (2001). *The places that scare you: A guide to fearlessness in difficult times.* Boston, MA: Shambhala.

Couture, P. (2003, January 7). *When public health and faith groups encounter each other: Overcoming obstacles.* Paper for the Carter Center Interfaith Health Working Group on Congregations and Public Health. Atlanta, GA: Carter Center.

Coyle, J. (2002). Spirituality and health: Towards a framework for exploring the relationship between spirituality and health. *Journal of Advanced Nursing, 37*(6), 589–587.

Donahue, M. P. (1985). *Nursing: The finest art, an illustrated history.* St Louis, MO: Mosby.

Dossey, B. M., & Keegan, L. (2013). Holistic nursing: A handbook for practice (6th ed.). Burlington, MA: Jones & Barton Learning.

Dossey, B. M. (1998). Florence Nightingale: A 19th century mystic. *Journal of Holistic Nursing, 16*(2), 111–165.

Droege, T., & Wenger, A. F. Z. (1997). *Starting point, empowering communities to improve health: A manual for training health promoters in congregational coalitions.* Atlanta, GA: Carter Center.

Eliopoulos, C. (2014). Invitation to holistic health: A guide to living a balanced life (3rd ed.). Burlington, MA: Jones & Bartlett Learning.

Frank, C. M. (1953). *Foundations of nursing.* Philadelphia, PA: Saunders.

Freeman, L. (2008). *Mosby's complementary and alternative medicine: A research-based approach* (3rd ed.). St Louis, MO: Mosby.

Freire, P. (1970). *Pedagogy of the oppressed.* New York, NY: Herder and Herder.

Gunderson, G. R. (1997). *Deeply woven roots: Improving the quality of life in your community.* Minneapolis, MN: Fortress Press.

Gunderson, G. R. (1998). Aligning assets for community health improvement. *Medical Journal of Allina, 7*(4), 2–5.

Klammer, C. M. (2006, January). Starting a church health ministry. *Clergy Journal,* 14–18.

Koenig, H. G. (2007). *Spirituality in patient care: Why, how, when, and what.* Philadelphia, PA: Templeton Foundation Press.

Koenig, H. G. (2008). *Medicine, religion, and health: How are they related and what does it mean?* West Conshhohocken, PA: Temple Press.

Leininger, M., & McFarland, M. R. (2002). Transcultural nursing: Concepts, theories, research and practice. (3rd ed.). New York, NY: McGraw Hill.

Macrae, J. (1995). Florence Nightingale's spiritual philosophy and its significance for modern nursing. *Image: Journal of Nursing Scholarship, 27*(1), 8–10.

McSherry, W., & Draper, P. (1998). The debates emerging from the literature surrounding the concept of spirituality as applied to nursing. *Journal of Advanced Nursing, 27*(4), 683–691.

Messikomer, C., & DeCraemer, W. (2002). The spirituality of academic physicians: An ethnography of a scripture-based group in an academic medical center. *Academic Medicine, 77*(6), 562–573.

O'Brien, M.A. (2014). *Spirituality in nursing: Standing on holy ground.* Burlington, MA: Jones & Bartlett Learning.

Oman, D., & Reed, D. (1998). Religion and mortality among the community-dwelling elderly. *American Journal of Public Health, 88*(10), 1469–1475.

Ott, B. B., Al-Khadhuri, B., & Al-Junaibi, S. (2003). Preventing ethical dilemmas: Understanding Islamic health care practices. *Pediatric Nursing, 29*(3), 227–230.

Patterson, D. (2006, March). The head bone's connected to the heart bone: Parish nurses as teachers. *Clergy Journal,* 21–24.

Reynolds, C. (2001). *Spiritual fitness.* London, England: Thorsons.

Sellew, G., & Nuesse, C. J. (1946). *A history of nursing.* St. Louis, MO: Mosby.

Simmons, P. (2000). *Learning to fall: The blessings of an imperfect life.* New York, NY: Bantam Books.

Skokan, L., & Bader, D. (2000). Spirituality and healing. *Health Progress, 81*(1), 1–8.

Solari-Twadell, P. A., & McDermott, M. A. (Eds.). (1999). *Parish nursing: Promoting whole person health within faith communities.* Thousand Oaks, CA: Sage.

Soloman, A. (2001). *The noonday demon: An atlas of depression.* New York, NY: Scribner.

Taylor, E. J. (2007). *What do I say? Talking with patients about spirituality.* Philadelphia, PA: Templeton Press.

Thich Nhat Hanh. (1998). *The heart of the Buddha's teaching: Transforming suffering into peace, joy, and liberation.* New York, NY: Broadway Books.

Thich Nhat Hanh. (2003). *Opening the heart of the cosmos: Insights on the Lotus Sutra.* Berkeley, CA: Parallax Press.

Tuck, I., Wallace, D., & Pullen, L. (2001). Spirituality and spiritual care provided by parish nurses. *Western Journal for Nursing Research, 23*(5), 441–453.

U.S. Department of Health and Human Services. (2003). *Standards for privacy of individually identifiable information*. Retrieved from http://www.hhs.gov/ocr/privacy/hipaa/news/2002/combinedregtext02.pdf

Wall, B. M., & Nelson, S. (2003). Our heels are praying very hard all day. *Holistic Nursing Practice, 17*(6), 320–328.

Walton, J. (1996). Spiritual relationships: A concept analysis. *Journal of Holistic Nursing, 14*(3), 237–250.

Watson, J. (2005). *Caring science as sacred science.* Philadelphia, PA: F.A. Davis.

Watson Caring Science Institute. (2013). Caring science theory and research. Retrieved from http://watsoncaringscience.org/about-us/caring-science-definitions-processes-theory/

Wenger, A. F. Z. (1998). Cultural openness, social justice, global awareness: Promoting transcultural nursing with unity in a diverse world. In P. Merilainen & K. Vehvilainen-Julkunen (Eds.), *The 23rd annual nursing research conference 1997, Transcultural nursing—Global unifier of care, facing diversity with unity* (pp. 162–168). Kuopio, Finland: Kuopio University Publications.

Winslow, G. R., & Winslow, B. W. (2003). Examining the effects of praying with patients. *Holistic Nursing Practice, 17*(4), 170–177.

Young, C., & Koopsen, C. (2011). *Spirituality, health, and healing: An integrative approach.* Sudbury, MA: Jones & Bartlett Learning.

Zinnbauer, B., Pargament, K., Cole, B., Rye, M. S., Butter, E. M., Belavich, T. G., . . . Kadar, J. L. (1997). Religion and spirituality: Unfuzzying the fuzzy. *Journal for the Scientific Study of Religion, 36*(4), 546–564.

Internet Resources

Arts & Faith: **http://www.filmsite.org/top100spiritual.html**

The Carter Center: http://www.cartercenter.org

Health Ministries Association: http://www.hmassoc.org

Healthy People 2020: http://www.healthypeople.gov/2020/default.aspx

International Parish Nurse Resource Center: http://www.parishnurses.org

Spirit-Health Connections: http://www.spirit-health.org

Wayne Oates Institute, a learning community for spiritual caregivers: http://www.oates.org

CHAPTER FOCUS

Holistic Framework

Historical Influences

Complementary Modalities: What Are They?

Natural Products

Manipulative and Body-Based Methods

Alternative Medical Systems

Energy Therapies

Mind–Body Interventions

Imagery

Herbal Therapies

Touch Therapy

Integrating Complementary Therapies into Community Nursing Care

Spirituality

Music Therapy

Potential Barriers to Use of Complementary Therapies

Complementary Health and Community Nursing Practice

The Right to Choose

Nursing Assessment

QUESTIONS TO CONSIDER

After reading this chapter, you will know the answers to the following questions:

1. What is complementary health?
2. How does a nurse know when to choose a complementary intervention?
3. What are barriers to using complementary therapy?
4. What are some of the most common complementary therapies?
5. How does the community health nurse evaluate the effectiveness of complementary therapy?

Civilizations have been using herbs, music, touch, and other "nonconventional" forms of healing for thousands of years. We are just beginning to discover the science behind these ancient healing systems and to include these healing methods into our scope of care.

CHAPTER 16

Complementary and Holistic Health

Margaret A. Burkhardt and
Lilianna K. Deveneau

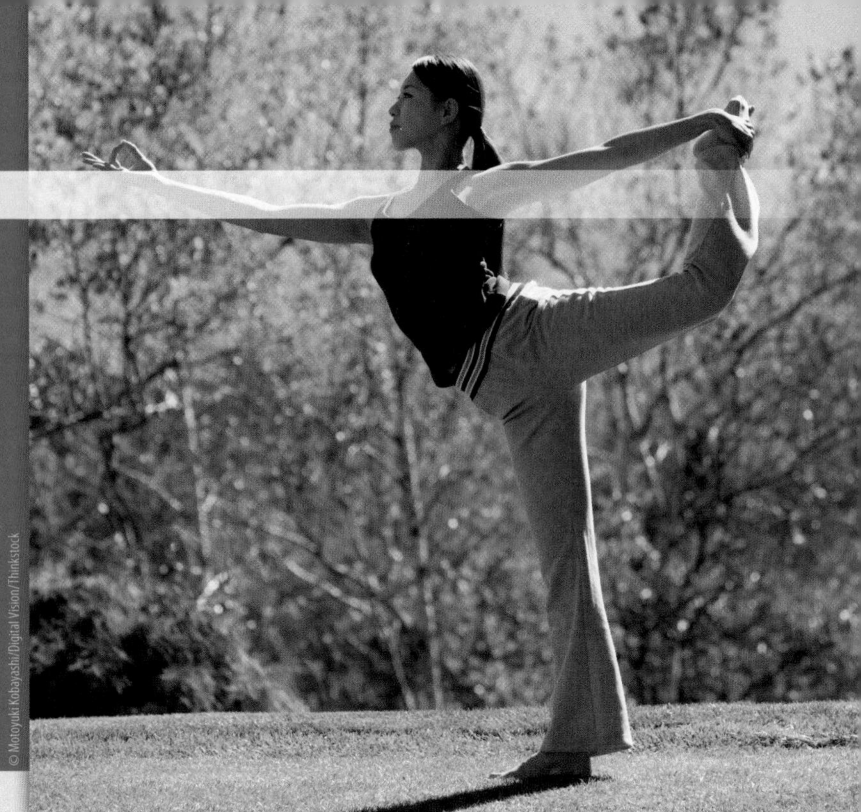

KEY TERMS

complementary health
healing
herbal and natural therapies
mind–body interventions
music therapy
Office of Alternative Medicine (OAM)
touch therapy

REFLECTIONS

Explain in your own words what "holistic" means to you. What has been your experience with complementary or alternative health practices?

THE "ICEMAN," DISCOVERED in the italian alps in 1991, is the oldest known member of the human family. His remains are dated to more than 5,000 years old. Medicinal herbs were among his preserved belongings. Could this simple remedy be due to a lack of scientific resources, or did the Iceman know secrets of the earth we are just now beginning to understand?

Alternative or unconventional therapies are becoming increasingly popular and more widely accepted in allopathic modalities, especially as research continues to explain why alternative approaches are beneficial. These methods are often termed *complementary* when used in addition to conventional therapies. In this chapter, the term *complementary therapy* is used regardless of the pattern of use, recognizing the need for healthcare providers to be open to exploring various approaches to health and healing to provide the best possible outcomes for patients.

> I begin to see that a man's got to be in his own heaven to be happy.
>
> —*Mark Twain*

Nurses within the community need to be familiar with various healing modalities used by their patients and aware of complementary modalities that may promote health, enhance healing, or contribute to unhealthy outcomes with patients. This chapter discusses a holistic framework for the integration of complementary therapies into care, complementary modalities, and assessment processes and ethical issues regarding **complementary health**. Selected complementary modalities that can be incorporated into community nursing care are discussed.

> Care and love are the most universal, the most tremendous, and the most mysterious of cosmic forces; they comprise the primal and universal psychic energy.
>
> —*Jean Watson*

> Dance is my therapy. Dance is my escape from real life. I can always forget my problems and be in a much better mood after ballet class. Dancing is fun. Dancing lets me express myself in a different way than words do.
>
> —*Tiffany, BSN, RN*

RESEARCH ALERT

This phenomenological study explored the meaning of spirituality among aging adults in Appalachia. Participants were adult volunteers ranging in age from 59 to 94 years old, in varying states of health, who lived independently in the community and at assisted living and skilled care facilities in an Appalachian community. Most of the participants were women. Data were collected through focus groups in which participants were asked open-ended questions about their perceptions of spirituality, spirituality and health, and the role of spirituality in helping them to cope. Data analysis revealed the themes of a conviction that God exists and acts in the lives of persons, calls them to action, and is a source of connection in times of loss. The data indicated that spirituality positively affects attitudes, especially as health declines, and that spirituality was of great importance in the lives of these elders. These participants expected empathetic and respectful health professionals who address both physical and spiritual concerns. Implications for nursing include the importance of incorporating spirituality into assessment and intervention with elderly and other patients.

Source: Lowry, L. W., & Conco, D. (2002). Exploring the meaning of spirituality with aging adults in Appalachia. *Journal of Holistic Nursing, 20*(4), 388–402.

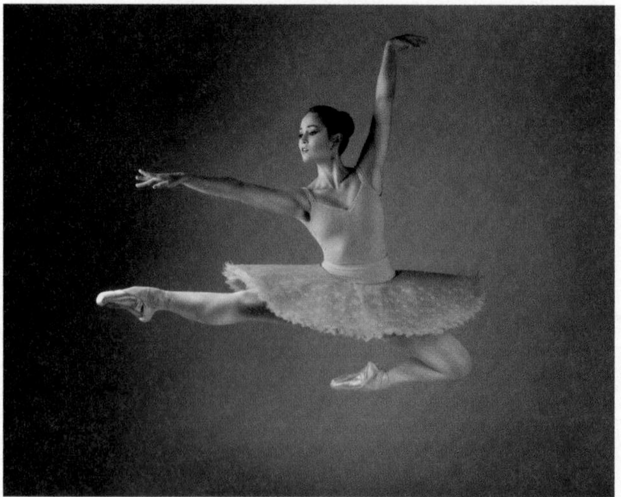

© Nanette_Grebe/iStock/Thinkstock

Holistic Framework

A holistic understanding of life that appreciates that each person is a bio-psycho-social-spiritual unity provides a framework for inclusion of complementary modalities into nursing care. Within a holistic framework, nurses are attentive to *healing* and to *curing* (Burkhardt, 1985; Burkhardt & Nagai-Jacobson,

2002; Quinn, 1989). Curing is a process that attends to disordered physical or psychological parts of a person, with a focus on disease processes and restoration of the integrity of a specific component (usually physiological) of a person. The allopathic approach focuses on curing by combating disease with techniques that produce effects different from those produced by the disease (Dossey & Guzzetta, 2005).

Healing, by contrast, acknowledges that disharmony in a whole person may be manifested as disease or illness and seeks to understand the totality of the lived experience for a person, taking into account the personal response to and meaning of the apparent disease or illness process (Burkhardt & Nagai-Jacobson, 1997b). Healing requires a relationship between the caregiver and care receiver that acknowledges common humanity and connectedness. Physical, emotional, and spiritual concerns are addressed within the healing relationship. Healing may be manifested as cure in one or more of the bio-psycho-emotional realms but can be present without a cure. Quinn (1989) aptly notes that, although diseases may be cured, people need healing. The desire to promote health, or the need for healing or curing, which is not being addressed by conventional approaches, often leads people to complementary modalities. Complementary or alternative therapies generally focus on body–mind–spirit integration through healing by an individual, healing between two individuals, or healing at a distance (Dossey & Guzzetta, 2005).

It is particularly important for nurses who work within the community to practice holistic nursing. Dealing with patients and families within their home environments enables nurses to appreciate cultural considerations in healing and to assess patients' use of complementary modalities. Because holistic nursing has the healing of the whole person as its goal, nurses work in therapeutic partnership with patients and families to integrate those modalities that best facilitate the patient's health and healing. Nurses also need to be aware of therapies that may be ineffective or cause potential harm when used alone or in combination with other modalities (Robison & Carrier, 2004). The American Holistic Nurses Association's description of holistic nursing presented in **Box 16-1**

RESEARCH ALERT

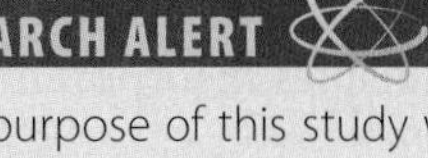

The purpose of this study was to determine the effect of laughter on natural killer cell activity and self-reported stress. The study was conducted in a community health center in a Midwestern city. The sample consisted of 33 healthy female volunteers who met specific inclusion and exclusion criteria that controlled for as many immunoresponsive factors as possible. Subjects were randomly assigned to experimental (humor) or control (distraction) groups. Experimental subjects viewed a humorous video, whereas subjects in the control group viewed a tourism video. Pre- and post-tests measured self-reported stress and arousal (Stress Arousal Check List), mirthful laughter (Humor Response Scale), and immune function (chromium-release natural killer cell cytotoxicity assay).

Findings of the study included a decrease in stress for subjects in the humor group compared with those in the distraction group, correlation between the amount of mirthful (overt) laughter and post-intervention stress measures in the humor group, and increased immune function in post-intervention subjects who scored greater than 25 on the Humor Response Scale. Although this study had some limitations, the findings suggest that mirthful laughter may reduce stress and improve natural killer cell activity, which is linked to enhanced immune response and, therefore, may be a useful cognitive behavioral intervention.

Source: Bennett, M. P., Zeller, J. M., Rosenberg, L., & McCann, J. (2003). The effect of mirthful laughter on stress and natural killer cell activity. *Alternative Therapies in Health and Medicine, 9*(2), 38–45.

BOX 16-1 American Holistic Nurses Association's Description of Holistic Nursing

Holistic nursing is defined as "all nursing practice that has healing the whole person as its goal" (American Holistic Nurses Association [AHNA], 1998, Description of Holistic Nursing, as cited in AHNA, 2014). Holistic nursing is a specialty practice that draws on nursing knowledge, theories, expertise, and intuition to guide nurses in becoming therapeutic partners with people in their care. This practice recognizes the totality of the human being—the interconnectedness of body, mind, emotion, spirit, social/cultural, relationship, context, and environment.

Holistic nurses may integrate complementary/alternative modalities (CAM) into clinical practice to treat people's physiological, psychological, and spiritual needs. Doing so does not negate the validity of conventional medical therapies, but serves to complement, broaden, and enrich the scope of nursing practice and to help individuals access their greatest healing potential.

The practice of holistic nursing requires nurses to integrate self-care, self-responsibility, spirituality, and reflection in their lives. This may lead the nurse to greater awareness of the interconnectedness with self, others, nature, and spirit. This awareness may further enhance the nurse's understanding of all individuals and their relationships to the human and global community, and permits nurses to use this awareness to facilitate the healing process.

Source: American Holistic Nurses Association, 2008. Used with permission.

provides a frame of reference for holistic nursing practice based on sound academic principles incorporating both the art and science of nursing.

> The part can never be well unless the whole is well.
>
> —*Plato*

Historical Influences

The United States is often referred to as a "melting pot" of persons from many different cultures, educational and socioeconomic backgrounds, and experiences. Therefore, it is imperative that we as nurses approach patients with a variety of healing techniques and an attitude of cultural acceptance. Healthcare practices have evolved (and continue to do so) from the healing traditions of both native peoples and those who have immigrated to this country, yet we often have preconceived notions of "acceptable" versus "inappropriate" treatment options well before the patient is ever consulted. Before the mid-1800s, practitioners from various healthcare systems, including allopathy, naturopathy, homeopathy, and botanics, were acknowledged as legitimate healers in the United States. Micozzi (1996) notes that the history of contemporary biomedicine as a scientific paradigm was as much influenced by social history as by scientific laws. Allopathic biomedicine began to predominate by the mid-1800s and gained further prominence by the late 1800s through state licensing laws sponsored by and lobbied for by the American Medical Association.

Dossey and Swyers (1994) note that the prominence of biomedicine was shaped in part by two important developments. One development was in the realm of scientific discoveries, such as the identification of specific organisms as the cause of particular disease states and the identification of substances and vaccines that ward off the effect of pathogens, which greatly influenced the direction of biomedicine. The other was the 1910 release of Abraham Flexner's report titled *Medical Education in the United States and Canada*, which was influential in upgrading medical education programs, enabling medical schools with a stronger biomedical orientation to receive more financial backing from philanthropic foundations. This, in turn, prompted the stifling of medical schools teaching theories other than biomedical regarding the origin of illness and appropriate therapies. What was considered scientific was defined by biomedicine's "way of knowing," which emphasized that knowledge about the world requires empiricism (Micozzi, 1996). Other paradigms were either relegated to the "fringe" or subsumed into the biomedical paradigm. Although biomedicine gained power and prestige and became the gold standard for health care, small numbers of naturopathic, homeopathic, chiropractic, and practitioners of other healing systems continued to provide care.

Over the past several decades, however, healthcare consumers have become more active in seeking care outside the biomedical system. Some of the factors that may have contributed to this phenomenon include the following:

- A shift away from infectious diseases as major causes of morbidity and mortality to health concerns that elude medical cure such as cancer, heart disease, hypertension, diabetes, and other chronic problems (Gordon, 1980)
- Increasingly depersonalized care and decreased personal control in healthcare decisions as a result of increased use of technology (Burkhardt & Nathaniel, 2002)
- A greater emphasis on self-care and personal responsibility for health
- A shrinking world that has allowed greater access to other cultures and their systems of healing
- Renewed appreciation that healing must address the whole body-mind-spirit person

Additionally, research is explaining the biomedical science behind ancient techniques that other cultures have intuited for centuries.

Although people have been using complementary therapies for years, the landmark study conducted by Eisenberg and colleagues (1993) documented an unexpected frequency of use of these therapies and caused the medical establishment to take note. The results of this national telephone survey of 1,539 adults indicated that one in three Americans of all sociodemographic groups used complementary therapies, and of those who used these therapies, 72% did so without informing their conventional healthcare provider. This study also indicated that people tended to use complementary modalities for chronic rather than life-threatening conditions. To identify trends in alternative medicine use in the United States, Eisenberg and colleagues (1998) conducted another national telephone survey of 2,055 English-speaking adults in 1997 asking about their use of 16 therapies. The therapies included relaxation techniques, herbal medicine, massage, chiropractic, prayer or spiritual healing by others, megavitamins, self-help groups, imagery, commercial diet, folk remedies, lifestyle diet, energy healing, homeopathy, hypnosis, biofeedback, and acupuncture. Results of this survey indicated that alternative therapy use increased from 33.8% in 1990 to 42.1% in 1997. Use of herbal medicine, massage, megavitamins, self-help groups, folk remedies, energy healing, and homeopathy increased the most.

In 2008, Barnes, Bloom, and Nahin reported that nearly four of every 10 adults surveyed had utilized CAM therapy within the past 12 months, with the most commonly used being nonvitamin, nonmineral natural products (17.7%) and deep breathing exercises (12.7%). Further, approximately one in nine children (11.8%) had used CAM in the past 12 months, with natural products being most common (3.9%), followed by chiropractic or osteopathic manipulation (2.8%). Finally, children whose parent(s) used CAM were almost five times as likely (23.9%) to use alternative medicine than children whose parent(s) did not (5.1%). This study also found that between 2002 and 2007 adult use of acupuncture, deep breathing exercises, massage therapy, meditation, naturopathy, and yoga increased, while CAM use for head and chest colds decreased 7.5%.

According to a 2010 survey conducted by the National Center for Complementary and Alternative Medicine (NCCAM) and AARP, 58% of people age 50 years or older who reported using complementary healthcare practices said they had discussed them with a healthcare provider (NCCAM, 2012). (See **Box 16-2**.)

In response to growing awareness and use of complementary therapies, the National Institutes of Health (NIH) created the **Office of Alternative Medicine (OAM)** in 1992. The OAM was established to facilitate scientific and fair evaluation of complementary modalities that can contribute to the health and wellbeing of many people and reduce barriers to awareness and availability of promising complementary therapies. In 1998, the OAM was elevated to the NCCAM, one of the 25 institutes and centers of NIH. NCCAM's mission is to conduct and support basic and applied research and training and to disseminate information on complementary and alternative medicine to practitioners and the public. The congressional mandate for the NCCAM provides for research training programs and a public information clearinghouse; however, the center is not a referral agency. The importance of research on and reliable information about complementary therapies is reflected in the increase in budget for the NCCAM that supports research and education on CAM.

BOX 16-2 Why Tell Your Healthcare Providers?

Giving your healthcare providers a complete outlook on your self-care helps you stay in control and allows them to act as partners in your care.

Some complementary health practices can have an effect on conventional medicine. For instance, the herb St. John's wort, often used for depression, has potentially dangerous interactions with a number of common prescription and over-the-counter medications. Talking to your healthcare providers will help ensure appropriate and safe care.

Your healthcare provider may be aware of new research regarding your CAM treatment and may be able to suggest other helpful CAM practices.

> What lies behind us and what lies before us are tiny matters compared to what lies within us.
>
> —*Ralph Waldo Emerson*

Complementary Modalities: What Are They?

Although the terms *alternative*, *complementary*, and *unconventional* are often used interchangeably in reference to nonbiomedical interventions, the term *complementary* best reflects the awareness that these therapies need to be considered adjuncts to—not replacements for—medical and surgical treatments. The definition of complementary modalities that was developed at the NIH/OAM Second Conference on Research Methodology in April 1995 notes that the broad domain of CAM encompasses all health systems, modalities, and practices other than those intrinsic to the politically dominant health system of a particular society or culture. Currently the NCCAM defines CAM as a group of diverse medical and healthcare systems, practices, and products that are not generally considered to be part of conventional medicine (NCCAM, 2013). CAM includes all practices and ideas self-defined by their users as preventing or treating illness or promoting health and wellbeing.

MEDIA MOMENT 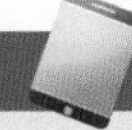

***Invitation to Holistic Health: A Guide to Living a Balanced Life* (2014) 3rd ed., Burlington, MA: Jones & Bartlett Learning**

—By Charlotte Eliopoulos

Dr. Eliopoulos provides an excellent overview of adopting a holistic lifestyle—for ourselves and our patients. This book is an extension of the AHNA's commitment to teach consumers measures to promote optimal health and wellbeing of the body, mind, and spirit. Eliopoulos compiles the knowledge and practical wisdom of nurses for health promotion and holistic wellness. Authored by health professionals who have the closest, most frequent contact with consumers and understand consumers best, this book presents practical health-promotion information in a unique manner, utilizing a holistic model. This book provides the practical "how to" information to enable consumers to safely and effectively use natural and complementary therapies. The public's skyrocketing interest in and use of alternative and complementary therapies make this aspect of the book particularly timely and relevant.

Each healing system (including biomedicine) has its own explanatory model that "summarizes the perceptions, assumptions, beliefs, theories, and facts that guide the logic of healthcare delivery" (Cassidy, 1996, p. 20). Some important distinctions between complementary and conventional medicine include differences in philosophical underpinnings, types of therapies offered, ways in which therapies are administered, and interactions between practitioner and patient (Cassidy, 1996; Dossey & Swyers, 1994). For example, in the biomedical model, the practitioner has traditionally been considered the authoritative expert who determines and designs care based on standardized treatments in which the patient has variable involvement. With complementary systems, treatments are more often individualized and developed in collaboration with patients who are acknowledged as having responsibility for their own healing processes. Complementary systems generally appreciate that humans have natural, built-in recuperative powers and often focus on therapies that enhance the patient's natural healing processes. Unifying threads that are common to most complementary healing systems include emphasis on the following:

- One's relationships, sense of values, place in society, and sense of self
- The role of spiritual values and religion in health
- The impact on health of consciousness manifested through thoughts, feelings, attitudes, emotions, values, and perceived meanings
- Diet, exercise, relaxation techniques, and modifications in lifestyle
- Utilization of whole foods and herbs rather than extracts (Dossey & Swyers, 1994)

Many of these threads are common parts of nursing practice as well, and conventional medicine is also beginning to pay more attention to them (Gordon, 2002; Sierpina, 2002).

NCCAM currently classifies complementary and alternative health practice into seven categories or domains, each of which contains subcategories designated as *CAM* (practices that are not commonly used, accepted, or available in conventional medicine), *behavioral medicine* (practices that may fall within the domain of conventional medicine), and *overlapping* (practices that can be in either subcategory). These categories with associated NCCAM classifications of alternative medicine practice are briefly summarized next. Given that the listing of specific modalities and therapies is updated and expanded on a regular basis, only a few selected examples are given here for each category. The reader is encouraged to visit the NCCAM website (http://nccam.nih.gov) for further information.

Natural Products

CAM options classified as natural products use substances found in nature such as foods, vitamins, herbs, and other plants. Although these substances are considered natural, their efficacy is as yet scientifically unproven. This field includes a wide assortment of drugs, biologic products, dietary supplements, and nutritional interventions used to prevent illness, maintain health, and reverse the effects of chronic disease.

The ingestion of herbal or botanical medicines was among the first attempts to improve the physical condition. The mummified "Ice Man" found in the Italian Alps in 1991, the oldest preserved human to date, had in his possession medicinal herbs. By the Middle Ages, thousands of botanical products had been discovered and utilized regularly. Further, all cultures and healing traditions have included the use of plants and plant products, and these are still a major component of indigenous populations all over the world.

Many of today's drugs have herbal origins, and about 25% of drugs dispensed from pharmacies have at least one active ingredient derived from plants. According to the World Health Organization (WHO), 80% of the world's population use herbal therapies for some aspect of their primary care. Because of U.S. Food and Drug Administration (FDA; 2014) regulations, herbal products can be marketed in the United States only as food supplements and cannot make any specific health claims.

The rise in chronic illnesses related to diet has prompted a shift in nutritional research in the United States toward dealing with the effects of nutritional excess and away from eliminating nutritional deficiency, and may be to blame for the rise in the popularity of natural products. The 2007 National Health Interview Survey (NHIS) found that nearly 18% of American adults had used a nonvitamin, nonmineral natural product, the most common of which was fish oil/omega-3 fatty acids, and more than 37% of children were administered echinacea (NCCAM, 2012). Though these methods are believed to be beneficial and even harmless, evidence indicates that inadequate intake of some micronutrients may increase risks of problems such as coronary artery disease, cancers, and birth defects, and that the required daily allowance for some minerals and vitamins may not be adequate to prevent chronic illnesses. Many alternative diets and dietary lifestyles that incorporate more fresh and freshly prepared fruits and vegetables and whole grains and legumes may offer greater resistance to illness.

Examples of interventions in this category include:

- Phytotherapy or herbalism—plant-derived preparations used for therapeutic and preventive purposes, such as Ginkgo biloba, echinacea, and green tea

- Special diet therapies—dietary approaches used as alternative therapies for particular risk factors or for chronic disease in general, such as vegetarian, Pritikin, and macrobiotic diets
- Orthomolecular medicine—products not covered in other categories that are used (usually in combinations and at high doses) as nutritional and food supplements for preventive or therapeutic purposes, such as ascorbic acid, coenzyme Q10 (CoQ10), and melatonin
- Cartilage products derived from sharks, chickens, and sheep, used for treating cancer; ethylene diamine tetraacetic acid (EDTA) chelation therapy, used for treating heart disease and preventing cancer; a liquid extract from mistletoe plants (*Iscador*), used to treat tumors
- Probiotics—found naturally in foods such as yogurt and also offered as a dietary supplement, these microorganisms are similar to those found naturally in the human digestive tract and aid in digestion

Manipulative and Body-Based Methods

Although contemporary biomedical providers tend to be distanced from physical contact with patients because of attitudes of reliance on diagnostic equipment and tests, as well as legal and time constraints, at one time physicians' hands were considered their most important diagnostic and therapeutic tool. Manual healing methods derive from the understanding that dysfunction of one area of the body can affect the function of other discrete and not necessarily connected body parts.

The NCCAM classification of manipulative and body-based methods focuses on therapies and systems that are based on movement or manipulation of one or more parts of the body, including soft tissues, bones and joints, and the circulatory and lymphatic systems. Examples of healing approaches found in this category include:

- *Spinal manipulation* is practiced by chiropractors, osteopathic and naturopathic physicians, and physical therapists. Practitioners use their hands or an instrument to apply controlled force to a particular joint of the spine. This treatment is used to relieve pain and pressure and to improve physical function, especially that caused by low back pain. Utilized by ancient Greeks, this therapy was incorporated into chiropractic and osteopathic medicine during the late 19th century (NCCAM, 2012).
- *Massage therapy* is defined as the pressing, rubbing, and manipulation of the muscles and soft tissues to relieve pain, rehabilitate sports injuries, reduce anxiety and depression, increase relaxation, combat stress, and promote general wellbeing. These tactics have existed for thousands of years (NCCAM, 2012). Swedish massage, Chinese Tui Na massage and acupressure, and body psychotherapy are all examples of this relaxing technique.

According to the 2007 NHIS, chiropractic/osteopathic manipulation and massage therapy ranked in the top 10 most popular CAM therapies among adults and children (NCCAM, 2012).

Movement Therapies

Movement therapy describes a broad range of Eastern and Western movement-based maneuvers and exercises used to promote physical, emotional, mental, and spiritual wellbeing. The Alexander technique is a practice that uses education and guidance to improve one's posture and movement to increase the body's overall functioning, and is used to treat low back pain and symptoms of Parkinson's disease. Pilates is also categorized as a type of movement therapy that uses a method of physical exercise to strengthen and build control of muscles, particularly those used for posture. Awareness of breathing and precise control of movements are key practices of Pilates, and often special equipment is needed. Feldenkrais uses physical coordination and a method of education to help the patient become more aware of how one's body moves through space and to improve physical functioning. Finally, Trager Psychophysical Integration applies a series of gentle rhythmic rocking movements to the joints to release tension and increase the body's range of motion. This technique is often used to treat chronic headaches. It also stresses the importance of physical and mental self-care to promote proper movement of the body (NCCAM, 2012).

Alternative Medical Systems

Worldwide, only 10–30% of human health care is delivered by conventional, biomedically oriented practitioners.

BOX 16-3 Tips for Talking to Your Providers

- When completing your patient history forms, include all therapies and treatments. Make a list in advance.
- Don't wait for your providers to ask. Be proactive about your health care.
- If you're considering a new CAM practice, ask your provider about its safety, effectiveness, and possible interactions with both prescription and nonprescription medications.

Source: NCCAM, 2012.

The remaining 70–90% of care varies from self-care according to folk principles to care sought within an organized healthcare system derived from traditions or practices that flow from paradigms of health and healing different from those associated with biomedicine. Some of these explanatory models have sound bases that have been developed, tested, and practiced over thousands of years. Because they derive from a different worldview, however, the processes and modes of action of many of these modalities are not understood within the biomedical paradigm.

The NCCAM classification *Alternative Medical Systems* addresses complete systems of theory and practice other than the Western biomedical approach. Many of these systems evolved apart from and earlier than the conventional medical system that dominates Western cultures. Examples of such systems include:

- Traditional Chinese medicine—includes acupuncture, herbal formulas, tai chi, diet
- Ayurvedic medicine and other traditional indigenous systems—include diet and herbal remedies, and emphasize body, mind, and spirit in both prevention and treatment
- Homeopathy—based on a belief that "like cures like" and uses highly diluted medicinal substances to treat symptoms
- Naturopathy—based on a belief that there is a natural healing power in the body that maintains and restores health, and uses various means to support this power, such as nutrition, lifestyle counseling, dietary and herbal supplements, exercise, and treatments from modalities like homeopathy and traditional Chinese medicine

The 2007 NHIS found that although a relatively small percentage of respondents said they had used Ayurveda or naturopathy, homeopathy ranked 10th in adult CAM use and fifth in use among children (NCCAM, 2012).

Energy Therapies

The therapies in this category involve the use of energy fields and are classified as either biofield therapies or bioelectromagnetic-based therapies. *Biofield* healing practices use subtle energy fields in and around the body for healing and health promotion, and generally operate under the belief that human beings are infused with subtle forms of energy. Examples of these therapies include healing touch (HT), reiki, light therapy, therapeutic touch (TT), and external qi gong. *Bioelectromagnetics* includes the unconventional use of electromagnetic fields for healing and health promotion. It is an emerging science that studies how living organisms interact with electromagnetic fields.

The understanding that electrical phenomena are found in all living organisms and that electrical currents in the body can produce magnetic fields extending outside the body is basic to this field of study. Exploration suggests that changes in the body's natural fields can produce physical and behavioral changes and that certain frequencies have specific effects on body tissues. Examples of energy therapies include pulsed fields, magnetic fields, and alternating or direct current fields (Cuellar, 2005; Cuellar, Rogers, & Hisghman, 2007).

The national health goals established in *Healthy People 2020* are designed to help bring the people of the United States to their full potential. The opportunities or objectives designated for achieving these goals relate to health promotion, health protection, and preventive services. Although the document does not address complementary modalities per se, many people use complementary therapies as part of their efforts to promote health and prevent illness. Most complementary modalities included in the NCCAM classification system relate to the goal of increasing the span of healthy life for people in this country. Appropriate use of complementary therapies and their practitioners may ultimately contribute to the goals of reducing health disparities. Because many complementary therapies focus on health promotion and illness prevention, appropriately integrating them into health care may promote access to preventive services for people across the United States. Although research on the role of many complementary modalities in health promotion and prevention has expanded in recent years, more validation of the efficacy of these therapies is needed. Because health-promotion strategies relate to individual lifestyle choices, nurses need to be particularly aware of choices people make regarding the use of complementary therapies in dealing with health promotion and illness prevention.

Traditional Healers

Traditional healers use methods based on indigenous theories, beliefs, and experiences that have been passed down through generations. Curanderos, espiritistas, hierberos/yerberos, Native American healers or medicine men, shamans, and sobadores are examples from various cultures (NCCAM, 2012).

Mind–Body Interventions

The belief that the mind plays an important role in the treatment of health and overall wellness has existed for more than 2,000 years (NCCAM, 2012). **Mind-body interventions** focus on the mind's capacity to affect the body and explore healing systems that make use of the interconnectedness of mind, body, and spirit. Most traditional healing systems acknowledge and incorporate the interconnectedness of mind–body–spirit, recognizing the power of each to affect the other. Since the 1980s, biomedicine has become more open to the awareness of the impact of the mind on the body, although exploring the role of spirituality in healing is still in its infancy. Mind–body–spirit interventions often enable patients to experience and express their illnesses in new and clearer ways, and to explore the meaning of their illnesses, which can have direct consequences on their health. Scientific exploration suggests that there is a complex interaction among the mind, neurological systems, and immune systems (psychoneuroimmunology) that can be affected by interventions in this category.

The NCCAM classification of mind–body interventions, which encompasses psychological, social, behavioral, and spiritual approaches to health, relates to this field of practice. Examples of CAM techniques and practices that are part of this category include:

- *Mind–body methods*—specific modalities incorporating awareness of mind–body interaction in healing, such as yoga, tai chi, imagery, mental healing, and creative outlets such as music, art, and dance. These techniques involve specific postures, rhythmic breathing, and focused attention. Often they are used to increase calmness and relaxation, improve psychological balance, cope with illness, increase flexibility and muscle tone, and relieve a variety of health conditions, particularly chronic illnesses (NCCAM, 2012).
- *Religion and spirituality*—the nonbehavioral aspects of religion and spirituality that relate to biologic function or clinical condition, such as nonlocality, meditation, prayer, forgiveness, and spiritual healing.
- *Social and contextual factors*—interventions that are social, cultural, symbolic, or contextual in nature, such as caring-based approaches like holistic nursing, intuitive diagnosis, and community-based approaches like certain Native American rituals.

Several mind and body therapies ranked among the top 10 CAM practices utilized by adults, according to the 2007 NHIS. The survey found 12.7% of adults had used deep-breathing exercises, 9.4% had practiced meditation, and 6.1% practiced yoga. Also included in the top 10 list were guided imagery and progressive relaxation (NCCAM, 2012).

MEDIA MOMENT 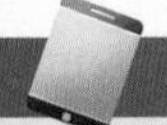

***The Spirit Catches You and You Fall Down* (1997)**

—By Anne Fadiman, New York, NY: Farrar, Straus and Giroux

When 3-month-old Lia Lee arrived at the county hospital emergency department in Merced, California, a chain of events was set in motion from which neither she nor her parents nor her doctors would ever recover. Lia's parents, Foua and Nao Kao, were part of a large Hmong community in Merced, refugees from the CIA-run "Quiet War" in Laos. The Hmong, traditionally a close-knit and fiercely independent people, have been less amenable to assimilation than most immigrants, adhering steadfastly to the rituals and beliefs of their ancestors. Lia's pediatricians, Neil Ernst and his wife, Peggy Philip, cleaved just as strongly to another tradition: that of Western medicine. When Lia Lee entered the American medical system, diagnosed as an epileptic, her story became a tragic case history of cultural miscommunication.

Integrating Complementary Therapies into Community Nursing Care

As noted previously, holistic care should be the goal of all nursing practice. Although holistic care presumes attention to physical, mental, emotional, and spiritual concerns, many look upon spirituality as complementary therapy. The tendency to view body and spirit as separate and unrelated entities (which persists within contemporary healthcare settings) supports the view that physical concerns are the prime focus of biomedicine and that spirituality has little or no place in biomedical care. However, the body, mind, and spirit are inextricably intertwined, and spirituality cannot be separated from physical and emotional health.

This section briefly discusses ways of integrating spirituality and selected complementary modalities into nursing care. When considering integrating any modality into practice, nurses need to address two fundamental concerns: (1) safety—the potential side effects and risks for harm when the therapy is used alone or in combination with other therapies, and (2) efficacy—the therapy's ability to produce the effect that it is intended to produce. The examples of complementary modalities presented here are chosen because they can be particularly valuable nursing interventions that clearly fall within nursing's domain of practice. Educational programs are available through which nurses can become certified practitioners of many of these therapies. Although it is within nursing's domain of practice to address diet, nutrition, and lifestyle changes, nurses must recognize that when such modalities are considered complementary or alternative, they are often based on nonorthodox systems of healing or are applied in unconventional ways. Nurses need to be aware that their patients are using these modalities, their reasons for using them, and potential risks and benefits.

The nursing role includes supporting that which promotes health and healing, advising caution where risks are involved, facilitating open communication about various options, and honoring the patient's right to choose. Nurses can become knowledgeable about and through training become practitioners of alternative healing modalities such as acupuncture, oriental medicine, homeopathy, and Ayurvedic medicine (Cuellar, 2005). Some aspects of other healing systems may be easily integrated into nursing care, such as use of particular acupressure points for relief of headaches or nausea. However, nurses need to be aware of the scope of practice stated in their state's nurse practice act and incorporate only those modalities that are within their scope of nursing practice.

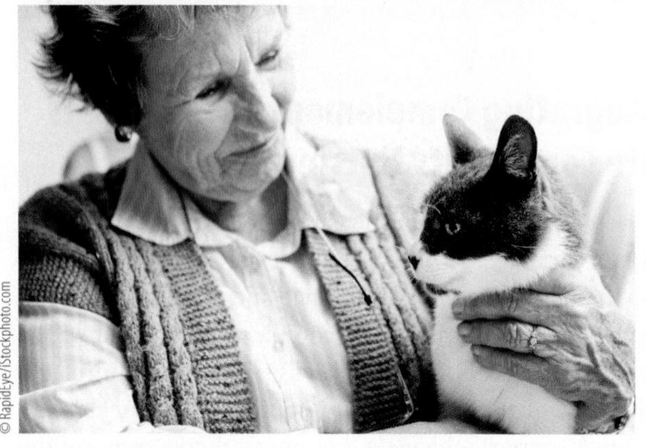

Complementary health research has consistently linked close human-pet relationships with improved health outcomes.

Spirituality

Spirituality is the essence of who one is, a unifying or animating force that permeates all of one's life and being. This essence is expressed in and through connectedness with one's self, with others, with nature, and with God or a Life Force. Although one's spirituality and relationship with God or Life Force is often nurtured and expressed through one's religious beliefs and practices, for many, spirituality transcends the boundaries of religion. Spirituality is connected to values and is vital to the process of discovering meaning and purpose in life. Spiritual issues are core life issues that are often related to mystery, suffering, forgiveness, grace, hope, and love (Burkhardt & Nagai-Jacobson, 1997a, 2002, 2005).

The nursing assessment of spirituality requires attentive listening, the ability to be fully present with the patient in this moment, and good communication skills. Assessment of spiritual concerns with patients includes exploration of issues of meaning and purpose; important values, beliefs, and practices; prayer or meditation styles; important relationships and their influence on the present circumstances; and desires for connection with religious groups or rituals. The process of assessment often is part of the intervention, because merely providing the opportunity for patients to talk of their spiritual concerns enables them to become more aware of their spiritual journey and its impact on present life experiences. Because people often use story and metaphor in expressing their spirituality and spiritual concerns, nurses can approach spirituality by encouraging people to tell their stories. In this process, nurses can gain insight into those connections that support and inspire a patient, relationships in need of forgiveness and healing, sources of strength, experiences that have given life meaning, and ways in which the person questions the meaning of life. Nurses can help patients attune to their spirituality by exploring and incorporating meaningful rituals into care such as sacred readings, drumming, and music; facilitating processes focused on mindfulness such as relaxation exercises, imagery, and paying attention to physical sensations; and fostering consideration of the place and meaning of prayer for patients and the ways they do or do not experience God or Life Force in their lives. Nurses need to be aware of their own spiritual perspectives to honor their own values and beliefs without imposing them on patients. Acts of compassion, selflessness, the use of social support, meditation, and contemplation are all characteristics of spirituality.

The word "gratitude" is derived from the Latin root gratia, meaning grace, gratefulness, and the beauty of giving and receiving. A grateful attitude toward life can lead to peace of mind, happiness, physical health, and deeper, more satisfying relationships. In a study of 65 adults (44 women, 21 men) with either congenital or adult-onset neuromuscular disease, participants were given a packet of 21 "daily experience rating forms" to be completed at the end of each day. Those in the gratitude condition (33 people) were asked to write five things they were grateful for before writing five hassles and up to five things that affected them. The control condition group (32 people) was only asked to complete five hassles and up to five things that affected them each day. Those in the gratitude condition had an increased amount and quality of sleep, increased positivity, greater optimism, and a sense of connectedness to others (Emmons & McCullough, 2003).

Journaling

Because the role of nurses is to care for others, it is critical to practice self-care. This includes creating the time and space to do so. Journaling is one way of accomplishing this. There is evidence that as a reflective and meditative activity, journaling can promote creativity, self-awareness, stress reduction and personal development.

Meditation

There are many types of meditation, the majority of which have been developed through religious and spiritual traditions. NCCAM (2010) describes meditation as learning to focus attention, to become mindful of thoughts, feelings, and sensations, and to observe them in a nonjudgmental way. This practice is believed to increase calmness, physical relaxation, and psychological balance. Most types of meditation share four common elements:

- A quiet location with as few distractions as possible
- A specific, comfortable position or posture—meditation can be done sitting, laying down, standing, walking, or in other positions
- A focus of attention—the meditator may focus on a mantra (a word or phrase that has personal meaning), an object, or breathing, for example
- An open attitude—this means allowing thoughts and distractions to come and go naturally without judging or focusing on them

Meditation used as CAM, as previously mentioned, is a type of mind–body medicine. People use meditation to alleviate various health problems, including anxiety, pain, depression, stress, insomnia, physical or emotional symptoms associated with chronic illnesses (heart disease, HIV/AIDS, and cancer) and their treatment, and overall wellness.

Some types of meditation may work by affecting the autonomic (involuntary) nervous system, which is responsible for organ and muscle regulation, controlling heartbeat, breathing, sweating, and digestion. The two major components of this are the sympathetic and parasympathetic nervous systems:

- The *sympathetic nervous system* aids in body mobilization and is responsible for the "fight or flight" reaction. This increases heart rate and breathing while restricting blood vessels.
- The *parasympathetic nervous system* causes the breathing and heart rate to decrease while dilating blood vessels and increasing the flow of digestive juices.

Meditation is believed to reduce sympathetic nervous system activity and increase parasympathetic nervous system functions (NCCAM, 2012).

Prayer

The experience of prayer or some form of connecting to the "beyond" is fundamental to human life and experience. The literature provides evidence indicating that prayer and religious devotion are associated with health outcomes (Burkhardt & Nagai-Jacobson, 2002; Dossey, L., 1993, 1996, 1997, 1998; Dunn & Horgas, 2000; Meisenhelder & Chandler, 2000; Walton & Sullivan, 2004). Dossey notes that research on intercessory prayer and distant intentionality indicate that open-ended, nondirective prayer such as "Thy will be done" or "whatever is best for all concerned" is more efficacious than prayers for particular outcomes. He also reminds us that prayer does not require scientific evidence for validation. Prayer is an appropriate nursing intervention, whether the nurse prays for or with patients or arranges for patients to have the quiet and privacy needed for prayer or meditation. Nurses who include prayer as part of their patient care need to remember that prayer has many forms and expressions and is culturally conditioned.

When nurses incorporate prayer for patients into their personal spiritual practices, they should not presume to know what the patient needs; rather, they should express prayer in terms such as, "whatever is for the patient's highest good." Nurses who wish to pray with patients should do so with the patient's permission and encourage patients to use their own forms and expressions of prayer. Very often, patients in healthcare institutions need nurses to help them make sacred space within daily routines to attend to their own prayer, either alone or with others.

Researchers are finding the benefits of prayer and spirituality are quantifiable. Results from several studies indicate that people with strong spirituality and/or religious beliefs heal faster from surgery, are less anxious and depressed, have lower blood pressure, and are much more able to cope with chronic illnesses such as arthritis, spinal cord injuries, diabetes, and cancer. One clinical study at Duke University found that of 232 older adults undergoing heart surgery, those who were religious and/or spiritual were three times less likely to die within 6 months after surgery than those who were not (Ikedo, Gangahar, Quader, & Smith, 2007).

Music Therapy

Music has been a vital part of all cultures and societies and has been linked with healing throughout history. Guzzetta (1997, 2005) notes that **music therapy** complements conventional therapies by providing patients with integrated body–mind experiences and by facilitating relaxation, self-healing, and active participation in health and recovery. Currently, music therapy is being used to treat insomnia (NCCAM, 2012), as music can promote relaxation and can produce changes in emotions, behavior, and physiology. Another benefit of music therapy is its accessibility and diversity; music can be used alone or in conjunction with prayer, meditation, relaxation exercises, and guided imagery.

Musical vibrations can help restore or maintain the body's regulatory function; can help reduce pain, anxiety, isolation, and psychophysiological stress; can enhance the immune system; and can facilitate development of self-awareness and help improve memory (Guzzetta, 1997, 2005).

Guzzetta (1997, 2005) reminds us that, when considering using music therapy with patients, nurses need to assess patients' music preferences, the importance of music in their lives, and the types of music that make them happy, sad, relaxed, tense, and so forth. Nurses must be aware that no one selection or type of music is best for all people or in all situations and that the patient's mood and preferences determine the types of music used and the goals of each session. Nurses can introduce patients to music therapy, initially guide them through the process, and help them develop their own healing scripts and music libraries. Guzzetta offers guidelines for incorporating music therapy into clinical settings and provides a script that nurses can use with patients during a music therapy session. Research conducted through the music therapy program at the University of Miami indicated that music contributed to an increase in levels of melatonin and human growth hormone (leading to better sleep patterns and fewer aches and pains) in Alzheimer's patients and that the combined use of music and guided imagery in clinical trials contributed to lower liver enzymes in patients with chronic hepatitis B and lower levels of stress hormones in healthy persons (Simonton, Cohen, Kumar, McKinney, & Tims, 1997).

ART CONNECTION 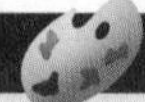

The Old Guitarist by Pablo Picasso: Art and Nursing

Jason Beasley, Senior BSN Nursing Student,
The University of Southern Mississippi

Art is a very powerful tool. It can express joy, hope, frustration, and many other human emotions in so many ways. Whether it is paint, crayon, clay, pencil, or charcoal, most people have a piece of art that they adore. *The Old Guitarist* by Pablo Picasso is the painting that I relate with health and grieving. The painting consists of an elderly man playing his guitar. The man's clothes are torn and dirty, but he plays. He looks like he does not have much longer to live, but he plays. His face tells a story of a hard life, but still he plays. To me, this painting symbolizes how people find ways to get through life. He looks as if he has nothing. I do not know what the history of the man was, but it looks as if he has endured his share of hardships. From what I see, he held on to his guitar—it is how he got through those hardships. He could have given up, just wasted away, but he has not. He is still playing—to play his guitar is to live.

My "guitar" is nature. There is nothing more enjoyable to me than going for a walk on a nature trail or through the woods. When my grandma died 3 years ago, I was torn apart. She was the first immediate family member of mine that passed away. I got very upset when I found out she had died. I left the house because I just did not want to be around anyone else at the time. I needed to be alone and process what was happening. I took a walk though the woods near our house as I had done so many times in my life. Walking through the woods, the trees, the birds, and the breeze . . . I just felt that everything had a reason. I am not a deeply religious person, but I am spiritual. I felt connected like I have never felt before. I reached one of the bigger pine trees, the one my niece had decided to decorate with ribbons. I sat down under the pine tree, and broke down into tears. How was I to deal with this, how was I supposed to deal with this? I did not understand death, was I supposed to understand death? I just did not understand why the physical body stopped and the spiritual soul was no longer here with me. I had so many questions that I knew nobody could answer. As I sat there, the breeze picked up again and I felt a sense of knowing. I knew that someone was out there keeping an eye on everything. I knew that my grandma was still with me, just not in physical form. And I knew that no matter what happened to me in the future or where I was, I could talk to her whenever I needed to. It was an awesome experience.

My grandpa passed away 2 weeks ago. Again, it was hard, but I knew how to deal with it a little better. It still was not easy, but my "guitar" this time was the Longleaf Trail. I rode my bicycle on the trail and just meditated on life. No, I did not find the secret to life, but I did find solace. I knew that I now had two people who truly loved me watching over me. That brought a peace to my soul that will never be replicated.

I feel that, like the guitarist in the painting, I need a "guitar" to hold on to. Everyone needs a "guitar" to support them through the tough times. Life is not fair or easy, but we must endure it. I cannot remember who said "the hardest thing in this world is to live in it," but the quote means more to me now. Rough things are going to come my way, as for us all, whether they are health, financial, or social problems. There is no way to avoid problems in life. You cannot just give up or pretend the problems are not there: Face the problems head on and keep your "guitar" close by. I hope that when I am older, I am still playing my "guitar." Not only to comfort myself, but to help others find their own "guitar."

Music therapy may focus on listening to music, moving to music, or participating in making music, either alone or with others. Community recreational drumming circles—an example of the latter—can be a therapeutic intervention in many community settings. Drumming has been a part of healing rituals in many cultures across the ages. Recreational drumming can promote self-expression, provide group support, decrease stress, enhance the immune system, and improve mood states (Bittman et al., 2001; Stevens, 2003).

Imagery

Imagery is a way of using the imagination and connecting with the more subtle aspects of inner experiences that may involve all senses—vision, taste, smell, touch, and hearing. Images, which can be considered a bridge between conscious processing of information and physiological change, can be produced by conscious as well as subconscious acts and may precede or follow physiological change (Dossey, B. M., 1997; Schaub & Dossey, 2005). Imagery enables access to our emotions and to our spiritual or higher self. Dossey (1997) describes several types of imagery: receptive, active, symbolic, process, correct biological, end-state, general healing, packaged, customized, and interactive guided imagery. Although nurses can use any type with patients to enhance their healing processes, they need to appreciate individual variations of images, colors, shapes, symbols, and meanings related to cultural diversity. Nurses can use imagery to help promote a sense of wellbeing with patients, encourage healthy behaviors, and help them modify their perceptions about their diseases, strengths, treatments, and healing capacities.

An example of a situation in which imagery can be incorporated into nursing care is with bone or wound healing. Before the session, in terms the patient can understand, the nurse describes the basic biological process involved in the healing. The imagery process begins with a relaxation exercise. While the patient is in a relaxed state, the nurse instructs the patient to imagine the natural process of healing that is occurring, helping the patient by quietly describing the elements of the healing process, and ultimately imagining oneself as fully healed and back to normal activities.

These techniques are used to release tension, teach the body to consciously produce the body's natural relaxation response (lower blood pressure and respiratory rates), reduce pain, and calm emotions. In the United States, the use of relaxation exercises is part of a comprehensive plan to treat, prevent, or reduce symptoms from an array of conditions, including stress, chronic pain and/or anxiety, insomnia, Irritable Bowel Syndrome (IBS), overactive bladder urges, nightmares linked to posttraumatic stress disorder (PTSD), depression, labor pains, cardiovascular disease, and side effects of chemotherapy (NCCAM, 2012).

Many resources are available for nurses who wish to develop skills in integrating imagery into nursing care (Achterberg, Dossey, & Kolkmeier, 1994; Dossey, B. M., 1997; Schaub & Dossey, 2005), including a nurses' certification program in interactive imagery sponsored by the AHNA and the Academy for Guided Imagery.

Herbal Therapies

Herbal and natural therapies, which have been used for healing in all cultures from before the time of written history, are becoming more common and are available in grocery stores and regular pharmacies. In fact, according to the 2007 NHIS, approximately 17% of adults use natural products including herbs, making this the most commonly used CAM therapy. The functions of herbal therapies range from the treatment, prevention, and/or alleviation of cancer, heart disease, diabetes, HIV/AIDS, food allergies, rheumatoid arthritis, and osteoarthritis (NCCAM, 2010). Although many natural and herbal preparations can enhance health and contribute to the prevention of disease, they are not necessarily safe just because they are natural (Duke, 1997; Murray, 1995). Because plants cannot be patented, limited research has been done in the United States on plants as medicinal agents, and there is a lack of standardization regarding the amount of the active ingredient of the plant that is in any particular herbal preparation (Murray, 1995). Although research on plants as medicinal agents is still in its infancy in this country, there is research to support the efficacy of many herbal and natural preparations (e.g., St. John's wort and Ginkgo biloba) that has been done in other countries (Murray & Pizzorno, 1998). Because many patients use herbs and other natural preparations, nurses need to become knowledgeable about common herbs, their uses, and potential interaction with pharmaceutical drugs.

For example, many people consider herbal supplements to be safe and without harmful effects because they are "natural." In reality, some herbal preparations can cause medical problems if they are used incorrectly, taken in large amounts, or taken with some pharmaceutical medications. Ephedra, for example, has been associated with increased blood pressure and stress to the circulatory system, causing sometimes fatal side effects. Because of this danger, dietary supplements containing ephedra have been banned by the FDA. Other supplements may have many health benefits and need to be used with careful consideration in only a few circumstances. For example, CoQ10 is made naturally by the body, helps cells produce energy, acts as an antioxidant, and stimulates the immune system. This dietary supplement can also reduce the body's response to the anticoagulant medication warfarin and can decrease insulin requirements for persons with diabetes (National Cancer Institute [NCI], 2014). People with these conditions who take CoQ10 must be carefully monitored.

Nurses need to ask about use of herbal and natural preparations in the same way they include discussion of other medications. Of particular importance is advising patients who take herbal preparations to read labels and buy only those that have standardized extracts of the active herb. Students are encouraged to explore the many good references available that discuss the healing benefits, side effects, and interactions of various herbal and natural preparations.

MEDIA MOMENT 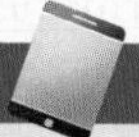

***Drumming on the Edge of Magic: A Journey into the Spirit of Percussion* (1990)**

—By Mickey Hart, with Jay Stevens,
New York, NY: HarperCollins

Mickey Hart, former drummer of the Grateful Dead, has written an illuminating history of drums from an insightful journey through ethnic drumming. The book is well referenced and documented, with research on the connection between drumming and human survival. This book is illustrated with ample photos and artwork from around the world and throughout history, including images of drumming circles and the various objects used for drumming. In this important seminal book on our human need for rhythm, Hart studies the emotional, spiritual, and physical effects of drums, ancient and new, on the human species. Those interested in incorporating drumming into wellness and health promotion will find this book an invaluable, classic resource.

Aromatherapy

Aromatherapy refers to the therapeutic use of the essential (concentrated) oils extracted from different parts of aromatic plants. The oils, which are widely available, may be applied to the body through massage or directly as a perfume, inhaled as mists, used as a compress, or mixed into an ointment. Although research on the health benefits of aromatherapy is in its infancy, use of this therapy shows promise in promoting relaxation; relieving stress, anxiety, pain, discomfort, insomnia, and restlessness; promoting wound healing; enhancing self-esteem; and stimulating immune function (Stevensen, 1996).

Researchers believe aromatherapy may work by sending chemical messages to the part of the brain that affects moods and emotions. Laboratory and animal studies have shown that certain essential oils have antibacterial, antifungal, antiviral, calming, or energizing effects. In addition, one study revealed that after essential oils were inhaled, markers of fragmented compounds were found in the bloodstream of the participants, suggesting that aromatherapy affects the body directly like a drug rather than indirectly such as through the central nervous system (NCI, 2012).

Although aromatic oils have been used for varied purposes for centuries, recent years have seen a resurgence in the use of aromatherapy among lay people as well as nurses. Robbins (1999) notes that aromatherapy is a safe therapy, with few adverse reactions reported in the literature, although its mechanisms of action and efficacy need further research. Robbins suggests that nurses who wish to consider using aromatherapy as an adjunct in nursing practice should have some formal training, use caution when using these oils with people with very sensitive skin or severe respiratory disorders, and be aware that most of these oils should not be ingested.

> If you can walk, you can dance. If you can talk, you can sing.
>
> —*Zimbabwe proverb*

Touch Therapy

Touch is essential for human survival and development. **Touch therapy** includes a broad range of hand techniques that a nurse can use on or near the body to support the patient's movement toward balance, wholeness, and optimal functioning (Keegan & Shames, 2005; Shames, 1997). Touch interventions used by nurses include both physical and energetic healing modalities such as therapeutic massage, TT, HT, acupressure, shiatsu, and reflexology. Massage (particularly of the back) has long been considered an important nursing intervention used to promote relaxation, relieve muscle discomfort, and stimulate circulation. Many books and educational programs are available for nurses who want to expand their skills with therapeutic massage.

TT, a noninvasive healing technique developed by a nurse, Dr. Delores Krieger (1979), involves touching with conscious intent to heal. In TT, the nurse works from a centered state using the natural sensitivity of the hands to assess the patient's energy fields and treat imbalances. HT (Hover-Kramer, 2001) is a collection of energy-based healing techniques, which, like TT, are noninvasive. The HT practitioner also works from a centered state to assist in making energy available to patients through application of systemic and localized techniques. In addition to promoting relaxation, decreasing anxiety, and balancing energy, research suggests that these therapies can enhance immune functioning (Olson et al., 1997), promote wound healing (Wirth, 1992), and decrease pain sensation (Lin & Taylor, 1998; Smith, 2001). Continuing education workshops, academic courses, and certification programs are available for nurses who wish to develop skills in these modalities. Acupressure, shiatsu, and reflexology are systems that use the application of pressure (with fingers, thumbs, or a blunt instrument) to specific points along energy pathways (meridians) of the body (acupressure and shiatsu) or in the feet or hands (reflexology). Continuing education workshops and certification programs are also available for nurses who wish to study these modalities.

DAY IN THE LIFE

In considering caring in the community, perhaps a case can be made for pure caring, in that it is noninstitutional, real-living situations in the community where the most authentic and yet demanding aspects of personal–professional caring become manifest. What the nurse offers first, by way of establishing relationship-centered care, is self: By this I mean bring one's whole self into the present. It is from this professional and philosophical orientation that authentic caring can be witnessed and experienced at its finest.

—Jean Watson, PhD, RN, FAAN, HNC, Distinguished Professor of Nursing, Endowed Chair in Caring Science, University of Colorado Health Sciences Center, Denver, Colorado

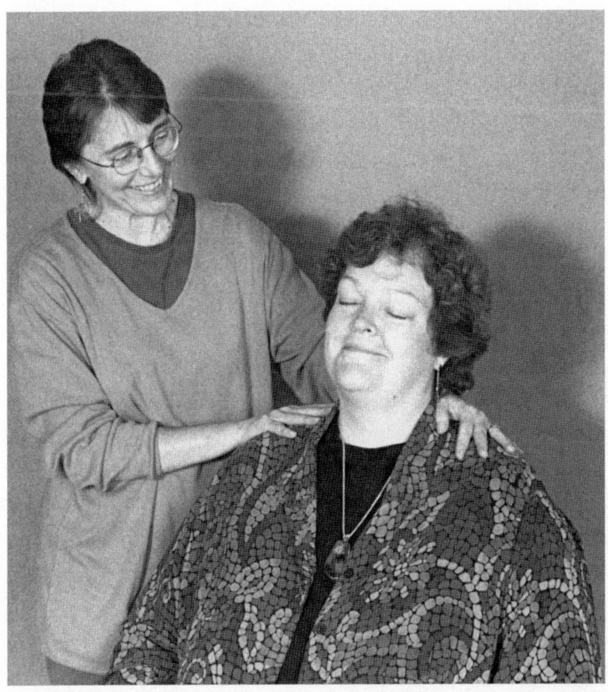

Dr. Margaret A. Burkhardt, chapter author, demonstrating healing touch with a patient.

Potential Barriers to Use of Complementary Therapies

Professional integrity requires nurses to take an honest look at potential barriers that may limit availability of and access to complementary therapies for patients and that may hinder the research into complementary therapies. Dossey and Swyers (1994) suggest that barriers to use of complementary therapies can be structural in nature or can relate to regulatory, economic, and belief systems. Structural barriers include problems caused by a lack of common classification systems and definitions between biomedicine and complementary modalities, difficulty in obtaining original research on complementary therapies because they are not published in English in scientifically reviewed literature, and lack of understanding of culturally based explanatory models. For example, a family may wish to obtain more information about the efficacy of an herbal preparation that they heard may help with their mother's chronic illness, but the major research is published in Chinese or German. Regulatory and economic barriers include current federal mechanisms for regulating medical research, which do not favor the evaluation of many forms of complementary treatments; the cost of conducting the necessary laboratory and clinical trials of a product or procedure; and the existence of state medical practice acts that limit the practice of healing arts to holders of medical licenses. An example of this barrier is the limited access to naturopathic physicians because they are not licensed in most states.

Belief barriers include ideological skepticism flowing from comfort with the status quo, belief that high-technology interventions are more effective, and attitudes that any modality other than biomedicine is unscientific.

These barriers include attitudes of conventional practitioners that consider use of herbal preparations, for example, rather than a medical intervention to be a waste of money because they have not been "scientifically" studied, even when the patient is experiencing benefit from the preparations. Although the work of NCCAM and other organizations is helping reduce these barriers, nurses need to be alert for situations in which patients experience limited access to or availability of complementary modalities (Cuellar, Cochran, et al., 2003).

The power relationship between the nurse and the patient can present barriers to the patient's use of complementary therapies. The nurse is in a role of power and authority derived from professional knowledge and skills. Persisting paternalistic attitudes within healthcare settings, which foster the dependent role for patients, may manifest as attitudes indicating that approaches to managing health concerns other than those proposed by the nurse are unacceptable and without sound basis. Consider, for example, a nurse who is very willing to support the physician's recommendation of surgery or strong narcotics for the management of severe pain but who is unwilling to discuss the patient's interest in trying acupuncture, declaring that such approaches are unreliable. When nurses assume that a patient's values and thought processes are the same as their own, they may believe that the only reasonable courses of action are those that they as nurses would choose. Such attitudes may prompt nurses to question the decision-making capacity of patients who choose complementary therapies in lieu of or in addition to conventional therapies or label them as noncompliant, both of which can present barriers to the patient's use of therapies that may enhance the healing process.

Complementary Health and Community Nursing Practice

Community health nurses must remember that decisions about health care are based on more than scientific expertise. Healthcare choices are influenced by a person's values, culture, and spiritual and other beliefs; evaluation of risks, benefits, and economic considerations; and effects on lifestyle and role. All of these areas must be considered in deliberations about health care. Cassidy (1996) writes, "cultural relativity is pivotal to the study of alternative medicine, because each alternative system of medicine provides a different set of ideas about the body, disease, and medical reality" (p. 12). Community nurses need to be particularly attentive to the influence of culture because emotional, psychological, aesthetic, interpersonal, and other dimensions of health concerns differ across cultures and belief systems, impelling certain actions and constraining others (Cuellar, Aycock, Cahill, & Ford, 2003; Cuellar, Cochran, et al.; 2003; O'Connor, 1996). Our culture teaches us the meaning of health; how to be sick; and when, how, and from whom to seek care.

Community nurses must be aware of the values, goals, and beliefs of personal culture (their own and that of their patients) as well as the culture of the biomedical system and of other healing systems as they develop healthcare plans with patients. With this awareness, nurses can be more alert for potential conflicts and negative value judgments that may interfere with integrating complementary modalities into care. Consider, for example, a situation in which a nurse learns that her patient with fibromyalgia is using herbs and vitamins recommended by a layperson who used kinesiology to determine what the patient needed. Recognizing that the culture of the biomedical system would find this process unscientific alerts the nurse to potential negative value judgments from the patient's biomedical practitioner regarding her choice and enables the nurse to consider ways to assist the patient in integrating the different modalities. Patients are more likely to discuss their complementary health practices with nurses who approach them with an openness to exploring and including different modalities in care than they are with nurses who place judgments on such modalities.

> They may forget what you said, but they will never forget how you made them feel.
>
> —*Carl N. Buechner*

The Right to Choose

Professional standards and codes of ethics direct nurses to respect each person and to value and support patient autonomy. Basic to autonomy are the ability to determine personal goals, the ability to decide on a plan of action, and the freedom to act on one's choice. Consequently, the principle of patient self-determination directs nurses to honor the right of persons to use modalities outside the realm of biomedicine in addressing their healthcare needs. When such choices are made, nurses may find it challenging to honor and respect the convictions derived from belief systems that underlie these choices, particularly when these beliefs are not understood or are contrary to their own. However, to deny such convictions in healthcare settings is "to deny the patient's very reality, sometimes risking serious psychological and emotional impact on patient and family alike, and always raising genuine ethical concerns about patient autonomy, provider beneficence, substituted judgment, and distributive justice" (O'Connor, 1996, p. 93). Attentiveness to patient values and desires for treatment options requires nurses to take seriously the patient's need for healing in addition to curing, and the contributions to health offered by other explanatory models. When nurses do not understand the other modality or question the efficacy or safety of the choice, they must explore these considerations with the patient. A nonjudgmental approach that is respectful of differing values and beliefs and alert for ethnocentric bias on the part of the nurse enhances joint exploration (Burkhardt & Nathaniel, 1996, 2002; Robison & Carrier, 2004).

DAY IN THE LIFE

BSN Nurse, Staff at an Inpatient Hospice Center

I work in a 12-bed, inpatient hospice center and consider holistic care to be critical in this specific setting. Our philosophy as a facility supports my holistic values, and we use music, poetry, art, garden walks, guided imagery, and meditation in our work with patients and their friends and family. Each room looks out to a garden setting and has ample artwork, which has been carefully chosen for color and comfort. I particularly enjoy working with music therapy, asking the patient and family for their favorite music, and then securing our two guitarists to play for the patients. I believe that patients who are in the last stages of their lives and who cannot communicate in any other way respond to music as a special healing intervention. I recall a patient with advanced cancer who was in late stage and was noncommunicative, slipping in and out of consciousness. Her family told me that she loved the music of the Beatles. The two guitarists played a few of her favorite songs and the patient actually mouthed the words to one song that I recall, "The Long and Winding Road." It was a moment I will hold dear to my heart always.

Nursing Assessment

To have a broad picture of the many factors affecting a patient's health and healing, nurses need to be aware of the various therapies being considered or used by patients. Community nurses need to develop the ability to incorporate discussion of complementary therapies into their nursing assessment in an open way, because patients may be hesitant to bring up the subject. Discussion may be prompted through open-ended questions such as "What do you do to take care of your health on your own?", "What other things have you tried (or thought about trying) for this health concern?", and "Sometimes people with your condition want to try other remedies, and I wonder if this is something that you have considered?" Another approach to opening a discussion of complementary therapies is to explore the use of specific modalities commonly used in your area with questions such as "Have you ever seen a (chiropractor, acupuncturist, herbalist, etc.) for that problem?", "Have you considered seeing the (*curandera*, medicine person, spiritual healer, etc.)?", or "Have you been using (special vitamins, a macrobiotic diet, herbal remedies, etc.) for your illness?"

Nurses must be knowledgeable about various modalities and therapies to effectively discuss their use with patients. Because of this, many nursing programs are now including courses on CAM and offering programs of study in holistic nursing (Fenton & Morris, 2003). Nurses need not subscribe to particular complementary therapies to effectively assess how patients use these therapies. Neither do nurses need to be practitioners of other modalities to discuss them with patients, any more than they need to be able to do surgery to discuss it. However, community nurses must be able to create an atmosphere that encourages a nonjudgmental assessment of all modalities being considered or used, with a goal of using whatever is beneficial for and will meet the needs of the patient and family (Cuellar et al., 2007).

Community nurses should become familiar with and develop at least a talking knowledge of complementary therapies that may be commonly used in their communities to be better able to discuss their use with their patients. Public education regarding CAM is essential to provide people with information on the risks and benefits of these therapies in the same way that risks and benefits of conventional therapies are discussed. Many therapies work as adjuncts to biomedical interventions, some may interact in unhealthy ways with particular biomedical treatments, and the efficacy of many modalities is not fully known.

When discussing choices with patients, nurses should draw on studies with which they are familiar in offering relevant information regarding particular therapies, allowing clinical and personal experience into the conversation in judicious ways, yet recognizing that the nurse never has all the pertinent information and that uncertainty is inherent in health choices (Hufford, 1996b). Based on their assessment and knowledge regarding particular therapies, nurses may find it appropriate to support or recommend some complementary modalities while discouraging the use of others.

Hufford (1996b) suggests that the patient has major responsibility for obtaining information regarding complementary therapies and making health choices in this regard. However, nurses need to have some knowledge about risks and benefits associated with these therapies. For example, although garlic may assist in lowering cholesterol, large doses can cause irritation to the digestive tract, which may result in some bleeding. Nurses should encourage patients to explore the validity of claims made about particular therapies and assist them in doing so, especially

MEDIA MOMENT

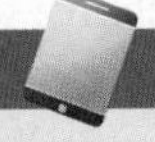

The Fisher King (1991)

A talk DJ inadvertently convinces a psychotic man to blow away restaurant patrons and himself when the psychotic man calls in for advice. After 3 years of wallowing in his remorse, he is attacked and almost set on fire, but a street person rescues him. The DJ finds out the transient is on a mission to find the Holy Grail and tries to repay his kindness with money. The transient has more hands-on assistance in mind and tries to convince the DJ to help him in his quest for the Grail.

if the nurse perceives the therapy to be potentially harmful for the patient. However, complementary modalities should not be discounted merely because they are not understood within the Western biomedical framework. When patients are interested in complementary therapies, nurses should help determine whether risks are involved. When the potential for significant risks exists and the patient is committed to using the therapy, the nursing goal is to minimize risks while maximizing treatment. If the patient does not have a strong commitment to the complementary modality, nurses should encourage ongoing discussion of known risks and benefits related to various options (Hufford, 1996a). As part of their assessments, nurses need to determine the congruency between patient and nursing goals regarding healing and curing; they also should review options considered viable by each as a means of meeting these goals. Maintaining an openness to working with traditional systems and their healers facilitates more effective and culturally congruent nursing and health care.

Conclusion

This chapter has discussed the use of complementary therapies within a holistic nursing frame of reference. Nurses must be aware that many people use complementary therapies in addition to biomedical interventions but often do not disclose this fact to their biomedical practitioners. Complementary modalities encompass all health systems, modalities, and practices other than those intrinsic to the politically dominant health system of a particular society or culture. Such therapies include all practices and ideas self-defined by their users as preventing or treating illness or promoting health and wellbeing. Many complementary modalities are based in cultural healing practices, which derive from different explanatory models than those of biomedicine.

Nurses need to be attentive to patient values and desires for treatment options, taking seriously the patient's need for healing as well as curing and the contributions to health offered by other explanatory models. If nurses do not understand the other modality or question the efficacy or safety of the choice, they should explore these considerations with the patient. Nurses need to be aware of the various therapies being considered or used by patients so that they are aware of the many factors affecting a patient's health and healing. Community nurses need to develop the ability to incorporate discussion of complementary therapies into assessment in an open way and work toward integration of complementary therapies with conventional interventions. Holistic nursing care implies attentiveness to spiritual concerns as well as to physical and emotional concerns. Prayer, imagery, music therapy, and touch therapy are examples of complementary modalities that can be incorporated into health care with patients in the community.

LEVELS OF PREVENTION

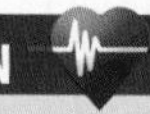

Primary: Teaching meditation techniques to class of pregnant parents

Secondary: Screening adults for hypertension and develop biofeedback classes for those at risk

Tertiary: Conducting yoga for adults with debilitating arthritis

HEALTHY ME

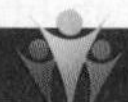

How do you calm down when faced with a stressful situation in nursing school (tests, clinical situations, etc.)? Try the approaches detailed in this chapter, such as meditation, relaxation exercises, and yoga to reduce the hazards of stress as a nurse.

Critical Thinking Activities

1. Explore the history, current practice, and research of a selected healing system other than biomedical medicine.
   - Compare and contrast the selected healing system with biomedical modalities relative to the explanatory model.
   - How are practitioners of the selected healing system educated, trained, and/or certified?
   - What are the roles of the practitioner and the patient in the selected healing system?
   - Describe how the selected healing system focuses on healing and curing.
2. Shawn is an outpatient oncology nurse who has cared for 32-year-old Kim during her 4 years of living with breast cancer. Kim has endured surgery and radiation and is currently undergoing another course of chemotherapy for recently discovered metastasis. Kim tells Shawn that she thinks the medical therapies are only making her sicker and that she has been doing a lot of reading about other ways of dealing with cancer. Kim says she is seriously considering discontinuing chemotherapy treatments and seeking healing through prayer and herbal remedies. She also indicates that she knows God can heal, but that if she is to die, she would rather die with dignity than be stuck in a hospital attached to machines. It is clear from what Kim says that she has

thoughtfully considered the various options with their risks and benefits. Shawn tells the physician about Kim's plans; the physician exclaims that Kim is "out of her mind" and suggests that family members be enlisted to persuade Kim to continue with conventional interventions.

- What do you think of Kim's plan?
- What personal values are evident in Kim's decision? How do you think you would respond if you were in Kim's situation?
- How can Shawn respond to Kim in a way that demonstrates respect for persons and supports her autonomy?
- What perspective is reflected in the physician's response?
- What ethical conflicts might occur?
- How might the nurse determine whether the family feels coerced?
- How do you think a holistic nurse would approach Kim and her care?

3. Talk with someone who uses a complementary health modality on a regular basis. Discuss why they use the modality, the benefits of the modality, whether they discuss the therapy with biomedical practitioners, the cost, and how they pay for the modality.

References

Achterberg, J., Dossey, B. M., & Kolkmeier, L. (1994). *Rituals of healing*. New York, NY: Bantam Books.

American Holistic Nurses Association. (2014). *What is holistic nursing?* Retrieved from http://www.ahna.org/About-Us/What-is-Holistic-Nursing

Barnes, P. M., Bloom, B., & Nahin, R. L. (2008). Complementary and alternative medicine use among adults and children, 2007. *National Health Statistical Report*, 10(12), 1–23.

Bennett, M. P., Zeller, J. M., Rosenberg, L., & McCann, J. (2003). The effect of mirthful laughter on stress and natural killer cell activity. *Alternative Therapies in Health and Medicine, 9*(2), 38–45.

Bittman, B. B., Berk, L. S., Felton, D. L., Westengard, J., Simonton, O. C., Pappas, J., & Ninehouser, M. (2001). Composite effects of group drumming music therapy on modulation of neuroendocrine-immune parameters in normal subjects. *Alternative Therapies in Health and Medicine, 7*(1), 38–47.

Burkhardt, M. A. (1985). Nursing, health and wholeness. *Journal of Holistic Nursing, 3*(1), 35–36.

Burkhardt, M. A., & Nagai-Jacobson, M. G. (1997a). Psychospiritual care: A shared journey embracing life and wholeness. *Bioethics Forum, 13*(4), 34–41.

Burkhardt, M. A., & Nagai-Jacobson, M. G. (1997b). Spirituality and healing. In B. M. Dossey (Ed.), *Core curriculum for holistic nursing* (pp. 42–51). Gaithersburg, MD: Aspen.

Burkhardt, M. A., & Nagai-Jacobson, M. G. (2002). *Spirituality: Living our connectedness*. Albany, NY: Delmar.

Burkhardt, M. A., & Nagai-Jacobson, M. G. (2005). Spirituality and health. In B. M. Dossey, L. Keegan, & C. E. Guzzetta (Eds.), *Holistic nursing practice* (4th ed., pp. 137–172). Sudbury, MA: Jones and Bartlett.

Burkhardt, M. A., & Nathaniel, A. K. (1996). Patient self-determination and complementary care. *Bioethics Forum, 12*, 24–30.

Burkhardt, M. A., & Nathaniel, A. K. (2002). *Ethics and issues in contemporary nursing* (2nd ed.). Albany, NY: Delmar.

Cassidy, C. M. (1996). Cultural context of complementary and alternative medicine systems. In M. S. Micozzi (Ed.), *Fundamentals of complementary and alternative medicine*. New York, NY: Churchill Livingstone.

Cuellar, N. (2005). Hypnosis for pain management in the older adult. *Pain Management Nursing, 6*(3), 105–111.

Cuellar, N., Aycock, T., Cahill, B., & Ford, J. (2003). The use of complementary and alternative medicine by African American and Caucasian American elders in a rural setting: A descriptive, comparative study. *BMC Journal of Complementary and Alternative Medicine, 3*(8).

Cuellar, N., Cochran, S., Ladner, C., Mercier, B., Townsend, A., Harbaugh, B., & Douglas, D. (2003). Depression and the use of conventional and non-conventional interventions of rural patients: A descriptive, comparative study. *Journal of the American Psychiatric Nurses Association, 9*(5), 151–158.

Cuellar, N. G., Rogers, A. E., & Hisghman, V. (2007). Sleep in the older adult: Evidenced-based research in complementary and alternative medicine (CAM). *Geriatric Nursing, 28*(1), 46–52.

Dossey, B. M. (1997). Imagery. In B. M. Dossey (Ed.), *Core curriculum for holistic nursing* (pp. 188–195). Gaithersburg, MD: Aspen.

Dossey, B. M., & Guzzetta, C. E. (2005). Holistic nursing practice. In B. M. Dossey, L. Keegan, & C. E. Guzzetta (Eds.), *Holistic nursing: A handbook for practice* (4th ed., pp. 5–37). Sudbury, MA: Jones and Bartlett.

Dossey, L. (1993). *Healing words*. New York, NY: HarperCollins.

Dossey, L. (1996). *Prayer is good medicine*. San Francisco, CA: HarperCollins.

Dossey, L. (1997). The return of prayer. *Alternative Therapies in Health and Medicine, 3*, 10–17, 113–120.

Dossey, L. (1998). *Be careful what you pray for . . . you just might get it*. San Francisco, CA: HarperCollins.

Dossey, L., & Swyers, J. P. (1994). Introduction. In National Institutes of Health, *Alternative medicine: Expanding medical horizons* (NIH Publication No. 94-066). Washington, DC: U.S. Government Printing Office.

Duke, J. A. (1997). *The green pharmacy*. Emmaus, PA: Rodale.

Dunn, K. S., & Horgas, A. L. (2000). The prevalence of prayer as a spiritual self-care modality in elders. *Journal of Holistic Nursing, 18*, 337–351.

Eisenberg, D. M., Kessler, R. C., Foster, C., Norlock, F. E., Calkins, D. R., & Delbanco, T. L. (1993). Unconventional medicine in the United States. *New England Journal of Medicine, 328*, 246–252.

Eisenberg, D. M., Rogers, B. D., Ettner, S., Appel, S., Wilkey, S., Van Rompay, M., & Kessler, R. C. (1998). Trends in alternative medicine use in the United States, 1990–1997. *Journal of the American Medical Association, 280*(18), 1569–1575.

Emmons, R. A., & McCullough, M. E. (2003). Counting blessings versus burdens: An experimental investigation of gratitude and subjective well-being in daily life. *Journal of Personality & Social Psychology, 84*(2), 377–389.

Fenton, M. V., & Morris, D. L. (2003). The integration of holistic nursing practices and complementary and alternative modalities into curricula of schools of nursing. *Alternative Therapies in Health and Medicine, 9*(4), 62–67.

Gordon, J. S. (1980). The paradigm of holistic medicine. In A. Hastings (Ed.), *Health for the whole person* (pp. 31–45). Boulder, CO: Westview Press.

Gordon, J. S. (2002). The White House Commission on Complementary and Alternative Medicine Policy: Final report and next steps. *Alternative Therapies in Health and Medicine, 8*(3), 28–31.

Guzzetta, C. E. (1997). Music therapy. In B. M. Dossey (Ed.), *Core curriculum for holistic nursing* (pp. 196–204). Gaithersburg, MD: Aspen.

Guzzetta, C. E. (2005). Music therapy. In B. M. Dossey, L. Keegan, & C. E. Guzzetta (Eds.), *Holistic nursing: A handbook for practice* (4th ed., pp. 617–640). Sudbury, MA: Jones and Bartlett.

Hover-Kramer, D. (2001). *Healing touch: A guidebook for practitioners* (2nd ed.). New York, NY: Delmar.

Hufford, D. J. (1996a). Ethical dimensions of alternative medicine. Presentation at the First Annual Alternative Therapies Symposium: Creating Integrated Healthcare. San Diego, CA, January 18–21.

Hufford, D. J. (1996b). Informed consent and alternative medicine. *Alternative Therapies in Health and Medicine, 2*, 76–78.

Ikedo, F., Gangahar, D. M., Quader, M. A., & Smith, L. M. (2007). The effects of prayer, relaxation technique during general anesthesia on recovery outcomes following cardiac surgery. *Complementary Therapy and Clinical Practice, 13*(2), 85–94.

Keegan, L., & Shames, K. H. (2005). Touch. In B. M. Dossey, L. Keegan, & C. E. Guzzetta (Eds.), *Holistic nursing: A handbook for practice* (4th ed., pp. 643–666). Sudbury, MA: Jones and Bartlett.

Krieger, D. (1979). *The therapeutic touch*. Englewood Cliffs, NJ: Prentice Hall.

Lin, Y. S., & Taylor, A. G. (1998). Effects of therapeutic touch in reducing pain and anxiety in an elderly population. *Integrative Medicine, 1*(4), 155–162.

Lowry, L. W., & Conco, D. (2002). Exploring the meaning of spirituality with aging adults in Appalachia. *Journal of Holistic Nursing, 20*(4), 388–402.

Meisenhelder, J. B., & Chandler, E. N. (2000). Prayer and health outcomes in church members. *Alternative Therapies in Health and Medicine, 6*, 56–60.

Micozzi, M. S. (1996). *Fundamentals of alternative and complementary medicine*. New York, NY: Churchill Livingstone.

Murray, M. (1995). *The healing power of herbs* (2nd ed.). Rocklin, CA: Prima.

Murray, M., & Pizzorno, J. (1998). *The encyclopedia of natural medicine* (2nd ed.). Rocklin, CA: Prima.

National Cancer Institute. (2012). Aromatherapy and essential oils (PDQ). Retrieved from http://www.cancer.gov/cancertopics/pdq/cam/aromatherapy/healthprofessional/

National Cancer Institute. (2014). Coenzyme CQ10. Retrieved from http://www.cancer.gov/cancertopics/pdq/cam/coenzymeQ10

National Center for Complementary and Alternative Medicine (NCCAM). (2010). Meditation: An introduction. Retrieved from http://nccam.nih.gov/health/meditation/overview.htm

National Center for Complementary and Alternative Medicine (NCCAM). (2012). Time to talk. Retrieved from http://nccam.nih.gov/timetotalk/forpatients.htm

National Center for Complementary and Alternative Medicine (NCCAM). (2013). Health information. Retrieved from http://nccam.nih.gov/health

O'Connor, B. B. (1996). Medical ethics and patient belief systems. *Alternative Therapies in Health and Medicine, 2*, 92–93.

Olson, M., Sneed, N., LaVia, M., Virella, G., Bonadonna, R., & Michel, Y. (1997). Stress-induced immunosuppression and therapeutic touch. *Alternative Therapies in Health and Medicine, 3*(2), 68–74.

Quinn, J. F. (1989). On healing, wholeness, and the Haelan effect. *Nursing and Health Care, 10*, 553–556.

Robbins, J. L. W. (1999). The science and art of aromatherapy. *Journal of Holistic Nursing, 17*(1), 5–17.

Robison, J., & Carrier, K. (2004). *Spirit and science of holistic health: More than broccoli, jogging, and bottled water. . . More than yoga, herbs, and meditation*. Bloomington, IN: AuthorHouse.

Schaub, B. G., & Dossey, B. M. (2005). Imagery. In B. M. Dossey, L. Keegan, & C. E. Guzzetta (Eds.), *Holistic nursing: A handbook for practice* (4th ed., pp. 567–614). Sudbury, MA: Jones and Bartlett.

Shames, K. H. (1997). Touch. In B. M. Dossey (Ed.), *Core curriculum for holistic nursing* (pp. 205–210). Gaithersburg, MD: Aspen.

Sierpina, V. S. (2002). Progress notes: A review of educational developments in CAM. *Alternative Therapies in Health and Medicine, 8*(8), 104–106.

Simonton, O. C., Cohen, D., Kumar, M., McKinney, C., & Tims, F. (1997). Music as a healing force. Presented at Second Annual Alternative Therapies Symposium: Creating Integrated Healthcare, Orlando, FL.

Smith, D. W. (2001). Pattern changes in people experiencing therapeutic touch, Phase II. Pandimensional pattern changes in healers and healees in a therapeutic touch series. *Rogerian Nursing Science News Online, 1*(1), 4–6.

Stevens, C. K. (2003). *The art and heart of drum circles*. Milwaukee, WI: Hal Leonard.

Stevensen, C. J. (1996). Aromatherapy. In M. S. Micozzi (Ed.), *Fundamentals of alternative and complementary medicine* (pp. 137–148). New York, NY: Churchill Livingstone.

U.S. Food and Drug Administration (FDA). (2014). Q & A on dietary supplements. Retrieved from http://www.fda.gov/food/dietarysupplements/qadietarysupplements/

Walton, J., & Sullivan, N. (2004). Men of prayer: Spirituality of men with prostate cancer. *Journal of Holistic Nursing, 22*, 133–151.

Wirth, D. (1992). The effect of non-contact therapeutic touch on the healing rate of full thickness dermal wounds. *Subtle Energies, 1*, 1–20.

CHAPTER FOCUS

Theoretical Bases
- Concepts
- Learning Theory
- Behavior Change Theory

The Health Education Process
- Assessment
- Planning
- Implementation
- Evaluation

Health Education in Communities
- Individuals, Families, and Groups
- Community
- Beyond Community

Ethical Issues in Health Education

QUESTIONS TO CONSIDER

After reading this chapter, you will know the answers to the following questions:

1. What is health education, and how does it differ in community settings?
2. What are behavioral concepts and theories in education?
3. How are behavioral concepts and theories used to provide direction for health education programs?
4. What are principles of education, and how can they be integrated into health education practice?
5. What are the various situations in community health nursing in which education for behavior change can be incorporated into nursing care at the individual, families, group, and community levels?
6. What are the ethical issues in health education that have emerged from the current healthcare environment?
7. How does health literacy play a part in the dynamics of health education?
8. How does cultural competency affect the way you teach?
9. What is the role of the nurse in shaping health behaviors of the learner?

CHAPTER 17

Health Education in the Community

Betty Sylvest and Lucy Bradley-Springer

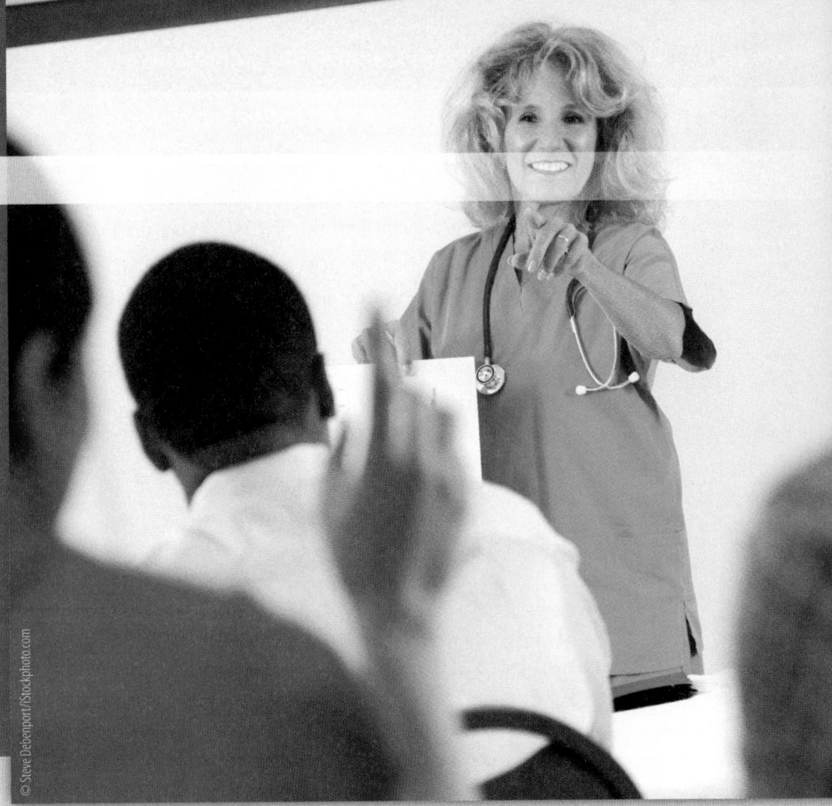

KEY TERMS

absolutism
adherence
advocacy
autonomy
barriers
behavior change
behavior change theories
benefits
cognitive dissonance
community-based teaching
discharge teaching
domains of learning
empowerment
health education
health literacy
learning goals and objectives
learning theories
motivation
paternalism
readiness
self-efficacy
teaching

> Be careful how you pronounce health promotion, lest the listener believe self-promotion to be your objective.
>
> —Mohan Singh

> Be careful of reading health books, you might die of a misprint.
>
> —Mark Twain

REFLECTIONS

You may ask, "Why should I teach? Why would I want to change people's behaviors? I went to nursing school to give patient care, not to teach. If I had wanted to teach, I would not have spent all this time learning to insert catheters and how to complete care plans." Teaching is essential to effective nursing care of individual patients, families, and communities. Teaching improves a population's health. Education positively influences health outcomes when patients experience fewer complications and faster recoveries; learn to care for themselves, increasing autonomy, accountability, and self-confidence; and are better prepared to resume their lives in a healthier state. Think about your own experiences. How do you learn best? Was it in a classroom or clinical setting? How did the teacher interact with the students?

> Wisdom is not a product of schooling, but the lifelong attempt to acquire it.
>
> —*Albert Einstein*

THE PURPOSE OF HEALTH education is to change behaviors that put people at risk for injury, disease, disability, or death. This may sound blunt, but whether you call it modifying behavior or influencing behavior (Rankin & Stallings, 2001, Rankin, Stallings, & London, 2005), it all boils down to the same thing: Nurses teach patients, families, groups, and communities with the primary goal of helping people to change behaviors in ways that focus on disease prevention, risk reduction, illness intervention, and health promotion. The mission of health education is to "reduce current and future suffering" by addressing "individual and social factors that contribute to health problems" (Guttman, Kegler, & McLeroy, 1996, p. i). This chapter explores the topic of health education: its theoretical bases, its application, the problems associated with it, and the community health nurse's role in health education.

Health education can increase the knowledge, skills, and confidence needed to make decisions about one's health. It improves continuity of care, decreases the risk of problem recurrence, and uses resources more efficiently. Educated patients and their families are better able to cope and more likely to recognize problems before they become severe. All of these benefits help nurses do their jobs because knowledgeable patients have fewer complications and present with fewer of the acute emergencies that require more complex care (Hunt, 1997). With the passage of the Affordable Care Act (ACA), health education will no longer be an optional intervention. All health organizations will be required to provide appropriate health education in order to remain financially viable.

While being prepared to offer much-needed education for individuals or groups, the healthcare provider must keep in mind the confidentiality of the person's health information. Electronic Medical Records (EMR) provide easy access to the person's past medical and educational records. The healthcare providers must keep in mind the number of individuals who have access to these records. Confidentiality is taught and mentored to nursing students from the beginning of their education. Patient privacy is taught throughout the curriculums. Students are taught about the Health Insurance Portability and Accountability Act of 1996 (HIPAA). Students must also be taught about the Health Information Technology for Economic and Clinical Health Act (HITECH Act or "The Act"). The ACT is part of the American Recovery and Reinvestment Act of 2009 (ARRA).

ARRA contains incentives related to health care information technology in general (e.g., creation of a national healthcare infrastructure) and contains specific incentives designed to accelerate the adoption of electronic health record (EHR) systems among providers. Because this legislation anticipates a massive expansion in the exchange of electronic protected health information (ePHI), the HITECH Act also widens the scope of privacy and security protections available under HIPAA; it increases the potential legal liability for noncompliance; and it provides for more enforcement (Health and Human Services HIPAA Survival Guide, 2013).

Educational literacy does not reflect health literacy. In a society where health insurance is not accessible to all, patient education that fits within the cultural beliefs and focuses on the healthcare literacy of the population within that cultural arena can decrease recidivism to primary care providers and ultimately to healthier lifestyles. The inability to read healthcare instructions leads to partial compliance/noncompliance with health care and leads to disparities in health care. **Health literacy** is defined as: "the degree to which individuals have the capacity to obtain, process and understand basic health information and services needed to make appropriate health decisions" (American Medical Association [AMA], 2007).

Heinrich (2010) poses that poor health status, adverse medical outcomes, ineffective management of chronic disease, and increased healthcare costs have been associated with low health literacy.

Initially, health education concentrated on crisis management ("What do you need to know now that you've got a colostomy?"). However, the healthcare system in the United States is evolving. The emphasis is now on cost containment, health maintenance, and managed care (Damrosch, 1991). Over the past decade, health education has had to adjust to support patient care in the midst of all these changes. Today health education includes disease prevention ("How do you keep from getting tuberculosis?" or "How can you decrease your risk of a stroke from hypertension?") and health promotion ("How can you change to a healthier diet?") in addition to continuing to deal with acute care issues.

Nurses do not have the luxury of relying on the saying "No time to teach" (London, 2012) as this is an integral part of the *Healthy People 2020* commission from the Office of the Assistant Secretary of Health (ASH). Financial cutbacks have led to decreased numbers of nurses to care for more acutely ill patients. Finding the time to do a thorough assessment of patient knowledge base as well as their health literacy levels is difficult at the least and impossible at the worst. Too frequently patients are sent home with printed discharge plans and instruction without the assessment of not only knowledge but an understanding of the instructions (London, 2012).

Healthy People 2020 provides a comprehensive set of national goals and objectives aimed at improving the health of all Americans for the 10-year period ending in 2020. Within the propositions of *Healthy People 2020*, there are 42 topic areas with nearly 600 objectives in which 1,200 measures are involved. As part of *Healthy People 2020*, a subset of factors called the Leading Health Indicators (LHI) have been identified as reflecting high-priority health issues and actions (see http://healthypeople.gov/2020/default.aspx).

APPLICATION TO PRACTICE 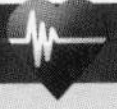

Case Study in Culturally Sensitive Health Literacy

Mr. Blanco is a married, 65-year-old Puerto Rican male who is an elementary school custodian. He dropped out of school at the age of 13 because he had to work to help support his family when his father died from uncontrolled hypertension. Mr. Blanco's reading skills in Spanish and English are weak. Mr. Blanco's son Manuel has interpreted for him during health visits in the past, but Manuel no longer lives at home and could not be reached.

Mr. Blanco was hospitalized related to an acute myocardial infarction. Staff gave him discharge instructions in written form (Spanish and English), and he was told to read about his new medication.

A short time later, Mr. Blanco was admitted to the emergency department via ambulance with bloody urine and black, tarry stools. Tests indicated Mr. Blanco had experienced a hemorrhagic stroke.

What could the nurse have done to help prevent this serious event? Did Mr. Blanco receive appropriate education? How did the healthcare system fail Mr. Blanco in relation to his learning needs?

Culturally Sensitive Teaching and Learning

Although nurses are not the only healthcare professionals who have patient teaching responsibilities, the knowledge, skills, and access to patients, especially in the community, make them particularly well suited to this complex task (Spellbring, 1991). Multiple disciplines interact with multiple culturally diverse groups. These groups are not only ethnically diverse but include those who have disabilities (physical or mental), those suffering from crisis-related situations such as returning military personnel, as well as gender-specific medical and mental health (gay, lesbian, transgender, etc.). The importance of understanding the cultures (and subcultures, i.e., African American, male, transgender) of those individuals receiving the teaching/learning is to allow nurses to build an educational plan that is best suited to the individual encompassing all aspects of the person (learner). There are too many possible subcultures to address all that the nurse will encounter.

First, the nurse must embrace the understanding of personal cultures and examine biases and stereotypes related to divergent cultures. The nurse must be able to set aside personal biases in order to provide the comprehensive education at the person's health literacy level that encompasses not only the disease process, the preventative actions necessary, as well as the actions that fit within the cultural norms specifically related to the person.

Nurses must allow the person to become more involved in developing a plan of action that is representative of what the person wants to learn or is willing to learn. A "patient engagement" (deBronkart, 2013) handbook was written to guide healthcare providers through avenues in which patients can and are becoming more knowledgeable and willing to be a part of the education process. Teaching the patient what the healthcare provider thinks is the right thing will be lost on a person who has other more immediate needs. Exploring with the person what is important to them will create a better atmosphere for learning, greater retention and adherence, as well as being more productive in an effort to improve health.

HEALTHY PEOPLE 2020 INITIATIVES 

The Office of the Assistant Secretary for Health (ASH) supports many initiatives, campaigns, and programs that promote the goals of public health, including

- Combating the Silent Epidemic of Viral Hepatitis: Action Plan for the Prevention, Care, and Treatment of Viral Hepatitis
- Ending the Tobacco Epidemic
- Healthcare-Associated Infections (HAI)
- HHS Initiative on Multiple Chronic Conditions
- Public Health System, Finance, and Quality Program (*Healthy People 2020*, 2014).

Theoretical Bases

When dealing with complex issues, it is wise to work from a theoretical base. Theories describe, explain, and predict behaviors within a functional framework (DiClemente, Crosby, & Kegler, 2002). Theories about health education and behavior change can help nurses understand behavior and thereby help them develop useful strategies that influence people's health.

> I'm going to learn to relax—even if I have to work at it 24 hours a day, seven days a week.
>
> —*Author unknown*

Concepts

Theories are based on concepts that are used to form the propositions that give structure to a theory. Some important concepts that support patient **autonomy** in health education are defined in **Table 17-1**. In addition, it would be helpful to discuss absolutism and paternalism, two concepts that have lost favor in health education not only because they tend to stifle autonomy, but also because they have not been found to be effective.

Absolutism is a tactic we have all used. When absolutism is used in health education, the teacher basically says, "This is what you must do." Absolutism requires absolute **adherence** to specific, prescribed strategies (Cates & Hinman, 1992). We have all done it because, as nurses, we know that smoking is not healthy and eating broccoli is. Absolute healthcare messages are usually well intentioned. They are

TABLE 17-1 Important Concepts for Health Education Theory

Concept	Definition
Advocacy	Process by which patients are informed and supported so that they can make the best decisions possible (Spellbring, 1991); advocacy is a primary nursing function.
Barriers	Those individually determined things that associate cost with a particular behavior (Palank, 1991); costs can be thought of in terms of money, time inconvenience, difficulty, risk, or interpersonal effort. Not having child care, for example, is a barrier for a mother who needs to attend a Narcotics Anonymous meeting.
Benefits	Those individually determined things that reinforce or reward a particular behavior (Palank, 1991); in other words, one person may see weight loss as a main benefit of exercise, but another may see meeting friends at the gym as the primary benefit.
Cognitive dissonance	Tension or discomfort that accompanies actions that oppose personal beliefs (Rankin & Stallings, 2001); for example, a person who lectures coworkers about good nutrition and then eats chocolate cake and feels guilty about it.
Empowerment	Process of helping people develop the abilities to understand and control their personal situations; can be applied at individual, group, and community levels (Israel, Checkoway, Schulz, & Zimmerman, 1994).
Motivation	Complex concept that refers to those "forces acting on or within an organism that initiate, direct, and maintain behavior" (Redman, 1997, p. 7).
Readiness	Motivation to perform a particular action at a particular time (Redman, 1997).
Self-efficacy	Personal conviction of ability to carry out specific behaviors in order to achieve a desired end (Damrosch, 1991; Palank, 1991); the "I know I can do this" feeling.

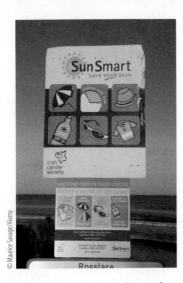

Public education campaign in Great Britain for prevention of skin cancer.

based on evidence that, if used consistently and correctly, the prescribed methods will make people healthier. The problem is that complete adherence to any behavior is difficult. Think, for instance, about the last time you tried to lose weight or start exercising regularly. Were you always able to meet your goals? Did you always skip dessert? Did you show up at the gym every morning? Demanding absolute compliance with absolute behaviors is risky because most people cannot meet such high standards. When they fail to meet these standards, they can lose confidence in their abilities to change and then give up (Strang, 1992). Maybe you have given up on some of your goals. Perhaps, you knew that missing a workout session or eating a piece of chocolate cake did not spell disaster. Ideally, you chalked it up to experience and moved forward in your behavior change program. If you didn't, maybe it was because you believed an absolutist message: Do it right or don't do it at all. One can see how this could make health education and behavior change difficult.

Absolutism is perpetuated in an atmosphere of paternalism. **Paternalism** occurs when healthcare providers (or other "experts") decide what the patient should do (Rankin & Stallings, 2001; Yu et al., 2007). Although this also is usually done with altruistic motives, it runs counter to the concept of promoting patient autonomy. Paternalism and absolutism demand compliance (adherence). Compliance carries the expectation that patients will do exactly what providers tell them to do. If they don't, they are labeled "noncompliant," a term that implies patient responsibility for failure (Rankin & Stallings, 2001). The nursing philosophy of holistic patient care supports individuals in their efforts to make health decisions and behavior changes. Absolutism, paternalism, and demands for strict compliance are all counter to this philosophy.

ENVIRONMENTAL CONNECTION

How does the learning environment affect our ability to learn rather than simply "be taught"?

Learning Theory

Much health education is based on **learning theories** that have been developed over the past several decades. These theories are usually familiar to nurses, but some of the more important learning theory contributions to health education are briefly discussed here. The behavioral theorists, including Pavlov, Thorndike, and Skinner, showed how teachers could connect a stimulus to a desired response. This leads to a conditioned change in behavior that occurs every time the stimulus is presented. A patient could, for instance, learn that brushing her teeth in the morning is associated with taking her birth control pill. Developmental theories, by comparison, state that individuals need to acquire competence at one level of a developmental process before moving to the next level. Piaget showed that children go through specific developmental stages in their intellectual abilities, Erikson defined the psychosocial stages of growth and development, and Maslow explained a hierarchy of human needs where basic needs (e.g., food and shelter) must be met before working on higher level needs (e.g., social connections and self-actualization). In addition, Rogers contributed the concept of learner-centered care in which the patient learns to make decisions and solve problems (Allender & Spradley, 2001; Hunt, 1997).

Adult learning theory provides important information for health education. This theory holds that motivation to learn is based on four assumptions (Knowles, Holton, & Swanson, 1998):

1. Adults perceive themselves to be self-directed: They want to have a say in what they learn.
2. Adults have a variety of life experiences and are insulted if these experiences are ignored: The wise teacher will build on these experiences.
3. Adults learn better when they see an immediate need: They are goal directed.
4. Timing education to coincide with an immediate need is more effective because the learner will see the immediate goal and be ready to learn.

Behavior Change Theory

Theories that specifically address behavior change and health education incorporate ideas from these learning theories. **Behavior change theories** provide direction for nurses who teach in a variety of situations. A brief overview of some of these theories is provided in **Table 17-2**.

TABLE 17-2 Overview of Selected Theories About Health Behavior

Theory and Key Components	Case Study
Health belief model: Individuals are more likely to take action to improve health if: • They perceive themselves to be at risk for a problem (susceptibility). • The problem is seen as serious enough to warrant action (severity, perceived threat). • The expected benefits of the action outweigh the anticipated costs (e.g., in terms of overcoming barriers related to time, effort, and money). • There is a personal sense of ability to perform the required actions (self-efficacy) (Charron-Prachnowik et al., 2001; Dutta-Bergman, 2004; Fertman & Allensworth, 2010; Jachna & Forbes-Thompson, 2005; Sharma & Ronas, 2011). *Revised health promotion model* (revised by Pender in 1996: • Perceived benefits of action (benefit) • Perceived barriers to action (barriers) • Perceived self-efficacy • Activity-related affect • Interpersonal influences (family, peers, providers, norms, support, models) • Situational influences (options, demand characteristics, aesthetics)	Nina's mother and sister both died of breast cancer. Nina took care of her mother during the terminal phases of the disease, and she has told friends, "That was the most horrible thing I ever had to do." Nina was concerned about her own risk, so she talked to her nurse practitioner (NP). The NP gave Nina information about breast cancer, did a breast examination, scheduled Nina for a mammogram, and taught Nina how to do breast self-examination (BSE). **Follow up:** Nina sees breast cancer as a terrible disease, and she feels that she may be at risk. She is motivated to protect her health but has trouble remembering to do BSE. Doing it actually frightens her: What if she should find a lump? At her next clinic visit, her NP provides Nina with a chart, watches her do BSE in the office, and discusses her concerns about finding a lump. The NP is able to assure Nina that she is doing everything right. Nina establishes a habit of BSE that works for her.
Harm reduction model: Health risks can be decreased by having patients ask, "What is healthier, safer, or less risky than what I am doing now?" and "Which steps am I willing and able to take to be healthier, safer, or less risky?" Basic principles include the following: • Most people are competent to make informed decisions about health behaviors; they are the only ones who know what will work for them in their specific situations. • Needs are diverse and can be met in diverse ways; offering people a spectrum of potential behaviors is better than demanding that they adopt an absolute requirement. • Incremental steps that provide chances for success work better than trying to make large, difficult changes where the risk of failure is high. • People may need social support, education, referrals, and assistance to make changes (Bradley-Springer, 1996; Brocato & Wagner, 2003).	Bob, who smokes two packs of cigarettes a day, arrives at an occupational health clinic for his annual physical. He tells the nurse that he exercises regularly and feels "as healthy as a horse." He denies any smoking-related problems, saying, "Smoking is my only vice and I really like it. It relaxes me. I tried to stop smoking once and it was a disaster, so why bother? But I am worried about smoking around my kids—they've been sick a lot lately." The nurse asks, "What do you think would be healthier for your kids?" Bob lists ideas ranging from quitting smoking altogether to not smoking in the house. The nurse then asks, "Which of these things do you think would work best for you?" Bob decides to try smoking only in his office at home where "the kids can't come anyway." **Follow up:** The nurse helped Bob explore his options without taking over and telling him what to do. He was then able to choose a behavior that he thought would work in his situation. Bob sees the nurse several months later and says, "Hey, you know how we talked about smoking only in my office to protect my kids? Well, it's working real well. The kids haven't been sick as often and I'm not smoking as much either. I'm down to a pack and a half a day." By helping Bob see his options and by not demanding that he quit smoking, the nurse gave him the support he needed to make positive changes. Bob will now feel good about talking to the nurse if he wants to make further changes.

Goal-setting theory: Setting goals can help people change health-related behaviors by focusing effort, persistence, and concentration on the goal. The following steps are used: • Determine the patient's commitment to change. • Analyze the tasks required to make changes: Complex tasks need to be broken down into subgoals (strategic analysis); simple tasks can be motivated by a simple goal. • Assess the patient's self-efficacy for performing required behaviors and help with skill development as needed. • Goals should be difficult enough to require significant effort; they should be optimistic as well as realistic. • Provide feedback on progress (Strecher et al., 1995).	At her last dental checkup, Ana's dentist pointed out that she had beginning gum disease and suggested that Ana start flossing. Ana said, "I know I should floss. I know how to do it. I floss for 2 to 3 days, but then I miss a day and I give up. I don't want to lose all my teeth like my mother did. I just can't keep it up." The dentist suggests that Ana set a goal of flossing every other day. **Follow up:** Ana was committed to making a change and already possessed the required skills. By suggesting a specific, attainable goal, the dentist provided additional motivation. At her next checkup Ana says, "It worked! I'm flossing almost every day now. When I miss a day it's not that big a deal because I know I will be able to floss the next day." During her oral examination, the dentist is able to tell Ana that her gums look much better.
Stages of change model: Focused around addictive and problem behaviors, there are six stages of changes: • Precontemplation • Contemplation • Preparation • Action • Maintenance • Termination	Alan finds himself passed out in the car on the side of the road. *Another blackout*, he thinks. What can he do to stop this from happening again? Alan decides to seek help. He calls Alcoholics Anonymous (AA) for help and completes the program. **Follow up:** Alan has been sober for 12 years and has a happy family and productive career. Alan realized his life was unmanageable and when he needed help, he sought it. Alan chose to follow the program, which led to success.
Theory of reasoned action: Behavioral intention to act is based on a combination of the following: • Personal beliefs and evaluations about what will happen if the behavior is used (perceived chance of success) • Personal attitudes and values about the behavior • Feelings about what key people (family, friends, and healthcare providers) in the person's life think about the behavior • Motivation to change behavior (Carter, 1990) • All things being equal, people are expected to act in accordance with their intentions (Miller, Wikoff, & Hiatt, 1992). ***Self-efficacy theory***: Self-efficacy is based on expectations about a course of action (Bandura, 1978; Soffer, 2009). Its four principal sources of information are: • Self-mastery of similarly expected behaviors (performance accomplishments) • Observation of successful expected behavior from others (vicarious experiences) • Verbal persuasion by others who believe in the person's ability to accomplish the behavior (verbal persuasion) • Self-judgment of physiological states of distress (emotional arousal) (Bandura, 1977)	Sue, a nursing student, has been dating Jack for 2 years. They plan to get married after she graduates. They have discussed having a family and agree that they do not want children for several years. Sue and Jack want to become sexually active. They visit the Student Health Center, where a nurse explains birth control options. Jack encourages Sue to use birth control pills (BCPs). Sue is worried because some of her friends have told her that BCPs caused them to gain weight. **Follow up:** Although Sue is worried about weight gain, she believes that BCPs are effective and easy to use. She is clear that she does not currently want a pregnancy. She has Jack's support. Sue rarely misses taking her vitamin pills, so she is sure that she can remember to take the pills every day. This model predicts that Sue is likely to use BCPs consistently and correctly.

TABLE 17-2 Overview of Selected Theories About Health Behavior (*continued*)

Theory and Key Components	Case Study
Social learning theory: Individual behavior, personal factors, and the environment create a triad of components that interact to influence health behaviors: • A change in one component of the triad has an effect on all components (reciprocal determinism). • Personal factors include behavioral capability, self-control, self-efficacy, internal reinforcements, emotional coping response, and a belief that performing a behavior will lead to expected outcomes. • The environment (everything external to the individual) and the situation (the individual's perception of the environment) provide opportunities to observe behaviors performed by others in the environment (vicarious learning) (Perry, Baranowski, & Parcel, 1990).	Jose is a depressed 13-year-old who just entered a new school. He hasn't made any friends at the new school, a problem he blames on being 20 pounds overweight. The people Jose admires most at school all seem to be thin. He also notices that they are active in after-school activities. Jose's mother reminds him that he is a good swimmer and encourages him to join the swim team. **Follow up:** Jose's desire to lose weight is influenced by the rewards that he sees being given to slim people. His perception of weight and his emotional response to it create a desire to change that is supported by his mother and his swimming ability. Jose knows that swimming can help. He tries out for the team and discovers that he can do the butterfly stroke better than anyone else. He joins the team, and in addition to exercising regularly and losing weight, Jose makes new friends and develops a more optimistic outlook.
Diffusion theory: New ideas, practices, or services (innovations) to improve health move from a resource (innovation developer) to the population (innovation users or adopters). Diffusion is more likely to occur if the innovation is cost-efficient, low risk, simple, flexible, and compatible with the social, economic, and value systems into which it is introduced. Innovations that are reversible (I can go back to where I was if I don't like it) and appear to be better than currently used methods have a better chance of being adopted. Diffusion can fail if the innovation does not work, if information about the innovation is not communicated well, if the potential user does not have the necessary resources for implementation, or if the innovation is in opposition to the user's value system. In addition, there may be a problem if components of the implementation process are abbreviated. An example of this would be when education about the innovation is omitted to save money. Maintenance of an innovation takes additional effort; without this, the adopted program can lose momentum and fade away (Orlandi, Landers, Weston, & Haley, 1990).	Injection drug users (IDUs) who do not share equipment to inject drugs are not at risk of infection with blood-borne diseases such as hepatitis B, hepatitis C, and human immunodeficiency virus (HIV). Activists in Metrotown, a community of 300,000, wanted to implement a needle and syringe exchange program (N/SEP) so that IDUs would have access to sterile injecting equipment. They gathered support from the city council, the health department, and law enforcement before setting up N/SEP sites around town. During the first week, only two IDUs brought in equipment to exchange. **Follow up:** Activists (resource) did a good job in Metrotown of involving the established power systems. No doubt they convinced all of these entities that N/SEPs would be cost-effective, simple, reversible, and better than allowing used injecting equipment to accumulate on the streets of the city. The activists were less effective in communicating the benefits of N/SEPs to the intended users of the program. IDUs need to know that obtaining sterile equipment will decrease the risk of disease, will be easily accessible, and will not put them at risk for being targeted by the police. Although Metrotown has made a difficult public health decision, it will not be successful unless the innovation diffuses to the intended users.

Social marketing theory: Public acceptance of programs to improve health can be enhanced through marketing techniques. Marketing functions on a number of well-developed principles: • Participants are offered benefits that are valued as being worth the cost (e.g., measured in effort, money, time). The consumer (patient) is the central concern. • Communication (in the form of advertising, public relations, direct marketing, promotion, and face-to-face encounters) is the key to getting information to the consumer. • The marketing process has six stages that occur in a cycle: (1) analysis; (2) planning; (3) development, testing, and refinement of the plan; (4) implementation; (5) assessment of effectiveness; and (6) feedback to analysis (completing the cycle). • Marketing strategies must be modified to function in situations in which social issues and health are the central concerns (Novelli, 1990).	Everyone at Russell High School (RHS) is shocked when three students, all with blood alcohol levels over the legal limit, are killed in a car accident. The principal forms a committee of students, teachers, and administrators to develop a program to decrease drunk driving. After assessing the situation at RHS, the committee proposes a plan to encourage the use of designated drivers. The program is kicked off at an assembly where student leaders (athletes, class officers, cheerleaders) describe the program. They all wear T-shirts that say, "I care about my friends. I'm a designated driver." Students are regularly reminded about the program in newspaper articles, intercom announcements, and student-led discussions in homeroom classes. **Follow up:** RHS used marketing strategies focused on consumers (students) to develop a program that would meet the objective to decrease drunk driving. Although the adults on the planning committee had some reservations about a program that seemed to condone drinking, they paid attention to the analysis provided by student representatives and approved the program. A survey done 3 months later showed that 40% of RHS students had been designated drivers, resulting in a significant decrease in drunk driving rates. An additional, unforeseen benefit was a decrease in the overall rate of drinking, a direct result of designated driving being seen as "cool."
Therapeutic alliance model (self-care): Addresses a shift of power from the provider in which a collaboration and negotiation partnership is developed and compares the components of: • Compliance (dependency) • Adherence (conforming) (Barofsky, 1978)	

The Health Education Process

Health education is a process of planned **teaching** and support activities that help people learn (Spellbring, 1991). The education process follows the format of the nursing process, including assessment, planning, implementation, and evaluation (Rankin & Stallings, 2001; Yu et al., 2007). While these steps are being taken, meticulous documentation should occur. This section presents detailed information about each step in the education process, but before that, some important general points about education need to be made.

The transtheoretical model, so called because it borrows from many other theories, provides new and helpful insights for health education. The central premise of the transtheoretical model is that people progress through a series of stages when they attempt to change behaviors. There are five stages of change: precontemplative, contemplative, preparation, action, and maintenance (Petty, Barden, & Wheeler, 2002, 2009). Progression through the stages is rarely linear. People will change their minds, will hesitate, and may relapse several times before behavior change is permanent. Ten processes are used to enhance progression through the stages of change:

1. Consciousness raising (increasing the level of awareness)
2. Dramatic relief (experiencing and expressing feelings)
3. Environmental reevaluation (assessing how the environment affects the situation)
4. Self-reevaluation (assessing how a person thinks and feels about the situation)
5. Self-liberation (believing in the ability to change)
6. Helping relationships (caring and trusting relationships)
7. Social liberation (seeing social changes that support personal changes)
8. Counter-conditioning (substituting more healthy behaviors for less healthy behaviors)
9. Stimulus control (restructuring the environment)
10. Reinforcement management (getting rewards)

Table 17-3 gives an overview of the transtheoretical model, including examples of the 10 processes and interventions appropriate in each stage.

TABLE 17-3 Overview of the Transtheoretical Model (Also Known as the Stages of Change Theory)

Precontemplative: Unaware of or unwilling to consider the problem; defensive about the change issue, resistant to information about the behavior, and reluctant to initiate a behavior change program; not considering change within the next 6 months; has little confidence in ability to change; sees many reasons not to change	During a routine physical, Sam, a 26-year-old lawyer, says, "You know, I was listening to the radio on the way over here and a woman was talking about having AIDS (consciousness raising). This whole thing scares me (dramatic relief). It's not just gay guys anymore. I know that I've had some risks, but the things I do are a part of my life and the people I hang with (environmental reevaluation)." **Stage-specific interventions:** Raise awareness of the issue through community-appropriate public education and media programs. Provide information and feedback to increase individual awareness of physical, social, economic, and psychological problems related to the commission or omission of specific behaviors. Discuss the positive aspects of change. Do not spend time discussing details of specific change tactics or programs: You're wasting your time if it is clear that the patient is not ready to think about changing.
Contemplative: Ambivalent; responds with "Yes, but ..."; may see reasons to change as well as reasons to remain the same; indecisive; aware that a problem exists and more open to information, but still unsure of ability to change; intends to change behavior within next 6 months	Sam's nurse encourages him to continue talking about his concerns and those behaviors that make him think he has been at risk. He says, "Well, I have some crazy friends. I go out with them every Saturday. We compare notes on how much sex we get. We dare each other to do things like using a prostitute or having anal sex or coming on to a gay guy. I'm not proud of some of the things I've done. Maybe I'm getting too old for this (self-reevaluation)." **Stage-specific interventions:** Tip the balance in favor of change. It is important to see this stage as the time when the patient will develop a commitment to change. It is still too early to look at strategies. The aim is to analyze risks and rewards of the behavior and to provide information. Clarify goals and discuss incentives to change. It is now time to emphasize negative aspects of not changing. A discussion of the risk for harm is appropriate.

Preparation: Expresses desire to do something to initiate change; some experimentation with new behaviors may already be occurring; thinks change may be possible; seriously planning change within next 30 days but has not set specific goals	When asked how this makes him feel, Sam responds by saying, with a sigh, "I guess I should think about being more careful. I don't want to get anything bad, especially AIDS. I need to change my act (self-liberation)." **Stage-specific interventions:** Now is the time to get down to details. Help the patient find change strategies that are acceptable, accessible, appropriate, and effective. Encourage the patient to experiment with a strategy: "Try it next time, see how you like it," or "Find out how your family/partner/friends react when you do it." Be available to the patient to discuss issues related to moving into the action stage. Help the patient establish specific objectives. In Sam's case, this could be limiting nights out with his friends to once a month.
Action: Engages in action to create desired change; feels developing confidence in self-efficacy; thinks reasons to change outweigh reasons not to; behavior modified to meet goal(s) for 6 months	Over the course of the next 6 months, Sam and the nurse meet several times to discuss his progress. During this time, Sam says, "I've talked about this with my friend Mia. She just listens and never acts like I'm a bad person even when I tell her bad things I've done (helping relationship). Since I've started talking about it, I've had people tell me that I'm right to be concerned and that I should be more careful—even some of my buddies agree (social liberation)." Sam begins to take specific actions to decrease his risks. He begins to use condoms and decides to have sex only when he wants to and not "on a dare" (counter-conditioning). **Stage-specific interventions:** Be aware that this is not an easy process. Support change efforts. Patients will need continuing encouragement, help with problem solving, and a place to simply vent frustrations.
Maintenance: Challenged to continue change; feels expanding self-efficacy; continues behavior change for more than 6 months	As Sam becomes comfortable with his new behaviors, he reports that other things are changing. He says, "I realized that my problems were related to my friends. They didn't understand why I wanted to change. They called me a wimp. So I decided to quit hanging out with them (stimulus control). The good thing is that I feel better about myself. Mia even told me that she's noticed that I seem happier (reinforcement management)." **Stage-specific interventions:** Help the patient maintain change. Problem solving and unconditional support for the patient are extremely important during this stage. Relapse-prevention efforts can include interactive discussions, role-playing, and "what if" sessions, in which the patient identifies risks for relapse and develops workable strategies.
Relapse (not a stage): An important event that can occur at any time in the change process; if relapse occurs, the patient may express anger and question ability to maintain change; may be embarrassed or ashamed; may blame self or others (including healthcare providers) for the relapse	Sam returns to clinic a year later. When asked about how he's doing, he blurts out, "I blew it. I ran into Jake a few weeks ago and we went for a drink. Before I knew it, we'd picked up a couple of women. I ended up in a strange apartment and no one ever thought about using condoms. I'm really embarrassed about this—especially after I made such a big deal out of being careful with my friends. Maybe I wasn't meant to be safe. Maybe I'm supposed to get the clap or HIV or something else that's just as bad. I can't even face Mia." **Stage-specific interventions:** Patients may get "stuck" in relapse if they resort to self-incrimination or self-blame. Help the patient renew the change process at an earlier stage without getting demoralized. Explain that relapse is common and may occur many times before behavior change is permanent. Point out specific instances of success that show the patient's abilities to change. Provide referral to needed services. Sam, for instance, may need a workup for sexually transmitted disease. Sam's nurse helps him understand the circumstance of his relapse: meeting Jake, having a drink, meeting the women, and so on. Sam and his nurse discuss the situation and role-play a similar situation so that he will feel better prepared if this should happen again. Sam also agrees to go to the STD clinic.

Source: Adapted from Bradley-Springer, L. (1996). Patient education for behavior change: Help from the transtheoretical and harm reduction models. *Journal of the Association of Nurses in AIDS Care*, *7*(Suppl.), 23–33.

MEDIA MOMENT

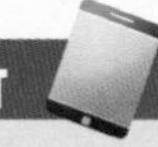

Good Will Hunting (1997)

Will Hunting (Matt Damon) is a genius who's living a rough life in South Boston, while being employed at a prestigious college in Cambridge as a janitor. He's discovered by a Fields Medal–winning professor, who tries to get Will to turn his life around with the help of therapist Sean Maguire (Robin Williams). Will begins to realize that there's more to himself than he thinks there is.

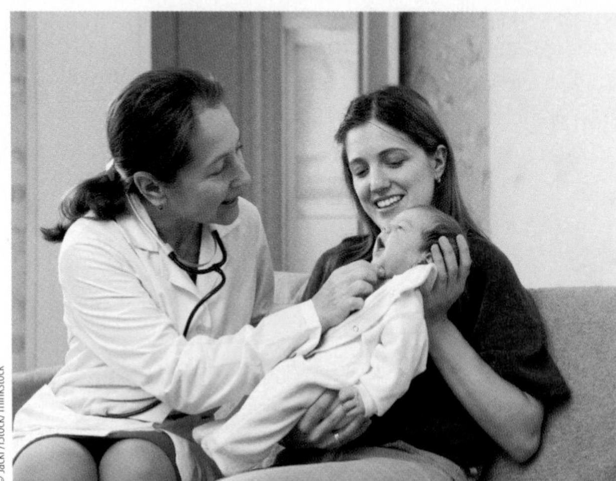

Nurse in the home setting educates new mother about newborn care.

Education is patient centered. An important question for the nurse to continually ask is, "How does *this* problem (e.g., diagnosis, stressor, need to change) affect *this* patient?" To truly make the process patient centered, nurses must remember that people live in complex social and culturally defined environments. Therefore, the involvement of family and significant others can help promote learning. In some cases, family involvement is essential, especially when health education is directed to children, patients with sensory deficits, or patients who are physically unable to perform the necessary skills (Yu et al., 2007). In general, involving others can provide social and emotional supports that help people make behavior changes (Rankin & Stallings, 2001). Unfortunately, patients do not always have healthy support structures, or they simply may not want others involved. In these cases, the nurse should not force the issue. Instead, referrals to community resources and support groups should be considered. Many cultural/subcultural patients will have no family support nor peer support depending on the subculture. Many patients who are transgender, gay, or lesbian have little support from family or from the community. Feelings of isolation or rejection override many attempts to educate related to a medical problem. My Brother's Keeper, Inc. (MBK) provides culturally-competent assistance to care services for transgender persons through the Community Guide Model for Linking Social Environment to Health. This organization's purpose is to assist transgender persons in locating community assistance for these persons to ensure access to health care (Lindsey, 2012). According to Bastable (2008), the roles of the nurse as an educator in health promotion are: (1) facilitator of change, (2) contractor, (3) organizer, and (4) evaluator.

Assessment

The task of assessment is to gather information. This can result in a huge amount of information that the nurse uses to determine needs and priorities. Obviously, educational needs cannot be determined without looking at the entire patient. Learning needs evolve from knowledge of the patient's overall health problems (actual and potential). In most cases, some of the needs discovered through assessment will have a cognitive, skill, or attitudinal component that must be addressed through education (Rankin & Stallings, 2001).

APPLICATION TO PRACTICE

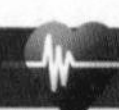

Case Study: Utilization of the Vulnerable Populations Conceptual Model to Access the Impoverished Elderly

A 78-year-old woman sees a nurse practitioner (NP) at a local clinic. The NP has been her primary provider for several years and is very familiar with her living situation. The NP is well aware of the sparse income of this individual. The NP finds cues that alert him to possible changes in the individual's lifestyle. Prior to this visit, the patient's hypertension and diabetes were well controlled. The laboratory results at this visit demonstrate that the conditions are not as well controlled. After further investigation, the NP learns that the woman was unable to afford the medication and had cut her medication back to three times a week instead of daily as prescribed.

What actions do you think the NP should take to assist this patient to regain the controlled status of her medical disease processes?

What teaching strategies might the NP employ to enhance the patient's understanding of the need for compliance?

Source: Meng, S. A., & Smith, M. A. (2013). Utilization of the vulnerable populations conceptual model to access the impoverished elderly. Mississippi Health Care Symposium on Cultural Competency: Pathways toward ending health disparities. Adapted from a Case Study by the authors.

As a student nurse, you went out into the community to teach an individual, a group, or an ethnic-centered population. Did you think about generational differences as specific populations? The impoverished elderly are a vulnerable population that must be addressed at their level of health literacy while taking into consideration the generational differences in the student's level of understanding and the elders' level of understanding. It is likely that the elderly population accepts what is told to them related to medical conditions and medication administration. This population has many differences such as decreased visual acuity, decreased hearing, and decreased mobility. The Vulnerable Populations Conceptual Model (VPCM) assesses for risk factors and addresses those factors in dealing with the impoverished elders:

> The VPCM shows the interrelationships and influences of resource availability, relative risk, and health status among the low-income elderly. Mortality and comorbidity rates are even higher in the impoverished elderly than in the financially secure elderly because of the presence of health disparities related to quality of care, access to care, and health outcomes. (Institute of Medicine, 2003)

How are teaching and learning affected by our fast-paced culture? Has personal (one-on-one) teaching become less important with the rise of the Internet? How does this affect the educator role of the nurse? Many of the persons with whom the community health nurse comes into contact for educational purposes have probably already explored the Internet for answers or information related to the subject being presented. The community health nurse must be aware of what can be found on the Internet so that erroneous information can be dispelled and correct information can be presented in a way that will allow the persons to make healthy choices for a healthy lifestyle. Social media venues such as Facebook, Twitter, Dingo, and so forth make information instantly accessible. This information is not always from reputable sources.

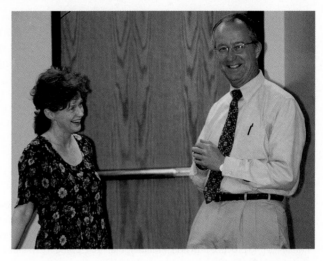

Chapter author Lucy Bradley-Springer and Kevin Morrisroe, RN , do a role-play on risk assessment at a class in New Mexico.

Assessment requires active nurse–patient interaction. This can be time-consuming, but the nurse can use assessment time to develop rapport with the patient and significant others (Redman, 1997, 2008). Building a good working relationship during this phase will increase the amount of information the patient reveals and will make the rest of the education process more enjoyable for both the patient and the nurse. This is especially important in community health settings where nurses need to establish long-term relationships with individuals in the community. **Table 17-4** lists some areas that need to be discussed during a health education assessment.

TABLE 17-4 Assessment Variables

What to Assess	Assessment Questions
• Patient understanding of the problem in question • Patient perception of need to change • Motivation to change: severity of problem and risks caused by the problem • Readiness to change • Self-efficacy • Perceived benefits to change • Perceived barriers to change • Psychosocial issues • Learning skills	• What do you think is the cause of this problem? • Why do you think it is happening now? • How does the problem affect you? • Has this problem limited your activities in any way? • How severe is the problem? Is it a short-term or a long-term problem? • What harm could this problem cause you? • What are the two to three main difficulties that you have because of this problem? • What do you fear most about the problem? • Why do you want to solve this problem? • What would you like to do about the problem in the next few days (weeks)? • What are the most important things that you would like to have happen? • How do you usually approach problems? • How would you like to approach this problem? • What do you think you can do about the problem? • Have you tried to deal with this problem before? If so, what did you do and how did it turn out?

TABLE 17-4 Assessment Variables (*continued*)

What to Assess	Assessment Questions
	• How would you feel if you solved this problem? • If you didn't have the problem, what would be better in your life? • What has kept you from dealing with this problem in the past? • Do you see things that may prevent your dealing with this problem? If so, what are they? • Who gives you the most support? Would you like this person to be in on our teaching sessions? • Also assess housing, economic status, educational background, community resources, cultural and religious contributions to health care, native language, and so on. • How do you learn best? Would you like reading materials or videotapes or group sessions or private counseling or . . . ?

Sources: Adapted from Kreuter, M. W., & Strecher, V. J. (1996). Do tailored behavior change messages enhance the effectiveness of health risk appraisal? Results from a randomized trial. *Health Education Research, 11*, 97–105; Palank, C. L. (1991). Determinants of health-promotive behavior: A review of current research. *Nursing Clinics of North America, 26*, 815–832; Rankin, S. N., & Stallings, K. D. (2001). *Patient education: Principles and practice* (4th ed.). Philadelphia, PA: Lippincott Williams & Wilkins; and Redman, B. K. (1997). *The practice of patient education*. St. Louis, MO: Mosby.

Data can be collected from a variety of sources, including direct observation, patient records, other members of the healthcare team, and professional literature. The best way to get the patient's point of view, however, is through an interactive interview. Patient disclosure of information is enhanced by the following tactics (Rankin & Stallings, 2001):

- *Establish an environment of trust*. This may require some time at the beginning of the conversation. Start by introducing yourself and telling who you are. ("Hi. I'm Faith Diaz, and I'm an RN from the home health agency.") Establish that you have experience in the area you will be addressing with the patient. ("I've been working with people who've had your kind of surgery for 2 years.") Describe the intention of the interview and make it clear that questions are asked to help the patient. As we all know, some of the questions that nurses need to ask can be embarrassing. Assure the patient that there are healthcare reasons for asking each question and that all answers are confidential.
- *Choose the right time*. Be sure that you have time to adequately assess the patient's needs. Ask if this is a good time for the patient. Be sure the patient is not in pain or anxious about an anticipated event. If you know that your time is short, introduce the assessment session by saying, "I know you are anxious about your wound care. I only have 15 minutes to spend with you right now and I need to ask you a few questions. Your answers will help me plan how I will teach you about your wound. I'll come back this afternoon, and we'll go over everything in detail. Do you think that will work for you?"
- *Choose the right place*. The location of an interview should be comfortable and private. If it is not, the patient (and the nurse) may concentrate more on the room temperature or the hard chairs or the constant interruptions than on the interview. If possible, do the interview on the patient's "home turf." This can be in the patient's home or a private room at the clinic. Asking questions in a known environment helps the patient feel safe (Hunt, 1997).
- *Use open-ended questions*. Going through a list of "yes/no" questions does not provide the depth of information needed to develop effective, individualized teaching plans. Asking the patient to describe her problems doing exercises after a mastectomy, for example, will get a lot of those "yes/no" questions answered without your even asking them. The patient will also benefit from the experience of telling her story to an interested listener. Remember, patients (as adult learners) have unique perspectives that they need to share with you and that you should build into your teaching plan.
- *Use active listening skills*. Ask for clarification, summarize, and use open body language (nod and smile; do not act like you have to leave). These listening skills enhance interactions and ensure that you understand the patient's meanings.
- *Assess reading and literacy level of patient*. Include an evaluation of the patient's literacy

level. Various tools are available, such as SMOG (Cutill, 2006; Demir, Ozsaker, & Ilce, 2008; McLaughlin, 1969).

When the interview is complete, summarize the main points and thank the patient for spending time with you. Tell the patient what you intend to do with the information and describe the next steps in the planning process. If you cannot continue the process at this time, tell the patient when you will return.

ETHICAL CONNECTION 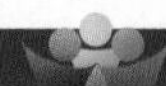

A high school student has requested information on pregnancy testing in the community. As a school nurse, you provide her with this information and educate her about the differences and quality of tests. The next day, the student's mother phones and tells you that she has found a pregnancy test kit in her daughter's room. The mother wants to know if you gave it to her daughter. How would you respond?

Planning

During planning, the nurse and patient discuss learning needs and potential goals. This is a negotiation process: The nurse provides input that the patient uses to make decisions about specific interventions. The result of this process is a list of learning objectives. In most cases, the list will not be too long, but some patients have many problems. In that case, it is best to prioritize the list by having the patient choose those problems (1) that are most pressing (cause the most discomfort for the patient) and (2) the patient is most willing to work on (an estimate of readiness). Limiting the teaching session to one or two objectives is less intimidating than trying to make a large number of changes at the same time (Kreuter & Strecher, 1996).

Based on the literacy assessment, the nurse should plan education appropriate for reading and comprehension level. For example, some patients may respond to visual materials presented according to reading level while others may prefer detailed explanations in written form. For example, reading materials can be assessed for readability using many word-processing programs for word count and using the widely used and accepted SMOG (Simple Measure of Gobbledygook) assessment tool. McLaughlin developed the easy-to-use readability formula in 1969, and the tool is now available online (http://www.harrymclaughlin.com/SMOG.htm). In health education materials, one size does not fit all (Cutill, 2006; Demir, Ozsaker, & Ilce, 2008; McLaughlin, 1969).

Learning goals and objectives are established in the initial part of the planning phase. Goals and objectives provide an agreed-upon direction for implementation and a guide for evaluation. Goals are broad statements of the desired outcome: "Jason will manage insulin administration to control his blood sugar," for example. Objectives are specific, detailed statements. They describe behaviors that will help meet a goal. They describe what the patient will do, define how it will be done, and prescribe time frames for task completion. Objectives for Jason could include the following:

1. Before he is discharged in 3 days, Jason will be able to list the signs and symptoms of high and low blood sugar.
2. By tomorrow, Jason will be able to test his blood for glucose with the equipment he will use at home.
3. By the day before discharge, Jason will be able to use a prescribed sliding scale to accurately draw up and inject insulin in the ordered doses at the ordered times.
4. Within a week after discharge, Jason will describe the benefits of controlling his blood sugar.

Notice that the objectives are specific and measurable. We will be able to tell when Jason accomplishes each objective (Rankin & Stallings, 2001).

Also notice that the objectives do not all look alike. That is because they address three different **domains of learning** (Redman, 1997). Some objectives refer to things that people need to know. These are called *cognitive objectives*. In Jason's case, the first objective asks him to know the signs of hyperglycemia and hypoglycemia. *Psychomotor objectives* refer to skills or behaviors. Jason will need to manipulate equipment (a skill) to meet the next two objectives. The final objective addresses an attitude: We want Jason to verbalize a positive outlook on his abilities. This objective occurs in the *affective* domain.

Knowing the type of objective helps the nurse and patient decide on teaching and learning methods. Jason may be able to learn the symptoms of hyperglycemia from a brochure, for instance, but he will need to practice drawing up insulin and injecting himself to really learn those skills. You cannot learn to give an injection by reading about it! **Table 17-5** provides an in-depth overview of the domains of learning and teaching methods appropriate to each domain.

The planning stage is not complete until the patient agrees to the goals, objectives, and teaching methods. Although Jason's plan looks good on the surface, he may have a morbid fear of sticking himself. In that case, the objectives and plan would need to be changed to have someone in his household learn the "sticking" skills (injections and finger sticks), but Jason should be able to

TABLE 17-5 Domains of Learning

Domain	Goals and Objectives	Teaching Methods	Application Case: Goal is to encourage breastfeeding in pregnant women who attend a low-income clinic
Cognitive subdomains			
Knowledge (to know)	To state, to list, to define, to recall, to name, to repeat	Lecture, one-on-one instruction, programmed instruction, videos or audio tapes, reading materials, questions and answers	Display breastfeeding posters in prominent places around the clinic. Run a continuous video on breastfeeding in the waiting room. Leave brochures and printed materials in examination rooms. Plan a series of lectures at a convenient time for patients.
Comprehension (to understand)	To explain, to label, to describe, to interpret	Lecture, one-on-one instruction, programmed instruction, video program, reading materials, learning guides, study questions	Arrange face-to-face sessions during prenatal visits; ask if patient has questions or concerns. Follow up educational activities by asking, "What difference could breastfeeding make for your baby?"
Application (to use)	To illustrate, to apply, to give examples	Demonstration, group discussion, simulation exercises, games, role-play, clinical practice	Demonstrate breast care and the process of breastfeeding using a simulation model or a video. Encourage partner participation in education.
Analysis (to identify elements)	To compare, to contrast, to differentiate, to debate, to question	Group discussion, games, group interaction, simulation exercises, role-play, case studies	Arrange small group sessions where women can discuss concerns about breastfeeding. Role-play issues that emerge from group discussions.
Synthesis (to use in new ways)	To assemble, to prepare, to create, to design, to formulate	Group projects, group discussion, simulation exercises, games, role-play, case studies	Invite women from the community who are successfully breastfeeding to discuss the process in small groups of pregnant women. Support breastfeeding efforts after delivery.
Evaluation (to judge)	To assess, to justify, to measure, to choose	Group discussion, guided imagery, role-play, self-evaluation worksheet	Ask women to share success stories related to breastfeeding. Provide questionnaire that helps patient assess values and fears about breastfeeding; follow up with a one-on-one discussion.
Psychomotor (to perform)	To assemble, to demonstrate, to control, to manipulate	Demonstration, practice with supervision, independent practice, return demonstration, role-play, simulation, clinical experience	Demonstrate breast care and the process of breastfeeding using a simulation model or a video. Provide guidance and positive reinforcement to women after delivery as they initiate breastfeeding with newborn.
Affective (to feel)	To tolerate, to accept, to defend, to adopt, to appreciate, to value	Group discussion, group project, simulation exercises, games, role-play, life experience	Encourage patient involvement. Reinforce positive statements about breastfeeding. Encourage attendance at group sessions where breastfeeding is discussed.

meet the other objectives and may eventually overcome his fears and learn the "sticking" skills himself.

MEDIA MOMENT 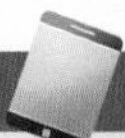

The Alchemist (1993)

By Paola Coelho, translated by Alan R. Clarke, New York, NY: HarperCollins

This tale of Santiago, a shepherd boy who dreams of seeing the world, is compelling in its own right, but gains resonance through the many lessons Santiago learns during his adventures. He journeys from Spain to Morocco in search of worldly success. Eventually, he makes his way to Egypt, where a fateful encounter with an alchemist brings Santiago at last to self-understanding and spiritual enlightenment. The story has the comic charm, dramatic tension, and psychological intensity of a fairy tale, but it's full of specific wisdom as well—about becoming self-empowered, overcoming depression, and believing in dreams.

MEDIA MOMENT 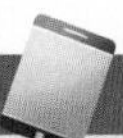

Dead Poets Society (1989)

Painfully shy Todd Anderson has been sent to the school where his popular older brother was valedictorian. His roommate, Neil, although exceedingly bright and popular, is very much under the thumb of his overbearing father. The two, along with their other friends, meet Professor Keating, their new English teacher, who tells them of the Dead Poets Society, and encourages them to go against the status quo. Each, in his own way, does so, and is changed for life. Robin Williams won an Academy Award for Best Actor in 1990 for his performance as Professor Keating.

Implementation

During implementation, the nurse and the patient use information from the assessment and planning stages to make decisions about learning activities. Learning activities must focus on the established objectives. Interventions are tailored to the patient's needs and abilities. Teaching plans are then put into action, but this is not a static process. The nurse continually observes and asks for feedback to track progress. The nurse should discuss any problems with the patient, modifying the plan as needs change. This is called *formative evaluation*: It helps the teacher adjust the format of the education as the teaching progresses. **Box 17-1** provides some general pointers to guide teaching.

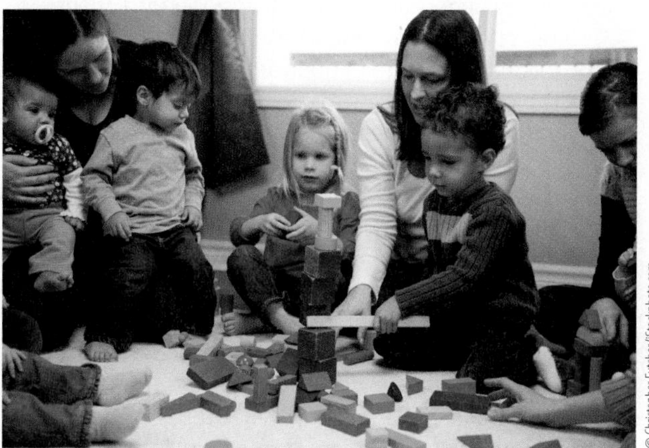

Groups may come together for a specific purpose, such as child care.

Evaluation

Evaluation is a process of gathering information to assess the extent to which learning objectives have been met—or not met. There are a number of ways to evaluate learning, but all evaluation methods should be based on the

BOX 17-1 Pointers for Health Education

- Assess readiness to learn. If the person is not ready to learn, then learning will not occur.
- Design teaching based on assessments of individual patients: needs, ability, knowledge base, learning styles, expectations, culture, language, readiness to learn, and so on.
- Develop educational objectives with input from the learner. Validate that the objectives are relevant to the learner's needs. Objectives serve as the basis for instruction and evaluation.
- Create a learning environment. It should be comfortable and free of distractions.
- Have an interpreter (cultural or linguistic) available if at all possible.
- Keep things simple.
- Focus on one issue at a time. Keep learning sessions short. Concentrate on outcomes that will be immediately obvious (e.g., feeling and looking better because of exercise rather than the more distant issue of preventing heart disease).
- Be sure written materials are appropriate. Keep sentences short. Use words a layperson can understand. Define medical words in simple terms. Use a font style and size that are easy to read. Use pictures and diagrams to clarify concepts.
- Be specific. "Lose weight," for instance, is not as effective as "Lose 2 pounds this week."

BOX 17-1 (continued)

- Avoid threatening messages that generate fear. Mild anxiety enhances learning, but high fear levels can lead to denial, tuning out the message, or inability to concentrate.
- Explain what you will be teaching and why it is important. This provides an "advance organizer" to keep sessions centered on the topic.
- Provide for success. Divide learning tasks into sequential learning units that start with easier concepts and build to more difficult ones. Encourage success at each level before progressing to more difficult tasks. This enhances self-efficacy and personal satisfaction.
- Follow up with the person in a week to assess continued understanding of what was taught. Patients can often repeat immediately what is taught but may forget or misinterpret upon arrival home.
- During follow up, ask the person: "Are you meeting your healthcare needs as planned? Are you taking the medication as prescribed?"
- Use a variety of teaching methods. People learn in different ways, and a combination of methods reinforces learning. Varying methods also keeps people involved.
- Provide visual learning materials. Seeing in addition to hearing enhances retention.
- Show the patient what is expected. Model behaviors to demonstrate how things are done.
- Skills (both verbal and physical) require practice. (For example, role-play communication skills, use a plastic model to teach self-catheterization techniques, or use syringes to practice drawing up insulin.)
- Involve all the senses in practice sessions. This reinforces learning on several levels.
- Provide immediate feedback that praises or corrects specific details during practice sessions. Highlight successes and express honest confidence in the learner's abilities to accomplish learning objectives. If you have doubts about the learner's abilities, do not give false praise. Instead, reassess with the learner and develop a new teaching plan.
- Develop mechanisms for support. Include family and friends in education as possible and as acceptable to the patient. Support groups that focus on specific issues have been shown to enhance learning while encouraging positive change and maintenance of newly developed behaviors.
- Discuss resources for further information and/or practice.
- Review major points of each learning session. Discuss plans for follow up, reinforcement, and expansion of learning experience.
- Keep learners involved: Ask for feedback and evaluation during teaching and learning.

Sources: Adapted from Allender, J. A., & Spradley, B. W. (2001). *Community health nursing: Concepts and practice* (5th ed.). Philadelphia, PA: Lippincott Williams & Wilkins; and Damrosch, S. (1991). General strategies for motivating people to change their behavior. *Nursing Clinics of North America, 26*, 833–843.

learning objectives. Objectives that are written with appropriate action verbs will tell you how to evaluate outcomes. An objective that says the learner will be able to list the steps in cardiopulmonary resuscitation (CPR), for instance, can be evaluated by asking her to write those steps on a piece of paper. If the objective states that the learner will be able to perform CPR, however, you will need to watch her perform the technique on a mannequin. Learning can be evaluated through quizzes, direct observation, physiological measures (Is the patient's blood pressure lower?), patient self-report and self-monitoring, or input from other healthcare team members (Redman, 1997, 2008).

The outcome of evaluation is a list of learning that has been accomplished as well as a list of those learning objectives that have not been met. *Summative evaluation* is a summary of what has occurred and is usually used as a summary of patient accomplishments when the nurse is closing out a case. More often, formative evaluation is used. As with the nursing process, information from formative evaluation feeds back to the assessment phase, and the teaching process repeats itself with new objectives, plans, and interventions until the patient and the nurse are satisfied with the final result (Rankin & Stallings, 2001).

Health Education in Communities

All nurses, regardless of work site or specialty, are expected to teach individuals and their families about health-related matters. Nurses who work in the community have additional opportunities to help people change behaviors for the improved health of aggregate populations. This section describes teaching efforts that can occur in community settings, including individual, group, and community education.

The availability of the Internet and ready access to social platforms and medical information allows individuals, groups, and communities to be knowledgeable regarding medical conditions before they are seen by the primary provider. Often, the provider must dispel information that was obtained from disreputable websites. Many who read about health on the Internet automatically think the information must be accurate and true. One important aspect of education is to first ask what

BOX 17-2 Social Networking Usage

- There are more Americans using the Internet; use is now up to 85% across the population, including 56% in people age 65+
- There has been a slight flattening of adoption curve, meaning the generations are starting to resemble each other more in their use of social networking sites
- As the Pew Internet team points out, Twitter use has doubled since November 2010, but it is still only 16% across the population—not as many people as one might think

This work was aimed at the use of Twitter (a social media venue), not the whole Internet use by generations.

To look at these numbers from a healthcare perspective, one has to look at total populations of users of social networking and Twitter rather than % Internet users, as these are reported.

Source: Adapted from: Social media adoption across the generations 2013 update. (Charts available at http://www.tedeytan.com/2013/or/22/13462#sthash.7xD9Xmut.dpuf)

the person knows or has read related to their medical condition or medication. It is of equal importance to ascertain what complementary and/or alternative medical treatments the person may have utilized. Homeopathic compounds are readily available to the public, and often people take something because a "friend" told them it helped them with a certain condition.

According to the Pew Research Center (2014), half of Internet users ages 50–64, and one in three users age 65 and older, use social networking sites. See **Box 17-2**.

The educator may find that persons stop taking prescribed medications because of something read on the Internet about a side effect that might occur. The educator must be cognizant of these actions and seek information from the person about possible misinformation and be ready to dispel any unwarranted information related to a medication or physical/mental condition.

Individuals, Families, and Groups

People live in groups, and the family is the most basic social group. For purposes of this discussion, the *family* is what the patient says it is. For some, family members are related by blood or marriage. For others, family members include close social (and sometimes sexual) ties with people who are not otherwise related. Families may be supportive or not supportive. They may be healthy or unhealthy. They may be large and extended or small and nuclear. Some people have rejected or cannot identify a family; others have been rejected by their families. Regardless of family process or content, the individual is greatly influenced by this first social unit.

One special group frequently not considered when discussing education related to medical or mental health are the veterans of the armed forces. Veterans return from foreign or domestic crises and must deal not only with the medical problems (sometimes life changing) but the mental and emotion toils as well. When nurses have a veteran as a patient, teaching this person in the same way you would teach a civilian would probably be less effective with the veteran. Veterans are offered services through the Veteran's Administration Medical System. According to the Gallup Poll of June 9, 2014, 87% of Americans responded that there needed to be an improvement in the way medical services are provided for the U.S. military veterans (Saad, 2014). As worldwide crises continue, the communities are welcoming back more and more veterans. It is imperative that nurses consider the special needs of the armed forces veterans. Assessing physical and mental needs of these persons can often be challenging to nurses who have had no exposure to the specific care needed by veterans.

A *group*, by comparison, is defined as people who interact as individuals to reach a common goal (Rankin & Stallings, 2001). Groups may come together for short periods to address one purpose (e.g., a bereavement support group) or they may be more stable over time with larger purposes (e.g., a local unit of Alcoholics Anonymous). Families and groups are important entities for community health nurses to recognize. Families and groups may need direct education (e.g., the nurse teaches a parent group how to take an infant's temperature or how to recognize the signs of adolescent suicide), or they may need to be included as a support system for an individual patient (e.g., the nurse includes family members in a discussion of safe food preparation for an immune-suppressed child). This chapter looks at two specific issues related to community education of individuals, families, and groups: discharge teaching and community-based teaching. The value of providing follow-up contact with the individual, family, group, or community cannot be overlooked. Immediate repetition or demonstration of what has been taught is important, but just as important, if not more so, is to follow up and make certain the learner has committed the education to memory and is utilizing the information to assist in achieving an optimal health status.

GLOBAL CONNECTION 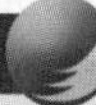

As a travel nurse, you are assigned to a public health department in a developing country with a low literacy rate. How will you adjust your role as educator in this setting?

Discharge Teaching

Discharge teaching happens in formal inpatient and outpatient care settings, but it provides a basis for community care. Discharge teaching has become more complex in recent years because of changes in the way health care is provided. People are discharged from acute care settings earlier, with less recuperation time. More procedures, including some that are quite complicated, are being done in outpatient settings. Hospitalization after delivery is usually 24 hours at most. All of these changes have led to people going home with more complex medications, treatments, pain, and anxiety. In addition, because the patient spends less time in the formal care setting, there is less time for teaching. This is further complicated by the fact that teaching must often happen in the immediate aftermath of a procedure, a time when patients tend to be most anxious and least able to attend to educational messages (Hunt, 1997). Discharge teaching also occurs in community settings such as home health, occupational settings, and school settings as nurses educate individuals about managing their own care.

Nurses can overcome these barriers with careful assessment and planning. If possible, some teaching should take place in the clinic, home, or community before the acute event; preoperative education and prenatal classes are good examples of this. In addition, community resources need to be identified in advance: Is the family willing and able to provide care? Will home health services be required? Are there other options? Assessing these needs and establishing early contacts can ensure that the individual is well prepared. Bringing the needed supports (e.g., responsible family members or homecare agencies) in early can decrease education time.

> To quit smoking is easy. I've done it hundreds of times.
>
> —*Mark Twain*
>
> Learning is what happens when what you thought would work doesn't.
>
> —*Unknown*

Education can then proceed through the teaching process as discussed earlier. Assessment should include a history of experiences that may influence this event, as well as individual and family coping mechanisms. Planning and implementation should be concise, clear, and supported by written information. Teaching should include demonstrations and return demonstrations for all treatments (e.g., dressing changes) and equipment (e.g., medication pumps). Follow-up telephone calls and referrals to community agencies for more intense follow up should be scheduled (Hunt, 1997). The bottom line is that patients should not feel that they are on their own at the time of discharge. Ideally, they should feel secure in their own abilities to provide self-care. If this is not possible, patients should know how to arrange for the support they will need at home.

Community-Based Teaching

The Centers for Disease Control and Prevention (CDC) has a Community Preventive Services Task Force established in 1996 with the charge to assess and provide information on wide ranges of decision makers on programs, services, and policies aimed at improving population health (CDC, 2014)

Discharge teaching provides information for patients who have been treated in a formal healthcare setting. More and more often, however, people need health education as a part of their daily lives. **Community-based teaching** can be complicated by a number of variables. The home setting itself can be difficult. The nurse will be on the patient's "home turf," and there may be distractions from family members (especially if there are children in the house). In addition, teaching equipment will need to be brought into the house by the nurse, and the nurse may need to address learning needs for a wider range in individuals. Health education in the home must also be carefully coordinated among various care providers. To make matters even more difficult, all this must be done in a limited amount of time (Hunt, 1997). However, there are major advantages to teaching in the patient's home:

- The nurse can assess the patient's environment and make changes in the teaching plan to compensate for problems and to take advantage of strengths to improve health and lead a healthy lifestyle even in less than optimal environments.
- The family can be more easily involved.
- The patient will usually be more comfortable in his or her own environment.
- The patient will be learning in the environment in which he or she will be using new information to perform new skills and behaviors.
- Home health nurses have the unique opportunity to provide education in a repetitive fashion and therefore improve cognitive learning opportunities. Repetition is necessary for some learners to maintain optimal retention of important information.
- Homecare providers also have the opportunity to assess the living conditions and form a plan that will assist the learner in obtaining the needed resources to improve health and lead a healthy lifestyle even in less than optimal environments.

Once again, application of the teaching process will help the nurse meet education goals. A most important step in community-based education is to keep the patient and significant others involved in the entire process from assessment to evaluation. This helps the nurse address those issues of highest concern, establish trust within the family setting, and provide the basis for further education. Nurses serve as case managers in the community: They are the professionals who are responsible for coordinating information between the patient and a variety of caregivers. In this process, nurses must cover objectives from each of the other care providers and integrate their orders with the needs of the patient and family. To accomplish this complex task, nurses need to be aware of community resources so that they can make appropriate referrals. The result should be that community-based patients feel comfortable with their self-care (or family-care) status. Patients should move toward independent care or toward the knowledge that care will be maintained by trusted family members and/or professional providers (Hunt, 1997).

One specific resource nurses need to be aware of is the American Nurses Association's (ANA) *HealthyNurse* program. Sachs and Jones (2013) discussed the development and function of the HealthyNurse program. Quoting ANA's president Daley, "When we model the healthiest behaviors ourselves it becomes easier to help our patients to do the best things for their health" (para. 4). ANA supports a healthy nurse who can focus on creating and maintaining a balanced physical, intellectual, emotional, social, spiritual, personal, and professional wellbeing. Supporting healthy nurses leads to nurses who are better able to assess the needs of the patient as well as develop a plan of care that is patient centered and role modeled by the nurse.

According to DeCola (2013) a healthy nurse promotes a healthy nation. ANA's concept of a healthy nurse includes five aspects that enable nurses to function at maximum potential: (1) Calling to care; (2) Priority to self-care; (3) Opportunity to serve as a role model; (4) Responsibility to educate; and (5) Authority to advocate (Sachs & Jones, 2013).

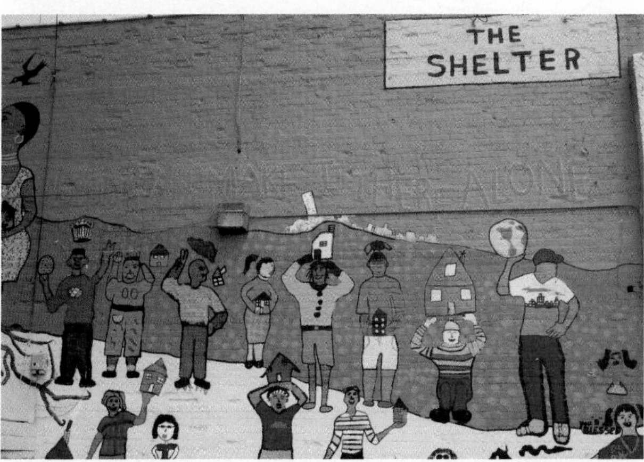

Mural on the wall of a community shelter in Tallahassee, Florida.

GOT AN ALTERNATIVE?

A nurse in the educator role will often be placed in situations where patients are more familiar with alternative and complementary therapies than the nurse is. How would you address this issue in a clinical setting?

Community

Community health learning occurs when knowledge, attitudes, and/or behaviors change within an entire community. Since the 1990s, major changes have been made in communities in areas such as seatbelt use, limitations on smoking areas in public spaces, and decreased tolerance of drunk driving. All of these changes came about when individuals in communities stood up and demanded safer and healthier environments. One such distraction that leads to unsafe driving habits and ultimately more frequent accidents within communities as well as more medical and mental distress would be the use of cell phones (mobile phones) when talking or texting while driving. Diverting one's attention while driving can lead to several injuries to one's self or to others in the vehicle or other vehicles. New laws have emerged that can lead to fines and possible arrest if stopped by law enforcement personnel (Garrison, 2014). Changes such as these often require legislative action; at other times, a shift in the community norm is all that has to occur. Nurses have not often taken full advantage of their positions in communities to influence change, but they should. Education and political action are within the realm of what nurses should and can do to improve the health of communities and the individuals in those communities.

Communities consist of groups of people who identify membership in the community. These people share commonalities in language, tradition, ritual, and ceremony. They share values and norms and exert influence over one another. They have emotional connections, common needs, and a commitment to the community to meet those needs. Community may occur within a geographic location (as in a neighborhood or a town) or may be connected by something other than geography (as in ethnic or age-specific groups). Community is defined by all of these connections, so people who merely live in close proximity may not be a community (Israel et al., 1994). An individual may have membership in more than one community and may have to deal with conflicting values from those communities. As you can see, a community has power that can affect **behavior change**. Although community support can be a powerful contribution to individual behavior change, lack of community support may doom an intervention to failure (Bigbee & Jansa, 1991). **Table 17-6** provides a case study to illustrate the process of community education.

TABLE 17-6 Community Education Process Case

Kris works as a school nurse at Center High School in a moderately sized Midwestern city. At a weekly team meeting, she tells her friend Sam, "I am so frustrated—we have five pregnant girls already this semester." Sam, who works at two middle schools, says, "You think that's bad? I have a case of chlamydia in a sixth grader!" Others add their comments until one says, "We clearly have a problem. What should we do?" The nurses decide to "do something about the risks of teen sexual activity." Because they already know the community well, the nurses decide to assess the problem by listing positive and negative community factors related to the problem of teen sexual activity and to use those assessments to plan interventions.

Assessment	Planning	Implementation	Evaluation
Positive factors: The community has a number of agencies that could be involved, including Planned Parenthood, Big Brothers/Big Sisters, the YMCA, churches, etc. Community schools have good reputations; most students graduate and many go to college. The state department of education supports a sex education curriculum based on harm reduction. School nurses have a ratio of 1:2,000 students. **Negative factors:** The school board (SB) supports and enforces an abstinence-only sex education curriculum as a result of pressure from a few vocal parents and one of the churches in the community. There are limited programs for students who are not succeeding in school and/or extracurricular activities. Most students come from families with working parents, and the majority has several hours of unsupervised time after school. Kris has had a number of students at her school tell her, "I want to get pregnant; it'd be cool." A survey of the nurses reveals 25 known teen pregnancies and 42 known cases of sexually transmitted diseases (STDs) in students over the past 24 months.	The nurses struggle with the question of what to do with the assessment information. After a long brainstorming session, they develop a plan. Each nurse will do the following: • Meet with his or her principal(s) to inform and educate about the problem • Attend the next two meetings of the SB and ask to have the topic of teen sexuality placed on the agenda • Encourage the use of the state's harm-reduction curriculum • Volunteer to teach sexuality classes in the 5th to 12th grades • Visit two to three community organizations (including churches) to discuss the problem, ask for support, and volunteer assistance to develop after-school programs	The nurses complete their assigned visits to the principals, SB, and local organizations. Each nurse reviews the state sex education curriculum and volunteers to teach classes at his or her assigned school(s).	**Summative evaluation:** All assignments are completed. **Formative evaluation:** All of the principals support the nurses' efforts. One principal asks about sexual abuse in students' families and peer relationships. The SB refuses to add the issue to the agenda. All of the nurses will teach sex education classes, but several principals and health teachers refuse to allow a harm-reduction curriculum until approval by the SB. Two churches and the YMCA are interested in setting up sports, games, and homework assistance programs after school. Planned Parenthood wants to develop a peer education program to address pressures to have sex to be "cool." **Follow up:** The nurses reassess the situation and plan for the next steps. The nurses will do the following: • Set up in-service programs for the nurses to learn about teaching a harm-reduction curriculum • Set up nurse counseling services for any student who wants to discuss issues privately—available to all students, but especially for students in abusive relationships • Continue attending SB meetings; encourage principals, teachers, and parents to add their support at those meetings • Collaborate with agencies as new programs are developed and encourage other agencies to consider developing their own programs

> There are some things you learn best in calm, and some in storm.
>
> —*Willa Cather*

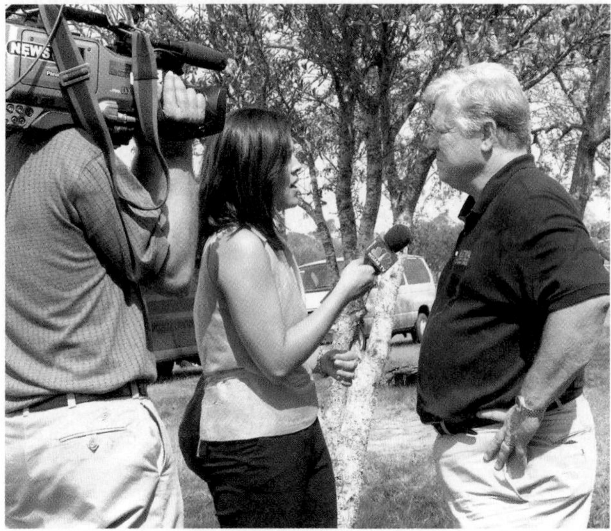

The media is underutilized by health professionals as a way to communicate critical information about a community's health and wellbeing. In this photo, Governor Haley Barbour of Mississippi speaks to the press about the Hurricane Katrina disaster health problems and plans for recovery.

Community Assessment

As with individual health education, health education at the community level starts with community assessment. As in individual education, this assessment needs to take into account the full spectrum of community variables. Individual behaviors take place within the context of community, and understanding this context can help nurses predict both barriers to and supports for behavior change (Israel et al., 1994). The nurse needs a clear idea of what the community is: How do people in the community define *health* and *health care*? What is the norm for nutrition, elimination, exercise, sleep, sexuality, reproduction, and coping with stress? How is intellect supported? How does the community perceive itself? How are roles and relationships established and supported? What does the community value? Which ethnic and cultural identities exist in the community? Which language(s) is(are) spoken? Which ceremonies occur? Which rituals are supported? How does the community share resources? Is there a sense of shared responsibility (Krozy, 1996)? Nurses can gather this information from community leaders, written histories and records, observations, consultations, and other community members.

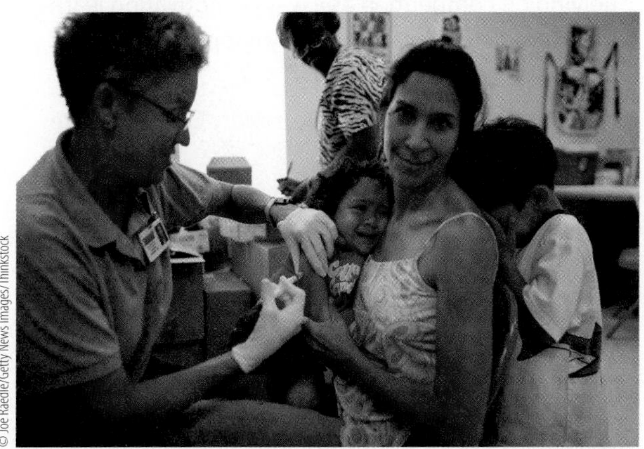

Community health nurses have limitless opportunities to educate parents about child care. Enlisting community lay volunteers in collaborative partnerships can be very effective in reaching specific populations.

> The illiterate of the twenty-first century will not be those who cannot read and write, but those who cannot learn, unlearn, and relearn.
>
> —*Alvin Toffler*

Communities, like individuals, experience stressors. These stressors range from daily hassles (as in ongoing arguments from businesses that want to limit government controls) to chronic problems (e.g., homelessness or air pollution) to major events (e.g., the closing of an industry) to cataclysmic events (e.g., an earthquake or flood) (Israel et al., 1994). Other community problems can include poverty, overpopulation, social injustice, lack of social organization, overcrowding (Carr, Lhussier, Wilkinson, & Gleadhill, 2008; Krozy, 1996; Yu et al., 2007), a history of powerlessness, and tensions created by inequity and discrimination (Israel et al., 1994). All of these contribute to community perceptions of powerlessness. Community empowerment, then, becomes a teaching strategy.

The good news is that communities also provide support for behavior change. The nurse should assess those things that enhance opportunities for education and change. These might include the emotional support given to community members who are trying to effect change. In addition, established agencies and services may already be available to support change. Information dissemination systems may be in place, and respected community members may be willing to sway opinion toward change (Israel et al., 1994).

Planning for the Community

The main point that needs to be made about community planning should be obvious: Planning requires community involvement (Andrade & Doria-Ortiz, 1995).

Shared decision making leads to better acceptance of change, support for the process, and commitment to programs that emerge from the process (Foran & Campanelli, 1995). Involving large portions of the community in planning can be difficult, but it is necessary. Representation should be sought from government, business, service, health care, and religious entities as well as from the individuals who will be targeted by the plan. Input can be gathered in community meetings, focus groups, and interviews with key informants. Opposing views must be sought, acknowledged, and considered in any planning activity (Krozy, 1996). Planning can then progress to setting educational goals and selecting an appropriate theory base, taking into account the strengths and weaknesses of the community.

Common broad-based goals for community health education are to (1) help people change unhealthy, unsafe, or risky behaviors; (2) equalize access to health and support services; and (3) decrease the incidence of preventable conditions that have negative effects on the community (Krozy, 1996). Goals and more specific objectives need to be established and agreed upon during the planning process. Consider using *Healthy People 2020* in this process. It delineates national goals for specific health issues targeted to at-risk populations (U.S. Department of Health and Human Services, 2011).

Foran and Campanelli (1995) identified the components of successful community health programs: They are flexible, they use ongoing evaluation to identify design problems as soon as possible, they use evaluation to guide change, they are valued by the community, and they evolve by incorporating new ideas and technologies as change occurs. Planners should understand all of these elements. And remember: Planning should include developing teaching interventions as well as evaluation tools.

Implementing Community Plans

Andrade and Doria-Ortiz (1995) encourage an implementation process that helps a community meet its own needs. This requires empowerment of community organizations, adequate resources and services to meet the needs of at-risk community members, and sufficient resources in the healthcare system. Programs and services (especially those targeted at underserved populations) must be available, accessible, acceptable, and accountable. Programs that do not meet these criteria will not succeed.

It is important to remember that community education and change are long-term processes—they do not happen overnight. Even after programs are established, there must be commitment to a continuing process of assessment, planning, implementation, and evaluation. Implementation will be enhanced if the process is participatory (members of the community are involved), cooperative, collaborative, empowering, and balanced. At its best, the process will promote group identification, reinforcing the idea of a shared fate and the need to look at more global aspects of health (Carr et al., 2008; Israel et al., 1994).

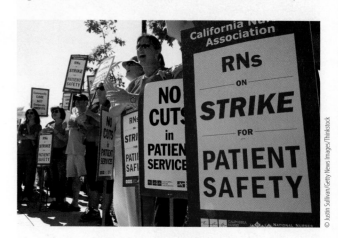

> Never underestimate that a small group of thoughtful, committed people can change the world; indeed, it's the only thing that ever has.
>
> —*Margaret Mead*

> Education is less and less a preparation for life and more and more a part of it.
>
> Our species thinks in metaphors and learns through stories.
>
> Relying on competition as a way of motivating learning eventually subverts not only cooperation but also the willingness to learn.
>
> —*Mary Catherine Bates*

The assessment and planning process will help nurses identify appropriate sites for community education. Where are the natural community networks? Are they centered on employment, recreational, religious, or commercial functions? Will organizations that are not viewed as healthcare agencies (e.g., schools and churches) get involved? Can early health-promotion programs be established in neighborhood elementary and middle schools? Are community colleges open to health education efforts? Will the justice system support health education for people who live in prisons, jails, and halfway houses? Establishing programs specific to people who congregate in these sites can promote education in ways that target at-risk individuals (Andrade & Doria-Ortiz, 1995; Carr et al., 2008).

How health education is implemented also depends on assessment and planning. It helps to have a theoretical base (see Tables 17-2 and 17-3), knowing that some models are better for community intervention than others. Diffusion theory and social marketing theory, for example, were developed from community-focused research. The transtheoretical model also includes components of community action. Common teaching strategies for community intervention include lectures, small group work, facilitated discussions, demonstrations, printed and audiovisual materials, simulation exercises, guided imagery, and social marketing (Krozy, 1996). The important thing to remember is that the teaching strategy needs to match the learning objective (see Table 17-5) as well as the developmental level of the audience.

Evaluating Community Programs

As stated earlier, evaluation is an ongoing process in health education. Formal evaluation should be planned, and informal evaluation should be acknowledged and used in the process. Formative evaluation is used throughout the process. Summative evaluation occurs at a set point when goals are expected to have been met. Effective evaluation determines progress toward goals and identifies goals that have not yet been met. Data from evaluation are used to do the following:

- Determine whether unmet goals are still a priority
- Plan interventions to address unmet goals
- Assess the impact of goals that have been achieved
- Assess evolving needs
- Establish new community goals and objectives

The community health education process is much like the individual teaching process (it is cyclical and progressive in nature), but it is more complicated.

Beyond Community

Nurses who are involved in community education activities realize that some problems are too big to deal with on a community level. Sometimes, changes need to be made at the level of state and federal governments. Political advocacy then becomes a part of the health education agenda. Nurses can educate communities about the political process to encourage input into legislative activities, knowing that communities with identified needs can often influence legislative outcomes.

BOX 17-3 Institute for Healthcare Improvement Open School: What Is the IHI Open School?

IHI Open School's goal is to be the "other school" with whom students can affiliate themselves, to act as a nonprofit organization established for the purpose of promoting patient safety and quality improvement in health care, to create projects that positively impact the community, and to inspire and train the future healthcare workforce to be skilled agents of change and to improve care at home, in the community, in the office practice, and throughout the hospital.

Our Mission

1. Inspire and train the future healthcare workforce to be skilled agents of change and to improve care at home, in the community, in the office practice, and throughout the hospital
2. Create quality improvement projects that beneficially impact the San Antonio community
3. To promote the importance of delivering the best care to our patients

Source: Institute for Healthcare Improvement. (2012). IHI Open School San Antonio. Retrieved from http://ihisanantonio.weebly.com/index.html

Some examples of community needs that have been addressed through legislative intent include drunk driving laws, water fluoridation bills, motorcycle helmet requirements, and funding for various initiatives ranging from school-based health education programs to needle and syringe exchange programs. Andrade and Doria-Ortiz (1995) recommend the following legislative actions to support the health of the Mexican American community: provide national health insurance to cover the working poor, cooperate with Mexico to provide health care in border communities, address high-risk diseases (e.g., diabetes and tuberculosis) and conditions (e.g., teen pregnancy and violence), increase Hispanic access to health professions schools, and ensure input from Hispanic communities into federal policy and legislative planning activities. Nurses can help communities achieve goals such as these.

New laws are being proposed by the government that will affect the country. For example, the law everyone knows as ObamaCare or ACA is officially the Patient Protection and Affordable Care Act. The Senate passed the bill on December 24, 2009, the House passed it on March 21, 2010, and President Obama signed it into law on March 23, 2010. Its provisions were upheld by the

Supreme Court on June 28, 2012. In this instance, the country is the "community."

Ethical Issues in Health Education

Health education on the surface seems like an appropriate and ethical thing to do. After all, how ethical would it be to withhold information that could relieve suffering, prevent pain, and avert disease? But health education has its own controversies. Some of these are discussed next; others will become obvious to you as you educate individuals and communities.

A major problem occurs when there are unexpected, negative consequences because of health education. These can be the result of erroneous, poorly planned, or improperly implemented education efforts (Guttman et al., 1996). For instance, suppose you want to teach a group of people who are newly diagnosed with cancer that there is hope. You ask four or five people with cancer to speak to your group. Unfortunately, several of the presenters are dealing with anger and depression because of their disease, and they take this opportunity to share their pain and frustration with the healthcare system. At the end of the session, your audience is likely to be confused (at the least) or to feel complete despair (at the worst). They may lose confidence in the ability to survive cancer treatment; they may even decide to forgo therapy altogether and "get it over with." Although this example is quite extreme, problems can occur even under ideal circumstances.

One of the primary concerns that nurses have to address is the fact that, in many ways, health education manipulates patients to change behaviors. Granted, the changes we seek (based on our assessment of the latest scientific evidence) are for the patient's benefit, but we are nevertheless clearly trying to influence change (Redman, 1997, 2008). This may be difficult for nurses to accept. We have, after all, been taught to respect individual autonomy. Manipulation, no matter how subtle, is hard to justify. This is not a reason to stop teaching or to stop advocating for policies such as motorcycle helmet laws. Instead, it is something that each nurse must weigh carefully before, during, and after health education programs. It also helps to differentiate manipulation from information dissemination. Giving a pregnant adolescent information on options, including the whole spectrum of choices involved in either continuing or terminating her pregnancy, for instance, is information dissemination that she can use to make an informed decision. Encouraging her to have an abortion, to give the infant up for adoption, or to have the baby and raise it herself is manipulation, especially if she makes her "informed" decision based on a lack of complete information that the nurse has failed to share.

Another issue is science itself and the rate at which knowledge expands (Redman, 1997). We have all heard patients say, "This is so confusing. How am I supposed to know what I should be doing? Last night there was a story on the news about how exercise can cause joint deterioration and here you are telling me that I need to exercise more!" Nurses have an obligation to keep up with advances in health care, but even nurses get confused. This all adds to the complex nature of education and reinforces the need to be able to read and critique research (see the following Research Alert for an example of a study about health education).

One of the social issues in patient education has to do with the growing gap between socioeconomic classes (Guttman et al., 1996; Redman, 2008). People who are

RESEARCH ALERT

The primary objective of this study was to assess the suitability and readability level of publicly available educational print resources related to physical activity (PA). Educational print resources related to PA ($n = 66$) were requested from organizations (e.g., professional, commercial, government, and educational). The suitability assessment of materials (SAM) and the Simple Measure of Gobbledygook (SMOG) readability appraisal were used to evaluate the suitability and readability of the PA resources. Of the 66 PA resources, suitability scores were superior in only 10 resources (15%), adequate in 36 resources (55%), and inadequate/not suitable in 20 resources (30%). The average reading grade level for the PA resources was a 10th grade level (S.D. = 1.82; Rg = 5th grade to 15th grade). Only 56.5% ($n = 35$) of PA resources depicted a primary PA recommendation that was consistent with the public health recommendation for PA. Results indicate that the majority of educational print resources related to PA have poor readability indices and inadequate to adequate suitability. Health educators developing educational print resources related to PA must ensure these resources conform to the highest suitability standards. This includes developing resources that contain information consistent with current public health recommendations and that can be utilized by all individuals regardless of health literacy status.

Source: Vallance, J., Taylor, L., & Lavallee, C. (2008). Suitability and readability assessment of educational print resources related to physical activity: Implications and recommendations for practice. *Patient Education & Counseling, 72*(2), 342–349.

financially secure are better equipped to act on advice to improve their health. Those without economic resources, however, often see health behaviors (e.g., exercise and eating well) as things they simply cannot afford. Poverty affects individuals' health, which further decreases their ability to earn a living or to get ahead. Nurses need to recognize that poor health practices may be related to social and economic barriers as much as they are related to a lack of knowledge, motivation, or positive attitudes. When this is the case, social and community solutions need to be explored rather than falling into the trap of victim blaming (Marantz, 1990). How appropriate, for instance, is it to blame an alcoholic for her liver disease? What if she was raised in a house where alcohol was used to deal with stress? What if her life has been filled with loss, abuse, and trauma? And what if her only solace is to sink into an alcoholic daze? Is this situation her fault? Maybe. Maybe not. Is she beyond help? No, but help is not easy to give if you blame the patient for her disability. Repetitious, ineffective teaching will not help the situation either.

Community health nurses must keep abreast of all legislature activities that are pending in the governing bodies of the country. Community members are exposed to many different ideas and are frequently unable to understand what the pending legislature might mean for them as an individual or as a community or country. Governmental bodies use social media networks to spread information quickly throughout the population. Popular or well-known platforms (i.e., sports or Hollywood stars) are used most often as they tend to have a great deal of influence on the behavior of the population. These avenues of exposure offer access to a greater number of individuals, families, groups, and communities to whom access would be problematic under political budgetary constraints. Individuals and families frequently place more importance on what is said by individuals in the social network than what is presented in news venues.

Sometimes, as a community health professional, the community health nurse may be required to enter specific areas that are designated to certain population-specific communities. This does not mean the community is labeled as a specific neighborhood for specific populations but that certain groups tend to live where there is less cultural stigma. A few of these might include communities of those individuals who have certain sexuality commonalities such as transgender or HIV/AIDS communities. The community health nurse must be able to distance personal feelings toward specific populations that have a stigma attached. There might be racial and ethnic groups where language is a barrier to education or where the specific group holds to the homeopathic treatments rather than the use of newer methods or treatment and/or medications. You as the nurse must find a way of allowing persons to have some control over their bodies while introducing them to and encouraging the use of more contemporary healthcare techniques. As the nurse, you must accept the individual's right to refuse some treatments. Sometimes, the nurse must allow the individual, family, group, and/or community to use the treatments they prefer while trying to assess the effectiveness of that alternative method of treatment. Trust is so important. If you as the nurse can gain the trust of the persons in the community, then the community may be more likely to become an active listener/learner.

A final ethical issue that deserves attention has to do with community and cultural norms (Guttman et al., 1996; Redman, 1997). We each bring cultural biases into our social interactions. This is true of nurses as well as of patients. In addition to all of their other cultures, nurses bring the culture of health care and scientific bias into every encounter. This makes it difficult for nurses to deal with situations in which, for example, we know that overweight children tend to grow up to be overweight adults, but the predominant culture believes that only "fat babies" are healthy. Nurses cannot ignore these conflicting values. They must instead use creative problem solving to develop acceptable solutions on a number of different levels. This can be a messy process with many trials and only a few successes. The alternative is to try to force the culture of science on people who are not going to accept it no matter how hard the nurse tries. So, why not take some chances? The outcome could be that new messages or teaching methods or solutions emerge, and that could be the best possible conclusion to a difficult situation.

Conclusion

Health education is an important intervention for nurses in all healthcare settings. The purpose of health education is to change behaviors and situations that put people at risk for injury, illness, disability, or death. It is a theory-based process that draws form learning theory as well as behavior change theory. The health education process is similar to the nursing process. It is appropriate in all clinical and community settings and can be applied to individuals, families, groups, and communities. Nurses may find that advocacy at the state and federal levels is required to make personal and community behavior change possible. Nurses must also be aware that health education poses some important ethical issues.

Elspeth Murray recites her poem that was included at the International Initiative in Mental Health Leadership Conference in Edinburgh, where she conducted poetry workshops.

This is bad enough
So please …
Don't give me
gobbledegook.
Don't give me
pages and dense pages
and
"this leaflet aims to explain … "
Don't give me
really dodgy photocopying
and
"DO NOT REMOVE
FOR REFERENCE ONLY."
Don't give me
"drafted in collaboration with
a multidisciplinary stakeholder
partnership consultation
short-life project working group."
I mean is this about
you guys
or me?
This is hard enough
So please:
Don't leave me
oddly none the wiser or
listening till my eyes are
glazing over.
Don't leave me
wondering what on earth that was about,
feeling like it's rude to ask
or consenting to goodness knows what.
Don't leave me
lost in another language
adrift in bad translation.
Don't leave me
chucking it in the bin
Don't leave me
leaving in the state I'm in.
Don't leave me
feeling even more clueless
than I did before any of this
happened.
This is tough enough
So please:
Make it relevant,
understandable –
or reasonably
readable
at least.
Why not put in
pictures
or sketches,
or something to
guide me through?
I mean how hard can it be
for the people
who are steeped in this stuff
to keep it up-to-date?
And you know what I'd appreciate?
A little time to take it in
a little time to show them at home
a little time to ask, "What's that?"
a little time to talk on the phone.
So give us
the clarity, right from the start
the contacts, there at the end.
Give us the info
you know we need to know.
Show us the facts,
some figures
And don't forget our feelings.
Because this is bad
and hard
and tough enough
so please speak
like a human
make it better
not worse.

You can contact me on elspeth@elspethmurray.com
http://www.elspethmurray.com/poems.htm

Critical Thinking Activities

1. Develop teaching plans for each of the following cases. Identify and use a theory base that can help guide the process. Discuss assessment, planning, implementation, and evaluation as a part of your process.
   - *Case 1*: Diane is a 48-year-old single mother who fractured her left wrist in a fall 3 weeks ago. The wrist was reduced in the hospital emergency department and set with a standard cast. Except for some pain and the need to modify a few of her activities, Diane has done well and feels that she will recover completely. Diane saw her NP for a regular checkup 3 days ago. The NP expressed concern about Diane's wrist and asked about the circumstances of the accident. When Diane described a situation that would not normally result in a fracture, the NP ordered a scan to assess bone density. The results show a 2.5% loss of bone mass. The NP orders exercise and dietary changes. Diane and her provider agree to try these tactics for 6 months before considering medications. Diane's 14-year-old son lives with her. Her 20-year-old daughter recently married and moved out of state. The rest of Diane's family lives 350 miles away. She is the co-owner of a business that builds office complexes, and she typically works 10 to 12 hours a day. When you question her about her current diet and exercise routines, she shrugs and says, "To tell you the truth, I'm way too busy to worry about those things. They just take up too much time."
   - *Case 2*: Janet, the nurse at Allen Elementary School, has documented 12 cases of head lice during the past week. Most of the affected students came from one 3rd-grade class, but two cases came from a 2nd-grade class, and one each came from a 5th-grade class and another 3rd-grade class.
   - *Case 3*: The nursing home in Sheridan County has a respite care center where families can leave elderly patients between the hours of 7 a.m. and 7 p.m. The program provides meals, organized activities, and nap facilities for 22 patients with various physical and cognitive disabilities. Families who use the service give positive feedback about improvements in their abilities to cope with the stresses of caring for elderly relatives in the home. Sheila is an 86-year-old woman with confusion and delusions who is a regular patient. Over the past week, Fred, the nurse manager, has noticed bruises around Sheila's wrists. Fred asks Sheila's daughter about the bruises, and she replies, "Oh, I guess she gets those from the restraints. She's started wandering around the house at night. I'm worried that she might fall and break a hip, so I talked to some of the other families at our last group meeting and several of them suggested that I tie Mama into bed at night."
   - *Case 4*: Community Care Center is a comprehensive outpatient healthcare facility that serves injection drug users. In addition to methadone treatment, the center provides counseling services, case management, first aid, and routine annual physical assessments. The physician who does the physicals is only in the center 2 days a week. She approaches Anita, the clinic nurse, and expresses concern about the number of chlamydia cases that she has diagnosed recently. She asks Anita, "What do you think we can do about this?" Although Anita agrees that the pattern the physician describes is an important concern, she worries about the ethical issues that could occur if the clinic takes any action. What ethical issues could develop? How can Anita address those issues for the clinic staff, patients, and surrounding community?

References

Allender, J. A., & Spradley, B. W. (2001). *Community health nursing: Concepts and practice* (5th ed.). Philadelphia, PA: Lippincott Williams & Wilkins.

American Medical Association. (2007). Health literacy and patient safety: Help patients understand. Policy H-160.931 Health Literacy. Retrieved from http://www.ama-assn.org/ama1/mm/367/healthlitclinicians.pdf

Andrade, S. J., & Doria-Ortiz, C. (1995). *Nuestro bienestar*: A Mexican-American community-based definition of health promotion in the southwestern United States. *Drugs: Education, Prevention, and Policy, 2*, 129–145.

Bandura, A. (1977). *Social learning theory.* Englewood Cliffs, NJ: Prentice Hall.

Bandura, A. (1978). Reflections on self-efficacy. In S. Rachman (Ed.), *Advances in behavior research and therapy* (Vol. 1., pp. 237–269). Oxford, England: Pergamon.

Barofsky, I. (1978). Compliance, adherence and the therapeutic alliance: Steps in the development of self-care. *Social Science and Medicine, 12*(5A), 369–376.

Bastable, S. B. (2008). *Nurse as educator: Principles of teaching and learning for nursing practice* (3rd ed.). Sudbury, MA: Jones and Bartlett.

Bigbee, J. L., & Jansa, N. (1991). Strategies for promoting health protection. *Nursing Clinics of North America, 26*, 895–913.

Bradley-Springer, L. (1996). Patient education for behavior change: Help from the transtheoretical and harm reduction models. *Journal of the Association of Nurses in AIDS Care, 7*(Suppl.), 23–33.

Brocato, J., & Wagner, E. F. (2003). Harm reduction: A social work practice model and social justice agenda. *Health and Social Work, 28*(2), 117–125.

Carr, S., Lhussier, M., Wilkinson, J., & Gleadhill, S. (2008). Empowerment evaluation applied to public health practice. *Critical Public Health, 18*(2), 161–174.

Carter, W. B. (1990). Health behavior as a rational process: Theory of reasoned action and multiattribute utility theory. In K. Glanz, F. M. Lewis, & B. K. Rimer (Eds.), *Health behavior and health education: Theory, research, and practice* (pp. 63–91). San Francisco, CA: Jossey-Bass.

Cates, W., Jr., & Hinman, A. (1992). AIDS and absolutism: The demand for perfection in prevention. *New England Journal of Medicine, 327*, 492–494.

Centers for Disease Control and Prevention (CDC). (2014). Morbidity and Mortality Weekly Report (MMWR). Atlanta, GA: Centers for Disease Control and Prevention.

Charron-Prachnowik, D., Sereika, S., Becker, D., Jacober, S., Mansfield, J., White, N., . . . Trail, L. (2001). Reproductive health beliefs and behaviors in teens with diabetes: Application of the expanded health belief model. *Pediatric Diabetes, 2*, 30–39.

Cutill, C. C. (2006). Do your patients understand? How to write effective healthcare information. *Orthopedic Nursing, 25*(1), 39–48.

Daley, K. A. (2013). HealthyNurse. *American Nurses Association*. Silver Springs, MA: American Nurses Association.

Damrosch, S. (1991). General strategies for motivating people to change their behavior. *Nursing Clinics of North America, 26*, 833–843.

deBronkart, R. D. (2013). Let patients help!: A patient engagement handbook—how doctors, nurses, patients and caregivers can partner for better care. North Charleston, SC: CreateSpace Independent Publishing Platform.

DeCola, P. R. (2013). HealthyNurse. American Nurses Association. Silver Springs, MA: American Nurses Association.

Demir, F., Ozsaker, E., & Ilce, A. O. (2008). The quality and suitability of written educational materials for patients. *Journal of Clinical Nursing, 17*(2), 259–265.

DiClemente, R. J., Crosby, R. A., & Kegler, M. C. (Eds.). (2002). *Emerging theories in health promotion practice and research: Strategies for improving public health*. San Francisco, CA: Jossey-Bass.

Dutta-Bergman, M. J. (2004). Primary sources of health information: Comparisons in the domain of health attitudes, health cognitions, and health behaviors. *Health Communication, 16*(3), 273–288.

Fertman, C. I., & Allensworth, D. D. (2010). Health promotion programs: From theory to practice. Retrieved from www.books.google.com/books?isbn=0470590211

Foran, M., & Campanelli, L. C. (1995). Health promotion communications system: A model for a dispersed population. *AAOHN Journal, 43*, 564–569.

Garrison, S. (2014). Law enforcement says texting ban has teeth. *The Daily Times*. Retrieved from www.daily-times.com

Guttman, N., Kegler, M., & McLeroy, K. R. (1996). Health promotion paradoxes, antimonies and conundrums. *Health Education Research, 11*(1), i–xiii.

Health and Human Services HIPAA Survival Guide (2013). Retrieved from http://www.hipaasurvivalguide.com/hitech-act-summary.php

Healthy People 2020. (2014). Centers for Disease Control and Prevention. Retrieved from http://www.cdc.gov/nchs/healthy_people/hp2020.htm

Heinrich, C. (2010). Health literacy: The sixth vital sign. *Journal of the American Academy of Nurse Practitioners, 24*(2012), 218–222.

Hunt, R. (1997). Teaching. In R. Hunt & E. L. Zurek (Eds.), *Introduction to community based nursing* (pp. 182–225). Philadelphia, PA: Lippincott.

Institute of Medicine. (2003). *Unequal treatment: Confronting racial and ethnic disparities in healthcare*. Washington, DC: National Academies Press.

Israel, B. A., Checkoway, B., Schulz, A., & Zimmerman, M. (1994). Health education and community empowerment: Conceptualizing and measuring perceptions of individual, organizational, and community control. *Health Education Quarterly, 21*, 140–170.

Jachna, C. M., & Forbes-Thompson, S. (2005). Osteoporosis: Health beliefs and barriers to treatment in an assisted living facility. *Journal of Gerontological Nursing, 31*(1), 24–30.

Knowles, M. S., Holton, E. F., & Swanson, R. A. (1998). *The adult learner* (5th ed.). Woburn, MD: Butterworth-Heinemann.

Kreuter, M. W., & Strecher, V. J. (1996). Do tailored behavior change messages enhance the effectiveness of health risk appraisal? Results from a randomized trial. *Health Education Research, 11*, 97–105.

Krozy, R. E. (1996). Community health promotion: Assessment and intervention. In S. H. Rankin & K. D. Stallings (Eds.), *Patient education: Issues, principles, practices* (3rd ed., pp. 245–271). Philadelphia, PA: Lippincott.

Lindsey, J. (2012). Transgender populations. Diversity Roundtable Case Studies. Mississippi Health Care Symposium on Cultural Competency: Pathways toward ending health disparities. Hinds Community College, Pearl, MS.

London, F. (2012). No time to teach: The essence of patient and family education for health care providers (4th ed.). CreateSpace Independent Publishing Platform. Retrieved from www.books.google.com

Marantz, P. R. (1990). Blaming the victim: The negative consequence of preventive medicine. *American Journal of Public Health, 80*(18), 186–187.

McLaughlin, G. H. (1969). SMOG grading: A new readability formula. *Journal of Reading, 12*(8), 639–646.

Miller, P., Wikoff, R., & Hiatt, A. (1992). Fishbein's model of reasoned action and compliance behavior of hypertensive patients. *Nursing Research, 41*, 104–109.

Novelli, W. D. (1990). Applying social marketing to health promotion and disease prevention. In K. Glanz, F. M. Lewis, & B. K. Rimer (Eds.), *Health behavior and health education: Theory, research, and practice* (pp. 342–369). San Francisco, CA: Jossey-Bass.

Orlandi, M. A., Landers, C., Weston, R., & Haley, N. (1990). Diffusion of health promotion innovations. In K. Glanz, F. M. Lewis, & B. K. Rimer (Eds.), *Health behavior and health education: Theory, research, and practice* (pp. 288–313). San Francisco, CA: Jossey-Bass.

Palank, C. L. (1991). Determinants of health-promotive behavior: A review of current research. *Nursing Clinics of North America, 26*, 815–832.

Pender, N. (1996). *Health promotion in nursing practice* (3rd ed.). Upper Saddle River, NJ: Pearson Education.

Perry, C. L., Baranowski, T., & Parcel, G. S. (1990). How individuals, environments and health behavior interact: Social learning theory. In K. Glanz, F. M. Lewis, & B. K. Rimer (Eds.), *Health behavior and health education: Theory, research, and practice* (pp. 161–186). San Francisco, CA: Jossey-Bass.

Petty, R. E., Barden, J., & Wheeler, S. C. (2002). The elaboration likelihood model of persuasion: Health promotions that yield sustained behavioral change. In R. J. DiClemente, R. A. Crosby, & M. C. Kegler (Eds.), *Emerging theories in health promotion practice and research: Strategies for improving public health* (pp. 71–99). San Francisco, CA: Jossey-Bass.

Petty, R. E., Barden, J., & Wheeler, S. C. (2009). The elaboration likelihood model of persuasion: Health promotions that yield sustained behavioral change. In R. J. DiClemente, R. A. Crosby, & M. Kegler (Eds.) *Emerging theories in health promotion, practice, and research* (pp. 185–214). San Francisco, CA: Jossey-Bass.

Pew Research Center. (2014). Pew Internet Social Networking. Retrieved from http://www.pewresearch.org/

Rankin, S. N., & Stallings, K. D. (2001). *Patient education: Principles and practice* (4th ed.). Philadelphia, PA: Lippincott Williams & Wilkins.

Rankin, S. H., Stallings, K. D., & London, F. (2005). Patient education in health and illness (5th ed.). Philadelphia, PA: Lippincott Williams & Welkins.

Redman, B. K. (1997). *The practice of patient education*. St. Louis, MO: Mosby.

Redman, B. (2008). When is patient education unethical? *Nursing Ethics, 15*(6), 813–820.

Saad, L. (2014). Most in U.S. Want to Prioritize Improving Veterans' Health. Retrieved from http://www.gallup.com/poll/171596/prioritize-improving-veterans-health.aspx

Sachs, A., & Jones, J. (2013). HealthyNurse. *American Nurses Association*. Silver Springs, MA: American Nurses Association.

Sharma, M., & Ronas, J. A. (2011). Theoretical foundations of health education and health promotion. (2nd ed.). Sudbury, MA: Jones & Bartlett Learning.

Soffer, A. (2009). Achievement goal theory and self-efficacy theory: Predicting the psychological effects of a New York Road Runners foundation running program. Ann Arbor, MI: ProQuest LLC.

Spellbring, A. M. (1991). Nursing's role in health promotion: An overview. *Nursing Clinics of North America, 26*, 805–814.

Strang, J. (1992). Harm reduction for drug users: Exploring the dimensions of harm, their measurement, and strategies for reductions. *AIDS and Public Policy Journal, 7*, 145–152.

Strecher, V. J., Seijts, G. H., Kok, G. J., Latham, G. P., Glasgow, R., DeVellis, B., . . . Bulger, D. W. (1995). Goal setting as a strategy for health behavior change. *Health Education Quarterly, 22*, 190–200.

U.S. Department of Health and Human Services. (2011). *Healthy People 2020*. Retrieved from http://www.hhs.gov/ash/initiatives/index.html

U.S. Department of Health and Human Services . (2014). http://www.healthypeople.gov/2020/default.aspx

Yu, M., Song, L., Seetoo, A., Cai, C., Smith, G., & Oakley, P. (2007). Culturally competent training program: A key to training lay health advisors for promoting breast cancer screening. *Health Education & Behavior, 34*(6), 928–941.

CHAPTER FOCUS

Types of Groups
Characteristics of Effective Groups
Common Goal
Collective Identity
Interdependent Interaction
Mutual Influence
Communication Within Groups
Group Roles
Shared Decision Making
Conflict Management
Group Leadership
Diversity
Dysfunctional Behavior
Sexual Harassment
Stages of Group Development
Group Maintenance Roles
Group Dissolution
Groups as Change Agents
Groups and Technology
Impact of Communication Technologies on the Work of Healthcare Groups in the Community
Evaluating Groups
Ethical Considerations

QUESTIONS TO CONSIDER

After reading this chapter, you will know the answers to the following questions:

1. What are group characteristics?
2. What are the stages of group development?
3. What kinds of functions do groups perform?
4. What are the different types of groups in which community health nurses might be involved?
5. How is group process evaluated?
6. What is group leadership? How does it apply in community health nursing?

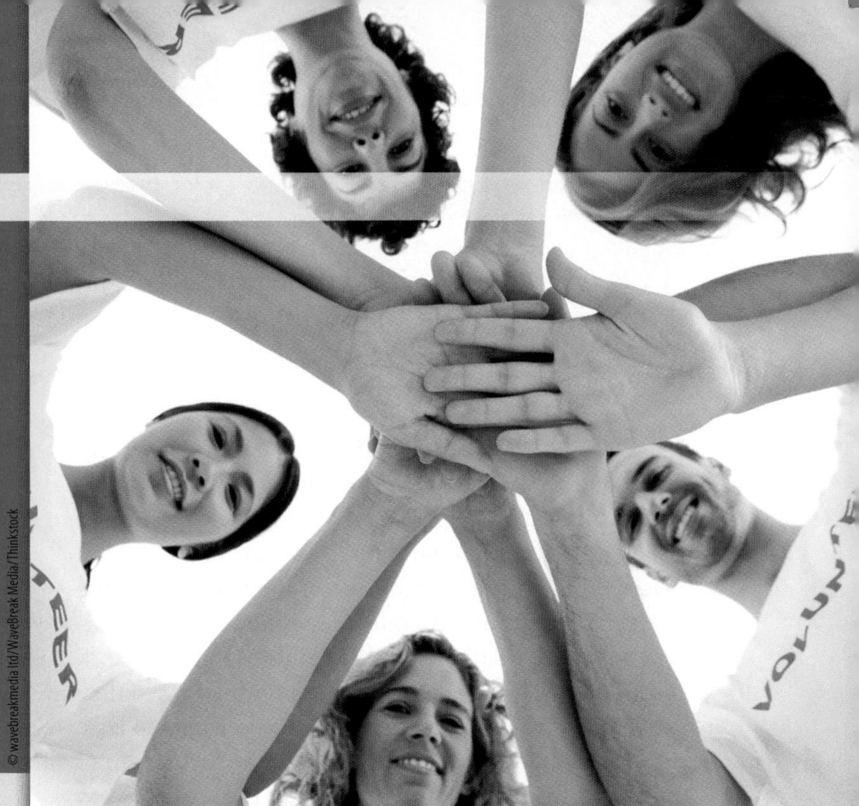

CHAPTER 18

Community and Group Communication

Grace Coggio and Lilianna K. Deveneau

KEY TERMS

asynchronous
coalitions
cohesion
convergence
decision making
emoticons
empowerment
group
impact evaluation
leadership
norms
open communication
outcome evaluation
participation
process evaluation
social presence
synchronous
synergy
virtual team

REFLECTIONS

Nurses work most of their professional lives in groups, and yet student nurses most frequently cite group work as their least liked part of nursing school. Human beings would not have survived without the formation of groups. How do you feel about working with a successful group that meets its goals? What are the differences between a successful group and a group that is inefficient and a time waster?

WORKING WITH GROUPS in community settings is an essential component of public health and community health nursing practices. The implementation of the Patient Protection and Affordable Care Act (ACA) has placed an increased emphasis on group work across the healthcare spectrum. As nurse practitioner and education specialist, Matthews (2012) points out, nurses work more effectively and efficiently in groups than when they work individually due to their "unique professional lens, expertise in team-based care, and patient partnerships". Nurses participate in a variety of groups that work toward achieving community health goals, and are members of work-related groups that often collaborate with others toward continued improvement of the healthcare system and the nursing profession. For example, community health nurses are contributing to community-based research teams and are helping to expand the capacity of community health initiatives, particularly among populations that may otherwise be difficult to access.

Research demonstrates that groups made up of individuals with a diversity of knowledge and skill sets perform more effectively and with greater efficiency than groups of people with similar skills (Saad, Damian, Benet-Martinez, Moons, & Robins, 2012), and interdisciplinary groups of healthcare professionals increasingly will be relied upon to "address and improve the health of populations" (Garr, Margalit, Jameton, & Cerra, 2012). To successfully achieve the population health promotion and restoration goals so central to community-based care, therefore, nurses participate in groups or teams that often include doctors, nutritionists, counselors, community leaders, and other community stakeholders. Even everyday community health practices, such as managing chronic disease and increasing immunization rates through education, have been improved by taking an interdisciplinary team approach.

Groups provide an advantage over working alone because they:

- Can accomplish tasks that often are not achievable by individuals
- Bring a wider range of resources, skills, and talents to contribute to solutions of complex health issues
- Provide a means of decision making that allows for multiple and sometimes conflicting views to be evaluated and synthesized
- Have the synergy of combined effort that surpasses the capacity of individuals to achieve community health goals

Given the emphasis on groups in community health initiatives, it is critical that nurses understand the basic concepts, leadership skills, and ethical considerations of working in groups. Drawing on a body of interdisciplinary research, including applicable theories that help guide nursing practice with groups, such as "Parse's Theory in Practice with a Group in the Community" (Kelley, 1995), this chapter focuses on the development, maintenance, and evaluation of effective group processes.

HEALTHY PEOPLE 2020 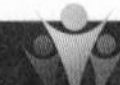

National Health Standards and Objectives

Collective Responsibility for Change

- *Healthy People 2000:* "While the responsibility for change lies with each of us, it also lies with all of us, and individuals cannot be expected to act alone" (U.S. Department of Health and Human Services [HHS], 1991, p. 85).
- *Healthy People 2010:* "Community health is profoundly affected by the collective behaviors, attitudes, and beliefs of everyone who lives in the community" (HHS, 2000; p. 3).
- *Healthy People 2020:* "On a practical level, it is a road map showing where we want to go as a nation and how we are going to get there—both collectively and individually" (HHS, 2008; p. 19).
- *Healthy Communities 2000:* "Improvements in public health require active community ownership and commitment" (American Public Health Association [APHA], 1991, p. xxiv).

Practice Partnerships Among Healthcare Providers and Others

- *Healthy People 2000:* "Practice can take the form of partnership with nonprofessionals in the pursuit of individual, family, and community health care. The effectiveness and efficiency of preventive services ... will be enhanced by such partnership" (HHS, 1991, p. 87).
- *Healthy People 2020:* "Get Involved!": "Consortium partners are the ones on the ground moving the Nation toward the *Healthy People 2020* goals and objectives every day." (HHS, 2013).

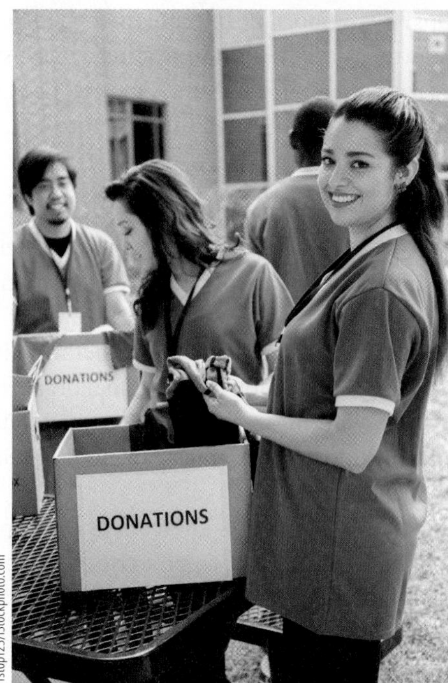

Student nurses often dislike working on group projects. Why is this a common "least favorite" part of nursing school?

Types of Groups

Throughout his or her career, a nurse will work with many types of groups, as well as recommend patients to join various groups. The type of groups one engages in is dependent upon the ultimate goal of that organization. These include increased mental and/or physical health, camaraderie, and gaining education and life skills to achieve overall wellness.

Educational or *learning* groups are designed to provide members with knowledge and understanding regarding a specific issue or area of need. These types of groups rely on each member to seek information (Bogenrieder & Nooteboom, 2004). The nurse's role in these groups is to provide structure and focus for group learning. The nurse may also be the educational provider (Toseland, 1995). Examples of educational groups include childbirth classes and diabetes education programs.

Support groups help members cope with situational crises, life transitions, and a variety of chronic health problems through the provision of emotional support, information, and guidance. Further, they rely on the sharing of

APPLICATION TO PRACTICE

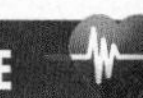

Working with Groups to Plan a Teen Health Clinic

J. C. Roberts, a school health nurse in an urban high school, runs a school-based education center targeting health problems affecting the student population. Lee Sorrel, a nurse in a nearby public health center, runs an after-school teen clinic to provide care for the same set of health problems. Although both nurses spent much time and energy implementing their respective programs, local teens are not using the services of either. After discussing their mutual frustration at a district nursing meeting, J. C. and Lee decide to work together. They form an advisory group made up of local teens to help them evaluate the two programs. The group learns the following:

- Students fear negative repercussions if teachers see them going into the health education center at school.
- Desired educational topics, such as safe sex and pregnancy prevention, cannot be offered by the health education center under existing school policy.
- Using a "problem-oriented" clinic has a negative social stigma among their peers.
- Many teens who might attend the health department clinic are working after school.

The group recommends a community-based program that includes social activities, health and education services, and job skills training. The nurse and advisory committee members initiate a coalition of community leaders and organizations that mobilizes resources for a comprehensive teen program at the local community center. The program is highly successful. Local teens are using a broader range of services than the school or health department were able to offer separately.

On a sheet of paper, list all the individuals (e.g., the two nurses, the teens), agencies, organizations, and community officials or representatives that should be part of the community coalition. Next to each, list examples of the knowledge, skills, and resources that each can potentially contribute to the pool of information that will be used as the basis for informed decision making.

1. Take a pencil and cover each entry, one at a time. What would be lost each time?
2. Look at each entry. What are the potential sources of power and influence for each?
3. Brainstorm a list of ground rules that would support shared leadership and decision making.
4. Look at the individuals, agencies, organizations, and community officials or representatives that you identified in the previous questions. Make a list of the potential sources and topics of conflict within this group.
5. Which, if any, detrimental effects to individuals and the group might result from these conflicts?
6. Which strengths might the group derive from these potential conflicts?
7. Brainstorm a list of ground rules that would support positive conflict management.

information (Wright & Bell, 2003). The nurse's role with support groups is to facilitate group interaction and process and to serve as a role model of acceptance (Schopler & Galinsky, 1993; Sharf, 1997; Yates, 1995). Examples of support groups are Alzheimer's disease caregiver groups, hospice bereavement groups, and breast cancer support groups.

> If I have seen farther than others, it is because I was standing on the shoulders of giants.
>
> —*Sir Isaac Newton*

Self-help groups are defined by self-governance and a common concern or problem. Group members provide one another with emotional support, information, education, social advocacy, and sometimes, material aid. High value is placed on experiential knowledge as a form of special understanding of a group member's experiences. Ongoing self-help participation provides a unique opportunity to give and receive simultaneously, which has been linked to benefits such as better psychosocial adjustment and increased longevity (Cohen, Gottlieb, & Underwood, 2000). Although nurses and other health professionals generally do not have a formal role in these groups, health professionals often make referrals to these groups (Humphreys, 1997; Ogborne, 1996; Schubert & Borkman, 1991; Social Policy Corporation, 1997; Stewart, 1990). Examples of self-help groups include Alcoholics Anonymous, Overeaters Anonymous, and Al-Anon.

Therapy groups provide treatment, most often professional, for people experiencing an emotional disturbance. The primary goal of these groups is to provide members with insight into themselves and help them change their behaviors. The nurse's role within these groups is therapeutic and involves role-modeling acceptance and caring, encouraging group **participation**, helping members explore the reasons behind their feelings and behavior, and providing structure and maintenance of group process (Clark, 1994; Corey & Corey, 1992). Examples might include therapy groups for people with depression, attention deficit disorder, post-traumatic stress disorder, or schizophrenia. After the terrorist attacks of September 11, 2001, and the Hurricane Katrina disaster, nurses often found themselves in need of support and therapy groups as a way of coming to terms and working through the grief of losing colleagues and patients in these disasters (Constantino & Smart, 2004).

Task groups focus on the achievement of a specific goal, and are therefore often time limited. When working in task groups, it is important to remember the five Cs for success: control, conflict, communication, consensus, and cohesion (Fernandez, 1997). Nurses may work in several different kinds of task groups throughout their career, including:

- *Professional organizations*. These include the American Nurses Association (ANA), the Fellows of the American Academy of Nursing, national response task forces like the American Red Cross, and international groups such as Doctors Without Borders. Reasons to join professional organizations include networking, education, peer recognition, and certification, all of which can aid in career advancement.
- *Business-oriented groups*. These focus on employee selection, career development, periodic training, and licensure.
- *Legal groups*. Because nurses are not just responsible for immediate but also long-term care, federal regulations require nurses to report suspicion of abuse. As a result, nursing staff may be required to work with local police and/or fire departments, social services, and judicial system officials. Complete honesty and cooperation in these groups are vital.
- *Community groups*. The roles of nurses expand to the care of the community. Advocacy, community organizing, health education, and political and social reform must also play a vital part in the responsibilities of nurses today (Kulbok, Thatcher, Park, & Meszaros, 2012). This not only encourages education and fosters healthy habits among community members, but also helps to ensure a sociological understanding of one's community and the specific issues community members face.

The nurse's role within task groups, which is to facilitate progress toward goal accomplishment, is determined by the membership position of the leader or group member (Kulbok et al., 2012). Examples of task groups include a community group to establish a recreation center or a group of teachers, parents, and the school nurse planning a health fair.

Focus groups provide a forum for obtaining data through group interviews about a variety of issues of concern to nurses and other health professionals. Although these groups have primarily been used in the business arena for marketing purposes, nurses and other health professionals are now using the approach to obtain information from patients about health services and needs. Another important aspect of focus groups is the presence of a moderator whose role is to create an encouraging

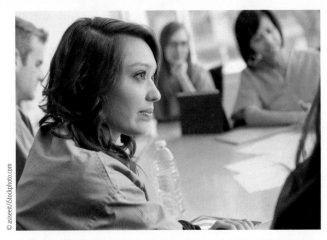

Participation means that all group members listen and are listened to, share in decision making, and contribute to the achievement of the group's tasks and objectives.

environment and to eliminate pressures to vote or respond in a specific way (McLafferty, 2004). Focus groups can help improve the planning and design of new programs, evaluate existing programs, and develop strategies, but should not be used to collect views held by the general public. The nurse's role within a focus group is to establish a nonthreatening and positive environment and to facilitate group process.

Complementary health groups meet a rising demand for complementary and alternative care services (Keyes, 2007). These groups focus on holistic health to promote and restore health through methods that are not available through conventional medicine. Examples include yoga, guided imagery/meditation, and tai chi.

Coalitions bring together people, organizations, community groups, factions, and constituencies in a working group to influence outcomes on a specific issue or problem to achieve a common goal. Advantages of coalitions include conservation of resources, potential to reach more people, greater credibility in numbers, enhanced information exchange, and cooperation among participating groups (Ford, Wells, & Bailey, 2004). The nurse's role may include chairperson, facilitator, or group member.

Team-building activities may be used to enhance the normal stages of group development and are an important aspect of managing groups. Team-building techniques may also be used when groups are experiencing conflict or failing to meet their goals.

Antai-Otong (1997) has identified four qualities that are present in successful teams:

- Open and effective communication
- Involved members who are committed to the team, understand team dynamics, and are emotionally invested in the team
- Clearly defined goals that identify member roles and responsibilities
- Trust and collegiality

RESEARCH ALERT

Focus groups were conducted in six Asian communities in Chicago to determine reasons for the downward trend in immunization rates among Asian American children. Participants ($n = 67$ [age range 7–15 years]) were paid a $25 stipend. Results indicated that barriers to immunization include cost, language, information, and records (lack of information, confusing immunization records, and uncertainty about records being up to date), difficulty in scheduling appointments and long waits to see doctors, and provider choice (participants weren't sure which doctors provided quality care). Recommendations include increasing awareness of free immunization services, decreasing language barriers, and providing immunization education materials to Asian American communities.

Source: Asian Health Coalition of Illinois. (2004). Identifying immunization barriers among Asian American children: Results and recommendations. Retrieved November 10, 2008, from http://www.cispiimmunize.org/resour/FAAP%20Presentations/Vickers.ppt

Characteristics of Effective Groups

Groups are central to the human experience. Not only are they necessary for performing complex tasks that require multiple participants, but they also are vital in meeting our need for inclusion and affection. Unique to a collection of individuals, such as people sitting together in an emergency department waiting area, groups consist of individuals who interact with one another in a manner that allows each person to influence and be influenced by every other person in the group (Shaw, Robbin, & Belser, 1981, p. 8). In contrast to those who simply wait to provide emergency care, the staff members who work together to address the needs of each patient are functioning as a *group*. The successful delivery of health services, whether within a hospital or across a community, requires the collaborative effort of groups.

A **group** can be defined as three or more people who interact with one another through a variety of communication-based processes to achieve a common goal. While the characteristics of a particular group are unique to its purpose for forming, the individuals who comprise it, and the situation or context, groups that work together effectively demonstrate the following: (1) a common goal, (2) a collective identity, (3) interdependent interaction, and (4) mutual influence.

Common Goal

In effective groups, individuals come together to achieve a shared goal or purpose. The purpose of *primary groups*, such as our nuclear family and circle of close friends, is to meet our need for affection, support, and a sense of belonging. Membership in these groups tends to remain constant over long periods of time, and interaction is typically at a more informal level. The purpose of *secondary* or *work-oriented groups* is to accomplish specific tasks, solve problems, or maintain necessary processes. A neonatal team delivering life-sustaining care to a premature infant is an example of a secondary group. These groups usually exist for shorter periods of time, and membership can change depending on the needs of the group. The goals of primary and secondary groups are not mutually exclusive. Our interactions with one another in work-oriented groups can also meet our need for close human connections, such as when a group of colleagues enjoys lunch together on a regular basis. And certainly there are times when primary group members work together to address problems or accomplish more specific tasks, such as friends forming a study group for an especially difficult anatomy class. Although they might satisfy multiple purposes for their members, effective groups exist to achieve a central goal.

Collective Identity

While groups are made up of unique individuals, the members are aware that they are part of a larger whole that is "the group." In other words, we know when we belong to a group because of the collective identity it gives us. A group's identity typically forms around its shared purpose and can be made explicit through a group name or title. A "Women's Health Network" might be one example. Collective identification also can be related to a common characteristic among the group members, such as being a breast cancer survivor in a "Bosom Buddies" group or having the same surname in a family group. To help sustain members' commitment to the group's goal and to one another, particularly when outside influences compete for their attention, effective groups develop a clear sense of "who we are."

Interdependent Interaction

Effective groups capitalize on one of the principal reasons for working with others rather than alone: to build on the diverse ideas and skill sets of the people who are brought together. More often than not, groups form to accomplish things that individuals simply cannot do, or would have a very difficult time doing, on their own. The reliance on one another, or interdependence, in accomplishing shared goals means that the success or failure of the group depends on the coordinated efforts of all of the members. In effective groups, collaborative interaction among all members of the group empowers the full contribution of everyone. It also encourages building on one another's strengths to produce high quality outcomes. The resulting dynamic of interdependent contributions, where the whole (what is produced by the group working together) is greater than the sum of its parts (what would be produced if each individual worked alone) is known as **synergy**. Even if it is possible for one person to complete a group's goal, it is the synergy of people working together interdependently that results in groups producing better solutions than what an individual working alone might produce (Cooren, 2004).

Mutual Influence

For synergy to happen successfully, members of a group must interact with one another in such a way that each member influences and is influenced by every other member of the group. Mutual influence is achieved when group members actively use verbal and nonverbal communication to exchange information and create shared meaning with one another. Shared understanding can be achieved *explicitly*, such as when a group member asks for clarification or nods in agreement when someone else expresses an idea. It also can be achieved *implicitly* by way of unstated norms governing group behavior. For example, a group might not establish official rules for how meetings will operate, yet everyone understands the expectation that they should arrive on time and fully prepared. **Norms** are the implicit "rules" that influence the behavior of group members. Because members can have a variety of assumptions about what is acceptable, effective groups make implicit norms explicit by developing written rules for how they will work together. When starting a new group, it is helpful to take some time to identify agreed-upon ground rules and to post them for easy reference. If someone then violates an explicit norm, the group can rely on the established rules when attempting to influence that person's behavior.

The number of people in a group can impact the degree of mutual influence among the members. The ideal group size for maximizing each member's ability to influence every other member is three to seven members. When groups grow larger than seven members, there is a tendency for influence to flow in one direction from the leader to the rest of the group or for mutual influence to be restricted to smaller subgroups that often form when group membership grows too large.

Communication Within Groups

Group Roles

Just as we assume various roles in our everyday lives depending on the situation and our relationships with those around us (e.g., student, daughter, friend, mentor), group members take on different roles to help their group achieve its goals. A group role is an expected pattern of communication behaviors consistently exhibited by a group member (Myers & Anderson, 2008). The types of roles members adopt range from task oriented, which emphasize the work the group needs to accomplish, to relational, which focus on team building and maintaining group harmony. In addition to group-focused roles, members also can adopt more individually oriented roles, which tend to be self-centered and disruptive rather than contribute to group processes.

Shared Decision Making

In effective groups, power and influence within the group are shared relatively equally. All members are involved in setting goals, gathering information, identifying alternative ways to achieve goals, and deciding on the plan of action. An assumption underlying shared **decision making** is that each group member has information of value that will contribute to informed decision making (Ward, 2006). Input is based on a group member's knowledge, skills, and access to needed resources, rather than on the member's formal title or position in the organization or community. For shared decision making to be effective, all group members should understand the following (Ramey, 1993):

- The nature of the goal and task being undertaken
- Alternative approaches and strategies for achieving the goal or accomplishing the task
- Potential consequences (positive and negative) of each alternative being considered
- The social, economic, and environmental costs of each alternative to individuals, families, and organizations in the community, as well as to the community as a whole

Conflict Management

One of the strengths of a group lies in its ability to bring together individuals and organizations that have diverse views about an issue or problem. With diversity, the potential for conflict is high, so conflict management is critical. Conflict that is not managed effectively can be harmful to individuals and can destroy group cohesion and productivity. In fact, negative, unsupportive, unpleasant, and uncooperative work environments are key factors of low retention rates in nursing. Moreover, a lack of peer cohesion, along with poor work relationships, are significant factors in nurse burnout (Roussel, 2011). This can poorly impact nurses' abilities to properly care for patients. However, conflict also has a high potential for promoting involvement in a group and increasing the creativity and quality of decision making. Therefore, effective groups view conflict as a source of potential strength and develop productive ways of managing and resolving conflict (Antai-Otong, 1997; Hamilton, 2011).

Group Leadership

Two **leadership** styles—democratic and autocratic—dominate approaches to group leadership. Although the leadership style is most closely associated with long-term learning and change, both styles have utility (Hickman, 1990; van Oostrum & Rabbie, 1995).

Democratic leadership, more commonly known as *participatory leadership*, refers to the approach that involves group members in all levels of information gathering, discussion, analysis, decision making, and evaluation. In a more restrictive form of democratic leadership, group members are presented with information as a basis for informed decision making. Participatory leadership builds group cohesion and contributes to individual and collective **empowerment**.

MEDIA MOMENT 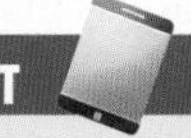

CSI: Crime Scene Investigation **(2000–present)**

This television show follows the nights of the detectives working at the Las Vegas Police Department Crime Scene Investigations bureau. As members of the second busiest crime lab in the United States, CSI officers use the best scientific and technical methods to solve puzzles and catch criminals.

A strength of participatory/shared leadership is that it builds a broad base of support for long-term change. A corresponding reality is that the decision-making and change processes will take longer to achieve.

Autocratic leadership, also known as *authoritarian leadership*, is the "top-down" style of leadership found in many healthcare settings. The authoritarian leadership style also is reflected in the approach to teaching, planning, and behavior change used by many educators in the health professions. Two advantages of this approach are the volume of information that can be transmitted in a short time and the speed with which change can be made. On the negative side, knowledge does not necessarily lead

TABLE 18-1 A Comparison of Leadership Styles

	Participatory Leadership	Authoritarian Leadership
Nurse's roles	Facilitator	Director
	Partner with expertise	Expert information provider
Group members' roles	Co-leaders	Recipients of information
	Partners with expertise	Providers of feedback
	Decision makers	Targets of change
Leadership actions	Ask questions	Tell/lecture
	Stimulate/guide discussion	Lead discussion
	Link to resource providers	Arrange for resources
Outcomes	Learning	Short-term change
	Empowerment	Knowledge expansion
	Sustained change	

to learning and growth, and changes made in this manner tend to be short-lived unless supported by major "selling" campaigns. **Table 18-1** offers a comparison of different leadership styles.

Both styles of leadership have some usefulness. When a decision must be made quickly or rapid change is essential, then a shift toward a more authoritarian leadership style may be indicated. For example, an infection control nurse might be working with a group of daycare center operators. During an outbreak of a communicable disease, the infection control nurse might *tell* the daycare operators what control measures they *must* adopt immediately to stop the outbreak (autocratic approach). However, in most group settings, the participatory leadership style is the preferred approach. For example, the infection control nurse might work with the group on a long-term basis to help the daycare operators develop and test the efficacy of a variety of strategies for preventing communicable diseases in their businesses (democratic approach). Furthermore, leadership style may be modified to fit with the capacities of group members. Factors such as age, physical or mental impairment, and physical disability may affect a group member's ability to engage in participatory or shared leadership (Cole, 1998; Seers & Woodruff, 1997; Toseland, 1995). Gender has also been demonstrated as a variable in leadership style. Men and woman may display different strategies in conflict resolution and consensus building (Currat & Michel, 2006).

Diversity

Diversity can refer to differences in one's cultural, racial, gender, age, disability, sexual orientation, or demographic background (Chen, Ren, & Riedl, 2010). To remain competitive in the global market of the 21st century, and to ensure equal care of patients from all over the world, workers must be highly specialized while working together in diverse teams. As nurses, you will be exposed to both patients and coworkers from various countries and experiences, as well as those with a variety of physical and emotional needs. Therefore, communication, particularly conflict management and decision making, becomes increasingly important in diverse groups.

Aside from personal growth, individuals exposed to opposing minority views consider more aspects of a situation, exert more effort in problem-solving, and are more likely to create solutions to problems. Furthermore, diversity in groups creates a greater capability for in-depth information processing, and the ability to manage a broader range of information (Mannix & Neale, 2006). Though challenging at times to question how one's own ideals and opinions differ from another's, the rewards are staggering, both personally and professionally, if we can learn to accept, respect, and consider one another for both our similarities and differences.

Dysfunctional Behavior

Dysfunctional behavior in groups serves an individual's needs while hindering those of the group. Some examples of these behaviors, according to Hamilton (2011), are as follows:

- Blocking: consistently putting down ideas and suggestions of others
- Aggression: insulting and criticizing, perhaps out of jealousy or dislike
- Dominating: monopolizing group interaction, usually due to preparedness
- Confessing: using the group as a soundboard for personal problems and feelings
- Special-interest pleading: representing the interests of another group, whether or not it relates to the topic being discussed
- Distracting: derailing focus of the group with jokes, inappropriate comments, or unnecessary movement of self or objects
- Withdrawing: failure to contribute to or pay attention to the meeting

To discourage these behaviors, Hamilton (2011) suggests creating an agenda or list of topics for the meeting to help keep all group members on track, assigning withdrawn members to specific tasks such as note-taking, asking specific questions, giving positive feedback, and by seating a person with potentially dysfunctional behaviors next to the leader of the group.

Reasons for nurses not engaging in critical conversations regarding their patients' care include disrespect from coworkers, lack of ability, and having little confidence that joining the conversation will result in a positive outcome. In order to advocate for patients, and for themselves, nurses must demonstrate cooperation, assertiveness, confidence, autonomy, and coordination (Raica, 2009).

Sexual Harassment

Workplace sexual harassment can generally be defined as verbal or nonverbal behavior with sexual content that is unwanted and negatively received by the target, and that leads to interference with the target's work (Diehl, Rees, & Bohner, 2012). Further, it can be either physical or nonphysical, and can be a single event or multiple instances. This is a widespread problem with significant legal, psychological, and economic consequences, particularly within nursing and healthcare fields (Bullough, 2004). Most sexual harassment in nursing comes from coworkers and supervisors, although other sources can be patients and/or their families (Bullough, 2004).

Studies have shown that victims who perceive the incident(s) as more severe are more likely to report the happenings to a supervisor (Bergman, Langhout, Palmieri, Cortina, & Fitzgerald, 2002). However, thanks to sexual harassment education, more instances, even the less pervasive ones, are being reported (Bergman et al., 2002) It is important to report any joke, touch, or comment that makes you feel uncomfortable and targeted. Not only do you have the right to feel safe and respected in your workplace, but the effects of sexual harassment are vast and damaging. These can include decreased satisfaction in one's job and professional relationships, loss of productivity, increased turnover rates, lower psychological wellbeing, more physical health problems, including symptoms of post-traumatic stress, substance abuse, absenteeism, and impaired intimacy and sexual functioning (Fitzgerald, Drasgow, Hulin, Gelfand, & Magley, 1997). Nurses also complain that sexual harassment creates an unsafe work environment that compromises the patients' quality of care. When the harasser is a colleague, necessary communication may be avoided, and the nurse may not ask that person for help to move or care for a patient, or relay important and perhaps time-sensitive information to the harasser. Moreover, errors in passing medication, drawing fluids, or handling surgical instruments can be dangerous and potentially deadly (Bullough, 2004). These examples demonstrate the potential risks of workplace sexual harassment, and outline reasons why sexual harassment should be reported immediately.

RESEARCH ALERT

Quality of life is a concern for people living with diagnoses of persistent mental illness. This project explored the meaning of quality of life for a group of persons attending a community center for persons with mental illness. Parse's human becoming practice method was used to guide the group process for eight men who met weekly with a nurse for 75- to 90-minute sessions over 10 weeks. The nurse's commitment to live true presence with the group enabled their expressions about life and the meanings of living with their particular struggles and joys, sufferings and hopes.

Source: Hee, N. C. (2004). Meaning of the quality of life for persons living with serious mental illness: Human becoming practice with groups. *Nursing Science Quarterly, 17*(3), 220–225.

CULTURAL CONNECTION

Not all cultures are comfortable in the open atmosphere of a group owing to the expectation of verbal participation by each member. Internet groups have been most successful with members of cultures that avoid confrontation and with persons who are more introverted.

RESEARCH ALERT

Cancer support groups are an important source of support for cancer patients. This research explored the views of 179 leaders of 184 cancer support groups in New South Wales, Australia. In the study, 416 members of 50 groups selected from the larger cohort completed questionnaires eliciting the importance of group processes, including leader qualities and satisfaction with group leadership. Members of nine groups participated in focus groups regarding effective group processes. The importance of the leaders was emphasized in all stages of the research. Fifty-nine percent of group leaders were currently experiencing a difficulty, primarily related to infrastructure or group process. Three characteristics of effective leaders were identified: educational qualities, facilitation skills, and personal qualities. Leadership in these self-help groups can be an often overlooked aspect in the successful management of help for patients with cancer.

Source: Butow, P., Ussher, J., Kirsten, L., Hobbs, K., Smith, K., Wain, G., . . . Stenlake, A. (2006). Sustaining leaders of cancer support groups: The role, needs, and difficulties of leaders. *Social Work in Health Care, 42*(2), 39–55.

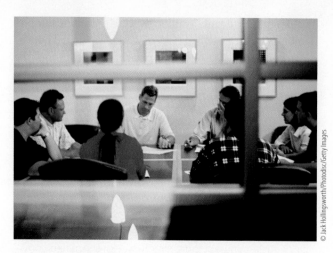
© Jack Hollingsworth/Photodisc/Getty Images

Communication by all group members is a critical attribute of a successful work group.

Stages of Group Development

Given that groups are made up of distinct individuals, no two groups are ever exactly the same, and we can't always predict what will happen during the course of a group's existence. Nonetheless, *Tuckman's Group Developmental Stages* model of small groups provides a framework for understanding what groups more commonly experience in their development (Tuckman & Jensen, 1977). The following discussion explains the Tuckman model and how communication affects each stage.

1. *Forming stage.* When individuals first come together in a group, they are typically uncertain of how they will work together or if they will get along. The initial focus of group work, therefore, involves both understanding the shared task or reason for being together and also assessing one another's level of commitment and willingness to work together. Communication at this stage is typically tentative and polite as members strive to make a good first impression while getting to know one another. These initial social tensions diminish as members interact to become better acquainted and gain more confidence in the group. Effective members work through the forming stage by exhibiting enthusiasm for the group's task and demonstrating genuine interest in working with everyone in the group.
2. *Storming stage.* As pressure to accomplish the group goal mounts, the "honeymoon phase" of forming typically gives way to disagreements and tensions over member roles and control. Questions of who will gain leadership status, which issues will be given attention, or who will have more influence during decision making often lead to conflict and some members becoming more assertive. Communication at this stage can become quite animated as members jockey to be heard by speaking louder, listening intently, and interrupting one another. Effective groups channel their conflict toward heightened engagement with one another and more fully exploring the issues they are addressing. Groups that cannot balance mutual respect and supportiveness with the disagreements that inevitably arise in group work have difficulty emerging from this phase of development. Becoming mired in the storming stage jeopardizes a group's ability to achieve its goals.
3. *Norming stage.* Groups address the imbalances of being overly cautious (forming) and overly confrontational (storming) by becoming comfortable with one another and establishing clear expectations for how to interact with one another. Communication during this stage is more open and addresses task and relational concerns. Effective groups address the tensions of conflict by developing norms (accepted patterns of behavior) for getting their work done and for maintaining their commitment to one another and the group. Groups will emerge from the norming stage as a result of their greater acceptance of one another and improved communication processes, and they will exhibit fluid work processes and high **cohesion**, which is the mutual attraction that unifies a group around a shared goal (Engleberg & Wynn, 2010).
4. *Performing stage.* At this stage of development, groups have optimized their processes to function at a high level of productivity. Through clear communication, active participation, and a willingness to adapt as needed, effective groups work toward the successful achievement of their goals.
5. *Adjourning stage.* Groups disband for multiple reasons, such as completion of a project or members moving on to other responsibilities; however, there is more to the process than simply no longer working together. After successful completion of a goal, effective groups take the time to celebrate their achievements and to solidify relationships with one another. Recognizing a job well done also brings satisfaction to the members and affirms their collaborative efforts. Positive closure sets the stage for future successful teamwork should the members ever work together again.

Stakeholder analysis is a technique often used to identify potential group members. In the example (planning teen health services) in the Application to Practice feature at the beginning of this chapter, two nurses initiated group

APPLICATION TO PRACTICE 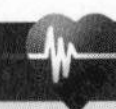

Health Needs of the Rural Elderly Population

Darla Parker, RN, BSN, works with a small home health agency that is located in a rural Appalachian community. Population in the county is estimated to be 13,798, with 2,578 people between the ages of 55 and 64. Another 3,459 people are older than 65. Demographic data indicate that the elderly population will continue to grow, with the "graying of America" and young adults leaving the area to find work. Chronic health problems among the older population of this county include high rates of cancer, especially late-stage diagnosed uterine and breast cancers, chronic lung diseases (including a high rate of black lung disease), and high rates of cardiovascular diseases. The incidence of cigarette smoking, sedentary lifestyles, and obesity are also high for this community.

In consultation with Shirley Janeff, director of the regional office on aging, Darla learned that a recent assessment of the community had found that a number of elderly citizens with chronic health problems were having difficulty getting access to needed healthcare resources. Results of this survey also showed needs for transportation, for home caregivers, and for help with the purchase of medications. Janeff said, "I think the problem is complex, but some of the problems we are encountering are related to changes in Medicare reimbursement policies that limit access to home health and also that people are simply not informed about the many resources available to them in the community." Darla responded, "I know we can't solve the problems with reimbursement at this time, but maybe we can do something to inform people about resources." When Darla returned to her office she talked with her supervisor about setting up a task force to investigate some possible solutions to these issues. Her supervisor, Mary Jane, agreed with the need to work on this issue and suggested that Darla proceed.

Two weeks later, Darla met with representatives of a variety of service agencies to develop some approaches to the documented needs of the elderly citizens of the community. After much discussion of the assessment data, the group decided to put on a health fair as one strategy to inform the community of the many resources in the area. At this first meeting, the group selected a date to coincide with Older Americans Month. They decided to hold it outdoors at the local county park, but they also identified another site in case of rain on the chosen date. The task force met two more times to complete planning for the event.

1. What are some factors Darla needs to consider when putting together a task force to plan this project? As you answer this question, think about the advantages and disadvantages of inviting various community and organizational representatives.
2. Once she has established the task force, what is Darla's role with the group? What are expected behaviors of the different possible roles she could assume?
3. At the first meeting, Darla is elected by the group to be the chairperson. What does it mean to be a leader? Describe leadership behaviors you would expect to see Darla exhibit.
4. Whenever a group of people comes together to work on an issue or a project, conflict is a possibility. How could Darla intervene with the group to control conflict and keep them moving toward their goal?

development by inviting some teens from the local high school to come together to form an advisory group. At the first meeting, the nurses may have used the technique of stakeholder analysis to identify other teens who might represent segments of the student population not included in the first meeting. Similarly, when the group expanded and formed a community coalition, stakeholder analysis would have been a useful way to identify potential coalition members (see **Box 18-1**).

Group Maintenance Roles

Group members fulfill the following roles when successfully keeping a group together:

- *Encourager*: The encourager complements the work of the gatekeeper by creating a climate of acceptance within the group so that members feel free to express themselves.

BOX 18-1 How to Conduct Stakeholder Analysis

1. Identify the specific issue, health topic, or problem that is the intended focus of the group.
2. List all agencies, organizations, and/or individuals who affect or are affected by the issue, health topic, or problem that is the intended focus of the group.
3. Narrow the list to a workable size by asking two questions about each potential participant:
   - What can this person, agency, or organization contribute to achieving this group's goal?
   - What will be lost if this person, agency, or organization does not participate in the group?
4. Refine the initial list, based on the answers in step 2, adding names and addresses of each person, agency, or organization that will be invited.
5. Invite each stakeholder to participate in the next group meeting.

- *Conflict manager*: As noted earlier, conflict is an inherent part of effective group functioning. The role of the conflict manager is to facilitate a tone of harmony and compromise in which individuals with strongly held beliefs and opinions can modify their personal views in favor of the greater good of the group. A strategy that is often effective in reducing tension is the appropriate use of humor.
- *Standard setter/tester*: When group relationships have broken down, the standard setter helps the group diagnose the situation and develop and implement standards of group behavior that will help correct the problem.

Group Dissolution

When a group has achieved its stated purpose and goals, it is faced with the decision of whether to dissolve or continue with new goals and objectives (Keyton, 1993). The dissolution stage can be tricky if the group has developed tangible assets. In some cases, a group may decide to merge with another group having similar purposes. Consensus building and conflict resolution are essential if group dissolution is to be achieved in a positive manner.

Groups as Change Agents

Much of the current knowledge about group dynamics and groups as agents of change originates in the social psychology research conducted by Kurt Lewin in the 1930s and 1940s. Lewin found that the traditional methods of education, such as lecturing and individual instruction, were effective in transmitting units of information but did not result in

MEDIA MOMENT 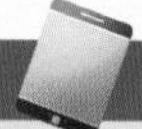

Survivor **(2000–present)**

In this competition/reality television show, a diverse group of contestants is stranded in a remote location with little more than the clothes on their backs. The contestants start off divided into two teams that compete against each other, with the losing team being forced to vote a member off. When the number of contestants is reduced to 10, the teams merge and it's everyone for himself or herself.

Groups and Technology

In the past few decades, we have seen unprecedented advances and a growth in applications for computer and mobile technologies. The vast and easily accessible array of communication technologies now at our disposal (e.g., instant messaging, videoconferencing, blogs) is having a pronounced effect on group processes. At the most fundamental, it means that people no longer need to gather face to face in the same location to get their work done. Nonetheless, relying on technology-based communication environments also means developing new ways of thinking about how we work together. Even perceptions of tried-and-true, face-to-face health care, such as a surgical team in an operating room, are being challenged with the advent of robotic surgeries and the ability of doctors and nurses to operate equipment from remote locations. This section explores some of the technologies impacting community health practices and offers suggestions for nurses to maximize their communication effectiveness when using them.

First, let's review some key terms for talking about group communication and technology:

- **Convergence** is a term used to describe the abundance of communication options at our disposal (face-to-face, phone, text, web, pictures, music, etc.) and how these choices blend and overlap in our day-to-day communication with one another.
- **Synchronous** tools allow for more immediate or real-time communication, such as talking on the phone; **asynchronous** tools allow for more delayed communication, such as sending an email or posting to a blog.
- **Social presence** describes the level of awareness people have of one another when communicating. Face-to-face communication is the highest in social presence because it incorporates all of our senses; we can see, hear, feel, and even smell the other as we strive for mutual meaning. Written or text-based communication is much lower in social presence due to the lack of nonverbal elements. Because the nonverbal component is so important to communication, we often attempt to increase the social presence of our written words by incorporating **emoticons**. These typed symbols represent emotion and are mean to enhance understanding, such as a colon and parenthesis to represent smiling or frowning. Unfortunately, they also can be misunderstood and instead might confuse your message. For example, does the smile emoticon represent happiness or sarcasm?
- **Virtual team** is a term used for groups that almost exclusively rely on technology when interacting with one another to achieve shared goals. Members of these groups often work across great geographical distances and multiple time zones, but they can also work in the same city and even

the same building. Regardless of how dispersed the members are, central to such groups is the use of interactive communication technologies rather than face-to-face meetings to get their work done.

Impact of Communication Technologies on the Work of Healthcare Groups in the Community

One of technology's principal benefits to community health groups is that it presents almost limitless opportunities for who can participate in the group. Close proximity no longer needs to be a deciding factor when forming groups. In other words, if a group needs diverse skill sets to address a problem, the expertise could be brought in from potentially anywhere in the world. An additional benefit of the digital environment for group work is that it is known to "level the playing field" among the members. The nonverbal cues that carry social meaning and give some people more status than others (e.g., gender, age, race/ethnicity, weight, and other distinctions) can inhibit the full contribution of "lower status" members. This is known as the *halo effect.* Because the halo effect is diminished online, physical characteristics are not as relevant as what someone actually has to contribute, and this ultimately can strengthen group communication (Madara, 1997).

Traditional technologies, such as video and teleconferencing, can be effective for facilitating group communication when members of the group aren't able to meet in the same location. Groupware programs, also known as electronic meeting systems or group support systems, give everyone the same platform for contributing to and managing group processes. These shared electronic spaces enable the sharing and organizing of information in ways that allow for everyone's review and are often used in conjunction with video/teleconferencing.

Teleconferencing, or conducting meetings from different locations via interconnected telephones, also allows for synchronous communication and multiple participants; however, the lack of nonverbal cues diminishes the social presence that aids in mutual understanding. This format is of particular disadvantage to those who are not native speakers of the language being used in the call. Also, turn taking is often difficult to navigate without visual cues, which can result in just a few people dominating the entire discussion.

Videoconferencing brings people in different locations together using a real-time video feed. This format allows for the nonverbal elements and synchronous communication of face-to-face meetings when opportunities for travel are limited. It is best used to provide information or specific training, particularly when a lot of people must be reached, for example when a new workplace policy is being explained to staff in multiple venues. While free videoconferencing programs are available, the expense of computers, an Internet connection, and an appropriate facility can make this option difficult to arrange for some group members. Also, the added value of social presence can be limited due to time lags in the video feed, equipment incompatibilities, image resolution issues, and the requirement that meeting participants be in a specific place at a specific time. However, continuing developments in mobile communication technologies that provide text, voice, and video connection (e.g., Skype, FaceTime, and Google Hangouts) increasingly allow people to connect from anywhere at anytime using multi-point calling via a smartphone or laptop with a webcam. While the video quality can be inconsistent, this option is continually becoming less expensive and more flexible for bringing a team together (Clemons, Sashidhar, & Row, 1993). It can be particularly useful during rapidly changing situations when individual group members are moving from location to location, such as during a community health emergency or crisis.

Indeed, technological advancements are providing a wealth of options for enhancing interactive communication among physicians, nurses, and other community health stakeholders who rely on one another to administer preventive care and treatment in the community. Online tools such as blogs, wikis, podcasts, rich site summary, (RSS), webinars, and social networking provide engaging spaces for the knowledge sharing and collaborative learning so essential to providing effective and responsive healthcare services (Griffin & de Leastar, 2009). It is important for members of community healthcare groups to recognize that such tools also can be effective for communicating with the people they are serving. For example, conference call coaching and online educational programs are being used by health workers to improve community immunization rates. Text messaging also is being used to support healthcare delivery processes, and texting-based interventions are effectively encouraging smoking cessation, weight management, and healthy pregnancies among specific patient populations in the community.

A potential downside to relying on communication technologies over face-to-face group work, particularly in the area of health care, is a diminishing of human connections and relationship development. Groups that are not colocated have a tendency to focus more attention on the task or work that needs to be done than on their relationships with one another. Given that group conflict tends to arise over issues concerning trust and communication style (Simons & Peterson, 2000), a lack of emphasis on how well team members identify with the group and get along with one another can negatively impact group functioning over time.

Much literature exists on how to maximize group processes when we rely almost exclusively on technology to achieve group goals. From the perspective of community health nursing, here are some key things to consider when working in this sort of group:

- Recognize potential disparities in language proficiency and comfort level with the technology being used. Because technology often brings together a diverse group of people, language and technology skills are not always at the same level. While a group might choose to communicate in English, keep in mind that it might not be the native language for everyone in the group. There is a tendency for those with greater fluency to dominate technology-based interactions. Also, don't assume that everyone is equally comfortable with the technology being used. A particularly quiet member might have a lot to contribute, but is unsure of how to participate in that environment.
- Coordinating work processes from a distance can get complicated given the asynchronous nature of the communication and the limited lines of sight (i.e., the ability to "see" what's going on in the environment of each member of the group). It is important, therefore, that every member shares leadership responsibility for maintaining group interdependence and synergy (Lipnack & Stamps, 2000, p. 218). This might include, but is not limited to, practicing **open communication**, sharing information with the whole group, and checking in with one another on a regular basis.

MEDIA MOMENT

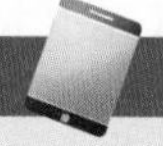

Lord of the Flies **(1954)**

By William Golding, London: Faber and Faber

William Golding's classic tale deals with a group of English schoolboys who are plane wrecked on a deserted island. At first, the stranded boys cooperate, attempting to gather food, make shelters, and maintain signal fires. Overseeing their efforts are Ralph, "the boy with fair hair," and Piggy, Ralph's chubby, wisdom-dispensing sidekick whose thick spectacles come in handy for lighting fires. Although Ralph tries to impose order and delegate responsibility, many in their number would rather swim, play, or hunt the island's wild pig population. Soon Ralph's rules are being ignored or challenged outright. His fiercest antagonist is Jack, the redheaded leader of the pig hunters, who manages to lure away many of the boys to join his band of painted savages. The situation deteriorates as the trappings of civilization continue to fall away, until Ralph discovers that, instead of being hunters, he and Piggy have become the hunted. This classic novel is an excellent example of a group's experiment to develop the perfect society from scratch.

> Be sincere; be brief; be seated.
>
> —*Franklin Delano Roosevelt, advice on being an effective speaker*

RESEARCH ALERT

This article explores contemporary women's perceptions of the experience of the menopausal process within the Western industrialized culture, describes and synthesizes the processes used by women to evaluate available information, and explores and facilitates processes used by women to envision and create change in their life world. An emancipatory group process was designed to facilitate dialogue between the investigator and nine women who met as a group eight times during a 10-week period in the home of one of the participants. Participants identified menses cessation as a time of change in all aspects of their lives. They employed decision making to cope with these changes and, as a result of the awareness that came through the research process, invited other women to celebrate the collective wisdom of women at all stages of life.

As demonstrated by this study, women experiencing menses cessation need information and time to process that information internally and in relation with others. Nurses can facilitate this process by providing knowledge, assisting women in decision making, and intervening in ways that contribute to a holistic quality of life for women.

Source: Timmerman, G. M. (2005). Commentary on "Navigating the journey to menses cessation." *Journal of Holistic Nursing, 23*(1), 51–53.

> I start with the premise that the function of leadership is to produce more leaders, not more followers.
>
> —*Ralph Nader*

GLOBAL CONNECTION

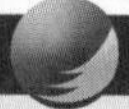

The Peace Corps works in groups in its efforts to improve the lives of residents of underdeveloped countries. The ability to work effectively as a group member under extreme conditions is a critical skill for selection as a Peace Corps volunteer.

> If your actions inspire others to dream more, learn more, do more, and become more, you are a leader.
>
> —*John Quincy Adams*

NOTE THIS!

Groupthink is a sociological phenomenon characterized by decision-making processes that are driven by consensus. The group tends to reject information or alternatives that do not fit with the group's original plan.

Evaluating Groups

Groups may be evaluated for process, impact, and outcome. **Process evaluation** often is focused on group dynamics and interactions. A useful tool for process evaluation is the *group interaction diagram*. The evaluator draws a circle that includes the initials of each member of the group. For each interaction, the evaluator draws an arrow from the person talking to the person being addressed. The direction and number of the arrows will show communication patterns within the group. In authoritarian groups, most of the interaction will be between the leaders and individual members of the group (**Figure 18-1**). In participatory groups, the direction of the arrows should be more evenly distributed (**Figure 18-2**). The diagram will also identify both nonparticipants and discussion dominators. It may be helpful to begin a new diagram when a new topic is introduced or after a major decision is made. Each diagram should be labeled clearly.

Impact evaluation focuses on intermediate behavior changes among group members or by those whose behavior the group is attempting to change. **Outcome evaluation** is based on the degree to which the group's goal and objectives have been met.

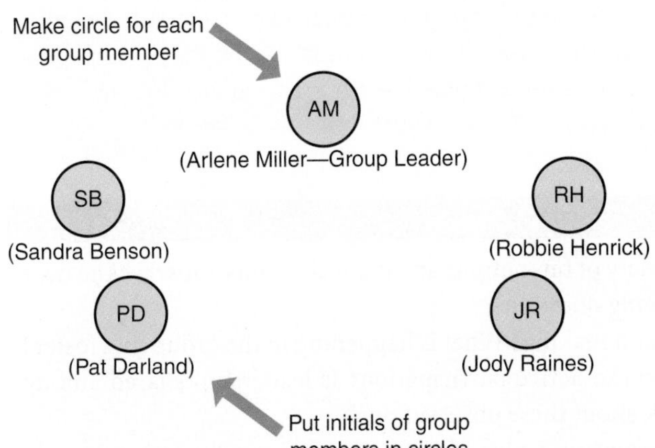

Figure 18-1 Beginning a process-recording diagram.

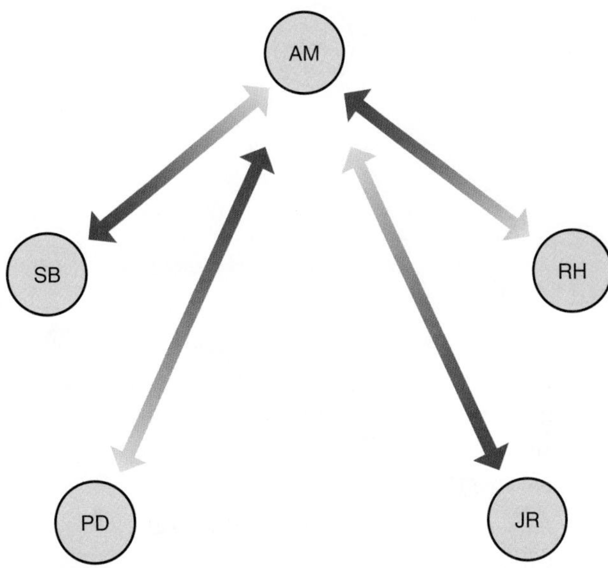

Figure 18-2 Process-recording pattern associated with authoritarian leadership.

NOTE THIS!

Groups of up to about seven members can take part in the same conversation. Beyond that number, it becomes progressively more likely that smaller groups will form and several conversations will take place.

Ethical Considerations

Group leadership brings with it some ethical considerations. Group leaders potentially have great power. Many of the world's belief systems warn of the corrupting effects of power that is not grounded in a set of higher moral values and a sense of responsibility. Furthermore, a skillful leader may be tempted to guide the group in the direction he or she believes is best for the group. Another consideration is that shared leadership, empowerment, and change will likely shift the existing balance of power. You also may face the dilemma of realizing that a group's actions or decisions may adversely affect individuals within the group or others in the community. Different approaches to ethical decision making will generate questions to guide reflective thinking. Some of these questions may include "How is my leadership style affecting the lives of the members of the group?" "Whose goals are being pursued?" "How is the balance of power being shifted?" "Who potentially benefits from this group's decisions and actions?" and "Who is potentially harmed?"

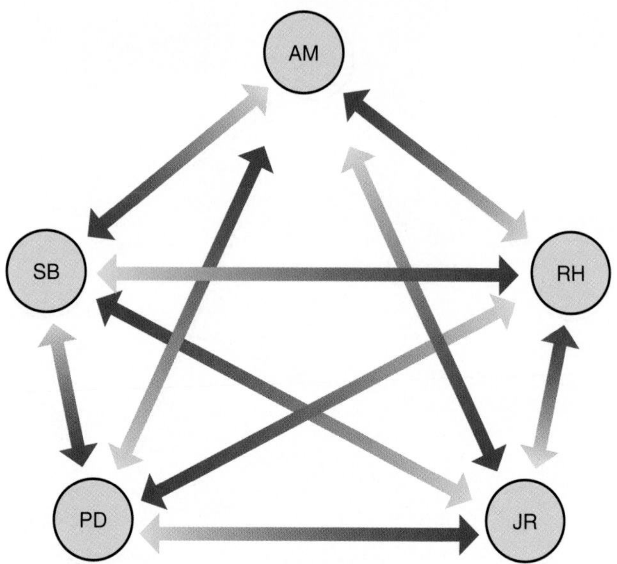
Discussion flows freely among all members of the group.
AM
SB
RH
PD
JR

Figure 18-3 Process-recording pattern associated with democratic leadership.

> When the best leader's work is done, the people say, "We did it ourselves."
>
> —*Lao-Tzu*

Conclusion

This chapter describes several types of groups encountered in nursing practice. Concepts, research, and strategies for effective nursing care of and with groups are discussed. Although the focus of this chapter has been on working with small, face-to-face groups, many of the concepts and skills are applicable to work with groups of all sizes, including community populations. For example, participatory leadership at the group level corresponds with the community development approach at the community level, and authoritarian leadership fits within the social planning model of community organization.

NOTE THIS!

Groups of more than 10 or 12 people have difficulty taking part in the same conversation unless one member assumes a leader role and regulates interaction so that everyone has a chance to contribute. Conversations directed to the group tend to become more formal at this size. Group members "address" the group rather than talk.

> We are not retreating—we are advancing in another direction.
>
> —*Oliver Bailey Smith*

> Treat people as if they were what they ought to be, and help them to become what they are capable of being.
>
> —*Goethe*

LEVELS OF PREVENTION 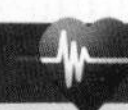

Primary: Teaching a class on exercise for high school teachers.

Secondary: Screening for diabetes among children at an elementary school.

Tertiary: Developing a support group for children who have been diagnosed with diabetes.

HEALTHY ME 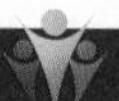

Working in groups sometimes is the least favorite part of being a nursing student. What is your experience working with groups for a common goal/assignment related to one's health and well-being? How can you use the content in this chapter to be a more effective and beneficial group member?

Critical Thinking Activities

1. As a student nurse, you are probably involved in a variety of on-campus and clinical groups. Observe the next meeting of one of these groups and answer the following questions:
   - Does everyone participate in discussions and decision making? What is happening in the group that fosters active participation? What are some of the barriers to active participation? Is leadership shared among various members of the group? What do you think about these observations?
   - In your community health nursing clinical group, brainstorm a list of ground rules for participation. Decide which ones you will adopt as a group. Post them and try them out at your next clinical group meeting. What are the outcomes of using these group rules?

- As a group, develop and implement some strategies for shared leadership. What are the outcomes?
- What are the sources of conflict within the group? Is conflict viewed as a potential strength or as something to be avoided? How is conflict managed? In your clinical group, brainstorm some ground rules for positive conflict management. Try them out. Do they work? Why or why not?

2. Observe the different roles played by members of groups in which you are participating as a student nurse.
   - What are the goal achievement and group maintenance roles played by each person in the group? Does one person play more than one role? Do two or more people play the same role?
   - What are the different strategies that you might use to assist a group in goal achievement and group maintenance?
3. In your community health nursing clinical group, take turns fulfilling each of the goal achievement and task maintenance roles.
   - Discuss your reactions and feelings related to each role. Evaluate one another's role performance. Which roles are most comfortable for you? Which roles do your classmates observe you performing most in other group settings?
   - Develop a list of facilitating questions for each role.
4. Interview a nurse who is facilitating a group over the Internet. (*Hint*: Some of the members of the nursing faculty may be conducting classes and groups using the Internet.)
   - How does this person facilitate group maintenance and goal attainment using the Internet?
   - With your classmates, brainstorm how you would modify your behavior and questions for each group role if you were using the Internet.
5. Observe the various learning situations (formal and informal settings) that you have been in. Think about the various teaching/learning approaches and activities that you have encountered.
   - Which approach(es) have involved you in reflection and critical thinking?
   - What is the relation between knowledge and behavior?
   - List 10 things that you know about health promotion but do not personally practice. Select one that you would like to target for change.
     - What are the driving and restraining forces that preserve your current behavior?
     - How could you work with others to initiate change?
     - How would a group approach fit with your proposed change?
   - List the groups in your community that fall into the category of groups that create or support change. How can you use these groups in nursing practice?
   - Make a list of health-related groups in your community. What is the purpose of each group? How does each group contribute to the health of individuals, families, or populations in your community?
   - Visit three of these groups. If possible, visit three different types of groups. Observe the behavior of group leaders. Which leadership styles are being used? How well do these leadership styles fit with the group's type and purpose? Which leadership style would you use with each group? Why?
6. There are many practical activities that must take place to ensure effective group meetings. Some of these activities may include arranging the time and place for the meeting, arranging the meeting room (e.g., lights, sound, seating, food, other resources, cleanup), inviting people to attend, setting the agenda, leading the meeting, taking minutes or notes (if appropriate), and evaluating outcomes. Select one type of group that might be found in one of your clinical settings. Make a table that has three columns. Label the first column "Practical Considerations." List all the specific activities that you can identify that would need to take place if your meeting is to be a success. Label the second and third columns "Participatory Leadership" and "Authoritarian Leadership." In the rows under each of these leadership styles, describe how you would ensure that the activities listed in the first column are carried out.
   - What are the similarities between the second and third columns? The differences?
   - What are the sets of skills needed for each of these leadership styles? Which of these skills do you already possess? Which self-directed learning activities might help you expand your skills and knowledge base for effective group leadership?
   - Which of these leadership styles are most comfortable for you? Why? What do you think about this?

Continued

Critical Thinking Activities (*Continued*)

7. You have been asked to develop an educational program about asthma for parents of elementary schoolchildren. One step you plan to use in developing the program is to bring together a focus group of parents to identify what they need to know.
   - Describe and explain the selection process you will use to identify participants for the focus group.
   - What is your role as the group leader (before, during, and after the meeting)?
   - How will you fulfill this role? What theories, concepts, and strategies will you use to guide your group leadership activities?
8. Observe the different ways that nurses work with groups in your community health clinical setting. Select one of these nurses and interview him or her.
   - Which types of groups does he or she work with?
   - What is his or her role with each group?
   - Which skills does he or she think are needed to work with these groups effectively?
   - What are the greatest challenges encountered when working with groups?
   - What advice would he or she give to student nurses who will be working with groups in the community?
   - Write a self-evaluation focused on working with groups. How effectively do you work in groups? Which group-related skills, knowledge, and experience do you already possess? How can you strengthen these during your remaining nursing education? After graduation?
   - Which additional group-related skills, knowledge, and experience do you need to develop as part of your nursing education to increase your group work? After graduation?

References

Antai-Otong, D. (1997). Team building in a health care setting. *American Journal of Nursing, 97*(7), 48–51.

Aspen Reference Group. (1997). *Community health education and promotion: A guide to program design and evaluation.* Gaithersburg, MD: Aspen.

Bergman, M. E., Langhout, R. D., Palmieri, P. A., Cortina, L. M., & Fitzgerald, L. F. (2002). The (un)reasonableness of reporting: Antecedents and consequences of reporting sexual harassment. *Journal of Applied Psychology, 87*(2), 230–242. doi: 10.1037/0021-9010.87.2.230

Bogenrieder, I., & Nooteboom, B. (2004). Learning groups: What types are there? A theoretical analysis and an empirical study in a consultancy firm. *Organization Studies, 25*(2), 287–313.

Bullough, V. L. (2004). Struggles of nurse practitioners. *Journal of Nursing Scholarship, 36*(95). doi: 10.1111/j.1547-5069.2004.4033_1.x

Chen, J., Ren,, Y., & Riedl, J. (2010). The effects of diversity on group productivity and member withdrawal in online volunteer groups. *Proceedings of the SIGCHI Conference on Human Factors in Computing Systems.* ACM.

Clark, N. (1994). *The nurse as group leader.* New York, NY: Springer.

Clemons, E. K., Sashidhar, P. R., & Row, M. C. (1993). The impact of information technology on the organization of economic activity: The move to the middle hypothesis. *Journal of Management Information Systems*, 9–35.

Cohen, S., Gottlieb, B. H., & Underwood, L. G. (2000). Social relationships and health. *Social Support Measurement and Intervention: A Guide for Health and Social Scientists*, 1–25.

Cole, M. (1998). *Group dynamics in occupational therapy.* Thorofare, NJ: Slack.

Constantino, J., & Smart, C. J. (2004). Death among us: Grieving the loss of a coworker is a group process. *American Journal of Nursing, 104*(6), 64.

Cooren, F. (2004). Textual agency: How texts do things in organizational settings. *Organization, 11*(3), 373–393.

Corey, M., & Corey, G. (1992). *Groups: Process and practice.* Pacific Grove, CA: Brooks-Cole.

Currat, T., & Michel, L. (2006). Groups and gender: The effects of a masculine gender deficit. *Group Analysis, 39*(1), 133–142.

Diehl, C., Rees, J., & Bohner, G. (2012). Flirting with disaster: Short-term mating orientation and hostile sexism predict different types of sexual harassment. *Aggressive Behavior, 38*(6), 521–531.

Engleberg, I. N., & Wynn, D. (2010). *Think communication.* Boston, MA: Pearson/Allyn & Bacon.

Fernandez (1997). White hat communications. All rights reserved. *THE NEW SOCIAL WORKER, 4*(1).

Fitzgerald, L. F., Drasgow, F., Hulin, C. L., Gelfand, M. J., & Magley, V. J. (1997). Antecedents and consequences of sexual harassment in organizations: A test of an integrated model. *Journal of Applied Psychology, 82*(4), 578.

Ford, E.W., Wells, R., & Bailey, B. (2004). Sustainable network advantages: A game theoretic approach to community-based health care coalitions. *Health Care Management Review, 29*(2), 159–169.

Garr, D. R., Margalit, R., Jameton, A., & Cerra, F. B. (2012). Commentary: Educating the present and future health care workforce to provide care to populations. *Academic Medicine, 87*(9), 1159–1160.

Griffin, L., & de Leastar, E. (2009). Social networking healthcare. *Wearable Micro and Nano Technologies for Personalized Health, 6th International Workshop on* IEEE.

Hamilton, C. (2011). *Communicating for results* (9th ed.). Boston, MA: Cengage Learning.

Hickman, P. (1990). Community health and development: Applying sociological concepts to practice. *Sociological Practice, 8*, 125–132.

Humphreys, K. (1997). Individual and social benefits of self-help groups. *Social Policy, 27*(3), 12–19.

Kelley, L. (1995). Parse's theory in practice with a group in the community. *Nursing Science Quarterly, 8*(3), 127–132.

Keyes, C. L. (2007). Promoting and protecting mental health as flourishing: A complementary strategy for improving national mental health. *American Psychologist, 62*(2), 95–108.

Keyton, J. (1993). Group termination: Completing the study of group development. *Small Groups Research, 24*(1), 84–100.

Kulbok, P. A., Thatcher, E., Park, E., & Meszaros, P. S. (2012). Evolving public health nursing roles: Focus on community participatory health promotion and prevention. *OJIN: The Online Journal of Issues in Nursing, 17*(2), 1.

Lipnack, J., & Stamps, J. (2000). *Virtual teams: People working across boundaries with technology* (2nd ed.). 2nd Edition. New York, NY: Wiley.

Madara, E. (1997). The mutual-aid self-help online revolution. *Social Policy, 27*(3), 20–27.

Mannix, E., & Neale, M. A. (2006). Diversity at work. *Scientific American Mind, 17*(4), 32–39.

Matthews, J., (2012). Role of professional organizations in advocating for the nursing profession. *OJIN: The Online Journal of Issues in Nursing, 17*(1), 3.

McLafferty, I. (2004). Focus group interviews as a data collecting strategy. *Journal of Advanced Nursing,* 48, 187–194. doi: 10.1111/j.1365-2648.2004.03186.x

Myers, S. A., & Anderson, C. M. (2008). *The fundamentals of small group communication.* Thousand Oaks, CA: Sage.

Ogborne, A. (1996). Professional opinions and practices concerning Alcoholics Anonymous: A review of the literature and a research agenda. *Contemporary Drug Problems, 23*(1), 93–105.

Raica, D. A. (2009). Effect of action-oriented communication training on nurses' communication self-efficacy. *Medsurg Nursing: Official Journal of the Academy of Medical-Surgical Nurses, 18*(6), 343–346.

Ramey, J. (1993). Group empowerment through learning formal decision making processes. *Social Work with Groups, 16*(1–2), 171–185.

Roussel, L. (2011). *Management and leadership for nurse administrators.* Sudbury, MA: Jones & Bartlett Learning.

Saad, D., Benet-Martinez, Moons, & Robins (2012). Multiculturalism and creativity. *Social Psychological and Personality Science, 4*(3).

Schopler, J. H., & Galinsky, M. J. (1993). Support groups as open systems: A model for practice and research. *Health and Social Work, 18*(3), 195–207.

Schubert, M. A., & Borkman, T. J. (1991). An organizational typology for self-help groups. *American Journal of Community Psychology, 19*(5), 769–787.

Seers, A., & Woodruff, S. (1997). Temporal pacing in task forces: Group development or deadline pressure? *Journal of Management, 23*(2), 169–186.

Sharf, B. (1997). Communicating breast cancer on-line: Support and empowerment on the Internet. *Women & Health, 26*(1), 65–84.

Shaw, Robbin, Belser. (1981). *Group dynamics: The psychology of small group behavior.* New York, NY: McGraw-Hill.

Simons, T. L., & Peterson, R. S. (2000). Task conflict and relationship conflict in top management teams: The pivotal role of intragroup trust. *Journal of Applied Psychology, 85*(1), 102.

Social Policy Corporation. (1997). The future of self-help. *Social Policy, 27*(3), 2–3.

Stewart, M. J. (1990). Professional interface with mutual-aid self-help groups: A review. *Social Science and Medicine, 31*(10), 1143–1158.

Toseland, R. (1995). *Group work with the elderly and family caregivers.* New York, NY: Springer.

Tuckman, B. W., & Jensen, M. A. C. (1997). Stages of small-group development revisited. *Group & Organization Management, 2*(4), 419–427.

U.S. Department of Health and Human Services (HHS). (1991). *Healthy People 2000: National health promotion and disease prevention objectives. Full report with commentary.* Washington, DC: U.S. Government Printing Office.

U.S. Department of Health and Human Services (HHS). (2000). *Healthy People 2010: Conference edition.* Washington, DC: U.S. Government Printing Office.

U.S. Department of Health and Human Services (HHS). (2008). *Phase I Report: Recommendations for the framework and format of Healthy People 2020.* Retrieved from http://healthypeople.gov/2020/about/advisory/PhaseI.pdf

U.S. Department of Health and Human Services (DHHS). (2013). *Healthy People 2020: Get involved.* Retrieved http://www.healthypeople.gov/2020/GetInvolved/default.aspx

van Oostrum J., & Rabbie, J. (1995). Intergroup competition and cooperation within autocratic and democratic management regimes. *Small Group Research, 26*(2), 269–295.

Ward, D. E. (2006). Complexity in group work. *Journal for Specialists in Group Work, 31*(1), 1–3.

Wright, K. B., & Bell, S. B. (2003). Health-related support groups on the Internet: Linking empirical findings to social support and computer-mediated communication theory. *Journal of Health Psychology, 8*(1), 39–54.

Yates, R. (1995). *Developing support groups for individuals with early-stage Alzheimer's disease.* Baltimore, MD: Health Professions Press.

UNIT 4

Common Community and Population Health Problems and Issues

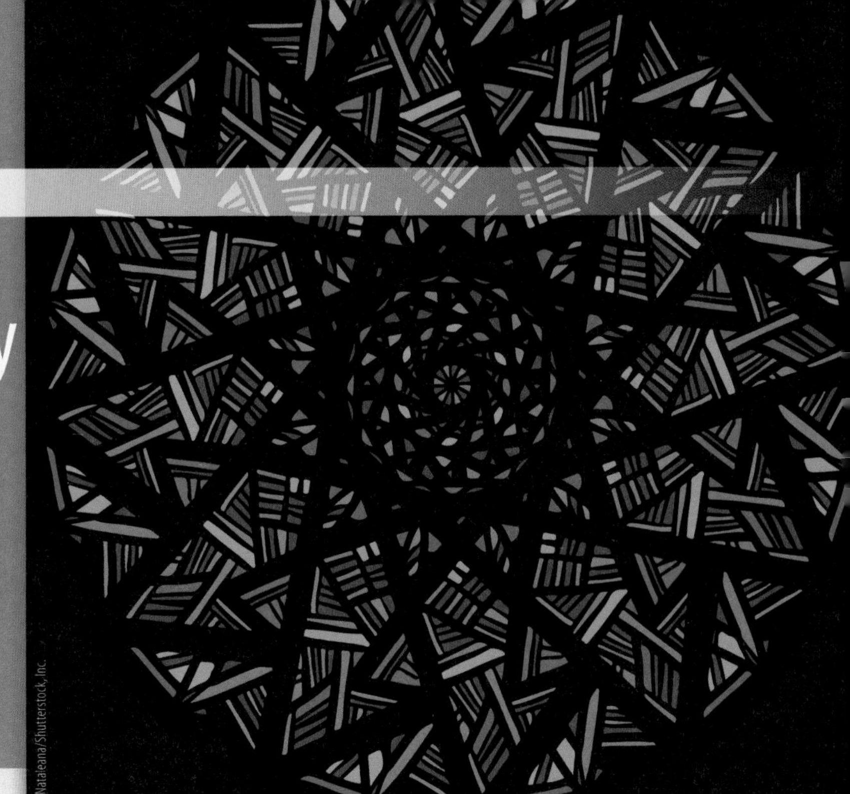
© Nataleana/Shutterstock, Inc.

CHAPTER FOCUS

The Nature of Disasters
- Definitions and Types of Disasters
- NA-TECH
- Disaster Characteristics
- Global Disaster Issues
- Natural Disaster Reduction
- Disaster as a Global Public Health Problem
- Populations at Risk in Disasters

Stages of Disaster

Disaster Planning
- Steps in the Disaster Process
- The Disaster Plan
- Disaster Management

Disaster Response
- Response and Recovery
- Levels of Disaster Response
- National Disaster Medical System
- Other Disaster Agencies
- Evacuation
- Rescue
- Triage
- Disaster Shelters

Role of the Community Health Nurse in Disasters
- General Functions of the Community Health Nurse
- Specific Nursing Approaches
- Shelter Management and Care

Disaster Recovery
- Effects on Survivors
- Special Survivor Populations: Elders and Children
- Collective Trauma: The Loss of Community
- Nurses' Reactions to Disasters
- Prevention Strategies for Nurses

QUESTIONS TO CONSIDER

After reading this chapter, you will know the answers to the following questions:

1. What are the categories and types of disasters community health nurses might deal with?
2. What are the variables by which disasters can be understood?
3. What is a global disaster?
4. Who are the populations most at risk in a disaster? Why?
5. What are the stages of disaster, and how does each stage affect both the disaster workers and the affected population?
6. What are the steps in the disaster process?
7. What are the characteristics of a disaster plan?
8. What are the common elements of a disaster plan?
9. What is disaster response? What are the different levels of response?
10. What is disaster triage? Why and how should it be implemented?
11. What is the role of the community health nurse in the disaster relief process?
12. Which specific approaches should a community health nurse use to mitigate human and material losses in a disaster?
13. What happens to the survivors in a disaster? How can a community health nurse promote recovery after a disaster?
14. Which factors can place individuals in a vulnerable position?
15. Why are children and the elderly at greater risk during a disaster? What can be done to intervene?
16. What are the sources of stress for the disaster workers, and how can they be managed?

Nurses are some of the first to respond during times of disaster. Think of recent events in New York City and New Orleans—do you know nurses who gave of themselves?

CHAPTER 19

Disasters in the Community

Karen Saucier Lundy and
Janie B. Butts

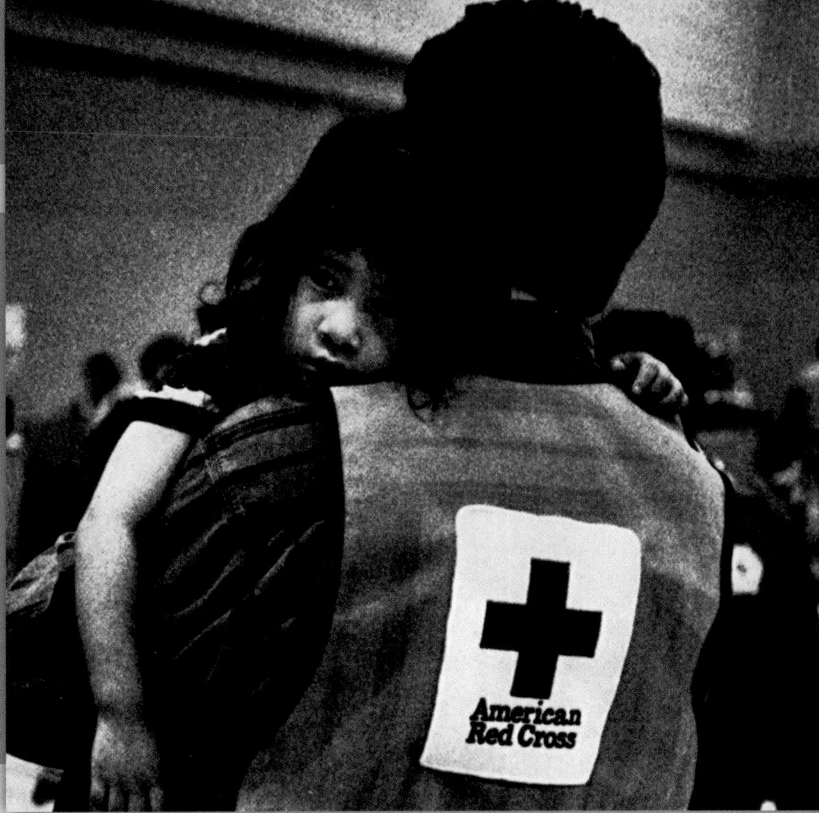

KEY TERMS

Department of Homeland Security (DHS)
disaster
disaster planning
disaster triage
emergency
emergency stage
human-generated (human-made) disasters
impact stage
interdisaster stage
level I response
level II response
level III response
level IV response
major disaster
National Disaster Medical System (NDMS)
natural disasters
posttraumatic stress disorder (PTSD)
predisaster stage
reconstruction (rehabilitation) stage
recovery
response

> Today our fellow citizens, our way of life, our very freedom came under attack in a series of deliberate and deadly terrorist acts.
>
> —President George W. Bush, following the September 11, 2001, terrorist attacks

> Crises, such as Hurricane Katrina and the unprecedented "disaster of disasters" in New Orleans, show society speeded up, its evolution compressed into a moment in time. The poor and dispossessed, the weak and the sick, always suffer disproportionately. And how society responds—or doesn't—is a reflection of its values, its way of organizing and caring for people.
>
> —Professor Jennifer Leaning, Harvard University, School of Public Health

> Noble souls, through dust and heat,
> Rise from disaster and defeat
> The stronger.
>
> —Henry Wadsworth Longfellow, "The Sifting of Peter," 1880

> Hurricane Katrina resulted in human loss that exceeded our imagination. The losses go beyond counting, as numbers of deaths, homes destroyed, and jobs and businesses lost cannot count the irreplaceable: lives cut short, health and quality of life compromised, a way of life permanently lost and cultures permanently altered. Individual stories capture these losses, but not the magnitude of the challenges that face us.
>
> —Betsy Foxman, 2006

REFLECTIONS

Think about the last time that you saw a television report on a terrorist event, such as the Boston Marathon bombings of 2013, or saw the devastation of a mass disaster, such as the tsunami that hit the Philippines in 2013 or Hurricane Sandy that hit the east coast of the United States in 2012. What went through your mind? If the context of the event were all outside the United States, would you have viewed it differently? If you had a personal experience with one of these disasters, did it change your view of the events? How can community health nurses help communities heal after a disaster? What are ways that we can all protect ourselves and our families and communities from the catastrophic health damage from disasters?

DISASTER! THE VERY WORD can evoke fear, panic, and a pounding heart. A major disaster occurs almost daily somewhere in the world: plane crashes, floods, hurricanes, tornadoes, fires, earthquakes, acts of terrorism, droughts, famines, and wars. Who among us can ever forget the images of the elderly and others dying in the New Orleans Superdome and Convention Center following Hurricane Katrina, people sitting on rooftops and on highways pleading to be rescued, Herculean rescues of patients from area hospitals, and bodies floating in the putrid water that literally covered the entire city of New Orleans? We will most likely never know the full impact on people's lives of dealing with the loss of those who died as a result of the flooding and coping with being transported to other states and shelters.

The community health nurse can assist communities in preparing for disasters such as Hurricane Katrina and limiting their damage in the aftermath. Communities can become stronger and healthier as a result. But what are the real threats of disaster? How can community health nurses be better prepared to strengthen communities in their responses to disasters? This chapter will help you answer these questions as you develop a better understanding of the nature of disasters and learn about the various levels of disaster preparedness in which community health nurses are involved. Start by reading about the familiar *Titanic* disaster of 1912 (**Box 19-1**) as an illustration of the role of preparedness in mediating the harmful effects of both natural and human-generated disasters.

BOX 19-1 The Making of a Disaster: The Sinking of the "Unsinkable" *Titanic*

Nondisaster or Interdisaster Phase

The *Titanic* was on its maiden voyage when it sank on April 14, 1912. The crown jewel of the White Star Line, the ship was a mammoth 46-ton British liner of incomparable luxury, three football fields long and eleven stories high, which was the world's largest and purportedly safest vessel on the water. On this maiden voyage, the *Titanic* had as its passengers both British and American aristocracy, along with immigrants coming to the "New World" with promises of a new life. The boat deck and bridge were 70 feet above water. According to White Star Line documentation, a "trial test" of 6 to 7 hours total was conducted 1 month before leaving Great Britain. This trial consisted of turning circles and compass adjustment; also, the ship sailed "a short time" at full steam, but never at full speed before passengers boarded.

The crew and officers of the *Titanic* (numbering 899) joined the ship a few hours before the passengers and went through only one drill: They lowered two lifeboats on starboard side into water. No evidence of crew duties being delineated as to task or role in event of disaster were noted by the U.S. Congress. Congressional hearings found that the crew did not know their "proper stations" or assignment until after passengers had already boarded in Queenstown, Ireland.

There were 1,324 passengers on board the ship, and together with 899 crew members, a total of 2,223 persons were on the maiden voyage of the *Titanic*. Congress found no evidence of passengers having any orientation in disaster procedures. There were lifeboats with capacity for 1,176 persons and life jackets for all persons on board. The *Titanic* was considered "unsinkable," having been constructed with special watertight bulkhead compartments that could be sealed off if the ship took on water. There was no evidence of a disaster plan or safety instructions posted or provided to passengers, nor were crew members prepared for their roles in the event of a disaster. The crew staffed the *Titanic* round the clock and had lookouts posted in the crow's nest for any water-related hazards.

Predisaster or Warning Phase

The *Titanic* had received several ice warnings on the third day of the voyage, and the captain noted them. On the day of the disaster, a warning message cited icebergs within 5 miles of the track that the *Titanic* was following, very near the place where the accident occurred. Congressional hearings revealed that despite repeated warnings, no general discussion took place among the officers, no conference was called to consider these warnings, and no heed was given to them. The speed was not reduced, the lookout was not increased, and the only extra vigilance noted was from the officer of the watch, who gave instructions to the lookouts to "keep a sharp lookout for ice." The speed of the ship had been gradually increased, and just before the collision, the ship was making her maximum speed of the voyage. Passengers had no advance knowledge of any possible risks of the ship related to the icebergs.

Impact Phase

At 10:13 p.m. on Sunday, April 14, the lookout signaled the bridge and telephoned the officer of the watch with this message: "Iceberg right ahead." The officer of the watch immediately ordered the quartermaster at the wheel to put the helm "hard astarboard" and reverse the engines. The *Titanic* immediately struck the ice, and the impact caused the vessel to roll slightly. The impact, which ripped a hole in the steel plating of the ship, was not violent enough to disturb the crew or passengers. During this time, the damage was reported by crew members from the boiler room related to water coming in; the captain began inspecting the ship for damage. Passengers were still not aware of the accident.

Emergency Phase

The reports by the captain after various inspections of the ship revealed that the compartments were rapidly filling with water and that the bow of the ship was sinking deeper and deeper. Through the open hatches, water promptly began overflowing into the other bulkheads and decks. No emergency alarm was sounded, no whistles were blown, and no systematic warning was given the passengers.

Within approximately 15 minutes after his inspection, the captain issued a distress call to ships in the area. The call was heard by several ships in the vicinity. The *Carpathia*, which was 58 miles away, responded to the distress signal by turning immediately toward the sinking ship. Other ships also attempted to sail toward the sinking ship but were too far away to be of any reasonable assistance. The closest ship, the *Californian*, was only 19 miles north of the *Titanic* but did not attempt to rescue the ailing ship. Proceedings indicate that the crew of the *Titanic* began firing distress rockets at frequent intervals and that the crew of the *Californian* saw them. The captain of the *Californian* failed to heed the warning signals and was chastised by Congress for "indifference or carelessness" and for not responding to the *Titanic*'s distress calls in accordance with the dictates of international usage and law.

The captain immediately gave the signal to retrieve the lifeboats, with the order to put women and children in the boats first. The proceedings report that the lack of preparation at this time was most noticeable. There was general chaos as passengers learned of the accident from each other, from some crew members who knocked on cabin doors, and from being awakened by the movement of people running on the ship:

> There was no system adopted for loading the boats; there was great indecision as to the deck from which boats were to be loaded; there was wide diversity of opinion as to the number of crew necessary to man each boat; there was no direction whatever to the number of passengers to be carried by each boat, and no uniformity in loading them. (Kuntz, 1998, p. 548)

In some boats, there would be only women and children; in others there would be an equal proportion of men and women. Only a few of the lifeboats were loaded to capacity; most were only partially loaded, which resulted in needless losses. If all of the lifeboats had been fully loaded at capacity for 1,176 persons, far more than the 706 persons who did survive could have reasonably been saved.

Furthermore, the proceedings noted that if the sea had been rough (which it wasn't), it is questionable whether any of the lifeboats would have reached the water without being damaged or destroyed. The lifeboats were suspended 70 feet above the water, and in the event of the ship's rolling (with a rough sea), the boats would have swung out from the side of the ship and then crashed back into the ship as they were being lowered. Also, had the survivors been concentrated in fewer boats once on the water, the crew could have returned and rescued more passengers.

Once the ship sank at 12:47 a.m., it broke in half and people died from drowning, exposure, and trauma; 1,517 persons died, 706 survived. Survivors of the *Titanic* reported rowing toward the lights of a ship in the distance, which has now been established as those of the *Californian*. There were questions about the way passengers were evacuated relative to whether they were in first-, second-, or third-class accommodation. Sixty percent of first-class passengers survived, 42% of second-class passengers survived, and only 25% of third-class passengers survived. These statistics suggest that there may have been a distinction in the warning and evacuation based on class accommodation. Twenty-five percent of the crew were saved.

The rescue of survivors came from the *Carpathia* crew and eventually from the crew of the *Californian*. After a thorough search, ships returned to New York and Nova Scotia with the survivors. A brief burial prayer service for the dead was held at 8:30 a.m. by the captain of the *Carpathia*. Public media notification occurred the evening of April 15, 1912.

Reconstruction or Rehabilitation Phase

The wreck of the *Titanic* represents in myth and reality a disaster beyond human comprehension at a time when

(*continues*)

BOX 19-1 *(continued)*

technological advances were seen as our defense against the disasters of nature. Because of lack of preparedness and lack of planning for ship disasters, technology could not have saved the passengers on the *Titanic*.

The recommendations that evolved from the *Titanic* hearings held by Congress in May 1912 were no less than revolutionary in terms of safety preparedness. One was that inspection certificates would be contingent on sufficient lifeboats to accommodate every passenger and every member of the crew. Inspection certificates that mandate these requirements would apply to all boats that carry passengers from ports of the United States. Lifeboats should be positioned in such a way that they would not be subject to damage from height related to water level. There would be no fewer than four members of the crew, trained in handling boats, on each lifeboat. All crew members assigned to this duty would be drilled in lowering and rowing the lifeboats not less than twice per month and the "fact of such drill or practice should be noted in the log." Recommendations also included assigning passengers to lifeboats before sailing and posting the shortest route to the lifeboats in each room. Two electric searchlights were to be present on boats carrying more than 100 passengers. A radio operator must be on duty at all times, 24 hours a day. And finally, all ships from that point on would be required to meet construction standards related to watertight compartments and hulls.

Source: Kuntz, T. (Ed.). (1998). *The Titanic disaster hearings: The official transcripts of the 1912 Senate investigation*. New York, NY: Pocket Books.

CULTURAL CONNECTION

Disaster nurses are often deployed outside of their regional home culture. Being prepared for the cultural values of the community experiencing the disaster is critical to the successful role of the disaster nurse using a holistic perspective.

When Hurricane Katrina made landfall on the Mississippi Gulf Coast and near New Orleans, Louisiana, in August 2005, Americans became keenly aware of how a natural disaster can threaten the health of an entire population. Through the images on television of people stranded on rooftops, trapped in the New Orleans Superdome in a makeshift disaster shelter, and facing the total destruction of the Mississippi Gulf Coast, we were all affected in some way from the ravages of this "disaster of disasters." More than 1,300 people died, many because of levee failures in New Orleans, and Hurricane Katrina earned the dubious distinction of being the worst natural disaster in U.S. history. Since the September 11, 2001, terrorist attacks on the World Trade Center, in Pennsylvania, and at the Pentagon, the U.S. public has become much more aware of the devastating national and global effects of terrorism as a current disaster threat. The United States has experienced a string of unprecedented disasters since the late 1980s, including major earthquakes, hurricanes, tropical storms, floods, landslides, volcanic eruptions, severe winter storms, and wildfires.

Outside the United States, the Indian Ocean tsunami occurred on December 26, 2004, following a 9.1-magnitude earthquake; it killed more than 200,000 people in Indonesia, India, Sri Lanka, Thailand, and many other countries as far away as South Africa. Entire towns and villages were swept away. In South Asia, more than 73,000 people died and tens of thousands were injured when an earthquake measuring 7.6 on the Richter scale struck Pakistan and other parts of the region in October 2004. The thousands who remained homeless continued to suffer disease and exposure to the elements from the aftermath of these two disasters, and the death toll continued to climb even 2 years later (Garheld & Hamid, 2006; Gospodinov & Burnham, 2008; Hassmiller, 2007; Telford & Cosgrave, 2007).

From 1999 to 2011, 1.2 million people were killed worldwide from natural disasters alone. In this same period, natural disasters such as earthquakes, tsunamis, hurricanes, floods, and volcanic eruptions adversely affected the lives of at least 2.7 billion people, with an economic price tag of at least $1.7 trillion dollars (see **Figure 19-1**). Floods continue to be the most common natural disaster in the world.

Natural disasters result in more deaths and property destruction in developing and least-developed countries. Most of the increase in natural disaster occurrence and damage was due to a combination of deforestation, greater population density in disaster prone areas and climate change, including global warming (EM-DAT: The OFDA/CRED International Disaster Database, 2012). See **Figure 19-2**.

Considered one of the strongest storms ever to make landfall, Typhoon Haiyan tore through the central Philippines November 8, 2013, killing nearly 6,000 people and displacing more than 3.6 million. The 13-foot storm surge and up to 235-mph wind gusts largely wiped out coastal cities and destroyed much of the region's infrastructure, such as roads, water and sanitation systems, and telecommunications lines. Just 3 weeks before Typhoon Haiyan hit Central Visayas, a magnitude-7.2 earthquake rocked the same region, killing 222 people, displacing 350,000, and damaging or destroying about 73,000 buildings. Thousands of displaced or homeless quake survivors still had not

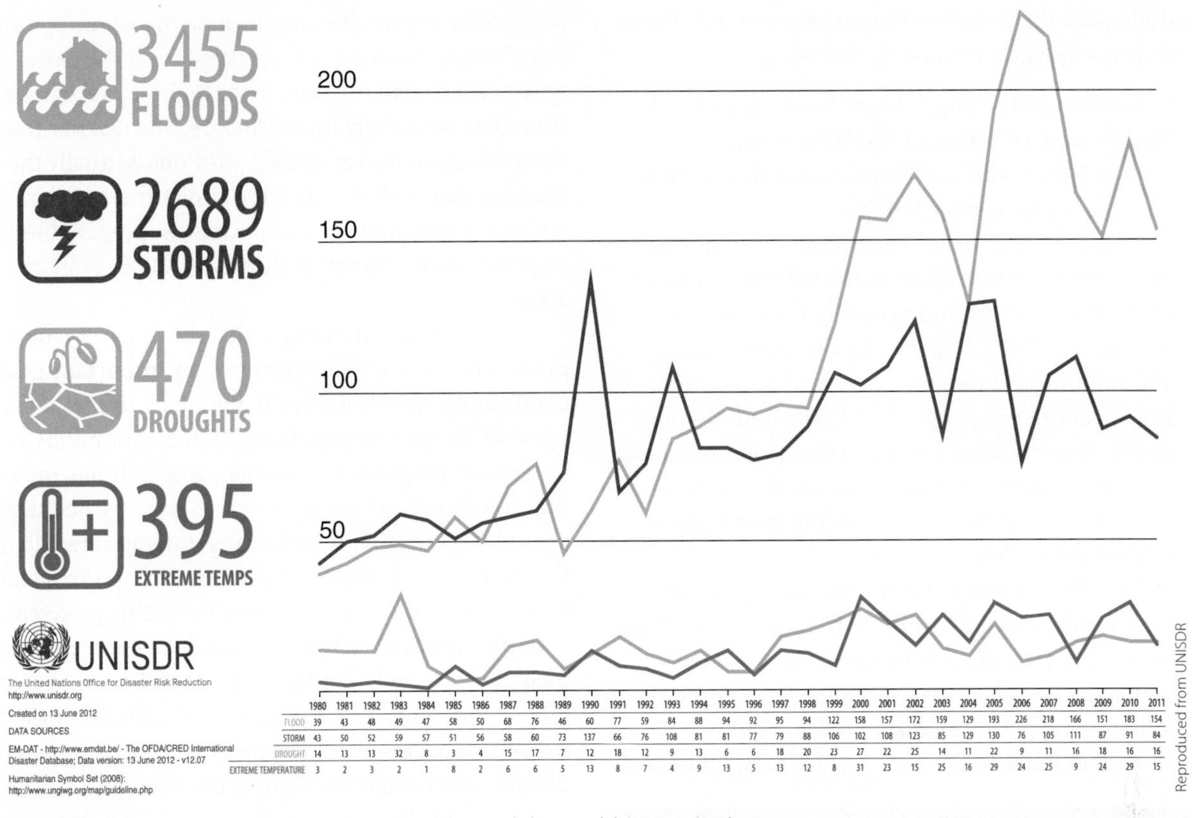

	1980	1981	1982	1983	1984	1985	1986	1987	1988	1989	1990	1991	1992	1993	1994	1995
FLOOD	39	43	48	49	47	58	50	68	76	46	60	77	59	84	88	94
STORM	43	50	52	59	57	51	56	58	60	73	137	66	76	108	81	81
DROUGHT	14	13	13	32	8	3	4	15	17	7	12	18	12	9	13	6
EXTREME TEMPERATURE	3	2	3	2	1	8	2	6	6	5	13	8	7	4	9	13

	1996	1997	1998	1999	2000	2001	2002	2003	2004	2005	2006	2007	2008	2009	2010	2011
FLOOD	92	95	94	122	158	157	172	159	129	193	226	218	166	151	183	154
STORM	77	79	88	106	102	108	123	85	129	130	76	105	111	87	91	84
DROUGHT	6	18	20	23	27	22	25	14	11	22	9	11	16	18	16	16
EXTREME TEMPERATURE	5	13	12	8	31	23	15	25	16	29	24	25	9	24	29	15

Figure 19-1 Number of climate-related disasters around the world (1980–2011).

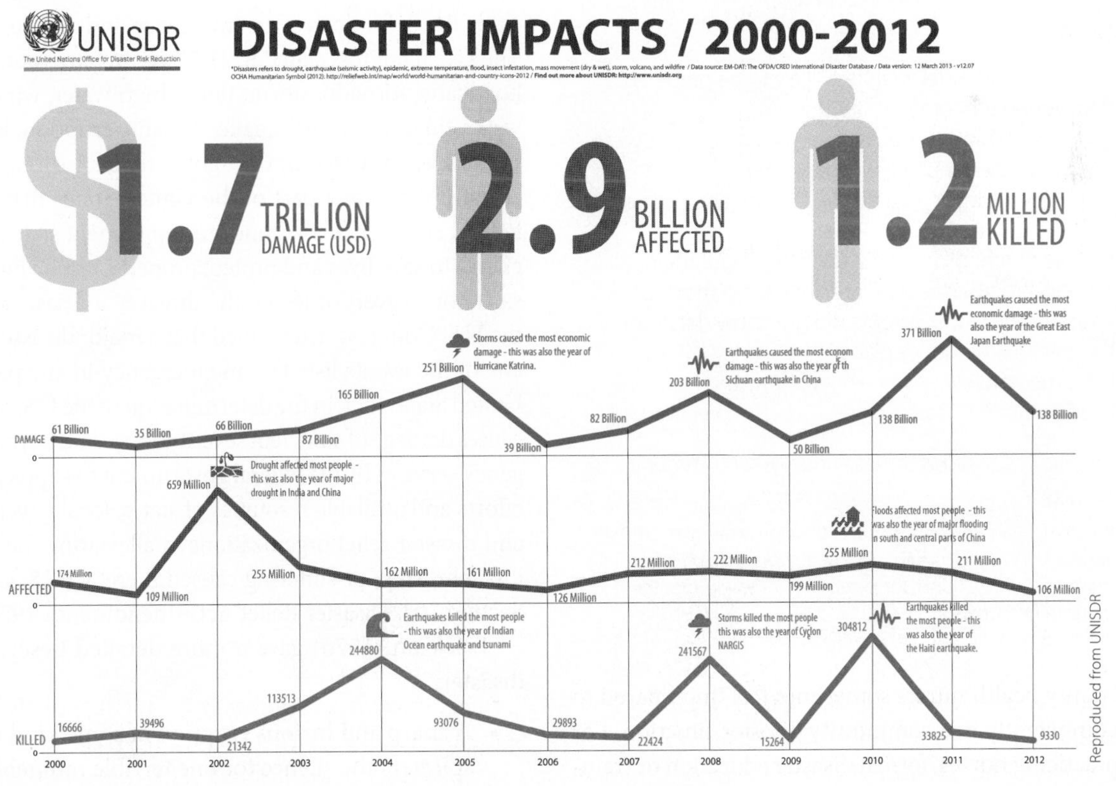

Figure 19-2 Disaster Impacts, 2000–2012.

found adequate shelter before Haiyan blew through. Other recent major disasters include the following:

- In October 2012, "Superstorm" Sandy devastated the U.S. eastern seaboard and large urban areas, such as New York City. Disaster assistance to New Jersey alone totaled $5.5 billion.
- In October 2013, the strongest cyclone to hit India in 14 years, Cyclone Phailin affected the livelihood of more than 13 million people in the country's northeast in 2013. Heavy rains and more than 150-mph winds brought widespread devastation. But fewer than 50 people died in the mid-October storm. Governments and aid organizations credited improved disaster preparedness and the early evacuation of about 1 million of the most vulnerable residents along the coast.
- In May 2013, a massive tornado, peaking at 210-mph winds, raked a 12-mile path through the Oklahoma City area, destroying homes and severely damaging two elementary schools. The twister killed 24 people. The week before, as many as 10 tornadoes touched down in North Texas, killing six.

NOTE THIS!

Why are we not prepared for a disaster?

Two-thirds of families still do not have basic emergency plans, even after 9/11 and Hurricane Katrina in 2005. A report sponsored by the Council for Excellence in Government also found:

- People 65 and older were less likely to be prepared than younger people.
- People with higher education and income levels were likely to be better prepared than others.
- Hispanics are less prepared than whites and African Americans.
- Parents of schoolchildren who know about their school's emergency plans are likely to be much better prepared, but most parents did not know details of the school emergency plans.
- Full-time employees who know about and have practiced company disaster plans are better prepared.

What are the implications of these findings for community health nurses?

Source: Peter D. Hart Research & Public Opinion Strategies. (2005). *The aftershock of Katrina and Rita: People not moved to prepare.* Washington, DC: The Council for Excellence in Government and the American Red Cross.

Community health nurses sometimes feel unprepared to react competently in a community disaster situation. For most practicing nurses, formal disaster education or training is not comprehensive. Therefore, the training that is received by nurses does not include the whole picture on levels of preparedness, which range from the basic emergency department response to the highest level of response from the community infrastructure. The disaster training that pertains to nurses' agency positions is usually the only training received, which often limits their understanding of the community's perspective on preparedness and response (Gospodinov & Burnham, 2008; Polivka et al., 2008).

Although the training delivered may not be comprehensive in many institutions, an important goal for community health nurses is for them to feel a greater sense of disaster preparedness. When community health nurses are prepared for disaster, research has indicated that communities benefit. Research has revealed that improved organization in delivering nursing care, planning the disaster response, and understanding the effects of disasters on families, communities, health professionals, and, ultimately, society can prevent or reduce the detrimental short- and long-term effects of disasters (Landesman, 2005; Noji, 1997; Plough et al., 2013). In essence, the community's health improves when it is prepared for disaster, even when the disaster doesn't come.

The Nature of Disasters

Definitions and Types of Disasters

Some of the many distinctions made between disasters include the definitions of an emergency and a major disaster. The U.S. Congress stated in 1974 that an **emergency** is any hurricane, tornado, storm, flood, high water, wind-driven water, tidal wave, earthquake, volcanic eruption, landslide, mudslide, snowstorm, drought, fire, explosion, or other catastrophe in any part of the United States that requires federal emergency assistance to supplement state and local efforts to save lives and protect property, public health, and safety or to avert or lessen the threat of a disaster. In 1974, the U.S. Congress determined that a **major disaster** may be any of the events listed as an emergency in any part of the United States that, in the determination of the U.S. president, causes damage of sufficient severity above and beyond emergency services by the federal government to supplement the efforts and available resources of states, local governments, and disaster relief organizations in alleviating the damage, loss, hardship, or suffering caused thereby (U.S. Congress, Section 102, Disaster Relief Act Amendments, 1974).

Erickson (1976) gave a more detailed description of disaster:

- A sharp and furious eruption of some kind that splinters the silence for one terrible moment and then goes away

- An event with a distinct beginning and a distinct ending that is by definition an extraordinary freak of nature, a perversion of the natural processes of life
- Doing a great deal of harm
- Sudden, unexpected, and acute

For the purposes of this chapter, a **disaster** is an event that causes human suffering and creates needs and demands exceeding the abilities of the community to cope without outside assistance. Most importantly, from a public health perspective, disasters are defined by what they do to people and, therefore, are relative to the context in which they occur. What results in a disaster in one community might not necessarily be considered a disaster in a different community (Landesman, 2005; Noji, 1997; Telford & Cosgrave, 2007). Disasters fall into two broad categories or types: **Natural disasters** arise from the forces of nature, such as hurricanes, tornadoes, earthquakes, and volcanic eruptions; **human-generated (human-made) disasters** are those in which the principal direct causes are identifiable human actions, deliberate or otherwise, such as the September 11 terrorist attacks. These two categories can be further subdivided into different types of disasters (**Box 19-2**).

NA-TECH

Although disasters can be grouped according to the stated definitions, in reality the distinction between natural and human-generated disasters is often blurred, because a natural disaster can trigger secondary disasters, such as explosions, fires, floods, and toxins released into the air after an earthquake. Such combination-type synergistic disasters are referred to as NA-TECH disasters; an NA-TECH disaster is a technological accident triggered by a natural event (natural-technological = NA-TECH). An example of an NA-TECH disaster occurred in the former Soviet Union when windstorms spread radioactive materials across the country, increasing by up to 50% the land area contaminated in an earlier nuclear disaster at Chernobyl. The flooding of New Orleans, after levee failure following landfall of Hurricane Katrina in Mississippi, is also an example of an NA-TECH disaster (Noji, 1997; Rebmann, Carrico, & English, 2008). On March 11, 2011, a 9.0-magnitude earthquake struck northeastern Japan, spawning an incredibly destructive tsunami that crippled the Fukushima Daiichi nuclear power plant. In the following year, much had changed; the effects of the disaster will most likely endure for many years to come. Nuclear power fell out of favor with the Japanese people, and confidence in the government was shaken. Japan mourned the confirmed deaths of more than 15,850 people, and still listed 3,287 as missing over a year later. Questions remain about rebuilding villages, cleaning up the nuclear exclusion zone, and deciding the future of nuclear power in Japan (Skirble, 2012).

As noted earlier, floods are the most common natural disaster in the world, accounting for more than one-third of all disasters from the late 1990s to the early 2000s. One example of a horrendous flood, although not necessarily a typical disaster, was the Mississippi River Flood of 1927, which has been cited as one of the worst natural disasters in U.S. history. In 1927, the Mississippi River swept across a geographic area larger than Massachusetts, Connecticut, New Hampshire, and Vermont combined and resulted in water as deep as 30 feet on the land, stretching from Illinois and Missouri south to the Gulf of Mexico and New Orleans. This flood forced almost 1 million people from their homes and resulted in thousands of deaths.

Many of the dead were still being pulled out of the Mississippi River at New Orleans even months after the flood. When more than 40,000 homes were destroyed close to where the dam broke in Mississippi, camps were set up in the Confederate National Park in Vicksburg. American Red Cross (ARC) nurses (see **Box 19-3**), nurses from the Mississippi State Department of Health, and nurses from other states were assigned to relief efforts for several months in the spring of 1927. A total of 383 nurses worked in the Mississippi flood disaster. Nurses worked in these refugee camps, battling typhoid and nutritional deficiencies such as pellagra. The waters from

BOX 19-2 Categories and Types of Disasters

Natural Disasters

- Meteorological: hurricanes, tornados, hailstorms, snowstorms, and droughts
- Topological: landslides, avalanches, mudslides, and floods
- Disasters that originate underground: earthquakes, volcanic eruptions, and tidal waves
- Bacteriological: communicable disease epidemics (e.g., Ebola virus) and insect swarms (e.g., locusts)

Human-Generated Disasters

- Warfare: conventional warfare (bombardment, blockage, and siege) and nonconventional warfare (nuclear, chemical, and biological; acts of terrorism), including mass refugee relocation
- Civil disasters: riots and demonstrations
- Accidents: transportation (planes, trucks, automobiles, trains, and ships); structural collapse (buildings, dams, bridges, mines, and other structures); explosion; fire; chemical (toxic waste and pollution); and biological (sanitation)

Sources: Modified from Garcia, L. M. (1985). *Disaster nursing: Planning, assessment, and intervention*. Rockville, MD: Aspen; Noji, E. K. (1997). *The public health consequences of disasters*. New York, NY: Oxford University Press.

BOX 19-3 An Early Field Test of the American Red Cross's Nurse Enrollment Campaign: The Purvis, Mississippi, Tornado of 1908

A devastating tornado hit the small town of Purvis, Mississippi in April 1908, injuring 200 persons. The American Red Cross had just undertaken its first major campaign to recruit and enroll nurses nationally for such disasters, and the Purvis tornado provided a "field test" of the newly developed communication system. In the end, a head nurse and 17 staff nurses were deployed from the District of Columbia, Philadelphia, and New York. These nurses managed tent hospitals and coordinated disaster relief for 3 weeks. Although the nursing was well done, recruitment and securement of nurses with the new system had been less than successful. The ARC staff had met with considerable difficulty locating the enrolled nurses and in the end had to recruit unenrolled, volunteer nurses outside the system. The disaster served to draw attention to the need for a more collaborative effort between nursing organizations together with the American Red Cross to develop a network of disaster preparedness through local volunteer nurses.

Source: Kernodle, P. (1949). *The Red Cross nurse in action 1882–1948.* New York, NY: Harper and Brothers.

the Mississippi did not recede for 3 months (Barry, 1997; Sabin, 1998).

Of course, a more recent flooding disaster occurred after Hurricane Katrina, when thousands of persons in New Orleans were left stranded after the levees broke, flooding the entire city with several feet of water. This unprecedented flooding left a major American city underwater for more than 4 weeks after the hurricane (Nigg, Barnshaw, & Torres, 2006). The major levee breaches in the city included breaches at the 17th Street Canal levee, the London Avenue Canal, and the wide, navigable Industrial Canal, which left approximately 80% of the city flooded. Flooding from the breaches put the majority of the city underwater for days, in many places for weeks (Boyer, 2005). Electricity and water were still not functioning in many of the hardest hit parts of the city as of 2007.

In another example, Colorado experienced torrential rain, floods, and mudslides in September 2012, resulting in catastrophic flooding along Colorado's Front Range, from Colorado Springs to Boulder County in the north. Boulder, Colorado was hit the hardest, with up to 20 inches (430 mm) of rain, which is comparable to Boulder County's average annual precipitation (20.7 inches, 525 mm). The floodwaters eventually spread across a range of almost 200 miles (320 km) from north to south, affecting 17 counties. Colorado experienced five deaths as a result of the flooding and more than 11,000 persons were evacuated from the mountainous area, including at least 1,750 people and 300 pets rescued by air and ground. Nearly 19,000 homes were damaged, and more than 1,500 were destroyed (Shank, 2013).

Disaster Characteristics

Disasters have different characteristics. Knowledge of these variables is necessary in disaster management and planning. Dynes, Quarantelli, and Kreps (1972) identified six variables by which disasters can be understood: predictability, controllability, speed of onset, length of forewarning, duration of impact, and scope and intensity of impact.

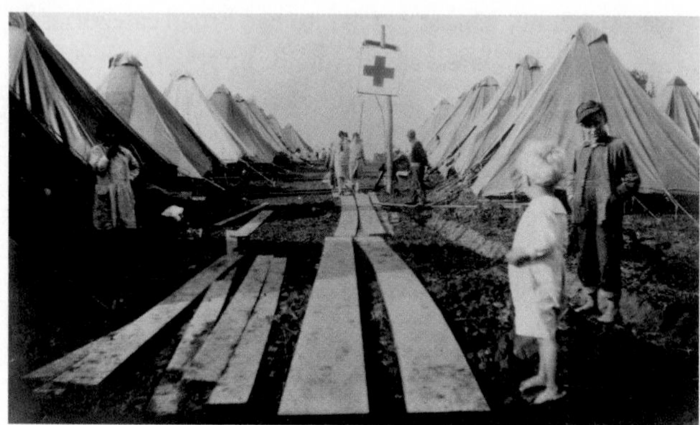

Public health nurse in disaster recovery during one of the worst natural disasters in the United States—the Mississippi River Flood of 1927.

DAY IN THE LIFE

David Lyon, nursing student who lost his family home on Mississippi Gulf Coast

The storm came on a Monday morning but we were not able to cross over the railroad tracks to see the destruction until 4 days later. It was a Friday and the first time the hospital allowed my mother, a nurse who rode out Katrina in a local hospital, to leave work. She had stayed during Katrina in her position as manager of nursing services at Memorial Behavioral Health in Gulfport, Mississippi. Although my family had evacuated, my mother worked during the entire hurricane and for 4 days afterwards. Mother said she wanted to try to get across the tracks and find our house. The guards were not officially allowing people to access their property at that point. The entire coast looked like a war zone and we feared the worst. We parked near the railroad crossing at the corner of Railroad Street and Cleveland Avenue. I walked with my mother up to the armed National Guard posted at the road access. A Humvee was parked to block traffic. My mother started talking to one of the soldiers, but wasn't able to get more than three words out before she lost her voice and began sobbing uncontrollably. She choked up, unable to talk through her grief, as she looked past the guards toward the destruction of our neighborhood. Our house was a full five blocks south of the tracks and I guess we had held out hope that we had been spared. I finally had to step in and speak for my mother, attempted to explain the situation, and asked what we had to do to get down there. I think it was probably my mother's sobbing more than my words that influenced the guard to let us through the barricade. He told us that we had 30 minutes to drive to our house, look at the wreckage, and drive back out. We drove down and spent about an hour there. The images of our neighborhood will always be imprinted on my brain; no words are adequate to describe the scene. When I think about that fated afternoon, all I can recall was my mother crying at the railroad crossing and having to be her voice, speaking for her. I cannot recall a time when I had seen my mother cry. I have seen her get misty over a sad ending to a movie, but never actually sob. This photo here is of our tragic discovery, the debris of our lives and what was lost forever.

—David Lyon, senior BSN nursing student
The University of Southern Mississippi College of Nursing

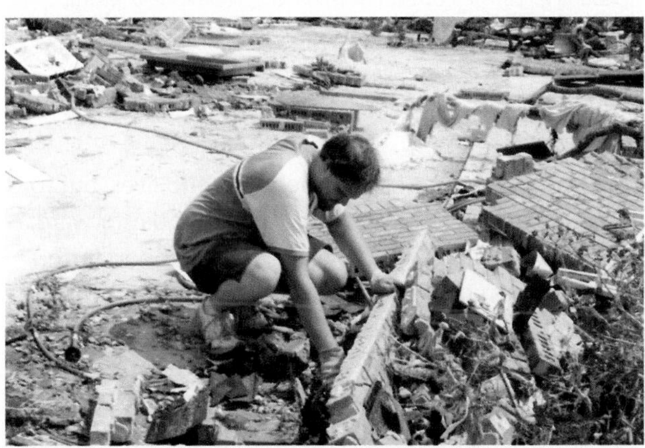

David Lyon, RN, BSN, sifts through the remains of his home after Hurricane Katrina.

THINK ABOUT THIS

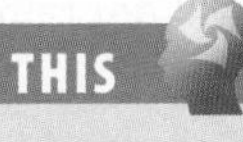

I helped rebuild communities in my home state of Gujarat after an earthquake in 2000, which killed 15,000 people and destroyed over a million homes. In India, one year after the earthquake in Gujarat, much of the affected areas had been rebuilt and the Indian government had given 100,000 INR (roughly US $2,250) to every family who had lost a loved one. That large sum is about two-thirds the average yearly income in India; the U.S. equivalent would be almost $30,000. The families of those who died during Hurricane Katrina have received nothing from their government.

When Martin Luther King, Jr., traveled to India, he was introduced to an audience he was about to address as "a fellow untouchable from the United States of America." He initially took great offense, but then thought about "twenty million of my brothers and sisters still smothering in an air-tight cage of poverty in an affluent society" and realized that, "Yes, I am untouchable" because he was African American. Many years after Martin Luther King's visit in New Orleans, I saw my "untouchable" brothers and sisters still living in these conditions.

Less than a year after the earthquake, Gujarat was back to normal, with people living in their own villages and cities. Here I stood on the land of the super power, the wealthiest nation in the world, where the debris of almost 40,000 homes remained unmoved nearly a year later. Ironically, the Federal Emergency Management Agency (FEMA) offered to sell its systems and services to India to aid in Gujarat after the earthquake. Seeing their results in New Orleans, I was glad India declined. The Indian government is far from perfect, but at least it recognized that it had a responsibility toward its people.

Martin Macwan is an advocate for the human rights of the people in India, founder of the Nasvarjan Trust, and 2000 winner of the Robert F. Kennedy Human Rights Award.

Source: Macwan, M. (2006). *Human Rights Day and Hurricane Katrina: "Untouchable" New Orleans*. BBSNews Special 2006. Retrieved from http://www.commondreams.org/views06/1208-33.htm

Predictability is influenced by the type of disaster. A hurricane has a high degree of predictability in industrialized countries. Earthquakes are considerably less foreseeable than floods. Although we often assume that disasters are rare occurrences, certain areas of the globe are clearly more prone to disasters, such as the flood plains of the Ohio River Valley or low-lying areas in Louisiana swamps. The Gulf Coast of Mississippi, Texas, Louisiana, Florida, and Alabama is vulnerable to the threat of hurricanes born from the warm waters of the Caribbean. Tornadoes are more common in Kansas, Texas, and Mississippi and less common in Utah and Idaho.

Controllability refers to the degree to which interventions can be used to control the disaster, such as using dams for flood control. Earthquakes, for example, have very little controllability.

Speed of onset is quick with floods and tornadoes, whereas hurricanes generally are slow to develop.

Length of forewarning is the period between warning and impact. Communities in the path of a hurricane may have the luxury of a 24-hour warning, whereas a tornado warning may provide only a few minutes of preparation.

Duration of impact also varies. A tornado may be on the ground for only a few minutes, whereas a flood's impact usually lasts for days. The worst combination of variables from the viewpoint of damage is the disaster that is rapid in onset, gives no warning, and lasts a long time. An earthquake with strong aftershocks is such a disaster and can also result in tsunamis.

Scope and intensity of impact refers to geographic and social space dimension. A disaster such as a tornado may be limited to a mile or two, whereas a flood may involve hundreds of miles. The population density of an area influences this variable and can lead to widespread consequences. An example of the effect of density can be seen in the Oklahoma City bombing, which was limited to a few city blocks but affected a large, dense population. The structure of New Orleans—also a densely populated urban area that is essentially trapped in a geographical "bowl"—led to devastating consequences when Hurricane Katrina struck, including the loss of thousands of lives and destruction of property that is taking years to repair. A disaster in a densely affected area can also result in disruption of community functions, depending on the number of persons involved and the geographic impact (Gamboa-Maldonado, Marshak, Sinclair, Montgomery, & Dyjack, 2012).

The World Trade Center and Pentagon attacks of 2001 have had global consequences, including U.S. military action and economic damage. Although the July 7, 2005, terrorist attacks on the London subway and buses were geographically limited, the population of the area was dense. Some 52 persons were killed and more than 700 injured in the deadliest attack in Great Britain since World War II; as with the 2001 U.S. attacks, the U.K. bombings had significant global political consequences (Ingram, Franco, Rio, & Khazai, 2006).

THINK ABOUT THIS 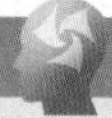

Hurricane Katrina: The Perfect Disaster?

Hurricane Katrina is one of the costliest and deadliest storms in U.S. history. Katrina was part of an unprecedented (and record-breaking) hurricane season, with 28 named storms (of which 15 became hurricanes), surpassing the previous record of 21 set in 1933. For the first time ever, the National Weather Service ran through an entire list of alphabetized proper names and resorted to naming hurricanes after Greek letters.

Levees failed in the city of New Orleans following Katrina's landfall on the Mississippi Gulf Coast, causing massive post-disaster flooding of the city of New Orleans. New Orleans was inundated with floodwaters for weeks in many areas after the storm. More than 1,300 people died in four states.

Katrina also exposed the nation's inadequate preparation for a disaster of this magnitude. Elders were left to die in nursing homes while they waited for transport, even though each nursing home was required by law to have transportation in place for evacuation. No one had counted how many transport companies existed or if the system might be easily overloaded. Disaster relief officials at the local, state, and federal levels were apparently unaware of the existence of frail and ill persons trapped in nursing homes and hospitals, so they focused their efforts on transporting the generally healthier, more visible group taking refuge in the Superdome. The number of elderly receiving in-home care, those who lived alone, and those with mental illness who lived on the street and were left stranded will probably never be accurately known.

Sources: Baum, D. (2006, August 16). Letter from New Orleans: The lost year. *The New Yorker;* Bourne, J. K. (2004, October). Gone with the water. *National Geographic*; Boyer, P. J. (2005, September 26). Letter from Mississippi: Gone with the surge. *The New Yorker*; Foxman, B., Camargo, C. A., Lillienfeld, D., Linet, M., Mays, V. M., McKeown, R., … Rothenberg, R. (2006). Looking back at Hurricane Katrina: Lessons for 2006 and beyond. *Annals of Epidemiology, 16*(8), 652–653; Kiewra, K. (2006, Winter). The eye of the storm: What lessons do Katrina and other humanitarian crises teach us about managing calamity? *Harvard Public Health Review*. Retrieved from http://www.hsph.harvard.edu/review/rvwwinter06_katrinaeye.html; Knabb, R. D., Rhome, J. R., & Brown, D. P. (2005, December 20). *Tropical cyclone report: Hurricane Katrina*. Miami, FL: National Hurricane Center; Waltham, R. (2005). The flooding of New Orleans. *Geology Today, 21*(6), 225–231.

> These terrorists kill not merely to end lives, but to disrupt and end a way of life. . . . From this day forward, any nation that continues to harbor or support terrorism will be regarded by the United States as a hostile regime. Our nation has been put on notice: We are not immune from attack. We will take defensive measures against terrorism to protect Americans. . . . Great harm has come to us. We have suffered great loss. And in our grief and anger we have found our mission and our moment. Freedom and fear are at war. . . . We will rally the world to this cause, by our efforts and by our course. We will not tire, we will not falter, and we will not fail.
>
> *—President George W. Bush, address to Congress on terrorism, September 20, 2002*

Shifting back to a global perspective, the 2004 Indian Ocean tsunami killed more than 200,000 people across South and Southeast Asia, including parts of Indonesia, Sri Lanka, India, and Thailand. This great undersea earthquake's epicenter, off the west coast of Sumatra, Indonesia, was the second largest earthquake ever recorded on a seismograph at (9.1 on the Richter scale) and was the longest duration of faulting ever observed, lasting between 8 and 10 minutes. It was large enough that it caused the entire planet to vibrate as much as half an inch and to minutely "wobble" on its axis by as much as 1 inch. The total energy released by this earthquake was equivalent to the explosion of 250 megatons of TNT. The shift of mass and massive release of energy very slightly altered the Earth's rotation. Although the exact amount is yet undetermined, theoretical models suggest the earthquake shortened the length of a day by 2.68 microseconds. It also triggered earthquakes in other locations as far away as Africa and Alaska in the United States (Ingram et al., 2006; Stein & Okal, 2005; Telford & Cosgrave, 2007).

Global Disaster Issues

As humans continue to migrate throughout the globe and population densities continue to increase in flood plains, along vulnerable coastal areas, and near faults in the Earth's crust, we can expect natural disasters to worsen and affect more people. The global community continues to witness complex emergencies resulting from the breakdown of traditional state structures, armed conflict, and the upsurge of ethnicity and micronationalism (Garheld & Hamid, 2006; Hayes, 2005; Noji, 1997; Rowitz, 2005; Stein & Okal, 2005; Telford & Cosgrave, 2007). One need look no further than today's newspaper headlines or watch a news network to find these political and cultural conflicts as they play out on a daily basis in disaster areas such as Bosnia, Syria, Darfur, Somalia, Rwanda, Chechnya, and Iraq, to name but a few. Because of these political and cultural upheavals, refugees have become a large and vulnerable population with complex health problems (Leaning & Guha-Sapir, 2013). Between 1965 and 2006, 90% of all natural disaster victims lived in Asia and Africa. The number of people affected (killed, injured, or displaced) by disasters worldwide rose from 100 million in 1980 to 157 million in 2005. By the mid-1990s, the number of refugees affected by a combination of natural and human-made disasters increased to an estimated 17 million throughout the world (International Strategy for Disaster Reduction [ISDR], 2006).

RESEARCH ALERT

The article discusses the impact of natural disasters and armed conflict on public health. It is stated that natural disasters and armed conflict have caused increases in mortality and morbidity. The growth in scale and scope of these events since 1990 is discussed. The effects of armed conflict and natural disasters on global public health progressed in the technical quality, normative coherence, and efficiency of the healthcare response.

Source: Leaning, J., & Guha-Sapir, D. (2013). Natural disasters, armed conflict, and public health. *New England Journal of Medicine, 369*(19), 1836–1842.

Earthquakes are global incidents that have been cited as causing the greatest number of deaths and the largest monetary loss of any type of natural disaster. The tragic 2004 earthquake that occurred in the Indian Ocean and the ensuing tsunami caused the deaths of more than 200,000 people, and the restoration of that area may take decades. This has further added to the poverty of these countries and to the already strained burden of immigration to other countries (Berz, 1984; Kumar et al., 2007; Telford & Cosgrave, 2007).

Not only are these displaced vulnerable populations at risk for serious health consequences, but the economic costs for their care are also devastating (Noji, 1997). As former United Nations (UN) Secretary General Boutros Boutros Ghali stated:

> There is no hard-and-fast division in terms of their [disasters'] effects on civilian populations between conflicts and wars, and natural disasters. Droughts, floods, earthquakes, and cyclones are just as destructive for communities and settlements as wars and civil confrontation. Just as preventive diplomacy can foresee and prevent the outbreak of war, so the effects of natural disasters can be foreseen and contained. (cited in Noji, 1997, p. xv)

Much of the destruction caused by natural disasters can be avoided. For almost every natural disaster in the world in the 1990s, an ounce of prevention or preparedness would have made a significant difference in terms of damage to persons and property (Noji, 1997, p. 7). Natural hazards, such as weather, earthquakes, and floods, are, in fact, only natural agents that transform a vulnerable condition into a disaster (Noji, 1997, p. 11).

People often do not know their limitations until they reach them. As technology has advanced and provided humans with opportunities to live in and explore the world without the territorial constraints of our ancestors, the probability that the future will be marked by periodic disasters is certainly increased. In many cases in recent disasters, building codes were ignored, communities were located in dangerous areas, warnings were not issued or followed, or plans were unknown to all community residents or were ignored (Noji, 1997).

We know much about the cause and nature of disasters, populations at risk, and the inevitable outcome when communities are not prepared for disasters. Such knowledge assists us in anticipating some of the effects that a disaster may have on the health of communities. Knowing how people are injured and killed in disasters is critical prerequisite knowledge for preventing or reducing injuries and deaths during future disasters (Noji, 1997). For example, although none of the advances in science and technology have done much to arrest the force of natural disasters, we often see them coming a few hours earlier and can measure their destructiveness with greater precision afterward. Yet those very advances have rendered us in many ways even more vulnerable to potential catastrophes, because persons often feel a false sense of security regarding the likelihood of serious threat from a disaster (Erickson, 1976). Persons in the New Orleans area hardest hit by Hurricane Katrina were living below sea level and were certainly accustomed to hurricane warnings, for example.

RESEARCH ALERT

Indian Ocean Tsunami, December 26, 2004

The 9.0-magnitude undersea earthquake occurred December 26, 2004. The earthquake generated a tsunami that was among the deadliest disasters in modern history. The tsunami wreaked devastation along the shores of Indonesia, Sri Lanka, South India, Thailand, Maldives, and other countries where waves of up to 30 meters hit the coast. Even areas as far as the coast of East Africa sustained damage and recorded fatalities. The World Health Organization (WHO) estimates that between 228,000 and 310,000 people died as a result of the tsunami, although an accurate count will never be known due to the number missing and destruction of the public health infrastructure in affected areas.

Sources: Garheld, R., & Hamid, A. Y. (2006). Tsunami response: A year later. *American Journal of Nursing, 106*(1), 76–79; Hassmiller, S. (2007). The 2004 tsunami. *American Journal of Nursing, 107*(2), 74–77; Kumar, M. S., Murhekar, M. V., Hutin, Y., Subramanian, T., Ramachandran, V., & Gupte, M. D. (2007). Prevalence of posttraumatic stress disorder in a coastal fishing village in Tamil Nadu, India, after the December 2004 tsunami. *American Journal of Public Health, 97*(1), 99–101; Telford, J., & Cosgrave, J. (2007). The international humanitarian system and the 2004 Indian Ocean earthquake and tsunamis. *Disasters, 31*(1), 1–28.

Natural Disaster Reduction

The UN General Assembly declared the 1990s to be the International Decade for Natural Disaster Reduction (IDNDR) and led the way in calling for a global, scientific, technical, and political effort to reduce the impact of catastrophic acts of nature (Advisory Committee IDNDR, 1987). The IDNDR was later renamed the International Strategy for Disaster Reduction (ISDR). This declaration came about because disasters and the number of their victims had increased in recent decades (Pickens, 1992; Rowitz, 2005). The UN has continued to meet yearly on this issue and, in June 2006, launched the 2006–2007 "Disaster Risk Reduction Begins at School" campaign.

When a natural disaster strikes, children are among the most vulnerable groups, especially those attending school in times of disaster. Disasters such as the October 2005 earthquake in Pakistan, in which more than 16,000 children died in schools that collapsed, or the 2006 mudslide on Leyte Island in the Philippines, where more than 200 school children were buried alive, are just a few tragic examples of why more needs to be done to protect our children during catastrophic events. The UN/ISDR secretariat and its partners made disaster risk education and safer school facilities the two key themes of the 2006–2007 World Disaster Reduction campaign. The "Disaster Risk Reduction Begins at School" initiative aimed to inform and mobilize governments, communities, and individuals to ensure that disaster risk reduction was fully integrated into school curricula in high-risk countries and that school buildings were built or retrofitted to withstand natural hazards. In all societies, children represent hope for the future. Because of their direct link to youths, schools are universally regarded as institutions of learning, for instilling cultural values, and for passing on both traditional and conventional knowledge to younger generations. Protecting our children during natural disasters, therefore, requires two distinct yet inseparable priorities for action: disaster risk education and school safety (ISDR, 2006).

The massive adverse impacts on the health of global populations resulting from disaster have now been recognized as a significant public health problem. Sudden-impact disasters, such as earthquakes and tornadoes, may result in large numbers of people killed, injured, or disabled for life; health facilities damaged or destroyed; and national healthcare development efforts in underdeveloped countries set back for years. As human societies have become denser as a result of the twin forces of urban migration and population growth, more people are now exposed and vulnerable to the hazards of disaster than ever before. Their increasingly sophisticated and technical physical infrastructure makes developed countries, such as the United States, even more vulnerable to destruction than in past generations. For instance, a major disaster could disrupt the computer networks of the federal government or some other large organization. Damage from both natural and technological disasters tends to be more and more extensive when proper planning and precautions are not taken. In the past 50 years, much has been learned about disasters and their aftereffects. Disaster preparedness involving careful and methodical planning does make a difference in mediating the destructive nature of disasters (Noji, 1997; Plough et al., 2013).

THINK ABOUT THIS

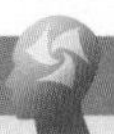

Healthcare needs of people in developing and underdeveloped countries experiencing violent conflict and disaster are similar. In such cases, nurses can play key roles in disease detection and control, social support, and rehabilitation. Nurses already provide much of the care in these situations because they are present on a daily basis, have key clinical and organizational skills, and have a high level of popular trust.

This commentary recommends that we can do more with systems training, disaster skill development, and participation in policy and research related to preventing and reducing the effects of disaster. Nurses are usually invisible, serving without discipline-specific orientation. The reasons for the lack of nursing's presence during disasters include unresolved ethical and political issues among nursing leaders regarding the role and image of nursing, humanist values, and relations between the profession and government. We are always the first on the scene and the last to leave, but rarely is our presence acknowledged in the press or official accounts of the disaster. Nightingale knew that better organization, autonomy, and recognition of the unique contribution that nurses make in times of war and disaster could do much to prevent further harm to damaged populations.

Source: Garfield, R., Dresden, E., & Rafferty A. (2003). Commentary: The evolving role of nurses in terrorism and war. *American Journal of Infection Control, 31*(3), 163–167.

> Begin at the beginning" the King said, gravely, "and go till you come to the end; then stop.
>
> —*Lewis Carroll's Alice's Adventures in Wonderland, 1865*

> Will you be a hero in your daily work? … We may give you an institution to learn in, but it is you who must furnish the heroic feelings of doing your duty, doing your best, without which no institution is safe.
>
> —*Florence Nightingale*

Disaster as a Global Public Health Problem

The Centers for Disease Control and Prevention (CDC) has led the way and has major responsibilities to prepare for and respond to public emergencies such as disasters. The CDC is also responsible for conducting investigations into the health effects and health consequences of disaster. The first major comprehensive research study of disasters was published in 1962 by Baker and Chapman in their book *Man and Society in Disaster.* Since then, many research centers have been established to study the health effects of disaster; among them are collaborative centers under the guidance and sponsorship of WHO and the Pan American Health Organization. The major aim of these research efforts is to assess risk for death and injury and to develop strategies for preventing or mitigating the impact of future disasters.

Disasters affect communities in myriad ways. Most effects are related to health, directly or indirectly (Noji, 1997). Communication lines, such as telephones, television, and Internet connections, may be disrupted, as well as transportation links, such as roads and methods of transportation. Public utilities (electricity, water, gas, and sewer) are often disrupted early in a massive disaster. A substantial number of persons may be without homes. Casualties may require medical and nursing care. Damage to food, damage to food preparation and sources, and lack of sanitation resources may create serious public health threats. A long-term effect is the community's possible destruction of its industrial or economic base. A detailed summary of disasters and public health is provided in **Box 19-4** and the health effects of disasters in **Box 19-5**.

BOX 19-4 Public Health Problems That May Result from Disasters

- Excessive deaths and injuries can tax the local health services and therapeutic capabilities, which may require external assistance.
- Destruction or disruption of acute care health facilities, such as clinics and hospitals, may leave services and resources unable to provide care to the injured from the disaster and predisaster patient population needs.
- Disruption of routine health services and preventive activities can lead to long-term consequences in terms of morbidity and mortality.
- Environmental hazards can lead to increased risks for communicable disease and injury from a damaged ecosystem.
- Psychological and social behavioral stressors, including panic, anxiety, neuroses, and depression, can be exacerbated.
- A shortage of safe, nutritional food sources may lead to severe nutritional deficiencies and sequelae in the very young and the very old.
- Displaced populations to overcrowded hospitals and shelter facilities may increase the dangers of communicable disease.

Sources: Adapted from Logue, J. N., Melick, M. E., & Hansen, H. (1981). Research issues and directions in the epidemiology of health effects of disasters. *Epidemiological Review, 3,* 140–162; and Noji, E. K. (1997). *The public health consequences of disasters.* New York, NY: Oxford University Press.

Box 19-5 Health Effects of Disasters

Physical

Sleep disturbance
Poor concentration
Back pain
Tachycardia
Poor diet

Psychological

Loss of self and relationships
Emotional pain
Brooding
Aggressive thoughts
Depression

Sociocultural

Loss of intimacy
Loss of sense of belonging to once claimed culture

Source: From Nurses' Role in World Catastrophic Events: War and Dislocation Effects on Serbian Australians by N. Procter and J. Cheek. In B. Neuman (Ed.) *The Neuman Systems Model* (3rd Int. ed.), pp. 119–131, 1995. Reproduced by permission.

Populations at Risk in Disasters

Not all persons in the world are equal regarding the probability of disaster occurrence or severity of consequences. The more vulnerable to a disaster a population is, the more serious the outcomes of injury and damage to persons and property (Garheld & Hamid, 2006; Mizutani & Nakano, 1989; Telford & Cosgrave, 2007). As far as individual health characteristics, persons with conditions that put them at risk, such as those with chronic diseases, elder persons, pregnant women, home health patients, the disabled, homebound persons, or children, are among the most vulnerable in any society concerning impact of disaster (FEMA, 2011). Industrialized countries are buffered from disasters by characteristics and abilities that are summarized in **Box 19-6**.

Stages of Disaster

Disasters can be divided into five chronological stages that require specific levels of prevention and levels of response at various points during each stage. Knowing the disaster stages will assist in the development of the disaster plan, role responsibilities, and the setting of priorities in each phase of the disaster plan. Refer to Box 19-1 about the 1912 Titanic disaster as an illustration of the stages of disaster. The stages of a disaster are as follows:

1. Nondisaster, or interdisaster, stage
2. Predisaster, or warning, stage
3. Impact stage
4. Emergency stage
5. Reconstruction, or rehabilitation, stage

BOX 19-6 Resources for Industrialized Countries

- Sophisticated technology to forecast storms
- Development and strict enforcement of codes for earthquake- and fire-resistant buildings
- Widespread mandatory use of communications networks to broadcast disaster warnings, alerts, and information about disaster preparedness
- Resources to provide timely and high-quality emergency health services and accommodation
- Contingency planning to prepare the population and public agencies for possible disasters
- Shelters for evacuation widely available and used by population

The low death rate associated with disasters in the United States, such as hurricanes Katrina and Rita (2005), Hugo (1989), Andrew (1992), and Georges (1998), earthquakes and wildfires in California, are evidence of the success of the United States' devotion of resources in disaster warning and recovery, which reduces the death risks to vulnerable populations (Noji, 1997; Rowitz, 2005). The following major factors contribute to the degree of vulnerability of populations:

- Human vulnerability resulting from poverty and social inequality
- Environmental degradation resulting from poor land use
- Rapid population growth, especially among the poor

It is estimated that 95% of the deaths that result from natural disasters occur among 66% of the world's poorest population. The poor are most at risk for greatest damage for the following reasons (EM-DAT, 2012):

- They are likely to live in substandard housing with little structural protection.
- They often live in coastal locations that are at high risk for disasters.
- They are likely to live in flood plains and other less desirable land.
- They are likely to live in substandard housing built on unstable geographic slopes.
- They are likely to live near hazardous industrial sites.
- They are not usually well educated about safe and appropriate life-saving behaviors and disaster preparedness.
- They are more dependent on others for transportation.

Source: Adapted from Garcia, L. M. (1985). *Disaster nursing: Planning, assessment, and intervention.* Rockville, MD: Aspen.

Disaster planning should begin before the disaster event. During the nondisaster stage (**interdisaster stage**), planning and preparation for a disaster include the two critical elements of disaster preparedness: (1) disaster training and education programs for the community and (2) the development of a disaster plan for all involved in the mitigation of a potential disaster (Noji, 1997; Rowitz, 2005). Mitigation is preventive in nature and is defined as action taken to prevent or reduce the harmful effects of a disaster on human health and property (Langan & James, 2004; Malilay, 1997). Included in this critical phase of primary prevention are assessment of hazards and risks, vulnerability analysis, inventory of existing resources for coping with a disaster (human, communication, and material), and the establishment of a disaster plan. Disaster planning is discussed in more detail later in this chapter.

A disaster is imminent during the warning stage (**predisaster stage**). The disaster plan, when available, is implemented, which includes early warnings based on predictions of impending disaster and mobilization as well as implementation of protective measures for the affected communities and populations (Garcia, 1985). Because primary prevention is the focus during this stage, disaster team members, officials, and emergency personnel prepare the population for disaster by providing information via multiple communication routes. Advisories and warnings are issued, and evacuation measures are taken where indicated. Mobilization can occur in the form of evacuation to shelters, preparation such as using sandbags around riverbanks to divert floodwaters, boarding up windows and tying down boats when a hurricane is forecast, moving to the basements or inner halls of homes and schools in the event of a tornado, or evacuating geographically vulnerable persons after volcano warnings. Healthcare workers may be placed on alert call for health facility staffing and disaster shelter management. The effectiveness of these protective measures will depend largely on the community's preparedness and contingency plans developed in the nondisaster phase (Leaning & Guha-Sapir, 2013; Noji, 1997).

Problems associated with such warnings include the fact that the communication systems may be inadequate in transmission and/or reception, or there may not be enough time to send warnings; in addition, the community must recognize the warning threat as serious and legitimate. Nevertheless, some people in the targeted community may deny the need for taking action based on previous experience with the specific disaster (e.g., persons who live on a fault line or on a coastline), and the occurrence of false alarms in the past can desensitize persons to appropriate reaction (Garcia, 1985; Janis & Mann, 1977; Rosenkoetter, Covan, Cobb, Bunting, & Weinrich, 2007).

The **impact stage** involves "holding on" and enduring the impact of the disaster. This stage may last from minutes (as in earthquakes, plane crashes, tornadoes, and bomb blasts) to days or weeks (hurricanes, floods, fire, and drought). People who are directly experiencing the disaster may be unable to comprehend the scope of the disaster (Garcia, 1985). If possible, disaster team members during the impact phase or immediately afterward should conduct a preliminary assessment and inventory of injuries and property damage so that the implementation of secondary prevention strategies of setting priorities can be set in motion. How much the impact affects community members depends on several factors: population density, the extent of the damage, the preparedness of the community, the extent of community resiliency, response to the consequences of the damage, and the organization of emergency response teams.

During the **emergency stage**, the community faces the consequences of the disaster's impact. This stage begins during the actual impact and continues until the immediate threat of additional hazards has passed (Garcia, 1985; Gibson, Theadore, & Jellison, 2012). Secondary prevention strategies are used to minimize damage and prevent further complications. This stage is divided into three parts—isolation, rescue, and remedy.

Isolation of the affected population can occur as a result of limited access (as a result of disaster damage, such as closed roads, downed trees, or building obstruction). The community members themselves must assume responsibility for their own needs relative to the disaster until outside help arrives.

ENVIRONMENTAL CONNECTION

Why was New Orleans a "disaster waiting to happen"?

The city of New Orleans sits below sea level. Why is this so? According to Tidwell, author of *Bayou Farewell*, the answer is the levees. The huge earthen river dikes that have kept the city dry and inhabitable for 300 years have also resulted in a virtual giant bathtub. Every great river delta in the world is shaped by two defining geological phenomena: One feature involves the flooding resulting from overflow, in this case, of the sediment-rich Mississippi River. This has created over the past 7,000 years a vast deltaic coast from the water-borne deposits composed of sediments and nutrients flowing from two-thirds of the United States. The second feature is subsidence, or sinking. The deposits of alluvial soil are extremely fine and unstable. Over time, they tend to compact, shrink in volume, and sink. This natural process of sediment deposit

(*continues*)

ENVIRONMENTAL CONNECTION *(continued)*

counterbalanced the sinking and resulted in net land building. By corseting the river with levees right out to the Gulf of Mexico's Continental Shelf, we are left with a sinking "bowl."

When French colonists first settled in Louisiana 300 years ago, vast, dense hardwood forests lay between what is now New Orleans and the Gulf of Mexico. There were freshwater marshes, endless saltwater wetlands, and a network of strong barrier islands. Today, all that land is essentially gone. Because of the levees and the "law of unintended consequences," New Orleans is a sunken, walled city, essentially jutting out exposed to the hurricane-prone Gulf of Mexico. Had Katrina struck 50 or 100 years ago, the destruction would not have been the same. In 2005 there were simply no land structures left to slow Katrina's deadly blow.

Every day, even without hurricanes, 50 acres of land in coastal Louisiana turn to water. Every 10 months, an area of land equal to Manhattan joins the Gulf of Mexico. It is the fastest disappearing landmass on Earth. This is why Katrina happened, why people drowned, lost their homes.

The entire coast of Louisiana, including New Orleans, began rapidly sinking, dropping 2–3 feet in the 20th century alone:

> It would be criminally irresponsible of us to fix a single broken window in New Orleans, pick up a single piece of debris, or fix a single cubic foot of levee without simultaneously committing as a nation to the massive plan to rebuild the entire Louisiana coast. To do one without the other is to simply set the table for the next nightmare hurricane.

Source: Tidwell, M. (2006). Exporting calamity: Katrinas for everyone. *World Watch, 19*(5), 43–45.

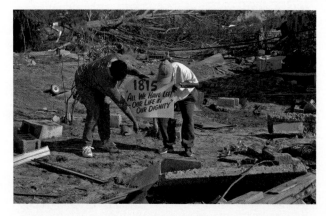

After a disaster, communities must come to terms with rebuilding their entire lives from the ground up. After Hurricane Katrina, these residents illustrate the shock of such devastation and the resilience of the human spirit.

Rescue begins when outside resources arrive and provide search-and-rescue operations. Community members are often harried, stressed, and nonproductive in this early stage. First aid, emergency medical assistance, and a command post for disaster management are established. Restoration of means of communication begins, and regional, state, federal, and voluntary organizations and agencies converge to meet the needs of the community.

Remedy begins with the establishment of organized, professional, and voluntary relief operations and organizations. The panic and confusion of the earlier phases tend to subside. Community members, disaster workers, and volunteers "get on with the task" of providing appropriate medical aid, clothing, food, and shelter to the affected population. The injured and ill are triaged, transportation becomes more organized, morgue facilities are established, reunions of family members become organized, and communication networks are established to provide early data on the disaster damage (Garcia, 1985). Later in the emergency stage, surveillance of public health effects (e.g., infectious disease, sanitation issues, safety concerns, and environmental fallout, such as flood debris and air pollutants) is put in place and interventions are developed (Wilson, 2006). When communities are well prepared and disaster plans are in place to help people know the "what, when, and how" of disasters for their population, both self-reliance and the effectiveness of early assistance can save lives and reduce injury during this critical period (Langan & James, 2004; Noji, 1997; Plough et al., 2013; Rowitz, 2005). At this stage, coordination of rescue efforts becomes critically important to execute and evaluate effectiveness.

The **reconstruction (rehabilitation) stage** begins when communities start the process of healing. Reconstruction or rehabilitation optimally restores the community to predisaster conditions (Noji, 1997). Health services are restored to normal. Damaged homes, facilities, and buildings are repaired and reconstructed. This period is also the time for evaluation and reflection by the community and disaster team members, community officials, and voluntary agencies, as lessons learned from the disaster are shared and documented (Noji, 1997). This period, which may combine secondary and tertiary prevention, may take days, months, or years, depending on the nature of the disaster, the response of the community, and the extent of the damages. For persons in the impact area, the recovery can be a long course and, in some cases, can be a lifelong readjustment to life and community living after the disaster (Garcia, 1985; Gibson et al., 2012; Wilson, 2006).

CULTURAL CONNECTION

A Manhattan Nurse Redefines "Normal" After 9/11

The word "normal" has taken on a whole new meaning for me. It is now normal for my heart to race when I hear a fire alarm or a siren, or to stop and look at the sky if I hear the engine of a plane that is loud. It is now normal for me to keep supplies in a closet at home for another possible attack; I have become familiar with anthrax, smallpox, and other diseases. I am not afraid to travel, but I am afraid that if I travel and another attack occurs I won't be able to get back to the people and things I love. For me, nothing will ever be the same.

Peter J. Ungvarski, MS, RN, FAAN, was a clinical nurse specialist in HIV infection and director of quality assessment and regulatory compliance at the Visiting Nurse Service (VNS) of New York at the time of the 9/11 terrorist attacks. Ungvarski was in his VNS office in Manhattan at 8:47 a.m. when the first plane, American Airlines Flight 111, crashed into Tower One of the World Trade Center.

Source: Reprinted from Association of Nurses in AIDS Care, 13(5), Ungvarski, P. J., Redefining the word "normal" in Manhattan, Page Nos. 21–24, Copyright 2002). 9/11:. Association of Nurses in AIDS Care, 13(5), 21–24., with permission from Elsevier.

In the wake of the September 11, 2001 disasters, people in New York City have reconstructed their lives in varied ways. Memorials have been held, artwork has been created, and a new community ethic of connectedness seems to have emerged. There appeared to be a need to invest in the future, to define and reach for goals, and to invest energy in plans to rebuild both the city and individual lives that had been personally touched by the trauma and loss. Klagsbrun (2002) suggests that by moving on in our personal lives, as well as in our communal lives, we are attempting to regain control over our destiny. Each person often reviews his or her own history and recognizes how the individual has overcome losses, difficulties of all kinds, pain, and failure and has succeeded in being able to go on.

RESEARCH ALERT

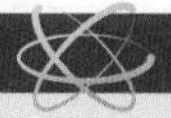

An emerging approach to public health emergency preparedness and response, *community resilience* encompasses individual preparedness and establishes a supportive social context in communities to withstand and recover from disasters. This article examines why building community resilience has become a key component of national policy across multiple federal agencies and discusses the core principles embodied in community resilience theory—specifically, the focus on incorporating equity and social justice considerations in preparedness planning and response. We also examine the challenges of integrating community resilience with traditional public health practices and the importance of developing metrics for evaluation and strategic planning purposes. Using the example of the Los Angeles County Community Disaster Resilience Project, the article discusses the authors' experience and perspective from a large urban county to better understand how to implement a community resilience framework in public health practice.

Source: Plough, A., Fielding, J. E., Chandra, A., Williams, M., Eisenman, D., Wells, K. B., ... Magaña, A. (2013). Building community disaster resilience: Perspectives from a large urban county department of public health. *American Journal of Public Health, 103*(7), 1190–1197.

It is during the rehabilitative phase that victims often suffer from posttraumatic stress disorder. **Posttraumatic stress disorder (PTSD)** is recognized by the American Psychiatric Association (APA) with the following symptoms and circumstances: The sufferer is a victim of an extremely distressing event who persistently reexperiences the event after it is over (compulsive and obsessive thoughts about details of the event), persistently avoids stimuli that remind the victim of the event, and experiences numbing of responsiveness and persistent symptoms of arousal not present before the trauma (APA, 2013). In conjunction with disaster, other symptoms include flashbacks, depression, inability to form close personal relationships, and sleep disturbances (Barker, 1989; Rhoads, Mitchell, & Rick, 2006). Florence Nightingale is thought to have suffered from PTSD after the Crimean War. This condition, once diagnosed, requires professional mental health intervention and follow up (Adams, 2007; Hyre, Ompad, & Menke 2007; Rebmann et al., 2008; Rhoads et al., 2006; Waters, Selander, & Stuart, 1992).

RESEARCH ALERT

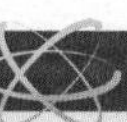

This study surveyed workers, truck drivers, heavy equipment operators, laborers, and carpenters about their work-related exposures and somatic and mental health symptoms after working on the cleanup and recovery efforts at the World Trade Center Disaster site following September 11, 2001. Respondents reported debilitating consequences of their work, being poorly prepared to work in a disaster,

(continues)

RESEARCH ALERT (continued) 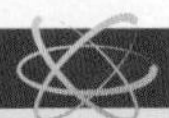

lacking protective equipment and training, and being overwhelmed by the devastation at the World Trade Center site.

Source: Johnson, S. B., Langlieb, A. M., Teret, S. P., Gross, R., Schwab, M., Massa, J., ... Geyh, A. S. (2005). Rethinking first response: Effects of the cleanup and recovery effort on workers at the World Trade Center disaster site. *Journal of Occupational and Environmental Medicine, 47*(4), 386–391.

Disaster Planning

A planned response to disasters must occur to lessen the terror of a disaster, to cushion the impact by providing care for the greatest number of potential survivors, and to increase society's ability to survive disasters and grow more self-sufficient and self-reliant in the process (Henderson, Inglesby, & O'Toole, 2002; Waeckerle, 1991). Clearly, the benefits of disaster planning for society today are more significant than ever as widespread disasters become more common and more costly, in both human and property terms.

Anticipating a disaster and planning for the possibility of multiple outcomes from disasters strengthen a community's adaptability. Consequently, the disaster team develops the ability to respond more quickly and more effectively in the face of disaster (Levy & Sidel, 2002; Muench, 1996). Another benefit to planning is the delineation of roles and responsibilities of the players in disaster preparedness. The result is less confusion over who does what and the roles of the multitude of organizations and volunteers once resources become available.

Once a disaster is imminent, it is too late to plan a response. Knowledgeable and experienced leaders and officials in the community should coordinate a clear community disaster plan for all contingencies. Such a plan must be as inclusive as possible, including input from health professionals; voluntary agencies; policymakers; officials from local, state, and federal levels, such as the civil defense and FEMA; emergency response system personnel; and all other components of the healthcare delivery system from acute care to home health to residential care, including medical and nursing schools (FEMA, 2006; Gospodinov & Burnham, 2008; Langan & James, 2004; Waeckerle, 1991).

Steps in the Disaster Process

When a major disaster has occurred, such as Hurricane Katrina in 2005, the president of the United States intervenes after the governor of the affected state requests the president to declare the area a major disaster. However, all major disaster declarations must follow certain steps (FEMA, 2006).

First, local government agencies, such as the mayor and civil defense, which includes neighboring communities and volunteer agencies, must respond. Second, if the local agencies become overwhelmed, the state responds at the governor's request through state agencies and the National Guard. Third, local, state, federal, and volunteer organizations make a damage assessment. Fourth, when state resources have been exhausted, the governor of the state makes a request to the president for a declaration of a major disaster. The governor bases this request on the already-completed damage assessment collected by the civil defense team and commits a certain amount of state funds and resources to the long-term recovery from the disaster. Fifth, FEMA evaluates the request and recommends action to the White House. Sixth, either the president gives the executive order for the declaration or FEMA informs the governor the request has been denied. The whole process may take only a few days. If the executive order is given, federal and financial resources are mobilized through FEMA for search and rescue and for the provision of basic human needs. Long-term federal programs are mobilized during this time.

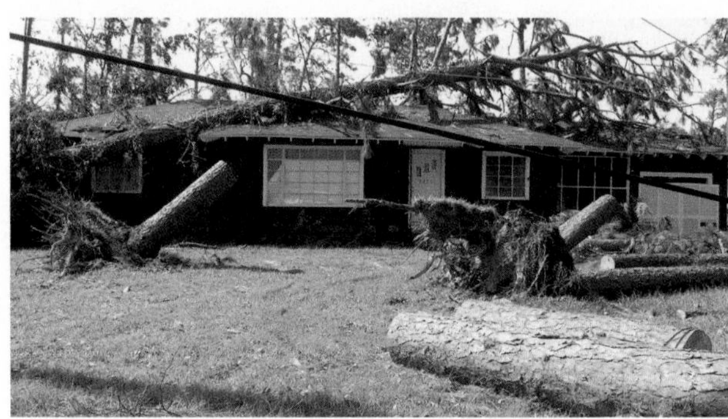

Tornados often leave a path of severe destruction, especially in densely populated urban areas.

ENVIRONMENTAL CONNECTION

"I'm a strong proponent of the restoration of the wetlands, for a lot of reasons. There's a practical reason, though, when it comes to hurricanes: The stronger the wetlands, the more [*sic*] likely the damage of the hurricane."

—President George W. Bush, discussing post-Katrina wetland improvements, New Orleans, March 1, 2007

A new report on the environmental effects of Hurricane Katrina in 2007 indicates that the Louisiana gulf coast is sinking. Findings a year after Katrina indicate that the coastline in southern Louisiana is gradually shifting, sliding ever so slowly into the Gulf of Mexico. The implication of this for future disaster risks is significant as engineers repairing the levees around New Orleans must now reconsider how this will affect previous plans to rebuild the levees. This lateral movement of land into the Gulf indicates that the bedrock under southern Louisiana southward has been triggered by deep underground faults that are slipping under the enormous weight of the sediment from the disaster as well as from the Mississippi River.

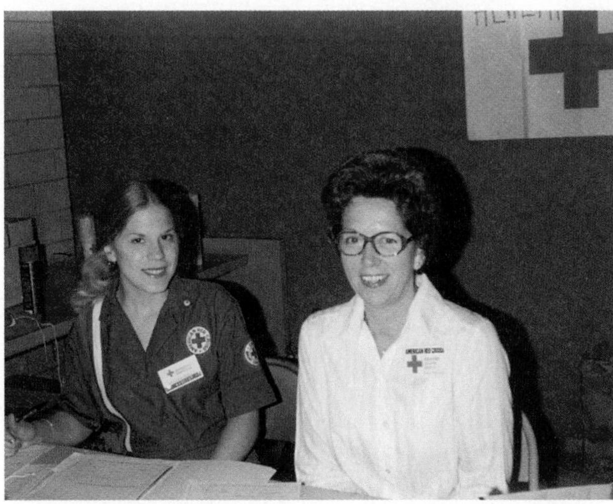

Chapter author Dr. Karen Saucier Lundy (left) at an American Red Cross shelter after Hurricane Allen in Galveston, Texas.

The Disaster Plan

The purpose of **disaster planning** is to reduce a community's vulnerability to the tremendous consequences of disasters and to prevent or minimize problems resulting from system damage associated with the disaster. Community health nurses are involved in disaster planning, as are other healthcare professionals in the community. Specific ways that a nurse can be more prepared for a disaster in his or her community are described in the next section (Drabek, 1986; Gospodinov & Burnham, 2008; Langan & James, 2004).

In a disaster, the usual strategies and process for providing care may not work. Deviating from a routine plan of care may present a few problems for nurses and other healthcare professionals when disaster occurs. Disaster health care is very different from daily nursing practice; it is not routine (even compared with emergency department services), and the philosophy of care is based on providing the greatest good for the greatest number. Abiding by this standard of care is often difficult for healthcare professionals, especially for those in routine practice settings who practice holistic care and provide optimal care to all who need services. The disaster plan is fundamental in the preparation of healthcare professionals (Waeckerle, 1991). Drabek (1986) identified general principles that can guide community health nurses who take part in disaster planning. These principles are listed in **Box 19-7**.

As Waeckerle (1991) has stated, "Disaster planning is an enormous undertaking" (p. 815). As in other areas of health care, enormous amounts of money are spent in the United States on disaster relief during the recovery period, yet few funds are made available for communities to use in disaster preparedness and disaster planning. This emphasis poses challenges in the development of a disaster plan. Although the disaster plan is usually developed from guidelines set forth by local, state, and

BOX 19-7 Principles to Guide Disaster Preparedness for All Persons Involved in Planning

- Measures used for everyday emergencies generally do not work in major disasters.
- Disasters are more uncertain, less predictable, with more unknowns, and citizens have little consensus on what needs to be done in a disaster.
- Laypersons are most likely to jump in and provide aid without direction and knowledge of prioritization and triage.
- Plan for specific population needs and consider "disaster planning" as a verb, which is ongoing, rather than as a noun, such as the limits of a written plan.
- Provide information regularly to the community to correct misconception through all forms of available media, including social media (Facebook, Twitter, etc.), television, newspapers, and in the virtual communities, such as blogging.
- Widespread looting and theft are actually quite uncommon.
- People should be given information and details about the extent of the disaster to enable them to take appropriate action, in contrast to the long-held belief of health workers that people will panic if they "know too much."
- Involve the entire community in the planning process, not just officials and emergency personnel.
- Such inclusion limits confusion about who does what and where the lines of authority are.
- Use routine working methods and procedures in the disaster plan, which will eliminate the need to learn new procedures and prevent confusion at the disaster site.
- Disaster plans should be flexible.
- Roles and responsibilities of team members should be identified by position or title, not by names of individuals, to avoid having to revise the plan when people change positions.

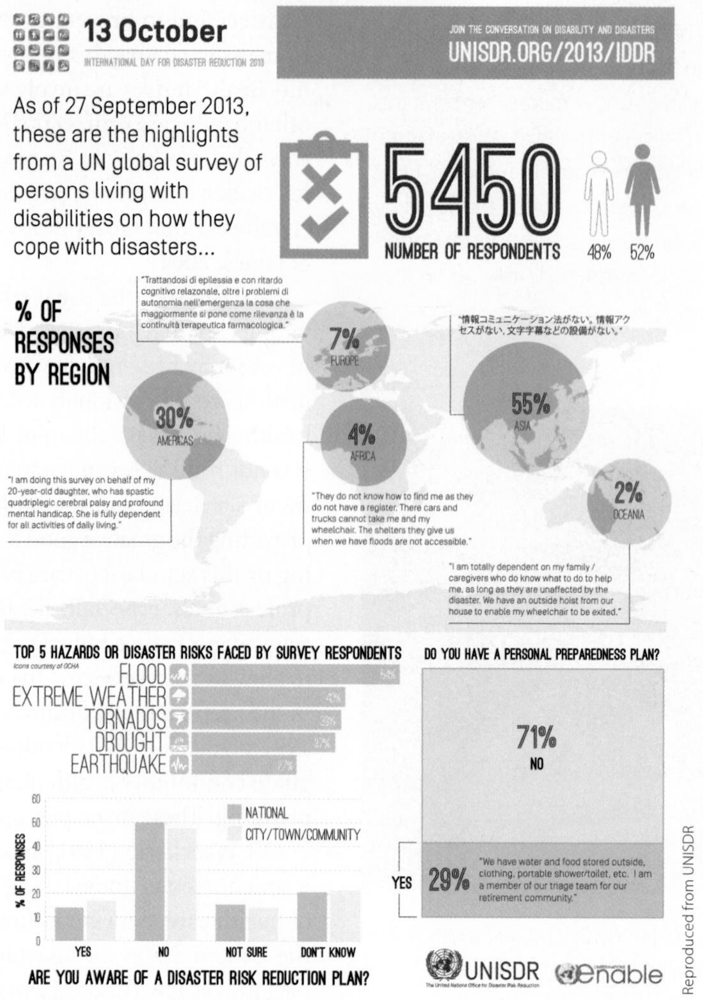

Figure 19-3

federal officials, communities are often on their own and must rely on local officials and volunteers to do much of the work when organizing a disaster plan and evaluating its validity through mock disaster drills (Gospodinov & Burnham, 2008).

Since the 2001 anthrax attacks on U.S. mail facilities and the emergence of the threat of smallpox bioterrorism, disaster plans must include much more detail on protocols for managing communicable diseases and chemical agents, most of which current healthcare professionals have never seen. Bioterrorism, germ warfare, and disaster/bioterrorism preparation have become common terms on news shows and in the vocabulary of the American public since September 11, 2001 (Porche, 2002). As the terrorist attacks in which anthrax spores were distributed through the U.S. Postal Service demonstrated, these threats are a means to produce fear and could potentially target unsuspecting individuals, but most citizens are unclear as to how to protect themselves. In addition to being prepared and educated about bioterrorist agents such as anthrax and smallpox, disaster planners need to prepare for even rarer infectious diseases that could be used in bioterrorism, such as *Brucellosis,* plague, tularemia, Q fever, and botulism. Additionally, chemical agents are substances that can injure and kill through a variety of mechanisms. Choking, blood, blister, or neural agents are the ones most likely to be used in a terrorist attack, because they will cause the highest rates of morbidity and mortality (Porche, 2002; Smith, 2000).

Garrett (2000) warns that the collapse of the public health infrastructure in the United States leaves us particularly vulnerable to such epidemics. Public health is the only viable protection against epidemics, whether natural or human made, and public health is responsible in most states for disaster planning. Since the 1980s, health departments have been chronically underfunded, according to Garrett (2000; see also Colias, 2005), because of their successes in the past century at keeping children immunized, the air breathable, factories safer, and citizens better educated about self-care. Disaster plans, however, must change as threats to the public's health evolve (see **Box 19-8**).

Characteristics of Disaster Plans

Through research into past disasters and the presence or absence of disaster plans, disaster specialists have determined common characteristics of effective disaster plans (Drabek, 1986; Ingram et al., 2006; Noji, 1997; Waeckerle, 1991):

- The disaster plan is based on a realistic assessment of potential problems that can happen, such as destruction to property, materials, and utilities; impairment of communication; and geographic isolation.
- Estimates of types of injuries that would result from the disasters most likely to occur in the area and the possible destruction of health facilities and alternative agency use are included in the plan.
- The plan is brief, concise, and inclusive of all who can provide disaster aid.
- The plan is organized by a timeline; it details the stages of a disaster, who must be involved, what must occur, and how each stage unfolds throughout the disaster process.
- The plan is approved by all agencies that provide authority endorsement, as well as sanctioned by those who have the most power to see that the plan is updated periodically and carried out when disaster strikes.
- The plan is regularly tested through mock drills and revised based on drill results.
- The plan is always considered a work in progress because needs and resources in a community relative to disaster preparedness change constantly.

NOTE THIS!

Online Resources for Disaster Preparedness

Pets and Disaster: Get Prepared

Developed with the Humane Society of the United States, this American Red Cross resource provides recommendations and specific suggestions on having a pet disaster plan: pet disaster supplies, what to do when a disaster threatens, and alternatives when pets are not allowed in shelters. For more information, visit http://www.redcross.org/prepare/disaster/pet-safety

Disaster Preparedness for People with Disabilities

This 46-page booklet is designed for use by anyone who has a disability or who works with, lives with, or assists a person with a disability. It has information on possible disaster effects, assessing personal needs and abilities, suggestions about forming a personal support network, and fill-in-the-blank checklists.

For more information, visit http://www.disastersrus.org/mydisasters/disability/disability.pdf

Facing Fear: Helping Young People Deal with Terrorism and Tragic Events

This curriculum supplement for teachers will help deal with children's concerns, fears, anger, and feelings when human-caused events occur. It is aligned with national standards in social studies, health, and language arts and available in four complete sets for teachers of grades K–2, 3–5, 6–8, and 9–12.

Terrorism: Preparing for the Unexpected

This is a brochure for the general public providing information about how to prepare for disasters of any type. It includes fundamental family disaster preparedness tips, what to do when disaster strikes, instructions on how to shelter in place and evacuation, and an abbreviated first aid primer.

For more information, visit http://www.redcross.org/images/MEDIA_CustomProductCatalog/m4440084_Terrorism.pdf

Your Family Disaster Plan

This 4-page brochure describes four steps to disaster safety—finding out what can happen, planning, preparing, and practicing.

For more information, visit http://www.fema.gov/pdf/library/yfdp.pdf

THINK ABOUT THIS 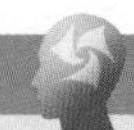

Children and Disasters: Protecting Our Future

How to teach children about disasters and their role in saving lives and livelihoods: An online game

The secretariat of the UN International Strategy for Disaster Reduction has created an online game aimed at teaching children how to build safer villages and cities against disasters. This initiative comes within the 2006–2007 World Disaster Reduction Campaign "Disaster Risk Reduction Begins at School." To access the game, go to www.stopdisastersgame.org

Common Elements of Disaster Plans

Although disaster plans should be targeted for the specific community, certain components should be included in all disaster plans. Each component may have more or less elaboration, detail, and specifics according to the needs of the community to which it applies. These components consist of authority; communication; supplies; equipment; human resources (health professionals, both acute and public health); emergency and disaster specialists; officials of government and voluntary agencies; engineers; weather specialists; community leaders, both lay and official; team coordination; transportation; documentation; record keeping; evacuation;

rescue; acute care; supportive care; recovery; and evaluation. Details of these components are summarized in Box 19-8.

Disaster Management

The goal of disaster management is to prevent or minimize death, injury, suffering, and destruction (Taggert, 1982). Disaster management by nature is an interdisciplinary, collaborative team effort (Sullivan, 1998); however, community health nurses are integral in planning for and responding to disasters. Specific community officials, such as those in civil defense, usually coordinate disaster management.

Once the civil defense efforts are begun, individuals overseeing these agencies carry out coordination of the many networks in the community disaster infrastructure. Some examples include the mayor, chief executive officer(s) of the local hospital(s), executive officer of the local American Red Cross chapter, the emergency medical system manager, and the emergency/triage physicians and nurses. Other agencies or resources and staff persons who make up the disaster team include local, state, and federal disaster management agencies; private relief organizations, such as churches and the Salvation Army; fire and police departments; political leaders who function under the mayor's administration; engineers, geologists, and meteorologists; sociologists, epidemiologists, and other researchers; community volunteers; and the media, including television news reporters, cable weather broadcasters, and radio communication persons (e.g., shortwave radio, HAM radio).

ETHICAL CONNECTION 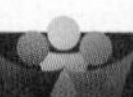

After the greatest natural disaster in American history, the U.S. government was often accused of being too slow in its response to the plight of abandoned residents in New Orleans after Hurricane Katrina in 2005. Often referred to as "an epic failure of the imagination," did the federal government, specifically FEMA, fulfill its mission, "to lead America to prepare for, prevent, respond to, and recover from disasters with a vision of 'A Nation Prepared'" to protect U.S. residents after disasters?

Disaster Response

Disaster response is a complex plan that is sometimes difficult to coordinate and carry out. All healthcare and other personnel should become knowledgeable about the disaster plan and their anticipated roles. As pointed out previously, regularly evaluating the performance of all involved personnel through mock disaster drills is an important function of community health nurses and other personnel involved in coordinating disaster response (Dixon, 1986; Neff & Kidd, 1993).

BOX 19-8 Common Elements of a Disaster Plan

- **Authority:** Issues warnings and official responses and is the central authority for disaster declarations and delegation
- **Communication:** Warnings to public and how communicated, whether by weather sirens, television, radio, police loudspeakers; includes chain of notification, rumor control, and restriction and access to the press in the disaster area
- **Equipment and supplies:** Sources and where located, usual and special needs, staging areas, and controlled access to supplies; dissemination of donated food, clothing, and storage
- **Human resources:** Health professionals, both acute and public health; emergency and disaster specialists; utility officials; officials of government and voluntary agencies; engineers; weather specialists; community leaders, both lay and official
- **Team coordination:** Central operations, staging area, chain of command
- **Transportation:** Traffic control, access and escape routes, control of risk to victims and rescuers related to transportation
- **Documentation:** Details of disaster plan, how and where disseminated; procedures for managing records of injuries, deaths, supplies, and agency reporting responsibilities; development of brief forms with minimal duplication
- **Evacuation:** Logistics and procedures, destiny of evacuees, and routes of escape
- **Rescue:** Search-and-rescue operations; details the removal of victims and immediate first aid, who is responsible, and what equipment is needed
- **Acute care:** Casualty collection points, triage, and detailed role descriptions of healthcare workers for immediate emergency care
- **Supportive care:** Shelter management
- **Recovery:** Postdisaster team meeting, debriefing, critical incident stress debriefing, press conferences, and reports to media
- **Evaluation:** Mock disaster drills and revision of disaster plan based on results

Response and Recovery

The disaster team's **response** is initiated during and after the impact stage of the disaster. Local, state, regional, national, federal, and volunteer agencies assist communities in need (FEMA, 2006). **Recovery** is a long-term process that occurs during the rehabilitation stage of the disaster. Sometimes, severe financial strain is placed on the local or state government during this time.

Levels of Disaster Response

Disasters are usually defined in terms of severity and levels of response required. Neff and Kidd (1993) identified four levels of disaster response, which are explained in the following paragraphs.

A **level I response** is limited to emergencies that require medical resources from the local hospital and community, such as minor injuries incurred in a local disaster, but also may include severe injuries incurred in multicar accidents or a plane crash. Occasionally, level I responses may include state and federal agency involvement (Neff & Kidd, 1993). In general, hospital and community resources are adequate to provide field and hospital triage, medical treatment, and stabilization for multiple casualties.

All hospitals maintain a written disaster plan that corresponds to the local civil defense and community disaster plan. Fundamental to all written level I hospital disaster plans is the assurance that a command post and chain of command will be established. Usually, the chief executive officer or a senior administrator of the hospital will be in command. Communication via telephones, cellular systems, and portable radios is limited to the commander, security, and other authorized personnel. Water conservation and backup generators are important considerations just in case they are needed. A smooth flow of patients depends on an efficient triage system in the field and within the hospital.

A **level II response** involves multiple casualties that require the use of multijurisdiction healthcare personnel and medical facilities across a specified region (Auf der Heide, 1989; Neff & Kidd, 1993). When more than one geographic jurisdiction is involved or required, the chain of command structure becomes unified for the sake of clarity, information flow, and minimization of duplications. Coordination and communication efforts among the agencies are emphasized at this response level.

When a mass-casualty disaster occurs, a **level III response** is required (Auf der Heide, 1989; Neff & Kidd, 1993). This level of disaster, such as occurred with Hurricane Andrew in South Florida in 1992 and the attacks on the World Trade Center and Pentagon in 2001, is so overwhelming that medical resources at the local and regional levels are exhausted. Consequently, state and federal agencies intervene.

A **level IV response** occurs when FEMA intervenes by providing financial and oversight assistance. FEMA is an independent agency that reports to the president of the United States. Level IV response efforts sometimes require an executive order from the president to declare the disaster a major disaster. (The presidential response to FEMA was discussed in the section "Disaster Planning.") From 1953 to early 2007, 1,688 disasters (an average of 30 per year) were declared by the president of the United States as level IV disasters (FEMA, 2011).

National Disaster Medical System

The **National Disaster Medical System (NDMS)** is a federally coordinated system that augments the United States' medical response capability. The overall purpose of the NDMS is to establish a single, integrated national medical response capability for assisting state and local authorities in dealing with the medical impacts of major peacetime disasters and to provide support to the military and the Department of Veterans Affairs medical systems in caring for casualties evacuated back to the United States from overseas armed conventional conflicts. The NDMS's efforts, such as recommendations and guidelines for disaster planning and response, filter down to state and local governments and officials, such as the civil defense office and the emergency medical services in the community (NDMS, 2006).

The National Response Plan utilizes the NDMS as part of the U.S. Department of Health and Human Services, Office of Preparedness and Response, under Emergency Support Function #8 (ESF #8), Health and Medical Care, to support federal agencies in the management and coordination of the federal medical response to major emergencies and federally declared disasters. These events may include any of the following situations.

- Natural disasters
- Technological disasters
- Major transportation accidents
- Acts of terrorism including weapons of mass destruction events

Nurses are involved at every level of the NDMS. Some of the functions of community health and other nurses include serving on the NDMS's national-level task force and board; decision making regarding guidelines and policies; disaster planning at the state and local levels; collaborating with other disaster team members on plans, procedures, and tasks; coordinating the disaster team at various locations within the community; triaging victims at community and hospital locations; and managing the care of victims.

ENVIRONMENTAL CONNECTION

New Orleans Residents and "Katrina Cough": Respiratory Problems After the Disaster

People returning to New Orleans and other flood-ravaged areas in 2005 exhibited a constellation of symptoms—coughs, sore throats, runny noses, and respiratory trouble—that health officials have named the "Katrina cough." The CDC attributes it mainly to the mold and contaminated dust left behind by the floodwaters that have been stirred up by cleanup and demolition work.

Although "Katrina cough" has not been associated with significant negative effects for the general population in New Orleans, it can be serious for people with asthma, respiratory illness, or compromised immune systems. In previous research studies of New York City residents in the aftermath of 9/11, early symptoms like coughs can exacerbate chronic health problems among people who are not protected from ongoing hazards. If Katrina cough follows the 9/11 pattern, more people are likely to become sick years after the disaster incident.

Following 9/11, numerous research studies have found that residents and workers at Ground Zero were exposed to asbestos, lead, glass fibers, concrete dust, and other toxins. The damage was caused not by a few days of rescue work, but by weeks and months of cleaning up the site or living nearby.

The aftermath of Katrina differs from 9/11 in the specific toxins that have been released into the environment. Residents who returned to their homes in New Orleans following Katrina were exposed to petroleum products, arsenic, lead, mercury, bacteria, and rampant mold. More than 16% of New Orleans children suffered from asthma, for example, according to the American Lung Association. They are at particularly high risk in mold-infested houses.

Although the U.S. Environmental Protection Agency (EPA) recommended that people who were involved in repairing homes in the post-Katrina New Orleans area wear protective equipment, like respirators, many were unable to purchase such equipment. Few retail businesses were open during the first 6 months following the disaster, which resulted in a severe shortage of the needed respirator mask model, called an N95, which filters about 95% of particulate matter and costs about $20 for a box of 20. Painters' masks offer no protection and can actually be worse than no mask at all because the material traps the debris inside the mask.

Links between post-disaster exposure, cancer rates, and other serious illnesses will not be known for years regarding exposed populations after 9/11 and Hurricane Katrina.

Sources: Schaffer, A. (2005). Katrina cough: The health problems of 9/11 are back. *Slate*. Retrieved from http://www.slate.com/articles/health_and_science/medical_examiner/2005/11/katrina_cough.html; EMS wire service. (2006, January). "Katrina cough" besets residents. *Emergency Medical Services, 35*(1), 16.

RESEARCH ALERT

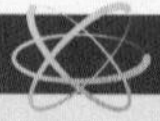

The Journal of Homeland Security and Emergency Management (*JHSEM*) was created to meet the needs of emerging issues on public health and disaster management. The journal features articles and important research on public health in the context of homeland security and emergency management. Issues have featured topics on diverse subjects, such as the effects of mass public outbreaks (e.g., pandemic flu and SARS) and secondary disasters, such as the flooding of New Orleans. By bridging health issues and homeland security and emergency management, *JHSEM* offers a forum where various fields can find common ground.

Source: The Journal of Homeland Security and Emergency Management (JHSEM).
Available online at http://www.bepress.com/jhsem

NOTE THIS!

Top U.S. States for Federal Declaration of Disaster

Texas	Alabama
California	Kentucky
Florida	Pennsylvania
New York	Ohio
Louisiana	Mississippi
Oklahoma	

Source: http://www.fema.gov/news/disaster_totals_annual.fema

Other Disaster Agencies

American and International Red Cross Disaster Services

The ARC is a humanitarian organization led by volunteers and guided by the Congressional Charter and the Fundamental Principles of the International Red Cross Movement (ARC, 2008). The ARC provides relief to victims of disasters and helps people prevent, prepare for, and respond to emergencies.

On May 21, 1881, Clara Barton and a group of her friends founded the ARC because of her commitment to and hard work with the mass casualties of yellow fever, dysentery, and many other infections during the Spanish–American War (ARC, 1990; Frantz, 1998). In gratitude for the efforts of the Red Cross nurses during the Spanish–American War, Cuba communicated the committed efforts of Clara Barton to important officials. A former schoolteacher and government worker from

Massachusetts, Barton was not actually a nurse. Nevertheless, her organizational skills were exceptional.

The unique contribution that Barton made to the worldwide Red Cross movement was her organization of volunteers to help disaster victims (ARC, 1990). America became the 32nd nation to support the Red Cross international treaty at the Geneva Convention in 1882. In 1900, the U.S. Congress granted the ARC its charter. The Red Cross nurses of the Spanish–American War were also responsible for the Congressional decision of 1901 to establish the Army Nurse Corps.

The ARC is composed of more than 1.2 million adult and youth volunteers. Many nurses are considered disaster volunteers. Community health nurses, for example, should take a voluntary leadership role in the ARC's disaster preparedness, response, and shelter management. Increasingly, ARC volunteers are being trained for technological disasters, such as those involving toxic chemicals, explosive materials, radiation, bioterrorism, and chemicals.

Salvation Army

William Booth founded the Salvation Army in London in 1865 (Salvation Army, 2014). The Salvation Army was founded on Christian principles. The Salvation Army Act of 1980 described this organization's mission as "the advancement of Christian religion … of education, the relief of poverty, and other charitable objects beneficial to society of the community of humanity as a whole" (Salvation Army, 2014).

During a disaster, the Salvation Army provides food, water, shelter, and clothing and helps trace families. With the goal of carrying out God's mission, Salvationists reach out to suffering and needy people by providing the word of God and basic human physical needs (Salvation Army, 2014).

New Nationwide Student Nurse Disaster Response Course

For more than 50 years, nursing students have been involved in helping the ARC deliver critical community services. Volunteering with the ARC is relevant to learning nursing skills and can lead to a lifelong opportunity for service.

Starting in January 2012, nursing programs across the nation became able to access a blended learning course, American Red Cross Disaster Health and Sheltering. This two-part, 4-hour awareness course introduces nursing students to how they could help in a disaster response and involves a tabletop exercise facilitated in the classroom by the nursing program instructor and a Red Cross nurse. Find out more about the course registration by contacting the local ARC chapter.

The ARC partners with nursing faculty to help students develop basic leadership skills; provide meaningful services; and help prepare for, prevent, and respond to emergencies (ARC, 2014). Some of the opportunities for nursing student involvement are described in "Helping Where It Counts" (ARC, 2010a) and "Make a Difference: Guidelines for Nursing Student Involvement in the American Red Cross" (ARC, 2010b).

Evacuation

Community health nurses, among many other healthcare personnel, need to realize that wild panic reactions are different from fleeing from a threat (Auf der Heide, 1989; Weeks, 2007). Mileti, Drabek, and Haas (1975) have noted that panic might occur but usually arises only when at least one of three conditions is present: (1) a perception of immediate danger, (2) an encounter with blocked escape routes, and/or (3) a feeling of being isolated. When panic occurs, it is usually of short duration and not contagious, depending on the response from the media (Auf der Heide, 1989).

ENVIRONMENTAL CONNECTION

What can we do to evacuate large numbers of people in advance of a major natural disaster?

After Hurricane Katrina, one of the primary problems cited by planning commissions was the inability to evacuate vulnerable populations. One of the solutions proposed by the state of Mississippi is the use of school buses and cafeterias. What solutions other than these might make mass evacuation more effective and save lives in natural disasters?

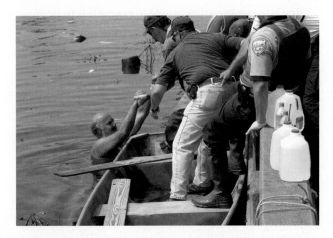

Hurricane Katrina created massive flooding after the storm when the levees failed. Residents were trapped in their homes or left alone in the water; many suffered and died as a result of the rising waters.

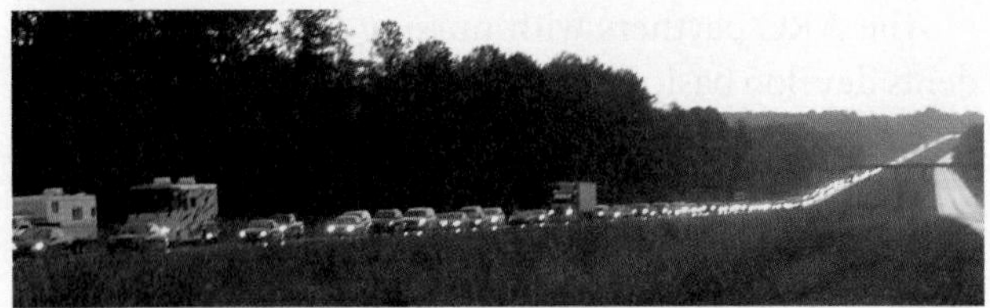

Disaster planning includes the rapid evacuation of large populations via U.S. interstate highways.

Evacuation traditionally has been a difficult task to carry out because of people's reluctance to evacuate (Langan & James, 2004; Quarantelli & Dynes, 1972; Wenger, James, & Faupel, 1985). There are several explanations for this reluctance. The primary reason for hesitancy is that some people do not believe that they are in danger. Another reason is that some people want to remain at the site to protect their property. Not wanting to evacuate until the family can be removed as a unit is another reason for hesitancy. The head of the household or another member may refuse to leave until other family members, who may also include dogs or other pets, are safe (Landesman, 2005; Saunders, 2007).

Besides demonstrating concern for human lives, FEMA is concerned for the lives of animals and, more specifically, the human–animal bond (FEMA, 2011; Lockwood, 1997; Rosenkoetter et al., 2007). Many people have developed close relationships with their pets. Lockwood (1997) has explored why animal owners will risk danger to themselves and not evacuate disaster areas without assurance of their animals' wellbeing; the most common responses are that people love their animals and treat them as part of the family. ARC shelters now include pet-friendly services for residents with pets.

The key to motivating people to evacuate is to improve warning effectiveness, which relies on several strategies (Auf der Heide, 1989; Rosenkoetter et al., 2007; Saunders, 2007). The credibility of the present warning and the validity of past evacuation warnings, for example, both influence a person's decision about whether to evacuate. Consistency and repetition of the warning by different sources of the evacuation command always increase the chance that a person will heed the warning. Commands to evacuate by agency and community officials are taken more seriously, which promotes the believability of the message. A clear, specific message to evacuate that is understood will yield better results. Finally, an effective strategy is to ensure a full range of protective actions, such as ample law enforcement officers on duty, for those people evacuating.

A significant problem in the evacuation of New Orleans residents prior to and during Hurricane Katrina was rooted in the Louisiana State Evacuation Plan. The plan left the means of evacuation up to individual citizens, parish governments, and private caretakers. Unfortunately, many private caretaking facilities relied on the same bus companies and ambulance services for evacuation and so were unable to function for this purpose. Fuel and rental cars were in short supply, and most forms of public transportation had been shut down well before the storm struck (Balinsky, 2003; Gospodinov & Burnham, 2008; Hayes, 2005; Kiewra, 2006; U.S. Congress, 2006).

Role of the Media

The mass media can be either a friend or a foe in the management of disasters (Dwyer & Drew, 2005; U.S. Congress, 2006). To enhance disaster response, the media can provide accurate information, convey instructions to the public, and stimulate donations from parts of the country not affected by the disaster. Conversely, the media may complicate the operations by putting a "feeding frenzy" spin on the facts (Haygood & Tyson, 2005). Reporters may make unreasonable demands on resources, facilities, and officials (Auf der Heide, 1989). Distortion of the facts, overreaction, and perpetuation of disaster myths are other factors that may interfere with the disaster response operations (Haygood & Tyson, 2005). For example, during the Hurricane Katrina disaster, rampant rumors about looting, homicides, mass uprisings, and deaths in the New Orleans Superdome proved to be unfounded, yet they dramatically affected both the communities experiencing the disaster and the general public's perceptions about the disaster.

MEDIA MOMENT

When the Levees Broke: A Requiem in Four Acts (2007)

Spike Lee commemorates the people of New Orleans with a 4-hour epic documentary about the destruction of the city of New Orleans from Hurricane Katrina and ill-fated disaster relief efforts. Lee doesn't just recount the events of late August 2005, but rather asks *why* they unfolded the way they did. Weaving interviews with news footage and amateur video, Lee uses the film to give meaningful voice to the people who were left behind. With a detached, unsentimental eye, he delivers a poignant account of a major moment in recent U.S. history. While offering no simple answers, you will be left with even more questions, such as "How could this unprecedented disaster involving a major U.S. city have happened in the United States?"

Good communication is vital during the evacuation operations (Yellowlees & MacKenzie, 2003). The Weather Bureau, social media, radio stations, television announcements, local sirens and announcements, and computers should be used to alert the public of the impending threat. Another key medium is the Emergency Broadcast System, which officials use to provide local, state, or national information and warnings. When the evacuation is in process, a large volume of requests place overwhelming demands on the media as well as on public officials of the city and county. One of the major findings of the 2006 U.S. Congress report on Hurricane Katrina, entitled *A Failure of Initiative: Final Report of the Select Bipartisan Committee to Investigate the Preparation for and Response to Hurricane Katrina,* was that critical problems in rescue efforts were related to communication technology breakdown, such as the destruction of cellular and relay towers, radio and television station destruction, and a lack of alternatives with such failure.

Rescue

The search-and-rescue mission is the most challenging part of disaster operations (Hayes, 2005; Saunders, 2007; Silverstein, 1984; Waeckerle, 1983, 1991). Searching for and rescuing disaster victims tax the physical capabilities and emotions of rescuers. Emotional demands can also be extremely traumatic to the rescuers, who may require psychosocial debriefing (Rhoads et al., 2006). Teams of healthcare personnel, fire and security officials, and volunteers comb the designated area many times in search of casualties. Once the casualties are located, quick triage actions are necessary. After the victims are categorized by way of triage, rescue workers need to continue to search the area for undiscovered injured people or dead bodies.

Triage

The triage system normally practiced in emergency departments across the country is not the same triage system used during a disaster (Kitt, Selfridge-Thomas, Proehl, & Kaiser, 1995; Waltham, 2005). Field (disaster) triage is used when mass casualties result from disaster. The initial triage that takes place in the field is called the primary triage. Secondary triage occurs at the point of entry into the medical facility. Tertiary triage occurs in the specified area where the patient is located, such as the emergency department, pediatrics, and so on. Home health agencies and community-based residential agencies also mandate the triage process in order to evacuate and manage these vulnerable populations.

Disaster triage allows healthcare personnel to identify the most salvageable patients so that treatment can be initiated immediately. Colored tags with symbols are attached to disaster victims so that healthcare personnel (Gospodinov & Burnham, 2008) can readily see level of triage (Kitt et al., 1995).

Several factors may affect the triage system (Dixon, 1986), such as the patient's general state of health. For example, an elderly person may have a poor cardiovascular status, which may decrease the person's survival expectation.

Another factor that may affect the outcome of triage is the healthcare worker's experience (or lack thereof) in triage and assessment. Lack of supplies or equipment is another factor. Not having proper supplies and equipment in sufficient quantities can adversely influence the disaster victim's triage status (Balinsky, 2003; Langan & James, 2004; Neff & Kidd, 1993; Weeks, 2007).

Disaster Shelters

Trained volunteers and/or ARC nurses manage shelters. When help is needed, the executive director of the affected local chapter of the ARC calls upon nurses and other volunteers. Shelters are opened by volunteers in the community through coordinated efforts of the ARC, the mayor, civil defense, and other officials of the community. Churches, schools, civic centers, and community centers may all be used as shelters.

APPLICATION TO PRACTICE 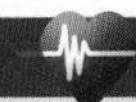

Thinking Critically . . . an Ethical and Management Nightmare from "Ground Zero" During Hurricane Katrina

Imagine you are the top nurse administrator at a large mental hospital in New Orleans after Hurricane Katrina hit. All hospitals in the metro area have evacuated and closed, with only your hospital remaining open. Nurses are having difficulty deciding which patients to care for, with a severe shortage of nurses and hundreds of patients pouring into the emergency department needing hospitalization. As a mental health facility, you do not have the resources for medical problems. Nurses are having ethical conflict over making decisions about which patients should be transferred via FEMA airlifts. They fear that their patients will be more at risk due to their fragile mental state if transferred. Food and water begin to run out after 2 days, and the morgue cannot take any more bodies. Rationing of basic supplies, food, and water has begun. Ice has run out and water from the flood remains in the halls and most patient rooms. A local television station is broadcasting from the hospital emergency department and has requested to enter the hospital for patient and nurse interviews. What actions should you take? Can you ask the station to stop broadcasting? Can you force them to do so? List the things that would be priority for you as nurse manager?

It is sometimes difficult to determine or anticipate shelter needs during disasters. The local ARC chapter depends on other ARC chapters, the mayor, and civil defense teams to report anticipated numbers of persons who are evacuating their premises and reporting to a shelter. In widespread disasters, shelters are opened in a number of areas that house local residents as well as victims who have traveled a long distance to escape more immediate danger. An example of a widespread disaster was Hurricane Camille in 1969, which traveled from the Mississippi Gulf Coast to North Mississippi and beyond. Persons in the most danger were on the Mississippi Gulf Coast, so they evacuated to cities and towns north of the coast, while the local residents of those areas also were evacuating their premises and relocating to the same shelters. In such instances, anticipating the correct number of shelter residents is difficult.

By the time Hurricane Katrina hit in 2005, 26 years later, ARC officials were better able to plan the evacuation route and anticipate how and when evacuees would most likely relocate. Even with mock disaster drills and extensive planning for facilitating disaster shelter triage of residents, the extensiveness of the affected disaster area (over many miles) meant that the system was ill prepared to handle the number and risk level of the evacuees from the New Orleans area (Nigg et al., 2006).

Good communication between city officials and remote areas regarding evacuation numbers must be a priority prior to the disaster, because communication is often hampered by the destruction of electricity, phone lines, and cell phone relay towers (Balinsky, 2003; Langan & James, 2004; Weeks, 2007). For each shelter, there is one team manager, at least one nurse volunteer, multiple people to keep records, and numerous volunteers trained to assist victims. Activities include keeping thorough records; coordinating meals; providing snacks, cots, blankets, and other essentials; providing health care, such as first-aid treatment and over-the-counter medications that have been authorized by a physician; acting as a liaison between victims and resource agencies and their families; and protecting the victims from harm by keeping alert to possible fire outbreaks, accidents, and other mishaps. When help is needed, the ARC coordinates mass recruitment of supplies, equipment, food, and shelter. For example, after the summer Midwest floods in 1993, Wal-Mart loaned the ARC a large warehouse, forklifts, and staff to expedite distribution of urgently needed supplies to the shelters (ARC, 1995). Other retail stores and pharmaceutical companies offered many supplies and a large amount of monetary assistance.

NOTE THIS!

Hurricane Camille

Hurricane Camille was a category 5 hurricane that hit the coasts of Mississippi, Alabama, and Louisiana with winds in excess of 200 mph. Hurricane Camille resulted in the deaths of 141 persons, 9,472 injuries, property loss and damage for 74,000 families, and more than $1 billion total damage. At the 30-year anniversary of the storm, the scars and influence of Camille still exist on the Mississippi Gulf Coast, where the most severe damage occurred. The storm produced 19-foot tidal waves in August 1969 and remains one of the deadliest storms of the 20th century.

Comments from Survivors

"Afterwards, it looked like we had been bombed. My house was 'caddy whompas' on its foundation. All you could hear were helicopters and people crying. It was the most horrible experience I have ever had."

"The thing that I remember were the dead cows on the beach."

"The beach looked like a holocaust. A woman slipping and sliding through mud and muck clutching a lifeless child to her chest."

Source: Hattiesburg American, August 14, 1994, p. 7A.

Role of the Community Health Nurse in Disasters

Why should community health nurses be involved in disasters? Aren't trauma and hospital nurses better qualified to work in disasters than nurses in the community? These are good questions—ones that many student nurses and practicing nurses alike may ask. Our ideas about disasters, including what happens and who is involved—both victims and rescuers—are often shaped by the media. The disaster movie formula developed as a major box office draw in the 1970s with such movies as the *Airport* series about jet liner crashes; *The Towering Inferno* (1974), about a burning skyscraper; *The Hindenburg* (1975), about the real-life zeppelin airship disaster of 1937; and *The China Syndrome* (1979), about a fictitious nuclear power plant accident, which became an eerie prelude to the actual Three Mile Island nuclear accident that same year. This trend in film has continued over the years, and U.S. and international moviegoers have been fascinated by disasters and continue to line up for movies such as *Armageddon* (1998), *Deep Impact* (1998), *The Day After Tomorrow* (2004), *Independence Day* (1996), and *Titanic* (1997), which became the highest grossing movie of all time (until 2009).

These movies, as well as television programs such as *Grey's Anatomy,* portray disasters as a backdrop for story lines and romances, heroes and villains, and greatly influence the way we visualize disasters. As a result, disaster planning and disaster preparedness are given very little attention. In truth, the most recent terrorist attacks on the World Trade Center and the Pentagon provided more specific details about actual recovery and effects of aftermath for the public through extensive media coverage. At least temporarily, the American public appears to be more aware about the need for preparedness for disaster.

Community health nurses are much better prepared than most other healthcare professionals are to manage disasters in the community, because emergency treatment and triage are but two of many activities that help people cope with disaster. Successful strategies often pair a community health nurse with a trauma nurse in the disaster setting. Among the major determinants of how effectively a disaster is managed are not only how well we carry out our individual roles in a disaster, but also how well we allow others to carry out their roles (Suserud & Haljamae, 1997; Weeks, 2007).

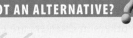

THINK ABOUT THIS

What would you do in a terrorist biological attack?

Assume you are a nurse administrator responsible for a large urban hospital when a biological terrorist attack occurs in your city. What precautions would you need to take? Think about things like quarantining patients, protecting the staff, decontaminating rooms and equipment, obtaining and securing antidotes, and monitoring the spread of disease. Do you think the same techniques would be applicable in a chemical or nuclear attack? What additional actions would you take in these circumstances?

GOT AN ALTERNATIVE?

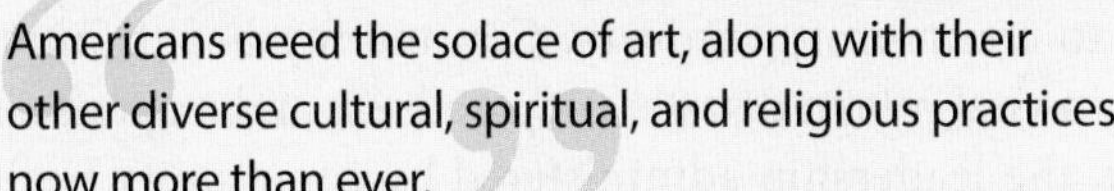

Americans need the solace of art, along with their other diverse cultural, spiritual, and religious practices, now more than ever.

—*Karen VanMeenen*

The Role of Art in Healing After the 9/11 Disaster

Art is created and viewed for pleasure, for distraction, to tell stories, to emote, for documentation purposes, as an educational tool, to channel creative energies, for the processing of personal experience and for healing. Artists have always responded to personal and political challenges with their own outpourings of creative practice—documenting their illnesses, celebrating their survival, working through their difficulties, calling for change. Artists and health professionals have long known the beneficial effects of creating and viewing artwork on an individual and a communal level (e.g., the success of the AIDS Quilt). Art can tell personal truths as well as allow viewers access to universal truths, universal experience.

Source: Van Meenen, K. (2001, November/December). Media art AS/IN therapy [special issue]. *Afterimage, 29*(3).

RESEARCH ALERT

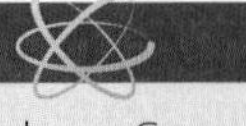

Emergency Preparedness Competencies for Public Health Nurses with Disaster Prevention: A Position Paper of the Association of State and Territorial Directors of Nursing

The Association of State and Territorial Directors of Nursing vision for emergency preparedness is that every community, family, and individual will have a comprehensive emergency preparedness plan that minimizes the consequences of disasters and emergencies and enables communities, families, and individuals to respond and recover. This position paper provides national and state policy guidance during emergencies to all public health nurses in the United States and its territories. Public health nurses bring critical experience to each phase of a disaster: mitigation, preparedness, response, and recovery. Public health nurses strive to achieve individual competencies so that they may better collaborate with others and contribute to emergency preparedness and response. Twelve Emergency Preparedness Competencies are listed in this position paper that will assist public health nurses with disaster prevention, planning, response, recovery, drills, exercises, and training. This position paper will be useful in clarifying the expertise that public health nurses can contribute to teams that serve to protect the health and safety of communities against disaster threats and realities.

Source: Jakeway, C. C., LaRosa, G., Cary, A., & Schoenfisch, S. (2008). The role of public health nurses in emergency preparedness and response: A position paper of the Association of State and Territorial Directors of Nursing. *Public Health Nursing, 25*(4), 353–361.

General Functions of the Community Health Nurse

Community health nurses, as well as other nurses, are involved in emergency treatment and triage during the impact stage of the disaster. Good physical assessment skills are vital for success. Only healthcare personnel highly skilled in assessment should perform the triage function. Most healthcare personnel are not trained in advanced assessment skills and cannot make acuity judgments proficiently.

Nursing is specialized, as are most health professions. As a result, community health nurses often are more knowledgeable about teamwork and interdisciplinary effort than nurses in other specialties are, because they rely on group efforts daily in community health nursing practice. Community health nurses are experts in program planning, community assessment, and group dynamics—all skills that are critical to the effective management of a disaster crisis. Because community health nurses are population focused, assessing and intervening with vulnerable populations are second nature to them.

Other functions that enable community health nurses to work effectively in disasters include working with the media to inform and educate, the use of public health interventions to minimize risks from communicable diseases, and the securing of community resources for victims. These functions are accomplished while coordinating multiagency efforts in the mediation of health risks at the disaster site. The background work of disaster management, for which community health nurses are perfectly suited, may not make it to the big screen, but such activities are what ultimately influence how well a community survives and heals from disaster.

Specific Nursing Approaches

A major goal of community health nurses is to be an asset to the community, not a burden. Specific approaches that community health nurses should take to mitigate human and material losses in a community disaster include the following strategies:

Personal preparedness:

- Be disaster-prepared and disaster-aware.
- Maintain your own emergency equipment, supplies, and skills.
- Be certain that your family knows what to do during a disaster, when to do it, who to call, and where to go.
- Use caution and prudence when selecting the location of your home.

Community involvement:

- Become familiar with local disaster plans and emergency evacuation procedures.
- Get involved in the political issues in your community that relate to disaster preparedness and recovery.
- Support leaders who choose long-term, focused solutions in loss reduction and emergency preparedness rather than those who choose shortsighted, politically expedient solutions.
- Help modify land use and develop ordinances that reflect the best knowledge of geography and water hazards.
- Support local emergency assistance organizations by serving on advisory boards.
- Assist in the education of the public in personal disaster preparedness.
- Visit schools to help prepare children for assuming the lifetime responsibility of being prepared for disasters in the community.

Professional preparedness:

- Become trained and certified in professional disaster nursing by the local ARC chapter.
- Get involved in the development of agency and community disaster plans.
- Attend continuing education classes and disaster skills updates to keep current in disaster management skills.
- Be supportive of administrative efforts to increase disaster preparedness.
- Write news stories, volunteer to speak at community meetings, write letters to the editor of local newspapers, and publish articles in nursing journals about the nursing role in disaster preparedness (Garcia, 1985; Gospodinov & Burnham, 2008).

Shelter Management and Care

Roles played by healthcare workers in disasters are critical to community recovery. Community health nurses play a vital role in disaster preparedness and response. In fact, the leadership administered by community health nurses may greatly affect the public's reception and comprehension of disaster education and warnings. See the Application to Practice feature about the Oklahoma City Bombing later in this chapter for examples of successful shelter management.

Neither the public nor many nurses realize the impact that nurses have before, during, and after a disaster (Gospodinov & Burnham, 2008; Landesman, 2005). The leadership role that community health nurses can take may prevent deaths and property damage.

ARC disaster nurses and other volunteers are often trained to coordinate and manage shelters, conduct tertiary triage within the shelter, and administer first aid to sick or wounded people. Currently, the ARC has a pool of more than 15,000 trained disaster volunteers, many of whom are nurses (ARC, 2006). With Hurricane Katrina, the number of disaster-trained nurses proved inadequate, and the ARC sought all RNs who could assist with the overwhelming number of shelters that were opened in the disaster area. These nurses were trained "on the spot" and were often asked to be on duty for much longer times owing to the magnitude of the disaster. Additionally, because of the large numbers of persons left homeless by Katrina, shelters in many areas remained open for months after the disaster.

DAY IN THE LIFE

Toni D. Frioux

Because of the tremendous response from caring volunteers at the Oklahoma City bombing disaster, the first critical step was to establish a centralized system to manage the number of individuals calling to report to the emergency site. Once established, we were able to schedule, validate licenses, and orient volunteers from the Oklahoma State Medical Association, Oklahoma Nurses Association, American Red Cross, hospitals, and other entities to the expectations and limitations of the bomb site.

There was tremendous generosity from everyone. Medical supplies, equipment, and medication were immediately available and continued to be delivered at the site for many days. Public health was responsible for centralizing and assuring that these supplies were used appropriately and responsibly by licensed providers. It was important to assure that the appropriate practice guidelines were in place.

Providing disaster services as a public health function doesn't end with just providing emergency services. Public health is also responsible for ensuring that volunteers who provide ongoing emergency health services are competent and properly licensed. It is important to be familiar with your state's nurse practice act and knowledgeable regarding any actions that might be needed to invoke licensure reciprocity in the event that the disaster is of such magnitude that volunteers arrive from other states or countries to assist.

Planning and ongoing networking with all players in the emergency response team are very important. While personnel may change, the fundamental needs in an emergency generally do not. Having a public health workforce that is prepared in disaster response is very beneficial.

Any coordination and networking that can be in place with state and local American Red Cross chapters prior to a disaster benefit both the public health agency and the American Red Cross.

—Toni D. Frioux, MS, CNS, ARNP, Chief, Nursing Service, Oklahoma State Department of Health

Volunteers are ready for immediate assignment for damage assessment, case management, and shelter management at a moment's notice. The ARC shelter manager, often a community health nurse, organizes and manages the shelter operations by fulfilling the roles of administrator, leader, and supervisor (Garcia, 1985; Saunders, 2007). The way the manager conducts operations affects the flow of operations and activities within the shelter. Functions of the manager include allocating space, obtaining supplies and equipment, scheduling staff, completing reports and records, and attending to problems. If the community health nurse volunteer happens to be the manager and the nurse on duty, the dual roles and functions can become overwhelming. Care should be coordinated by application of the nursing process. Good assessment and planning skills are among the most important functions of the community health nurse volunteer. Interventions in this setting include preventing disease and illness, providing emotional support, protecting health, and providing intermittent, temporary care to this vulnerable population. With Hurricane Katrina, residents were often displaced from their homes and family, which made the housing issue much more challenging. Many residents in these shelters did not know if they had a home to return to, nor did they know where their families were. Because of the rapid evacuation of survivors from the New Orleans and Mississippi Gulf Coast, many had nothing except the clothes on their backs, no medication, and few necessities for self-care. As in most disasters of this severity, elders, patients with chronic physical and mental problems, and children accounted for a large number of the evacuees (Garcia, 1985; Gospodinov & Burnham, 2008).

NOTE THIS!

What Is the American Red Cross?

The American Red Cross is a voluntary, nonprofit organization that responds to all disasters, regardless of size and scope. The Federal Emergency Management Agency (FEMA) is a federal agency under the Department of Homeland Security. FEMA responds when a disaster has received a presidential declaration. FEMA is involved with community recovery, such as repairing and building bridges and public buildings and assisting in security of disaster areas; ARC provides humanitarian aid to individuals. Nurses have always been a cornerstone for the provision of services by the American Red Cross. Historically, Red Cross nurses have provided their assistance during times of disaster and conflict beginning with the 1889 Johnstown flood and the 1888 yellow fever epidemic. Jane Delano formally established the Red Cross Nursing Service in 1909. Red Cross nursing has also had a major role in the historical evolution of nursing and nursing leadership in the United States with many Red Cross

(continues)

NOTE THIS! (continued)

nurses, including Jane Delano, Clara Noyes, Julia Stimson, and others playing strategic roles in the development of American nursing.

Today more than 30,000 nurses continue to be involved in paid and volunteer capacities at all levels and in all service areas throughout the American Red Cross. These activities consist of:

- Providing direct services such as local disaster action teams, health fairs, volunteering in military clinics and hospitals, blood collection teams, and first aid stations
- Teaching and developing courses in cardiopulmonary resuscitation (CPR) and first aid, automated emergency defibrillator (AED), disaster health services, nurse assistant training, babysitting, and family care giving
- Acting in management and supervisory roles including chapter and blood services region executives
- Functioning in governance roles such as local board member to national board of governors

Source: American Red Cross. (2014). *Disaster services.* Retrieved from http://www.redcross.org/services/disaster

Then and now ... perspectives on disaster

> The detection and control of saboteurs are the responsibilities of the FBI, but the recognition of epidemics caused by sabotage is particularly an epidemiologic function.... therefore any plan of defense against biological warfare sabotage requires trained epidemiologists alert to all possibilities and available for call at a moment's notice, anywhere in the country.
>
> —*Alexander Langmuir, 1952, Founder of the Centers for Disease Control and Prevention (CDC) Epidemiological Investigation Service (EIS) Program*

Anticipation of certain problems will facilitate the operations and care of the community health nurse volunteer. For instance, in the shelter population, the nurse should expect some everyday, normal occurrences, which will include chronically ill people who are dependent on medications and equipment, normal episodes of illness and infection, communicable disease, and emotional stress reactions. Evaluation of the shelter population should be ongoing, including one-on-one conferences with shelter families and staff members. In the Hurricane Katrina example, the ARC was able to use advanced technology to keep up-to-date shelter resident rosters all over the affected area, which assisted nurses in helping residents locate their families in shelters located throughout the United States.

Disaster Recovery

Toffler (1970), in his classic study *Future Shock*, described future shock as "the response to overstimulation" (p. 344). He described numerous examples of stress in situations requiring constant change; among them are persons in disasters. Toffler described persons who experienced a disaster as being trapped in environments that are rapidly changing, unfamiliar, and unpredictable. Results of such situations can be devastating, even for the most stable and well-prepared person. Victims of disasters may be hurled into anti-adaptive states and be incapable of the most elementary decision making (Toffler, 1970). Evidence of this reaction can be seen in pictures of a woman, after a destructive earthquake, strolling down a dangerous, debris-filled road with a dead or wounded baby in her arms, her face blank and numb, appearing impervious to the danger around her. Persons can be overwhelmed and become paralyzed as familiar objects and relationships are transformed. Where a person's house once stood, a tornado can within minutes change the environment into an unrecognizable pile of rubble and gushing water pipes. The Oklahoma City bombing destroyed life and property within minutes, replacing familiar landmarks with images of unimaginable horror and destruction.

Simple acts taken for granted hours before, such as making a telephone call or pouring a cup of coffee, are no longer appropriate or possible. Signs, sounds, and other psychological and cultural cues surround disaster victims without meaning, without recognition during and immediately after the impact. Every word, every action, every movement is characterized by uncertainty. Even in a crowd, victims often experience a sense of isolation and loneliness, abandonment, and an overwhelming sense of loss of the world as they know it. Confusion, disorientation, and distortion of reality occur spontaneously; fatigue, anxiety, tenseness, and extreme irritability follow. Apathy, emotional withdrawal, and pessimism result when victims develop a sense of little hope for the future or when they see themselves as never being safe or stable again (Toffler, 1970).

After a major disaster, such as Hurricane Andrew in Homestead, Florida, and Hurricane Katrina on the Mississippi Gulf Coast and New Orleans, Louisiana, healthcare facilities are often disabled or destroyed. Recovery may take years, and the community is often faced with inadequate or nonexistent health services. This is often referred to as the "disaster after the disaster"—catastrophic community changes that can hamper recovery efforts and further damage a community's health. The havoc wrought by a major disaster affects the lives of healthcare facilities' staff, patients, and the community for many years after the initial disaster.

For example, a year after Hurricane Andrew struck Homestead, Homestead Hospital had lost 70% of its employees, many of whom had worked tirelessly through the disaster. Charity care spiked from 11% of patients to 26%. The hospital went from years of profitability to an $8 million loss. Additionally, demographic shifts in the community created challenges for the hospital. Many senior citizens left the community, never to return; replacing them were young families attracted by the affordable, federally funded housing market. These demographic changes are common after a hurricane, especially in coastal areas that attract large numbers of retirees. In addition to losing Medicare dollars and adding more Medicaid-insured families, hospitals often have to completely reorganize their services to meet the needs of the post-disaster community (Colias, 2005).

NOTE THIS!

Children, Terrorism, and Disasters: Web Resources

Society's most vulnerable population, children, is at a greater risk for developing health problems as a result of terrorism and disasters. Additionally, exposure to media coverage about disasters and other catastrophic events can have adverse emotional and psychological effects for children. The American Academy of Pediatrics has an area on its website dedicated to children, terrorism, and disasters. The website helps pediatricians, parents, community leaders, and others prepare for and meet children's needs during a disaster. Examples of information available include the following:

- Family Readiness Kit: Preparing to Handle Disasters
- The Youngest Victims: Disaster Preparedness to Meet Children's Needs
- AAP resources, federal resources, and medical journal and report information on topics such as biological, chemical, and nuclear agents
- How to communicate with children in the wake of a disaster

See http://www.aap.org/terrorism

In Their Own Words: 9/11 Parents Help Other Parents and Schools with Lessons Learned

Through the constructive advice of experienced parents, this publication discusses emergency planning for schools. The events of September 11, 2001 and its aftermath have challenged health, environment, and education agencies to understand how children are different from adults in relation to environmental hazards, and how schools are different from offices in terms of their responsibilities for the occupants and the demands on the facilities.

See http://www.healthyschools.org/documents/INTHEIROWNWORDS.pdf

School Nurse Role in Bioterrorism Emergency Preparedness and Response

It is the position of the National Association of School Nurses that school nurses should be designated and recognized as first responders to mass casualty emergencies, including those resulting from bioterrorist events. School nurses should be trained in protection, detection, and treatment of victims of such events and in the command and control management techniques of the logistics of such a situation. The strategic position of well-prepared nurses within the school environment has significant potential for minimizing the effects of a bioterrorist attack in school settings and, subsequently, in the community at large.

See http://www.nasn.org/Portals/0/positions/2005psbioterrorism.pdf

How Schools Can Become More Disaster Resistant: Resources for Parents and Teachers

FEMA recommends the following actions for all school officials:

- Identify hazards likely to happen to your schools.
- Mitigate the hazards.
- Develop a response plan, including evacuation route.
- Plan for coping after a disaster.
- Implement drills and family education.

See http://www.fema.gov/kids/schdizr.htm

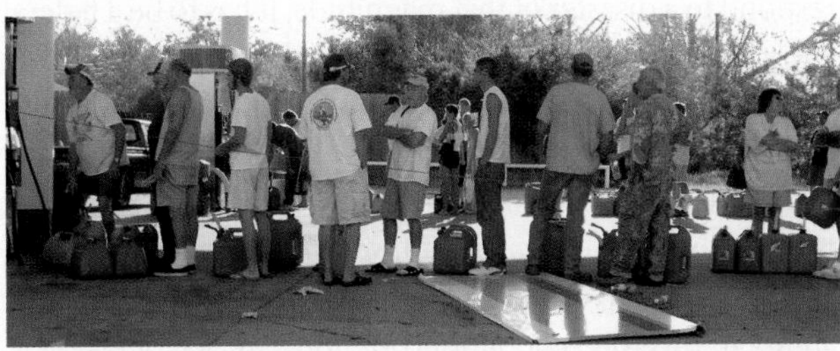

Fuel shortages often accompany major disasters and add to the stress of recovery.

NOTE THIS!

The Bush–Clinton Fund for Hurricane Katrina recovery

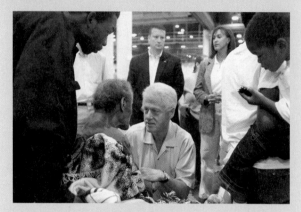

Former Presidents Bill Clinton and George H. W. Bush have paired up to raise funds for the hurricane disasters via the Bush–Clinton Katrina Fund and had raised $100 million as of 2006.

The Bush–Clinton Katrina Fund is made possible by contributions received from donors throughout the nation and the world in response to Hurricane Katrina. The fund was set up to provide grants for medium- to long-term recovery needs in the affected areas. In December 2005, Presidents George H. W. Bush and William J. Clinton allocated $20 million from the Bush–Clinton Katrina Fund (BCKF) for local and regional faith-based organizations located in the affected areas prior to Hurricane Katrina in Alabama, Louisiana, and Mississippi. The fund sought applications from religious organizations to assist in rebuilding houses of worship and to cover costs for temporary relocation. The BCKF seeks to make a distinct impact on the unmet needs of the affected region in the following areas: financial self-sufficiency, economic opportunity, and quality of life.

Hurricane Katrina was a wake-up call for hospitals throughout the Gulf Coast region, according to Brian Keeley, CEO of Baptist Health South Florida in Coral Gables, Florida. "My conclusion is that it's beyond the capability of the municipal or state government to adequately respond to a disaster of that magnitude. It has to be a federal effort, and we've seen firsthand that it takes a long time to get them in here" (cited in Colias, 2005, p. 44). Baptist Health is spending millions to ensure that all of its hospitals in the Gulf Coast area can withstand a Category 5 hurricane—that is, have diesel storage, backup water and air-conditioning systems, reinforced windows, hurricane shutters, and the ability to turn on generator power for 2 weeks.

In the classic study *Everything in Its Path,* sociologist Kai Erickson (1976) described the 1972 Buffalo Creek flood and its aftermath in terms of disaster impact and the destruction of community. This study provided a detailed and analyzed view of a disaster and the resulting conflict between individualism and dependency, self-assertion and resignation, and self-centeredness and community orientation. The results of this devastating disaster included loss of community connection, declining morality, rise in crime, and the rise in out-migration from the sudden loss of neighborhood and community. Organized disaster activity was largely provided by outsiders.

Collective deaths, like those in a disaster, do not permit persons to set up the usual barriers between the living and the dead, as is customary in the deaths of the hospital, where "death is screened from view, sanitized, muffled, tidied up" (Erickson, 1976, p. 169). In disaster, "death lies out there at its inescapable worst. There are no wreckers to rush the crushed vehicle away, no physicians to shroud death in a crisp white sheet or to give it a clean medical name, no undertakers to wash away the evidence of death and to knead out the creases of pain or fear … and the sight does not go away easily" (Erickson, 1976, p. 169).

Effects on Survivors

When death is experienced on a wide scale, such as in a disaster, survivors often experience guilt as a result of their own survival (Erickson, 1976). They may even come to regret their own survival, when others around them were killed in what seems like a meaningless and capricious way, in part because "they cannot understand by what logic they came to be spared" (p. 170). Survivor guilt has often been described in disaster research literature. Lifton (1967), in his classic study of the psychological effects of the atomic bomb in Hiroshima, found that survivors described the open eyes of corpses as evoking guilt: It was as if the eyes were saying, "Why me, why not you?"

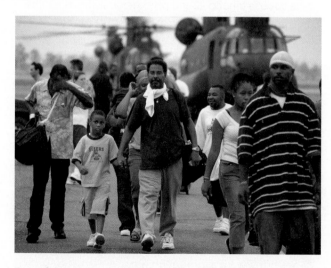

One of the consequences of a major disaster, such as Hurricane Katrina, is the challenge of keeping families together.

NOTE THIS!

Four years after 9/11, thousands of people who worked at Ground Zero or lived in lower Manhattan were still sick with respiratory problems and other illnesses because of the contaminants they were exposed to. Some did not respond to standard medications and were unable to work. The total impact on the population from these toxins will most likely remain unknown for years.

Lifton and Olson (1976) identified five major elements that may be found in some type of combination in all disasters. Psychological difficulty or maladaptive response is more likely to occur if all five elements are found in a single disaster, as in the Buffalo Creek flood. The five elements are suddenness of the event, human callousness in causation (human-made rather than natural causation), continuing relationship of survivors to the disaster, isolation of the community, and totality of destruction.

The experience of the disaster can have both short- and long-term effects on mental health and functioning, such as dissociation, depression, and PTSD (Gerrity & Flynn, 1997). Refer to Box 19-5 for other health effects associated with disasters. Meichenbaum (1994) has compiled from disaster research a list of factors that can place individuals in a vulnerable position for developing psychological problems when all five of Lifton and Olson's (1976) elements are present in a disaster:

- Objective and subjective characteristics of the disaster, such as proximity of the victim to the disaster site, the duration, the degree of physical injury, and the witnessing of grotesque, graphic scenes
- The characteristics in the community of the post-disaster response and recovery environment, such as cohesiveness of community and disruption of social support systems
- The characteristics of the individual or group—for example, elders, unemployed persons, single parents, children, those with previous history of mental disorders, and those with marital conflict before the disaster

NOTE THIS!

More than 5 million people's livelihoods were affected during Hurricane Katrina in 2005. Fifty percent experienced moderate to severe psychological distress.

RESEARCH ALERT

Those who lived through Hurricane Katrina in August 2005, especially residents of New Orleans and the Mississippi Gulf Coast, were at risk for developing PTSD and most suffered some degree of emotional distress from trauma and loss. People who watched the disaster unfold on television have also reported symptoms of emotional distress, even if they did not experience the disaster personally. This article provides an extensive review of previous studies about PTSD in disaster survivors, and the etiology of traumatic stress disorders. The authors provide specific guidance for all nurses in the identification of PTSD and appropriate nursing interventions to promote healing from the horror of disaster.

Source: Rhoads, J., Mitchell, F. A., & Rick, S. (2006). Posttraumatic stress disorder after Hurricane Katrina. *Journal for Nurse Practitioners, 2*(1), 18–26.

NOTE THIS!

An estimated 35,000 workers—who responded from all across the country after the worst terrorist attacks on U.S. soil on September 11, 2001—were exposed to concrete dust that may have contained asbestos, lead, fiberglass, and other particles released when the twin towers of the World Trade Center collapsed after being hit by two hijacked aircraft.

Most studies on the aftermath of disasters have reported that the first reaction of survivors is a state of dazed shock and numbness. The "disaster syndrome" consists of classic symptoms of mourning and bereavement on a communitywide scale: grief for lost community members and homes and grief for lost culture and familiar surroundings (which will never be the same again, no matter what form the recovery takes). To make this reaction worse, government and rescue workers often control access to the disaster area, keeping residents from their own homes and cleaning up wreckage without consulting the community members. Often, such work by disaster workers, although necessary, further distances the survivors from their need to be a part of the recovery process and exacerbates feelings of loss of control caused by the disaster itself. People may experience symptoms of PTSD, such as intense fear, helplessness, and horror. Research has found that many persons who survived Hurricane Katrina as well as those who watched the disaster unfold on television experienced one or more common stress reactions for several days and possibly weeks (Sloand, Ho, Klimmek, Pho, & Kub, 2012). Affected individuals may experience temporary psychological reactions, cognitive responses, physical complaints,

BOX 19-9 Words of Wisdom from Nurses Working the Oklahoma City Bombing

I realized that in the midst of the organized chaos, I had found the focus which nurses have had since Florence Nightingale, when she attended wounded soldiers of the Crimean War. I found that my degree of specialization no longer mattered. I had become a trauma nurse for one patient when he needed me.

—*Melissa Craft, RN*

These memories are hard to forget. But I will remember the strength and goodness that could not be extinguished even by such devastation. For its part, nursing as a caring profession was made manifest during this time.

—*Karen Bradford, RN*

Source: Left: Used by permission of Melissa Craft, RN, PLO, AOCN. Right: From Karen Bradford "The many graces of Oklahoma City nurses" (1996), *Reflections, 22*, (1), 10–12. Reproduced by permission.

or changes in psychosocial behavior that cause them to avoid large crowds or social activities where they might have to recall the event. While PTSD is always a risk, most persons affected by Hurricane Katrina will most likely experience only mild, normal stress reactions (Adams, 2007; Hyre et al., 2007; Rhoads et al., 2006).

Among the symptoms of extreme trauma that can affect an entire society (such as the Oklahoma City bombing, the September 11 terrorist attacks, and Hurricane Katrina) is a sense of vulnerability, a feeling that one has lost a certain natural immunity to misfortune, a growing conviction that the world is no longer a safe place to be (see **Box 19-9**). A lingering thought grows into a prediction of sorts: If this can happen, something even more terrible is bound to happen—the line has been crossed (Erickson, 1976). **Box 19-10** describes an example of the far-reaching effects of the Chernobyl disaster, which continues to threaten the wellbeing of affected communities.

BOX 19-10 The Chernobyl Nuclear Disaster: Will It Ever Be Over?

On April 26, 1986, a reactor blew up in Chernobyl in the former Soviet Union, resulting in an explosion that threw out 100 million curies of dangerous radionuclides to surrounding areas of the Ukraine, Belarus, and Russia. The World Health Organization estimates that 4.9 million persons were affected, making it the largest nuclear disaster in history. The results: Livestock, vegetables, grains, the soil, and the environment continue to be hazardous for human existence, although a large population still inhabits these areas. Cancers (including rare pediatric cancers and leukemia), chromosomal damage, and stress-related disorders plague the region and result in premature death and disability among all age groups. Scientists even now do not know how long the nuclear danger will remain or if the region will be safe to live in ever again.

Source: Edwards, 1994. Michael W. Edwards/National Geographic Image Collection.

Special Survivor Populations: Elders and Children

Children are at special risk during a disaster because of their immaturity—they have not yet developed adult coping strategies and do not yet have the life experiences to help them understand what has happened to them. In addition, we know that children rely on routine and consistency in their environment, relationships, and home life for a sense of security and identity. These areas are often disrupted in a disaster. Problems can emerge at school and last for much longer periods when compared with adults (Dugan, 2007; Gerrity & Flynn, 1997). Children may suffer from fears, phobias, sleep disorders, nightmares, excessive dependence, fear of being alone, hypersensitivity to noise and weather conditions, and regression, such as thumbsucking, bedwetting, and "baby talk" or stuttering (Kumar et al., 2007; Laube & Murphy, 1985; Sloand et al., 2012).

RESEARCH ALERT

The purpose of this study was to explore the experiences of nurse volunteers caring for children after the Haiti earthquake in January 2010. Design and methods: This descriptive qualitative study using in-depth interviews focuses on the experiences of 10 nurse volunteers. Results: Four themes emerged: hope amid devastation, professional compromises, universality of children, and emotional impact on nurses. Practice implications: Nurses who volunteer after natural disasters have rich personal and professional experiences, including extremes of sadness and joy. Nurse volunteers will likely need to care for children. Nurses and humanitarian agencies should prepare for the unique challenges of pediatric care.

Source: Sloand, E., Ho, G., Klimmek, R., Pho, A., & Kub, J. (2012). Nursing children after a disaster: A qualitative study of nurse volunteers and children after the Haiti earthquake. *Journal for Specialists in Pediatric Nursing, 17*(3), 242–253.

Elders often experience significant depression and despair from losing homes and being uprooted from familiar surroundings. Many of the elderly will have already lost primary family members and friends before the disaster. Among their valuables are family photos and mementos, Bibles, and keepsakes. Loss of this sort has a considerably greater effect on elders than others. There are also the compounded problems of more chronic diseases and health problems among this population, making them more vulnerable to disaster stress (Gerrity & Flynn, 1997). Disorientation and memory disturbances have also been noted in this population (Laube & Murphy, 1985). Refer to Box 19-5 to review health effects in disasters.

Simple intervention methods, such as group work for children and elders and short-term counseling immediately after the disaster, have proven quite effective in helping the recovery process. Community health nurses are in an excellent position to intervene with these vulnerable populations. Community health nurses must be able to locate children and elders so that immediate action can be taken. The most likely place to find these populations is in community shelters.

Recovery teams to assist the community in looking within for healing energy have also used traditional healers and informal community resource persons effectively. Women's associations, community development schemes, family welfare workers, and church volunteers have all had significant success in mobilizing community resources to promote community healing and recovery. Such strategies reduce the need for outside resources and help the community regain its stability using its own assets of solidarity (Richman, 1993).

MEDIA MOMENT

The 9/11 Terrorist Attacks from a Child's Perspective

My Country Fights Terrorism: The Terror Begins

On September 11, 2001, four American planes on their way to California were hijacked by 14 terrorists. The terrorists flew two of the planes into the World Trade Center Twin Towers in New York City and the sound of two 110-story buildings thundering down filled the city. One of the planes flew into the Pentagon and the last one crashed in Pennsylvania that officials think was headed for the White House. Over 5,000 people were killed when the Twin Towers fell. Children lost their mothers and fathers in a split second on that horrible day. Firefighters were killed finding and rescuing people and many bodies are still missing. Many people still need our help in donating blood to the hospitals in New York City and they need our prayers to help them get well again and to never forget this horrible day.

September 30, 2001
Parker Lundy, Age 10
Fifth Grade
Excerpt from an essay for Mrs. Kim Watts Evans
English composition class
Purvis Middle School
Purvis, Mississippi

Collective Trauma: The Loss of Community

Erickson (1976) detailed not only the loss of the sense of community, which occurs in a mass disaster, but also the loss of communality, which consists of a network of relationships that make up their general human surround. Communality can be described as a "state of mind shared among a particular gathering of people" (p. 189). In a sense, this community is one that cushions the pain, provides a context for intimacy, represents morality, and serves as the repository of old traditions and culture.

When a disaster demolishes a community, people find that they no longer have the collective reservoir of pooled resources, both physical and emotional, from which to draw. Communities act as a:

> cluster of people acting in concert and moving to the same collective rhythms who allocate their personal resources in such a way that the whole comes to have more humanity than its constituent parts. In effect, people put their own individual resources at the disposal of the group—placing them in the communal store and then drawing on that reserve supply for the demands of everyday life. (Erickson, 1976, p. 194)

APPLICATION TO PRACTICE 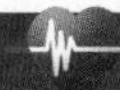

The Oklahoma City Bombing, April 19, 1995

On the morning of April 19, 1995, the Alfred P. Murrah Federal Building in Oklahoma City was the site of a devastating terrorist bombing. In addition to federal employees and other government workers, the building was the site of a daycare center. Because of the effectiveness of the city's disaster plan, rescue and recovery began within minutes after the explosion. Oklahoma experiences frequent, deadly tornadoes throughout the state and consequently maintains a highly organized disaster planning response. Initial priorities the morning of the bombing included getting people out of the building, triaging injuries, and transporting the injured to six nearby hospitals. Nurses in hospitals, home health agencies, and public health and other facilities in the community quickly responded to the needs of the victims.

(continues)

APPLICATION TO PRACTICE (*CONTINUED*) 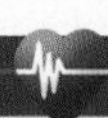

By midafternoon of that day, the four trauma departments had seen 40 to 80 persons each. Victims were transported by ambulances, private vehicles, cabs, and vans. A family communication center was quickly set up at a local church, 5 miles from the bomb site, by the American Red Cross and FEMA. This center, which "wrapped its arms around the families of the victims of the blast," provided mental health professionals, hospice nurses, psychiatric nurses, and counselors 24 hours a day for 2 weeks after the bombing. The medical examiner's office communicated with the families of the victims there, and rescue workers from the bomb site frequently reported back to the families concerning the progress of the search teams.

A play area for children was set up, and the Salvation Army provided comfort services, including food and clothing. Pets were brought by local groups to provide solace for the victims. A Native American healer was present for tribal members. Toll-free numbers were provided by the state mental health department for direct and indirect victims' use to prevent and treat posttraumatic stress disorder. Support groups were set up, television talk shows featured survivors and disaster workers, and articles were printed in the local newspapers, all directed toward giving the people of Oklahoma a chance to talk through the horror of their collective experiences. The city's convention center became a huge hostel that fed, clothed, and housed thousands of rescue workers during this period. Roses and chocolates appeared on the pillows of disaster workers, stress management was available, massages were provided for sore muscles, and there was "always a listening ear for sore souls."

Nurses were involved at all levels of the disaster, including triage at the command center, accompanying surgeons as they removed the legs of a child in the bombed building, providing grief counseling for the families of victims and for the disaster workers themselves, providing direct care at hospitals to the injured, and visiting the families of victims in their homes for forensic identification and later on as follow up.

According to Wilson (1996), an "important reason why the people here worked so well was because of disaster planning. When people live in an area that is nicknamed 'tornado alley,' they plan for disaster" (p. 24). "Though we will never rectify the loss of life incurred in a disaster by planning ahead, we can be ready to mobilize the resources to make all of us a little less vulnerable" (p. 25).

Source: Wilson, J. S. (1996). Healing Oklahoma's wounds. *Home Healthcare Nurse, 14*(1), 23–25.

When a community is destroyed, people find themselves without the reservoir of support on which they have relied in the past. They find that they are almost empty of feeling, empty of affection, and empty of confidence and assurance. Residents feel abandoned, often expressing feelings of fear, apathy, and demoralization. Comments from survivors often reflect despair: "I thought this was the end of the world" or "It looked like Dooms Day" (Erickson, 1976, p. 199).

> Whoever fights monsters should see to it that in the process he does not become the monster. And when you look into the abyss, the abyss looks into you.
>
> —*Nietzsche*

Nurses' Reactions to Disasters

Nurses should attend to the needs of the disaster workers themselves during and after a disaster to reduce the possibility of producing secondary victims. Rescue personnel are often reluctant to take breaks to replenish food, water, and rest when time is of essence in the search and recovery phase when they are needed. Nevertheless, nurses should be firm in reminding workers that, to remain useful, they must not exhaust themselves in the process. Seeing that workers are rotated and providing rest, nourishment, and relaxation for the rescuers should be considered essential responsibilities of the community health nurse.

Nurses often experience the same disturbing, and sometimes dramatic, emotional problems as those found in their patients who were victims. Nurses may experience difficulty

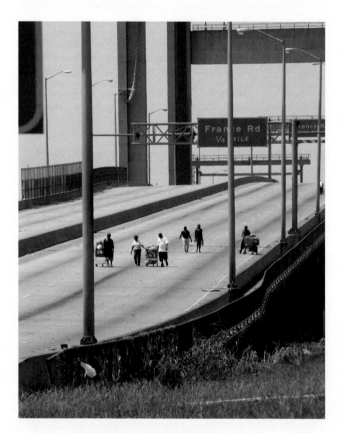

Residents in New Orleans sought refuge and disaster rescue on interstate highways after Hurricane Katrina.

concentrating, fatigue, irritability, insomnia, and other unique symptoms of stress. Unique symptoms may include depersonalization of the victim, a macabre sense of humor, hypervigilance, and excessive unwillingness to disengage or leave the disaster scene or the helping role (e.g., refusal to leave after the arrival of a relief shift) (Gerrity & Flynn, 1997; O'Boyle, Robertson, & Secor-Turner, 2006; Rhoads et al., 2006). Reactions of nurses are magnified when the nurse is a member of the affected community and when the nurse may have endured property and community damage, as well as stress related to family wellbeing. According to Laube (1992), nurses should be considered "normal persons reacting in a very normal manner to an abnormal condition" (p. 19).

A qualitative study conducted by O'Boyle, Robertson, and Secor-Turner (2006) found that nurses who work in hospitals that are designated as receiving sites during public health emergencies continue to express a "fear of abandonment" regarding their work assignments during a major disaster. The nurses in the study reported concerns about their own safety, fear of nursing colleagues refusing to work, failure to have a clear chain of command, and the stress of working in a chaotic environment without adequate preparation. Clearly, there is much work to be done on a national basis to involve all nurses in all healthcare settings with disaster planning and preparedness—not just the administrative staff in selected facilities.

Sources of stress for the disaster nurse can be generally classified into three categories:

- Event stressors—the trauma and fatigue associated with the extreme intensity of the disaster event, of the highest intensity if the nurse lives in the affected community and has family who are potential victims
- Occupational stress—stress related to role conflict, role overload, and role confusion
- Organizational stressors—factors that emerge from the organizational response itself, multiagency demands, and the complex tangle of bureaucracy that emerges in a major disaster (Hartsough & Myers, 1985)

With every disaster victim treated, nurses often experience an unconscious fear that the victim could just as easily have been one of their loved ones.

RESEARCH ALERT

This study examined associations between alcohol use and PTSD symptoms among Red Cross workers who responded to the September 11, 2001 terrorist attacks against the United States. Seven hundred seventy-nine Red Cross paid and volunteer staff who responded during the first 3 months were randomly assigned to receive one of four questionnaire packets. Women made up 64% of the sample. The sample was chosen from an ARC mailing list of all paid and volunteer staff ($n = 6{,}055$ with valid addresses) who participated in the disaster relief operations in response to the 9/11 attacks. This study is based on the fourth group, which received the alcohol questionnaires. The researchers found that overall, traumatic stress symptoms and alcohol use were low. Hyperarousal and intrusion symptoms on the Impact of Events Scale-Revised (IES-R) were associated with alcohol consumption, hazardous alcohol consumption, and change in alcohol consumption when controlling for age, gender, and worksite. Positive associations between intrusion and avoidance scores and hazardous consumption were stronger for younger participants. Individuals who reported increasing or decreasing alcohol use had higher IES-R scores than did those who maintained their normal rate of alcohol consumption, though effects were stronger for increasing alcohol use. Associations between alcohol variables and avoidance symptoms were minimal. The results suggest that there is a functional relation between posttraumatic stress symptoms and alcohol consumption. The study suggests that efforts to cope with traumatic stress symptoms may manifest in either increases or decreases in alcohol consumption.

Source: Gaher, R., Jacobs, G., Meyer, D., & Johnson-Jimenez, E. (2005). Associations between alcohol use and PTSD symptoms among American Red Cross disaster relief workers responding to the 9/11/2001 attacks. *American Journal of Drug & Alcohol Abuse, 31*(2), 285–295.

DAY IN THE LIFE

Dr. Jerri Laube

How did you become interested in disaster research?

In 1970 I was fresh out of my master's program at the University of Colorado and was asked by the local American Red Cross Chapter in Dallas to give a talk to their nurses on the psychological effects of disaster. I thought they wanted me to talk about the psychological effects of disaster on nurses (later I learned that they just wanted the effects in general). I had no experience so I went to the library to research the subject and found only one reference specific to the effect on nurses—Jeannette Rayner's article written in 1958. By generalizing from publications about army nursing, plus Rayner's article, I managed to meet my assignment but felt a great need for an in-depth study of the psychological effects of disaster on nurses. I later wrote a small grant to the American Red Cross for funding to survey nurses' reactions in a recent tornado close to home. While waiting on that response, Hurricane Celia hit the coast of Texas. I immediately called and requested that I be sent to that

(continues)

DAY IN THE LIFE (*CONTINUED*)

area. This was granted and I was on site within 24 hours of the disaster. That study was published in *Nursing Research*. I later broadened my area of study to cover all healthcare providers in disaster. Not long after my first study, I was invited to be a part of a task force to revise the Disaster Act to include assistance for psychological aspects of disaster. That was completed and has been carried forth ever since.

Should BSN nurses be prepared in disaster response and recovery?

Students in baccalaureate programs should have classes and simulated experience in reducing the impact of disaster. If available, collaboration with the local Red Cross chapter is ideal. Nursing students who take their courses can earn hours toward Red Cross certification, thus shortening the time after graduation to become a Red Cross nurse.

Why do you believe BSN nurses should be prepared in disaster nursing?

Nurses are uniquely qualified by the nature or their education and experience. Nurses are prepared to work with the whole patient—physically and psychologically. They work both in crisis and chronic conditions, which is necessary because a disaster victim, definitely in crisis, may also have a chronic illness. Thus, they have the basic qualifications. Updating their knowledge and skills should continue through workshops and disaster drills sponsored by/through their place of work.

—Jerri Laube, RN, PhD, FAAN

Dr. Jerri Laube is co-author, with Dr. Shirley A. Murphy, of *Perspectives on Disaster Recovery* (1985, Appleton-Century-Crofts)

Nurses are educated to maintain professional composure in any type of stressful situation, even in the face of grief, suffering, and death. This composure has been termed "detached concern" by Coombs and Goldman (1973). Detached concern is the adaptive ability to care for critically ill and injured patients while maintaining an acceptable emotional detachment. Research has revealed that nurses function effectively in disasters, and very few have long-term emotional difficulties after the disaster. Chubon's (1992) study of nurses who worked during the Hurricane Hugo disaster in Florida supported the findings of previous studies—namely, nurses continued to function effectively in their work roles despite their emotional responses. In this research study, nurses' functioning was generally consistent with their predisaster work patterns. Sources of stress were consistently related to the safety of their own loved ones and family. Suggested interventions were (1) to bring outside nurses from other home health agencies to care for assigned patients until the local nurses stabilize their own family situations and (2) to make mental health resources available in the immediate postrecovery period for the nurses in the agency.

In Laube's (1973) study of the Hurricane Celia disaster, the majority of nurses functioned in their role without impairment from anxiety. Research into excessive physical demands has identified major stressors that nurses may experience during disasters, such as concerns for personal safety, inadequate supplies, seeing people suffer and not being able to meet basic needs of all, hurt children, disorganization, and concern for their own family's welfare (Waters et al., 1992).

Family roles seem to play a critical part in the nurse's response to disaster. Healthcare workers who are from the disaster area experience exceptional stress; not only must they work through their own reactions to and losses of the community from the disaster, but they also must resolve the family/community role conflict (Adams, 2007; Hyre et al., 2007; Rhoads et al., 2006; Waters et al., 1992; Weeks, 2007). In other words, when the wellbeing of the nurse's family is jeopardized, professional effectiveness decreases and stress becomes more likely to affect the nurse's role. This finding means that relying on outside disaster workers is indicated early in the course of disasters and should continue until the local healthcare providers can be assured of their own family's safety (Laube & Murphy, 1985).

Stuhlmiller (1996) suggests that, because nurses are typically involved with suffering and disruption of lives of their patients, they may actually be in a better position than other disaster workers to mediate the effects of the disaster. By participating in debriefings, nurses begin healing themselves even as they help others begin their own process of healing. Stuhlmiller contends that we often assume that workers are at risk for posttraumatic stress and proceed with negative assumptions about how they should react. By doing so, we unwittingly hamper their "natural restorative capacities" (p. 19). In other words, looking for the negative effects may overshadow the positive outcomes on which nurses tend to focus—the positive outcomes that come from helping people in extreme need.

"Disasters challenge self-understanding and meanings just as illness does ... what the rescuers need most then is what nurses are particularly good at providing. Nurses can foster emotional recovery and growth by attending to what approaches work best and by acknowledging the validity of the person's expressed pain, fear, and grief" (Laube, 1973, p. 19). Such a view is consistent with Laube's (1973) conclusion that, even with all of the possible stressors nurses face during disasters, studies consistently reveal that nurses' responses to disaster do not interfere with their effectiveness as professionals.

Because of these findings, it can be concluded that nurses are extremely vulnerable to PTSD in the aftermath of a disaster. See the Research Alert feature that describes nurses' reactions and feelings during and after Hurricane Hugo and Box 19-9, which consists of actual quotes from nurses who expressed their feelings about their work in a disaster.

Prevention Strategies for Nurses

By becoming prepared for a disaster through specialized training and anticipatory stress counseling, nurses can reduce the damage of a disaster to self (see **Box 19-11**). Simple measures such as appreciating the intensity of emotions and dealing with them; taking breaks; eating nutritious foods in the form of smaller, more frequent meals; avoiding drinking large amounts of caffeine and alcohol; exercising; and sleeping as much as possible have given nurses the added strength to not only survive but actually flourish in a disaster. Seldom can as much attention be given to the victims as the nurse believes is necessary (Weeks, 2007).

Although nurses seem to be effective in mediating stressors in the disaster setting, they are certainly not immune to possible ill effects. Based on her research into the 1989 Loma Prieta earthquake in California, Laube (1992) has suggested that prevention programs for disaster workers should be included in disaster preparedness. For primary-level prevention, a crisis team should work with the disaster staff before a disaster strikes. This crisis team should include a social worker, minister, psychiatric nurse, and other mental health professionals as available. It should have input into the disaster plan and be included in disaster drill critiques and debriefing. At a secondary level of prevention, the same team should be highly visible during the impact of the disaster. Its members could provide emotional support and monitor the emotional stability of workers, intervening as necessary. At the tertiary level of prevention, after the disaster, the team should take an active role in organizing and conducting mandatory disaster debriefing sessions. Counseling referrals should be made at this time, and nurses should have input into the critique of the disaster plan's effectiveness related to worker response and recovery (Laube, 1992). Such strategic interventions can prevent burnout and emotional casualties of the healthcare provider.

BOX 19-11 Be Red Cross Ready...for a Disaster

1. Have a disaster kit that includes the following:
   - Flashlight
   - Battery-powered or hand-crank radio
   - Extra batteries of various sizes
   - First aid kit
   - Seven-day supply of medications
   - Copies of personal and financial documents
   - Store at least 3 days' supply of food, water, and other supplies in your family disaster kit.
   - Emergency contact information
   - Extra cash
   - Maps
   - Extra car and house keys
   - Check disaster kit every 6 months and replace expired items
   - Keep cell phones charged
2. Make a family disaster plan:
   - Discuss with all family members what to do during an impending disaster.
   - Develop a family plan that includes roles for each member and let all family members know where the disaster kit is located.
   - Learn how and when to turn off utilities and how to use fire extinguishers.
   - Develop escape routes from house and area, including a common meeting place for family members.
   - Include pets and their safe evacuation in the plan.
3. Remain informed and vigilant about emergency preparedness:
   - Identify sources in the community for information about disasters.
   - Know your geographical region and the associated risk factors for disasters in your area.
   - Consider taking an American Red Cross disaster preparedness class and/or a first aid course.

RESEARCH ALERT

Chubon was in the midst of an ethnographic study of home care nurses' job stress when Hurricane Hugo struck the South Carolina coast in 1989. The home health agency was heavily damaged by wind and water and was uninhabitable for more than a week. Because the nurse researcher had observed the nurses for 10 weeks before the hurricane, she was able to collect data about their response to the disaster in the context of their usual role of home health nurse. The nurses in the agency were simultaneously victims and caregivers for their home health patients. They experienced grief, anger, and frustration about their losses, as well as conflict between family responsibilities and work responsibilities. Chubon's work supported the findings of previous studies in which nurses continued to function effectively in their work roles despite their emotional responses. Because baseline data were available before the hurricane struck, this study indicated that the nurses' functioning was generally consistent with their predisaster work patterns. Sources of stress consistently related to the safety of their own loved ones and family. Suggested interventions were (1) to bring outside nurses from other home health agencies to care for assigned patients until the local nurses could stabilize their own family situations and

(continues)

RESEARCH ALERT (*CONTINUED*) 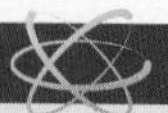

(2) to make mental health resources available in the immediate postrecovery period for the nurses in the agency.

Source: Chubon, S. J. (1992). Home care during the aftermath of Hurricane Hugo. *Public Health Nursing, 9*(2), 97–102.

LEVELS OF PREVENTION 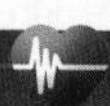

Primary: involves warnings, preparation, and a disaster plan, including educating the population about appropriate disaster response. These interventions are aimed at reducing the probability of disease, death, and disability resulting from a disaster.

Secondary: includes the immediate identification of disaster problems and the implementation of measures to treat and prevent their recurrence or complications.

Tertiary: involves rehabilitation of disaster victims and the community to an optimal functional level, with permanency of change from the disaster being assumed. The goal during rehabilitation is to minimize further damage resulting from the disaster.

AFFORDABLE CARE ACT (ACA) 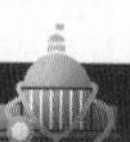

Section 5210 establishes a Ready Reserve Corps with the Commissioned Corps for service in times of national emergency. It authorized $50 million each year for fiscal years 2010–2014.

Section 5314 authorizes the Secretary to address workforce shortages in state and local health departments in applied public health epidemiology and public health laboratory science and information, including expansion of the Epidemic Intelligence Service.

Conclusion

Disasters are increasing in number and severity each year, so community health nurses need to be adequately prepared to deal with them. Lillian Wald, a famous nursing theorist and community activist, responded to her societal needs by developing the Henry Street Settlement House in 1893. At the time, Wald stated, "Nurses not only serve the individual but also promote the interest of a collective society" (as cited in Kippenbrock, 1991, p. 209). This statement also applies today, especially in the face of disasters.

Being prepared for future disasters means that community health nurses must plan disaster care for multicultural populations. The hallmark of American society is multiculturalism (Sobier, 1995). The major disaster goal for nurses now and in the future is to retain maximum wellness of individuals and populations in communities (Procter & Cheek, 1995). Learning to work with appropriate resources and placing emphasis on specific approaches to enhance individuals, families, and communities are integral to protection and healing from a disaster.

Melanie Dreher (1996), past president of Sigma Theta Tau International, pointed out that nurses are very resilient and can be called everyday heroes. Numerous nurses have performed heroic acts, such as Nightingale, Alcott, and Cavell. Dreher contended that nurses with "heroine" status are recognizable by traits and actions: "They define their life's work not in terms of paychecks, working conditions, and employment benefits, but in terms of the number of lives saved, families in crisis who were counseled, and patients comforted" (p. 5).

Critical Thinking Activities

1. Based on the Application to Practice feature on the Oklahoma City bombing, answer the following questions:
   - What were the primary, secondary, and tertiary prevention disaster interventions carried out by nurses during the Oklahoma City bombing?
   - Identify activities in each of the stages of disaster recovery.
   - Give examples of the three categories of stressors that disaster nurses faced in Oklahoma.
   - Identify the components of the Oklahoma City disaster plan. What would be your recommendations for the disaster team?
2. How can community health nurses better prepare individuals for the present and future threat of bioterrorism and terrorism?

HEALTHY ME 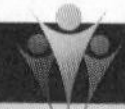

Be prepared for a disaster and consider volunteering as an ARC disaster nurse. Make sure you and your family have a disaster plan and kit ready at all times. See Box 19-11, "Be Red Cross Ready."

References

Adams, L. M. (2007). Mental health needs of disaster volunteers: A plea for awareness. *Perspectives in Psychiatric Care, 43*(1), 52–54.

Advisory Committee on the International Decade for Natural Hazard Reduction. (1987). *Confronting natural disasters: An international decade for natural hazard reduction.* Washington, DC: National Academies Press.

American Psychiatric Association (APA). (2013). *Diagnostic and statistical manual of mental disorders* (5th ed.). Washington, DC: American Psychiatric Publishing.

American Red Cross (ARC). (1990). *A history of helping others* (ARC Publication No. 4627). Washington, DC: ARC National Headquarters.

American Red Cross (ARC). (1995). *Disaster is everybody's business* (ARC Publication No. 5061). Washington, DC: ARC National Headquarters.

American Red Cross (ARC). (2006). *A year of healing: The American Red Cross response to Hurricanes Katrina, Rita and Wilma—One year report.* Washington, DC: Author.

American Red Cross (ARC). (2008). *About us.* Retrieved from http://www.redcross.org/about-us/

American Red Cross (ARC). (2010a). *Helping where it counts: Student nurse volunteers.* Retrieved from http://www.redcross.org/images/MEDIA_CustomProductCatalog/m4440167_HelpingStudentNurse.pdf

American Red Cross (ARC). (2010b). *Make a difference: Guidelines for nursing student involvement in the American Red Cross.* Retrieved from http://www.redcross.org/images/MEDIA_CustomProductCatalog/m4440168_MakeADifferenceGuide.pdf

American Red Cross (ARC). (2014). Nursing students. Retrieved from http://www.redcross.org/support/volunteer/nurses/students

Auf der Heide, E. (1989). *Disaster response: Principles of preparation and coordination.* St. Louis, MO: Mosby.

Baker, G., & Chapman, R. (1962). *Man and society in disaster.* New York, NY: Basic Books.

Balinsky, W. (2003). The home care emergency response to the September 11 tragedy. *Caring, 22*(9), 38–40.

Barker, E. (1989). Care givers as casualties. *Western Journal of Nursing Research, 11*, 5.

Barry, J. M. (1997). *Rising tide: The great Mississippi flood of 1927 and how it changed America.* New York, NY: Simon & Schuster.

Baum, D. (2006, August 16). Letter from New Orleans: The lost year. *The New Yorker.*

Berz, G. (1984). Research and statistics on natural disasters in insurance and reinsurance companies. *Geneva Papers on Risk and Insurance, 9*, 135–157.

Bourne, J. K. (2004, October). Gone with the water. *National Geographic.*

Boyer, P. J. (2005, September 26). Letter from Mississippi: Gone with the surge. *The New Yorker.*

Chubon, S. J. (1992). Home care during the aftermath of Hurricane Hugo. *Public Health Nursing, 9*(2), 97–102.

Colias, M. (2005, October). The disaster after the disaster. *Hospitals and Health Networks,* 36–44.

Coombs, R. H., & Goldman, L. J. (1973). Maintenance and discontinuity of coping mechanisms in an intensive care unit. *Social Problems, 20*, 3.

Dixon, M. (1986). Disaster planning—Medical response: Organization and preparation. *American Association of Occupational Health Nurses, 34*(12), 580–584.

Drabek, T. E. (1986). *Human system response to disaster: An inventory of sociological findings.* New York, NY: Springer-Verlag.

Dreher, M. C. (1996, First Quarter). Heroism. *Reflections,* 4–5.

Dugan, B. (2007). Loss of identity in disaster: How do you say goodbye to home? *Perspectives in Psychiatric Care, 43*(1), 41–46.

Dynes, R. R., Quarantelli, E. L., & Kreps, G. A. (1972, December). *A perspective on disaster planning, TR-77* (pp. 6–8). Washington, DC: Defense Civil Preparedness Agency.

Dwyer, J., & Drew, C. (2005, September 29). Fear exceeded crime's reality in New Orleans. *New York Times.*

Edwards, M. (1994, August). Living with the monster—Chernobyl. *National Geographic,* 186, 2.

EM-DAT: The OFDA/CRED International Disaster Database. (2012). Brussels, Belgium: UCL. Retrieved from http://www.emdat.be/

Erickson, K. (1976). *Everything in its path: Destruction of community in the Buffalo Creek flood.* New York, NY: Simon & Schuster.

Federal Emergency Management Agency (FEMA). (2006). *The federal disaster declaration process and disaster aid programs: Response and recovery.* Retrieved from http://www.fema.gov/hazard/dproc.shtm

Federal Emergency Management Agency (FEMA). (2011). *Emergency Management Institute (EMI) Overview.* Retrieved from http://training.fema.gov/History/

Foxman, B., Camargo, C. A., Lillienfeld, D., Linet, M., Mays, V. M., McKeown, R., ... Rothenberg, R. (2006). Looking back at Hurricane Katrina: Lessons for 2006 and beyond. *Annals of Epidemiology, 16*(8), 652–653.

Frantz, A. K. (1998). Nursing pride: Clara Barton in the Spanish–American War. *American Journal of Nursing, 98*(10), 39–41.

Gamboa-Maldonado, T., Marshak, H., Sinclair, R., Montgomery, S., & Dyjack, D. T. (2012). Building capacity for community disaster preparedness: A call for collaboration between public environmental health and emergency preparedness and response programs. *Journal of Environmental Health,* 75(2), 19–29.

Garcia, L. M. (1985). *Disaster nursing: Planning, assessment, and intervention.* Rockville, MD: Aspen.

Garheld, R., & Hamid, A. Y. (2006). Tsunami response: A year later. *American Journal of Nursing, 106*(1), 76–79.

Garrett, L. (2000). *Betrayal of trust: The collapse of global public health.* New York, NY: Hyperion.

Gerrity, E. T., & Flynn, B. W. (1997). Mental health consequences of disasters. In E. K. Noji (Ed.), *The public health consequences of disasters* (pp. 101–121). New York, NY: Oxford University Press.

Gibson, P., Theadore, F., & Jellison, J. B. (2012). The Common Ground Preparedness Framework: A comprehensive description of public health emergency preparedness. *American Journal of Public Health, 102*(4), 633–642.

Gospodinov, E., & Burnham, G. (Ed.). (2008). *The Johns Hopkins and Red Cross and Red Crescent public health guide in emergencies* (2nd ed.). Geneva, Switzerland: International Federation of Red Cross and Red Crescent Societies.

Hartsough, D. M., & Myers, D. G. (1985). *Disaster work and mental health: Prevention and control of stress among workers.* Rockville, MD: National Institute of Mental Health.

Hassmiller, S. (2007). The 2004 tsunami. *American Journal of Nursing, 107*(2), 74–77.

Hayes, B. (2005). Natural and unnatural disasters. *American Scientist,* 93(6), 496–499.

Haygood, W., & Tyson, A. S. (2005, September 15). It was as if all of us were already pronounced dead. *Washington Post.*

Henderson, D. A., Inglesby, T. V., & O'Toole, T. (2002). *Bioterrorism: Guidelines for medical and public health management.* Chicago, IL: American Medical Association Press.

Hyre, A., Ompad, D., & Menke, A. (2007). Symptoms of posttraumatic stress disorder in a New Orleans workforce following Hurricane Katrina. *Journal of Urban Health, 84*(2), 142–152.

Ingram, J. C., Franco, G., Rio, C. R., & Khazai, B. (2006). Post-disaster recovery dilemmas: Challenges in balancing short-term and long-term needs for vulnerability reduction. *Environmental Science & Policy,* (7/8), 607–613.

International Strategy for Disaster Reduction (ISDR). (2006). *2006–2007 World Disaster Risk Reduction Campaign: Disaster Reduction Begins at School.* Geneva, Switzerland: United Nations Inter-agency Secretariat for the International Strategy for Risk Reduction.

Jakeway, C. C., LaRosa, G., Cary, A., & Schoenfisch, S. (2008). The role of public health nurses in emergency preparedness and response: A position paper of the Association of State and Territorial Directors of Nursing. *Public Health Nursing, 25*(4), 353–361.

Janis, I. L., & Mann, L. (1977, June). Emergency decision making: A theoretical analysis of responses to disaster warnings. *Journal of Human Stress,* 35–48.

Kiewra, K. (2006, Winter). The eye of the storm: What lessons do Katrina and other humanitarian crises teach us about managing calamity? *Harvard Public Health Review.* Retrieved from http://www.hsph.harvard.edu/review/rvwwinter06_katrinaeye.html

Kippenbrock, T. A. (1991). Wishing I'd been there. *Nursing and Health Care, 12*(4), 209.

Kitt, S., Selfridge-Thomas, J., Proehl, J. A., & Kaiser, J. (1995). *Emergency nursing: A physiologic and clinical perspective* (2nd ed.). Philadelphia, PA: Saunders.

Klagsbrun, S. C. (2002). A mental health perspective on 9/11. *Journal of the Association of Nurses in AIDS Care, 3*(5), 67.

Knabb, R. D., Rhome, J. R., & Brown, D. P. (2005, December 20). *Tropical cyclone report: Hurricane Katrina.* Miami, FL: National Hurricane Center.

Kumar, M. S., Murhekar, M. V., Hutin, Y., Subramanian, T., Ramachandran, V., & Gupte, M. D. (2007). Prevalence of posttraumatic stress disorder in a coastal fishing village in Tamil Nadu, India, after the December 2004 tsunami. *American Journal of Public Health, 97*(1), 99–101.

Landesman, L. Y. (2005). *Public health management of disasters: The practice guide* (2nd ed.). Washington, DC: American Public Health Association.

Langan, J. C., & James, D. C. (2004). *Preparing nurses for disaster management.* Upper Saddle River, NJ: Prentice Hall.

Laube, J. (1973). Psychological reactions to nurses in disaster. *Nursing Research, 22,* 343–347.

Laube, J. (1992). The professional's psychological response in disaster: Implications for practice. *Journal of Psychosocial Nursing, 30*(2), 17–22.

Laube, J., & Murphy, S. A. (1985). *Perspectives on disaster recovery.* Norwalk, CT: Appleton-Century-Crofts.

Leaning, J., & Guha-Sapir, D. (2013). Natural disasters, armed conflict, and public health. *New England Journal of Medicine, 369*(19), 1836–1842.

Levy, B. S., & Sidel, V. W. (2002). *Terrorism and public health: A balanced approach to strengthening systems and protecting people.* New York, NY: Oxford University Press.

Lifton, R. J. (1967). *Death in life: Survivors in Hiroshima.* New York, NY: Random House.

Lifton, R. J., & Olson, E. (1976). The human meaning of disaster. *Psychiatry, 39,* 1–7.

Lockwood, R. (1997). *FEMA: Through hell and high water: Disasters and the human–animal bond.* Washington, DC: FEMA and the Humane Society of the United States.

Logue, J. N., Melick, M. E., & Hansen, H. (1981). Research issues and directions in the epidemiology of health effects of disasters. *Epidemiological Review, 3,* 140–162.

Malilay, J. (1997). Floods. In E. K. Noji (Ed.), *The public health consequences of disasters* (pp. 287–301). New York, NY: Oxford University Press.

Meichenbaum, D. (1994). *Disasters, stress and cognition.* Paper presented for the NATO Workshop on Stress and Communities, Chateau da Bonas, France, June 14–18, 1994.

Mileti, D. S., Drabek, T. E., & Haas, J. E. (1975). *Human systems in extreme environments: A sociological perspective* (Monograph No. 21). Boulder, CO: Program on Technology, Environment, and Man, Institute of Behavioral Science, University of Colorado.

Mizutani, T., & Nakano, T. (1989). The impact of natural disasters on the population of Japan. In J. I. Clarke, P. Curson, S. L. Kayastha, & P. Nag (Eds.), *Population and disaster.* Cambridge, MA: Basil Blackwell.

Muench, J. (1996). Disaster training pays off for Juneau nurses. *Alaska Nurse, 46*(5), 1.

National Disaster Medical System (NDMS). (2006). *Department of Health and Human Services, Office of Preparedness and Response.* Washington, DC: U.S. Government Printing Office. Retrieved from http://www.phe.gov/preparedness/Pages/default.aspx

Neff, J. A., & Kidd, P. S. (1993). *Trauma nursing: The art and science.* St. Louis, MO: Mosby.

Nigg, J. M., Barnshaw, J., & Torres, M. R. (2006). Hurricane Katrina and the flooding of New Orleans: Emergent issues in sheltering and temporary housing. *Annals of the American Academy of Political & Social Science, 604,* 113–128.

Noji, E. K. (1997). *The public health consequences of disasters.* New York, NY: Oxford University Press.

O'Boyle, C., Robertson, C., & Secor-Turner, M. (2006). Nurses' beliefs about public health emergencies: Fear of abandonment. *American Journal of Infection Control, 34*(6), 351–357.

Pickens, S. (1992). The decade for natural disaster reduction. *Nursing & Health Care, 13,* 192–195.

Plough, A., Fielding, J. E., Chandra, A., Williams, M., Eisenman, D., Wells, K. B., ... Magaña, A. (2013). Building community disaster resilience: Perspectives from a large urban county department of public health. *American Journal of Public Health, 103*(7), 1190–1197.

Polivka, B., Stanley, S., Gordon, D., Taulbee, K., Kieffer, G., & McCorkle, S. (2008). Public health nursing competencies for public health surge events. *Public Health Nursing, 25*(2), 159–165.

Porche, D. J. (2002). Biological and chemical bioterrorism agents. *Journal of the Association of Nurses in AIDS Care, 13*(5), 57–64.

Procter, N. G., & Cheek, J. (1995). Nurses' role in world catastrophic events: War dislocation effects on Serbian Australians. In B. Neuman (Ed.), *The Neuman systems model* (3rd ed., pp. 48–70). Norwalk, CT: Appleton & Lange.

Quarantelli, E. L., & Dynes, R. R. (1972, February). When disaster strikes (it isn't much like what you've heard about or read about). *Psychology Today,* 72.

Rebmann, T., Carrico, R., & English, J. F. (2008). Lessons public health professionals learned from past disasters. *Public Health Nursing, 25*(4), 344–352.

Rhoads, J., Mitchell, F. A., & Rick, S. (2006). Posttraumatic stress disorder after Hurricane Katrina. *Journal for Nurse Practitioners, 2*(1), 18–26.

Richman, N. (1993). After the flood. *American Journal of Public Health, 83*(11), 1522–1524.

Rosenkoetter, M. M., Covan, E. K., Cobb, B. K., Bunting, S., & Weinrich, M. (2007). Perceptions of older adults regarding evacuation in the event of a natural disaster. *Public Health Nursing, 24*(2), 160–168.

Rowitz, L. (2005). *Public health for the 21st century: The prepared leader.* Sudbury, MA: Jones and Bartlett.

Sabin, L. (1998). *Struggles and triumphs: The story of Mississippi nurses.* Jackson, MS: Mississippi Hospital Association Foundation.

Salvation Army. (2014). *About us: What is the Salvation Army?* Retrieved from http://www.salvationarmyusa.org/usn/about

Saunders, J. M. (2007). Vulnerable populations in an American Red Cross shelter after Hurricane Katrina. *Perspectives in Psychiatric Care, 43*(1), 30–37.

Shank, J. (2013, September). From Boulder, Colorado: Notes on a thousand-year flood. *Atlantic Monthly,* pp. 23–27.

Silverstein, M. E. (1984). *Triage decision trees and triage protocols.* Washington, DC: FEMA Headquarters.

Skirble, R. (2012). After Japan, experts rethink costs, safety of nuclear power. *Voice of America.* Retrieved from http://www.voanews.com/content/after-japan-experts-wonder-if-nuclear-power-is-safe-economical-142061263/179604.html

Sloand, E., Ho, G., Klimmek, R., Pho, A., & Kub, J. (2012). Nursing children after a disaster: A qualitative study of nurse volunteers and children after the Haiti earthquake. *Journal for Specialists in Pediatric Nursing, 17*(3), 242–253.

Smith, P. (2000). Terrorism awareness: Weapons of mass destruction: Part I, Chemical agents. *Internet Journal of Rescue and Disaster Medicine, 2*(1).

Sobier, R. (1995). Nursing care for the people of a small planet: Culture and the Neuman systems model. In B. Neuman (Ed.), *The Neuman systems model* (3rd ed.). Norwalk, CT: Appleton & Lange.

Stein, S., & Okal, E. A. (2005). Speed and size of the Sumatra earthquake. *Nature,* 434, 581.

Stuhlmiller, C. M. (1996, First Quarter). Studying the rescuers. *Reflections,* 18–19.

Sullivan, T. J. (1998). *Collaboration: A health care imperative.* New York, NY: McGraw-Hill.

Suserud, B., & Haljamae, H. (1997). Acting at a disaster site: Experiences expressed by Swedish nurses. *Journal of Advanced Nursing, 25*(1), 155–162.

Taggert, S. D. (1982). *Emergency preparedness manual.* Salt Lake City, UT: University of Utah.

Telford, J., & Cosgrave, J. (2007). The international humanitarian system and the 2004 Indian Ocean earthquake and tsunamis. *Disasters, 31*(1), 1–28.

Toffler, A. (1970). *Future shock.* New York, NY: Random House.

U.S. Congress. (2006). *A failure of initiative: Final report of the Select Bipartisan Committee to Investigate the Preparation for and Response to Hurricane Katrina.* Washington, DC: U.S. Government Printing Office.

Waeckerle, J. F. (1983). The skywalk collapse: A personal response. *Annals of Emergency Medicine, 12,* 651.

Waeckerle, J. F. (1991). Disaster planning and response. *New England Journal of Medicine, 324,* 815–821.

Waltham, R. (2005). The flooding of New Orleans. *Geology Today, 21*(6), 225–231.

Waters, K. A., Selander, J., & Stuart, G. W. (1992). Psychological adaptation of nurses post-disaster. *Issues in Mental Health Nursing, 13,* 177–190.

Weeks, S. M. (2007). Mobilization of a nursing community after a disaster. *Perspectives in Psychiatric Care, 43*(1), 22–29.

Wenger, D. E., James, T. F., & Faupel, C. E. (1985). *Disaster beliefs and emergency planning.* New York, NY: Irving.

Wilson, J. F. (2006). Health and the environment after Hurricane Katrina. *Annals of Internal Medicine, 144*(2), 153–156.

Wilson, J. S. (1996). Healing Oklahoma's wounds. *Home Healthcare Nurse, 14*(1), 23–25.

Yellowlees, P., & MacKenzie, J. (2003). Telehealth responses to bioterrorism and emerging infections. *Journal of Telemedicine & Telecare,* 9(Suppl 2), S80–S82.

CHAPTER FOCUS

The Problem of Communicable Disease
Transmission of Infectious Agents
- Chain of Infection
- Routes of Infection
- Susceptibility Versus Immunity

Communicable Disease Prevention
- Primary Prevention
- Secondary Prevention
- Tertiary Prevention

Control of Diseases
- Vaccine-Preventable Diseases
- Routine Vaccinations Indicated for Adults

Emerging and Reemerging Infectious Diseases
- Healthcare-Associated Infections
- Food-Borne Diseases
- Vector-Borne Diseases
- Zoonoses
- Hantavirus
- Parasitic Diseases
- Bioterrorism
- HIV/AIDS
- Tuberculosis
- The HIV/TB Connection

Global Disease Eradication Efforts

QUESTIONS TO CONSIDER

After reading this chapter, you will know the answers to the following questions:

1. What is the current infectious disease threat both in the United States and worldwide?
2. What are the reasons for the emergence of new diseases and the reemergence of diseases previously under control?
3. What are the factors that make up the chain of infection?
4. What are the different types of immunity?
5. How do vaccines aid in the prevention of communicable disease?
6. What is the role of the community health nurse in the prevention and treatment of infectious disease?
7. What are the incidence and prevalence of reviewed communicable diseases?

Throughout the world, the eruption and spread of new and old communicable diseases once again threaten the survival of our species.

CHAPTER 20

Communicable and Infectious Disease

Cathy Keen Hughes and
Sharyn Janes

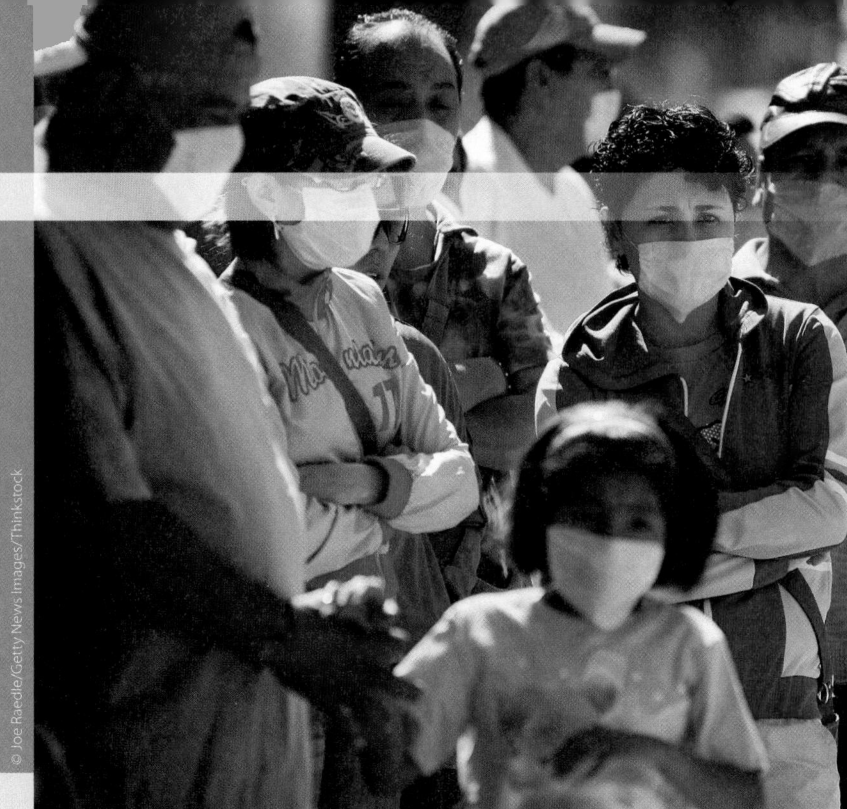

KEY TERMS

acquired immunity
active humoral immunity
agent
fomites
herd immunity
immunity
incubation period
isolation
passive immunity
pathogenicity
period of infectivity
personal surveillance
quarantine
reservoir
segregation
vector
virulence
zoonoses

> The single biggest threat to man's continued dominance on the planet is the virus.
>
> —Joshua Lederberg, Nobel Laureate

> The microbe is nothing; the terrain is everything.
>
> —Louis Pasteur

REFLECTIONS

Many communicable diseases, such as tuberculosis (TB) and syphilis, have made a "comeback" in the United States after many decades of dormancy. What has changed about the "terrain" of infectious diseases in recent years? What is the relationship between culture and communicable disease? How does the continued high rate of AIDS in Africa affect the health of U.S. populations? In this chapter, you will learn about the importance of communicable disease prevention and treatment in community health.

The Problem of Communicable Disease

Communicable disease, or infectious disease, has always been a focus of community health nursing practice. In fact, at the end of the 19th century, when public health nursing emerged as a nursing specialty, communicable diseases were the leading cause of illness and death. During the early years of the 20th century, nurses continued to care for large numbers of adults and children who were sick or dying from a wide variety of infectious diseases. The typhoid epidemic in the early 1900s and the great influenza pandemic of 1918, which killed 20 million people worldwide (Centers for Disease Control and Prevention [CDC], 1998), are just two examples of infectious diseases that caused enormous suffering and death. TB was a leading killer until well into the 1930s and 1940s, when TB sanitariums were overflowing. Nursing students in hospital schools in bigger cities were routinely tested for antibodies against TB, and most of those who came from rural areas tested positive. After a year in the urban hospital wards of the 1930s and 1940s, it was almost a certainty that nursing students would test positive for TB (Garrett, 1994).

CULTURAL CONNECTION

Think about how specific cultural groups define "hygiene." Can a culture's values about food preparation, personal hygiene, and childcare practices influence a group's risk for communicable disease transmission? How can public health nurses intervene appropriately considering a patient's cultural values when teaching about infectious disease control and prevention?

The development of antibiotics, particularly penicillin, in the mid-1940s curbed the spread of bacterial infections and significantly decreased the number of deaths from infectious diseases like TB and typhoid fever. Vaccinations against diseases such as polio, whooping cough, and diphtheria, along with urban sanitation efforts and improved water quality, dramatically lowered the incidence of infectious diseases (CDC, 1998). So although infectious disease still took an enormous toll on the rest of the world, a shift in leading causes of morbidity and mortality from infectious diseases to chronic diseases in industrialized nations like the United States caused attention to be focused on chronic conditions such as heart disease, cancer, and diabetes. Antibiotics became the "wonder drugs" of the latter half of the 20th century, and modern medicine triumphed—or so we thought.

As early as the 1950s, penicillin began to lose its effectiveness against infections caused by *Staphylococcus aureus*. In 1957, and again in 1968, new strains of influenza originating in China rapidly spread throughout the world. During the 1970s, several new diseases were identified in the United States and elsewhere, including Legionnaires' disease, Lyme disease, toxic shock syndrome, and Ebola hemorrhagic fever. The 1980s brought human immunodeficiency virus/acquired immune deficiency syndrome (HIV/AIDS) and a resurgence of TB, which rapidly spread throughout the world. By the 1990s, it was apparent that the threat of infectious disease was again a global reality (CDC, 1998).

Now that we are in the second decade of the 21st century, we are again faced with infectious diseases that challenge medical and nursing practice. Some are old and familiar, like TB and influenza, and others are new and unfamiliar, like Ebola, severe acute respiratory syndrome (SARS), avian flu, and hantavirus. Many of the new challenges are viral in origin, but the overuse and misuse of antibiotics over the last half-century have also caused drug-resistant and often fatal strains of bacterial infections to emerge (**Box 20-1**). Conflict zones, which disrupt access to medical and preventive care and may create mass migrations of people who may wind up living in crowded and unsanitary makeshift refugee camps, can be particular breeding grounds for disease. For example, in October 2013, the World Health Organization (WHO) Global Alert Response (GAR) was alerted to clusters of acute flaccid paralysis (AFP) cases in Syria, which has been the center of significant internal fighting since 2011. This outbreak could represent the first polio cases in Syria since 1999 and is likely directly related to the lapse of access to preventive vaccines due to the Syrian civil war (WHO, 2013a).

BOX 20-1 Facts About Antibiotics and Antibiotic Resistance

- Alexander Fleming, a Scottish scientist, discovered the first antibiotic in 1928.
- Antibiotics became widely available in the 1940s.
- Two million pounds of antibiotics were produced in the United States in 1954. Today, more than 50 million pounds are produced.
- Antibiotics work by either killing bacteria or inhibiting their growth. They do not work on viral infections.
- People consume more than 235 million doses of antibiotics yearly. The CDC estimates that 20% to 50% of that use is unnecessary.
- Antibiotic resistance occurs when bacteria causing a specific infection are not destroyed by the antibiotics taken to halt the infection. Unnecessary and improper use of antibiotics promotes the spread of antibiotic-resistant bacteria.

Source: Data from CDC. (2013a). Vaccines and preventable diseases. Retrieved from http://www.cdc.gov/vaccines/vpd-vac/default.htm

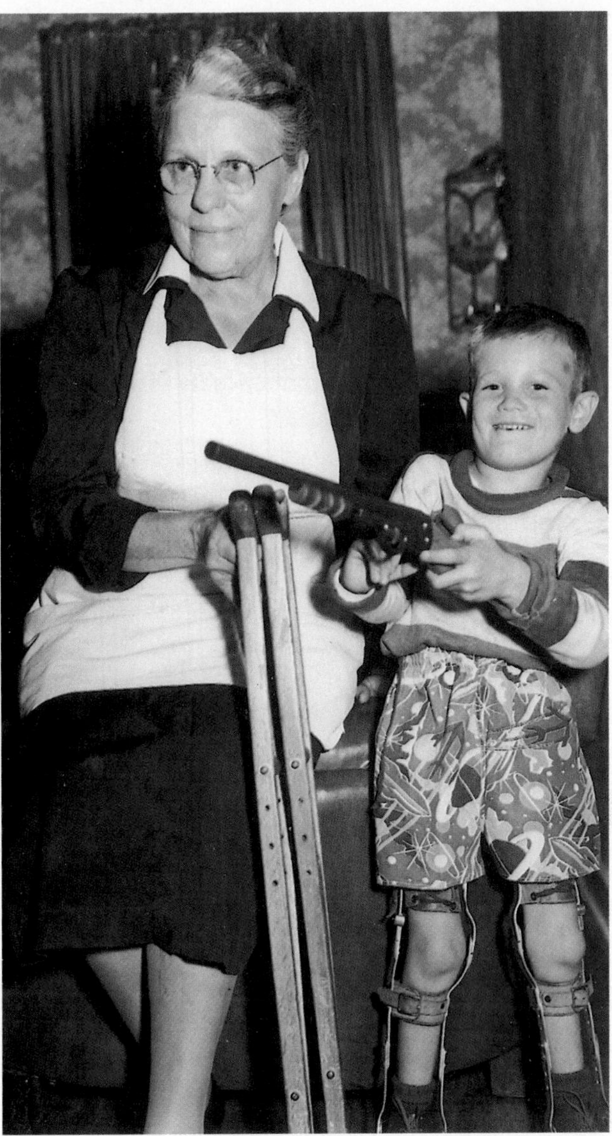

A home visit provided the public health nurse with an opportunity to assess a child with polio in familiar surroundings (circa 1951).

The entire world is becoming much more vulnerable to the eruption and spread of both new and old infectious diseases. Infectious disease is a global problem brought about by recent dramatic increases in the worldwide movement of people, goods, and ideas. Not only are people traveling more, but they are traveling more rapidly and going to more places than ever before (Mann, 1994). The United Nations (UN, 2013) estimates that there are over 232 million international migrants worldwide. Every year more than 800 million people travel by air (U.S. Department of Transportation, 2013). At least 66 million people from around the world visit the United States each year. Currently, more than 17 million people throughout the world die each year from infectious diseases (Fauci, Touchette, & Folkers, 2005), with children disproportionately impacted. Some of the contributing factors are the emergence of new diseases, reemergence of diseases previously thought to have been contained, mass population shifts, and economic and social globalization. Control of many of these emerging and reemerging infectious diseases has become a global public health problem because of the lack of new, effective vaccines and therapeutic drugs, or because drugs that offered successful treatment in the past have become resistant to new strains of existing microorganisms (Heymann, 2004).

> In the old days, our neighbors were Canada and Mexico. Nowadays, with the frequency and speed of air travel, our neighbors are Sri Lanka and Paraguay, you name it.
>
> —*Jeffrey Koplan, Former CDC Director*

To address the increasing threat of infectious diseases, nurses must understand the problem from global and historical perspectives. There are many roles for nurses in the battle against infectious diseases. From a community health nursing perspective, primary and secondary prevention concepts must guide nursing practice. A holistic approach that includes health education, environmental health, political action, human rights, and cultural competency is the key. Communicable disease is, after all, not a new concept. Microbes have been an enemy of humans since ancient times. They did not disappear just because science developed drugs and vaccines or because Europeans and Americans cleaned up their cities and towns, and they certainly will not go away when humans choose to ignore or downplay their existence (Garrett, 1994). This chapter describes the present-day threat of infectious diseases and explores the role of community health nurses. Selected objectives related to communicable diseases are provided in the *Healthy People 2020* box.

HEALTHY PEOPLE 2020 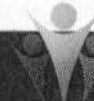

Objectives Related to Communicable Diseases

Education

- ECBP-2.7 Increase the proportion of elementary, middle, and senior high schools that provide comprehensive school health education to prevent health problems in unintended pregnancy, HIV/AIDS, and STD infection
- ECBP-7.8 Increase the proportion of college and university students who receive information from their institution on HIV/AIDS and sexually transmitted infections

Food Safety

- FS-1 Reduce infections caused by key pathogens transmitted commonly through food
- FS-2 Reduce the number of outbreak-associated infections due to Shiga toxin-producing *Escherichia coli* O157, or *Campylobacter*, *Listeria*, or *Salmonella* species associated with food commodity groups
- FS-3 Prevent an increase in the proportion of nontyphoidal *Salmonella* and *Campylobacter jejuni* isolates from humans that are resistant to antimicrobial drugs
- FS-4 Reduce severe allergic reactions to food among adults with a food allergy diagnosis
- FS-5 Increase the proportion of consumers who follow key food safety practices
- FS-6 Improve food safety practices associated with foodborne illness in foodservice and retail establishments

Healthcare-Associated Infections

- HAI-1 Reduce central line–associated bloodstream infections (CLABSIs)
- HAI-2 Reduce invasive healthcare-associated methicillin-resistant *Staphylococcus aureus* (MRSA) infections

HIV

Diagnosis of HIV Infection and AIDS

- HIV-1 Reduce new HIV diagnoses among adolescents and adults
- HIV-2 Reduce new (incident) HIV infections among adolescents and adults
- HIV-3 Reduce the rate of HIV transmission among adolescents and adults
- HIV-8 Reduce perinatally acquired HIV and AIDS cases

Death, Survival, and Medical Health Care After Diagnosis of HIV Infection and AIDS

- HIV-9 Increase the proportion of new HIV infections diagnosed before progression to AIDS
- HIV-10 Increase the proportion of HIV-infected adolescents and adults who receive HIV care and treatment consistent with current standards
- HIV-11 Increase the proportion of persons surviving more than 3 years after a diagnosis with AIDS
- HIV-12 Reduce deaths from HIV infection

HIV Testing

- HIV-13 Increase the proportion of persons living with HIV who know their serostatus
- HIV-14 Increase the proportion of adolescents and adults who have been tested for HIV in the past 12 months
- HIV-15 Increase the proportion of adults with tuberculosis (TB) who have been tested for HIV

HIV Prevention

- HIV-16 Increase the proportion of substance abuse treatment facilities that offer HIV/AIDS education, counseling, and support
- HIV-17 Increase the proportion of sexually active persons who use condoms
- HIV-18 Reduce the proportion of men who have sex with men (MSM) who reported unprotected anal sex in the past 12 months

Immunization and Infectious Diseases

- IID-1 Reduce, eliminate, or maintain elimination of cases of vaccine-preventable diseases
- IID-2 Reduce early onset group B streptococcal disease
- IID-3 Reduce meningococcal disease
- IID-4 Reduce invasive pneumococcal infections
- IID-5 Reduce the number of courses of antibiotics for ear infections for young children
- IID-6 Reduce the number of courses of antibiotics prescribed for the sole diagnosis of the common cold
- IID-7 Achieve and maintain effective vaccination coverage levels for universally recommended vaccines among young children
- IID-8 Increase the percentage of children aged 19 to 35 months who receive the recommended doses of DTaP, polio, MMR, Hib, hepatitis B, varicella, and pneumococcal conjugate vaccines

- IID-9 Decrease the percentage of children in the United States who receive 0 doses of recommended vaccines by age 19 to 35 months
- IID-10 Maintain vaccination coverage levels for children in kindergarten
- IID-11 Increase routine vaccination coverage levels for adolescents
- IID-12 Increase the percentage of children and adults who are vaccinated annually against seasonal influenza
- IID-13 Increase the percentage of adults who are vaccinated against pneumococcal disease
- IID-14 Increase the percentage of adults who are vaccinated against zoster (shingles)
- IID-15 Increase hepatitis B vaccine coverage among high-risk populations
- IID-16 Increase the scientific knowledge on vaccine safety and adverse events
- IID-17 Increase the percentage of providers who have had vaccination coverage levels among children in their practice population measured within the past year
- IID-18 Increase the percentage of children under 6 years of age whose immunization records are in a fully operational, population-based immunization information system (IIS)
- IID-19 Increase the number of states collecting kindergarten vaccination coverage data according to CDC minimum standards
- IID-20 Increase the number of states that have 80% of adolescents with two or more age-appropriate immunizations recorded in an IIS among adolescents aged 11 to 18 years
- IID-21 Increase the number of states that use electronic data from rabies animal surveillance to inform public health prevention programs
- IID-22 Increase the number of public health laboratories monitoring influenza virus resistance to antiviral agents
- IID-23 Reduce hepatitis A
- IID-24 Reduce chronic hepatitis B virus infections in infants and young children (perinatal infections)
- IID-25 Reduce hepatitis B
- IID-26 Reduce new hepatitis C infections
- IID-27 Increase the proportion of persons aware they have a hepatitis C infection
- IID-28 Increase the proportion of persons who have been tested for hepatitis B virus within minority communities experiencing health disparities
- IID-29 Reduce tuberculosis (TB)
- IID-30 Increase treatment completion rate of all tuberculosis patients who are eligible to complete therapy
- IID-31 Increase the percentage of contacts to sputum smear–positive tuberculosis cases who complete treatment after being diagnosed with latent tuberculosis infection (LTBI) and initiated treatment for LTBI
- IID-32 Increase the proportion of culture-confirmed TB patients with a positive nucleic acid amplification test (NAAT) result reported within 2 days of specimen collection

Source: U.S. Department of Health and Human Services. (2013). *Healthy People 2020: Topics and Objectives A-Z.* Retrieved from http://healthypeople.gov/2020/topicsobjectives2020/default.aspx

ENVIRONMENTAL CONNECTION

How you travel can make you sick!

Infectious disease outbreaks aboard commercial cruise ships have become increasingly common. The CDC (2014a) has documented more than two decades' worth of incidents, usually involving diarrheal diseases. Transmission occurs via a number of routes: by food and person-to-person contact, as well as persistence of virus despite sanitization onboard, including introductions of new strains and seeding of an outbreak on land. Increased awareness of the problem—not to mention adverse publicity that affects the carriers when outbreaks occur—has led to intensified efforts to combat disease outbreaks, including significant procedural updates to the Vessel Sanitation Program (VSP) Operations Manual in 2011 (CDC, 2014a). Nevertheless, each year dozens of ships carrying 100 or more passengers experience an illness outbreak; four such outbreaks were recorded in the first two months of 2014 alone. The causative organisms in the vast majority of cases are Noroviruses (NoV), which have been positively identified in 82% of cases since 2010 and are potentially implicated in an additional 12% of cases where the pathogen involved is unknown (CDC, 2014a).

Noroviruses are the most common cause of infectious acute gastroenteritis and are transmitted feco-orally through food and water, directly from person to person, and by environmental contamination. These viruses are often responsible for protracted outbreaks in closed settings, such as cruise ships, nursing homes, and hospitals.

Although illness outbreaks on cruise ships were not unknown prior to 2002, that year had an unusually high level of disease outbreak incidence. According to the CDC's (2014a) Vessel Sanitation Program data, 21 separate incidents of cruise ship illness outbreaks involving 16 different ships from 11 different cruise lines were recorded for the year—more than five times the 2001 count. A 2005 study described one particularly tenacious outbreak in which a cruise ship recorded an elevated number of persons with acute gastroenteritis symptoms reporting to the ship's infirmary (84 [4%] of 2,318 passengers) during a 7-day vacation cruise from Florida to the Caribbean in November 2002 (Isakbaeva et al., 2005). According to federal regulations, when the incidence of acute gastroenteritis among passengers and crew exceeds 3%, an outbreak is declared and requires a formal

(continues)

ENVIRONMENTAL CONNECTION (*continued*)

investigation. The outbreak continued on the subsequent cruise (cruise 2), after which the vessel was removed from service for 1 week of aggressive sanitization. Despite cleaning, gastroenteritis also developed in 192 (8%) of 2,456 passengers and 23 (2.3%) of 999 crew members on the following cruise (cruise 3).

Epidemiologists began an investigation on cruise 1 and collected stool specimens from persons with gastroenteritis on this cruise and the next five cruises. All 2,318 passengers on cruise 1 were surveyed to determine dates of illness onset, symptoms, cabin locations, activities, and food consumption. Additionally, a sanitary inspection of the ship was performed. A case-control design was used, and all passengers in whom illness developed early in the cruise (days 3 and 4) after embarkation (defined as day 1) and with passengers who became ill later (day 5) were included in the study. Controls were systematically selected among passengers who reported no symptoms of gastroenteritis throughout the entire cruise. The number of acute gastroenteritis cases on the subsequent five cruises was monitored, and researchers collected fecal specimens from ill persons on all six cruises. During the shipboard investigation, researchers also obtained stool specimens from ill persons in a long-term care facility affected by an outbreak of acute gastroenteritis, in which the index patient was a passenger who returned ill to the facility after disembarking from a cruise.

In this investigation, epidemiological analysis suggested an initial food-borne source of infection with subsequent secondary spread from person to person, while molecular analysis provided several new insights into disease transmission. Application of genetic sequencing documented persistence of the same strain onboard between cruises by detecting identical sequences in stool samples from ill passengers before and after 1 week of the vessel's cleaning. Although these findings suggest that environmental contamination may have helped perpetuate the outbreak, infected crew members could have also been a reservoir of infection between cruises.

Molecular fingerprinting of detected viruses confirmed several introductions of new strains aboard, which underscores the difficulty in controlling outbreaks of NoV on cruise ships. Sequence analysis provided evidence that an outbreak of NoV in the care facility was caused by a person returning ill from an outbreak-affected cruise.

Like other outbreaks of viral gastroenteritis on cruise ships, this outbreak affected several hundred people, was transmitted by multiple modes, and recurred on subsequent cruises. Multiple routes of NoV transmission have been documented in other reports, such as that of an outbreak of gastroenteritis among football players, in which initial food-borne transmission of virus and secondary person-to-person spread were demonstrated. Outbreaks of gastroenteritis aboard cruise ships are similar to those in other closed and crowded settings where identifying and interrupting multiple routes of transmission have proved particularly challenging.

This investigation suggested that efforts to control gastroenteritis outbreaks on cruise ships should address all possible modes of NoV transmission, including food-borne, environmental persistence, and person-to-person spread. Such measures should include extensive disinfection, good food-and-water-handling practices, isolating ill persons, providing paid sick leave for ill crew, and promoting handwashing with soap and water among passengers and crew. Developing strategies and incentives to dissuade symptomatic passengers from boarding may also minimize opportunities to introduce new strains aboard. Cruise ship outbreaks with less than 3% of passengers reporting ill should be considered for investigation because they may contribute substantial information on the transmission and epidemiological characteristics of NoV, which could be used to develop control strategies and prevent future outbreaks on land and at sea.

Sources: Centers for Disease Control and Prevention (CDC). (2014a). Vessel Sanitation Program. Retrieved from http://www.cdc.gov/nceh/vsp/default.htm; Isakbaeva, E. T., Widdowson, M.-A., Beard, R. S., Bulens, S. N., Mullins, J., Monroe, S. S., ... Glass, R. I. (2005, January). Norovirus transmission on cruise ship. *Emerging Infectious Disease, 11*(1). Retrieved from http://www.cdc.gov/ncidod/EID/vol11no01/04-0434.htm

MEDIA MOMENT 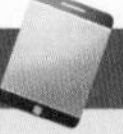

Plague Among the Magnolias: The 1878 Yellow Fever Epidemic in Mississippi (2009)

By Deanne Stephens Nuwer, Tuscaloosa, AL: The University of Alabama Press

This book explores the social, political, racial, and economic consequences of the 1878 yellow fever epidemic in Mississippi. A mild winter, a long spring, and a torrid summer produced conditions favoring the *Aedes aegypti* mosquito and its spread of yellow fever.

Transmission of Infectious Agents

The role of nurses in the control of infectious disease through prevention and treatment is based on an understanding of ways in which diseases are transmitted from one person to another. *Transmission* is "any mechanism by which an infectious agent is spread from a source or reservoir to a person" (Benenson, 1995, p. 544). There are three general modes of transmission: direct, indirect, and airborne. The importance of handwashing in any environment cannot be stressed enough. Following guidelines for handwashing with soap and water as well as the appropriate use of hand sanitizer is an example of a way to decrease transmission to others. Using soap and water with handwashing is the preferred intervention, especially if *Clostridium difficile* is the known or suspected organism, because alcohol-based products do not kill *C. difficile* spores (CDC, 2012a; Cohen et al., 2010).

Chain of Infection

The chain of infection is defined as the minimum requirements for an infectious or communicable disease to occur. Six factors make up the chain of infection: (1) an etiological agent or pathogen, (2) a source or reservoir of infection, (3) a means of escape from the source or reservoir (portal of exit), (4) a mode of transmission, (5) a portal of entry into the new host, and (6) a susceptible host.

The causative **agent** or pathogen is any substance or factor that can cause disease. Agents may be bacteria, virus particles, chemicals, or any other plant or animal substance that can cause illness, disease, disability, or death. Causative agents differ both in their ability to cause disease and in their ability to cause serious illness. **Pathogenicity** refers to the agent's capacity to cause disease in an infected host, whereas **virulence** defines the ability of the agent to produce serious illness. For example, both botulism and *Salmonella* are highly pathogenic agents (they can easily cause disease), but botulism is much more virulent (it causes more severe disease).

The source of infection, or **reservoir**, is the habitat or medium in which the agent lives and/or multiplies. Reservoirs can be living things (e.g., humans, animals, insects) or inanimate objects (e.g., food, intravenous [IV] fluids, feces, surgical instruments, stuffed animals) that are conducive to the maintenance or growth of the agent. Reservoirs of infection are human beings, animals, and environmental sources. Humans become reservoirs of infection when the infectious agent has entered the body and established itself. There are three levels of infection in humans: (1) colonization, (2) inapparent infection, and (3) clinically overt disease.

Colonization occurs when the agent is present on the surface of the body or in the nasopharynx and multiplies at a rate sufficient to maintain its numbers without producing any identifiable evidence of a reaction in the person. Inapparent infection (subclinical infection) occurs when the agent is not only present but multiplies in the human reservoir. In an inapparent infection, the agent causes a measurable reaction; however, it does not cause the human to have symptoms of illness. Inapparent infections are usually identified only through laboratory testing (Benenson, 1995; Merrill & Timmreck, 2013). Finally, clinical disease occurs when the agent is present in the human and causes physical symptoms. The time interval between initial contact with an infectious agent and the first appearance of disease symptoms is the **incubation period** (Benenson, 1995). The communicable period, or **period of infectivity**, is the time during which an infectious agent may be transferred directly or indirectly from an infected person to another person, from an infected animal to humans, or from an infected person to animals. All infected persons, including those with colonization, are reservoirs for the agent. Animal reservoirs are mainly domestic animals and rodents.

Zoonoses are animal diseases that are transmissible to humans under natural conditions. Animals transmit the disease directly to humans, but these diseases usually are not transmitted from human to human. Examples of zoonoses are bovine TB, rabies (although theoretically it can be transmitted by humans), and anthrax. Environmental reservoirs also transmit directly to humans. An example of an environmental reservoir is hookworm in soil. Inanimate objects such as food, surgical instruments, and human feces can also be reservoirs for diseases.

The agent leaves the reservoir through a portal of exit. Portals of exit and portals of entrance are similar. They include the following: respiratory, oral, gastrointestinal, reproductive, IV, urinary, skin, conjunctival, and transplacental (Merrill & Timmreck, 2013).

The last factor in the chain of infection is a susceptible host. The agent must enter a human host who is vulnerable to the specific disease agent. Susceptibility can be related to factors such as age, immunological status, lifestyle habits, or the presence of other infectious diseases or chronic illnesses.

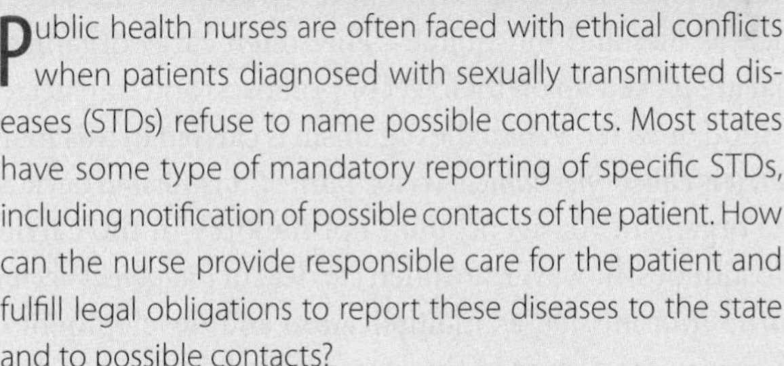

ETHICAL CONNECTION

Public health nurses are often faced with ethical conflicts when patients diagnosed with sexually transmitted diseases (STDs) refuse to name possible contacts. Most states have some type of mandatory reporting of specific STDs, including notification of possible contacts of the patient. How can the nurse provide responsible care for the patient and fulfill legal obligations to report these diseases to the state and to possible contacts?

Routes of Infection

The agent then must be transmitted to the next susceptible host through a mode of transmission. Transmission can be direct, indirect, or airborne (see **Table 20-1**).

Direct transmission consists of the direct and immediate transfer of an infectious agent from one infected host or reservoir to a portal of entry in the new host. This may be through direct contact that occurs through biting, kissing, or sexual intercourse or by direct projection of droplet spray into the conjunctiva of the eye or mucous membranes

TABLE 20-1 Classification of Major Infectious Diseases by Mode of Transmission

Airborne Respiratory Diseases	Intestinal Discharge Diseases	Open Sores or Lesion Diseases	Zoonoses or Vector-Borne Diseases	Fomite-Borne Diseases
Chickenpox	Amoebic dysentery	AIDS	African sleeping sickness	Anthrax
Common colds	Bacterial dysentery (shigellosis) (staphylococcal)	Anthrax		Chickenpox
Diphtheria		Erysipelas	Encephalitis	Common colds
Influenza		Human papillomavirus	Lyme disease	Diphtheria
Measles	Cholera	Gonorrhea	Malaria	Influenza
Meningitis	Giardiasis	Scarlet fever	Rocky Mountain spotted fever	Meningitis
Pneumonia	Hepatitis	Smallpox		Poliomyelitis
Poliomyelitis	Hookworm	Syphilis	Tularemia	Rubella
Rubella	Poliomyelitis	Tuberculosis	Typhus fever	Scarlet fever
Scarlet fever	Salmonellosis	Tularemia	Yellow fever	Streptococcal throat infections
Smallpox	Typhoid fever			
Throat infections	Poliomyelitis			
Tuberculosis			Tuberculosis	
Whooping cough				

Source: Merrill, R. M., & Timmreck, T. C. (2013). *Introduction to epidemiology* (6th ed.). Burlington, MA: Jones & Bartlett Learning.

of the eye, nose, or mouth. The projection of droplet spray occurs with sneezing, coughing, talking, singing, or spitting and is usually limited to a distance of approximately 1 meter (Benenson, 1995; Merrill & Timmreck, 2013).

Indirect transmission usually occurs through a vector or by a vehicle. A vector is some form of living organism, usually an animal or an arthropod. Arthropods are insects such as flies and mosquitoes. Flies often carry organisms that are picked up on their feet or proboscis and transferred to food or water. When the organism is carried in this manner, it is called *mechanical vector-borne transmission* because the organism (or agent) does not multiply in the carrier. Mosquitoes, however, are often carriers of *biological vector-borne transmission* as multiplication and development of the organism occurs in the mosquito before the organism is transmitted to the new host through a bite (or inoculation). An example of this type of vector-borne disease is the transmission of malaria via the bite of a mosquito.

Vehicle-borne transmission is defined as transmission via contaminated inanimate objects, called **fomites**, which serve as an intermediate means by which an infectious agent is transported and introduced into a susceptible host through an appropriate portal of entry (Benenson, 1995; Merrill & Timmreck, 2013). Examples of fomites are toys, bedding, soiled clothes, surgical instruments, and contaminated IV fluids. An example of a vehicle-borne disease is *Salmonella,* which can be transmitted from a kitchen countertop contaminated while thawing raw chicken for dinner.

Airborne transmission occurs through droplet nuclei and dust, which are particles suspended in the air in which microorganisms may be present. Droplet nuclei result from the evaporation of fluid from droplets disseminated by coughing, talking, or sneezing between one infected person and another host. Droplet nuclei can remain suspended in the air for long periods in a dry state. During this time, some droplet nuclei retain their infectivity, while others lose their infectivity or virulence. The particles are very small and are easily breathed into the lungs, where they are retained. When these particles reach the terminal air passages, they begin to multiply and an infection begins in the new host (Benenson, 1995; Merrill & Timmreck, 2013). Pulmonary TB and legionellosis (Legionnaires' disease) are two illnesses that are transmitted by droplet nuclei.

Dust particles in which microorganisms may be present can also become airborne and thus can be breathed into the lungs and cause infection. Contaminated bedding and clothes are examples of objects that can create dust that may carry infectious microorganisms from one infected person to another host. Dust particles contaminated with deer mouse feces may be one way to transmit hantavirus to human hosts.

The cycle of transmission can be broken by breaking the chain of infection—by eliminating the agent, eliminating the reservoir of infection, eliminating transmission at the portal of exit or the portal of entry, or eliminating susceptible hosts.

Susceptibility Versus Immunity

For a disease to be transmitted, the new host must be susceptible to that disease. The concept of immunity forms the basis of understanding host resistance to disease. **Immunity** is the increased resistance on the part of the host to a specific infectious agent (Valanis, 1999). There are two types of acquired immunity found in humans: active and passive (Atkinson & Wolfe, 2003).

Acquired immunity can occur after having had the disease or through vaccination. If a person is infected with the disease (with or without clinical signs and symptoms), the disease agent stimulates the body's natural immune system. However, if the person is inoculated with the agent (in a killed, modified, or variant form), the vaccination artificially stimulates the immune system (see **Box 20-2** for a list of vaccine-preventable diseases). Both methods of acquired immunity result in active humoral immunity because the human body produces its own antibodies when the immune system is stimulated. **Active humoral immunity** is based on a B-lymphocyte response, which results in immunity that lasts for several years with diseases such as tetanus or a lifetime with diseases such as measles or mumps (Atkinson & Wolfe, 2003; Benenson, 1995). **Passive immunity** can be acquired either through the transplacental transfer of the mother's immunity to a disease to her unborn child or from the transfer of already-produced antibodies into a susceptible person (such as the use of immune serum globulin for persons exposed to hepatitis A). Passive immunity is based on a cellular, T-lymphocyte sensitization. Passive immunity is of short duration, lasting from days to months (Benenson, 1995; Merrill & Timmreck, 2013).

Herd immunity is the resistance of a population or group to the invasion and spread of an infectious agent (Benenson, 1995; Merrill & Timmreck, 2013). Herd immunity is based on the level of resistance a population has to a communicable disease because of the high proportion of group members in the population who cannot get the disease because they have been previously vaccinated (see **Box 20-3** for a list of potential new vaccines) or have previously had the disease. Jonas Salk, one of the developers of the polio vaccine, suggested that if 85% of the population were immunized against polio (the herd immunity level), a polio epidemic would not occur (Merrill & Timmreck, 1998). Herd immunity provides barriers to the direct transmission of infection through a group or population, because the lack of susceptible individuals in the population stops the spread of infection.

BOX 20-2 Vaccine-Preventable Diseases

Anthrax	Pertussis
Cervical cancer (HPV)	Pneumococcal pneumonia
Chickenpox (varicella)	Polio
Diphtheria	Rabies
Haemophilus influenzae	Rotavirus
Hepatitis A	Rubella
Hepatitis B	Shingles (Herpes zoster)
Influenza	Smallpox
Japanese encephalitis	Swine flu (H1N1)
Lyme disease	Tetanus
Measles	Typhoid
Meningococcal infections	Tuberculosis
Mumps	Yellow fever

Source: Data from CDC. (2013a). Vaccines and preventable diseases. Retrieved from http://www.cdc.gov/vaccines/vpd-vac/default.htm

Communicable Disease Prevention

One of the foundations of public health is the prevention and control of communicable disease. Merrill & Timmreck (1998) states that the three key factors in the control of communicable disease are as follows:

1. The removal, elimination, or containment of the cause or source of infection
2. The disruption and blockage of the chain of disease transmission
3. The protection of the susceptible population from infection and disease

Approaches to the control of communicable disease should be based on the levels of prevention—primary, secondary, and tertiary.

BOX 20-3 Vaccines 2010–2014

- Group B Streptococci with perinatal morbidity and mortality
- Vaccines for Alzheimer's disease
- Vaccines against smallpox and anthrax
- HIV vaccine
- DNA vaccine focused on parasitic diseases
- Alternate approaches to delivery of vaccines (intramuscular, intradermal, intranasal, etc.)

Source: Immunization Action Coalition. (2014). Potential New Vaccines 2014–2010. Retrieved from http://www.immunize.org/journalarticles/toi_poten.asp

Primary Prevention

Primary prevention activities are targeted at intervening before the agent enters the host and causes pathological changes. This level of prevention attempts to increase the host's resistance, inactivate the agent (source of infection), or interrupt the chain of infection.

A major focus of primary prevention is on increasing the resistance of the host. This can be accomplished through health education and/or immunization. Health education can target many subjects to increase the resistance of the host. It can identify a variety of activities that will improve the host's resistance, such as frequent handwashing, proper nutrition, adequate rest, and proper attire. Immunization is another method of primary prevention that increases the host's resistance. Education of the public by the news media as an early warning to avoid contaminated foods is considered primary prevention if the individual or population of an area has not consumed the food.

Immunization uses vaccines that are obtained either from the agent in a killed, modified, or variant form or from fractions or products of the agent (Merrill & Timmreck, 2013; Valanis, 1999). Vaccines are available for many common infectious diseases. See Box 20-2 for a list of vaccine-preventable diseases and Box 20-3 for vaccines in development.

Inactivating the agent involves stopping the agent by chemical or physical means. The protection of food has become particularly important in the last few years, with frequent food-borne illness outbreaks occurring as a result of improper storage, preparation, and handling. Proper temperatures must be maintained to inactivate the agent when storing, preparing, and cooking food. Proper food handling, which includes handwashing during preparation, is also important. Many bacterial agents (e.g., staphylococci, salmonellae, and *E. coli*) can contaminate food and make the consumers of the food extremely sick. Irradiation of food (particularly beef and vegetables) has been suggested as a method of control, but this continues to be vigorously debated. Chemical methods are also used to inactivate agents. Chemical methods are used to chlorinate water supplies and to treat sewage, as well as to disinfect infectious or potentially infectious materials.

A common method of breaking the chain of infection is environmental control. Environmental control is aimed at providing clean and safe air, food, milk, and water; managing solid waste (garbage) and liquid waste (sewage); and controlling vectors (insects and rodents). Environmental control may target the reservoir, such as chlorination of a water supply. Environmental control may also be aimed at destroying the vector that transports the agent. One way a community may target the vector is to spray swamp areas (known to serve as reservoirs) with an insecticide to prevent mosquito-borne viral encephalitis. However, when this method is used, care must be taken to preserve the ecosystem as much as possible. Another method of breaking the chain of transmission is to encourage good personal hygiene and use of protective clothing. Methicillin-resistant *S. aureus* (MRSA) is an increasingly difficult nosocomial infection seen on medical and surgical floors in hospitals and in nursing homes. Healthcare providers must protect themselves and their patients by using proper hygiene and standard precautions when caring for all patients. Structural changes in public restrooms, such as eliminating entrance doors and providing automated faucets and hand-dryers, reduce the opportunity for the host to have contact with an agent.

Primary prevention also includes restricting the spread of infection to human reservoirs and preventing the spread to other susceptible human hosts (Valanis, 1999). The four most commonly used methods are isolation, quarantine, segregation, and personal surveillance.

Isolation is the separation of infected persons during the period of communicability (Benenson, 1995; Merrill & Timmreck, 2013; Valanis, 1999). These infected persons may be under one of several different types of isolation: strict isolation, contact isolation, respiratory isolation, TB isolation, enteric precautions, and drainage/secretion precautions.

Quarantine is the restriction of healthy persons who have been exposed to a person with a communicable disease during the period of communicability. These persons are considered contacts of the infected human host. Quarantine prevents further transmission of the disease during the incubation period if the healthy contacts should become infected. Quarantine usually occurs for the longest usual incubation period of the disease. Quarantine is rarely if ever used today; however, before vaccination for diphtheria, it was often used in the United States.

Segregation is another method to control the spread of communicable disease. It is used to separate and observe a group of people who are infected with a specific disease. Segregation has been used in some countries to separate HIV-infected individuals from the general public in an effort to control the spread of AIDS. The United States still has public health laws that allow the segregation of persons with TB; however, those laws are rarely enforced, although in the early part of the 20th century, persons with TB were segregated from the general public in hospitals known as *sanitariums*. With the advent of new drug therapies and treatment, these sanitariums are no longer necessary.

Personal surveillance is close medical or other supervision of contacts and identified carriers of a specific disease without restricting their personal movement (Benenson, 1995). For example, public health officials continue to require personal surveillance of persons known to have had TB and to be carriers of typhoid.

As distinct from personal surveillance, disease surveillance is the continuing investigation of the incidence and spread of a disease relevant to effective control (Benenson, 1995). Public health surveillance is the systematic collection, analysis, interpretation, dissemination, and use of health information. Surveillance and data systems provide information on morbidity, mortality, and disability. Surveillance information is used to plan, implement, and evaluate public health programs to control communicable disease. To provide maximum benefits, surveillance data must be accurate, timely, and available in useful form (Merrill & Timmreck, 2013; U.S. Department of Health and Human Services [HHS], 1991).

Although successful disease surveillance involves collaboration among federal, state, and local agencies, the U.S. Public Health Service (PHS) takes a leading role. PHS activities include collecting and analyzing health information at the national, regional, and, when possible, state and local levels; providing data to federal, state, and local agencies for further analysis or use; assisting states and local agencies in conducting public health surveillance and evaluating data; and coordinating a network of federal, state, and local public health surveillance for diseases of public health importance (HHS, 1991). Since 1961, the CDC has been collecting and publishing data on nationally reportable diseases. While reporting of communicable diseases at the national level is voluntary, reporting communicable diseases at the state level is required. Each state health department determines which diseases are reportable in order to address state-specific issues (Merrill & Timmreck, 2013). Infectious diseases that are currently reported by most states are presented in **Table 20-2**. State health departments require physicians, dentists, nurses, allied health practitioners, and medical examiners to report any disease listed as reportable by their specific state. Some states may require that any reportable diseases also be reported by laboratory directors and administrators of hospitals, clinics, nursing homes, schools, and nurseries. Several social media sources and apps are available for mobile devices for tracking SARS, TB, influenza, and general use (CDC, 2013b).

Secondary Prevention

Secondary prevention activities are targeted at detecting disease at the earliest possible time to begin treatment, stop progression, and initiate primary prevention activities to protect others in the community (Merrill & Timmreck, 2013). Secondary prevention in infectious disease contributes to primary prevention because it restricts the infection to the human reservoir and prevents its spread to other susceptible individuals. Case finding and health screening are common activities used to accomplish this task. An example of case finding is following up on food handlers who may be infected during an outbreak of hepatitis. Screening for new cases of diseases can significantly decrease the spread of infection. Examples include screening for TB through tuberculin testing to detect and treat cases of TB among new immigrants, screening for herpes simplex virus type 2 in pregnant women to prevent infection of the infant during the birth process, screening for several sexually transmitted infections (STIs) as a requirement for marriage licenses in some states, and administering gamma-globulin or immune serum after exposure to hepatitis. Surveillance of disease and early detection of an outbreak of communicable diseases are also considered secondary prevention measures. Examining the outbreak from an epidemiological standpoint is important to determine any factors that may have changed within the agent, host, or the environment in which the disease occurred. This is applicable to the individual, population, and system levels.

Health education also plays a significant role in secondary prevention, because it provides education about signs and symptoms, which enables individuals to identify illness and seek care early. Knowledge of health risk behaviors that contribute to the spread of disease may influence infected individuals to modify their behavior and thus assist in the prevention of the spread of disease.

GLOBAL CONNECTION

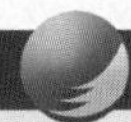

An influenza pandemic of the type that ravaged the globe in 1918 and 1919 could kill as many as 62 million people today, with 96% of the deaths occurring in developing countries, according to WHO. The illness caused by the 1918 virus was largely untreatable. There were no antiviral drugs, no mechanical ventilators to help people breathe, and no antibiotics to treat bacterial pneumonias that often set in after the viral infection. All are available now and would reduce the death toll, although some interventions would be in short supply during a pandemic.

Historical accounts suggest that what became known as Spanish flu emerged at an Army camp in Kansas in early March 1918 and was carried to Europe by American troops. The infection circulated in Europe before undergoing a change early the next fall that made it unusually lethal. It spread around the world and was brought back to the United States, where it killed hundreds of thousands of Americans in October and November 1919. The disease continued to circulate until early 1920, with virtually everyone on Earth eventually being exposed to the virus.

The global death toll from the pandemic is unknown, though rough estimates put mortality in the range of 50 to 100 million.

Sources: Barry, J. (2004). *The great influenza: The epic story of the 1918 pandemic*. New York, NY: Viking Publications; PBS film series: The American experience. (1998). *Influenza 1918*. Retrieved from http://www.pbs.org/wgbh/amex/influenza/

TABLE 20-2 Nationally Notifiable Infectious Conditions in the United States, 2014

Anthrax	Meningococcal disease
Arboviral diseases, neuroinvasive and non-neuroinvasive	Mumps
Babesiosis	Novel influenza A virus infections
Botulism	Pertussis
Brucellosis	Plague
Chancroid	Poliomyelitis, paralytic
Chlamydia trachomatis infection	Poliovirus infection, nonparalytic
Cholera	Psittacosis
Coccidioidomycosis	Q fever
Congenital syphilis*	Rabies, animal
Cryptosporidiosis	Rabies, human
Cyclosporiasis	Rubella
Dengue virus infections	Rubella, congenital syndrome
Diphtheria	Salmonellosis
Ehrlichiosis and anaplasmosis	Severe acute respiratory syndrome–associated coronavirus disease
Giardiasis	
Gonorrhea	Shiga toxin-producing *Escherichia coli*
Haemophilus influenzae, invasive disease	Shigellosis
Hansen's disease	Smallpox
Hantavirus pulmonary syndrome	Spotted fever rickettsiosis
Hemolytic uremic syndrome, post-diarrheal	Streptococcal toxic-shock syndrome
Hepatitis A, acute	Syphilis*
Hepatitis B, acute	Tetanus
Hepatitis B, chronic	Toxic shock syndrome (other than streptococcal)
Hepatitis B, perinatal infection	Trichinellosis
Hepatitis C, acute	Tuberculosis
Hepatitis C, past or present	Tularemia
HIV infection (AIDS has been reclassified as HIV Stage III)	Typhoid fever
Influenza-associated pediatric mortality	Vancomycin-intermediate *Staphylococcus aureus* and vancomycin-resistant *Staphylococcus aureus*
Invasive pneumococcal disease	
Legionellosis	Varicella
Leptospirosis	Varicella deaths
Listeriosis	Vibriosis
Lyme disease	Viral hemorrhagic fever
Malaria	Yellow fever
Measles	

*Beginning January 1, 2014, Congenital Syphilis and Syphilis appear as separate categories of conditions, whereas previously they were combined within the Syphilis category.

Source: Data from CDC. (2014b). National Notifiable Diseases Surveillance System (NNDSS): 2014 National notifiable infectious conditions. Retrieved from http://wwwn.cdc.gov/NNDSS/script/ConditionList.aspx?Type=0&Yr=2014

Tertiary Prevention

Tertiary prevention limits the progression of disability (Merrill & Timmreck, 2013; Merill & Timmreck, 1998). Hearing impairment from frequent ear infections, paralyzed limbs from polio, impaired vision from severe conjunctivitis, and shingles are just a few of the possible disabilities resulting from infectious disease. Treatment of symptoms and rehabilitation vary with each specific disease. Also, interventions focused on individuals and populations living with blindness from congenital rubella, the status of chronic disease of AIDS, and the effects of post-polio syndrome are considered tertiary prevention.

Control of Diseases

Vaccine-Preventable Diseases

Immunization is one of the most accepted and cost-effective preventive health practices in the United States. Since the 1950s, vaccines have prevented countless days of illness and hundreds of thousands of deaths. Most healthcare providers take for granted the rarity of vaccine-preventable diseases; many healthcare providers will never see a child with diphtheria, measles, or polio. This chapter focuses on the vaccine-preventable diseases of adults and the need for adults to be immunized against them.

Adult immunization is extremely important. Each year in the United States alone, at least 45,000 adults die from complications resulting from influenza, pneumonia, or hepatitis B, despite the availability of safe and effective vaccines to prevent these diseases. Vaccine coverage depends, in some respects, upon which vaccine is being discussed for which age group. For example, in 2012, 56% of adults in the United States were immunized against influenza, while only 41.5% of children under 17 received a flu shot; in contrast, 55% of adults had a tetanus vaccine (Williams et al., 2014), compared to 85% of infants and 75% of school-age children.

Hepatitis

Viral hepatitis encompasses several distinct infections. All are hepatatrophic and have similar clinical presentations. However, they differ in their cause and in some clinical, pathological, immunological, and epidemiological characteristics. Their prevention and control also vary (Benenson, 1995; CDC, 2012b, 2013c, 2013d, 2013e; Heymann, 2004). See **Figure 20-1** and **Figure 20-2**.

Hepatitis A virus (HAV) HAV is a highly contagious viral infection of the liver. In the 1990s, an average of 27,000 cases annually were reported in the United States (Atkinson & Wolfe, 2003). In 2010, a change was noted in the recorded cases of acute symptomatic HAV, with 1,670 cases reported and an incidence rate of 0.6/100,000. This reflects the lowest recorded rate. An estimated annual number of new infections, including underreporting and asymptomatic infections for 2010, was 17,000 (CDC, 2013c). See **Table 20-3**.

HAV is the most common vaccine-preventable disease in travelers (National Foundation for Infectious Diseases, 2002b). HAV is found in the stool of infected people. The mode of transmission is person to person by the fecal–oral route. The infection is passed on by infected persons who do not wash their hands after having a bowel movement and contaminate everything they touch. Outbreaks have been related to contaminated water and to food prepared by food handlers who are infected with HAV. People can also become infected with HAV by eating contaminated raw shellfish, fruits, or vegetables (Heymann, 2004). See **Figure 20-3**, **Figure 20-4**, and **Figure 20-5**.

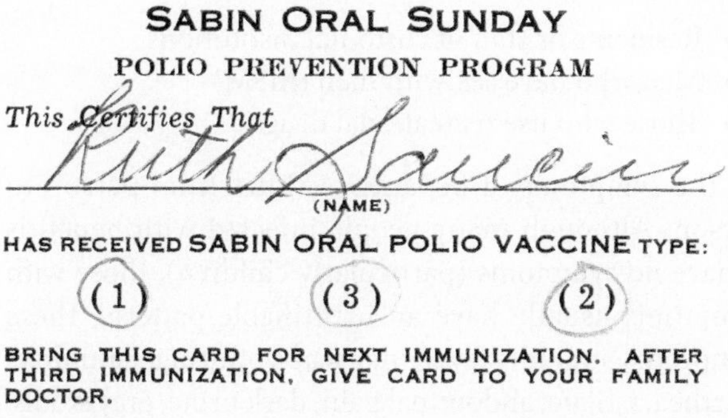

SABIN ORAL SUNDAY
POLIO PREVENTION PROGRAM
This Certifies That
(NAME)
HAS RECEIVED SABIN ORAL POLIO VACCINE TYPE:
(1) (3) (2)
BRING THIS CARD FOR NEXT IMMUNIZATION. AFTER THIRD IMMUNIZATION, GIVE CARD TO YOUR FAMILY DOCTOR.

Courtesy of UNAIDS

Figure 20-1 Vaccination card for polio prevention program, circa 1956.

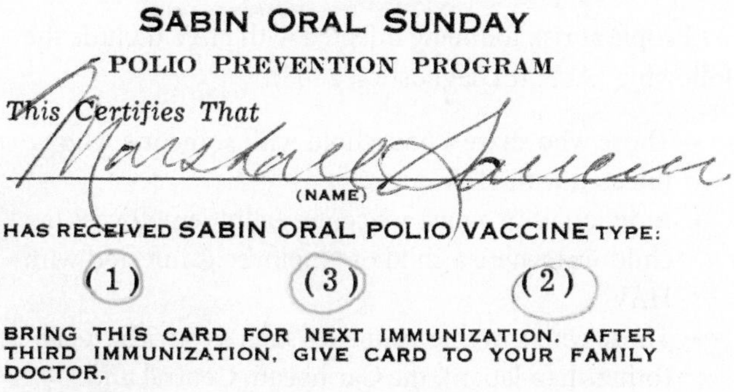

SABIN ORAL SUNDAY
POLIO PREVENTION PROGRAM
This Certifies That
(NAME)
HAS RECEIVED SABIN ORAL POLIO VACCINE TYPE:
(1) (3) (2)
BRING THIS CARD FOR NEXT IMMUNIZATION. AFTER THIRD IMMUNIZATION, GIVE CARD TO YOUR FAMILY DOCTOR.

Courtesy of UNAIDS

Figure 20-2 Vaccination card for polio prevention program, circa 1956.

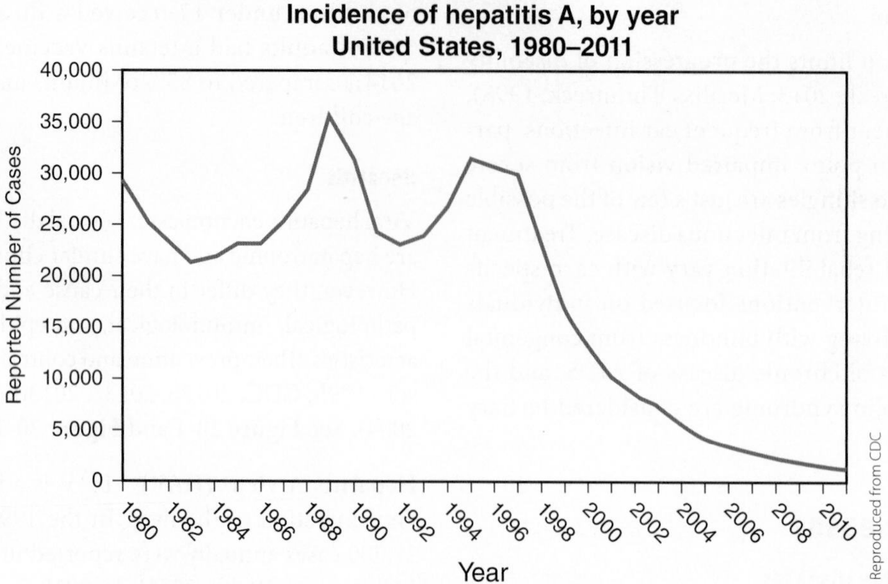

Figure 20-3 Disease burden from viral hepatitis A in the United States.

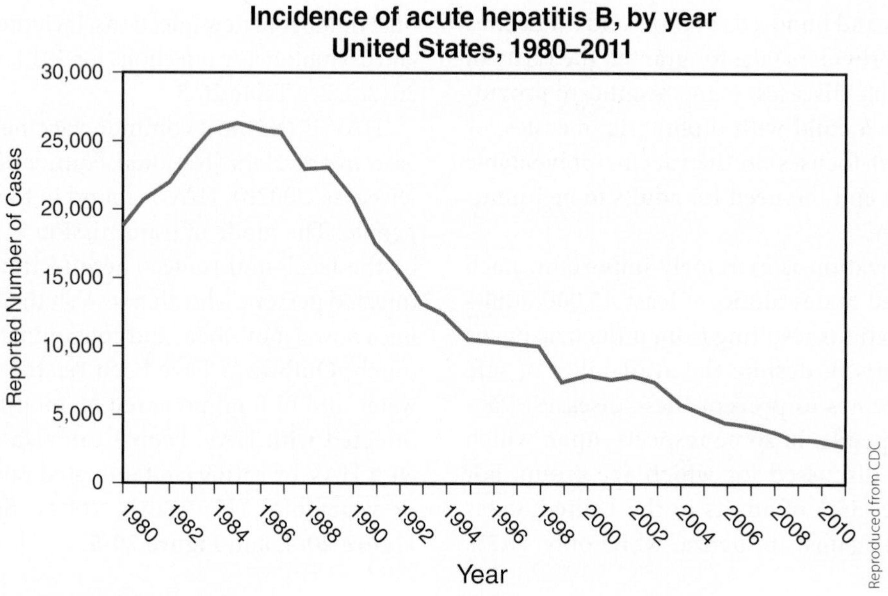

Figure 20-4 Disease burden from viral hepatitis B in the United States.

People at risk for being infected with HAV include the following (Abbott Diagnostics, 2008):

- Those who share a household with someone who is infected with HAV
- Individuals in a daycare center (adult employees or children) where a child or employee is infected with HAV
- Those who travel to countries such as Africa, Asia (other than Japan), the Caribbean, Central and South America, Eastern Europe, the Mediterranean basin, and the Middle East
- Residents or staff of custodial institutions
- Men who have sex with men (MSM)
- Those who use recreational drugs

The symptoms of hepatitis A differ from person to person. Although many people infected with hepatitis A have no symptoms (particularly children), those with symptoms usually have an identifiable pattern. These symptoms include fever, nausea, vomiting, jaundice, diarrhea, fatigue, abdominal pain, dark urine, gray stools, and loss of appetite. Respiratory symptoms, joint pain, and rash occasionally occur (CDC, 2012c).

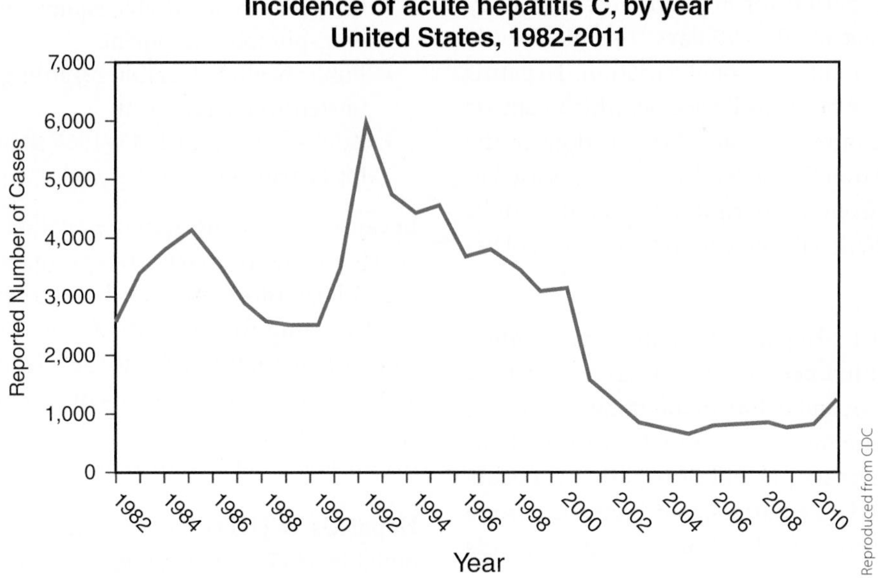

Figure 20-5 Disease burden from viral hepatitis C in the United States.

The incubation period is from 15 to 50 days, with the average time being approximately 28 days. The period of infectivity is during the last half of the incubation period, up to and including a few days after the onset of jaundice (Benenson, 1995; Heymann, 2004).

Hepatitis A is prevented through the following means (Benenson, 1995; CDC, 2013c; Heymann, 2004):

- Vaccination with the hepatitis A vaccine (with an initial injection providing protection for up to 1 year, with a booster dose [6 to 12 months after the first dose] providing prolonged protection)
- Education of the public about good sanitation and proper hygiene, with careful emphasis on handwashing
- Proper water and sewage treatment
- Education of employees in child daycare centers about the need for thorough handwashing after every diaper change and before feeding children or eating
- Immunization of child daycare employees
- Cooking shellfish to the proper temperature (85–90°C, or 185–190°F)
- Immunization with the hepatitis A vaccine of all travelers going to developing countries

NOTE THIS!

In the 10-state outbreak of hepatitis A in May 2013, 162 people were confirmed ill after eating a product containing pomegranates exported from Turkey. There were no reported deaths (CDC, 2013d).

Hepatitis B (HBV) Hepatitis B is also a highly contagious virus that infects the liver. It is caused by the hepatitis B virus (HBV), which infects approximately 300,000 Americans annually. In the United States, more than 1 million people are chronically infected with HBV. In 2009, there were an estimated 38,000 new cases of HBV (CDC, 2012b). Globally, there are an estimated 350 million chronic HBV carriers (Abbott Diagnostics, 2008). WHO estimates that more than 2 billion people have been infected with HBV worldwide. Each year about 600,000 people die from HBV-related causes (WHO, 2013b). In 1990, routine HBV vaccination was implemented in the United States. Since that time, rates of HBV infection have decreased by approximately 82% in the United States (CDC, 2012b).

The virus is found in the blood and body fluids of infected people. All persons who test positive for the hepatitis B antigen are potentially infectious. The mode of transmission can be person to person through sexual contact, through direct contact with blood or blood products resulting from sharing of needles or razors, and from infected mother to infant during the birthing process. Hepatitis B is often described as a silent disease because it infects many people without making them feel ill. Infants are usually asymptomatic, and small children usually have a milder case of the disease. When symptoms do occur, the infected person will often complain of flulike symptoms, with loss of appetite, nausea and vomiting, stomach cramps, and extreme fatigue, which may progress to jaundice. Hepatitis B can progress to fulminating hepatic necrosis and death (Atkinson & Wolfe, 2003; CDC, 2012b; Heymann, 2004).

The incubation period for hepatitis B is 45 to 180 days, with an average of 60 to 90 days. This disease occurs worldwide with little seasonal variation. Hepatitis B is prevented by the hepatitis B vaccine, which consists of a series of three intramuscular (IM) injections of the hepatitis B vaccine over 6 months. This vaccine is used to protect everyone, from newborn infants to older adults (Heymann, 2004; National Foundation for Infectious Diseases, 2002c).

Hepatitis C (HCV) Hepatitis C is also a viral infection of the liver. It has been referred to as *parenterally transmitted hepatitis,* and before blood donor screening it was the most common cause of post-transfusion hepatitis worldwide. Ninety percent of hepatitis C occurrence in Japan, the United States, and Western Europe is a result of exposure to blood or other body fluids (Holtzman, 2014).

Hepatitis C virus (HCV) is found worldwide. WHO estimates that up to 3% of the world's population is infected with HCV (Holtzman, 2014). In the United States, hepatitis C has infected an estimated 3.2 million people (1.8% of the U.S. population) with incidence in 2010 of 17,000 new cases (CDC, 2012c). Its occurrence is highest in IV drug users and hemophilia patients; moderate in hemodialysis patients; low in heterosexuals with multiple partners, homosexual men, healthcare workers, and family members of HCV patients; and lowest in volunteer blood donors (Benenson, 1995; CDC, 2010). The reservoir for the virus is humans. The mode of transmission is indirect, spread through contaminated needles and syringes; however, this accounts for fewer than 50% of the infected cases in the United States. Transmission rates through household contact and sexual activity appear to be low, and perinatal transmission is uncommon. The route of transmission cannot be identified in more than 40% of infected patients (Benenson, 1995).

The incubation period of hepatitis C is from 2 weeks to 6 months, with most cases occurring within 6 to 9 weeks after infection. Most infected individuals with hepatitis C are asymptomatic (up to 90%); this includes even those with chronic disease (CDC, 2013e; Heymann, 2004). The most common symptoms are fatigue, nausea, vague abdominal discomfort, and jaundice. Severity ranges from inapparent cases (approximately 75%) to rare fulminating, fatal cases (Benenson, 1995).

Prevention measures for hepatitis C include the following (Abbott Diagnostics 2008; CDC, 2010; CDC, 2013e):

- Universal screening of blood and blood products
- Effective use of standard precautions and barrier techniques
- Sterilization of reusable equipment and destruction of disposable equipment
- Public health education regarding the risks of using unsterilized equipment
- Adults born from 1945–1965 should be tested once for Hepatitis C

Because there is no vaccine against hepatitis C, prevention is the primary strategy against the virus. New secondary interventions have been recommended for screening for Hepatitis C for those persons born from 1945–1960 (CDC, 2013e). In the United States, approximately three-fourths of all chronic HCV infections among adults are noted in the population born from 1945–1960 (Smith et al., 2012).

Hepatitis D (HDV) Hepatitis D virus (HDV), first noted in 1977 and also known as "delta," is a defective, single-stranded RNA virus that requires the helper function of HBV to replicate. HDV is found worldwide, but its prevalence varies. Because it requires the HBV to replicate and to infect cells, it occurs either epidemically or endemically in populations with high rates of HBV infection (Benenson, 1995; Heymann, 2004). Places where HDV is found to be endemic are Africa, southern Italy, Romania, parts of Russia, and South America. Populations that have high rates of hepatitis D include hemophiliacs, drug addicts, people with frequent blood exposures, residents in homes for the developmentally disabled, and male homosexuals.

Humans serve as the reservoir for hepatitis D. The modes of transmission are similar to those of hepatitis B, with direct contact with blood or blood products the most efficient. Sexual transmission is less efficient than that of hepatitis B, and perinatal transmission is rare.

The onset of hepatitis D is usually abrupt, with signs and symptoms similar to those of hepatitis B. Hepatitis D varies from being self-limiting to progressing to chronic hepatitis. It can be acquired either as a co-infection with hepatitis B or as a superinfection in persons with chronic HBV infection (CDC, 2004). When it is acquired as a co-infection, the person has a greater risk of severe acute disease, with a 2% to 20% chance of fulminant hepatitis. Chronic HBV carriers who acquire hepatitis D as a superinfection have a greater chance of developing chronic HDV infection. The superinfection with HDV has been found to increase the development of chronic liver disease with cirrhosis in 70% to 80% compared with 15% to 30% of patients with HBV alone (Abbott Diagnostics, 2008).

The incubation period is approximately 2 to 8 weeks. Peak infectivity is thought to occur just before the onset of the illness. Symptoms are similar to those of hepatitis

B and are identified as joint pain, abdominal pain, loss of appetite, nausea and vomiting, fatigue, and jaundice. No vaccine exists for HDV. The method of control is immunization with the hepatitis B vaccine; however, this is effective only in persons who are not already infected with HBV. For those infected with HBV, avoidance of any possible exposure to HDV is the only preventive measure (Abbott Diagnostics, 2008; Heymann, 2004).

Hepatitis E Hepatitis E is similar to hepatitis A in that there is no evidence of a chronic form. The fatality rate for hepatitis E is also similar to that of hepatitis A, except in pregnant women during the third trimester, when the fatality rate may reach 20% (CDC, 2012d). Hepatitis E virus (HEV) is transmitted by the fecal–oral route. Transmission may also (rarely) occur with infected blood products and from pregnant woman to the fetus. Globally, of all HEV-related deaths, 65% occur in East and South Asia. Half of the population in Egypt over age 5 is serologically positive for HEV (WHO, 2014a).

Contaminated water from feces of infected humans is the most commonly documented vehicle of transmission. Person-to-person transmission (seen in hepatitis A) does not appear to be a mode of transmission in hepatitis E, because secondary household cases are not common during outbreaks. The attack rate is highest in young adults; cases are uncommon in children and the elderly (Benenson, 1995; CDC, 2012d).

The reservoir is human beings, although an animal reservoir is possible. In the United States, as well as in most other industrialized countries, hepatitis E cases have been documented only among travelers returning from HEV-endemic areas (Benenson, 1995). HEV is endemic in Mexico, Central America, Asia, North Africa, the Middle East, and a few sub-Saharan African countries along the western coast (Abbott Diagnostics, 2008).

The incubation period is 15 to 64 days, with the mean incubation period ranging between 26 and 42 days (Benenson, 1995; Heymann, 2004). Symptoms of hepatitis E include loss of appetite, nausea and vomiting, fever, fatigue, and abdominal pain. Many people who contract HEV have no symptoms. Prevention of hepatitis E relies primarily on the provision of clean water. Hygiene practice must be strict among travelers to prevent contracting hepatitis E when traveling in developing countries, such as avoiding drinking water and beverages with ice, uncooked shellfish, and uncooked fruits and vegetables (Abbott Diagnostics, 2008; CDC, 2012d). There is no vaccine and no identified treatment at this time; thus, prevention is very important. System-level interventions include developing policies and maintaining standards for public water supplies and proper disposal of sanitary waste. World Hepatitis Day is observed annually on July 28.

Influenza

Influenza is another vaccine-preventable disease important in adults. "The flu" is an extremely contagious viral infection of the nose, throat, and lungs. In temperate zones, epidemics occur in the winter season, and in tropical zones, they occur during the rainy season. Influenza derives its importance from the rapidity with which epidemics occur, the high morbidity rate, and the severity of the complications that result from the infection. Annual influenza epidemics account for 3 to 5 million cases of severe illness and 250,000 to 500,000 deaths worldwide each year (WHO, 2014b). During major epidemics, the most severe illnesses and deaths occur in the elderly population and in those with debilitating diseases.

In fact, influenza deaths in the United States increased substantially in the last few decades partly because of the general aging of the population (Thompson et al., 2003). On average, 114,000 people are hospitalized and 36,000 deaths occur from influenza annually in the United States (Goldrick, 2004).

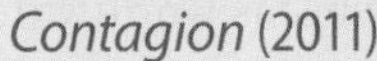

MEDIA MOMENT

Contagion (2011)

When a businesswoman traveling from overseas contracts a deadly virus, her family and medical researchers race against time to identify the cause of the disease and isolate a vaccine. Meanwhile, the social repercussions of the rapidly spreading mystery illness lead to chaos in the sick woman's community—and social breakdown proves as contagious as the disease.

Contagion Movie: Fact and Fiction in Film http://www.cdc.gov/features/contagionmovie/

CDC's Disease Detectives: Contagion, the Movie: Hollywood's Take on Disease Detectives http://www.cdc.gov/24-7/savinglives/disease_detectives/contagion_hollywood.html

Contagion The Movie: A NewPublicHealth Q&l; A with Barbara Reynolds http://www.rwjf.org/en/blogs/new-public-health/2011/09/contagion-the-movie-a-newpublichealth-qa-with-barbara-reynolds.html

There are three types of influenza viruses: A, B, and C. Type A, associated with widespread epidemics and pandemics, causes moderate to severe illness and affects all age groups; type B, associated with regional or widespread epidemics, generally causes milder disease than type A

APPLICATION TO PRACTICE 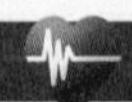

You are a nurse in a neighborhood-based clinic. In October, Mrs. Clark, a 75-year-old woman, comes into the clinic for her regular yearly physical examination. Mrs. Clark is in good health overall, with relatively few minor complaints. Last year, as part of her yearly visit, Mrs. Clark had been given an influenza vaccination. During this visit, however, Mrs. Clark tells you that she does not need to be vaccinated against influenza because she had gotten her "flu shot" last year. She also said, "I don't want the flu shot this year because I know somebody who got sick from it. I don't want to get sick."

1. Should you convince Mrs. Clark to get the influenza vaccination this year? Why or why not?
2. What other vaccines should you consider offering to Mrs. Clark?
3. What are the patient education considerations for Mrs. Clark?
4. What influenza-focused information can you offer Mrs. Clark?

and primarily affects children; and type C, associated with sporadic and minor localized outbreaks, is rare and has not been associated with epidemic disease (Atkinson & Wolfe, 2003; Benenson, 1995). Occurrence is worldwide. The United States has an epidemic almost every year with type A, type B, or sometimes with both A and B.

Influenza symptoms are fever, myalgia, headache, sore throat, dry cough, and some gastrointestinal symptoms, such as nausea, vomiting, and diarrhea. Humans are the primary reservoir, with swine and avian reservoirs as likely breeding grounds for new strains. Avian influenza (H5N1) is discussed further under zoonoses later in this chapter. The mode of transmission is airborne, which is aerosolized or droplet material from the respiratory tract. The incubation period is very short, ranging from 1 to 3 days. People are infectious from 1 to 2 days before onset of symptoms to 4 to 5 days after onset (CDC, 2013g; Heymann, 2004).

Most cases of influenza are preventable through a vaccine. Because the virus changes from year to year, it is necessary to be vaccinated yearly. The following people should receive a yearly vaccine: people 65 years and older, people with chronic disease (cardiac and/or respiratory), people who are immunocompromised, pregnant women who will be in their second or third trimester during the flu season, residents in long-term care facilities, healthcare workers, persons who are morbidly obese, and adolescents receiving long-term aspirin therapy (CDC, 2013g).

GLOBAL CONNECTION 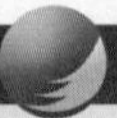

Although clean water is taken for granted in the United States, most of the world's population does not have access to sanitary water. This poses a formidable challenge in the control of water-borne diseases—especially dysentery, which is a major cause of high morbidity and mortality rates throughout the world.

Pneumococcal Disease

Pneumococcal disease is an acute bacterial infection. It is characterized by a rapid onset with shaking chills, fever, pleural pain, a productive cough, dyspnea, tachycardia, anorexia, malaise, and extreme weakness. Its onset is not as rapid in the elderly, and the first evidence is usually by x-ray examination. In infants and young children, the onset may be characterized by fever, vomiting, and convulsions. Pneumococcal disease is most severe in infants and elders, with higher death rates in both groups. The mortality rate is 5% to 10% with antibiotic therapy but can be as high as 60% for infants in developing countries where antibiotics are unavailable. The infectious agent is *Streptococcus pneumoniae* (pneumococcus). Its occurrence is worldwide, with peaks in the winter and early spring in temperate zones. However, it occurs in all climates and in all seasons (Benenson, 1995; Heymann, 2004).

The reservoir for pneumococcal disease is humans, and pneumococci are often found in the lungs of healthy people worldwide. The mode of transmission is airborne through droplets spread either by direct transfer or by indirect transfer when droplets have recently contaminated articles of clothing or bedding with discharge from the respiratory track. Person-to-person transmission is common. The incubation period may be as short as 1 to 3 days.

Pneumococcal disease can be prevented in children and adults through vaccination with polyvalent vaccine. One immunization lasts most adults a lifetime against almost all the bacteria that cause pneumococcal disease. The following adults should be vaccinated: people 65 and older, because risk of infection and fatality rates increase with age; people with chronic diseases; people who are immunosuppressed; and residents of long-term care facilities.

Routine Vaccinations Indicated for Adults

All adults should be protected against many of the same diseases as adolescents and children. The tetanus and diphtheria (Td) vaccine should be given to all adults (**Table 20-4**).

TABLE 20-4 Recommended Adult Immunization Schedule, All, by Vaccine and Age Group, 2013

Vaccine Type	20–26 Years	27–59 Years	60–64 Years	65 Years and older
Human papillomavirus (HPV) women	3 doses age 20–26	------------	------------	------------
Human papillomavirus (HPV) men	3 doses age 20–21	------------	------------	------------
Meningococcal	1 or more doses lifetime	1 or more doses lifetime	1 or more doses lifetime	1 or more doses lifetime
Influenza	Every year	Every year	Every year	Every year
Pneumococcal (polysaccharide)	------------	------------	------------	1 dose
Tetanus, diphtheria, pertussis (Tdap)	Get Tdap once, Td booster every 10 years	Get Tdap once, Td booster every 10 years	Get Tdap once, Td booster every 10 years	Get Tdap once, Td booster every 10 years
Measles, mumps, rubella (MMR)	1–2 doses lifetime	1–2 doses lifetime to age 55	------------	------------
Varicella (chickenpox)	2 doses lifetime	2 doses lifetime	2 doses lifetime	2 doses lifetime
Zoster (shingles)	------------	------------	1 dose lifetime	1 dose lifetime
Hepatitis A	2 doses lifetime	2 doses lifetime	2 doses lifetime	2 doses lifetime
Hepatitis B	3 doses lifetime	3 doses lifetime	3 doses lifetime	3 doses lifetime

Source: Data from CDC. (2013f). Recommended immunizations for adults by age. Retrieved from http://www.cdc.gov/vaccines/schedules/easy-to-read/adult.html

It is important for adults to be immunized against diphtheria and tetanus because 1 of every 10 people who get diphtheria will die from it (Heymann, 2004), and 40 to 60 cases of tetanus occur each year, resulting in at least 10 deaths. Almost all reported cases of tetanus occur in people who are inadequately immunized (Atkinson & Wolfe, 2003).

Adults born before 1957 do not usually require the measles, mumps, and rubella vaccine because most of these adults have acquired immunity as a result of having the diseases during childhood. However, all adults born after 1957 should be immunized (see Table 20-4). Women of childbearing age should be given the rubella vaccine unless they have documentation of immunization after their first birthday. Currently, approximately 12 million women of childbearing age are susceptible to rubella. If rubella occurs during pregnancy, severe birth defects, miscarriages, and stillbirths can result (Atkinson & Wolfe, 2003; National Foundation for Infectious Diseases, 2002a). Although laboratory evidence of rubella immunity is acceptable, a stated previous history of rubella is unreliable and should not be accepted as proof of immunity. Before giving rubella immunization, the nurse should determine the likelihood of pregnancy during the next 3 months. The nurse should discuss with the woman her plans for reliable birth control during the following 3 months. Although there is no evidence that the rubella vaccine or other live viruses cause birth defects, the possibility exists. Thus, healthcare providers should not give any live vaccine to women known to be pregnant (Atkinson & Wolfe, 2003).

All adults without a reliable history of varicella disease (chickenpox) should receive the varicella vaccine. Adults who are either at highest risk for susceptibility or at high risk for exposing people to varicella should be targeted for varicella immunization (see Table 20-4). These adults include teachers, college students, military personnel, healthcare workers, and family members of immunocompromised persons. Although varicella is not considered a serious disease of childhood, adults

GOT AN ALTERNATIVE?

Many complementary health practices, such as yoga and meditation, can reduce stress and anxiety, thereby enhancing the immune system and reducing the risk of contracting an infectious disease.

are 25 times more likely to die from the disease. Adolescents and adults who develop varicella are 10 times more likely to require hospitalization and/or develop pneumonia, bacterial infections, and encephalitis (Atkinson & Wolfe, 2003; National Coalition for Adult Immunization, 2009).

Emerging and Reemerging Infectious Diseases

Infectious diseases continue to be a problem for all people, regardless of age, gender, lifestyle, ethnicity, or socioeconomic status. New and mutated infectious diseases that have the potential to cause suffering and death and impose an enormous financial burden on individuals and society are always emerging. Two examples occurred in 1997, when a new strain of influenza that had never been seen in humans began to kill previously healthy people in Hong Kong and strains of *S. aureus* with diminished susceptibility to vancomycin were reported in both Japan and the United States. If scientists cannot replace antibiotics that are losing their effectiveness, some diseases may become untreatable, as they were in the pre-antibiotic era (CDC, 1998).

Emerging infectious diseases are diseases that have appeared for the first time or that have occurred before but are appearing in populations where they had not previously been reported. Reemerging infectious diseases are familiar diseases caused by well understood organisms that were once under control or declining but are now resistant to common antimicrobial drugs or are gaining new footholds in the population and increasing in incidence (Dzenowagis, 1997; National Institute for Allergy and Infectious Diseases, 2010).

Concern about emerging and reemerging infectious diseases prompted a 1992 report issued by the Institute of Medicine (IOM) of the National Academy of Sciences (NAS). The report, *Emerging Infections: Microbial Threats to Health in the United States,* concluded that emerging and reemerging infectious diseases are a major threat to the health of Americans and challenged the U.S. government to take action. The IOM (1992) report defined emerging or reemerging infectious diseases as those diseases whose incidence had increased within the last 2 decades of the 20th century or threatened to increase in the near future. Modern conditions that favor the spread of disease are listed in the Environmental Connection feature.

As a result of the IOM (1992) report, in 1994 the CDC and other healthcare groups launched a national effort to support public health efforts to control the negative impact of infectious diseases. As funds became available, the CDC, in partnership with the IOM, state and local health departments, medical and public health professional associations, and international organizations, implemented a plan of prevention strategies to address these disease threats. The four major goals of the plan and the implications for nursing are surveillance, applied research, prevention and control, and infrastructure (CDC, 1994).

ENVIRONMENTAL CONNECTION

Modern Demographic and Environmental Conditions That Favor the Spread of Infectious Diseases

- Global travel
- Globalization of the food supply and centralized processing of food
- Population growth and increased urbanization and overcrowding
- Migration due to wars, famines, and other artificial or natural disasters
- Political refugees and war
- Irrigation, deforestation, and reforestation projects that alter the habitats of disease-carrying insects and animals
- Human behaviors, such as intravenous drug use and risky sexual behavior
- Increased use of antimicrobial agents and pesticides, hastening the development of resistance
- Increased human contact with tropical rain forests and other wilderness habitats that are reservoirs for insects and animals that harbor unknown infectious agents

Source: CDC. (1998). *Preventing infectious diseases: A strategy for the twenty-first century*. Atlanta: U.S. Department of Health and Human Services.

Healthcare-Associated Infections

Healthcare-associated infections (HAIs), also known as nosocomial infections, are acquired by patients while being treated for other conditions in a healthcare setting. According to the CDC, an estimated 2 million HAIs occur annually, resulting in 90,000 deaths. The number of HAIs is steadily increasing with a financial burden of $4.5 billion per year (Kestel, 2006). CDC (2013h) released a landmark report, *Antibiotic Resistance Threats in the United States, 2013*, which "gives a first-ever snapshot of the burden and threats posed by the antibiotic-resistant germs having the most impact on human health." Included are antibiotic-resistant categories for microorganisms with threat levels as urgent, serious, and concerning. Nurses should be aware of these threats and active in prompt reporting.

Staphylococcus aureus, often referred to as "staph," is one of the leading causes of nosocomial (hospital-acquired) infections and is the most common cause of skin infections in the United States. Most of these skin infections are minor and can often be treated without antibiotics. Staph bacteria are commonly carried on the skin or in the noses of healthy people. At any given time 25% to 30% of the population can be colonized with *Staphylococcus aureus* without showing any signs of illness. However, staph bacteria can also cause severe illness (such as surgical wound infections, bloodstream infections, catheter-associated urinary tract infections, and pneumonia) in people who have weakened immune systems (CDC, 2014c).

MRSA

MRSA is a type of staph that is resistant to antibiotics called beta-lactams, which include methicillin and other more common antibiotics such as oxacillin, penicillin, and amoxicillin. Over the years, the number of staph infections caused by MRSA has grown steadily from 2% in 1974 to 63% in 2004 (CDC, 2014c) making it one of the most common nosocomial infections. Vancomycin has been successful in treating MRSA until the last few years. Increasing numbers of vancomycin-intermediate *S. aureus* (VISA) with partial resistance to vancomycin and vancomycin-resistant *S. aureus* (VRSA) have been reported. Before the advent of antibiotics, *Staphylococcus aureus* infections were often fatal. Healthcare providers are concerned that increasing antibiotic resistance may again make staph a leading cause of death (CDC, 2011a; Todd, 2006). Persons at risk for vancomycin-resistant enterococcal (VRE) infections include those with recent vancomycin therapy, comorbidities of diabetes or renal disease, previous infections with MRSA, and those with urinary catheters.

Until the late 1990s, MRSA was confined to patients with weakened immune systems who were being treated for other illnesses in hospitals or other healthcare settings. A new form of MRSA, known as community-acquired MRSA, began occurring in otherwise healthy people in the community (CDC, 2014c; Krisberg, 2006). Community-acquired MRSA, genetically different from hospital-acquired MRSA, accounts for about 10% of all MRSA infections and is still treatable with a variety of antibiotics, although antibiotic-resistant strains are being identified (Gorwitz et al., 2006). While most community-acquired MRSA infections are mild, severe invasive conditions such as necrotizing pneumonia and empyema, osteomyelitis, and necrotizing fasciitis have occurred (Gorwitz et al., 2006; Krisberg, 2006). Community-acquired MRSA has been reported in a variety of populations, groups, and environmental settings. Its genetic distinction indicates that the organism is mutating and evolving rapidly (Krisberg, 2006), which may make it more virulent, more able to affect people with healthy immune systems, and more easily transmitted (CDC, 2014c). These infections may occur in the community, but most deaths are in the nursing home and hospital settings. In addressing tracking and prevention strategies and estimating HAIs in 2013, an "estimated 30,800 fewer MRSA infections occurred in the United States compared with 2005" (Dantes et al., 2013, p. 1970). Another emerging HAI is carbapenem-resistant Enterobacteriaceae (CRE), which have high levels of resistance to antibiotics. Examples of Enterobacteriaceae include *Klebsiella* species and *E. coli* that can become carbapenem resistant. With the increased antibiotic resistance, these are more difficult to treat and have increased mortality rates by up to 50% (CDC, 2013i). One type of CRE infection has been reported in medical facilities in 42 states since the early 2000s. CRE quality improvement staff education includes dedicated staff, patient rooms, and equipment and improved use of gown and gloves (CDC, 2013j).

Primary prevention is the best form of defense against all forms of MRSA. Good handwashing is critical in both hospital and community settings. As always, nurses in all healthcare settings should use standard precautions when exposed to any open skin lesions or wounds. People in the community with skin infections need to be monitored for MRSA and all community members should be informed of the potential risk for MRSA and taught proper handwashing techniques and good general hygiene (CDC, 2014c).

Food-Borne Diseases

Infections caused by food-borne parasites or viruses are common. In 2011, in the United States, 49 million people got sick from food-borne diseases, and more than 3,000 died. In recent years, food-borne illness has become one of the fastest growing threats to community health in the United States (CDC, 2013k; Hoffman et al., 2005; Mahon et al., 1999; NAS, 2005). Much of the reason for this is that enormous quantities of food are being produced in central locations and then being widely distributed to all parts of the country (Mahon et al., 1999). There have also been sharp increases in the number and types of food being imported from other countries (NAS, 2005). In response to these factors, the National Food Safety Initiative

(NFSI) was created in 1997 to improve the safety of the nation's food supply (CDC, 2013l). The NFSI ended in 2001, but the CDC has institutionalized its funding and activities as an ongoing food safety program (Hoffman et al., 2005), which is known as the Foodborne Diseases Active Surveillance Networks, or FoodNet. The health care for people with food-borne illnesses can be very expensive. The yearly cost for food-borne illnesses in the United States is $6.9 billion in medical costs and lost productivity (NAS, 2005).

Foods can serve as a medium for growing bacterial pathogens or as a passive vehicle for transferring parasitic or viral pathogens. Although most food-borne infections are directly related to foods of animal origin such as meat, fish, shellfish, poultry, eggs, and dairy products (Kaferstein & Meslin, 1998), foods of plant origin can also be contaminated. Many food-borne bacterial diseases have emerged or increased since the 1990s. Some of the factors that bring about the multiplication and distribution of these bacteria in food are poor hygienic practices at the animal husbandry, slaughterhouse, and food-processing levels as well as poor food preparation practices.

Prevention

There are three measures of protection against food-borne pathogens (Kaferstein & Meslin, 1998):

1. Prevention of contamination of food
2. Prevention of growth of pathogens
3. Prevention of the spread and survival of pathogens

First, the quality of food at the production level must be improved. The environmental conditions under which food animals are raised and the use of fertilizers and pesticides for food plants must be monitored and controlled.

Second, food-processing technology must be improved and used to prevent the survival and spread of food pathogens. Pasteurization, sterilization, and irradiation contribute significantly to food safety by reducing or eliminating disease-causing organisms.

Third, all food handlers must be educated in the principles of safe food preparation. This is probably the most critical line of defense, because most food-borne diseases are a result of one or more of the following (Kaferstein & Meslin, 1998):

- Insufficient cooking of food
- Preparation of food too many hours before it is eaten, along with improper storage
- Use of contaminated raw food
- Cross-contamination where food is prepared
- Food preparation by infected persons

From a systems approach, FoodNet reports annually on the changes in the number of people sickened with food-borne infections that have been confirmed by laboratory tests. Food-borne diseases monitored through FoodNet include infections caused by the bacteria *Campylobacter*, *Listeria*, *Salmonella*, Shiga toxin–producing *E. coli* O157 and non-O157, *Shigella*, *Vibrio*, and *Yersinia*, and the parasites *Cryptosporidium* and *Cyclospora*. Reporting may be found on the CDC website (CDC, 2013l).

Nurses' Roles in Prevention Because many cases of food-borne diseases are a result of mishandling food in the home, community health nurses who visit families in their homes are in an excellent position to provide education for the persons in a family who are responsible for food handling and preparation (Kaferstein & Meslin, 1998). It is important to stress safety in all stages of food handling. This includes: (1) what to look for when purchasing food at the store or market, (2) how to store food in the home, (3) the importance of good handwashing and clean utensils and surfaces for food preparation, and (4) proper cooking techniques (CDC, 2011c; Dols, Bowers, & Copfer, 2001). School nurses can be successful in reducing the incidence of food-borne infections by educating children in the schools about the concepts of food safety. Educating children is not only an effective way to communicate safe food-handling procedures to parents, but also a way to implant the principles of safe food preparation in the minds of future adults (Kaferstein & Meslin, 1998). School nurses should monitor school food programs and educate school food services personnel about proper handling and storage of foods. Educational programs should also be provided for teachers because of the amount of "food treats" that are served in the classrooms, especially in elementary schools.

Common Food-Borne Diseases in the United States

The top three pathogens contributing to food-borne illness are, in order of highest estimates, norovirus, *Salmonella*, and *Clostridium perfringens*. These three pathogens have been noted in illnesses resulting in hospitalization. *Salmonella*, *Toxoplasma gondii*, and *Listeria monocytogenes* are most frequently noted in fatal food-borne illnesses (CDC, 2011c; CDC, 2013l; Scallan et al., 2011).

Campylobacteriosis Campylobacteriosis, caused by bacteria of the genus *Campylobacter*, is one of the most common diarrheal diseases in the United States. The symptoms (diarrhea, abdominal pain, fever, nausea, and vomiting) usually develop within 2 to 5 days after exposure and typically last 1 week. Most people infected with *Campylobacter* will recover with no treatment except for drinking plenty of fluids for the diarrhea. However, in more severe cases, an antibiotic such as azithromycin or fluoroquinolones can be used. Most cases of campylobacteriosis are a result of handling or eating raw or undercooked poultry. Most cases occur as isolated, sporadic events, although small outbreaks have been reported. More than 10,000 cases are reported to the CDC each year. However, because many cases are undiagnosed or unreported, campylobacteriosis is estimated to affect more than 1.3 million people every year (CDC, 2013m; Potter, Kaneene, & Hall, 2003). Rarely, some persons, after experiencing illness with *Campylobacter*, may have long-term consequences of arthritis or Guillain-Barré syndrome—approximately 1 in 1,000 (CDC, 2013m).

Listeriosis Listeriosis, caused by the bacterium *Listeria monocytogenes,* has been recognized as a serious public health problem in the United States. The symptoms are fever, muscle aches, and sometimes nausea or diarrhea. If the infection spreads to the nervous system, headache, stiff neck, confusion, loss of balance, or seizures can occur. *L. monocytogenes* is found in a variety of raw food, such as uncooked meats and vegetables, as well as in processed foods that become contaminated after processing. The disease primarily affects pregnant women, newborns, and adults with weakened immune systems. An estimated 1,600 people become ill from listeriosis each year, and 260 of them die. Most deaths occur among immunocompromised and elderly patients. Infected persons are treated with antibiotics. However, even with prompt treatment some infections can result in death (CDC, 2013n, 2013o; Scallan et al., 2011).

Salmonellosis Salmonellosis, caused by many different kinds of *Salmonella* bacteria, is a diarrheal disease that has been known for more than 100 years. The symptoms (diarrhea, fever, and abdominal cramps) usually develop within 12 to 72 hours after exposure and usually last 4 to 7 days. Salmonellosis usually does not require any treatment, but if the patient becomes severely dehydrated or the infection spreads from the intestines to other body parts, rehydration with IV fluids and antibiotic therapy may be necessary. *Salmonella* can be transmitted to humans by eating foods contaminated with animal feces. Many raw foods of animal origin are frequently contaminated, but fortunately, thorough cooking kills *Salmonella.* Foods may also be contaminated by the unwashed hands of an infected food handler. Approximately 40,000 cases of salmonellosis are reported in the United States each year, but the actual number of cases may be 30 or more times greater (CDC, 2013p). Most recent outbreaks in 2011 to 2013 can be traced to poultry farms and handling of small turtles (CDC, 2013q, 2013r). Also, an outbreak in 473 persons infected in 41 states (with no deaths) was traced to small turtles with shell size less than 4 inches, which originated from two turtle farms in Louisiana. Pet owner alerts were issued and farms monitored.

***Escherichia coli* O157:H7** *Escherichia coli* O157:H7 is a leading cause of food-borne illness. *E. coli* O157:H7 is one of the hundreds of strains of the bacterium *E. coli.* Most strains of *E. coli* are harmless and live in the intestines of healthy humans and animals, but *E. coli* O157:H7 produces a powerful toxin that can cause severe illness. The combination of letters and numbers in the name refers to specific markers on the surface of the bacterium that distinguish it from other types of *E. coli.* The symptoms of *E. coli* O157:H7 are bloody diarrhea and abdominal cramps, although sometimes there are no symptoms. Most people recover in 5 to 10 days without antibiotics or other specific treatment. In about 8% of infections, particularly among young children and elders, hemolytic uremic syndrome (HUS) develops. This complication causes destruction of the red blood cells and kidney failure. HUS is a life-threatening condition usually treated with blood transfusions and kidney dialysis. With intensive care treatment, the death rate for HUS is 3% to 5%. Many persons with HUS have permanent abnormal kidney function and may require long-term dialysis. Most cases of *E. coli* O157:H7 are associated with eating undercooked, contaminated ground beef; drinking raw milk; or swimming in or drinking sewage-contaminated water (CDC, 2013s).

Three recent major *E. coli* outbreaks in the United States were traced to a variety of food sources: raw sprouts, frozen prepared food products such as pizzas and quesadillas, and ready-to-eat packaged salads. The first of these occurred in early 2012, in which 29 persons in 11 states with confirmed *E. coli* illness reported eating raw sprouts at a specific restaurant chain in the week prior to illness (CDC, 2013t). The second case, which occurred in May 2013 (CDC, 2013u), was traced to a Georgia food-processing plant; the subsequent recall extended to products produced over a nearly 2-year period. That outbreak involved 35 persons from 19 states, with 31% of ill persons hospitalized; there were no deaths, but two victims experienced HUS. The final episode, in November 2013, was an outbreak in which 33 people reported illness in four states (CDC, 2013v). All confirmed consuming ready-to-eat salads produced by a California company. Of those affected, 32% were hospitalized but no deaths were reported. HUS was reported in two victims.

Vector-Borne Diseases

A **vector** is an "animal, particularly an insect, that transmits a disease-producing organism from a host to a noninfected animal" (Agnus, 2004). Vector-borne diseases were responsible for more human disease and death from the 17th century through the early 20th century than all other causes combined (Gubler, 1998). In the late 1800s, mosquitoes were discovered to transmit such diseases as malaria, yellow fever, and dengue from human to human. By 1910, other major vector-borne diseases, such as African sleeping sickness, plague, Rocky Mountain spotted fever, Chagas disease, sandfly fever, and louse-borne typhus, had been shown to be transmitted by blood-sucking arthropods (Gubler, 1998).

Primary prevention interventions are focused on personal protection and vector controls. They include wearing of long sleeves and long pants, DEET-treated bed nets, use of insect repellant; having intact screens on doors and windows, limiting outdoors exposure from dusk to dawn, and emptying sources of standing water outside. Through a global effort during the 20th century, most of the vector-borne diseases in the world had been effectively controlled, primarily by the elimination of arthropod breeding sites and limited use of chemical insecticides.

However, the benefits of vector-borne disease control programs were short lived. Vector-borne diseases such as Lyme disease and malaria began to emerge and reemerge in different parts of the world during the 1970s, and the numbers of cases have greatly increased since then. Although the reasons for the resurgence are complex and poorly understood, two factors have been identified: (1) the diversion of financial support and subsequent loss of public health infrastructure and (2) reliance on quick-fix solutions such as insecticides and drugs (Gubler, 1998).

Malaria

Malaria is one of the oldest known diseases, with the first recorded case appearing in 1700 b.c. in China. In ancient Chinese, it was called "the mother of fevers" ("The mother of fevers," 1998). Malaria is the most important of all vector-borne diseases because of its global distribution, the numbers of people affected, and the large numbers of deaths (CDC, 2012e; Gubler, 1998). Worldwide, 8% of all deaths of children younger than 5 years of age are attributed to malaria. Each year, approximately 350–500 million people are infected by it, and as many as 1 million children (WHO, 2005a).

Today, cases of malaria are reported in 107 countries throughout the world. Although more than 60% of cases and 80% of deaths occur in sub-Saharan Africa, the disease is also found in parts of Asia, the western Pacific, and Central and South America. An estimated 3.3 billion people live in areas at risk of malaria transmission (CDC, 2012e). Air travel has brought the disease to the doorsteps of industrialized countries, resulting in increased illness and death among travelers to areas with endemic disease (Nchinda, 1998). (See **Box 20-4**.) Although malaria is not endemic to the United States, it is the most common imported disease in the United States. Although malaria is not a widespread problem in the United States, nurses should be alert for imported malaria infection in their patients who travel abroad. In 2011, approximately 2,000 cases of malaria were diagnosed and treated in the United States. The majority of persons had traveled to regions with malaria transmission, with the most having visited sub-Saharan Africa (CDC, 2012e).

Malaria in humans is caused by a protozoon of the genus *Plasmodium* and the four subspecies, *falciparum, vivax, malariae,* and *ovale* (Nchinda, 1998). *P. falciparum* causes the most severe form of the disease in humans (Molyneux, 1998; Yin, 2006). The disease is transmitted through the bite of *Anopheles* mosquitoes (CDC, 2012e; Marsh & Waruiru, 1998; Nchinda, 1998). Once inside the human host, the malaria organism enters the bloodstream and travels directly to the liver, where it hides and multiplies. After about 2 weeks, the newly produced organisms burst out of the liver into the bloodstream, where they attack red blood cells. These new malaria organisms rapidly reproduce in the bloodstream over the next few days until there are tens of millions of them. It is at this point that

BOX 20-4 Factors Contributing to the Resurgence of Malaria

- Increased resistance of malaria organisms to drugs currently used for treatment
- Civil wars in many countries, forcing large populations to relocate to different geographic regions
- Changing rainfall patterns and water development projects (e.g., dams, irrigation systems), which create new mosquito breeding places
- Poor economic conditions resulting in reduced health budgets and inadequate funding for drugs
- Changes in mosquito biting patterns, from indoor to outdoor biters

Source: Nchinda, T. C. (1998). Malaria: A reemerging disease in Africa. *Emerging Infectious Diseases, 4*(3), 398–403.

the human host begins to feel symptoms of illness (CDC, 2012e; Marsh & Waruiru, 1998).

The first signs of illness are usually fever and malaise, often accompanied by a severe headache. At this stage of the illness, many people think they are experiencing the flu. Other malaria symptoms, such as vomiting, diarrhea, or coughing, might lead nurses or other healthcare providers to suspect gastric upset or respiratory infection. Malaria is a great imitator, making it important for nurses to suspect any fever as a potential case of malaria for patients who have recently traveled to a country where the disease is known to exist. Early diagnosis and rapid treatment are the keys to the secondary prevention efforts necessary to keep the disease from progressing to a complicated or severe state (CDC, 2011b; Marsh & Waruiru, 1998). No malaria vaccine is available at this time; instead, those traveling to areas where malaria is endemic are encouraged to take the recommended drug prophylaxis. Drug choices include atovaquone/proguanil (Malarone), chloroquine, doxycycline, mefloquine, or primaquine, but the choice is influenced by the country destination, personal health status, and frequency of dosage (CDC, 2011b).

Lyme Disease

In the 1990s, Lyme disease was listed as the most important emerging infection in the United States, accounting for 90% of vector-borne illness (Herrington et al., 1997). First identified in 1975, when unusually high numbers of children living in Lyme, Connecticut, were diagnosed with juvenile arthritis, the annual number of reported cases of Lyme disease increased to 23,305 cases reported in 2005 for a national average of 7.9 cases per 100,000 population. In the 10 states where Lyme disease is most common, the average was 31.6 per 100,000 (CDC, 2013w). In the United States in 2012, Lyme disease was the seventh most commonly reported disease in the Nationally Notifiable Disease database and the most commonly reported of all of the vector-borne illnesses. Reporting is noted in 13 of the 50 states. Reported confirmed cases of Lyme disease in 2003–2012 ranged yearly from a low of 19,804 in 2004 to a high of 29,959 confirmed cases in 2009 (CDC, 2013w).

The disease is caused by infection with the spirochete *Borrelia burgdorferi,* transmitted by infected *Ixodes scapularis* ticks in Northeastern, Midwestern, and Southern states and *I. pacificus* on the West Coast (CDC, 2013x). (See **Box 20-5**.) These ticks generally feed on white-tailed deer and the white-footed mouse. Most cases of human illness occur in late spring and summer when ticks are most active and people spend more time outdoors (CDC, 2013x).

BOX 20-5 States with the Highest Incidence of Lyme Disease, 2012

	Cases per 100,000
New Hampshire	75.9
Maine	66.6
Vermont	61.7
Delaware	55.3
Massachusetts	51.1
Connecticut	46.0
Pennsylvania	32.5
New Jersey	30.8
Wisconsin	23.9

Source: Data from CDC. (2013w). Lyme disease: Statistics. Retrieved from http://www.cdc.gov/lyme/stats/index.html

The symptoms of Lyme disease are multistage and multisystem. Early disease symptoms include a red rash resembling a bull's eye forming over the tick bite and systemic flulike symptoms such as headache, muscular aches and pains, and fatigue. If untreated, symptoms can progress to include heart problems such as an irregular heart rate, shortness of breath, or dizziness; neurological problems such as meningitis, Bell's palsy, numbness, pain, weakness in the limbs, or poor muscle coordination; and arthritis that shifts from joint to joint, with the knee being most commonly affected. About 60% of untreated patients develop chronic arthritis (CDC, 2013x).

Most cases of Lyme disease can be treated with antibiotic therapy. The earlier the treatment is begun, the more successful the treatment will be. However, early diagnosis is difficult because many of the disease symptoms mimic those of other disorders, and the distinctive bull's-eye rash is absent in 20–30% of those infected (CDC, 2013x). It is important for the nurse to interview patients presenting with flu symptoms thoroughly to determine whether possible exposure to deer ticks could have occurred, particularly in warm weather months. After the initial 2–4 week antibiotic therapy for Lyme disease, 10–20% of patients experience post-treatment Lyme disease syndrome. They may report lingering muscle aches, joint aches, pain, and fatigue. Some of these symptoms may last longer than 6 months. Ongoing research is being conducted to further evaluate this condition (Barbour, 2012; CDC, 2013y).

RESEARCH ALERT 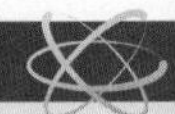

Campylobacter jejuni is one of the most common causes of bacterial gastroenteritis in the United States. Including undiagnosed and unreported cases, it is estimated to affect more than 2 million people annually, with its costs estimated to be between $1.3 billion and $6.2 billion.

This prospective, matched case-control study was implemented to determine the risk factors for *C. jejuni* enteritis in rural communities. It was hypothesized that exposure to food animals is a major risk and that the odds of infection change with exposure to different species. Study participants were selected from among all new cases of *C. jejuni* reported to the Michigan Department of Community Health during the 1-year period from October 2000 to October 2001. Each case subject was matched with two control subjects according to specified criteria. All participants completed a self-administered postal questionnaire.

The results of the data analysis indicated that contact with farm animals was a significant risk factor. Specifically, the caring for and raising of poultry increased the odds for the disease seven times more than the odds associated with husbandry of other species known to be reservoirs of *C. jejuni*. The study concluded that an estimated 18% of *C. jejuni* cases occurring in rural areas are attributable to poultry husbandry.

Source: Potter, R. C., Kaneene, J. B., & Hall, W. N. (2003). Risk factors for sporadic *Campylobacter jejuni* infections in rural Michigan: A prospective case-control study. *American Journal of Public Health, 93*(12), 2118–2123.

West Nile Virus (WNV)

WNV is a *Flavivirus* commonly found in Africa, West Asia, and the Middle East. The first case of West Nile virus was discovered in the West Nile District of Uganda, Africa, in 1937. It first appeared in Egypt and Israel in the 1950s, where it was recognized as a cause of severe human meningoencephalitis. In recent years, it has emerged in the temperate regions of Europe and North America, with the first case in the United States occurring in 1999. In 2013, there were 2,318 cases of WNV infections including 105 deaths, which occurred in 48 states and the District of Columbia (CDC, 2013z).

The virus is spread by infected mosquitoes and can infect humans, horses, many types of birds, and a few other kinds of animals (CDC, 2013aa).

Humans generally experience a mild form of the disease, characterized by flu-like symptoms that typically last only a few days and do not appear to cause any long-term negative effects. However, in less than 1% of cases, humans can develop severe neurological diseases—West Nile encephalitis, West Nile meningitis, or West Nile meningoencephalitis. Among those with severe illness, case fatality rates range between 3% and 15% and are highest among elderly patients (CDC, 2013aa; Petersen & Marfin, 2002).

Zoonoses

Many of the infectious diseases that have emerged or reemerged in the past few years have been zoonotic. Zoonoses are diseases that are caused by infectious agents that can jump from species to species—jumping from vertebrate animals to humans (Agnus, 2004; Murphy, 1998). Vector-borne diseases can also be considered zoonotic because they are indirectly transmitted from animal reservoirs to human reservoirs via another living source, usually insects. Throughout time, humans have interacted with the other animals that share the Earth. Whether domesticated work animals, animals raised or hunted for food, family pets, or unwanted household pests, animals and their products are an integral part of our daily lives (Meslin & Stohr, 1998). A variety of both domestic and wild animals carries viruses, bacteria, or parasites that can be transferred to humans either through direct contact with the animals and their waste products or through food products of animal origin (Heymann, 1998). About half of all microorganisms known to infect humans come from animals. Since the 1980s, scientists have identified more than 40 new infectious diseases, most of which have come from animals (Baylor College of Medicine, 2014; WHO International Health Regulations (n.d.). Zoonotic diseases seem to be increasing at a rapid pace for several reasons: Global human populations are increasingly bringing people into closer contact with animal populations; modern air travel has made it possible to travel to the other side of the world in a matter of hours; enormous environmental changes have been brought about by human activity; and bioterroristic activities are increasing, and the infectious agents of choice are usually zoonotic (CDC, 2007; Murphy, 1998).

Hantavirus

Hantavirus pulmonary syndrome was first recognized in the southwestern United States in 1993 when several deaths occurred from acute respiratory distress syndrome (CDC, 2012f).

Initial symptoms include fever plus muscle aches and pains, and may include gastrointestinal upset and headache. Late symptoms occur 4–10 days after initial symptoms and include respiratory difficulty as the lungs fill with fluid. As of January 2007, 460 cases were reported in 30 states, with 35% of cases resulting in death (CDC, 2012f).

Deer mice are the primary reservoir hosts for the southwestern states, along with cotton rats and rice rats in the Southeast and white-footed mice in the Northeast. Infection can occur when saliva or feces particles are inhaled in aerosol form during direct contact with the rodents or when dried materials contaminated by rodent excreta are loosened, directly introduced into open wounds or eyes, or ingested in contaminated food or water. Humans can also become infected through rodent bites (CDC, 2012f). Avoidance of contact with most rodent populations is the best way to prevent infection and control disease. Risks can be controlled through environmental hygiene practices that deter rodents from inhabiting home and work environments (CDC, 2012f). In 2012, there were 10 confirmed cases of hantavirus infection in Yosemite National Park; nine with persons staying at the Signature Tents Cabins in Curry Village in the park and probable exposure of one person while hiking nearby (CDC, 2012f).There is no specific treatment, cure, or vaccine for hantavirus. If infected individuals are diagnosed early, they can be intubated and receive oxygen therapy. However, if the individual experiences full respiratory distress without being treated, it is too late to begin oxygen therapy and the infected person usually dies (CDC, 2012f).

Avian Influenza

Since 2003, the WHO has been monitoring the progress of avian influenza, also known as bird flu, a highly pathogenic influenza virus found in parts of eastern Asia that has the potential to cause a major pandemic. As of early 2007 only a few cases had been reported in humans, with transmission occurring primarily from birds to humans. However, the high mortality rate and lack of effective treatment or vaccines for avian influenza have health professionals concerned that the virus could mutate and become transmissible from human to human. As more and more migratory birds carry the infection to western Asia, Africa, and other parts of the world, it could prove to be a serious threat to human health and wreak the kind of worldwide devastation caused by the 1918 Spanish influenza epidemic that killed more than 50 million people and created social, economic, and political havoc (CDC, 2014d; Schwartz, 2006).

Pet Diseases

Pets, especially cats and dogs, are considered members of the family by many people worldwide. People give their pets names, share their food, and sometimes even share their beds with them, all in exchange for unconditional love (De Menezes Brandao & Anselmo Viana da Silva Berzins, 1998). Unfortunately, pets can be a source for zoonotic diseases. However, if pets are well nourished, properly vaccinated, and regularly examined by a veterinarian, there is little to fear (CDC, 2013bb; Chomel, 1998).

Cat-scratch fever, caused by *Bartonella henselae,* is generally a benign local inflammation of the lymph nodes transmitted through a break in the skin caused by a cat scratch. However, in people with weakened immune systems, it causes bacillary angiomatosis, a life-threatening vascular disease in which tumors are formed from blood cells. The organism is transmitted from cat to cat primarily by fleas (CDC, 2013bb; Chomel, 1998).

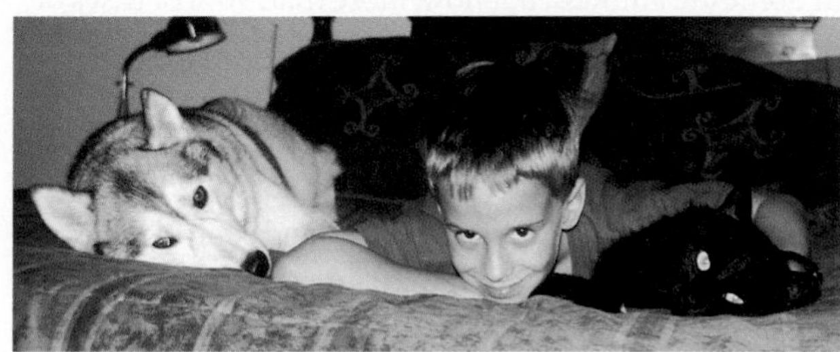

In American households, pets are members of the family. Children are especially vulnerable for exposure to infectious agents carried by pets.

In countries where plague is endemic, cats can become infected or carry fleas from infected rodents they may have killed. Several cases of bubonic and pneumonic plague in humans in the United States have been associated with pet cats (CDC, 2013bb; Chomel, 1998).

Pets can carry infectious agents such as *Campylobacter* or *Salmonella,* which can cause diarrheal and gastrointestinal illness. Puppies and kittens with diarrhea pose the greatest risk. Reptiles are also carriers of a wide variety of *Salmonella* species. Pet turtles and iguanas have been linked to several severe, and even fatal, cases of *Salmonella* among young children worldwide. It is easy to see why handwashing is extremely important after handling pets and before eating (CDC, 2013r; Chomel, 1998).

Rabies

Rabies is probably the best known and most feared of the zoonoses because the disease is almost always fatal in humans once symptoms occur. WHO estimates that more than 55,000 deaths from rabies occur a year, but the figure may actually be higher because of the large number of deaths worldwide that go unreported. In the United States, the number of rabies-related deaths has declined from more than 100 annually in 1900 to only one or two per year in the 1990s. Modern prevention efforts have proven almost 100% effective, with U.S. deaths occurring only in people who do not recognize their risk and fail to seek medical treatment (CDC, 2013cc).

The virus is usually transmitted through bites from infected animals, but in rare cases, it can also be transmitted through infected licks on mucous membranes, inhaled infected bat secretions, and corneal transplants from undiagnosed human donors. Reservoirs for infection are domestic dogs and cats as well as many wild animals such as skunks, raccoons, foxes, wolves, and bats (Wilde & Mitmoonpitak, 1998). Before 1960, most rabies cases were in domestic animals, but now, more than 90% of cases occur in wild animals (CDC, 2013cc). Efforts by U.S. wildlife agencies have helped control rabies in wild animal populations in recent years.

Although human rabies deaths in the United States are rare, the public health costs to prevent and control rabies exceed $300 million a year. These costs include vaccinations for pets and other domestic animals, animal control programs, maintenance of rabies laboratories, and medical costs related to rabies post-exposure prophylaxis (RPEP) treatment for humans bitten by at-risk animals (CDC, 2013cc).

After entering the host, the rabies virus multiplies slowly at the portal of entry. It then invades the surrounding nerve tissue and slowly migrates to the spinal cord and brain. Once there, it multiplies, causing a rapid death. The incubation period can range from a few days to many years (CDC, 2013cc; Wilde & Mitmoonpitak, 1998). Rabies in humans is preventable by immediately cleansing all animal bites with soap and water and using rabies immune globulin and vaccine as indicated (Benenson, 1995; Heymann, 2004; Wilde & Mitmoonpitak, 1998). Current rabies vaccinations are the best protection for pets and other domestic animals, thus significantly reducing the risk of exposure for humans. In 2013, one death was confirmed from rabies, which was contracted through organ transplantation done more than a year prior. The CDC reports only one other person to have died from the same raccoon-type rabies virus in the last 50 years (CDC, 2013dd).

Parasitic Diseases

Parasitic diseases, although more common in developing countries, have been on the rise in recent years in the United States. According to *Webster's Dictionary* (Agnus, 2004), a *parasite* is an animal that lives on or in an organism of another species, from which it derives sustenance or protection without benefit to, and usually with harmful effects on, the host. The most common parasites are helminths (worms and flukes) and one-celled protozoans.

Helminths

Pinworm infection (enterobiasis) occurs worldwide and is the most common helminth intestinal infection in the United States, with the highest prevalence in school-aged children, followed by preschoolers. The prevalence is low in adults except for mothers of infected children. Pinworm infection often results in no symptoms, but in some persons, there may be perianal itching and disturbed sleep. Diagnosis can be made by applying cellophane tape to the perianal region early in the morning before bathing or defecating. Transmission occurs by direct transfer of infective eggs from the anus to the mouth or indirect transfer through contaminated clothing, bedding, food, or other fomites. Treatment with oral vermicides and disinfection of clothing and bedding are usually effective (Benenson, 1995; Heymann, 2004).

Roundworm infection (ascariasis) occurs worldwide, with the highest prevalence in children between 3 and 8 years of age living in moist, tropical countries. Typically, no symptoms occur. Live worms, passed in stools or occasionally through the mouth or nose, are often the first sign of roundworm infection. Transmission occurs by ingestion of infective eggs from soil contaminated with human feces or from uncooked produce contaminated with soil containing infective eggs; it is not transmitted directly from person to person. Treatment with oral vermicides is usually effective (Benenson, 1995; Heymann, 2004).

Hookworm infection (ancylostomiasis) is widely endemic in tropical and subtropical climates but can also occur in temperate climates. Approximately 2 billion people are estimated to be infected with hookworms (WHO, 2014c). In persons with heavy infections, there is severe iron deficiency, which leads to severe anemia. Children with heavy, long-term infection may have hypoproteinemia and may be delayed in physical and mental development. Light hookworm infections generally produce no clinical symptoms. Diagnosis is made by finding hookworm eggs in feces. Transmission occurs by larvae in the soil penetrating the skin, usually of the foot. The larvae then enter the bloodstream and travel to the lungs, where they enter the alveoli and migrate up the trachea to the pharynx. They are swallowed and reach the small intestine, where they develop into mature half-inch worms in 6 to 7 weeks. They attach to the intestinal wall and suck blood. Treatment with vermicides is usually effective (Benenson, 1995; CDC, 2008a; Heymann, 2004).

Protozoans

Giardiasis Giardiasis is a disease caused by *Giardia lamblia,* a microscopic, one-celled parasite that lives in the intestines of humans and animals. This parasite is found in every part of the United States and every region of the world. In recent years, giardiasis has become one of the most common water-borne diseases in the United States. Transmission is through the fecal–oral route or through ingestion of contaminated food or water from swimming pools, lakes, rivers, springs, ponds, or streams. The most common symptoms of giardiasis are diarrhea, abdominal cramps, nausea, fatigue, and weight loss. Symptoms usually appear within 1 to 2 weeks after exposure and generally last 2 to 6 weeks, but they can last longer (CDC, 2008b; Heymann, 2004).

Persons at risk for giardiasis are childcare workers, children in diapers who attend daycare centers, international travelers, hikers, campers, or anyone who drinks untreated water from a contaminated source. Because chlorine does not kill *G. lamblia,* several community outbreaks have been linked to contaminated community water supplies (CDC, 2008b; Heymann, 2004).

RESEARCH ALERT 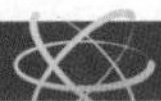

Government-sponsored research from 2006 found that the mutated, drug-resistant "superbugs" that are causing an increasing number of hospital infections and deaths can live for weeks on bed linens, on computer keyboard covers, and under acrylic fingernails. *Staphylococcus aureus,* a methicillin-resistant strain, is usually harmless and very common, found on skin or in the noses of about 30% of all people. In hospitals, methicillin-resistant *S. aureus* (MRSA) can cause serious and sometimes deadly infections, including necrotizing fasciitis or "flesh-eating" disease. Only vancomycin administered intravenously can treat MRSA. Computer keyboards can contaminate the fingers, bare or gloved, of a nurse or physician, who could then transfer bacteria to patients.

Source: Centers for Disease Control and Prevention. (2007). *MRSA in healthcare settings.* Retrieved from http://www.cdc.gov/mrsa/healthcare/

Giardiasis is difficult to diagnose and may require examination of several stool specimens over several days. The pharmacological treatment for giardiasis is metronidazole (Flagyl). Nurses can help prevent giardiasis outbreaks in their communities by teaching patients in community settings to wash their hands after using the bathroom and before handling food, to wash and peel all raw vegetables and fruits, and to avoid drinking water from any source unless it has been filtered or chemically treated (Benenson, 1995; CDC, 2008b; Heymann, 2004).

Cryptosporidiosis Cryptosporidiosis, often called *crypto,* is a disease caused by *Cryptosporidium parvum,* a microscopic, one-celled parasite. Although not a new disease in the developing world, cryptosporidiosis made its first major appearance in the United States in 1993 when 400,000 people became ill with diarrhea after drinking contaminated water. Today, crypto is still a major threat to the U.S. water supply. Transmission is through the fecal–oral route or through ingestion of food or water contaminated with stool, including water in recreational parks or swimming pools (CDC, 2008c; Heymann, 2004).

Immunocompromised persons are most at risk for crypto infection, particularly HIV-positive persons or persons receiving chemotherapy for cancer treatment. Other persons at risk for infection are childcare workers, children in diapers who attend daycare centers, persons exposed to human feces by sexual contact, and caregivers of persons infected with crypto. The most common symptoms are watery diarrhea and cramps, which in some cases can be severe. Weight loss, nausea, vomiting, and fever may also occur (CDC, 2008c; Guerrant, 1997; Heymann, 2004).

Currently, no cure exists for crypto, but some drugs (e.g., paromomycin) may reduce the severity of the symptoms. Oral rehydration powders and sports drinks can help prevent dehydration. Nurses can help at-risk populations reduce their risk by teaching them to wash their hands often with soap and water; to avoid sex that involves contact with stool; to avoid touching farm animals; to avoid touching the stool of pets; to wash and/or cook food; to be careful when swimming in lakes, rivers, pools, or hot tubs; to drink safe water; and to take extra precautions when traveling, particularly to developing countries (CDC, 2008c; Heymann, 2004).

Bioterrorism

A bioterrorism attack occurs when viruses, bacteria, and other infectious agents are used to deliberately cause illness or death in people, animals, or plants. Infectious agents make perfect instruments of destruction. They self-propagate, adapt easily, jump international borders effortlessly, and it takes only a small amount to wreak havoc on a nation's healthcare system. Agents used for biowarfare are living organisms or toxins secreted by living organisms (Drexler, 2002). The anthrax outbreaks in the United States during the fall of 2001 proved that bioterrorism could be a significant threat to public health (CDC, 2006).

Many infectious agents found in nature can be used even more effectively as biological weapons when altered to increase their ability to cause disease, resist current medications, and spread more rapidly in the environment (CDC, 2006). In a bioterrorist attack, health officials might not notice until too late. Pathogens require an incubation period to multiply in the body before triggering symptoms. It could be days or weeks before the first signs of disease are apparent and even longer to identify outbreaks as an epidemic. By the time an epidemic situation is established, it may be impossible to determine the triggering event or events (Drexler, 2002).

Bioterrorism agents kill by causing suffocating pneumonia, septic shock, massive bleeding, or paralysis. The CDC divides bioterrorism agents into three categories, depending on how easily they can spread and the severity of the illness they can cause. Category A agents include organisms or toxins that are considered the highest risk to public and national security because they can be easily spread or transmitted from person to person and result in high death rates. They have the greatest potential for major public health impact, because they can cause public panic and social disruption and require special action for public health preparedness (CDC, 2006; Drexler, 2002). Category B agents are the second highest priority because they are moderately easy to spread, result in moderate illness and low death rates, and require specific enhancements of the CDC's laboratory capacity and enhanced disease monitoring. Category C agents are the third highest priority because they are easily available, easily produced and spread, and have the potential for high morbidity and mortality rates and major public health impact. The agents include emerging pathogens that could be engineered for mass spread in the future (CDC, 2006). See **Box 20-6** for the diseases listed under each category.

BOX 20-6 Categories of Bioterrorism Agents/Diseases

Category A

- Anthrax (*Bacillus anthracis*)
- Botulism (*Clostridium botulinum* toxin)
- Plague (*Yersinia pestis*)
- Smallpox (*Variola major*)
- Tularemia (*Francisella tularensis*)
- Viral hemorrhagic fevers (filoviruses [e.g., Ebola, Marburg] and arenaviruses [e.g., Lassa, Machupo])

Category B

- Brucellosis (*Brucella* species)
- Epsilon (toxin of *Clostridium perfringens*)
- Food safety threats (e.g., *Salmonella* species, *Escherichia coli* O157:H7, *Shigella*)
- Glanders (*Burkholderia mallei*)
- Melioidosis (*Burkholderia pseudomallei*)
- Psittacosis (*Chlamydia psittaci*)
- Q fever (*Coxiella burnetii*)
- Ricin toxin (from *Ricinus communis* [castor beans])
- Staphylococcal enterotoxin B
- Typhus fever (*Rickettsia prowazekii*)
- Viral encephalitis (alphaviruses [e.g., Venezuelan equine encephalitis, eastern equine encephalitis, western equine encephalitis])
- Water safety threats (e.g., *Vibrio cholerae, Cryptosporidium parvum*)

Category C

- Emerging infectious diseases such as Nipah virus and hantavirus

Source: CDC. (2014e). Bioterrorism Agents/Diseases. Retrieved from http://www.bt.cdc.gov/agent/agentlist-category.asp

Response to a bioterrorism event will require a rapid deployment of limited public health resources. The health of America's communities will depend on the nation's public health workforce. This workforce includes physicians, nurses, environmental health scientists, health educators, laboratory personnel, and managers, supplemented by other professionals, first responders, and volunteers who will form the public health frontline of defense. Preparation in the core competencies of bioterrorism and emergency preparedness is essential for agencies and communities to respond appropriately. The most common agents for nurses to have a working knowledge of include anthrax, botulism, plague, smallpox, and tularemia (CDC, 2014e). Nurses should be familiar with the aspects of drug administration for the following commonly prescribed medications in the event of an act of bioterrorism: tetracycline, doxycycline, streptomycin, gentamycin, chloramphenicol, and ciprofloxacin. Factors such as the exposed person's age and weight, pregnancy status, drug allergies, and the agent exposed are evaluated to determine the appropriate medications and possible routes of administration (oral [PO], intramuscular, or IV). Anthrax, botulism, and tularemia have no person-to-person transmission. The vaccine for anthrax is available for high-risk populations such as lab and mortuary workers, first responders, and the military. Extensive partnerships are required among federal, state, and local agencies; educational institutions; and professional organizations to ensure a systematic approach to education and training (CDC, 2002). The CDC (2012g) Strategic National Stockpile (SNS) has stockpiled medications for the American public in the event of a public health emergency or bioterrorism attack. Medication may be delivered by open or closed "points of distribution" (PODs). The public should be encouraged to prepare for such circumstances as they would for any other disaster—by getting a kit, making a plan, and staying informed.

HIV/AIDS

The most significant emerging disease in the world since the 1980s is HIV/AIDS. AIDS is the life-threatening, late clinical stage of infection with HIV. The disease was first recognized as a distinct syndrome in 1981, and the virus was first isolated in 1983 (Benenson, 1995; Heymann, 2004).

As of December 2013, the number of people currently infected with HIV was about 1.1 million. Cumulatively, about the same number of people have been diagnosed with AIDS (the immunodeficiency disorder that is caused by HIV infection) since the disease was first identified. The rate of infection has stabilized at about 50,000 new cases per year. The total number of deaths from AIDS in the United States was 636,000 at the end of 2013 (CDC, 2013ee). Worldwide, the number of adults and children estimated to be living with HIV is about 35.3 million (UNAIDS, 2013), but new infections have declined since 2001. In 2012, approximately 260,000 children were newly infected with HIV—a decline of nearly 50% since 2001—and an overall decrease of 33% in new HIV infections (from about 3.4 million in 2001 to about 2.3 million in 2012) has been observed as well (UNAIDS, 2013). An estimated 1.6 million deaths occurred in 2012, a decrease of about 31% since 2005 (UNAIDS, 2013).

HIV can be transmitted from person to person through unprotected sexual contact, through direct contact with blood or blood products through sharing needles or razors, and from mother to baby during gestation or the birthing process (Benenson, 1995; Heymann, 2004).

Tuberculosis

TB is one of the leading causes of death worldwide from an infectious agent. Approximately 2 billion people to one-third of the world's population are infected with TB, with about 860,000 new cases and 1.3 million deaths occurring in 2012 (WHO, 2014d).

Historically, TB has been one of the great scourges of humankind. It was a leading killer in the United States until the advent of antibiotics in the 1950s. For the next 30 years, TB was on a steady decline, at least in the developed countries (American Association for World Health [AAWH], 1998; CDC, 2005). The 1980s, however, saw a sharp increase in TB cases, which has been primarily the result of the development of multidrug-resistant (MDR) strains of the disease (AAWH, 1998; CDC, 2005). Other reasons for the upsurge include the spread of TB in institutional living facilities such as shelters and correctional facilities, a declining public health infrastructure, increased immigration from regions where TB is endemic, and the HIV/AIDS pandemic (Clark, Cegielski, & Hassell, 1997).

The number of reported TB cases in the United States has shown a steady decline, with fewer than 10,000 cases reported in 2012 (CDC, 2013ff), but the rate of decline has been slowing each year since 2000. The greatest concern now is that various strains of TB are showing resistance to multiple antibiotic drugs (multidrug-resistant or MDR-TB). Cases are still high among high-risk groups such as the incarcerated, the homeless, elders, and HIV-infected persons, as well as underrepresented racial and ethnic groups and immigrants from countries with high TB rates and inadequate control measures (AAWH, 1998; CDC, 2013ff).

TB is caused by *Mycobacterium tuberculosis* and is transmitted by droplets in the air. It usually affects the lungs (pulmonary), which accounts for 75% of all cases, although other body organs may be involved (extrapulmonary) about 25% of the time. TB can live in an infected person's body and not cause illness. This is called *inactive* TB or latent TB. Approximately 5% of people with inactive TB develop active TB or TB disease later in life. Only about 10% of all persons infected with TB actually develop active TB. Symptoms of active TB include fatigue, weight loss, fever, chills, and night sweats. Symptoms of pulmonary TB also include a persistent cough, chest pain, and bloody sputum (CDC, 2013ff).

TB is both preventable and curable. Prevention is focused on treating persons with inactive TB infection prophylactically with anti-TB medications such as isoniazid (INH) for 6 to 12 months. It is extremely important for infected persons to complete the preventive therapy treatment both to prevent progression to active disease and to prevent the development of drug-resistant organisms (CDC, 2013ff).

Treatment for persons with active TB disease commonly includes such drugs as INH, rifampin, pyrazinamide, ethambutol, and streptomycin. These drugs are usually prescribed in various combinations. It is important that persons with active TB take the medication therapy prescribed for at least 6 months (CDC, 2013ff).

MDR-TB may occur when medications are not taken consistently for the 6 to 12 months necessary to completely destroy the *M. tuberculosis* organism. In some U.S. cities, more than 50% of TB patients fail to complete their prescribed course of therapy. Many of these patients are homeless persons, drug addicts, or other persons living in poverty, who may not be reliable about taking their medications. Many individuals with TB may feel better after only a few weeks of therapy and stop taking their medications because of unpleasant side effects. MDR-TB is difficult and complicated to treat. Inappropriate treatment can have life-threatening results. Depending on the combination of alternative drugs needed, treatment can last as long as 2 years and be very costly (CDC, 2013ff). Globally in 2012, WHO reported that 450,000 persons developed MDR-TB (WHO, 2014d).

The best method of treatment for persons in high-risk circumstances is directly observed therapy (DOT). DOT is a community-based prevention program in which a nurse or other healthcare provider is paired with a person infected with TB to ensure that the patient follows the prescribed treatment plan. DOT programs have been successful in curing 95% of patients with pulmonary TB (Torres, 1998) and have the potential to save millions of lives worldwide ("DOTS: A breakthrough," 1998).

> If I were going to imagine a real terror it would be a deadly virus that kills 100% of its victims, but incubates so slowly, say a decade, that millions of people are infected before they know it. It would be a virus that is transmitted sexually, attacking young adults while it takes advantage of our social inhibitions and bigotry about sex.
>
> —*Dr. Joe McCormick, Chairman, Community Health Sciences Department, Aga Khan University, Pakistan*

THINK ABOUT THIS 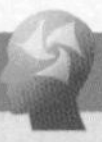

The CDC's most important achievements in 2013 were the outbreaks that didn't happen, the diseases that were stopped before they crossed our borders, and the countless lives saved from preventable chronic diseases and injuries.

> While our biggest successes may be the bad things that did not happen, careful assessment of what we did well—and what we might do better—is essential for continued success,
>
> —*CDC Director Tom Frieden, MD, MPH*

The HIV/TB Connection

WHO estimates that globally about 13 million people of the 35.3 million people living with HIV are co-infected with HIV and latent TB. In countries with high HIV prevalence, up to 80% of people with TB test positive for HIV (WHO, 2005b). Worldwide, TB is the leading killer among people infected with HIV. TB is listed as an AIDS-defining opportunistic infection for people who are infected with HIV. TB often occurs early in the course of HIV infection and may be the first indication that a person has HIV ("HIV-Related Conditions," 1999; CDC, 2012h; WHO, 2013c).

Early diagnosis and treatment of TB are critical for HIV-infected patients because the risk for drug-resistant TB is higher among people with HIV infection compared with other groups (Moore, McCray, & Onorato, 1999; "Prevention and Treatment of Tuberculosis," 1998; WHO, 2013c). For people with HIV infection, the death rate for MDR-TB is as high as 80%. Because TB symptoms are the same as the symptoms for many other HIV-related opportunistic infections, TB is easy to overlook initially. HIV-infected patients may not react to tuberculin skin testing because their immune systems are suppressed ("HIV-Related Conditions," 1999). The three "I"s for HIV/TB are intensified case finding, isoniazid, and infection control. A comprehensive health history is an essential tool for assisting nurses and other healthcare providers to identify TB exposure risks in HIV-infected patients.

The Bill and Melinda Gates Foundation partners with WHO in supporting many targeted health prevention, control, and eradication programs (WHO, 2013d). Some of the global programs focused on health are HIV/TB; poliomyelitis; human African trypanosomiasis; rabies; maternal, newborn, and child health; clean water; and global vaccines.

Global Disease Eradication Efforts

Despite the emergence and reemergence of infectious diseases in recent years, significant advancements in the elimination or eradication of some diseases that have existed for centuries have occurred through a united global effort. The eradication of smallpox by 1979 is thought to be the greatest triumph of modern public health (Garrett, 1994). WHO, in collaboration with other international public and private health organizations, has targeted six other communicable diseases for eradication in the beginning of the 21st century. These diseases are polio, maternal and neonatal tetanus, measles, leprosy, guinea worm disease, and lymphatic filariasis. According to WHO, these crippling and sometimes deadly diseases can be eliminated in parts of the world and even completely eradicated worldwide within a generation. The methods being used to accomplish this goal are immunization and vaccination, drug therapy, community training, health education, and national disease surveillance efforts (Wittenberg, 1998).

Conclusion

Community health nurses have played a significant role in the prevention, control, and treatment of communicable disease throughout recent history. Nurses' skills and knowledge will continue to be a vital part of global eradication efforts well into the 21st century.

AFFORDABLE CARE ACT (ACA) 

Medicare payments to acute care and other facilities will be based on quality measures, not number of patients served. Payments will be reduced for hospital-acquired infections or excessive readmissions.

LEVELS OF PREVENTION 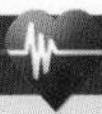

Primary: Appropriate handwashing

Secondary: Use of isolation for patients with communicable diseases

Tertiary: Rehabilitation for patients with AIDS

Critical Thinking Activities

1. As a nurse working with WHO, what actions would you take to eliminate the reservoir for a vector-borne disease such as malaria? What kind of actions would you take to eliminate the reservoir for an airborne disease such as legionellosis?
2. Discuss the differences between active immunity and passive immunity. Give two examples of each kind of immunity. How long does immunity last for each example?
3. Identify one infectious disease and discuss primary, secondary, and tertiary prevention methods appropriate for that disease at the community level.
4. Compare and contrast the five viral types of hepatitis. Identify similarities and differences regarding the following:
   - Occurrence in the world
   - Infectious agent
   - Reservoir
   - Incubation period
   - Methods of control

HEALTHY ME 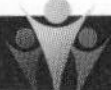

Don't get sick on cruise ships: Protect yourself. Over the past few years, outbreaks of gastroenteritis or Noroviruses have afflicted hundreds of people, especially aboard cruise ships where confined living conditions allow the virus to spread rapidly.

Whether you're at home or traveling, you can fend off Norovirus with these tips:

- Wash your hands frequently with soap and water, particularly before and after meals, and keep your hands away from your face and mouth.
- Every so often, use alcohol-based hand sanitizers.
- Don't share eating utensils or drinking glasses.
- Avoid eating uncooked food.
- Wash fruit and vegetables before consumption.
- If you're traveling, drink only bottled water.
- If you're planning a trip and are older than 65 or have a weakened immune system, your healthcare provider can suggest additional precautions.

References

Abbott Diagnostics. (2008). *Hepatitis learning guide.* Retrieved from http://my.abbottdiagnostics.com/AssetsVerify?locale=au&asset=/viewFile.cfm%3Ffile%3Dlearning_hepatitis.pdf

Agnus, M. E. (2004). *Webster's new world college dictionary* (4th ed.). New York, NY: Macmillan.

American Association for World Health (AAWH). (1998). *TB alert.* Washington, DC: Author.

Atkinson, W., & Wolfe, C. (Eds.). (2003). *Epidemiology and prevention of vaccine-preventable diseases* (7th ed.). Atlanta, GA: Centers for Disease Control and Prevention.

Barbour, A. (2012). Remains of infection. *Journal of Clinical Investigation, 122*(7), 2344–2346.

Baylor College of Medicine, Department of Molecular Virology and Microbiology. (2014). Emerging infectious diseases. Retrieved from https://www.bcm.edu/departments/molecular-virology-and-microbiology/index.cfm?pmid=16501

Benenson, A. S. (Ed.). (1995). *Control of communicable diseases manual* (15th ed.). Washington, DC: American Public Health Association.

Centers for Disease Control and Prevention (CDC). (1994). *Addressing emerging disease threats: A prevention strategy for the United States.* Atlanta, GA: U.S. Department of Health and Human Services.

— (1998). *Preventing infectious diseases: A strategy for the twenty-first century.* Atlanta, GA: U.S. Department of Health and Human Services.

— (2002). *Centers for Public Health preparedness.* Atlanta, GA: U.S. Department of Health and Human Services.

— (2004). *Viral hepatitis D fact sheet.* Atlanta, GA: U.S. Department of Health and Human Services.

— (2005). *Questions and answers about TB.* Atlanta, GA: U.S. Department of Health and Human Services.

— (2006). *Bioterrorism.* Atlanta, GA: U.S. Department of Health and Human Services.

— (2007). *Division of Vector-Borne Infectious Diseases.* Atlanta, GA: U.S. Department of Health and Human Services.

— (2008a). *Hookworm infection.* Retrieved from http://www.cdc.gov/ncidod/dpd/parasites/hookworm/factsht_hookworm.htm

— (2008b). *Giardiasis.* Retrieved from http://www.cdc.gov/ncidod/dpd/parasites/giardiasis/factsht_giardia.htm

— (2008c). You can prevent *cryptosporidiosis.* Retrieved from http://www.cdc.gov/hiv/resources/brochures/crypto.htm

— (2010). *Viral hepatitis C fact sheet.* Retrieved from http://www.cdc.gov/hepatitis/hcv/pdfs/hepcgeneralfactsheet.pdf

— (2011a). Healthcare associated infections: Vancomycin-resistant *Enterococcus* (VRE) infection. Retrieved from http://www.cdc.gov/HAI/organisms/vre/vre-infection.html

— (2011b). Drugs to use to prevent malaria. Retrieved from http://www.cdc.gov/malaria/travelers/drugs.html

— (2011c). CDC estimates of foodborne illness in the United States. Retrieved from http://www.cdc.gov/foodborneburden/2011-foodborne-estimates.html#illness

— (2012a). *Epidemiology and prevention of vaccine-preventable diseases.* Atlanta, GA: U.S. Department of Health and Human Services.

— (2012b). Hepatitis B FAQs for health professionals. Retrieved from http://www.cdc.gov/hepatitis/HBV/HBVfaq.htm

— (2012c). The ABCs of hepatitis. Retrieved from http://www.cdc.gov/hepatitis/Resources/Professionals/PDFs/ABCTable.pdf

— (2012d). Hepatitis E information for the health professionals. Retrieved from http://www.cdc.gov/hepatitis/HEV/index.htm

— (2012e). Malaria facts. Retrieved from http://www.cdc.gov/malaria/about/facts.html

— (2012f). Hantavirus. Retrieved from http://www.cdc.gov/hantavirus/outbreaks/yosemite-national-park-2012.html

— (2012g). Strategic National Stockpile (SNS). Retrieved from http://www.cdc.gov/phpr/stockpile/stockpile.htm

— (2012h). TB and HIV coinfection. Retrieved from http://www.cdc.gov/tb/topic/TBHIVcoinfection/default.htm

— (2013). Seasonal influenza. Retrieved from http://www.cdc.gov/flu/about/disease/high_risk.htm

— (2013a). Vaccines and preventable diseases. Retrieved from http://www.cdc.gov/vaccines/vpd-vac/default.htm

— (2013b). Social media tools. Retrieved from http://www.cdc.gov/mobile/

— (2013c). Hepatitis A information for health professionals. Retrieved from http://www.cdc.gov/hepatitis/HAV/HAVfaq.htm#general

— (2013d). Multistate outbreak of hepatitis A virus infections linked to pomegranate seeds from Turkey (final update). Retrieved from http://www.cdc.gov/hepatitis/Outbreaks/2013/A1b-03-31/index.html

— (2013e). Hepatitis C information for health professionals. Retrieved from http://www.cdc.gov/hepatitis/HCV/HCVfaq.htm

— (2013f). Recommended immunizations for adults by age. Retrieved from http://www.cdc.gov/vaccines/schedules/easy-to-read/adult.html

— (2013g). Seasonal influenza: Flu basics. Retrieved from http://www.cdc.gov/flu/about/disease/index.htm

— (2013h). Antibiotic resistance threats in the United States, 2013. Retrieved from http://www.cdc.gov/drugresistance/threat-report-2013/

— (2013i). Carbapenem-resistant Enterobacteriaceae (CRE). Retrieved from http://www.cdc.gov/HAI/organisms/cre/

— (2013j). Vital signs. Making healthcare safer. Stop infections from lethal CRE germs now. Retrieved from http://www.cdc.gov/vitalsigns/HAI/CRE/

— (2013k). CDC estimates of foodborne illness in the United States. Retrieved from http://www.cdc.gov/foodborneburden/2011-foodborne-estimates.html

— (2013l). Foodborne Diseases Active Surveillance Network (FoodNet). Retrieved from http://www.cdc.gov/foodnet

— (2013m). National Center for Emerging and Zoonotic Infectious Diseases: *Campylobacter*. Retrieved from http://www.cdc.gov/nczved/divisions/dfbmd/diseases/campylobacter/

— (2013n). *Listeria* (Listerosis) statistics. Retrieved from http://www.cdc.gov/listeria/statistics.html

— (2013o). Vital signs: Listeria illnesses, deaths, and outbreaks—United States, 2009–2011. *Morbidity and Mortality Weekly Report, 62*(22), 52.

— (2013p). *Salmonella*. Retrieved from http://www.cdc.gov/salmonella/general/index.html

— (2013q). Multistate outbreaks of multidrug-resistant *Salmonella* Heidelberg infections linked to Foster Farms brand chicken. Retrieved from http://www.cdc.gov/salmonella/heidelberg-10-13/index.html

— (2013r). Salmonellosis. Retrieved from http://www.cdc.gov/salmonella/small-turtles-03-12/index.html

— (2013s). CDC estimates of foodborne illness in the United States. Retrieved from http://www.cdc.gov/foodborneburden/2011-foodborne-estimates.html

— (2013t). Multistate outbreak of Shiga toxin-producing *Escherichia coli* O26 infections linked to raw clover sprouts at Jimmy John's restaurants (final update). Retrieved from http://www.cdc.gov/ecoli/2012/O26-02-12/index.html

— (2013u). Multistate outbreak of Shiga toxin-producing *Escherichia coli* O121 infections linked to Farm Rich brand frozen food products (final update). Retrieved from http://www.cdc.gov/ecoli/2013/O121-03-13/index.html

— (2013v). Multistate outbreak of Shiga toxin-producing *Escherichia coli* O157:H7 infections linked to ready-to-eat salads (final update). Retrieved from http://www.cdc.gov/ecoli/2013/O157H7-11-13/index.html

— (2013w). Lyme disease: Statistics. Retrieved from http://www.cdc.gov/lyme/stats/index.html

— (2013x). Lyme disease. Retrieved from http://www.cdc.gov/lyme/

— (2013y). Post-Treatment Lyme Syndrome. Retrieved from http://www.cdc.gov/lyme/postLDS/

— (2013z). West Nile Virus. Preliminary Maps & Data for 2013. Retrieved from http://www.cdc.gov/westnile/statsMaps/preliminaryMapsData/index.html

— (2013aa). FAQ: General questions about West Nile Virus. Retrieved from http://www.cdc.gov/westnile/faq/genQuestions.html

— (2013bb). Healthy pets, healthy people. Retrieved from http://www.cdc.gov/healthypets/

— (2013cc). Rabies. Retrieved from http://www.cdc.gov/rabies/index.html

— (2013dd). Questions and answers—Human rabies due to organ transplantation, 2013. Retrieved from http://www.cdc.gov/rabies/resources/news/2013-03-15.html

— (2013ee). HIV/AIDS: Basic statistics. Retrieved from http://www.cdc.gov/hiv/basics/statistics.html

—(2013ff). Trends in tuberculosis, 2012. Retrieved from http://www.cdc.gov/tb/publications/factsheets/statistics/TBTrends.htm

— (2014a). Vessel Sanitation Program: Outbreak updates for international cruise ships. Retrieved from http://www.cdc.gov/nceh/vsp/surv/gilist.htm

— (2014b). National Notifiable Diseases Surveillance System (NNDSS): 2014 National notifiable infectious conditions. Retrieved from http://wwwn.cdc.gov/NNDSS/script/ConditionList.aspx?Type=0&Yr=2014

— (2014c). Methicillin-resistant *Staphylococcus aureus* (MRSA) infections. Retrieved from http://www.cdc.gov/mrsa/

— (2014d). Highly pathogenic avian influenza A (H5N1) virus. Retrieved from http://www.cdc.gov/flu/avianflu/h5n1-virus.htm

— (2014e). Bioterrorism agents/diseases, A-Z. Retrieved from http://emergency.cdc.gov/agent/agentlist-category.asp

Chomel, B. B. (1998). Diseases transmitted by pets. *World Health, 51*(4), 24–25.

Clark, P. A., Cegielski, J. P., & Hassell, W. (1997). TB or not TB? Increasing door-to-door response to screening. *Public Health Nursing, 14*(5), 268–271.

Cohen, S. H., Gerding, D. N., Johnson, S., Kelly, C. P., Loo, V. G., McDonald, L. C., … Wilcox, M. H. (2010). Clinical practice guidelines for *Clostridium difficile* infection in adults: 2010 update by the Society for Healthcare Epidemiology of America (SHEA) and the Infectious Diseases Society of America (IDSA). *Infection Control and Hospital Epidemiology, 31*(5), 431–455.

Dantes, R., Mu, Y., Belflower, R., Aragon, D., Dumyati, G., Harrison, L. H., . . . Fridkin S. (2013). National burden of invasive methicillin-resistant *Staphylococcus aureus* infections, United States. *JAMA Internal Medicine, 173*(21), 1970–1978.

De Menezes Brandao, M., & Anselmo Viana da Silva Berzins, M. (1998). When does a pet become a health hazard? *World Health, 51*(4), 20–21.

Dols, C. L., Bowers, J. M., & Copfer, A. E. (2001). Preventing food- and water-borne illnesses. *American Journal of Nursing, 101*(6), 24AA–24HH.

DOTS: A breakthrough in TB control. (1998). *World Health, 51*(2), 14–15.

Drexler, M. (2002). *Secret agents: The menace of emerging infections.* Washington, DC: Joseph Henry Press.

Dzenowagis, J. (1997). Using electronic links for monitoring diseases. *World Health, 50*(6), 8–9.

Fauci, A. S., Touchette, N. A., & Folkers, G. K. (2005). Emerging infectious diseases: A 10-year perspective from the National Institute of Allergy and Infectious Disease. *Emerging Infectious Diseases, 11*(4). Retrieved from http://wwwnc.cdc.gov/eid/article/11/4/04-1167.htm

Garrett, L. (1994). *The coming plague. Newly emerging diseases in a world out of balance.* New York, NY: Farrar, Straus and Giroux.

Goldrick, B. A. (2004). Influenza 2004–2005. What's new with the flu? *American Journal of Nursing, 104*(10), 34–38.

Gorwitz, R. J., Jernigan, D. B., Powers, J. H., Jernigan, J. A., & Participants in the CDC Convened Experts Meeting on Management of MRSA in the Community. (2006). Strategies for clinical management of MRSA in the community: Summary of an experts meeting convened by the Centers for Disease Control and Prevention. Retrieved from http://www.cdc.gov/mrsa/pdf/MRSA-Strategies-ExpMtgSummary-2006.pdf

Gubler, D. J. (1998). Resurgent vector-borne diseases as a global health problem. *Emerging Infectious Diseases, 4*(3), 442–449.

Guerrant, R. L. (1997). Cryptosporidiosis: An emerging, highly infectious threat. *Emerging Infectious Diseases,* 3(1).

Herrington, J. E., Campbell, G. L., Bailey, R. E., Cartter, M. L., Adams, M., Frazier, E. L., … Gensheimer, K. F. (1997). Predisposing factors for individuals' Lyme disease prevention practices: Connecticut, Maine, and Montana. *American Journal of Public Health, 87*(12), 2035–2038.

Heymann, D. L. (1998). Zoonoses—disease passed from animals to humans. *World Health, 51*(4), 4.

Heymann, D. L. (2004). *Control of communicable diseases manual* (18th ed.). Washington, DC: American Public Health Association.

HIV-related conditions. Focus on: Tuberculosis. (1999, June/July). *HIV Frontline. A Newsletter for Professionals Who Counsel People Living with HIV*, 37, 6.

Hoffman, R. E., Greenblatt, J., Matyas, B. T., Sharp, D. J., Esteban, E., Hodge, K., & Liang, A. (2005, January). Capacity of state and territorial health agencies to prevent foodborne illness. *Emerging Infectious Diseases, 11*(1). Retrieved from http://www.cdc.gov/ncidod/eid/vol11no01/04-0334.htm

Holtzman, D. (2014). Infectious diseases related to travel: Hepatitis C. CDC Health Information for International Travel 2014. New York, NY: Oxford University Press.

Institute of Medicine. (1992). *Emerging infections: Microbial threats to health in the United States.* Washington, DC: National Academies Press.

Isakbaeva, E. T., Widdowson, M.-A., Beard, R. S., Bulens, S. N., Mullins, J., Monroe, S. S., … Glass, R. I. (2005). Norovirus transmission on cruise ship. *Emerging Infectious Diseases, 11*(1). Retrieved from http://wwwnc.cdc.gov/eid/article/11/1/04-0434.htm

Kaferstein, F. K., & Meslin, F. X. (1998, July/August). Keeping foods of animal origin safe. *World Health, 51*(4), 28–29.

Kestel, F. (2006). Preventing HAIs. *Advance for Nurses* (Florida ed.), *7*(16), 25–26.

Krisberg, K. (2006, September). Public health responding to new threat of staph infections. *The Nation's Health: The Official Newspaper of the American Public Health Association,* pp. 1, 12.

Mahon, B. E., Slutsker, L., Hutwagner, L., Drenzek, C., Maloney, K., Toomey, K., & Griffin, P. M. (1999). Consequences in Georgia of a nationwide outbreak of *Salmonella* infections: What you don't know might hurt you. *American Journal of Public Health, 89*(1), 31–35.

Mann, J. M. (1994). Preface. In L. Garrett (Ed.), *The coming plague. Newly emerging diseases in a world out of balance.* New York, NY: Farrar, Straus and Giroux.

Marsh, K., & Waruiru, C. (1998). What is malaria? *World Health, 51*(3), 6–7.

Merrill, R. M., & Timmreck, T. C. (1998). *An introduction to epidemiology* (2nd ed.). Boston, MA: Jones and Bartlett.

Merrill, R. M., & Timmreck, T. C. (2013). *Introduction to epidemiology* (6th ed.). Burlington, MA: Jones & Bartlett Learning.

Meslin, F. X., & Stohr, K. (1998). Animals that infect humans. *World Health, 51*(4), 5.

Molyneux, M. (1998). Severe malaria. *World Health, 51*(3), 8–9.

Moore, M., McCray, E., & Onorato, I. M. (1999). Cross-matching TB and AIDS registries: TB patients with HIV co-infection, United States, 1993–1994. *Public Health Reports, 114*, 269–277.

The mother of fevers. (1998, March/April). *World Health, 51*(2), 12–13.

Murphy, F. A. (1998). Emerging zoonoses. *Emerging Infectious Diseases, 4*(3), 429–435.

National Academy of Sciences (NAS). (2005). *Addressing foodborne threats to health: Policies, practices, and global coordination: Workshop summary.* Retrieved from http:/www.nap.edu/catalog/11745.html

National Coalition for Adult Immunization. (2009). *Facts about adult immunization.* Bethesda, MD: Author.

National Foundation for Infectious Diseases. (2002a). *Facts about adult immunization.* Retrieved from http://www.nfid.org/_old/factsheets/adultfact.html

National Foundation for Infectious Diseases. (2002b). *Facts for hepatitis A for adults.* Retrieved from http://nfid.org/_old/factsheets/he;aadult.html

National Foundation for Infectious Diseases. (2002c). *Facts about hepatitis B for adults.* Retrieved from http://www.nfid.org/_old/factsheets/hepbadult.html

National Institute for Allergy and Infectious Diseases (NIAID). (2010). Emerging and re-emerging infectious diseases: Introduction and goals. Retrieved from http://www.niaid.nih.gov/topics/emerging/Pages/introduction.aspx

Nchinda, T. C. (1998). Malaria: A reemerging disease in Africa. *Emerging Infectious Diseases, 4*(3), 398–403.

Petersen, L. R., & Marfin, A. A. (2002). West Nile virus: A primer for the clinician. *Annals of Internal Medicine, 137*(3), 173–179.

Potter, R. C., Kaneene, J. B., & Hall, W. N. (2003). Risk factors for sporadic *Campylobacter jejuni* infections in rural Michigan: A prospective case-control study. *American Journal of Public Health, 93*(12), 2118–2123.

Prevention and treatment of tuberculosis among patients infected with human immunodeficiency virus: Principles of therapy and revised recommendations. (1998, October 30). *Morbidity and Mortality Weekly Report, 47*(RR-20), 5.

Scallan, E., Hoekstra, R. M., Angulo, F. J., Tauxe, R. V., Widdowson, M-A, Roy, S. L., … Griffin, P. M. (2011). Foodborne illness acquired in the United States—major pathogens. *Emerging Infectious Diseases, 17*(1), 7–15. Retrieved from http://www.ncbi.nlm.nih.gov/pmc/articles/PMC3375761/

Schwartz, R. D. (2006). Pandemic flu preparedness and response in corrections facilities. *Infectious Diseases in Corrections Report, 9*(10), 1.

Smith, B. D., Morgan, R. L., Beckett, G. A., Falck-Ytter, Y., Holtzman, D., Teo, C. G., … Ward, J. W. (2012). Recommendations for the identification of chronic hepatitis C virus infection among persons born during 1945–1965. *Morbidity and Mortality Weekly Report*, 61(RR04), 1–18. Retrieved from http://www.cdc.gov/mmwr/preview/mmwrhtml/rr6104a1.htm

Thompson, W. W., Shay, D. K., Weintraub, E., Brammer, L., Cox, N., Anderson, L. J., & Fukuda, K. (2003). Mortality associated with influenza and respiratory syncytial virus in the United States. *Journal of the American Medical Association, 289*(2), 179–186.

Todd, B. (2006). Beyond MRSA: VISA and VRSA. *American Journal of Nursing, 106*(4), 28–30.

Torres, M. (1998, July). Tuberculosis update. *National Council of La Raza Center for Health Promotion Fact Sheet.*

UNAIDS. (2013). *2013 Global Fact Sheet.* Retrieved from http://www.unaids.org/en/resources/campaigns/globalreport2013/factsheet/

United Nations, Department of Economic and Social Affairs, Population Division. (2013). Trends in international migrant stock: The 2013 revision—migrants by age and sex. Retrieved from http://esa.un.org/unmigration/TIMSA2013/documents/MIgrantStocks_Documentation.pdf

U.S. Department of Health and Human Services (HHS). (1991). *Healthy People 2000: National health program and disease prevention objectives*. Washington, DC: U.S. Government Printing Office.

U.S. Department of Health and Human Services (HHS). (2013). *Healthy People 2020: Topics and Objectives A-Z*. Retrieved from http://healthypeople.gov/2020/topicsobjectives2020/default.aspx

U.S. Department of Transportation (USDOT). (2013). Total passengers on U.S airlines and foreign airlines: U.S. flights increased 1.3% in 2012 from 2011. Bureau of Transportation Statistics Press Release No. BTS 16-13. Retrieved from http://www.rita.dot.gov/bts/press_releases/bts016_13

Valanis, B. (1999). *Epidemiology in health care* (3rd ed.). Stamford, CT: Appleton & Lange.

Wilde, H., & Mitmoonpitak, C. (1998). Canine rabies in Thailand. *World Health, 51*(4), 10–11.

Williams, W. W., Lu, P.-J., O'Halloran, A., Bridges, C. B., Pilishvili, T., Hales, C. M., & Markowitz, L. E. (2014). Noninfluenza vaccination coverage among adults—United States, 2012. *Morbidity and Mortality Weekly Report, 63*(05), 95–102. Retrieved from http://www.cdc.gov/mmwr/preview/mmwrhtml/mm6305a4.htm

Wittenberg, R. L. (1998). From the president. Efforts toward eliminating seven diseases from the globe. *American Association for World Health Quarterly, 12*(2), 2.

World Health Organization (WHO). (2005a). World malarial report 2005. Retrieved from http://rbm.who.int/wmr2005/

— (2005b). Key TB and TB/HIV facts and figures. Retrieved from http://www.who.int/3by5/en/facts.pdf

— (2013a). Report of suspected polio cases in the Syrian Arab Republic. Retrieved from http://www.who.int/csr/don/2013_10_19_polio/en/index.html

— (2013b). Hepatitis B fact sheet. Retrieved from http://www.who.int/mediacentre/factsheets/fs204/en/

— (2013c). HIV-Associated TB Facts 2013. Retrieved from http://www.who.int/tb/challenges/hiv/tbhiv_factsheet_2013_web.pdf

— (2013d). The Bill and Melinda Gates Foundation. Retrieved from http://www.who.int/trypanosomiasis_african/partners/gates/en/

— (2014a). Hepatitis E fact sheet. Retrieved from http://www.who.int/mediacentre/factsheets/fs280/en/

— (2014b). Influenza (seasonal): Fact Sheet No. 211. Retrieved from http://www.who.int/mediacentre/factsheets/fs211/en/

— (2014c). Soil-transmitted helminth infections. Retrieved from http://www.who.int/mediacentre/factsheets/fs366/en/

— (2014d). Tuberculosis: Fact Sheet No. 104. Retrieved from http://www.who.int/mediacentre/factsheets/fs104/en/

— WHO International Health Regulations (n.d.). Retrieved from http://www.who.int/ihr/about/10things/en/

Yin, S. (2006). Special section: Malaria. In M. M. Kent & S. Yin, *Population Bulletin: Controlling Infectious Diseases, 61*(2), 14–16. Washington, DC: Population Reference Bureau.

CHAPTER FOCUS

Scope of the Problem
Common STIs
- Human Papillomavirus (HPV)
- Chlamydia
- Gonorrhea
- Syphilis
- Herpes Simplex Virus (HSV)

Health Consequences of STIs
- Cancers
- Reproductive Health Problems
- Health Consequences for Pregnant Women and Infants
- Health Consequences for Men

HIV/AIDS
- Scope of the Problem
- Populations at Risk for HIV/AIDS

STIs and the U.S. Healthcare System
- Health Services
- Screening and Prevention

The Role of Community Health Nurses

QUESTIONS TO CONSIDER

After reading this chapter, you will know the answers to the following questions:

1. How are STIs affecting global health?
2. What are some of the most common STIs in the United States?
3. What are some of the major health consequences of STIs?
4. How is the HIV/AIDS pandemic affecting global health?
5. What are some of the populations at risk for HIV in the United States and why?
6. How is the U.S. healthcare system handling the overload of sexually transmitted diseases and HIV/AIDS?
7. What is the role of the nurse in the diagnosis and treatment of STIs and HIV/AIDS?
8. What are some of the prevention efforts being done by communities?
9. What is the role of the community health nurse in prevention efforts?
10. How has the risk of STIs/HIV affected the health of older Americans?

Sexual activity is a way to express intimacy and positive emotions, enable reproduction, and provide physical pleasure, but it also can be associated with potentially harmful consequences. The undesired outcomes from sexual activity include unintended pregnancies and sexually transmitted infections (STIs), including infection with the human immunodeficiency virus (HIV), which can lead to acquired immune deficiency syndrome (AIDS). STIs have been described as America's "hidden epidemic," because the rates of some STIs are now higher than they were a few decades ago and the United States has the highest rates of STIs in the industrialized world.

CHAPTER 21

Sexually Transmitted Infections and HIV/AIDS

Cathy Keen Hughes

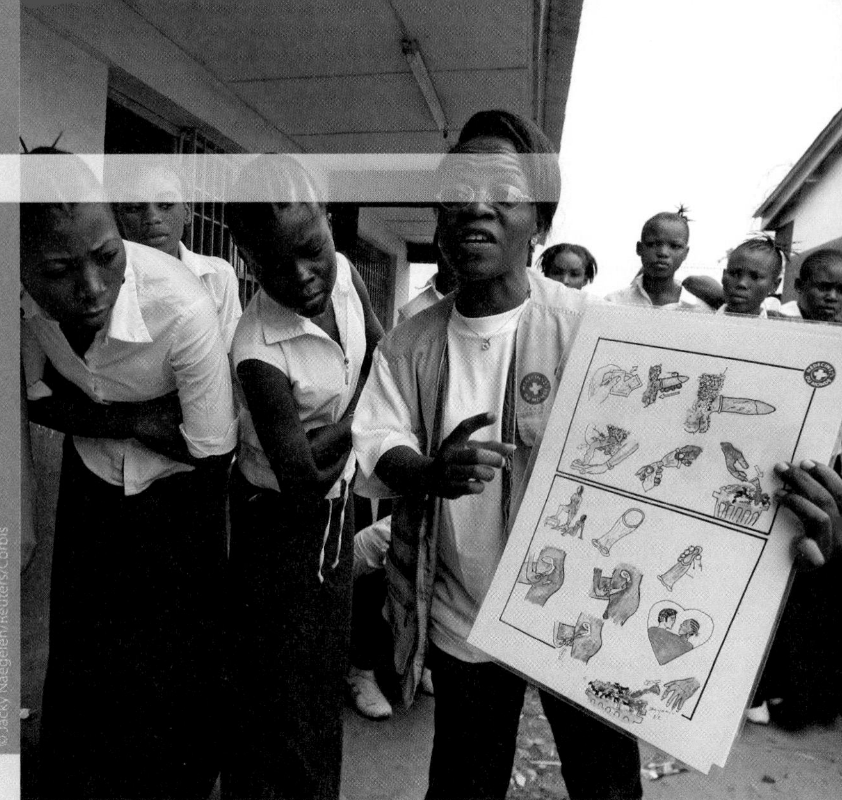

KEY TERMS

acquired immune deficiency syndrome (AIDS)
chlamydia
gonorrhea
herpes simplex virus (HSV)
human immunodeficiency virus (HIV)
human papillomavirus (HPV)
Ryan White CARE Act
sexually transmitted infections (STIs)
syphilis

> Nonetheless, he knew that the tale he had to tell could not be one of final victory. It could only be the record of what had had to be done, and what assuredly would have to be done again in the neverending fight against terror and its relentless onslaughts, despite their personal afflictions, by all who, while unable to be saints but refusing to bow down to pestilences, strive their utmost to be healers.
>
> —Albert Camus, *The Plague*

REFLECTIONS

Camus wrote these words long before the appearance of HIV/AIDS. Does it have meaning for the HIV epidemic? What does it say to you as a nurse? Can you refuse to bow down and strive to be a healer in an epidemic that has so many moral, political, and ethical undertones?

Scope of the Problem

Sexually transmitted infections (STIs)—also known in medical literature as sexually transmitted diseases (STDs)—affect people of all socioeconomic levels, races, ethnicities, genders, ages, and religions. There is no such thing as a "typical" STI patient. STIs are almost always transmitted from one person to another during sexual intercourse. They are transmitted most efficiently during anal or vaginal intercourse and less efficiently during oral intercourse. Some STIs, such as hepatitis B and HIV, can also be transmitted parenterally and are particularly problematic among intravenous drug users who share injection equipment. In some cases, a pregnant woman can transmit an STI to her infant prenatally, during birth, or postnatally during breastfeeding, as happens with HIV, for example.

The estimates of annual incidence (new infections) of STIs in 2008 were 20 million cases, with a prevalence of 100 million cases. Total medical costs of STIs are estimated at $16 billion dollars (Centers for Disease Control and Prevention [CDC], 2013a). Against this backdrop of high STI rates, some subpopulations have higher STI incidence rates than average. In most parts of the United States, sexually active adolescents have high rates of STIs, particularly chlamydia, regardless of their race or socioeconomic status. In addition, men who have sex with men (MSM), especially young men, generally have higher rates of STIs. STIs are also common among persons who use illicit drugs, including both injection drug users (IDUs) and non-IDUs. The presence of an STI greatly increases the risk of HIV transmission during sexual activity.

Common STIs

The terms *STI* or *STD* in the literature refer to infectious organisms that can be transmitted during sexual contact and cause dozens of different clinical presentations. Five of the most common STIs are described briefly in the following sections and in **Table 21-1**. HIV/AIDS is discussed separately later in this chapter.

Human Papillomavirus (HPV)

Human papillomavirus (HPV) is one of the most common STIs in the world, occurring across all socioeconomic levels. Approximately 79 million American are currently infected, with an estimated 14 million Americans newly infected each year. HPV is so common that nearly all sexually active persons will get at least one type of HPV at some point in their lives (CDC, 2013a). Almost half of all HPV infections in the United States occur in women between 15 and 25 years old. Of the more than 100 known types of HPV, 40 are spread through sexual contact. Low-risk types of HPV cause genital warts (condylomata acuminata). High-risk types of HPV can cause vaginal, cervical, and anal cancers (Markowitz et al., 2007).

Genital warts are very contagious. Approximately two-thirds of people who have sexual contact with a person with genital warts will develop warts, usually within 3 months of exposure. In women, warts can occur inside and outside the vagina, on the cervix, or around the anus. In men, warts can occur on the tip or shaft of the penis, on the scrotum, or around the anus. Left untreated, genital warts may disappear or may grow into a raised fleshy

TABLE 21-1 Snapshot of STIs/STDs in United States in 2011

STI	Cases	Rate per 100,000	Changes
Chlamydia	1,412,791	457.6	Increased 8% since 2010
Gonorrhea	321,849	104.2	Increased 4% since 2010 Decreased 11.7% overall 2007–2011
Syphilis (P&S)	13,900	4.5	Unchanged since 2010
Syphilis (Congenital)	360	8.5	Decreased 7% since 2010 Decreased 20% since 2008

Source: Data from CDC. (2013c). *Sexually Transmitted Disease Surveillance 2012*. Retrieved from http://www.cdc.gov/sTD/stats12/default.htm

growth with a cauliflower-like appearance. Because there is no way to predict whether warts will disappear or grow, people who suspect that they have genital warts should seek treatment (CDC, 2010; Markowitz et al., 2007). In 2006, the U.S. Food and Drug Administration (FDA) approved a vaccine for HPV for females ages 9–26 years for the prevention of cervical cancer. Vaccines are now available for primary prevention of types of HPV that are linked with 70% of cervical cancers in females and 90% of genital warts for both genders. The three-dose series is recommended for:

- Females age 11–26, especially those with compromised immune systems and those not fully immunized earlier
- Males age 11–21 or to age 26 for MSM (gay or bisexual men) or those with compromised immune systems and those not fully immunized earlier

The primary goal of treatment is removal of the warts. Although there is no cure for HPV, treatment can induce wart-free periods. Treatment varies with each individual case and is guided by the preference of the patient, the experience of the healthcare provider, and the available resources. Like many other STIs, HPV often has no visible symptoms. It is estimated that nearly 50% of people infected with HPV are unaware of their infection and the risk of transmission to others.

Examination of sex partners is not necessary because chance of reinfection is minimal, and in the absence of a cure, treatment to reduce transmission is not realistic. However, sex partners should be counseled about the implications of having a partner who has HPV. Because there is no cure for HPV, patients and sex partners should be aware that the patient might remain infectious after the warts are gone. Condom use may decrease the risk of infection but does not eliminate it (CDC, 2010, 2013b).

Chlamydia

Chlamydia, caused by *Chlamydia trachomatis,* is the most commonly reported notifiable disease and the most common bacterial STI in the United States. It is estimated that as many as 2.5 million Americans are infected each year. Because many infections are asymptomatic, however, it is difficult to determine exact infection rates. The prevalence is higher in women younger than 25 years of age. Women are frequently reinfected if their sex partners are not treated (CDC, 2010, 2013c). Chlamydia screening is recommended for all sexually active women younger than 25.

If symptoms occur, they usually appear within 1 to 3 weeks after exposure. Early signs of chlamydia include abnormal genital discharge or painful urination. However, these symptoms often are ignored because they are so mild. Chlamydia can be transmitted during vaginal, anal, or oral sex with an infected partner. Pregnant women may pass the infection to their newborns during delivery, leading to neonatal eye infections or pneumonia (CDC, 2010, 2014a). Untreated, chlamydia can cause pelvic inflammatory disease (PID), which may lead to infertility or risk of ectopic pregnancy (CDC, 2014a).

Chlamydia is completely curable if diagnosed before complications occur. The antibiotics most commonly used are a 1-day course of azithromycin or a 7-day course of doxycycline. Persons should abstain from sex for 7 days if they receive single-dose therapy and use latex condoms after (CDC, 2010, 2014a).

Gonorrhea

Gonorrhea, a bacterial infection caused by *Neisseria gonorrhoeae,* is spread through vaginal, anal, or oral sexual activity with an infected partner. Pregnant women can pass the infection to their newborns during delivery, leading to eye infections or life-threatening blood infections in their babies. The early symptoms are often mild, and many women never develop symptoms. If symptoms occur, they usually appear within 2 to 10 days after exposure. Initial symptoms in women include pain or burning with urination and yellow or bloody vaginal discharge. Men usually experience a penile discharge and burning with urination that may be severe. Symptoms of rectal infection include anal itching, discharge, or painful bowel movements (CDC, 2010, 2014b).

Gonorrhea is the second most commonly reported notifiable disease in the United States. Rates are highest in three groups: women age 15–20 and 21–24 years, and men age 21–24 years. After a 74% decline between 1975 and 1997, the rates of gonorrhea remained steady for 10 years. Rates in 2006–2007 were the lowest since reporting began, but steadily increased from 2009–2011 (CDC, 2013c).

Gonorrhea is becoming increasingly resistant to antibiotics, resulting in more expensive treatment because the usual options are no longer effective. As recently as 1976, almost all gonorrhea infections could be cured with penicillin (Aral & Holmes, 1991), but increasingly widespread drug resistance has meant that once effective medications often do not work (CDC, 2013c). Currently, dual therapy with cefixime and azithromycin is recommended for effective treatment of gonorrhea. Partners of infected individuals should also be treated. Because gonorrhea often occurs simultaneously with a chlamydial infection, combination therapy with cefixime and doxycycline or azithromycin is often effective. Since dual therapy for gonorrhea and chlamydia was initiated, the incidence of chlamydia has decreased significantly in some populations. Routine cotreatment may possibly help to hinder the development of

TABLE 21-2 The Five Ps Approach to Effective Clinical Interviewing to Identify STI Risk Factors

Partners	❑ Do you have sex with men, women, or both? ❑ In the past few months, how many sex partners have you had? ❑ In the past 12 months, how many sex partners have you had?
Prevention of pregnancy	Are you or your partner trying to get pregnant? If no, what are you doing to prevent pregnancy?
Protection from STIs	What do you do to protect yourself from STIs and HIV?
Practices	To understand your risks for STIs, I need to understand the kind of sex you have had recently: ❑ Have you had vaginal sex, meaning penis in vagina? ❑ If yes, do you use condoms never, sometimes, or always? ❑ Have you had anal sex, meaning penis into rectum/anus? ❑ If yes, do you use condoms never, sometimes, or always? ❑ Have you had oral sex, meaning mouth on penis or vagina? For condom answers: ❑ If never, why don't you use condoms? ❑ If sometimes, in which situations or with whom, do you not use condoms?
Past history of STIs	❑ Have you ever had an STI? ❑ Have any of your sex partners had an STI?
Additional questions to identify HIV	Have you or any of your sex partners ever injected drugs?

Source: Reproduced from CDC. (2010). Sexually transmitted diseases treatment guidelines, 2010. *Morbidity and Mortality Weekly Report, 55*(RR–11).

microbial-resistant strains of gonorrheal infections (CDC, 2010). As more antimicrobial strains continue to evolve, the CDC has warned that clinicians may run out of treatment options.

Syphilis

Syphilis is a systemic disease caused by *Treponema pallidum*. The disease progresses through three stages, with different clinical presentations at each stage. The three stages, with some of the most common clinical symptoms, are:

1. Primary infection: ulcer or chancre at the infection site
2. Secondary infection: rash, mucocutaneous lesions, and adenopathy
3. Tertiary infection: cardiac, neurological, ophthalmic, auditory, liver, or bone damage

Latent syphilis is defined as the periods when patients are seropositive but have no signs or symptoms. Treatment of latent syphilis is important to halt the progression of the disease. Although most associated with tertiary infection, central nervous system disease can occur at any stage of syphilis. Persons diagnosed with syphilis showing any neurological symptoms such as ophthalmic or auditory symptoms, cranial nerve palsies, and signs and symptoms of meningitis should have a cerebrospinal fluid examination. Severe dementia can occur if syphilis infection is left untreated (CDC, 2014c; Heymann, 2009).

Pregnant women should be screened for syphilis in the early stages of pregnancy because early treatment of the mother's syphilis infection has a high success rate in preventing the baby from acquiring congenital syphilis. In communities in which the prevalence of syphilis is high or for patients at high risk, serological testing should also be done at 28 weeks' and 32 weeks' gestation and at delivery. No infant should leave the hospital or birthing center without the mother having been screened for syphilis at least once during pregnancy. Children born with congenital syphilis can have birth defects affecting all systems, including severe neurological abnormalities (CDC, 2010).

Benzathine penicillin G, given intramuscularly, has been an effective treatment for syphilis for many years. It is a cure in the early stages of syphilis and helps slow disease progression and prevent complications in later stages. Dosage and duration of treatment depend on the stage and severity of the disease. For nonpregnant patients with penicillin allergies, doxycycline or tetracycline can be used. However, patients with poor treatment compliance histories or those who are pregnant should be desensitized and treated with penicillin. All sexual partners should be identified and treated (CDC, 2010, 2013c).

After remaining at a steady level through the 1970s and into the 1980s, syphilis increased substantially from 1987 to 1990, then began to decrease once again (CDC, 2013c). From 1990–2000 in the United States, the primary and secondary syphilis rates declined 89.7%. By 2000, the incidence and prevalence rates of primary and secondary syphilis were the lowest since reporting began in 1941. Since then, however, syphilis rates have steadily increased. The highest increases were seen primarily in males, with a rate increase of 8.5%, up from 4.7 per 100,000 in 2004 to 5.1 per 100,000 in 2005. The rate of reported cases for females also increased for the first time in more than 10 years. Additionally, the syphilis rates for African Americans have increased steadily since 2004 after a decade of steady decline. The rate declined during 2010–2011 in the overall population except in men (CDC, 2013c).

Herpes Simplex Virus (HSV)

Sexually transmitted **herpes simplex virus (HSV)** infection is widespread and produces intermittent painful ulcers. Although the ulcers can be treated, the underlying infection persists and ulcers recur. This is of concern because HSV can be transmitted to a sex partner even in the absence of a genital ulcer and can also be passed from an infected mother to her newborn during childbirth. Approximately 776,000 new cases of HSV occur each year in the United States. This prevalence estimate means that one of every five women and one of every nine men in the United States will become infected with HSV during their lifetimes (CDC, 2010, 2013c, 2014d).

There are two types of HSV, both of which can cause genital herpes. HSV type 1 most often causes fever blisters and cold sores around the mouth area, but it can cause genital herpes as well. HSV type 2 generally causes genital lesions, but it can also cause sores around the mouth. Eighty percent of people with genital herpes never develop symptoms or do not recognize them. If symptoms do occur, they will usually appear within 2 weeks after exposure. The first episode of ulcers usually lasts 2 to 4 weeks. Early symptoms include genital itching or burning; pain in the legs, buttocks, or genital area; and vaginal discharge. Later symptoms include lesions inside the vagina or in the urinary tract. Small red bumps occur first, followed by blisters, and then painful sores. However, as already mentioned, many people with HSV type 2 infections are unaware of the infection because they never develop symptoms, or the symptoms are mild and may be mistaken for a rash or other skin condition (CDC, 2010, 2014d).

Genital herpes cannot be cured, but it can be controlled with acyclovir. Treatment with acyclovir also reduces the risk of transmission to sexual partners. A baby born with herpes can develop encephalitis, severe rashes, and eye problems. Early treatment with acyclovir greatly reduces serious complications in infants. Delivery by cesarean section also greatly reduces the risk of newborn infection (CDC, 2014d).

Health Consequences of STIs

Most people are not aware of the long-term health consequences of STIs other than HIV/AIDS. There are several reasons why STIs rarely command attention or concern. Many STIs are without symptoms and go undetected until years after infection, when serious sequelae appear. Many of the major adverse outcomes that do occur from STIs likewise arise years after the initial infection, so the connection is not made between the original infection and the later consequence, except for the awareness that HIV infection leads to AIDS. Viral STIs, in particular, often result in lifelong infection for which there is no cure at present. Public discourse is also hampered by the stigma of STIs. Finally, many people—including health providers—find it difficult to discuss sexual behavior openly and comfortably. This can make it difficult for a health provider to take a patient's sexual history or to counsel a patient effectively about his or her sexual health.

Cancers

The relationship between STDs and several types of cancer has only recently been recognized by the public. Some cancer-related STIs include HPV, hepatitis B, and human herpes virus type 8. In fact, HPVs are now recognized as the major cause of cervical cancer. An estimated 10,000 women in the United States are diagnosed with cervical cancer every year, and approximately 4,000 die from it. Worldwide, nearly half a million women develop cervical cancer each year, with nearly 250,000 dying from the disease. Studies show that HPV may also be involved in cancers of the anus, vulva, and vagina. A few types of oropharyngeal and penile cancer have been linked to certain types of high-risk HPV infections as well (National Cancer Institute [NCI], 2012). The two HPV vaccines on the market today are the first and only primary prevention interventions available at this time for cervical cancer (CDC, 2012a). Approximately 17,000 women and 9,000 men are affected by HPV with cancers. Cancers may be of the penis, oropharynx, cervix, vulva, and vagina. One percent of all sexually active adults in the United States has genital warts at any given time (CDC, 2012a).

Reproductive Health Problems

Many reproductive health problems are the consequence of unrecognized or untreated STIs. Such reproductive health problems may be short term, as is the case for PID, pregnancy complications, or epididymitis, or long term, such as infertility.

Gonorrhea and chlamydia infections are the most common causes of PID in women (CDC, 2014e). PID occurs when bacteria move upward from the vagina or cervix into the uterus, fallopian tubes, and other reproductive organs. If left untreated, PID can lead to serious complications that may include infertility, ectopic pregnancy, internal abscesses, and chronic pelvic pain. More than 50% of all preventable infertility in women is a result of STDs (CDC, 2013c). Each year in the United States, more than 1 million women develop PID, with 100,000 becoming infertile and more than 150 dying. A large proportion of ectopic pregnancies are believed to be due to PID.

Prompt and appropriate treatment of PID can help prevent complications. Because of the difficulty in identifying the agent infecting the internal reproductive organs, PID is usually treated with at least two antibiotics that are effective against a wide range of microorganisms. Treating STIs early can prevent PID. Yearly chlamydia screening is recommended for all sexually active women younger than age 25 and for all older women with risk factors such as new or multiple sex partners (CDC, 2010, 2013c).

Health Consequences for Pregnant Women and Infants

STIs create many complications for pregnant women and their infants. Pregnant women with STIs can transmit the infections prenatally, during birth, or after birth. Common STIs that are known to create adverse outcomes in pregnant women and their babies include chlamydia, gonorrhea, syphilis, cytomegalovirus, genital herpes, and HIV (CDC, 2013d).

The harmful effects for babies include stillbirth, low birth weight, conjunctivitis, pneumonia, neonatal sepsis, neurological impairments, blindness, deafness, acute hepatitis, meningitis, chronic liver disease, and cirrhosis. To prevent many of these problems, pregnant women should be screened for STIs starting early in the pregnancy, with testing being repeated close to delivery, if necessary. Pregnant women should be treated for STIs occurring in pregnancy and infants can be treated if infection is found at birth (CDC, 2013d).

Health Consequences for Men

The consequences of some STIs are similar in both men and women. HPV, for example, is associated with penile and anal cancers in men, although both are less common than cervical cancer among women. Most people are not aware that STIs produce long-term problems such as infertility for men, but the health burden of chancroid, chlamydia, gonorrhea, HIV, and syphilis is high among men as well as among women.

HIV/AIDS

By impairing and eventually destroying the immune system, **human immunodeficiency virus (HIV)** progressively eliminates the body's ability to fight infections and certain cancers. A badly weakened immune system is unable to fight off microbes that would not cause illness in a healthy person. These life-threatening diseases are called *opportunistic infections* and are generally the first sign that an HIV-infected person has progressed to **acquired immune deficiency syndrome (AIDS)**. AIDS is the end stage of HIV disease, which includes the whole spectrum of HIV infection, from initial infection with the virus to clinical AIDS and eventual death. HIV is found in semen, vaginal secretions, blood, and human milk. This virus does not live outside the body and can be transmitted only through unprotected anal, vaginal, or oral sex; contaminated needles for injection drug use; contaminated blood products; or from an infected mother to her infant during pregnancy or delivery or through breastfeeding. The most common route of transmission is sexual contact (Heymann, 2009).

In 1993, the criteria for an AIDS diagnosis were amended to include three additional opportunistic infections (invasive cervical cancer, tuberculosis, and recurrent pneumonia) with a positive HIV antibody test and/or a CD4 blood cell count of 200 cells/mm^3. Before 1993, a positive HIV antibody test and a diagnosis of 1 of 23 specific opportunistic infections were the only criteria for an AIDS diagnosis. As a result, AIDS cases were undercounted before 1993.

HEALTHY PEOPLE 2020 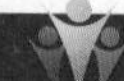

Objectives Related to Sexually Transmitted Diseases

- STD-1 Reduce the proportion of adolescents and young adults with *Chlamydia trachomatis* infections
- STD-2 Reduce *Chlamydia* rates among females aged 15 to 44 years
- STD-3 Increase the proportion of sexually active females aged 24 years and under enrolled in Medicaid

plans who are screened for genital *Chlamydia* infections during the measurement year

- STD-4 Increase the proportion of sexually active females aged 24 years and under enrolled in commercial health insurance plans who are screened for genital *Chlamydia* infections during the measurement year
- STD-5 Reduce the proportion of females aged 15 to 44 years who have ever required treatment for pelvic inflammatory disease (PID)
- STD-6 Reduce gonorrhea rates
- STD-7 Reduce sustained domestic transmission of primary and secondary syphilis
- STD-8 Reduce congenital syphilis
- STD-9 Reduce the proportion of females with human papillomavirus (HPV) infection
- STD-10 Reduce the proportion of young adults with genital herpes infection due to herpes simplex type 2

Source: U.S. Department of Health and Human Services. (2014a). Sexually Transmitted Diseases. Retrieved from http://www.healthypeople.gov/2020/topicsobjectives2020/overview.aspx?topicid=37

Scope of the Problem

Since its discovery in 1981, HIV/AIDS has had a devastating effect in the United States and throughout the world. In 2010, an estimated 1.1 million people were living with HIV in the United States; almost 50,000 of these were newly diagnosed in 2011 (CDC, 2013e). The cumulative number of AIDS deaths in the United States has reached more than 635,000, and globally nearly 30 million (CDC, 2013f). AIDS death rates increased during the first 15 years of the epidemic and were highest in the mid-1990s. Since then, the death rates have dropped significantly, primarily due to the standardized treatment with highly active antiretroviral therapy (HAART). HIV prevalence is currently at its highest level and continues to rise each year. The only exception to the steady rise in prevalence occurred in the mid-1990s, before the introduction of HAART, when the annual number of deaths exceeded the number of new HIV infections. The increasing prevalence of HIV/AIDS is partially due to the availability of effective treatment options, which has reduced HIV-related morbidity and mortality (CDC, 2013f; Kaiser Foundation, 2006).

> And that was the day that we knew, oh! In the world there is a new disease called AIDS. I thought surely this will be the greatest war we ever fought. Surely many will die. And surely we will be frustrated, unable to help. But I also thought the Americans will find a treatment soon. This will not be forever.
>
> —*Dr. Jayo Kidenya, Bukoba, Tanzania, 1985*

MEDIA MOMENT 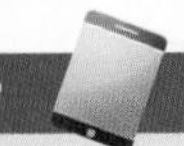

And the Band Played On (1993)

This is the story of the discovery of HIV. The film relives events from the early days in 1978, when numerous homosexuals in San Francisco began dying from unknown causes, to the identification of the human immunodeficiency virus by French and U.S. scientists in 1984. It is based on the book by Randy Shilts.

The Normal Heart (2014)

This TV movie adaptation of the mostly autobiographical play of the same name by Larry Kramer focuses on the HIV/AIDS crisis in New York between 1981 and 1984. Mark Ruffalo plays a writer turned activist who attempts to raise awareness of the new epidemic.

An overview of HIV/AIDS in other parts of the world is even more serious. It is estimated that there were more than 35 million people worldwide living with HIV in 2012 (World Health Organization [WHO], 2014). More than 95% of them live in developing countries, where social, economic, cultural, and political conditions that contribute to the spread of the virus are more prevalent. The most frightening concern for worldwide prevention and treatment efforts is the fact that more than half of all HIV-infected people, especially in developing countries, do not know they are infected. Sadly, in the absence of an affordable cure, most of the people in the world living with HIV will die within a decade (Johnson, 2007; UNAIDS, 2013).

The introduction of the "triple-drug cocktails" (various combinations of antiretroviral drugs and protease inhibitors, called HAART) in 1996 caused a significant drop in new AIDS cases and AIDS deaths in the United States. These drug therapies have enabled persons infected with HIV to live longer, more healthful lives by slowing the progression of HIV infection into AIDS and lowering the death rate from AIDS complications. Combination drug therapy can improve the ability of the drugs to control HIV so well that in many cases the viral load becomes so low that HIV cannot be detected in the blood. HAART may also significantly decrease the incidence of drug resistance in HIV patients when strict compliance to drug treatment regimes is maintained (Goodroad, 2003).

Unfortunately, HAART, which has been very effective in controlling HIV disease progression in the United States, is not available to most of the people infected with HIV in the rest of the world. The high cost of the drugs exceeds the healthcare budgets of developing countries, where the majority of HIV-infected persons live.

Treatment is problematic in the United States as well. The cost of HAART is prohibitive for many uninsured

BOX 21-1 Ryan White Comprehensive AIDS Resources Emergency CARE Act

This act was signed into law by the U.S. Congress on August 18, 1990, to improve the quality and availability of care for people with HIV/AIDS and their families. It is managed by the Health Resources and Services Administration (HRSA), an agency of the U.S. Department of Health and Human Services. HRSA's HIV/AIDS Bureau administers programs under four titles and Part F:

1. Title I—provides grants to metropolitan areas that are disproportionately affected by the HIV epidemic. Grants are awarded to the chief elected official and are used to fund services such as outpatient health care; support services like case management, home health and hospice care, housing and transportation assistance, nutrition services, and day care and respite care; and inpatient case management services that expedite discharge and prevent unnecessary hospitalization.
2. Title II—provides grants to the states and territories to provide services for people living with HIV/AIDS. Some of these services include home and community-based health care and support services; continuation of health insurance coverage; pharmaceutical treatments through an AIDS Drug Assistance Program; local organizations that assess needs and organize and deliver HIV services in collaboration with healthcare providers; and direct health services.
3. Title III—supports outpatient HIV early-intervention services for low-income, medically underserved people in existing primary care systems. Educational, clinical, and psychological services are provided for prevention, treatment, and support through community and migrant health centers, homeless programs, local health departments, family planning centers, and so on. Small time-limited grants are also available to prepare organizations to plan for the development of HIV early-intervention services or to provide capacity building for organizations to develop, enhance, or expand their capabilities to provide HIV primary care services.
4. Title IV—provides comprehensive, community-based, family-centered services for women, children, adolescents, and families. A special focus for Title IV is to help identify HIV-positive pregnant women and connect them to health care. A large percentage of the people served are from poor, minority families with limited access to housing and transportation.
5. Part F—provides funding for special programs and services related to HIV/AIDS. Examples include:
   - Special Projects of National Significance (SPNS) Program—supports the development of innovative models of HIV/AIDS care designed to address minority and hard-to-reach populations.
   - AIDS Education and Training Center Program—a national network of 15 centers that provide HIV/AIDS education and training for healthcare professionals.
   - HIV Dental Programs—(1) The Dental Reimbursement Program assists institutions with accredited dental or dental hygiene programs by defraying their unreimbursed costs associated with providing oral health care to people with HIV. (2) The Community-Based Dental Partnership Plan provides increased access to oral health services for HIV-positive individuals while providing education and clinical training for dental care providers, especially those located in community-based dental practices and clinics.

Source: HRSA, 2009. Legislation: Ryan White Care Act. Retrieved from http://www.hab.hrsa.gov/abouthab/legislation.html

and underinsured patients. **Ryan White CARE Act** funding (**Box 21-1**), which was enacted in 1990 and reauthorized in 1996, 2000, and 2006 is providing the necessary drugs for some, but the number of patients needing treatment is increasing while funding is not. In 2009, the Ryan White CARE Act was expanded to include additional resources for women, children, and ethnic minorities (Health Resources and Services Administration [HRSA], 2009).

Populations at Risk for HIV/AIDS

The HIV/AIDS pandemic has affected different populations in different ways around the world. In the United States and Europe, HIV/AIDS has been primarily a male disease, with high rates of infection among homosexual and bisexual men, IDUs, and their sexual partners. In the early years of the U.S. epidemic, hemophiliacs were also infected at high rates because of contaminated blood products used in the production of factor VIII. However, after April 1985, when testing of the blood supply for HIV antibodies was initiated, the incidence of HIV in this population greatly declined and has remained low. In the rest of the world, however, the male-to-female HIV infection ratio has always been nearly equal, with transmission primarily through heterosexual contact (Vuylsteke, Sunkutu, & Laga, 1996). In recent years, we have seen new trends in HIV/AIDS infection in industrialized nations like the United States. Although infection rates remain high among homosexual and bisexual men, IDUs, and their sexual partners, the numbers of women, adolescents, and members of underrepresented ethnic groups, particularly African Americans and Latinos, have risen at alarming rates (CDC, 2013g; HRSA, 2009).

Men Who Have Sex with Men (MSM)

The fact that AIDS was first identified in 1981 in the American homosexual, Caucasian, male population, and was, in fact, called *gay-related immune deficiency syndrome* (GRID) for a short time, greatly affected the way it was perceived worldwide (Coxon, 1996; Shilts, 1987).

Because homosexual behavior is stigmatized in most societies, efforts aimed at prevention or treatment were limited early in the pandemic. However, gay organizations such as the Gay Men's Health Crisis Center in New York City and ACT UP (AIDS Coalition to Unleash Power) were formed at the beginning of the U.S. epidemic and were instrumental in providing information and influencing HIV/AIDS policy.

The efforts of the gay population to spread the prevention message resulted in reported behavioral changes among gay, white males, with a subsequent drop in HIV/AIDS diagnoses during the late 1980s and 1990s. However, recent surveillance data show an increase in HIV/AIDS incidence for this group. MSM still continue to account for the largest number of people living with AIDS by risk group (CDC, 2013h). It would be a mistake to think that high-risk behaviors are no longer a problem for MSM. Young men who have never lived in a world without HIV and who are possibly motivated by the success of HAART, which has minimized negative perceptions of HIV infection, are engaging in unprotected intercourse with greater frequency. This may be partly due to their misguided perceptions that HIV/AIDS is a disease of older gay men or that their peers are not practicing safer sex (CDC, 2013h).

Men of color account for and represented more than three-fourths of all estimated new HIV infections annually from 2008 to 2010 (CDC, 2014f). Many ethnic minority men have poor access to health care because of poverty and lack of health insurance. In addition, MSM of color must cope with many different types of stigma—for being a minority, for engaging in sexual activity with other men, and for being HIV positive. As a consequence, many ethnic minority MSM fear condemnation from their families, communities, and service providers. Men of color become infected at earlier ages than whites and are more likely to be diagnosed later in the disease process. Many minority MSM do not self-identify as gay or bisexual, meaning that prevention messages aimed at the gay community are often ineffective. They are often reluctant to seek services at organizations perceived to be gay oriented (CDC, 2014f; HRSA, 2008).

Community prevention programs must continue to address the needs of MSM, particularly young gay and bisexual men and especially men of color within this group. The involvement of social and political leaders in the community is important to be able to overcome cultural barriers related to homophobia and stigmatization. Prevention efforts must be geared to both uninfected and infected MSM, because research shows that HIV-infected MSM are continuing to practice high-risk sexual behavior. Treatment and prevention of other STIs are critical for this population because studies of MSM who are treated in STI clinics have shown consistently high rates of HIV infection (CDC, 2013h).

Ethnic Minority Populations

In recent years, HIV/AIDS has disproportionately affected the African American and Hispanic/Latino communities in the United States. African Americans account for up to 44% of new HIV infections in the United States. This is particularly significant considering that African Americans make up only 12% of the total U.S. population (CDC, 2014g). In 2010, Hispanics/Latinos comprised 21% of the new HIV infections. The rate of new HIV infections for Hispanics/Latinos (27.5%) was three times the rate for whites (8.7%) (CDC, 2013i).

Although African American and Hispanic/Latino populations are disproportionately affected by HIV/AIDS, this is not meant to suggest that individuals are at high risk for HIV/AIDS just because they are members of ethnic minority groups. Community prevention efforts for HIV/AIDS must consider not only the multicultural nature of U.S. society, but also social and economic factors such as poverty, unemployment, and poor access to health care that disproportionately affect ethnic minority populations.

Social barriers also play a significant role in blocking HIV/AIDS education efforts in ethnic communities, especially in African American and Hispanic communities, where HIV/AIDS is still identified with homosexuality and drug use. Until HIV/AIDS prevention and treatment efforts gain support from the community, including churches and political leaders, HIV/AIDS will continue to affect ethnic minority groups in disproportionate numbers (CDC, 2013i, 2014g).

Illicit Drug Users

Although the estimated number of new HIV/AIDS cases among IDUs has steadily decreased since 2001, injection drug use continues to contribute to the spread of HIV disease in significant proportions. Its impact on HIV transmission goes far beyond the circle of those who inject drugs. Sexual partners of IDUs are at high risk for HIV infection, as well as babies born to mothers who are IDUs or who have had sex with IDUs. Use of non-injection drugs, such as "crack" cocaine, also contributes to the spread of HIV/AIDS when drug users trade sex for drugs or money, or when they engage in risky sexual behavior that they would not engage in if not under the influence of drugs (CDC, 2013j, 2013k).

Substance abuse prevention is strongly related to HIV prevention, so comprehensive community-based programs must provide information, skills, and support for reducing risks for both. Community HIV/AIDS prevention programs require a wide range of approaches, including the following (National Institute on Drug Abuse [NIDA], 2008):

- Initial drug use prevention
- Street outreach programs
- Access to high-quality substance abuse treatment programs
- HIV prevention programs in correctional facilities
- Comprehensive health care for HIV-infected drug users
- HIV risk-reduction counseling for drug users and their sex partners

Effective substance abuse treatment programs that assist people to eliminate drug use not only eliminate the risk of HIV transmission through contaminated needles, but also reduce the risk of engaging in behaviors that contribute to the risk for sexual transmission. Unfortunately, the need for substance abuse treatment in the United States greatly outweighs the ability to provide it. There is a long waiting list for admission to available drug treatment programs and U.S. laws exist that restrict the possession, distribution, or sale of any drug injection equipment. The U.S. government bans the use of federal funds for needle exchange programs that allow IDUs to exchange dirty needles for clean ones to reduce the transmission of HIV. Scientific studies have provided sufficient evidence that needle exchange programs, when combined with a comprehensive prevention program, reduce HIV transmission without increasing drug use (CDC, 2013j).

The absence of needle exchange programs and insufficient numbers of substance abuse treatment programs make efforts aimed at HIV prevention for IDUs even more critical. IDUs should be taught to use sterile needles and to never reuse needles. But if using sterile needles is not always possible, IDUs should be taught to clean their needles with a chlorine bleach and water solution between uses. However, it should be noted that cleaning needles with bleach is not as safe as using sterile needles (NIDA, 2008).

Adolescents and Young Adults

Worldwide, greater and greater numbers of adolescents and young adults are infected with HIV. Approximately 42% of new HIV infections worldwide in 2010 were in persons 15–24 years old, with twice as many females as males affected (UNAIDS, 2012). Adolescents in developing countries, particularly Sub-Saharan Africa, are most affected, but the risk is high for teens in industrialized countries, too.

In the United States and Canada, HIV is spreading, with 26% of all new infections in the United States in 2010 occurring in young people between the ages of 13 and 24 (Kaiser Foundation, 2013). The majority (75%) of new diagnoses in this age group were in persons between the ages of 20 and 24 years old (CDC, 2011). Sexual exposure accounts for the majority of adolescent HIV infections. For young men, the biggest sexual risk is homosexual contact; for young women, it is heterosexual contact. Adolescents engage in multiple high-risk behaviors, often associated with drug and alcohol use. Alcohol and other drug use are common among high school students, often leading to high-risk sexual behavior. The 2011 CDC Youth Risk Behavior Surveillance Report (CDC, 2012b) shows that nearly 48% of all high school students have had sexual intercourse by the time they have reached 12th grade, with 12th-grade females slightly (6.3%) more likely to have had sexual intercourse than their male peers. Nearly one in four sexually active 12th graders have had four or more sex partners; 60.2% reported consistent condom use (CDC, 2012b).

Adolescents are difficult to engage in the care needed for the diagnosis and treatment of HIV disease. They often believe they are invincible and tend to deny they are at risk. This belief may cause them to engage in high-risk behavior, delay HIV testing, or delay or refuse treatment when they have tested positive for HIV. When adolescents are treated by healthcare providers for other reasons, HIV risk is seldom discussed. Recent studies show that fewer than half of adolescents with histories of "survival sex" (sex to earn money to live on the street), injection drug use, same-gender sexual behavior, or prior STI infection seek treatment or help for these HIV-related issues. Thus, prevention is the key weapon in reducing the incidence of adolescent HIV/AIDS (CDC, 2011).

Behavioral science has shown that young people respond best to a balance of different approaches to prevention. To be effective, a wide range of activities must be implemented in communities. For example, school-based programs must include kindergarten through 12th-grade education programs that address not only HIV prevention but also prevention of STIs, unintended pregnancy, and tobacco and drug use and programs that encourage healthy eating and physical exercise. School programs should address social norms that regulate gender roles, develop good decision-making skills, and increase self-esteem and self-efficacy. Other community-based programs to reach teens not in school are needed for homeless and runaway youth, juvenile offenders, or school dropouts (CDC, 2013e).

Women

In 2010, women accounted for 20% of new HIV infections, with black women making up 64% of these (Kaiser Foundation, 2014). The "feminization of AIDS" is a result of many different factors—biological, social, economic, and political—that interact differently for women and men.

More than 3 decades into the epidemic, gender inequality and the low status of women remain two of the major forces driving the spread of HIV/AIDS. Global responses to HIV have only just begun to address the social, cultural, legal, and economic factors that put women at risk for HIV infection and make treatment efforts more difficult. Women and girls traditionally have had less access to education and HIV information, have experienced inequality in marriage and sexual relationships, and have been the primary caregivers in their families and communities. Poverty is highly correlated with high rates of HIV. Worldwide, women are more likely than men to be poor with no source of personal income and no legal rights to property or inheritance (UNAIDS, 2013).

Violence is also a significant risk factor for women. Domestic violence is considered private—even normal—in many cultures. Laws protecting women in these societies are nonexistent, weak, or poorly enforced (UNAIDS, 2013). Rape is often used as a weapon for subjugation in war and armed conflict situations, especially in relation to "ethnic cleansing." International commitments are being made to improve the status of women, but in many areas of the world efforts have been small scale and haphazard (UNAIDS, 2013).

Worldwide, most women are infected with HIV through heterosexual contact. Women are more biologically vulnerable to HIV than men, because the physiology of the female reproductive tract makes women two to four times as likely as men to acquire HIV during heterosexual sexual intercourse. In addition, cultural, legal, religious, and economic factors often limit the amount of control many women have over their own bodies, putting them at increased risk for HIV infection. For example, condom requests by women are often misinterpreted by male partners as an indication of mistrust or infidelity, leading to loss of the male partner or domestic violence. Women with minimal education and job skills are often unable to negotiate safer sex practices because of economic dependence on their partners for both themselves and their children (HRSA, 2011; UNAIDS, 2013). Cultural and economic factors also mean that many women do not have access to preventive care and early treatment, resulting in their later diagnosis and earlier death from HIV/AIDS. Research, prevention, and care activities for women have been slow to develop, even though the number of women infected in the developing world has been equal to the number of men infected since the beginning of the pandemic. Much of this may be related to the unequal role and status of women worldwide. Another factor may be that, until recently, the proportion of cases of AIDS in women in the industrialized world, where most of the research is conducted, was much lower than for men.

Currently, the female condom is the only female-initiated HIV prevention method available. It is bulkier and more expensive than male condoms and has been poorly marketed. Its obvious presence makes it more likely to be rejected by male partners during intercourse. An effective microbiocide would be a big breakthrough in the search for female-controlled HIV prevention not detectable by males. "First-generation" candidate microbiocides are currently being tested in large-scale efficacy trials in Africa and Asia. A microbiocide that is only 60% effective could potentially prevent as many as 1 million new HIV infections per year. Research is under way to develop "second-generation" microbiocides with higher efficacy rates for future testing (UNAIDS, 2013).

With an effective microbiocide still years in the future, community HIV-prevention efforts need to emphasize interventions aimed at women. Conventional education programs that address male and female condom negotiation and use, routine HIV testing, and drug abuse still need to be implemented, but programs that address domestic abuse, self-esteem, and self-efficacy need to be developed and implemented as well. In addition, more community-supported domestic crisis centers, daycare facilities, educational and job training programs, and support groups specifically for women at risk need to be established. High-quality care for women living with HIV must address not only their medical and physical needs, but also their economic needs, their relationships, their culture, their emotional needs, and their spiritual needs. In other words, a systems approach is needed to address all aspects of a woman's life (Aranda-Naranjo, Barini-Garcia, Pounds, & Davis, 2005).

ETHICAL CONNECTION 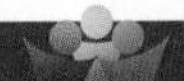

In a study of HIV-risk behaviors, sexual orientation, and sexual abuse, surveys were used from five school-based cohorts in Seattle, Washington, and British Columbia. Secondary analyses were done on surveys of more than 800,000 adolescents conducted between 1992 and 2003. An HIV-risk scale of seven items assessed risky sexual behaviors and injection drug use. Self-identified sexual orientations included heterosexual, bisexual, and gay/lesbian. Analyses of covariance were conducted separately by gender and were adjusted for age and sexual abuse when comparing means.

Gay/lesbian and bisexual adolescents had higher mean age-adjusted risk scores compared with heterosexual adolescents. When controlled for sexual abuse history, mean scores were two to four times higher among abused students than among nonabused students in each sexual orientation group. The study concluded that sexual minority adolescents reported higher HIV risk behaviors, and higher

(continues)

ETHICAL CONNECTION (*continued*)

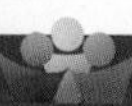

prevalence of sexual victimization may partially explain these risks.

What are the ethical implications for community health nurses when working with high school students in at-risk, abusive relationships?

Source: Saewyc, E., Skay, C., Richens, K., Reis, E., Poon, C., & Murphy, A. (2006). Sexual orientation, sexual abuse, and HIV-risk behavior among adolescents in the Pacific Northwest. *American Journal of Public Health, 96*(6), 1104–1110.

THINK ABOUT THIS

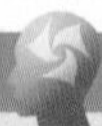

"Ninety-two percent of women carry lip protection. Ten percent of women carry HIV prevention."

—American Foundation for AIDS Research (AmFAR), public service slogan, 2004

Children

UNAIDS and WHO estimate that, throughout the world, approximately 3.3 million children younger than 15 years of age have been infected with HIV since the epidemic began in 1981. Many of them were infants born to HIV-positive mothers. Because HIV infection progresses quickly in children, most HIV-infected children younger than age 15 have progressed to AIDS, and most of these have died. In several African countries, the under-5 mortality rate rose from 2% in 1990 to 6.5% in 2003, adding another devastating consequence to the HIV epidemic (Child and Adolescent Health and Development [CAH], 2005; WHO, 2013).

Although the number of people receiving HAART in low- and middle-income countries has more than tripled since the end of 2001, the fact remains than only one person in 10 in Africa and one in seven in Asia in need of treatment received it in 2005. While international efforts to provide adequate treatment and prevention programs are moving faster, the HIV infection rate is still sprinting far ahead of providers' efforts. Worldwide, fewer than one in five people at risk for HIV infection has access to basic prevention services and only one in 10 people living with HIV has been tested and is aware that he or she is infected (WHO, 2013). Without HAART, the infection rate for children born to mothers with HIV is between 25% and 30%; with HAART, the infection rate for children born to mothers with HIV is less than 2%. It is obvious that comprehensive prevention, treatment, and support programs have nearly eliminated HIV transmission from mothers to their babies in industrialized countries. Some healthcare professionals believe that having a life-saving treatment that is available only to a privileged few is the highest form of human cruelty.

In addition to bringing suffering and death for those infected, the HIV/AIDS epidemic has had another devastating consequence: 13 million children around the world have lost their mothers or both parents to HIV/AIDS. AIDS orphans have become a major problem in the developing world. In parts of Africa, grandparents whose adult children have succumbed to HIV/AIDS are raising as many as 30 grandchildren with very few resources. In other families, children younger than 12 are struggling to care for dying parents and to raise younger siblings after their parents have died. With the family wage-earners dead or dying, these fragmented families are sinking further into abysmal poverty. The intense psychological stress already experienced from dealing with poverty and illness is intensified by the stigma associated with HIV/AIDS. Increasingly, these children must withdraw from school, losing any opportunities for acquiring the knowledge and skills needed to create sound families and living environments for the future (CAH, 2005).

Older People

A growing number of people age 50 years and older in the United States are living with HIV infection. People age 55 and older account for almost one-fifth (19%, or 217,000 people) of the estimated 1.1 million people living with HIV infection in the United States in 2010. Making an initial AIDS diagnosis in older people is common, with half of all people older than 50 with AIDS having been infected for less than a year. Of new HIV infections in 2010, 5% were among the older population (55 and older) with white men accounting for 36% of this total, black men (24%), black women (15%), Hispanic/Latino men (12%), and 4% each in white women and Hispanic/Latino women. In 2011, older adults accounted for 24% of those diagnosed with AIDS. AIDS was the 10th leading cause of death among men and women ages 50–54.

Older adults are infected through the same high-risk behaviors as young adults, though they may not be aware that they are at risk for HIV/AIDS. Having a new diagnosis of HIV means a later start to treatment, possible existing comorbidities, and a shorter HIV-to-AIDS interval. Healthcare providers do not always test older adults for HIV and STIs. Today, HIV/AIDS has shifted from caring for the dying to caring for the aging. Preventive care and regular screenings for body mass index (BMI), diabetes, blood pressure, cholesterol, osteoporosis, smoking, alcohol use, substance abuse, depression, and risk factors and current sexual history are part of holistic health care for this population (CDC, 2013l).

Few HIV education campaigns target older Americans (AIDS InfoNet, 2014; CDC, 2013l; Gottesman, 2005; National Association of HIV Over Fifty [NAHOF], 2007). The older population is steadily growing larger with the maturing of the Baby Boomer generation. Social norms about divorce, sex, and dating are changing, and erectile dysfunction drugs such as sildenafil (Viagra) are facilitating a more active sex life for older adults (NAHOF, 2007). Heterosexual women age 50 and older are most in need of the HIV-prevention message. Most stop using protection because pregnancy is no longer a concern. After menopause, however, decreased lubrication and thinning vaginal walls put them at higher risk for HIV transmission (Gottesman, 2005; CDC, 2013l).

Rates of HIV infection (not AIDS) are difficult to determine in the older population because older people are not routinely tested, early misdiagnosis is common, and the immune system naturally weakens with age (NAHOF, 2007). Healthcare and service providers—and often older people themselves—do not realize that elders have many of the same risk factors as other populations, including having unprotected sex (homosexual and heterosexual) and using illicit drugs. Healthcare providers are often reluctant to initiate discussions related to sexuality with their older patients (AIDS InfoNet, 2014; NAHOF, 2007).

HAART seems to work as well in older people as it does in younger people in controlling viral loads, for both newly infected people and people who were diagnosed and began treatment before age 50 and then got older. However, T-cell levels do not recover as quickly in older people and treatment side effects may be more frequent. Older people generally have other chronic health conditions that require medications that may adversely interact with HAART (AIDS InfoNet, 2014; NAHOF, 2007).

DAY IN THE LIFE

Yes, it's true life can be scary, but life can also be exciting, thrilling, and fabulous. And to be honest with you, I would much rather have life than the alternative. I don't regret this disease. It's taught me some valuable lessons—helped me face some exciting and new challenges and introduced me to some charming people. All of which never would have happened had it not been for this disease. It's true I may die tomorrow. But if I do die, I'm going to die happy, without regrets. If I had to live my life all over again, I wouldn't change a thing. I'd take it all—AIDS included. I don't have HIV, I have AIDS and I am proud of who I am. And I am proud of the person I am going to become. My name is Rob Lanier and I have AIDS and I am alive. I am alive! I am alive!

—Rob Lanier died in 1995, at the age of 28

STIs and the U.S. Healthcare System

Health Services

STI care is often lacking outside of dedicated STI clinics. Community outreach for STI prevention programs has increased, but cuts in funding have limited many of the services offered. Public health clinics cannot reach all of the people who need STI care, and greater effort is needed to stimulate and encourage private providers to take sexual histories, screen for asymptomatic infections, and provide a range of STI services in their practices. More recently, managed care organizations have emerged as a dominant organizational framework for medical care across much of the United States, particularly for the more disadvantaged segments of the population, and could serve many individuals at risk for STIs. However, STI and HIV prevention and testing are not generally included in routine services.

Screening and Prevention

People often do not know they are infected with STIs because they do not have or do not recognize symptoms. Studies of STI screening outside of healthcare settings (e.g., in jails, workplaces, and other community-based settings) reveal that a large number of persons with gonorrhea and chlamydia have no symptoms or signs of infection (CDC, 2013c).

The fact that gonorrhea and chlamydia so often do not produce any symptoms has many implications for community health nursing, because no matter how effectively access to healthcare is enhanced, many of these silent infections will go undetected and untreated unless screening and treatment are provided in nontraditional settings. Even though asymptomatic individuals will not access health care specifically for STI testing or treatment, they do visit a variety of healthcare settings for other purposes. There are many opportunities to identify and treat asymptomatic but infected persons in healthcare settings when they present for other unrelated problems (e.g., in emergency departments, in family planning clinics, during routine or sports physicals, during immunization visits) and in non-healthcare settings such as schools and jails.

HEALTHY PEOPLE 2020 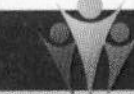

Objectives Related to HIV

- HIV-1 Reduce new HIV diagnoses among adolescents and adults
- HIV-2 Reduce new (incident) HIV infections among adolescents and adults

(continues)

- HIV-3 Reduce the rate of HIV transmission among adolescents and adults
- HIV-4 Reduce new AIDS cases among adolescents and adults
- HIV-5 Reduce new AIDS cases among adolescent and adult heterosexuals
- HIV-6 Reduce new AIDS cases among adolescent and adult men who have sex with men
- HIV-7 Reduce new AIDS cases among adolescents and adults who inject drugs
- HIV-8 Reduce perinatally acquired HIV and AIDS cases

Death, Survival, and Medical Healthcare After Diagnosis of HIV Infection and AIDS

- HIV-9 Increase the proportion of new HIV infections diagnosed before progression to AIDS
- HIV-10 Increase the proportion of HIV-infected adolescents and adults who receive HIV care and treatment consistent with current standards
- HIV-11 Increase the proportion of persons surviving more than 3 years after a diagnosis with AIDS
- HIV-12 Reduce deaths from HIV infection

HIV Testing

- HIV-13 Increase the proportion of persons living with HIV who know their serostatus
- HIV-14.1 Increase the proportion of adolescents and adults who have been tested for HIV in the past 12 months
- HIV-14.2 Increase the proportion of men who have sex with men who have been tested for HIV in the past 12 months
- HIV-14.3 Increase the proportion of pregnant women who have been tested for HIV in the past 12 months
- HIV-14.4 Increase the proportion of adolescents and young adults who have been tested for HIV in the past 12 months
- HIV-15 Increase the proportion of adults with tuberculosis (TB) who have been tested for HIV

HIV Prevention

- HIV-16 Increase the proportion of substance abuse treatment facilities that offer HIV/AIDS education, counseling, and support
- HIV-17 Increase the proportion of sexually active persons who use condoms
- HIV-18 Reduce the proportion of men who have sex with men who reported unprotected anal sex in the past 12 months

Source: U.S. Department of Health and Human Services. (2014b). HIV. Retrieved from http://www.healthypeople.gov/2020/topicsobjectives2020/overview.aspx?topicid=22.

What's New?

In 2012, the FDA approved a label indication for a new pre-exposure prophylaxis (PrEP) drug combination: tenofovir disoproxil fumarate (TDF) 300 mg combined with emtricitabine (FTC) 200 mg, to prevent sexual transmission of HIV in MSM, sexually active heterosexual women and men, and intravenous drug users. This new therapy is used in addition to comprehensive prevention services. Watch the CDC website for updates (CDC, 2013k).

The Role of Community Health Nurses

To prevent the spread of STIs, it is not enough to screen for and treat infections; community nurses also need to be able to help individuals change their behavior by counseling about how to prevent infections and reinfections. It is not who one is but what one does that determines whether a person becomes infected or reinfected with an STI. Screening and treating infections are effective for current infections, but unless individuals can be helped to change their behavior, they may continue to behave in ways that put them at risk for further infections.

A number of different behaviors can be targeted at reducing infections: increasing the seeking of appropriate health care, improving patients' adherence to medication and cooperation with efforts to notify their partners of possible infection, reducing the rate of partner change, and lowering the number of sex partners. Increasing consistent and correct condom use can prevent some infections, such as gonorrhea and HIV, but is less effective with other STIs such as HPV. The most effective counseling interventions are those that are directed at a specific behavior. Perhaps the most difficult task facing community health nurses is identifying the behaviors that warrant change for specific patients and matching their intervention to the patients' readiness to change behavior.

Decisions about the behaviors in need of change should be based on a careful assessment of the patient's sexual and drug-use history. Although many nurses are uncomfortable taking such histories, most patients view sexual and drug histories as an expected part of a medical examination. At the very least, information should be gathered about the number and type of sexual partners (regular and occasional partners), types of sex practiced, condom use (with regular and occasional partners), use of both injected and noninjected drugs, and in the case of IDUs, information about their use of sterile syringes and disinfection of shared injection paraphernalia. It is only by taking such histories that behaviors that are placing the patient at risk can be identified. These behaviors should then be the target of the nursing intervention (CDC, 2010).

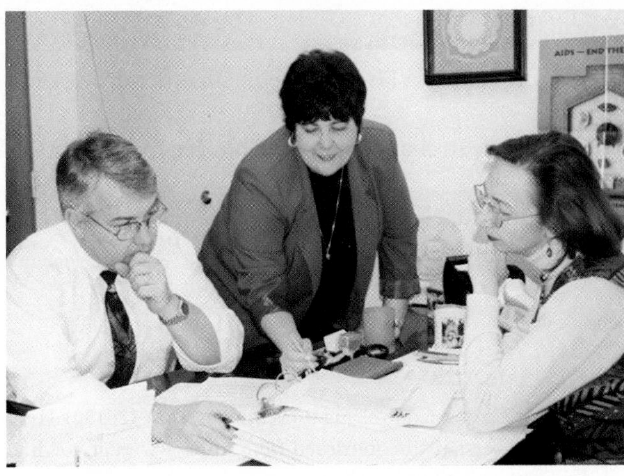

Dr. Sharyn Janes (center) plans a statewide HIV education program for healthcare providers with Craig Thompson (left), Director of the STI/HIV Division of the Mississippi State Department of Health, and Cheryl Hamill, RN, Director of the Resource Center of the Delta Region AIDS Education and Training Center at the University of Mississippi Medical Center.

RESEARCH ALERT

This study examined the effects of an HIV prevention intervention on women's condom-use behaviors. The community-level intervention targeted sexually active women of child-bearing age in four different inner-city communities. At the beginning of the study, nearly 70% of the participants did not intend to use condoms with their sexual partners. After 2 years of theory-based and culturally specific intervention activities, increases in talking with partners about condoms and attempting to use condoms with partners were significantly larger in the intervention communities than in comparison communities. The results of this study show that (1) large-scale community interventions can be implemented successfully in low-income, inner-city neighborhoods; (2) many women were still not using condoms, which confirms the necessity for relevant, effective prevention interventions that target women; and (3) a community-level intervention can affect women's condom-use behavior. To be successful in low-income neighborhoods, interventions must address social, economic, and cultural issues that affect the target population's access to information and its ability to focus on health-related behaviors.

Source: Lauby, J. L., Smith, P. J., Stark, M., Person, B., & Adams, J. (2000). A community-level HIV prevention intervention for inner-city women: Results of the women and infants demonstration projects. *American Journal of Public Health, 90*(2), 216–222.

Conclusion

STIs are a hidden epidemic with enormous health and economic consequences in the United States. They remain hidden because so many Americans are unable to address sexual health issues openly and because of the biological and social characteristics of these diseases.

All Americans have a vested interest in STI prevention, because every community is affected by STIs and everyone directly or indirectly pays for the costs of these diseases.

STIs are public health problems that lack easy solutions, because they are rooted in fundamental human behavioral and social problems. Despite the barriers to open discussion of sexuality, there are prevention programs that are effective and that can be implemented on a local level.

Ultimately, multifaceted approaches are needed at the individual and community levels to produce the best results. Although no intervention is perfect, together they can have a synergistic and positive impact on lowering the disease burden in this country. Subpopulations such as adolescents and disenfranchised adults will need special attention and outreach efforts.

To develop more effective STI treatment and prevention in the United States will require full participation by the public and private sectors. Community health nurses can be key stakeholders in modifying how STI services are provided and by accepting new responsibilities to ensure that the hidden epidemic of STIs in this country is addressed.

AFFORDABLE CARE ACT (ACA) 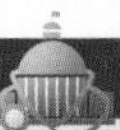

The ACA directs the HHS Secretary to convene a national public/private partnership for the purpose of conducting a national prevention and health promotion outreach and educational campaign (funding not to exceed $500 million). In addition, the HHS Secretary shall provide guidance to states regarding preventive services available to Medicaid enrollees.

LEVELS OF PREVENTION 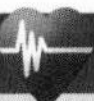

Primary: Mass media campaign on the use of condoms for reduction of STIs

Secondary: Screenings for gonorrhea in an incarcerated population

Tertiary: Assisting patients who have AIDS with symptom management and medication protocol initiation

HEALTHY ME 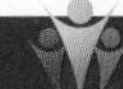

If you are in an intimate relationship, what precautions are you using to protect against becoming infected and spreading STI diseases? Do you talk to your partner about protection prior to intimacy?

Critical Thinking Activities

1. What are some of the reasons the United States has vastly higher rates of STIs compared with other developed countries?
2. How can you, as a community health nurse, play an important role in changing the STI burden in the United States?
3. How comfortable are you with talking about sexual health and sexual behavior with your family? With your friends? With your patients?

References

AIDS InfoNet. (2014). Older people and HIV fact sheet. Retrieved from http://aidsinfonet.org/fact_sheets/view/616?lang=eng

Aral, S. O., & Holmes, K. K. (1991). Sexually transmitted diseases in the AIDS era. *Scientific American, 264*, 62–69.

Aranda-Naranjo, B., Barini-Garcia, M., Pounds, M. B., & Davis, R. (2005). Addressing cultural issues to improve quality of care. In J. R. Anderson (Ed.), *A guide to clinical care of women with HIV.* Washington, DC: Health Resources and Services Administration.

Centers for Disease Control and Prevention. (2010). Sexually transmitted diseases treatment guidelines, 2010. *Morbidity and Mortality Weekly Report, 59*(RR–12).

Centers for Disease Control and Prevention (CDC). (2011). Fact sheet: HIV among youth. Retrieved from http://www.cdc.gov/hiv/pdf/library_factsheet_HIV_amongYouth.pdf

Centers for Disease Control and Prevention (CDC). (2012a). HPV Vaccine Information for Clinicians - Fact Sheet. Retrieved from http://www.cdc.gov/std/hpv/stdfact-hpv-vaccine-hcp.htm

Centers for Disease Control and Prevention (CDC). (2012b). *Youth Risk Behavior Surveillance—United States,* 2011. Retrieved from http://www.cdc.gov/mmwr/pdf/ss/ss6104.pdf

Centers for Disease Control and Prevention (CDC). (2013a). Fact Sheet: Incidence, prevalence, and cost of sexually transmitted infections in the United States. Retrieved from http://www.cdc.gov/std/stats/sti-estimates-fact-sheet-feb-2013.pdf

Centers for Disease Control and Prevention (CDC). (2013b). Genital HPV infection - Fact Sheet. Retrieved from http://www.cdc.gov/std/HPV/HPV-factsheet-March-2014.pdf

Centers for Disease Control and Prevention. (2013c). *Sexually Transmitted Disease Surveillance 2012.* Atlanta: U.S. Department of Health and Human Services. Retrieved from http://www.cdc.gov/sTD/stats12/default.htm

Centers for Disease Control and Prevention (CDC). (2013d). STDs & pregnancy - CDC fact sheet. Retrieved from http://www.cdc.gov/std/pregnancy/stdfact-pregnancy.htm

Centers for Disease Control and Prevention (CDC). (2013e). *Today's HIV/AIDS epidemic.* Retrieved from http://www.cdc.gov/nchhstp/newsroom/docs/hivfactsheets/todaysepidemic-508.pdf

Centers for Disease Control and Prevention (CDC). (2013f). Diagnoses of HIV infection in the United States and dependent areas, 2011. Retrieved from http://www.cdc.gov/hiv/library/reports/surveillance/2011/surveillance_Report_vol_23.html

Centers for Disease Control and Prevention (CDC). (2013g). HIV/AIDS basic statistics. Retrieved from http://www.cdc.gov/hiv/basics/statistics.html

Centers for Disease Control and Prevention (CDC). (2013h). Fact sheet: HIV among gay, bisexual, and other men who have sex with men. Retrieved from http://www.cdc.gov/hiv/risk/gender/msm/facts/index.html

Centers for Disease Control and Prevention (CDC). (2013i). HIV incidence. Retrieved from http://www.cdc.gov/hiv/statistics/surveillance/incidence/

Centers for Disease Control and Prevention (CDC). (2013j). HIV and substance use in the United States. Retrieved from http://www.cdc.gov/hiv/risk/behavior/substanceuse.html

Centers for Disease Control and Prevention (CDC). (2013k). Update to interim guidance for preexposure prophylaxis (PrEP) for the prevention of HIV infection: PrEP for injecting drug users. *Morbidity and Mortality Weekly Report, 62*(23), 463–465. Retrieved from http://www.cdc.gov/mmwr/preview/mmwrhtml/mm6223a2.htm

Centers for Disease Control and Prevention (CDC). (2013l). HIV Among older Americans. Retrieved from http://www.cdc.gov/hiv/risk/age/olderamericans/index.html

Centers for Disease Control and Prevention (CDC). (2014a). Chlamydia fact sheet. Retrieved from http://www.cdc.gov/std/chlamydia/stdfact-chlamydia.htm

Centers for Disease Control and Prevention (CDC). (2014b). Gonorrhea fact sheet. Retrieved from http://www.cdc.gov/STD/gonorrhea/STDFact-gonorrhea.htm

Centers for Disease Control and Prevention (CDC). (2014c). Syphilis fact sheet. Retrieved from http://www.cdc.gov/STD/syphilis/STDFact-syphilis.htm

Centers for Disease Control and Prevention (CDC). (2014d). Genital herpes fact sheet. Retrieved from http://www.cdc.gov/STD/herpes/STDFact-herpes.htm

Centers for Disease Control and Prevention (CDC). (2014e). Pelvic inflammatory disease (PID)—CDC fact sheet. Retrieved from http://www.cdc.gov/STD/PID/STDFact-PID-Detailed.htm

Centers for Disease Control and Prevention (CDC). (2014f). HIV among African American gay and bisexual men. Retrieved from http://www.cdc.gov/hiv/risk/racialethnic/bmsm/facts/index.html

Centers for Disease Control and Prevention (CDC). (2014g). HIV Among African Americans. Retrieved from http://www.cdc.gov/hiv/risk/racialethnic/aa/facts/index.html

Child and Adolescent Health and Development (CAH), World Health Organization. (2005). HIV/AIDS. Publisher: WHO.

Coxon, A. P. M. (1996). Male homosexuality and HIV. Section I: Behavior changes among homosexual men. In J. Mann & D. Tarantola (Eds.), *AIDS in the world II* (pp. 252–254). New York, NY: Oxford University Press.

Goodroad, B. K. (2003). Managing antiretroviral therapy. In C. Kirton (Ed.), *ANAC's core curriculum for HIV/AIDS nursing* (2nd ed., pp. 51–63). Thousand Oaks, CA: Sage.

Gottesman, N. (2005, July/August). HIV over 50. *AARP Magazine.* Retrieved from http://www.aarpmagazine.org/

Health Resources and Services Administration (HRSA), HIV/AIDS Bureau. (2008). Men of color who have sex with men and HIV/AIDS in the United States. Retrieved from ftp://ftp.hrsa.gov/hab/MSMofcolor.pdf

Health Resources and Services Administration (HRSA), HIV/AIDS Bureau. (2009). Legislation: Ryan White Care Act. Retrieved from http://www.hab.hrsa.gov/abouthab/legislation.html

Health Resources and Services Administration (HRSA), HIV/AIDS Bureau. (2011). Women and the Ryan White HIV/AIDS Program. Retrieved from http://hab.hrsa.gov/livinghistory/issues/Women-And-Aids.pdf

Heymann, D. L. (2009). *Control of communicable diseases manual* (18th ed.). Washington, DC: American Public Health Association.

Johnson, T. D. (2007). Millions around world observe, pay respects on World AIDS Day. *The Nation's Health: The Official Newspaper of the American Public Health Association,* December 2006/January 2007, p. 22.

Kaiser Foundation. (2006). *AIDS at 25: An overview of major trends in the U.S. epidemic.* Washington, DC: Kaiser Family Foundation.

Kaiser Foundation. (2013). *The HIV/AIDS epidemic in the United States.* Retrieved from http://kff.org/hivaids/fact-sheet/the-hivaids-epidemic-in-the-united-states/

Kaiser Foundation. (2014). *Women and HIV/AIDS in the United States.* Retrieved from http://kff.org/hivaids/fact-sheet/women-and-hivaids-in-the-united-states/

Markowitz, L. E., Dunne, E. F., Saraiya, M., Lawson, H. W., Chesson, H., & Unger, E. R. (2007). Quadrivalent human papillomavirus vaccine: Recommendations of the Advisory Committee on Immunization Practices (ACIP). *Morbidity and Mortality Weekly Report, 56*(RR-02), 1–24. Retrieved from http://www.cdc.gov/mmwr/preview/mmwrhtml/rr5602a1.htm

National Association of HIV Over Fifty (NAHOF). (2007). HIV and older adults educational tip sheet. Publisher: NAHOF.

National Cancer Institute (NCI). (2012). Human papillomaviruses and cancer: National Cancer Institute fact sheet. Retrieved from http://www.cancer.gov/cancertopics/factsheet/Risk/HPV

National Institute on Drug Abuse (NIDA). (2008). Principles of HIV prevention in drug-using populations. Retrieved from http://archives.drugabuse.gov/POHP/

Saewyc, E., Skay, C., Richens, K., Reis, E., Poon, C., & Murphy, A. (2006). Sexual orientation, sexual abuse, and HIV-risk behavior among adolescents in the Pacific Northwest. *American Journal of Public Health, 96*(6), 1104–1110.

Shilts, R. (1987). *And the band played on: Politics, people, and the AIDS epidemic.* New York, NY: Penguin.

UNAIDS. (2012). Fact Sheet: Adolescents, young people and HIV. Retrieved from http://www.unaids.org/en/media/unaids/contentassets/documents/factsheet/2012/20120417_FS_adolescentsyoungpeoplehiv_en.pdf

UNAIDS. (2013). *UNAIDS Report on the Global AIDS Epidemic 2013.* Retrieved from http://www.unaids.org/en/media/unaids/contentassets/documents/epidemiology/2013/gr2013/UNAIDS_Global_Report_2013_en.pdf

U.S. Department of Health and Human Services. (2014a). Sexually transmitted diseases. Retrieved from http://www.healthypeople.gov/2020/topicsobjectives2020/overview.aspx?topicid=37

U.S. Department of Health and Human Services. (2014b). HIV. Retrieved from http://www.healthypeople.gov/2020/topicsobjectives2020/overview.aspx?topicid=22

Vuylsteke, B., Sunkutu, R., & Laga, M. (1996). Epidemiology of HIV and sexually transmitted infections in women. In J. Mann & D. Tarantola (Eds.), *AIDS in the World II* (pp. 97–109). New York, NY: Oxford University Press.

World Health Organization (WHO). (2013). Ten facts on HIV/AIDS. Retrieved from http://www.who.int/features/factfiles/hiv/en/

World Health Organization (WHO). (2014). Global health observatory: HIV/AIDS. Retrieved from http://www.who.int/gho/hiv/en/

CHAPTER FOCUS

The Nature of Substance Abuse as a Community Health Problem
- Definitions of Substance Abuse
- Scope of Substance Abuse
- Impact of Substance Abuse on Society
- Impact of Substance Abuse on the Individual

Risk Factors for Substance Abuse
- Society's Influence
- The Family's Influence
- The Workplace's Influence
- Personal Factors

Nursing Assessment
- Nurses' Attitude Self-Assessment
- Drug History
- Recognizing the Signs of Substance Abuse

Interventions
- Society's Response
- Interventions with Special Populations

QUESTIONS TO CONSIDER

After reading this chapter, you will know the answers to the following questions:

1. What is the scope of substance abuse in the community?
2. What are the most commonly abused drugs?
3. What are the community health consequences of substance abuse?
4. What are the risk factors associated with substance abuse?
5. How does a nurse's self-awareness relate to addressing the problem of substance abuse in the community?
6. How are primary, secondary, and tertiary prevention strategies implemented in the community?
7. What are specific intervention strategies for various age groups in the prevention of substance abuse?
8. Which specific population groups are most at risk for substance abuse?
9. What is the role of the community health nurse in substance abuse prevention in schools and in the workplace?

The top public health problems in the United States are linked with substance abuse. Research about the risks for substance abuse (such as age, gender, and culture) can guide community health nurses in developing effective prevention interventions for vulnerable populations.

CHAPTER 22

Substance Abuse and Misuse as Community Health Problems

Judith A. Barton, Jean A. Haspeslagh, and Marshall Parker Lundy

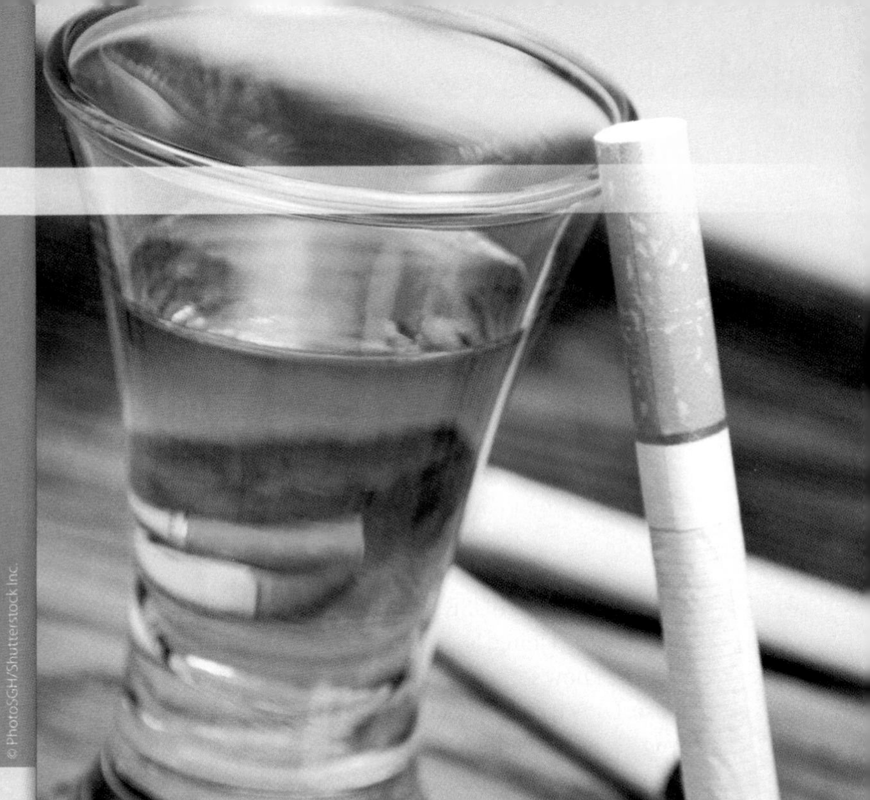

KEY TERMS

addiction
alcoholism
comprehensive school health
dependence
interdiction
primary prevention
return to work contract
secondary prevention
social control
social modeling theory
substance abuse
supply
tertiary prevention

REFLECTIONS

Macduff: What three things does drink especially provoke?
Porter: Marry, sir, nose-painting, sleep and urine. Lechery, sir, it provokes and unprovokes. It provokes the desire, but it takes away the performance; therefore, much drink may be said to be an equivocator with lechery; it makes him and it mars him; it sets him on, and it takes him off, it persuades him, and disheartens him, makes him stand to and not stand to, in conclusion, equivocates him in a sleep, and, giving him the lie, leaves him.

—William Shakespeare, *Macbeth, Act 2, Scene 3*

After reading the quotation from *Macbeth*, how would you interpret Shakespeare's "picture" of how alcohol affects a person? Would you identify this description as abuse or overuse of alcohol? Why or why not?

SUBSTANCE ABUSE AS A MAJOR public health problem in the United States affects society on multiple levels. All of us know someone who has been affected by substance abuse. Directly or indirectly, every community is affected by drug abuse and addiction, as is every family. The abuse of drugs in all forms takes a tremendous toll on societies and communities. This includes healthcare expenditures, lost earnings, and costs associated with crime and accidents. Community health nurses are faced with the costs and consequences of substance abuse from homelessness to child and family abuse. The top health problems of the community can often be directly linked to substance abuse: cancer, cardiovascular disease, human immunodeficiency virus (HIV)/acquired immune deficiency syndrome (AIDS), drug abuse, accidents, and violence. Drug addiction and substance abuse are preventable. Effective primary prevention efforts in the community involve families, schools, communities, and the media. Although many events and cultural factors affect drug and substance abuse trends, research consistently demonstrates that drug education can be effective to help youth and the public to understand the risks of drug abuse. The community health nurse is in an ideal position to assist communities in efforts to enhance protective factors and reverse or reduce risk factors in the population. In this chapter, risks associated with substance abuse and addictions are explored and protective factors that affect all populations are identified. Variables, such as age, gender, ethnicity, culture, and environment, are examined in the context of the role of the community health nurse.

THINK ABOUT THIS 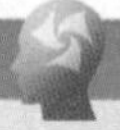

Every form of addiction is bad, no matter whether the narcotic be alcohol or morphine or idealism.

—Carl Gustav Jung

Dependence or **addiction** is present when there are physiological symptoms that occur with withdrawal of the substance. However, the important thing to remember is that, whether the individual is experiencing dependence or is "merely" overusing or misusing drugs, the effects on the person and the community are similar.

The Nature of Substance Abuse as a Community Health Problem

Definitions of Substance Abuse

When speaking of substance abuse, one finds a number of terms used in the literature, including *substance abuse, chemical dependence,* and *addiction.* In this chapter, *substance abuse* is used to cover the broad spectrum of abuse of alcohol and other drugs, including dependence and addiction. **Substance abuse** is the use of any drug (alcohol, street drugs, or prescription and over-the-counter medications) that results in a loss of control over the amount taken and when it is taken. It also includes continuation of drug use regardless of the consequences (physical, social, and psychological). Misuse of prescription drugs and over-the-counter drugs is a form of substance abuse often encountered in the community. **Box 22-1** lists the major classes of abused drugs.

ETHICAL CONNECTION 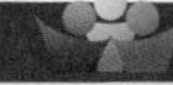

Addiction should never be treated as a crime. It has to be treated as a health problem. We do not send alcoholics to jail in this country. Over 500,000 people are in our jails who are nonviolent drug users.

—Ralph Nader

Scope of Substance Abuse

The use and abuse of alcohol and other drugs contribute to one of the major public health problems facing society today. The use and abuse of alcohol and other drugs are widespread across all races and ethnic groups in society; furthermore, someone you know at work could be using drugs (**Box 22-2**). Alcohol use and abuse are occurring at a younger age, making the need for prevention programs

BOX 22-1 Major Classes of Abused Drugs

Sedative-Hypnotics
- Central nervous system depressants
- Benzodiazepines
- Barbiturates
- Alcohol

Psychostimulants
- Amphetamines and methamphetamines
- Cocaine

ADD Rx drugs for ADHD (Adderal, Ritalin, Vivanse)

Opioids/Opiates
- Codeine
- Heroin
- Morphine

Hallucinogens
- LSD ("acid") and LSD-like drugs (mescaline, psilocybin)
- MDMA ("ecstasy") and MDMA-like drugs

Inhalants
- Glue
- Solvents
- Aerosols
- Nitrous oxide
- Gasoline

Cannabinoids
- Marijuana
- Hash
- THC

Nicotine
- Tobacco
- Smokeless tobacco

Phencyclidine (PCP)

in schools essential. For young people going off to college, the military, or first jobs, their newly found independence also includes new peer pressures to drink, smoke, or use recreational drugs. In addition, as persons live longer and experience more chronic health problems, they are faced with an existence that includes the use of multiple drugs. Along with the benefits associated with improved pharmacological management of chronic conditions, it is necessary to acknowledge the problems associated with the misuse of these same agents.

BOX 22-2 Most Drug Users Are in the Workforce

The stereotype of poor, unemployed people as users of illicit drugs is not borne out by the findings of a 2012 Substance Abuse and Mental Health Services Administration (SAMHSA) study. Of the 21.5 million illicit drug users 18 year of age or older in 2012, 14.6 million (67.9%) were employed either full or part time. Indeed, nearly 60% of workers noted that they could easily obtain or use illicit drugs during the workday, and nearly 13% reported having encountered a coworker who was impaired by illicit drugs within the preceding 12 months.

Sources: SAMHSA. (2012). *Results from the 2012 National Survey on Drug Use and Health: Summary of National Findings*. Retrieved from http://www.samhsa.gov/data/NSDUH/2012SummNatFindDetTables/NationalFindings/NSDUHresults2012.pdf; Frone, M. R. (2012). Workplace substance use climate: Prevalence and distribution in the U.S. workforce. *Journal of Substance Use, 71*(1), 72–83.

Illicit Drug Users

An estimated 23.9 million Americans used some form of illicit drugs in 2012 (SAMHSA, 2012). This number indicates that 9.2% of the population 12 years of age and older used an illicit drug in the month prior to the National Survey on Drug Use and Health (NSDUH) conducted by SAMHSA (2012). By comparison, the number is greatly reduced from its highest level in 1979, when the estimate was that 25 million or 14.1% of Americans used illicit drugs.

Marijuana continues to be the most commonly used illicit drug in the United States. In 2012, 18.9 million people used marijuana, and 5.4 million of these were daily or near-daily users of marijuana (SAMHSA, 2012). By contrast, 1.6 million people used cocaine, hallucinogens were used by 1.1 million persons, psychotherapeutics (prescription-type) by 1.6 million persons, inhalants by 500,000 persons, and heroin by 300,000 persons (SAMHSA, 2012). Youths ages 12–17 had a substance use rate of 10.1%, an increase from the 2008 rate of 9.3% (SAMHSA, 2012). Men continue to have higher rates of illicit drug use than women do, and men are more likely to consume multiple types of drugs (SAMHSA, 2012). The rates of illicit drug use in metropolitan areas are higher than in nonmetropolitan areas. Illicit drug use rates remain highly correlated with educational status. Among young adults 18 and older, those who had not completed high school had the highest rates of current use (11.1%), whereas college graduates had the lowest rate (6.6%). Illicit drug use for African

Americans (11.3%) was similar to that for whites (9.2%) and Hispanics (8.3%) (SAMHSA, 2012).

Use of Alcohol

Alcohol and fermented spirits have been used throughout history. Alcohol use is a part of American culture. Approximately 52.1% of persons (age 12 and older) report having consumed alcohol in the past year (SAMHSA, 2012). (See **Box 22-3**.) Binge drinking (5 or more drinks on the same occasion in the past month) was highest among adults age 21–25 years old, with 45.1% reporting binge drinking of alcohol in the month prior to the survey (SAMHSA, 2012). Alcohol use tends to be more moderate among African Americans than among other racial/ethnic groups. Men's use of alcohol was greater than women's use. Although the overall rate of alcohol use is lower in rural areas than in metropolitan areas, the rates of binge drinking and heavy alcohol use in rural areas were similar to the rates in nonrural areas. In contrast to the pattern for illicit drugs, the higher the level of education, the more likely the current use of alcohol (National Center for Health Statistics, 2007). It should be noted, however, that some of this use relates to a popular belief in the health benefits of consumption of red wine, which has been a topic of considerable scientific research and public interest (Aleixandre, Aleixandre-Tudó, Bolaños-Pizzaro, & Aleixandre-Benavent, 2013).

BOX 22-3 Age and Alcohol Use by Youth

Age	Percentage of Users
12–13 years	2.2%
14–15 years	11.1%
16–17 years	24.8%
18–20 years	45.8%
21–25 years	69.2%
Binge drinking	
12–20 years	15.3% (5.9 million)
Heavy drinking	
12–20 years	4.3% (1.7 million)
Youth driving under the influence of alcohol	
16–17 years	4.7%
18–20 years	12.8%

Source: SAMHSA. (2012). *Results from the 2012 National Survey on Drug Use and Health: Summary of National Findings.* Retrieved from http://www.samhsa.gov/data/NSDUH/2012SummNatFindDetTables/NationalFindings/NSDUHresults2012.pdf

Use of Tobacco and Nicotine

Tobacco use continues to be a major public health concern, with 70 million current smokers in the United States. This actual number of tobacco smokers represents a smoking rate of 29.2% for those 12 and older. Current smokers were more likely than nonsmokers to be heavy drinkers and illicit drug users. In addition, an estimated 3.5% of the population are current users of smokeless tobacco (SAMHSA, 2012).

The smoking rate among young adults ages 18 to 25 increased from 34.6% in 1994 to 39.5% in 2003 but declined slightly to 38.1% in 2012. Among 12- to 17-year-olds, cigarette smoking—by far the most common means of tobacco use—declined from 13% in 2002 to 6.6% in 2012, a decrease of almost 50% (SAMHSA, 2012). Smoking rates are similar among different races and ethnic groups. Males had higher rates of smoking than females—33% versus 20.9% (SAMHSA, 2012). Lower educational attainment was correlated with higher tobacco use (SAMHSA, 2012). However, novel tobacco products such as flavored cigarettes and smokeless nicotine alternatives ("e-cigarettes") may alter these trends in the near future. A 2014 study of U.S. middle and high school students found that among those who smoked, those using flavored products reported lack of intention to quit (59.7%) at a considerably greater rate than those who used unflavored products (49.3%) (King, Tynan, Dube, & Arrazola, 2014). Another recent study suggests that e-cigarettes, which essentially bypass tobacco altogether for delivery of nicotine, may nevertheless encourage use of conventional tobacco-based cigarettes among adolescents (Dutra & Glantz, 2014).

Youthful Illicit Drug Users

The Monitoring the Future study (National Institute on Drug Abuse [NIDA], 2007) concluded that illicit drug use by middle and high school students continues to decline. Past-year prevalence of illicit drug use has fallen by 44% among 8th graders since the peak year of 1996. From 2006 to 2007, the percentage of 8th graders reporting lifetime use of any illicit drug declined from 20.9% to 19.0%. As of 2012, this percentage has continued to decline to 18.5%. Past-year prevalence fell 27% among 10th graders and 15% among 12th graders since the peak year of 1997. As of 2012, the past-year prevalence rates among 10th and 12th graders have remained relatively steady since 2009, with rates of 36.8% and 49.1%, respectively (NIDA, 2012).

Marijuana is still the most widely used illicit drug among the nation's youth, although its use continues to decline. Although there was evidence of some decline in alcohol use at the 8th, 10th, and 12th grade levels, 49.5% of all high school seniors reported being drunk at least once in the 30-day interval preceding the survey (NIDA, 2012).

Overall, the conclusions of the 1998 NIDA survey of illicit drug use among youth were promising. The study points out that behaviors change very slowly, and often only after there has been some reassessment by young people about the dangers of drugs and how acceptable they are in the peer group. Other effects include more attention being paid to drug issues by community groups, parents, government, and the media.

ENVIRONMENTAL CONNECTION

The Poor Man's Cocaine: Methamphetamine as a Public Health Threat

The Drug

Methamphetamine (in all of its forms—powder, crystal, or pills) is a powerfully addictive stimulant that affects the central nervous system. It is easy to make using inexpensive materials such as pseudoephedrine, paint thinner, kerosene, battery acid, brake cleaner, and lye. The final product may or may not be a "pure" methamphetamine (meth). Because of its stimulant effects, other drugs such as cocaine, marijuana, heroin, and alcohol are often used to bring the person down from the stimulant effects.

The User

Methamphetamine (meth) use has increased to approximately 1.2 million users (SAMHSA, 2012), and that rate continues to rise. Notable populations in which methamphetamine use is growing include white- and blue-collar workers, prostitutes, long-haul truckers, and runaway youth.

Methamphetamine users can be identified by signs such as agitation, rapid speech, decreased appetite, and insomnia. Physical manifestations include dilated pupils, elevated blood pressure, irregular pulse, chest pain, shortness of breath, and elevated temperature. Users may exhibit sudden episodes of violent behavior, intense paranoia, and hallucinations. Drug exposure doesn't readily wear off and is highly addictive from first use.

The Environment

Manufacturing of methamphetamine is not limited to urban areas. There has been a rapid increase in use of this drug in rural areas of the South, Southwest, and Midwest. Clandestine laboratories routinely dump waste materials into fields, streams, and sewage systems. Waste materials include ignitable, corrosive, and reactive toxic chemicals that present a high risk for explosions, fires, and toxic fumes. Toxic fumes make houses and buildings uninhabitable. Estimates for cleanup are approximately $2,000 to $4,000 per site. Meth labs produce materials that are toxic byproducts (lye, sulfur with acid, camping fuel, ether), and these toxins are dumped outside in rural areas where pets and wild animals—as well as children—may happen upon them.

Strict control of at least some of the ingredients used to "cook" meth has occurred at both national and state levels. Medications including the ingredient pseudoephedrine (which is found in over-the-counter allergy and cold medications) are now sold behind the counter, and limited in supply for individual purchase. In 2005, Congress passed the Combat Methamphetamine Epidemic Act, which states that purchasers of these products must present identification and can be tracked by signature.

Implications

Users of methamphetamine are at increased risk of engaging in behaviors that place them at greater risk for HIV/AIDS and sexually transmitted diseases. Research has also indicated that the use of methamphetamine slows the user's response time (21% slower than nonusers), a phenomenon that is especially evident in tasks requiring working memory, immediate storage of information, and mental calculations (National Institute on Drug Abuse & Drug Enforcement Administration, 2008).

Neglect of children is also an issue when methamphetamine enters SAMSHA, 2012 the picture. Authorities have found that 20% of meth labs had children present when the makers were manufacturing the drug. Children in households where meth is being manufactured are not only at risk of abuse and neglect, but also face risks from effects of toxic chemicals; as many as 55% of children removed from meth labs tested positive for such toxins (Messina, Marinelli-Casey, West, & Rawson, 2007).

Children are often present in meth labs while the drug is being cooked; thousands are being exposed to the highly addictive drug and its toxic byproducts. The drug's ingredients—acids, bases, metals, solvents, and salts—soak into fabrics and porous surfaces and produce toxic gases that find their way into ventilation systems. People, pets, and toys may all become contaminated in these "home meth labs." Following are some of the toxic substances often used in the preparation of methamphetamines:

- Acetone, acetic acid, vinegar
- Alcohol, isopropyl
- Ammonia, anhydrous, farm fertilizer
- Benzene, dye, varnish
- Ether, starter fluid
- Ethyl ether, computer dust-off
- Freon
- Hydrochloric acid/muriatic acid, iron ore processing, concrete cleaner
- Iodine crystals, antiseptic

(continues)

ENVIRONMENTAL CONNECTION (*continued*)

- Lithium metal, batteries
- Red phosphorus, match striker plates
- Sulfuric acid battery acid
- Toluene brake cleaner fluid
- Trichloroethane gun scrubber

Impact of Substance Abuse on Society

Alcohol is associated with over 100,000 preventable deaths each year, and that alcohol costs taxpayers over $185 billion annually. Healthcare costs related to smoking are estimated at $75 billion (Goodman, 2004). The annual financial losses to victims of alcohol-related violence (approximately 500,000 persons annually) total more than $400 million, while the average victim of such violence pays $1,500 out of pocket for related medical expenses (Goodman, 2004).

The National Highway Traffic Safety Administration (2007) reported that alcohol was involved in most traffic fatalities. The Drug Enforcement Administration (DEA) of the U.S. Department of Justice (2011) reported that alcohol abuse was a factor in 4 in 10 violent crimes and that approximately 4 in 10 criminal offenders reported using alcohol at the time they committed their offense. The National Justice Institute asserts that abuse of alcohol and other drugs by criminal offenders, parolees, and probationers contributes to 80% of crime in the United States. In incidents of spouse abuse, alcohol use by the offender was documented in 75% of reported cases.

RESEARCH ALERT

This research provides an overview on prescription drug abuse and highlights a number of related legislative and policy initiations in response to this growing epidemic. Prescription drug abuse has emerged as the nation's fastest growing drug problem. Deaths from prescription pain medicine in particular have reached epidemic proportions throughout the United States. This article underscores the importance of a multifaceted approach to combating prescription drug abuse and concludes with implications for nursing.

Source: Phillips, J. (2013). Prescription drug abuse: Problem, policies, and implications. *Nursing Outlook, 61*, 78–84.

Impact of Substance Abuse on the Individual

The effects of substance abuse on the individual are many and range from loss of a job and loss of relationships to major health problems. Substance abusers find themselves at greater risk for death as a result of auto accidents and violence (suicide and homicide), and numerous health problems. They are also more likely to develop chronic health problems such as central nervous system neuropathy, impaired cognition, cardiovascular disease, hypertension, and chronic gastrointestinal problems, including gastritis. Acute and chronic pancreatitis and liver disease are often associated with alcohol abuse. Nutritional deficiencies and anemia are often identified and are a result of not only poor dietary habits but more importantly the physiological changes that result from abuse of alcohol and other drugs.

Although low self-esteem is a common characteristic exhibited by the person who abuses substances, no personality factors or other behaviors have reliably differentiated substance abusers from other individuals. It would appear that low self-esteem appears to be more a result of the substance abuse rather than a causative factor (West & Kinney, 1996, p. 28). After reviewing psychological theories related to substance abuse, Goldsmith (1997, p. 6) concluded that the idea that there is an addictive personality is a myth. It appears that the depression, anxiety, and lack of self-esteem are as much a result of the substance use as they are causative factors. Zwickler (2004) indicates childhood sexual abuse increases the risk for drug dependence in adult women.

Participation in high-risk behaviors such as intravenous drug use and promiscuous sexual activity put the substance abuser at greater risk for acquiring sexually transmitted diseases. There are associated high rates of positive tests for HIV in high-risk groups, which include intravenous drug users, "sex workers" (i.e., prostitutes), and those who have multiple sex partners. Individuals who are using illicit drugs and need to find ways to pay for their drugs often turn to prostitution to help support their habit, placing them in this high-risk group.

ETHICAL CONNECTION

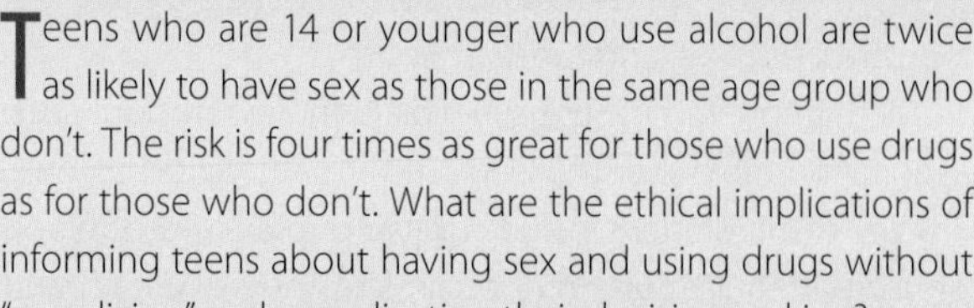

Teens who are 14 or younger who use alcohol are twice as likely to have sex as those in the same age group who don't. The risk is four times as great for those who use drugs as for those who don't. What are the ethical implications of informing teens about having sex and using drugs without "moralizing" and complicating their decision making?

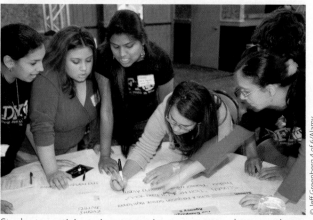

© Jeff Greenberg 4 of 6/Alamy

Students participate in a campaign to prevent substance abuse.

MEDIA MOMENT 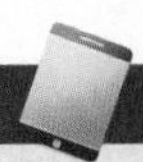

Breaking Bad (2008–2013)

High school chemistry teacher Walter White, diagnosed with terminal lung cancer, decides to secure his family's financial future before he dies by starting a methamphetamine lab. With a former student as his partner, he enters the dark, dangerous world of illicit drug dealing at the same time he is juggling family responsibilities and cancer treatment. Over the series' five seasons, Walter maintains a double life in the face of illness, conflict with local crime gangs, police investigations, and his family's suspicion.

Risk Factors for Substance Abuse

Society's Influence

Media Influences

Societal factors that influence the use and abuse of alcohol and other drugs are all around us. Television, social media, and movies present the use of alcohol and tobacco as glamorous, a rite of passage, something the sophisticated person does. The Research Alerts on the pages that follow highlight recent studies on the potential influence of the media on substance use in our society.

Advertisements tell us we need a break, we need to relax and unwind, and what better way than by having a drink, taking an antidepressant, or having a smoke? We live in a fast-paced world where people are encouraged not to feel. Ads remind us that if it hurts, take something; if you are stressed, have a drink, take a pill, smoke another cigarette.

Societal Attitudes

Attitudes toward legal and illegal substances, abuse of substances, and interventions and treatment for drug-addicted individuals vary according to society, community, ethnicity, social status, gender, and time. In other words, substance abuse is a socially constructed concept. Sometimes drug use is considered okay, and other times it is not okay. For example, the use of amphetamines or tranquilizers by a businessperson might be considered a matter of personal judgment, but the use of the same drugs by a young person who wishes to experience their effects produces much more emotion. Society's influence can again be seen when one looks at alcohol, which was actually prohibited in the United States through a constitutional amendment—the Eighteenth Amendment, passed by the U.S. Congress in 1920. After 13 years of unsuccessful efforts to enforce the law, Prohibition was repealed. Currently, tobacco use is increasingly being viewed as deviant, and those individuals and groups who use tobacco are experiencing stigmatization and subsequent discrimination.

RESEARCH ALERT

Portrayal of Substance Use in the Media

This study examined the frequency and nature of substance use in the most popular movie rentals and songs of 1996 and 1997. The intent was to determine the accuracy of public perceptions about extensive substance use in media popular among youth. Because teenagers are major consumers of movies and music, there is concern about the potential for media depictions of tobacco, alcohol, and illicit drugs to encourage use.

The study examined the 200 most popular movie rentals and 1,000 of the most popular songs from 1996 and 1997. Substances included in the study were illicit drugs, alcohol, tobacco, and over-the-counter and prescription medicines. The researchers examined what was used, by whom, how often, under what circumstances, and with what consequences.

Findings revealed that 98% of the movies studied depicted illicit drugs, alcohol, tobacco, or over-the-counter and prescription medicines. Fewer than half (49%) of the movies portrayed short-term consequences of substance use, and only 12% depicted long-term consequences.

The major finding from the song analysis was the dramatic difference among music categories (country, alternative rock, hot 100, rap, and heavy metal), with substance references being most common in rap. Illicit drugs were mentioned in 63% of rap songs versus about 10% of the lyrics in all other categories.

Source: Kelly, K., & Donohew, L. (1999). Media and primary socialization theory. *Substance Use and Misuse, 34*(7), 1033–1045.

DAY IN THE LIFE

Alcoholism and other drug addictions are equal-opportunity diseases—women and men, young and old, all walks of life are affected. Addiction is a complex disease of mind, body, and soul.

The chronic nature of alcoholism and other drug addiction is often what gets in the way of understanding and awareness. There continue to be many myths about this illness and much stigma attached to alcoholics and addicts.

The Betty Ford Center, in addition to having over 38,000 women, men, and their families participate in our treatment programs, offers unique training opportunities. Licensed professionals and students take part in the Professional in Residence Program, which is an experiential, hands-on program.

(continues)

DAY IN THE LIFE (*continued*)

Nurses, in particular, who are often on the frontline of intervention and treatment, have been eager participants in this training experience.

There is no question that our national drug policy is failing. I believe that is because the majority of emphasis continues on interdiction rather than treatment and prevention. This failure has even led to calls of legalization. Legalization would be an invitation to young people to use drugs. This would be a disaster. We need to change the emphasis of our national programs.

—Betty Ford, founder of the Betty Ford Center

Source: Betty Ford, personal communication, October 25, 1999.

Substance Abuse as a Criminal Activity or as a Disease

Alcoholism in American culture has been defined as a chronic disease manifested by repeated drinking causing injury to the drinker's health and/or social or economic functioning. Alcohol for individuals 21 years of age and older is legal in the United States. Alcoholism is being defined as a chronic disease, which has shifted alcohol-related problems from the category of sin or crime to the category of sickness. Nevertheless, many in our society tend to stereotype the alcoholic as a skid row derelict. Consequently, many persons who regularly drink to excess do not seek treatment because they do not see themselves as fitting that stereotype. Although excessive use of alcohol has been viewed as a disease, the excessive use of other psychoactive drugs in our society has not (Carroll, 2000).

Currently, there is some movement toward defining alcohol and drug addiction as meeting the criteria for a disability under the Americans with Disabilities Act (ADA). The medical community is taking leadership in this movement. The American Medical Association (AMA) and the American Society of Addiction Medicine (ASAM) are particularly concerned about managed care denials for individuals with drug addictions. Although it appears that our society is far from decriminalization of illicit drug use or the legalization of drugs, there is a growing concern about the prevention and treatment of drug addiction. The Research Alert that discusses current substance abuse treatment policy is based on the attitude that substance abuse is a criminal activity to deter rather than a disease to treat. The conversation with Betty Ford, former President Ford's wife, contributed especially for this nursing text, discusses addictions and the need for more emphasis on treatment of addictions as a disease.

Cultural Influences

Research has demonstrated that peer pressure, particularly for youth, is highly correlated with the use of illicit substances. If peer pressure to use substances is joined with other cultural influences, the risk of use becomes even stronger. For example, Goldsmith (1997) found that first use of alcohol and drugs often occurs in a social setting, suggesting that peer pressure and positive social/group attitudes about using substances, availability of the drugs, and pro-use norms in the community contribute to substance abuse.

Think about the many cultural influences for and against the use and potential abuse of drugs in the United States. Will the restriction of billboards promoting the glamour of cigarette smoking reduce the use of tobacco? Will smoking rates continue to decline as more and more public facilities restrict use? Are the current movement by the National Organization for the Reform of Marijuana Laws and the resurgence of the use of marijuana in Hollywood movies going to have an influence on the use of marijuana in our society?

MEDIA MOMENT 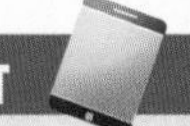

Miller, R. W., & Carroll, K. M. (2006). *Rethinking substance abuse: What the science shows and what we should do about it.* New York, NY: Guilford Press.

This book reviews what we know and do not know about substance abuse from biological, psychological, and social perspectives and the existing research outcomes regarding treatments for substance abuse. This edited text represents diverse neurobiological genetic and social-environmental perspectives and weighs in on possibilities for future effective treatments for substance abuse.

The Family's Influence

Although in modern society many of the socialization functions of the family have been taken over by other institutions such as schools, churches, or the media, the family remains a significant agent of socialization. Parents normally take care to monitor their offspring's behavior and pass on the language, values, norms, and beliefs of their culture. Research in the area of adolescent substance abuse has demonstrated that the family can have a positive effect in reducing the risk of initiation into alcohol, tobacco, and other drug use among children and youth (Goodman, 2004; Hahn, 1993; Hahn & Rado, 1996; Hahn, Simpson, & Kidd, 1996). For example, a young man who is raised in a family where all the male role models drink heavily will most often follow their lead. The opposite is also true—the person who is raised in a family or culture where there are strong prohibitions against drinking may be more inclined to experiment with alcohol at a later time, hopefully when he or she is more mature and will not end up abusing alcohol. Research continues to indicate that young people surveyed indicated parental disapproval of drug use was a very important factor influencing their decision to abstain from drug use (Bauman et al., 2001; Hawkins, Catalano, & Arthur, 2002; Kelly, Darke, & Ross, 2004; Kosterman, Hawkins, Haggerty, Spoth, & Redmond, 2001; Van Ryzin, Fosco, & Dishion, 2012).

The family can play a role in either maintaining a family member's escalation into substance abuse or the recovery from substance abuse. Non-substance-abusing family members initially experience emotions such as anger, fear, resentment, guilt, and shame when they first recognize that a spouse or child is a substance abuser. Because many people in our society view substance abuse as a character weakness, non-substance-abusing family members often share in the stigma (i.e., discrediting and discrimination) imposed on the substance abuser. Literature indicates spouses and parents most likely have inaccurate knowledge about the extent of their spouse's or child's substance abuse activities and therefore are inclined to show a great deal of tolerance of untoward behavior among family members, often taking a long time to acknowledge that a problem exists. In most cases, families attempt to cope with the abuser's problem; however, in some cases, the problem is dealt with by means of divorce or ejection of the adolescent (Barton, 1991; Kelly et al., 2004; Weinberg & Vogel, 1990).

A family history of alcoholism or addiction as well as biochemical and genetic factors also make certain family members more sensitive to the effects of substances. Research in this area, although not totally confirming, is becoming more definitive as to the correlation between familial alcoholism and offspring alcoholism (Hill, 1998). In addition, the problem of drug dependence during pregnancy is known to lead to babies who show withdrawal symptoms (Schneider et al., 1996) and the concern could be that these children will exhibit tendencies toward substance abuse in their youth and adult lives.

The Workplace's Influence

Current illicit drug use differed by employment status in 2012 (SAMHSA, 2012). Among adults aged 18 or older, the rate of current illicit drug use was higher for those who were unemployed (18.1 percent) than for those who were employed full time (8.9 percent), employed part time (12.5 percent), or "other" (6.3 percent) (which includes students, persons keeping house or caring for children full time, retired or disabled persons, or other persons not in the labor force. The percentage of adults employed full time who were current illicit drug users increased between 2011 (8 percent) and 2012 (8.9 percent).

Substance abuse in the workplace is a concern for both employers and consumers of products and services. This includes such things as the cost of intervention, treatment, and absenteeism, as well as reduced productivity. How substance abuse is viewed in the workplace is important. Does management send a message that drinking and using drugs in the workplace are unacceptable? Does management simply avoid confronting the issue of substance abuse with the stand that "We don't have anyone on our staff who does that"? Failure to acknowledge that substance abuse can be a problem in the work environment is itself a problem that can lead to further risk for employees.

Acknowledgment that substance abuse can be a problem for many workers, creation of health promotion and prevention programs, and policies related to treatment for workers will put all workers on alert that the demands of work require workers to deal with their substance abuse problem.

MEDIA MOMENT 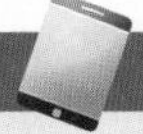

Maria Full of Grace (2004)

This movie is the conflicted and terrifying story of an atypical drug-running "mule." Maria Alvarez (Catalina Sandino Moreno) is a smart, independent 17-year-old girl from Colombia who agrees to smuggle a half-kilo of heroin into the United States for a shot at a normal existence in the magical land of "El Norte"—where she imagines the city streets must be paved with gold. It provides insight into the illegal drug trade and demand in the United States.

Personal Factors

Substance abuse affects people of all ages, socioeconomic groups, and occupations. **Box 22-4** lists populations vulnerable to substance abuse. Young people remain the most vulnerable to substance abuse, with the highest rate of illicit drug use occurring in those younger than 20 years of age, while only a small portion of illicit drug use occurs in the over-50 group. There appears to be little difference between whether the individual lives in an urban or rural setting.

According to a 2003 household survey (SAMHSA, 2004), the use of illicit drugs appears to be higher in young people who have dropped out of high school and is lowest in college graduates. Similarly, although 60% of individuals

BOX 22-4 Vulnerable Populations

- Children and adolescents
- High school dropouts
- People with dual diagnoses
- People with family history of alcoholism/addiction
- Unemployed individuals
- College students

BOX 22-5 Individual Risk Factors

- Family history of substance abuse
- Genetic/biochemical factors
- Prenatal exposure
- Psychiatric disorders

use alcohol, the group most likely to binge or fall into the heavy drinking category tends to be individuals between 18 and 35 years of age who have not completed high school. Alcohol use is also strongly associated with illicit drug use.

When looking at risk factors for alcoholism and addiction, it is essential to consider such things as the biochemical and genetic factors that make one individual more sensitive to the effects of drugs, prenatal exposure to drugs, and preexisting or coexisting psychiatric disorders. **Box 22-5** provides a list of individual risk factors nurses should be alert to during any assessment.

Research has indicated that there is no one clear-cut cause for substance abuse disorders. It has been found that for many people, a family history of alcoholism or addiction is a red flag indicating that the risk of becoming addicted or dependent on alcohol and/or other drugs is greater. It would stand to reason, then, that babies who were born addicted because of maternal drug abuse will be at a higher risk for developing substance abuse problems should they experiment with alcohol or other drugs when they are older.

The existence of preexisting or coexisting psychiatric disorders may also contribute to substance abuse. Anthenelli (1997) found evidence that persons with both a psychiatric diagnosis and a substance abuse problem are not uncommon. Persons with antisocial personality disorders, schizophrenia, and bipolar disorders are at greater risk for developing a substance abuse disorder. Goldsmith (1997) emphasized that "alcohol exaggerates both mood disorders and anxiety and that alcohol and drugs cause organic mood and organic anxiety disorders" (p. 6).

In an age when families are often scattered and talking with a neighbor appears to be a lost art, the sharing and receiving of emotional support is difficult for many people in our society. The image of rugged individualism, self-reliance, and high achievement often discourages people from allowing others to see their vulnerability and leads them to seek other ways of dealing with emotional pain. For some individuals, using alcohol or other drugs becomes their way of coping with their emotional pain. What results is a vicious cycle in which the person experiences emotional pain, uses alcohol or drugs to relieve that pain, experiences emotional pain related to consequences of substance abuse, and turns back to the substance to dull the emotional pain.

ETHICAL CONNECTION 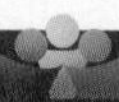

E-cigarettes

Will e-cigarettes cause more or fewer people to smoke? The answer matters. Cigarette smoking is still the single largest cause of preventable death in the United States, killing about 480,000 people a year.

GLOBAL CONNECTION 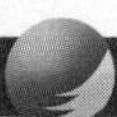

Opium production in Afghanistan rose 60% in 2006, after the U.S. invasion of Iraq. According to the United Nations, 6,100 tons of opium is enough to make 610 tons of heroin. The supply of heroin is outstripping heroin users' demands by one-third.

Nursing Assessment

Nurses' Attitude Self-Assessment

For community health nurses to work effectively with substance abusers, it is important that they develop an awareness of their own issues and attitudes about substance abuse. The nurse's attitudes regarding use of legal and illicit drugs, about those people who use or abuse drugs, and past experiences with substance abuse/abusers need to be assessed.

One of the first areas of self-awareness that needs to be addressed is what feeling the nurse has about the use of alcohol, tobacco, and recreational drugs. Questions to ask oneself include the following:

- What do I believe about the use of alcohol, tobacco, and recreational drugs? Is it morally wrong?
- Is it okay to use alcohol and tobacco but not marijuana or other recreational drugs? Marijuana but not any other illegal drugs?
- Is the use of any mind-altering substance up to the individual's freedom of choice?

The second area that one needs to examine is one's attitude about the substance abuser:

- How do I feel about the person who uses and abuses alcohol, tobacco, or other drugs?
- Is that person just weak-willed, immoral, or undisciplined, or ill and in need of treatment?
- Is the answer to the substance abuse problem punishment and incarceration?

Third, the community health nurse must look carefully at how past experiences with substance abuse/abusers may have influenced attitudes toward those individuals who abuse substances. Nurses should ask themselves the following questions:

- Have I known someone who abused alcohol or other drugs? How did their substance abuse affect me and my relationship with them?
- Was I raised in an alcoholic or addicted family? What did this mean to me? Have I received any assistance in dealing with my own issues?
- Have I ever lost someone who was important to me as a result of substance use?
- Have I ever been physically, sexually, or emotionally abused by someone who was abusing alcohol or other drugs?

For some people, asking and answering these questions may bring up uncomfortable, painful feelings. If this occurs, it is important that available resources be used to work through those feelings. For those individuals who have never shared their experiences, working with substance abusers may be difficult unless those unresolved issues are addressed. Failure to do so may result in the nurse's unconsciously avoiding interactions, being judgmental, and failing to be therapeutic when working with this population.

Drug History

One of the nurse's critical tasks when substance abuse is suspected is to conduct a drug history, taking note of the drugs of choice, the route of administration, the amount used, the frequency of use, and polysubstance use. **Box 22-6** summarizes key elements to address in a drug history. Information regarding the initiation of drug use, including the age and drugs first used, is important. Drug histories may need to be repeated to get a more accurate picture of what drugs have been used and how often. The substance abuser may give inaccurate information initially for a number of reasons: confusion because of drugs, fear, lack of trust, and uncertainty regarding what drugs were taken. The latter is often a problem with street drugs because the purity of these substances is often questionable.

BOX 22-6 Key Elements in a Drug History

- Which drug/drugs have been taken? In what combination?
- Which route was used to administer the drug (e.g., injection, intravenous, oral, sniffed, smoked)?
- How much of the drug was taken?
- What is the frequency of drug use?
- When was the drug last taken?
- At what age did drug use begin?

Recognizing the Signs of Substance Abuse

To address substance abuse issues, it is essential that the nurse recognize that abuse of drugs is multifaceted, with a variety of substances being used either singularly or in combination (see Box 22-1 for a list of major classes of abused drugs). The community health nurse needs to be aware of those major drug groups that are subject to abuse. In addition, for community health nurses, knowledge regarding the signs of substance abuse is essential if they are to recognize such abuse early so that intervention can be planned. Efforts must be made to detect the problem as soon as possible. Common signs indicative that an individual may be abusing one or more substances are found in **Boxes 22-7** and **22-8**.

Interventions

Society's Response

Society today is increasingly responding to the problems associated with substance abuse in a two-pronged approach: politically and as a healthcare issue. In the past, the political response to substance abuse was focused on punishment for the use or supplying of illicit drugs. Indeed, the acquisition and sale of illicit drugs continue to be the focus, with emphasis on law enforcement and punishment. Prevention is key and the need for a "balanced" program that addresses not only the **supply** (i.e., support to developing countries to put an end to their drug market) and **interdiction** (i.e., to stop drug trafficking at U.S. borders) issues, but also prevention, education, and treatment. The strategies recognize substance abuse problems as being international and long term, and as such they must be addressed with realistic programs that support families, schools, and communities and that include the international aspects of drug control.

BOX 22-7 Indicators of Possible Substance Abuse: Common Signs Across Categories

- Changes in attendance patterns (school or work)
- Change in mood or attitude (e.g., self-discipline, work habits, efficiency)
- Poor physical appearance
- Association with known substance abusers
- Heightened secrecy
- Borrowing of money

Source: Adapted from Carroll, C. (2000). *Drugs in modern society* (5th ed.). Dubuque, IA: Brown & Benchmark.

BOX 22-8 Specific Indicators of Possible Substance Abuse Across Categories of Psychoactive Drugs

Narcotics
- Lethargic, drowsy behavior
- Restlessness
- Constricted pupils and red, watery eyes
- Loss of normal appetite
- Equipment such as syringes and bent spoons as well as "track" marks on arms, hands, or legs

Depressants
- Behavior similar to alcohol intoxication
- Headaches, irritability, and anxiety
- Confusion and memory impairment
- Insomnia
- Impaired motor skills
- Faulty judgment, moody

Stimulants
- Extended wakefulness, irritability, hostility
- Dilated pupils
- Flushed skin, palpitations, increased sweating
- Chronic runny nose

Marijuana
- Intoxicated-type behavior
- Dulling of attention, lethargy
- Distorted sense of time and distance
- Seeds and shreds of plant material in pockets

Psychedelic (Hallucinogens)
- Difficulty in communicating
- Profound changes in thinking patterns or mood
- Trancelike states or fearful behavior
- Nausea, chills, flushing, and sweating

Phencyclidine (PCP)
- Amnesia
- Noncommunicative with blank, staring eyes
- Increased insensitivity to pain
- Profound changes in thinking and mood

Source: Adapted from Carroll, C. (2000). *Drugs in modern society* (5th ed.). Dubuque, IA: Brown & Benchmark.

These strategies do recognize that persons who are addicted need assistance. They hold individuals accountable for their negative behaviors but offer treatment that can help change those self-defeating destructive behaviors.

Healthy People 2020 has recognized the seriousness of substance abuse and has identified 21 objectives related to alcohol and other drugs and 20 specifically focused on tobacco. Much of the emphasis in the objectives is placed on youth and decreasing the use and abuse of alcohol, tobacco, and other drugs within this group. One of the biggest needs identified in *Healthy People 2020* is access to culturally, linguistically, and age-appropriate service, education, and research necessary to meet the objectives. In addition, it is recognized that ongoing research must be undertaken to identify changes, evaluate the effectiveness of interventions and programs, and determine where further emphasis is needed. See the *Healthy People 2020* feature for selected objectives.

MEDIA MOMENT

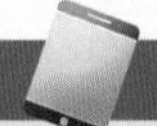

Days of Wine and Roses (1962)

While this film is dated, it provides an outstanding portrayal of alcoholism and its consequences for a married couple, both of whom are trying to outdrink the other.

Becoming familiar with the indicators of potential substance abuse is important for nurses, particularly those who work in primary care or community settings because it is at these nonstigmatizing medical settings (as opposed to drug abuse treatment centers) that the substance abuser may first make contact with healthcare professionals.

The assessment process, however, is not always straightforward. The early stages can be difficult to recognize. The psychological, social, and physical manifestations vary widely, depending on the particular substance or substances used, the amount used or the frequency of use, and factors such as age and the physical health of the user (Grant & Hodgson, 1991).

Primary Prevention

Primary prevention involves the *prevention* of diseases or conditions through protective factors as well as through health-*promotion* activities. In the case of substance abuse, the first level of intervention pertains to activities that are begun before drug abuse occurs. Typical primary prevention techniques include education for responsible decision making, knowledge of risk factors, legislation and law enforcement, interdiction activities, and programs to strengthen resistance to substance abuse (Carroll, 2000).

HEALTHY PEOPLE 2020 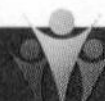

Objectives Related to Substance Abuse and Tobacco Use

Substance Abuse

- SA-1 Reduce the proportion of adolescents who report that they rode, during the previous 30 days, with a driver who had been drinking alcohol
- SA-2 Increase the proportion of adolescents never using substances
- SA-3 Increase the proportion of adolescents who disapprove of substance abuse
- SA-4 Increase the proportion of adolescents who perceive great risk associated with substance abuse
- SA-5 (Developmental) Increase the number of drug, driving while impaired (DWI), and other specialty courts in the United States
- SA-6 Increase the number of states with mandatory ignition interlock laws for first and repeat impaired driving offenders in the United States

Screening and Treatment

- SA-7 Increase the number of admissions to substance abuse treatment for injection drug use
- SA-8 Increase the proportion of persons who need alcohol and/or illicit drug treatment and received specialty treatment for abuse or dependence in the past year
- SA-9 (Developmental) Increase the proportion of persons who are referred for follow-up care for alcohol problems, drug problems after diagnosis, or treatment for one of these conditions in a hospital emergency department (ED)
- SA-10 Increase the number of Level I and Level II trauma centers and primary care settings that implement evidence-based alcohol screening and brief intervention (SBI)

Epidemiology and Surveillance

- SA-11 Reduce cirrhosis deaths
- SA-12 Reduce drug-induced deaths
- SA-13 Reduce past-month use of illicit substances
- SA-14 Reduce the proportion of persons engaging in binge drinking of alcoholic beverages
- SA-15 Reduce the proportion of adults who drank excessively in the previous 30 days
- SA-16 Reduce average annual alcohol consumption
- SA-17 Decrease the rate of alcohol-impaired driving (.08+ blood alcohol content [BAC]) fatalities
- SA-18 Reduce steroid use among adolescents
- SA-19 Reduce the past-year nonmedical use of prescription drugs
- SA-20 Reduce the number of deaths attributable to alcohol
- SA-21 Reduce the proportion of adolescents who use inhalants

Tobacco Use

- TU-1 Reduce tobacco use by adults
- TU-2 Reduce tobacco use by adolescents
- TU-3 Reduce the initiation of tobacco use among children, adolescents, and young adults
- TU-4 Increase smoking cessation attempts by adult smokers
- TU-5 Increase recent smoking cessation success by adult smokers
- TU-6 Increase smoking cessation during pregnancy
- TU-7 Increase smoking cessation attempts by adolescent smokers

Health Systems Changes

- TU-8 Increase comprehensive Medicaid insurance coverage of evidence-based treatment for nicotine dependency in states and the District of Columbia
- TU-9 Increase tobacco screening in healthcare settings
- TU-10 Increase tobacco cessation counseling in healthcare settings
- TU-11 Reduce the proportion of nonsmokers exposed to secondhand smoke
- TU-12 Increase the proportion of persons covered by indoor worksite policies that prohibit smoking
- TU-13 Establish laws in states, District of Columbia, territories, and tribes on smoke-free indoor air that prohibit smoking in public places and worksites
- TU-14 Increase the proportion of smoke-free homes
- TU-15 Increase tobacco-free environments in schools, including all school facilities, property, vehicles, and school events
- TU-16 Eliminate state laws that preempt stronger local tobacco control laws
- TU-17 Increase the federal and state taxes on tobacco products
- TU-18 Reduce the proportion of adolescents and young adults in grades 6 through 12 who are exposed to tobacco marketing
- TU-19 Reduce the illegal sales rate to minors through enforcement of laws prohibiting the sale of tobacco products to minors
- TU-20 (Developmental) Increase the number of states and the District of Columbia, territories, and tribes with sustainable and comprehensive evidence-based tobacco control programs

Source: HHS. (2014). *Healthy People 2020: Substance Abuse Objectives.* Retrieved from http://www.healthypeople.gov/2020/topicsobjectives2020/objectiveslist.aspx?topicId=40

APPLICATION TO PRACTICE 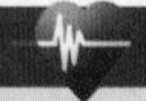

A nurse at a university health services clinic has noticed a high number of females from sororities coming into the clinic complaining of "hangover" symptoms during the rush season. She begins to compare the numbers with the year before and finds a 200% increase in the number of females who have presented with alcohol-related symptoms. The nurse would like to do a population assessment of the sororities at the university and plan educational programs and interventions related to responsible and safe alcohol use.

1. Who should the nurse contact first to begin the assessment process?
2. What kind of demographic information would the nurse need to know in the planning of appropriate interventions?
3. Are there other professionals and laypersons who need to be involved in educational interventions for this population group?
4. How should the sororities be involved with the assessment, planning, and intervention related to safe alcohol use?
5. What kinds of evaluation measures could the nurse use to determine intervention effectiveness?

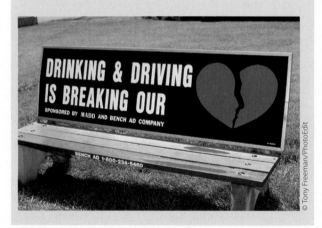

© Tony Freeman/PhotoEdit

One example of a primary prevention program conducted on a community level is the Kansas City comprehensive community program for drug abuse prevention with high- and low-risk adolescents. The program targeted early adolescent children within the community, because research has demonstrated that this is the first risk period for onset of drug use. The program targeted multiple agencies within the community—schools, parents, community leaders, and mass media. Drug use resistance skills training took place for adolescents in grades 6 or 7, parent–school organizations set agendas to review school prevention policies, and parents were trained in positive parent–child communication; community leaders were organized into a drug abuse prevention task force; and considerable media coverage was given to the program. Research on the outcomes of the program indicates that the community-based prevention program was effective in reducing cigarette smoking and marijuana use at the 9th- and 10th-grade levels (3 full years after delivery of the school-based program). The program did not demonstrate a significant reduction in the use of alcohol by 9th and 10th graders who had participated in the program. However, the program was equally effective with both high- and low-risk adolescents. Overall, the program suggests that social/behavioral approaches to prevention that are addressed to whole populations can be effective and that prevention effects can be enduring (Johnson et al., 1990).

Programs that involve students in the design of a prevention campaign have two advantages. First, students are mobilized to become involved in the prevention of substance abuse among peers; second, the messages in health educational materials will be relevant to the population. For example, at the University of Colorado at Boulder, students in journalism classes had a unique assignment: to create an ad campaign aimed at college students that emphasizes responsible drinking. Students in the class knew that their peers would not respond to fear tactics because college-age youth still have a tendency to think that nothing tragic will happen to them. The class decided it would be best to focus on social issues like sexually transmitted diseases and poor sexual performance. The students created six print and voice ads that appeared in newspapers, buses, and movie theaters as well as on a local radio station ("Drinking—get real," 1998).

ETHICAL CONNECTION 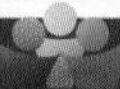

Campaigns featuring slogans such as "Drug-Free Zones" and "We are a drug-free school" have been common for the past several years in U.S. schools—and yet teens are more likely to abuse nonprescribed and over-the-counter drugs and marijuana than alcohol today. Recent research shows an alarming trend among teens involving the use of caffeinated "energy" drinks such as Volt mixed with cough syrup or other high-alcohol drinks. While alcohol use is down in general among teens, use of prescription drugs, marijuana, and methamphetamine is up. Are we sending the right message to teenagers that drugs—even those that preserve and save lives—are bad and wrong? What are alternatives to this approach?

Community health nurses can and will be more involved in participating in population-focused intervention such as the previously mentioned programs. In addition, preventing the initial use of illicit substances or intervening to prevent further escalation of illicit substance use by our nation's youth before they move into adulthood should be a goal for all community health nurses who work with youth and their families. This goal is especially true for school health nurses, public health nurses, and nurses working in community-based primary care settings. Efforts to prevent a public health problem before it begins or arresting it quickly in the early stages is far more effective than waiting until a substance abuse problem is firmly established. Remember, always include prevention strategies and keep substance abuse assessment criteria in mind whenever you are working with youth.

Secondary Prevention

Secondary prevention efforts are focused on the early stages of substance abuse. The goal of secondary prevention is *to detect and arrest substance abuse* before the individual becomes physically addicted and the problem becomes a chronic condition.

Efforts are made to detect the problem as soon as possible and to begin treatment so that the condition does not progress. Health professionals need training in substance abuse as a significant health problem. Nurses and other health professionals need knowledge of high-risk populations and indicators of possible substance abuse, skills in assessment for the problem, and knowledge of interventions at the individual, family, and community levels. The primary aims of the assessment are outlined in **Box 22-9**.

Box 22-9 Secondary Prevention: Primary Aims of Substance Abuse Assessment

- To meet the goal of secondary prevention with early detection and referral
- To obtain as much accurate information as possible about the individual's substance(s) use (frequency, amounts)
- To identify the factors associated with substance abuse, such as physical illnesses and social and psychological problems
- To identify the strengths and weaknesses of the individual and his or her family and ability to cope with and assist in the management of the problem

Source: Adapted from Grant, M., & Hodgson, R. (Eds.). (1991). *Responding to drug and alcohol problems in the community.* Geneva, Switzerland: World Health Organization.

After early detection and a beginning willingness on the part of the individual and his or her family to break the silence of denial, the next task involves getting the substance abuser into treatment to prevent physiological addiction. Perhaps the entire family is in a crisis state. The nurse would be involved, along with a healthcare team, in crisis intervention with the family. It is no longer wise or necessary to assume that the individual needs to "hit bottom" before he or she can be helped. Indeed, it is detrimental for the individual and the family to receive help only after the loss of physical and mental health, family and friends, employment, and self-respect. The substance-abusing individual needs to initiate treatment. Persuading the individual to do so at an early stage in substance abuse is difficult but can be accomplished. If possible, intervention is best implemented through a coalition of a healthcare team and family members of the substance abuser. Planning for an actual confrontation is often the best way to "shock" the individual into seeking treatment. Depending on the circumstances, the best time for confrontation is when the substance abuser's defenses are low—for example, shortly after the loss of a job, a drunk-driving arrest, a warning from a physician about a health problem, or the threat of a divorce (Carroll, 2000).

Tertiary Prevention

The third level of prevention, **tertiary prevention**, is initiated during later or advanced stages of substance abuse. Tertiary interventions include physical, mental, and social treatment procedures; detoxification; institutionalization; or outpatient drug-maintenance programs. You will find community health nurses working in all aspects of tertiary care. Many hospitals have drug treatment units. County mental health services sponsor detoxification centers where nurses are needed to do medical assessments, counseling, and referral. A major role for community health nurses in tertiary care is case or care management involving ongoing assessment and care coordination among the various services a chronic substance abuser may need in order to slowly move toward a potential recovery.

THINK ABOUT THIS 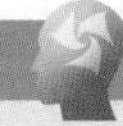

Caffeine is the most used drug in the world, followed by alcohol. Cigarette smoking and misuse of over-the-counter and prescribed drugs are common drug abuse issues. As a society, why do we focus on illegal drug use more than on the most commonly abused drugs? How do the media affect our ideas concerning drug use and abuse? What are your own opinions about drug use, misuse, and abuse?

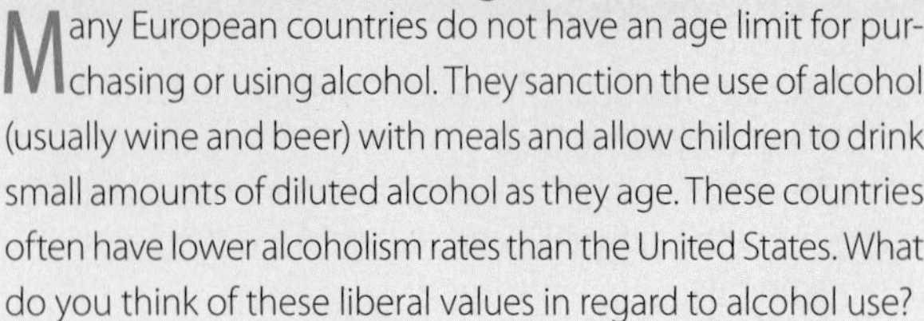

CULTURAL CONNECTION

Many European countries do not have an age limit for purchasing or using alcohol. They sanction the use of alcohol (usually wine and beer) with meals and allow children to drink small amounts of diluted alcohol as they age. These countries often have lower alcoholism rates than the United States. What do you think of these liberal values in regard to alcohol use?

BOX 22-10 Tertiary Prevention: Partial Listing of Substance Abuse Treatment Options

Drug-Free Treatments

- Therapeutic community
- Self-help groups such as Alcoholics Anonymous and Narcotics Anonymous
- Psychotherapy, including cognitive, behavioral, supportive-expressive, and family therapy
- Behavioral therapy specifically aimed at prevention of relapse

Drug-Based Treatments

- Methadone maintenance for heroin addicts
- Naltrexone (nonaddicting narcotic antagonist, also used in treating alcoholism)
- Antabuse (blocks alcohol metabolism)
- Mifepristone (reduces severity of cognitive deficiencies associated with chronic alcohol withdrawal)
- Psychoactive medication when indicated
- Heroin clinics for chronic addicts (primarily in Europe)

Source: Carroll, C. (2000). *Drugs in modern society* (5th ed.). Dubuque, IA: Brown & Benchmark.

The primary goal of tertiary prevention is *to prevent reactivation* of substance-abusing behaviors (Carroll, 2000). Many health authorities now view dependence on alcohol or other drugs as a chronic, relapsing disease. As such, drug dependence is often marked by a return of the substance abuse problem. Some professionals believe that it is more reasonable to think in terms of remissions (a lessening or reduction of the problem and its associated symptoms) rather than a cure (NIDA, 1998). **Box 22-10** is a partial listing of potential tertiary treatment programs.

Although treatment is the focus of tertiary prevention, it is essential that common barriers to treatment be removed or reduced. Emotional support must be available. This is a primary intervention area for community health nurses because all nurses receive education and experience in interpersonal interaction with caring as a philosophical base. Financial support must be ensured through social policies that promote workplace drug assistance programs or through job counseling, job training, and a return to employment. Child care may also be an important treatment enhancer.

Interventions with Special Populations

Children and Adolescents

Youthful deaths and substance abuse Three-quarters of all deaths among school-age youth and young adults in the United States result from four causes: auto accidents, other unintentional injuries, homicide, and suicide. Research has also shown that Native Americans, African Americans, males, and those youths with the least education and income are at greater risk of both overall and injury-specific youth mortality (SAMHSA, 2012). Furthermore, many of these unintentional injury deaths are associated with substance abuse (Mezzich et al., 1997; National Highway Traffic Safety Administration, 2007). It is particularly disturbing that U.S. suicide rates are highest among persons 15 to 24 years of age and in those older than 65 years of age. The association between suicide and the abuse of alcohol and other drugs is also a significant problem as highlighted in data gathered from the Drug Abuse Warning Network (DAWN), a large-scale drug abuse data collection system sponsored by NIDA. DAWN records substances linked with emergency department admissions in various metropolitan areas of the United States. According to the DAWN report on annual trends in total drug-related episodes in emergency departments (SAMHSA, 2012), the most commonly reported motive for taking a substance was suicide.

Specific prevention programs for children and adolescents The type of substance abuse prevention program most often used in schools has been either the presentation of factual information about the dangers of substance use (fear-arousal) or "affective" education to enhance self-esteem, responsible decision making, and social development. One program that is very popular in school districts and communities is the Drug Abuse Resistance Education (DARE) program. The DARE curriculum is organized into classroom sessions conducted by a police officer, coupled with activities taught by the regular classroom teacher. DARE combines the fear-arousal approach with the affective educational approached just described.

MEDIA MOMENT

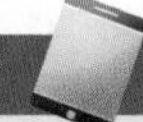

28 Days (2000)

Sandra Bullock stars in this movie about a 28-day rehab center and a patient's struggles to stay sober.

Despite the long tradition of these two approaches to prevention of substance abuse among youth, it is abundantly clear from scientific research that these approaches have only a short-term effect (Botvin & Botvin, 1992; Resnicow & Botvin, 1993). Why do these approaches fail to prevent substance abuse among youth? First, they fail to address the psychosocial factors promoting substance use, particularly peer pressure. Second, although the affective programs attempt to reduce the intrapsychic motivations to engage in substance use, the methods used are inadequate in that they do not place enough emphasis on skills training using behavior-change techniques (Botvin & Botvin, 1992).

Literature in the area of substance abuse prevention is abundant. However, there is a consensus in the literature that substance use prevention must begin early and that drug use resistance programs (in particular programs that use peer influences) are far superior to programs that focus on information and general affective programs involving self-esteem enhancement and problem-solving skills (Bukoski, 1997; National Highway Traffic Safety Administration, 2007).

Families

Many of the studies on families and illicit substance use by youths within the family are based on **social modeling theory**. Using this perspective, Fleming, Brewer, Gainey, Haggerty, and Catalano (1997) examined the relationship among parental drug use, bonding to parents, and child substance use. The families in this study were headed by substance abusers in methadone treatment for opiate addiction. The results of this study support the social development model and suggest that family interventions for preventing substance use in children of substance abusers should focus on reducing parental drug use and promoting bonding to parents who are abstinent.

Social control through parental involvement with youth is a second area of research that has been conducted on families as a risk factor in substance abuse in youth. In a study of male narcotic addicts, Nurco and Lerner (1996) found that an intact family structure and parental disapproval of misbehavior by subjects were identified as significant deterrents to later addiction. Aseltine (1995) studied the reciprocal associations of family and peer relations and adolescent drug use over time. In this study, parental social control (e.g., being alert, having rules) was found to be stronger at the initiation stages of drug use but weaker than peers at maintenance. Parents may also indirectly help in the prevention of adolescent drug use by acting as friendship "gatekeepers," thereby preventing youths from associating with other youths who are using drugs.

RESEARCH ALERT

In an analysis of family structure and substance abuse risk, the Center on Addiction and Substance Abuse found that children living in two-parent families who have a fair or poor relationship with their father are at 68% higher risk of smoking, drinking, and using drugs compared with all teens living in two-parent households. The average teen living in a household headed by a single mother is at 30% higher risk compared with all teens in two-parent households. The results of this survey emphasized that "parent power" is the key to preventing drug use by children and youth.

Source: Center on Addiction and Substance Abuse. (1999). *CASA survey: Many dads AWOL in the battle against teen substance abuse.* Retrieved from http://www.casacolumbia.org

A third area of research on family and risk factors for substance abuse is the influence of family functioning and drug use. Researchers at Arizona State University followed 179 adolescents, ages 11 to 15, over a 3-year measurement period. All youth entered into the study as nonusers of illicit drugs. Over the 3-year measurement period, 88 initial abstainers began to use substances. Results showed that older adolescents and adolescents from disorganized home environments were more likely to initiate substance use than younger adolescents and those from homes high in family organization that exhibited good communication and good problem solving (Hussong & Chassin, 1996). The Research Alert summarizing a study from the Center on Addiction and Substance Abuse highlights the importance of having fathers involved in family functioning.

Family-focused interventions The family has been viewed as a target of nursing care since the time of Florence Nightingale. The practice of nursing in the United States began in family homes. There has been a return to the importance of family nursing in the 21st century as health-care finance reform is moving health care back into community settings. How do nurses intervene with families in which one or more members of the family has a substance abuse problem? Craft and Willadsen's (1992) investigation into nursing interventions related to family provides a taxonomy of general nursing interventions that are appropriate to use with substance-abusing families. **Table 22-1** provides a list of generalized family-focused interventions to use when caring for a family in which one or more members has a substance abuse problem. It is important to note that these interventions fall within the practice domain of nursing. Often, nurses feel that they do not have the practice skills to deal with a family in which one or more members have a substance abuse problem. Nurses do have skills

TABLE 22-1 Family Nursing Interventions and Their Defining Activities

Nursing Intervention	Defining Activities
Family support	Promotion of family interest and goals
Family process maintenance	Minimization of disruption in family environment
Family integrity promotion	Promotion of family cohesion and unity
Family involvement	Promoting all family members in problem solving their situation of having one or more family members with a substance abuse problem
Family mobilization	Utilization of family strengths to influence substance-abusing member(s) in positive direction
Caregiver support	Provision of necessary information, advocacy, and emotional support
Family therapy	Interaction with the family as a change agent to move family toward a more productive way of living
Sibling support	Helping family understand the need to provide support (and attention) to nonabusing sibling when another sibling is the substance-abusing family member
Parent education	Assistance to parents to understand effects of different substances and theories on causes of substance abuse

Source: Adapted from Craft, M. J., & Willadsen, J. A. (1992). Interventions related to family. *Nursing Clinics of North America, 27*(2), 517–531.

in family support, education, facilitation of problem solving, and so on, which should be and are effective nursing interventions to be used when a family needs nursing care for a substance abuse problem. (See **Box 22-11**.)

Schools

Although there has been a downward trend in adolescent substance use since 1996, schools are definitely a target for substance abuse prevention. Indeed, the critical period for initial experimentation with one or more drugs and the subsequent development of regular patterns of use typically spans the beginning to middle adolescent years (SAMHSA, 2012).

The movement known as **comprehensive school health** is a broad strategy for improving student health. This movement views education and health as highly integrated. The movement proposes that healthy children learn better and cautions that no curriculum can compensate for deficiencies in student health status (Kann et al., 1995). The goal of the movement is to improve student risk behaviors in the areas of alcohol and other drugs, unintentional injuries, tobacco, diet, physical activity, and sexual intercourse (Symons, Cinelli, James, & Groff, 1997). Despite growing support for the movement among parents, communities, and the federal government, local school leaders, who are under tremendous pressure to improve academic achievement, and other political stakeholders often remain unconvinced that improving student health represents a means to achieve improved academic outcomes. Instead, the current primary approach toward students with substance abuse behaviors is to discipline

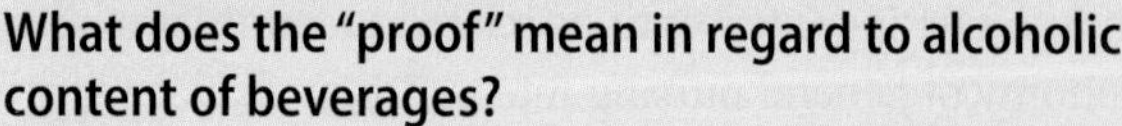

What does the "proof" mean in regard to alcoholic content of beverages?

Proof comes from the process of unloading cargo of whiskey when merchants had only one way to tell the strength of the liquor they were carrying. They mixed a spoonful of whiskey with a pinch of gunpowder. When a lighted match was dropped into the mixture, it ignited with an audible "proof." This would only happen if the alcohol mixture was 50% or more by volume. Today, proof is defined as twice the alcohol content by volume. Whiskey that is 100 proof is 50% alcohol.

BOX 22-11 HELP! What Do I Do When I Get the Call That My Daughter or Friend Has Been Arrested on Drug Charges?

1. Don't panic—stay calm.
2. Talk with the authorities and find out the charges and the details of what occurred.
3. Don't argue, challenge, or become defensive—it won't help.
4. Talk with an attorney about options. If you can't afford one, the court will appoint one.
5. If you need to get a bail bonds person, pick one carefully. Don't use the first one who approaches you. Ask others to recommend an honest, reliable bail bonds person.
6. Take a friend with you to the hearings so you have moral support.
7. Don't attempt to talk with the person being charged until you have permission from the authorities/court.
8. Don't panic—stay calm.

the offenders—suspending or expelling students, thus putting the youth at more risk for academic failure and future life difficulties. Adults working with children need to teach them how to identify and express their feelings. They should provide a healthy adult–child relationship, especially with children of substance-abusing parents (SAMHSA, 2012).

Workplace

Substance abuse in the workplace is a concern for both employers and consumers of products and services. Failure to address substance abuse in the workplace affects not only the person abusing substances, but also coworkers. It has been found to be a frequent factor in workplace violence (SAMHSA, 2012). In communities without occupational health nurses, the community health nurse is sometimes called on to provide employers with assistance in the development of programs to address workplace substance abuse problems. In addition to the signs of substance abuse found in Boxes 22-7 and 22-8, signs specifically found in the workplace are listed in **Box 22-12**.

To deal effectively with substance-abusing employees, it is necessary to take some proactive measures. For this to occur, it is important to consider not only the needs of the company but also the legal issues, equal employment opportunity laws, the National Labor Relations Act, drug-free workforce rules and regulations, the ADA, Department of Transportation drug testing rules and regulations, and just-cause dismissal regulations (Naegle, 1993).

It is important to develop policies and processes for dealing with substance use and abuse in the workplace. Many times, nurses will be asked to participate in committees that develop these policies, particularly policies that are being developed by their own employers. These policies should be provided to new employees and periodically reviewed with all employees to ensure that they fully understand the policies and how the policies affect them. Any substance abuse policy needs to include a statement regarding drug testing. This statement needs to include when drug testing will be done (e.g., on employment, randomly). It should also include how the testing will take place, who will do it, how the security of the specimen will be maintained, who will pay for the testing, and how confidentiality of results will be handled.

BOX 22-12 Workplace Signs of Potential Substance Abuse

- Decreased productivity or work fall off
- Decreased quality of job performance
- Increased work-related injuries, accidents, or illness
- Increased absenteeism, especially just before or after days off (e.g., holidays or vacations)
- Increasingly longer breaks and meal times

For any drug policy to be effective, the employers, management personnel, and supervisory personnel should become familiar with what alcoholism, addiction, and substance abuse are; how to recognize them; and how to handle an employee experiencing such problems. Often, it is the community health nurse who is called on to assist in providing educational programs regarding substance abuse.

Many employers turn to community-based employee assistance programs (EAPs) to address the issue of substance-abusing employees. For EAPs to be effective, it is essential that any service, counseling, or intervention be kept separate from supervision of employees, with maintenance of confidentiality critical. The nurse working in a community-based EAP needs to be sure that policies and procedures regarding follow up with supervisors who refer employees for assistance are handled in such a way that the employee's confidentiality is maintained. Reviewing policies and procedures regularly and being sure that they are in compliance with governmental rules and regulations are essential, and the nurse will often be actively involved in this process.

Rural

Approximately one-quarter of all Americans and of the total elderly population live in rural areas. Farm foreclosures and the declining farm economy are stressors faced by those living in rural communities. In addition, rural communities are aging, with all of the health concerns associated with getting older.

Limited income, unemployment, and poverty are added stressors for rural families. Although illicit drug use does not appear to be as much of a problem in rural communities, high alcohol consumption and tobacco use, especially smokeless tobacco, are concerns. Attempts at establishing and carrying out prevention programs in rural communities are directly related to the rural nature of these communities. Key factors that the community health nurse needs to consider in planning for this population include the following: a shortage of healthcare providers, geographic distance, isolation, transportation, access, rural economy, a shrinking tax base, and issues of stigmatization (**Box 22-13**).

For substance abuse prevention programs to be effective in rural communities, they must be accessible and available at neutral sites such as schools, churches, and community centers. Prevention efforts need to target those groups at greatest risk. Smoking and the use of

BOX 22-13 Factors to Consider When Planning Rural Substance Abuse Intervention Programs

- Geographic distance
- Transportation
- Rural economy
- Shortage of healthcare providers
- Shrinking tax base
- Isolation
- Access
- Issues of stigmatization

smokeless tobacco are of particular concern in rural communities. Information about the health effects of smokeless tobacco should be made available and included in any drug prevention program. Potential users need to be made aware of not only the addictive nature of smokeless tobacco but also the long-term health effects. **Box 22-14** is a summary of the health effects of dipping and chewing smokeless tobacco, which is a particular problem in rural communities.

Because depression and alcohol abuse can be coexisting conditions in rural communities, programs that provide for self-esteem building, decreased negative self-talk, building of support networks, and identification of accessible resources are needed. The community health nurse is often the person who is called on to plan, develop, and sometimes conduct these programs. The nurse may also become involved in planning and implementing groups for rural women conducted through the church, planning and implementing men's groups at the volunteer fire department hall, or arranging support groups for all substance abuse prevention efforts.

Neighborhoods

The communities and neighborhoods where people live, work, play, and raise their families are important areas for addressing the problems associated with substance abuse. Interventions that are focused on the substances (drugs) are often aimed at eliminating the accessibility of drugs, limiting the sale of alcohol and tobacco, and providing education regarding the health effects of tobacco and drug use. Efforts to discourage and prevent substance abuse in neighborhoods have been found to be effective means of providing intervention to people where they live. See **Box 22-15** regarding community action for addressing youth.

BOX 22-14 Health Effects of Smokeless Tobacco

- Oral cancer
- Gum problems
- Loss of teeth
- Heart problems

For many individuals, the idea of using official agencies (e.g., hospitals, clinics, health departments, social welfare agencies) is unpleasant. Fear of authority and prior experiences that might have been embarrassing or upsetting often discourage the use of such agencies, making it difficult to accept intervention and treatment.

People prefer contacts with community health nurses in their own neighborhoods. Neighborhood programs that actively involve residents have been shown to be highly effective in drug prevention efforts. The community health nurse is often asked to assist in the development of such a program. The first step the nurse needs to take is to assess the neighborhood. Six questions need to be asked (Office of Substance Abuse Prevention, 2004):

1. Do convenience stores, liquor stores, and gas station minimarts in your neighborhood check identification of people purchasing alcohol and tobacco? Do they sell beer in six-packs, not singles?
2. Do bars and restaurants in the neighborhood refuse service to intoxicated patrons? Make sure intoxicated patrons get rides home? Promote nonalcoholic drinks during happy hours?
3. Do employers in your neighborhood have a policy on alcohol use? Do they require nonalcoholic beverages to be served at social events they sponsor? Do they refuse to pay for alcoholic drinks at business meals? Do they provide for transportation, if needed, after social events where alcohol is served?
4. Can you find health messages about alcohol and tobacco use on local radio and TV stations?

BOX 22-15 Community Action

Parents

- Talk with children
- Provide boundaries before problems occur
- Set family rules

Educators

- Address early aggressive behavior and poor conduct
- Provide support for the learner who is struggling

Community

- Assess community risks
- Plan for prevention services, early intervention, and family counseling

Source: NIDA. (2003). NIDA-funded research drives revision of guide to prevention programming. Retrieved from http://www.drugabuse.gov/NIDA_Notes/NNVol18N4/tearoff.html

5. Is there a communitywide policy that prevents alcohol- and drug-related problems at sporting events, rock concerts, and other large community gatherings?
6. Do local schools, universities, and sports centers accept advertising for alcoholic beverages or tobacco that is displayed at the sports arenas or in the program?

It is important that community health nurses not only assume a role in promoting neighborhood involvement, but also become actively involved themselves. The community health nurse can assist with as well as encourage others to take the following six steps:

1. Write letters to support legislation on alcohol and drug policy.
2. Join a coalition of organizations involved with alcohol and drug policy.
3. Organize educational programs about alcohol- and drug-related programs.
4. Work with the media on developing health messages regarding alcohol, tobacco, and drug use.
5. Work with community organizations to implement alcohol-safe policies for large community events.
6. Set up programs to monitor the granting of new alcohol licenses.

The community health nurse is seen as a leader and role model within the community. As a role model, it is important that residents see nurses taking proactive roles in drug prevention efforts. When issues related to substance abuse arise, nurses should take the lead in informing elected officials about the need to support legislation and programs for prevention and treatment. Write and call your political leaders, urging action. Ask others to also contact their elected officials. It is also important to activate supporters of prevention programs regarding legislation about substance abuse prevention, especially if there is a threat to such programs. Meet with elected officials and speak about your concerns. If necessary, mobilize the community to take action regarding substance abuse through letter writing, petitions, and other positive actions to make the neighborhood needs known.

Women

Walton-Moss and Becker (2000) reported that 45% of the women they surveyed used alcohol, 26% used tobacco, and 13% used drugs. Use of drugs (illicit or prescription) and alcohol by women is not a new phenomenon, but the response to women who are substance abusers is often different than it is for their male counterparts. In the 1980s, it was reported that women who were alcoholics were considered sicker, wives of alcoholics were considered enablers, and husbands of alcoholic wives were looked at with respect for putting up with their wives' problems (Sandelowski, 1981). Things are beginning to change, but some issues still need to be addressed when working with the problems associated with substance abuse in women. Women's drug use differs from men's in that they often use prescription drugs in combination, are less likely to have a stable relationship/marriage, and most often have children living with them. Zwickler (2004) reported a study from the Medical College of Virginia Commonwealth University in which there was a high incidence of childhood sexual abuse in women who are drug dependent. How these women view themselves is an important factor in addressing issues of their substance abuse. The Research Alert addresses the issue of pregnant women and substance abuse.

Most treatment programs use a model that was developed when the majority of persons receiving treatment were men. Women tend to be hesitant about entering treatment programs that use confrontation and mixed-sex groups. For substance-abusing women, who often have experienced abuse (physical and verbal) from men, verbalizing their vulnerability in a mixed group is difficult, if not impossible. Low self-esteem is an issue for this population. A second contributor was related to the effects of "violent

RESEARCH ALERT

In-depth interviews were conducted with 60 pregnant or postpartum women who were crack cocaine users to better understand the issues and problems these women face. Findings suggested fears about bearing a drug-dependent baby and/or concerns about losing custody were very real. Guilt, fear, and pressure to take action were common feelings. The women initially dealt with the threats to their self-esteem by delaying acknowledging the pregnancy and seeking care. However, once they did acknowledge the pregnancy, they attempted to make the best of the situation by decreasing drug use, trying to improve their diet, and trying to avoid conflict and worry. When healthcare providers were perceived as threatening custody of the child, they tried to avoid the healthcare system and "relied on their own self-care to optimize pregnancy outcomes" (p. 212).

For the community health nurse, it is essential that the nurse recognize the fears and concerns of the substance-abusing pregnant woman and provide avenues for entry into care that support the mother-to-be and foster trust and safety rather than fear and distrust.

Source: Kearney, M., Murphy, S., Irwin, K., & Rosenbaum, M. (1995). Salvaging self: A grounded theory of pregnancy on crack cocaine. *Nursing Research, 44*(4), 208–213.

THINK ABOUT THIS 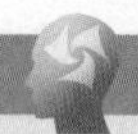

Florence Nightingale first published information about an association between health and music. Country music portrays human emotions in the rawest and most vivid of terms and has been described as a "three-minute soap opera." Watch the music video "Little Rock," performed by Collin Raye and written by Tom Douglas (1994), which depicts alcohol and family abuse and provides a visual resource for Al-Anon at the end of the video (http://youtu.be/eRv0jVZtdbY).

Think about the concepts that are explored in this song: abuse, child trauma, family dysfunction, violence, alcoholism, and recovery:

- Explore the issue of alcoholism, recovery, and relationships as depicted in this song and music video.
- How did you feel about the man's situation? Is he likely to maintain sobriety? Why or why not?
- How did you feel the child experienced the abuse?
- What role does religion play in this song?
- Is there a nurse's role in this scenario?

relationships and inability of the women to recognize this area as a contributor to their alcohol/drug abuse." Providing same-sex groups where the women feel safe and supported and are received in a nonjudgmental manner is helpful in facilitating the treatment process. The same-sex groups also provide the opportunity for women to openly discuss relationship issues. Williams (2004) found intervention with women is often more successful if they are first treated with one-on-one sessions before moving into group therapy.

Treatment issues related to the pregnant woman and to women with children need to be addressed. The highest incidence of substance abuse in pregnant women is found in women younger than 25 years of age, with a large percentage of these women being unmarried. A major problem is the lack of treatment programs geared to caring for women who are pregnant and using drugs or for women with children who are using drugs.

Community health nurses need to focus their attention on two areas when addressing the problems associated with substance abuse in women: education and advocacy. First, educating women about the effects of alcohol and drug use is essential, especially with young women who are of childbearing age. Knowledge about the effects of drug use on the unborn child is essential for young women to make informed decisions (Kinney, 1996). Second, it is essential that the community health nurse take an advocacy position and lobby for treatment programs that adequately provide for women with young children, addressing such issues as child care, treatment for the pregnant woman, and physical and sexual abuse. Community health nurses have an obligation to keep informed about which programs are most effective in treatment and prevention of substance abuse and its associated problems if they are to meet the needs of this special population. Williams (2004) indicated women prefer community-based programs that use a holistic approach that addresses women's multiple social roles and needs such as clothing, food, and daycare. These programs need to be convenient and "comfortable."

Elders

Substance abuse in the elderly population is often a hidden problem. It has been estimated that by the year 2030, the fastest growing segment of the population will be persons older than 85 years of age. Fewer than 50% of elders live in institutions, and at least half of older people have some health problems. According to the 2002 National Survey on Drug Use and Health, this group has the lowest rate of illicit drug use and the highest use of over-the-counter drugs. Prescription medication use is also a reality for 60% to 78% of the older population. One of the major concerns with this population results from the adverse effects of drug–drug and drug–alcohol interaction, leading to an increased risk for illness, injury, and death (**Table 22-2**).

Adams and Kinney (1996) suggest that even minimal alcohol use/abuse can be a problem for the older person. The problem in part is due to alcohol interaction with other prescription drugs, as well as the physiological changes that are associated with aging, such as impaired absorption and excretion of those substances (Meiner, 1997). For example, alcohol use by an older person who is taking a nonsteroidal anti-inflammatory agent increases the likelihood of gastrointestinal bleeding. Problems such as these are further complicated by the movement of former prescription medications into the over-the-counter category.

It is essential that the community health nurse recognize the potential for problems, because it is often the nurse who must sort out the elder's shoebox of prescription and over-the counter medications and make sense of what that individual is really taking. Therefore, it is important that the nurse recognize the possibility that alcohol use/abuse could be a complicating factor.

For the elderly population with multiple chronic health problems, additional factors that may contribute to alcohol and drug abuse are limited income, inadequate instructions regarding their medications and alcohol interaction, and poor follow up. Community health nurses must carefully assess the older person's medication regimen and determine how well it is being followed.

When attempting to determine whether there is a substance abuse problem, the family and friends of the elder

TABLE 22-2 Common Alcohol–Drug Interactions to Look for in the Elderly	
Drug Category	**Interaction/Effect**
Antibiotics	Nausea, vomiting, headache, possible seizures, reduced effectiveness of the medication
Anticoagulants	Acute alcohol consumption = increased risk of hemorrhage Chronic alcohol consumption = reduced blood thinning effect and potential for blood disorder
Antidepressants	Increased sedative effects, elevated blood pressure
Antidiabetic medications	Nausea, headache Acute alcohol consumption = prolonged effect Chronic alcohol consumption = decreased effect
Cardiovascular medications	Dizziness, fainting, reduced effectiveness of some antihypertensives

are often the first to identify the potential problem. Nelson (1998) reported that the elderly most at risk for a substance abuse problem are those who are "widowed, single, living in disadvantaged areas, blue-collar workers, and those with criminal records" (p. 28). Nelson also indicated that older women have the potential to develop drinking problems later in life as a result of such factors as outliving their spouses and having a higher poverty rate. Community health nurses, especially those who work with the elderly in their homes, need to be aware of the potential for a substance abuse problem and provide necessary referral should the problem be identified. An effective treatment program must take into consideration the health problems and necessary medications to treat those problems when planning care. When working with the elder who has a substance abuse problem, it is important for the community health nurse to recognize that this person is a survivor and to build on that strength when planning care. Any intervention planned by the community health nurse must include contact for the elder with other people and assistance in identifying ways to provide meaningful activity for the elder.

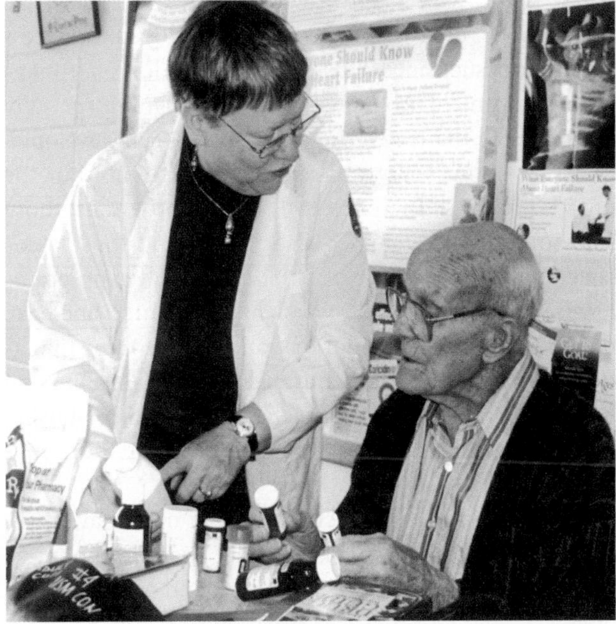

Chapter author Dr. Jean Haspeslagh assists an elder patient with understanding multiple drug interactions.

Primary prevention efforts should focus on teaching about age-specific dangers of alcohol use, particularly in relation to medications that are being taken. Presently, there are no safe guidelines for drinking for older adults. Prevention programs need to include content that reviews medications and their appropriate use, problems associated with mixing medications and alcohol, mixing prescription and over-the-counter medications, and proper disposal of medications (see **Box 22-16**). The Office of Substance Abuse Prevention suggests that programs encouraging responsible use of medications be implemented. It encourages having "dumping contests" (i.e., a contest for throwing away outdated and no longer used medications). We need to remember that prevention efforts are not just for the young and that our elderly also need our assistance if they are to avoid problems with substance misuse and abuse.

Nurses and Other Healthcare Professionals

Nurses and other healthcare professionals are another group at risk for substance abuse problems. Accuracy of reports of substance abuse in the general population of nurses and healthcare providers is difficult to determine, because denial is a key component of alcoholism and substance abuse, related to these issues, lessening the likelihood of accurate self-reporting in surveys. The American Nurses Association has estimated that approximately 6% to 8% of nurses have a substance abuse problem (Kinney,

BOX 22-16 Need to Knows for Elders

1. Some medications don't mix well with other medications, including over-the-counter (OTC) medications and herbal remedies.
2. Many medications do not mix well with alcohol.
3. Medications for sleep, pain, or depression make use of alcohol unsafe.
4. If there is no history of a drinking problem, one drink a day is the recommended limit (12 ounces of beer, 1.5 ounces of distilled spirits [hard liquor], or 5 ounces of wine).
5. Keep lists of all medications from all doctors. Include all regularly used OTC drugs and herbal remedies. Update as doses or medications change.
6. Have your doctor review all of your medications once a year.

Sources: Center for Substance Abuse Treatment (CSAT). (2001). *Aging, medicine and alcohol;* U.S. Department of Health and Human Services (HHS). (2004). *As you age: A guide to aging, medicines, and alcohol.* [Brochure]. Rockville, MD: Author.

NOTE THIS!

Bhutan became the first country in the world to ban the sale of tobacco.

1996). In addition, there is a high rate of smoking among nurses (see **Table 22-3**).

Because substance abuse in nurses affects not only the nurse but also those who receive health care and those who work with the nurse, it is important that community health nurses recognize the issues associated with nurses who abuse substances. Community health nurses will encounter substance-abusing nurses and other healthcare professionals in the community both as patients and as colleagues. Factors influencing how you may respond can be found in **Box 22-17**.

As with any chronic condition, recognition that the condition exists is the first step toward rehabilitation. Signs of substance abuse in nurses range from mood swings to blackouts. **Box 22-18** presents a list of indicators of substance abuse that may be noticed in a nurse's job performance. Deteriorating work performance is often one of the later signs of the problem. One recovering nurse reported that even at the peak of her active drug use, she continued to receive good performance evaluations from her supervisor. During that time, she was never confronted about her performance even though she was experiencing blackouts (periods when she was unable to recall what happened).

A number of programs have been developed to address the needs of substance-abusing nurses. In addition to community treatment programs and EAPs, programs specially designed for the recovering nurse have been developed to assist the nurse toward recovery and to monitor the nurse's progress. There are two types of programs: those sponsored by state nurses associations and those associated with state boards of nursing. The latter programs have legal power, provide oversight to the nurse, and have power to grant permission to work with certain stipulations (requirements) that must be met to retain a nursing license. Such programs ensure that the substance-abusing nurse is meeting those requirements placed on the license to practice.

Nurses returning to active nursing must have a **return to work contract.** This contract protects the nurse and the agency employing the nurse, and ultimately the

TABLE 22-3 Profile of Registered Nurses Who Smoke

15% of RNs smoke.	
10–14% of nursing students smoke.	
By specialty:	
Mental health/psychiatry	23%
Gerontology	18%
Emergency room	18%
Pediatrics	8%
Oncology	7%

Source: Data from http://www.tobaccofreenurses.org

BOX 22-17 Factors Influencing Responses to Substance-Abusing Nurses

- Prior experience with someone else who is a substance abuser
- Holding a view that a nurse is a "superhuman being" who should be able to avoid such behavior
- Holding a strong moralistic view of substance abuse as being morally wrong
- Feeling anger at anyone who would "steal" medication from patients
- Feeling fear and anxiety that this could easily happen to themselves

BOX 22-18 Indicators of Possible Substance Abuse in Nurses

Any Substance

- Frequent medication errors
- Poor documentation—illogical, sloppy, illegible
- Patient complaints
- Withdrawal, isolation—removing self from professional committees and organizations
- Signs out more controlled substances than others
- Volunteers to work extra hours or assignments that provide access to drugs

Narcotics

- Incorrect counts of controlled substances
- Large amounts of drugs wasted
- Significant variation in quantity of drugs required on the unit when that nurse is working
- Discrepancies between patient's and nurse's reports of pain
- Patient reports of ineffective pain medication only when suspected nurse gives the medication
- Patient complaints of pain or restlessness only when the suspected nurse is working

Sources: Crosby, L., & Bissell, L. (1989). *To care enough.* Minneapolis, MN: Johnson Institute; Haspeslagh, J. (1990). Recovering nurses' perceptions of job re-entry. Unpublished Ph.D. dissertation. Louisiana State University Medical Center, New Orleans; Sullivan, E., Bissell, L., & Williams, E. (1988). *Chemical dependency in nursing.* Menlo Park, CA: Addison-Wesley.

patients. This contract should include the stipulations for returning to work, the length of time for the stipulations, frequency of random drug screens, restrictions on license, required group and individual counseling sessions, and written reports. **Box 22-19** is a list of resources that provide information on return to work contract requirements.

MEDIA MOMENT 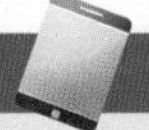

Philip Morris, the largest cigarette maker in the United States, began running advertisements in 2006 discouraging Hollywood from using its products on the big screen, citing studies that have shown cinematic portrayals of tobacco use can entice children to smoke.

Richmond-based Philip Morris USA ran advertisements in *Daily Variety, Hollywood Reporter,* and other trade publications imploring moviemakers: "Please Don't Give Our Cigarette Brands a Part in Your Movie."

Haspeslagh (1990) found that returning to work was a process during which the recovering nurse could either cope successfully or relapse. The time when nurses are most vulnerable for relapse is between 3 months and 1 year after treatment. There are three factors that put recovering nurses at risk for relapse: not working their aftercare program, not going to aftercare/support groups, and only doing what is required for their license or family, not for themselves. She also found that nurses who had the support of colleagues and supervisors who were knowledgeable about substance abuse and relapse were more likely to not relapse. For community health nurses, it is important to be able to recognize issues associated with substance abuse in nurses and other healthcare professionals. It is essential for the nurse to understand the importance of confronting substance abuse in nurses and to provide support for the returning recovering nurse. It is imperative that the community health nurse be cognizant of the signs of relapse and the proper steps to take if a coworker begins to take that walk down the path to relapse.

BOX 22-19 Resources for Return to Work Contract Requirements

Crosby, L., & Bissell, L. (1989). *To care enough* (pp. 255–260). Minneapolis, MN: Johnson Institute.

Durburg, S., & Werner, J. (1989). Re-entering the professional practice environment. In M. R. Haack & T. L. Hughs (Eds.), *Addiction in the nursing profession* (pp. 119–171). New York, NY: Springer.

Maher-Brisen, P. (2007). Addiction: An occupational hazard in nursing. *American Journal of Nursing, 107*(8), 78–79.

Naegle, M. (1993). *Substance abuse education in nursing* (vol. 3, pp. 231–235). New York, NY: National League for Nursing.

Conclusion

Substance abuse is a major public health concern. Community health nurses have a responsibility to address this problem as both healthcare professionals and private citizens. Looking at yourself and identifying your own issues and biases regarding the substance abuser is the first step to developing and providing appropriate care for those populations affected by substance abuse. The nurse must take an active role in assessment and early identification of persons at risk for substance abuse. Planning and implementing prevention programs is a primary role for community health nursing practice. Working with community leaders in the planning and implementation of programs that address the issues of drugs and youth, programs for women and children, drug-related crime, and community-focused prevention programs must be addressed if the *Healthy People 2020* objectives are to be achieved.

LEVELS OF PREVENTION 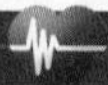

Primary: Education for elementary students about the risks of alcohol and tobacco use

Secondary: Screening high school students for tobacco use

Tertiary: Leading smoking cessation classes for high school students and faculty

Critical Thinking Activities

1. In a state legislative session, the state legislature passed three bills related to alcoholic beverages. One bill set a zero tolerance level (when tested, no level of alcohol can be present) for intoxicated adolescents picked up by authorities. The second bill raised the alcohol level allowed in beer sold in the state, thus allowing for a stronger beverage. The third bill permitted the establishment of microbreweries in the state.
   - What kind of message do these three bills send?
   - If you were a resident of this state, how would you react?
   - What do you see as the major issue(s) related to the passage of these three bills?
   - Which moral and ethical dilemmas can you identify?
   - Which options are available to address these issues?
2. You are a community health nurse working in home health. One day your patient's daughter tells you the following about one of the agency's home health aides:

   I really like Mrs. Green—she is a good person and has so many responsibilities, but I need to tell you she does tend to fall asleep when she is staying with dad. Last week he said that he thought he smelled alcohol on her breath but couldn't be sure. I've noticed she has been late coming to work more and more. Monday, when she came, she had a number of bruises and looked like she might have fallen down. I hate to complain, but I'm concerned about dad's safety. I also like Mrs. Green and am concerned about her.
   - How would you respond to the daughter?
   - What should the agency do about Mrs. Green? Why?
   - What is your responsibility?
   - How would you feel in this situation?

HEALTHY ME 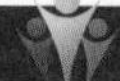

How have your attitudes about alcohol and other mind-altering substances changed since you began nursing school?

References

Adams, W., & Kinney, J. (1996). The elders. In J. Kinney (Ed.), *Clinical manual of substance abuse* (2nd ed.). St. Louis, MO: Mosby.

Aleixandre, J. L., Aleixandre-Tudó, J. L., Bolaños-Pizzaro, M., & Aleixandre-Benavent, R. (2013). Mapping the scientific research on wine and health (2001–2011). *Journal of Agricultural and Food Chemistry, 61*(49), 11871–11880.

Amaro, H. (1999). An expensive policy: The impact of inadequate funding for substance abuse treatment. *American Journal of Public Health, 89*(5), 657–659.

Anthenelli, R. (1997). A basic clinical approach to diagnosis in patients with comorbid psychiatric and substance use disorders. In N. Miller (Ed.), *The principles and practice of addictions in psychiatry* (pp. 119–126). Philadelphia, PA: Saunders.

Aseltine, R. H. (1995). A reconsideration of parental and peer influences on adolescent deviance. *Journal of Health Social Behavior, 36*(2), 103–121.

Barton, J. A. (1991). Parental adaptation to adolescent drug abuse: An ethnographic study of role formulation in response to courtesy stigma. *Public Health Nursing, 8*(1), 39–45.

Bauman, K. E., Foshee, V. A., Ennett, S. T., Pemberton, M., Hicks, K. A., King, T. S., & Koch, G. G. (2001). The influence of a family program on adolescent tobacco and alcohol. *American Journal of Public Health, 91*(4), 604–610.

Botvin, G. J., & Botvin, E. M. (1992). Adolescent tobacco, alcohol, and drug abuse: Prevention strategies, empirical findings, and assessment issues. *Developmental and Behavioral Pediatrics, 13*(4), 290–301.

Bukoski, W. J. (Ed.). (1997). Meta-analysis of drug abuse prevention programs. *NIDA Research Monograph*, 170.

Carroll, C. (2000). *Drugs in modern society* (5th ed.). Dubuque, IA: Brown & Benchmark.

Center for Substance Abuse Treatment (CSAT). (2001). *Aging, medicines and alcohol* [Brochure]. Rockville, MD: Author.

Center on Addiction and Substance Abuse. (1999). *CASA survey: Many dads AWOL in the battle against teen substance abuse.* Retrieved from http://www.casacolumbia.org

Centers for Disease Control and Prevention. (2011, November). Prescription painkiller overdoses in the US. Retrieved from http://cdc.gov/vitalsigns/painkilleroverdoses

Craft, M. J., & Willadsen, J. A. (1992). Interventions related to family. *Nursing Clinics of North America, 27*(2), 517–531.

Crosby, L., & Bissell, L. (1989). *To care enough.* Minneapolis, MN: Johnson Institute.

Drinking—get real. (1998, December). *The Coloradan*, p. 2.

Durburg, S., & Werner, J. (1989). Re-entering the professional practice arena. In M. Haack & T. Hughs (Eds.), *Addiction in the nursing profession* (pp. 119–171). New York, NY: Springer.

Dutra, L. M., & Glantz, S. A. (2014, March 6). Electronic cigarettes and conventional cigarette use among US adolescents: A cross-sectional study. *JAMA Pediatrics.* doi: 10.1001/jamapediatrics.2013.5488. [Epub ahead of print]

Fleming, C. B., Brewer, D. D., Gainey, R. R., Haggerty, K. P., & Catalano, R. F. (1997). Parent drug use and bonding to parents as predictors of substance use in children of substance abusers. *Journal of Child and Adolescent Substance Abuse, 6*(4), 75–86.

Frone, M. R. (2012). Workplace substance use climate: Prevalence and distribution in the U.S. workforce. *Journal of Substance Use, 71*(1), 72–83.

Goldsmith, R. J. (1997). The integrated psychology for addiction psychiatry. In N. Miller (Ed.), *The principles and practice of addictions in psychiatry* (pp. 3–10). Philadelphia, PA: Saunders.

Goodman, A. (2004). Passive smokers unite. *Cure, 3*(1), 64–67.

Grant, M., & Hodgson, R. (Eds.). (1991). *Responding to drug and alcohol problems in the community.* Geneva, Switzerland: World Health Organization.

Hahn, E. J. (1993). Parental alcohol and other drug (AOD) use and health beliefs about parent involvement in AOD prevention. *Issues in Mental Health Nursing, 14*, 237–247.

Hahn, E. J., & Rado, M. (1996). African American head start parent involvement in drug prevention. *American Journal of School Health, 20*(1), 41–51.

Hahn, E. J., Simpson, M. R., & Kidd, P. (1996). Cues to parent involvement in drug prevention and school activities. *Journal of School Health, 66*(5), 165–170.

Haspeslagh, J. (1990). Recovering nurses' perceptions of job reentry. Unpublished Ph.D. dissertation. Louisiana State University Medical Center, New Orleans.

Hawkins, J. D., Catalano, R. F., & Arthur, M. (2002). Promoting science-based prevention in communities. *Addictive Behaviors, 90*(5), 1–26.

Hill, S. Y. (1998). Alternative strategies for uncovering genes contributing to alcoholism risk: Unpredictable findings in a genetic wonderland. *Alcohol, 16*(1), 53–59.

Hussong, A., & Chassin, L. (1996). Substance use initiation among adolescent children of alcoholics: Testing protective factors. *Journal of Studies on Alcohol, 58*(3), 272–279.

Johnson, C. A., Pentz, M., Weber, M., Dwyer, J. H., Baer, N., MacKinnon, D. P., … Flay, B. R. (1990). Relative effectiveness of comprehensive community programming for drug abuse prevention with high-risk and low-risk adolescents. *Journal of Consulting and Clinical Psychology, 58*(4), 447–456.

Kann, L., Collins, J. L., Pateman, B. C., Small, M. L., Ross, J. G., & Kolbe, L. J. (1995). The School Health Policies and Programs (SHPPS): Rationale for a nationwide status report on school health programs. *Journal of School Health, 65*(8), 291–294.

Kearney, M. H., Murphy, S., Irwin, K., & Rosenbaum, M. (1995). Salvaging self: A grounded theory of pregnancy on crack cocaine. *Research, 44*(4), 208–213.

Kelly, E., Darke, S., & Ross, J. (2004). A review of drug use and driving: Epidemiology impairment, risk factors, and risk perceptions. *Drug Alcohol Review, 23*(3), 319–344.

Kelly, K., & Donohew, L. (1999). Media and primary socialization theory. *Substance Use and Misuse, 34*(7), 1033–1045.

King, B. A., Tynan, M. A., Dube, S. R., & Arrazola, R. (2014). Flavored-little-cigar and flavored-cigarette use among U.S. middle and high school students. *Journal of Adolescent Health, 54*(1), 40–46.

Kinney, J. (1996). *Clinical manual of substance abuse* (2nd ed.). St. Louis, MO: Mosby.

Kosterman, R., Hawkins, J. D., Haggerty, K. P., Spoth, R., & , C. (2001). Preparing for the drug free years: Session-specific effects of a universal parent-training intervention with rural families. *Journal of Drug Education, 31*(1), 47–68.

Maher-Brisen, P. (2007). Addiction: An occupational hazard in nursing. *American Journal of Nursing, 107*(8), 78–79.

Meiner, S. (1997, July). Polypharmacy in the elderly. *Advance for Nurse Practitioners,* 29–33.

Messina, N., Marinelli-Casey, P., West, K., & Rawson, R. (2007, March 22). Children exposed to methamphetamine use and manufacture. *Child Abuse and Neglect.* doi: 10.1016/j.chiabu.2006.06.009

Mezzich, A. C., Giancola, P. R., Tarter, R. E., Lu, S., Parks, S. M., & Barrett, C. M. (1997). Violence, suicidality, and alcohol/drug use involvement in adolescent females with a pyschoactive substance use disorder and controls. *Alcoholism Clinical and Experimental Research, 21*(7), 1300–1307.

Naegle, M. (1993). *Substance abuse education in nursing* (vol. 3). New York, NY: National League for Nursing.

National Center for Health Statistics. (2007). *Health: With chartbook on trends of the health of Americans.* Hyattsville, MD: Author.

National Highway Traffic Safety Administration. (2007). *Traffic Safety Facts Research Note* (Rep. No. DOT HS 810 821). Washington, DC: U.S. Department of Transportation.

National Institute on Drug Abuse (NIDA). (1998). *Monitoring the future—1998.* Rockville, MD: Department of Health and Human Services.

National Institute on Drug Abuse (NIDA). (2003). NIDA-funded research drives revision of guide to prevention programming. Retrieved from http://www.drugabuse.gov/NIDA_Notes/NNVol18N4/tearoff.html

National Institute on Drug Abuse. (2007). *Monitoring the future: National survey results on drug use, overview of key findings.* Bethesda, MD: Author.

National Institute on Drug Abuse. (2012). *Monitoring the future Study: Trends in prevalence of various drugs.* Retrieved from http://www.monitoringthefuture.org/pubs/monographs/mtf-vol1_2012.pdf

Nurco, D., & Lerner, M. (1996). Vulnerability to narcotic addiction: Family structure and functioning. *Journal of Drug Issues, 26*(4), 1007–1025.

Office of Substance Abuse Prevention. (2004). *Prevention Plus: Tools for creating and sustaining drug-free communities.* Rockville, MD: Department of Health and Human Services.

Phillips, J. (2013). Prescription drug abuse: Problem, policies, and implications. *Nursing Outlook, 61,* 78–84.

Resnicow, K., & Botvin, G. (1993). School based substance use prevention programs: Why do effects decay? *Preventive Medicine, 22,* 484–490.

Robinson, T. N., Chen, H. L., & Killen, J. D. (1998). Television and music video exposure and risk of adolescent alcohol use. *Pediatrics, 102*(5), 1201–1209.

Sandelowski, M. (1981). *Women, health, and choice.* Englewood Cliffs, NJ: Prentice Hall.

Schneider, C., Fischer, G., Diamant, K., et al. (1996). Pregnancy and drug dependence. *Wiener Klinisch Wochenschrift, 108*(19), 611–614.

Substance Abuse and Mental Health Services Administration (SAMHSA). (2012). *Results from the 2012 National Survey on Drug Use and Health: Summary of National Findings.* Retrieved from http://www.samhsa.gov/data/NSDUH/2012SummNatFindDetTables/NationalFindings/NSDUHresults2012.pdf

Sullivan, E., Bissell, L., & Williams, E. (1988). *Chemical dependency in nursing.* Menlo Park, CA: Addison-Wesley.

Symons, C., Cinelli, B., James, T. C., & Groff, P. (1997). Bridging student health risks and academic achievement through comprehensive school health programs. *Journal of School Health, 67*(6), 220–227.

U.S. Department of Health and Human Services (HHS). (2004). *As you age: A guide to aging, medicine, and alcohol* [Brochure]. Rockville, MD: Author.

U.S. Department of Health and Human Services (HHS). (2014). *Healthy People 2020: Substance abuse objectives.* Retrieved from http://www.healthypeople.gov/2020/topicsobjectives2020/objectiveslist.aspx?topicId=40

U.S. Department of Justice, Drug Enforcement Administration. (2011). *Drugs of abuse.* Retrieved from http://www.justice.gov/dea/docs/drugs_of_abuse_2011.pdf

Van Ryzin, M. J., Fosco, G. M., & Dishion, T. J. (2012). Family and peer predictors of substance use from early adolescence to early adulthood: An 11-year prospective analysis. *Addictive Behaviors, 37*(12), 1314–1324.

Walton-Moss, B., & Becker, K. (2000). Women and substance use disorders. *Primary Care Practitioner, 4*, 290–302.

Weinberg, T. S., & Vogel, C. (1990). Wives of alcoholics: Stigma management and adjustments to husband–wife interaction. *Deviant Behavior, 11*, 331–343.

West, D., & Kinney, J. (1996). Overview of substance use and abuse. In J. Kinney (Ed.), *Clinical manual of substance abuse* (pp. 17–39). St. Louis, MO: Mosby.

Williams, J. S. (2004). Researchers adopt HIV risk prevention program for African American Women. *NIDA News, 19*(1).

Zwickler, P. (2004). Childhood sexual abuse increases risk for drug dependence in adult women. Retrieved from http://archives.drugabuse.gov/NIDA_Notes/NNVol17N1/Childhood.html

CHAPTER FOCUS

From Criminal Justice to Public Health
Defining and Explaining Violence
Types of Violence in U.S. Society
- Violence in the Family
- Human Sex Trafficking
- Youth Violence
- Workplace Violence
- Mass Violence and War

Interventions to Prevent Violence
- Microlevel Interventions: Individuals and Families
- Mesolevel Interventions: Community Structures
- Macrolevel Interventions: Society and Culture

QUESTIONS TO CONSIDER

After reading this chapter, you will know the answers to the following questions:

1. How does a public health approach to violence differ from a criminal justice approach?
2. What are the forms of behavioral violence?
3. What are the forms of structural violence?
4. What are the factors that contribute to violent behavior?
5. Which populations are at greater risk for violence?
6. What is the typical pattern of abuse episodes in family violence?
7. What are the forms of violence among youths?
8. Which factors contribute to youth violence?
9. What roles do nurses have in relation to the global issue of the violence of war?
10. Which primary, secondary, and tertiary interventions contribute to the prevention of violence?

Nearly 2 million people worldwide lose their lives to violence each year, making violence a leading cause of death for people between the ages of 15 and 44.

CHAPTER 23

Violence and the Community

Sherry Hartman, Lilianna K. Deveneau, and Ann Thedford Lanier

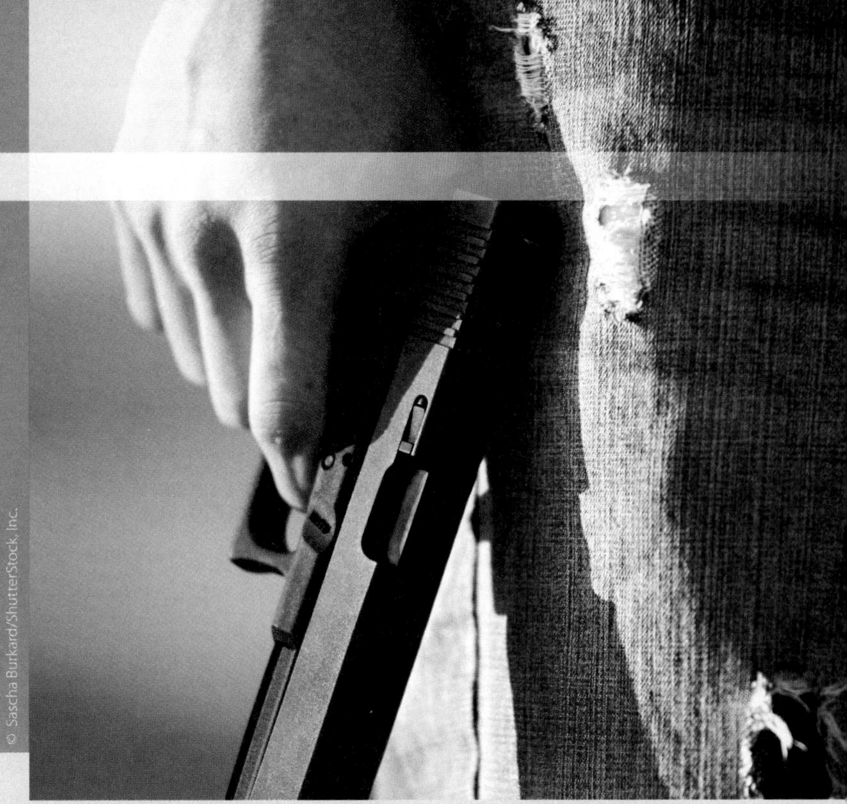

KEY TERMS

abuse
behavioral violence
collective violence
cyberbullying
cycle of abuse
interpersonal violence
intimate partner violence
learned helplessness
learned hopefulness
self-directed violence
structural violence
survivors

REFLECTIONS

When there is light in the soul, there is beauty in the person
When there is beauty in the person, there is harmony within the home
When there is harmony within the home, there is order in the nation
When there is order in the nation, there is peace in the world.

—*Lao Tzu*

I Have Been Thinking

I have been thinking about violence. I have been thinking about an airplane full of terrified women and men and children smashing into a tower full of unsuspecting women and men who were just sipping their morning coffee. I have been thinking of the burning people jumping from the 100th floor, jumping for their lives. I have been thinking about the hundreds of firefighters and police officers who were lost, crushed under a collapsing tower. I have been thinking about a husband waiting in his office for 14 hours for his wife who worked on the 104th floor, his wife who had not called, who was probably never going to call, and yet he was still waiting. I was thinking of the man who called his mother from the hijacked plane to tell her he loved her, to remember he loved her. I have been thinking about the debris and the dust on New Yorkers' shoes and how shocked we are here in America, how protected we have been. I have been thinking about all the war-torn countries I have been to, Bosnia, Kosovo, Israel, Afghanistan, and the dust on the peoples' shoes and the debris. I have been thinking about the people who were driven to hijack airplanes with knives and box cutters and fly them through buildings, who were ready, eager to lose their lives to hurt other people. I have been thinking about why, what would make people want to do that. I have been thinking about the words "retaliation" and "punishment" and "act of war." I have been thinking about violence, what it feels like to be nothing to someone else. What it feels like to be a consequence of someone else's disassociated rage, disconnected fury. I have been thinking about the cycle of hurt for hurt, nation against nation, tit for tat. I have been thinking about how deeply something else is required. I have been thinking about the courage it requires to think about something other than violence as a response to violence. I am thinking about the complexity of this and the loneliness of this and the helplessness and the sorrow that would be felt in the space where violence once was and the grief. I have been thinking that for those of us who are living on the planet right here, right now, we must live in this dangerous space, allowing the helplessness, the grief, the sorrow to create new wisdom that can and will and must free us from this terrible prison of violence. I urge you, each one of you—fall into this space, weep, be lost, let go, die into the grief—inside the emptiness and the pain it will be revealed.

—Eve Ensler, playwright, author of *The Vagina Monologues*, "Stop the Violence.
Spread the Word. Join Us," www.vday.org September 12, 2001

How has violence touched your life? Where were you on September 11, 2001? Have you or someone close to you ever been the victim of violence? After reading Eve Ensler's "I've Been Thinking," can you imagine "feeling the consequence of someone else's disassociated rage"? Do you think that we can ever think about "something other than violence as a response to violence"? How can nurses lead communities to nonviolent solutions—in schools, in churches, in the workplace?

Violence is one of the leading causes of death in all parts of the world (Centers for Disease Control and Prevention [CDC], 2014a). On an average day worldwide, one person is killed from homicide each minute, one person commits suicide every 40 seconds, and 35 people are killed each hour due to armed conflict (CDC, 2014a). In the United States alone, 24 people per minute are victims of rape, sexual assault, or stalking (CDC, 2014a). Further, violence accounts for 5.8 million (10%) global deaths with nearly twice as many males affected as females (World Health Organization [WHO], 2010); however, for each individual who dies because of an act of violence, there are many more who are injured and who suffer a wide range of physical, mental, sexual, and reproductive health problems. Violence places major economic burdens on national governments worldwide, costing countries billions of U.S. dollars each year to pay for health care, law enforcement, and lost productivity, while simultaneously accounting for a reduction in income or overall financial wellbeing in families and communities affected by the death or injury of even just one member (WHO, 2010).

Various forms of violence, such as torture, human trafficking, violence against women, violence against children, and harmful traditional cultural practices, have been long recognized as human rights issues. But only recently have we begun to realize that, when human rights are respected, protected, and fulfilled, the underlying societal conditions that foster violent behavior are controlled. Many of the risk factors common to many forms of violence, such as poverty, unemployment, gender inequality, racial discrimination, and weak economic and social safety nets, are closely linked to human rights, such as the right to equality and freedom from discrimination, the right to education, the right to an adequate standard of living, and the right to social security (WHO, 2014d).

From Criminal Justice to Public Health

Violence has been a part of humankind's world at least since recorded history. Our oldest texts are rife with tales of violence at individual and collective levels. In more recent history, violent behavior has been regarded as a social problem having moral overtones, with prevention efforts focused on tertiary prevention through imprisonment, capital punishment, and sometimes psychosocial rehabilitation. Violence has remained primarily a criminal justice issue of deviant and antisocial behavior (WHO, 2002). In discussing interpersonal violence, Hawkins (1999) commented that "one of the widely noted developments of the past decade is the trend toward viewing interpersonal aggression and violence as a public health concern rather than as a matter to be handled exclusively by the criminal justice system" (p. 87). It was in the 1980s that the CDC initiated efforts to prevent injuries from violence by using a public health approach. Both a rapid rise in homicide rates in the United States and a growing acceptance by public health workers of the importance of behavioral factors in the etiology of disease and injury encouraged the efforts. Violence was becoming a "behavior-based epidemic that kills and injures as certainly as a disease of the flesh" (Jones, 1993, p. 9). It became accepted that the nation needed to have more than a criminal justice approach to violence.

Criminal justice approaches, however, continue to attend to violence with secondary and tertiary interventions after violence has occurred. A public health approach does not imply that violence is only or mainly a problem of health or that responsibility for solutions lies with health professionals. It provides a multidisciplinary, scientific approach that uses the methods of epidemiology to study how primary prevention strategies can reduce violence (CDC, 2014b; Mercy, Rosenberg, Powell, Broome, & Roper, 1993). A public health approach implies the belief that violence is a learned behavior and, therefore, can be changed and prevented. Describing the scope of the problem, identifying risk and protective factors, evaluating interventions, and implementing promising community programs are the components of the CDC approach to prevention.

Nurses have long played a role in addressing the trauma of violence and its health consequences and continue to be highly involved. In 1991, the American Nurses Association (ANA) issued a statement about physical violence against women that reflected the important nursing research that had been done in the area. In recognition of the magnitude of the health problems related to violence, several other nursing organizations have since issued position statements on violence. Violence against women, children, and elders in familial or intimate relationships was given special emphasis as a form of violence with high incidence and prevalence resulting in morbidity and mortality and requiring healthcare interventions.

This chapter provides a public health approach to violence and examines many varieties of its expression. Some forms will be more common and will be familiar from courses focusing on women's health, children's health, and mental health. The emphasis here is on populations at risk and interventions directed to communities and populations. The broader context within which violence occurs and the complex interplay of individuals with their larger community and with society need to be understood in order to take on the task of reducing harm from violence.

Defining and Explaining Violence

Depending on the discipline and purposes of inquiry, conceptualizations and explanations of violence vary. The most common and narrow definition of violence is of physical harm at an interpersonal level. The WHO (2014a) definition of violence is among the most comprehensive: "the intentional use of physical force or power, threatened or actual, against oneself, another person, or against a group or community, that either results in or has a high likelihood of resulting in injury, death, psychological harm, maldevelopment, or deprivation." This definition can be broken down further in relation to the victim–perpetrator relationship and to ensure more accurate care (WHO, 2014a):

- **Self-directed violence** refers to violence in which the perpetrator and the victim are the same individual and is subdivided into *self-abuse* and *suicide*.
- **Interpersonal violence** refers to violence between individuals, and is subdivided into *family* and *intimate partner violence* and *community violence*. The former category includes child maltreatment, intimate partner violence, and elder abuse, while the latter is broken down into *acquaintance* and *stranger*

violence and includes youth violence, assault by strangers, violence related to property crimes, and violence in workplaces and other institutions.
- **Collective violence** refers to violence committed by larger groups of individuals and can be subdivided into social, political, and economic violence.

Proposed explanations of individual **behavioral violence** include biological causes such as instinct, heredity, lesions of the brain, drugs and alcohol, and various neurochemical causes such as increased testosterone or lowered serotonin. In psychological theories, violent behavior is sometimes further distinguished as "emotive" aggression, as seen in crimes of passion, and "instrumental" aggression governed by rewards and punishments stimulated by a number of personal or material gains such as power, status, money, and sex. Developmental approaches look to early life experiences and parental relationships that develop violence potential. Related to this is the belief that violence is learned in the family from the social role models, which may sanction physical punishment and the privacy of family interactions.

Personality or character disorders in which the person is inadequate in coping and communications is another perspective. In the cases of child and elder abuse, stress, inadequacy, and frustration from the dependency of the child or elder influence the abuser's choice in using violence.

THINK ABOUT THIS

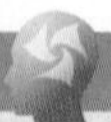

Many believe that violence is an innate feature of society. What do you think? How does violence on a personal level compare to societal violence? As a nurse, what is your idea of violence? How have your ideas been influenced by your family, personal experiences, and violence in the media? Can community health nurses use primary prevention efforts to affect violence at the personal level and the societal level?

Violence is not simply a problem that plagues individuals, but societies as a whole. One reason for this is the nature of **structural violence**. This can be defined as social, political, and cultural institutions that systematically deny some people their basic human needs, which constitute a structural violation of human rights (Ho, 2007). These often remain unnoticed, as they are taken for granted in one's culture and become expected. Gilligan (1997) describes it as "the increased rates of death and disability suffered by those who occupy the bottom rungs of society, as contrasted with the relatively lower rates experienced by those above them" (p. 192). Structural violence is a product of

GLOBAL CONNECTION

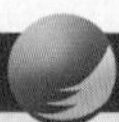

The Other Victims of War: A Nurse's Experience in a Refugee Camp

As a new graduate, I felt unprepared for my role as a nurse in Thailand, working with Cambodian refugees. We carried walkie-talkies and knew the warning signal to leave the camp if the North Vietnamese were entering the area. The very thought of deserting these gentle people, after spending months with them, seemed impossible. Equally impossible was the task of screening the recipients for food, by age. Only women and children under 6 were to be fed. Man's inhumanity to man was everywhere. I looked into the faces of children who had survived hell. How could I say they were too old to eat? A photographer for a U.S. magazine asked me if I wanted to come along into the jungle for pictures. I started to follow, only to have a still small voice remind me that I wasn't in New Jersey anymore and that those paths led to places no one should have to see.

—Anne Troy, RN, FNP, refugee relief worker, Cambodia, 1982

society's collective human choices and values, such as how to distribute available resources and services for violence prevention and treatment.

Figure 23-1 shows the relationship between behavioral and structural violence. There are several implications of the model for understanding violence. First, there are reciprocal effects of the micro-, meso-, and macrosystem levels on each other. Individual behavior is affected by all levels: personal characteristics and the environment of institutions and culture. The top level is the most obvious, overt form of violence that we can see and assess. The second two levels refer to the unseen, covert forces that guide thoughts, words, and actions. These can be forces or situations that in subtle ways hinder health, growth, and development of individuals or certain groups of individuals. For example, at the institutional or mesosystem level, policies for reporting domestic violence have the potential to put the victim at greater harm from retaliation by the abuser. Because there are no policies requiring assessment, training, or screening, women often remain undiagnosed for domestic violence. Until recently, in many states, it was legal for a husband to rape his wife. Many of the barriers to access to health care are the result of bureaucracy and oppressive social policy and are examples of structural violence at the institutional level.

Like the young fish who asks the wise, old fish, "So what is this 'ocean' I hear others talking about?", individuals live

DAY IN THE LIFE

The Work of Forensics: The Care of the SANE Nurse

Anne Troy, RN, LNC, SANE

A 30-minute response time was required, from the first beep, to arrival at the emergency department (ED) outpatient unit. Thirty minutes to steel oneself against vicarious trauma. Bridging a victim's journey from attack through treatment required empathy, courage, and spiritual fortitude. Sometimes it was barely enough time to pray and will those qualities into action before pushing open the exam door. This night, I faced a frail woman, barely 20, with tears drenching the exam table. "He made me do those things," she whispered as the detective left to give us privacy. I found myself shocked and overwhelmed as she retold the horror of her abduction into a city park.

We were to learn this was not his first rape. As DNA provided the evidence, the circumstantial facts solidified into a sordid history of serial raping. He would drop his girlfriend off at a local college and use her car to abduct, by gunpoint, women as they walked from bus stops or shopped for their families. If he had applied for nursing school, there would have been nothing to warn of his deviant behavior by his social presentation. Well spoken and well loved by a courtroom full of family, who still believe him innocent, he gave no indication of his intent by his appearance.

As this woman consented to a forensic exam, I ensured the chain of evidence was maintained and vaginal swab samples were dried before boxing and taping. As I reviewed the prophylactic medications we could provide, I anticipated her despair as I offered the human immunodeficiency virus (HIV) medication. Instead, as her mother came screaming into the exam room, she stood and whispered in my ear, "I'm HIV positive; don't tell my mom. I hope he got it from me." I couldn't share her sense of retaliation as I sorted through my reeling emotions. Most rapists are known to their victims, so he didn't fit the statistical profile. However, all rapists repeat the act and I feared for his future victims, should he have acquired HIV from his present attack.

I offered her new clothing, as we bagged hers for collection of leaves and possible fiber evidence. I talked to her several times prior to going to court. She did not want to return to the hospital for any follow-up appointments. I focused on her guilt about her son and provided for their follow-up counseling.

As I entered the court, I was ushered into a room with the three victims waiting to testify. I was an expert witness and planned on testifying about the chain of evidence. Two of the victims sat alone with sweatshirts pulled to cover their faces. They had not acknowledged each other. Their shame and fear was still haunting them. I told them all quietly how much I, and every woman in our city, thanked them for their bravery in facing this perpetrator. I told them that because of what they were about to do in court, my daughter was safer on the street. I reminded them not to allow the rape to define them or their life. I was proud that, as women, they were strong in spite of the personal cost. Slowly, the sweatshirts came down and we talked instead of whispered. I was proud of the role of nursing in helping women find their way back. Our voices united and he received three consecutive life sentences. There wasn't joy, as his family collapsed in agony. Our work of prevention has just begun. The time, before the beeper goes off again, is the time I am desperately working in to stop the insanity.

their lives surrounded and affected by the forces represented by the macrosystem. This desensitization is reflected in our youth culture. Today's young people struggle to even identify their exposure to violence as they are bombarded daily with misogynist messages in music and videos. This is also shown in unconscious acceptance of inequalities and deprivations, such as differential infant mortality rates, premature death, or lack of political representation. These indicate the excess suffering of some groups over others. Seldom, however, are the forces leading to this type of suffering referred to as *violence.*

> You cannot shake hands with a clenched fist.
>
> —*Indira Gandhi*

According to Van Soest (1997), the pattern of thinking that is most revealing is the continued easy acceptance of threat or use of violence as a method of social control and an appropriate method of problem solving.

One example of the cultural propensity to use force and attack to solve problems is the frequent characterization of health and social problems as an enemy that becomes an opponent to engage in battle, as "war" is waged against drugs and violence. Just as the child who experiences violence is thought to learn to respond with violence, some believe that meeting violence with violence at the structural and cultural levels also breeds a cycle of violence. Gilligan (1997) explains how the horrific violence committed by the prisoners he worked with may seem senseless if studied in isolation. Combining the insights of psychiatry with a public health approach to violence, he believes their violent acts have a logic when seen as a response to structural violence of social conditions that stimulate shame and guilt. He details how these emotions lead to violent acts that are counterviolence to the social conditions of structural violence. He lists poverty, race, age discrimination, and gender asymmetry as the most important of these.

Box 23-1 is based on the work of Potter (1999), who reviewed the research on violence and classified influences based on an ecological model. In public health terms, these can be viewed as factors associated with the risk of violent behaviors. From this perspective, the presence or absence of certain factors or circumstances determines the likelihood of instigating violence. This compilation is not an exhaustive list of the various influences that have been studied related to violence, nor do the influences always lead to violence. A complex interaction between individuals, their varied environments, and existing social ills combine to lead to violence.

BOX 23-1 Risk Factors Related to Violent Behavior

Microsystem

Individual

- Prenatal and perinatal factors
- Neurobiology and genetics
- Substance abuse
- Hormones—cortisol, testosterone, serotonin
- Premature, special-needs children
- Male sex
- Temperament
- Low IQ
- Slow language development
- Processing and attributing hostile intent
- Attention deficit/hyperactivity disorder
- Conduct disorder
- Poor social skills
- Lack of sympathy/empathy
- Low self-esteem
- High stress levels
- Alcohol and/or drug use
- Younger than 30 years of age
- Head trauma

Family, peers, school, and religious communities

- Physical and/or sexual abuse or neglect
- Witness of violence in home
- Rejection by peers
- Witness peer fighting/homicides
- Free access to weapons
- Inadequate coercive posting
- Single female head of household
- Disadvantaged schools
- Bullied
- School dropout
- Gang activity
- Spiritual alienation

Mesosystem

- Collective powerlessness in neighborhood/community
- Collective sense of confusion in transient neighborhoods
- Gentrification of neighborhoods
- Overcrowding/demolition of housing projects
- Substandard, high-cost rental units
- White flight to suburbs
- Poor economy with joblessness
- Oppressive work environment
- Lack of access to health care in general, and substance abuse rehabilitation and mental health therapy in particular

Macrosystem

- Poverty
- Income inequality—minimum wage is not a living wage
- Community instability—political corruption
- Exposure to dramatic violence in media (TV, music, film)
- Economic activities supporting violence such as gun and drug trafficking and prostitution
- Declining public assistance programs
- Denigration of minorities, gays, ethnic groups, refugees, and people with disabilities
- Organizational structures that maintain and tacitly support violence against women
- Pornography of women legal and considered erotica
- Changes in gender roles that produce fear of power loss in males
- Tacit acceptance of violence to resolve conflict: war and weapons, child punishment, and death penalty
- Rigid stereotypes of roles of men and women
- Correctional facilities as economic base to communities
- Inequity of justice for poor and people of color

Source: Based on Potter, L. B. (1999). Understanding the incidence and origin of community violence: Toward a comprehensive perspective on violence prevention. In T. P. Gullotta & S. J. McElhaney (Eds.), *Violence in homes and communities: Prevention, intervention, and treatment.* Thousand Oaks, CA: Sage.

Types of Violence in U.S. Society

Violence in the Family

> War, to sane men at the present day, begins to look like an epidemic insanity, breaking out here and there like the cholera or influenza, infecting men's brains instead of their bowels.
>
> —*Ralph Waldo Emerson, Miscellanies, 1884*

Family violence is a pervasive and often lethal problem of epidemic proportions, with far-reaching challenges and consequences in communities, nations, and worldwide. Family violence is often silent and hidden from view—a family secret. It physically, emotionally, financially, and spiritually devastates victims and their children. It also lays the foundation for the continuation of violence, as many abusers were once abused themselves. It threatens the stability of the family and violates communities' safety and economies by costing billions of dollars annually in medical expenses, sick leave, absenteeism, and nonproductivity (Davey & Davey, 1998; Office for Victims of Crime, 2013; Waters et al., 2004).

> The right to swing my fist ends where the other man's nose begins.
>
> —*Oliver Wendell Holmes*

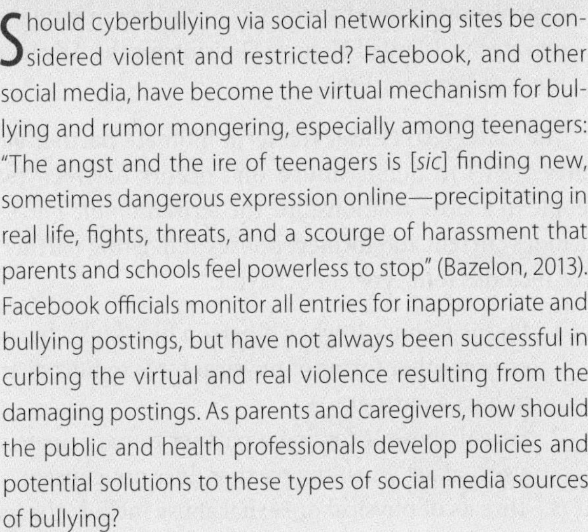

ETHICAL CONNECTION

Should cyberbullying via social networking sites be considered violent and restricted? Facebook, and other social media, have become the virtual mechanism for bullying and rumor mongering, especially among teenagers: "The angst and the ire of teenagers is [*sic*] finding new, sometimes dangerous expression online—precipitating in real life, fights, threats, and a scourge of harassment that parents and schools feel powerless to stop" (Bazelon, 2013). Facebook officials monitor all entries for inappropriate and bullying postings, but have not always been successful in curbing the virtual and real violence resulting from the damaging postings. As parents and caregivers, how should the public and health professionals develop policies and potential solutions to these types of social media sources of bullying?

> The invention of nuclear weapons has changed everything—except the way we think. . . . We shall require a substantially new manner of thinking if mankind is to survive.
>
> —*Albert Einstein*

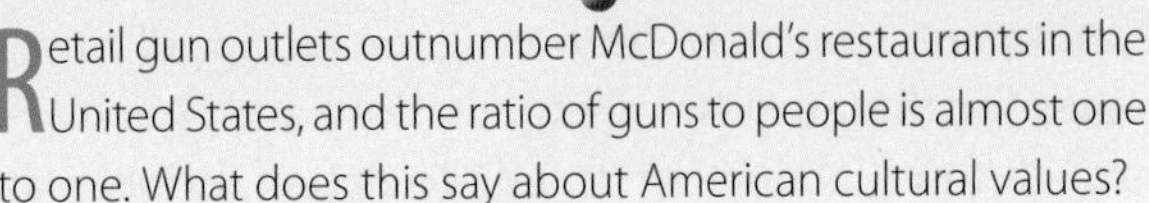

CULTURAL CONNECTION

Retail gun outlets outnumber McDonald's restaurants in the United States, and the ratio of guns to people is almost one to one. What does this say about American cultural values?

There is growing recognition that family violence is a major health problem for women and children in the United States and around the world. Family violence presents unique challenges and opportunities for healthcare providers. Because victims of family violence and their children are found across healthcare services, as are nurses, nurses are in unique positions to assess and identify those affected by family violence. As such, nurses, especially community health nurses, have the opportunity to be leaders in the prevention of family violence. Nursing approaches to domestic violence have an advocacy orientation that can be absent from other healthcare professions. Research has shown that healthcare professionals can contribute to further subjugation of domestic violence victims. In many cases, those victimized by violence are viewed as a deviant group. Those victimized are often members of disenfranchised groups, minority or ethnic groups, and/or women and children. Professionals may try to distance themselves from such groups and their problems by holding the belief that it is the problem of an "other" or deviant group. Many nurses who work and research in this area are believed by some to have avoided the victim blaming that is characteristic of some disciplines. Their research has grown out of clinical, grassroots concerns that have developed an activist agenda and a recognition of **survivors'** needs for empowerment (Campbell, Harris, & Lee, 1995; Donovan & Vlais, 2005; UNIFEM, 2003).

According to Campbell, Harris, and Lee (1995), there are three main theories useful for exploring family violence. The first emphasizes the abuser and the possible behavioral or psychopathological causes, such as mental illness, developmental disability, or substance abuse. In the family violence model, "the cycle of violence," with its use of force, is created when violence is learned in childhood and transmitted across generations. The third theory speculates that stressful situations precipitate violence.

For example, violence arises when adults are unable to cope appropriately with the stress of unemployment or caring for a dependent elder. Children with special needs can increase stress and potential abuse (U.S. Department of Health and Human Services [HHS], 2008).

Human Sex Trafficking

Human sex trafficking is the most common form of modern-day slavery (Walter-Rodriguez & Hill, 2011). Activities related to human sex trafficking refer to the recruitment, transport, harboring, or receipt of human beings for the purpose of exploitation, and is achieved through force, abduction, fraud, deception, bribery, and the abuse of power. Sex trafficking involves abducting people, particularly children, and transporting and prostituting them. They are held captive, often through force and drugs to deter their escape. Many of the children being trafficked are runaways or "throw-away youths," and are often not properly cared for and may even be homeless. However, they are also sought out in malls and other crowded public places by captors who lure their victims with expensive gifts, money, attention, and the promise of independence and wealth. The average target age of girls is 12–14 years, and the target age range for boys is 11–13 years (Walter-Rodriguez & Hill, 2011). However, traffickers are known to prey on children as young as 9 years old (U.S. Department of Education, 2013). The United Nations estimates 1.2 million children are trafficked each year globally. Grown women, particularly those who are homeless and/or prostitutes, are also easy targets of sex traffickers. Human trafficking is currently one of the most profitable endeavors of organized crime, and the fastest growing (U.S. Department of Justice, 2013).

Cases of human trafficking have been reported in all 50 states; Washington, DC; and all U.S. territories (U.S. Department of Education, 2013). In 2000, Congress passed the Trafficking Victims Protection Act, the first of many comprehensive federal laws to address sex trafficking, with a significant focus on the international dimension of the problem (Walter-Rodriguez & Hill, 2011). These allow task forces to monitor and combat trafficking through the use of tools that had not been available before such laws were passed (U.S. Department of State, 2013).

Victims of human trafficking, particularly children, may exhibit the following characteristics (U.S. Department of Education, 2013):

- Chronically running away
- Making references to frequent travels to other cities
- Bruises or other signs of physical trauma
- Malnourishment
- Inappropriate dress
- Inappropriate level of knowledge regarding sexual activity

The child or other suspected trafficked person should be tested for sexually transmitted infections (STIs). If you suspect the patient has been abused or trafficked, immediately contact law enforcement and, if necessary, Child Protective Services, and ensure the patient is protected and accompanied at all times.

Violence Against Women

"Violence against women is a pervasive global public health problem of epidemic proportions, requiring urgent action," WHO (2013) asserts. This phenomenon is known by many names: *spouse abuse, wife abuse, wife beating, battering, marital assault, woman battery, domestic violence, dating violence, and intimate partner violence.* These terms are sometimes used interchangeably, and occasionally, a term is used to refer to a specific problem (e.g., *family violence* to indicate wife and children are being battered). There are also many behavioral and legal definitions of violence against women, which sometimes makes it unclear what is meant by each term. This lack of clarity can lead to inconsistencies in healthcare providers' identification and interventions as well as differences in research terminology and even legal policies, procedures, and laws.

In 1995, the Fourth World Conference on Women, held in Beijing, developed a platform for action on violence against women and defined it as follows:

> Violence against women: any act of gender-based violence that results in, or is likely to result in, physical, sexual, or psychological harm or suffering to women, including threats of such acts, coercion, or arbitrary deprivation of liberty, whether occurring in public or private life. (United Nations Division for the Advancement of Women, 1995)

The CDC (2011) uses the term **intimate partner violence** (IPV) to define **abuse** that occurs between two people in a close relationship. The term *intimate partner* includes current and former spouses and dating partners. IPV includes four types of behavior:

1. Physical abuse is when a person hits, kicks, burns, or uses other forms of physical force to hurt or try to hurt a partner.
2. Sexual abuse is forcing a partner to participate in a sexual act when the partner does not consent.
3. Threats of physical or sexual abuse include the use of words, gestures, weapons, or other means to communicate the intent to cause harm.

4. Emotional abuse is threatening a partner or his or her possessions or loved ones, or harming a person's sense of self-worth. Stalking, name-calling, intimidation, and isolation are some examples.

More than 35% of women worldwide have experienced either physical and or sexual IPV or non-partner sexual violence, and most violence against women is from an intimate partner. Worldwide, nearly one in three women have experienced IPV, and 38% of all murders of women are a result of IPV (WHO, 2013). Most abusive relationships are male batterers of female victims; however, the reverse may be true. IPV also occurs in gay and lesbian relationships.

Violence cuts across all of society, all ethnic and cultural groups, and all educational and socioeconomic levels. Three types of batterers have been described based on the severity of their violence, who they direct violence toward, and their degree of personality disorder. Some batter with less severity and only within the family; others use more violence, mostly in the family, and show some signs of distress and emotional instability; and the most severe batterers are violent outside the family and often demonstrate criminal activity, alcohol and drug abuse, and antisocial personality disorder (Hotzworth-Monroe & Stuart, 1994). More attention has been given to the characteristics of male batterers than to abused women, because these characteristics have been found to be more helpful in assessing risk of partner violence. Batterers are not a homogeneous group and vary greatly in their profiles. However, there are some generalities (Neighbors et al., 2010). Batterers often suffer from low self-esteem and have a need to use power and control tactics over victims. They usually minimize their own behavior, justify it as "normal," or blame the victim for the violence. They tend to be more jealous, abusive to children, and sexually aggressive toward partners. After battering episodes, batterers manipulate by offering remorse, loving words, and promises to change—anything to gain control over the partner. This is known as the **cycle of abuse**. Substance abuse often is involved in partner violence.

For some women, IPV can lead to **learned helplessness**. Women are viewed as helpless, passive victims who restrict their behaviors because they lose the ability to predict whether their actions will be effective. What is viewed as helplessness is just the reality of a situation in which resources to enable escape are inadequate. As isolation from support continues, abuse escalates, leaving a previously confident woman struggling not to believe it is partly her fault. Women logically try to protect themselves and their children, but police response, child care, shelter, education and employment opportunities, and community support are lacking or are already overwhelmed.

An approach that counters learned helplessness in women draws on the societal expectation that women must be responsible for maintaining relationships. Relationship hope is present in women in general, and **learned hopefulness** in battered women is their belief that the perpetrator will change behavior or personality. The concept explains why women stay with or return to abusers, especially if the abusers enroll in treatment programs. **Box 23-2** outlines the signs that may indicate a women is the victim of IPV.

Women experiencing IPV can not only have physical and psychological issues, but also have higher rates of

BOX 23-2 Indicators of Occurrence of Intimate Partner Violence

- Recurrent trauma history
- Proximal injuries, such as to head, neck, torso, breast, abdomen, or genitals
- Patterned, multiple, or bilateral injury
- Poor explanations or no explanations for injuries
- Concealing or acting ashamed of injuries
- Delay in seeking treatment for injury with wounds in various stages of healing
- Physical injury during pregnancy, especially to abdomen or breasts
- Signs of depression: flat affect, failure to make eye contact, mood swings, poor hygiene
- Other psychological cues such as suicidal thoughts, anxiety, difficulty sleeping, panic attacks
- Alcohol or substance abuse symptoms
- Chronic pain with no known cause
- Seeking medical care for minor problems to maintain contact with healthcare professionals
- Missing scheduled appointments or only coming for acute care
- Overly protective, controlling partner who visits healthcare professionals with patient and refuses to leave his or her side

Sources: Cassidy, K. (1999). How to assess and intervene in domestic violence situations. *Home Healthcare Nurse, 17,* 665–671; Centers for Disease Control and Prevention (CDC). (2011). *The National Intimate Partner and Sexual Violence Survey: 2010 Summary Report.* Retrieved from http://www.cdc.gov/violenceprevention/nisvs/2010_report.html; Scott-Tilley, D. (1999). Nursing interventions to prevent domestic violence. *American Journal of Nursing, 99*(10), 24–27.

other health problems as well, including being 16% more likely to have a low-birth-weight baby, more than twice as likely to have an abortion, almost twice as likely to experience depression, and in some places more than one and a half times more likely to acquire HIV than women who have not experienced IPV (WHO, 2013). Moreover, women who have experienced IPV are almost twice as likely to have alcohol abuse issues and are one a half times more likely to acquire syphilis, chlamydia, or gonorrhea (WHO, 2013).

The medical care, mental services, and lost productivity costs of IPV were estimated in 2003 as $8.3 billion (CDC, 2003). According to WHO (2013), "The health sector must play a greater role in responding to IPV and sexual violence against women." They emphasize an urgent need to integrate issues relating to violence in clinical training. This will allow nurses the opportunity to provide emotional support and connect women to other sexual and reproductive health services, mental health services, emergency services, and HIV testing. New guidelines set by WHO (2013) emphasize:

- Importance of training all levels of healthcare workers to recognize risk factors of IPV and appropriate responses
- How to ask about violence in a private, confidential, and safe setting
- Creation of referral systems to ensure related services
- Implementation of these practices into nursing curricula and training

The prevalence statistics found in **Box 23-3** have been obtained from numerous studies. There are few national sources of epidemiological data on IPV. Most states collect data from law enforcement agencies. Although these sources provide information on trends, it is generally believed that domestic violence is seriously underreported and severely underdiagnosed by healthcare providers.

DAY IN THE LIFE

Nurses historically have been in a key position to assess and prevent domestic violence. We typically spend more time with patients and their families than any other healthcare professional. We are with people at all the important times in their lives and can see how patients and families interact with each other. National surveys also have shown that patients trust nurses and are likely to confide in us.

. . . We cannot let another year go by without having a strong, nationwide educational and assessment program to educate healthcare professionals to assess for domestic violence and work with women to promote their health and safety.

After all, asking the right questions won't hurt women. Not asking those questions certainly will.

—Patricia Underwood, PhD, RN, Secretary of the American Nurses Association, 1999

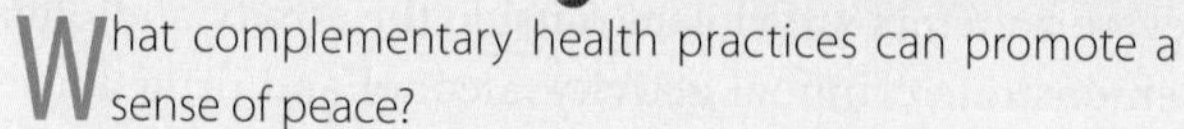

What complementary health practices can promote a sense of peace?

Female Genital Mutilation WHO (2014b) has estimated that between 100 and 140 million girls and women worldwide have been subjected to female genital mutilation (FGM). There are four types of FGM (WHO, 2014b):

1. Clitoridectomy—partial or total removal of the clitoris and/or prepuce
2. Excision—partial or total removal of the clitoris and labia minora, with or without excision of the labia majora
3. Infibulation—narrowing of vaginal orifice through the creation of a seal by cutting and repositioning

BOX 23-3 Facts About Intimate Partner Violence

- About 4.8 million intimate partner victimizations occur each year among U.S. women age 18 and older. Men are the victims of about 2.9 million intimate partner assaults (CDC, 2011).
- Intimate partner violence resulted in nearly 1,600 deaths in 2004. Of these deaths, 75% were female and 25% were male (CDC, 2011).
- Intimate partner violence costs billions of dollars every year in medical care, mental health services, and lost productivity (CDC, 2011).
- Intimate partner violence occurs across all populations, irrespective of social, economic, religious, or cultural group. However, young women and those below the poverty line are disproportionately affected (Heise & Garcia-Moreno, 2002).
- As many as 324,000 women each year experience intimate partner violence during pregnancy (Gazmarian et al., 2000).
- Forty-four percent of women murdered by an intimate partner had visited an emergency department within 2 years of the homicide, 93% of whom had at least one injury visit (Crandall, Walters, Kernic, Holt, & Rivara, 2004).

the labia minora and/or labia majora, which may also involve excision of the clitoris
4. All other harmful procedures to female genitalia for nonmedical purposes, including pricking, piercing, incising, or scraping

FGM is reported all over the world but is most prevalent in western, eastern, and northeastern Africa; some countries in Asia and the Middle East; and among certain immigrant communities in North America and Europe. Growing migration rates have increased the number of girls and women who may be at risk of this horrendous practice, as FGM is sometimes adopted by new groups and new areas after migration and displacement through the introduction to the practice by neighboring groups. This is sometimes performed as an attempt to preserve one's ethnic identity and increase the possibility of intermarriage between other similar ethnic groups who submit their girls and women to FGM (WHO, 2014b).

This painful practice is almost always performed on minors, and therefore violates the rights of the child. These procedures are often supported by women and men, usually without question, as anyone who does not conform to this cultural practice may face condemnation, ostracism, harassment, or even death. Girls who have not been mutilated are often seen as unclean and unfit to marry, because women believe FGM enhances a man's sexual pleasure while restraining her own, which is thought to ensure marital fidelity and prevent sexually deviant behavior. As marriage is often essential in securing one's social and economic future in these cultures, the social pressure and fears of stigma and social rejection are often believed to outweigh the negative health risks, thus continuing the tradition. In some cultures, there are even incentives such as coming of age celebrations, gifts, and promises of entry into secret societies of women who vow to continue the practice. Therefore, FGM has become an important cultural identity, upheld by local and traditional leaders such as government officials, religious leaders, elders, and even medical personnel (WHO, 2014b).

Cultural beliefs notwithstanding, FGM has proven harmful effects but no known benefits to physical health. The harms include the following:

- A girl's legs may be bound together for days or weeks after
- Trauma
- Pain and bleeding
- Chronic physical and psychological problems: infections, chronic pain, decreased sexual enjoyment, posttraumatic stress disorder (PTSD)
- Higher incidence of cesarean section and postpartum hemorrhage
- Increased death rates of newborns:15% higher with clitoridectomy, 32% increase with excision, and 55% increase with infibulation
- An estimated additional one to two babies per 100 births die due to FGM

Evidence has shown that, despite these health risks, FGM is increasing in a number of countries, particularly that performed by medical professionals. In fact, in some countries, it has become a routine practice to mutilate a newborn girl immediately after birth. Possible reasons for medical staff to mutilate girls include:

- Economic gain
- Pressure by clients and society
- Sense of duty to community
- Upholding cultural traditions
- Attempting to reduce risks of infection and complications

However, even when performed by healthcare professionals, the procedure is not necessarily less severe or painful, nor the conditions more sanitary. In fact, there is no evidence that supports the belief that performing FGM in hospitals lowers health risks (WHO, 2014b).

Healthcare providers must never perform FGM and should face serious consequences including risk of one's medical license being withdrawn for doing so. Further, medical staff—particularly nurses—can play a key role in the prevention of FGM by providing women and girls with information regarding sexual and reproductive health and through community outreach and women's empowerment. Studies show a close link between women's ability to exercise control over their lives and their belief that FGM should not be performed (WHO, 2014b). Therefore, it is crucial to educate and empower women, the primary performers of FGM, to promote lasting social change that will increase the quality of life for women, children, and men (WHO, 2014c).

Violence Against Children

Violence involving children includes all types of abuse and neglect resulting in harm to children younger than 18 years of age. There are four common types of abuse:

1. *Physical abuse* occurs when a child's body is injured by hitting, kicking, shaking, burning, or other forms of physical force.
2. *Sexual abuse* involves engaging a child in sexual acts such as fondling, rape, and exposing a child to any sexual activity.
3. *Emotional abuse* refers to any behavior that harms a child's self-worth or emotional wellbeing. Examples include name-calling, shaming, rejection, withholding love, and threatening.

4. *Neglect* is the failure to meet a child's basic needs, which include housing, food, clothing, education, and access to health care (CDC, 2012a).

In 2011, an estimated 3.7 million referrals of child abuse were received by state and local agencies—slightly more than 7 referrals per minute (CDC, 2013a). Of the child victims, 79% experienced neglect, 18% suffered physical abuse, 9% endured sexual abuse, and 10% experienced other types of violence such as emotional abuse or lack of supervision (CDC, 2013a). Further, most victims (81%) were abused by a parent (CDC, 2013a). Although families living in poverty and single-parent families are at increased risk, all socioeconomic levels and family patterns experience violence. **Box 23-4** shows some of the risk factors associated with child abuse.

Studies estimate up to one in five children experience some form of violence in their lifetime, which contributes to slowing a country's economic and societal development (CDC, 2014c). The economic cost to society of child maltreatment ending in the death of the child has been calculated at a staggering $1,272,900 per death, taking into account the costs associated with healthcare, legal system, and criminal justice costs; lost productivity; and other economic factors (Fang, Brown, Florence, & Mercy, 2012). Even less extreme cases carry significant economic and social consequences, with a total lifetime economic burden of both fatal and nonfatal child abuse in the United States estimated at $124 billion based on data from 2008 (Fang et al., 2012).

Consequences of abuse for survivors can be lifelong and vary depending on the nature of the act, the child's age, and the general environment. These can include impaired physical and mental health, poor school performance, and job and relationship difficulties. Physical harm can include disability or disfigurement, sexually transmitted diseases, and pregnancy in older children. Extreme stress can disrupt early brain development and can negatively affect the development of the nervous and immune systems. Children who are abused are at much higher risk for health problems as adults. These problems may include alcoholism, depression, drug abuse, eating disorders, obesity, sexual promiscuity, smoking, suicide, and certain chronic diseases (CDC, 2013a).

The abolition of child abuse begins with changing the public's perception of acceptable behavior. In Sweden, for example, corporal punishment of children became outlawed in 1979. Since then, the rate of child injury and violence has decreased in the past decades by nearly 80% in boys and 75% in girls (WHO, 2013). Additionally, creating safe, stable, and nurturing relationships can reduce the occurrence of childhood violence, reduce the negative effects of child abuse, reduce health disparities, and create a positive effect on the child's overall wellness (CDC, 2014c).

> If we have no peace, it is because we have forgotten that we belong to each other.
>
> —*Mother Teresa*

Table 23-1 lists behavioral and physical signs of child abuse. **Box 23-5** provides information for educating parents on protecting their children from abuse. The enactment of "Megan's Law" requires sex offenders to register and notify the community they are residing in, to allow parents the opportunity to protect their children. Some experts are concerned that there is no consistent tool used

BOX 23-4 Key Facts About Child Physical and Sexual Abuse

- Girls are sexually abused three times more often than boys.
- Surveys show at least 20% of women and 5% to 16% of men experienced sexual abuse as children.
- Two percent of all forms of confirmed abuse occurred in daycare or foster care settings.
- The most vulnerable age for sexual abuse is 7 to 13 years.
- Children are mostly abused by adults related to them or known to their families; however, as many as 30% may be by strangers.
- Children are more likely to be physically abused by their fathers than by their mothers, and more severe abuse is committed by men.
- Mothers who are victims of domestic violence are more likely to abuse their children.
- There is a dramatic increase in adolescents who commit sexual aggression against other children.
- Single-parent families and families in poverty are at increased risk of abuse.
- Younger and less educated parents are at greater risk to abuse their children than older or more educated parents.
- Families in which prenatal care was absent or inadequate or in which the mother is depressed are at greater risk.

Sources: Aron, L. Y., & Olsen, K. K. (1997). Efforts by child welfare agencies to address domestic violence. *Public Welfare*, 4–13; Tjaden, P., & Thoennes, N. (2000). *Full report of the prevalence, incidence, and consequences of violence against women: Findings from the National Violence Against Women Survey* (NJC 183721). Washington, DC: National Institute of Justice.

TABLE 23-1 Physical and Behavioral Indicators of Child Abuse

	Physical Indicators	Behavioral Indicators
Physical abuse	Unexplained bruises (in various stages of healing) Unexplained burns, especially cigarette burns or immersion burns Unexplained fractures, lacerations, or abrasions Swollen areas Evidence of delayed or inappropriate treatment for injuries	Self-destructive Withdrawn and/or aggressive, behavioral extremes Arrives at school early or stays late as if afraid to be at home Chronic runaway (adolescents) Complains of soreness or moves uncomfortably Wears clothing inappropriate to weather to cover body Bizarre explanation of injuries Apprehensive when other children cry
Physical neglect	Abandonment Unattended medical needs Consistent lack of supervision Consistent hunger, inappropriate dress, poor hygiene Lice, distended stomach, emaciated Inadequate nutrition	Regularly displays fatigue or listlessness, falls asleep in class Steals food, begs from classmates Reports that no caretaker is at home Frequently absent or tardy Self-destructive School dropout (adolescents) Extreme loneliness and need for affection
Sexual abuse	Sexual abuse may be *nontouching:* obscene language, pornography, exposure; or *touching:* fondling, molesting, oral sex, intercourse Torn, stained, or bloody underclothing Pain, swelling, or itching in genital area Difficulty walking or sitting Bruises or bleeding in genital area Venereal disease Frequent urinary or yeast infections	Withdrawn, chronic depression Excessive seductiveness Role reversal, overly concerned for siblings Poor self-esteem, self-devaluation, lack of confidence Peer problems, lack of involvement Massive weight change Suicide attempts (especially adolescents) Hysteria, lack of emotional control Inappropriate sex play or premature understanding of sex Threatened by physical contact, closeness Unwilling to change clothes in front of anyone Exhibits fantasy or babylike behavior Frequent nightmares High level of unexplained anxiety
Emotional abuse	Emotional abuse may be name-calling, insults, putdowns, etc., or may be terrorization, isolation, humiliation, rejection, corruption, ignoring Speech disorders Delayed physical development Substance abuse Ulcers, asthma, severe allergies	Habit disorder (sucking, rocking, biting) Antisocial, destructive Neurotic traits (sleep disorders, inhibition of play) Passive and aggressive, behavioral extremes Delinquent behavior (especially adolescents) Developmentally delayed Fire setting Cruelty to animals

Sources: Miller, K., & Knutson, T. (1997). Reports of severe physical punishment and exposure to animal cruelty by inmates convicted of felonies and by university students. *Child Abuse and Neglect, 21,* 59–82;

BOX 23-5 Intervention with Parents: Teaching Tips for Child Safety

- Know everything you can about your children's activities and friends. Monitor children's activities and participate with them. Do not allow children to play alone in fields, on playgrounds, or in other dangerous or isolated areas.
- Teach your children about strangers.
- Teach your children to refuse anything from strangers, including money, gifts, and rides. Know where new items come from.
- Teach your children how to safely enter home alone. Teach them how to pretend you are home and how to answer the phone if they are alone.
- Teach your children to keep a safe distance from strangers and not to give strangers directions or help. Adults need to get help from other adults.
- Use secret codes with your children (for use when they may need to positively identify each other or ask for help).
- Do not let your children go to public places, especially restrooms, alone. Develop a family plan stressing where to meet if lost, when you are away from home. Do not have children meet you in the parking lot.
- Do not place your children's names on their clothing or on the outside of their possessions.
- Teach your children to say NO to "touches" on the part(s) of their bodies covered by a swimsuit.
- Teach your children to say NO, to TELL SOMEONE, and to GET AWAY if someone bothers them.
- Join with other concerned parents to set up safety systems for your neighborhood.
- Teach your children about secrets and that some "secrets" have to be told if children and their parents are to be kept safe.

Source: Project SAFE, HISD, and the Child Abuse Prevention Network, Houston, TX.

to establish the perpetrator's risk of re-offending. Each state has the discretion to determine which offenders are subject to registration and notification (Zevitz & Faikas, 2000).

Violence Against the Elderly

The current elder population is the largest in the history of civilization. As our aging population increases, the need for understanding and preventing elder abuse becomes more pressing than ever. In fact, the global population of people age 60 years and older is expected to more than double from 605 million in 2000 to approximately 1.2 billion in 2025 (WHO, 2012). Elder abuse can be compared with child abuse regarding the dependent situation of the victim. Elders who are abused are frail and often mentally or physically impaired. They have a special relationship with and are dependent on a family member or caregiver. Federal definitions of elder abuse, neglect, and exploitation were first used in the 1987 amendments to the Older Americans Act. Categories of abuse include domestic abuse, institutional abuse, self-abuse, and neglect. State statutes define these with various degrees of specificity. As with children, abuse takes the forms of physical, sexual, financial, and emotional abuse; neglect; and abandonment. Elders are also at risk for financial or material exploitation. Abuse can be both unintentional and extensional. Perpetrators are most often family members.

Caring for frail elders can be difficult and stressful. Elders who are mentally or physically impaired are especially needy of special care that the family or caregiver is ill equipped to provide. Skills and resources in the form of family or financial support may be lacking. Increased stress and poor coping combine to lead to stress. The more impaired and dependent the elder is, the greater the likelihood of maltreatment. Adult children who abuse are often dependent on the parent themselves because of their own mental, social, emotional, or financial problems. Abuse signals their response to their own inadequacies. As with other forms of abuse, the learned behavior is passed through the generations as children who were abused learn and reciprocate when a parent becomes vulnerable.

APPLICATION TO PRACTICE 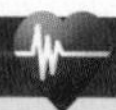

Childhood sexual abuse is a particularly heinous form of violence, with implications for all healthcare workers, especially nurses. Research reveals that the negative symptomatology associated with sexual abuse, such as borderline pathology, behavior problems, depression, suicidal ideation, drug abuse, sexual problems, and self-mutilation attempts, are more frequently reported in sexually than physically abused adolescents.

As nurses, we are in a unique situation not only to report cases of suspected sexual abuse, but also to assist in the treatment of these children. This may include accurate assessment of the victim and family, provision of a safe environment, support of positive coping strategies, as well as monitoring of symptomatology and implementation treatment protocols. In this manner, nurses have an opportunity to be a positive and dynamic force in a potentially devastating situation.

—*Susan Rick, DNS, RN, CNS*

MEDIA MOMENT 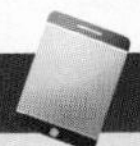

Anger Management (2003)

Overworked and undervalued Dave Buznik is a businessman whose life seems stuck in second gear. His boss would just as well step on him as acknowledge the fact that Dave does all the work while the boss takes the credit. He has a pacifist nature that always gets the best of him, causing him to avoid conflict whenever possible. But matters get worse for Dave when he can't take action and lets everything just sit. When a misunderstanding aboard an airplane lands Dave in court, the only way out is through the therapy of Dr. Buddy Rydell, a psychiatrist and anger management expert. While the unconventional Buddy seems harmful and psychotic, he might just be Dave's only solution to a problem that seriously needs to be addressed. Adam Sandler (Buznik) and Jack Nicholson (Rydell) star in this film.

Often, caregivers are themselves elderly and are unable to care for another.

There are no federal laws providing protective services and shelters for elderly victims, but all 50 states have such legislation. These laws establish guidelines for reporting and investigating suspected abuse and vary widely in terms of age and circumstances for eligibility. In many states, separate laws exist to cover long-term care and other institutions. All states have laws authorizing a long-term care ombudsman program, which is a requirement for receiving federal funds. They are advocates for those residing in long-term care.

Definition and Types of Elder Abuse WHO (2012) states that elder abuse is:

> a single or repeated act, or lack of appropriate action occurring within any relationship where there is an expectation of trust, which causes harm or distress to an older person. Elder abuse can take many forms including physical, psychological, and sexual abuse; financial exploitation; neglect and self-neglect; medication abuse; abandonment; scapegoating; and marginalization of older people in institutions or social and economic policies.

According to the CDC (2013b), 1 in 10 elders reported abuse or maltreatment in the past year. However, elders are often hesitant to report these incidents due to fear that the abuse will continue or become worse, fear that the caretaker will abandon him or her, or fear that the caretaker will face legal ramifications, particularly if the person caring for the elder is a family member or friend.

Risk factors that may increase the potential of elder abuse include (WHO, 2012):

- Individual factors—dementia of elder, mental disorders of elder or caretaker, alcohol or other substance abuse in abuser, gender of victim such as an elderly female widow or cultures in which women have lower social status
- Relational factors—abuser's dependence on elder, history of poor family relations, increased burdens on caretakers
- Sociocultural factors—depiction of elder people as frail, weak, and dependent; erosion of intergenerational bonds; systems of inheritance affecting the distribution of power; migration of young couples, leaving elders alone; lack of funds to pay for elderly care
- Institutional factors—low standards for healthcare and welfare services and facilities, poorly trained and/or overworked staff, policies favoring institutions rather than residents

Because of the lack of data regarding the rate of elder abuse, particularly in nursing homes and other long-term care facilities, it is difficult to properly assess the problem. However, a survey of U.S. nursing home staff indicates rates may be much higher than originally anticipated. According to WHO (2012), 36% of those surveyed witnessed at least one incident of physical abuse of an elderly patient in the previous year. Yet perhaps most concerning is that 10% of those surveyed committed acts of physical violence toward at least one elder patient, and 40% admitted to psychologically abusing their clients.

In an attempt to address and reduce this tragic and unacceptable behavior, the National Adult Protective Services Association (NAPSA, 2013) advocates for the following:

- Accurate and uniform data at both state and national levels to allow trends to be tracked and studied
- Uniform definitions of abuse and standard measures for reporting abuse
- Training on the identification of abuse for potential reporters of abuse, including municipal agents, postal service workers, utility workers, and hospital discharge planners
- Increased number of reports, investigations, and substantiation that may lead to increased local, state, and national interventions and education efforts targeted toward the abuse of older adults

Finally, WHO (2012) recommends the following preventions and interventions to help reduce the risk and rate of elder abuse:

- Screening of potential victims
- Mandatory reporting to authorities

BOX 23-6 Indicators of Elder Abuse

Physical Abuse

- Bruises, black eyes, lacerations, and rope marks
- Bone fractures
- Open wounds and punctures
- Untreated injuries in various stages of healing
- Sprains, dislocations, and internal injuries/bleeding
- Broken eyeglasses/frames
- Physical signs of being subjected to punishment—flinching when approached
- Laboratory findings of medication overdose or underutilization of prescribed drugs
- An elder's report of being hit, slapped, kicked, or mistreated
- An elder's sudden change in behavior
- Caregiver's refusal to allow visitors to see an elder alone

Sexual Abuse

- Bruises around the breasts or genital area
- Unexplained venereal disease or genital infections
- Unexplained vaginal or anal bleeding
- Torn, stained, or bloody underclothing
- An elder's report of being sexually assaulted or raped

Emotional/Psychological Abuse

- Being emotionally upset or agitated
- Being extremely withdrawn and uncommunicative or nonresponsive
- Unusual behavior usually attributed to dementia (e.g., sucking, biting, rocking)
- An elder's report of being verbally or emotionally mistreated

Neglect

- Dehydration, malnutrition, untreated bed sores, or poor personal hygiene
- Unattended or untreated health problems
- Hazardous or unsafe living condition/arrangements (e.g., improper wiring, no heat, or no running water)
- Unsanitary and unclean living conditions (e.g., dirt, fleas, lice on person, soiled bedding, fecal/urine smell, inadequate clothing)
- An elder's report of being mistreated

Abandonment

- The desertion of an elder at a hospital, nursing facility, or other similar institution
- The desertion of an elder at a shopping center or other public location
- An elder's report of being abandoned

Financial or Material Exploitation

- Sudden changes in bank account or banking practice, including an unexplained withdrawal of large sums of money by a person accompanying the elder
- The inclusion of additional names on an elder's bank signature card
- Unauthorized withdrawal of the elder's funds using the elder's ATM card
- Abrupt changes in a will or other financial documents
- Unexplained disappearance of funds or valuable possessions
- Substandard care being provided or bills unpaid despite the availability of adequate financial resources
- Discovery of an elder's signature being forged for financial transactions or for the titles of his or her possessions
- Sudden appearance of previously uninvolved relatives claiming their rights to an elder's affairs and possessions
- Unexplained sudden transfer of assets to a family member or someone outside the family
- The provision of services that are not necessary
- An elder's report of financial exploitation

Source: National Center on Elder Abuse (2008). Frequently asked questions. Retrieved from http://www.ncea.aoa.gov/faq/index.aspx

- Move resources to allotted Adult Protective Services
- Self-help groups for victims and abusers
- Safehouses and emergency shelters for victims
- Caregiver support such as stress management, respite care, and more thorough training

Patterns of Behavior in Family Violence

Many individuals who use violence in their intimate relationships grew up in homes where they saw violence between adults and were abused themselves. Many saw frequent drug abuse by adults. They themselves often abuse alcohol and other drugs. They have little experience with men and women dealing successfully with each other to solve problems nonviolently. They tend to have rigid ideas about men's and women's roles. Many do not use violence outside of the home, and some have no criminal record before a family violence incident. They find approval for their behavior in daily life through media, entertainment, and sports events, as well as from peers.

For batterers, family violence is often a pattern of behaviors directed at a victim. It is not an isolated event. It is a pattern of multiple episodes of a variety of abusive acts, which occur over the course of the familial relationship. In each episode, there is often a buildup of tension, followed by a violent episode, followed by remorse, gifts, and attention. Each episode builds on the last and sets the stage for future events. Some perpetrators use a particular set

BOX 23-7 Examples of Abusive Behaviors Occurring in Families

Physical Abuse: Inflicting injury or illness, withholding necessities of health

- Spitting
- Scratching
- Biting
- Grabbing
- Shaking
- Choking
- Twisting
- Slapping
- Pushing
- Restraining
- Burning
- Punching
- Using weapons
- Inappropriate use of drugs
- Inappropriate use of physical restraint
- Force feeding
- Withholding food, medications, assistive devices

Sexual Abuse: Coercing any sexual contact without consent, undermining sexual identity

- Coerced sex
- Unwanted touching
- Sexual assault or battery
- Rape
- Sodomy
- Coerced nudity
- Sexually explicit photographing
- Forced prostitution
- Undermining sexuality by criticizing desirability

Psychological Abuse: Instilling fear, isolating, undermining sense of self-worth

- Verbal assaults
- Insults
- Threats
- Destruction of pets or property—punching holes in walls
- Intimidation
- Humiliation
- Harassment
- Isolation from family or friends
- Withholding transportation and/or phone access
- Isolation from regular activities
- Silent treatment
- Ongoing accompaniment
- Constant "checking up"
- Restricting entry or exit from home
- Spiritual designation
- Threatening to take the children
- Jealousy

Economic Abuse: Taking funds, making financially dependent

- Cashing checks without authorization
- Forging signature on checks
- Stealing money or possessions
- Deceiving into signing any financial documents
- Improper conservatorship, guardianship, or power of attorney
- Controlling financial resources
- Accumulating bills for which victim is responsible
- Preventing concentration at work by visits or phone calls

of abusive behaviors repeatedly, whereas others use a wide variety of behaviors randomly. These abusive and coercive behaviors take several different forms, including physical, sexual, psychological, and economic. **Box 23-7** provides examples of abusive behaviors occurring in families.

ENVIRONMENTAL CONNECTION

How does the physical environment of schools either promote or decrease violence in school children? What are ways that school nurses can implement primary health strategies in school health programs to decrease the "culture of violence" in today's school system?

Youth Violence

Scope of the Problem

For public healthcare providers, there is growing concern over the victimization and violent behavior of children and youth, which continues to be a source of overwhelming injury, death, and cost. In 2011, for example, more than 700,000 young people 10–24 years of age were treated in EDs for nonfatal injuries sustained from assaults (CDC, 2012b). Youth violence is described as harmful behaviors that can start early and continue into young adulthood. The young people involved can be victims, offenders, or witnesses to the violence. Youth violence includes a wide range of behaviors and actions. Some behaviors,

BOX 23-8 Facts About Youth Violence in the United States

- In 2010, 4,828 young people ages 10 to 24 were murdered—an average of 13 each day.
- Of these homicide victims, 86% were male and 14% were female.
- Homicide is the second leading cause of death for young people ages 10 to 24 years old.
- Of these deaths, 82.8% involved a firearm.
- Homicide rates among non-Hispanic African American males 10 to 24 years of age (51.5 per 100,000) exceed those of Hispanic males (13.5 per 100,000) and non-Hispanic white males (2.9 per 100,000) in the same age group.
- In 2011, 707,212 young people ages 10 to 24 were treated in emergency departments for injuries sustained from violence.

Source: Centers for Disease Control and Prevention. (2012b). *Youth violence facts at a glance.* Retrieved from http://www.cdc.gov/violenceprevention/pdf/yv-datasheet-a.pdf

such as bullying, slapping, or hitting, often cause more emotional harm than physical harm. Other violent acts, such as robbery, assault, or rape can lead to serious injury or even death. Many young people seek medical care for violence-related injuries. Some injuries, like gunshot or stab wounds, can lead to lasting disabilities. Violence can have a powerful effect on the health and wellbeing of entire communities by increasing healthcare costs, decreasing property values, and disrupting social services. The cost of youth violence exceeds $16 billion dollars each year (CDC, 2012b). **Box 23-8** presents further evidence on the problem of youth violence.

School Violence

Schools are increasingly associated with youth violence, including assaults, bullying, shootings, and bomb threats, making violent events against youths at school a growing health concern. Whether children turn their aggression against others or toward themselves, the increasing climate of violence is evident. As the baseline of violence rises, the chance of deadly incidents increases. Society demands that our schools be safe for our children, yet as the NOTE THIS! feature shows, schools are not always safe places. In fact, a 2011 U.S. national survey of youth in grades 9–12 produced alarming results: 20% of those surveyed reported being bullied at school at least once in the previous 12 months, and 16% reported being bullied electronically (via email, chat rooms, websites, or text messages), with results being twice as high for females than for males. Further, 33% admitted to being in a physical fight in the previous 12 months, and a shocking 17% reported carrying a weapon (gun, knife, or club) to school on one or more days in the 30 days preceding the survey (CDC, 2012c). This percentage was almost four times higher for males (26%) than females (6.8%), with 8.6% of surveyed males specifically admitting to bringing a gun to school. Finally, 7% of surveyed students confessed to being threatened or injured with a weapon on school property at least one time in the 12 months preceding the survey, and 6% admitted to skipping school on one or more days in the preceding 30 days because they felt unsafe on the way to and from school or while at school. This demonstrates the prolific nature of youth violence and its impact on student health and performance, illustrating why more must be done to eradicate youth violence (CDC, 2012c).

In recent years, bullying has become a major problem associated with violence in schools. Though universal, bullying behavior did not become a research or policy issue until the late 1990s. The fact that bullied children became revenge killers brought to light the need to address this form of violence (McGee & DeBernardo, 1999). The CDC (2012c) reported the following:

- Young people who bully are more likely to smoke, drink alcohol, get into fights, vandalize property, skip school, and drop out of school.
- Sixty percent of boys who were bullies in middle school had at least one criminal conviction by the age of 24.
- Among the student perpetrators of school-associated homicides, 20% were known to have been victims of bullying.
- 160,000 students go home from school early on any given day because they are afraid of being bullied.

Box 23-9 outlines the risk factors for youth or school violence.

Cyberbullying

Another, more pervasive form of youth violence is **cyberbullying**, also known as electronic bullying. This involves using technology such as email, social media sites, chat rooms, text messages, and websites to harass, intimidate, belittle, and torture another person. Some cyberbullying episodes resulted in suicides by the victims, both male and female, some as young as 12 years of age. Because of the immediacy and spectrum of technology, cyberbullying

BOX 23-9 Risk Factors for Perpetrators of Youth Violence

Individual

- History of violent victimization
- Attention deficit, hyperactivity, or learning disorders
- History of early aggressive behavior
- Association with delinquent peers
- Involvement in gangs
- Involvement with drugs, alcohol, or tobacco
- Low IQ
- Poor academic performance
- Low commitment to school or school failure
- Poor behavioral control
- Deficits in social, cognitive, or information-processing abilities
- High emotional stress
- Antisocial beliefs and attitudes
- Social rejection by peers
- Exposure to violence and conflict in the family
- Lack of involvement in conventional activities

Relationship

- Harsh, lax, or inconsistent disciplinary practices
- Low parental involvement
- Low emotional attachment to parents or caregivers
- Low parental education and income
- Parental substance abuse or criminality
- Poor family functioning (e.g., communication)
- Poor monitoring and supervision of children

Community/Societal

- Diminished economic opportunities
- High concentration of poor residents
- High level of transiency
- High level of family disruption
- Low levels of community participation
- Socially disorganized neighborhoods

Source: Centers for Disease Control and Prevention. (2013d). *Youth violence: Risk and protective factors.* Retrieved from http://www.cdc.gov/violenceprevention/youthviolence/riskprotectivefactors.html

NOTE THIS!

Facts About School Violence in the United States

A nationwide survey during the 2010–2011 school year reported:

- 32.8% of students had been in a physical fight, and 12% had been in a physical fight on school property in the 12 months before the survey.
- 20% of students reported bullying on school property; 16% reported electronic bullying in the 12 months before the survey.
- 7% of teachers reported being threatened with injury or being physically attacked by students.
- 5.4% of students carried a weapon on school property in the 30 days preceding the survey. Weapons included guns, knives, or clubs.
- 7.4% of students were threatened or injured on school property in the 12 months preceding the survey.
- 7.8% of students attempted suicide one or more times in the 12 months preceding the survey.
- 5.9% reported feeling unsafe enough at school or en route to school that they avoided attending one or more days in the 30 days before the survey.
- 25.6% of students were offered, sold, or given an illegal drug on school property in the 12 months preceding the survey.

Source: Centers for Disease Control and Prevention. (2012c). Youth risk behavior surveillance—United States, 2011. *MMWR, Surveillance Summaries, 61*(SS–4). Retrieved from http://www.cdc.gov/mmwr/pdf/ss/ss6104.pdf; Centers for Disease Control and Prevention. (2013c). *Understanding school violence fact sheet.* Retrieved from http://www.cdc.gov/violenceprevention/pdf/school_violence_fact_sheet-a.pdf

THINK ABOUT THIS

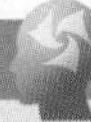

The effects of hate crime on any particular community are not limited to bleeding victims in the ED of the hospital or scenes from school shootings. Why hate crimes? Why now? And what can nurses possibly do to prevent them from occurring?

The significance of hate crimes to the community goes beyond the physical injuries of the victims. If you do not believe that hate crimes affect you and your community, consider the following questions: Did your perception of safety in your school change after the first time you heard about shootings at school? Did it the second? What about the third, and all the times after that? Have you ever changed your behavior in an effort to avoid potential harm that might come to you based on some personal characteristic of yours? Is there anywhere in your community that you avoid because you do not "belong

(*continues*)

THINK ABOUT THIS (*continued*)

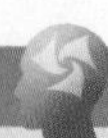

there" and fear that harm would come to you if you went there? These are just a few of the ways that hate crime shapes our perceptions of safety, the ways in which we interact, and our actions toward each other.

Is there anything about you that someone else might not like? Anything about your physical nature: the color of your skin, your gender, any disability? What about your sexual orientation or practices, your ethnic or national origin or that of your family, or your religious practices? Remember, this is not asking about your tolerance of others; this is asking about the potential tolerance of others toward you.

In short, the answer is that there are always people out there who will react negatively toward you based on some personal characteristic of yours. It does not have to be logical, it does not have to be justified, and it does not have to be out in the open.

It is human nature to reject what makes us uncomfortable or what we do not understand and seek the company of others like ourselves. The more positive expression of this tendency is demonstrated within social circles: With common interests or shared characteristics, more can be accomplished as a group. People of the same religious faith gather together to practice that faith and celebrate its tenets, those who share fondness for a sport find others to play with or observe with, and those who share characteristics such as being parents of small children or having the same disability find support and advice in each other's company. Nurses are always being reminded that there is strength in numbers; by joining together, nurses can influence legislation and make changes in the way things are done. People are more powerful in groups.

Neutrality is also possible. An individual may "agree to disagree" with someone else on some point of difference, if there are other points they share. An example of this would be friendship between people of different religious faiths. Neither person is expected to relinquish his or her beliefs; neither one is "right" or "wrong." If they are willing to seek out points of sharing and commonality rather than focus on differences, people from widely differing groups can also share strength and enrich each other's experience. This is a true expression of tolerance: acceptance of others based not on their similarity to oneself, but on the merits of their own characteristics.

The dark side of this aspect of human nature emerges when the characteristics of one's own group are considered the only correct ones. It is not enough to associate with others like oneself. Those who are different are less trustworthy, dangerous, less human. The discomfort felt when in the presence of someone different from this "norm" leads to action against that individual. Those who are different must be kept out, moved away, eliminated. There are untold millions of examples of this intolerance in human history; all people, of all cultures, share in this inheritance.

This is the origin of hate crimes. One of the aphorisms of Hippocrates is, "Of two pains existing at the same time, but not in the same place, the stronger obscures the other." Hatred in this case is the stronger pain, drawing attention from its quieter companions, fear of the other, fear of the unknown, fear of what is different.

This fear is intolerable, and the reaction of the individual is hatred for the thing that has caused this discomfort. The hatred is louder, obscuring the existence of the fear, but the fear is there.

At present, the federal statute regarding hate crimes is 18 U.S.C. §245, which covers the threat, attempt to use, or use of force to injure, intimidate, or interfere with "any person because of his race, color, religion, or national origin" who is participating in one of six federally protected activities. These are (1) enrolling in or attending a public school or public college; (2) participating in or enjoying a service, program, facility, or activity provided or administered by any state or local government; (3) applying for or enjoying employment; (4) serving in a state court as a grand or petit juror; (5) traveling in or using a facility of interstate commerce; and (6) enjoying the goods or services of certain places of public accommodation.

The Hate Crimes Prevention Act of 1999 eliminates the "federally protected activities" requirement because some cases that have satisfied juries as to bias motivation had to be dismissed because the victims were not involved in one of the six protected activities. This act also adds gender, perceived or actual sexual orientation, and disability to the list of bias motivations. Other attempts at legislation with similar intent were the Violent Crime Control and Law Enforcement Act of 1994 and the Bias Crimes Compensation Act of 1993, neither of which made it into law.

Are you surprised? Many members of the public assume that any crime motivated by bias can be prosecuted as a hate crime; with a vague sense that there are "hate crime laws," they believe the issue to be closed. There are also misperceptions of the purpose of hate crimes legislation.

If bias against a certain religion is the motivation for killing someone, is the victim any less dead than if the action had taken place during a robbery? Aren't they both murder, which is against laws that already exist? Is it less heinous if the victim was at home rather than participating in one of the six federally protected activities? Is it more wrong to kill someone who is in one group than someone who is in another? Why should the motivation for the act or the identity of the victim make any difference in the prosecution? The answers are: no, yes, no, no, and please pay attention, because that comes next.

Burt Neuborne, the John Norton Pomeroy Professor of Law at the New York University School of Law, testified before the Senate on May 11, 1999, in support of the Hate Crimes Prevention

Act of 1999 (S. 622). He stated, "The First Amendment does not protect violence merely because it is motivated by hatred. No principle of First Amendment law shields a violent offender against increased punishment because the crime was motivated by group hatred." The two things to note here are "increased punishment" and "group hatred." Remember the nature of prejudice: Another group of people is perceived as a threat. Neuborne contended that the heavier penalties for hate crimes would act as a deterrent against activities of hate and that hate crimes legislation would have "educational value" because it singles out the unacceptability of organized bias crimes. Murder is a crime; the perpetrator should be punished. But if the murder is part of the program of a hate group, should that group not also be punished? What if the murderer is not a member of a hate group but singles out victims with certain characteristics?

The victims of random crime are no less valuable than the victims of hate crime; that is not the reason different penalties are sought. The reason that hate crimes are different from other crimes is that existing laws punish random actions, while hate crime laws seek to punish organized activities of hate, whether they are the actions of hate groups or of individuals.

Nurses can have an effect on hate crimes and the communities they damage. The politics of difference can have a chilling effect on the pursuit of justice; by authoring or monitoring legislation, nurses can promote politics of equity. The 104th Congress asked the Library of Congress to make federal legislative information available via the Internet. Beginning in January 1995, this information has been available through Thomas, a service of the Library of Congress. This is one online source that should remain current for many years to come; the URL is http://thomas.loc.gov. By using this resource, nurses can follow the progress of federal legislation.

Nurses can also work to promote tolerance in their communities. If fear is the basis for prejudice, then understanding and information are the countermeasures. This is not something that can be imposed from outside. Peace comes from partnering with the community. It is important to respect the concerns of the members of the community and help them to move toward their own acceptance and tolerance of others. To that end, I offer this quotation from C. S. Lewis:

> For every one pupil who needs to be guarded from a weak excess of sensibility there are three who need to be awakened from the slumber of cold vulgarity. The task of the modern educator is not to cut down jungles but to irrigate deserts. The right defence against false sentiments is to inculcate just sentiments. By starving the sensibility of our pupils we only make them easier prey to the propagandist when he comes. For famished nature will be avenged and a hard heart is no infallible protection against a soft head (p. 27, *The Abolition of Man*).

Written for educators in 1944, this is relevant for nurses working with the community now; fear and mistrust have created deserts that separate people from each other, and the apathy that grips the population must be akin to the slumber of which Lewis wrote. Promoting tolerance of diversity and providing learning opportunities form the best protection against hard hearts; the "soft heads" will never be any less soft until efforts are made to improve the situation.

—Regina Hood Posey, RN, MSN

is not restricted to in-person contact and can therefore occur any time, day or night. Unlike traditional bullying, it can be anonymous and therefore difficult to track. Another consequence of this for the victim, aside from increased fear and paranoia, is the extreme difficulties in removing the messages or images from the Internet. In recent years, media outlets have highlighted a number of instances in which cyberbullying involved posting embarrassing photos or videos of individuals engaged in alcohol use or sexual situations—including cases of outright rape or gang-rape.

With the significant increase in technology over the past few decades, it is easy to see how electronic bullying can be so prevalent in our culture. Sixty-nine percent of teens own a computer or smartphone, and of those, 80% are active on social media sites, with 7.5 million Facebook users under the age of 13 years. Technology is now integrated into children's lives earlier than ever, with 1 in 3 children ages 3–5 years using the Internet every day, and 1 of every 2 U.S. children ages 6 to 9 having daily Internet access. Further, teens send an average of 60 texts per day. As the use of technology has continued to grow, so have suicide rates in children; from 1985 to 2007, suicides in girls ages 15–19 rose by 32%; even more disturbing, the rate in girls 10–14 years old rose 76% (Patchin & Hinduja, 2013). This demonstrates the importance of monitoring tech use in children.

The CDC's 2011 youth risk survey (CDC, 2012c) found 16% of high school students (grades 9–12) were electronically bullied in the past year; a review of multiple other studies suggests the rate is more accurately placed at about 21% (Patchin & Hinduja, 2013). Studies also show that bullied students are twice as likely to commit suicide than non-bullied children, and that 1 in 5 students who have been cyber-bullied contemplate suicide, with 1 in 10 actually attempting to kill themselves. According to stopbullying.gov, a website of the HHS (2013), students who are bullied electronically are also more likely to:

- Use alcohol/drugs
- Skip school
- Be bullied in person
- Receive poor grades
- Have low self-esteem
- Have more health problems

In fact, 3 million students are absent from school each month in the United States because they fear bullying, and yet only about two in five victims of cyberbullying will report this abuse to their parents or guardians. Witnesses of electronic bullying are also highly unlikely to report the abuse: 90% of surveyed teens who witnessed online bullying say they ignore it. Therefore, it is the responsibility of parents and guardians, faculty members, and healthcare providers to ask children if they are experiencing any form of bullying, and to provide support while putting a stop to the bullying, recruiting the help of law enforcement if necessary. Doing so may save a life.

NOTE THIS!

A 2013 cyberbullying survey that canvassed more than 10,000 persons 13–22 years of age (average age 16 years) found:

- 7 in 10 have been victims of cyberbullying
- 37% experience cyberbullying on a highly frequent basis
- 20% are experiencing extreme cyberbullying on a daily basis
- Young males and females are at equal risk of cyberbullying
- Young people are twice as likely to be cyber-bullied on Facebook than on any other social network
- 54% of young people using Facebook reported that they have experienced cyberbullying on the network
- Facebook, Ask.FM, and Twitter were found to be the most likely sources of cyberbullying
- Cyberbullying has catastrophic effects upon the self-esteem and social lives of up to 70% of young people

Source: Ditchthelabel.org. (2013). The annual cyberbullying survey. Retrieved from http://www.ditchthelabel.org/downloads/the-annual-cyberbullying-survey-2013.pdf

Gangs

The growth of youth gangs in the past decades is a major concern, especially with the expansion of gang activity in rural and suburban communities and in cities where gangs did not previously exist. A 2008 survey found that 32.4% of all cities, suburban areas, towns, and rural areas in over 3,300 jurisdictions experienced gang problems, an increase of 15% from 2002 (Egley, Howell, & Moore, 2010). Larger cities and suburban counties have seen the greatest rise in activity, but rural areas are not immune. As gangs migrate across the country, they bring with them drugs, weapons, and criminal activity. In recent years, gangs have become more sophisticated and aggressive in their use of violence and intimidation practices. They threaten our schools, our children, and our homes. As gang members relocate, they establish new branches of their gang in the new locale, bringing gang activity to areas without previous gang activity or entering into deadly conflict with local gangs (Bureau of Justice Assistance, 2005).

Gangs are the primary distributors of illicit drugs throughout the United States and around the world. Gang members have become efficient in their use of computers and technology. Devices such as cell phones, navigation systems (e.g., GPS), and laptop computers, are being used to communicate, facilitate criminal activity, and avoid detection by law enforcement. In some communities, colors, tattoos, and outward acknowledgment of gang membership are less visible as gangs try to hide from law enforcement. In other communities, gang affiliation is flaunted as an intimidation weapon, or gangs are uniting to facilitate stronger networks for criminal activity. Often, community leaders refuse to acknowledge that gang activity exists. Community denial of gang activity is a gang's greatest ally (Bureau of Justice Assistance, 2005).

New immigrant populations in the United States are vulnerable to gang formation because immigrants are often isolated in communities because of language and employment difficulties. Hispanic gangs flourish as a means of providing their communities with support and protection. Asian gangs, however, often victimize Asian communities, as the community members may be less likely to report crimes to police (Bureau of Justice Assistance, 2005).

Gun Control

Firearms are the second leading cause of traumatic death in the United States and the second leading cause of death overall for Americans ages 15 to 24. In 2010, 4,828 young people in America 10 to 24 years old were victims of homicide, an average of 13 children per day. Of those, 83% were killed with a firearm (CDC, 2012b). For every gun-related death there are nearly three nonfatal gun injuries treated in EDs each year (Violence Policy Center, 2008). This results in an estimated $16 billion per year in combined medical and

BOX 23-10 Highlights of the National Crime Victimization Survey

- Firearm-related homicides declined 39%, from 18,253 in 1993 to 11,101 in 2011.
- Nonfatal firearm crimes declined 69%, from 1.5 million victimizations in 1993 to 467,300 victimizations in 2011.
- Firearm violence accounted for about 70% of all homicides and less than 10% of all nonfatal violent crime from 1993 to 2011.
- From 1993 to 2011, about 70% to 80% of firearm homicides and 90% of nonfatal firearm victimizations were committed with a handgun.
- Males, blacks, and persons ages 18 to 24 had the highest rates of firearm homicide from 1993 to 2010.
- About 61% of nonfatal firearm violence was reported to the police from 2007–2011.

Source: Planty, M., & Truman, J. L. (2013). Firearm violence, 1993–2011. U.S. Department of Justice/Bureau of Justice Statistics. Retrieved from http://www.bjs.gov/content/pub/pdf/fv9311.pdf

work loss costs (CDC, 2012b). In addition to smoking and drinking, owning and using firearms have become a part of youthful experimentation. Ease of access has contributed to the situation, and interest in public policy on gun control has become more intense. It is notable that this reality comes *despite* significant improvement in the national rate of firearm violence between 1993 and 2011 (see **Box 23-10**).

The United States is losing too many children to gun violence. Each year, more children and teens die from gunfire than from cancer, pneumonia, influenza, asthma, and HIV/AIDS combined. In a single year, at least 3,000 children and teens are killed by gunfire in the United States. That is one child every 3 hours, eight children every day, and more than 50 children every week. In addition, four to five times as many children and teens suffer from nonfatal firearm injuries each year. American children are more at risk from firearms than the children of any other industrialized nation. In one year, firearms killed no children in Japan, 19 in Great Britain, 57 in Germany, 109 in France, 153 in Canada, and 5,285 in the United States. American children are 16 times more likely to be murdered with a gun, 11 times more likely to commit suicide with a gun, and 9 times more likely to die from a gun accident than children in 25 other industrialized nations combined (National Education Association [NEA], 2005).

The NEA submitted a letter to Vice President Biden on reducing gun violence on January 4, 2013 after 20-year-old Adam Lanza opened fire in Sandy Hook Elementary School in Sandy Hook, CT, killing 20 children and 6 staff members on December 14, 2012. This tragedy was the second deadliest mass shooting in American history, following the Virginia Tech Massacre in 2007.

According to the National Association of Mental Health Program Directors, states cut $4.35 billion in public mental health spending from 2009–2012. However, despite multiple school shootings and attempts following the Sandy Hook tragedy, the U.S. government has not yet passed any new legislation in an effort to prevent such devastating events from occurring.

When a gun is present in a home, the risk of homicide and suicide is greatly increased for those residing there. In 2001, 55% of suicides were committed with a firearm (Anderson & Smith, 2003). Some studies indicate that increased concentration of firearms (indicated by permits issued, new sales, or surveys of ownership) is associated with increased firearm robbery, assault, and homicide. Both the ANA and the American Public Health Association have been long-time advocates for policy proposals to decrease access to guns.

Dating Violence

Dating violence is defined as physical, sexual, or psychological violence within a dating relationship (CDC, 2006a, 2006b, 2013). Dating violence is a serious problem in the United States, because 72% of teens are already dating by the time they are in the 8th and 9th grades. Many adolescents do not report dating violence because they are afraid to tell friends and family. But the fact is that teens experience dating abuse more often than other age groups. According to the CDC, one in four adolescents experience verbal, physical, emotional, or sexual abuse each year, and one in 11 have been physically hurt by someone they were dating. Among teens, boys often start the violence and use greater force. Girls are more likely than boys to

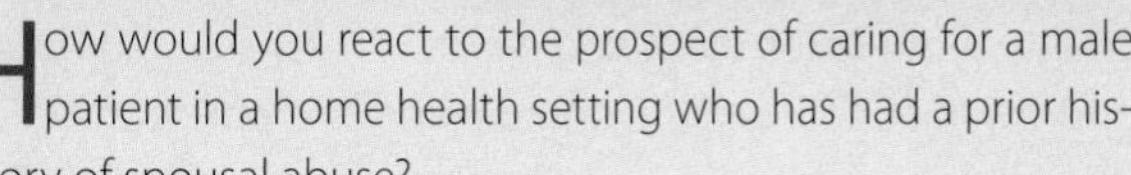

How would you react to the prospect of caring for a male patient in a home health setting who has had a prior history of spousal abuse?

be victims of sexual abuse. Studies show that teens who abuse their dating partners are more depressed, have lower self-esteem, and are more aggressive than peers (CDC, 2006c, 2013d).

Dating violence has a negative effect on health throughout life. Teens who experience dating violence are more likely to do poorly in school and often engage in unhealthy behaviors like drug and alcohol abuse. The anger and stress that victims feel may lead to depression, eating disorders, and even suicide. Abused high school students are three times more likely than their nonabused peers to experience dating violence later in college or the workplace. In adulthood, they are more likely to be involved in IPV (CDC, 2006c, 2013d).

Teens need to understand that we can only change what we can acknowledge. A forum is needed where teens can learn facts about dating violence and practice resistance skills. The idea that oral sex is not sex has influenced the decision-making skills of youths as young as in middle school. Both sexes need to have knowledge of the deleterious consequences resulting from the present culture of permissiveness. Studies have shown that early maturation can place women at risk because they become targets for older youth (Wiesner & Ittel, 2002). Nurses can support parents in their pivotal role in helping their teen-aged children postpone sexual activity and decrease their risk of rape by making wise choices about alcohol and drugs and avoiding physical intimacy when dating or with friendly acquaintances.

Suicide

Suicide is the 11nth leading cause of death in the United States. Although suicide occurs in all age groups, it is the second leading cause of death among 25–34 year olds and the third leading cause of death among 15–24 year olds (CDC, 2007b, 2012c). More than 90% of suicides in the United States are among whites. Gay and lesbian youth are two to three times more likely to commit suicide, pointing to issues of sexual identity and experienced abuse as risk factors for suicide (Van Wormer, Wells, & Boes, 2000). Males take their own lives at nearly four times the rate of females, although women attempt suicide two to three times as often as men (Levay & Valente, 2003). Firearms are the most commonly used method of suicide among males, while poisoning is the most common method for women (CDC, 2007b).

In addition to prevention efforts to screen and counsel those at risk for suicide, nurses will be involved with the families and friends of those who both succeed and fail at suicide attempts. Families and friends experience anger and guilt over the suicide event and often are unable to discuss it. Nurses intervene during the immediate shock phase and assist with the eventual integration of the event into the survivors' lives.

Causes of Youth Violence

The theories on causation of youth violence are similar to those cited earlier for violence in general and to family violence. The focus with youth is on the early development of aggressive behavior and the tendencies for it to be exhibited at earlier ages. The escalation of violence may, as proposed earlier, be due to societal factors that have made youth aggression more destructive than in the past (see Box 23-9). Easy access to handguns is also a factor. A second strong social factor is the increasing violence in the media. Television, movies, and video games have been declared culprits. Technology such as the Internet and satellite and cable television gives children greater access to a wide range of violent images.

Research studies indicate a strong correlation between television violence and violent behavior, both immediately and long term (Huesmann & Taylor, 2006). The critical period for lasting harm is childhood. The American Academy of Pediatrics (2013) recommends that parents limit television watching to 1 or 2 hours daily and keep televisions out of children's bedrooms and suggests a "family home use plan" for all media. Exposure to violent video games is associated with a decrease in empathy (Funk, Baldacci, Pasold, & Baumgardner, 2004). Cultural norms,

MEDIA MOMENT

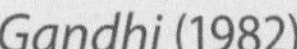

Gandhi (1982)

This film describes the life and times of Mahatma Gandhi, the Indian political leader who managed to free his country from British rule using peaceful means, giving hope and inspiration for generations to come. This epic won eight Academy Awards.

THINK ABOUT THIS

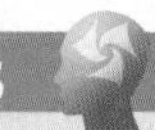

Gun Control

Nurses debate the question: Are tighter gun control restrictions the answer to the epidemic of violence in schools, workplaces, and communities?

Yes

There is some truth in the slogan, "Guns don't kill people, people kill people"; nevertheless, people without access to guns are more often than not stymied in their murderous impulses, whether those impulses arise from a distorted perception of reality or from evil. Of course, a substantive cure for the epidemic of violence in our country includes meaningful employment for all, better mental health programs, warm and welcoming families for all children, improved educational systems, increased serenity, and the uprooting of all forms of bigotry. But while we as people are struggling to bring all these about, ought we not, at the very least, do what is within our immediate grasp? It is within our current legislative and enforcement power to (1) make illegal the sale and possession of those particular guns for which the purpose is to kill lots of people quickly; (2) make the ownership of all guns as traceable as that of the automobile; and (3) disqualify for gun ownership persons who have committed felonies or given evidence of potential harm to themselves or to others. For reasons of public health and the common good we restrict entry into school for children who have not been immunized. It seems only common sense that we also restrict the possession of firearms in an effort to control the public health menace of easy killing.

—Mary Margaret Mooney, DNSc, ARNP, FAAN, Dubuque, Iowa

No

I do not believe that tighter gun control restriction is the answer to the epidemic of violence in our schools, workplaces, and communities. I do not believe the answer is that simple. Violence in our society is a multilevel problem. We need to start with education at an early age to help our children deal with anger. Our children today are taught to handle their anger with violence, as evidenced in modern television, movies, and video games. The average child lacks the skills to deal with his or her frustrations. Television and movies show adults being rude and nasty to others, and this is perceived as being funny. Hitting and fighting back (getting revenge) are displayed as the right thing to do. We need to educate our children to respect others. Parents of today are often overwhelmed with material concerns and lack the energy to teach their children respect of others. Other concerns are seen as more important. Education regarding respect for others is needed at a young age, as well as how to deal with one's anger. Proper channeling of one's frustration will help prevent some of the violence in our society today. We, as healthcare providers, should stress the importance of stress management for our patients. We should also write our legislators to give our opinion of the violence on television and in the movies. We need to change the way our society views aggression and seek ways to help the public deal with it.

—Daria Napierkowski, MSN, RN, Stanhope, New Jersey

Source: Kaleidoscope. (1999). *The American Nurse, 31*(5), 4.

group norms, and family characteristics also are important in determining the effects of media violence on children's aggressive behavior. Violent portrayals most likely to influence behavior are those that show social approval, result in reward, are perceived as real, and are fast paced (Jason, Hanaway, & Brackshaw, 1999). The industry has taken steps to solve some of these issues, with rating of media and blocking options. These steps, however, only regulate content; they do not improve the material viewed by children. Parents must still play a large role and need assistance in understanding the industry classifications of films and videos and obtaining information on film and game content. They must be encouraged to monitor both the time spent and the content of viewing by children (Jason et al., 1999).

Workplace Violence

Although concerned about those who are victims of violence, nurses are increasingly aware of their own vulnerability in the workplace. Workplace violence, like domestic violence, is not new but has been hidden by much denial. It is an emerging field of study. Workplace violence exists on a continuum from verbal abuse to physical assault to homicide. It includes homicide, beatings, rape, assault, battery, theft, robbery, threats, harassment, and intimidation (McClure, 1999; Occupational Safety and Health Administration [OSHA], 2002).

Sexual harassment is one of the most common forms of workplace violence. This can include unwelcome sexual advances, requests for sexual favors, and other verbal or physical harassment. Both victims and harassers may be male or female, and they can be the same sex. The costs of sexual harassment include:

- Sick leave and time away from both one's office and workplace
- Decreased productivity
- Increased job turnover through quitting, firing, and transfers
- Legal fees
- Health consequences—sleep difficulties, depression and/or anxiety, PTSD, drug/alcohol use, weight-related problems
- Poor staff morale
- Damaged company reputation

Though sexual harassment is one of the most discussed forms of on-the-job violence, homicide is among the most pervasive. Nurses face violence from coworkers, patients, and patients' family and friends. Risk factors that increase the chance of injury to healthcare workers include the prevalence of guns and other weapons among patients or their visitors, the increased use of hospitals by the criminal justice system for criminal holds and acute care of violent individuals, the increased number of acute and chronically mentally ill patients being released from the hospital without proper follow up, low staffing levels, isolated work with patients, and a lack of training in recognizing escalating hostile behavior and proper safety and de-escalation techniques (Emergency Nurses Association, 2011).

Perpetrators of violence can be frustrated or threatened coworkers, random thieves, or disgruntled patients. An average of 20 people a week are murdered while working, and it is estimated that 2 million more are assaulted annually. Retail establishments open at night have the highest rates of homicide. According to the estimates of the Bureau of Labor Statistics (BLS), in 2012, nonfatal injuries stemming from intentional violence by another person occurred among nursing assistants at a rate of 30.4 per 10,000 workers. This rate is much higher than the rate of 7.2 per 10,000 nonfatal violence-related injuries for all private-sector industries workers (BLS, 2012). In 2009, more than 50% of emergency center nurses experienced violence by patients on the job. There were 2,050 assaults and violent acts reported by registered nurses (RNs) requiring an average of 4 days away from work. Of these acts, 1,830 resulted in injuries inflicted by patients or residents (Emergency Nurses Association, 2011).

Patients are most often responsible for these assaults, but their friends and family members can also be violent. Jobs in health care, education, and social services are the settings at highest risk of violence for women. The leading cause of occupational death for women is violence. These statistics show that nurses are a population at particular risk for workplace violence.

Some risk factors are the same for all work settings and include an increasingly violent society, availability of handguns and other weapons, and high-crime neighborhoods. Also included for all work settings are organizational characteristics such as negative management practices; a culture at work that creates pressure for performance; poor staffing, hiring, and retention practices; and increased diversity in the workforce, which can create conflict over differences (McClure, 1999; OSHA, 2002). Parents should monitor the workplaces of their children, because certain jobs, such as convenience store clerk, may be subject to robbery or even murder.

Risk factors specific to nursing situations include the presence of money and drugs, working alone as well as on nights and holidays, poorly lit parking lots, and open exits and entrances. Untrained security guards can add to escalating interactions or fail to respond in a timely manner. EDs and psychiatric units are two of the highest risk work areas for nurses. Also, reduced staffing levels and sicker patients with shorter lengths of stay increase the frustration levels of patients and families. The release of more acutely and chronically ill patients has increased the number of potentially dangerous patients in community health settings and EDs.

On October 28, 2002, three nursing professors at the University of Arizona were murdered in full view of their students, by a nursing student. Subsequently, protocols for identifying and intervening with at-risk-for-violence students were developed (Stauffer, 2002).

DAY IN THE LIFE

Nurses care for victims of violence, perpetrators, and witnesses to violent acts. The experiences of nurses who care for those affected by violence in many parts of the world point out the pervasive nature of violence. In addition, nurses themselves are at risk for violence in their personal lives, in their communities and, unfortunately, in their places of work. Violence in nursing is seldom discussed, and if it is, it is in hushed tones and with a "thank goodness it is not me" sentiment. Nurses care for and about others. It's why you are a nurse; it's why I am a nurse. We are courageous, but we don't have to suffer indignities or harm to do our jobs. All we need is respect for our professional work and to be safe. It is little enough to ask.

—Eleanor J. Sullivan, RN, PhD, FAAN, President, Sigma Theta Tau, International Nursing, Honor Society of Nursing, 1999–2000

Source: Sullivan, E. J. (1999). President's message, *Reflections, 25*(3), 4.

NOTE THIS!

The United States leads the industrialized world in the number of homicides per capita. In 2011, the rate of U.S. homicides was 4.7 per 100,000, compared to 1.6 in Canada, 1.2 in the United Kingdom, and 0.8 in Germany. Japan's rate of homicide is less than 10% of the U.S. rate. At the same time, the United States also has one of the highest rates of incarceration in the world, both among industrialized nations and developing countries, estimated at 707 per 100,000.

Sources: International Centre for Prison Studies. (2014). *World prison brief: Highest to lowest.* Retrieved from http://www.prisonstudies.org/highest-to-lowest

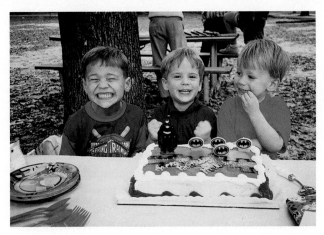

Male children raised in the United States embrace action figures who often use violence to triumph over their foes.

Posttraumatic Stress Disorder (PTSD)

After experiencing a traumatic event, a patient is immediately assessed for any physical damage. However, far too frequently there is no psychological assessment. Yet PTSD can occur with any traumatic event. This is a reaction of "fight or flight" that persists more than 30 days after the threat has been removed. Though the disorder is commonly associated with war veterans, PTSD can result from physical or sexual assault, stalking, mugging, car accidents, natural disasters, child abuse, train wrecks, plane crashes, or any other violent event (National Institute of Mental Health [NIMH], 2014). PTSD is fairly common, with one in 30 adults suffering from this condition each year (NIMH, 2014). Therefore, nurses should address the possibility of developing PTSD with all patients who have endured a traumatic event. Further, the person who experiences PTSD may be the one who was exposed to the threat, a witness of the event, or even a loved one of the person who was present for the trauma.

When faced with terror or danger, the parts of the brain responsible for less critical body functions (memory, emotion, and reasoning processes) are essentially turned off. This allows the body to use all energy for survival, such as increasing the heart rate to supply more blood to the muscles, allowing the body to run faster, and an increase in the amount of stress hormones released to help fight infection and stop bleeding in case of a wound. These prevent traumatic experiences from being properly processed in the brain. People living with PTSD are less able to access these experiences, because the normal functions of emotion remain deeply affected by the event (National Alliance on Mental Illness [NAMI], 2011). Further, research has shown that experiencing trauma can change the way our brains function, particularly with severe or repeated exposure. This may create scenarios in which a person can feel the event is reoccurring again and again (NAMI, 2011).

Symptoms Symptoms generally begin to appear directly after the event or trauma, but may take many months or years to surface. They may also wax and wane over several years. The *Diagnostic and Statistical Manual of Mental Disorders, 5th Edition* (DSM-V) criteria require the symptoms to be active for at least 1 month after the event, including a decline in areas of normal functioning such as occupational, social, emotional, or psychical (NAMI, 2011).

According to NAMI (2011), there are three categories of symptoms for PTSD. A person may experience one or more of the following:

1. Persistent re-experiencing—recurrent flashbacks or nightmares, recurring and pervasive images or memories of the event, intense distress toward reminders of the trauma, physical reactions to triggers that resemble or symbolize the event
2. Avoidance/numbness responses—efforts to avoid feelings/triggers associated with the trauma, including places, people, or activities that serve as a reminder, inability to recall important aspects of the event, feelings of detachment or estrangement from others, restricted range of feelings, difficulty thinking about or preparing for long-term future because the person doesn't believe he or she will be alive for a normal lifespan
3. Hyperarousal responses—difficulties falling or staying asleep, outbursts of anger or irritability, difficulties concentrating, exaggerated startle response

Numbing and avoidance techniques are associated with a worse and prolonged prognosis.

People with PTSD also often suffer from other conditions simultaneously, including depression, anxiety, sleep disorders, and substance abuse. Research shows that 21–43% of people with PTSD will develop a long-term substance abuse problem, compared to 8–25% of the general population (NAMI, 2011).

Triggers Triggers are anything that reminds the person of the event. These can be difficult to identify, and may change throughout a person's lifetime as more memories of the trauma are uncovered. Examples may include particular scents such as perfume or deodorants, a specific make and model of a car, the amount of lighting (such as candlelight), shouting or yelling, an article of clothing, a watch or other jewelry, or certain weather conditions. Often people suffering from PTSD do not expect certain triggers to have an effect on their physical and mental state. Seeking help through therapy may help people living with PTSD to identify and address their triggers in an attempt to regain power and control in their lives and conquer their fears.

Children and PTSD Because of a child's growing brain, traumatic events during childhood and adolescence have a profound impact on their developing mind, body, and sense of self and security. Children can carry these negative effects of trauma well into their adult lives. One major cause of PTSD in children is child abuse. More than 1 million reports of child abuse/neglect are received by Child Protective Services each year in the United States. Children who experience chronic physical, sexual, or emotional abuse are at a much greater risk of developing PTSD, and struggle in many areas of their lives (NAMI, 2011).

Due to the transitory nature of a child's brain, symptoms of PTSD are often expressed differently than in adults. According to NAMI (2011), these can include:

- Difficulties regulating emotions
- Difficulties establishing and maintaining relationships
- Inability to control aggression
- Low self-esteem and poor performance in school
- High rates of substance abuse throughout their lifetime
- Increased risk of developing psychiatric illnesses throughout their lifetime, including borderline personality disorder, dissociative disorder, and eating disorders well into adulthood

Gender and PTSD Studies suggest women experience PTSD at more than twice the rate of men. This may be due to several factors, including the increased likelihood women will experience a traumatic event such as stalking, physical abuse, sexual abuse, psychological abuse, or rape. Also, research suggests men are much less likely to admit to or discuss symptoms of PTSD. A survey of male troops in Iraq and Afghanistan found a correlation between PTSD and exposure to combat. Yet of those who met the criteria for diagnosis, only 38–45% expressed interest in receiving help. This was due to fear of being treated differently, fear of retaliation, and fear of appearing weak (NAMI, 2011). However, another study suggests women in the military were more than twice as likely to develop PTSD symptoms than their male counterparts. Again, the increased risks of women suffering sexual harassment is believed to play a large role (NAMI, 2011). More research is needed to determine whether there are gender differences that influence a person's risk of experiencing PTSD.

Treatment The first step in the treatment of PTSD is for nurses and other healthcare professionals to warn at-risk patients of the signs and symptoms of PTSD upon treatment of the initial trauma. Educating the patient on possible symptoms will allow him or her to understand what to look for, what are "normal" and "abnormal" responses to the trauma, and therefore seek help sooner.

Group therapy, psychotherapy, and cognitive behavioral therapy have all been shown to be useful forms of treatment. Medications, such as mood stabilizers, beta blockers, and sleep aids may be used to supplement therapy to help reduce anxiety, depression, and sleep problems. Service dogs are also becoming increasingly common forms of treatment, particularly for veterans. These animals can not only provide a form of pet therapy; they also can serve as social buffers, encourage exercise, and be a great de-escalation tool in times of stress, giving the brain a break from hypervigilance. Finally, comprehensive and alternative techniques, such as yoga, aquatic therapies, and meditation, are becoming popular forms of treatment for people with PTSD (NAMI, 2011).

Resilience Not all who experience traumatic events will develop PTSD. It is therefore just as important to study those who are resilient as those who are in need of treatment. The following have been shown to reduce the likelihood of developing PTSD and/or reduce the frequency and intensity of symptoms, and should be encouraged by healthcare professionals (NAMI, 2011):

- Being open about and accepting of the trauma
- Seeking support from friends and family
- Finding a support group
- Feeling good about one's own actions while facing danger
- Having or developing healthy coping strategies

Mass Violence and War

Modern nursing was born in the battlefields of the Crimean War when Florence Nightingale revolutionized the care of the soldiers in that battle. History since that time has been marked by continuous instances in which nurses have served the wounded in battle. Nursing also has a history of peace activism among its historical leaders (Temkin, 1997). It has only been in the very recent past that public health professionals, including nurses, have begun to view the violence of war as a proper social ill to address in the public health model of prevention. When violence was first recognized as a public health issue in the 1980s, very little was written in public health literature on the violence of war. Groups of health professionals did have divisions of professional organizations or independent groups that had a special interest in peace, but war was not brought to the forefront until more recently.

Levy and Sidel (1997) introduced the first comprehensive examination of the relationship between war and public health. They documented the public health consequences of war, roles of health professionals, and prevention interventions. There have been cautions in social science literature about the overextension of preventive health measures to inappropriate areas, or the inappropriate role of health sciences (usually referring to medicine) as the "social guardian of morality." However, there seems to be a growing number who believe that identifying risks, developing interventions to lower risk, and implementing the interventions are possible for war. Conscious steps can be taken to measure and reduce the risk of arms, mass violence, and conflict (Foege, 1997). Mass violence of war can be claimed as a legitimate inclusion on community health prevention agendas. Amnesty International and Human Rights Watch, for example, investigate and monitor for suffering and abuse in people across the world.

MEDIA MOMENT

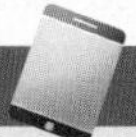

A History of Violence (2005)

In Millowbrook, Indiana, mild-mannered Tom Stall owns a diner and has a calm life with his beloved wife Edie Stall, his teenage son Jack, and his little daughter Sarah. His life turns upside down when he kills two cold-blooded killers in his diner to protect his waitress, becoming a local hero and being shown on the front page of the newspaper and on TV. The mobster Carl Fogarty comes to the town calling Tom "Joey Cusack" and telling everyone that he was a former hitman. When Carl and his men threaten his family, Tom defends them, and violence is released in a chain reaction.

Epidemiology of War

The health consequences of war are both direct and indirect. **Box 23-11** details major health consequences of warfare. Nightingale is recognized as the first to do statistical analyses on the management of mass casualties during war (Nightingale, 1954). In recent decades, rates of mortality attributable to war have risen. World War II caused the death of 3% of the world's population of the time. The former Soviet Union lost 10% of its population in that war and the United States lost 0.3%. The number of civilian deaths in war has risen such that in 1990 civilian deaths accounted for 90% of all deaths in war. The rate of wounding during combat has decreased from 97 per 1,000 troops in the Civil War to 27 per 1,000 in World War II. Indirect effects indicate that more deaths follow from wars than occur during war itself. These deaths result from breakdown of the normal systems of sanitation, food, and other supplies and the lack of available medical care. One measure of the burden of disease, disability-adjusted life years (DALYs), combines death and suffering. In looking at the global burden of disease, violence ranked second

BOX 23-11 Mass Violence and War: Scope of the Health Problem

Physical Health

- Increased mortality from direct violence, famine, disease
- Malnutrition from lowered food production, poverty, displacement
- Physical trauma of wounded, maimed, disfigured
- Epidemics from lowered vaccination rates and overcrowding
- Increased human immunodeficiency virus (HIV) rates from soldiers' sexual abuse and rape

Psychological Health

- Persistent threat of attack
- Grief from loss of family, homes, land, possessions
- Witnessing of atrocities
- Capture and torture
- Forced to perform violence and condone violence

Soldiers' Post-Combat Health

- Interpersonal and family violence
- Suicide
- Addiction
- Posttraumatic stress
- Alienation
- Psychic disintegration

Impact on Health Determinants

- Flight from homes creates displaced persons, abandoned and orphaned children
- Economic crisis—national resources spent on defense—no money for food, required health services, infrastructures
- Diminished health care—costs prohibitive, delivery systems destroyed, access to remaining healthcare system is reduced or dangerous
- Limited time and focus on parenting, caregiving as safety, basic needs, and avoidance of attack predominate
- Schools destroyed—access to education decreased and illiteracy increased, compromising both personal health education and future health manpower systems
- Health workers' morale and income decreased, thus lowering quality of health care
- Massive environmental destruction and increased hazards

only to respiratory disease in DALYs lost, representing its disease burden on the world (World Bank, 1993).

Nursing adopted a resolution in 2001 at the American Academy of Nurses meeting addressing the issue of torture. After the Abu Ghraib prison incident, it became apparent that the profession must make a contribution in preventing inhumane treatment of prisoners (Glittenberg, 2003). No torture is justified. Presently, the United States, Israel, Russia, and other nations are on the front line in the war on terrorism. The suicide bombers who attacked on September 11, 2001, left the United States with anticipation of future attacks (Lee, 2004). Nursing assumed a role of caring for the survivors and the caregivers at Ground Zero. In military branches across the United States, nurses are activated and essential to the present effort in the war on terrorism.

Roles of Nurses Related to War

Levy and Sidel (1997) list the following war-related activities for nurses: surveillance and documentation of the health effects of war and factors causing war, education and awareness-raising programs on the health effects of war, advocacy of preventive policies and actions, and direct action to prevent war and its consequences, such as participation in nonviolent conflict resolution and building trust. The last role requires skills that many expert community health nurses develop. These skills include refinement of interpersonal communication skills; knowledge of conflict processes at the individual, group, and community levels; understanding and using theories of conflict and conflict resolution; clarification of the history and origins of a conflict situation; and a humanitarian commitment to the pursuit of just, peaceful conflict resolution.

The Research Alert feature illustrates the work of nurses that focuses on the experiences of war refugees. Care is provided by nurses to war refugees either by traveling to serve in relief missions or through contact with refugees who come to the United States. Refugees present unique health problems related both to previous traumatic experiences and to marginalization from the mainstream society (Allotey, 1998).

Community health nurses who work with refugee populations must manage feelings of anger, frustration, guilt, and loneliness; sleeplessness; and recurring images of suffering. Following resettlement in countries that grant asylum, refugees often experience depression symptoms related to both premigration and postmigration

RESEARCH ALERT 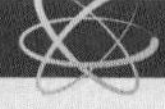

The purpose of this study was to investigate the ways in which children ages 10 to 17 who have grown up amid violence "make sense" of their experiences. The interpretive methods used gave voice to individual experiences but placed them within the socially constructed political, economic, and cultural context in which violence is allowed. The children's exposure to violence was conceptualized, then, not as a private or individual problem, but as a public problem demanding social change.

Dialogue, reflection, and critique—methods of critical research—guided the data collection and analysis of data from 16 children of war and 16 children of battered women. All had witnessed violence but were no longer living with violence.

It was typical for the children of battered women to have no warm memories or happy moments to hold on to. Violence for them had been an everyday part of their lives in subtle and not so subtle ways. In contrast, for the children of war, the violence marked a temporary disruption in their previously happy lives.

Both groups had profound feelings of betrayal. For those who suffered war, the betrayal was from outside the home by those previously viewed as friends. The children of battered women felt betrayed from within their homes by those who were to protect them. Similar emotions of sadness, anger, and confusion were felt by both groups, but those of battered women also experienced shame and embarrassment.

Their experiences of suffering revealed the distinct ways in which war and abuse or women are socially and politically constructed. Both were in battlefields, but the battlefields of war were publicly declared and fought. They were justified, rationalized, and given legitimacy in the world. International bodies set up rules for the regulation of war. These are rules for all to abide by. In contrast, the violence directed toward women and children was conducted in secrecy, the privacy of their homes, and without rules of fair play. Rules were set by the perpetrators.

The stories of the children showed their capacity to find surprising resources. They had self-confidence, hope, and optimism for things to be better. Their "escapes" made them feel lucky, but they felt they were unlikely to forget what had happened to them.

The author concluded that although the children showed remarkable insight and strength, they faced many challenges. In spite of common conceptions that children cannot talk about deeply troubling experiences, the research demonstrated that children want to discuss their experiences and welcome the opportunity.

Source: Berman, H. (1999). Stories of growing up amid violence by refugee children of war and children of battered women living in Canada. *Image: Journal of Nursing Scholarship, 31*(1), 57–63.

HEALTHY PEOPLE 2020 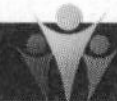

Selected objectives related to injury and violence prevention:

- IVP-1 Reduce fatal and nonfatal injuries
- IVP-2 Reduce fatal and nonfatal traumatic brain injuries
- IVP-3 Reduce fatal and nonfatal spinal cord injuries
- IVP-4 Increase the number of states and the District of Columbia where 90% of deaths among children age 17 years and under that are due to external causes are reviewed by a child fatality review team
- IVP-5 Increase the number of states and the District of Columbia where 90% of sudden and unexpected deaths to infants are reviewed by a child fatality review team
- IVP-6 Increase the proportion of states and the District of Columbia with statewide emergency department data systems that routinely collect external-cause-of-injury codes for 90% or more of injury-related visits
- IVP-7 Increase the proportion of states and the District of Columbia with statewide hospital discharge data systems that routinely collect external-cause-of-injury codes for 90% or more of injury-related discharges
- IVP-8 Increase access to trauma care in the United States
- IVP-8.1 Increase the proportion of the population residing within the continental United States with access to trauma care
- IVP-8.2 Increase the proportion of the land mass of the continental United States with access to trauma care

Violence prevention objectives:

- IVP-29 Reduce homicides
- IVP-30 Reduce firearm-related deaths
- IVP-31 Reduce nonfatal firearm-related injuries
- IVP-32 Reduce nonfatal physical assault injuries
- IVP-33 Reduce physical assaults
- IVP-34 Reduce physical fighting among adolescents
- IVP-35 Reduce bullying among adolescents
- IVP-36 Reduce weapon carrying by adolescents on school property
- IVP-37 Reduce child maltreatment deaths
- IVP-38 Reduce nonfatal child maltreatment
- IVP-39 Reduce violence by current or former intimate partners
- IVP-39.1 Reduce physical violence by current or former intimate partners
- IVP-39.2 Reduce sexual violence by current or former intimate partners
- IVP-39.3 Reduce psychological abuse by current or former intimate partners
- IVP-39.4 Reduce stalking by current or former intimate partners
- IVP-40 Reduce sexual violence
- IVP-40.1 Reduce rape or attempted rape
- IVP-40.2 Reduce abusive sexual contact other than rape or attempted rape
- IVP-40.3 Reduce non-contact sexual abuse
- IVP-41 Reduce nonfatal intentional self-harm injuries
- IVP-42 Reduce children's exposure to violence
- IVP-43 Increase the number of states and the District of Columbia that link data on violent deaths from death certificates, law enforcement, and coroner and medical examiner reports to inform prevention efforts at the state and local levels

experiences. Interventions for these symptoms and other health-related problems are particularly sensitive to the need for culturally congruent care (International Council of Nurses [ICN], 2008).

Interventions to Prevent Violence

Recognition of violence as a public health issue is a relatively recent development. Those who practice or do research in the field readily admit that knowledge of causes and risk factors, and thus of prevention, are only beginning to be developed. Interventions related to violence can be directed to all three system levels—micro, meso, and macro—that were shown in Figure 23-1. In addition, such interventions can be representative of the three areas of prevention: primary, secondary, and tertiary. Following the public health approach to the problem, interventions are efforts to break the causal chain between potential violence and actual violence. Although much more needs to be discovered about the complicated interplay of causes of violence, the factors identified in Box 23-1 and discussed throughout the chapter represent a summary of those factors that guide current intervention strategies. At the micro level, characteristics that put individuals at risk for perpetration (e.g., use of alcohol by batterers) or victimization (e.g., children in unstable homes) can be targeted for screening and group prevention activities. Similarly, as we know more about societal influences on development and expression of violence, macrolevel interventions directed toward laws, education, and media images are implemented. See the *Healthy People 2020* feature for selected objectives related to violence.

Currently, healthcare practitioners' response to violence is sometimes criticized. This is related to the fairly recent recognition of violence as not just a criminal justice problem, but also as a health behavior problem. In 1999 the membership of the American Association of Colleges of Nursing (AACN) approved their position statement on domestic violence and delineated necessary competencies for nurses to provide high-quality care to victims of violence. Education efforts are prevalent among all healthcare workers to raise their awareness and increase assessment and screening for abuse. Studies have indicated that physicians and nurses seldom routinely inquire about abuse. Even when treating the injuries of abused patients, psychosocial assessment or safety issues are most frequently not addressed. Although the healthcare response needs to be improved, there are many ways in which community health nurses do currently initiate and collaborate in violence interventions. These are described in the following sections, according to level of intervention.

Microlevel Interventions: Individuals and Families

Community health nurses are confronted with individuals who have experienced violence in all of the many community-based settings in which they live and work. Nurses in home health, schools, clinics, religious communities, homeless shelters, and other community sites will encounter victims and potential victims of violence. Those who work in institutional settings also design protective programs for individuals who are members of populations at risk such as frail and vulnerable nursing home residents, daycare residents, and coworkers at risk for workplace violence.

Primary Prevention

Primary intervention strategies focus on strengthening the resistance of vulnerable individuals. Such efforts, including encouraging interest and involvement in school, can be successful and should begin as early as possible before young people adopt violent beliefs and behaviors (Hawkins, 1999). The general population of youth can be targeted, and outreach to high-risk youth can also be extended to those who engage in physical fights, those with criminal records or history of inflicting or receiving violent injuries, drug users, gang members, and school dropouts. Relocated youth from immigrant, refugee, and mobile communities, as well as those with emotional or mental problems, are also at risk (CDC, 2013c; ICN, 2008).

Collaborative interventions by nurses in schools, daycare settings, after-school programs, and community youth organizations include nonviolent conflict resolution training, mediation training, coping and stress management training, life and social skills training, self-esteem and ethnic pride enhancement, mentoring programs, parenting classes, and personal safety classes that include gun safety (Jones & Selder, 1996). As part of the team that is implementing programs, nurses can ensure that gender-specific issues of power and control in male–female relationships, date rape, other dating violence, and attitudes toward women are added to the often gender-neutral and male–male focus of programs.

Young people should be taught the risk factors or "red flags" that warn of potential abusive relationships. Programs such as "Safe Dates" can offer a countercultural message of self-respect and protect against tolerance of abuse (Foshee, Bauman, & Everett, 2004).

Nurses in New Orleans have posted notices in bars during Mardi Gras warning that sex with an intoxicated person is sex with someone incapable of consent, or rape. Young people should realize that the number one date rape drug is alcohol and they are giving it to themselves. Instruction is also needed regarding the long-term consequences of so-called "harmless" drugs like ecstasy (McGuire, 2000; Morgan, 2000).

Although early intervention with youth is an optimal time for prevention, the same factors are the target for modification when working with those who are older and in situations of potential violence. Other developmental periods such as marriage, pregnancy, and retirement present opportunities for prevention by service providers. An elder's registration for Medicare could provide an opportunity for health and social service interventions to support healthy family adapting (Institute of Medicine, 1999). Further primary prevention strategies include coping, self-esteem development, early drug and mental illness treatment, realistic parenting expectations, enhanced family bonding, and development of alternatives to the use of violence for conflict resolution. The nurse should also encourage avoidance and/or protection in situations conducive to violence such as bars, high-crime areas, presence of guns in homes, lone work situations, or use of alcohol in dating situations. Individual and family counseling and referral are appropriate.

Some programs have screening protocols to assess for the potential for abuse among pregnant mothers in overburdened families and to initiate home visits for those at high risk (Southern Regional Children's Advocacy Center, 1998). Hawaii's Healthy Start program of home-based

GOT AN ALTERNATIVE?

Anger management classes have effectively used meditation, yoga, biofeedback, and other self-management techniques that teach men and women how to mediate anger before violence occurs.

services is targeted at families at risk for child abuse and neglect and uses lay home visitors trained and supervised by professional health providers. Parental attitudes toward children and parent–child interaction patterns show measurable benefits. Programs to prevent elder abuse include efforts to reduce caregiver stress by ensuring respite care, daycare, and homemaker and aid services to the family.

Secondary Prevention

Secondary prevention involves actions that are taken when violence and abuse are present. Goals include identifying the fact of abuse and intervening to aid the victim. Often, the only, or the first, practitioners to come into contact with victims are healthcare providers. One pressing issue is the need to increase the recognition, diagnosis, and assessment of violence by these professionals. Support for such assessment was provided when the Joint Commission set standards, in 1992 and 1994, for assessment protocols in EDs, alcohol abuse centers, ambulatory care centers, and all inpatient and outpatient facilities accredited by the organization. Such protocols have been developed and implemented by nurses for specific organizations (Campbell & Dienemann, 1999). General guidelines for routine screening that were released by the Family Violence Prevention Fund (FVPF, 1999) have had the support of the ANA; the CDC has also produced a set of screening instruments (Basile, Hertz, & Back, 2007). The FVPF guidelines recommend routine screening of all women older than 14 years of age, whether or not symptoms or signs are present and whether or not the provider suspects abuse has occurred. Examples of questions for screening are shown in **Box 23-12**.

In cases of sexual assault, increasing numbers of nurses are becoming specialized as sexual assault nurse examiners (SANEs). Their work is specialty work in forensic nursing. They work closely with law enforcement in collecting and preserving evidence of crimes. Their role is special in that they are trained to perform the necessary technical procedures during examinations, and at the same time, they counsel and provide support in a patient's time of crisis. SANEs provide consistency as they follow up with victims of assault at monthly intervals to review lab results and assess psychological and spiritual healing. SANEs have qualified as expert witnesses in court and have been instrumental in the conviction of perpetrators.

Reporting of abuse to authorities is a mandated task of healthcare providers on behalf of victims. Healthcare providers in all 50 states and in the District of Columbia are required to report confirmed or suspected instances of child abuse. Most states require reporting of suspected abuse of the elderly, and state laws and procedures should be known. Mandatory reporting in the case of adults who have injuries due to domestic violence is an ongoing legal issue. At present, most states have some type of reporting of all patients who have injuries as a result of domestic violence. Some states have mandatory reporting by healthcare providers in instances in which the patient has an injury that appears to have been caused by a gun, knife, firearm, or other deadly weapon. Some states require reporting when there is reason to believe the patient's injury may have resulted from an illegal act. Other states mandate reporting when the health provider believes injuries resulted from an act of violence. Still other states require mandatory reporting when domestic violence or adult abuse is suspected (NEA, 2005).

Laws such as those described in the previous paragraph are somewhat controversial. Some contend more harm is done than good. Ethically, there are those who argue that such mandates violate patient autonomy. The stereotype of a passive/helpless victim is perpetuated. It is argued that partner abuse is not considered the same as elder abuse (cases in which there are vulnerable victims). Another potential harm is to the healthcare provider–patient relationship by violating confidentiality and overriding informed

BOX 23-12 Recommended Questions to Screen Women for Family Violence

Framing questions

- Because violence is so common in many people's lives, I've begun to ask all of my patients about it.
- I'm concerned that your symptoms may have been caused by someone hurting you.

Direct questions

- Are you in a direct relationship with a person who physically hurts or threatens you?
- Did someone cause these injuries? Was it your partner/husband?
- Has your partner or ex-partner ever hit you or physically hurt you?
- Has your partner or ex-partner ever threatened to hurt you or someone close to you?

Source: Family Violence Prevention Fund (FVPF). (1999). *Preventing domestic violence: Clinical guidelines on routine screening.* San Francisco, CA: Author; Centers for Disease Control and Prevention (CDC). (2012d). *Understanding intimate partner violence fact sheet.* Retrieved from http://www.cdc.gov/violenceprevention/pdf/ipv_factsheet-a.pdf. Used by permission of Family Violence Prevention Fund.

BOX 23-13 Domestic Violence Assistance Programs

- Safety planning for women and children
- Help obtaining protection orders
- Support and advocacy during interviews with law enforcement, medical personnel, and legal representation
- Someone to go to court with victims
- Pretrial services
- Assistance with crime victim compensation claims
- Services for children
- Transitional housing
- Assistance and advocacy with employers regarding safety in the workplace and retention of employment
- Supportive services of clothing, food, shelter, transportation, education
- Job training or job relocation
- Counseling
- Child care
- Safety planning and other daily living needs

consent of patients. There are also arguments that such reporting affects women's safety by discouraging care. Women fear risk of retaliation to themselves or their children by perpetrators, or perpetrators may restrain women from seeking care. Also, until better resources in the form of shelters, counseling, and even effective law enforcement of policy and procedures are, in fact, in place, reporting gives women false hopes of help and assistance. Nurses need to deliberate carefully and consider the patients' best interests when making a decision to report abuse. The decision should be made jointly.

Victims of abuse need to be protected from further abuse, and this may require placement of children in foster care and of victims of domestic violence in shelters or safe houses. **Box 23-13** outlines interventions that may be needed by victims of domestic violence and their children. For reasons discussed previously, some victims may choose not to leave the abusive situation. The nurse should support and assist the patient in decision making. Contingency plans and shelter information should be provided. Interventions can also be directed at treatment for the perpetrators of abuse. Nurses can act as facilitators in group treatment sessions or make referrals to group programs or couples counseling. It must be taken into account that couples counseling may increase the woman's danger in the relationship. Often, such counseling may be court ordered. Approaches to content vary but usually address at least anger management, skill building, and resocialization. Dropout and resistance are common in such programs. Assessment protocols for male batterers exist currently (Kropp & Hart, 2000).

Tertiary Prevention

Many of the same strategies that help build resistance to the use of violence are also used to rehabilitate and prevent further incidence of abuse. Education, counseling, skill building, modification of unsafe situations, stress reduction, support, and guidance are all part of the rehabilitative efforts directed toward victims and abusers. Research has shown that women can predict their risk of injury at a 96% accuracy rate. A woman's predictions should be given serious attention (Wiesz, Tolman, & Saunders, 2000).

Mesolevel Interventions: Community Structures

Prevention at this level is focused on broader factors in the larger community that contribute to violence or encourage the presence of violence. Such interventions recognize the general belief that violence prevention will not be successful unless coordinated, comprehensive, multidisciplinary, community-based approaches are initiated. These efforts must address the broader service system issues and move away from fragmented efforts. One term often used to describe such interventions is *community development,* which is action to enhance the ability of communities to meet the needs of its members. Communities are characterized as having more or less community efficacy or competence. Structures and programs must be coordinated.

One step that is needed to motivate coordinated action toward a community problem is the recognition that the problem exists. **Box 23-14** outlines steps nurses can take to raise community awareness of the problem of domestic violence. Nurses working with the community often must become involved in outreach activities to promote healthier communities through partnerships with other groups, including citizens. Such work is long term, and results are often not immediate. To optimize community resources, all residents, organizations, agencies, institutions, and other components of the community must be included in the response. This makes the community response prevention and intervention oriented, not just crisis oriented.

Because each community is unique, each has different needs and resources, which means the ways to access a communitywide response to violence will be varied. What works in one community might very well not work in another. Also, consider that often there are communities within communities. For example, a neighborhood might

BOX 23-14 Interventions to Raise Awareness About Domestic Violence in the Community

- Organize a bumper-sticker slogan contest for the community reflecting the needs of that area.
- Ask men in the community to speak out against domestic violence and use their influence as workers and community members to let other men know that violence against women and children is wrong and will not be tolerated.
- Challenge radio stations' disparaging remarks about women. Offer to speak on violence issues to the public.
- Personally speak out about domestic violence and refuse to listen to anyone make derogatory jokes or comments about women.
- Review your community's newspaper for articles on domestic violence and determine whether there is victim-blaming language included in the articles. Speak with the newspaper editor periodically to discuss your findings and offer solutions.
- Organize a fundraising effort for your local family violence shelter.
- Assess businesses' employee assistance programs and determine if community businesses offer help and referrals for employees who are victims of domestic violence. If not, offer information detailing options for referrals.
- Spearhead multidisciplinary coalitions in the community to address primary prevention issues with adolescents.

have a Jewish ethnic group and an Italian ethnic group, each with its own traditions and sense of community. There are also self-contained communities such as Native American reservations (see the following Research Alert), prisons, religious neighborhoods, community colleges, and senior universities. Self-contained communities may have different governing principles, needs, and resources than the community at large.

Collaboration and partnership of community citizens, institutions, and organizations are essential in establishing a communitywide response to domestic violence. Citizens must have ownership of the response and see themselves as playing a significant role in articulation and attainment of the response vision. Support of the members includes the support of the key leaders (both formal and informal) in the community. These are the people who are highly regarded for their knowledge and contributions to the community. Nurses can identify these leaders by doing the following:

- Getting to know the community before any decisions are made that will impact citizens
- Finding out where women in the community go for help when needed
- Asking for advice and support from coworkers who live in the community
- Asking for advice and support from others who provide direct and supportive services to individuals living in the community
- Volunteering in a community-based organization

After community leaders are identified, meetings and ongoing communication are necessary to develop a common definition of violence and common goals. This step will prevent the development of conflicting interventions and thus tension between participants. For instance, traditional services for battered women and their abused children have not been coordinated and are often in conflict regarding the goals of their interventions. A wide range of interventions, initiatives, and cooperative effort is possible, limited only by the imagination and commitment of the nurse and community participants.

One outcome of awareness interventions in the community may be an increase in the demand for individual advocacy and supportive services of violence programs. Work has been suggested, for example, to improve such areas as police response, enforcement of present laws, and safer situations for reporting of cases of abuse. Community services need to be in place that increase social and psychiatric services for at-risk youth, expand alcohol and drug treatment services for pregnant and parenting women, and increase educational and employment opportunities. Child protective agencies need an increased capacity to assist patients through the provision of training, funding, and appropriate caseload assignments. Safe environments need to be created through increased surveillance, such as metal detectors at schools, and increased policing in high-crime neighborhoods. Recreational facilities and programs for youth need to be available. Research supports a direct relationship between neighborhood characteristics and adolescent outcomes. Living in a high-risk neighborhood can double the incidence of behavioral and academic problems (Halpern-Felsher et al., 1997; Kalil & Eccles, 1998).

Macrolevel Interventions: Society and Culture

Policy issues dominate the types of interventions that nurses undertake at the macrosystem level of intervention. These interventions go far beyond reducing the virulence of the perpetrator (agent) or strengthening the victim (host) to recognize the preconditions (environment) underlying events of violence. Action at this level is directed at large-scale efforts to address poverty, income disparity, prejudice, sexism, ageism, media violence, handgun control, and the culture of violence. These prevention efforts are attempts to change society's norms and values related to those factors that contribute to and allow violence to occur.

Risk factors for violence, such as binge drinking, can be mitigated by increasing alcohol taxes, maintaining and enforcing the minimum drinking age, and implementing education programs routinely (Cook & Moore, 2002; Holden et al., 2000). Faith-based connections in a community are found to be successful in helping to curtail neighborhood violence (Lee & Bartkowski, 2004; Osgood & Chambers, 2000). Religious involvement promotes civic volunteerism and a social justice mentality that benefits the entire community (Becker & Dhingia, 2001).

Policy can be promoted and legislated that moves change in the right direction. Nurses, nursing organizations, and coalitions of other healthcare providers lobbied successfully for the comprehensive Violence Against Women Act passed in 1994 that promotes protection of women in many areas. Global history reflects the suffering that can be inflicted on entire populations if good citizens remain complacent. Jews in Europe during the Holocaust, large groups of people in Bosnia and Cambodia who endured ethnic cleansing, African Americans under Jim Crow laws in the Southern United States, and blacks under apartheid in South Africa are some examples of the groups who suffered in the 20th century. These groups, among others, should serve as reminders of the need for constant vigilance against hatred and violence.

RESEARCH ALERT 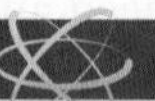

Both of these studies sought to determine the extent of domestic violence (physical only) experienced in Native American populations. Outcomes were improved documentation of the severity and high prevalence of domestic violence in the communities. In the Apache group, depression and PTSD symptoms were highly associated with domestic violence. Among the Navajo, receipt of government assistance (low socioeconomic status) was associated with greater rates of domestic violence.

Sources: Fairchild, D. G., Fairchild, M. W., & Stoner, S. (1998). Prevalence of adult domestic violence among women seeking routine care at a Native American health care facility. *American Journal of Public Health, 88*(10), 1514–1517; Hamby, S. L., & Skupien, M. B. (1998). Domestic violence on the San Carlos Apache reservation. *The IHS Primary Care Provider, 23*(8), 102–105.

Conclusion

Community health nursing can seem daunting to some because of the broad perspective that community health nurses must address in taking on a population focus. Community health nurses, by virtue of their cooperative work with many disciplines, need to develop multiperspectival and multilingual skills. They learn to understand and communicate in many different ways (Diekemper, SmithBattle, & Drake, 1999). All public health problems challenge nursing, but the problem of violence by its very nature may be the most challenging. Alleviating all of the many forms of violence to have health, wellbeing, and peace for individuals in communities may be the ultimate prevention project. The challenge has been compared with the biblical task of "taking on Goliath" because of how large it looms (Hartman, Lundy, & Janes, 1997). The following thoughts by the leader, Vaclav Havel, of the peaceful "Velvet Revolution" in the former Czechoslovakia give encouragement:

> *Hope,* in this deep and powerful sense, is not the same as joy that things are going well, or willingness to invest in enterprises that are obviously headed for success, but rather an ability to work for something because it is good, not just because it stands a chance to succeed . . . definitely not the same thing as optimism. It is not the conviction that something will turn out well, but the certainty that something makes sense, regardless of how it turns out. (Havel, 1991, p. 181)

LEVELS OF PREVENTION 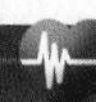

Primary: Teaching a class for parents on appropriate nonviolent disciplinary childcare practices

Secondary: Assisting students who have reported observing abuse at home with appropriate intervention with school authorities and counseling parents about nonviolent ways to interact with each other

Tertiary: Once abuse has been verified, referring patients to appropriate social, community, and legal resources

HEALTHY ME 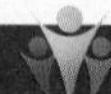

How do you handle stress? When you feel angry, how do you feel and what actions do you take to resolve the conflict? What are healthier ways to reduce stress and avoid situations where anger and violence may result?

Critical Thinking Activities

1. Consider the following quotations from two famous people. How do you interpret them and how are they related?
   "The deadliest form of violence is poverty."
   —Mohandas Gandhi
   "The most violent element in society is ignorance."
   —Emma Goldman
2. Consider the following quotation: "Those worthy gentlemen who look upon war, if successful, as a cause of opulence and prosperity might with equal justice ... look upon the loss of a leg as a cause of swiftness" (Jeremy Bentham, 1987/1843). Should war properly be considered an "ailment" of humankind, and if so, is it "curable"? How would you put military action into a prevention framework? Or could you?
3. For questions 3 and 4, read: Sidel, V. W. (1997). The roles and ethics of health professionals in war. In B. S. Levy & V. W. Sidel (Eds.), *War and public health.* New York, NY: Oxford University Press.
   Potential ethical conflicts exist when health professionals and war intersect:

   - Conflict between caring for personnel of their own military force versus opposing forces or civilians who may need their care
   - Conflict between combatant and noncombatant roles for health personnel
   - Conflict between obligation to serve one's country in the military and broader obligation to prevent war

   Discuss these dilemmas with a military nurse and ask how he or she resolves these obligations.
4. Discuss the criticism of caring for victims of war as making war more tolerable.

References

Allotey, P. (1998). Traveling with "excess baggage": Health problems of refugee women in Western Australia. *Women and Health, 28*(1), 63–81.

American Academy of Pediatrics. (2013). Policy statement: Children, adolescents, and the media. *Pediatrics, 132*(5), 958–961.

American Association of Colleges of Nursing. (1999). *Violence as a public health issue.* Washington, DC: Author.

American Nurses Association (ANA). (1991). *Position statement: Physical violence against women.* Washington, DC: Author.

Anderson, R. N., & Smith, B. L. (2003). Deaths: Leading causes for 2001. *National Vital Statistics Report, 52*(9), 1–86.

Aron, L. Y., & Olsen, K. K. (1997). Efforts by child welfare agencies to address domestic violence. *Public Welfare* (Summer), 4–13.

Basile, K. C., Hertz, M. F., & Back, S. E. (2007). *Intimate partner violence and sexual violence victimization assessment instruments for use in healthcare settings: Version 1.* Atlanta: Centers for Disease Control and Prevention, National Center for Injury Prevention and Control. Retrieved from http://www.cdc.gov/ncipc/pub-res/images/ipvandsvscreening.pdf

Bazelon, E. (2013). How to stop the bullies. *The Atlantic.* Retrieved from http://www.theatlantic.com/magazine/archive/2013/03/how-to-stop-bullies/309217/

Becker, P. E., & Dhingia, P. W. (2001). Religious involvement and volunteering: Implications for civil society. *Sociology of Religion, 62,* 315–335.

Bentham, J. (1987). A plan for a universal and perpetual peace. In H. P. Kainz (Ed.), *Philosophical perspectives on peace* (pp. 128–136). Athens, OH: Ohio University Press. (Originally published in 1843).

Bureau of Justice Assistance. (2005). *2005 national gang threat assessment.* Washington, DC: Author.

Bureau of Labor Statistics. (2012). Nonfatal occupational injuries and illnesses requiring days away from work, 2012. Retrieved from http://www.bls.gov/news.release/pdf/osh2.pdf

Campbell, J. C., & Dienemann, J. (1999, June). *Symposium on violence against women.* Presentation at Sigma Theta Tau International Research Conference, London, England.

Campbell, J. C., Harris, M. J., & Lee, R. K. (1995). Violence research: An overview. *Scholarly Inquiry for Nursing Practice, 9,* 105–126.

Cassidy, K. (1999). How to assess and intervene in domestic violence situations. *Home Healthcare Nurse, 17,* 665–671.

Centers for Disease Control and Prevention (CDC). (2003). *Costs of intimate partner violence against women in the United States.* Retrieved from http://www.cdc.gov/violenceprevention/pdf/ipvbook-a.pdf

Centers for Disease Control and Prevention. (2006a). Physical dating violence among high school students—United States, 2003. *Morbidity and Mortality Weekly Report, 55,* 532–535.

Centers for Disease Control and Prevention. (2006b). *Dating abuse fact sheet.* Retrieved from http://www.cdc.gov/ncipc/dvp/DatingViolence.htm

Centers for Disease Control and Prevention. (2006c). *Understanding teen dating abuse fact sheet.* Retrieved from http://www.cdc.gov/injury

Centers for Disease Control and Prevention. (2007). *Suicide facts at a glance.* Retrieved from http://www.cdc.gov/injury

Centers for Disease Control and Prevention (CDC). (2011). *The National Intimate Partner and Sexual Violence Survey: 2010 summary report.* Retrieved from http://www.cdc.gov/violenceprevention/nisvs/2010_report.html

Centers for Disease Control and Prevention (CDC). (2012a). *Understanding child maltreatment fact sheet.* Retrieved from http://www.cdc.gov/violenceprevention/pdf/cm_factsheet2012-a.pdf

Centers for Disease Control and Prevention. (2012b). *Youth violence facts at a glance.* Retrieved from http://www.cdc.gov/violenceprevention/pdf/yv-datasheet-a.pdf

Centers for Disease Control and Prevention. (2012c). Youth risk behavior surveillance—United States, 2011. *MMWR, Surveillance Summaries 2012, 61* (no. SS-4). Retrieved from www.cdc.gov/mmwr/pdf/ss/ss6104.pdf

Centers for Disease Control and Prevention (CDC). (2012d). *Understanding intimate partner violence fact sheet.* Retrieved from http://www.cdc.gov/violenceprevention/pdf/ipv_factsheet-a.pdf

Centers for Disease Control and Prevention. (2013a). *Child maltreatment facts at a glance.* Retrieved from http://www.cdc.gov/violenceprevention/pdf/cm-data-sheet-2013.pdf

Centers for Disease Control and Prevention. (2013b). *Fact sheet: Understanding elder abuse.* Retrieved from http://www.cdc.gov/violenceprevention/pdf/em-factsheet-a.pdf

Centers for Disease Control and Prevention. (2013c). *Understanding school violence fact sheet.* Retrieved from http://www.cdc.gov/violenceprevention/pdf/school_violence_fact_sheet-a.pdf

Centers for Disease Control and Prevention. (2013d). *Youth violence: Risk and protective factors.* Retrieved from http://www.cdc.gov/violenceprevention/youthviolence/riskprotectivefactors.html

Centers for Disease Control and Prevention (CDC). (2014a). *Injury prevention and control: Data and statistics (WISQARS™).* Retrieved from http://www.cdc.gov/injury/wisqars/index.html

Centers for Disease Control and Prevention (CDC). (2014b). *Violence prevention.* Retrieved from http://cdc.gov/ncipc/dvp/prevention_at_CDC.htm

Centers for Disease Control and Prevention (CDC). (2014c). *Cost of child abuse and neglect rival other major public health problems.* Retrieved from http://www.cdc.gov/violenceprevention/childmaltreatment/economiccost.html

Cook, P. J., & Moore, M. J. (2002). The economics of alcohol abuse and alcohol control policies: Price levels, including excise taxes, are effective at controlling alcohol consumption. *Health Affairs, 21*, 120–133.

Crandall, M., Walters, A. B., Kernic, M. A., Holt, U. L., & Rivara, F. P. (2004). Predicting future injury among women in abusive relationships. *Journal of Trauma, Injury Infection, and Critical Care, 56*(4), 906–912.

Davey, D. B., & Davey, P. A. (1998, Nov/Dec). Domestic violence today. What nursing students should know. *Imprint*, 41–43.

Diekemper, M., SmithBattle , L., & Drake, M. A. (1999). Bringing the population into focus. A natural development in community health nursing practice: Part I. *Journal of Public Health Nursing, 16*(1), 3–9.

Donovan, R. J., & Vlais, R. (2005). *VicHealth review of communication components of social marketing/public education campaigns focusing on violence against women.* Melbourne, Australia: Victorian Health Promotion Foundation.

Egley, A., Jr., Howell, J. C., & Moore, J. P. (2010). Highlights of the 2008 National Youth Gang Survey. Retrieved from https://www.ncjrs.gov/pdffiles1/ojjdp/229249.pdf

Emergency Nurses Association. (2011). *Emergency department violence survey study, November 2011.* Retrieved from http://www.ena.org/practice-research/research/Documents/ENAEDVSReportNovember2011.pdf

Family Violence Prevention Fund (FVPF). (1999). *Preventing domestic violence: Clinical guidelines on routine screening.* San Francisco, CA: Author.

Fang, X., Brown, D. S., Florence, C. S., & Mercy, J. A. (2012). The economic burden of child maltreatment in the United States and implications for prevention. *Child Abuse & Neglect, 36*(2), 156–165.

Foege, W. (1997). Arms and public health. In B. Levy & V. Sidel (Eds.), *War and public health.* New York, NY: Oxford University Press.

Foshee, V. A., Bauman, K., & Everett, S. (2004). Assessing the long-term effects of the safe dates program. *American Journal of Public Health, 94*(4), 619–624.

Funk, J. B., Baldacci, H. B., Pasold, T., & Baumgardner, J. (2004). Violence exposure in real life, video games, television, movies, and the Internet: Is there desensitization? *Journal of Adolescence, 27*, 23–39.

Gazmarian, J. A., Peterson, R., Spiz, A. M., Goodwin, M. M., Saltzman, L. E., & Marks, J. S. (2000). Violence and reproductive health: Current knowledge and future research directions. *Maternal and Child Health Journal, 4*(2), 79–84.

Gilligan, J. (1997). *Violence. Reflections on a national epidemic.* New York, NY: Vintage Books.

Glittenberg, J. (2003). The tragedy of torture: A global concern for mental health nursing. *Issues of Mental Health Nursing, 24*(6–7), 627–638.

Halpern-Felsher, B. L., Connell, J. P., Spencer, M. B., Aber, J. L., Duncan, G. J., Clifford, E., . . . Seidman, E. (1997). Neighborhood and family factors predicting educational risk and attainment in African American and White children and adolescents. In T. Brooks-Gunn, G. J. Duncan, & J. L. Avet (Eds.), *Neighborhood poverty: Context and consequences for children,* (Vol. *1*, pp. 146–173). New York, NY: Russell Sage Foundation.

Hartman, S., Lundy, K. S., & Janes, S. (1997, June). *Taking on Goliath: Nursing's response to violence.* Paper presented at Association of Community Health Nursing Educators' Annual Spring Institute, Vancouver, British Columbia, Canada.

Havel, V. (1991). *Disturbing the peace.* New York, NY: Random House.

Hawkins, D. (1999). Preventing adolescent health-risk behaviors by strengthening protection during childhood. *Archives of Pediatrics and Adolescent Medicine, 153*, 226–234.

Heise, L., & Garcia-Moreno, C. (2002). *Violence by intimate partners: World report on violence and health.* Geneva, Switzerland: World Health Organization.

Ho, K. (2007). Structural violence as human rights violation. *Essex Human Rights Review, 4*(2), 1–16.

Holden, H. A., Gruenwold, P. J., Ponicki, W. R., Treno, A. J., Grube, J. W., Saltz, R. F., ... Roeper, P. (2000). Effect of community-based interventions on high risk drinking and alcohol-related injuries. *Journal of the American Medical Association, 284*, 2341–2347.

Hotzworth-Monroe, A., & Stuart, G. L. (1994). Typologies of male batterers: Three subtypes and the differences among them. *Psychological Bulletin, 116*(3), 476–497.

Huesmann, L. R., & Taylor, L. D. (2006). The role of media violence in violent behavior. *Annual Review of Public Health, 27*, 393–415.

Hyde-Nolan, M. E., & Juliao, T. (2011). Theoretical basis for family violence. In R. S. Fife & S. Schrager (Eds.), *Family violence: What healthcare providers need to know*. Sudbury, MA: Jones & Bartlett Learning.

Institute of Medicine. (1999). *Violence and the American family; Report of a workshop. Next steps: A guide to effective action.* Washington, DC: National Academies Press.

International Centre for Prison Studies. (2014). *World prison brief: Highest to lowest.* Retrieved from http://www.prisonstudies.org/highest-to-lowest

International Council of Nurses (ICN). (2008). *Nursing matters. ICN on displaced persons: A global challenge*. Published position paper, ICN.

Jason, L. A., Hanaway, L. K., & Brackshaw, E. (1999). Television violence and children: Problems and solutions. In T. P. Gullotta & S. J. McElhaney (Eds.), *Violence in homes and communities: Prevention, intervention, and treatment* (pp. 133–156). Thousand Oaks, CA: Sage.

Jones, F. C., & Selder, F. (1996). Pyschoeducational groups to promote effective coping in school-aged children living in violent communities. *Issues in Mental Health Nursing, 17*, 559–571.

Jones, L. (1993, November 26–28). Can a doctor stop the violence? *USA Weekend*, p. 9.

Kalil, A., & Eccles, J. S. (1998). Does welfare affect family process and adolescent adjustment? *Child Development, 69*, 1597–1613.

Kropp, P. R., & Hart, S. (2000). The spousal assault risk assessment (SARA) guide: Reliability and validity in adult male offenders. *Law and Human Behavior, 24*, 101–118.

Lee, C. (2004, April). Most say they are less safe since 9/11. *Washington Post*, p. A3.

Lee, M. R., & Bartkowski, J. P. (2004). Civic participation, regional subcultures and violence: The differential effects of secular and religious participation on adult juvenile homicide. *Homicide Studies, 7*, 1–35.

Levay, S., & Valente, S. (2003). *Human sexuality.* Sunderland, MA: Sinaurer.

Levy, B. S., & Sidel, V. W. (1997). *War and public health.* New York, NY: Oxford University Press.

McClure, L. F. (1999). Origins and incidence of workplace violence in North America. In T. P. Gullotta & S. J. McElhaney (Eds.), *Violence in homes and communities: Prevention, intervention, and treatment* (pp. 71–99). Thousand Oaks, CA: Sage.

McGee, T. P., & DeBernardo, C. R. (1999). The classroom avenger: A behavioral profile of school based shootings. *Forensic Examiner, 8*, 16–18.

McGuire, P. (2000). Long-term psychiatric and cognitive effects of MDMA use. *Toxicology Letters, 112*, 153–156.

Mercy, J. A., Rosenberg, M. L., Powell, K. E., Broome, C. V., & Roper, W. L. (1993). Public health policy for preventing violence. *Health Affairs, 12*(4), 7–29.

Miller, K., & Knutson, T. (1997). Reports of severe physical punishment and exposure to animal cruelty by inmates convicted of felonies and by university students. *Child Abuse and Neglect, 21*, 59–82.

Morgan, M. J. (2000). Ecstacy (MDMA): A review of possible persistent psychological effects. *Psychopharmacology, 152*, 230–248.

National Adult Protective Services Association (NAPSA). (2013). National policy and advocacy. Retrieved from http://www.napsa-now.org/policy-advocacy/national-policy/.

National Alliance on Mental Illness. (2011). Understanding and coping with PTSD. Retrieved from http://www.nami.org/Content/ContentGroups/Programs/Family_to_Family/PTSD_Module_Pevised_Feb_2011.pdf

National Center on Elder Abuse. (2006). *The 2004 survey of state adult protective services: Abuse of adults 60 years of age and older.* Washington, DC: Author.

National Center on Elder Abuse. (2008). *Frequently asked questions.* Retrieved from http://www.ncea.aoa.gov/faq/index.aspx

National Education Association. (2005). *NEA Health Information Network statistics: Gun violence in our communities.* Retrieved from http://www.neahin.org/programs/schoolsafety/gunsafety/statistics.htm

National Institute of Mental Health (NIMH). (2014). What is post-traumatic stress disorder? Retrieved from http://www.nimh.nih.gov/health/topics/post-traumatic-stress-disorder-ptsd/index.shtml

Neighbors, C., Walker, D. D., Mbilinyi, L. F., O'Rourke, A., Edleson, J. L., Zegree, J., & Roffman, R. A. (2010). Normative misperceptions of abuse among perpetrators of intimate partner violence. *Violence Against Women, 16*(4), 370–386.

Nightingale, F. (1954). Notes on matters affecting the health of the British army. In F. Nightingale, *Selected Writings, 1820–1910.* New York, NY: Macmillan.

Occupational Safety and Health Administration. (2002). *OSHA fact sheet: Workplace violence.* Washington, DC: U.S. Department of Labor.

Office for Victims of Crime/Office of Justice Programs. (2013). Domestic and family violence. Retrieved from http://ovc.ncjrs.gov/topic.aspx?topicid=27

Osgood, D. W., & Chambers, J. M. (2000). Social disorganization outside the metropolis: An analysis of rural youth violence. *Criminology, 38*, 81–115.

Patchin, J. W., & Hinduja, S. (2013). *Cyberbullying prevention and response: Expert perspectives.* New York, NY: Routledge.

Planty, M., & Truman, J. L. (2013). Firearm violence, 1993–2011. U.S. Department of Justice/Bureau of Justice Statistics. Retrieved from http://www.bjs.gov/content/pub/pdf/fv9311.pdf

Potter, L. B. (1999). Understanding the incidence and origin of community violence: Toward a comprehensive perspective on violence prevention. In T. P. Gullotta & S. J. McElhaney (Eds.),

Violence in homes and communities: Prevention, intervention, and treatment. Thousand Oaks, CA: Sage.

Scott-Tilley, D. (1999). Nursing interventions to prevent domestic violence. *American Journal of Nursing, 99*(10), 24–27.

Sidel, V. W. (1997). The roles and ethics of health professionals in war. In B. S. Levy & V. W. Sidel (Eds.), *War and public health*. New York, NY: Oxford University Press.

Southern Regional Children's Advocacy Center. (1998). *Healthy families—North America*. SRCAC: Author.

Stauffer, T. (2002, November 3). University of Arizona tries to limit student threats. *Arizona Daily Star*. Retrieved from http://www.AZstarnet.com

Temkin, E. (1997). Nurses and the prevention of war: Public health nurses and the peace movement in World War I. In B. S. Levy & V. W. Sidel (Eds.), *War and public health*. New York, NY: Oxford University Press.

Tjaden, P., & Thoennes, N. (2000, November). *Full report of the prevalence, incidence, and consequences of violence against women: Findings from the National Violence Against Women Survey* (NJC 183721). Washington, DC: National Institute of Justice.

UNIFEM. (2003). *Making a difference: Strategic communications to end violence against women*. New York, NY: United Nations Development Fund for Women.

United Nations Division for the Advancement of Women. (1995). *Beijing declaration and platform for action: Strategic objectives and actions: Violence against women*. Retrieved from http://www.un.org.womenwatch/daw/beijing/platform

U.S. Department of Education. (2013). *Human trafficking of children in the United States: A fact sheet for schools*. Retrieved from http://www2.ed.gov/about/offices/list/oese/oshs/factsheet.html

U.S. Department of Health and Human Services. (2008). *Child maltreatment 2006*. Washington, DC: Government Printing Office.

U.S. Department of Justice. (2013). *Anti-human trafficking task force initiative*. Retrieved from https://www.bja.gov/ProgramDetails.aspx?Program_ID=51

U.S. Department of State. (2013). *Human trafficking: U.S. government response*. Retrieved from http://www.state.gov/j/tip/response/index.htm

Van Soest, D. (1997). *The global crisis of violence: Common problems, universal causes, shared solutions*. Washington, DC: National Association of Social Workers.

Van Wormer, K., Wells, J., & Boes, M. (2000). *Social work with lesbians, gays, and bisexuals: A strengths perspective*. Boston, MA: Allyn & Bacon.

Violence Policy Center. (2008). *National Rifle Association information. Gun violence in America*. Retrieved from http://www.vpc.org/nrainfo/phil.html

Walter-Rodriguez, A., & Hill, R. (2011). Human sex trafficking. *FBI Law Enforcement Bulletin*. Retrieved from http://www.fbi.gov/stats-services/publications/law-enforcement-bulletin/march_2011/human_sex_trafficking

Waters, H., Hyder, A., Rajkotia, Y., Basu, S., Rehwinkel, J. A., & Butchart, A. (2004). *The economic dimensions of interpersonal violence*. Geneva, Switzerland: World Health Organization.

Wiesner, M., & Ittel, A. (2002). Relations of pubertal timing and depressive symptoms to substance use in early adolescence. *Journal of Early Adolescence, 22*, 5–23.

Wiesz, A., Tolman, R., & Saunders, D. (2000). Assessing the risk of severe domestic violence: The importance of survivors' predictions. *Journal of Interpersonal Violence, 15*, 75–90.

World Bank. (1993). *World development report, 1993*. New York, NY: Oxford University Press.

World Health Organization (WHO). (2002). *World report on violence and health*. Geneva, Switzerland: Author.

World Health Organization (WHO). (2010). *Injuries and violence: The facts*. Geneva: Author. Retrieved from http://whqlibdoc.who.int/publications/2010/9789241599375_eng.pdf?ua=1

World Health Organization (WHO). (2012). *Interesting facts about ageing*. Retrieved from http://www.who.int/ageing/about/facts/en/

World Health Organization (WHO). (2013). *Global and regional estimates of violence against women: Prevalence and health effects of intimate partner violence and non-partner sexual violence*. Retrieved from http://apps.who.int/iris/bitstream/10665/85241/1/WHO_RHR_HRP_13.06_eng.pdf

World Health Organization (WHO). (2014a). *Definition and typology of violence*. Retrieved from http://www.who.int/violenceprevention/approach/definition/en/

World Health Organization (WHO). (2014b). *Female genital mutilation: Fact sheet*. Retrieved from http://www.who.int/mediacentre/factsheets/fs241/en/

World Health Organization (WHO). (2014c). *Female genital mutilation and other harmful practices*. Retrieved from http://www.who.int/reproductivehealth/topics/fgm/prevalence/en/

World Health Organization (WHO). (2014d). *Violence, health, and human rights*. Retrieved from http://www.who.int/violence_injury_prevention/violence/activities/human_rights/en/

Zevitz, R. G., & Faikas, M. (2000). *Sex offender community notification: Assessing the impact in Wisconsin*. Washington, DC: Institute of Justice.

Appendix: A Day in the Life of a Nurse Who Faces Violence: Prison Nursing

Miriam Cabana, RN, MSN, GNP

The nurse supervisor turned onto the blacktop road that ribboned through the 22,000-acre southern prison. As the expansive horizon of flat delta land passed on her short drive to the prison hospital, she recalled the conversation with her husband earlier in the day. He was the warden of the prison and had mused that the full moon usually means some form of violence would erupt within the prison units and that it was an "ideal" time for an escape attempt. She knew he was diligent in his efforts to protect the community as well as to maintain a safe environment for those incarcerated, which often included protecting them from violence inflicted on each other; and he shared her strong opinion about society's obligation to provide inmates with access to safe, competent health care. At the very least, there would be more physical altercations among the inmates or increased somatic complaints screened by phone from the emergency department. She instinctively knew her evening shift would be busy. Oh, for the days in her nursing career that the "full moon" myths were associated only with increased birth rates!

The transition between shifts for both nursing and security personnel was smooth. Predictably, several inmates remained in the large holding room with barred windows and door waiting their turn to see the physician. They were the last patients of the scheduled sick call. Once their assessment, diagnostic tests, or treatments were completed, the hospital correctional officers assigned to transportation would return them in handcuffs and a secured van to their respective housing units. The phone rang constantly and required the nursing supervisor and a second RN to screen the calls from officers in the housing units who reported the inmate complaints, requests for medications and refills, accidents, or any unusual behavior or symptoms observed by the officers. The nurses made the decision that required assessment in the emergency department, and two hospital officers would pick up the inmate and bring him to the hospital. The licensed practical nurse (LPN) and two emergency medical technicians (EMTs) assisted the physician. Finally, at around 8:00 p.m., the nursing supervisor realized that the phone calls were becoming less frequent. She always felt like she was playing Russian roulette, hoping she and her staff asked the right questions or were receiving accurate replies for accurate phone assessments.

The loud ring from the "red" emergency phone jarred everyone into a state of readiness. The phone was connected to the warden's office, the central security office, and the hospital emergency department, so that all key personnel were alerted with the dialing of a single number. The ominous sound always meant an emergency of some description. As nursing and security staff gathered at the doorway to listen, the nursing supervisor quickly picked up the receiver. The excitable, stuttering voice on the other end was barely intelligible. It was obvious the officer was in trouble and had to be coaxed by the security chief to report the housing unit number. The nursing supervisor had heard the word "stabbing" and the unit number. Suddenly, she heard the quivering male voice on the other end cry out, "Oh my God, he's gonna kill all of us!" before the line went dead. She immediately dispatched one of the two life-support ambulances. The second ambulance was on its way to another far-flung maximum security housing unit so the RN, a former critical care unit nurse, could assess an inmate complaining of severe chest pain. The supervisor instructed the transportation officer and RN to report to the scene of the stabbing as soon as the assessment was completed unless the inmate required further monitoring in the emergency department. She and the remaining nursing and security personnel then put into action the plan they had developed as a team shortly after her arrival. The two major trauma rooms and the staff were ready to receive victims of violence within minutes after the departure of the ambulance. The physician on call was on her way to the hospital to await their arrival.

The radio was crackling with orders and the relaying of information from security. The ambulance crew was unable to enter the housing unit until the violent rampage had been quelled and the drug-crazed inmate had been subdued by the E-squad, officers who received continuous training in confronting violence within the prison and searching for escaped felons. She could hear and feel the palpable fear and chaos; the number of victims could not be immediately determined and could not be reached because the perpetrator wielded a homemade knife, daring the officers to come near him or the victims. She had never been so close to violence. The ambulance crew described the horror of the scene to her as they arrived with the first victim removed from the unit: a young male with multiple stab wounds to the chest. A second physician was called for assistance because two other victims were reportedly arriving. She and the physician worked quickly to start IVs, insert chest tubes, and stabilize the first victim for transport to a hospital intensive care unit 30 miles away. The second victim arrived with cardiopulmonary resuscitation (CPR) in progress; he had been stabbed in the back repeatedly, then literally picked up and flipped over and stabbed in the face, chest, and abdomen. Each time his chest was compressed, blood gushed from the multiple wounds, which totaled more than 50. After a grueling hour, the inmate, in his early 20s, was pronounced dead. She had never seen so much blood. Linens were soaked with the warm, moist liquid that continued to drip from the sides of the stretcher on which the inmate lay, and one could not avoid the pools of blood on the floor.

She silently wondered what could provoke such a hideous act of violence. She choked back the tears of anger, fear, and bewilderment. There were no family or friends to mourn or to console, because the family would be notified by phone. Her past experiences and education had not prepared her for the little value placed on life within prison and the potential for raw violence within human beings. She gently covered him with a clean sheet as she remembered her husband's frequent rebuttal to her complaints about late-night phone calls from inmates' parents: Everybody here is some mother's baby.

She entered the corridor and knew the pounding of her heart could be heard over the din of the animated conversations between officers and healthcare personnel. She managed to assign staff to transport the first victim to the hospital and to prepare the body of the deceased victim for the funeral home before she retreated into the quiet conference room. She could not control the violent shaking of her entire body or the feeling of revulsion that manifested as an overwhelming nausea. She knew what she had to do; but for the first time since she had become a nurse, she doubted her ability to be nonjudgmental. How could she provide care for someone who had committed such a senseless act of violence? The respect for the individuality of patients and human worth had been the foundation of her 20-year nursing career; yet, for the first time, she questioned her own ability to follow these beliefs. She also had to confront her paralyzing fear for the safety of her family as well as her own safety in her world of nursing. Finally she was able to leave the conference room and enter the noisy clinical area. Still shaking, she took a deep breath and picked up the chart of the next patient to be assessed: the inmate who had stabbed the first two patients and had brought violence into her world that night.

UNIT 5

Vulnerable Populations

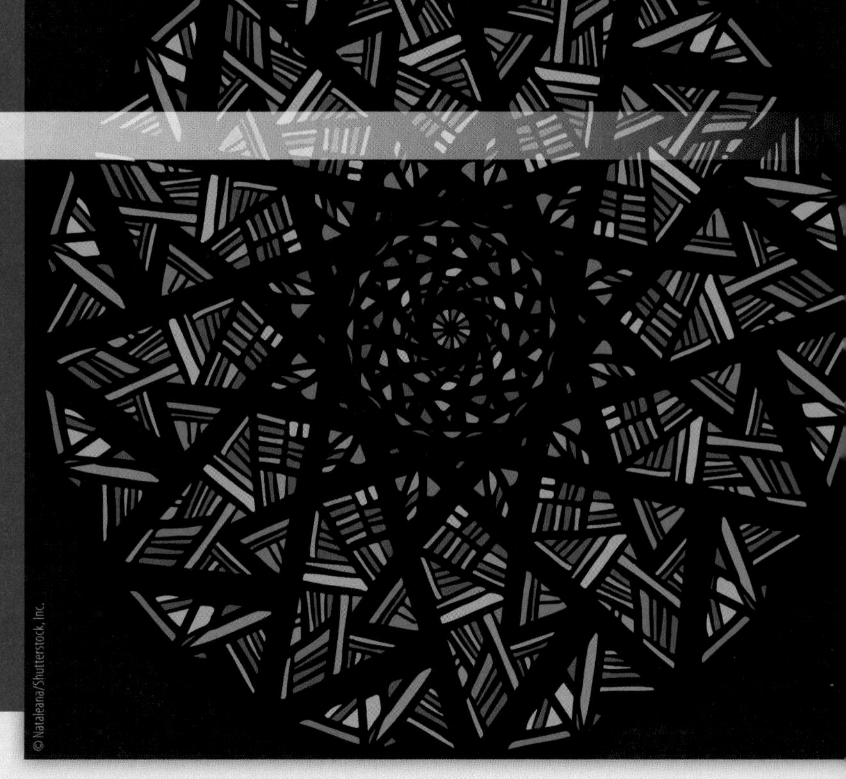

CHAPTER FOCUS

Basic Concepts Related to Risk and Vulnerability
- Social Determinants
- Risk
- Vulnerability
- Persons with Special Needs
- Vulnerable Populations

Web of Causation: The Interrelationship Social Determinants, Risk and Vulnerability

Poverty: Impact on Risk and Vulnerability
- Historical Perspectives
- Cultural Perspectives
- Policy Perspectives
- Health-Related Perspectives
- Community Perspectives

Vulnerable Populations with Special Needs
- Children and Adolescents
- Elders
- Underrepresented Ethnic Groups
- Uninsured and Underinsured Populations
- Disenfranchised Populations

Nursing Considerations
- Limited Access to Care
- Ethical and Legal Considerations
- Patients' Strengths and Resources

Nursing Roles
- Case Manager
- Educator and Counselor
- Advocate and Activist
- Collaborator and Partner
- Researcher

QUESTIONS TO CONSIDER

After reading this chapter, you will know the answers to the following questions:

1. What are social determinants and how do they impact health status?
2. What is vulnerability?
3. What are the risk factors that contribute to vulnerability and poor health?
4. What is the relationship between poverty and vulnerability?
5. What are some examples of vulnerable populations?
6. What are some characteristics of specific vulnerable populations?
7. How can nurses intervene to bring about positive health outcomes for vulnerable populations?

Community health nurses traditionally have been recognized as crusaders and advocates for populations described as vulnerable and at risk. Compared with the general population, persons in these groups are at great risk for experiencing disparities in access and uneven quality of care, which contributes to poorer health outcomes.

CHAPTER 24

Vulnerability in Community Populations: An Overview

Angeline Bushy

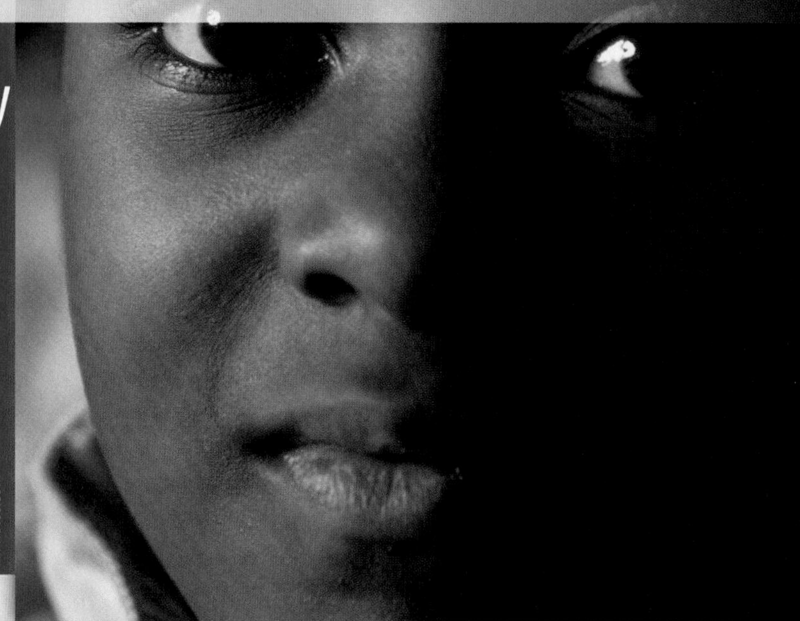

© Photos.com

KEY TERMS

access to health care
at risk
disadvantaged
disenfranchised
hardiness
health disparity
impoverished
medically indigent
near poor
neighborhood poverty
persistent poverty
poverty index
risk
social determinants
underinsured
uninsured
vulnerability
vulnerable families
vulnerable populations
working poor

> What a devil art thou, Poverty! How many desires—how many aspirations after goodness and truth—how many noble thoughts, loving wishes toward our fellows, beautiful imaginings thou hast crushed under thy heel, without remorse or pause!
>
> —Walt Whitman

> To be shelterless and alone in the open country, hearing the wind moan and watching for day through the whole long weary night; to listen to the falling rain, and crouch for warmth beneath the lee of some old barn or rick, or in the hollow of a tree; are dismal things—but not so dismal as the wandering up and down where shelter is, and beds and sleepers are by thousands; a houseless rejected creature.
>
> —Charles Dickens

> Loneliness and the feeling of being unwanted is the most terrible poverty.
>
> —Mother Teresa

REFLECTIONS

What does it mean to feel vulnerable? Have you experienced times in your life when things seemed hopeless? How did this affect your health? Vulnerability is a complex concept and related to health and social risks of specific populations. As a student nurse, how do you view those who are poor, disenfranchised, and stigmatized by society?

HEALTHY PEOPLE 2020 (U.S. Department of Health and Human Services [HHS], 2011) notes that social determinants can impact health status and lists specific objectives for illness prevention and health promotion that target populations described by some as at risk and vulnerable. Specifically cited are the poor, homeless, very young, elderly, adolescents who are pregnant, severely mentally ill persons, substance abusers, victims of abuse, and the disabled. Also targeted in this policy-guiding document are persons at risk for, or who already have, communicable diseases, specifically human immunodeficiency virus (HIV), hepatitis B virus (HBV), and other sexually transmitted diseases. The interaction effect of multiple risk factors results in comorbidity among people who are vulnerable. Therefore, the epidemiological web of causation model is useful for nurses to understand the interrelationship of risks and vulnerability. Poverty is a recurring theme and an important intervening factor in health status but surely not the only one. Furthermore, nurses must examine patients' hardiness and level of resilience, their strengths, access to community resources, and social support systems, because these can counterbalance other risk factors that promote vulnerability.

Basic Concepts Related to Risk and Vulnerability

The concepts of social determinants of health, risk, and vulnerability can be difficult for nurses to fully understand in relation to the multiple factors inherent in these terms. Moreover, not all people experience these factors in the same way. While one person may thrive after experiencing certain risks, for example, another individual may have less favorable outcomes. Essentially, understanding the interrelationship of these three concepts is influenced by personal beliefs, cultural values, and societal attitudes about dependency. The terms *social determinants*, *risk*, and *vulnerability* often are interchanged in health policy discussions and in the nursing literature. Even though these three concepts are interrelated, there are some differences in their meanings (Bushy, 2013; Marmot & Wilkinson, 1999; Merriam-Webster Dictionary, 2014a, 2014b).

Social Determinants

Since the early 2000s, the term **social determinants** has come into use in health policy and nursing literature. Essentially, social determinants are conditions of the environment into which people are born, live, work, play, worship, and age that can affect health status, functioning, and quality of life. Social determinants include contextual attributes of "place" (e.g., built and physical environment, social and economic conditions, resources) that exist in various settings where individuals function (e.g., school, church, recreational venues, worksite, and neighborhood). The concept of place further alludes to a community's preferred patterns of social engagement that can impact individuals', families', and whole communities' sense of wellbeing (Marmot & Wilkinson, 1999; McDavid-Harrison & Dean, 2011). Resources, on the one hand, that enhance quality of life can have a positive influence on health status. Conversely, the lack of certain resources could be detrimental to wellbeing and impact the health status of individuals, families, and communities (Centers for Disease Control and Prevention [CDC], 2011; Institute of Medicine [IOM], 2002; Secretary's Advisory Committee on Health Promotion and Disease Prevention [SACHPDP], 2011; World Health Organization [WHO], 2008).

Examples of place-based resources that could impact health include adequate and affordable housing, access to quality education, assurance of public safety, availability of healthy food, a continuum of local emergency and healthcare services, and the built environment that is free from threatening toxins (e.g., air, water, noise, infrastructures; CDC, 2011; IOM, 2002). The manner in which an individual, family, and community experience place (i.e., risk), as it influences health and health status, is inherent in the notion of social determinants. Examples of place-related social determinants (risks) include, among others:

- Availability of resources to meet basic daily needs (safe housing, food, water, air)
- Socioeconomic conditions (access to economic and employment opportunities versus high unemployment, concentrated poverty, and the stressful repercussions associated with these events)
- Access to quality and appropriate health-related services
- Access to quality education and job training
- Availability of community-based resources that support opportunities for employment, social support, lifelong learning, and leisure time activities
- Transportation options and public safety (exposure

to crime and social disorder, presence of community decay, lack of community cohesiveness)
- Supportive social norms and attitudes (e.g., without discrimination, racism, mistrust of government, residential segregation)
- Literacy levels
- Access to mass media and emerging technologies such as the Internet and social media (e.g., digital divide)

In other words, policies and a built environment that positively influence social and economic conditions can support change in individual behaviors; ultimately, over time they can improve and sustain the health of a family and a community.

Healthy People 2020 (HHS, 2011) specifies social determinants of health as one of its four overarching goals (SACHPDP, 2011). Topic areas related to this goal focus on creating social and physical environments that promote optimal health for populations. Advances are needed not only in health care, but also in education, childcare/childrearing, housing, business, law, media, community planning, transportation, and agriculture. When a community (or subgroup/subpopulation) experiences deficits in one or more of these dimensions (risks), everyone in the group becomes more susceptible (vulnerable) to an outcome that could ultimately result in a **health disparity**. Risks that contribute to a health-related disparity include among others, disadvantageous socioeconomic status, unhealthy lifestyle behaviors, low self-esteem, a sense of powerlessness, and hopelessness. Age, race, ethnicity, and gender are demographic variables that might diffuse (or enhance) the potential for a particular outcome or sometimes, even, a group health disparity. Conversely, intervening to diffuse one or more of these variables (risks) could reduce or even eliminate a particular disparity (Agency for Healthcare Research and Quality [AHRQ], 2010; National Partnership for Action, 2011; National Prevention and Health Promotion Strategy, 2011).

> Poverty is the parent of revolution and crime.
>
> —*Aristotle*

Risk

The term **risk** emerges from writings on the natural history of diseases (Merriam-Webster Dictionary, 2014a). In epidemiological models, risk refers to health conditions that result from the interaction of many factors, including a person's genetic makeup, lifestyle, and the physical and social environments in which he or she lives and works. The effect of the integration of multiple factors subsequently makes it more or less likely that a person will develop a particular health problem.

Vulnerability

The term **vulnerability** has its origins in the Latin word *vulnerare,* which means "to wound." Broad definitions of the term include the notion of susceptibility to injury and lack of protection from danger—that is, a potential for physical attack and being insufficiently defended; being liable to censure and criticism; or being more liable to succumb to persuasion and temptation. More specifically, in reference to health policy and community health nursing, vulnerability refers to a person or group that is more likely to develop a health-related problem and have more serious outcomes stemming from exposure to multiple risks (Merriam-Webster Dictionary, 2014b).

> Poverty is an anomaly to rich people. It is very difficult to make out why people who want dinner do not ring the bell.
>
> —*Walter Bagehot*
>
> Anyone who has struggled with poverty knows how extremely expensive it is to be poor.
>
> —*James Baldwin*

Persons with Special Needs

Individuals with special needs often are forgotten, discounted, or misunderstood and may or may not be **at risk**, vulnerable, or disenfranchised. In most cases, the community and families of persons with special needs have additional challenges in meeting their healthcare needs, which may be emotional, economic, physical, or social in nature (CDC, 2011).

Vulnerable Populations

It is important to stress that the vulnerable are not a homogeneous group, but rather represent all segments of society. **Vulnerable populations** are a (sub)group that shares common risks or combinations of risk factors; one that is pervasive is poverty or low socioeconomic status (HHS, 2008; 2011). Vulnerability implies that, compared with the general population, some people are more sensitive to risk factors; this can affect their health, usually for the worse. Those who are vulnerable are particularly sensitive to risks that originate from economic, physical, social, biological, and genetic factors, along with their lifestyle behaviors. Rarely does one risk factor act in isolation, as shown in the web of causation model (see **Figure 24-1**). For example,

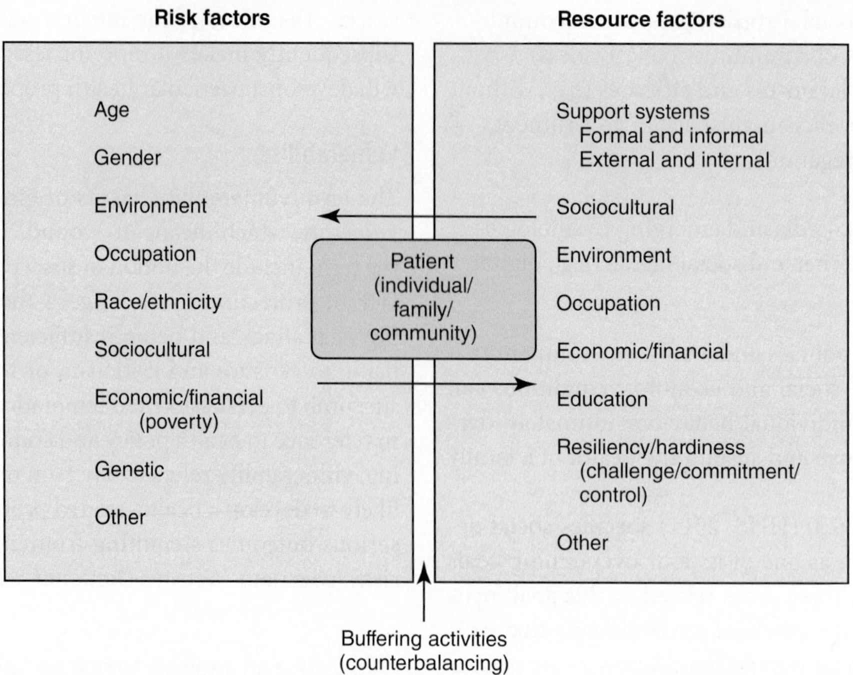

Figure 24-1 Web of causation model.

a person with a chronic mental illness or a physical disability, such as a seizure disorder or respiratory condition that is difficult to manage, may not be able to maintain a full-time job. Therefore, the person probably will not have a regular or adequate salary. In turn, this has an impact on his or her ability to secure adequate and/or safe housing, essential health care, and pharmacological services, and may prevent the person from pursuing further education to seek a job that will pay a higher wage. Associated with chronic symptoms and the inability to be financially self-sufficient, the person may experience chronic depression and lowered self-esteem. To deal with the seemingly overwhelming emotional issues, and in an effort to self-manage the physical symptoms, the person may resort to using over-the-counter medications or alcohol or increase the dosage of prescribed medications. The interaction of these multiple risks results in the person becoming even more susceptible (vulnerable) to additional factors that can negatively impact his or her health status (Bushy, 2013).

Vulnerable families is another phrase often found in the health policy literature. These families are at particular risk because of the intensity or clustering of multiple stressors associated with unanticipated life events and normal maturational changes. Examples of families at high risk and who are particularly vulnerable to future health problems include those who have a member who is chronically ill or disabled, has a chronic mental illness, or abuses alcohol or other mind-altering substances. Families with a pregnant teenager also are considered vulnerable. Special or unexpected events can promote vulnerability, too, such as a family member receiving a diagnosis of a fatal disease, the sudden death of a child, unemployment, and natural or manmade disasters such as a devastating fire, flood, hurricane, tornado, or earthquake. Trauma-related events such as auto accidents, domestic violence, sexual abuse, and violent crimes also predispose a family, as well as a community, to subsequent physical, emotional, and social problems. An increasing combination of intense and multiple stressors (risks) coupled with the depletion of resources can push the family or a community beyond its ability to cope, hence intensifying vulnerability (Bushy, 2013; Kulig, 2000; Leight, 2003). Therefore, nurses in community health practice must closely listen to patients to learn about their personal stories. What words are used to describe a health problem in relation to their lifestyle and activities of daily living? Understanding the patient's perspective is essential for instructing, counseling, advocating, developing, and evaluating nursing interventions that are deemed appropriate and acceptable by a targeted population (Leininger, 1997).

Web of Causation: The Interrelationship Social Determinants, Risk and Vulnerability

From the preceding discussion it becomes obvious that numerous antecedents (risks) contribute to vulnerability. It also fits the web of causation model that is used in epidemiology to understand and approach health and illness.

This schematic model can assist nurses in the community to understand the interrelationship among multiple factors that contribute to the choices made by individuals, families, and communities that ultimately affect their health status. Factors commonly associated with vulnerability that could be included in a web of causation model include disadvantaged socioeconomic status, lifestyle behaviors, low self-esteem, feelings of powerlessness, and disenfranchisement. Consistent with the web of causation model, the interaction among individual assets, social assets, and demographic factors contributes to a higher likelihood of poorer versus better health. Moreover, age, race, ethnicity, and gender are demographic variables associated with variations in health outcomes. Even more noteworthy is the role that social, economic, and cultural factors play in developing vulnerability or resilience. The web of causation is a useful tool for determining areas where nursing interventions can most effectively be focused to prevent or manage particular risks that predispose a person, family, or even a community to a particular health risk (see Figure 24-1).

For example, a variation that results from genetic predisposition is breast cancer. Or, for instance, race and ethnicity are associated with an intricate set of socioeconomic variables that correlate to chronic illnesses such as hypertension, diabetes, and cardiovascular diseases. Health disparities are examined in greater detail later in this chapter. Individual assets include skills and resources that contribute to one's ability to be economically self-sufficient, such as education and employment. Social assets are characteristics of one's social network that provide emotional and instrumental support, such as family structure, friendship ties, neighborhood connections, and religious organizations. These are but a few of the many risk factors and intervening variables that contribute to vulnerability and resilience (Kulig, 2000).

In applying the web of causation model to teenage pregnancy, for example, nurses in community health settings are able to reflect on the multiple factors that contribute to this costly public health problem. It is important to emphasize that this problem cannot be viewed from an isolated perspective such as not using birth control or the lack of morals of teenage girls. The risk factor of **disadvantaged** status partly is attributable to adolescents' lack of physical and emotional maturity, which predisposes them to impulsive lifestyle choices and poorer pregnancy outcomes than women who are several years older. Low self-esteem is another characteristic shared by many adolescents, resulting in some emulating peers to feel accepted. Unprotected sex is a risky lifestyle behavior that often is fostered by the use of mind-altering substances such as alcohol and street drugs. These behaviors increase the risk of exposure to communicable infections such as HIV, hepatitis, and other sexually transmitted diseases, all of which contribute to less than optimal pregnancy outcomes.

Risky lifestyle behaviors are reinforced or discouraged by community as well as family attitudes regarding sex education and family planning in school curricula. Low socioeconomic status is closely related to level of education and employment opportunities, characteristics that are common themes among adolescent parents. Poverty persists because a young, single mother cannot get a job that provides an adequate salary to support herself, much less a family. As for political and social factors, these are reflected in policies related to public assistance programs (welfare) and childcare programs. Ultimately, these can enable, or deter, an adolescent from obtaining the necessary skills to secure a job that can provide an adequate wage to support a family (HHS, 2008, 2012).

Essentially, adolescent pregnancy is a complex problem involving many risk factors that makes a highly susceptible group even more vulnerable. Moreover, it has a direct impact on the children of adolescent parents, who are the adults of the future. The interaction of these factors and many others are determinants in the rate of adolescent pregnancies in a particular community. Other vulnerable groups similarly are caught up in a web of causation composed of many risk factors.

Poverty: Impact on Risk and Vulnerability

Poverty is closely associated with risk, even though it is not the only contributing factor to vulnerability. Being poor affects the health and wellbeing of individuals of all ages as well as families and communities. Although it often is hidden in a community, poverty exists even within areas that seem affluent. Poverty significantly contributes to other health risk factors, thereby increasing the vulnerability of all community residents, especially other poor residents (HHS, 2008, 2011).

Most health professionals and policymakers contend that poverty is associated with poorer health. Yet one of the greatest obstacles in addressing the problem is the multitude of definitions and individual perspectives about poverty and who truly is "poor." Almost everyone has an idea about poverty; however, it tends to be a relative concept based on personal experiences and cultural values. To understand the meaning of poverty and its impact on the daily lives of families, community health nurses should first examine their own perspectives about the issues and their personal beliefs in relation to others' views. The self-appraisal process can be an effective approach to glean insights on what being poor can mean to others, especially vulnerable patients and their families. In addition, the self-appraisal should reflect on social, cultural, and environmental factors and consider how they contribute to poverty for a particular at-risk group, such as the homeless, single parents, elderly, children, or persons infected with a communicable disease. Insights about another's life situation can go a long way to helping nurses become more accepting and nonjudgmental when working with patients whose personal choices and life situations are different from their own.

THINK ABOUT THIS 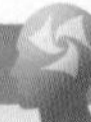

How do changing labels and language influence community nurses and care for vulnerable populations, such as those in poverty?

Historical Perspectives

It also can be useful for nurses to understand the historical evolution of society's attitudes about poverty and people who are poor and dependent. Historically, people in the United States have been rather ambivalent in their views on the topic. Over the centuries, two common themes consistently emerge: a strong work ethic and religious/moral beliefs. When our nation was first established, the view of poverty held by some groups was that it was a temporary condition that could and would be overcome with commitment and hard work. Then, citizens believed that poor people were worthy of assistance and displayed a sense of responsibility to help the needy. The notion that poverty could be a permanent state did not fit with the ideals of our founding fathers, however, who embraced self-sufficiency and individual achievement. Therefore, people were willing to help others who were afflicted with poverty, but it was assumed that persons in need would be on their own, sooner rather than later.

With the Industrial Revolution at the end of the 19th century, the public's frame of reference changed about poverty and assisting those in financial need. At that time, the prevailing attitude was that poor and dependent persons were deserving of their plight in life. Affluence was seen as a moral issue. In other words, it was a just reward for hard-working individuals and a punishment for those who did not work hard. This perspective corresponded with the lack of public assistance programs for the poor and disadvantaged in our nation. In fact, it was not until the mid-1930s, after the Great Depression, that the Social Security program went into effect in the United States. The Medicare program, which focused on the health care of the elderly, went into effect about 30 years after that.

Ambivalence toward the poor and dependent continues even today. Persons who are seen as "temporarily" poor are considered to be worthy of public assistance. This view became a central theme in the 1995 debates leading to the enactment of U.S. welfare reform legislation in 1996. Since then, eligibility criteria have become quite stringent as to who does and who does not qualify for public assistance and for how long. Since then, caring for the poor has shifted from the federal government to the state governments and to the private sector. The long-term effect of the welfare-to-work legislation has been mixed. On the one hand, the actual number of recipients of welfare has dropped in most states in the short term. On the other hand, there has been an increase in the number of families that are classified as "near-poor" and children living in poverty, many of whom are single mothers with children. In turn, this means that persons receiving public assistance may need to move out of their community to develop the necessary work skills and to obtain employment, often part-time and at the minimum wage. For some, it means leaving behind family and other support systems. The situation can become even more complicated because childcare, in many instances, is nonexistent or inadequate for women who must work outside of the home. Another approach to help reduce the cost of public assistance to single mothers with children has been a concerted effort to ensure that child support is paid by fathers who are not present in the home. In brief, long-range consequences for vulnerable families of the welfare-to-work program remain to be seen. Current public sentiment for the most part is to reduce financial entitlements to people who are perceived as not wanting to help themselves.

Cultural Perspectives

The meaning of poverty and the approaches taken to deal with it are culturally based and vary widely among societies and individuals. Often, the cultural beliefs of a particular subgroup or community may conflict or even contradict public sentiment. For example, some people give poverty spiritual relevance by believing that poor people on earth will earn riches in heaven. Still others view most aspects of poverty quite negatively and believe that if poor people would get motivated and work for a living they would be better off and others wouldn't have to support them and their children for the rest of their lives (Leininger, 1997).

Professional groups describe poverty in terms related to the culture of their various disciplines. For instance, social scientists often use the term **impoverished** to describe a variety of conditions related to the lack of a home, relationships, or material possessions. This term also can refer to limited educational, occupational, and financial resources. Healthcare providers tend to define poverty in terms of not having sufficient financial resources to meet basic living expenses such as food, clothing, shelter, transportation, and health care. Therefore, adequate or inadequate financial resources can either counterbalance or intensify other risk factors that contribute to vulnerability (Leight, 2003).

CULTURAL CONNECTION

Roessel is a Navajo writer and photographer and author of *Kinaalda: A Navajo Girl Grows Up*. Although this is a children's book, it provides insights for all adolescents about the importance of ritual in the milestones of womanhood. The main character, Celinda McKelvey, looks like a typical 13-year-old American, and most of the time she lives like one, but her roots are deep in the Navajo nation. With her family, she returns to the reservation to solemnize and celebrate her change from girl to woman. The ceremony, called Kinaalda (Dine or Navajo for "puberty"), marks the coming-of-age for a Navajo girl and is usually held once a Navajo girl has her first menstrual period. Celebrated outdoors and in the family hogan, it consists of 2 days of prayer, ritual, feasting, running, and rejoicing. Celinda mixes the traditional (a handwoven dress) with the new (store-bought clothing) while avoiding processed foods, such as sugar. She blesses her relatives and is blessed by them. She mixes a huge cake, made in part from cornmeal she has ground herself, dedicated to the sun god, and shared with all who attend the Kinaalda. Roessel's text describes Celinda's preparations and the ceremony itself and relates the ancient myth of Changing Woman, the most honored of all Navajo Holy People.

Think about how the Kinaalda ritual honors adolescent fertility in contrast to the negative societal views about teen sexuality and pregnancy. What are implications for community health nurses in caring for adolescent females as a vulnerable population?

Source: Roessel, M. (1993). *Kinaalda: A Navajo Girl Grows Up*. Minneapolis, MN: Lerner Publishing Group.

Policy Perspectives

The federal and state governments use an absolute economic standard to delineate poverty based on the criteria of an "adequate living wage" for a family with a certain number of members (HHS, 2012). People who fall below this standard are considered poor; hence, they qualify for public assistance programs. This standard is referred to as the **poverty index**, which is determined by calculating the cost of specific goods and services within a given timeframe. The federal poverty index takes into consideration the cost of food for a minimum/adequate diet for an individual. This rate is then adjusted for the number (size) and ages of members in a household and place of residence. In 2012, for example, the poverty threshold for a family of four was $23,050. In other words, a family of four whose income falls below this economic index is considered poor; those above the threshold are not. Families who have a slightly higher income sometimes are referred to as the **near poor**. Poverty guidelines are issued by the HHS and revised annually based on the consumer price index. Subsequently, the guidelines are used to determine whether a person or family qualifies for assistance or services under a particular federal or state entitlement program, such as Medicaid, WIC, Head Start, State Children's Health Insurance Program (S-CHIP), and Pell educational grants. The U.S. Bureau of the Census uses this index for statistical purposes to compare national, state, and county socioeconomic and other quality-of-life factors (National Center for Health Statistics, 2012).

There is some question as to the adequacy of the federal poverty index as a tool used in determining services for poor families. Standards that are used to derive the index are disputed, in particular by health professionals. Criticism centers on conceptual and measurement approaches that are used to calculate the index, specifically the diet plan and substance indicators. These are proposed to be an adequate measure of poverty. A broader measure is recommended by advocates for the poor, because the standard of living that is offered by the financial resources of the poverty index is far from adequate. Others suggest that reluctance to revise the poverty index has political implications. In other words, if new measures are adopted or higher inflation adjustments are used, substantially more people would be added to the national poverty rolls. No one in federal and state governments, particularly elected officials, wants to be held responsible for an increase in the number of people receiving public assistance. Regardless, community health nurses will often encounter the poverty index and poverty thresholds, because these have implications for planning, coordinating, and evaluating services for at-risk patients who are vulnerable and also poor.

Economists and policy developers use the phrase **persistent poverty** to categorize individuals, families, communities, and counties that are very poor for an extended time. For instance, a number of rural counties across the United States have been classified as having persistent poverty for nearly half a century. In persistent poverty families, poverty is transmitted from one generation to another. Community planners talk about **neighborhood poverty**, which refers to geographically defined urban areas that characteristically are poor, with substandard housing and high levels of unemployment. Essentially, each person, family, community, and professional discipline has a perspective on the definition, cause, and cure of poverty. A community health nurse may find these frames of reference useful in examining personal attitudes and biases about poverty, people who are poor, and the risks that promote and sustain vulnerability.

Health-Related Perspectives

Compared with those with a higher socioeconomic status, health care generally is less available and accessible to the poor, as evidenced by wide health disparities, especially among underrepresented ethnic groups (HHS, 2008, 2012). For example, the poor have higher rates of infant mortality, complex health problems, and physical limitations resulting from chronic illness. Furthermore, they are hospitalized three times more often than people in higher income brackets. Common hospital admission diagnoses for the poor are asthma, diabetes, hypertension, and other chronic illnesses that in many instances could be better managed with education and routine health care.

Low socioeconomic status can have an impact on the health of people in other ways, too. For example, some types of cancer have significantly higher morbidity and mortality rates among people who are poor, especially if they are members of an underrepresented ethnic group. Likewise, poor people are more vulnerable to trauma-induced injuries and death by violence. Injuries to children in poor families most often are associated with fires, drowning, and suffocation. In impoverished communities, infant mortality rates create additional acute and chronic health concerns. Also, there is a higher incidence of adolescents who become parents. Patterns of risk exposure that contribute to vulnerability continue throughout adulthood, as evidenced by a higher incidence of chronic diseases that are not managed, trauma-related injuries, and early death. Even though low socioeconomic status is not a direct cause of vulnerability, it certainly is a stressor that can intensify the impact of other risk factors.

Community Perspectives

Rural and urban communities of all sizes and cultures have poor people in their midst. Poor communities and neighborhoods share several commonalties, including a higher proportion of underrepresented ethnic groups and single mothers, higher rates of unemployment, and lower wages for those who are employed. In poor communities, children in single-parent households are poorer in income and other resources compared with counterparts in communities with higher average family incomes (National Center for Health Statistics, 2012). People of color who also are poor are more likely to experience violence, discrimination, and police brutality than more affluent counterparts. Other correlates of poverty include increased rates of communicable disease (especially tuberculosis and HIV), premature death, occupational hazards, unsafe housing, and homelessness. Especially unfortunate correlates for impoverished children include delayed development, depression, anxiety with increased incidences of separation from families, and placement in foster care. Using the web of causation model, nurses can visualize how poverty intensifies other risk factors that contribute to and sustain vulnerability in an individual, family, and community.

Poor neighborhoods have higher rates of crime and substance abuse with lower-quality levels of education. Housing often is less than adequate—sometimes even deplorable. Community health nurses should not be surprised to find poor individuals and families living in condemned buildings, on the street, in cardboard boxes, under highway viaducts, in stalled vehicles, or in storage sheds. It is not unusual for poor families to be intermittently homeless. Substandard living conditions result in residents being exposed to a range of environmental hazards (risks), including inadequate heating, sanitation, and bathing facilities; vermin and other pests; and unsafe drinking water. Poor neighborhoods are more likely to be situated near highly industrialized areas, landfills, and toxic waste sites and have gang-related activity. Thus, living in a poor neighborhood poses an additional risk that contributes to increased morbidity and mortality independent of an individual's lifestyle, behaviors, and occupation.

Living in a resource-depleted environment affects vulnerability in other ways, too. Poor people continually are faced with multiple risks associated with chronic stressors such as frustration over employment options, inadequate and unsafe housing conditions, repeated exposure to violence and crime, inadequate childcare assistance, and the insensitive attitudes of health and social service agencies. Bombardment of stressful situations on an already vulnerable patient, family, or community perpetuates feelings of powerlessness, hopelessness, and helplessness; poor self-esteem; anxiety; chronic depression; and physical illness. It is not unusual for an individual, family, neighborhood, or community to become immobilized. In other words, they do not have the ability to effectively respond to even the routine activities of daily living. They go from crisis to crisis and try to cope as best they can. As coping abilities are strained by unpredictable and unrelenting events, vulnerable individuals, families, and communities lose their ability to master multiple stress-producing situations, which can be a detriment to their health.

Vulnerable Populations with Special Needs

There are many at-risk vulnerable populations with special needs in this nation. The needs of the vulnerable populations that are receiving the most public attention are discussed here—specifically, children, elders, underrepresented ethnic groups, women, the **disenfranchised**, and the **uninsured** and **underinsured**. As mentioned earlier, at-risk individuals usually experience comorbidity and fall into more than one of these groups, thereby intensifying their degree of vulnerability.

ENVIRONMENTAL CONNECTION

The Year After the Perfect Disaster

A year after Hurricane Katrina devastated the city of New Orleans, the Brookings Institution tracked reconstruction efforts with a "Katrina Index." The 1-year report by the Brookings Institution found some signs of life and hope in the metropolitan area of New Orleans. The housing market was making slow gains, with home rehabilitation and demolition proceeding and rentals on the rise; many hospitals and schools had reopened and there was some indication that tourists were slowly returning to the French quarter. Yet, fewer than half of all bus and streetcar routes were running, only a third of the region's restaurants and grocers had reopened, as had fewer than a quarter of childcare centers. Gas and electricity were flowing into 40% and 60%, respectively, of homes and businesses that received those services before the hurricane struck in August of 2005. Six months after the hurricane, the city's labor force had dropped by a third, from 633,759 to 429,469. As of August 2006, it stood at just 444,153, and the unemployment rate was rising faster than the growth of the labor force.

Hurricane Katrina posed a special threat to vulnerable populations, such as the poor, elders, children, and people with disabilities. How can the lessons learned from this disaster assist community health nurses better reduce the environmental risks for vulnerable populations in U.S. urban areas such as New Orleans?

Source: Liu, A. (2006). *Building a better New Orleans: A review of and plan for progress one year after Hurricane Katrina*. Brookings Institution. Retrieved from http://www.brookings.edu/metro/pubs/20060822_katrinaes.pdf

Children and Adolescents

Compared with adults, nearly twice as many children live in poverty. In recent years, the number of adults and elderly living in poverty has decreased, while the number of children living in poverty has increased dramatically. Of all persons in the United States who are poor, nearly 40% are younger than 18 years of age, and about 11% are older than 65. One in five American children younger than 6 years of age and one in four children younger than 18 is poor. Children in single-parent households are twice as likely to be poor as those who live in two-parent homes. Of all children who are poor, about one-third are African American. In recent years, poverty among Latinos has increased more than any other group. Native American children, however, probably are the poorest and the most likely to be in substandard living conditions, especially those who live on Indian Reservations (HHS, 2008, 2011, 2012; National Center for Health Statistics, 2012; U.S. Bureau of the Census, 2012). Despite these statistics, many Americans do not see poverty as a major problem for children.

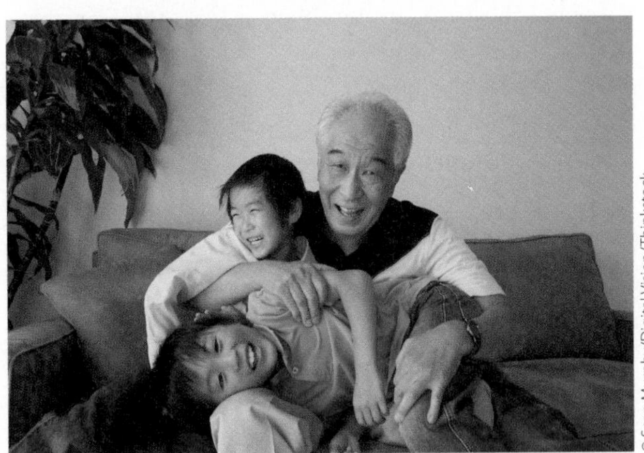

Elders and children have greater risks for many diseases.

Dr. Jocelyn Elders, a former U.S. Surgeon General, has stated that many of these children are members of the 5-H Club; that is, they are hungry, homeless, hugless, hopeless, and without health care. Furthermore, low income, low educational level, and low-wage occupations correlate with infant mortality, low birth weight, birth defects, and infant deaths (HHS, 2008, 2011). Poverty also increases the risk in young children for developing chronic diseases, trauma-induced injuries and death, developmental delays, poor nutrition, inadequate immunizations, iron deficiency anemia, and elevated serum lead levels. Compared with nonpoor children, their poor counterparts are more likely to go hungry and suffer from fatigue, dizziness, irritability, headache, and ear infections. Poor children have a higher prevalence of upper respiratory infections, weight loss, inability to concentrate, and absenteeism from school. The youngest are at the greatest risk and are more vulnerable to developmental delays associated with inadequate nutrition and lack of routine preventive health care.

As for disadvantaged adolescents, usually they do not have the opportunity to acquire the skills and knowledge that are associated with success in adulthood. Correspondingly, they lack a sense of personal mastery and self-esteem. Compared with more affluent teens, those who are poor are more likely to have below-average academic skills and subsequently to drop out of school (National Center for Health Statistics, 2012).

MEDIA MOMENT 

Selected Films About Vulnerable Populations

To Kill a Mockingbird (1962)

Based on the Pulitzer Prize-winning novel by Harper Lee published in 1960, the film won numerous awards and is considered one of the most important films of the 20th century. The film and novel are loosely based on Lee's observations of her family and neighbors, as well as an event that occurred near her hometown in 1936, when she was 10 years old. The story takes place in a small Southern town and was one of the first to deal with the serious social issues of rape and racial inequality.

ATL (2006)

This film chronicles the lives of teenagers in Atlanta and the challenges of inner-city living. The film presents a rare portrait of male parents raising their children alone under harsh conditions with hope for the future.

A Boy's Life (HBO Films, 2004)

This film documentary by award-winning filmmaker Rory Kennedy presents a dramatic and unflinching portrait of the disturbing family and social forces that have influenced the life of a 7-year-old boy from the Mississippi delta. From his grandmother and single mother (who conceived Robert as a result of a rape at age 16) along with his therapist and school officials, viewers are presented with various opinions of the boy's destructive behavior. Social, cultural, family, and environmental influences emerge as contributing variables in this excellent film about a vulnerable family, hope, and possibility in the face of seemingly insurmountable conditions.

Regardless of their race, poor adolescents are about six times more likely to have children than their nonpoor counterparts. A number of reasons are cited for this demographic variance, including lack of knowledge about sexual development and practicing safe sex, limited access to family planning services, and lack of responsible adult role models. With welfare reform, there are restrictions on the length of time that one can receive public assistance. During this timeframe, the welfare recipient is expected to make significant life changes that will lead to financial independence. Most often, this entails the person's completing the necessary education to obtain a job. Usually, these are entry-level positions in the service industry offering the minimum hourly wage. Many times, it is only a part-time job that does not provide health insurance benefits. With the passage of the Affordable Care Act (ACA) in 2010, more patients have access to affordable insurance through public exchanges. Although female single parents may eventually be removed from states' welfare rolls, they often do not make an adequate living wage to support themselves and their children. Community health nurses should be aware that poor money management skills, along with the costs of childcare, contribute to the problem of sustained poverty among single-parent families. A variety of innovative programs are being implemented across the nation to help address the special needs of vulnerable children and adolescents, such as after-school recreational programs and employer-sponsored childcare services. Community health nurses have an important role in health promotion, anticipatory guidance, and illness prevention strategies in these initiatives.

Elders

Elderly persons constitute another vulnerable group who are at risk (HHS, 2008, 2012). Many of them live on fixed incomes, have chronic health problems, live alone, and are unable to manage their own affairs. For example, elders in many instances do not have transportation because they do not own a vehicle, cannot drive, and have no access to public transportation or anyone to transport them. The elderly who are in long-term care or extended care facilities are particularly vulnerable because of the additional stress (risk) of being displaced from their home and family. Even though the poverty rate among elders has decreased since the 1980s and early 1990s, many experience numerous risks that predispose them to health problems, including environmental, nutritional, and sociocultural factors. The decline in poverty is partly attributable to changes in Social Security benefits, coupled with the increased availability of other federal and state entitlement programs that focus on the elderly population. A few elders, even though they are eligible for entitlement benefits, are not aware that these programs exist, and others may not know how to access these services. This phenomenon occurs most often in rural areas, where a person may be socially or geographically isolated, and among individuals who cannot speak or read English or for whom English is their second language. Elderly people who are members of underrepresented ethnic groups, particularly African Americans, Latinos, and Native Americans, tend to experience higher rates of chronic illness, which contributes to the health disparities that have been identified within these groups.

Underrepresented Ethnic Groups

Race and ethnicity are related to risk and vulnerability (National Center for Health Statistics, 2012). Similar to poverty, the factors of race and ethnicity do not operate in isolation. People of color who are also poor are more likely to be exposed to other risk factors, which interact negatively to affect the health status of their communities. (The predominant underrepresented ethnic groups in the United States are African Americans, Latinos/Hispanics, Asian Americans, Native Americans, and Alaska Natives.) Although health status in the United States improved throughout the 20th century, disparities still exist across various segments of the population. Health disparities among underrepresented ethnic groups are rooted in economic, environmental, and socioeconomic circumstances (National Center for Health Statistics, 2012).

RESEARCH ALERT

A primary goal of welfare reform was to overcome welfare dependency through the promotion of work and the setting of lifetime limits. While at first glance, this goal may have appeared reasonable for young recipients, it does not address the needs of older recipients, particularly women. Based on in-depth interviews with welfare recipients in four impoverished rural Appalachian counties over a 4-year timespan (1999–2001; 2004), this article evaluates the experiences of older women as they confront the changes brought on by welfare reform legislation. Findings suggest that impoverished older women in isolated rural communities experience multiple crises as they attempt to negotiate the "new" welfare system. As a result of spatial inequality, limited social capital, and the effects of ageism, they have tremendous difficulty meeting even their most basic needs.

Source: Henderson, D., & Tickmayer, A. (2008). Lost in Appalachia: The unexpected impact of welfare reform on older women in rural communities. *Journal of Sociology and Social Welfare, 35*(3), 153–171.

Essentially, those having a low socioeconomic status and fewer years of education do not fare as well in terms of morbidity, mortality, injuries, exposure to environmental hazards, and access to health care as do those with more financial resources and higher educational backgrounds. However, it is not race or ethnicity that is the primary contributor to these poor outcomes, but lower socioeconomic status. In comparing the gap in life expectancies between African Americans and Caucasians in the United States, gaps (disparities) have been associated with socioeconomic status rather than race. Thus, members of certain subsets of the population are at higher risk or are more vulnerable to poor health than the population as a whole, and these vulnerabilities have much to do with economic and social circumstances. The view that health is an outcome of both personal assets, such as heredity and lifestyle, and social and environmental context (e.g., access to health care, healthy living and working environments, access to nutritious foods) is not a new one but is receiving increasing attention in policy and research arenas (National Center for Health Statistics, 2012).

GLOBAL CONNECTION 

"Keep, ancient lands, your storied pomp!" cries she
With silent lips. "Give me your tired, your poor,
Your huddled masses yearning to breathe free,
The wretched refuse of your teeming shore.
Send these, the homeless, tempest-tossed, to me;
I lift my lamp beside the golden door."

Emma Lazarus (1849–1887), U.S. poet.
Written for inscription on the Statue of Liberty.

Based on Bushy's (2013) definition of vulnerable and marginalized populations, why are the immigrants in this poem by Lazarus vulnerable?

Healthy People 2020 has a goal of elimination of "the disparities in six areas of health status experienced by racial and ethnic minority populations while continuing the progress we have made in improving the overall health of the American people." These six areas are infant mortality, cancer screening and management, cardiovascular disease, diabetes, HIV and acquired immune deficiency syndrome (AIDS), and immunizations. *Healthy People 2020* (HHS, 2011) calls for a reduction in health disparities between the majority population and special populations in the United States, particularly for people of color. Communities that are particularly vulnerable are those in persistent poverty counties, especially Native Americans living on reservations, African Americans living in the rural South, and migrating farm workers of Latino origin. Many in these communities experience living standards and health outcomes that compare with those in Third World countries.

Uninsured and Underinsured Populations

Even though vulnerable populations are more likely to need healthcare services, many are not able to access them (Leight, 2003). A number of reasons are cited for this phenomenon (**Box 24-1**), but one of the most problematic is the lack of healthcare insurance. Prior to the implementation of the ACA of 2010, more than 45 million people in the United States did not have health insurance benefits. Three groups are particularly affected by escalating healthcare costs and reductions in service within a community—the elderly, poor children, and growing numbers of individuals who do not have health insurance or do not receive public assistance, specifically Medicaid (National Center for Health Statistics, 2012). Of these, some may

BOX 24-1 Select Dimensions of Limited Access to Care

- Lack of adequate healthcare insurance
- Inability to pay for services
- Language and cultural barriers
- Inequitable distribution of healthcare providers (more often in inner cities and remote rural counties)
- Geographic and social isolation
- Challenges associated with transportation and communication infrastructures (great distances to providers, poor travel conditions, lack of telephone services)
- No public transportation
- Inconvenient hours to see patients at clinics or health centers
- Insensitive attitudes by healthcare providers toward patients who are poor or of another racial/ethnic/cultural background

qualify for public assistance, but the family does not have the ability to apply or lacks the motivation to do so. Some of the **medically indigent** fall in the category of **working poor** or near poor. That is, there are working adults in the family, but they do not have enough money to purchase healthcare insurance, yet their income is too high (above the federal poverty index), so they are disqualified from obtaining public assistance. A number of families have health insurance but do not have adequate coverage (underinsured) with low reimbursement rates, high prescription drug costs, and high copayments,

Although the elderly, poor children, and the near poor have been in the public spotlight, other populations are also affected. As cost-containment strategies are implemented by employers, many employees find that portions of their insurance benefits have been reduced or eliminated. Families often assume they have adequate coverage until a family member experiences a catastrophic illness or chronic disability, and subsequently they are confronted with excessive medical expenses. Community health nurses should also be sensitive to the fact that the working poor/near poor are likely to underuse preventive services. For many of them, illnesses often go untreated until there is an acute manifestation of symptoms or an emergency. This behavior has implications for designing, implementing, and evaluating nursing services that target at-risk vulnerable groups and populations with special needs.

Disenfranchised Populations

Some people who are disenfranchised may be vulnerable, but that is not necessarily true in all cases. Disenfranchisement refers to feelings of separation from mainstream society. When this phenomenon occurs, an individual or group does not experience an emotional connection with the rest of society. The disenfranchised include the chronically and/or mentally ill, the homeless, prisoners, persons with HIV/AIDS, refugees, and immigrants. Some veterans of the war in Iraq and Afghanistan, for example, are disenfranchised as a result of serving in the military for wars not fully supported by the American public. The current conflicting political environment, exacerbated by posttraumatic stress disorders that often develop as a result of intense combat experiences, contributes to their feelings of isolation from society.

Nursing Considerations

Limited Access to Care

At-risk and vulnerable individuals, families, and populations tend to have numerous nursing care needs. For example, poor health conditions often are exacerbated because the vulnerable, especially those who also are poor, have limited access to healthcare professionals and primary healthcare services (HHS, 2008, 2011). **Access to health care** infers more than having health services available in a neighborhood or a community. Existing healthcare or social services must fit with the needs and preferences of the population for these to be deemed as acceptable and appropriate. Achieving "fit of service" implies that community health nurses must partner and work with the community. The following strategies have been found useful in designing appropriate and acceptable services for vulnerable patients in diverse settings:

- Getting to know the community and working with residents to identify what services are needed and the best way to provide those services
- Scheduling clinic visits for patients at times that are convenient for vulnerable populations, such as after finishing field work or at times when public transportation is operational
- Having bilingual nurses available in the healthcare facility for the convenience of patients who do not speak English
- Having staff members who reflect the cultural, racial, and ethnic background of the patients who use the healthcare facility
- Ensuring that all employees are sensitive to the plight of others, especially the poor and those having other belief systems. This may involve offering sensitivity programs for employees
- Demonstrating a nonjudgmental attitude when working with people who are poor and of another culture

Ethical and Legal Considerations

There are innumerable ethical and legal issues accompanying poverty and providing care to vulnerable and at-risk populations (Bushy, 2013). Community health nurses often find themselves in key positions to advocate for vulnerable populations and help them effectively solve their problems and become contributing members of society. Associated with this responsibility are ethical and legal considerations that must be understood. One of the most common ethical issues encountered is the allocation of scarce resources. At the core of this value-laden issue are a number of questions. For example, who is most needy, worthy, or deserving to receive scarce resources? Who decides? Where does enabling dependent behavior end? Where does helping the needy to become more self-sufficient start? As resources become scarcer, grappling with ethical issues will become paramount in our society, especially when designing nursing services for vulnerable populations in medically underserved regions.

There also is an array of corresponding legal issues associated with poverty. For instance, poor neighborhoods often experience more violence and crime. Consequently, legal situations may arise related to maintaining confidentiality versus reporting criminal activity that nurses may encounter, such as domestic abuse, child neglect, and gang- and drug-related activities. Community health nurses are encouraged to become familiar with ethical and legal issues related to their nursing practice and to reflect on approaches to prevent and deal with such situations in an appropriate manner.

ETHICAL CONNECTION 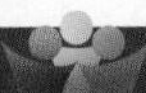

The current debate about immigrants, refugees, and undocumented workers in the United States involves passionate and conflicting views among U.S. citizens. Political debates often result in few solutions that are acceptable to the public, regardless of the public's beliefs and values. What are the ethical implications of our ideas about who deserves health care and other social services? How do these ideas affect our ability to provide care for all?

Patients' Strengths and Resources

Successful nursing interventions build on resources that are available to and acknowledged by the patient. Moreover, health promotion research focuses on factors that contribute to health and maintain long-term wellbeing. Specifically, negative risk factors must be balanced against health-enhancing factors such as hardiness and support systems. The concepts of hardiness and support systems are best understood as interfacing catalysts, one enhancing the effects of the other.

Hardiness

Hardiness is a term used to describe aspects of human resilience (Kabasa, 1979; Low, 1996). Theoretically, hardiness alludes to a combination of factors that keep some people from developing a problem, even with exposure to a health risk. It is identified as a potential intervening factor in individuals and families (perhaps communities, too) who seem to overcome the most adverse conditions and still lead meaningful lives. For example, hardiness may be a factor in why some persons with HIV infections survive for decades, whereas others become very ill or even die within a short time after becoming infected. Dimensions of the concept of hardiness include control, commitment, and challenge. The interrelationship among the three dimensions is the essence of hardiness. Essentially, faced with stressful life events, the hardy person will attempt to change or modify the event (control) into something that is consistent with his or her life purpose (commitment), which will result in learning and personal growth (challenge). There may be additional aspects related to all three dimensions that are relevant to community health nursing, in particular that of "control," or the lack of it, among at-risk and vulnerable groups.

Support Networks

Support networks also can be counterbalancing and mediating forces to risk factors that contribute to vulnerability. Support can be formal or informal in nature. Furthermore, there is no prescription as to who should be included in the individual's support network that could include family, friends, neighbors, and others in the community. Preference and use of support varies by individuals, families, and communities and is culturally defined. For instance, some cultures have extensive social support networks, as is the case for many Native American, African American, and Latino families. The extent of these networks often becomes evident when a patient visits the clinic or is hospitalized, accompanied by a contingent of relatives representing several generations. Such an extensive network is not the case for everyone, however. Community health nurses will find that some patients are unable to identify even one person in their support network. For these people, the healthcare system becomes even more significant.

For example, a middle-aged homeless man, recently released from prison after being incarcerated for several decades, lost all contact with his family. In another case, a 25-year-old homosexual man was diagnosed with HIV/AIDS in a large city located in another state. Upon visiting his parents in a very small town, he told them about his diagnosis and how the infection probably was acquired. They responded by asking him never to come back to their home or their town, because their religious belief system did not condone homosexuality. More than likely they would be extremely ashamed if the community found out about their son's diagnosis or sexual orientation. Increasingly, many faith communities are identifying and supporting vulnerable congregation members. Parish nurses, along with other community health nurses, assume a variety of roles in developing and sustaining support networks for the most vulnerable individuals, families, and populations.

Nursing Roles

Nurses in community health settings assume a variety of roles in coordinating services and developing interventions for at-risk and vulnerable individuals, families, and communities. When developing a plan of care, it is important for nurses not only to assess the multiple risk factors, but also to identify mediating resources, such as an individual's, a family's, or a community's resiliency and the quantity and quality of their support networks. Assessment goes beyond helping to identify formal and informal resources, however. It implies the use of specific nursing roles, including advocate, activist, case manager, educator, counselor, partner, collaborator, and researcher. The roles change when developing, implementing, and evaluating interventions to fit vulnerable patients' particular needs and preferences.

Case Manager

A case manager is another role for nurses who work with patients having special needs. This role usually involves the nurse in partnership with an individual patient. Case management is a process in which services are organized and coordinated to meet a patient's particular needs and to use scarce resources more effectively. In community health nursing centers, case management for a patient can extend over a very long period, sometimes months or even years. Moreover, case managers will find that the need for formal and informal services often increases in intensity and complexity as patients are exposed to other health risks and stressful situations. Nurses in the role of case manager, especially those working with vulnerable patients who experience multiple risks, must ensure that needed services are used and care plans are modified to reflect changes. Effective case management requires a broad knowledge base of nursing roles, formal resources, and informal community support networks and an innate ability to integrate all three. Case managers are crucial in preventing and resolving confusion that can arise when patients have multiple members on their healthcare teams. Confusion is especially problematic among patients in very large agencies. Inherent in case management are the activist and advocacy roles described later, along with the nurse educator and counselor roles (Bushy, 2013).

Educator and Counselor

Two other important, often overlapping roles for nurses are teacher and counselor. People might change risky lifestyle behaviors if they learn about their detrimental impact on their health. Education can be one of the most cost-effective and noninvasive interventions to inform consumers, regardless of their socioeconomic status, about pharmacotherapy protocols, health promotion, stress management, developmental events, and changing life roles. For instance, education, accompanied by counseling interventions, can be used by nurses in supporting patients through the grief process; in adjusting to anticipated, and unanticipated, life events; and for improving communication skills between family members and with health professionals. Education and counseling, in some instances, can be used to teach high-risk patients to ask appropriate questions of investigating agencies they encounter. The educator and counselor roles are important to enable patients to locate and access community resources. However, nurses cannot do it all alone. Community-focused interventions must be developed to expand a nurse's span of effectiveness using resources that are available and acceptable to the client and his or her family system (Bushy, 2013).

GOT AN ALTERNATIVE?

Models, such as the Eden Alternative, have presented a theoretical basis for attempting to create a therapeutic environment by bringing live-in animals and plants into the nursing home. This research article reports on the implementation and assessment of an intervention termed the "Living Habitat," which applies concepts from the Eden Alternative model. Implemented on a 32-bed unit of a large urban nursing home, the Living Habitat offered numerous plants, a parakeet to any resident who requested one, and two cats and a dog for the unit. A baseline assessment of residents ($n = 26$) was conducted prior to the introduction of the animals and plants, and follow-up data were obtained 6 months after the intervention began. Results indicate that, following the introduction of the Living Habitat, residents higher in cognitive status became more positively engaged with their environment but reported a decreased sense of control. Residents who had greater affinity for pets also became more positively engaged with their environment. System interventions for implementing the "Living Habitat" project are discussed.

What are specific ways that community health nurses can use this research in working with vulnerable populations, such as homebound elders?

Source: Ruckdeschel, K., & Van Haitsma, K. (2001). The Impact of live-in animals and plants on nursing home residents: A pilot longitudinal investigation. *Alzheimer's Care Quarterly*, *2*(4), 17–28.

Advocate and Activist

In the role of advocate, the nurse must first be sensitive to the healthcare needs of the vulnerable individual, family, or community, in addition to having a broad knowledge of community resources and how to access them. The nurse also must possess the ability to communicate in a professional manner with and for a patient to coordinate a continuum of services. Persistence is needed on the part of the nurse when acting on behalf of a vulnerable patient. Time and patience often are necessary to maintain contact with these patients and direct them to the appropriate resources. Political activism at the local, state, and national levels is another aspect of the advocacy role. Nurses can make a difference in the lives of those who are vulnerable and poor by getting involved in the policy arena and by working with elected officials. Community health nurses are in positions to work with public and private entities to provide the necessary resources for new or more comprehensive services. An example of this is using formal and informal opportunities to discuss issues relevant to public health with legislators and policymakers. Remember, during these interactions the nurse is seen first and foremost as a professional role model having expert power. Nurses in community health practice are in a unique position to advocate for improving the economic and health status of vulnerable populations and for those having special needs (Bushy, 2013).

ETHICAL CONNECTION 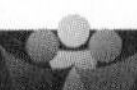

The Digital Divide: Are the poor part of the technology revolution?

In 2012, 97% of children whose family income was $75,000 or more per year had computers in their homes, while 58% of children whose family income was less than $15,000 per year had computers at home. White and Asian/Pacific Islander children (65% and 63%) were more likely to have Internet access than black or Latino children (49% and 44%).

If information is power and the poor have limited access to the vast resources available online through the Internet, what are the ethical issues related to resource allocation and technology? How does this influence community health nursing care of vulnerable populations?

Advocacy involves representing special consumer groups to regulatory organizations and even local health commissions. The nurse advocate publicly supports and sometimes opposes federal and state initiatives. Advocacy may entail grassroots lobbying for legislation that provides a financial safety net for people with catastrophic costs that are not covered by Medicare or health insurance. Sometimes, it involves a nurse testifying against the views of an elected official who does not support a safe house for abused women, or a residential home for the mentally challenged, or a halfway house for youth offenders. The overall goal of a nurse advocate is to represent vulnerable populations and help these patients solve problems and develop appropriate solutions for their concerns. Advocacy and activism do not mean taking care of, enabling, or promoting long-term dependency. They are about teaching people how to help themselves by developing greater resilience and more effective coping skills to deal with their concerns.

Collaborator and Partner

Nurses can collaborate with providers from community-based agencies and citizen groups to address the particular concerns of vulnerable and at-risk populations with special needs to create a seamless continuum of care. Nurses in community health settings must learn to partner with administrators and others from institutions outside the healthcare system, specifically education, housing, and employment bureaus. Collaboration can be useful to extend and enhance scarce resources, especially in medically underserved and persistent poverty communities. Nurses should also learn to collaborate with private and not-for-profit entities on community projects that focus on the needs of groups who are at risk for poor health outcomes. Even if community health nurses are not involved directly in partnerships, they can serve as liaisons or facilitators to promote collaboration between community groups. The challenge for community health nurses is to become as proficient in partnering/collaborating roles as in direct caregiving skills (Bushy, 2013).

Researcher

The role of the nurse as a researcher has become very important in recent years. The needs of vulnerable and at-risk

ART CONNECTION 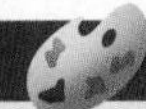

The Dutch painter, Van Gogh, often depicted poor, working class persons who worked in rural areas in his paintings. Locate one of his paintings and describe why these populations would meet the definition of vulnerability.

RESEARCH ALERT

Driving while distracted: Teens with attention deficit hyperactivity disorder and auto accidents

This research provides compelling evidence that attention deficit hyperactivity disorder (ADHD) is associated with significantly increased risks for various adverse outcomes while driving, including increased traffic citations (particularly speeding), motor vehicle crashes for which the driver is at fault, repeated crash occurrences, and more severe crashes as determined from dollar damage and likelihood of bodily injuries from the crash. Teens with ADHD are more likely to have their licenses suspended and even fully revoked. Research further suggests that these driving risks cannot be accounted for by the comorbid disorders likely to be associated with ADHD, such as oppositional defiant disorder (ODD), conduct disorder (CD), depression, or anxiety, or by lower than normal levels of intelligence. Teens diagnosed with ADHD have almost four times more auto accidents as those without the disorder. They receive three times more speeding violations than those without ADHD and are more likely to have auto accidents resulting in bodily injury. The author offers some explanation of how the disorder conveys such increased risks. The findings of studies indicate that ADHD interferes with the basic operational components of driving by means of the impairments it produces in attention, resistance to distraction, response inhibition, slower and more variable reaction time, and the capacity to follow rules that may compete with ongoing sensory information. Those with attention deficit disorder/hyperactivity disorder are more easily distracted and when placed in situations that require critical moment-to-moment concentration, such as driving a car, may be at a greater risk for accidents involving driving. Added to the risk of driving is the use of music players and cell phone/smart phones, which has moved these "tools of distraction" from the home to the car. Parents of teens with ADHD should be advised about these heightened risks and encouraged to take steps that may reduce them, including the consideration of more graduated licensing for adolescents with ADHD and the possible use of stimulant medication in teens with ADHD while they are operating a motor vehicle.

How can the community health nurse apply this research to practice with this vulnerable population?

Source: Barkley, R. (2004). Driving impairments in teens and adults with attention-deficit/hyperactivity disorder. *Psychiatric Clinics of North America,* Volume 27, Issue 2, Pages 233–260.

populations can be significant, and there are no easy answers to meet them, especially in communities with seemingly few resources. There is an urgent need for nursing research on implementing and evaluating interventions that can be used with vulnerable and medically underserved segments of society. In many instances, vulnerable populations with special needs must first be identified, because they may be hidden or forgotten. In addition, outcome studies are needed to measure the health-related effects of existing community-based nursing interventions within a targeted population. Nurse scholars report that the sky is the limit for studying health concerns of particular populations that experience multiple risk factors that promote vulnerability. Likewise, there is a need for evidence-based and cost-effective nursing practice models that target selected at-risk groups and lead to favorable health outcomes (Bushy, 2013; Cole & Fielding, 2007; McDavid-Harrison & Dean, 2011).

AFFORDABLE CARE ACT (ACA)

As of September 2010, all new health insurance plans, including Medicare, Medicaid, and government-sponsored market insurances, have been required to include recommended preventive services and immunizations to which no deductible and copayments can be applied.

LEVELS OF PREVENTION

Primary: Provide health teaching to a group of seniors in a nutrition program concerning healthy eating choices on a limited income.

Secondary: Develop a screening program for senior adults at a local church for hypertension and diabetes.

Tertiary: Staff a disaster shelter for special needs populations, such as those who are disabled and are dependent on specialized equipment.

Conclusion

This chapter examined the issues surrounding risk and vulnerability and their impact on health. Definitions were examined along with risk factors that contribute to vulnerability and poor health status. *Healthy People 2020* objectives (HHS, 2011) specifically address the factors that contribute to health disparities among vulnerable groups, including the homeless, children, elders, pregnant adolescents, the chronically mentally ill, substance abusers, victims of abuse, and those with disabilities. Community health nurses should be aware that vulnerability is precipitated by a multitude of interrelated risk factors. Perhaps the one risk that most exacerbates the effect of others is poverty. In other words, not having enough money to procure safe housing, adequate nutrition, preventive health care, and the education to develop the skills to work in a job that provides a living wage all can contribute to level of vulnerability. Community health nurses must learn to accept, respect, and understand how these risk factors contribute to vulnerability and influence a patient's lifestyle and healthcare behaviors. Sensitivity entails recognizing health risks and the person's, family's, or community's strengths and resources when designing a holistic nursing care plan.

Critical Thinking Activities

1. How do you define poverty? Which words are used in your family when talking about poor or dependent families and individuals?
2. Which characteristics or attributes do you associate with a family or individual who is poor? On which experiences or situations do you base your ideas? Family? Friends? Classmates? Personal experience?
3. Which sorts of resources are available in your community to address the needs of the poor or vulnerable? Make a list of formal and informal resources to refer to when referring patients. If possible, contact one or two agencies or providers to discuss the criteria that are used to determine who can receive entitlements.
4. Interview an elderly person or a single mother who is on a fixed income that is provided by an entitlement program, such as Social Security or a welfare-to-work program. Ask the person to share personal insights on what it means to be dependent, with very limited financial resources. What at-risk or vulnerable group does the person fall into? Is this group cited in *Healthy People 2020*? How does the person/family feel about public services that they are enrolled in, and how do they describe healthcare providers' attitudes toward them or their family?
5. Ask someone you know to share his or her life story with you. Identify risk factors that contribute to vulnerability. Which strengths and resources are used to cope with those risk factors? Describe the person's health care–seeking behaviors when he or she needs professional care for a health problem. What suggestions does the person have to make healthcare services more accessible? Reflect on potential ethical and legal implications that contribute to vulnerability in this person's lifestyle. How can these best be addressed?
6. Learn about partnership models in your community. Ask local school officials, the ministerial association, law enforcement, and public safety officials if similar initiatives exist. Describe these and share your findings with peers. Develop strategies to give credit to the partners, and encourage other groups to assume a proactive role in dealing with the special populations who are at risk in your area; for instance, interview participants for the school newspaper or invite them to speak to peers.
7. Describe attributes of health-promoting social determinants in a community. Reflect on your own community in which you live and work. Describe the absence of health-promoting social determinants and the impact this has had on the people who live in this community.

NOTE THIS!

A new nurse-led initiative between the American Academy of Nursing entitled "Have You Ever Served?" and the National Association of State Directors of Veterans Affairs (NASDVA) has resulted in a new program that nurses can use to assess and intervene with the vulnerable group of military veterans and their families. This program uses a pocket clinical guide for nurses to use when assessing associated risks for all populations of military and veteran age groups. For more information on how to implement this program and improve health care for veterans, service members, and their families go to HaveYouEverServed.com.

HEALTHY ME

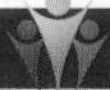

Think of a time when you felt vulnerable, whether your life was threatened or your health was threatened, without means to receive treatment or care. How did you react? Where did you seek assistance? How did you feel about being vulnerable?

References

Agency for Healthcare Research and Quality (AHRQ). (2010). 2009 national healthcare quality and disparities reports. Retrieved from http://www.ahrq.gov/qual/qrdr09.htm

Bushy, A. (2013). Risk, vulnerability, social, determinants and health disparities. In C. Winters (Ed.), *Rural nursing: Concepts, theories and practice* (4th ed.). New York, NY: Spring Publications.

Centers for Disease Control (CDC). (2011). CDC health disparities and inequalities report—United States, 2011. Retrieved from http://www.cdc.gov/mmwr/pdf/other/su6001.pdf

Cole, B., & Fielding, J. (2007). Health impact assessment: A tool to help policy makers understand health beyond health care. *Annual Review of Public Health, 28*, 393–412. Retrieved from http://www.annualreviews.org/doi/abs/10.1146/annurev.publhealth.28.083006.131942

Institute of Medicine (IOM). (2002.) Disparities in health care: Methods for studying the effects of race, ethnicity, and SES on access, use, and quality of health care. Retrieved from http://www.iom.edu/~/media/Files/Activity%20Files/Quality/NHDRGuidance/DisparitiesGornick.pdf

Kobasa, S. C. (1979). Stressful life events, personality, and health: An inquiry into hardiness. *Journal of Personality and Social Psychology, 37*(1), 1–11.

Kulig, J. C. (2000). Community resiliency: The potential for community health nursing theory development. *Public Health Nursing, 17*(5), 374–385.

Leight, S. B. (2003). The application of a vulnerable populations conceptual model to rural health. *Public Health Nursing, 20*(6), 440–448.

Leininger, M. (1997). Transcultural nursing research to transform nursing education and practice: 40 years. *Image: Journal of Nursing Scholarship, 29*(4), 341–347.

Low, J. (1996). The concept of hardiness: A brief but critical commentary. *Journal of Advances in Nursing, 24*(3), 588–590.

Marmot, M., & Wilkinson, R. (Eds.). (1999). *Social determinants of health.* Oxford, UK: Oxford University Press.

McDavid-Harrison, K., & Dean, H. (2011). Guest editorial: Use of data systems to address social determinants of health: A need to do more. *Public Health Reports, 126*(3), 1–6. Retrieved from http://www.publichealthreports.org/issueopen.cfm?articleID=2718

Merriam-Webster Dictionary. (2014a). Risk. Retrieved from http://www.merriam-webster.com/definition/risk

Merriam-Webster Dictionary. (2014b). Vulnerability. Retrieved from http://www.merriam-webster.com/definition/vulnerability

National Center for Health Statistics. (2012). Summary Health Statistics for U.S. Adults: National Health Interview Survey, 2011. Retrieved from http://www.cdc.gov/nchs/data/series/sr_10/sr10_256.pdf

National Partnership for Action. (2011). HHS action plan to reduce racial and ethnic health disparities. Retrieved from http://www.minorityhealth.hhs.gov/npa/files/Plans/HHS/HHS_Plan_complete.pdf

The National Prevention and Health Promotion Strategy. (2011). *The national prevention strategy: America's plan for better health and wellness*. Retrieved from http://www.cdc.gov/features/preventionstrategy/

U.S. Bureau of the Census. (2012). Washington, DC: Government Printing Office. Retrieved from http://www.census.gov

U.S. Department of Health and Human Services (HHS). (2008). *Health United States: 2007*. Hyattsville, MD: Author. Retrieved from http://www.cdc.gov/nchs/hus.htm

U.S. Department of Health and Human Services (HHS). (2011). *Healthy People 2020*. Hyattsville, MD: Author. Retrieved from http://www.healthypeople.gov/2020/default.aspx

U.S. Department of Health and Human Services (HHS). (2012). *2012 HHS poverty guidelines*. Retrieved from http://aspe.hhs.gov/poverty/12fedreg.shtml

World Health Organization, Commission on Social Determinants of Health (WHO). (2008). Closing the gap in a generation: Health equity through action on the social determinants of health. Retrieved from http://whqlibdoc.who.int/publications/2008/9789241563703_eng.pdf

CHAPTER FOCUS

Rural Populations
- Definitions of Rural
- Rural Population Characteristics
- Perspectives and Stereotypes
- Issues, Concepts, and Populations

Urban Populations
- Health and Social Problems
- Programs for Healthier Urban People
- Urban Sprawl and Health

The Homeless Population
- Scope of the Problem
- Definitions of Homeless People
- Historical Perspective
- The Health Problems of Homeless People

Caring for Urban and Homeless People
- Use Leadership Skills
- Be Committed
- Be an Advocate
- Use Available Resources
- Foster Communication and Trust
- Assess the Problem
- Plan and Give Care

QUESTIONS TO CONSIDER

After reading this chapter, you will know the answers to the following questions:

1. What are the various definitions of rural health?
2. How do rural populations differ from urban populations?
3. Which lifestyles and behaviors of rural adolescent populations put them at risk for illness or injury?
4. Which specific characteristics of rural life increase isolation for rural elders?
5. Which specific cultural characteristics of migrant workers provide a challenge for community health nurses?
6. What are the differences between rural and urban homeless populations?
7. What are the major factors contributing to homelessness today?
8. How is poverty related to homelessness?
9. What is the Healthy Cities movement?
10. What is the Federal Emergency Relief Administration?
11. What was the first federal legislation specifically passed to aid the homeless?
12. What are barriers to health care for the homeless?
13. What are some of the most common health problems of the homeless?
14. What is the role of the community health nurse in addressing the needs of urban homeless persons?

Living in urban areas often means "living in one's car." Poverty in urban populations has been the source of many problems that have developed in cities, especially stress, hunger, communicable diseases due to overcrowding, violence and crime, homelessness, and inadequate housing.

CHAPTER 25

Rural, Urban, and Homeless Populations

Janie B. Butts and Gale A. Spencer

KEY TERMS

access to health care
agricultural hazards
confidentiality
culture
Federal Emergency Relief Administration (FERA)
ghetto counterculture
Healthy Cities
homeless
housing
intentional injury
isolation
lifestyle
metropolitan statistical areas
migrant farm workers
rural–urban continuum
sexual activity
Stewart B. McKinney Homeless Assistance Act of 1987
substance use and abuse
unintentional injury
urban population

> "City life is millions of people being lonesome together."
>
> —Henry David Thoreau

REFLECTIONS

The farmer is a hoarded capital of health, as the farm is the capital of wealth; and it is from him that the health and power, moral and intellectual, of the cities came.

He stands close to Nature; he obtains from the earth the bread and the meat. The food which was not, he causes to be.

The city is always recruited from the country.

The men in cities who are the centers of energy, the driving-wheels of trade, politics or practical arts, and the women of beauty and genius, are the children or grandchildren of farmers, and are spending the energies which their fathers' hardy, silent life accumulated in frosty furrows, in poverty, necessity and darkness.

Put him on a new planet and he would know where to begin; yet there is no arrogance in his bearing, but a perfect gentleness. The farmer stands well on the world.

The first farmer was the first man, and all historic nobility rests on possession and use of land.

—Ralph Waldo Emerson, Chapter VI, "The Farmer," in *The Complete Works of Ralph Waldo Emerson*, ed. Edward Waldo Emerson. Boston, MA: Houghton Mifflin, 1903–1904.

What is your image of farming and rural communities? We often associate rural areas with stereotypical images of unsophisticated people without the advantages and resources of their more fortunate and affluent urban counterparts. How does this perspective influence the way nurses care for this population? What does Emerson mean that the farmer "was the first man" and that "it is from him that the health and power, moral and intellectual, of the cities came"?

If you have lived in or visited an urban area, what have you observed about the culture, people's behavior, and those who find themselves homeless?

Most people reading this chapter will have never experienced being "homeless." What are your impressions of those who are on the streets begging for change, rummaging through garbage cans, or talking to themselves? Why as nurses do we avoid taking positions that involve the homeless?

Rural Populations

Definitions of Rural

Rural has multifaceted definitions based on geographic, demographic, sociological, and economic perspectives. A simple definition of rural is "country." If you do not see many houses or buildings but instead you see nature—mountains, plains, forests, or other scenery—you are in a rural area. This definition is based on geography and the environment. It is the most subjective definition. Eighty-four percent of the land area in the United States is considered nonmetropolitan, and 97.3% of the land area in the United States is rural (U.S. Department of Agriculture [USDA], 2008). Only 19.3% of the total U.S. population lives in those rural areas (U.S. Census Bureau, 2010). Although this is a small percentage of the population, people living in these areas have many special health needs. Community health nurses are a significant source of health care for rural people. When the characteristics of a place are taken into consideration, sociological ideas are applied to the definition. The availability of services such as libraries, colleges, newspapers, transportation, and health care affect people's perceptions regarding how urban or rural life seems. One commonly used definition of rural combines demographics and proximity to services. Proximity to services is assumed when a place is near an urbanized center. The **rural–urban continuum** (USDA, 2013) is a coding system that describes counties by both population and proximity to services. The continuum identifies **metropolitan statistical areas** (MSAs) as one or more counties that are considered metropolitan. Counties that are not in MSAs are either micropolitan or nonmetropolitan, but they range on a continuum based on their urbanization, population, and adjacency to an MSA (see **Figure 25-1**). For instance, counties in North Carolina are described as follows (North Carolina Rural Health Research and Policy Analysis Center, 1998):

- Urbanized, adjacent to MSA (4)
- Urbanized, not adjacent to MSA (5)
- Less urbanized, adjacent to MSA (6)
- Less urbanized, not adjacent to MSA (7)
- Thinly populated, adjacent to MSA (8)
- Thinly populated, not adjacent to MSA (9)

Examples of rural counties are provided in Figure 25-1 and are given numbers according to their urbanization and adjacency to an MSA. There are three categories of metro counties; they are included in the MSA and are numbered in the schematic as 1–3 (USDA, 2013).

Economists have defined rural counties in terms of their economic base. This way of defining a rural area helps in predicting the impact of events. For example, if

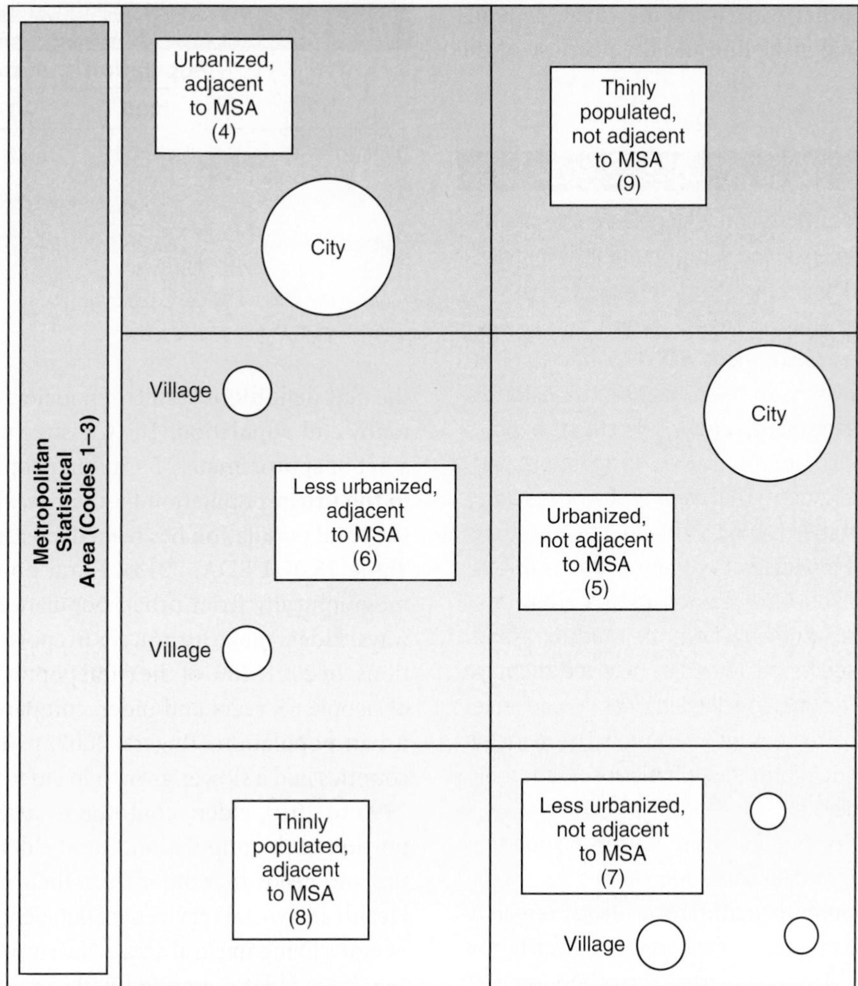

Figure 25-1 Schematic of rural counties.

an area is dependent on farming and the weather interferes with crop growth, economists can project earnings and losses for the region. When the major income of an area declines, it can be expected that services (e.g., car sales, new construction) in that area will also suffer. Some types of counties defined by their economic base include the following:

- Farming-dependent counties (440 total, 403 nonmetro): remotely located, sparsely populated, geographically concentrated in the Midwest
- Mining-dependent counties (128 total, 113 nonmetro): most are in the South or West
- Manufacturing-dependent counties (905 total, 585 nonmetro): account for 31% of the nonmetropolitan population; three-fifths are in the Southeast, with a more urban orientation
- Government-dependent counties (381 total, 222 nonmetro): approximately 75% are state and local government jobs, whereas 25% are federal; evenly distributed across the country
- Services-dependent counties (340 total, 114 nonmetro): serve as centers for trade, services, or recreation; evenly distributed across the country
- Nonspecialized counties (948 total, 615 nonmetro): may have economic activities such as construction, agricultural services, forestry, or fisheries; found across the country, but most are in the South (Cook & Mizer, 1994; USDA, 2005)

Using all of the definitions together will help community health nurses get the most complete picture of the area. Combining the concepts of population density, resources, access and distance to services, and predominant economic base guides the nurse in identifying the barriers to health and health care.

In general, rural areas are sparsely populated, isolated from services, and have limited services from which to choose. Rural people sometimes have multiple roles such as farmer, judge, rotary president, and church elder. This is because there are fewer people to fulfill all the necessary functions of a community.

There are many other ways to define rural, depending on the professional discipline and the purpose of the definition.

RESEARCH ALERT 

This research study used a convenience sample of 100 migrant farm workers living temporarily in a migrant worker center in El Paso, Texas, to determine the use of complementary herbal remedies for health and illness. A structured interview instrument was designed to elicit information about reasons for medicinal herb use, forms in which herbs were ingested, serious side effects experienced, location of purchase, effectiveness of treatment, and use of allopathic medications. The majority of workers used herbal remedies or other natural products because they believed them to be more effective than pharmaceuticals and because of tradition. Most learned about herbal remedies from a relative—primarily from their mother—and the majority who used herbal remedies believed them to be very helpful in treating specific illnesses. No adverse reactions to any herbal remedy were reported. The majority of participants did not inform their physicians about their use of herbal remedies.

Implications for community health nurses include the need to maintain up-to-date knowledge about the use of herbal remedies among migrant farm workers, research about these remedies' use, and interactions with traditional interventions. By showing an understanding of and sensitivity to the use of these remedies, healthcare providers will be able to conduct more comprehensive health assessments of migrant workers and their families and provide them with more culturally competent care.

Source: Poss, J., Pierce, R., & Prieto, V. (2005). Herbal remedies used by selected migrant farmworkers in El Paso, Texas. *The Journal of Rural Health, 21*(2), 187–191.

Twenty-six different definitions of *rural* were used by authors who published articles in *The Journal of Rural Health* between 1993 and 1995 (Ricketts & Johnson-Webb, 1997). It is important to know what definition is being used when evaluating literature or programs. An area that an author defines as rural may have more services available than the community for which you are planning interventions.

Rural Population Characteristics

In 2010, the U.S. Census Bureau (2010) found that 19.3% of the U.S. population resided in rural areas, while the Office of Management and Budget (OMB) classified 23% as nonmetropolitan (USDA, 2008). The introduction of the new definitions resulted in major shifts in rural geography and population. The Census Bureau estimates that a net of approximately 5 million people have been added to the urban population by the new definitions and that the rural population has been decreased by 3 million; see **Table 25-1** (USDA, 2013). Rural populations differ demographically from urban populations in the following ways. Elders make up a larger proportion of rural populations. In 2001, 20% of the rural population was composed of people 65 years and older, compared with 15% of the urban population (Rogers, 2002, p. 30). Although rural counties had a slower growth in elderly populations from 1990 to 2010, elders continue to make up a larger proportion of the population. Rural elders have characteristics and needs that differ from their urban counterparts. Health and social services are deficient for 25% of all older persons living in rural areas. Nearly 6% of rural elders are age 75 or older compared with 5% of urban elders. The older population found in rural areas is predominately white (**Table 25-2**). The older population is concentrated in the rural South (45%), with a substantial older population also found in the rural Midwest (31%). Rural elders are more likely to be married than their urban counterparts (61% rural to 57% urban). However, widowhood increases with age, and by age 75, 41% of rural women are likely to be widowed. Rural elders are also more likely to assess their health as fair or poor, with 37% of rural elders reporting health problems compared to 32% of urban elders (Rogers, 2002, p. 31).

TABLE 25-1 Regional Population Change 2000–2010

	Population (thousands)		
	2000	2010	% Change
United States	281,421	308,745	9.7%
Rural (nonmetro)	19,132	19,484	1.8%
Urban (metro)	262,290	289,261	10.3%

Source: Data from U.S. Census Bureau, 2011a.

TABLE 25-2 Persons Age 60 and Older by Race/Ethnicity and Residence, 2001

	Rural/Nonmetro	Urban/Metro
White/ non-Hispanic	92%	84%
Hispanic	2%	6%
African American	6%	10%

Source: Data from March 2006 Current Population Survey (CPS) data file.

There are also key ethnic differences in elder populations living in rural and urban areas. The following are just a few of these differences (USDA, 2008, p. 35):

- Elders who are members of underrepresented ethnic groups make up a smaller proportion of the elderly population living in rural than in urban areas.
- Rural African American elders are more likely to be widowed and live alone than their urban counterparts.
- Elders who are members of underrepresented ethnic groups in rural areas are less educated and less healthy than white elders living in both rural and urban areas.
- Elders who are members of underrepresented ethnic groups living in rural areas tend to be poorer than their urban counterparts.

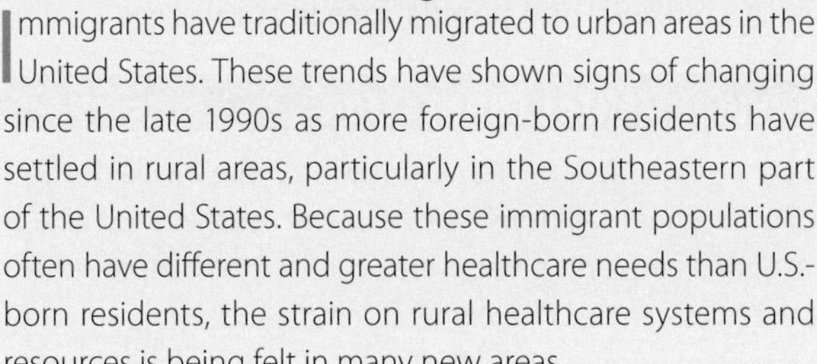

CULTURAL CONNECTION

Immigrants have traditionally migrated to urban areas in the United States. These trends have shown signs of changing since the late 1990s as more foreign-born residents have settled in rural areas, particularly in the Southeastern part of the United States. Because these immigrant populations often have different and greater healthcare needs than U.S.-born residents, the strain on rural healthcare systems and resources is being felt in many new areas.

The rural population of the United States is predominately non-Hispanic white, which represents 81.5% of the rural population and 73% of the urban population. Hispanics represent 12% of the urban population and 6.3% of the rural population (USDA, 2014). Although African Americans make up approximately 14% of the urban population, they account for only 8.4% of the rural population (Klein, Karchner, & O'Connell, 2002; USDA, 2014). (See **Figure 25-2**.) Poverty is more extensive in rural areas. In 2002, the poverty rate was 14% in rural areas and 12% in urban areas (USDA, 2004). The poverty gap of 2 to 3 percentage points between rural and urban areas remained quite stable and is also evident when poverty is analyzed by family structure, ethnicity, race, and age (USDA, 2004). However, in rural areas, 26% of the residents live in households with income just above the poverty guideline (**Box 25-1**), compared with 18% of urban households (Connor, Rainer, Simcox, & Thomisee, 2007; USDA, 2004). This fact makes rural residents vulnerable to downturns in the national or regional economies, as well as to personal or family economic setbacks.

Based on the 2000 Census, ethnic and racial minorities make up 17% of the urban (nonmetro) U.S. population. The rural (nonmetro) ethnic and racial minority populations are growing in all 50 states. The U.S. poverty rates are higher

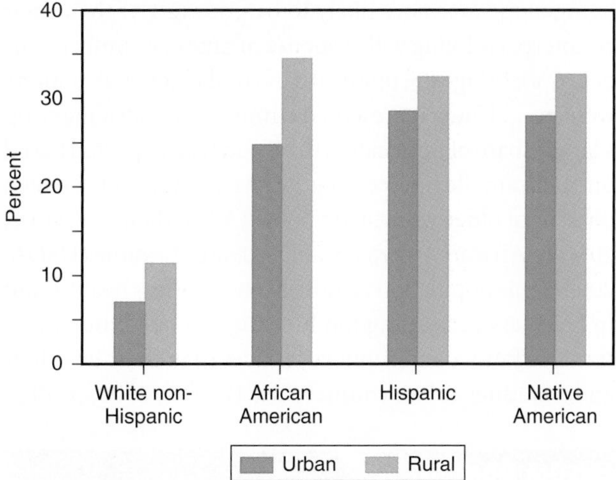

Figure 25-2 Comparison of rural–urban poverty rates by race/ethnicity.

Sources: Data from U.S. Department of Agriculture, 2000; Annual Social-Economics Supplement to the current population survey.

for rural minority populations than for non-Hispanic whites. Rural children also live in poverty at higher rates than do urban children. In 2002, 2.6 million children living in rural nonmetro areas were poor, constituting 36% of the rural poverty population in the United States. One out of every five children living in a nonmetro area was poor. Forty-six percent of all non-Hispanic black children were poor, and 43% of nonmetro Native American children were poor (USDA, 2004, p. 3). The majority (62%) of rural poor children lived in single-parent families, and females headed 55% of these families (USDA, 2008, p. 83).

Rural elders also have a substantially higher poverty rate than urban elders (13% rural to 9% urban). This rate essentially was the same as that of working adults. Poverty is more pronounced among older women, elders living alone, and the oldest old. Women 60 years and older living in rural areas in 2000 were more likely to be poor than older men (15% of women versus 11% men). Rural elders

BOX 25-1 What Does the Poverty Guideline Mean?

Poverty guidelines are the minimum income level needed by a family or individual to meet basic needs of food, shelter, clothing, and other essential goods and services. The official poverty guidelines are adjusted for family size and are set by the U.S. Department of Health and Human Services (HHS) for use by all federal agencies. They are adjusted every year for inflation. In 2014, the poverty guideline was $23,850 for a family of four, and $11,670 for a single individual.

Source: Data from DHHS. (2008). 2008 HHS poverty guidelines. Federal Register, 73(15), 3971–3972.

living alone are more likely to be poor (28%) than their counterparts living with a spouse or another family member (6%); by age 85, one-third of rural elders living alone were poor. Underrepresented ethnic groups also make up a larger share of poor elders than would be expected based on their smaller percentage of the population. Sixteen percent of older women are poor; 14% of them are white, 40% are African American, and 34% are Hispanic (USDA, 2008). This population is more likely to be less healthy and to have less access to good housing, adequate nutrition, transportation, and support services than their healthier and wealthier urban counterparts (USDA, 2008, p. 40).

MEDIA MOMENT 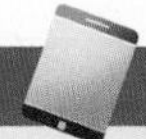

Places in the Heart (1984)

Sally Field won her second Academy Award for Best Actress as a young widow living in Depression-era Waxahachie, Texas, who is determined to keep her small farm by growing cotton on her land. Danny Glover and John Malkovich (playing a blind man) are excellent as hired hands who try to help her make a go of it. Director Robert Benton also won an Oscar for his bittersweet screenplay.

THINK ABOUT THIS 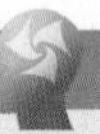

The Farmer

He bends to the order of the seasons, the weather, the soils and crops, as the sails of a ship bend to the wind. He represents continuous hard labor, year in, year out, and small gains. He is a slow person, timed to Nature, and not to city watch.

—Ralph Waldo Emerson

Perspectives and Stereotypes

The word *rural* means many different things to people. It may bring to mind a place where a person can be close to nature and a place where people rely on honesty and hard work. To others, *rural* may be a place where tiny trailers surrounded by rusting automobiles express the poverty of country life. Learning about our personal biases and preexisting ideas is a lifelong process. We learn as professional nurses to put aside our impressions to give the best care possible to our patients. Even when we try to overcome our biases about people, however, these thoughts may still underlie our behaviors. Constantly confronting what we think and asking where these beliefs come from will always enlighten our behaviors. Recognizing the power of the media and the biases expressed in them helps us stay alert to subtle influences in our lives.

Issues, Concepts, and Populations

Rural life is associated with certain issues and concepts that nurses need to be aware of when caring for rural populations. Because rural populations are diverse, it is difficult to find similarities for discussion. For example, elderly Amish people present very different health needs than elderly coal miners. For this reason, special at-risk populations are discussed in relation to more broad issues and concepts found in rural life. See the *Healthy People 2020* feature for objectives related to rural life. Some of the more important issues and concepts identified in rural health care are **lifestyle, isolation, culture, housing, confidentiality,** and **access to health care.** These concepts serve as the framework for the following discussion of at-risk populations in rural areas. Each concept is identified and related to a selected at-risk population. These examples can be integrated into your own experience and study of issues, concepts, and populations in rural areas.

ENVIRONMENTAL CONNECTION

Rural residents are often exposed to more pesticides and other chemical toxins than are urban residents due to agricultural and farming activities. Which kinds of preventive strategies can community health nurses include as part of routine physical examinations that take into account these higher risks?

Lifestyle: Adolescents

Health behaviors and lifestyle profoundly affect the health of all people. Rural people especially lack opportunities for health promotion and health education because of limited access to healthcare providers. Although rural adolescents face many of the same health problems as adolescents in urban areas, they also face unique barriers to health promotion, which include limited access to appropriate health services (Connor et al., 2007; HHS, 1991, 2000). There is a limited amount of research specifically on the health status of rural adolescents; however, the risks that have been identified for all adolescents will be discussed as they relate to rural adolescents and rural lifestyle. These risks include **unintentional injury** from bicycles and automobiles, particularly in combination with alcohol consumption; **intentional injury**, including homicide, suicide, and dating violence; **substance use and abuse** and its related consequences of delinquency and human immunodeficiency virus (HIV); and **sexual activity**, with the risks of sexually transmitted diseases and unintended pregnancy (Fahs et al., 1999; Foster & Frazier, 2008; Johnson et al., 2008; Spencer & Bryant, 2000). One additional risk for rural adolescents that is not identified for urban adolescents is that of **agricultural hazards** (Harvey, 2008).

Unintentional Injury Unintentional injuries are responsible for more deaths in children than from any other cause. In addition, a substantial proportion of childhood hospitalizations and emergency department visits are attributable to unintentional injury (Grossman, 2000). The age-adjusted death rate for unintentional injury in the most rural counties is 86% higher than the corresponding rate in suburban or metropolitan areas (Eberhart & Pamuk, 2004).

Unintentional injuries are found to occur most often when driving or riding in a moving vehicle, whether it is a bicycle, all-terrain vehicle (ATV), snowmobile, or automobile. Bicycle helmets have been proven to be effective in preventing head injuries, but many adolescents still are not using helmets. In rural areas, bicycles may be the only source of transportation because of poverty, isolation, or multiple roles of family members who must share one car (U.S. Department of Labor, Bureau of Labor Statistics, 2008). Thus, bicycle safety issues are of great importance. There may also be more hazards in the rural areas because there are no designated bicycle paths, which results in riding on country roads. The roads are often rough and have no shoulders to allow the rider to get out of the way of automobile and truck traffic.

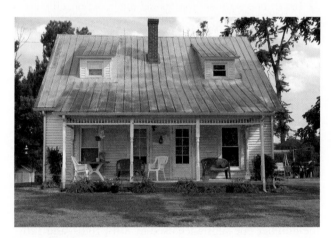

An example of rural housing.

Automobile driving behaviors of adolescents have always been of concern in rural areas. Past studies by Kidd and Holton (1993) and Grossman (2000) found that risky driving practices in rural areas were correlated with alcohol use, risk-taking motivations, a low grade-point average in school, age of 15 to 19 years, and male gender. Rural adolescents often drive all types of vehicles at a much younger age than in urban areas because they can drive without a license on private property. In addition, poor roads and using the car to cruise for entertainment put rural adolescents at greater risk. More recently, McGehee, Raby, Carney, Lee, and Reyes (2007) studied 26 U.S. rural teen drivers, ages 16 to 17, to determine if equipping their vehicles with an event-triggered video device, which was designed to capture 20-second clips of the forward and cabin views whenever the vehicle exceeded lateral or forward threshold accelerations, would improve safety incidents of teen rural drivers. To implement the study, the researchers combined this video technology with parental weekly safety reviews. Results indicated a significant decrease in events for the more at-risk teen drivers.

ATVs and snowmobiles are also more common in rural areas. These vehicles represent special safety risks because of exposure of the rider, likelihood of turnover, limited safety requirements, and rough terrain. Muellman, Walker, and Edney (1993) investigated the magnitude of difference in death rates between rural and urban areas. Age-adjusted unintentional injury death rates were higher in rural areas, with motor vehicle accidents being the main contributor (U.S. Department of Labor, Bureau of Labor Statistics, 2008).

Intentional Injury Violence resulting in intentional injury most often results from the use of firearms. Intentional injuries can be against oneself or against others. In fact, firearm suicide rates alone changed during the 1990s from urban areas to a trend toward rural counties (Branas, Nance, Elliott, Richmond, & Schwab, 2004). In one study by Brent and colleagues (1993), access to a gun by an adolescent was associated with suicide, thus increasing the risk of intentional injury to oneself. In another study by Rausch, Sanddal, Sanddal, and Esposito (1998), the researchers found that deaths in a rural pediatric practice have changed from the 1980s to the 1990s. Deaths related to suicide and homicide have increased; and injuries related to firearms increased during the 1990s. Eberhardt and Pamuk's (2004) study found the age-adjusted suicide rate among rural residents 15 years and older is 37% higher than that for suburban residents. Alcohol and other risk behaviors such as carrying weapons have been correlated with violence against others. In a study by Spencer and Bryant (2000), high school students in rural school districts were found to carry a weapon to school and in the community more often than students in urban or suburban school districts. It might be expected that the rural students would carry guns in the community more often because hunting is an acceptable sport in rural areas. The significant differences found between rural, urban, and suburban students carrying weapons to school is of concern, particularly in light of the several school shootings in small rural communities and suburbs that have occurred in recent decades.

Dating violence is most frequently studied in college populations; however, a study by Symons, Groer, Kepler-Youngblood, and Slater (1993) examined self-reported incidence of dating violence in rural adolescents. This study found that most of the students had been involved in at least one incident of dating violence, and one-fourth of the students had been involved in dating violence two or more times. Dating violence, including date rape, occurs more often than expected in high school students. However, most adolescents are not able to accurately label date rape even when they can clearly report the incident (Fahs et al., 1999). Violent behavior was found in the reported studies to be correlated with adolescents who took more drug risks, carried weapons, were involved in fights, and who were more likely to be victimized (Johnson et al., 2008; Spencer & Bryant, 2000).

RESEARCH ALERT

All-terrain vehicles (ATVs) are a popular form of transportation and recreation for youth, especially for farm-related activities. This study was developed to determine differences in ATV-related behaviors, exposures, risk factors, and injuries between farm youth and their nonfarm peers. A cross-sectional study design was used, and a survey was administered to 652 youths in agricultural education programs throughout the state of Arkansas. A majority (60%) of students had operated ATVs within the past month. Cross-tabulations found that farm youth who rode ATVs were more likely to be white and male, to own a three-wheel ATV, and to ride more often with a single rider. Risk factors for sustaining an ATV-related injury were related to frequency of use, number of persons on the ATV, and use of a helmet. Farm youth were less likely to use a helmet and to ride on a road.

Source: Jones, C. S., & Bleeker, J. (2005). A comparison of ATV-related behaviors, exposures, and injuries between farm youth and nonfarm youth. *The Journal of Rural Health, 21*(1), 70–73.

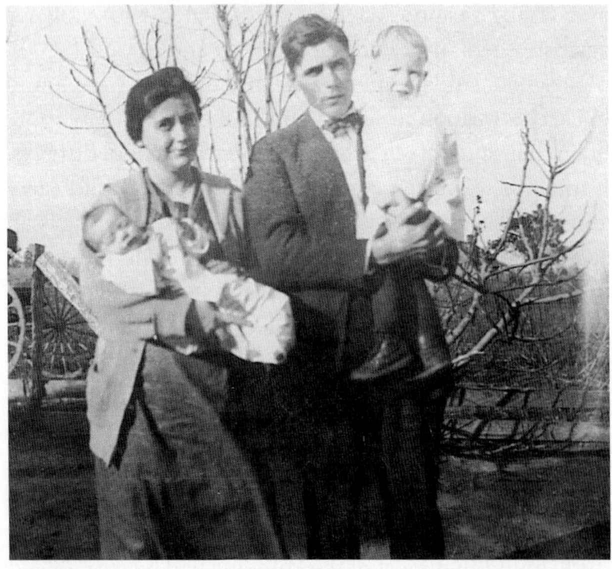

Families in rural settings during the early part of the twentieth century experienced a high infant and maternal mortality rate.

Substance Use

Substance use and *abuse* are terms often used to discuss tobacco, alcohol, and other drugs. Most available research has found that smoking cessation is much more successful among those who started smoking after the age of 13. Few differences were found between urban and rural adolescents in rates of smoking. However, in a study of upstate New York adolescents, smoking was found to be significantly higher in rural adolescents than in their urban counterparts, with 58% of the rural adolescents indicating use of tobacco, compared with 43% of the urban adolescents (Atav & Spencer, 2002). From the data collected in this study, the parents of the rural adolescents were not as well educated, and many smoked themselves, making the behavior more acceptable (Atav & Spencer, 2002; Hartley, 2004). These adolescents also spent more time without parental supervision, which would also allow them to smoke without parental censure.

ETHICAL CONNECTION 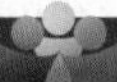

Home health nurses in rural areas often visit patients who know one another. How should the home health nurse respond when a patient asks about the condition or wellbeing of another patient the nurse is visiting?

> The nation that destroys its soil, destroys itself.
>
> —*Franklin D. Roosevelt*

Rural adolescents appear to have alcohol use rates higher than the national average. Though the use of alcohol in adolescents has decreased over the past 5 years, alcohol use still increases significantly as adolescents get older and is the number one substance used by 8th-, 10th-, and 12th-grade students (National Institutes of Health [NIH], 2013). Adolescents in rural areas often participate in large outdoor drinking parties in secluded areas that are not monitored by adults. Older adolescents often initiate younger adolescents to these parties by getting them drunk. Many older adolescents reportedly purchase alcohol for younger adolescents (Atav & Spencer, 2002; Wagenaar et al., 1993). Although cocaine and methamphetamine use has been on the increase by rural adolescents, use of other drugs, especially marijuana, by adolescents continues to be a more common problem (Fahs et al., 1999; Pruitt, 2009). In fact, by the time adolescents reach the age of 17, 68% can buy marijuana within 1 day, 62% have friends who use marijuana, and 58% have been solicited to buy marijuana (Atav & Spencer, 2002). Anabolic steroids appear to be used equally in both rural and urban areas (Whitehead, Chillag, & Elliot, 1992).

Sexual Activity

The birth rate has been declining over the past several years. However, even with this decline, every year more than 1 million adolescents give birth. Of these births, approximately 200,000 occur to teens in rural areas (Yawn & Yawn, 1993). In rural areas, more unmarried mothers are likely to be adolescents. The Centers for Disease Control and Prevention (CDC) Division of Reproductive Health (2013), in partnership with the Office of the Assistant Secretary for Health (OASH), has proposed a program called the President's Teen Pregnancy Prevention Initiative (TPPI) to reduce teen pregnancy and address the disparities in teen pregnancy rates, with a large focus on African American and Latino/Hispanic teens, ages 15 to 19. Goals of this program are to reduce the rates of teen pregnancies and births, increase teen access to evidence-based and evidence-informed programs to prevent pregnancy, increase linkages between teen pregnancy prevention programs and community-based clinical services, and educate stakeholders about resources needed and strategies to reduce pregnancy rates in teens.

Births to unmarried adolescent mothers are a community problem because they require additional support from community agencies. This support takes the form of additional economic resources from welfare agencies or from families who do not have monies to finance a new family unit, and from schools who must teach not only academic subjects to the young mother but parenting skills. Many rural schools have found that the best way to keep adolescent mothers in school is to provide home tutoring for them during the later stages of the pregnancy and childcare later at the school. Although both require additional funds from the community, they are cost-effective because these services often make the difference between young mothers finishing or not finishing high school. Many rural schools have found that having the school nurse participate in teaching child care as part of the curriculum for adolescents returning to school with their babies enhances parenting and assists in preventing additional teen pregnancies.

Community health nurses are often the healthcare professionals most consistently seen by rural adolescents during their pregnancies. This requires community health nurses to serve in the following roles:

- Educators to prepare the adolescent and her family for the changes that will occur throughout the pregnancy
- Counselors regarding family concerns and disagreement regarding the pregnancy
- Advocates for services for the adolescent and her newborn

Research conducted on sexually transmitted diseases in both rural and urban adolescent populations found no differences. A study of rural and urban high school students by Svenson, Varnhagen, Godin, and Salmon (1992) found no differences in knowledge, attitudes, and behaviors regarding sexually transmitted diseases. Engaging in risky behaviors such as unprotected intercourse was also not found to be different between the two groups. However, the 1997 study by Spencer, Atav, and Collins found that sexual activity was significantly different between urban and rural adolescents. Rural adolescents reported sexual activity beginning at a younger age (9.6% of rural adolescents reported being 11 years or younger at age of first intercourse compared with 7.4% of urban adolescents). Participation in sexual activity was also significantly different between rural and urban adolescents, with 49% of rural adolescents stating they participated in sexual activity, compared with 35% of urban adolescents. Many rural school districts do not address the issue of sexually transmitted diseases or teen pregnancy because of the more conservative nature of the school boards, whose members are representatives of these districts. Community health nurses and school nurses must be advocates in rural communities for health education on these topics to be introduced in the school and at community-sponsored activities such as church groups, scouts, or 4-H clubs (Atav & Spencer, 2002; Connor et al., 2007).

MEDIA MOMENT

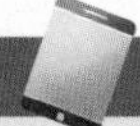

Cold Comfort Farm (1995)

When Flora Poste (Kate Beckinsale), a young society woman in London in the 1930s, becomes suddenly orphaned, she's forced to take up residence with a group of her unsophisticated, oddball relatives at their farm. Despite protests from the bedridden, iron-willed matriarch of the farm, the aspiring lass tries to achieve some semblance of order and class in the house—and in her own life. The cast also includes Eileen Atkins, Ian McKellen, and Joanna Lumley. Both urban and country folk learn from each other in this offbeat satire about life under difficult conditions.

NOTE THIS!

Seventy percent of federally designated medically underserved areas in the United States are rural.

Urban populations have higher rates of alcohol and more illegal drug use than rural areas, with the exception of use of methamphetamine. Missouri law enforcement officers found more than 2,700 "meth labs" in 2004—more than any other

(*continues*)

NOTE THIS! (continued)

state. Rural areas are becoming havens for small-time "cooks" of meth for several reasons:

- Rural areas provide cover for the pungent chemical odors from meth labs.
- Rural areas are populated with many abandoned buildings, such as farmhouses and barns on remote roads. Some of these buildings house methamphetamine labs, which can often operate undetected.
- Anhydrous ammonia is one of the key ingredients in producing meth. It is readily available in rural areas because farmers use this chemical as fertilizer.

Methamphetamine use in rural areas is being affected in the following ways:

- Rural areas are dealing with the cleanup of toxic methamphetamine lab sites, which have a severe impact on the environment. Each pound of methamphetamine produced releases poisonous gas into the atmosphere and creates 5 to 7 pounds of toxic waste. In addition, many meth lab operators dump the toxic waste down household drains, in fields and yards, or on rural roads.
- Children are being endangered. Children who are around areas of meth labs are exposed to toxic chemicals that present significant health and environmental risks. According to research by the federal government, in 2003, 60% of children removed from lab sites had methamphetamine in their systems.

"Meth orphans" include children who are in foster care as a result of one or both parents being in either jail or dead due to methamphetamine use or children being born to mothers addicted to the drug. Their number is growing at an alarming rate. The number of grandparents raising their grandchildren because of this problem is also growing. According to law enforcement officials, the rise in arrests of methamphetamine users in rural America created 3,000 meth orphans in 2003.

Injury to EMS personnel can occur when first responders arrive at a meth site and deal with hazardous substances as well as people under the influence of meth who may be violent, agitated, and unpredictable. The same is true of police and other officials who are involved with responding to illegal meth labs; they are also vulnerable to toxic exposure.

Rural health resources are seldom adequate to accommodate these new health threats, which are becoming a serious public health problem for the entire United States.

Source: Substance Abuse and Mental Health Services Administration, U.S. Department of Health and Human Services. (2008). *The DASIS report: Trends in methamphetamine/amphetamine admissions to treatment, 1993–2003*. Retrieved from http://oas.samhsa.gov/2k6/methTx/methTX.cfm

RESEARCH ALERT

Survey data were collected from a random sample of teens working on farms in North Carolina. The teens ranged in age from 14 to 17. The researchers analyzed the data for farm-based hazard exposure and injury. The sample consisted of 141 teens (72% male) whose mean age was 16.6 years. The data indicated that these North Carolina teens were exposed to significant safety hazards throughout their farming experience. The teens in the sample were exposed to tractors, large animals, all-terrain vehicles, farm trucks, and rotary mowers. More than one-third of the sample was exposed to pesticides and tobacco harvesting equipment. Commonly reported injuries ranged from insect stings to cuts, burns, and falls.

Source: Schulman, M. D., Evensen, C. T., Runyan, C. W., Cohen, L. R., & Dunn, K. A. (1997). Farm work is dangerous for teens: Agricultural hazards and injuries among North Carolina teens. *The Journal of Rural Health, 13*(4), 295–305.

Agricultural Hazards

Adolescent workers on farms are at particular risk of injury as a result of the hazardous nature of agriculture and the lack of safety regulations (see Research Alert). Estimates indicate that approximately 20% of all fatalities in the United States each year occur on U.S. farms. Because the Occupational Safety and Health Administration (OSHA) regulates only businesses employing 11 or more people and the majority of family farms have a small labor force, children/adolescents working on farms are not subject to regulatory protections. Older adolescents and males have higher injury and death rates than do younger adolescents and females. The traditional division of labor by gender on the farm also is an important social influence on work hazards and injury rates. With increasing age, adolescents are channeled into gender-specific tasks, such as males using machines and females doing household tasks (Bartlett, 1993; USDA, 2004; Waller, 1992).

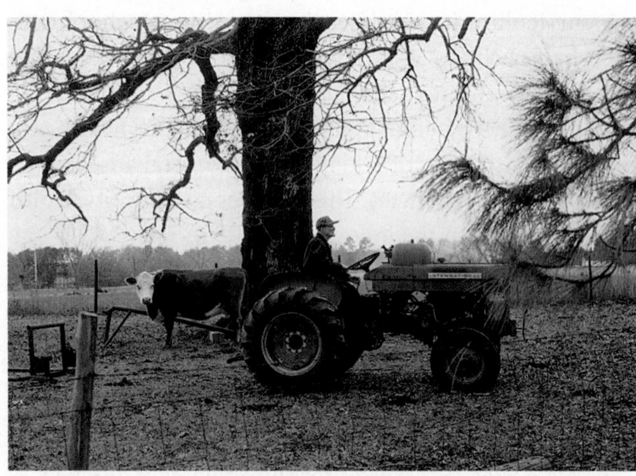

Tractor accidents are a leading cause of injuries in rural areas.

Community health nurses need to find ways to target rural adolescents for health promotion. One way is to work with school nurses in junior and senior high schools to advocate for current information to be included in school health curricula. Many rural schools are linked with the Internet, which can be a way to engage many adolescents in innovative health programming. Clubs, church youth groups, scouts, and 4-H are other arenas where young adolescents in rural areas gather, and many of these groups are often in need of programs for these teens. Community health nurses often are members of the rural community and are asked to present programs on health; they should take full advantage of these opportunities.

Isolation: Rural Elders

Isolation is fundamental to rural life. Isolation encompasses the ideas of sparse population, limited contact with others, greater distances between people, and limited transportation. Sometimes, people choose the isolation of rural life because they feel it gives them independence and opportunity for self-sufficiency. Isolation is neither a positive nor negative feature, but a reality that community health nurses need to take into account when planning and implementing health care.

Elderly people in rural areas present challenges to community health nurses that arise from both the isolation of rural life and the isolation of elderly life. Multiple losses, both physical and psychosocial, add to the isolation elderly people can experience. Physical changes of normal aging can contribute to isolation. Sensory losses such as diminished hearing and vision result in distancing from the normal experience of life. Decreased mobility resulting from skeletal changes and disease may cause elderly people to stay at home. Fear of falling and other safety issues limit social interaction. Loss of friends because of relocation and death limit opportunities for human connections. Disease processes further isolate elders. For example, diabetes requires a special diet and frequent blood glucose testing and insulin injections, which may prohibit participation in some social events.

Other problems that rural people experience can be more complex if they are older. On average, rural elders have approximately 22% lower incomes than metropolitan elderly because of lower social security payments, smaller savings, fewer opportunities for part-time work, and infrequent enrollment in Supplemental Security Income (SSI) (Krout, 1994; National Center for Farmworker Health, 2003; Rogers, 2002). Most (80%) rural elders own their homes, but these homes are likely to have been built before 1940. These homes may lack modern heating, plumbing, and insulation and may be in need of other repairs. Rural elders often need to relocate, but there are limited alternative housing opportunities in rural areas. Their houses may resell at a low price, creating another financial loss for the rural elder.

Elderly people residing anywhere may find themselves unable to drive their own cars. Lack of alternative transportation in rural areas is a problem that has wide-reaching effects on rural people. Elders have difficulty obtaining supplies, accessing health care, and meeting psychosocial needs.

Many research studies have been conducted that examine the unique characteristics and needs of this at-risk population. Community health nurses are challenged to design interventions that recognize the independence of older rural people but maintain their safety and health. Community-based services for rural elders must meet the criteria of availability, accessibility, awareness, acceptability, affordability, appropriateness, and adequacy. Parish nurse programs have had great success in rural areas because they meet these criteria. Nurses serve church members by "organizing health fairs, writing health articles for church newsletters, making presentations, providing blood pressure screening, referring to community health and social service resources, making home visits, and coordinating support groups" (Mockenhaupt & Muchow, 1994, p. 195). Healthcare providers must find a way to reduce the isolation experienced by rural elders by providing transportation, enhancing communication systems, and creating additional opportunities to bring elders together (Cosby et al., 2008; Ziller, Coburn, Anderson, & Loux, 2008).

GOT AN ALTERNATIVE?

The use of herbs for health and medicinal use is common among rural and migrant populations. These natural remedies are seldom discussed with medical and nursing professionals, according to research. What is the role of the community health nurse in regard to complementary and medicinal herbal use among rural residents in the promotion of health?

Culture: Migrant Farm Workers

Migrant farm workers—any farm workers outside their own country—are a unique culture arising from ethnic backgrounds and a distinctive lifestyle. The migrant farm worker population is estimated to be approximately 5 million (HHS, 1990; Lambert, 1995; Sandhaus, 1998; USDA, 2004). Even though there is a trend toward decreasing numbers of migrant farm workers in the United States, more than half of the U.S. farm workers are undocumented immigrants (Taylor, Charlton, & Yúnez-Naude, 2012). There are three primary streams in which they travel. The West Coast and midcontinent (or central) streams consist mostly of people of Mexican heritage. The East Coast stream is the most ethnically diverse, consisting of African Americans, Haitians, Puerto Ricans, whites, and some Mexican Americans (Lambert, 1995; Smith & Gentry, 1987).

Migrant farm workers "follow the crops." That is, they move north with the spring, living in temporary housing for days or weeks. The housing is often substandard and crowded, from shacks to mobile homes, rarely with furnishings. Sanitation and drinking water provision are also variable and often not available in the fields where the migrants work. Entire families make the season-long trip, with those who are unfit for fieldwork (elders and preteens) caring for the young children. Some areas make an effort to provide schooling for the young children, even though it is summer. Farm work provides the income that the family lives on for the entire year. Pay is hourly, at or below minimum wage, and for only the duration of the farming season.

Often, local communities react with hostility toward migrant farm workers because the workers are commonly seen as markedly different and potential carriers of disease. Thus, living apart from the local communities, this population is vulnerable to isolation and neglect. Fear of deportation, poverty, and limited education only serves to intensify feelings of distrust. Migrant workers form cohesive communities of their own based on language, food, music, religion, social interactions, and beneficial folk practices. It is critical that community health nurses acknowledge their cultural differences and include family and social support networks when planning care for this population (Sandhaus, 1998).

In addition to understanding the culture of migrant farm workers, healthcare providers are confronted with their difficult healthcare needs. The major healthcare problems include women's health issues, high infant mortality, delayed immunization, poor dental health, mental health problems, substance abuse, family violence, malnutrition, diabetes, hypertension, respiratory illness (especially tuberculosis), anemia, and parasites. The infant mortality rate for migrant workers is 25 times higher than the U.S. national average. Parasitic infections occur 11 to 59 times more often in migrant workers than in the general population. Deaths from tuberculosis, influenza, and pneumonia are 25% higher. The life expectancy for migrant workers is 49 years, compared with a national average of 75 years (Sandhaus, 1998). Occupation-specific health problems are also worse for migrant workers than for other farm workers. These problems include risk of motor vehicle accident caused by high annual mileage, pesticide exposure, poor sanitation, farm accidents, skin diseases, and frequent and severe heat and cold exposures (Rust, 1990; Sandhaus, 1998). The fact that the population does not stay in one place for very long interferes with diagnosis, follow up, and referral for any health problem (Harvey, 2008; Ziller et al., 2008).

Community health nurses have led the way in designing healthcare delivery models that respond to cultural differences, mobility, and the fundamental healthcare needs of migrant farm workers. Recognizing that migrant farm workers cannot rely on the consistency of one healthcare provider to oversee care, nursing models that emphasize education, self-care, empowerment, and responsibility for one's own health have found success with this population (Poss & Meeks, 1994; Stein, 1993; Watkins, Larson, Harlan, & Young, 1990). Successful programs often include mobile clinics with hours appropriate to migrant work schedules, sensitivity to cultural preferences, bilingual workers, and use of lay workers and peers.

The health care of migrant farm workers must be supported at the local, state, and national levels. With the identified health concerns of migrants ranging from infant mortality to communicable disease, funds must be found to support the following:

- The provision of adequate and accessible health care
- Adequate living wages
- Migrant education programs

Housing: Homeless People

Poverty in rural areas is most reflected in available housing. Rural homes are in worse condition than those in urban areas. Some have incomplete plumbing facilities, and others have structural problems such as inadequate heating, faulty electric, leaking roofs, and holes in the walls. Home ownership, however, is higher in rural areas than in urban areas. These two facts combined lead to rural homelessness. People have difficulty finding adequate housing to rent.

Homelessness in urban populations has been extensively examined, but little attention has been given to the problem of homelessness in rural populations. Research studies at both the state and national levels have noted that rural homelessness appears to be growing (First, Rife, & Tooney, 1990; Fitchen, 1991; Lindsey, 1995). The Housing Assistance Council, a Washington advocacy group, estimates up to 12.5% of homeless persons in the United States live in rural areas (USDA, 2004). The National Rural Health Association (NRHA, 1996) defines a family as homeless if they have no fixed place of residence. This includes living temporarily in shelters, with friends or relatives, in informal church-sponsored arrangements, in automobiles, in abandoned buildings, on the street, in campgrounds, and in the case of farm families facing imminent eviction (NRHA, 1996, p. 1).

Homeless families are the largest growing subgroup of the homeless (Bassak, 1991; Helvie, 1999; Lindsey, 1995). Homeless families are often single-parent families with the mother as head of household. Approximately 3.5% of poor workers in rural areas have at least three barriers to earning a livable wage: low educational level, female head of household, and a child younger than 6 years old at home (USDA, 1997). These workers are at grave risk of becoming homeless. Wagner, Menke, and Ciccone conducted a study in 1995 to examine the health of rural homeless families. Their study found the following similarities to previous urban studies:

- Most families were female headed.
- The ethnic distribution of homeless families mirrored the percentage of poor people in the area under study.
- Poverty was more extensive in rural than in urban areas as a greater percentage of the population was below the poverty line, and thus poverty was more difficult to escape.

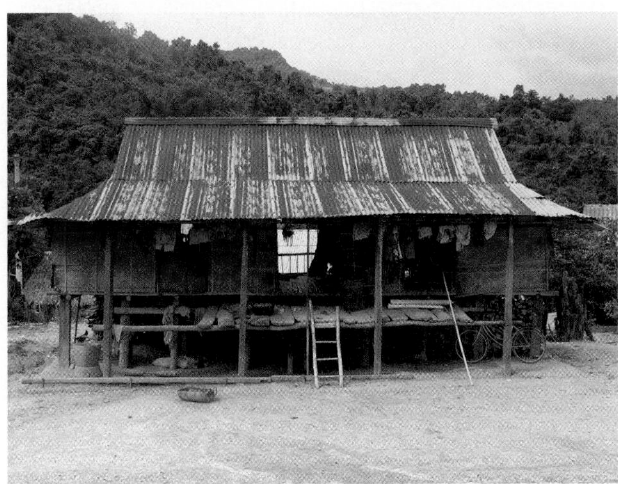

Housing in rural areas is often substandard.

Wagner, Menke, and Ciccone (1995) also found the following differences between rural and urban homeless families:

- The average number of rural homeless children was lower than reported in urban studies.
- Rural families were more likely to have been homeless for 4 to 12 months, which is longer than found for urban homeless families.
- Rural families were more likely to have doubled up with another family, which has been found to mask the degree of homelessness present in rural areas.
- Fewer rural families were found to stay in shelters, which may be attributed to the fact that fewer shelters were available.

Community health nurses who practice in rural areas are likely to encounter homeless families daily. These nurses must have an understanding of the needs of rural homeless families and be prepared to provide accessible, adequate, and appropriate care. This is not a simple task because homeless rural families are not easily identifiable, and each family will have different needs based on the length of time that they have been homeless. Case management has been found to be a particularly helpful tool in assisting homeless families or those who are near homeless find solutions. Rural community health nurses acting as case managers are challenged to identify which services (healthcare or social services) are available in the community, to creatively piece together other types of services available to fill in the gaps that exist, and to make these services acceptable to the families.

Multidisciplinary teams are often created to meet the needs of homeless families identified in the rural area. These teams may be composed of healthcare professionals, clergy, local politicians, community organizations, and other social support groups available in the rural community. The community health nurse is in a perfect position to develop and lead these teams as a member of the community who is knowledgeable about community support systems and able to broker a coalition of various community members.

The need for housing for homeless families in rural areas is at crisis proportion. With the number of poor, single-parent families that are now found to be homeless, affordable housing must be a prime concern for rural policy.

GLOBAL CONNECTION 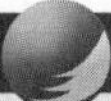

Half of the world's population lives in rural areas.

APPLICATION TO PRACTICE 

As a community health nurse, you are running the once-a-week well-child clinic in a rural town. As you call in the first young mother, Mrs. Boone, you recognize the strong odor of dirty clothing, soiled diapers, and unwashed children. Mrs. Boone sits down and places her youngest child, a small, pale girl, on her lap. The other two children, boys who appear to be preschool age, sit quietly on the floor at the end of the room. Mrs. Boone and the three children all are wearing grimy clothes. Mrs. Boone looks at the floor and says, "We come over from the emergency room—they sent us over here because we don't have health insurance and the baby is sick. The nurse in the emergency room said you would see us even if we don't have no money."

You ask, "Tell me what's been going on," as you take a seat opposite Mrs. Boone.

"We just come here last week from Little County with my boyfriend. We're staying with his brother but we've got to find another place to live because there isn't enough room.

(continues)

APPLICATION TO PRACTICE (*Continued*)

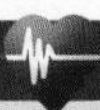

A couple of days ago Melanie—that's the baby's name—started being real fussy and she feels hot. She didn't sleep at all last night and kept us all awake. My boyfriend got real mad and told me to do something about her. Kids drive him crazy. Anyway, it seemed like she was pulling on her ear. She had the same thing about a month ago, and we got some medicine from the nurse where we lived before and it got better. Can you give me some medicine?"

You ask, "What was wrong with Melanie when the nurse saw her, and what kind of medicine did she get?"

"The nurse said her ear was infected and gave her some kind of medicine for the infection and for the fever. I gave her the medicine until she felt better. I lost the rest of the bottle when we were getting ready to move or I could have given her the rest of it now. I've really got to do something to make her be quiet—she is driving my boyfriend crazy."

The older of the two boys on the floor begins to whine, "I'm hungry." Mrs. Boone quickly turns to him and yells, "I told you to be quiet. Shut up before I smack you."

You take a deep breath and begin to get a health history on Mrs. Boone and the children. Mrs. Boone tells you that Melanie, the youngest, is 18 months old. The other two children, Travis and Jack, are 3 and 5, respectively. Mrs. Boone is 19. She did not finish high school but got married at 14, when she found that she was pregnant with Jack. She has been at home with the children, and her husband had been supporting the family with his earnings from two part-time jobs. About 2 months ago, her husband abandoned her and the children; she does not know where he is. Mr. Boone does not believe in welfare and has not let Mrs. Boone apply for any government assistance. After Mr. Boone left, Mrs. Boone managed to get some emergency food from a church food pantry and was thinking about applying for emergency assistance from welfare. Instead, she met her current boyfriend, Ashford, about 4 weeks ago, and they decided to come to Big County to see if they could find work. Mrs. Boone states that both the boys are quite healthy but that Melanie has been sick on and off since birth.

After you examine Melanie, you find that she has an ear infection and anemia. There is no money for medication for Melanie's ear infection.

1. What should you do?
2. Would you consider this family homeless?
3. What community supports should be sought to help them?

> Those who labor in the earth are the chosen people of God, if ever he had a chosen people.
>
> —*Thomas Jefferson*

RESEARCH ALERT

This study sought to examine the relationships among stress, caregiver burden, and the health status of rural caregivers and to assess whether caregiver burden and stress predict the physical health status of caregivers in the rural setting. The study's descriptive-correlational design utilized a convenience sample of 63 rural caregivers. The subjects self-reported their perceptions of stress, burden, and health status using the Zarit Caregiver Burden Interview Scale, Lifestyle Appraisal Questionnaire, and the health status question from the National Health Interview Survey.

The relationships among stress, burden, and health status in rural caregivers were significantly related ($p < 0.05$), and caregivers were found to have higher rates of obesity, hypertension, and cardiovascular disease and to rate their health as poorer than the general population. Caregivers complained of experiencing uncomfortable physical symptoms and sleep disturbances. Significant variance in health status ($p < .05$) was accounted for by the model variables of stress and caregiver burden. Significant variance ($p < .05$) in caregiver burden was accounted for by the model variables of caregiver age and employment status. Caregivers who provided care for individuals with low levels of functioning experienced greater levels of caregiver burden and reported a poor health status. These findings should be considered when planning care for the chronically ill and their caregivers.

Source: Sanford, J. (2004). Unpublished doctoral dissertation, University of South Alabama, Mobile, AL.

Access to Health Care: Agricultural Workers

Agricultural workers are exposed to distinct health risks. The annual occupation-related death rate for all workers is 9 per 100,000 workers, but the death rate for farmers is 42 per 100,000 (Gerberich, 1995). Compared with blue-collar and white-collar workers, farmers have a higher rate of amputations, arthritis, cardiovascular disease, ischemic heart disease, hypertension, skin cancer, chronic respiratory diseases, asthma, and back pain (Schenker, 1996). Farmers are exposed to excessive noise from machinery. They sometimes resist wearing the protective equipment required because it is bulky and hot and prevents them from hearing mechanical problems and warning cries (Marvel, Pratt, Marvel, Regan, & May, 1991). Entanglements in machinery, falls, and electrocution are common injuries (Ehlers, Connon, Themann, Myers, & Ballard, 1993). Agricultural chemical hazards for farmers include pesticides, fertilizers, fumes, solvents, and sanitizing solutions. They can also experience minor to major allergic reactions to chemicals, but also of importance is an increased risk for certain types of cancer, particularly lymphomas, leukemia, and other cancers of the prostate, brain, cervix, and stomach (Mills, Dodge, & Yang, 2009). The workers also experience respiratory diseases from dusts, gases, and chemicals, which are prevalent in farm work. Exposure to these hazards can occur during almost all the phases of farm work. Work with animals creates risk for communicable diseases and injury.

Mental health is a serious problem for farmers. They report high stress levels caused by the responsibilities placed on one person, the risks in farm work, the necessity to maintain a great store of current knowledge, and the unpredictability of factors such as the weather, market prices, and land value. Suicide rates for farmers are nearly twice that of the general population (Ehlers et al., 1993; Fraser et al., 2005).

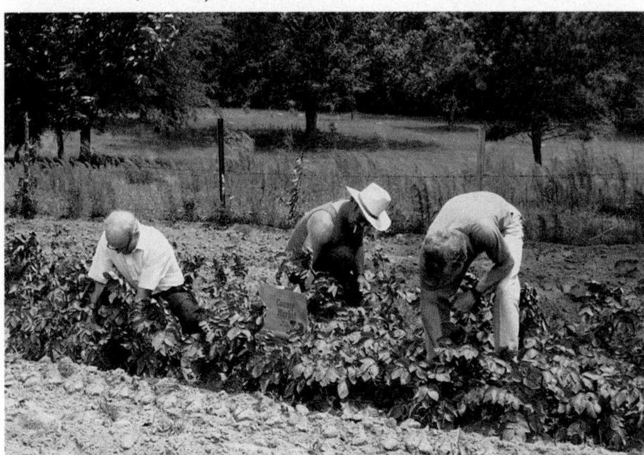

Agriculture is the main industry in many rural areas.

HEALTHY PEOPLE 2020 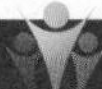

Objectives Related to Rural Life

Access to Care

- AHS-4 Increase the number of practicing primary care providers
- AHS-5 Increase the proportion of persons who have a specific source of ongoing care
- AHS-6 Reduce the proportion of persons who are unable to obtain or delay in obtaining necessary medical care, dental care, or prescription medicines

Cancer

- C-20 Increase the proportion of persons who participate in behaviors that reduce their exposure to harmful ultraviolet (UV) irradiation and avoid sunburn

Environmental Health

Water Quality

- EH-4 Increase the proportion of persons served by community water systems who receive a supply of drinking water that meets the regulations of the Safe Drinking Water Act
- EH-5 Reduce waterborne disease outbreaks arising from water intended for drinking among persons served by community water systems
- EH-6 Reduce per capita domestic water withdrawals with respect to use and conservation

Toxics and Waste

- EH-10 Reduce pesticide exposures that result in visits to a healthcare facility
- EH-11 Reduce the amount of toxic pollutants released into the environment
- EH-21 Improve quality, utility, awareness, and use of existing information systems for environmental health
- EH-22 Increase the number of states, territories, tribes, and the District of Columbia that monitor diseases or conditions that can be caused by exposure to environmental hazards

Infrastructure and Surveillance

- EH-20 Reduce exposure to selected environmental chemicals in the population, as measured by blood and urine concentrations of the substances or their metabolites
- EH-23 Reduce the number of new schools sited within 500 feet of an interstate or federal or state highway

Injury and Violence Protection

Unintentional Injury Prevention

- IVP-8 Increase access to trauma care in the United States
- IVP-30 Reduce firearm-related deaths
- IVP-31 Reduce nonfatal firearm-related injuries

Occupational Safety and Health

- OSH-1 Reduce deaths from work-related injuries
  - OSH-1.1 Reduce deaths from work-related injuries in all industries
  - OSH-1.2 Reduce deaths from work-related injuries in mining
  - OSH-1.3 Reduce deaths from work-related injuries in construction
  - OSH-1.4 Reduce deaths from work-related injuries in transportation and warehousing
  - OSH-1.5 Reduce deaths from work-related injuries in agriculture, forestry, fishing, and hunting
- OSH-2 Reduce nonfatal work-related injuries
- OSH-8 Reduce occupational skin diseases or disorders among full-time workers

Source: HHS, 2011.

Farm families also experience special risks. Farm wives often help on the farm and have jobs out of the home. Children are at very high risk of injury on the farm. Approximately 300 children die every year on U.S. farms, and thousands more are injured (National Committee for Childhood Agricultural Injury Prevention, 1996). Farm family members demonstrate higher than expected rates of some cancers, respiratory illnesses, and adverse reproduction outcomes (Ehlers et al., 1993). Finally, migrant farm workers are exposed to all of the same risks, but potentially without the knowledge, skills, and safety equipment that are recommended.

Many farmers face an issue of access to health care. Distance from metropolitan areas and services is definitive of rurality. Travel may be over poor roads and involve geographic barriers. When one bridge is out, the travel necessary to get to the next bridge may be prohibitive.

THINK ABOUT THIS 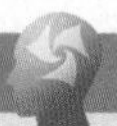

> Farming looks mighty easy when your plow is a pencil and you're a thousand miles from the corn field.
>
> —*Dwight D. Eisenhower*

Farmers define *health* as "the ability to work" (Lee cited in Weinert & Long, 1994). Because farmers may be indispensable to their work, they push themselves to work when they are ill or injured. They will seek health care only when they are unable to ignore the health problem. Under these circumstances, farmers often seek health care in almost an emergency state. Sometimes, they need a higher level of care because they wait until the health problem demands action. Because they are self-employed, farmers may forgo buying health insurance for themselves and their families. Furthermore, there is no law that requires smaller farmers as employers to insure their workers. Lack of insurance also may inhibit farm workers from seeking health care. With the passing of the Affordable Care Act in 2010, more workers are able to purchase insurance through the state and federal markets.

Emergency rescue of farmers presents several barriers. Farmers work independently and their absence may not be noticed for several hours. Notification systems to call for emergency help are sporadic through rural America. The terrain and distance may delay rescue vehicles.

Healthcare delivery to farmers and other rural residents requires innovation that recognizes their special needs. Mobile clinics, flexible hours, prevention and screening programs, and networks for peer education and assistance are possibilities. Throughout the country, there are agricultural health and safety centers that provide grant funding, report research findings, and support community health workers' efforts to protect farm workers.

Rural life is often idealized as one of peacefulness and health. Although there are rewards associated with rural living, research is just beginning to reveal the realities of healthcare needs in this population. Healthcare planners and providers must develop innovative, acceptable programs and educate healthcare providers to give accessible, acceptable, appropriate, and better than adequate care.

Community health nurses lead the way in understanding diverse rural populations and communities by recognizing the effects of lifestyle, isolation, culture, poverty/housing, confidentiality, specific health needs, and access to health care. The community nurse is capable of reaching these unique populations because often the nurse is part of the rural culture and is accepted as an insider by the people for whom he or she cares.

Country Lanes

One more time we walk down a country lane
Not the same as when the children were small
They would dance ahead just within view
Threatening to fall or run into poison ivy
This time we walk—much slower—talk
Much less of children's clothes and scratched knees
Amber leaves rick—deep among our feet
Smoke from the dying fire of fall
Soft and blue above our heads
Our voices low—whispering the years away.

—*Ann Thedford Lanier*

RESEARCH ALERT

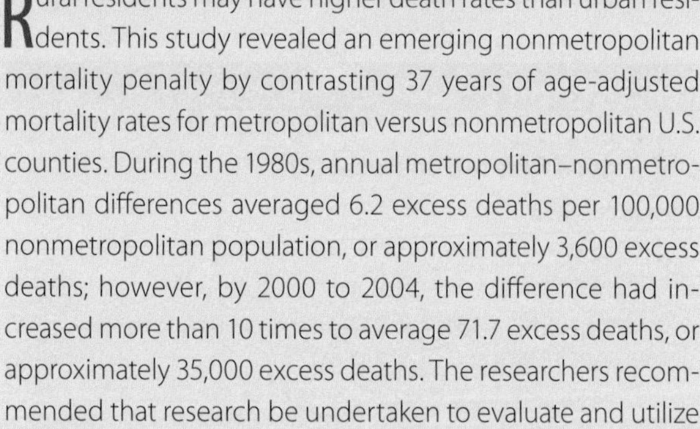
Rural residents may have higher death rates than urban residents. This study revealed an emerging nonmetropolitan mortality penalty by contrasting 37 years of age-adjusted mortality rates for metropolitan versus nonmetropolitan U.S. counties. During the 1980s, annual metropolitan–nonmetropolitan differences averaged 6.2 excess deaths per 100,000 nonmetropolitan population, or approximately 3,600 excess deaths; however, by 2000 to 2004, the difference had increased more than 10 times to average 71.7 excess deaths, or approximately 35,000 excess deaths. The researchers recommended that research be undertaken to evaluate and utilize these preliminary findings of an emerging U.S. nonmetropolitan mortality penalty.

Source: Cosby, A., Neaves, T., Cossman, R., Cossman, J., James, W., Feierabend, N., . . . Farrigan, T. (2008). Preliminary evidence for an emerging nonmetropolitan mortality penalty in the United States. *American Journal of Public Health*, *98*(8), 1470–1472.

Urban Populations

People who live in urban areas are under siege. Community health nurses traditionally have been accustomed to solving difficult health and social problems in various populations. Today, problems associated with urban and homeless people pose challenges requiring every skill that can be mustered by community health nurses. Strong community leadership for dealing with these problems is essential. Community health nurses can be the leaders on the forefront in preventing and managing these problems. Urban communities are exposed to diseases, health disorders, violence, crime, hunger, poverty, drug abuse, and homelessness at alarming rates. Although homelessness is a problem in both rural and urban areas, most homeless people exist in urban areas.

An **urban population** is at least 50,000 people in an incorporated or unincorporated area (U.S. Conference of Mayors, 2006; U.S. Department of Commerce, 2002). Cities have continued to increase in population as people—especially young adults—have migrated to cities from rural areas in hopes of fulfilling their dreams of success. With the promise of wealth and a new way of life, young people are charmed, sometimes only to find disappointment in their careers, poverty, and stress (Darbyshire, Muir-Cochrane, Fereday, Jureidini, & Drummond, 2006; Goldstein & Kickbusch, 1996; Salomonsen-Sautel et al., 2008; Wehler et al., 2004). Some have been unable to find jobs. Not only do many people migrate to the city, but many people are born and remain in the city for the duration of their lives. Low income and unemployment perpetuate urban poverty and its problems. With a rapidly growing population, urban officials cannot keep pace with the needs of the people. A majority of urban problems are associated with rapid growth, such as diminishing supplies of clean water, air pollution, crime and violence, poverty, diseases, overcrowding, racial discrimination, and inadequate housing.

Health and Social Problems

People in urban areas face many stressors that are different from those in rural areas. Although some of the same problems exist in rural areas, the health and social problems associated with living in urban areas usually are more pronounced. Poverty in urban populations has been the source of many problems that have developed in cities, especially hunger, health problems, communicable diseases because of overcrowded conditions, violence and crime, homelessness, and inadequate housing. Lack of steady employment is a major problem. However, many Americans continue to view government support for the poor as the main cause of the social problems in the United States. As a result, the public and many governmental policymakers have increasingly rejected such programs. The consequence of these attitudes has been a deterioration of health and welfare programs for poor people (Jones, 2006).

Racial discrimination remains an unsettling issue. A "color line," described by Lewis (1993, p. 251), has caused whites and nonwhites to remain segregated. Data from a 5-year American Community Survey (U.S. Census Bureau, 2011b) showed that 13.5% of the U.S. population lived in poverty between 2006 and 2011. Major income and healthcare differences exist between whites and nonwhites overall. Poverty and overcrowding in nonwhite populations have been linked to the exacerbation of communicable diseases (Jones, 2006).

ETHICAL CONNECTION+

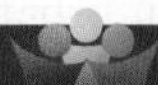

Historically, the nursing metaparadigm has been used to describe four concepts of nursing knowledge (person, environment, health, and nursing) that reflect beliefs held by the profession about nursing's context and content. The authors offer an assessment of the metaparadigm as it applies to community and public health nursing in urban settings and offer an amendment of the metaparadigm to include the central concept of social justice. Each of the metaparadigm concepts and the central concept of social justice are discussed as they apply to a model of urban health nursing, teaching, research, and practice.

Source: Schim, S. M., Benkert, R., Bell, S. E., Walker, D. S., & Danford, C. A. (2007). Social justice: Added metaparadigm concept for urban health nursing. *Public Health Nursing, 24*(1), 73–80.

MEDIA MOMENT

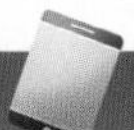

Dark Days (2000)

Documentarian Marc Singer focuses his camera on a group of homeless people who live deep underground in an abandoned New York City railroad tunnel. By day, they scavenge for food on the mean streets of Manhattan. At night, they retreat to the tunnel, where they have built huts out of scrap metal, plastic, and plywood, which are equipped with electricity, furniture, working kitchens, and a sense of community.

Poverty in inner cities also is linked to a poor quality of life and increased health problems among adults of all ages (Jones, 2006; Polednak, 1997; U.S. Conference of Mayors, 2006). A substantially higher infant mortality rate among nonwhites has been found in metropolitan areas (Corburn, 2004; Gamst et al., 2006; Polednak, 1997; Wehler et al., 2004). Lack of access to health care, poor prenatal care, adolescent pregnancy, substance abuse, and an overall poor quality of life are consequences of poverty.

Causes of mortality among African Americans and other nonwhites in urban areas included cardiovascular diseases, renal diseases, and homicides at higher rates than whites (Cheung & Hwang, 2004; Salomonsen-Sautel et al., 2008; Wenzel, Tucker, Elliott, & Hambarsoomians, 2007).

In the latter part of the 20th century, the movement of people to the suburbs contributed to higher rates of obesity, less community cohesiveness, and higher stress due to greater driving commutes, less time for exercise, and greater isolation of families.

Ghetto counterculture is a term that has been used to label a phenomenon in urban America (Massey & Denton, 1993, p. 48). Ghetto counterculture is used to describe the racial segregation that has taken place in residential areas. This residential segregation has created nonwhite urban underclass communities, producing "concentration" effects in these areas (p. 48). The concentration of nonwhites in high-poverty areas, such as inner cities, has resulted in a spiraling decline in the human condition. Rap music has evolved as a musical expression of ghetto life.

RESEARCH ALERT

The efficacy of a nurse case-managed intervention was evaluated in subsamples of participants with one of the following characteristics: female gender, African American, recruited from a homeless shelter, a history of military service, lifetime injection drug use, daily alcohol and drug use, poor physical health, and a history of poor mental health. The purpose of this study was to determine whether a nurse case-managed intervention with incentives and tracking would improve adherence to latent tuberculosis infection treatment in subsamples of homeless persons with characteristics previously identified as predictive of nonadherence. A study was conducted with 520 homeless adults residing in 12 homeless shelters and residential recovery sites in the Skid Row region of Los Angeles from 1998 to 2003. Study results revealed that daily drug users, participants with a history of injection drug use, daily alcohol users, and persons who were not of African American race had particularly poor completion rates, even in the nurse case-managed intervention program (48%, 55%, 54%, and 50%, respectively). However, the intervention achieved a 91% completion rate for homeless shelter residents and significantly improved latent tuberculosis infection treatment adherence in 9 of 12 subgroups tested, including daily alcohol and drug users, when potential confounders were controlled using logistic regression analysis.

Source: Nyamathi, A., Nahid, P., Berg, J., Burrage, J., Christiani, A., Aqtash, S., … Leake, B. (2008). Efficacy of nurse case-managed intervention for latent tuberculosis among homeless subsamples. *Nursing Research, 57*(1), 33–39.

Concentration effects lead to increased social problems such as crime and drugs, physical deterioration of buildings, poor access to healthcare facilities and other services, and fewer quality educational opportunities. Respiratory infections, tuberculosis (TB), skin infections, and many other illnesses occur in concentrated areas. The Research Alert highlights the public health threat of adult pertussis in urban people.

Another health problem associated with urban living in the United States is the reemergence of communicable diseases, such as measles. The CDC (2005) has documented a 20-fold increase in measles since 1990, which is largely attributed to failure to vaccinate children in accordance with established public health guidelines. However, it is important to note that vaccine coverage in children may be uneven; a recent study found that less than 8% of counties surveyed met the objective of 90% coverage for diphtheria, tetanus, and pertussis vaccine among children ages 19–35 months, but 93% did meet this objective for polio vaccine coverage and 86% met the goal for measles-mumps-rubella (MMR) vaccinations (Smith et al., 2011). One study of flu vaccine coverage in inner-city children noted a disparity between the likelihood of vaccination in African American (50%) versus Latino (31%) children that may be influenced by English proficiency in the parents (Uwemedimo, Findley, Andres, Irigoyen, & Stockwell, 2012).

Other health problems have emerged in recent years. Contamination of community water supplies has contributed to many outbreaks of infectious diseases in urban areas, such as the *Cryptosporidium* outbreak in a California water park in 2004 that sickened over 250 people (Wheeler et al., 2007). There has been the reappearance of plague, cholera, and dengue fever in many parts of the world, especially in the "mega-cities" of 10 million or more people (United Nations, 2005).

Programs for Healthier Urban People

Healthy People 2020 specifies four major goals to improve the health of Americans (HHS, 2010). One of these goals is to achieve health equity and eliminate health disparities. Although the goals do not specifically mention urban populations, they can be applied to urban populations. A large percentage of the population in inner cities is nonwhite. Mortality, morbidity, and lack of healthcare and healthcare gaps between whites and nonwhites in the United States increased. Access and utilization continue to soar among nonwhites, especially in inner cities (HHS, 2000). As a result, several national health programs have been targeted at African Americans and other underrepresented ethnic groups. Many of the national programs have stemmed from the Public

Health Service. Community health nurses are in an excellent position to help manage these health programs or coordinate the health care.

The **Healthy Cities** movement was initiated by the World Health Organization (WHO) in Europe in 1984. It was brought about by a speech given at an international meeting in Canada with a theme that "health is much more than medical care" (International Healthy Cities Foundation ([IHCF], 2002). Soon after the initiation of Europe's Healthy Cities project, others followed, including programs in Canada, the United States, Latin America, Africa, and Asia.

The IHCF was established in August 1994 (IHCF, 2002). From the beginning, this organization was envisioned by global advisory boards as a dynamic interconnection of people, organizations, and networks involving many disciplines and interest groups. The goal of IHCF and WHO is to increase the level of health for all citizens of the world.

IHCF's mission is to facilitate linkages among people, issues, and resources to support the development of the Healthy Cities movement (IHCF, 2002). With this mission in mind, IHCF developed an infrastructure of three programs: communications, resource tools, and training and advisory services. Many people at various levels are involved in IHCF, including partners from public health and safety; educators; religious groups; alcohol and drug programs; and community groups focusing on civil and human rights, volunteerism, housing, labor, business, environment, occupation, and more. Virtually every discipline on the global front has a voice in IHCF.

WHO recognized that urban cities held almost half the world's population. Through the Healthy Cities program, local individuals and local resources are recruited to work together to identify and help resolve health problems in their community. There are numerous participating cities throughout the United States and the world. In the Healthy Cities program, attention is given to modifying the physical, social, and economic environment of the community to improve the health of individuals. One of the first major United States cities to launch a Healthy Cities project was Boston. Since the movement's inception in 1992, Boston has served as a leader of the Healthy Cities movement in the United States. After an extensive evaluation of the Healthy Boston project, the Office of Community Partnerships realized that the project had been very successful in reaching its goals, which were to create a collective community voice, serve as a catalyst to optimize services, create new partnerships, embrace multicultural and collaborative values, embrace health issues, and create healthy communities. Only four recommendations for improvement came from the evaluation. One of those recommendations was for the improvement of leadership development and more support for coalitions. Community health nurses could fill this role by becoming leaders and providing support and coordination of health and political coalitions. Community health nurses need to realize the potential healthy outcomes for urban populations when a Healthy Cities project has been successfully undertaken.

At the IHCF Conference in Athens, Greece, in June 1998, the third phase of the Healthy Cities movement was launched. Jo Asvall, WHO's Regional Director for Europe, stated at this conference, "WHO is emphasizing the diversity and seriousness of urban health issues and the need for action at the local level" (WHO, 1998, p. 1). At this conference, the members evaluated outcomes and the impact of the movement for the previous 10 years.

Several other programs have been specially targeted at the African American population in inner cities, such as the Harlem Health Connection and the Safe Kids/Healthy Neighborhoods Injury Prevention Program in Harlem (Polednak, 1997). African American inner-city churches and community groups have also been committed to improving living conditions in urban areas.

Urban development projects across U.S. cities have provided health opportunities for urban populations. Improving the health outcomes of these people through better access to health care with an emphasis on health promotion and prevention of disease is a result of urban development efforts. Many problems still exist, but the urban development efforts of communities are becoming beneficial to the urban residents. Many of these projects start at the grassroots level and are coordinated and managed by city officials and community leaders.

One urban development project that began at the local level and has spread rapidly throughout the United States is the Atlanta Project, which has now become The America Project (Berger, 2007; Biven, 2002; TAP, 1995). This project was developed by President Jimmy Carter in an effort to promote hope and healing and to unite the Atlanta people to improve the quality of life in neighborhoods. The success of the project spread quickly throughout the United States and has been adopted by many major city officials. The project's mission required several elements for success, which included having a vision, planning well, empowering the community, collaborating, volunteering, and communicating effectively.

West (1994) emphasized that young African American urban people are faced with despair and are fighting the forces of death, destruction, and disease. With consistent efforts, programs such as the Healthy Cities movement and other urban development programs can provide the resources for health promotion and healing. Community health nurses have a responsibility to become involved in urban policymaking, urban development projects, and urban health care (Corburn, 2004; Lowe, 2008).

Urban Sprawl and Health

Urban health efforts in the late 1990s and into the 21st century have initiated research and programs that focus on the "built environment"—such as architecture and locations of stores, schools, and community services. One such example is the study of urban sprawl and its connection to physical activity, obesity, stress, and mental health issues. Urban sprawl occurs as large numbers of urban residents move to the suburbs. These suburbs are characterized as decentralized, automobile-dependent neighborhoods, often called "bedroom communities." The built environment most associated with urban areas includes the inferior air quality of workplaces, street layout, presence or absence of sidewalks, walkable streets, and population density. When populations move out of the central city, fewer businesses, such as local grocery stores, are within walking distances for this already vulnerable population. Given that many urban poor are dependent on mass transit, health is affected through poorer nutrition, obesity, and less attention to preventive care (Corburn, 2004; Lopez & Welker-Hood, 2007). Urban sprawl affects nurses as well. Long hours at work and long commutes decrease exercise possibilities and contribute to greater stress and poor nutritional choices (Lopez & Welker-Hood, 2007).

The Homeless Population

Today the United States is faced with overwhelming social problems, including the tragedy of the homeless. Although estimates of numbers of homeless people change from day to day, the U.S. Department of Housing and Urban Development (2013) estimates that almost 700,000 people experience homelessness on any given night in the United States. Of those, approximately almost 240,000 are people in families. Knowing exactly how many people in the United States are homeless on a daily basis is difficult to determine. The most predominant reason people are homeless in the United States is because they cannot find affordable housing. Interwoven throughout the homeless population are the social problems of substance abuse, racism, violence, limited education, crime, and poverty (Gamst et al., 2006; North, Eyrich, Pollio, & Spitznagel, 2004; Washington, 2002; Wehler et al., 2004). A new culture of homeless people has emerged. The number and composition of homeless people during the last 2 decades of the 20th century have grasped the attention of the American people and have continued to plague us as a society. We exhibit attitudes ranging from "blaming the victim" to feeling helpless in doing anything about this serious social problem. The individuals comprising the homeless populations are no longer the "skid row bums," "hobos," and "tramps" found years ago. Now women, adolescents, families with children, and elderly people represent a large portion of the homeless population (Baum & Burnes, 1993; Gamst et al., 2006; Wenzel et al., 2007).

The homeless lifestyle is a barrier to good health practices and thus leads to more prevalent health problems (Galea & Vlahov, 2002; Meadows-Oliver, 2006). Community health nurses play a vital role in breaking down the barriers that prevent positive health practices in this new culture of homeless women, men, and children. As we will see later, outreach to nontraditional service locations and case management are key strategies on which community health nurses can focus (Bolland & McCallum, 2002; Cousineau, Wittenberg, & Pollatsek, 1995; Rosenblum, Magura, Kayman, & Fong, 2005). Although the *Healthy People 2020* objectives do not specifically address the issue of homelessness, they address all of the conditions, problems, and population groups affected.

Rescue Mission

They'll sit like that for hours
for a ticket away from
their hunger rack ribs
with their shirts off
in summer lined up
as if waiting on
Buck Rogers' next
scuffle
those racks look
like evil fingers
closing around
empty innards
when the bell chimes
Jesus saves
and the door flings open
they file in like boys
returning from an
exhausting recess
it's bread that saves now
as they sit quietly
almost broken of old habits
although a few
(perhaps toothless?)
still neatly trim
the crust away

—*James A. Lopresti*

MEDIA MOMENT 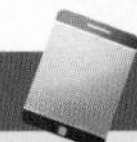

Homeless in America (2004)

This documentary chronicles the world of the homeless and shatters myths about our ideas of what it means to live on the streets.

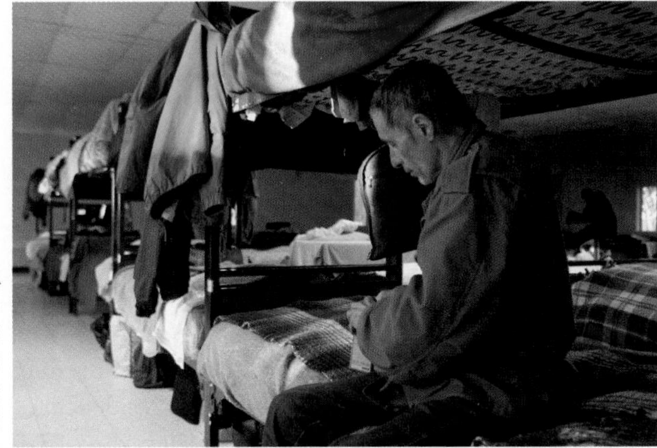

Homeless clinics in inner-city locations can provide essential care for the homeless population.

TABLE 25-3 Characteristics of Homeless People in 2011–2013	
Individuals	64%—62% male, 38% female
	19% were employed
	13% were veterans
	22% under 18
Families	36%
Resources	22% of persons needing assistance did not get it
	71% of surveyed cities reported turning away families with children due to lack of beds
Race and ethnicity	37% are African American
	42% are Caucasian
	8% are Hispanic
	5% are other single races
	7% are multiracial
Health	30% of adults were severely mentally ill
	3% were HIV positive
	17% were physically disabled
	16% were victims of domestic violence

Sources: U.S. Conference of Mayors, 2013; SAMHSA, 2011.

Scope of the Problem

Cities all across the United States—and globally—have unmet needs for shelter and food. The homeless population is located in both urban and rural areas, although the largest numbers are in urban areas. Women, adolescents, substance abusers, families with children, and people with mental illness or who are deinstitutionalized make up the homeless population (HHS, 2003; Interagency Council on the Homeless, 2000; Lezak & Edgar, 1996). The estimate of homeless children is 100,000 at any given day or night (Institute of Medicine, 1988). Still more astounding are the facts that each year 30% to 50% of all homeless people are families with children and 7% of all homeless people are children (Darbyshire et al., 2006). (See **Table 25-3**).

A problem exists in counting accurate numbers of homeless people because of the "one point in time" reference. The group of homeless persons may be different people and different numbers from one night to another. During a 7-day period in March 1987, statistics revealed that more than 600,000 homeless people sought shelter from the outside environment (Burt & Cohen, 1989). During the 2000 Census, the U.S. Department of Commerce (2002) attempted to gather statistics on numbers of homeless people. The department was unable to obtain specific numbers across the country but gathered data in certain cities over a specific number of days and nights. In 2010, however, the Census Bureau produced a report canvassing use of group homes, emergency shelters, and transitional shelters that accounted for 209,000 people in emergency shelters and almost 8 million persons in group quarters (U.S. Census Bureau, 2012). Currently, the U.S. Conference of Mayors studies specific U.S. cities every year to draw conclusions about the scope of the problem and characteristics of the population of homeless people.

Researchers have estimated the number of homeless people across the United States, suggesting that the number of individuals experiencing homelessness is even greater than previously expected. In the latter part of the 1980s, as many as 9.32 million persons were believed to have been homeless at least once (Culhane, Dejowski, Ibanex, Needham, & Macchia, 1993; Interagency Council on the Homeless, 2000; Link et al., 1995). Even more disturbing is the fact that families are the fastest growing segment of the homeless population (National Coalition for the Homeless, 2009). **Box 25-2** delineates the composition of homeless people.

The estimated number of homeless people does not include the growing segment of people who are on the verge of homelessness (Interagency Council on the Homeless, 2000). More than 1 million families are on waiting lists for public housing at any given time. Many more people have moved in with friends or relatives. Increasing numbers of people are paying more than half their income for rent, making them at risk for homelessness at any time.

BOX 25-2 Who Are the New Homeless People?

- Single adults unaccompanied by children
- Single mothers with children
- Families with children
- Individuals who have been deinstitutionalized
- Persons who are diagnosed with mental illness
- Runaway and throwaway youths
- Abandoned children
- Unemployed, impoverished adults
- Immigrants
- Veterans—both women and men
- Elderly people

NOTE THIS!

In 2009, the *average* real income of working poor people was $9,151. In that year, the so-called "poverty line" was set at $10,956 for a single individual, and $21,954 for a family of four.

Source: U.S. Census Bureau. (2009). Poverty thresholds 2009. Retrieved from http://www.census.gov/hhes/www/poverty/data/threshld/thresh09.html; National Alliance to End Homelessness. (2011). Average real income of working poor people by state—State of homelessness 2011. Retrieved from http://www.endhomelessness.org/library/entry/average-real-income-of-working-poor-people-by-state-state-of-homelessness-2

CULTURAL CONNECTION 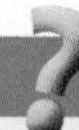

Rural and urban poverty rates have narrowed in the proportion of the populations who are poor—16.6% versus 14.9%, respectively, in 2010.

African Americans have been effectively frozen out of suburbs by racial covenants, discriminatory mortgage practices, and racial bias since the 1950s. Whites have benefited from access to low-cost suburban homes, low interest rates on government-subsidized home mortgages, and publicly funded transportation projects linking their suburban homes to unemployment recreation and commercial centers.

I don't think Dr. King helped racial harmony, I think he helped racial justice. What I profess to do is help the oppressed, and if I cause a load of discomfort in the white community and the black community, that in my opinion means I'm being effective, because I'm not trying to make them comfortable. The job of an activist is to make people tense and cause social change.

—The Reverend Al Sharpton

Definitions of Homeless People

An official definition of **homeless** was offered by the federal government in the Stewart B. McKinney Homeless Assistance Act of 1987 (U.S. Congress, House, 1987). Any individual lacking a fixed, regular, and adequate nighttime residence is defined as a homeless person. The definition includes any individual with a primary nighttime residence at shelters, missions, welfare hotels, and public or private places not designated for sleeping quarters. Any person needing institutionalization but instead residing in an institution providing only temporary residence for homeless people is also considered homeless. **Box 25-3** provides an insight into the way the term *homeless* has been used in the past.

Other definitions of homeless include individuals with no mailing address or place to sleep; people who sleep outdoors on streets or in parks, at train stations, at subways, underground, or in cars; and people on the verge of homelessness (Bean, Stefl, & Howe, 1987; Benda & Dattalo, 1988; Interagency Council on the Homeless, 2000; Phillips, Pauley, & Rudolph, 1997; Rivilin, 1986; Stark, 1987).

DAY IN THE LIFE

Donald, a Homeless Man in Gulfport, Mississippi

"You never know, it could be your brother … out there needing your help."

Nurse: Donald, you told me you were from New York and that you came here. Do you have any family down here?

Donald: No, no family at all. Like a bird I fly south for the warm weather. This time in New York right now it's freezing and it's really crowded in the line of business I'm in.

Nurse: What line of business is that?

Donald: I do a little everything. I am over here now a couple of days 'cause people give me a lot of yard work over here, and they feed me, give me a little change of clothes. I sprinkle a little water on myself.

Nurse: You don't find this weather cold down here right now? It's like 40-something degrees out here.

Donald: Yeah, it's like 40-something degrees here and maybe 20-something degrees in New York City. I'm pretty well prepared: I got about four layers of clothing on. Most of the time down here, I have to strip some of this off.

Nurse: Well, let me ask you something, Donald. Like I explained to you, I'm a nurse and I'm studying health care. Where do you go when you get sick—how do you go about getting some help, about seeing a doctor?

Donald: Well, most of the hospitals here, they've been all right, they direct me to the emergency room ... they'll fix you up, say if I just have a cold.

Nurse: Well you look fairly young anyway ...

Donald: Yeah, I am in pretty good health.

Nurse: Well, I see that you got some stuff with you.

Donald: This is just basic essentials, you know—sneakers, a little change of clothes. I have my blanket; I have been running into some cold nights. I have some utensils, and things, nothing much, just everyday homeless persons' things. People give me this, I go to shelters. I have been lucky to catch a few shelters down here, but you know last night it was a little crowded and I had to stay outside, but I am pretty much prepared for it.

Nurse: How long do you plan to stay down here?

Donald: As long as business is good. I say that as long as I can make a meal, work somewhere, and make a meal, I'll stay.

Nurse: You say you don't have any family down here, but do you have any family up in New York?

Donald: I have a sister, last address unknown. I don't bother anybody; I am self-sufficient; I try to take care of myself; I don't ask for much; I lead a simple life.

Nurse: Like I said before, if I ask you anything personal and you don't want to answer, you don't have to. Do you drink any alcohol?

Donald: Very little, very little ... like my sign reads here "Will work for food," it doesn't say, "for alcohol." ... Now occasionally I have been known to take a good sip—it warms the innards.

Nurse: How about the people who you meet at the shelters: Do you notice that they drink much alcohol?

Donald: The majority of them are heavy wine drinkers. Well, they drink whatever they can get a hold of, anything that's over 1% alcohol they drink it.

I am basically a loner. I travel alone. I've been all over this country. I've been by myself, I've been making it.

Nurse: You're not scared out on the roads ... the violence?

Donald: Yeah, there's times I'm scared, but, you know, luckily people know I don't have anything. They don't bother me. I have run into a lot of good people. They just don't bother me ever.

Nurse: Was there anything you think would be helpful for me to know about people who live on the roads?

Donald: Yes, if you could get to talk to some more people or if more people would talk openly, I think that you would find that the homeless situation is really bad and people who could lend a hand in any kind of way, just donating some old clothes to Salvation Army or Goodwill, they should really look into it. I think the states should look more into the homeless situation 'cause it's really out there and it's really bad. It could be your brother, one of your relatives—out there needing your help.

—Interviewer: James Ryan, RN, MSN, ANP

Ryan found Donald under a freeway underpass in Mississippi holding a sign that said "Will work for food."

Homelessness has also been described in terms of three stages (Belcher, Scholler-Jaquish, & Drummond, 1991). *Episodic homelessness* characterizes people who live below the poverty line and who are on the verge of homelessness or may actually experience one or more episodes of homelessness for short periods. *Temporary homelessness* describes people who have recently become homeless but still view themselves as part of their community. *Chronic homelessness* describes people who have adopted their state of being as a way of life and have declined in social status, financial status, and interpersonal and family connections.

Historical Perspective

The Beginning of Homelessness in America

As long as can be remembered, homeless people have been inhabitants of America (Institute of Medicine, 1988). English people who settled on North American soil segregated themselves by classes. The workers and the more affluent people gave assistance to poor people (Trattner, 1984). During the 1600s, colonists adopted England's ideology and many principles of England's law, which was written to protect the welfare of families and communities. Therefore, adult white men, "free" African Americans, and Indians were left to wander aimlessly and beg for food, clothing, and other assistance. The only individuals who warranted assistance at that time were white women, children, and disabled people.

As the mid-1800s approached, a new generation of poor people surfaced in the United States during the industrialization and farming era. Sporadic and transient labor became essential (Hoch & Slayton, 1989). Most of the homeless populations consisted of men because they were the providers and often had to leave home to find work. Some who traveled the land by railways to look for transient work were labeled as "hobos." Other men who sought transient work on foot were labeled as "tramps." Then there were "bums," who usually traveled by railways, stole from others, and begged for money and food. The Civil War and migration to the West created another mass of homeless people, who were labeled "cowboys," "Indian scouts," and "gold seekers" (Hoffman, 1953).

Not long after the turn of the 20th century, "skid rows" surfaced in major cities, where homeless and indigent people gathered for food, assistance, and word-of-mouth information at diners, bars, mission homes, and old hotels. Most of these people were older white men. The skid row population fluctuated with the status of the U.S. economy (Momeni & Wiegand, 1989). Shantytowns, where homeless people colonized, sprang up across the United States after the crash of the stock market in 1929. The skid row population continued to increase until World War II brought new jobs.

Societal and Governmental Influences Through the 1970s

Because manifestations of mental illness place persons at high risk for homelessness, a large proportion of the homeless population was believed to be mentally ill in the 1800s. In 1890, New York was the first state to enact a law allowing the state government to assume full responsibility for individuals classified as the "insane poor" (Anderson, 1934).

A federal plan was not initiated until 1933, when the **Federal Emergency Relief Administration (FERA)** supplied food, shelter, clothing, money, jobs, and health care to homeless individuals (Anderson, 1940). In 1935, FERA was replaced by the Works Progress Administration federal program, which was aimed at creating jobs only for people who could meet strict residency standards. Because a residence was required to receive assistance, homeless people were not included in this plan.

GLOBAL CONNECTION 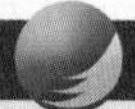

The primary factor that influences a country's growth is industrialization. The more industrialized the country, the greater the urban growth.

In 1800, only 3% of the world's population lived in cities. Today, half of the world's population lives in cities, and 75% of people in the world's industrialized nations live in cities. Without the Industrial Revolution, this urbanization of the world could not have taken place.

RESEARCH ALERT

Links between homelessness and ill health are well established. However, homeless people are less likely to access traditional health care owing to administrative barriers and the hostility of healthcare professionals. For this reason, more flexible modes of healthcare delivery, including nurse-led care, have been explored. There has been a rapid increase in innovative nursing roles since the 1990s, and the literature suggests that a clear role definition, good interprofessional working relationships, and supportive cultures are some of the features that ensure role effectiveness.

A large study exploring new roles in nursing and midwifery in Northern Ireland identified an innovative nurse-led approach in meeting the needs of single homeless people. The aim of this paper was to explore the effectiveness of this role using a public health framework. A case study design was used that incorporated semi-structured interviews with analysis of secondary sources and a period of observation. Results demonstrated that the role fitted within a public health framework in that it involved assessment of needs, skills to meet those needs, facilitation of access to care, partnership working, health promotion, health protection and influencing policy, and strategy development. The conclusion is that the role met the set criteria for innovative nursing roles. Furthermore, such a practitioner meets the criteria for advanced nursing practice, providing evidence of effective nurse-led care that meets the health agenda of targeting inequalities in health.

Source: Poulton, B., McKenna, H., Keeney, S., Hasson, F., & Sinclair, M. (2006). The role of the public health nurse in meeting the primary health care needs of single homeless people: A case study report. *Primary Health Care Research & Development, 7*(2), 135–146.

The 1940s and World War II created new jobs and decreased poverty and homelessness for a few years, but the 1960s brought a substantial increase in the homeless population. In 1963, the Community Health Centers Act was enacted, which deinstitutionalized approximately 430,000 people with mental illness (Rossi, 1989). These people were released from the institutions in which they resided, and many of them had nowhere to live and no job. Deinstitutionalizing thousands of people was cited as a humane act but detrimentally expanded the homeless population.

The combination of deinstitutionalization and the declining economy in the 1970s forced courts to rule on homelessness for the first time. In 1972, the U.S. Supreme Court ruled that vagrancy was no longer a crime (Cook, 1979). The Court also declared that governmental assistance provided only to people who claimed a permanent residence was unconstitutional. In the same decade, the New York Supreme Court ruled that homeless people should be provided a clean place to sleep, nutritious food, supervision, and security. Efforts were made to comply with the court ruling. Many, but not all, homeless people in New York were given assistance.

Societal and Governmental Influences in the 1980s

The state of New York's move toward improving homeless conditions contributed to the federal government's actions toward homeless programs. Several other major events occurred in the United States during the 1980s that drove the federal government into action to provide federal assistance (Interagency Council on the Homeless, 2000). A dramatic increase in poverty and the shrinking of affordable housing were major forces that led to the homeless epidemic.

Racial discrimination in the job market presented another concern. By 1985, less than 45% of African American men ages 16 to 24 were able to find employment, compared with 70% of white men of the same age range (Interagency Council on the Homeless, 2000). Other situations that contributed to homelessness and poverty were substance abuse, disabilities, chronic health problems, and changes in the family structure that led to a shift toward female-headed households.

Also in the 1980s, a shift in the labor market from a focus on goods production to a focus on services caused plants to relocate or close and farms to shrink or cease to operate. Laborers were no longer in high demand. Rather, the demand was for highly skilled and educated people. A way of life had disappeared; jobs were gone; a new culture of homeless people existed.

The combined tensions created by all of these problems placed at-risk people at serious disadvantages and thus strained many households to the point of homelessness.

Table 25-4 provides a list of governmental activities during the 1980s. Historically, the assistance offered by government programs and local groups has provided only immediate relief and has failed to address the long-term problems of homelessness (Fuchs & McAllister, 1996). The **Stewart B. McKinney Homeless Assistance Act of 1987** and the grass-roots efforts of local relief groups were instrumental in prompting the federal government to make a commitment to reduce homelessness (Interagency Council on the Homeless, 2000).

> There is nothing new about poverty. What is new is that we now have the techniques and the resources to get rid of poverty. The real question is whether we have the will.
>
> —*Martin Luther King, Jr., 1968*

Societal and Governmental Influences in the Late 1990s and Early 21st Century

Many programs were born during the 1990s. Once the initial Stewart B. McKinney Homeless Assistance Act of 1987 was developed, the program branched into numerous programs throughout the federal government (Interagency Council on the Homeless, 2000). **Table 25-5** outlines a few of those programs. By 1994, the McKinney programs had expanded to $1.2 billion. Numerous non-McKinney programs also were created. Today, almost a dozen of these

TABLE 25-4 Governmental Activities for Homeless People in the 1980s

Date	Activities of the 1980s
1982	The Community for Creative Non-Violence in Washington, DC, estimated that 2.2 million Americans lacked shelter.
1982	The U.S. Conference of Mayors reported that the demand for emergency services for the homeless far outweighed the capabilities to provide services. In fact, only 43% of the demand was met.
1983	The Emergency Food and Shelter (EFS) Program of the Federal Emergency Management Agency (FEMA) allocated $100 million to the U.S. Department of Agriculture's Temporary Emergency Food Assistance Program (TEFAP) to reduce the impact of the homeless crisis.
1984 to 1987	FEMA allocated $325 million for continued relief. Other agencies that allocated money for relief efforts included the Health and Human Services Emergency Assistance Program and the HUD Community Development Block Grant Program.
1987	The Stewart B. McKinney Homeless Assistance Act was enacted to provide emergency shelters, job training, and other assistance to homeless people, providing $490 million.
1988	The National Resource Center on Homelessness and Mental Illness was established by the Policy Research Associates (PSA) to provide on-site technical assistance, targeted workshops, publications, databases, and instant access to homeless people with mental illness.

TABLE 25-5 Governmental Activities for Homeless People in the 1990s and Early 21st Century

Date	Activities of the 1990s and Early 21st Century
1992	Funding was set aside to provide rental assistance to 4,750 disabled homeless households annually for 3 years.
1993	President Clinton committed to make homelessness a top priority in the White House.
1994	The Interagency Council on the Homeless published a proposal to reduce the homeless population. The main objective was to find "a decent home and a suitable living environment" for every American, which would become known as the "continuum of care." The reality was that the council hoped to reduce homelessness by one-third.
1995	President Clinton proposed a reorganization of the HUD McKinney programs under a single account. Homeless projects continued as a high priority in the Oval Office.
1995	President Clinton vetoed the balanced budget bill, which would have cut federal welfare by $81.5 billion and virtually eliminated homeless assistance programs provided by the McKinney Act. The President's budget proposed consolidating three runaway and homeless programs. The budget also focused on disadvantaged groups, including veterans and other homeless people.
1995	The National Law Center on Homelessness and Poverty published a report that evaluated NIMBY (not in my backyard) opposition to services for homeless people in 36 jurisdictions across the United States.
1995	Funding was set aside to provide rental assistance to 15,000 homeless households annually for 5 years.
2003	U.S. Department of Health and Human Services published *Ending Chronic Homelessness: Strategies for Action* with specific ways that the federal and state governments could increase flexibility and limit restrictions on health and social services to the homeless.
2010	Affordable Care Act of 2010 passed into law.

non-McKinney programs target homeless people. Many federal programs, although not targeted at the homeless, provide indirect assistance to homeless people. The McKinney Act has been the major federal vehicle to assist homeless people (Interagency Council on the Homeless, 2000).

The 1990s brought about unprecedented growth and complexity in the homeless population. As a result, nurses, social workers, agencies, and others have gained rich, abundant experiences in trying to manage homelessness. The same social problems leading to homelessness persist: declining wages, poor education, persistent illiteracy, racial discrimination, chronic health problems, violence, crime, and poverty.

Americans must face that even as new programs have sprung up, the problem of homelessness has grown because economic, health, and social forces are ever present. Organizations have historically looked for easy solutions to seemingly unresolvable problems. Homelessness remains a problem without an easy solution, just as it has always been. The United States is now faced with even more complex human problems: newer, stronger, and more addictive drugs, such as heroin and cocaine; socially stigmatizing infections such as tuberculosis, sexually transmitted diseases, and HIV; and decline of family support, which means that relatives often do not take in family members needing assistance anymore. **Box 25-4** delineates several factors that may contribute to an individual's homelessness.

THINK ABOUT THIS 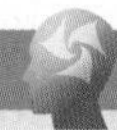

How Could a Nurse Ever End Up Homeless?

What if you, as a nurse, were laid off and could not find a position that accommodates your small children? Eventually, child support disappears (if it ever existed). You are living from month to month and eventually are evicted from your apartment. Through an unfortunate turn of events, you end up without relatives or friends who can take you in for more than a few days.

Now imagine yourself on the streets or living out of your car. Your car breaks down; you do not have the money to repair it. You are essentially living on the streets, putting the children in the car at night. The area around you becomes unsafe for the children but you cannot move the car. Soon, you are bathing your children in public bathrooms, such as those in subway stations, gas stations, and McDonald's restaurants. As the children grow dirtier and their clothes more worn, these options seem to close down due to the owners' reactions and denial of your use of their facilities.

Your days are spent looking for work. Even with an RN license, the work history interruption and your unkempt appearance (no professional clothes and lack of bath facilities) leave you with few or no options. You have to leave your children alone while job hunting, which exposes them to violence and sexual abuse. Your days begin to run together.

You and the children spend hours each day looking for food in garbage cans and McDonald's trash.

You find homeless shelters, but they are often riskier for yourself and your children than being on the streets owing to the risk of theft and the shelters' limited hours. You find yourself trusting no one, having no friends, and living in constant fear that you or your children will be attacked or raped. People pass you on the street and make disparaging remarks, such as "Get a job," turn their eyes away, or run you off from the place where you are sleeping. Police ticket you for vagrancy. You cease to care about what others think of you.

This could not happen to you, you think, right? Neither did the nurse.

Source: This is based on an actual case from Dr. Karen Saucier Lundy's personal experience in an urban homeless shelter. The nurse had a master's degree and three children ranging in age from 6 to 12 and was interviewed in a homeless shelter. The nurses in that shelter never saw her again.

The Health Problems of Homeless People

Common Health Problems

Homelessness in the United States translates into major health problems. People who are homeless are faced with myriad health problems, which fall into three basic categories: health problems that contribute to a state of homelessness, health problems that are the consequence of homelessness, and treatment of health problems that is complicated by homelessness (Institute of Medicine, 1988).

The first category involves health problems that contribute to a state of homelessness. Most people with chronic health problems that lead to a state of homelessness suffer from lack of employment because of their disabling state of health (Berne, Dato, Mason, & Rafferty, 1993; Corburn, 2004; Institute of Medicine, 1988; Wehler et al., 2003). These homeless persons usually do not have a support network of family members and friends. Chronic schizophrenia, dementia, and personality disorders are examples of mental illnesses that may actually contribute to a state of homelessness and financial insecurity. Relationships with family and friends may become excessively strained when an individual's ability to cope with everyday life situations diminishes. Family members may become so stressed trying to deal with everyday problems that they abandon or throw out the mentally ill family member into the streets.

Individuals with acquired immune deficiency syndrome (AIDS) may become homeless when they are no longer able to work because of illness and opportunistic infections (Institute of Medicine, 1988). They often lose their houses or apartments and face overwhelming medical expenses. Living on the street or in a shelter becomes a way of life for them. Alcoholism, drug dependency, and other disabling health problems (e.g., accidental injuries or degenerative diseases) may lead to similar life situations. In 15 studies on alcoholism in the homeless population (as cited in Rossi, 1989), 33% of homeless people abused alcohol and were homeless as a result of alcoholism (Rosenblum et al., 2005; Salazar et al., 2007; Salomonsen-Sautel et al., 2008).

The second category includes many disorders and illnesses that result from living on the streets or in shelters. Examples of physical problems include skin and blood vessel diseases, respiratory disorders and infections, malnutrition, parasitic infestations, foot and lower extremity problems, physical assault, rape, trauma, periodontal disease, tooth decay, degenerative joint disease, sexually transmitted diseases, cirrhosis, and hepatitis (Institute of Medicine, 1988). Psychological and social problems that may be triggered include personality disorders, alcohol and drug dependence, prostitution, poor oral and body hygiene, hunger, adolescent pregnancy, developmental and learning delays in children, violence, criminal convictions, depression, low self-esteem, and other mental illnesses (Institute of Medicine, 1988; Interagency Council on the Homeless, 2000; Rossi, 1989). **Table 25-6** reflects specific health problems associated with homelessness.

Skin, blood vessel, and traumatic problems that homeless people experience are often related to strenuous walking and wandering, inadequate clothing, improper fitting of shoes, and exposure to infections and parasites. Some of these problems include venous stasis, varicose veins, peripheral vascular disease, cellulitis, skin ulcerations, skin infestations, bruises, contusions, lacerations, abrasions, abscesses, and burns of all severities (Cheung & Hwang, 2004; Gamst et al., 2006; Rossi, 1989).

Communicable diseases affect scores of homeless people and are cause for a major public health concern (Rossi, 1989). Living on the streets or in shelters subjects homeless people to poor sanitary conditions, poor hygiene, and inadequate, if any, sleeping quarters. Communicable

BOX 25-3 Use of the Term "Homeless"

In the latter part of the 1970s, the term *homeless* became a trendy way to refer to individuals living on the streets or in shelters (Interagency Council on the Homeless, 2000). At that time, homeless individuals were predominantly males who had been deinstitutionalized. The term was popularized by proponents as a way to describe homeless people in a nonstigmatizing, nonjudgmental way. However, the term became synonymous with "bums." A new kind of homelessness has placed a strain on the use of the term. Since that time, poverty has brought families, women, and children in record numbers to face homelessness.

TABLE 25-6 Common Health Problems of Homeless People

Classification	Specific Health Problems
Skin and traumatic disorders	Skin ulcerations
	Skin infestations (e.g., lice, scabies, worms)
	Peripheral vascular disease, varicose veins
	Cellulitis
	Carbuncles
	Bunions, corns
	Abrasions, lacerations
	Wounds
	Bruises, contusions
	Sprains, strains
	Burns
Acute disorders/diseases	Tuberculosis, pneumonia, influenza, asthma
	Bladder and renal infections
	Female-specific genitourinary infections
	Male-specific genitourinary infections
	Diabetes mellitus complications
Chronic disorders/diseases	Psychosocial disorders/problems
	Cancer of all types
	Endocrine disorders (e.g., diabetes mellitus)
	Anemia and other nutritional deficiencies
	Eye, ear, mouth, and dental disorders
	Cardiovascular disorders (hypertension, heart, and circulatory disorders)
	Arthritis and other musculoskeletal disorders
	Pregnancy
	HIV/AIDS and other sexually transmitted diseases
	Seizures and other neurological disorders
	Obstructive pulmonary disease
	Gastrointestinal disorders
Mental illnesses	Personality disorders
	Criminal convictions
	Jail, prison, or detention sentencing
	Drug and alcohol abuse
	Lack of family or friends support system
	Poverty

Source: From *Down and Out in America: The Origin of Homelessness*, by Rossi, 1989. Used by permission.

diseases (e.g., tuberculosis) are easily transmitted in these living conditions.

The third category results from complications associated with the treatment of acute or chronic health problems in homeless people (Institute of Medicine, 1988). One major chronic disease that is complicated by inadequate treatment is diabetes mellitus. Daily injections and a diabetic exchange diet are difficult, if not impossible, to maintain while homeless. Protecting syringes from theft or contamination, for example, is challenging.

BOX 25-4 Why Are People Homeless?

- Poverty
- Changes in the labor market from focus on goods production to services
- Lack of affordable housing
- Devaluation of the dollar and devaluation of federal income assistance
- Unemployment
- Street violence, domestic violence, and crime
- Crisis in families; abuse, neglect, and incestuous relationships
- Lack of kin support
- Mental illness
- Deinstitutionalization
- Substance abuse
- Socially stigmatizing infectious diseases (e.g., HIV, tuberculosis)

Sources: Interagency Council on the Homeless. (2000). *The federal plan to break the cycle of homelessness.* Washington, DC: Department of Housing and Urban Development; Jahiel, R. I. (Ed.). (1992). *Homelessness: A prevention-oriented approach.* Baltimore, MD: Johns Hopkins University Press; Sumerlin, J. R., & Bundrick, C. M. (1997). Research on homeless men and women: Existential-humanistic and clinical thinking. *Psychological Reports, 80,* 1303–1314; Susser, E., Struening, E., & Conover, S. (1987). Childhood experiences of homeless men. *American Journal of Psychiatry, 144,* 1599–1601.

Hypertension, renal disease, liver disease, peripheral vascular disease, and schizophrenia are other chronic problems that are complicated by homelessness. Inability to follow the prescribed medical regimen, lack of money to cover medical and health expenses, or inability to follow the prescribed dietary regimen complicate these health problems.

Homeless families have similar acute and chronic physical and mental problems. Homeless children also are at risk for developing chronic physical disorders (Forchuk, Russell, Kingston-MacClure, Turner, & Dill, 2006). In a study conducted by Wright and Weber (1987), 16% of the homeless children were reported to have a variety of chronic physical disorders. Some of the most common disorders included asthma, anemia, and malnutrition. Some other disorders reported at high rates were various types of respiratory infections, skin infections, ear and eye infections, dental problems, and gastrointestinal problems.

In another study of homelessness in New York City in 1985 (Chavkin, Kristal, Seabron, & Guigli, 1987), the infant mortality rate of the homeless population (24.9 per 1,000 live births) was more than twice the overall infant mortality rate in New York City (12 per 1,000 live births). In the same study, the researchers found that homeless pregnant women were more likely to give birth to infants of low weight than nonhomeless pregnant women.

HIV transmission is a primary concern for all homeless people, especially homeless adult and adolescent women. In a survey of homeless adults who were entering a storefront medical clinic, 69% were found to be at risk for acquiring HIV infection because of several at-risk behaviors: unprotected sex with multiple partners, injection drug use, sex with a partner who injects drugs, or exchanging sex for money or drugs, primarily crack (St. Lawrence & Brasfield, 1995). Safe, intimate relationships may be difficult, if not impossible, for homeless people to maintain because of drug use, mental illness (Darbyshire et al., 2006), violence, survival sex (sex in exchange for food, money, or drugs), and transient living conditions. In their survey, Fisher, Hovell, and Hofstetter (1995) found that 91% of homeless women experienced battery and 56% experienced sexual assault. Cheung and Hwang (2004) found that homeless women younger than age 45 had higher death rates than older women. Deaths among younger women often approach or are equal to those of homeless men.

Rescue Mission 2

They gather themselves in groups of twelve
around shakey cardtables
some unvarnished wood
and others metal and formica
they're here for another supper
for some the last one
before they lean slowly
toward another side of town
here they all gather at the Riverside mission
apostles of the alleys
sheltered in boxes and
doorways opened onto the
promised streets and rails
lord, are these bones hungry
these tweeds and wools shine
but not with grace from the father
a dull halo of wear
in the seat where a man
can rub thin with contact
from concrete and unpainted benches
and still turn the other cheek
some bring their own wine
refusing the coffee or tea
and milk can no longer faithfully
support these crumbling bones

(*continues*)

(continued)
no one will be betrayed here
though some have thought of a sellout
at times for thirty cents to luck
onto more wine or cigarettes
the bread is passed around again
wholly for the sake of one's almighty health
a man's got to eat to save himself
though the word wasn't made flesh
enough to bless them with a small
taste of steak
after supper they file out on
the thin soles of unpolished shoes
the moon rests like a large stone
rolled to close a room where a brother
waits with a good steak, new tweed
a cigarette and a rousing story of
how when he was hungry there was always
someone to share their bread

—*James A. Lopresti*

THINK ABOUT THIS 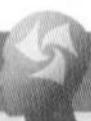

The urban giants: Population of the 10 largest megacities (more than 10 million residents) in the world by ranking

1. Tokyo, Japan (37.2 million)
2. Delhi, India (22.6 million)
3. Mexico City, Mexico (20.5 million)
4. New York City, United States (20.3 million)
5. Shanghai, China (20.2 million)
6. São Paulo, Brazil (19.9 million)
7. Mumbai, India (19.7 million)
8. Beijing, China (15.5 million)
9. Dhaka, Bangladesh (15.4 million)
10. Calcutta, India (14.4 million)

Source: United Nations, 2012.

Homeless mothers have been a forgotten population in terms of research or published literature. Berne and colleagues (1993) noted that homeless mothers traditionally have waited to seek health care until their conditions developed into emergency situations. Chronic stressors, physical and sexual abuse, lack of family ties, poverty, lack of coping abilities, domestic violence, street violence, overcrowded conditions, poor hygiene, and poor nutrition predispose homeless mothers to chronic physical, social, and mental problems. Tuberculosis, depression, sexually transmitted diseases, HIV/AIDS, drug abuse, prostitution for money or drugs, and poor parenting skills often result (Austin, Andersen, & Gelberg, 2008; Cooke, 2004; Wehler et al., 2004).

Adolescents are also vulnerable to a variety of social and health problems, including violence, prostitution, drug abuse, and physical and mental disorders (Meadows-Oliver, 2006). The following Research Alert summarizes research findings about homeless youth and their exposure to and involvement in violence while living on the streets.

A study of women veterans indicates an alarming overrepresentation of women among homeless veterans. This trend has been attributed to the increasing numbers of women serving in military conflicts, such as in Iraq (Gamache, Rosenheck, & Tessier, 2003).

The accumulation of problems that homeless people experience is overwhelming to say the least. Reducing or alleviating homelessness is critical to the general health and human condition in our society. Public policies are needed to meet two goals: to reduce or combat the short-term problems of pain and suffering in homeless individuals and to address the long-term problems by reducing the risk of becoming homeless. By becoming a political advocate for the basic rights and health of the homeless population, community health nurses can help create or change public policies involving homelessness.

Barriers to Health Care

Researchers have repeatedly indicated that lack of access is a major barrier to health care for homeless people (Corburn, 2004; Hunter, Getty, Kemsley, & Skelly, 1991; Snowden & Yamada, 2005; Vijayaraghavan et al., 2012; Wood & Valdez, 1991). Homeless people cannot afford health insurance and, not surprisingly, homeless people experience even more problems in accessing health care than nonhomeless people with or without insurance. Homeless people typically do not have a regular family practitioner. They seek care from emergency departments more often than poor people who are not homeless. Homeless people may also be discouraged from obtaining healthcare services or even turned away by healthcare personnel from private clinics (Freeman et al., 1987). Other barriers to health care include the following (Flynn, 1997; Forchuk et al., 2006; Hatton, 1997; Institute of Medicine, 1988; Nyamathi, Flaskerud, & Leake, 1997; Percy, 1995):

- Lack of systematic communication with healthcare professionals
- Lack of transportation to a healthcare facility
- Lack of social and family support
- Psychological depression; hard-to-reach homeless people
- Lack of motivation by the homeless person to seek health care

RESEARCH ALERT

A survey of 432 youth between the ages of 13 and 23 years old, who were homeless or at imminent risk for homelessness, revealed that males and females were exposed to equally high levels of violence on the streets. Females were more likely to have been sexually assaulted but less likely to report it or report any other violent acts. Ethnic identity was not a significant predictor of exposure to violence. The overall findings revealed that these youth were exposed to violence at a significantly higher level than other youth in national surveys.

Source: Kipke, M. D., Simon, T. R., Montgomery, S. B., Unger, J. B., & Iversen, E. F. (1997). Homeless youth and their exposure to and involvement in violence while living on the streets. *Journal of Adolescent Health, 20*, 360–367.

ETHICAL CONNECTION 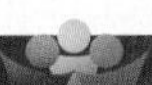

As community health nurses, do we have a moral obligation to care for the homeless as part of the public's health? Such individuals are difficult to locate, they are transient, and their problems are deep-seated and complex. Should we instead concentrate on those populations where preventive health care can be more effective?

Caring for Urban and Homeless People

Community health nurses function on all three levels of prevention—primary, secondary, and tertiary—regarding the care of urban and homeless aggregate populations. Homeless people have generated a culture all their own, enriched with diverse customs and backgrounds that should be taken into consideration when managing care for them (Acosta & Toro, 2000; Corburn, 2004; Family and Youth Services Bureau, 1994; Lowe, 2008). Managing health and social problems for urban and homeless individuals and populations is among the most challenging functions of the community health nurse.

Homeless people suffer from myriad emotional and physical ups and downs. The Research Alert that follows reflects a summary of research findings on the experiences of homeless female-headed families.

Both young and old homeless people need what everyone needs—opportunities, advantages, and services that help them live healthier lives. Ed DeBerri, as the Assistant Director at the National Resource Center on Homelessness and Mental Illness (1997), stated that the most effective programs and policies have human dignity as their guiding principle. Through hands-on experience with homeless individuals, DeBerri learned five important principles about homeless people and their needs.

First and foremost, DeBerri (1997) found that homeless people have talents, needs, and desires. They want to be shown respect for who they are and what they know. Second, shelters and case management traditionally have not been sufficient to prevent the problems of homelessness or to end homelessness. Housing, financial support, and social and family support are needed to improve the conditions. Third, providing comprehensive health care, social services, and housing can reduce homelessness. Fourth, helping to find work for homeless individuals is essential. Homeless people need to feel productive and useful, just like all people. Fifth, new resources need to be developed and used creatively; then the successes of these programs need to be publicized.

RESEARCH ALERT

Homeless families are at high risk for severe physical, emotional, and social health problems. Eighty-five percent of all homeless families are headed by single women. Sixteen of these women were asked to describe their experiences of being the head of the homeless family. The themes that emerged were loss of freedom, a sense of being different, feeling down, maternal survival (motherhood), and living under pressure. They described being homeless as a nightmare, not knowing what will happen to them or where they will be from day to day.

Source: Menke, E. M., & Wagner, J. D. (1997). The experience of homeless female-headed families. *Issues in Mental Health Nursing, 18*, 315–330.

These five principles also can be applied to the care of urban populations. Drawing on the strengths of urban or homeless individuals and the resources available in the community will enable community health nurses to implement appropriate interventions that can actually work. An example of drawing on the strength of a homeless person would be to find a homeless person who can sew and asking him or her to teach a group of people in the shelter how to mend their clothes. Another example is to recruit a person from the shelter to teach good hygiene and handwashing techniques to the children in the shelter. The community health nurse's interventions will help create social and economic viability, build diversity in skills and resources, strengthen the community, and contribute to healthier people in the community.

Use Leadership Skills

Become an enthusiastic leader and an encourager. Being committed to enthusiastically leading the way in solving problems for urban and homeless people will help others catch on, pitch in, and follow. Once others start contributing their time and efforts into this mission, specialized expertise areas will start to develop among the workers. Acting as a leader and encourager can be used at all three levels of prevention. One example of using excellent leadership skills is when, upon recognizing the need for a community health center, the community health nurse promotes and sells the idea to key people in the community and political officials, leads the way in planning and organizing, and then coordinates the activities. Before long, the nurse's dream will be realized through hard work and commitment.

Be Committed

Be committed to make a difference in the community. To properly intervene, community health nurses first need to be committed enough to help make a difference in the community. A high level of commitment will facilitate nurses' care of urban and homeless patients in the community. In fact, all three levels of prevention interventions will follow more easily if commitment to make a difference in the community has already been established. Commitment from community health nurses translates to hope and healing among the urban and homeless populations.

A paramount example of one person's commitment to make a difference is former President Jimmy Carter. The Atlanta Project (TAP) was initiated by Carter in 1991 (TAP, 1995). The central mission of this project was to bring the "two Atlantas" (the affluent and poverty groups) together to improve the quality of life in Atlanta's neighborhoods, especially urban areas. TAP has been somewhat successful since its induction in decreasing the gap between the rich and the poor. In fact, Carter became committed to spreading TAP to all of America, thus becoming The America Project. By 1995, more than 100 official delegations from numerous cities across America had begun modeling their urban enhancement and development programs after TAP (Berger, 2007; Biven, 2002).

> Even Fuji is without beauty to one who is hungry and cold.
>
> —*Japanese saying*

GLOBAL CONNECTION 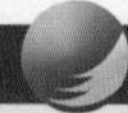

Changes in the growth of the world's cities: How more cities grow and join the "Million People" club

1900: 16 cities had more than 1 million residents.
1975: 195 cities had more than 1 million residents.
1995: 364 cities had more than 1 million residents.
2015: 564 cities projected to have 1 million residents.

Sources: Haub, C. (2002). Has global growth reached its peak? *Population Today, 30*(6), 6; Haub, C. (2003). *2003 world population data sheet of the Population Reference Bureau.*

Be an Advocate

Become a political advocate for preventing homelessness and the problems associated with the urban population. Intervention at this level is primary prevention, which involves taking political action. Talking to politicians and speaking out in favor of prevention of homelessness and the problems associated with urban populations are essential to effecting change in the community. Even more important is for community health nurses to speak out in numbers through their professional organizations, such as the American Nurses Association and the American Public Health Association, and encourage new public policies to be adopted. Being a united voice through large numbers of community health nurses is powerful and grabs the attention of politicians across the country.

In becoming politically involved, community health nurses need to remember not to become overwhelmed or take on too many issues at one time. It is more effective to concentrate on one or two problems at a time. Promoting ideas and attitudes and selling a political viewpoint or solution can go a long way toward reducing the problems associated with homelessness or the urban poverty population. Writing letters to local, state, and federal officials and congressional members is an effective way to capture attention. Other ways include presenting concerns at public meetings, getting elected as a lobbyist through organizations, interacting with members of Congress on a one-on-one basis, and publicizing the needs and concerns of these populations through brochures, newspapers, radio, and television.

Use Available Resources

Draw on every federal and community resource available to you. Community health nurses should realize that to make a difference they need to network with other agencies and draw on existing community and federal resources. The management of care involved in this level of intervention is secondary prevention. Drawing on federal and community resources to provide outreach programs mandates that the community health nurse maximize the use of collaborative partnerships with disciplines and agencies within the community.

One of the fundamental elements that contributed to the success of TAP was its personnel's realizing that everything and every resource needed to make a difference in Atlanta was within reach. Mark O'Connell, then president of the United Way of Metro Atlanta, speaking about one solution for improving urban life, stated, "The answer is in how we use the resources we already have and in how we value people" (TAP, 1995). In this regard, community health nurses can equate O'Connell's statement about valuing people to caring about urban and homeless people, which takes a high level of commitment to help with improving the community.

Local resources can help supply meals, hygiene products, clothing, and even health care. Food missions, local free clinics, churches, Salvation Army, and American Red Cross are valuable resources that the community health nurse can use. State and federal resources can be drawn upon for financial, health, education, and shelter programs, as well as other types of programs. Medicare, welfare, Medicaid, Head Start, and food stamps include a variety of state and federal programs that can be used.

Vagrant

he floated like a guppy once
didn't need to care
didn't care to need
it's all there in the sac
the warmth and cushion
the belly always filled first
but he still had to let go
though stubborn; a caesarian
and make his way in the world
there was a breast for a spell
and he grew into a plump little
pear on buttermilk bisquits and gravy
he stole apples and squash
sneaking in and hiding the plunder
in the crowded cupboards
it doesn't take long for years
to rot and ripe and rot again
and jobs came and went
why, once not long back he even
sold carnations—fullblown white ones—
on street corners for change
he's shrunk and wrinkled like a
sunbaked codfish now
wandering from mission to mission
turning up on doorsteps like some
crazy orphaned bouquet of lillies-of-the-valley
not caring to need
not needing to care

—*James A. Lopresti*

GOT AN ALTERNATIVE?

One of the threats to health for the homeless is related to their feet, due to standing for long periods of time, poor footwear, and exposure to adverse environmental conditions. One successful strategy that homeless shelter clinics have utilized in the past to promote their services has been to offer whirlpool footbaths. Once in the clinic, the community health nurse can use the time with the patient to assess and offer assistance in other health areas.

MEDIA MOMENT

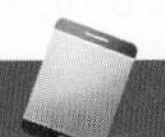

House of Sand and Fog (2003)

This film is about the concept of "home" and the lengths to which people will go to preserve it. An alcoholic woman who has been dumped by her husband, Kathy Nicolo (Jennifer Connelly) finds her family house in the California hills seized in foreclosure and put up for public auction by a local sheriff deputy (Ron Eldard). An exiled Iranian Air Force colonel (Ben Kingsley) sees Nicolo's house as his family's dream home and quickly snaps it up. Trouble is, Nicolo is obsessed with getting the house back and goes to extreme measures to reclaim it. This film is about family, cultural issues, alcoholism, and redemption. An emotional rollercoaster, this outstanding movie covers the full range of human reactions to isolation and fear of homelessness.

Foster Communication and Trust

Develop open communication and trust among the urban and homeless populations. A climate of open communication and trust is pivotal to developing an environment of security and support. Violations of trust and conveying a false sense of security have serious consequences and should be avoided when interacting with urban and homeless people. Nurses need to remember not to make promises of hope that will never be met. Trust is built on truth, reliability, and open communication. For a leader to be effective, trustworthiness is critical. Following through on a project or goal and being dependable are ways that the community health nurse can establish trust and open communication.

Assess the Problem

Develop and practice good assessment skills. For primary prevention, assessment is aimed at identifying factors that play a role in the problems of urban living and problems that contribute to homelessness. At this level of prevention, community health nurses need to assess the political structure of the city and state resources available in the community at all levels of government.

NOTE THIS!

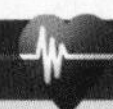

Homeless as a term was first used in 1981 by Mitch Snyder and Robert Hayes to describe the growing number of persons living in boxes and eating out of garbage cans in urban areas as a result of the worst recession in half a century.

Source: Jencks, C. (1994). *The homeless*. Cambridge, MA: Harvard University Press.

APPLICATION TO PRACTICE

Descent of a Woman: From Rags to Riches to Rags

By age 26, Nadine had a husband, three healthy sons, a prosperous clothing boutique in New York's trendy Soho district, and a lifestyle she had always wanted. Her life as a child was saddened by the abandonment of her mother, who turned to drugs and prostitution. Nadine, by age 8, was herself experiencing the effects of alcohol. Later, she turned to marijuana and cocaine, often smoking marijuana with her father.

She temporarily cleaned up her life. But taking care of a family and attending to a business with all its financial demands resulted in too much pressure for Nadine. Nadine and her husband sometimes experimented with cocaine as they celebrated their newfound success. The drugs, the money, and the success pushed Nadine and her husband to vicious fights. Soon the money was gone. Nadine left her family. Nadine's drug use became excessive—from pot and cocaine to, finally, a powerful addiction to heroin. The drug had so much power over her that she turned to prostitution to support a $100-a-day habit.

When she had exhausted all of her resources, her boyfriend (a drug pusher) introduced her to "the condo," an underground subway escape in New York where thousands of homeless people live to stay high on drugs and to escape life, family, and the law. People refer to the underground people as the "mole people." After unsuccessfully trying drug rehabilitation 20 times, Nadine felt she had hit rock bottom. She had even been pronounced clinically dead once in an emergency department in New York.

> She joined a band of drug addicts descending under an iron plate literally into the bowels of New York city, down 13 metal steps, then around and around a grimy concrete staircase . . . just a few blocks and a world away from her old life. Instead of a bathroom . . . the subway tracks were her toilet.
>
> The kitchen? Whatever they could beg, borrow, or steal. And this soot-filled platform right next to the roaring train, her bedroom. [Under New York] there's another city. . . . This one has about 45,000 people in it . . . the homeless who are sleeping underground. (Phillips, Pauley, & Rudolph, 1997, p. 16)

After a long time living homeless and like a mole underground, Nadine's break came. She crossed paths with Renny Chun, a journalist. Chun pushed Nadine, through numerous contacts, to rehabilitation. Nadine wanted help but was afraid of being sober and of failure. She desperately wanted to see her sons, which provided her the strength she needed to kick the habit cold turkey. Now Nadine lives one day at a time and hopes to never be in the condo again. She reunited for a short while with her sons. *Dateline NBC* reported that she was seeking legal visiting rights for the future. Nadine's courage has helped her to be clean and sober today and hopefully tomorrow.

Underground living is a reality for homeless people in major cities where subway escapes exist. Rudolph (Phillips, Pauley, & Rudolph, 1997) discussed the nightmare that Nadine experienced and related the magnitude of the problem of the underground. Nadine took Rudolph and the television viewers to "the condo" to see the drug addicts lying with the rats, the human waste, the garbage, and the sewer. She noticed that the same people she had previously known were still underground.

1. What are some factors, psychological and external, that led Nadine to homelessness? As you answer this question, think about her life as a child and as an adult.
2. What health problems/infections would you anticipate Nadine to have while exposed to underground living? As a prostitute? As a homeless person? If Nadine had been homeless in your city, list resources that would have been available to her.
3. How would you, as a community health nurse, help Nadine? Include how you could intervene using a holistic approach. Include as many physical, psychosocial, cultural, developmental, and spiritual factors that you should take into consideration when planning Nadine's care.

Source: Phillips, S. (Announcer), Pauley, J. (Announcer), & Rudolph, L. (Reporter). (1997, August 19). *Dateline NBC*. New York, NY: National Broadcasting System. Transcript from Burrelle Publishing, Livingston, NJ.

THINK ABOUT THIS 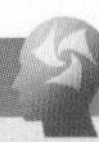

Can our cities be saved? Here are 25 ways to improve urban health:

1. Reclaim dangerous neighborhoods.
2. Discover the effects of stress in the lived environment.
3. Build learning communities.
4. Understand the local culture.
5. Reach out to immigrants.
6. Target cancer prevention efforts.
7. Keep on the offensive.
8. Use community health workers.
9. Eliminate disparities in health.
10. Broaden diabetes treatment.
11. Unleash positive peer pressure.
12. Nurture connectedness.
13. Anticipate expanding needs.
14. Understand HIV-risk behaviors.
15. Take aim at illegal gun sales.
16. Highlight stores' healthy foods.
17. Give back to cities.
18. Train mental health mentors.
19. Start a school of science.
20. Undo the trauma of violence.
21. Rebuild aging infrastructure.
22. Clear the air.
23. Roll out injury prevention.
24. Prepare for home emergencies.
25. Share your insights.

Read the article from the publication below for more detail about successful research-based urban health interventions. Select one of the preceding options and identify one way that community health nurses can influence a city's health. Who would you involve in your efforts?

Source: John Hopkins Public Health (Magazine of the Johns Hopkins Bloomberg School of Public Health), Fall 2006, pp. 14–53.

Plan and Give Care

Develop and implement an effective plan of care. Planning care for urban and homeless populations means that community health nurses will need to focus on basic life care needs as well as population needs. First, short-term and long-term goals need to be identified at the primary, secondary, and tertiary levels. Needs should also be prioritized from most urgent human needs to least urgent.

However, an effective plan of care is futile if the plan does not lead to action on the part of the community health nurse and other community resource providers. Actually following through with an effective plan goes back to maintaining a high level of commitment. Resource agencies and people are available and ready to help. The community health nurse must be committed to finding these resources and then using them. Although referral agencies are critical to good outcomes for homeless people, community health nurses need to realize the importance of the nursing role. The community health nurse provides a continuity of care that no other discipline offers. While providing continuity, the nurse's quality of care has an excellent chance to improve health and holistic outcomes for the person.

Critical Thinking Activities

1. Richford, New York, is a community with a population of approximately 1,150. Most of the residents work elsewhere, and those who do not are mostly self-employed in farming. There is no local industry, grocery store, hotel, bank, library, school, or police department. There is one outreach clinic operated by a hospital system about 30 miles away, and a volunteer fire/EMS department. There is a closer community hospital (22 miles), but the residents prefer traveling the 30 miles to the metropolitan area for health services. There is very limited public transportation (twice daily stops) and no taxi services. According to the rural–urban continuum, in which type of county is Richford located? How does this understanding affect your health planning?
2. A rural community health nurse has been asked to participate on a community task force to develop a plan to stop underage drinking in the community. The task force receives $10,000 from its state senator to be used in the development and implementation of the plan. If you were the community health nurse, what would your role be as community health educator and consultant for this group?
3. Think about Nadine's state of homelessness as described in the Application to Practice feature. Consider her desire for drugs and the life she was living during her period of homelessness. What views/attitudes should you, a community health nurse, take as a logical and ethical approach toward Nadine?

4. Discuss the way each of the following six ethical principles might apply to Nadine, her situation, and her health care:

Autonomy	Privacy
Freedom	Beneficence
Veracity	Fidelity

5. John, 36 years old, is a homeless man with a history of intravenous drug use and AIDS. He is wasting away and has multidrug-resistant tuberculosis. He went to the free neighborhood health clinic where you work, presenting with fever, cough, and purulent blood-tinged sputum. As a community health nurse, discuss four health outcomes that John and you would plan for his care. Give the rationale for each.
6. Discuss some therapeutic communication strategies the community health nurse might use with a single mother with two children, all of whom are homeless. The mother has a crack addiction, and you have reason to believe that she swaps sex for drugs while the children, ages 2 and 8, are left alone on the street.
7. Select nursing interventions at the primary, secondary, and tertiary levels for an elderly homeless female with a history of congestive heart failure and insulin-dependent diabetes mellitus. Include interventions that address the holistic nature of the individual.
8. Yolanda, a 16-year-old homeless African American adolescent, has presented to a shelter for food, clothing, and sleep. You are the community health nurse assisting her. You learned through your assessment that she has had morning sickness and has been very sick, to the point that she slept on the streets for 7 nights because she did not have the strength to walk 2 miles to the shelter. She had become dehydrated and weak. She admitted to using crack cocaine on a regular basis and stated that she could not control her desire to use the drug. She has not seen a family practitioner for her morning sickness and dehydration or to receive a pregnancy test. She thinks that she is at least 3 months pregnant by a young man she met on the streets. He has since been imprisoned for selling drugs. She ran away from home several months ago to escape a poor family relationship with her mother.
    - Based on what you have learned about Yolanda, list the risk factors that may have contributed to Yolanda's homelessness and her situation.
    - Knowing that shelter care would not be enough for Yolanda, what would be your plan of care for her? Include resources, social support, family, and other agencies you may use.
    - Yolanda receives medical attention and is stabilized for now. What can you do in the first few days at the shelter to instill in Yolanda a sense of competence, a sense of usefulness, a sense of belonging, and a sense of power and control? Include cultural considerations and values.
    - What barriers will Yolanda face when she makes any decisions concerning her wellbeing? Obtaining a primary practitioner? Returning to her environment? Returning to school?

References

Acosta, O., & Toro, P. A. (2000). Let's ask the homeless people themselves: A needs assessment based on a probability sample of adults. *American Journal of Community Psychology, 28*, 343–366.

Anderson, N. (1934). *Homeless in New York City*. New York, NY: Board of Charity.

Anderson, N. (1940). Highlights of the migrant problem today. *Proceedings of the National Conference of Social Work*. New York, NY: National Conference of Social Work.

Atav, A. S., & Spencer, G. A. (2002). Health risk behaviors among rural, suburban, and urban adolescents: A comparative study. *Family & Community Health, 23*(2), 1–18.

Austin, E., Andersen, R., & Gelberg, L. (2008). Ethnic differences in the correlates of mental distress among homeless women. *Women's Health Issues, 18*(1), 26–34.

Bartlett, P. F. (1993). *American dreams, rural realities: Family farms in crisis*. Chapel Hill, NC: University of North Carolina Press.

Bassak, E. L. (1991). Homeless families. *Science America, 265*(6), 66–74.

Baum, A. S., & Burnes, D. W. (1993). *A nation in denial: The truth about homelessness*. Boulder, CO: Westview Press.

Bean, G., Stefl, M., & Howe, S. (1987). Mental health and homelessness: Issues and findings. *Social Work, 32*, 411–416.

Belcher, J. R., Scholler-Jaquish, A., & Drummond, M. (1991). Three stages of homelessness: A conceptual model for social workers in health care. *Health and Social Work, 16*(2), 87–93.

Benda, B. B., & Dattalo, P. (1988). Homelessness: Consequence of a crisis or long-term process? *Hospital and Community Psychiatry, 39*, 884–886.

Berger, J. (2007). "There is tragedy on both sides of the layoffs:" Privatization and the urban crisis in Baltimore. *International Labor & Working-Class History, 71*, 29–49.

Berne, A. S., Dato, C., Mason, D. J., & Rafferty, M. (1993). A nursing model for addressing the health needs of homeless families. In G. D. Wegner & R. J. Alexander (Eds.), *Readings in family nursing*. Philadelphia, PA: Lippincott.

Biven, W. C. (2002). *Jimmy Carter's economy: Policy in an age of limits*. Chapel Hill, NC: University of North Carolina Press.

Bolland, J. M., & McCallum, D. M. (2002). Touched by homelessness: An examination of hospitality for the down and out. *American Journal of Public Health, 92*, 116–118.

Branas, C. C., Nance, M. L., Elliott, M. R., Richmond, T. S., & Schwab, C. S. (2004). Urban-rural shifts in intentional firearm death: Different causes, same results. *American Journal of Public Health, 94*(10), 1750–1755.

Brent, D. A., Perper, J. A., Moritz, G., Baugher, M., Schweers, J., & Roth, C. (1993). Firearms and adolescent suicide. A community case control. *American Journal of Diseases in Children, 147*(10), 1066–1071.

Burt, M., & Cohen, B. (1989). *America's homeless: Numbers, characteristics, and the numbers that serve them*. Washington, DC: Urban Institute.

Centers for Disease Control and Prevention (CDC). (2005). *National Immunization Survey: A User's Guide for the 2005 Public-Use Data File*. Retrieved from http://www.cdc.gov/nis/pdfs/nispuf05_dug.pdf

Centers for Disease Control and Prevention (CDC). (2013). Teen pregnancy prevention 2010–2015: Integrating services, programs, and strategies through communitywide initiatives: The President's Teen Pregnancy Prevention Initiative. Retrieved from http://www.cdc.gov/teenpregnancy/PreventTeenPreg.htm

Chavkin, W., Kristal, A., Seabron, C., & Guigli, P. (1987). The reproductive experience of women living in hotels for the homeless in New York City. *New York State Journal of Medicine, 371*, 10–13.

Cheung, A. M., & Hwang, S. W. (2004). Risk of death among homeless women: A cohort study and review of the literature. *Canadian Medical Assessment Journal, 170*(8), 1243–1247.

Connor, A., Rainer, L. P., Simcox, J. B., & Thomisee, K. (2007). Increasing the delivery of health care services to migrant farm worker families through a community partnership model. *Public Health Nursing, 24*(4), 355–360.

Cook, P. J., & Mizer, K. L. (1994, December). *The revised ERS county typology: An overview.* Rural Development Research Report Number 89. Economic Research Service, U.S. Department of Agriculture.

Cook, T. (Ed.). (1979). *Vagrancy: Some new perspectives*. New York, NY: Academic Press.

Cooke, C. L. (2004). Joblessness and homelessness as precursors of health problems in formerly incarcerated African American men. *Journal of Nursing Scholarship, 36*(2), 155–160.

Corburn, J. (2004). Confronting the challenges in reconnecting urban planning and public health. *American Journal of Public Health, 94*(4), 541–545.

Cosby, A., Neaves, T., Cossman, R., Cossman, J., James, W., Feierabend, N., ... Farrigan, T. (2008). Preliminary evidence for an emerging nonmetropolitan mortality penalty in the United States. *American Journal of Public Health, 98*(8), 1470–1472.

Cousineau, M. R., Wittenberg, E., & Pollatsek, J. (1995). *Study of the health care for the homeless program*. (HV 4505). Bethesda, MD: U.S. Department of Health and Human Services, Bureau of Primary Health Care.

Culhane, D. P., Dejowski, E. F., Ibanex, J., Needham, E., & Macchia, I. (1993). *Public shelter admission rates in Philadelphia and New York City: The implications of turnover for sheltered population counts*. Washington, DC: Fannie Mae Office of Housing Research.

Darbyshire, P., Muir-Cochrane, E., Fereday, J., Jureidini, J., & Drummond, A. (2006). Engagement with health and social care services: Perceptions of homeless young people with mental health problems. *Health and Social Care in the Community, 14*(6), 553–562.

DeBerri, E. (1997). Listening to the voice of homelessness. *Access, 9*(1), 2.

Eberhardt, M. S., & Pamuk, E. R. (2004). The importance of place of residence: Examining health in rural and nonrural areas. *American Journal of Public Health, 94*, 1682–1686.

Ehlers, J. K., Connon, C., Themann, C. L., Myers, J. R., & Ballard, T. (1993). Health and safety hazards associated with farming. *American Association of Occupational Health Nursing Journal, 41*(9), 414–421.

Fahs, P. S. S., Smith, B. E., Atav, A. S., Britten, M. X., Collins, M. S., Morgan, L. L., & Spencer, G. A. (1999). Integrative research review of risk behaviors among adolescents in rural, suburban, and urban areas. *Journal of Adolescent Health, 24*(4), 230–243.

Family and Youth Services Bureau. (1994). *Guide to enhancing the cultural competence of runaway and homeless youth programs*. Silver Spring, MD: U.S. Government Printing Office.

First, R. J., Rife, J. C., & Tooney, B. G. (1994). Homelessness in rural areas: Causes, patterns, and trends. *Social Work, 39*(1), 97–108.

Fisher, B., Hovell, M., & Hofstetter, C. R. (1995). Risks associated with long-term homelessness among women: Battery, rape, and HIV infection. *International Journal of Health Services, 25*, 351–369.

Fitchen, J. M. (1991). Homelessness in rural places: Perspectives from upstate New York. *Urban Anthropology and Studies of Cultural Systems, 20*(2), 177.

Flynn, L. (1997). The health practices of homeless women: A causal model. *Nursing Research, 46*(2), 72–77.

Forchuk, C., Russell, G., Kingston-MacClure, S., Turner, K., & Dill, S. (2006). From psychiatric ward to the streets and shelters. *Journal of Psychiatric & Mental Health Nursing, 13*(3), 301–308.

Foster, P., & Frazier, E. (2008). Rural health issues in HIV/AIDS: Views from two different windows. *Journal of Health Care for the Poor & Underserved, 19*(1), 10–15.

Fraser, C., Smith, K., Judd, F., Humphreys, J., Fragar, L., & Henderson, A. (2005). Farming and mental health problems and mental illness. *International Journal of Social Psychiatry, 51*(4), 340–349.

Freeman, H. E., Blendon, R. J., Aiken, L. H., Sudman, S., Mullinix, C. F., & Corey, C. R. (1987). Americans report on their access to care. *Health Affairs, 6*(1), 6–18.

Fuchs, E., & McAllister, W. (1996). *A continuum of care: A report on the new federal policy to address homelessness* (HUD Contract No. DU100C000018360). Washington, DC: Department of Housing and Urban Development, Center for Urban Policy.

Galea, S., & Vlahov, D. (2002). Social determinants and the health of drug users: Socioeconomic status, homelessness and incarceration. *Public Health Reports, 117*(1), 5135–5145.

Gamache, G., Rosenheck, R., & Tessier, R. (2003). Over representation of women veterans among homeless women. *American Journal of Public Health, 93*(7), 1132–1135.

Gamst, G., Herdina, A., Mondragon, E., Munguia, F., Pleitez, A., Stephens, H., ... Cuéllar, I. (2006). Relationship among respondent ethnicity, ethnic identity, acculturation, and homeless status on a homeless population's functional status. *Journal of Clinical Psychology, 62*(12), 1485–1501.

Gerberich, S. G. (1995). Prevention of death and disability in farming. In H. H. McDuffie, J. A. Dosman, K. M. Semchuk, S. A. Olenchock, & A. Senthilselvan (Eds.), *Agricultural health and safety.* Boca Raton, FL: Lewis.

Goldstein, G., & Kickbusch, I. (1996). *A healthy city is a better city. World Health Organization*. Geneva, Switzerland: World Health Organization.

Grossman, D. C. (2000). The history of injury control and the epidemiology of child and adolescent injuries. *Future Child, 10*(1), 23–52.

Hartley, D. (2004). Rural health disparities, population health, and racial culture. *American Journal of Public Health, 94*(10), 1675–1677.

Harvey, P. (2008). Community work injuries: Country style. *Australian Journal of Rural Health, 16*(5), 321–321.

Hatton, D. C. (1997). Managing health problems among homeless women with children in a transitional shelter. *Image: Journal of Nursing Scholarship, 29*(1), 33–37.

Helvie, C. O. (1999, Spring). Nursing the homeless—A vulnerable population. *American Public Health Association Public Health Nursing Newsletter*, pp. 8–9.

Hoch, C., & Slayton, R. A. (1989). *New homeless and old: Community and the skid row.* Philadelphia, PA: Temple University Press.

Hoffman, V. F. (1953). *The American tramp, 1870–1900.* Unpublished master's thesis. Chicago, IL: University of Chicago.

Hunter, J. K., Getty, C., Kemsley, M., & Skelly, A. H. (1991). Barriers to providing health care to homeless persons: A survey of providers' perceptions. *Health Values, 15*(5), 3–11.

Institute of Medicine. (1988). *Homelessness, health and human needs.* Washington, DC: National Academies Press.

Interagency Council on the Homeless. (2000). *The federal plan to break the cycle of homelessness.* Washington, DC: Department of Housing and Urban Development.

International Healthy Cities Foundation (IHCF). (2002). *What is the Healthy Cities movement?* Retrieved from http://www.healthycommunitiesinstitute.com/international-foundation/

Jahiel, R. I. (Ed.). (1992). *Homelessness: A prevention-oriented approach.* Baltimore, MD: Johns Hopkins University Press.

Jencks, C. (1994). *The homeless.* Cambridge, MA: Harvard University Press.

Johnson, A., Mink, M., Harun, N., Moore, C., Martin, A., & Bennett, K. (2008). Violence and drug use in rural teens: National prevalence estimates from the 2003 Youth Risk Behavior Survey. *Journal of School Health, 78*(10), 554–561.

Jones, T. (2006). Resilience in homeless adults: A review of literature. *Journal of the National Black Nurses Association, 17*(1), 36–44.

Kidd, P. S., & Holton, C. (1993). Driving practices, risk-taking motivations, and alcohol use among adolescent drivers: A pilot study. *Journal of Emergency Nursing, 19*(4), 292–296.

Kipke, M. D., Simon, T. R., Montgomery, S. B., Unger, J. B., & Iversen, E. F. (1997). Homeless youth and their exposure to and involvement in violence while living on the streets. *Journal of Adolescent Health, 20*, 360–367.

Klein, S. J., Karchner, W. D., & O'Connell, D. A. (2002). Interventions to prevent HIV-related stigma and discrimination: Findings and recommendations for public health practice. *Journal of Public Health Management & Practice, 8*(6), 44–53.

Krout, J. A. (1994). An overview of older rural populations and community-based services. In J. A. Krout (Ed.), *Providing community-based services to the rural elderly* (pp. 3–18). Thousand Oaks, CA: Sage.

Lambert, M. I. (1995). Migrant and seasonal farm worker women. *Journal of Obstetric, Gynecologic, & Neonatal Nursing, 24*(3), 265–268.

Lewis, D. L. (1993). *W. E. B. DuBois: Biography of a race, 1868–1919.* New York, NY: Henry Holt.

Lezak, A. D., & Edgar, E. (1996). *Preventing homelessness among people with serious mental illnesses: A guide for states.* (HHS Publication No. 3106). Rockville, MD: U.S. Department of Health and Human Services, Center for Mental Health Services.

Lindsey, A. M. (1995). Physical health of homeless adults. *Annual Review of Nursing Research, 13*, 31–61.

Link, B., Phelan, J., Breshan, M., Stueve, A., Moore, R., & Susser, E. (1995). Lifetime and five-year prevalence of homelessness in the United States: New evidence on an old debate. *American Journal of Orthopsychiatry, 65*, 347–354.

Lopez, R., & Welker-Hood, K. (2007, January). Environment, health, and safety: Urban sprawl and the built environment. *American Nurse Today.*

Lowe, S. (2008). It's all one big circle: Welfare discourse and the everyday lives of urban adolescents. *Journal of Sociology & Social Welfare, 35*(3), 173–194.

Luhby, T. (2012, June 21). Income inequality in America: Worsening wealth inequality by race. *CNNMoney.* Retrieved from http://money.cnn.com/2012/06/21/news/economy/wealth-gap-race/index.htm

Marvel, M. E., Pratt, D. S., Marvel, L. H., Regan, M., & May, J. J. (1991). Occupational hearing loss in New York dairy farmers. *American Journal of Industrial Medicine, 20*, 517–531.

Massey, D. S., & Denton, N. A. (1993). *American apartheid: Segregation and the making of the underclass.* Cambridge, MA: Harvard University Press.

McGehee, D. V., Raby, M., Carney, C., Lee, J. D., & Reyes, M. L. (2007). Extending parental mentoring using an event-triggered video intervention in rural teen drivers. *Journal of Safety Research, 38*, 215–227.

Meadows-Oliver, M. (2006). Homeless adolescent mothers: A metasynthesis of their life experiences. *Journal of Pediatric Nursing, 21*(5), 340–349.

Menke, E. M., & Wagner, J. D. (1997). The experience of homeless female-headed families. *Issues in Mental Health Nursing, 18*, 315–330.

Mills, P. K., Dodge, J., & Yang, R. (2009). Cancer in migrant and seasonal hired farm workers. *Journal of Agromedicine, 14*(2), 185–191.

Mockenhaupt, R. E., & Muchow, J. A. (1994). Disease and disability prevention and health promotion for rural elders. In J. A. Krout (Ed.), *Providing community-based services to the rural elderly* (pp. 183–201). Thousand Oaks, CA: Sage.

Momeni, J. A., & Wiegand, G. (1989). *Homelessness in the United States*. New York, NY: Greenwood Press.

Muellman, R. L., Walker, R. A., & Edney, J. A. (1993). Motor vehicle deaths: A rural epidemic. *Journal of Trauma, 35*(5), 717–719.

National Alliance to End Homelessness. (2011). Average real income of working poor people by state—State of homelessness 2011. Retrieved from http://www.endhomelessness.org/library/entry/average-real-income-of-working-poor-people-by-state-state-of-homelessness-2

National Center for Farmworker Health (NCFH). (2003). *Overview of American's farmworkers*. Retrieved from http://www.ncfh.org/aaf_01.php

National Center for Farmworker Health (NCFH). (2012). *Facts about farmworkers*. Retrieved from http://www.ncfh.org/docs/fs-Facts%20about%20Farmworkers.pdf

National Coalition for the Homeless. (2009). Homeless families with children. Retrieved from http://www.nationalhomeless.org/factsheets/families.html

National Committee for Childhood Agricultural Injury Prevention. (1996). *Children and agriculture: Opportunities for safety and health*. Marshfield, WI: Marshfield Clinic.

National Institutes of Health (NIH). (2013, December). *Monitoring the future survey, overview of findings for 2013*. National Institute on Drug Abuse. Retrieved from http://www.drugabuse.gov/monitoring-future-survey-overview-findings-2013

National Rural Health Association (NRHA). (1996). *The rural homeless: America's lost population*. Kansas City, MO: Author.

North, C. S., Eyrich, K. M., Pollio, D. E., & Spitznagel, E. L. (2004). Are rates of psychiatric disorders in the homeless population changing? *American Journal of Public Health, 94*, 103–108.

North Carolina Rural Health Research and Policy Analysis Center. (1998). *Mapping rural health: The geography of health care and health resources in rural America*. Chapel Hill, NC: Author.

Nyamathi, A., Flaskerud, J., & Leake, B. (1997). HIV-risk behaviors and mental health characteristics among homeless or drug-recovering women and their closest sources of social support. *Nursing Research, 46*, 133–137.

Percy, M. S. (1995). Children from homeless families describe what is special in their lives. *Holistic Nursing Practice Journal, 9*(4), 24–33.

Phillips, S. (Announcer), Pauley, J. (Announcer), & Rudolph, L. (Reporter). (1997, August 19). *Dateline NBC*. New York, NY: National Broadcasting System. Transcript from Burrelle Publishing, Livingston, NJ.

Polednak, A. P. (1997). *Segregation, poverty, and mortality in urban African Americans*. New York, NY: Oxford University Press.

Poss, J. E., & Meeks, B. H. (1994). Meeting the health care needs of migrant farmworkers: The experience of the Niagara County Migrant Clinic. *Journal of Community Health Nursing, 11*(4), 219–228.

Pruitt, L. R. (2009). *The forgotten fifth: Rural youth and substance abuse*. Davis, CA: University of California Press. Retrieved from http://www.windham.k12.me.us/wsd_hs/Rural%20Youth%20and%20Substance%20Abuse.pdf

Rausch, T. K., Sanddal, N. D., Sanddal, T. L., & Esposito, T. J. (1998). Changing epidemiology of injury-related pediatric mortality in a rural state: Implications for injury control. *Pediatric Emergency Care, 14*(6), 388–392.

Ricketts, T. C., & Johnson-Webb, K. D. (1997). *What is "rural" and how to measure "rurality": A focus on health care delivery and health policy*. Chapel Hill, NC: Federal Office of Rural Health Policy, North Carolina Rural Health Research and Policy Analysis Center, Cecil G. Sheps Center for Health Services Research.

Rivilin, L. G. (1986). A new look at the homeless. *Social Policy, 16*(4), 3–10.

Rogers, C. C. (2002). Rural health issues for the older population. *Rural America, 17*(2), 30–35.

Rosenblum, A., Magura, S., Kayman, D., & Fong, C. (2005). Motivationally enhanced group counseling for substance users in a soup kitchen: A randomized clinical trial. *Drug & Alcohol Dependence, 80*(1), 91–103.

Rossi, P. H. (1989). *Down and out in America: The origin of homelessness*. Chicago, IL: University of Chicago Press.

Rust, G. S. (1990). Health status of migrant farmworkers: A literature review and commentary. *American Journal of Public Health, 80*(10), 1213–1217.

St. Lawrence, J. S., & Brasfield, T. L. (1995). HIV risk behavior among homeless adults. *AIDS Education and Prevention, 7*, 22–31.

Salazar, L., Crosby, R., Holtgrave, D., Head, S., Hadsock, B., Todd, J., & Shouse, R. L. (2007). Homelessness and HIV-associated risk behavior among African American men who inject drugs and reside in the urban south of the United States. *AIDS & Behavior, 11*, S70–77.

Salomonsen-Sautel, S., Van Leeuwen, J., Gilroy, C., Boyle, S., Malberg, D., & Hopfer, C. (2008). Correlates of substance use among homeless youths in eight cities. *American Journal on Addictions, 17*(3), 224–234.

Sandhaus, S. (1998). Migrant health: A harvest of poverty. *American Journal of Nursing, 98*(9), 52–54.

Schenker, M. B. (1996). Preventive medicine and health promotion are overdue in the agricultural workplace. *The Journal of Public Health Policy, 17*(3), 275–305.

Schulman, M. D., Evensen, C. T., Runyan, C. W., Cohen, L. R., & Dunn, K. A. (1997). Farm work is dangerous for teens: Agricultural hazards and injuries among North Carolina teens. *The Journal of Rural Health, 13*(4), 295–305.

Smith, L. S., & Gentry, D. (1987). Migrant farm workers' perceptions of support persons in a descriptive community survey. *Public Health Nursing, 4*(1), 21–28.

Smith, P. J., Singleton, J. A., & National Center for Immunization and Respiratory Diseases; Centers for Disease Control and Prevention (CDC). (2011). County-level trends in vaccination coverage among children aged 19–35 months—United States, 1995–2008. *MMWR Surveillance Summary, 60*(4), 1–86.

Snowden, L. R., & Yamada, A.-M. (2005). Cultural differences in access to care. *Annual Review of Clinical Psychology, 1*, 143–166.

Spencer, G. A., Atav, A. S., & Collins, M. S. (1997). *A comparison of health risk behaviors of rural, suburban and urban adolescents* [Unpublished manuscript]. Binghamton, NY.

Spencer, G. A., & Bryant, S. A. (2000). Dating violence: A comparison of rural, suburban, and urban teens. *Journal of Adolescent Health, 27*(4).

Spencer, G., & Bryant, S. (2000). Dating violence: A comparison of rural, suburban, and urban teens. *Journal of Adolescent Health, 27*(5), 302–305.

Stark, L. (1987). A century of alcohol and homelessness: Demographics and stereotypes. *Alcohol, Health and Research, 11*, 8–13.

Stein, L. M. L. (1993). Health care delivery to farmworkers in the southwest: An innovative nursing clinic. *Journal of the American Academy of Nurse Practitioners, 5*(3), 119–124.

Sumerlin, J. R., & Bundrick, C. M. (1997). Research on homeless men and women: Existential-humanistic and clinical thinking. *Psychological Reports, 80*, 1303–1314.

Susser, E., Struening, E., & Conover, S. (1987). Childhood experiences of homeless men. *American Journal of Psychiatry, 144*, 1599–1601.

Svenson, L. W., Varnhagen, C. K., Godin, A. M., & Salmon, T. L. (1992). Rural high school students' knowledge, attitudes, and behaviors related to sexually transmitted diseases. *Canadian Journal of Public Health, 83*(4), 260–263.

Symons, P. Y., Groer, M. W., Kepler-Youngblood, P., & Slater, V. (1993). Prevalence and predictors of adolescent dating violence. *Journal of Child and Psychiatric Nursing, 7*, 14–23.

Taylor, J. E., Charlton, D., & Yúnez-Naude, A. (2012). The end of farm labor abundance. *Applied Economic Perspectives and Policy, 34*(4), 587–598.

The America Project (TAP). (1995). *Because there is hope: Gearing up to renew urban America*. Atlanta, GA: Carter Collaboration Center.

Trattner, W. I. (1984). *From poor law to welfare state: A history of social welfare in America* (3rd ed.). New York, NY: Free Press.

United Nations. (2005). *United Nations Statistical Yearbook*. New York, NY: United Nations Publication.

U.S. Census Bureau. (2009). Poverty thresholds 2009. Retrieved from http://www.census.gov/hhes/www/poverty/data/threshld/thresh09.html

U.S. Census Bureau. (2010). 2010 Census Urban and Rural Classification and Urban Area Criteria. Retrieved from https://www.census.gov/geo/reference/ua/urban-rural-2010.html

U.S. Census Bureau. (2011a). *Population distribution and change: 2000 to 2010*. Retrieved from http://www.census.gov/prod/cen2010/briefs/c2010br-01.pdf

U.S. Census Bureau. (2011b). Areas with concentrated poverty: 2006–2010. American Community Survey. Retrieved from http://www.census.gov/prod/2011pubs/acsbr10-17.pdf

U.S. Census Bureau. (2012). The emergency and transitional shelter population: 2010. Retrieved from http://www.census.gov/prod/cen2010/reports/c2010sr-02.pdf

U.S. Conference of Mayors. (2006). *Hunger and homelessness survey: A status report on hunger and homelessness in America's cities*. Retrieved from http://www.usmayors.org/hungersurvey/2005/HH2005FINAL.pdf

U.S. Congress, House. (1987). *Stewart B. McKinney Homeless Assistance Act, conference report to accompany H.R. 558*. Washington, DC: 100th Congress, First Session.

U.S. Department of Agriculture (USDA). (1997). *Rural Conditions and Trends, 8*(2).

U.S. Department of Agriculture (USDA). (2004). *Rural development research report: Rural poverty at a glance* (Publication No. 100). Economic Research Service. Retrieved from http://www.ers.usda.gov/publications/rdrr-rural-development-research-report/rdrr100.aspx#.U8gLKBYxodI

U.S. Department of Agriculture (USDA). (2005). *Measuring rurality: 2004 county typology codes*. Economic Research Service. Retrieved from http://webarchives.cdlib.org/sw1tx36512/http://www.ers.usda.gov/briefing/rurality/typology/

U.S. Department of Agriculture (USDA). (2014). *Population and migration*. Retrieved from http://www.ers.usda.gov/topics/rural-economy-population/population-migration.aspx#.U8gOxxYxodI

U.S. Department of Agriculture (USDA). (2013). *Rural-Urban Continuum Codes, 2013*. Retrieved from http://www.ers.usda.gov/data-products/rural-urban-continuum-codes.aspx

U.S. Department of Agriculture (USDA). (2008). *What is rural?* Retrieved from http://www.nal.usda.gov/ric/ricpubs/what_is_rural.shtml

U.S. Department of Commerce. (2002). *2000 census of population: General population characteristics, United States*. Washington, DC: Department of Health and Human Services, U.S. Government Printing Office.

U.S. Department of Health and Human Services (HHS). (1990). *Atlas of state profiles*. Washington, DC: Author.

U.S. Department of Health and Human Services (HHS). (1991). *Healthy people 2000*. Washington, DC: Author.

U.S. Department of Health and Human Services (HHS). (2000). *Healthy people 2010: Conference edition*. Washington, DC: U.S. Government Printing Office.

U.S. Department of Health and Human Services (HHS). (2003). *Strengthening homeless families: An annotated resource guide for homeless shelters*. Washington, DC: U.S. Government Printing Office.

U.S. Department of Health and Human Services (DHHS). (2010). *Healthy People 2020: Conference edition*. Washington, DC: U.S. Government Printing Office.

U.S. Department of Housing and Urban Development. (2013). Homeless assistance. Retrieved from http://portal.hud.gov/hudportal/HUD?src=/program_offices/comm_planning/homeless

U.S. Department of Labor, Bureau of Labor Statistics. (2008). *Occupational outlook handbook, 2008–2009 edition: Agricultural workers*. Retrieved from http://www.bls.gov/opub/mlr/2008/06/cls0806.pdf

Uwemedimo, O. T., Findley, S. E., Andres, R., Irigoyen, M., & Stockwell, M. S. (2012). Determinants of influenza vaccination among young children in an inner-city community. *Journal of Community Health, 37*(3), 663–672.

Vijayaraghavan, M., Tochterman, A., Hsu, E., Johnson, K., Marcus, S., & Caton, C. L. (2012). Health, access to health care, and health care use among homeless women with a history of intimate partner violence. *Journal of Community Health, 37*(5), 1032–1039.

Wagenaar, A. C., Finnegan, J. R., Wolfson, M., Anstine, P. S., Williams, C. L., & Perry, C. L. (1993). Where and how adolescents obtain alcoholic beverages. *Public Health Reports, 108*(4), 459–464.

Wagner, J. D., Menke, E. M., & Ciccone, J. K. (1995). What is known about the health of rural homeless families? *Public Health Nursing, 12*(6), 400–408.

Waller, J. A. (1992). Injuries to farmers and farm families in a dairy state. *Journal of Occupational Medicine, 34*(3), 414–421.

Washington, T. A. (2002). The homeless need more than just a pillow, they need a pillar: An evaluation of a transitional housing program. *Families in Society, 83*, 183–188.

Watkins, E. L., Larson, K., Harlan, C., & Young, S. (1990). A model program for providing health services for migrant farmworker mothers and children. *Public Health Reports, 105*(6), 567–575.

Wehler, C., Weinreb, L. F., Huntington, N., Scot, R., Hosmer, D., Fletcher, K., ... Gundersen, C. (2004). Risk and protective factors for adult and child hunger among low-income housed and homeless female-headed families. *American Journal of Public Health, 94*, 109–115.

Weinert, C., & Long, K. (1994). Rural health and health seeking behaviors. *Annual Review of Nursing Research, 12*, 65–92.

Wenzel, S., Tucker, J., Elliott, M., & Hambarsoomians, K. (2007). Sexual risk among impoverished women: Understanding the role of housing status. *AIDS and Behavior, 11*(6 Suppl.), 9–20.

West, C. (1994). *Race matters*. New York, NY: Vintage.

Wheeler, C., Vugia, D. J., Thomas, G., Beach, M. J., Carnes, S., Maier, T., ... Werner, S. B. (2007). Outbreak of cryptosporidiosis at a California waterpark: Employee and patron roles and the long road towards prevention. *Epidemiology and Infection, 135*(2), 302–310.

Whitehead, R., Chillag, S., & Elliot, D. (1992). Anabolic steroid use among adolescents in a rural state. *Journal of Family Practice, 35*(4), 401–405.

Wood, D., & Valdez, R. B. (1991). Barriers to medical care for homeless families compared with housed poor families. *American Journal of Diseases of Children, 145*, 1109–1115.

World Health Organization Regional Office for Europe (WHO). (1998). *International healthy cities conference: Athens, 20–23 June 1998*. Retrieved from http://www.euro.who.int/__data/assets/pdf_file/0007/90664/E93730.pdf

Wright, J. D., & Weber, E. (1987). *Homelessness and health*. New York, NY: McGraw-Hill.

Yawn, B. P., & Yawn, R. A. (1993). Adolescent pregnancies in rural America: A review of the literature and strategies for primary prevention. *Community Health, 16*(1), 36–45.

Ziller, E., Coburn, A., Anderson, N., & Loux, S. (2008). Uninsured rural families. *The Journal of Rural Health, 24*(1), 1–11.

CHAPTER FOCUS

Sexual Behavior and Pregnancy Rates
- Teen Birth Rates: How Does the United States Compare?
- Teen Sexual Activity in the United States

Factors Contributing to Adolescent Pregnancy
- Developmental Stage
- Social and Environmental Factors

Impact of Adolescent Pregnancy
- Psychosocial and Health Outcomes of the Mother
- Impact on the Family
- Impact on the Adolescent Father
- Psychosocial and Health Outcomes of the Newborn

Role of the Nurse
- Primary Prevention
- Adolescent Pregnancy Prevention Community-Based Programs
- Program Evaluation
- Secondary and Tertiary Prevention

QUESTIONS TO CONSIDER

After reading this chapter, you will know the answers to the following questions:

1. Which factors contribute to adolescent pregnancy?
2. What are the health outcomes for adolescent mothers?
3. What is the effect of adolescent pregnancy on the family?
4. How are adolescent fathers affected by their partner's pregnancy?
5. What are the health outcomes for babies born to adolescent mothers?
6. What kinds of community-based prevention programs are available?
7. What are effective interventions to promote the role and involvement of the teen father?
8. What is the role of the community health nurse in primary, secondary, and tertiary prevention efforts for adolescent pregnancy?
9. What are policy implications of research findings for teen pregnancy prevention?
10. How can the community nurse who works with teens use research data in the prevention of teen pregnancy?

Parenting classes help teen mothers bond with their babies.

CHAPTER 26

Adolescent Pregnancy

Loretta Sweet Jemmott and
Karen Saucier Lundy

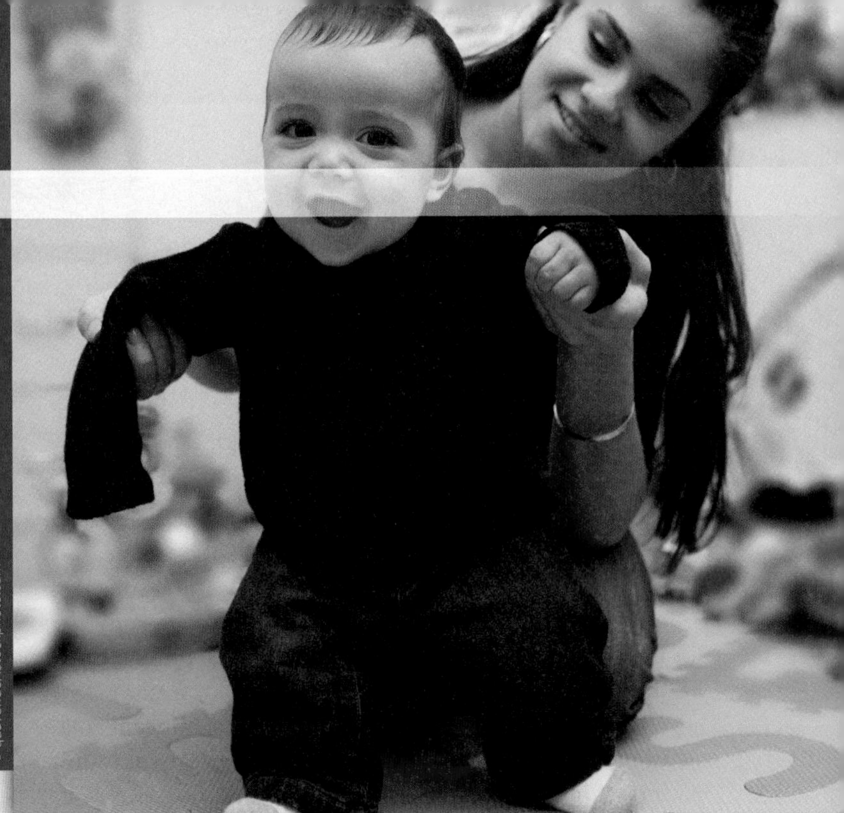

KEY TERMS

- abortion
- abstinence
- acculturation
- adolescent fathers
- adoption
- childhood victimization
- condoms
- contraception
- family dynamics
- gynecological age
- health outcomes
- low birth weight (LBW)
- prenatal care
- primary prevention
- repeat pregnancy
- secondary prevention
- tertiary prevention

> Ours is not the task of fixing the entire world all at once but of stretching out to mend the part of the world that is within our reach. Any small, calm thing that one soul can do to help another soul, to assist some portion of this poor suffering world, will help immensely. It is not given to us to know which acts, or by whom, will cause the critical mass to tip toward an enduring good.
>
> —Clarissa Pinkola Estes

REFLECTIONS

Adolescent pregnancy is a modern public health issue. Prior to the 20th century, females were married and bearing children in their early teens as a societal norm. In many parts of the world, this is still an accepted cultural pattern. Think about your own beliefs and feelings about teenage pregnancy. How do they affect your nursing care of this vulnerable population?

ADOLESCENT PREGNANCY AFFECTS individuals across all ethnic groups, socioeconomic classes, and geographic boundaries in the United States. Despite our investment of significant amounts of attention, time, research, and money on prevention efforts, the results remain discouraging, as adolescent pregnancy rates in the United States remain higher than those in all other industrialized countries.

Community health nurses can play a significant role in reducing the incidence of adolescent pregnancy and improving the quality of **health outcomes** of adolescent mothers, their children, and communities overburdened by this problem. By implementing creative interventions that address adolescents, families, and the community, community health nurses can play critical roles at all levels of prevention—primary, secondary, and tertiary alike.

In this chapter, adolescent pregnancy is examined by reviewing the contributing factors and key variables and considering the impact of pregnancy on the adolescent, family, schools, community, and society. The role of community health nurses at all levels of prevention is presented.

Sexual Behavior and Pregnancy Rates

More than 47% of high school students in the United States are sexually active (Centers for Disease Control and Prevention [CDC], 2012). The incidence of unplanned pregnancy and sexually transmitted diseases (STDs) statistically correlates to the early onset of sexual activity (Collins et al., 2004). Although there has been a decline in the teenage pregnancy rate since the 1990s, the United States continues to have the highest teen pregnancy rate in the industrialized world (Hoffman, 2006). One of every three teenage girls will become pregnant. More than 400,000 babies are born to teen mothers in the United States annually (CDC, 2012), and 80% of these teen mothers are unmarried (Hoffman, 2006).

The 2011 Youth Risk Behavior Survey (CDC, 2012) revealed that adolescent sexual activity was more prevalent among black adolescents (60%) than among white (44%) or Hispanic (49%) adolescents. The survey also revealed that 6.2% of high school students had their first sexual intercourse prior to age 13 and 15.3% had had sexual intercourse with more than four partners.

Teen Birth Rates: How Does the United States Compare?

The 1990s and 2000s have seen declines in the U.S. teen birth rate of nearly 40% (Kearney & Levine, 2012). Much of this has taken place recently; in 2004, the U.S. teen birth rate was 41.1 births per 1,000 teens aged 15–19; by 2012, that number had decreased to 29.4 per 1,000 teens (Martin, Hamilton, Osterman, Curtin, & Matthews, 2013). Even so, the United States still ranks fairly high in comparison to other industrialized nations: the U.S. teen birth rate is twice the teen birth rate in Canada (14.2), almost triple that of Germany (9.8) and France (10.2), and more than six times higher than Japan's (4.9) (Planned Parenthood Foundation [PPF], 2012). See **Figure 26-1**.

Teen Sexual Activity in the United States

The Youth Risk Behavior Survey (YRBS) was developed by the CDC in 1990 to monitor teen sexual behavior, tobacco and alcohol use, and other behaviors. The survey is conducted every 2 years and provides data on 9th- through 12th-grade students in public and private schools in the United States. The figure reflects the most recent data available (from 2011). At that time 47.4% of all high school students reported they had had sexual intercourse. The percentage of high school students who had had sex decreased by 13.1% between 1991 and 2011 (from 54% to 47.4%).

NOTE THIS!

- Three of four teens used a method of contraception during their first intercourse.
- Eleven percent of teen females and 5% of teen males report that their first sexual intercourse was unwanted.
- Teenage females are more than twice as likely to have experienced forcible sexual intercourse versus teen males (11.8% vs. 4.5%).
- Hispanic and African American females ages 15–19 have more than twice as many births per 1,000 (46.3 and 43.9, respectively) than non-Hispanic white teens (20.5).

Sources: Martinez, G., Copen, C. E., & Abma, J. C. (2011). Teenagers in the United States: Sexual activity, contraceptive use, and childbearing, 2006–2010 National Survey of Family Growth. *Vital and Health Statistics, 23*(31); U.S. Department of Health and Human Services. (2013a). Trends in teen pregnancy and childbearing: Teen births. Retrieved from http://www.hhs.gov/ash/oah/adolescent-health-topics/reproductive-health/teen-pregnancy/trends.html; CDC. (2012). Youth risk behavior surveillance—United States, 2011. *Morbidity and Mortality Weekly Report, 61*(SS–4). Retrieved from http://www.cdc.gov/mmwr/pdf/ss/ss6104.pdf

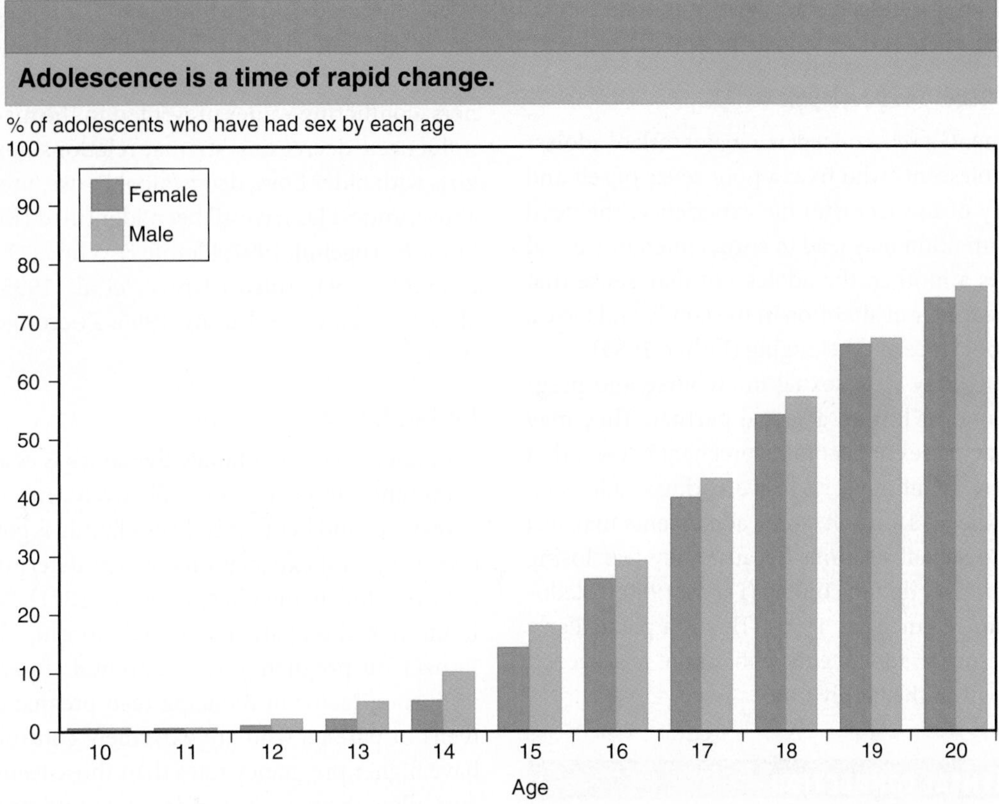

Figure 26-1 Teen sexual activity.

Source: Alan Guttmacher Institute. (20062013). Facts on American teens' sexual and reproductive health. Washington, DC: Author. Available online: http://www.guttmacher.org/pubs/fb_ATSRH.html

Factors Contributing to Adolescent Pregnancy

Many factors have been associated with adolescent pregnancy. Factors including earlier age of onset of puberty, earlier age of initiation of intercourse, nonuse or inconsistent use of contraceptives, lack of knowledge about sex and conception, developmental age, early risk-taking behaviors such as smoking and alcohol/drug use (CDC, 2012; Kaiser Family Foundation, 1998; Kandel, 1990; Ventura, Abma, Mosher, & Henshaw, 2006; Whitbeck, Conger, & Simons, 1993), and social/environmental status all contribute to an increased risk for teenage pregnancy. For the community health nurse to develop appropriate interventions to prevent adolescent pregnancy, it is essential to understand the contributing factors.

Developmental Stage

Adolescence is a time of uncertainty and experimentation, as young people strive to develop their identity in preparation for adulthood. For many young people, it is a time of sexual experimentation. This experimentation is in response to the adolescents' physical, hormonal, cognitive, and psychosocial development. Unfortunately, the consequences of such experimentation far too often include increased risk of pregnancy.

Psychosocial Development

Adolescent psychosocial development progresses through three stages: early, middle, and late adolescence. Early adolescence (ages 11 to 13) is characterized by turmoil stemming from physical changes and emotional fluctuation influenced by changing hormone levels (Drake, 1996). In this stage, adolescents are often seeking control, may show defiance to authority figures, and may use sex as an outlet for the expression of their perceived control (Drake, 1996; Flavell, Miller, & Miller, 1993). Middle adolescence (ages 14 to 16) is characterized by development of self-identity and sexual identity. In search of their identity, adolescents may imitate the behaviors they see around them from media, older peers, parents, and other adults (Foster, 1997; Males, 1993). Late adolescence (ages 17 to 20) is characterized by the adaptation of self-identity and development of coping strategies that will be used in adulthood (Drake, 1996). Adolescents who do not have a strong self-identity and sexual identity may not be able to assert themselves and apply coping strategies such as the sexual negotiation skills that are used with a sexual partner (Flavell et al.,

1993). As a result, adolescents may give in to sexual pressure from their peers and sexual partners.

Intrapersonal Issues and Development

The development of self-concept is a major task of adolescence. For adolescents who have a poor sense of self and have a history of unsuccessful life experience, the need for love and attention may lead to sexual intercourse and pregnancy. As a mother, the adolescent may sense that she will be the center of attention in the family and have a feeling of importance and belonging (Fisher, 1984).

Adolescents may view sexual intercourse and pregnancy as a bond or link to a sexual partner. They may believe that having sex or becoming pregnant is a way that they can ensure a continued, exclusive, caring relationship with that partner. As a result, some adolescents may feel pressured into sexual relations because they fear losing their partner if they do not comply (Davis, 1980; Toledo-Dreves, Zabin, & Emerson, 1995). This is a particularly important factor for adolescents who do not feel needed or cared for within the family unit.

ENVIRONMENTAL CONNECTION

Consider the following possible environmental threats affecting adolescent pregnant teens:

- Tanning booths
- Secondhand smoke
- Occupational hazards, such as in fast food restaurants
- Cosmetic and hair products
- Alcohol and substance abuse

How do these environmental hazards pose threats to this population?

In general, pregnancy as a strategy to compensate for unmet needs, to have self-esteem, or to assert independence is not particularly beneficial or successful. Parenting provides ample opportunity for failures, which are not helpful to adolescents already faced with repeated failures in their lives. An infant cannot meet all the nurturing expectations of the adolescent and has significant nurturing and attention needs of its own.

Social and Environmental Factors

Environment significantly influences adolescent ideas about sexual intercourse and pregnancy and their consequences. Each society has implied messages about sexuality, social behavior, and pregnancy. The clarity of the messages the community provides influences the sexual behaviors and expectations of its members (Foster, 1997). Several social and environmental factors have been identified as contributing to the high rates of adolescent pregnancy in the United States. Influences from family, culture, socioeconomic status, peers, sexual partners, conflicting values presented in the media, feminist influences, decreasing stigma, relationships of younger girls with older boys, drugs/alcohol use, previous sexual abuse, and STDs have all been identified (Kenney, Reinholtz, & Angelini, 1997; Plouffe & White, 1996; Robinson & Frank, 1994; Toledo-Dreves et al., 1995; Ventura et al., 2006; Widom & Kuhns, 1996; Zoccolillo, Meyers, & Assiter, 1997).

The Family of the Adolescent

An understanding of **family dynamics** is essential for the community nurse to work effectively with the pregnant adolescent and her family. Every family is governed by its own rules and expectations, which determine expected behavior for its members (Bowen, 1971). Miller (2002) found that close parent–child relationships have a direct impact on pregnancy risk. Parental supervision is an important factor in reducing teen pregnancy. However, teens of parents who are extremely controlling tend to have higher pregnancy rates than those teens whose parents allow them a sense of freedom and privacy (Miller, 2002). Miller (2002) stresses the importance of supportive parental relationships and appropriate monitoring of teens' activities.

Problems occur when there is poor communication and conflicting messages about sex and pregnancy (DiIorio, Hockenbeery-Eaton, Maibach, Rivero, & Miller, 1996). Adolescents may hear mixed messages from the family, which often come from the family's own discomfort and embarrassment about sex and pregnancy. As a result, adolescents may perceive affirming attitudes about adolescent sexuality.

The Ethnicity/Culture of the Adolescent

Differences in culture may affect the family and peer reactions to adolescent pregnancy, which in turn influence an adolescent's perception of pregnancy. Many factors contribute to cultural identity, and it is not suggested that all members of a particular cultural group will behave in an identical fashion; however, the community nurse must be aware of and sensitive to cultural influences on adolescent pregnancy.

Mainstream American culture has a negative view toward adolescent pregnancy, yet the rates of adolescent pregnancy remain higher in the United States than in other industrialized nations (Desmond, 1994; Trad, 1999). Hoffman (2006) and Jemmott and Jemmott (2007) gave the same information (U.S. pregnancy rates are highest among the world's industrialized nations).

The existence of many subcultures and various culturally based beliefs may contribute to the higher rates of adolescent pregnancy. For example, in traditional, patriarchal Latino culture, females are expected to respond to male demands, and marriage and motherhood/fatherhood are viewed as catalysts to adulthood (Orshan, 1996). As a result, Latino adolescents may have a positive attitude toward pregnancy that, according to one study (Lau, Lin & Flores, 2014), may be as much as three times more likely than in white adolescents and 50% higher than in African American adolescents (see Research Alert). However, the extent to which these common culturally based beliefs affect attitudes toward pregnancy may depend on the adolescent's level of acculturation. **Acculturation** is a dynamic, multidimensional phenomenon in which the ideals and beliefs of one culture are incorporated into that of another (Orshan, 1996; Reynoso, Felice, & Shragg, 1993). Acculturated American Latino adolescents from traditional Latino families may receive contradictory sexual messages from mainstream American society and the more traditional messages of their Latino culture.

ETHICAL CONNECTION

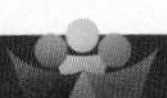

A 15-year-old female presents at the school nurse office with a request for a pregnancy test. She tells you that she has been involved with a 35-year-old male friend of her parents and fears that she is pregnant. Her pregnancy test is positive. As the school nurse, what are specific state legal and ethical considerations that you need to know in order to provide appropriate nursing care for this patient? What would you do initially to counsel this patient? What are the ethical implications of this scenario?

GLOBAL CONNECTION

How is teen pregnancy viewed in third world and developing countries around the world? As a travel nurse, would your nursing care be different in cultures where early pregnancy is valued and promoted by these global communities?

RESEARCH ALERT

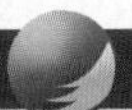

This research study used data from the National Survey of Family Growth (2002 and 2006–2008 cycles) to identify sociodemographic correlations with positive pregnancy attitude among sexually active U.S. teen females. Bivariate and multivariable analyses were performed to assess for associations of contraceptive history, sexual education and behavior history, medical services history, and family and sexual attitudes with a positive pregnancy attitude. Among the 975 adolescent females surveyed, 15% reported a positive pregnancy attitude; these females were significantly ($p < 0.05$) more likely to have public insurance (43% vs. 20%), to be poor (33% vs. 10%), to have reached menarche at an earlier age (12 years old vs. 13 years old), and to ever have had HIV testing (35% vs. 23%) compared with those reporting a negative pregnancy attitude. Teens who reported an older age of menarche and/or higher family income had reduced likelihood of a positive attitude toward pregnancy. Teens with a negative perception of pregnancy were significantly more likely to have ever been forced to have sex (10%) than teens with a positive pregnancy attitude (1%). Multivariable analyses found that race/ethnicity strongly affected the likelihood of positive perceptions of pregnancy: Latina teens had three times more likelihood of positive outlook toward pregnancy, and African American adolescents had double the odds of a positive pregnancy attitude compared with adolescent females of other races.

Source: Lau, M., Lin, H., & Flores, G. (2014). Pleased to be pregnant? Positive pregnancy attitudes among sexually active adolescent females in the United States. *Journal of Pediatric and Adolescent Gynecology*, 27(4), 210–215.

> Just saying 'No' prevents teenage pregnancy the way 'Have a nice day' cures chronic depression.
>
> —*Faye Wattleton, past president of Planned Parenthood*

To the adolescent who is developing an identity, these conflicting views may lead to inconsistent feelings about sexual activity and contraceptive use and subsequent risk-taking sexual behavior. For example, positive or ambivalent perception of pregnancy has been shown to correlate with less consistent condom use in sexually active adolescent and young adult females (Miller, Trent, & Chung, 2014).

Similarly, African American adolescents who grow up in single-parent families may receive mixed messages about adolescent pregnancy. These adolescents may see a pattern of intergenerational out-of-wedlock teen pregnancies but hear disapproving messages about adolescent pregnancy from parents, media, and school (CDC, 2006; Desmond, 1994; Jemmott, Jemmott, & O'Leary, 2007). Compounding the issue, there may be poor communication between the adolescent and parent about sexual issues.

Cultural influences are not limited to adolescents in minority cultures. Caucasian adolescents may also be influenced by cultural issues. In some European American cultures, discussion about sex and pregnancy is taboo. Adolescents who live in these environments may look to their peers and the media for rules of acceptable sexual conduct. Uneducated peers may provide misinformation. The media often depict sex as being disconnected from sexual responsibility, such as contraception and STD protection, with romanticized and idealized images of sexual behavior (Ventura et al., 2006).

Socioeconomic Factors

Teens whose parents talked openly with them about sex were more likely to delay becoming sexually active. When these teenagers did become sexually active, they were more likely to practice protected sex. Several components of the parent–child relationship appeared to affect teen sexual behavior: family closeness, parental monitoring and supervision, and parent–child communication (Blake, Simkin, Ledsky, Perkins, & Calabresa, 2001). Family levels of education, income, and social standing in the community also appear to influence teen sexual behavior (Kirby, 2001). Miller (2002) proposed that single and divorced parents' more permissive sexual conduct increased the adolescents' probability of becoming sexually active at a younger age. Miller (2002) also cited an earlier onset of sexual activity and unprotected sex in neighborhoods with higher crime rates. Girls who have lived in foster care are more likely to become teen mothers. Children of mothers who had first intercourse at an early age are more likely to also be sexually active at an early age (Miller, 2002).

The Adolescent's Peers

One of the single most influential factors in adolescent sexual activity and pregnancy is the influence of peers (Coyle et al., 1996). Formation of peer groups and an increased need for peer acceptance are normal developmental milestones of adolescence. However, this increased need for acceptance may cause adolescents to give in to the requests of their peers or imitate the actions of their peers, which may include sexual experimentation and risky sexual behavior. Moreover, sexual information is often exchanged by adolescent peers and may lead to misconceptions and result in unintended pregnancy. The ready availability of technology, particularly cell phones, tablets, and computers, complicates peer sexual interactions by introducing text and video components of sexual behavior; use of technology by teens to exchange intimate photos and videos as well as "sexting" is associated with higher rates of sexual activity.

The attitudes, or perceived attitudes, of teens' peers regarding sexual activity greatly influence the teens' own concepts. This tendency to follow a pattern of behavior similar to that of peers relates to the decision to become sexually active and also to the use of condoms among those teens who choose to become sexually active (Kirby, 2001).

The Adolescent's Sexual Partner

It is important to understand the male partner of female adolescents because female adolescent sexual activity often is submissive to male sexual desire (Blythe & Diaz, 2007; Heavey, Moysich, Hyland, Druschel, & Sill, 2008; Jemmott & Jemmott, 1990). In addition, the typical contraceptive methods on which adolescents rely before seeking prescription contraceptives are male methods, such as condoms, oral sex, status, and coitus interruptus (Blythe & Diaz, 2007; Morrison, 1985).

Male attitudes toward contraceptive use, especially **condoms**, have been described as negative (Jemmott & Jemmott, 1990, 1992; Jemmott, Jemmott, & Fong, 1998; Morrison, 1985; Sorensen, 1973). For instance, many males view condom use unfavorably because they believe it reduces the pleasure or spontaneity of sexual activities. Adolescent males commonly believe that **contraception** is a female's responsibility (Blythe & Diaz, 2007; Jemmott & Jemmott, 1990). Even so, use of contraceptives is increasing; between 2006 and 2010, 86% of female teens and 93% of male teens reported using contraceptives of some kind during their most recent sexual encounter (Martinez et al., 2011). Since 1990, the birth rate has declined nearly 42%, in large part due to improved contraceptive use among teens (Santelli, Lindberg, Finer, & Singh, 2007).

Little attention has been paid to the age of sexual partners of adolescents. It has been reported that the majority of male sexual partners of adolescent females are approximately 5 years older (average age 20 to 24) (Alan Guttmacher Institute [AGI], 2013; Jemmott et al., 2007; Lemay, Cashman, Elfenbein, & Felice, 2007), with only 30% of adolescent pregnancies resulting from **adolescent fathers**. Adolescent females may view their relationships with older partners as providing an escape from poverty, a show of defiance, a display of sexuality, and a boost to self-esteem. However, adolescent females with an incomplete perception of self may not feel able to negotiate and assert sexual boundaries, such as condom use with their older partners, and may submit to the older partner's sexual demands. Consequently, many adult–adolescent relationships result in an adolescent pregnancy (Kalmus, Davidson, Cahall, Laraque, & Cassell, 2003; Toledo-Dreves et al., 1995).

THINK ABOUT THIS

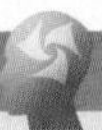

Social costs related to teen pregnancy are far reaching:

- Teen mothers are more likely to drop out of school; only half of teen fathers who have children before age 18 finish high school or get a GED.
- Teen mothers are more likely to remain unmarried and live in poverty.
- Of the approximately 10 million adolescent males aged 12–16 in 1996, 10% became fathers before age 20.
- Babies born to teen mothers are more likely to have a low birth weight.
- Babies born to teen mothers are more likely to experience abuse and neglect.
- Babies born to teen mothers are more likely to enter the welfare system.
- Daughters of teen mothers are more likely to become teen mothers, and sons of teen fathers are more likely to become teen fathers.
- Daughters of absent fathers are more likely to engage in early sexual intercourse and have increased risk of adolescent pregnancy.
- Taxpayers saved $8.4 billion in 2008 due to the approximately 42% decline in the teen birth rate between 1991 and 2008.

Sources: AGI (2013). Fact sheet: Facts on American teens' sexual and reproductive health. Retrieved from http://www.guttmacher.org/pubs/FB-ATSRH.html; Ellis, B. J., Bates, J. E., Dodge, K. A., Fergusson, D. M., Horwood, L. J., Pettit, G. S., & Woodward, L. (2009). Does father absence place daughters at special risk for early sexual activity and teenage pregnancy? *Child Development, 74*(3), 801–821; Hoffman, S. D. (2006). *By the numbers: The public costs of teen childbearing*. Washington, DC: National Campaign to Prevent Teen Pregnancy.

RESEARCH ALERT

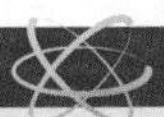

Almost half of high school–aged teens in the United States have had sexual intercourse. Researchers have examined the time and place that teens are more likely to first have sex.

Where Do Teens Have Sex for the First Time?

Two-thirds (68%) of 16- to 18-year-olds reported in 2000 that they first had sexual intercourse in their family home, their partner's family home, or a friend's house. More than one in five (22%) reported that their first sexual encounter occurred in their family homes. Only 4% reported having sex for the first time in a vehicle and 3% in a hotel, park, or outdoors.

When Do Teens Have Sex for the First Time?

More than two-thirds (70%) of teens report having their first sexual experience in the evening or night (3 p.m. to 7 a.m.). The time breaks down as follows for timing of first intercourse:

- 42% during the hours between 10 p.m. and 7 a.m.
- 28% during the hours between 6 p.m. and 10 p.m.
- 15% during the hours between 3 p.m. and 6 p.m.
- 14% before 3 p.m.

Research indicated that there is no significant difference between the time of year or month when teens have sex for the first time. Teens appear to have the first sexual encounter as often during the school year as during summer vacation.

Source: Cohen, D. A., Farley, T. A., Taylor, S. N., Martin, D. H., & Schuster, M. A. (2002). When and where do youths have sex? The potential role of adult supervision. *Pediatrics, 110*(6), 110–116.

MEDIA MOMENT

Listen to these popular songs about unplanned pregnancy. What messages do they send to adolescent females?

- "Papa Don't Preach" —Madonna
- "Baby Mama" —Fantasia Barrino
- "There Goes My Life" —Kenny Chesney
- "Brenda's Got a Baby" —Tupac
- "With Arms Wide Open" —Creed
- "I Ain't Goin' Down" —Shania Twain
- "Backseat of a Greyhound Bus" —Sara Evans
- "Red Rag Top" —Tim McGraw

Adolescent males have similar risk factors for pregnancy as their female peers. Often, adolescent males struggle with development and may attempt to demonstrate independence, belong to peer groups, and demonstrate physical and sexual maturity by engaging in sexual activity. As adolescents, males may also lack future-oriented thinking and concrete thinking abilities. Together, these factors contribute to increased potential for participating in risky sexual behaviors that may lead to pregnancy. Adolescent males may also view pregnancy as a catalyst toward manhood and may purposely have unprotected intercourse. In the African American community, the risk for an adolescent-fathered, teenage pregnancy may be higher. The mean age for sexual initiation among African American males has been estimated to be as low as 11.1 years

(Blythe & Diaz, 2007; Jemmott, 1993; Jemmott & Jemmott, 1990; Terry-Humen & Manlove, 2003).

Substance Use Among Adolescents

Several studies have found that the use of alcohol or drugs during sexual activity is associated with risky sexual behavior, such as intercourse with multiple partners and failure to use condoms (Cavazos-Rehg et al., 2010a; Jemmott & Jemmott, 2007). Alcohol and drug use may change the nature of the sexual behavior in which people engage because logic and good judgment are clouded and inhibitions are loosened when people are "high" or because intoxication provides an excuse to engage in risky behavior (Crowe & George, 1989; Fortenberry, Orr, Katz, Brizendine, & Blythe, 1997; Jemmott & Jemmott, 2007; Kokotailo, Langhough, Cox, Davidson, & Fleming, 1994). However, there is a second, simpler explanation of the relationship between alcohol and drug use and risky sexual behavior. Adolescents who use alcohol and drugs more frequently than their peers may also engage in more sexual activity than their peers; consequently, they may engage in more risky sexual activity compared with their peers. A 2010 study confirmed that those at highest risk, substance-using adolescents with multiple partners, were least likely to use any form of contraception (Cavazos-Rehg et al., 2010b). An even more troubling aspect of this association is that teens' behavior often doesn't change when they encounter consequences such as pregnancy; one study noted that not only were teen girls engaged in substance use at higher risk of pregnancy, they were at an even greater risk of having multiple pregnancies during adolescence (Cavazos-Rehg et al., 2010a).

Sexual and Physical Abuse of Adolescent Females

Childhood victimization may be linked to promiscuity and adolescent pregnancy. Adolescent females who were physically and/or sexually abused may be more likely to initiate sexual intercourse at a younger age, use drugs and alcohol, and engage in more promiscuous relationships than nonabused adolescents (CDC, 2012; Kenney et al., 1997). Childhood abuse has been associated with low socioeconomic status, unemployment, family dysfunction, substance use, and psychological dysfunction. Because many of the risk factors for childhood abuse are interrelated and linked to adolescent pregnancy, it is difficult to separate the effect of each factor in a child's environment that may influence behavior (Fiscella, Kitzman, Cole, Sidora, & Olds, 1998).

Adolescents who have experienced physical or sexual abuse may use sex in an effort to attain loving nonabusive relationships or may view pregnancy as a way out of the abusive environment at home (Widom & Kuhns, 1996). However, the adolescent who has not fully developed emotionally may not be in the position to be assertive and use sexual negotiation skills, leaving him or her at greater risk for experiencing further sexual exploitation by present and future partners.

Knowledge Deficit Regarding Sex, Conception, and Contraception

The increased sexual activity among adolescents has not been accompanied by increased knowledge about sexual function, procreation, or birth control. Studies indicate that many adolescents remain woefully ignorant about conception and the menstrual cycle (Blythe & Diaz, 2007; Darabi, Jones, Varga, & Hourse, 1982; Davis & Harris, 1982; Jemmott & Jemmott, 1990; Jemmott et al., 2007; Landry, Bertrand, Cherry, & Rich, 1986; Villarruel, Jemmott, Jemmott, & Ronis, 2007). In addition to lack of information on sex and conception, adolescents lack correct information on birth control methods and the correct use of contraceptives (Collins et al., 2004; Morrison, 1985; Pollack, 1992; Ventura et al., 2006). A 2008 study by the nonpartisan research center Child Trends also found that about 20% of males had their first sexual intercourse before having any form of sex education, and that these males were significantly (50%) less likely to use a condom (Manlove, Ikramullah, & Terry-Humen, 2008).

Even though contraceptive information has become more available, many adolescents do not use birth control on a regular basis (**Box 26-1**). Adolescents generally engage in sexual intercourse for some time before obtaining reliable contraception. Reluctance to obtain and use contraception is associated with certain attitudes and psychological and social factors. Stevens-Simon, Kelly, Singer, and Cox (1996) reported that adolescents' attitudes include "I don't mind getting pregnant" or "I want to get pregnant." Adolescents who feel this way may neglect to use contraception or be inconsistent users of contraception.

Impact of Adolescent Pregnancy

Adolescent pregnancy has significant, far-reaching consequences. Pregnancy can affect the adolescent's health, development, education, socioeconomic status, and, ultimately, future. The family and community may also feel the effects because the majority of adolescents are unwed, live with their families, and depend on public assistance (Coley & Chase-Lansdale, 1998). In addition to psychosocial and economical outcomes, the adolescent mother experiences physical consequences that may affect her health.

Psychosocial and Health Outcomes of the Mother

Pregnancy is a time of increased demands on a woman's body. These demands can be harmful to a developing

BOX 26-1 Why Adolescents Don't Use Contraception

- I didn't mind getting pregnant.
- I wanted to get pregnant.
- I didn't know how to get birth control.
- I didn't think that I could get pregnant.
- I wanted to have a baby so my boyfriend would love me.
- I was afraid my family would find out.
- I was afraid of the side effects.
- I didn't want to appear to my partner to be prepared to have sex.
- I wasn't planning to have sex.
- I thought my boyfriend was sterile.
- I didn't know how to use birth control.
- I thought my partner would be angry with me if I used birth control.
- I wanted a baby to love.
- I thought other people would find out that I was using birth control.
- It's hard to talk to my partner about birth control.
- My boyfriend wanted me to get pregnant.
- My partner didn't want to use birth control.
- Using a condom interferes with sexual pleasure.
- I was embarrassed about using birth control.
- I just did not get around to it.
- Birth control can be expensive.
- Getting birth control is inconvenient.

Sources: Adapted from AGI, 1981; Howard & McCabe, 1992; Jemmott & Jemmott, 1990, 1992; Jemmott, Jemmott, & Fong, 1998; Loda, Speizer, Martin, Skatrud, & Bennett, 1997; Zelnik & Kantner, 1979.

adolescent, especially if there is no focus on the increased needs of pregnancy such as nutrition and rest. In general, adolescents experience greater health problems with pregnancy than do women older than 20 years of age. The consequences are especially severe to the youngest adolescents, those 12 to 15 years of age (Chedraui, 2008; Hoffman, 2006; Levy, Perhats, Nash-Johnson, & Welter, 1992; Trad, 1999).

Adolescents are at greater risk for developing pregnancy-induced hypertension and toxemia (AGI, 1981), anemia, nutritional deficiencies, and urinary tract infections (Bulcholz & Gol, 1986; Chedraui, 2008; Wilson, Alio, Kirby, & Salihu, 2008; Zeck, Walcher, Tamussino, & Lang, 2008). Adolescent girls are more likely to deliver prematurely, experience rapid or prolonged labor, develop abruptio placentae, or have fetal or maternal infections (Mott, 1990; Zeck, Bjelic-Radisic, Haas, & Greimel, 2007).

NOTE THIS!

One of every five pregnant adolescents is physically and/or sexually abused (hitting; unwanted touching, sexual advances, and intercourse) by a family member or partner during her pregnancy. Nurses need to assess adolescents, their partners, and their families for signs of abuse.

Lack of Prenatal Care

One of the major reasons for negative health outcomes for mothers and infants is lack of **prenatal care**. More pregnant adolescents delay seeking prenatal care, access less prenatal care, or do not receive regular care as often as adult women (Cockey, 1997; Geronimus, 1986; Hoffman, 2006). The same teenagers at greatest risk for pregnancy—those from poor families—are also at greatest risk for poor prenatal care. This lack of care contributes to poorer health outcomes for both mother and infant. Most adolescents do not receive prenatal care in the first trimester, with nearly 20% accessing care in the last trimester only. In general, this group tends to be more illness-oriented than prevention-oriented in their health practices. The reasons for this delayed initiation of prenatal care are varied and include denial of the pregnancy, lack of knowledge, lack of access to health care, concern about concealing the pregnancy, developmental immaturity (Cockey, 1997; Hoffman, 2006; Zuckerman, Walker, Frank, Chase, & Hamburg, 1984), and an orientation toward concrete, present-centered reasoning (Geronimus, 1986).

Repeated Pregnancy

Several studies have shown that many young mothers have more than one child during their teen years. Obtaining exact numbers is difficult because U.S. Census data do not report **repeat pregnancy** rates, but estimates range from 15% to 60%, depending on the study (Brown, Saunders, & Dick, 1999; Cavazos-Rehg et al., 2010a; CDC, 2012; Cockey, 1997; Hoffman, 2006).

Adolescent mothers who have repeat pregnancies continue to be at higher risk for poor outcomes. Although it might be reasonably assumed that adolescent mothers would be savvier in a second pregnancy, seeking and receiving more timely prenatal care, this is often not the case. One study examined the outcomes of first and second adolescent pregnancies among Caucasian and African American teenagers. The results revealed that a poor outcome in the first pregnancy was associated with a three times greater risk of repeating that outcome in the second pregnancy. The recurrence rate of preterm delivery was especially severe for African American adolescents (Blankson et al., 1993; SmithBattle, 2007; Tocce, Sheeder, & Teal, 2008; Wilson et al., 2008). These results are critical because they provide a specific target for the **secondary prevention** efforts of nurses working in the community.

NOTE THIS!

- One in eight adolescents ages 15–19 years in the United States becomes pregnant each year.
- One-half of all initial adolescent premarital pregnancies occur within the first 6 months after initiation of coitus; 20% occur in the first month alone.
- Media images of adolescent pregnancy often show minority adolescent teens, but adolescent pregnancy is not only a minority issue. Caucasian teenagers consistently account for the largest percentage of adolescent pregnancies and births (AGI, 1994, 2013; Pittman & Adams, 1988).
- Approximately one in seven Caucasian adolescents, one in four African American adolescents, and one in four Latino adolescents are mothers by age 19.

Psychosocial Outcomes

Although pregnancy can become a stimulus for positive growth in an adolescent, generally the results are more negative than positive. Motherhood or fatherhood in the adolescent years can cause severe disruption in the normal psychosocial development of adolescents. Pregnancy places an additional psychosocial burden on teenagers, who are already attempting to cope with the normal maturational crisis of adolescence (Bulcholz & Gol, 1986; Trad, 1999).

Adolescents typically cope with the confusion and conflict in their lives by finding safety and acceptance in their peer groups. However, adolescent parents, especially mothers, may find themselves isolated from their peer groups at a critical time in their development. The degree of isolation may vary depending on the norms accepted by different cultural peer groups.

A primary goal of adolescence is attainment of independence. Although pregnancy may enhance independence in some ways by forcing the adolescent to take charge of a difficult situation, this forced rapid ascension into adulthood certainly is not without negative consequences. After delivery, as adolescent parents cope with the demands of a new infant, their own needs and desires are no longer first priority. The increased stress of being an adolescent parent can lead to more self-doubt, uncertainty, loneliness, and helplessness. The adolescent's inability to effectively cope with these feelings is reflected in the increased incidence of child abuse and neglect within this cohort (Ispa, Sable, Porter, & Csizmadia, 2007; Lieberman, 1980; Marshall, Buckner, & Powell, 1991).

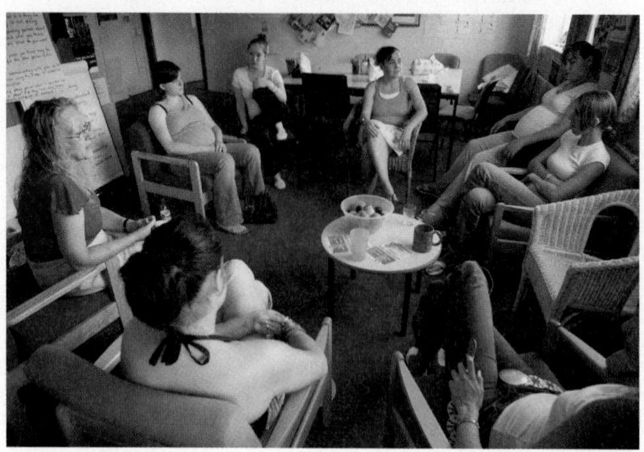

Adolescent parents typically need more structured education focusing on newborn care, parenting skills, and fostering developmentally appropriate interactions.

DAY IN THE LIFE

A Teen Mother

This teenage mom was 17 when she had her first child. She married the father of the child, finished high school, and is pursuing a college education.

On learning I was pregnant, I was really sad. My world was coming to an end. Many changes took place. My boyfriend and I both wanted to finish high school. So we were married and moved in with my in-laws.

After the baby was born, we graduated and soon moved into a trailer. I was overwhelmed with the responsibility. I lost so much sleep I thought I would never feel rested again!

We made the choice to stay married and I chose to go on to college against all odds. Now that college graduation is only a little over a year away, and I've grown up a lot, my future has hope! It has taken us more than 3 years, but I can truthfully say the last 4 months have been happy for us as a family.

Two major factors that have helped me keep from giving up on education and my marriage were the support of my mother and the teen-mom support group leader who became a real friend to me. They gave me something to hang on to and hope for when the winds of strife seemed capable of blowing me over.

After almost 4 years, we are beginning to see ourselves as a family mostly because of two concepts learned in the support group. The first was that I realized decisions in life were mine to make. I was responsible for my life. The second concept was learning how to effectively communicate love to my husband and son. He and I are the two people in the world that will love our son more than anyone else. We are partners in our responsibility for his nurturance, guidance, and support. How different my life might have been if I had not involved myself with this community service.

Source: Contributed by Arlene McFarland, DNSc, RN, from her weekly column, "Family Matters" in the Fort Payne (Alabama) *Times Journal*, May 5, 1998. Reprinted with permission.

MEDIA MOMENT

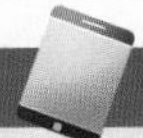

Movies About Adolescent and Unplanned Pregnancy

Juno (2007)
Knocked Up (2007)
Junebug (2005)
For Keeps (1988)
Saved (2004)
Riding in Cars with Boys (2001)

Education and Economic Disruption

Adolescents who become pregnant are less likely than their non-pregnant peers to complete their education. For example, whereas 90% of women who delay childbearing beyond adolescence complete a high school education, only 70% of adolescent mothers ultimately reach this goal. Without a complete education, many adolescent mothers find employment opportunities out of their reach and rely on low-paying jobs or public assistance programs (AGI, 1994; CDC, 2012; Grogger & Bronars, 1993; Rolleri, Wilson, Paluzzi, & Sedivy, 2008).

Impact on the Family

An unplanned adolescent pregnancy can seriously jeopardize quality of life not only for the young mother and infant but also for their extended families. Families are often called on to shoulder considerable economic and emotional burdens. The strain on the family is often intensified because adolescent mothers are more likely to live in single-parent households. The long-term impact on the family is unknown, but as families compensate to deal with adolescent pregnancy, they may normalize the experience and set the stage for future adolescent pregnancy. From generation to generation, this trend may develop into a cycle. The children of adolescent parents are at increased risk of perpetuating the cycle by becoming adolescent parents themselves and dropping out of school.

Impact on the Adolescent Father

For every adolescent conception that occurs outside marriage, there is a father as well as a pregnant mother, yet there is limited research focusing on adolescent males who become fathers. The impact of adolescent pregnancy has been largely focused on adolescent females despite the obvious involvement of males. Even though adolescent males are the fathers in only 30% of adolescent pregnancies, it is important for the community health nurse to address the problem of teenage pregnancy with this group. Adolescent fathers may be more at risk for continued educational and social problems (Fletcher & Wolfe, 2011). Fagot, Pears, Capaldi, Crosby, and Leve (1998) found that adolescent fathers had more arrests and substance use problems than did nonfathers of the same age. The adolescent father's reaction to the pregnancy, his own psychosocial developmental issues and needs, and his behavior as a young father are critical to developing positive health outcomes for the child and impacting the behaviors of these young men before adulthood.

The adolescent father's reaction to the pregnancy is a crucial factor in determining what role he will play in the pregnancy and delivery and in the child's life. Some adolescent males react positively, but others do not. Reactions to pregnancy are influenced by many factors, including family reaction, peer group reaction, and relationship with the mother of the child. Another factor that may influence the reaction is the developmental stage of the father, because many may not be able to cope effectively with a pregnancy. Problems that affect the adolescent male revolve around the acknowledgment of the child, his financial responsibility, his school commitment, and his work situation (Albert, 2004; Lowe, 2008; Males, 1993). Adolescent fathers report feeling frightened and disturbed by the responsibilities and neglected in the decision-making process, although few abandon the mother during pregnancy. Unfortunately, the young father may abandon the adolescent mother after pregnancy.

Regardless of the good intentions of most men, the fate of most adolescent fathers is similar to that of teenage mothers. Most are ill prepared to assume the role of fatherhood, and few relish the opportunity. Generally, having come from poor, relatively uneducated backgrounds, they experience serious social and economic disadvantages compared with young men who postpone fatherhood until a later age (Ispa et al., 2007; Lowe, 2008; Sonenstein, Stewart, Lindberg, Pernas, & Williams, 1997). Most of the fathers lack the necessary skills to provide a stable home environment for their families even if they want to. In short, poverty is the tie that binds most adolescent fathers and mothers. Although some manage to cope with their situation, continue educational and vocational pursuits, and mature into self-sufficient, productive members of society, the odds are stacked against them.

HEALTHY PEOPLE 2020 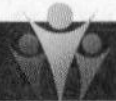

Selected Adolescent Pregnancy Primary Prevention Goals

- FP-8 Reduce pregnancies among adolescent females
  - FP-8.1 Reduce pregnancies among adolescent females age 15 to 17 years
  - FP-8.2 Reduce pregnancies among adolescent females age 18 to 19 years
- FP-9 Increase the proportion of adolescents age 17 years and under who have never had sexual intercourse
  - FP-9.1 Increase the proportion of female adolescents age 15 to 17 years who have never had sexual intercourse
  - FP-9.2 Increase the proportion of male adolescents age 15 to 17 years who have never had sexual intercourse
  - FP-9.3 Increase the proportion of female adolescents age 15 years and under who had never had sexual intercourse
  - FP-9.4 Increase the proportion of male adolescents age 15 years and under who had never had sexual intercourse
- FP-10 Increase the proportion of sexually active persons age 15 to 19 years who use condoms to effectively prevent pregnancy and to provide barrier protection against disease
  - FP-10.1 Increase the proportion of sexually active females age 15 to 19 years who use a condom at first intercourse
  - FP-10.2 Increase the proportion of sexually active males age 15 to 19 years who use a condom at first intercourse
  - FP-10.3 Increase the proportion of sexually active females age 15 to 19 years who use a condom at last intercourse
  - FP-10.4 Increase the proportion of sexually active males age 15 to 19 years who use a condom at last intercourse
- FP-11 Increase the proportion of sexually active persons age 15 to 19 years who use condoms and hormonal or intrauterine contraception to effectively prevent pregnancy and to provide barrier protection against disease
- FP-12 Increase the proportion of adolescents who received formal instruction on reproductive health topics before they were 18 years old
  - FP-12.1 Increase the proportion of female adolescents who received formal instruction on abstinence before they were 18 years old
  - FP-12.2 Increase the proportion of male adolescents who received formal instruction on abstinence before they were 18 years old
  - FP-12.3 Increase the proportion of female adolescents who received formal instruction on birth control methods before they were 18 years old
  - FP-12.4 Increase the proportion of male adolescents who received formal instruction on birth control methods before they were 18 years old
- FP-13 Increase the proportion of adolescents who talked to a parent or guardian about reproductive health topics before they were 18 years old
  - FP-13.1 Increase the proportion of female adolescents who talked to a parent or guardian about abstinence before they were 18 years old
  - FP-13.2 Increase the proportion of male adolescents who talked to a parent or guardian about abstinence before they were 18 years old
  - FP-13.3 Increase the proportion of female adolescents who talked to a parent or guardian about birth control methods before they were 18 years old
  - FP-13.4 Increase the proportion of male adolescents who talked to a parent or guardian about birth control methods before they were 18 years old

Source: U.S. Department of Health and Human Services. (2013b). *Healthy people 2020: Topics and objectives—family planning.* Retrieved from http://www.healthypeople.gov/2020/topicsobjectives2020/objectiveslist.aspx?topicId=13

Psychosocial and Health Outcomes of the Newborn

Infants born to adolescents are at risk for various health problems as a result of complications with the adolescent mother's pregnancy and with the birth. These health problems include the increased incidence of preterm deliveries (before 38 weeks' gestation), increased incidence of **low-birth-weight (LBW)** infants (birth weight of less than 2,500 g), and increased incidence of perinatal morbidity and mortality (Abma, 2001; Blankson et al., 1993; Leppert, Namerow, & Barker, 1986; Miller, 2002; Ventura et al., 2006).

There has been considerable debate over whether young maternal age alone is an independent risk factor for complications, and the results are still unclear (DuPlessis, Bell, & Richards, 1997; Hoffman, 2006). More recent research suggests that other mediating factors (e.g., low socioeconomic status, poor prenatal care, race/ethnicity, unfavorable sociocultural circumstances) play a critical role (Hoffman, 2006; Plouffe & White, 1996; Yoder & Young, 1997). One recent study found that infants whose fathers were present and involved in the pregnancy fared better than those whose fathers were absent, suggesting that the social support offered by a partner provided benefits for the neonate (Alio, Mbah, Grunsten & Salihu, 2011).

Role of the Nurse

It is apparent that pregnancy during the adolescent years presents some unique risks and special needs for the adolescent, her pregnancy, and her infant. Obviously, **primary prevention** of pregnancy is a crucial component of any adolescent intervention program. For effective primary prevention intervention success with teen females and males, the community health nurse must consider developmental, cultural, and socioeconomic issues as well as values in the community. However, if young girls become pregnant, it is imperative that they receive secondary and tertiary preventive care, including adequate prenatal care coupled with long-term postpartum follow up to ensure a healthy outcome for both mother and child. Community health nurses, because of their expertise in assessment, health teaching, and program development, are well suited to this task. Their accessibility to adolescent populations places them in a pivotal position to play a significant role in the delivery of care before sexual activity, during pregnancy, and during long-term follow up with the parents and child.

Healthy People 2020 addresses specific goals for adolescent pregnancy prevention (see the *Healthy People 2020* box for selected objectives). The community health nurse may use these national objectives to guide the development of individual, local, and regional nursing interventions.

> The majority of adolescents behave as if their states were that of moratorium. That is, adolescence is a time for experimenting with how one might want to be as an adult.
>
> —*Rew, 1998*

Primary Prevention

Because primary prevention is a critical component of effective community health nursing, there are tremendous opportunities for nurses to address the multifaceted problem of teen pregnancy and make important contributions to developing and implementing interventions to reduce the incidence of adolescent pregnancy. **Table 26-1** provides a list of issues to be considered when planning nursing interventions. An example of primary prevention is education and counseling for adolescents about sexual health issues, including, but not limited to, pregnancy prevention, family life education, family planning, and the postponement of pregnancy into adulthood. A comprehensive program in primary prevention targeting adolescent pregnancy includes four goals:

1. Delaying or halting participation in sexual activity
2. Providing access to contraception and sufficient knowledge and skills to use contraception appropriately
3. Strengthening life goals and encouraging long-term planning
4. Educating teens about the relationship between all risky behaviors (i.e., substance abuse) and risk for teen pregnancy

Some prevention programs focus selectively on one goal, whereas others address all four.

One task in primary prevention is contraceptive education targeted at both males and females, encouraging adolescents to practice responsible sexual behavior. For adolescents to use contraceptives (including condoms) consistently, they need not only the correct knowledge on how to use the method, but also technical skills on how to use them correctly and on how to negotiate contraceptive use, especially condoms, with their partners (Jemmott et al., 2007). Adolescents need confidence and self-efficacy in their ability to use contraceptive methods, and the desired method must be available and accessible (Cook, Erdman, & Dickens, 2007). Finally, adolescents need positive attitudes toward contraceptive use, especially condoms (Jemmott & Jemmott, 1992; Jemmott et al., 1998). Community health nurses should carefully explore an adolescent's knowledge base and correct any misconceptions about birth control methods. This is the important first step in providing adolescents with clear, accurate directions regarding the use of birth control. Some recent trends in contraceptive use among adolescents are encouraging (Jemmott, Jemmott, Hutchinson, Cederbaum, & O'Leary, 2008; Santelli et al., 2007; Villarruel et al., 2007). For example, two-thirds of adolescents reportedly use some form of contraception at first intercourse, with a significant increase in prevalence of use at first intercourse among 15- to 19-year-old females (AGI, 1994, 2013). Kahn, Brindis, and Glei (1999) claim that more than 1 million adolescent pregnancies were averted in 1995 because of consistent contraceptive use. These pregnancies would have led to approximately 480,000 live births, 390,000 abortions, 120,000 miscarriages, 10,000 ectopic pregnancies, and 37 maternal deaths.

CULTURAL CONNECTION

Recent news about young teens in a conservative Mormon community in Texas marrying older men and bearing children prior to age 18 resulted in national controversy. Due to allegations of polygamy, hundreds of children were taken from these families by the state of Texas in 2008. Community health nurses should respect cultural differences in families and yet, when community norms are threatened, this can cause conflict in our roles as advocates. Read about the culture of various religions and their values about teen mothers. How can these differences be respected in the care of all families while recognizing the health risks of early pregnancy for females?

TABLE 26-1 Considerations for Nursing Interventions

Issue	Considerations
Adolescent father	• Acknowledge the risk factors for adolescent fatherhood and encourage involvement in the prenatal and postnatal periods. In speaking with adolescent males, it is important for the nurse to identify and assess beliefs and diagnose problems that may be specific to the adolescent male. • Personalize interventions to adolescent males, both in terms of preventing adolescent pregnancy through responsible sex and in terms of coping with the consequences of being a young father. Interventions that positively affect adolescent fathers may indirectly benefit their partners by enhancing partner support (Roye & Balk, 1996). • Talking in a nonthreatening, engaging manner with the male adolescent will facilitate effective communication that will address risk factors and beliefs and promote healthy outcomes for the father, mother, their families, and their child (Roye & Balk, 1996; Sonenstein et al., 1997). • Stress male responsibility in birth control. • Increase his role in pregnancy and child care. • Improve his parenting skills and support his lifestyle changes (completing school, job training, and working).
Developmental stage	• Nurses who are knowledgeable about factors in adolescent development can better design developmentally appropriate primary interventions to prevent pregnancy, STDs, and HIV in their community. • Recognize the developmental tasks and stages of adolescence so as to understand the influence that those developmental factors have on adolescent sexual behavior. Consider the biophysical, cognitive, and psychosocial theories of development. • Answer questions and educate the adolescent about physical development and sexual issues.
Culture/ethnicity	• Assess and diagnose each adolescent patient and family to develop culturally sensitive interventions that are tailored to address cultural factors that affect sexual behavior, contraception, and potential pregnancy.
Peer	• Take advantage of the powerfully influential peer group to reach adolescents, as trained peer educators may be utilized to deliver safer sex and abstinence messages.
Intrapersonal	• Be aware that the adolescent is in a stage where he or she is developing self-identity and self-esteem, and that the adolescent may utilize sexual activity and pregnancy to bolster his or her identity.
Attitudes	• Explore nonjudgmentally the adolescent's attitudes about pregnancy.
Socioeconomic	• Assess the adolescent's economic situation and intervene to connect the adolescent and family with needed community resources.
Sexual abuse	• Identify adolescents in potentially abusive situations and assess both the adolescent and the adolescent's family for abuse.
Positive health	• Conduct home visits to adolescents during pregnancy and after birth to improve pregnancy outcomes and infant health status and to delay repeat pregnancies (Olds, 1992; Olds, Henderson, & Kitzman, 1994; Olds, Henderson, Tatelbaum, & Chamberlin, 1988).

The two most popular methods of contraception used by adolescents have traditionally been the birth control pill and the condom. Although it is beyond the scope of this chapter to fully discuss contraceptive options, it is particularly important for nurses working with adolescents to recognize the type of methods, side effects, and potential barriers that influence contraceptive choice.

Considering the variety of factors that contribute to an adolescent's increased risk for pregnancy, it is clear that there is not just one reason why teens become pregnant.

However, there are clear solutions and programs. These solutions and programs differ according to their target and the problem identified.

HEALTHY PEOPLE 2020 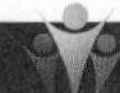

Selected Maternal, Infant, and Child Health Goals with Secondary and Tertiary Prevention Implications for Adolescent Pregnancy

Morbidity and Mortality

- MICH-1.1 Reduce the rate of fetal deaths at 20 or more weeks' gestation
- MICH-1.2 Reduce the rate of fetal and infant deaths during perinatal period (28 weeks' gestation to 7 days after birth)
- MICH-1.3 Reduce the rate of all infant deaths (within 1 year)
- MICH-1.4 Reduce the rate of neonatal deaths (within the first 28 days of life)
- MICH-1.5 Reduce the rate of postneonatal deaths (between 28 days and 1 year)
- MICH-5 Reduce the rate of maternal mortality
- MICH-6 Reduce maternal illness and complications due to pregnancy (complications during hospitalized labor and delivery)
- MICH-7.1 Reduce cesarean births among low-risk women with no prior cesarean births
- MICH-8 Reduce low birth weight (LBW) and very low birth weight (VLBW)
- MICH-9 Reduce preterm births

Pregnancy Health and Behaviors

- MICH-10 Increase the proportion of pregnant women who receive early and adequate prenatal care
- MICH-11 Increase abstinence from alcohol, cigarettes, and illicit drugs among pregnant women
- MICH-12 Increase the proportion of pregnant women who attend a series of prepared childbirth classes
- MICH-16.6 Increase the proportion of women delivering a live birth who used contraception to plan pregnancy
- MICH-19 Increase the proportion of women giving birth who attend a postpartum care visit with a health worker

Source: U.S. Department of Health and Human Services. (2013c). *Healthy people 2020: Topics and objectives Maternal, infant, and child health*. Retrieved from http://www.healthypeople.gov/2020/topicsobjectives2020/objectiveslist.aspx?topicId=26

Adolescent Pregnancy Prevention Community-Based Programs

A comprehensive review of adolescent pregnancy prevention research reveals many successes and failures.

Box 26-2 Characteristics of Effective Adolescent Pregnancy Prevention Programs

Effective programs should do the following:

- Focus clearly on reducing one or more sexual behaviors that lead to unintended pregnancy or HIV/STD infection.
- Incorporate behavioral goals, teaching methods, and materials that are appropriate to the age, sexual experience, and culture of the students.
- Be based on theoretical approaches that have been demonstrated to be effective in influencing other health-related risky behaviors.
- Last long enough to allow participants to complete important activities.
- Provide basic, accurate information about the risks of unprotected intercourse and methods of avoiding unprotected intercourse.
- Employ a variety of teaching methods designed to involve the participants and have them personalize the information.
- Include activities that address social pressures related to sex.
- Provide models of and practice in communication, negotiation, and refusal skills.
- Select teachers or peers who believe in the program and then provide them with training, which often includes practice sessions.

Source: National Campaign to Prevent Teen Pregnancy. Used by permission.

Kirby (1997) concludes that programs with positive outcomes share important characteristics (**Box 26-2**). There is no clear agreement on what exact combination of these elements makes up the ideal prevention program. Clearly, programs must be tailored to match the needs of the particular target population (Blythe & Diaz, 2007). Ideally, members of the target population, the family, and the community should be involved in the program development and implementation (Grobler, Botma, Jacobs, & Nel, 2007). There is a pressing need for prevention programs that are culturally sensitive and relevant, addressing the norms, attitudes, and beliefs of the target population (Cook et al., 2007). There are various types of programs with different approaches to pregnancy prevention, such as peer education, life options, working with parents, and working in schools and other community settings, including faith communities (Flynn, Budd, & Modelski, 2008; Kalmus et al., 2003).

NOTE THIS!

The U.S. Department of Health and Human Services' Office of Adolescent Health has a comprehensive, searchable list of evidence-based programs for prevention of teen pregnancy, available online at http://www.hhs.gov/ash/oah/oah-initiatives/teen_pregnancy/db/tpp-searchable.html

Lessons Learned

Important lessons have been learned in the area of adolescent pregnancy prevention. For example, although some prevention efforts focus solely on the importance of **abstinence** from sexual intercourse, the bulk of current evidence indicates that this approach is not successful in delaying the onset of intercourse (Kohler, Manhart & Lafferty, 2008; Rosenbaum, 2009; Trenholm et al., 2008; Williams & Thompson, 2013). Furthermore, education alone is generally not sufficient to change risky behavior such as inconsistent contraceptive use (Flynn et al., 2008; Howard & Mitchell, 1993; Kalmus et al., 2003). Multidisciplinary programs are needed that combine elements such as sexuality education, enhanced negotiation and communication skills, and access to services and contraceptives (AGI, 1994; Flynn et al., 2008; Howard & Mitchell, 1993; Kalmus et al., 2003; Plouffe & White, 1996). Finally, although some have expressed concern that sexuality education and/or contraceptive distribution might encourage sexual activity among teens, recent research reviews have concluded that the opposite is actually true (Flynn et al., 2008; Jemmott & Jemmott, 2007; Kirby, 1997; Kirby et al., 1993).

Peer Education Approach

The peer education model shows great promise for use in adolescent pregnancy prevention because the peer group is a common source for information about sex. In this model, peers are trained to lead prevention programs within their peer group. Community health nurses may serve as trainers and facilitators in these programs. Some of the advantages of peer education are that it provides positive role models, reinforces norms, empowers youth, and encourages personal responsibility (Albert, 2004; Coyle et al., 1996; Schaffer, Jost, Pederson, & Lair, 2008).

Life Option Approach

A promising approach that is worthy of additional study is implementing programs that shift the focus to enriching an adolescent's life options across the board by addressing concerns such as academic performance, self-esteem, substance abuse, and long-term goal realization (Albert, 2004; Schaffer et al., 2008). These programs may include one-on-one mentoring and role modeling with successful adults, community service participation, remedial education, tutoring services, counseling by both professional and peer groups, self-worth enhancement techniques, and exposure to new experiences to expand life options (e.g., concerts, museums, travel). This approach attempts to expand an adolescent's future goals and expectations by improving educational and employment prospects. Because future-oriented, goal-directed adolescents are less likely to become pregnant, the expected result is a reduction in the rate of adolescent pregnancies. Although this approach does not directly address adolescent pregnancy, it targets many of the factors that contribute to an adolescent's risk for unintended pregnancy (Abma, 2001; Hoffman, 2006; Kirby, 1997; Loda et al., 1997; Rolleri et al., 2008). Because the community health nurse is familiar with the community and its members, he or she may serve as a trusted mentor, educator, community liaison, and coordinator of such programs. In addition, for these programs to be effective, community health nurses must be aware of programs and resources that target adolescents in a broader sense, not only in terms of pregnancy prevention and contraception.

> Adolescence is a period of rapid changes. Between the ages of 12 and 17, for example, a parent ages as much as 20 years.
>
> —*Author Unknown*

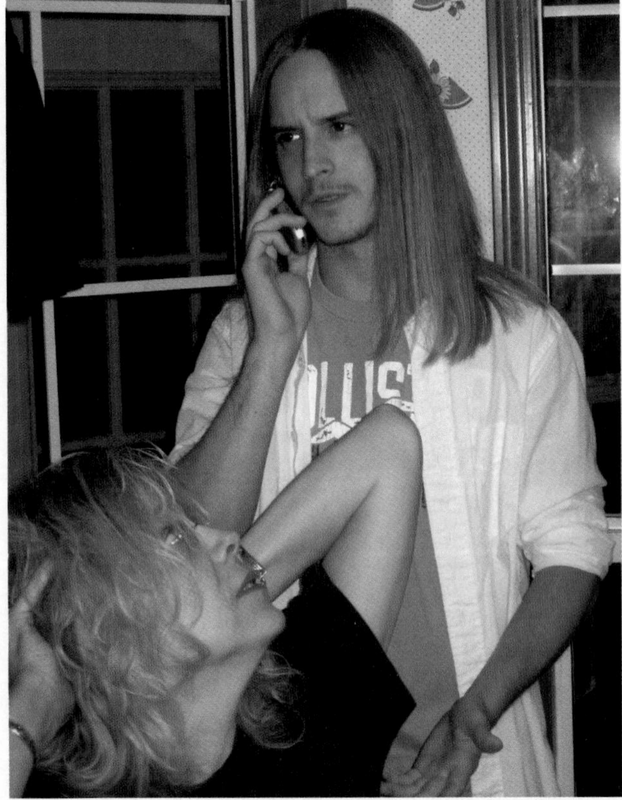

Working with Parents and Adults

Community health nurses may work with parents and other adults significant to the adolescent, such as adult

BOX 26-3 Ten Tips for Parents to Help Their Children Avoid Teen Pregnancy

1. Be clear about your own sexual values and attitudes.
2. Talk with your children early and often about sex, and be specific.
3. Supervise and monitor your children's behaviors, setting rules, curfews, standards, and other limitations.
4. Know your children's friends and their families.
5. Discourage early, frequent, and steady dating.
6. Take a strong stand against your daughter dating a significantly older boy; don't allow your son to develop an intense relationship with a much younger girl.
7. Help your teenager to have options for the future that are more attractive than early parenthood.
8. Let your kids know that you value education highly.
9. Know that your kids are influenced by the media; pay attention to what they are watching, listening to, and reading.
10. Develop strong, close relationships with your children at an early age.

Source: National Campaign to Prevent Teen Pregnancy. Used by permission.

relatives, teachers, coaches, and neighbors. Recent research indicates that parents may be one of the most significant factors in preventing the onset of teen sexual behavior. This approach may be a promising avenue for prevention because parents and significant adults influence the behavior of adolescents, including sexual behavior, in their everyday interactions (Kirby, 2001; Miller, 2002). Although there is no single way for parents to effectively communicate with their children, the nurse may suggest that parents follow the guidelines provided by the National Campaign to Prevent Teen Pregnancy outlined in **Box 26-3**.

School-Based Programs

A large number of pregnancy prevention programs target teens through school programs. Some of the programs in school may include sex education, family life education, and contraception education. Sex education is provided by some private schools and by public schools in approximately 75% to 80% of the United States; however, most family life programs are offered at the junior or senior high school level as an elective course, which means they do not reach many adolescents and cannot target those at greatest risk (Grobler et al., 2007). Also, most sex education teachers have little training in sex education, and it is not their primary focus. In school systems with school nurses, the nurse is involved in both sex and family life education (Lederman & Mian, 2003). Nurses can also provide factual sex education to teenagers as they provide other health services. Nurses are effective sex educators because they are equipped to provide sexual content in a factual, nonjudgmental approach. They are also proficient at encouraging and guiding patient discussion, characteristics helpful in addressing sex education with adolescents (Jemmott et al., 2008). These and other school-based programs receive limited funding, and access is limited for most students. However, school-based programs operate within a highly politicized environment. Decisions to include or exclude certain program elements within school-based programs may be made in an effort to minimize controversy rather than to maximize positive outcomes. As a result, community health nurses may need to broaden the focus of their prevention efforts beyond the domain of the school to the community at large.

Working in Various Settings

Rather than limit the discussion of sexuality and pregnancy prevention to any one setting or a particular type of visit, community health nurses are uniquely positioned to seize opportunities to provide education and implement prevention in numerous settings. These settings, such as family planning clinics, primary healthcare clinics, school health clinics, community-based health clinics, churches, and teen centers are all ideal settings for adolescent pregnancy prevention, even when the adolescent does not present for contraceptive services. Interventions targeting adolescents who use the services of family planning clinics appear to be particularly promising in that they can effectively reach a high-risk group, adolescent females (and potentially their partners) who come to the clinic for a pregnancy test. These clinics are logical sites because of the population that they serve: More than 60% of adolescents younger than 17 use family planning clinics, and more than 82% of young African American adolescents use them. In addition, they provide the opportunity to reach a population of vulnerable, high-risk adolescents at a timely moment (CDC, 2012; Delphisheh et al., 2007; Zabin & Clark, 1981; Zabin, Emerson, Ringers, & Sedivy, 1996). Some research groups have also explored the possibility of using technology such as social media websites or text messaging to provide educational resources for adolescents, finding that teens expressed a wish for resources that met three criteria: accessibility, trustworthiness, and resources that could be considered "safe", that is, that protect the user's privacy and confidentiality, are nonthreatening, and pose no risk of exposure to content such as pornography (Selkie, Benson, & Moreno, 2011).

Program Evaluation

Evaluation is an important part of the nursing process. Programs must be continually evaluated and modified by the community health nurse to ensure their effectiveness and appropriateness for preventing adolescent pregnancy. New prevention programs are constantly in the process of being designed; however, because few programs are carefully and consistently developed and evaluated, efforts may be wasted on interventions that are not effective. One measure of a sound design is the incorporation of theory in the design. Community nurses should have a knowledge base that includes an understanding of various behavioral theories such as the health belief model (Becker, 1974), social cognitive theory (Bandura, 1986), and the theory of reasoned action (Azjen & Fishbein, 1980). These theories can be used to understand the factors that encourage or discourage health-promotion behaviors and can guide both program design and evaluation. The lack of meaningful program evaluation is a major defect in the primary prevention of adolescent pregnancy. Evaluation by the community health nurse is critical not only to identify ineffective programs or program elements but also to identify effective interventions and provide the impetus for replication and reevaluation in a different population. An effective prevention intervention is one that makes positive behavioral changes in measurable outcomes such as decreased incidence of early sexual intercourse or unprotected sex, or decreased number of sexual partners.

Secondary and Tertiary Prevention

Prevention efforts may not reach all adolescents because the risk of pregnancy may not be associated with extremely negative outcomes (Stevens-Simon et al., 1996). Therefore, the community health nurse must implement secondary and **tertiary prevention** techniques. In secondary and tertiary prevention, the community health nurse focuses attention on the health care, prevention needs, and long-term development of pregnant adolescents and adolescents who are already young mothers or fathers, with an emphasis on continuing their education to reduce the social and economic risks that can affect their future (**Table 26-2**). Secondary prevention efforts are designed to promote healthier outcomes from adolescent pregnancy (see **Figure 26-2**). These efforts are aimed at improving participation in prenatal care, childbirth preparation, and parenting activities. Interventions may include early detection of pregnancy, options counseling, prenatal care, childbirth education, parenting education, and safer sex education. Community health nurses may also be involved on a more global scale in

TABLE 26-2 Secondary and Tertiary Prevention: Nursing Intervention

Issue	Considerations for Nursing Interventions
Early detection	• Identify pregnant adolescents early in their pregnancies. • Recognize factors linked to failure to receive early diagnosis and care.
Pregnancy options	• Assess knowledge about pregnancy options. • Be sensitive to the factors that influence the mother's decision. • Assess the support the adolescent receives throughout the pregnancy. • Facilitate therapeutic relationships with the adolescent mother and father and their social support networks. • Include the father of the baby. A comprehensive assessment should include identification of his attitudes, emotional reactions, plans for education, and plans for involvement with the pregnancy, his partner, and the child. • Provide options counseling.
Prenatal care	• Encourage early and consistent prenatal care to reduce neonatal and maternal complications. • Teach the adolescent and her partner about the special needs of pregnancy. • Assess barriers to adolescent prenatal care. • Provide health screening assessments, counseling, and education for pregnant patients.
Adolescent father	• Encourage the father's participation in prenatal visits. • Invite the father to prenatal classes, encourage questions and participation in prenatal visits, and acknowledge the father's role as a partner in the pregnancy. • Encourage fathers to participate in the delivery.
Parenting education	• Assess knowledge about parenting. • Provide education about positioning and handling of infants, nutrition, hygiene, elimination, growth and development, immunization, and recognition of illnesses. • When doing health teaching, it is important to be sensitive to the ethnicity and culture of the patient and integrate those considerations into the care of the infant.

Postpartum care	• Focus on the standard postpartum areas as well on specific concerns of the adolescent, such as body image, weight loss, and fatigue. • Assess the adolescent's adjustment to her new role and the emotional support systems available to her. • Provide a health assessment of both the mother and the infant, newborn care education and supervision, prenatal education on growth and development and parenting skills, review of role adjustment and available supports, and sex education and birth control information. • Encourage the adolescent to continue developing as an individual (e.g., to continue education, participate in some social activities, and explore relationships with peers) and at the same time increase the adolescent's proficiency and confidence in parenting.
Support	• Assess physical and emotional support available. • Refer adolescents to other possible resources, such as parenting programs, cooperative daycare programs, or programs that pair the new mother with an older adolescent mother with a successful experience.
Status of the newborn	• Provide a newborn assessment/well-baby check. • Assess for signs of adequate maternal–infant bonding. • Provide information about child care.
Sexual activity and contraceptive use	• Assess adolescents' plans for sexual activity and need for contraceptive methods. • Initiate discussion about birth control while the adolescent is pregnant so that both partners have an opportunity to identify contraceptive and safer sex methods that they will use after the pregnancy. • Provide instruction on condom use during pregnancy in your discussion of disease prevention in pregnancy. • Help adolescents explore the risks involved if they have sex without adequate protection. • Help the adolescent select the most appropriate form of contraception from several alternatives. • If the adolescent has already used birth control, it is helpful to identify the method, how it was used, and the reason for discontinuance. • Make sure that the adolescent is aware of community resources (family planning clinics) where she may be supplied with contraceptives. • Encourage clinic attendance, promote access to contraception, and provide referrals to appropriate contraceptive services. When counseling individuals or teaching sex education classes, emphasize the importance of contraceptive use by all sexually active adolescents. • Monitor compliance and encourage cooperation with adolescents.

secondary prevention efforts by working to increase pregnant adolescents' access to care. These efforts may include developing policies relevant to adolescent pregnancy in various organizations, working through coalitions and in other professional organizations.

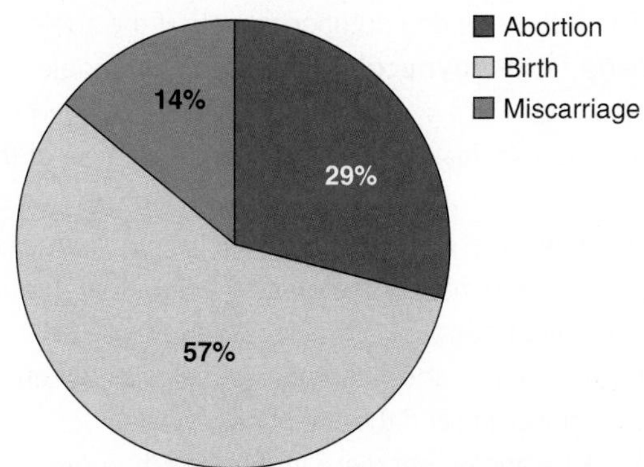

Figure 26-2 Teen pregnancy statistics.

Source: Alan Guttmacher Institute. (2013). Facts on American teens' sexual and reproductive health. Washington DC: Author. Available online: http://www.guttmacher .org/pubs/fb_ATSRH.html

- More than one-quarter (26%) of all teen pregnancies end in abortion; 15% end in miscarriage; the remainder end in birth.
- Black women have the highest teen pregnancy rate (117 per 1,000 women ages 15–19), followed by Hispanics (107 per 1,000) and non-Hispanic whites (43 per 1,000).
- The pregnancy rate among black teens decreased by 48% between 1990 and 2008, more than the overall U.S. teen pregnancy rate declined during the same period (42%).
- Eighty-two percent of teen pregnancies are unplanned; they account for about one in five of all unintended pregnancies annually.

- Nearly 7% of all 15- to 19-year-old females become pregnant annually.
- Two-thirds of teen pregnancies occur among 18 to 19 year olds.

Source: Alan Guttmacher Institute. (2013). *Fact sheet: American teens' sexual and reproductive health.* Washington DC: Author. Retrieved from http://www.guttmacher.org/pubs/fb_ATSRH.html

Early Detection

A goal for the community health nurse is to identify pregnant adolescents early in their pregnancies, because many teens wait until they are visibly pregnant before they initiate prenatal care. Factors such as shame, denial, self-esteem issues, low value and knowledge of health, limited access to care, lack of future-oriented thinking, and lack of symptoms have all been linked to failure to receive early diagnosis and care (Baker, 1996; Lee & Grubbs, 1995; Thompson, Powell, Patterson, & Ellerbee, 1995). Community health nurses can work to identify teens early in their pregnancies by using community outreach techniques such as advertisement for prenatal services in malls, schools, public transportation, and churches.

Options Counseling

In counseling the pregnant adolescent, the nurse must be aware that the adolescent's decisions about her pregnancy and subsequent pregnancy prevention will affect both the adolescent mother and her entire family. Once pregnancy is confirmed, the adolescent faces an important decision about her options, which include **abortion** (**Table 26-3**), **adoption**, or keeping the baby. The nurse has the responsibility to provide (or refer to someone who will provide) the adolescent with information about pregnancy options. Among adolescents, the most common outcome (59%) is a live birth. Only 1 in 20 pregnant adolescents chooses to place her infant for adoption, whereas 26% of adolescent pregnancies end in abortion (Ventura et al., 2006).

The community health nurse must recognize that many factors play a role in the decision the adolescent makes about the pregnancy. These factors may include cultural and religious upbringing, family attitude toward the pregnancy (perceived or real), partner attitude, community values and norms, and state law. Partner age plays an important role, as data have shown that adolescent females with younger partners tend to terminate their pregnancies at a higher rate than adolescent females with adult partners (Collins et al., 2004; Hoffman, 2006).

TABLE 26-3 Adolescents and Abortion in the United States

- There were 192,000 abortions among 15- to 19-year-olds in 2008.
- Twenty-six percent of pregnancies among females ages 15–19 ended in abortion in 2008, compared with 21% among all women.
- The reasons teens give most frequently for having an abortion are concerns about how having a baby would change their lives, inability to afford a baby now, and feeling insufficiently mature to raise a child.
- Thirty-eight states (as of April 2014) require that a minor seeking an abortion involve her parents in the decision.
- Six in 10 minors who have abortions do so with at least one parent's knowledge. The great majority of parents support their daughter's decision to have an abortion.

Source: Data from Alan Guttmacher Institute. (2013). *Fact sheet: American teens' sexual and reproductive health.* Washington DC: Author. Available online: from http://www.guttmacher.org/pubs/fb_ATSRH.html

Prenatal Care

Once an adolescent decides to continue the pregnancy, effort is directed toward ensuring a healthy outcome for the mother and infant. Early initiation and regular continuance of prenatal care significantly reduce the risk for both adolescents and their infants. The nurse should educate the adolescent and her partner about the special needs of pregnancy as they relate to adolescence, such as the following:

- Special nutritional needs (**Box 26-4**)
- Physical changes and demands of pregnancy

BOX 26-4 Adolescent Pregnancy and Nutrition Requirements

The nutritional needs of the pregnant adolescent are often different from those of adult women. Many adolescents are experiencing rapid physical growth and maturation during their teenage years. Pregnancy increases the nutritional requirements of the adolescent.

The recommended nutritional goals of the adolescent depend on the **gynecological age** of the adolescent. Adolescents with a gynecological age less than or equal to 2 years have increased nutritional needs because of their own physical growth requirements. When the gynecological age is less than 2 years, the nutritional requirements of a pregnant teen may compete with the nutritional requirements of the fetus.

Gynecological age = number of years between the chronological age and the age of menarche

Because adolescent diets are often high in salt, sugar, and fatty foods, and low in protein, vitamins, and minerals, the nurse must be diligent about assessing and diagnosing deficits in the pregnant adolescent's diet.

- How pregnancy affects the female adolescent's growth and development
- Emotional changes during pregnancy for both parents
- What to expect during delivery
- Preterm labor
- Signs and symptoms of pregnancy complications

Programs that address barriers to adolescent prenatal care have demonstrated positive outcomes, including reduced neonatal and maternal complications (CDC, 2012; Delpisheh et al., 2007; Rogers, Peoples-Sheps, & Suchindran, 1996; Yoder & Young, 1997).

Prenatal care services that prove successful in getting teenagers to use and comply with the overall program of care are those that provide an accepting, caring atmosphere and work to reduce obstacles to beginning or continuing care. These results have been in comprehensive community-based programs with a heavy outreach and educational emphasis, using multidisciplinary healthcare teams, especially community health nurse involvement, and home visits. The community health nurse acts as the case manager of prenatal care and sees that patients are provided with needed services. The nurse is the team member who spends the most time with the adolescent, providing most of the health screening assessments, counseling, and education for pregnant patients.

Prenatal programs should also aim to improve the quality and duration of the father–child relationship. Community health nurses can assist in these efforts by encouraging the father's participation in prenatal visits. Most fathers are curious and interested in the process of gestation and delivery but are uncomfortable asking questions and hesitant in interacting with healthcare providers. The community health nurse can invite the father to prenatal classes, encourage questions and participation in prenatal visits, and acknowledge the father's role as a partner in the pregnancy. Fathers can be encouraged, but not forced, into participation in the baby's delivery.

Three types of programs offer prenatal care to adolescents: private medical services, public health clinic programs, and school-based prenatal programs. The choice of program depends on the accessibility and the financial circumstances of the adolescent and her family. Private medical services are provided by physicians in single or group practices or are associated with health maintenance organizations. These services are available to people who have a medical insurance plan or can afford to pay. Public health clinic programs are for families without insurance or the financial resources to pay for prenatal care (Schaffer, Goodhue, Stennes, & Lanigan, 2012). School-based programs provide services in connection with other school-run clinic services or in separate schools designed for the exclusive use of pregnant adolescents (Olds, 1992). School-based prenatal services provide a comprehensive approach to care and are usually found in large school districts with high rates of adolescent pregnancy.

RESEARCH ALERT

American Indian adolescent pregnancy rates are high, yet little is known about how Native youth view primary pregnancy prevention. This study was meant to identify pregnancy prevention strategies from the perspectives of urban Native youth to inform program development. Native Teen Voices (NTV) was a community-based participatory action research study in Minneapolis, Minnesota. Focus groups were convened with Native youth who had never been involved in a pregnancy. Participants were asked what they would do to prevent pregnancy if they were in charge of programs for Native youth. Respondents' recommendations were identified and categorized across age and sex cohorts. Participants in all cohorts emphasized the following themes: Show the consequences of adolescent pregnancy, develop more pregnancy prevention programs for Native youth in schools and community-based organizations, improve access to contraceptives, discuss teen pregnancy with Native youth, and use media to reach Native youth. Native youth perceived limited access to comprehensive pregnancy prevention education and contraceptives. They suggested a variety of mechanisms to address gaps in sexual health services and emphasized enhancing school-based resources and involving Native peers and elders in school and community-based adolescent pregnancy prevention initiatives.

Source: Garwick, A., Rhodes, K., Peterson-Hickey, M., & Hellerstedt, W. (2008). Native teen voices: Adolescent pregnancy prevention recommendations. *Journal of Adolescent Health*, *42*(1), 81–88.

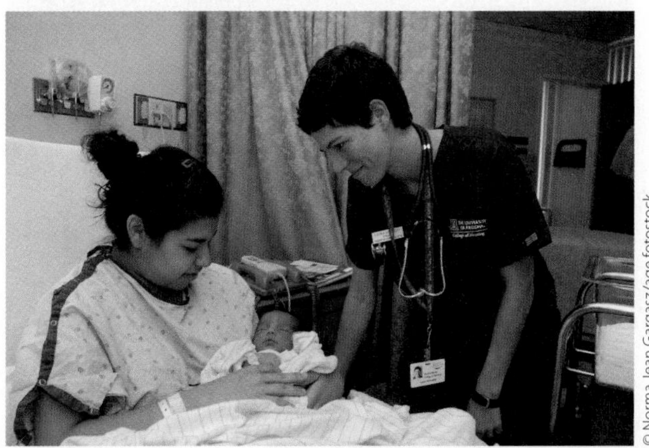

Nurse role modeling appropriate infant care with teen mother.

Transition from Prenatal to Postpartum Care

After delivery of the baby, the focus is on postpartum care, which varies widely in scope and duration of services. All prenatal programs provide a postpartum check for the mother. A well-baby check is included in most services, although a private obstetrical practice may rely on the mother to make her own arrangements for all infant care. The most extensive postpartum care is delivered in community programs that rely heavily on nurses. These programs usually include the following:

- Health assessment of both the mother and infant
- Newborn care education and supervision
- Prenatal education on growth and development and parenting skills
- Review of role adjustment and available supports
- Sex education and birth control information
- Promotion of the role of continuing education to reduce future risks for the teen mother and father

One valuable component of these programs is the emphasis on regular contact with the new mothers, starting the first week after delivery. Studies show that regular nurse visits reduce anxiety and increase infant health as measured by fewer accidents and emergency department visits (Olds, 1992; Olds et al., 1994; Schaffer et al., 2012). Mothers experience many concerns or problems before the first scheduled clinic or physician visit. Earlier contacts allow the adolescent and nurse to address these issues and reduce anxiety. Contact need not always be in person; some care can be provided by telephone monitoring of the new mother and newer technology such as email reminders.

Parenting Education and Contraceptive Education

Adolescent parents typically need more structured education focusing on newborn care, parenting skills, and fostering developmentally appropriate interactions. Discussion about birth control should also be initiated while the adolescent is pregnant so that both partners have an opportunity to identify contraceptive methods that they will use after the pregnancy. The community health nurse is in a unique position to provide these services at a group or individual level and to promote continuity of care that focuses on the new family.

MEDIA MOMENT 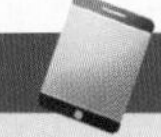

Dear Diary, I'm Pregnant: Teenagers Talk About Their Pregnancy (1997)

Annrenee Englander, Vancouver, BC: Annick Press.

This book is the result of interviews with women who became pregnant during adolescence. Englander demonstrates through first-person narratives (by the women interviewed) the experiences of many teens who become pregnant. Women of differing race, ethnicity, and income levels provide a more well-rounded view of the adolescent pregnancy experience. In these different narratives, you are able to see how each teen had to make difficult decisions about the pregnancy and her life, sometimes with limited support.

The Pregnancy Project (2013)

Gaby Rodriguez: Simon & Schuster.

Gaby Rodriguez was a straight-A student who had a secret—she *wasn't* pregnant. As part of a school project, 17-year-old Gaby faked her pregnancy to see (and document) how her peers and others in her community responded. Her reason for undertaking this deception—which ultimately sparked international headlines—was simple: She'd been told all her life that she was predestined to teen motherhood because her mother, as well as all her siblings, had become parents during adolescence. Gaby was the only one who was on a path toward college due to her success in school. Would her "pregnancy" change people's minds about her? Would it alter the way they talked to her, thought about her, treated her? And what would happen once the secret was revealed? *The Pregnancy Project* tells Gaby's story in her own words.

Kids Having Kids: Economic Costs and Social Consequences of Teen Pregnancy, 2nd edition (2008)

Saul D. Hoffmann and Rebecca A. Maynard, Baltimore, MD: Urban Institute Press.

Kids Having Kids is a book of essays by experts in the field of adolescent pregnancy. Revised and updated from the original 1997 edition, this edition includes a chapter on teen pregnancy interventions. This book takes a look at the problem of adolescent pregnancy and estimates the economic and social effects of adolescent pregnancy on the teen, her child, her family, the community, and the U.S. economy. It provides an in-depth look at the long-term consequences of adolescent pregnancy as well.

Health and Psychosocial Status of the Mother

At a minimum, the mother should have a 6-week postpartum examination. Some community health programs start home visits at about 2 weeks postpartum. The physical assessment should focus on the standard postpartum areas as well as on specific concerns of the adolescent, such as body image, weight loss, and fatigue. In addition, the nurses should assess the adolescent's adjustment to her new role and the emotional support systems available to her. Adjusting to the role of parent during adolescence is difficult. Conflict is not unusual. Family members may expect the adolescent to instantly become an adult and mother, or the opposite, to remain a child and allow her parents to assume all the responsibilities for the infant. Ideally, the adolescent should be encouraged to continue developing as an individual (e.g., to continue her education, participate in some social activities, to explore relationships with peers). The adolescent mother needs support in increasing her proficiency and confidence in parenting and integrating her new responsibilities into her daily routine. She may be juggling school, social activities, and infant care. Fatigue and stress are common.

GOT AN ALTERNATIVE?

Pregnant adolescents are often fearful of gaining weight and losing their relatively new female shape. Exercise, such as yoga and aerobics, often appeal to this group and can promote a healthy pregnancy, with proper professional supervision.

The community health nurse can help the new mother look at the immediate family, other relatives, significant others, and the father of the infant and his family for support. The adolescent mother could also be referred to other possible resources, such as parenting programs, cooperative daycare programs, or programs that pair the new mother with an older adolescent mother who has had a successful experience. Even if support systems are adequate, the family may need some help in understanding and supporting the adolescent as a maturing individual (Zeck et al., 2007). Adequate physical and emotional support, along with health teaching and realistic expectations for their children, successfully reduce the incidence of abuse and neglect from at-risk mothers (Abma, 2001; East, Reyes, & Horn, 2007; Marshall et al., 1991; Olds, 1992; Olds et al., 1994; Olds et al., 1988).

MEDIA MOMENT

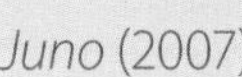

Juno (2007)

Academy Award winner Ellen Page plays a 16-year-old high school student (Juno) suddenly faced with an unexpected pregnancy after a one-time sexual encounter with her good friend. Juno faces the pregnancy with a pragmatic attitude and intent to control her and her unborn baby's future. She ultimately decides to find a suitable couple to adopt her baby, choosing a closed adoption and the prospect of never seeing her child again. This film explores the complexities of adolescent pregnancy and the family.

APPLICATION TO PRACTICE 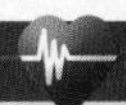

You are a school nurse at Oak Hills High School. You have carefully followed several of your students who have become pregnant and helped them find resources for support both during and after their pregnancies. You have noticed, however, that several of your students have decided to discontinue breastfeeding. In speaking with Arlene Johnston, a 15-year-old sophomore with a 3-month-old son, Antonio, you find out that she is also reconsidering breastfeeding. She understands the benefits of breastfeeding and is able to discuss them with you. Both Arlene and her mom think that breastfeeding is good for Antonio. However, upon further questioning, you discover that her new partner, Sam, and her friends at school think that breastfeeding is "nasty." Arlene feels embarrassed that her friends know she breastfeeds and she is afraid that she will lose her friends and boyfriend.

1. Which factors in Arlene's (and the other adolescents') cognitive development support her decision to discontinue breastfeeding?
2. How can you address this to continue to promote Arlene's breastfeeding of Antonio?

You decide that one means to addressing attitudes toward breastfeeding is to address the attitudes of all students at Oak Hills High.

1. Consider different ways that you, as the school (community) health nurse, can address the students at Oak Hills High.
2. Which special considerations apply for such an intervention?

Sexual Activity and Contraceptive Use

Ideally, the idea of future contraception should be introduced as part of the prenatal program. The adolescent must decide whether she will continue sexual activity after delivery and must be encouraged to be honest with the nurse about her decision. Sometimes, the mother is no longer involved with the father of the infant and announces that she does not intend to be sexually active or to have another child. In this case, the adolescent mother should be helped to explore the risks involved if she changes her mind without adequate protection. Once an adolescent has been pregnant, she risks repeating the situation (AGI, 1981; Brown et al., 1999; CDC, 2006).

Access to and regular use of birth control is the goal of contraceptive services for adolescents. Family planning clinics and private physicians are one source; school-based clinics are a more recent effort. Community health nurses can encourage clinic attendance, promote access to contraception, and provide referrals to appropriate contraceptive services when counseling individuals or teaching sex education classes. The nurse must emphasize the importance of contraceptive use by all sexually active adolescents.

Health Status and Care of the Newborn

In addition to the usual newborn assessment, the community health nurse should look for signs of adequate maternal–infant bonding. Evidence of attachment includes calling a child by name, cuddling, talking to the infant, and demonstrating an interest in infant care and development. Adolescents often demonstrate difficulty in bonding simply because they have had no previous experience with infants and are afraid to do anything. Sometimes, another person has assumed the role of caregiver and the adolescent becomes an observer rather than caregiver. Bonding can be assessed in clinic settings, but home visits by the community health nurse allow for a more accurate picture of the nature and scope of the mother–infant relationship and the relationship of the adolescent father with the mother. Considering the current trend of short postpartum length of stay, the community health nurse has the opportunity to observe the interaction among the infant, teenager, father, and other caregivers for a longer time than nurses in the clinical setting.

Tertiary Prevention

Tertiary prevention efforts may include prevention of additional adolescent pregnancies, support of positive parent–infant interaction, support groups for adolescent parents, and programs that support adolescents while they pursue educational goals. The techniques discussed previously that are used in primary prevention may be used

BOX 26-5 Key Ideas

- Adolescent pregnancy is a nationwide problem, affecting more than 1 million adolescents per year in the United States—a higher rate than in other industrialized countries.
- Adolescent pregnancy transcends ethnic, racial, and cultural boundaries.
- Repeat pregnancies for adolescents are of great concern, because half of all pregnant adolescents will have a repeat pregnancy in 2 years.
- Pregnant adolescents and their children experience more complications with pregnancy and have poorer health outcomes.
- Adolescent parents may have increased psychological stress and disruption of psychosocial development. They may also have incomplete education, poor success in the job market, and higher dependence on public funds. As a result, the community and the families of adolescent parents may experience increased economic and social stress.
- Adolescent males have similar risk factors for pregnancy to their female peers. However, adolescent males (and issues particular to them) are frequently overlooked in the literature. The impact of fatherhood on adolescent boys and inclusion of fathers in the maternity and postpartum experience is an important and new phenomenon to increase father involvement.
- Pregnant adolescents and their infants are at greater risk for developing medical complications (e.g., hypertension, toxemia, anemia, low birth weight, stillbirth, and infant mortality) than are older women and their infants.
- There is no single factor that causes adolescent pregnancy, but an awareness of the personal, environmental, and social contributing factors allows the community health nurse to appropriately assess, diagnose, plan, and evaluate interventions for adolescents and their families.
- Many contraceptive options are available for the adolescent. The nurse must have an awareness of the potential barriers that the adolescent may encounter in using contraception consistently and effectively.
- The ideal manner in which to prevent the complications associated with adolescent pregnancy is to prevent pregnancy from occurring. Primary prevention efforts need to focus on the special developmental needs of adolescence, emphasize the importance of peer groups, and occur in various settings to effectively promote behavior change. Programs that include sex education, contraceptive information, and access to contraceptive services have been found to delay sexual activity and increase contraceptive use in sexually active adolescents. Successful prevention programs share important characteristics that should be considered in program development.
- The nurse should develop secondary prevention programs that include interventions that have been documented to reduce medical complications and promote healthy outcomes for the pregnant adolescent and her newborn infant, including promoting early initiation of prenatal care, childbirth education, and nutrition counseling.
- Tertiary prevention programs are largely rehabilitative—that is, they provide a variety of support services for new mothers and their infants to reduce health risks for both mother and child and to increase the chances that the mother will continue her education. Prevention programs may include activities that promote education completion, psychosocial development, and development of career goals.
- The overall goal of the community health nurse is to prevent adolescent pregnancy, promote healthy outcomes of adolescent pregnancy, prevent repeat pregnancies, and foster positive long-term development of adolescents and their children.

to prevent repeat pregnancies in adolescents. The nurse may work collaboratively with organizations that provide support such as child care and allowing adolescent parents to complete and pursue further education. Other nursing interventions may include long-term child development education and parenting classes. Programs that foster maternal education, father involvement, and increased self-esteem show significant promise for better maternal and infant development (Diehl, 1997; Hoffman, 2006; Roye & Balk, 1996).

Conclusion

Despite the proliferation of prevention efforts, adolescent pregnancy is a significant and enduring community health problem. It has been linked to various problems such as increased poverty, decreased educational attainment, increased psychological stress, potential isolation from peers, and increased reliance on public funds. Multiple pregnancies among adolescents are not uncommon and are particularly disturbing because the negative effect of pregnancy increases dramatically.

Many factors contribute to adolescent pregnancy, and community health nurses must be aware of potential risk factors and understand the complex interaction of these factors. Without this awareness and understanding, the nurse will not be able to adequately perform the nursing process to develop and evaluate age-appropriate, culturally sensitive, convenient, comprehensive, and affordable interventions that will meet the special needs of adolescents. It is clear that unless community health nurses and other health professionals make an effort to provide information, few adolescents will actively seek out nurses or other professionals as resources. Nurses are well suited to address the issues of adolescent pregnancy. The professional roles in schools, clinics, screening programs, health departments, and community outreach centers provide access to at-risk populations. Community health nurses have the opportunity, sensitivity, and commitment to work to achieve positive outcomes for adolescents and their children.

Beyond the scope of care to individuals, community health nurses are sensitive to the community in which they practice. Community health nurses are uniquely equipped to assess communities, identify needs and special risk groups, and formulate solutions (see **Box 26-5**). Nurses have an obligation to meet the special needs of pregnant adolescents by designing programs, organizing community support, and advocating for funding and policy changes to enhance positive health outcomes for adolescents and their infants.

BOX 26-6 Websites of Interest

Organization/Service	Website
Advocates for Youth, Teen Pregnancy Prevention Initiative	http://www.advocatesforyouth.org/pregnanc.htm
Alan Guttmacher Institute	http://www.agi-usa.org
Ask NOAH (New York Online Access to Health) About Pregnancy	http://www.noah.cuny.edu/pregnancy/pregnancy.html (information in both English and Spanish)
National Campaign to Prevent Teen Pregnancy	http://www.teenpregnancy.org
Planned Parenthood Federation of America	http://www.plannedparenthood.org

Critical Thinking Activities

1. What are the social norms and cultural beliefs about adolescent pregnancy and sexuality in your community? How do you think that these beliefs affect adolescent behavior?
2. What strategies can the community health nurse implement to help the pregnant adolescent and her family cope with the changes in the family structure?
3. You are planning a pregnancy prevention intervention for adolescents in your community. Identify program characteristics that you might include in your intervention that have been shown to be effective in adolescent pregnancy prevention programs.
4. It is important for the community health nurse to be aware of community resources to appropriately refer patients. What resources are available in your community for pregnant adolescents? Adolescents with children? Adolescent fathers?
5. Does your school district provide child care for adolescents with children? Do you believe it should? Why?

LEVELS OF PREVENTION

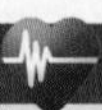

Primary: Teaching middle school students about the risks of teen pregnancy for both males and females

Secondary: Community class for pregnant teens on optimal nutrition during pregnancy

Tertiary: Home visit to mother of premature infant to discuss developmental delay and appropriate interventions for family

HEALTHY ME

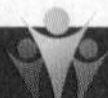

As a teenager, what are/were your standards and self-protection for having sex in terms of primary prevention? Have they changed since you have been in nursing school?

AFFORDABLE CARE ACT

The Affordable Care Act of 2010 provides funding to replicate evidence-based teen pregnancy prevention program models through the Personal Responsibility Education Program (PREP), administered by the Family Youth Service Bureau (FYSB) and the U.S. Department of Health and Human Services.

Source: http://www.hhs.gov/ash/oah/adolescent-health-topics/reproductive-health/teen-pregnancy/tpp-program.html

References

Abma, J. C. (2001). *Sexual activity and contraceptive practices among teenagers in the United States, 1988 and 1995*. Hyattsville, MD: U.S. Dept. of Health and Human Services, Centers for Disease Control and Prevention, National Center for Health Statistics.

Alan Guttmacher Institute (AGI). (1981). *Teenage pregnancy: The problem that hasn't gone away*. New York, NY: Author.

Alan Guttmacher Institute (AGI). (1994). *Sex and America's teenagers*. New York, NY: Author.

Alan Guttmacher Institute (AGI). (2013). Fact sheet: Facts on American teens' sexual and reproductive health. Retrieved from http://www.guttmacher.org/pubs/FB-ATSRH.html

Albert, B. (2004). *With one voice 2004: America's adults & teens sound off about teen pregnancy*. Washington, DC: The National Campaign to Prevent Teen Pregnancy.

Alio, A. P., Mbah, A. K., Grunsten, R. A., & Salihu, H. M. (2011). Teenage pregnancy and the influence of paternal involvement on fetal outcomes. *Journal of Pediatric and Adolescent Gynecology*, *24*(6), 404–409.

Azjen, I., & Fishbein, M. (1980). *Understanding attitudes and predicting social behavior*. Englewood Cliffs, NJ: Prentice Hall.

Baker, T. J. (1996). Factors related to the initiation of prenatal care in the adolescent nullipara. *Nurse Practitioner*, *21*(2), 29–42.

Bandura, A. (1986). *Social learning theory*. Englewood Cliffs, NJ: Prentice Hall.

Becker, M. H. (1974). The health belief model and personal health behaviors. *Health Education Monographs*, *2*, 324–508.

Blake, S., Simkin, L., Ledsky, R., Perkins, D., & Calabresa, J. (2001). Effects of a parent–child communications intervention on young adolescents' risk for early onset of sexual intercourse. *Family Planning Perspective*, *33*(2), 52–62.

Blankson, M. L., Cliver, S. P., Goldenberg, R. L., Hickey, C. A., Jin, J., & Dubard, M. B. (1993). Health behavior and outcomes in sequential pregnancies of black and white adolescents. *Journal of the American Medical Association*, *269*(11), 1401–1403.

Blythe, M., & Diaz, A. (2007). Contraception and adolescents. *Pediatrics*, *120*(5), 1135–1148.

Bowen, M. (1971). The use of family theory in clinical practice. In J. Haley (Ed.), *Changing families*. New York, NY: Grune & Stratton.

Brown, H. N., Saunders, R. B., & Dick, M. J. (1999). Preventing secondary pregnancy in adolescents: A model program. *Health Care for Women International*, *20*(1), 5–15.

Bulcholz, E. S., & Gol, B. (1986). More than playing house: A developmental perspective on the strengths in teenage motherhood. *Theory and Review*, 347–357.

Cavazos-Rehg, P. A., Krauss, M. J., Spitznagel, E. L., Schootman, M., Cottler, L. B., & Bierut, L. J. (2010a). Associations between multiple pregnancies and health risk behaviors among U.S. adolescents. *Journal of Adolescent Health*, *47*(6), 600–603.

Cavazos-Rehg, P. A., Krauss, M. J., Spitznagel, E. L., Schootman, M., Peipert, J. F., Cottler, L. B., & Bierut, L. J. (2010b). Type of contraception method used at last intercourse and associations with health risk behaviors among U.S. adolescents. *Contraception*, *82*(6), 549–555.

Centers for Disease Control and Prevention (CDC). (2006). *Youth risk behavior survey*. Atlanta: U.S. Department of Health and Human Services.

Centers for Disease Control and Prevention (CDC). (2012). Youth risk behavior surveillance—United States, 2011. *Morbidity and Mortality Weekly Report, 61*(SS-4). Retrieved from http://www.cdc.gov/mmwr/pdf/ss/ss6104.pdf

Chedraui, P. (2008). Pregnancy among young adolescents: Trends, risk factors and maternal-perinatal outcome. *Journal of Perinatal Medicine, 36*(3), 256–259.

Cockey, C. D. (1997, June). Preventing teen pregnancy. It's time to stop kidding around. *Lifelines*, 32–40.

Coley, R. L., & Chase-Lansdale, P. L. (1998). Adolescent pregnancy and parenthood. Recent evidence and future directions. *American Psychologist, 53*(2), 152–166.

Collins, R., Elliott, M., Berry, S., Kanouse, D. E., Kunkel, D., Hunter, S. B., & Miu, A. (2004). Watching sex on television predicts adolescent initiation of sexual behavior. *Pediatrics, 114*(3), 280–289.

Cook, R., Erdman, J., & Dickens, B. (2007). Respecting adolescents' confidentiality and reproductive and sexual choices. *International Journal of Gynecology & Obstetrics, 98*(2), 182–187.

Coyle, K., Kirby, D., Parcel, G., Basen-Engquist, K., Banspach, S., Rugg, D., & Weil, M. (1996). Safer choices: A multicomponent school-based HIV/STD and pregnancy prevention program for adolescents. *Journal of School Health, 66*(3), 89–94.

Crowe, L. C., & George, W. H. (1989). Alcohol and human sexuality: Review and integration. *Psychological Bulletin, 102*, 374–386.

Darabi, K. F., Jones, J., Varga, P. L., & Hourse, M. (1982). Evaluation of sex education outreach. *Adolescence, 17*(65), 57–64.

Davis, K. A. (1980). *A theory of teenage pregnancy in the U.S. adolescent. Pregnancy and childbearing*. Washington, DC: U.S. Department of Health and Human Services.

Davis, S. M., & Harris, M. B. (1982). Sexual knowledge, sexual interests, and sources of sexual information of rural and urban adolescents from three cultures. *Adolescence, 18*(66), 471–492.

Delpisheh, A., Kelly, Y., Rizwan, S., Attia, E., Drammond, S., & Brabin, B. (2007). Population attributable risk for adverse pregnancy outcomes related to smoking in adolescents and adults. *Public Health, 121*(11), 861–868.

Desmond, A. M. (1994). Adolescent pregnancy in the United States: Not a minority issue. *Health Care for Women International, 15*(4), 325–331.

Diehl, K. (1997). Adolescent mothers: What produces positive mother–infant interaction? *Maternal Child Nursing, 22*, 89–95.

DiIorio, C., Hockenbeery-Eaton, M., Maibach, E., Rivero, S., & Miller, K. (1996). The content of African American mothers' discussions with their adolescents about sex. *Journal of Family Nursing, 2*(4), 365–382.

Drake, P. (1996). Addressing developmental needs of pregnant adolescents. *Journal of Obstetric, Gynecologic, & Neonatal Nursing, 25*(6), 518–524.

DuPlessis, H. M., Bell, R., & Richards, T. (1997). Adolescent pregnancy: Understanding the impact of age and race on outcomes. *Journal of Adolescent Health, 20*, 187–197.

East, P., Reyes, B., & Horn, E. (2007). Association between adolescent pregnancy and a family history of teenage births. *Perspectives on Sexual & Reproductive Health, 39*(2), 108–115.

Ellis, B. J., Bates, J. E., Dodge, K. A., Fergusson, D. M., Horwood, L. J., Pettit, G. S., & Woodward, L. (2009). Does father absence place daughters at special risk for early sexual activity and teenage pregnancy? *Child Development, 74*(3), 801–821.

Fagot, B., Pears, K., Capaldi, D., Crosby, L., & Leve, C. (1998). Becoming an adolescent father: Precursors and parenting. *Developmental Psychology, 34*(6), 1209–1219.

Fiscella, K., Kitzman, H. J., Cole, R. E., Sidora, K. J., & Olds, D. (1998). Does child abuse predict adolescent pregnancy? *Pediatrics, 101*(4 Pt. 1), 620–624.

Fisher, S. M. (1984). The psychodynamics of teenage pregnancy and motherhood. In M. Sugar (Ed.), *Adolescent parenthood*. Jamaica, NY: Spectrum Publications.

Flavell, J. H., Miller, P. H., & Miller, S. A. (1993). *Cognitive development* (3rd ed.). Englewood Cliffs, NJ: Prentice Hall.

Fletcher, J. M., & Wolfe, B. L. (2011). The effects of teenage fatherhood on young adult outcomes. *Economic Inquiry, 49*. doi: 10.1111/j.1465-7295.2011.00372.x. Retrieved from http://publichealth.yale.edu/news/archive/2011/81271_Teenage%20Fatherhood.pdf

Flynn, L., Budd, M., & Modelski, J. (2008). Enhancing resource utilization among pregnant adolescents. *Public Health Nursing, 25*(2), 140–148.

Fortenberry, J. D., Orr, D. P., Katz, B. P., Brizendine, E. J., & Blythe, M. J. (1997). Sex under the influence. *Sexually Transmitted Diseases, 24*(6), 313–319.

Foster, H. W. (1997). The campaign to prevent teen pregnancy. *Journal of Pediatric Nursing, 12*(2), 120–121.

Geronimus, A. (1986). The effects of race, residence and prenatal care on the relationship of maternal age to neonatal mortality. *American Journal of Public Health, 76*(12), 1412–1421.

Grobler, C., Botma, Y., Jacobs, A., & Nel, M. (2007). Beliefs of grade six learners' regarding adolescent pregnancy and sex. *Curationis, 30*(1), 32–40.

Grogger, J., & Bronars, S. (1993). The socioeconomic consequences of teenage childbearing: Finding from a natural experiment. *Family Planning Perspectives, 25*(4), 156–161, 174.

Heavey, E., Moysich, K., Hyland, A., Druschel, C., & Sill, M. (2008). Female adolescents' perceptions of male partners' pregnancy desire. *Journal of Midwifery & Women's Health, 53*(4), 338–344.

Hoffman, S. D. (2006). *By the numbers: The public costs of teen childbearing.* Washington, DC: National Campaign to Prevent Teen Pregnancy.

Howard, M., & McCabe, J. A. (1992). An information and skills approach for younger teens: Postponing sexual involvement program. In B. C. Miller, J. T. Card, R. L. Paifoff, & J. I. Peterson (Eds.), *Preventing adolescent pregnancy.* Newbury Park, CA: Sage.

Howard, M., & Mitchell, M. E. (1993). Preventing teenage pregnancy: Some questions to be answered and some answers to be questioned. *Pediatric Annals, 22*(2), 109–118.

Ispa, J., Sable, M., Porter, N., & Csizmadia, A. (2007). Pregnancy acceptance, parenting stress, and toddler attachment in low-income black families. *Journal of Marriage & Family, 69*(1), 1–13.

Jemmott, L. S. (1993). AIDS risk among black male adolescents: Implications for nursing intervention. *Journal of Pediatric Health Care, 7*, 3–11.

Jemmott, L. S., & Jemmott, J. B., III. (1990). Sexual knowledge, attitudes, and risky sexual behavior among inner-city black male adolescents. *Journal of Adolescent Research, 5*, 346–369.

Jemmott, L. S., & Jemmott, J. B., III. (1992). Increasing condom-use intentions among sexually active inner city black adolescent women: Effects of an AIDS prevention program. *Nursing Research, 41*, 273–279.

Jemmott, L. S., & Jemmott, J. B., III (2007). Applying the theory of reasoned action to HIV risk reduction behavioral interventions. In A. Icek, D. Albarracin, & R. Hornik (Eds.), *Prediction and change of health behavior: Applying the reasoned action approach* (pp. 93–100). Mahwah, NJ: Lawrence Erlbaum Associates.

Jemmott, J., Jemmott, L., & Fong, G. (1998). Abstinence and safer sex HIV risk-reduction interventions for African American adolescents: A randomized controlled trial. *Journal of the American Medical Association, 279*(19), 1529–1536.

Jemmott, L., Jemmott, J., Hutchinson, M., Cederbaum, J., & O'Leary, A. (2008, March). Sexually transmitted infection/HIV risk reduction interventions in clinical practice settings. *JOGNN: Journal of Obstetric, Gynecologic, & Neonatal Nursing, 37*(2), 137–145.

Jemmott, L. S., Jemmott, J. B., & O'Leary, A. (2007). Effects on sexual risk behavior and STD rate of brief HIV/STD prevention interventions for African American women in primary care settings: Effects on sexual risk behavior and STD incidence. *American Journal of Public Health, 97*, 1034–1040.

Kahn, J. G., Brindis, C. D., & Glei, D. A. (1999). Pregnancies averted among U.S. teenagers by the use of contraceptives. *Family Planning Perspectives, 31*(1), 29–34.

Kaiser Family Foundation. (1998). *National survey of teens: Teens talk about dating, intimacy and their sexual experiences*. Menlo Park, CA: Author.

Kalmus, D., Davidson, A., Cahall, A., Laraque, D., & Cassell, C. (2003). Preventing sexual risk behaviors and pregnancy among teenagers: Linking research and programs. *Perspectives on Sexual and Reproductive Health, 35*, 87–93.

Kandel, D. B. (1990). Early onset of adolescent sexual behavior and drug involvement. *Journal of Marriage and the Family, 52*, 783–798.

Kearney, M. S., & Levine, P. B. (2012). Why is the teen birth rate in the United States so high and why does it matter? *Journal of Economic Perspectives, 26*(2), 141–166.

Kenney, J. W., Reinholtz, C., & Angelini, P. J. (1997). Ethnic differences in childhood sexual abuse and teenage pregnancy. *Journal of Adolescent Health, 21*(1), 3–10.

Kirby, D. (1997). *No easy answers: Research findings on programs to reduce teen pregnancy* (Summary). Washington, DC: The National Campaign to Prevent Teen Pregnancy.

Kirby, D. (2001). Understanding what works and what doesn't in reducing adolescent sexual risk-taking. *Family Planning Perspectives, 33*(6), 276–281.

Kirby, D., Resnick, M. D., Downes, B., Kocher, T., Gunderson, P., Potthoff, S., ... Blum, R. W. (1993). The effects of school-based health clinics in St. Paul on school-wide birthrates. *Family Planning Perspectives, 25*(1), 12–16.

Kohler, P. K., Manhart, L. E., & Lafferty, W. E. (2008). Abstinence-only and comprehensive sex education and the initiation of sexual activity and teen pregnancy. *Journal of Adolescent Health, 42*(4), 344–351.

Kokotailo, P. K., Langhough, R. E., Cox, N. S., Davidson, S. R., & Fleming, M. F. (1994). Cigarette, alcohol and other drug use among small city pregnant adolescents. *Journal of Adolescent Health, 15*, 366–373.

Landry, E., Bertrand, J., Cherry, F., & Rich, J. (1986). Teenage pregnancy in New Orleans: Factors that differentiate teens who deliver, abort, and successfully contracept. *Journal of Youth and Adolescence, 15*, 259–274.

Lau, M., Lin, H., & Flores, G. (2014). Pleased to be pregnant? Positive pregnancy attitudes among sexually active adolescent females in the United States. *Journal of Pediatric and Adolescent Gynecology, 27*(4), 210–215.

Lederman, R., & Mian, T. (2003). The parent–adolescent relationship education (PARE) program: A curriculum for prevention of STDs and pregnancy in middle-school youth. *Behavioral Medicine, 3*(29), 33–41.

Lee, S. H., & Grubbs, L. M. (1995). Pregnant teenagers' reasons for seeking or delaying prenatal care. *Clinical Nursing Research, 4*(1), 38–49.

Lemay, C., Cashman, S., Elfenbein, D., & Felice, M. (2007). Adolescent mothers' attitudes toward contraceptive use before and after pregnancy. *Journal of Pediatric & Adolescent Gynecology, 20*(4), 233–240.

Leppert, P. C., Namerow, P. B., & Barker, D. (1986). Pregnancy outcomes among adolescents and older women receiving comprehensive prenatal care. *Journal of Adolescent Health Care, 7*, 112–117.

Levy, S. R., Perhats, C., Nash-Johnson, M., & Welter, J. F. (1992). Reducing the risks in pregnant teens who are very young and those with mild mental retardation. *Mental Retardation, 30*(4), 195–203.

Lieberman, E. J. (1980). *The psychological consequences of adolescent pregnancy and abortion: Adolescent pregnancy and childbearing.* Washington, DC: U.S. Department of Health and Human Services.

Loda, F. A., Speizer, I. S., Martin, K. L., Skatrud, J. D., & Bennett, T. A. (1997). Programs and services to prevent pregnancy, childbearing, and poor birth outcomes among adolescents in rural areas of the Southeastern United States. *Journal of Adolescent Health, 21*, 157–166.

Lowe, S. (2008). It's all one big circle: Welfare discourse and the everyday lives of urban adolescents. *Journal of Sociology & Social Welfare, 35*(3), 173–194.

Males, M. (1993). School-age pregnancy: Why hasn't prevention worked? *Journal of School Health, 63*(10), 429–432.

Manlove, J., Ikramullah, E., & Terry-Humen, E. (2008). Condom use and consistency among male adolescents in the United States. *Journal of Adolescent Health, 43*(4), 1–9.

Marshall, E., Buckner, E., & Powell, K. (1991). Evaluation of a teen parent program designed to reduce child abuse and neglect and to strengthen families. *Journal of Child Adolescent Psychiatric and Mental Health Nursing, 4*(3), 96–100.

Martin, J. A., Hamilton, B. E., Osterman, M. J. K., Curtin, S. C., & Matthews, T. J. (2013). Births: Final data for 2012. *National Vital Statistics Report, 62*(9). Retrieved from http://www.cdc.gov/nchs/data/nvsr/nvsr62/nvsr62_09.pdf#table02

Martinez, G., Copen, C. E., & Abma, J. C. (2011). Teenagers in the United States: Sexual activity, contraceptive use, and childbearing, 2006–2010 National Survey of Family Growth. *Vital and Health Statistics, 23*(31). Retrieved from http://www.cdc.gov/nchs/data/series/sr_23/sr23_031.pdf

Miller, B. (2002). Family influences on adolescent sexual and contraceptive behavior. *Journal of Sex Research, 39*, 22–26.

Miller, W. B., Trent, M., & Chung, S. E. (2014). Ambivalent childbearing motivations: Predicting condom use by urban, African-American, female youth. *Journal of Pediatric and Adolescent Gynecology, 27*(3), 151–160.

Morrison, D. (1985). Adolescent contraceptive behavior: A review. *Psychological Bulletin, 98*, 538–568.

Mott, S. (1990). Adolescence. In S. Mott, S. James, & A. Sperhac (Eds.), *Care of children and families*. Redwood City, CA: Addison-Wesley.

Olds, D. (1992). Home visitation for pregnant women and parents of young children. *American Journal of Diseases of Children, 146*(6), 704–708.

Olds, D., Henderson, C., & Kitzman, H. (1994). Does prenatal and infancy nurse home visitation have enduring effects on qualities of parental caregiving and child health at 25 to 50 months of life? *Pediatrics, 93*(1), 89–98.

Olds, D., Henderson, C., Tatelbaum, R., & Chamberlin, R. (1988). Improving the life-course development of socially disadvantaged mothers: A randomized trial of nurse home visitation. *American Journal of Public Health, 78*(11), 1436–1445.

Orshan, S. A. (1996). Acculturation, perceived social support, and self-esteem in primigravida Puerto Rican teenagers. *Western Journal of Nursing Research, 18*(4), 460–473.

Pittman, K., & Adams, G. (1988). *Teenage pregnancy: An advocate's guide to the numbers*. Washington, DC: Children's Defense Fund.

Planned Parenthood Foundation (PPF). (2012). Fact sheet: Pregnancy and childbearing among U.S. teens. Retrieved from http://www.plannedparenthood.org/files/PPFA/pregnancy_and_childbearing.pdf

Plouffe, L., & White, E. W. (1996). Adolescent obstetrics and gynecology: Children having children—Can it be controlled? *Current Opinion in Obstetrics and Gynecology, 8*(5), 335–338.

Pollack, A. E. (1992). Teen contraception in the 1990s. *Journal of School Health, 62*(7), 288–293.

Rew, L. (1998). The adolescent. In N. C. Frisch & L. E. Frisch (Eds.), *Psychiatric mental health nursing*. Albany, NY: Delmar.

Reynoso, T. C., Felice, M. E., & Shragg, G. P. (1993). Does American acculturation affect outcome of Mexican-American teenage pregnancy? *Journal of Adolescent Health, 14*, 257–261.

Robinson, R. B., & Frank, D. L. (1994). The relation between self-esteem, sexual activity, and pregnancy. *Adolescence, 29*(113), 26–35.

Rogers, M. M., Peoples-Sheps, M. D., & Suchindran, C. (1996). Impact of a social support program on teenage prenatal care use and pregnancy outcomes. *Journal of Adolescent Health, 19*, 132–140.

Rolleri, L., Wilson, M., Paluzzi, P., & Sedivy, V. (2008). Building capacity of state adolescent pregnancy prevention coalitions to implement science-based approaches. *American Journal of Community Psychology, 41*(3/4), 225–234.

Rosenbaum, J. E. (2009). Patient teenagers? A comparison of the sexual behavior of virginity pledgers and matched nonpledgers. *Pediatrics, 123*(1), e110–e120.

Roye, C. F., & Balk, S. J. (1996). The relationship of partner support to outcomes for teenage mothers and their children: A review. *Journal of Adolescent Health, 19*, 86–93.

Santelli, J., Lindberg, L., Finer, L., & Singh, S. (2007). Explaining recent declines in adolescent pregnancy in the United States: The contribution of abstinence and improved contraceptive use. *Contemporary Sexuality, 41*(7), 8–12.

Schaffer, M., Jost, R., Pederson, B., & Lair, M. (2008). Pregnancy-free club: A strategy to prevent repeat adolescent pregnancy. *Public Health Nursing, 25*(4), 304–311.

Schaffer, M. A., Goodhue, A., Stennes, K., & Lanigan, C. (2012). Evaluation of a public health nurse visiting program for pregnant and parenting teens. *Public Health Nursing, 29*(3), 218–231.

Selkie, E. M., Benson, M., & Moreno, M. (2011). Adolescents' views regarding uses of social networking websites and text messaging for adolescent sexual health education. *American Journal of Health Education, 42*(4), 205–212.

SmithBattle, L. (2007). Legacies of advantage and disadvantage: The case of teen mothers. *Public Health Nursing, 24*(5), 409–420.

Sonenstein, F., Stewart, K., Lindberg, L., Pernas, M., & Williams, S. (1997). Practical advice and program philosophy. In *Involving males in preventing teen pregnancy* (pp. 153–174). Washington, DC: Urban Institute Press.

Sorenson, D. (1973). *Adolescent sexuality in contemporary America*. New York, NY: World Press.

Stevens-Simon, C., Kelly, L., Singer, D., & Cox, A. (1996). Why pregnant adolescents say they did not use contraceptives prior to contraception. *Journal of Adolescent Health, 19*, 48–53.

Terry-Humen, E., & Manlove, J. (2003). Just who is having sex before age 15? Dating and sexual experience among middle school youth: Analysis of the NLSY97. In B. Albert, S. Brown, & C. M. Flanigan (Eds.), *14 and younger: The sexual behavior of young adolescents (Full Report)*. Washington, DC: The National Campaign to Prevent Teen Pregnancy.

Thompson, P. J., Powell, M. J., Patterson, R. J., & Ellerbee, S. M. (1995). Adolescent parenting: Outcomes and maternal perceptions. *Journal of Obstetric, Gynecologic, & Neonatal Nursing, 24*(8), 713–717.

Tocce, K., Sheeder, J., & Teal, S. (2008). The road to repeat adolescent pregnancy is paved with good intentions. *Contraception, 78*(2), 176–176.

Toledo-Dreves, V., Zabin, L. S., & Emerson, M. (1995). Duration of adolescent sexual relationships before and after conception. *Journal of Adolescent Health, 17*, 163–172.

Trad, P. V. (1999). Assessing the patterns that prevent teenage pregnancy. *Adolescence, 34*(133), 221–240.

Trenholm, C., Devaney, B., Fortson, K., Clark, M., Bridgespan, L. Q., & Wheeler, J. (2008). Impacts of abstinence education on teen sexual activity, risk of pregnancy, and risk of sexually transmitted diseases. *Journal of Policy Analysis and Management, 27*(2), 255–276.

U.S. Department of Health and Human Services (HHS). (2013a). Trends in teen pregnancy and childbearing: Teen births. Retrieved from http://www.hhs.gov/ash/oah/adolescent-health-topics/reproductive-health/teen-pregnancy/trends.html

U.S. Department of Health and Human Services. (2013b). *Healthy people 2020: Topics and objectives—Family planning.* Retrieved from http://www.healthypeople.gov/2020/topicsobjectives2020/objectiveslist.aspx?topicId=13

U.S. Department of Health and Human Services. (2013c). *Healthy people 2020: Topics and objectives—Maternal, infant, and child health.* Retrieved from http://www.healthypeople.gov/2020/topicsobjectives2020/objectiveslist.aspx?topicId=26

Ventura, S., Abma, J., Mosher, W., & Henshaw, S. (2006). *Recent trends in teenage pregnancy in the United States 1990–2002.* Hyattsville, MD: National Center for Health Statistics.

Villarruel, A., Jemmott, J., Jemmott, L., & Ronis, D. (2007). Predicting condom use among sexually experienced Latino adolescents. *Western Journal of Nursing Research, 29*(6), 724–738.

Whitbeck, L. B., Conger, R. D., & Simons, R. I. (1993). Minor deviant behaviors and adolescent sexual activity. *Youth and Society, 25*(1), 24–37.

Widom, C. S., & Kuhns, J. B. (1996). Childhood victimization and subsequent risk for promiscuity, prostitution, and teenage pregnancy: A prospective study. *American Journal of Public Health, 86*(11), 1607–1612.

Williams, S., & Thompson, M. P. (2013). Examining the prospective effects of making a virginity pledge among males across their 4 years of college. *Journal of American College Health, 61*(2), 114–120.

Wilson, R., Alio, A., Kirby, R., & Salihu, H. (2008). Young maternal age and risk of intrapartum stillbirth. *Archives of Gynecology & Obstetrics, 278*(3), 231–236.

Yoder, B. A., & Young, M. K. (1997). Neonatal outcomes of teenage pregnancy in a military population. *Obstetrics & Gynecology, 90*(4), 500–506.

Zabin, L. S., & Clark, S. D. (1981). Why they delay: A study of teenage family planning clinic patients. *Family Planning Perspective, 13*, 205–217.

Zabin, L. S., Emerson, M. R., Ringers, P. A., & Sedivy, V. (1996). Adolescents with negative pregnancy test results: An accessible at-risk group. *Journal of the American Medical Association, 275*(2), 113–117.

Zeck, W., Bjelic-Radisic, V., Haas, J., & Greimel, E. (2007). Impact of adolescent pregnancy on the future life of young mothers in terms of social, familial, and educational changes. *Journal of Adolescent Health, 41*(4), 380–388.

Zeck, W., Walcher, W., Tamussino, K., & Lang, U. (2008). Adolescent primiparas: Changes in obstetrical risk between 1983–1987 and 1999–2005. *Journal of Obstetrics & Gynaecology Research, 34*(2), 195–198.

Zelnik, M., & Kantner, J. F. (1979). Reasons for nonuse of contraception by sexually active women age 15–19. *Family Planning Perspectives, 11*(5), 289–296.

Zoccolillo, M., Meyers, J., & Assiter, S. (1997). Conduct disorder, substance dependence, and adolescent motherhood. *American Journal of Orthopsychiatry, 67*(1), 152–157.

Zuckerman, B. S., Walker, D. K., Frank, D. A., Chase, C., & Hamburg, B. (1984). Adolescent pregnancy: Biobehavioral determinants of outcome. *Journal of Pediatrics, 105*(6), 857–863.

CHAPTER FOCUS

The Unique Role and Perspective of Psychiatric–Mental Health Nursing in Caring for the Public's Health

Definitions of Mental Health

History of Mental Health in the Community

- Early Humanitarian Reform in Mental Health
- Community Mental Health Reform in the 1960s
- Legislation Impacting Mental Health

Historical Context for Professional Nursing

History and Spirit of Psychiatric–Mental Health Nursing in the Community

- State of the Science of Psychiatric–Mental Health Nursing
- Levels of Psychiatric–Mental Health Nursing Practice

Individuals and Population Groups Needing Psychiatric–Mental Health Services

Current Assessment of the Public's Mental Health Status

- Ethics of Psychiatric–Mental Health Services

Psychiatric–Mental Health Nursing's Roles and Phenomena of Concern

- Guiding Philosophical and Theoretical Frameworks for Mental Health Nursing

Models for Psychiatric–Mental Health Nursing Practice

- Public Health Model
- Primary Care Model
- Primary Mental Health Care Model
- Using Reflection in Nursing Education and Practice
- Using a Phenomenological Perspective: Understanding the Public's Mental Health Lived Experience, One Person at a Time

The Future of Psychiatric–Mental Health Nursing Practice

QUESTIONS TO CONSIDER

After reading this chapter, you will know the answers to the following questions:

1. What is the definition of *mental health in the community*?
2. What is the history of community mental health nursing?
3. What is the current mental health status of Americans?
4. What are some of the conceptual and theoretical frameworks for psychiatric–mental health nursing?
5. What are some of the models for psychiatric–mental health nursing practice?
6. What will psychiatric–mental health nursing practice be like in the future?

Given contemporary life in society with its constant state of change, it is imperative that nurses in psychiatric–mental health take self-care and caring for one another seriously. Nurses must develop self-care strategies that ensure they enjoy balanced, healthy, meaningful lives.

CHAPTER 27

Psychiatric Care and Mental Health in the Community

Sarah Steen Lauterbach and John Hodnett

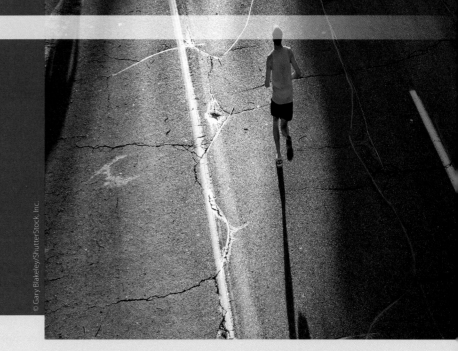

KEY TERMS

advocacy
community mental health centers (CMHCs)
mental health
phenomena of concern
phenomenology
presence
prevention
psychiatric–mental health nursing
seriously mentally ill
universal human experiences

REFLECTIONS

Much madness is divinist sense
To a discerning eye;
Much sense the starkest madness.
'Tis the majority
In this, as all, prevails.
Assent, and you are sane;
Demur,—you're straightway dangerous,
And handled with a chain.

—*Emily Dickinson*

Mental health is a neglected area of public health. Community health nurses work within a holistic framework and address the entire spectrum of a community's health. After reading Emily Dickinson's poem, reflect on your own ideas about what contributes to mental wellbeing.

THE IDEA OF MENTAL HEALTH in this chapter is embedded within cultural, social, political, and economic contexts of the time, and within a historical—and contemporary—perspective. The chapter presents psychiatric–mental health (P-MH) conditions and treatment as being contextually bound, and ultimately responding to the state of knowledge and science surrounding mental health. Additionally, the influence of nursing history and professional **psychiatric–mental health nursing** practice are relevant to the idea of mental health. Mental health and illness play a key role in determining the state of the public's health. This chapter examines the American public's mental health and illness continuum, using current information—that is, demographic, population, and epidemiological data.

Although population and numerical data are tremendously useful, it is also important to use qualitative, humanistic perspectives and lenses in assessing and understanding mental health. Conceptual frameworks, interdisciplinary theory, nursing theory, philosophical perspectives, and models for reflective practice are particularly useful in understanding current care and practice.

The central context used for defining the scope of P-MH nursing is the state of knowledge and research and nursing's historic role in social reform and activism. Receiving particular emphasis in the chapter is the unique contribution made by P-MH nursing to professional nursing. Specifically, this contribution lies in articulating for professional nursing a primary role in facilitating and developing therapeutic relationships with persons, families, groups, and populations at risk. It is rooted in Hildegard Peplau's (1952) nursing work and text, *Interpersonal Relations in Nursing*. This classic work established therapeutic relationships as a primary focus, underpinning the entire nursing discipline. Her intent was to involve the patient in actual care, not as a passive recipient, but to actively develop a therapeutic nurse–patient relationship to establish a comfortable place for the patient/client to gain strength and emotional wellbeing. The multiple theoretical perspectives nursing uses contribute to its unique role, which will be discussed in detail in this chapter. The focus on facilitating and developing relationships underpins nursing in every care context and role, and is proposed to serve as a primary task for all nurses. It underlies nursing's potential role in promoting health and wellness, preventing disability and dysfunction, and treating and restoring the mental health of the public.

Public health policy and care provision need to be inclusive of mental health, and P-MH services and treatments need to be mainstreamed into the primary healthcare system. Currently, the private-public split in P-MH care establishes and promotes disparities in the public's mental health. Public programs carry the burden of serving the chronically and **seriously mentally ill** (SMI) with inadequate resources. The inequity and disparities relate to access, quality, and cost of care, and they have direct effects on mental health, especially for vulnerable groups. The dual nature of the P-MH care system serves to further impoverish vulnerable and at-risk populations, such as the homeless, incarcerated SMI, and people with both physical and mental disabilities. It is time for the overarching goals of *Healthy People 2020* of improving mental health through preventive measures and accessible services to be taken seriously. Responsible, ethical, social, and health policy reform continues to be drastically needed. With the passage of the Affordable Care Act (ACA) of 2010, federal healthcare reform now includes mandatory coverage of mental health services.

This chapter includes textual contributions from creative writers, artists, and public figures as reflective of classic struggles that many humans face. Many of the

AFFORDABLE CARE ACT 

The ACA, federal healthcare reform, now includes mandatory coverage of mental health services. All marketplace insurance plans cover mental health and substance abuse services as an essential health benefit. Other provisions of the ACA related to mental health and substance abuse include coverage for treatment of preexisting conditions and no lifetime or yearly dollar limits for mental health and substance abuse services.

Source: https://www.healthcare.gov/do-marketplace-insurance-plans-cover-mental-health-and-substance-abuse-services/

most accomplished people who have made tremendous contributions to science, literature, and art have lived with serious mental health conditions. Their contributions and wisdom have been very helpful in articulating what it is like to be human. These sources are especially informative for healthcare professionals and the public in understanding what it is like to live with mental health and/or illness. Additionally, the comments of students are included as they reflect on their growing awareness and understanding of mental health and illness and learn what it is like to provide therapeutic healing care and relationships.

Universal human phenomena are discussed as still in need of research and public policy attention. Many common human conditions and experiences need to be explored by using reflection to explicate the meanings in experiences. These conditions are often involved in the etiology of P-MH problems and dysfunction. Conditions and experiences particularly needing exploration include dealing with loss, death, change, anxiety, stress, crisis, inadequate coping, depression, and disappointment. Reflection offers an opportunity to enhance understanding through reflecting on meanings in experiences. As understanding grows, enhanced care and treatment potentially become better informed and facilitated.

Quiver of Fear

Quiver of fear down the spine
    Black towers of
    Never ending hallways

Florescent lit
White coated men

Come Daddy.
    Why?

There is no merciful prayer,
    No merciful answer
    Not for me
    Not for you.

—*Ann Thedford Lanier*

The Unique Role and Perspective of Psychiatric–Mental Health Nursing in Caring for the Public's Health

The unique and special contribution of psychiatric nursing in caring for the public's mental health comes from the specialty's history, commitment, and expertise in therapeutic communication and relationship development. The P-MH nurse engages in *therapeutic use of self*, a concept that involves the nurse becoming and being an *instrument of care*. Through using self in communication therapeutically, and through using expert relationship-building knowledge, "We can, literally, become the healing environment" (Quinn, 1992).

Becoming the healing environment in caring for the public's mental health often involves providing both very vulnerable people and functional people with basic human needs for trust, support, and security, as well as specialty treatment and care. Many P-MH nurses see the specialty as underpinning all of nursing, with professional nursing literally becoming the healing environment and being the instrument of care in each nursing encounter regardless of specialty or practice arena.

The patient–nurse relationship is developed over time and is cultivated through the development of a trusting rapport. The trusting rapport is evolved through the nurse's ability to understand the client's perspective of his or her issues and feelings. Additionally, the relationship is fostered through the nurse's reflecting the client's feelings and body language (i.e., active listening), thereby gaining complete understanding of the client's present state. The patient is heard and understood with the nurse having a true comprehensive understanding, not merely from supposition. Weger, Castle, and Emmett (2010) describe active listening as having "unconditional acceptance and unbiased reflection" (p. 35) between a client and therapist/nurse.

Nursing's professional commitment to holistic care, providing the public with a holistic, caring presence, is actualized in the P-MH concept of relationship. The focus on providing comfort care—caring for persons in the present as well as in the future—provides a temporal relationship in caring for the public that is unique to nursing. Nursing caring involves *doing for*, *being with*, *helping*, and *healing through relationships* when the person is incapable of self-care. The nursing focus is on understanding a person's history using strengths and resources to address areas of needed change.

Presence is another concept used to describe nursing work. *Being fully present for another*, with an intention to facilitate and promote healing and comfort, and *being with* people are nursing intentions and goals. It is critical that the nurse understands the experience from the perspective of the person in need of care. In being fully present, often the nurse must look at and explicate past personal experiences, biases, and attitudes.

Self-reflection is a critical activity and process in P-MH nursing. Reflective education and practice activities are provided throughout this chapter. Through reflection, the nurse is able to become more aware of, and use bracketing to put aside, personal material consciously so that the nursing presence is focused on those in need. Reflection and bracketing become critical in understanding the person. Reflection and bracketing pre-understandings and biases, values, and attitudes make it possible for the nurse to become fully present in caring for the mental health needs of the other.

In P-MH nursing, the nurse is involved with implementing treatment programs, and with facilitating, developing, and using groups and the therapeutic milieu. The context of caring for persons 24/7 puts P-MH nurses in a similar role to nurses in other nursing specialties. Nurses assist people in their activities of daily living (ADLs). P-MH patients often have difficulty in navigating through self-care routines. Similarly, in chronic care, self-care deficits are often the norm.

The nurse is often the point person in case management of mental health patients. The P-MH nurse has a history of accepting responsibility for and demonstrating a long-term commitment for care. P-MH nursing has an ethic of responsibility for caring for persons, especially vulnerable groups and populations over the lifespan. Follow-up care, communication, and partnering with other disciplines and agencies are critical to providing comprehensive, holistic care.

Finally, nursing work is often very private, especially when considering the stigma attached to and attitudes of many people toward people suffering from mental health problems. Just as cancer was once a dreaded, stigmatized condition, mental health problems are often associated with stigma. Education and research, along with improvements in treatment, should eventually eliminate this phenomenon that surrounds mental health care. Further, knowledge and understanding must be consciously implemented and planned.

Nursing often involves body work, up close and personal. In P-MH, the personal aspects of the disease often involve lack of ability to function or problematic behaviors and symptoms. Mental health symptoms are often complex and difficult to manage or control. This unique vantage point taken by the caregiver provides the P-MH nurse with an opportunity to know the person intimately and, therefore, makes the nursing role potentially sensitive and complicated. Nurses are involved with people who experience alterations in health and, in many cases, intolerable suffering.

As stated earlier, in P-MH nursing the therapeutic relationship is the primary instrument of care. It is through

APPLICATION TO PRACTICE

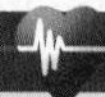

Reflective Education and Practice Exercise 1

Caring for Self

The idea of caring for self was a hard concept for me to undertake. I've always been a person who enjoyed helping others, and often would get so caught up in others that self could be considered a foreign thing at times. It is sometimes easier to avoid looking at myself and my own problems by making other people the focus of my attention.

However, when this assignment began, I wanted to make a legitimate effort to look at my needs, and the areas where I needed improvement.... There were several areas that needed to be addressed, including the need for appropriate amounts of sleep, leisure, and relaxation. I found these to be very important, especially when going through the mental health clinical experiences. I was feeling drained and would go home and just sleep for hours and hours, sometimes not waking until the next morning. I recognized that this was an ineffective coping method for the stress I felt. To combat those feelings, I started doing meditation and prayer on the mornings of the clinical or when I knew I would have a challenging day. Doing these activities completely changed my attitude and the experiences that I had. During the rest of my clinicals, I was much more mentally and emotionally prepared to learn what the experience had to teach me, and I slept soundly at night, not during the day.

—BSN nursing student

As we all know, nursing school is no walk in the park. It has to be one of the most difficult, time-consuming things I've ever had to go through in my life. I've never had to work as much or as hard as I have for these classes. I realize, however, that during these trying times, I need to take care of myself as well as working for the grades I am attempting to achieve. . . . In my life after college, I hope to live as much of a holistic life as possible: I want to go to work, exercise regularly, and eat well. I think that when working in health care, it is important to be healthy yourself—otherwise, you might be contradictory. If you tell your patient to do something like exercise a few times a week, and you yourself don't do it, then it makes you look bad. Of course, I want to exercise for my life . . . I want to live a long, happy life so I need to take care of the body I have because it's the only one I'll get.

—BSN nursing student

the development and maintenance of relationships with people over time that nursing P-MH work is accomplished.

Nurses learn from the beginning of the nursing educational experience that therapeutic use of self and communication are critical in intervention and healing. Through the proximity of nursing involved in intimately engaging in patients' lives, the nurse can become a role model for relationships and communication. The P-MH nurse mentors, guides, coaches, and assists persons in becoming more fully functional.

To become a fully functioning P-MH nurse requires that opportunities provided by nursing education and nursing practice for self-reflection are fully embraced. Reflection is a process through which one's awareness of values, perceptions, and meanings in life experience is enhanced. Through reflection, there is an enhanced understanding of self and others, a heightened awareness of meanings in experiences, and potential for taking action.

Knowing, a concept introduced by Parse (1998), is a process through which the nurse–patient relationship evolves. In her Human Becoming Theory, Parse identifies the nurse as a not-knowing stranger and advocates establishing a relationship with the client without judgment or preconceived notions. The nurse enters the role in practice as a stranger to the client and listens to the client's perception of his or her reality, which is the real meaning of reality. The nurse joins the client in true presence of his or her reality and makes no judgments, but makes witness of changing health patterns (Parse, 1998).

Human becoming is lived on a continuum. During the therapeutic relationship, new themes or problems may emerge and the process will adjust to assist the client with those needs. Parse (1998) refers to these newly identified issues as paradoxes and believes these paradoxes are true to human becoming and living (Bunkers, 2002). Surmounting these paradoxes develops synchronized movement and rhythm, which propels the client into human becoming. Entering a therapeutic relationship and experiencing true presence with a client indicates unquestioned trust between the client and nurse.

> No temper could be more cheerful than hers, or possess, to a greater degree, that sanguine expectation of happiness which is happiness itself.
>
> —*Jane Austen, 1775–1817*

To care for others fully, the nurse must first care for self (Lauterbach & Becker, 1996; Lauterbach & Becker Hentz, 1998, 2005). This issue is especially important considering the nursing shortage. Many see nursing as an oppressed profession, with nurses' burnout further threatening the public's health. Given today's stresses, it is imperative that nurses in P-MH take self-care and caring for one another seriously. Nurses—P-MH nurses in particular—must develop self-care strategies that ensure they enjoy balanced, healthy, meaningful lives. Self-care is no longer just a choice or a nice thing to do, but rather a necessity. Otherwise, nurses' and the public's care and safety will suffer, stress and anxiety will be exacerbated, and personal feelings of security will be unattainable for nurses. The reader is referred to the boxes throughout this chapter, which focus on reflection, journaling, and caring for self.

In summary, through interaction and development of relationships, P-MH nursing is committed to caring and facilitating healing for persons, families, groups, communities, populations, nations, and the planet/environment. It is through the context of helping relationships that nurses respond to and care for self and others, interacting with patient systems, other professions, and community partners in a diversity of health and human life contexts.

Definitions of Mental Health

Definitions of mental health in literature range from a focus on the absence of disease to the attainment of one's potential.

> Everything has been figured out, except how to live.
>
> —*Jean Paul Sartre, 1905–1980*

Concepts of mental health and illness have changed drastically over the last few centuries. In the 15th century the mentally ill were thought to be witches "possessed" by demons. Some cultures historically regarded persons with psychiatric conditions as worthy of great respect, as having uncanny abilities and as visionaries. At one time, mental illness was thought to be caused by a lesion or physical injury to the brain. If no objective injury or lesion was found, mental illness was thought to be a defect in morality and character.

Since the early 1900s, identifying the mentally ill has been the focus of psychiatry. Great efforts were made toward the diagnosis and treatment of specific mental disorders and conditions. The development of the *Diagnostic and Statistical Manual of Mental Disorders* (*DSM*; now in its 5th revision) by the American Psychiatric Association (APA) since the 1950s (APA, 1980, 1987, 1992, 2000, 2013) has contributed to differentiation and research. Designated as "the decade of the brain," the focus of research in the 1990s has contributed to a more comprehensive understanding of biological determinants of behavior (Hedaya, 1996). The major psychiatric milestones of the 20th century included the development of the diagnostic manual and assessment procedures; psychotherapy, including psychoanalysis; developmental theories; behavioral, cognitive, and psychological foci for psychotherapy, including crisis intervention, short-term, group, family, and long-term therapy; psychopharmacology; and knowledge concerning the biological determinants of behavior.

The definition of **mental health** is still in need of our attention and continued thinking in nursing. Many believe that the focus on biology has obscured, once again, the understanding of mental illness or mental health. The view of mental health in this chapter encompasses the notion that mental health involves connection of body, mind, and spirit, in mental and physical wholesomeness. The concept of "balance" is common in holistic literature. Mental health is further viewed as involving a process through which a (w)holistic balance between mind, body, and spirit (of individuals, families, groups, communities, and the public at large) is pursued through meaningful life activities. The mentally healthy person seeks experiences that promote wellbeing, productivity, and happiness as fully as possible given the particular situational contexts and limitations.

This notion of health is consistent with the aim of phenomenological inquiry. The ultimate aim of phenomenology is to assist persons, through understanding, to "become fully human." Nursing has historically embraced a role with caring that has focused on maximizing human potential. A focus on maintaining harmony and balance is needed in many areas of human endeavor and experience: in meaningful work, occupation, or pursuit; in relationships with loved ones, significant others, and in social relationships, friendships, and work relationships; in meaningful relaxation, leisure, balanced nutrition, and fitness activities; and in having a respect and responsibility for the planet and world.

Mental illness or dysfunction, although it exists more in vulnerable population groups, is not wholly a respecter of vulnerability. There have been and currently are many gifted as well as ordinary people who have periodic mental health issues and conditions. The arts and sciences are filled with examples of brilliant and revolutionary contributions from people who had mental health problems. For example, the symbolist artist Edvard Munch, born in 1863, was an alcoholic and experienced depression throughout his life. His work focuses on themes of life and death and his experience with mental illness. The lithograph *The Scream* is one of his most important and popularized pieces. Of particular interest are three other works, *Anxiety*, *The Sick Child*, and *Death in the Sickroom*. As a young child, Munch experienced the death of his mother, and when he was 14, his sister died. *Death in the Sickroom* depicts the family scene years earlier.

History of Mental Health in the Community

Mental disorders are conditions that impair thinking, mood, and/or behaviors and are a leading cause of disability. Mental disorders are often more generically referred to as *mental illness*.

In the United States today, the public community mental health program has been the primary model of care for people with serious mental illness. Beginning in 1963, President John F. Kennedy raised awareness of and attention to mental health with the Community Mental Health Centers Act. Federal funds were committed for the construction and staffing of **community mental health centers (CMHCs)**, using the catchment area concept, which distributed mental health services throughout states all over the country. Today these programs provide access to a range of services that before this legislation were nonexistent.

Community mental health development was closely associated with legislation. **Box 27-1** describes the major mental health legislative efforts and their influence on the development of mental health services. Understanding that community mental health is a humanitarian reform is seen when considering the early reform history of mental health. It is still in need of reform today.

Early Humanitarian Reform in Mental Health

Early treatment for people with mental illness was both cruel and inhumane. In 1843, Dorothea Dix, a school teacher, started the reform movement for the treatment of criminals, the mentally ill, and later, victims of the Civil War. Her work led to the establishment of asylums dedicated to humane treatment for the mentally ill. States built institutions for housing and treating persons with severe mental disorders. Intended as a humane movement, the establishment of asylums that housed large numbers of patients and were operated with little knowledge and information about either cause or cure of mental illness was, in retrospect, anything but humane. Within a few years, these large state institutions provided the only mental health treatment and grew to be overcrowded. Patients were not discharged to families in communities that had no treatment services. Psychiatric treatment was limited to somatic therapies and did very little to handle difficult symptoms. The asylum population continued to grow as new people were admitted and the long-term residential population grew. It was not uncommon for "back ward" patients to have stays of 20 to 40 years. The asylum became the home.

BOX 27-1 Mental Health Legislation and Its Influence on Mental Health Services

1935	Social Security Act Shifted care for ill people from state to federal government
1943	National Institute of Mental Health Established as one of the Institutes of Health, where funds for research and development were committed to mental health
1955	Mental Health Study Established Joint Commission on Mental Illness and Health Led to the transformation of state hospitals to establishment of CMHCs
1963	Community Mental Health Centers Act Marked beginning of CMHCs and deinstitutionalization of large psychiatric hospitals
1960s	Funds were committed from federal government for grants for education for mental health disciplines, including nursing; stipends were made available for traineeships for undergraduate and graduate nursing students; gradually these were less frequent and finally were no longer available
1975	Developmental Disabilities Act Addressed rights of developmental disabilities and provided for similar actions for individuals with mental disorders
1977	President's Commission on Mental Health Reinforced importance of community-based services, protection of human rights, and national health insurance for mentally ill persons
1978	Omnibus Reconciliation Act Rescinded much of the 1977 commission's provisions and shifted funds for all health programs from federal to state governments in the form of block grants
1986	Protection and Advocacy for Individuals with Mental Illness Act Legislated advocacy programs for mentally ill persons
1990	Americans with Disabilities Act Prohibited discrimination and promoted employment opportunities for people with disabilities, including mental disorders
1996	Mental Health Parity Act Required that dollar limits on mental health benefits be no lower than dollar limits on medical and surgical benefits of group health insurance plans.
2008	Mental Health Parity and Addiction Equity Act Required group health plans and health insurance providers to ensure that financial requirements and treatment limitations for mental health and substance use disorder benefits were equal to those of medical/surgical benefits.
2010	Affordable Care Act (ACA) The goals of the ACA were to increase the quality and affordability of health insurance, reduce the number of uninsured by expanding public and private insurances, and reduce healthcare costs to individuals and the government.

Source: Adapted from Stanhope, M., & Lancaster, J. (2014). *Public health nursing: Population-centered health care in the community* (8th ed.). Maryland Heights, MO: Mosby.

Community Mental Health Reform in the 1960s

The CMHC movement, a century after Dorothea Dix's reform efforts, was another mental health reform movement. Some progress had been made in mental health science and treatment. The development of psychopharmacology was a milestone in treatment reform. Previously untreatable conditions were opened to the possibility of treatment. Since the early 1900s, psychotherapy had also been the focus of scholarship from several disciplines, including psychiatry, psychology, social work, and nursing. Psychotherapies that developed included long- and short-term and crisis intervention with individuals, groups, and families.

The CMHC movement was short-lived as the ideal solution to mental health care. Currently, large numbers of patients discharged from the state institutions and those who would have required institutional care in years past are residing in communities. A large number of the homeless population in urban centers are chronically mentally ill. They continue to have exacerbating mental conditions

BOX 27-2 Vulnerable Populations

- Young and old
- Experiencing developmental transitions—adolescence, childbirth, aging, family transitions
- Experiencing work and vocational problems and transitions
- Unemployed
- Part of the growing population of the very old, older than 85, elderly
- Living in poverty
- Single parents of young children
- Adolescent parents
- Grandparents in parenting roles because adult children are suffering with dysfunction
- Uneducated
- Isolated and marginalized
- Dealing with learning and attention deficits, having disabilities
- Minority populations
- Lesbian, gay, bisexual, and transgender
- Depressed
- Angry
- Acutely or chronically ill
- Present and prior incarceration
- Have been victims of human and environmental abuse
- Victims of oppressive political systems seeking asylum
- Populations experiencing stress, crisis, and change
- Immigrants
- Survivors of sexual assault, rape, molestation, and associated violence
- Military veterans and families

and experience environmental stresses, including the stress of meeting basic needs (i.e., food, water, and shelter). This group of homeless, chronically mentally ill is especially vulnerable.

Legislation Impacting Mental Health

> Mental illness is the last great stigma of the twentieth century. Most people treat someone with a mental illness as if it's their fault or as if they can just snap out of it.
>
> —*Tipper Gore*

As individuals were discharged from state mental institutions, private fee-for-service psychiatric services sprang up quickly in communities all over the country. Although care and a full range of treatment services are now more easily accessible within the community, there is inequity in access as a result of economic issues. Often, the families of the SMI are unable to do what is necessary to ensure continuity of care or to get any care.

The inequity in access and economics of mental health care and physical care continues to dominate the environment of mental health care. Within most communities, supportive services have been developed, primarily by the consumer movement, to meet particular support needs of the general population. **Box 27-2** identifies vulnerable populations who are in need of preventive, health-promotion, and specialized treatment. **Box 27-3** provides a list of support services and groups available in many communities.

Beginning with the consumer movement of the 1970s, the groups focusing on support and psychoeducational

BOX 27-3 Support Groups

- Compassionate friends: focus on death, bereavement, and loss (spouses, sudden infant death syndrome, perinatal, sibling)
- Cancer support: focuses on variety of phenomena, including breast cancer and ostomy
- Caregivers support group: for caregivers of elderly, cancer, mentally ill
- Infertility support: for couples experiencing infertility
- Parents Without Partners
- Suicide survivors
- Addictions Anonymous: for alcohol, gambling, exercise, shopping, food
- Smoking cessation: including smokeless tobacco
- Families of murdered victims
- Families of seriously mentally ill
- Medication follow up and education: for patients and families
- Parenting groups: for parents of adolescents, learning disabilities, autism, incarcerated
- Grandparenting
- Homeless mothers
- Diabetes education
- Alzheimer's family support: including Parkinson's
- Fibromyalgia support
- Cardiac: Mended Hearts
- Organ donor support group: families of donors and recipients of organs
- Physical disabilities support
- Homeless mothers and families support
- Survivors of sexual assault, rape, and molestation
- Military veterans groups

APPLICATION TO PRACTICE 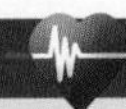

Reflective Education and Practice Exercise 2

Therapeutic Use of Self in Nursing Relationships

I could not believe how unsure and anxious I was about my first therapeutic conversation in the mental health nursing course. Never before had I even considered what to say in relationships. And then, all of a sudden I was very uncomfortable. I realized that most of my interactions with patients in the first course were all about me . . . not focused on the patient at all. I talked about my family, being a student, and whatever came into my mind.

Until mental health, I hadn't really thought about the differences in helping or therapeutic relationships. The course came at a good time for all of us, since we are just beginning the really hard nursing clinicals. All of us had made similar mistakes, continually chatted with patients, and unaware of their real needs. The realization that it really matters what you say to mental health patients really hit home. It really made me think. All of a sudden, it seemed important to know and understand something about the condition a mental patient has in order to respond in a helpful therapeutic way. After the class, when we discussed the differences in therapeutic and social relationships, I felt completely like a fish out of water. I realized that therapeutic communication involved more than just having a nice conversation. It demands a thoughtful, careful approach to be used along with very careful listening. I realized that this would be harder than I had expected.

After the first couple of weeks in post-conferences, where much of the discussion was focused on therapeutic interactions, I finally began to be more comfortable. By using active, careful listening and taking time to respond, I realized that if I made mistakes, I could always correct a response. I am confident that my communication with all patients, regardless of where I work, will be much improved by the experience of analyzing interactions with patients in mental health.

—BSN nursing student

issues with particular conditions have grown. These groups are available to the public, are listed in telephone directories, are promoted on the Internet, and are advertised on varying community bulletin boards.

Mental health programs offer many services to the SMI. **Box 27-4** lists examples of mental health services available in a CMHC in Mississippi.

Increasingly, community programs are being called to provide consultation to schools and communities in dealing with sensitive issues needing professional mental health attention. See the *Healthy People 2020* feature for a list of the priority areas elsewhere in this chapter. Even though mental health and mental disorders are listed separately, it is clear that mental health underpins many other priority areas, such as those listed in preventive services and health promotion.

Inpatient services for the SMI are still provided by the state hospital system. Patients experiencing acute problems or acute exacerbations of chronic conditions are usually housed within jails in holding facilities, which usually have consultative psychiatric services. Despite attempts to build in continuity and access to care, reforms

BOX 27-4 Community Mental Health Services

Services

- Seriously mentally ill day treatment
- Acute partial hospitalization for seriously mentally ill
- Children's services
- Adult day care
- Day Treatment Club House: for those with chronic conditions who live in the community
- Alcohol and chemical addictions programs
- Outpatient follow up
- Group living
- Military services

Possible Treatment Modalities Available in These Programs

- Resocialization, remotivation, and life skills assistance
- Social services
- Psychological services, including testing
- Medical services management and referral
- Psychopharmacological management
- Occupational therapy
- Recreational therapy
- Group, family therapy, and individual therapy
- Outreach and home visiting
- 12-step program
- Vocational rehabilitation
- Psychotherapy, long and short term
- Intensive outpatient programs

are needed in all systems that use holding facilities rather than inpatient treatment facilities. Inpatient services for the private system exist within relative geographic access in most communities. However, as cost-containment measures have been instituted, inpatient care is often too brief. Insurance and economics are currently the greatest barriers in gaining access to comprehensive, appropriate, and timely care in both the private and public systems. The expense of mental health services impedes service delivery to those who need it most and are unable to pay out of pocket for the services.

MEDIA MOMENT

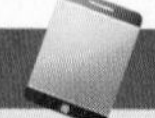

A Beautiful Mind (1998)

Sylvia Nasar, New York, NY: Simon & Schuster

This book about the brilliant mathematician and Nobel Laureate John Nash, who lapses into schizophrenic psychosis at the height of his career and remains there for 30 years, gives the reader an impression about what the experience of living with a serious mental illness is like. It also describes the extraordinary effort that returning to his theoretical work requires. At times, Nash thinks he can escape the ravages of time, picking up where he left off. And there are days when he cannot work; other days when he is full of remorse. The film that is based on the text is also informative and gives one a virtual experience of auditory and visual hallucinations. Chronicity and long-term disability accompany schizophrenia. The book also addresses the effects of illness on Nash's family, his community of scholars, and his life's work.

Historically, payment sources for mental health have been limited with higher copayments and stricter limitations, such as limited visits, lifetime limits on outpatient and inpatient days of treatment, and lower percentages of coverage. The Mental Health Parity Act of 1996 was the first legislative attempt to level differences between mental health coverage and medical/surgical coverage. However, it targeted group plans with 50 or more participants (Barry, Huskamp, & Goldman, 2010).

In an effort to further overcome limitations, The Mental Health Parity and Addiction Equity Act (MHPAEA), a component of the Emergency Economic Stabilization Act of 2008, equalized the insurance benefits between medical mental health and addiction treatment and the benefits for medical/surgical coverage (Barlas, 2013; & Barry et al., 2010). Although it provided a starting point for future legislation, the MHPAEA mostly impacted larger group insurance plans.

The most profound legislation, although controversial, was the ACA of 2010. The ACA augmented the MHPAEA by expanding eligibility of Medicaid recipients and by the development of state health insurance exchange plans. Nevertheless, provisions were made within the ACA for either partial or complete compliance with the plan, based on the type of insurance coverage (Cummings, Lucas, & Druss, 2013). Furthermore, the ACA is being implemented incrementally over several years, and the true impact of this legislation is unknown at this time.

Historical Context for Professional Nursing

Nursing as a profession was part of a social reform movement, with professional roots in "women's suffrage, abolition, missionary work, and social reform" (Lynaugh & Brush, 1999, p. xi). Professional nursing represents the emergence of women from a private role to a public, humanitarian role, caring for the public's suffering and illness just as they had traditionally cared for their own families. In a classic study of American nursing during the period 1850–1945, Reverby (1987) stated, "nursing's contemporary difficulties are shaped by the factors that created its historical obligations to care in a society that refuses to value caring" (p. i).

Nightingale (1859) defined nursing as the finest of the fine arts, stating that the role of nursing is to "put the patient in the best possible condition for nature to work upon him." Close to 100 years later, Virginia Henderson declared,

> As a nurse, I try to do for [patients] what they would do for themselves if they had the strength, the will, and the knowledge that a nurse has. And I try to do it in such a way that I don't make them dependent on me, any more than is necessary. (Baer, 1990, interview with Virginia Henderson)

Nursing is defined by the authors of this chapter as an open, caring art, spirit, human science, holistic practice, and discipline that uses a commitment to research, knowledge, humanity, education, the creative arts, and peace to facilitate, transform, actualize human potential, and promote wellness and healing for all people and the planet in the present, future, and beyond. Nursing work, according to Wolf (1988), is work that is both "sacred and profane." It is personal, involves up-close and personal work, is private, and often involves body work. In many cases, it is surrounded by an atmosphere of phenomenological silence (Lauterbach, 2003). Nursing work is very hard and is often physically and mentally challenging, especially in P-MH.

It often involves caring for the most vulnerable, without resources, or using methods that have not been researched, or using untested, reliable treatments. Nursing often involves dealing with tremendous human suffering, as well as hope and opportunity for improving the human condition. In mental health, nursing involves *knowing*, *caring for*, and *being with* persons whose lives have often been dominated and altered forever by acute exacerbations in mental functioning, change, dysfunction, and serious mental illness.

> I come to present the strong claims of suffering humanity. I come to place before the Legislature of Massachusetts the condition of the miserable, the desolate, the outcast. I come as the advocate of helpless, forgotten, insane men and women; of beings sunk to a condition from which the unconcerned world would start with real horror.
>
> —*Dorothea Dix, memorial to the Legislature of Massachusetts, 1843*

History and Spirit of Psychiatric–Mental Health Nursing in the Community

As influenced by the social, political, and economic forces and the tenor of the times, the dilemma faced by modern nursing is highlighted by P-MH nursing. P-MH nurses care for persons and populations suffering from mental conditions that do not resolve readily. They care for those who experience the devastating effects of tormenting, chronic mental conditions, often over the course of a lifetime. The asylum movement actually began and continued as a social reform movement. P-MH nurses care for people who represent a growing "Third World" community residing within America's borders. Mentally ill citizens include many of the United States' vulnerable, oppressed, disenfranchised, ethnic, and often hopeless people.

Box 27-5 identifies important events in the history of P-MH nursing. Hildegard Peplau is considered the founder of P-MH nursing; she is referred to fondly as "the mother of psychiatric nursing." Interestingly, she was one of the first nursing theorists, and her book *Interpersonal Relations in Nursing* has been translated into more than 50 languages. The text was ready for publication in 1949, but Peplau was unable to find a publisher who would publish it with a female nurse as the sole author. She refused to seek out a first author who was a physician and finally was able to publish the book under her own name in 1952.

Orlando's 1961 text, *The Dynamic Nurse–Patient Relationship*, is another classic work that has been used in nursing education—not only in P-MH nursing, but in foundations and skills courses. Travelbee's (1971) *Intervention in Psychiatric Nursing* continued the work on relationships; her major contribution was in her conceptualization of the *therapeutic use of self*. Other work related to the thesis that the nurse is the primary instrument of nursing and therapeutic care includes Quinn's (1992) conceptualization of the healing environment. The authors of this chapter and many other nursing faculty have used the classic works of Peplau, Orlando, Parse (1998), and Travelbee in developing guidelines for reflection on developing therapeutic relationships in undergraduate and graduate students in nursing. Such therapeutic relationships underpin all of nursing, regardless of specialty or practice level.

The experience of P-MH nurses today is reflective of the struggles of the profession as a whole and of the struggles of women around the world. The nursing profession needs to bring a heightened awareness and consciousness of the phenomenon of misogyny, the hatred of women.

BOX 27-5 Important Events in Psychiatric Nursing History, 1773–1955

1773	First mental hospital in the United States established in Williamsburg, Virginia
1846	First use of the term *psychiatry* by physicians attempting to upgrade the status of their work with the mentally ill
1882	First school for psychiatric nurses (or mental health nurses) established at the McLean Asylum in Somerville, Massachusetts
1913	Johns Hopkins Hospital included psychiatric nursing in the course of study for general nurses
1920	Publication of the first psychiatric nursing textbook, *Nursing Mental Diseases*, by Harriet Bailey
1946	Passage of the National Mental Health Act, which established the National Institute of Mental Health (NIMH)
1948	Publication of the Brown Report, which recommended that psychiatric nursing be included in general nursing education
1952	Publication of *Interpersonal Relations in Nursing* by nurse theorist Hildegard Peplau
1955	National League for Nursing made psychiatric nursing a requirement for accreditation of basic nursing programs

Source: Adapted from Frisch, H., & Frisch, L. (1998). *Psychiatric mental health nursing*. Albany, NY: Delmar.

This phenomenon demands attention, awareness, and global critical action. Other oppressed marginal people are also worthy of attention. The Research Alerts in the chapter highlight work investigating the experiences of women, oppressed people, and vulnerable groups within society who need attention and mental health intervention.

Though short-lived, the CMHCs established in the mid-1960s through the late 1970s provided P-MH nurses with opportunities to develop significant roles for themselves in **advocacy**, community liaison building, consultation, crisis stabilization, case management, medication management, research, and education, as well as to develop the role of therapist in working with individuals, families, and groups.

Unfortunately, the P-MH nurses and professionals involved with the CMHC reform movement experienced lost hopes and dreams as the needed mental health care revolution and reform failed to materialize. Many nurse researchers who were originally involved in the CMHC movement took other paths as the movement all but disappeared. Through the application of partisan politics in the early 1980s, the U.S. federal government established block grants for states to administer mental health services. With that act, the federal oversight role, along with the CMHC movement, was abolished.

Deinstitutionalization of the large public asylums and state hospitals began with the development of CMHCs and was finally completed by the late 1970s, just in time for the state block grants to take over the public mental health program. In response to this trend, a new group of private psychiatric hospitals sprang up. Mental health care for the private hospitals became a lucrative business, which further motivated privatization of mental health treatment. The state-funded public programs, in turn, began shouldering the primary burden of caring for the SMI, those without financial resources, and/or the uninsured.

The public–private split in mental health care exists today, and P-MH care remains desperately in need of revolution and reform. While the United States is advanced in technology for physical care, there is a gap in research into and knowledge of mental health care. Further, for a large number of state and federal professionals and residential care providers, caring for the nation's most seriously ill and incarcerated population is often considered an undesirable assignment. As a consequence, the most seriously ill are cared for by the least educated, least supported healthcare providers.

State of the Science of Psychiatric–Mental Health Nursing

The 1990s were considered the decade of the brain, during which great strides were made in understanding the biological component of mental disorders and functioning and developing drugs to treat these conditions. Atypical antipsychotic medications have continued to be developed and, although they are not without adverse consequences, have provided some hope for relief of symptoms. Long-term studies of these drugs are still needed. The weight gain associated with use of many antidepressants and antipsychotics has been associated with the development of type 2 diabetes. Clearly, there is a continuing need for research. Complementary and alternative modalities are in great need of research as well.

There is a growing need for public education focused on anxiety, stress and coping with stress, depression, integration of complementary and alternative therapies with traditional approaches, and assisting in people developing balanced lives. Large-scale community violence and terror experiences in the United States in the mid- to late 1990s have continued to be of national concern. The Oklahoma City bombings; school violence in Pearl, Mississippi, and Columbine, Colorado; bombings at the Boston marathon; and continuing community experiences related to sniper and perpetrator violence have produced significant anxiety in the general population. In the aftermath of the threats to national security following the terrorist attacks on September 11, 2001, large-scale community education and intervention programs are needed. The aftermath of the war on terrorism, the Iraq war, and the continuing concern about terrorism and violence have caused great stress for those serving in the U.S. military, their families, the rest of the country, and the world. Further, widespread corporate scandals and unethical practices exposed around the same time as the 2001 terrorist attacks and discoveries in 2013 of inequities in the U.S. Internal Revenue Service have further threatened personal as well as national security for many U.S. residents. The notion of safety in the United States and all over the world, as terrorists' takeover of a Russian elementary school demonstrates, has been altered forever.

There is also a need for further exploration of human and basic sciences and research in the areas of treatment, prevention, and health promotion. Nursing research and the social sciences disciplines have begun to make significant contributions to our understanding of the person and experience of mental illness. A growing body of literature is devoted to evidence-based practice and outcome-focused research. Nevertheless, there is an unmet need for research that identifies qualitative outcomes and qualitative evidence for practice. The growing wealth of research literature delves into both quantitative and qualitative research and studies new methodologies. Both foci add to the knowledge and understanding of the human condition and human experience.

Additionally, there is a growing need for development of and research into integrative complementary alternatives in mental health treatment. Many people suffering with depression, anxiety, or stress use complementary and alternative therapies, often exclusively. In addition, professional groups that face undue stress because of the nature of their work or the state of the profession, such as nursing, need to research the stress related to the practice discipline. Further, research findings related to human phenomena need to be shared directly with the public, as it often has direct practice application, particularly research emerging from qualitative methodologies.

Research carried out using qualitative perspectives offers new understanding of the human experience. Phenomenological research uncovers and discovers meanings in human lived experience and leads to better understanding of the human experience. Ethnography offers an understanding of the culture and mores that surround human experience and phenomena. Grounded theory seeks to explicate the basic human process underlying human experience. Narratives and stories, in "their own words" accounts, and naturalistic settings further inform and serve to fully describe the human experience. Quantitative studies, using large random population samples, have the potential for generalizing findings

RESEARCH ALERT

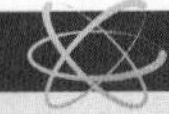

Using street ethnography while interviewing homeless men in San Francisco and St. Louis, researchers examined the nexus and interaction between homelessness and incarceration. Among the men in the study, crimes of desperation, aggressive policing, and close proximity of homeless men and many ex-cons created a strong likelihood of incarceration and re-incarceration. For incarcerated men, time inside eroded employability, family ties, and other defenses against homelessness. For several men, homelessness had occurred for the first time following release from prison or jail. The following phrase is worthy of close scrutiny: "[the] homelessness/incarceration cycle, more powerful than the sum of its parts, a racialized exclusion/punishment nexus which germinates, isolates, and perpetuates lower-class male marginality" (p. 500).

Where the plight of homeless women is different from that of homeless men, the homeless/incarceration cycle for women is different in that "historically, poor women have been positioned differently vis-á-vis the law" (p. 502).

For the homeless, untreated mentally ill, this phenomenon is in need of continued scrutiny.

Source: Gowan, T. (2002). The nexus: Homelessness and incarceration in two American cities. *Ethnography*, *3*(4), 500–534. This special issue of the journal *Ethnography* is entitled "In and Out of the Belly of the Beast: Dissecting the Prison."

APPLICATION TO PRACTICE

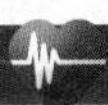

Reflective Education and Practice Exercise 3

Constructing a Multigenerational Genogram

Sometimes the things you think you know the most about are the things that can teach you so much. When the family assessment was assigned, I was sure that I already knew everything there was to know about my family. Yet, as I began to talk to my parents, grandparents, aunts, and uncles, I realized that there are many stories, traits, and patterns that run throughout. I learned new things about people I thought I knew everything about. . . . But, most importantly, researching my family allowed me to learn new things that I may have never had the opportunity to learn. I am lucky to have grandparents who know about family medical history and, even better, who know about the traditions that our family is based on. . . . The things I have learned are not only valuable to me personally, but will also be priceless in my career as a nurse. This was an opportunity to see family in a whole new light, to analyze relationships and see patterns among members. I learned the effect that one conflict in a relationship can have on an entire family. I also learned the value of having family close by. This assignment has allowed me to see the big picture . . . to see how much family can impact a person, especially in hard times. This will be precious in helping to treat patients.

—BSN nursing student

The first and most obvious pattern in my family is for men and women on my mother's side to be alcoholics or to marry alcoholics. . . . I mention this because they have impacted me in ways that I myself do not even understand. . . . So, I unwittingly followed the pattern set by my mother and grandmother. I married a recovering alcoholic . . . I love my family. The strength of character, although it may not be obvious from what I have reported, is a predominant theme. Despite their faults, [my family members] have overcome many trials of faith and I have learned from the stories they tell.

—BSN nursing student

Conducting the analysis was pretty simple. It is easy to see the trends that flow through our family. . . . It brought my attention to many of the health issues in my family. Any nurse should be aware of family histories. Creating a genogram can be a good way to give tips on preventing certain diseases that run in a patient's family.

—BSN nursing student

APPLICATION TO PRACTICE 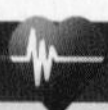

Reflective Education and Practice Exercise 4

Student Reflection: Journaling

The first time I approached journaling was 12 weeks ago. At that point I was still trying to grasp an understanding of what it was I was trying to accomplish through the journaling process. Now, 12 weeks later, I have a greater appreciation of what journaling can do. It has helped me grasp some of the thoughts that fly rapidly through my head, and turn them into something legible that I can view. The whole process has helped me understand my thought processes and turn the abstract into a somewhat tangible reality.

—Nursing student

Journaling has also helped me to express my thoughts and feelings, which is something I have persistently had a problem with. Even to this day, I struggle in sharing with others when I am having trouble either in my personal life or in my life as a student. I tend to keep issues bottled up inside, but those around me can clearly see that something is bothering me. This lack of communication has affected some of my relationships in the past and present, but journaling has provided me with a means of expression.

—Nursing student

to the population at large. Each methodology scrutinizes a slice of human experience and, when combined with other perspectives, plus triangulation of methods and data-collection strategies, presents a fuller understanding of human experience.

Many P-MH phenomena have been investigated by advanced practice nurses to date, including the work of the following authors: Becker (1991); Becker Hentz (1994); Douglas (2004); Frank (1987); Hutchinson (1986); Lauterbach (1992, 1995, 2003); Lesser, Koniak-Griffin, and Anderson (1999); Lesser, Oakes, and Koniak-Griffin (2003); Lesser, Tello, Koniak-Griffin, Kappos, and Rhys (2001); Munhall (2007); Munhall and Boyd (1993); and Swanson-Kaufmann (1983). All of these authors are advanced practice P-MH nurses involved with qualitative inquiry.

Loss, change, and bereavement, along with stress and anxiety, are universal human phenomena that involve human suffering. These conditions often underlie mental health conditions. As examples of **universal human experiences**, they occur throughout the lifespan and require specific and general resources for coping and resolution. Research into these and other universal human experiences is of particular interest to P-MH nursing. Lauterbach's (1992, 1995, 2003) doctoral and follow-up research, for example, focused on perinatal loss—specifically, on uncovering meanings surrounding mothers' experience with having a wished-for baby die.

Levels of Psychiatric–Mental Health Nursing Practice

P-MH nursing practice includes practice at basic and advanced levels. The basic levels included in **Box 27-6** are registered nurses (RNs) who have associate or baccalaureate degrees. There are still a small number of RNs in practice who were trained in diploma programs. Currently, assistive-level personnel in public institutions provide most of the day-to-day supportive care and assistance for patients. These personnel are called mental health technicians (techs), patient care assistants, or a

BOX 27-6 Psychiatric–Mental Health Nursing: Areas of Practice

Basic-Level Functions

- Health promotion and health maintenance
- Intake screening and evaluation
- Case management
- Preventive management of a therapeutic environment
- Self-care activities
- Psychobiological interventions
- Health teaching, including psychoeducation
- Crisis intervention
- Counseling
- Community action
- Advocacy

Advanced-Level Functions

- Psychotherapy
- Psychobiological interventions
- Medication management and prescriptive authority (in some states)
- Clinical supervision/consultation
- Consultation/liaison building

Source: Adapted from Nurses for a Healthier Tomorrow. (2008). *Psychiatric-mental health nursing*. Retrieved from http://www.nursesource.org/psychiatric.html

APPLICATION TO PRACTICE 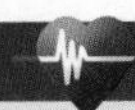

Reflective Education and Practice Exercise 5

Attending a Support Group

I have tried my best to apply some of the steps that I acquired from attending the AA meeting to my eating habits. I have been on Weight Watchers off and on throughout the semester. I find myself feeling so much lighter and healthier when I stay on it. It is hard to eat healthy today when every restaurant is pushing "biggie size." With technological advances, energy expenditures are not promoted. It is much easier to say yes to the food that tempts me than to the food that is good for me. All of my life I have had to watch my weight, but all I seem to watch is it go up! I have found, though, that journaling about it helps me express my feelings instead of eating them away. Hopefully, I will continue to stay motivated and will not allow myself to become a statistic.

—Nursing student

Sitting in on a CA and AA meeting was a quick way to learn about their general purposes, the audience, and group procedures and process. The content of the discussion presented a picture of life as a drug user. Although each person's story was unique, several themes surfaced. The prevailing themes were the bondage to the drug, feelings of total defeat, and enslavement to the drug. Drug use had had a marked impact on their work performance, which usually led to their unemployment. They exploited family and friends to maintain their addiction. Many spoke about how their drug-using friends abandoned them when they faced trouble or prison.

The group process impressed me the most. The meetings seemed to be desperately needed by the members. In both meetings, people were eager to participate and share their lives and situation. Those who were clean offered their experiences and encouragement. Mutual respect for each other was high. When one man picked up his chip, there was applause and encouragement and celebration. . . .

This experience was highly beneficial to me. As a nurse, I can confidently recommend such support groups to drug-abusing patients. As a nursing student, I have a better grasp of mental health concepts. As an FSU [Florida State University] student, the sad stories I heard warn of the horrors of drug and alcohol abuse. As a friend, I have a better understanding of the life and struggles that drug users experience.

—BSN nursing student

similar designation. Private programs and institutions often have technicians who have college degrees. Medication supervision is provided by an RN with an associate or baccalaureate degree, or by a licensed practical nurse (LPN).

Nurses at the advanced practice level have master's degrees in nursing and may also have doctoral degrees. Specialization in the clinical area of P-MH is available at the master's level, with board certification available as a clinical specialist (CS) since the late 1970s and 1980s and for the nurse practitioner (NP) since the early 2000s. The nurse practice act (NPA) of the state determines whether prescriptive privileges and independent practice are available for the advanced-practice-level nurse. Additionally, some P-MH nurses earn multiple degrees and obtain additional credentials, such as nurse practitioner, clinical nurse specialist, licensed clinical social worker, or licensed professional counselor, to provide more advanced levels of care.

An example of a relatively new specialty role, which has emerged from the P-MH specialty, is that of forensic nursing. This specialty area integrates nursing and forensic science in bridging the gap between the healthcare and criminal justice systems. As a response to the increasing epidemic of violence, this specialty attempts to meet care needs of both victims and perpetrators. Although it is quite different in scope and purpose from the P-MH clinical specialty and nurse practitioner role, this specialty is of growing interest to nursing. Board certification is becoming available for advanced practice nurses in forensic roles.

Increasingly, there is a need for primary mental health care within primary care organizations. Many P-MH nurse practitioners work in primary care practice settings, such as college healthcare programs. **Prevention** and early intervention are key to reducing the ultimate societal and human costs in treating mental disorders. Over time, many disorders escalate out of control because they are overlooked and/or undertreated. Providing timely, appropriate, and supportive care for people who experience common human problems such as trauma, loss, or anxiety, or for those who experience intolerable suffering seems to be critical in preventing patterns of dysfunctional and inadequate coping.

Public education remains an area of great unmet need. This need has been partially addressed by the National Alliance for the Mentally Ill (NAMI) and state mental health associations, but much remains to be accomplished. Reducing the resistance to treatment and societal stigma attached to mental health problems through education, research, and knowledge-based treatment should be a *Healthy People* public health goal.

HEALTHY PEOPLE 2020 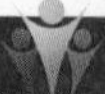

Objectives Related to Mental Health and Mental Disorders

Mental Health Status Improvement

- MHMD-1 Reduce the suicide rate
- MHMD-2 Reduce suicide attempts by adolescents
- MHMD-3 Reduce the proportion of adolescents who engage in disordered eating behaviors in an attempt to control their weight
- MHMD-4 Reduce the proportion of persons who experience major depression episodes
  - MHMD-4.1 Reduce the proportion of adolescents age 12–17 who experience major depressive episodes
  - MHMD-4.2 Reduce the proportion of adults age 18 years and older who experience major depressive episodes

Treatment Expansion

- MHMD-5 Increase the proportion of primary care facilities that provide mental health treatment on site or by paid referral
- MHMD-6 Increase the proportion of children with mental health problems who receive treatment
- MHMD-7 Increase the proportion of juvenile residential facilities that screen admissions for mental health problems
- MHMD-8 Increase the proportion of persons with serious mental illness who are employed
- MHMD-9 Increase the proportion of adults with mental health disorders who receive treatment
  - MHMD-9.1 Increase the proportion of adults age 18 years and older with serious mental illness who receive treatment
  - MHMD-9.2 Increase the proportion of adults age 18 years and older with major depressive episodes who receive treatment
- MHMD-10 Increase the proportion of persons with co-occurring substance abuse and mental disorders who receive treatment for both disorders
- MHMD-11 Increase depression screening by primary care providers
  - MHMD-11.1 Increase the proportion of primary care physicians who screen adults age 19 years and older for depression during office visits
  - MHMD-11.2 Increase the proportion of primary care physicians who screen youth age 12–18 years for depression during office visits
- MHMD-12 Increase the proportion of homeless adults with mental health problems who receive mental health services

Source: U.S. Department of Health and Human Services. (2014). *Mental health and mental disorders*. Retrieved from http://www.healthypeople.gov/2020/topicsobjectives2020/objectiveslist.aspx?topicId=28

RESEARCH ALERT 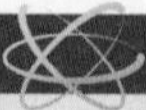

Research has provided us with a better understanding of the experience of obsessive–compulsive disorder (OCD). Using a phenomenological perspective, the author of one study investigated the lived experience of the phenomenon of OCD, a personality disorder according to the *DSM-IV-R*. In its severe form, OCD is similar to the psychoses, in that it completely dominates the conscious experience with obsessive thoughts and compulsions that are directed to lessening the anxiety, and it renders the person unable to function in activities of daily living or work.

This work and the text of which it is a part represent a collection of writings aimed at explicating and understanding the human experience. The researcher author uses subjects' descriptions "in their own words." The beauty of this qualitative method and research is that *knowing about* and *understanding* the condition have direct practice applications.

Source: Haase, M. (2002). Living with "obsessive compulsive disorder." In M. van Manen (Ed.), *Writing in the dark: Phenomenological studies in interpretive inquiry*. London, England: Althouse Press.

Nursing is an art; and if it is to be made an art, Requires as exclusive a devotion, as hard a preparation;

As any painter's or sculptor's work;

For what is the having to do with dead canvas or dead marble,

Compared with having to do with the living body—

The temple of god's spirit?

It is one of the fine arts;

I had almost said, the finest of Fine Arts.

—*Florence Nightingale*

HEALTHY PEOPLE 2020 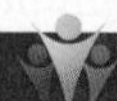

Highlights of *Healthy People 2010* Progress Review: What did we accomplish in the first decade of the 21st century?

Nearly half of all Americans will meet the criteria for a mental disorder at some time in their lives, with first onset usually in childhood or early adolescence.

More than 25% of adult Americans have at least one mental disorder, and approximately 5% have three or more.

The four most widespread disorders are anxiety disorders, mood disorders, impulse disorders, and substance disorders.

Mental disorders are a leading cause of disability, absenteeism, and lost productivity in the workplace.

Emerging factors contributing to the prevalence of mental illness in the United States include an aging population and the large proportion of veterans returning from Iraq and Afghanistan with posttraumatic stress disorder, depression, and anxiety.

To help address the increased risk of male veterans dying by suicide, a national suicide hotline is being made available to veterans. Options for providing telephone crisis counseling and referrals to active duty military personnel and their families are also being explored.

Advances in research have shown that depression and certain cognitive losses are not an inevitable part of aging. This should lead to improved diagnostic precision and enhance the provision of age-appropriate treatment.

Too few primary care providers are trained to recognize depression and the variety of disabilities associated with it.

Five states have legislated parity in insurance benefits for treatment of mental disorders and physical illnesses.

The provision of mental health services in schools provides an opportunity for early intervention. For example, the city of Baltimore, through collaboration with local universities, is able to offer the services of full-time mental health professionals in more than 60 of its public schools.

Source: Adapted from U.S. Department of Health and Human Services. (1999). *Healthy People 2000: Mental health and mental disorders progress review.* Retrieved from http://www.cdc.gov/nchs/about/otheract/hp2000/mentalhlth.htm

RESEARCH ALERT 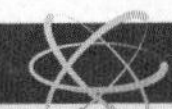

This article examines the health-related issues of the spouses of deployed military personnel who are living in community settings. It focuses on increasing the knowledge of healthcare providers regarding the stressors these spouses may experience and providing resources in case they may require extra support and assistance. Suggestions of possible community health nursing interventions in dealing with these spouses and the role of nurse practitioners in their coping strategies are discussed.

Source: Tollefson, T. (2008). Supporting spouses during a military deployment. *Family & Community Health, 31*(4), 281–286.

Individuals and Population Groups Needing Psychiatric–Mental Health Services

Mental health and mental disorders are included in *Healthy People 2020* as part of health promotion; the *Healthy People 2020* features provided in this chapter identify mental health problems and populations in need. Parents with young teens are aware of this growing population of youth who are encountering very serious substance use, including cigarettes, smokeless tobacco, an incredible variety of inhalants, abuse of prescription mood-altering drugs, cocaine, crack, crystal meth, hallucinogens, and daily use of marijuana, coupled with alcohol. In addition, the epidemics of rape, violence, sexual assault, legal entanglements, and pregnancy among school-aged children and teens are, from the perspective of the youth, much greater than statistics demonstrate. The pattern of misuse and abuse that is reflected in the aforementioned behaviors, along with a recognition of problems with anxiety, depression, and attention to school and learning, warrant careful investigation, research, and concurrent social action. Many of the behaviors are seen by professionals as attempts to self-medicate. However, research is needed to identify factors that are associated with and contribute to "using" behaviors. We need to understand more about these human phenomena.

A growing number of individuals and populations is at risk and in need of primary mental health nursing and specialized P-MH. This reflects the growing consumer and public recognition that specialized support is needed to cope with particular human phenomena and experiences. **Box 27-7** lists universal human experiences that are often in need of special support and crisis or continuing care. The potential direction and roles for P-MH nursing will focus on assisting persons and groups in handling living through difficult human experience.

BOX 27-7 Common Human Experiences

- Loss, death, separation
- Crisis
- Relationships with significant others—family, friends, work, society
- Anxiety
- Sadness, depression, and mood conditions
- Developmental eras and transitions—individual, family, group, societal
- Illness—acute and chronic
- Stress and coping
- Coping with rapid social changes
- Violence and war

As a focal phenomenon, changes in the American family warrant particular attention. A growing number of children grow up in single-parent homes, usually with the father absent. There are changes in the structure and function of families. Single parents and working women are growing aggregates. This combined with poverty serves to compound vulnerability.

The growing elderly population with cognitive impairments, institutionalized elders, and those with Alzheimer's disease and their families further reflect the concept of compounding vulnerability. More work, more research, and more preventive efforts are needed for serious mental health conditions and diagnoses, such as schizophrenia, which involve exacerbations of acute symptoms of distress and disturbance. This population represents a large number of persons and families who experience periods of acute exacerbation of chronic illness. Other chronic illnesses, such as diabetes, have patterns involving crisis and management and need P-MH nursing attention.

> We are more alike, my friends,
>
> than we are unalike.
>
> We are more alike, my friends,
>
> than we are unalike.
>
> —*Maya Angelou*

APPLICATION TO PRACTICE

Reflective Education and Practice Exercise 6

The Shelter Experience

. . . as you looked around, you could see some people with very definite mental illnesses, and there were some whom you couldn't really decide if they had an illness or not. . . . It was interesting because when I looked around at the people there, I didn't see just the people; I saw individual stories . . . stories that I wanted to learn about, but did not want to intrude. . . . Maybe if I volunteered more of my time, they would become able to trust me and then possibly confide in me. One will never know unless the time is dedicated. . . .

—BSN nursing student

Each experience in life presents us with a unique situation to observe and learn from. The Shelter is no exception. Approaching the experience was intimidating, much like the first experience at Florida State Hospital. But, by simply participating, sitting back and watching the people who call this their home offered many insights into a side of life I have never considered before.

As I arrived at The Shelter, I surveyed what was around me: hand-me-down blankets, well-worn clothes, used towels and sheets. I smelled the smells of people who had not bathed in days. I smelled tobacco, so strong that it made my eyes water. I wondered how anyone could live there.

Soon the people who lived there taught me an important lesson. This life was better than sleeping in a cardboard box on the streets, and better than freezing out in cold weather. When they began to file into The Shelter, I realized as they signed in that they were real people. There were women released from jail to find their homes repossessed, women who had nowhere else to go. There were men with families, men who had been kicked out of their homes, men who fought for their country and came home to nothing. I realized that they were thankful to have a place to sleep, to be safe, where they didn't have to worry about someone taking the few things they carried in their bag.

It became obvious that the life they had lived had taken a toll on them. Physically they seemed drained. Their hands showed scars and years of work with no care. Many were sick, coughing, and were grateful for a glass of water. Mentally, many were plagued with illness. One man hid in a corner. Many were alcoholic. Each person who came through the door had a story.

This experience changed my attitude toward the homeless. Many are employed, working long hours and not getting paid enough to get back on their feet. They have hopes and dreams and goals like the rest of us. Perhaps the biggest eye opener for me was the way they interacted with each other. They were careful to see that the older men had extra blankets, or were able to have their special mat, or that everyone got a blanket. They joked and laughed and told stories about their families and experiences. This experience was perhaps one of the most meaningful experiences in my life. Two nights with these people drastically changed my ideas. It made me realize that many are trying their hardest to survive and to make it on their own. In the meantime, they are grateful and appreciative of the care received. I will take away a compassion for those who have been humble enough to admit that they need help and have graciously accepted it.

—BSN nursing student

To be homeless and not to have any place to go is an overwhelming reality to many people in our society. That notion is difficult for me to comprehend. How could someone not have family or friends who would love him or her unconditionally and give [the person] simple shelter? Where can such people go? The Shelter is one place. It is an unconditional place that will accept anyone and only ask the residents to obey limited rules for their own safety and the safety of others. The Shelter provides the basic needs of residents. . . . In this place they can be treated with respect. Some of the new residents were unsure at first, but they quickly felt comfortable. The residents were thankful for everything and they expressed it openly. . . .

My experience at The Shelter was humbling. It made me appreciate my family in many different ways. I also felt like helping at The Shelter made a small difference in the lives of homeless people. Leaving The Shelter, I felt like I needed to do much more, and I plan to volunteer again in the future. They say that most of us are only a couple of paychecks away from living on the streets. What a scary thought!

—BSN nursing student

RESEARCH ALERT 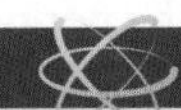

This article reviews literature and data supporting the links between substance abuse and men's violence toward women partners. It also examines critical issues in treatment for men who batter and discusses particular treatment issues for black men who abuse substances and batter women partners.

Common explanations of substance abuse and violence discussed are disinhibition owing to lower brain functioning caused by substance use, cognitive distortion, learned disinhibition, disavowal of responsibility ("It was the alcohol"), and power and control.

Effective treatment needs to involve an integration of services and agencies, and a coordinated effort by all involved, including the community. The following elements were identified as critical in helping black men change their behavior:

- Confront and take ownership of the problem and associated negative behavior
- Challenge the current method of addressing problems in their lives
- Identify other models for life and problem solving
- Develop alternative life codes of conduct
- Build the capacity to problem-solve in challenging situations

Further, it is important to view black men's partner violence not only as a personal problem, but also as a larger social community problem. Women's abuse occurs within the context of the larger society and cultural group. A lower tolerance for partner violence in the community is needed.

When considering a population-focused approach to the problem of substance abuse and violence, this theoretical exploration has implications for other human phenomena. Substance abuse is often related to criminal behavior, and it is a critical component in other relationship problems, health-related conditions, morbidity, and mortality.

Source: Bennett, L., & Williams, Oliver, J. (2003). Substance abuse and men who batter. *Violence Against Women*, *9*(5), 558–575.

Current Assessment of the Public's Mental Health Status

Mental disorders occur across the lifespan and affect people from all racial, ethnic, and geographic areas. They affect both genders and cut across all socioeconomic groups. The present scope of the problem of mental health is daunting. In the United States, approximately 26.2% of the population is affected by some type of mental disorder, and 6% of the population is plagued with a serious

RESEARCH ALERT 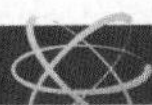

The purpose of this study was to systematically review qualitative research that addresses how people live with suicidality or recover a desire to live. Suicide is a pressing social and public health problem. Much emphasis in suicide research has been on the epidemiology of suicide and the identification of risk and protective factors. Relatively little emphasis has been given to the subjective experiences of suicidal people, but this is necessary to inform the care and help provided to individuals. A systematic review of the literature and thematic content analysis of findings was conducted. The findings were extracted from selected papers and synthesized by way of content analysis in narrative and tabular form. Twelve studies were identified. Analysis revealed a number of interconnected themes: the experience of suffering, struggle, connection, turning points, and coping. Living with or overcoming suicidality involves various struggles, often existential in nature. Suicide may be seen as both a failure and a means of coping. People may turn away from suicide quite abruptly through experiencing, gaining, or regaining the right kind of connection with others. Nurses working with suicidal individuals should aspire to be identified as people who can turn people's lives around.

Source: Lakeman, R., & FitzGerald, M. (2008). How people live with or get over being suicidal: A review of qualitative studies. *Journal of Advanced Nursing*, *64*(2), 114–126.

mental illness (NIMH, n.d.). These population figures show few differences from the results of Leighton, Harding, Macklin, MacMillan, and Leighton's 1963 study, which found that SMI typically affects the impoverished (low-socioeconomic-status) population.

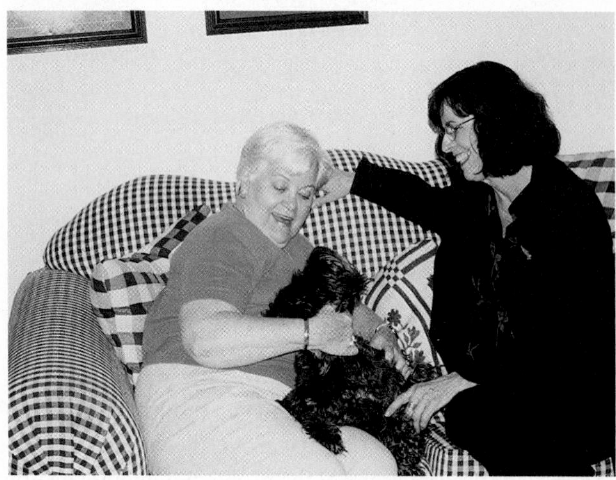

Dr. Sarah Steen Lauterbach, chapter author, in an encounter with an elder patient.

In the United States, more than 57 million people have a diagnosis of mental disorder. Approximately 13% of children and adolescents between ages 9 and 17 years have a diagnosable mental disorder. Serious emotional disturbances in this population often lead to school failure, alcohol or illicit drug use, violence, or suicide.

Casey (2012) reported the worldwide prevalence of dementia in 2000 was 24.3 per million of the population and estimated its growing to 81.1 per million of the population by 2040. Similarly, Dilworth-Anderson, Pierre, and Hilliard (2012) estimated that by 2030, the number of people age 65 years and older in the United States is expected to double, reaching about 71 million individuals or about 20% of the U.S. population. This expected growth of the older population, coupled with the resulting suggestion from Casey's (2012) study that a person's risk of developing dementia doubles every 5 years, will result in the number of those living with dementia proportionately increasing.

There are multiple types of dementia; at times, the exhibited symptoms overlap. The most common form of dementia, Alzheimer's disease (discovered by Dr. Alois Alzheimer in 1906), accounts for 60–80% of dementias and is the sixth leading cause of death in the United States (Alzheimer's Association, 2013a). The remaining 20–40% of dementias consist of less frequently occurring dementia types, including vascular dementia, mixed dementia, dementia with Lewy bodies, Parkinson's disease, frontotemporal dementias (primary progressive aphasia, Pick's disease, and progressive supranuclear palsy), Creutzfeldt-Jakob disease, normal-pressure hydrocephalus, Huntington's disease, and Wernicke-Korsakoff syndrome (Alzheimer's Association, 2013b).

Serious mental illnesses (SMIs) such as schizophrenia, mood disorders (major depression and bipolar disorder), and severe anxiety disorders (obsessive–compulsive disorder and panic disorder) can be, and often are, enormously disabling. Schizophrenia affects 2.4 million people, approximately 1.1% of the population. Affective (mood) disorders affect roughly 9.5% of the population. Major depression affects approximately 6.7%, bipolar disorder affects approximately 2.6%, and dysthymic disorder affects approximately 1.5% of the population, with men and women being equally affected. A high rate of suicide is associated with mood disorders. Anxiety disorders (panic disorder, obsessive–compulsive disorder, posttraumatic stress disorder (PTSD), and phobia) are more common than other disorders and affect as many as 40 million people in the United States annually (NIMH, n.d.).

Rates of the most severe forms of SMI have been estimated to be between 2.6% and 2.8% of adults ages 18 and older during any given year. Only 25% of these individuals obtain help for their condition through the heathcare system. In contrast, 60–80% of all persons with heart disease seek and receive care. More importantly, 40% of people with SMI do not receive help from either general or specialty mental health providers, and most do not receive any help. Of those ages 9–17 years who have a mental disorder, 27% receive help from the health sector, but 20% of children and adolescents with mental disorders use only mental health services in their schools. Comorbidity (more than one mental disorder existing at the same time) is a growing problem and requires specialized treatment and understanding, such as is needed for concomitant depression and substance abuse.

There are great disparities in the occurrence of mental disorders in the population and treatment opportunities. Disparities in P-MH treatment merely serve to increase and compound disparities in the occurrence of mental disorders within a population. Since the early 1980s, with the changes in allocation of funds in block grants and oversight of the federal government to states, private P-MH hospitals have served the insured; state programs have served the SMI population. Additionally, within healthcare systems, there are marked differences in how disorders present themselves, and how they are prevented, diagnosed, and treated by gender, racial, ethnic groups, and age. Depression affects twice as many women as men, but women who are poor, have little formal education, are unemployed or on welfare, and live in rural areas are more likely to experience depression than women in the general population. Many of these women have no access to health care or are underserved. This gender gap in care and disorder is seen from adolescence on.

Suicide is one of the leading causes of death in the population ages 15–24 years. Suicide attempts are more common in females; however, more men die from suicide, with the greatest rate of suicide being in white males 85 years of age and older (NIMH, n.d.). Recently, attention has focused on the increasing suicide rate for returning war veterans of the Middle Eastern conflict. Research has consistently shown that approximately 90% of all people who kill themselves have a mental disorder, a substance abuse problem, or combination of these disorders. Suicide is sometimes associated with a copy-cat phenomenon. This phenomenon is also seen in violent acts involving the taking of hostages, situations of school violence, and terrorism acts. Examples of this phenomenon are threats of violence, and some cases of actual shootings, such as those that followed the 2012 Sandy Hook Elementary School massacre. Although much is known about suicide prevention, it is increasingly evident that violence needs particular research support.

Marginal, oppressed individuals and groups, for example, are at risk of perpetrating violent acts on society. Fundamentalism in politics, religion, and social programs, where only one solution is considered the "right" solution, seems to breed violence. Multicultural and reflective perspectives offer strategies to understand experiences from the perspective of the other. This phenomenon needs particular attention, as terrorism has been an increasingly global problem since the dawn of the 21st century.

Following violent societal acts, such as the September 11, 2001 terrorist attacks, or other large-scale crises, such as the Hurricane Katrina disaster, experiences of severe anxiety and depression increase. PTSD is an acute anxiety disorder that develops as a response to overwhelming anxiety. Following the Vietnam War, PTSD proved debilitating for many returning veterans and their families. In military personnel returning from the Iraq war, approximately 16% have PTSD, although this disorder is probably grossly underreported.

Following the September 11, 2001 terrorist attacks, there was an increase in anxiety and depression in the general population, and a much higher incidence of anxiety and depressive symptoms in survivors, individuals who were relatively close in geographic proximity to the events, and individuals who had family members and friends who lost their lives. For recovery workers, the direct and protracted nature of the rescue and recovery made them especially vulnerable. Data from the Mount Sinai School of Medicine's evaluation of 9/11 rescue and recovery workers and volunteers, many of whom worked 4 months of 8-hour workdays, indicated that 51% met threshold criteria for a clinical mental health evaluation. The top three emotionally related disabilities were in the area of problems with social life, work, and home life. More than a decade after these events, the nation continues to deal with bereavement and coping with change and loss. The feeling of safety, security, and freedom in everyday life seems gone forever (Centers for Disease Control and Prevention, 2004).

Another population group needing special attention and understanding is the homeless population. Approximately 25% of the homeless in the United States have a SMI. Although new approaches and attention have been focused on this group, the population remains especially vulnerable. Treatment is not enough for this population: A complex array of human services, health care, and affordable housing solutions is needed to address their problems. Further, homeless shelters are often very restrictive in who they will serve and how long housing is provided, and they are top heavy with rules about who can gain admission and use services. For example, many refuse to give shelter to a person under the influence of alcohol. For a person in a small city in northern Florida living on minimum wage, it would require 96 hours of work per week to afford a one-bedroom apartment. About one-fourth of shelter residents have jobs and return to the shelter for housing and meals. They see the shelter as a primary group, similar to that of a family. In fact, many refer to the shelter as "home" and as being "family."

Violence in the United States has reached epidemic levels. More than 100,000 youths are placed in U.S. juvenile justice facilities annually. There is an increasing trend in childhood violent deaths, with infant homicides considered to be fatal child abuse. Males are more often perpetrators, and African Americans are more than five times as likely as whites to be murdered. Factors such as low income, racism and discrimination, and lack of education and employment opportunities are associated with greater rates of violence. In addition, substance use and abuse, including use of illicit drugs and alcohol, are often associated with violence.

There is a growing concern about the increase in personality disorders in the general larger population. Of special concern is the growing number of individuals with antisocial personality disorders and their lack of response to psychosocial therapies and treatment. There is a need for research in all disorders, but particularly in personality disorders that are listed under Axis II diagnoses. The person with antisocial personality does not experience anxiety, which is often used as part of therapy and is associated with learning. Such an individual does not experience distress or assume responsibility for his or her acts and behavior. This general lack of anxiety or distress, coupled with feeling no responsibility, is common among forensic residents in prisons and mental health units. These individuals do not experience discomfort or guilt from behaviors that harm or take away the rights and privileges of another. In fact, the pleasure taken in another's suffering is a common feature of their disorders.

Statistics and rates of mental disorders, although impressive on their own, need to be personalized. Numerical data need personalized interpretations. Such figures do not inform alone, nor do they tell the human story behind the condition. Each statistic represents a person, an individual—someone's child, spouse, father or mother, sibling, or friend. Each person represented suffers often unbearable pain and anxiety, along with failed hopes and dreams, as do all of the people connected to that person, such as the family, community, coworkers, or social group.

Ethics of Psychiatric–Mental Health Services

Inequity that exists around mental health care impoverishes a group of people who are already at risk. Furthermore, the cost of services is a factor in access and serves to compound risk in an already vulnerable population. This is in direct conflict with prevention concepts and health promotion, which require delicate timing and appropriate intervention within the least restrictive environment. The right to fair and equal mental health treatment is a human rights issue. Interestingly, the community mental health movement was concurrent with the civil rights movement in the United States and was just about as successful.

MEDIA MOMENT 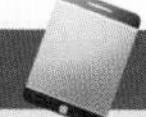

Portrayal of Mental Illness and Psychiatric Conditions in Media

Embedded within a mental health nursing course can be opportunities for planned, structured reflective exercises. The following films are examples of audiovisual materials that have been used for in-class or outside-class viewing. These films, combined with reflective journaling, dialogue, and class discussion, help develop the skills needed in reflective nursing practice. The following list includes only a few of the many excellent films that can be used to support the development of reflective practice:

American Beauty (1999)
As Good as It Gets (1997)
Asylum (1972)
A Beautiful Mind (2001)
Black Swan (2010)
The Bucket List (2007)
Clean, Shaven (1993)
The Days of Wine and Roses (1962)
Eternal Sunshine of the Spotless Mind (2004)
Extremely Loud and Incredibly Close (2011)
50 First Dates (2004)
Fight Club (1999)
Fried Green Tomatoes (1991)
Garden State (2004)
Girl, Interrupted (1999)
The Girl with the Dragon Tattoo (2011)
The Hours (2002)
House of Cards (1993)
House of Sand and Fog (2003)
Leaving Las Vegas (1995)
Little Miss Sunshine (2006)
The Machinist (2004)
Matchstick Men (2003)
Melancholia (2011)
Memento (2000)
Misery (1990)
Nurse Betty (2000)
One Flew Over the Cuckoo's Nest (1975)
Ordinary People (1980)
Prozac Nation (2001)
Rain Man (1988)
Reign Over Me (2007)
Silver Linings Playbook (2012)
A Single Man (2009)
The Talented Mr. Ripley (1999)
Three Faces of Eve (1957)
Tuesdays with Morrie (1999)
What About Bob? (1991)
What's Eating Gilbert Grape (1993)
When a Man Loves a Woman (1994)

Whose Life is it, Anyway? (1981) *Wit* (2001) Student reflection focused on *The Three Faces of Eve* (1957)

I have always been fascinated with split personalities. This movie helped me see that behind the turmoil of all these personalities vying for control was a suffering young lady in need of help. It is easy in situations where someone is disturbed to want to probe and inspect the mind, forgetting that there is a person who is affected by that mind. The movie gave me a greater understanding of the disorder and the suffering of another human being.

—BSN nursing student

Where civil rights and care are much improved today, there is great need for equity and mainstreaming of mental health services into the healthcare system of services.

Mental health problems, in contrast to physical health problems, are often very complex, involving an interaction of many factors, including heredity, culture, social class, living conditions, lifestyle, family relationships, occupation, and economic and political factors. There are often unrecognized mental health issues surrounding and involved with physical health and illness conditions that, if treated along with the physical illness, would promote a healthier adjustment.

The separation of mental health services from other health services creates problems of access to treatment. Problems occur both for those with major or chronic and debilitating mental health conditions and for those who have symptoms that, if treated appropriately at the time, would contribute to the recovery, health, and wellbeing of the person.

Psychiatric–Mental Health Nursing's Roles and Phenomena of Concern

The preceding discussion is particularly important in understanding the complexities of the art and science of P-MH nursing care. The American Nurses Association (ANA, 1994) identified a list of actual or potential mental health problems, presented in **Box 27-8**, that comprise **phenomena of concern** for P-MH nursing. These include phenomena presented earlier as universal human experiences in need of attention, care, and research. Basic-level functions of P-MH nursing presented previously are inclusive of both prevention and promotion activities as well as treatment and intervention activities. Advanced-level functions further delineate the specialty and therapist role of the advanced practice P-MH nurse.

The P-MH nursing role includes health promotion, health maintenance, health teaching, community action, and advocacy; however, this area encompasses one of the greatest needs in community mental health program development. Currently, nurses in practice within community programs function primarily as managers of care, overseeing care, administering medication, and maintaining records. Community action and advocacy activities are often limited. Some nurses are involved in developing and maintaining the therapeutic milieu, but staffing issues are prevalent throughout the private and public programs.

Missing from the list of functions is the nurse's key role in providing continuity of care. The nurse's unique role and position with persons and groups over time provide opportunities for support and intervention that others on the treatment team simply do not have. In addition, the commitment to using strengths of people and active involvement of those cared for place nursing in a key position.

Since the beginning of modern nursing, the concept of *prevention as intervention* has been a key concept of public health care. The unique vantage provided by the nursing perspective, nursing presence, and the temporality of this role is often underused in therapeutic relationships with individuals, groups, and communities. This is an area in need of attention in both public and private programs.

The P-MH nurse of the 21st century has assumed more coordinating, collaborative, and case management activities than ever before. At the same time, the role encompasses direct service and therapeutic interventions with

BOX 27-8 Psychiatric–Mental Health Nursing's Phenomena of Concern

Actual or potential mental health problems of patients pertain to the following:

- The maintenance of optimal health and wellbeing and the prevention of psychobiological illness
- Self-care limitations or impaired functioning related to mental and emotional distress
- Deficits in the functioning of significant biological, emotional, and cognitive systems
- Emotional stress or crisis components of illness, pain, and disability
- Self-concept changes, developmental issues, and life process changes
- Problems related to emotions such as anxiety, anger, sadness, loneliness, and grief
- Physical symptoms that occur along with altered psychological functioning
- Alterations in thinking, perceiving, symbolizing, communicating, and decision making
- Difficulties in relating to others
- Behaviors and mental states that indicate the patient is a danger to self or others or has a severe disability
- Interpersonal, systemic, sociocultural, spiritual, or environmental circumstances or events that affect the mental and emotional wellbeing of the individual, family, or community
- Symptom management, side effects/toxicities associated with psychopharmacological intervention and other aspects of the treatment regimen

Source: © 2007 ANA, APNA, and IPNA. *Psychiatric Mental Health Nursing: Scope and Standards of Practice.* Silver Spring, MD: Nursesbooks.org. Reprinted by permission.

individual and groups within services and programs in a variety of locations—within community agencies and the home. The role of nursing in the public's mental health needs continued assessment and evaluation.

In primary mental health care environments, basic-level P-MH nurses are key professionals who are ideally positioned to assume a variety of roles in multiple settings ranging from acute inpatient to community settings. They are often the only member of the healthcare team who has knowledge to monitor general health as well as mental health needs and care and who possesses the knowledge of the impact of comorbid illnesses on the clinical presentation of the mental disorder (see **Box 27-9** for leading health indicators). They are prepared in early identification of problems, including preventive intervention, primary prevention, and health promotion. They possess skills in assessment, social intervention, and psychoeducational processes connected with understanding illness and experience of mental illness, and also have knowledge of symptom management, pharmacology, and rehabilitation. The advanced practice P-MH nurse is prepared to manage the care of persons, including monitoring medications.

Guiding Philosophical and Theoretical Frameworks for Mental Health Nursing

The purposes of theory are description, explanation, prediction, and control of human phenomena. In addition, nursing theory serves the purpose of providing understanding of human experience and phenomena. Nursing, as a practice discipline until the latter part of the 20th century, operated based on theories related to a biological model of health. It also used interdisciplinary theory. In addition, the use of practice experience as described in the discussion of "tacit understanding" provided a basis for nursing intervention. Nurses have always borrowed and "cut and pasted" theory, sometimes without enough concern for the relevance or "fit." Increasingly, with the development of qualitative research that focuses on developing theory and quantitative research, which requires a theoretical structure, clarity, and operationalization of concepts, mid-level nursing theory is being developed. The 1960s and 1970s were the decades for development of nursing grand conceptual models (**Table 27-1**). In addition, the development of doctoral programs in nursing has provided the impetus for theory analysis, theory derivation, and theory construction. Advanced-level P-MH nurses have been involved in theory development, which can be seen in the dissertations and writings of several qualitative nurse researchers, including Becker (1991), Hutchinson (1986), Lauterbach (1992, 1995), Swanson-Kaufmann (1983), and Swanson (1993). Aguilera's (1998) classic nursing text is in its eighth edition and is almost universally used in nursing education curricula that teach crisis intervention. Aguilera's model of crisis intervention assesses the presence of balancing factors.

More recently, writings from P-MH nurses such as Boyd (1988), Lauterbach and Becker (1996), Lauterbach and Becker Hentz (1998, 2005), Munhall (1994, 2007), Munhall and Boyd (1993), and others also embrace the philosophy of phenomenology. Jean Watson's writings and contributions identify caring as the central focus of nursing (Morrow, 2014). There is need for continuing theory development in P-MH nursing. Researchers and scholars such as Janice Morse and her colleagues' (1997) symposium on the Comfort Project and other qualitative nurse researchers show potential for theory development.

Models for Psychiatric–Mental Health Nursing Practice

The writings of educator John Dewey in the early 1900s, who was a friend and colleague of Isabel Stewart, then Chair of the Department of Nursing at Teachers College, Columbia University, are informative. The 1938 writings of Horace Mann (Cremin, 1957) are appropriate considering his views on the value of universal education as the "great equalizer" of human conditions, the "balance wheel of the social machinery," and the creator of wealth undreamed of. He believed that poverty would disappear as an educated

BOX 27-9 Leading Health Indicators in *Healthy People 2020*

- Access to health services
- Clinical preventive services
- Environmental quality
- Injury and violence
- Maternal, infant, and child health
- Mental health
- Nutrition, physical activity, and obesity
- Oral health
- Reproductive and sexual health
- Social determinants
- Substance abuse

Source: U.S. Department of Health and Human Services. (2014). Leading Health Indicators. Retrieved from http://www.healthypeople.gov/2020/LHI/default.aspx

TABLE 27-1 Chronology of Conceptual Models in Nursing, 1950–1986

Year	Author	Key Emphasis, Publication, and/or Model
1952	Hildegard E. Peplau	*Interpersonal Relations in Nursing*
1960	Faye Abdellah	Client's problem is focus of nursing care
1961	Ida Jean Orlando	*The Dynamic Nurse–Patient Relationship*
1964	Ernestine Wiedenbach	*Clinical Nursing: A Helping Art*
1966	Virginia Henderson	*The Nature of Nursing*
1966	Lydia Hall	*Nursing Care—Use of Self*
1967	Myra E. Levine	*Four Conservation Principles of Nursing*
1970	Martha Rogers	*Science of Unitary Human Being*
1971	Imogene King	General Systems Framework
1971	Dorothea Orem	Self-care framework for model
1971	Joyce Travelbee	*Therapeutic Use of Self*
1974	Betty Neuman	Systems Model
1976	Sr. Callista Roy	Adaptation Model
1976	Josephine G. Paterson & Loretta T. Zderad	Existential philosophical foundation of nursing
1978	Madeleine M. Leininger	Caring and transcultural perspectives
1980	Dorothy E. Johnson	Behavioral System Model
1981	Rosemarie Rizzo Parse	*Man-Living–Health*
1985	Jean Watson	*Nursing: Human Science and Human Care*
1986	Margaret Newman	*Health as Expanding Consciousness*
1989	Patricia Benner and Judith Wrubel	Caring is central to the essence of nursing

public discovered new "treasures of natural and material wealth." Mann also stated, "a nation cannot remain ignorant and free." Education is the key to an informed public and underpins P-MH nursing practice at all levels.

Public Health Model

The traditional public health model includes all levels of prevention: primary, secondary, and tertiary. It has been a viable model for P-MH nursing practice. Central to this model is the critical role of public education. This model uses concepts of mental health and illness, epidemiology, and population-focused statistics in assessing mental health needs and risks. Population statistics, when combined with knowledge of mental health issues, are useful in identifying populations vulnerable to experiencing dysfunction.

Currently, the major thrust of U.S. mental health care is toward secondary prevention efforts, providing treatment and minimizing disability. There is a need for research and funding in all areas of prevention, but particularly within primary prevention. The following primary prevention activities are in need of public policy inquiry and research: mental health promotion and dysfunction prevention; holistic, meaningful, mind–body wellness activities; personal and community education; acquisition of effective coping skills; wholesome early attachments and healthy lifelong relationships; facilitating environments conducive to meaningful work and mental and physical health; and finally, self-empowerment. There is a need for large-scale community studies of stress and crisis conditions.

Secondary prevention activities are the major thrust of care and include early diagnosis and intervention, accessible services, and timely, appropriate treatment. One of the most important contributions of the community mental health movement of the 1960s and since has been the development of crisis intervention services. This, combined with the consumer movement of the 1970s, has made a significant contribution to support services for individuals and communities. Still, major primary prevention work is needed to address the conditions and environments that create and perpetuate interpersonal crises. Situational crises, which are superimposed on predicted developmental crises, further create risk, but with proper attention, they can be addressed. Consumer involvement has been helpful in the development of suicide prevention programs, services for rape crisis and victim recovery, and other phenomena needing support and therapeutic intervention. However, more research into crisis prevention, intervention, and impact of crises on life is needed. The phenomenon of human abuse and violence needs to be researched and better understood. Where treatment usually is focused on the victim, more work is needed in addressing the treatment and rehabilitation of the perpetrator, facilitating a violence-free environment. Phenomena need to be reconceptualized and investigated as a community and social phenomenon as well as an individual phenomenon.

Tertiary care has been the focus of community mental health programs and currently provides most of the care for the SMI public, including state hospitalization. The community mental healthcare system includes a range of community-based services addressing a full range of needs and particular groups needing care. These programs address ongoing and acute exacerbations of conditions and chronic care. Activities aimed at rehabilitation and reducing the discomfort and suffering associated with particular mental health problems need research.

Community studies of health have provided information that is potentially useful in articulating nursing's future role in community mental health. Early studies such as Hollingshead and Redlich's (1958) work associated social class and mental health. Studies that also show the promise of stress and education include Folkman and Lazarus's (1980) analysis of coping in a middle-aged community. Antonovsky's (1979, 1987) work on health focuses on "salutogenesis," the origins of health, and "what healthy people have in common." This mid-level theory, along with Selye's (1956, 1974) classic work on the biological model of stress and the work of Benson (1975, 1984), have contributed much to the field. The value of theories such as these comes from the combination of the idea of the connection between mental and physical health and a sociological model for conceptualizing stress.

CULTURAL CONNECTION 

Domestic violence is of concern throughout the world and is present in all economic, racial, and ethnic groups. The status of women and the oppression of women in economic, social, and political roles are underlying causes of such violence. Intimate-partner violence is a major public health issue for all women and for people who are oppressed. There is a great need for healthcare providers to be culturally aware and competent to provide services and intervention. The dual discrimination that black women face predisposes them to black male aggression. Further, the cultural and spiritual conditions trap battered black "women into silence, submission, and continued victimization" (p. 535).

There are also structural, cultural, and situational issues surrounding the violence. The structural context is defined as the macro-level structural arrangements and social conditions that have a direct effect on access to opportunity and the quality of life. Intergenerational exposure to racial and gender oppression is a major feature of many black men's experience. Chronic unemployment and underemployment have profound effects on black women and children.

The cultural-community context provides the socialization that black men have, which instills in them views similar to the white male views about their superiority over women. Subordinated masculinity for black men and other lower class men has prompted many of them to redefine masculinity in a manner consistent with the context of their subordinated status. For all these reasons, black women wives and girlfriends are at increased risk for becoming victims of black men committing violent crimes against them.

The situational context is that most intimate-partner violence occurs close to home, between 6:00 p.m. and midnight. It typically occurs within the normal context of everyday life.

Although no single program can eliminate this violence, successful efforts might include early intervention in the form of school retention programs, high school–based programs providing job readiness, low-interest loans for education, and placement centers for employment in inner cities. When black men are employed, they are less available on the street—organizing their daily activities, rather than hanging out and getting in trouble with their wives or girlfriends, which in turn increases the likelihood of conflict.

Source: Hampton, R., Oliver, W., & Magarian, L. (2003). Domestic violence in the African American community: An analysis of social and structural factors. *Violence Against Women*, *9*(5), 533–557.

Primary Care Model

Since the beginning of modern nursing, nursing has offered two different perspectives for the focus of care: caring for the individual and caring for the needs of populations. There is often tension between these two different perspectives. This is especially true for P-MH nursing, where the individual often is seen as the identified patient but in reality reflects dysfunction within a family, community, or larger social system. Taking the example of the state of the mental health care system within the nation, there is dichotomization, stigma, and economic differences within systems providing physical care and mental health care.

Privatization of mental health care, reimbursement differences between physical and mental care, and the current contrast with public mental health care's focus on tertiary care are reflective of sentiment and thinking in a society that values economics and physical care over mental health.

Nursing has traditionally been able to provide care to both individuals and groups, using both paradigms for providing care: the public health model and person-focused or family-centered model. Nurses have seen the need for the current "illness care" system to be transformed into a "health care" system.

Primary health care is increasingly being viewed as synonymous with provision of health care (Haber & Billings, 1995). If this concept is to be fully actualized, then primary care will necessarily have to include mental health care. Whether this concept will be fully realized is doubtful. Rather than being a reactive profession, nursing needs to take a position for advocating planned change, advocating for the right for each citizen to have responsive, quality mental health care alongside responsive quality health care. Access to the healthcare system needs to include both.

Primary Mental Health Care Model

Increasingly, the discussion of a primary mental health care model is being proposed as a model for delivering community-based, comprehensive P-MH nursing (Haber & Billings, 1995). It has the potential to integrate the two traditional models of care and positions nursing in a key role to meet the needs of individuals and communities. There is need for continued dialog between psychiatric nurses themselves, represented by the Coalition of Psychiatric Nursing Organizations (COPNO), including the ANA Council on Psychiatric Mental Health Nursing, the American Psychiatric Nursing Association (APNA), and the International Society of Psychiatric–Mental Health Nurses (ISPN), which includes the following divisions:

- Association of Child and Adolescent Psychiatric Nurses (ACAPN)
- International Society of Psychiatric Consultation-Liaison Nurses (ISPCLN)
- Society for Education and Research in Psychiatric–Mental Health Nursing (SERPN)
- Adult and Geropsychiatric–Mental Health Nurses (AGPN)

Primary care roles need to be conceptualized to include providing P-MH care within frontline health care and should include more than case management of the large population of psychiatric patients receiving tertiary and chronic P-MH care.

GLOBAL CONNECTION 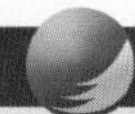

The publication of *Nurses of All Nations* marked the 100th anniversary of the International Council of Nurses (ICN). This text is the culmination of more than a decade of scholarly inquiry, research, and planning. The first chapter, entitled "Above All Other Things—Unity," begins by identifying the roots of the ICN in "women's suffrage, abolition, missionary work, and social reform" (p. xi). The text is organized around five perspectives that trace ICN's 100-year history: self-image; race, class, and gender; meaning(s) attached to professional nursing; nursing diplomacy; and friendship. In 1997, the president of ICN, Kirsten Stallknecht (from Denmark), urged nurses to continue to stress "humanity," regardless of whether governments or others do, urging nurses to demonstrate their values (p. 198). In addition to urging nurses to demonstrate concern for public health, ICN has since its inception been concerned about the "special" needs of women around the globe. The history of ICN and professional nursing worldwide reflects the history of women in society.

Unity, as a theme for nursing, is of particular interest for the chapter authors. Nursing's history is also a history of friendships. Unity is a critical phenomenon in past, current, and future nursing work. We acknowledge that often nurses fail to provide individual and collective support to one another, even as care is provided the public. Nursing work is often anxiety provoking, sensitive, and private; involves human suffering; and is often surrounded by a phenomenological silence. It is imperative that nurses value and provide care for themselves and for one another to provide the care the public needs and deserves.

Source: Bush, B. L., Lynaugh, J. E., Boschma, G., Rafferty, A. M., Stuart, M., & Tomes, N. J. (1999). *Nurses of all nations: A history of the International Council of Nurses 1899–1999*. Philadelphia, PA: Lippincott.

NOTE THIS!

Primary Mental Health Care: A Model for Psychiatric–Mental Health Nursing

Haber and Billings (1995) stated that primary care is increasingly becoming synonymous with the provision of health care. In addition to discussing roles of basic- and advanced-level nursing practice in primary mental health care, these authors state that anxiety disorders, depression, and substance abuse are among the most commonly misdiagnosed categories in primary healthcare practice. In addition, they propose that the boundaries of mental health care delivery must be redefined and expanded from a specialty focus to a primary mental healthcare model. Furthermore, they state that nurses are beginning to find their niche in nontraditional settings.

Using Reflection in Nursing Education and Practice

Throughout this chapter are many references to P-MH nursing's use of reflection as a critical activity in nursing education and practice. Becoming a reflective practitioner is especially critical in P-MH nursing. It is imperative that self-reflection be developed early in the educational experience and continued throughout nursing practice.

Reflective practice involves a bending back of attention to self and others and to the therapeutic encounter. Reflection takes place throughout the nursing encounter.

> We do not see things as they are, we see them as we are.
>
> —*Talmud*

It involves carefully attending to and focusing on the other and the experience itself. It includes the unfolding interaction, focusing on the *content* of communication, the possible meanings, and the unfolding communication *process*. By using a reflective and thoughtful, attentive posture, it becomes possible to "see" much more fully the meanings in the experience of another. This practice increases awareness and leads to greater understanding of the other. As a result of this enhanced understanding, the nursing process can be more fully, appropriately, and timely implemented and evaluated.

Many examples of reflective activities have been provided that have been particularly useful in nursing education and in P-MH nursing practice. Reflection on personal attitudes, feelings, and values, as well as reflection on life and educational experience, is a critical process in nursing education; it is a critical process in becoming a nurse.

Using publications and teaching experiences (Lauterbach & Becker, 1996; Lauterbach & Becker Hentz, 1998, 2005), reflection is introduced and used in nursing courses and elective university courses in several nursing programs. Since the early 1990s, reflective practice has been integrated into human sciences disciplines and practice. In nursing education, reflective practice and activities have become critical strategies to enhance learning. The following are examples of the types of reflective education and practice activities used for this purpose. Student reflections are included in the Application to Practice features throughout the chapter.

Journaling to Learn: A Strategy to Develop the Art, Science, and Practice of Reflection in Nursing

Journaling has been used as an educational strategy in P-MH nursing and other nursing and elective courses. Reflective activities have been developed that are geared toward increasing awareness of meanings in self and in others. Through journaling, students become aware of their own attitudes, values, and biases regarding mental illness. Journaling has been used as a critical activity in developing a habit of reflection, using informal yet disciplined writing. It has helped to create a greater depth of awareness and more expansive breadth of understanding. This activity has been especially helpful in developing therapeutic communication and relationships in P-MH nursing courses where students are placed in a variety of settings, including community programs and civil and forensic units in a state mental hospital.

Self-reflection activities have been and continue to be developed in the following areas: understanding the family as it moves through time, with an emphasis on changing family structures, functionality, family process, patterns of health and illness, and patterns of stress and coping; caring for persons who are residents in The Shelter in a small Southern city, including the homeless SMI residents; and serving as observer-participants in support groups. In addition, class material, films, and other mental health materials were used as focal topics for guided reflection. Students kept a weekly clinical journal and wrote a short reflection and critique of the course experiences at three times during the semester. The written reflective critique was found to be especially helpful in students' continued reflection and processing of experiences.

ETHICAL CONNECTION

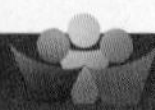

Costello and Dunaway have focused on "threatened egotism" as a major condition of violent behavior. Where the social sciences in the last several years have attempted to test the hypothesis that low self-esteem is associated with violent behavior, this research addresses the association between inflated self-esteem and violent behavior. The researchers conducted a preliminary test with participants from a small junior and senior high school in a Southern city. Their results showed that egotism is positively associated with violent and nonviolent delinquency and that the relationship holds when a number of important predictors of violent behavior are controlled, including self-control and social control.

Substance use is often associated with a person developing an excessive self-focus, inflated self-esteem, or narcissism. This may be a contributing factor in the development of egotism, where inflated self-esteem and excessive self-focus prevent the person from developing appropriate, reality-based self-esteem.

Are there ethical implications of this research linking inflated self-esteem and delinquency? As nurses we tend to focus on promoting self-esteem in patients. How would you plan nursing intervention in a school setting using these findings?

Source: Costello, B. J., & Dunaway, R. G. (2003). Egotism and delinquent behavior. *Journal of Interpersonal Violence, 18*(5), 572–590.

Reflecting on Experiences with the Homeless

While assisting at The Shelter, the students helped check residents in for the evening, provided supplies for bath and personal care, and assisted with the evening meal. They had brief interactions focused on these activities. Students found this experience to be especially transformative.

Reflecting on Support Group Experiences

Students in the following nursing courses attended and wrote reflective papers on their support group experience: the core P-MH clinical course, an RN/BSN concepts course, an elective university-wide substance abuse course, and a university-wide required communication course. Examples of groups attended were Alcoholics Anonymous, (AA), Al-Anon, Narcotics Anonymous (NA), Alzheimer's Support, Caring for the Caregiver, Hospice and Palliative Care, Cancer Support, Victims of Violent Crimes, Breast Cancer Survivors, and Mothers Against Druck Driving.

Reflecting on Family Experiences: Constructing a Multigenerational Family Genogram

The concept of family has been explored in nursing courses in several nursing programs, including P-MH nursing courses, an RN/BSN concepts course, a communication course, and a substance abuse course. The students were required to construct a multigenerational genogram of their own family going back three generations. They identified issues related to health and illness, stress and coping patterns, family structure, and family process using a family systems theory framework. Through focusing on issues and family process in their own family, students became more self-aware and understanding of the issues in their own lives that needed attention. They also developed an understanding of family processes that was applicable to their nursing practice. Students became more aware of the complexity of issues in working with patients and their families. In working with SMI patients and forensic SMI residents, they understood the care and needs of this population group, who cry out for a revolution in care. They saw the profound impact of SMI on the family.

Self-as-Patient Clinical Reflection: Caring for Self

Self-as-patient clinical activities have been included in several courses in a variety of nursing programs. This activity was used in a professional development course, in the first theory course in the nursing curriculum, in P-MH nursing courses, and in a variety of holistic nursing courses. Students used a personal journal for reflection, and conducted an assessment of and identified priorities for care in the following areas: personal health issues and status, patterns of stress and coping, nutrition, rest and leisure, relaxation, fitness, and family relationships. A plan of care focused on areas of need, priority, and interest. At the end of the semester, students shared their work in several formats, including posters and portfolio, oral presentations, and a written paper about the experience.

Therapeutic Use of Self: Clinical Reflection

Using guidelines developed for a focus on therapeutic use of self (TUS), students in several courses in several nursing curricula have been introduced to the concept of using the self therapeutically. The thesis underlying this approach is that the nurse is an instrument of healing and care. TUS activities have been used in P-MH nursing, communication, and substance abuse courses, for example. Reflecting on interactions with patients has been especially informative to students. Immediately following these interactions, students recalled the verbatim conversation and wrote process recordings. Interactions were processed and analyzed in post-conferences using the readings and theories underlying human development, therapeutic communication, and relationship development. The reflection on conversations with patients helped students identify possible interpretations of the conversation and possible meanings as they reflected on their use of therapeutic communication strategies. Such guided reflective activities help students learn to critically process, evaluate, and identify appropriate, effective communication strategies.

> I always said that mental health got what was left over after everybody else in the health field got what they wanted.
>
> *—Rosalyn Carter, who as first lady served as co-chair of the President's Commission on Mental Health and championed the rights of those with mental illness*

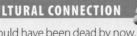

CULTURAL CONNECTION

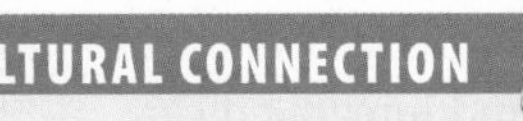

I could have been dead by now, you know, I was gang related, on drugs, really big time. Like now, I'm not gang related. I have, next month, one year clean with drugs. You just change (as a father) automatically. And when you see your son crying or you see your son smiling at you it's like, oh, I want to be at home with him . . . all the time I have to spend, I spend with my family now.

—Robert, age 19 (fictitious name)

Using a Phenomenological Perspective: Understanding the Public's Mental Health Lived Experience, One Person at a Time

Phenomenology as a philosophical human science and research perspective has been embraced by P-MH nurses as a perspective for understanding human experience. Max van Manen (1990) stated that phenomenology is the "study of the lifeworld—the world as experienced rather than as conceptualized, categorized, or reflected upon" (p. 9). It is the observation and experience of lived experience as it happens, as presented to our consciousness. It involves seeking for meaning in everyday, commonplace experiences. The writings of nurse researcher Munhall (1994) and others have further developed phenomenology as a perspective that provides a vantage point for "knowing" others and as a research methodology. In P-MH nursing, this perspective is especially illuminating. Therefore, personal reflection aids the nurse in becoming a more thorough, comprehensive healthcare provider.

Understanding underpins the nursing process from the beginning assessment, planning, and therapeutic intervention and evaluation. Sartre (1984/1967) asserted that the goal of literature, or the written word, is "to reveal the world and particularly to reveal man to other men so that the latter may assume full responsibility before the object which has been thus laid bare" (p. 18). Likewise, he stated, "If you name the behavior of an individual, you reveal it to him; he sees himself. And since you are at the same time naming it to all others, he knows that he is seen at the moment he sees himself" (p. 16). Insight and understanding in therapeutic encounters are enhanced for both nurse and patient.

Phenomenology as a perspective in P-MH practice offers strategies for uncovering meanings in lived experiences. It reveals meanings and insight to the patient and the nurse about what it is like to be a person with the particular experience. Understanding is the ultimate goal of using a phenomenological perspective. The nurse who uses a phenomenological perspective has a goal of facilitating the patient's personal understanding of behavior, of understanding more fully the patient's experience, and of helping others to understand through better communication and more coordinated and integrated care.

A phenomenological stance in nurse caring and relating involves listening carefully, imagining what it is like to be the other person with the experience, and being open to multiple meanings attributed to experience. It requires listening carefully for themes that emerge in the descriptions and paying attention to their emergence in therapeutic conversations. From a phenomenological perspective, we learn about the meaningful, relevant experiences from the perspective of the person in focus.

To understand the person requires that we listen actively to the patient's experiences and elicit rich descriptions of life experience. Often, the novice nurse fails to fully glean an understanding of the patient because of not taking the time, or hastily jumping to conclusions, or simply not being comfortable with the meanings underlying the descriptions and stories.

This perspective also helps in discovering themes in universal human experiences as well as discovering uniqueness and differences in people and experiences. Further, living through a difficult experience is common to many mental health patients and their families. In developing phenomenologically focused therapeutic relationships, the nurse develops a deeper, broader understanding of persons and differences among and between people. This broadened understanding contributes to the development of consciousness. There is a need for a public consciousness regarding the status of mental health care and the growing disparities in needs and care for particular population groups. For nursing, this recognition could potentially facilitate planning, developing, and participating in social and human advocacy with renewed and fuller understanding.

A quote by the poet T. S. Eliot (1936) describes the temporal nature of human experience: "Time present and time past are contained in time future . . . And time future contained in time past" (p. 175). The understanding and insight gleaned from every therapeutic relationship and encounter are intimately connected to past and future experiences for each nurse and patient. Through the process of caring for and of understanding one person, the nurse affects the experience of all those connected to the person, and the encounter leads to a potentially transformative relationship for many.

The Future of Psychiatric–Mental Health Nursing Practice

Current P-MH nursing practice operates within the managed care, cost-containment drive behind health care. A growing number of persons, groups, and communities are not receiving care, do not have basic needs met, and are being lost between services and programs. Preventive care is still in need of development. P-MH nurses need to be integrated into primary healthcare environments and community-based programs, such as schools, daycare programs, parenting programs, and self-help and support programs. Most importantly, there is need for P-MH advocacy in the area of health policy and healthcare planning.

Increasingly, communities are experiencing acts of violence. Since the September 11, 2001 terrorist attacks, there has been national security anxiety and depression. Following the invasion of Iraq, there has been heightened anxiety, depression, and PTSDs among the population. Grandparents are parenting their dysfunctional adult children's children. The future looks bleak as the future grandparents are today's dysfunctional adults. Within this day of information and technology, the growing Third World vulnerable populations, within the larger affluent American society, are cause for concern. Unless we support and care for all our populations' needs, health, and human rights, including shelter, nutrition, and meaningful life, the health and happiness of the public are threatened. Caring comprehensively for a multicultural population and world is key.

RESEARCH ALERT 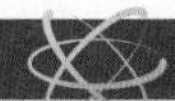

An ethnographic approach was selected to generate an explanatory model for minority young offenders in the juvenile justice system receiving mental health services. Thirty (10 female, 20 male) youths between the ages of 13 and 17 years participated. Five themes were identified in the group: a desire for caring and stable families, lack of personal control, a love–hate relationship with school, feeling depressed and hopeless, and "it's better to be tough than sick." These youths felt they had no control over their lives. Reliance on peers (gangs) was commonly used as a means of protecting themselves when they had no reliable family. Expressions of sadness and anxiety were common, and the youths were regressed, appearing very childlike as they expressed themselves. They were secretive about their mental health problems and expressed distrust of counselors even though they needed to talk to someone and indicated that they might use mental health services if they could be assured of confidentiality. This study concluded that further research is needed about this phenomenon.

Source: Shelton, D. (2004). Experiences of detained youth offenders in need of mental health care. *Journal of Nursing Scholarship, 36*(2), 129–133.

MEDIA MOMENT 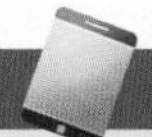

"Never doubt that a small group of thoughtful, committed citizens can change the world: Indeed, it is the only thing that ever has."

—Margaret Mead

On Civic Responsibility

In his address during *Inequality Matters* on June 3, 2004, at New York University, Bill Moyers ended his broadcast with the following:

"What we need is a mass movement of people like you. Get mad, yes—there's plenty to be mad about. Then get organized and get busy. This is the fight of our lives."

See http://www.inequalitymatters.org

On October 28, 2008, the Mental Health Parity and Addiction Equity Act was passed with bipartisan support. This ensures that more than one-third of all Americans will be able to receive equal coverage for mental and physical illnesses. The law went into effect January 1, 2010. This represents a major accomplishment for mental health coverage for Americans. See http://www.nami.org

Conclusion

"There, but by the grace of God, go I." This phrase is often used when referring to those suffering from mental illness. Often very little separates those with a P-MH condition and those without such a disorder. Accidents of birth, geography, culture, and the tenor of the times are all factors contributing to the distinction between *those who have* and *those who have not*. Mental health epidemiology demonstrates that *those who have not* are also those who have a greater risk of having a mental disorder. Equal opportunity lies in the accident of birth.

Today, as in the past, mental illness, disorder, and dysfunction are surrounded by a pervasive atmosphere of misunderstanding and social stigma. The stigma is fueled by a lack of knowledge, scientific advances, and reliable treatment and cure. Further, little value is assigned to mental health and treatment of P-MH disorders, and an impoverished and universal lack of public understanding is all too common.

Stigma has been attached to many serious illnesses, such as cancer, in the not too distant past. Over time, however, research and scientific advances in physical health have greatly expanded our knowledge base and treatment options, resulting in positive outcomes and ultimately diminishing stigma.

Even though the 1990s were considered the decade of the brain, and many advances were certainly made in treatment modalities, there is still a lack of reliable, tried-and-true treatments for mental health disorders. We know more about the biological basis of many mental conditions, and we have developed many new psychopharmacological agents that target specific symptoms and produce fewer negative side effects. Nevertheless, we have a long way to go in translating the research into effective treatment. We have not invested the time, energy, and intellectual and economic resources needed to do so.

It was not until the 1950s, with the advent of psychiatric medications, that many troublesome mental health symptoms were treated. Until then, the reliance on somatic therapies, such as hydrotherapy, insulin shock, and physical restraints, produced even more fear and stigma in association with these disorders.

Mental health problems are often very complex and have roots in social, economic, and political injustices, as well as in problematic behavior patterns. We have made progress in greatly enhancing the treatment of serious episodes and acute exacerbations of chronic mental conditions. With knowledge and treatment success has come a greater openness and acceptance of mental illness. However, our work has just begun. We must take on the *lack of parity* for mental health care and physical health care for research and treatment. It is only by achieving equity in the research and science underpinning mental disorders that treatment success and understanding will occur.

As members of a specialty, P-MH nurses continue to lead the way in developing reflective practice strategies for nursing and other disciplines. We continue to support the public in experiencing better mental health and self-actualization through developing timely, targeted, and critical interventions. We continue to advocate for the development of therapeutic, facilitative environments and relationships for treatment to thrive. We continue our efforts to revolutionize mental health care and advocate for its status to be equal to physical health care in terms of research support, with affordable, quality, accessible treatment for all people. We hope to ensure the improvement of the public's mental health by caring for people, one person at a time, including self, in families and groups, populations, and nations.

HEALTHY ME

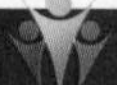

What ways do you 'de-stress' as a student in nursing school? Are these activities healthy or unhealthy? Do they work for you in the long term? What have you learned from this chapter as a way of coping in healthy ways with the mental and emotional strains of being in nursing school?

LEVELS OF PREVENTION

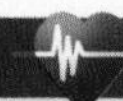

Primary: Teaching a class on how appropriate nutrition and a consistent exercise program can promote mental health

Secondary: Leading a group at a senior center on recognizing the symptoms of depression

Tertiary: Teaching a class for mental health center residents on the necessity of medication and therapeutic compliance

Critical Thinking Activities

1. Consider what is it like to experience the following:
   - Serious mental illness, such as schizophrenia, mania, or depression
   - Paranoid feelings, to the degree that you know that if you do not take medication, you will get sicker and sicker
   - Feeling that the medication dulls your attention, which helps you stay vigilant; feeling that something bad will happen if you let down your guard
2. What is it like to experience the following?
   - Having no one who you feel understands you and likes you just the way you are
   - Having no friends
   - Experiencing your little brother's death after he was sick so long with leukemia
   - Watching your dad begin to drink heavily in the evenings
   - Feeling fat, even though you ate only lettuce today, weigh 105 pounds and are 5 feet, 7 inches tall
   - Wanting and feeling very independent but still being told by your parents what time you must come in
3. What is it like to experience the following?
   - Wanting your parents to stop fighting
   - Wanting your parents to get back together even though you remember how awful it was before they separated
   - Being devastated when your dad moved out
   - Living with your mom, who works too hard and still does not have enough money even though she gets some child support
   - Visiting your dad, who has forgotten what it is like to have anyone, much less a child, around
4. What is it like to experience the following?
   - Being so depressed that you simply are too tired to get out of bed
   - Feeling that you have nothing to live for
   - Feeling that the world and your family would be better off if you just died
   - Being 17 and suddenly discovering that you had lost all your dreams and goals

References

Aguilera, D. (1998). *Crisis intervention: Theory and methodology* (8th ed.). St. Louis, MO: Mosby.

Alzheimer's Association. (2013a). Alzheimer's facts and figures. Retrieved from http://www.alz.org/alzheimers_disease_facts_and_figures.asp

Alzheimer's Association. (2013b). Types of dementia. Retrieved from http://www.alz.org/dementia/types-of-dementia.asp

American Nurses Association (ANA). (1994). *A statement on psychiatric–mental health clinical nursing practice and standards of psychiatric–mental health clinical nursing practice*. Washington, DC: American Nurses Publishing.

American Psychiatric Association (APA). (1980). *Diagnostic and statistical manual of mental disorders* (3rd ed.). Washington, DC: Author.

American Psychiatric Association (APA). (1987). *Diagnostic and statistical manual of mental disorders* (3rd ed., rev.). Washington, DC: Author.

American Psychiatric Association (APA). (1992). *Diagnostic and statistical manual of mental disorders* (4th ed.). Washington, DC: Author.

American Psychiatric Association (APA). (2000). *Diagnostic and statistical manual of mental disorders* (4th ed., rev.). Washington, DC: Author.

American Psychiatric Association (APA). (2013). *Diagnostic and statistical manual of mental disorders* (5th ed.). Washington, DC: Author.

Antonovsky, A. (1979). *Health, stress, and coping*. San Francisco, CA: Jossey-Bass.

Antonovsky, A. (1987). *Unraveling the mystery of health: How people manage stress and stay well*. San Francisco, CA: Jossey-Bass.

Baer, E. (1990). *Editor's notes. Nursing in America: A history of social reform, a video documentary*. New York, NY: National League for Nursing Press.

Barlas, S. (2013). Update on mental health benefits and substance use disorder services under the Affordable Care Act. *Psychiatric Times*. Retrieved from http://www.psychiatrictimes.com/articles/update-mental-health-benefits-and-substance-use-disorder-services-under-affordable-care-act

Barry, C. L., Huskamp, H. A., & Goldman, H. H. (2010). A political history of federal mental health and addiction insurance parity. *Milbank Quarterly*, *88*(3), 404–433. doi:10.1111/j.1468-0009.2010.00605.x

Becker, P. (1991). *Perspectives of ethical care: A grounded theory approach*. Ann Arbor, MI: University Microfilms International Dissertation Service.

Becker Hentz, P. (1994). Out of silence. In P. Munhall (Ed.), *In women's experience* (pp. 27–46). New York, NY: National League for Nursing Press.

Bennett, L., & Williams, O. J. (2003). Substance abuse and men who batter. *Violence Against Women*, *9*(5), 558–575.

Benson, H. (1975). *The relaxation response*. New York, NY: Avon Books.

Benson, H. (1984). *Beyond the relaxation response*. New York, NY: Times Books.

Boyd, C. (1988). Phenomenology: A foundation for nursing curriculum. In *Curriculum revolution: Mandate for change*. New York, NY: National League for Nursing Press.

Bunkers, S. S. (2002). Lifelong learning: A human becoming perspective. *Nursing Science Quarterly*, *15*(4), 294–300.

Bush, B. L., Lynaugh, J. E., Boschma, G., Rafferty, A. M., Stuart, M., & Tomes, N. J. (1999). *Nurses of all nations: A history of the International Council of Nurses 1899–1999*. Philadelphia, PA: Lippincott.

Casey, G. (2012). Alzheimer's and other dementias. *Kai Tiaki Nursing New Zealand*, *18*(6), 20–24.

Centers for Disease Control and Prevention. (2004). Physical health status of world trade center rescue and recovery workers and volunteers—New York City, July 2002–August 2004. *Morbidity and Mortality Weekly Report*, *53*(35), 807–812. Retrieved from http://www.cdc.gov/mmwr/preview/mmwrhtml/mm5335a1.htm

Costello, B. J., & Dunaway, R. G. (2003). Egotism and delinquent behavior. *Journal of Interpersonal Violence*, *18*(5), 572–590.

Cremin, L. (1957). *The republic and the school: Horace Mann on the education of free man*. New York, NY: Teachers College University Press.

Cummings, J. G., Lucas, S. M., & Druss, B. G. (2013). Addressing public stigma and disparities among persons with mental illness: The role of federal policy. *American Journal of Public Health*, *103*(5), 781. doi:10.2105/AJPH.2013.301224

Dilworth-Anderson, P., Pierre, G., & Hilliard, T. S. (2012). Social justice, health disparities, and culture in the care of the elderly. *Journal of Law, Medicine & Ethics*, *40*(1), 26–32. doi: 10.1111/j.1748-720X.2012.00642.x

Douglas, D. (2004). The lived experience of loss: A phenomenological study. *Journal of the Psychiatric Nurse's Association*, *10*(1), 9–15.

Eliot, T. S. (1936). *Collected poems 1909–1962*. New York, NY: Harcourt, Brace & World.

Folkman, S., & Lazarus, R. (1980). An analysis of coping in a middle-aged community sample. *Journal of Health and Social Behavior*, *21*(3), 219–239.

Frank, D. (1987). The health experience of a single woman having a child through AID. Presented at the 8th Annual Research Symposium, Gamma Zeta Chapter, Sigma Theta Tau International, UNC, Greensboro & Northwest AHCC, April 2, 1987.

Frisch, H., & Frisch, L. (1998). *Psychiatric mental health nursing*. Albany, NY: Delmar.

Gowan, T. (2002). The nexus: Homelessness and incarceration in two American cities. *Ethnography*, *3*(4), 500–534.

Haase, M. (2002). Living with "obsessive compulsive disorder." In M. van Manen (Ed.), *Writing in the dark: Phenomenological studies in interpretive inquiry*. London, England: Althouse Press.

Haber, J., & Billings, C. (1995). Primary mental health care: A model for psychiatric–mental health nursing. *Journal of the American Psychiatric Nurses Association*, *1*(5), 154–163.

Hampton, R., Oliver, W., & Magarian, L. (2003). Domestic violence in the African American community: An analysis of social and structural factors. *Violence Against Women*, *9*(5), 533–557.

Hedaya, R. (1996). *Understanding biological psychiatry*. New York, NY: W. W. Norton.

Hollingshead, A., & Redlich, F. (1958). *Social class and mental disorder*. New York, NY: Wiley.

Hutchinson, S. (1986). Grounded theory: The method. In P. Munhall & C. Oiler (Eds.), *Nursing research: A qualitative perspective*. New York, NY: National League for Nursing Press.

Lauterbach, S. (1992). *In another world: A phenomenological perspective and discovery of meaning in mothers' experience of death of a wished-for baby*. Ann Arbor, MI, University Microfilms International Dissertation Service.

Lauterbach, S. (1995). (Issue Ed.). The experience of loss. *Holistic Nursing Practice, 9*(3).

Lauterbach, S., & Becker, P. (1996). Caring for self: Becoming a self-reflective nurse. *Holistic Nursing Practice, 10*(2), 57–68.

Lauterbach, S. S. (2003). Phenomenological silence underlying sensitive human phenomena. *International Journal for Human Caring, 7*(2).

Lauterbach, S. S., & Becker Hentz, P. (1998). Becoming a reflective nurse: Caring for self (pp. 97–107). In C. E. Guzetta (Ed.), *Essential readings in holistic nursing*. New York, NY: Aspen.

Lauterbach, S. S., & Becker Hentz, P. (2005). Journaling to learn: A reflective nursing education strategy to develop the nurse as person and person as nurse. *International Journal of Human Caring, 9*(1), 48–59.

Leighton, D., Harding, J., Macklin, D., MacMillan, A., & Leighton, A. (1963). *The character of danger: Psychiatric symptoms in selected communities*. New York, NY: Basic Books.

Lesser, J., Koniak-Griffin, D., & Anderson, L. R. (1999). Depressed adolescent mothers' perceptions of their own maternal role. *Issues in Mental Health Nursing, 20*, 131–149.

Lesser, J., Oakes, R., & Koniak-Griffin, D. (2003). Vulnerable adolescent mothers' perceptions of maternal role and HIV risk. *Health Care Women International, 24*(6), 513–528.

Lesser, J., Tello, J., Koniak-Griffin, D., Kappos, B., & Rhys, M. (2001). Young Latino fathers' perceptions of paternal role and risk for HIV/AIDS. *Hispanic Journal of Behavioral Sciences, 23*(3), 327–343.

Lynaugh, J. E., & Brush, B. L. (1999). *Nurses of all nations: A history of the International Council of Nurses, 1899–1999*. Philadelphia, PA: Lippincott.

Morrow, M. (2014). Caring science, mindful practice: Implementing Watson's human caring theory, by K. Sitzman and J. Watson. *Nursing Science Quarterly, 27*(3), 263–264. doi: 10.1177/0894318414534468

Morse, J. (1997, December 1–6). *The comfort project*. Presentation at 75th Anniversary Sigma Theta Tau Conference, Indianapolis, IL.

Munhall, P. (1994). *Revisioning phenomenology: Nursing and health science research*. New York, NY: National League for Nursing Press.

Munhall, P. (2007). *Nursing research: A qualitative perspective* (4th ed.). Sudbury, MA: Jones and Bartlett.

Munhall, P., & Boyd, C. (1993). *Nursing research: A qualitative perspective*. New York, NY: National League for Nursing Press.

Nasar, S. (1998). *A beautiful mind*. New York, NY: Simon & Shuster.

National Institute of Mental Health. (n.d.). The numbers count: Mental disorders in America. Retrieved from http://www.nimh.nih.gov/health/publications/the-numbers-count-mental-disorders-in-america/index.shtml?LS-2659

Nightingale, F. (1859). *Notes on nursing: What it is and what it is not*. New York, NY: Dover.

Nurses for a Healthier Tomorrow. (2008). *Psychiatric-mental health nursing.* Retrieved from http://www.nursesource.org/psychiatric.html

Orlando, I. J. (1961). *The dynamic nurse–patient relationship: Function, process, and principles.* New York, NY: G. P. Putnam.

Parse, R. R. (1998). The human becoming theory: The was, is, and will be. *Nursing Science Quarterly, 10*(1), 32–38.

Peplau, H. (1952). *Interpersonal relations in nursing.* New York, NY: G. P. Putnam.

Quinn, J. F. (1992). Holding sacred space: The nurse as healing environment. *Holistic Nursing Practice, 6*(4), 26–36.

Reverby, S. (1987). *Ordered to care: The dilemma of American nursing 1850–1945.* New York, NY: Cambridge University Press.

Sartre, J. (1984, orig. 1967). *Existentialism and human emotions.* Sacramento, CA: Citadel Press.

Selye, H. (1956). *The stress of life.* New York, NY: McGraw-Hill.

Selye, H. (1974). *Stress without distress.* New York, NY: Signet.

Shelton, D. (2004). Experiences of detained young offenders in need of mental health care. *Journal of Nursing Scholarship, 36*(2), 129–133.

Stanhope, M., & Lancaster, J. (2014). *Public health nursing: Population-centered health care in the community* (8th ed.). Maryland Heights, MO: Mosby.

Swanson, K. (1993). Nursing as informed caring for the wellbeing of others. *Image: The Journal of Nursing Scholarship, 45*(4), 352–357.

Swanson-Kaufmann, K. (1983). *The unborn one: A profile of the human experience of miscarriage.* Ann Arbor, MI: University Microfilms International Dissertation Service.

U.S. Department of Health and Human Services (HHS). (1999). *Healthy People 2000: Mental health and mental disorders progress review.* Retrieved from http://www.cdc.gov/nchs/healthy_people/hp2000/reviews/mental_health

U.S. Department of Health and Human Services (HHS). (2014). Mental health and mental disorders. Retrieved from http://www.healthypeople.gov/2020/topicsobjectives2020/overview.aspx?topicid=28

van Manen, M. (1990). *Research on lived experience: Human science for action-sensitive pedagogy.* New York, NY: SUNY Press.

Weger Jr., H., Castle, G. R., & Emmett, M. C. (2010). Active listening in peer interviews: The influence of message paraphrasing on perceptions of listening skill. *International Journal of Listening, 24*(1), 34–49. doi:10.1080/10904010903466311

Wolf, Z. (1988). *Nurses' work: The sacred and the profane.* Philadelphia, PA: University of Pennsylvania Press.

CHAPTER FOCUS

Issues and Public Policies Affecting Individuals with Chronic Illnesses and Disabilities

Chronic Illness and Disabilities in the United States

Defining Disability and Chronic Illness

- International Classification of Functioning, Disability, and Health (ICF)
- Understanding the Differences Between Disability and Chronic Illness
- Needs of Those with Chronic Illness and Disability

Caregivers for Individuals with Chronic Conditions

- Prevention Measures

Vulnerable Populations

- Disability
- Experiences of Populations with Chronic Illnesses and Disabilities

Caring for Persons with Long-Term Health Problems

Quality of Life in Disability and Chronic Illness

The Chronic Care Model

Stages of Adjusting to a New Form of Disability

- People with Disabilities
- The Experience of a New Disability
- Disability Diversity in Society

Roles for Community Health Nurses

- Change Agent
- Advocate
- Professional Caregiver

Role Models

- Interdisciplinary Roles and Responsibilities

Financing Costs of Chronic Illness

- The Future of Managed Care for People with Disabilities
- Racial Disparities in Health Care in Chronic Illness and Disability

Self-Determination: The Patient as Partner

Sensitivity in Community-Based Caring

- Gender-Specific Considerations

Issues Community Health Nurses Encounter

- Supporting Community-Based Caregivers
- Palliative and Hospice Care
- Institutionalization
- Health Promotion in Chronic Illness and Disability

Community Living Needs of People Who Have Disabilities

- Homes of Their Own
- An Accessible Community
- Meaningful Work
- Relationships
- Recreation
- Transition from Education to Work and Living in the Community
- Rehabilitation
- Medical Technology
- Nonmedical Assistive Technology
- Assistance Animals

Ethical Issues Related to Disabilities

The Role of Community Health in Chronic Illness and Disability Care in the Future

QUESTIONS TO CONSIDER

After reading this chapter, you will know the answers to the following questions:

1. What are the reasons for the increase in chronic and disabling conditions in the United States?
2. Which population groups are most vulnerable in regard to chronic illness and disabilities?
3. How do chronic illness and disability differ?
4. How do the concepts of paradox and loss relate to the experience of chronic and disabling illnesses?
5. What are current and future roles of the community health nurse in caring for persons with chronic and disabling illnesses?
6. How does the financing of chronic illness and disabilities affect persons with chronic illness?
7. What are specific challenges in caring for diverse groups with chronic illness and disabilities?
8. How are the health issues of caregivers of the chronically ill and those with disabilities related to nursing management?
9. What is hospice care?
10. What role do institutions play in the management of chronically ill and individuals with disabilities?
11. What are the legal protections for a person with chronic illness or disabilities?
12. How should we communicate with a person with chronic illness or disabilities?
13. What are community living needs related to caring for a population with chronic illness or disabilities?
14. Which services are available for persons with chronic illness or disabilities?
15. Are there ethical issues that influence the care of persons with chronic illness or disabilities?

Chronic illness and disabilities are among the most important issues within our healthcare system in the 21st century. With the population of the United States growing older, combined with advances in care, more people are living longer with chronic and disabling conditions. The move toward comprehensive community services for individuals with chronic and disabling health issues has greatly expanded the role of the community health nurse serving these populations.

CHAPTER 28

Chronic Illness and Disability

Edith Hilton and Valerie Rachal

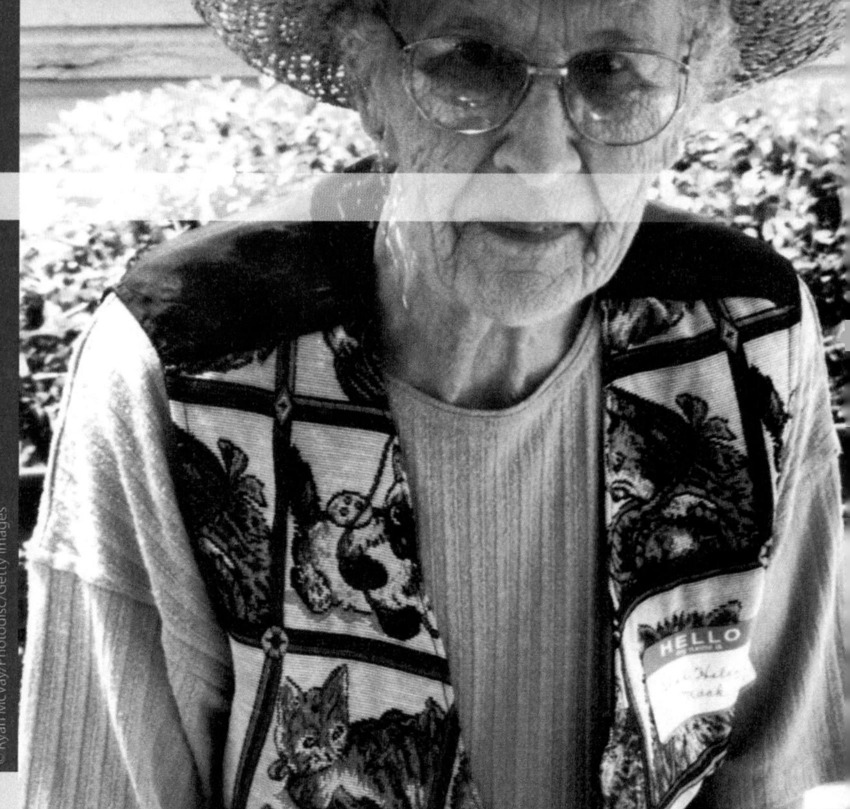

KEY TERMS

adjustment and acceptance
anger and depression
assistive technology device
case management
chronic care model
chronic illness
chronic sorrow
congregate housing
denial
developmental disability
disability
geriatric depression
handicap
home health care
impairment
informed consent
medical assistive devices
mental impairment
people-first language
person-centered planning
personal care attendant
physical impairment
power
rehabilitation
respite care
shock
sick role

CHRONIC ILLNESS AND DISABLING conditions are among today's most pressing challenges. In 2012, 117 million adults, almost half of all Americans, lived with at least one chronic illness, and this does not include the roughly 32 million children with chronic illnesses ranging from asthma (nearly 7 million) to developmental disabilities (nearly 10 million) to less common conditions like type 1 diabetes (around 200,000) (Centers for Disease Control and Prevention [CDC], 2014). Chronic disease accounts for 70% of all deaths in the United States (CDC, 2008a). As our society ages and the number of individuals with chronic illness increases, growing demands on existing healthcare infrastructures and resources will challenge long-standing values that have been shifting during the past century. The magnitude of human suffering that chronic illness and disability cause is difficult to grasp or describe. Because of the complexity of the experiential component of living with an incurable state or condition, and because recent medical and technological advances have extended the life expectancy of many persons with these conditions, research into chronic illness and disability is drawing broader interest. Since the beginning of the 2000s, there has been an upsurge in interdisciplinary research focused on quality of life. Much attention is currently directed at improving the life quality of individuals with chronic conditions and helping others to modify current health practices that contribute to the onset of chronic illness and disability. Once these conditions develop, they require daily self-care and management (Improving Chronic Illness Care [ICIC], 2008). The number of individuals with chronic conditions and disability is projected to increase substantially during the first half of the 21st century.

Many people with disabilities and chronic illnesses face difficulties accessing health care. In recent years, several key public policy initiatives have been undertaken to reduce such barriers. Implementation of the Affordable Care Act (ACA) has offered an opportunity for millions of uninsured or underinsured persons to obtain healthcare coverage they can afford without facing the prospect of denials due to preexisting conditions. In addition, policymakers have sought to increase access to Medicare and Medicaid health insurance for disability income recipients who return to work, with the goal of reducing disincentives to find employment. Community health nursing is poised as the key healthcare profession to integrate knowledge of the healthcare needs of people with disabilities and chronic conditions with the challenging needs related to full inclusion into society. This chapter considers chronic illness and disability with a global lens that highlights individuals and groups for the purpose of improving health and health care and identifying areas of future research. Roles and activities of community health nurses are explored in this context as well.

Issues and Public Policies Affecting Individuals with Chronic Illnesses and Disabilities

In the 1950s, chronic illness and disabling conditions were identified as the major challenge of the era (Mayo, 1956). Now, in the 21st century, new challenges are confronting society and community health nurses. In great measure, new immigration patterns, sophisticated emerging technological applications, utilization of increasingly scarce healthcare resources, and increases in healthcare knowledge are all affecting the outcomes of those with chronic illness and disability. Increased public awareness of and interest in quality-of-life research provide affected individuals with reference points wherein they can make informed decisions about treatment options that reflect their experiences as patients and as consumers.

Changing societal expectations of chronic illnesses and disability have provided the impetus for the broad expansion of community health nursing services since the beginning of the 21st century. Since 2000, new populations have developed from survivor groups—that is, groups comprising those who lived through previously untreatable illnesses. The driving forces for this change include social, technological, economic, political, and environmental factors (Wilson & Satterfield, 2007). The prevalence of chronic illness will only increase as the population ages. In response to the Americans with Disabilities Act (ADA), the American public has fewer reservations and clearer expectations about chronically ill or disabled individuals remaining at or returning to employment, given that the ability to manage symptoms associated with chronic processes improves constantly. Disease management including "broad, long-term approaches that encompass a diverse array of programs and services designed to promote the wellbeing of individuals, families, and communities" is a clearly articulated goal in many states (Klein, Cruz, O'Donnell, Scully, & Birkhead, 2005).

NOTE THIS!

President George H. W. Bush signed the Americans with Disabilities Act on July 26, 1990, the landmark law that advanced the rights of persons with disabilities.

One example of this emerging trend is human immunodeficiency virus (HIV) and acquired immune deficiency syndrome (AIDS), which are now considered chronic diseases. Health departments are intensely involved in prevention efforts aimed at limiting the spread of HIV and AIDS; they are also involved in extensive management of human services including hospice care, nursing homes, AIDS adult day care, and home health care for those affected by HIV/AIDS (Klein et al., 2005). Currently, the public's concern about HIV/AIDS is falling due in part to the powerful multi-drug regimens of antiretroviral therapies (Jaffe, 2004). Disease management is increasingly important to community health nurses who are focusing their efforts on outcomes, maintenance, and reinforcing the importance of individuals knowing their HIV status.

Local and global efforts to address preventive, acute, and chronic health problems are facing increasing scrutiny from many quarters. Old ways of thinking are being discarded, while more workable solutions to conditions not previously identified are increasingly sought. Researchers from various continents face both similar and different issues that urgently demand their attention, consideration, and resolution. Old, unresolved health problems such as malnutrition, contagious diseases such as tuberculosis and pertussis, and newer diseases including severe acute respiratory syndrome (SARS) pose challenges for globally scattered populations as well as those found locally. Paradoxically, existing travel has opened the world to far-reaching advances and has fostered information sharing but, because of numerous sources of contagion worldwide, has catapulted the traveling public into harm's way.

When considering the present and future health needs of the public, chronic diseases are of utmost importance. Many stem from acute processes, others from lifestyle choices, and still others from genetic disorders or entrenched poverty, both in the United States and globally. Nurses working in the community are in prime positions to positively affect the quality of life of those whom they serve. Nurses working in the local and global communities must be aware of problems whose solutions lie within the environment and existing systems. They must also be aware of their important role as advocates for the nation's health and equip themselves with reliable information and critical thinking abilities. To identify barriers to change that affect access to health care and disparities within and among various racial, ethnic, gender, and age-specific groups, community health nurses must think in different ways and seek new solutions to persistent problems.

CULTURAL CONNECTION

Cultural differences exist regarding the family's role in managing chronic disease. For example, some Native American tribes seek the authority of the tribal healer prior to using Western medications or interventions. The community health nurse should determine how these influences will affect the patient's management of his or her chronic disease based on the totality of the patient's life and family.

Community health nurses have an important role in present and future efforts to curtail such potential chronic and disability conditions, such as childhood obesity, and supporting an active lifestyle through education and increasing public awareness of the risks and comorbidities associated with this condition. According to Meadows (2009), community health nurses are valued for their adaptability and willingness to provide care in many settings, including community health clinics, churches, homeless shelters, and schools. These nurses provide comprehensive care to patients within their homes, at organized events such as health fairs, and at agencies and institutions serving people who have particular health needs.

Advanced practice nurses in communities improve access to care and lower costs at nurse-managed clinics on college campuses and at primary and secondary schools. They develop and implement corporate wellness programs, thereby supporting the health and productivity of employees and their organizations. In industry, they identify, assess, and manage risk to provide a balance between workplace hazards and employee behaviors, helping to develop policies and procedures to enhance safety. In a systematic review of the literature published in the *British Medical Journal* (2002), Horrocks, Anderson, and Salisbury found no differences in the quality of care between physicians and nurse practitioners (NPs) and noted that NPs spent more time with their patients and had higher patient-satisfaction ratings.

Nurse-run clinics have cared for the poor since social reformer Lillian Wald established the Henry Street settlement in 1893. Nurse-managed health centers are especially important to those with chronic illnesses and disability by providing affordable health care that is critical to the target population. Quality of care is an important value in the vision of care in the clinics and has been found to provide care of excellent quality to underserved patients.

Using education as a vehicle to empower community health initiatives, collaborative efforts between community members, faith-based initiatives, and healthcare professionals have proven valuable in assessing participants' knowledge of modifiable risk factors in leading to chronic disease in African Americans (Lewis-Washington & Holcomb, 2010). According to the CDC (2014), chronic illnesses present three major health problems in the United States: cardiovascular disease, stroke, and diabetes. Nonmodifiable risk factors such as age, race, gender, family history, and genetic predisposition leading to these diseases were considered. In a study assessing participants' knowledge of modifiable risk factors, including smoking, hypertension, obesity, high cholesterol, physical inactivity, and unhealthy eating habits, Lewis-Washington and Holcomb (2010) were able to assess the effect of knowledge gained on lifestyle practices from population-specific educational program development in religious institutions inside underserved communities.

Nurses in community health work with diverse partners and providers to address complex challenges in the community. Nowhere is this more evident than in current efforts to identify, reach, treat, and help the elderly effectively manage their chronic and disabling conditions and health problems while remaining at home. "Aging in place" has taken on new importance as older adults seek ways to maintain their independence, autonomy, and optimal health. Nurses in this specialty area of practice must highlight not only their clinical skills but also their critical thinking, advocacy, and analytical abilities to best address the health needs of the communities they serve. As the needs of individuals within the community change, community health nurses must adapt to provide responsive, appropriate care. The care is typically provided within the residence of the individual or in a combined residence of several elderly people who reside together for the purpose of companionship, shared expenses, fellowship, similar tastes and lifestyles, and to pool resources and avoid some of the issues commonly associated with nursing home living. Services are made available to those who are homebound or for whom mobility may be difficult.

Home health care is a community-based nursing service offered in the client's home or assisted living residence that provides both acute and chronic care. The homebound clients may be experiencing an exacerbation in chronic illness, may be extremely debilitated by age or illness, or may be dying. According to Gerber (2012), care is individualized for the client, and teaching family and friends who are caregivers is an important part of the care plan. Those with chronic illnesses such as diabetes, mobility impairments, or vascular disease will require assistance with drawing blood, changing urinary catheters, and filling medication boxes and insulin syringes. Home health nurses can also help by providing supervision to home healthcare aides. Care focuses on managing diseases or wellness such as nutrition, exercise, aging, family developmental tasks, spirituality, sexuality, and stresses associated with disability, aging, and chronic illness. Teaching health promotion to those with chronic illness is an important emphasis, because health promotion is essential to building on existing strengths and maintaining optimal functional abilities.

This chapter considers chronic illness and disability with a global lens that highlights individuals and groups for the purpose of improving health and health care and identifying areas of future research. Roles and activities of community health nurses are explored in this context as well.

> The world is full of suffering. Birth is suffering, decrepitude is suffering, sickness and death are sufferings. To face a man of hatred is suffering, to be separated from a beloved one is suffering, to be vainly struggling to satisfy one's needs is suffering. In fact, life that is not free from desire and passion is always involved with suffering.
>
> —*Buddha*

Chronic Illness and Disabilities in the United States

Chronic diseases and disabling conditions form the cornerstone of anticipated healthcare needs for this century (see **Box 28-1**). Until prevention becomes universally accepted and incorporated into the daily practices of all, nursing practice in the community will continue to involve caring for those in whom chronic diseases developed from unresolved acute processes. The health burden of chronic disease is staggering, not only in physical and emotional loss, but also in its economic costs. Chronic diseases account for more than three-fourths of all healthcare expenditures, or in excess of $1 trillion annually.

Chronic diseases have replaced many of the devastating epidemics of the 18th, 19th, and 20th centuries. Because contagion and disease transmission routes and vectors for many illnesses are known, the mystery of their occurrence is diminished. However, epidemics persist; tropical, viral, bacterial, and parasitic infections continue to affect destitute populations in poorly developed countries. Some disabling diseases for which effective prevention exists have re-emerged in recent years, often as a result of local or regional conflicts that make vaccination difficult or impossible; this situation has been seen, for example, in Syria, where the civil war that erupted in 2011 has produced a large-scale polio outbreak (World Health Organization [WHO], 2013). Worldwide, HIV/AIDS, malaria, and tuberculosis are acknowledged as paramount health concerns and have been aggressively attacked on many fronts with sustained efforts (Molyneux, 2004). The H1N1 pandemic, or "swine flu," which killed more than 18,000 people in 214 countries in 2009–2010,

BOX 28-1 Conditions Included in Chronic Illness and Disability

The following frequently encountered conditions are included in the expanding list of chronic illnesses and disabilities:

- Alzheimer's disease
- Amyotrophic lateral sclerosis (ALS)
- Arthritis
- Asperger's syndrome
- Asthma
- Attention deficit hyperactivity disorder (ADHD)
- Autism and autism spectrum disorders
- Bipolar disorder
- Blindness
- Cancer
- Cerebral palsy
- Childhood obesity
- Chronic kidney disease
- Chronic obstructive pulmonary disease
- Congestive heart failure
- Deafness and hard-of-hearing
- Depression
- Developmental disability
- Diabetes mellitus
- Down syndrome
- Epilepsy
- Fetal alcohol spectrum disorder (FASD)
- Glaucoma
- HIV/AIDS
- Hypercholesterolemia
- Hypertension
- Learning disability
- Macular degeneration
- Mental illness
- Multiple sclerosis
- Muscular dystrophy
- Nicotine addiction
- Obesity
- Osteoporosis
- Posttraumatic stress disorder (PTSD)
- Spina bifida
- Spinal cord injury
- Traumatic brain injury and stroke

demonstrates that health emergencies may arise without warning (WHO, 2010). Most of these conditions produce chronic illness or disabled states after the acute phase is past, so the long-term consequences of present-day contagion are enduringly evident and, in many cases, catastrophic.

THINK ABOUT THIS

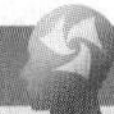

Migraine headaches affect an estimated 6 million Americans and are believed to afflict from 5% to 10% of the world's population. The Greek physician Hippocrates (460–357 B.C.) described the pains of a migraine episode. Pliny the Elder (A.D. 23–79), the Roman medical writer, refers to the symptoms we now know as migraine. The term *migraine* is originally derived from the Greek word *hemicrania,* which means "half of the head." The head pains of migraine are attributed to biochemical changes causing nausea, vomiting, irritability, visual impairment, and unsteady gait.

Millions of dollars are wasted and needless suffering is experienced by patients who are misdiagnosed or who resort to jaw reconstruction, neck surgery, hormonal manipulation, and sinus surgery in an effort to "cure" the migraine headache. Too often migraine headaches are lumped together with other forms of head pain. Also, patients often seek relief from nontraditional forms of intervention.

Migraine headaches are often labeled as psychological disorders; in actuality, they are the result of a chronic condition that can be controlled and effectively treated when considered the result of a chronic neurological disorder, influenced by hereditary factors, hormones, and particular "trigger" influences in diet and the environment. Although migraine is one of the most painful and frustrating disorders known, it is relatively benign and not life-threatening. Most migraineurs (migraine sufferers) function well even while the symptoms are coming on. Not until they are overcome by the fatigue, head pain, and nausea do they become functionally "disabled."

Effective prevention and early-intervention, nonnarcotic treatments are available now that allow the migraine sufferer to live a normal life. Complementary and self-care environmental management focusing on a holistic approach to migraine prevention offers the best control for this debilitating chronic condition.

Among those who have been tormented by the disorder in history are Joan of Arc, Charles Darwin, Sigmund Freud, Thomas Jefferson, Frederic Chopin, Saint Paul, Julius Caesar, Immanuel Kant, Lewis Carroll, Ulysses S. Grant, Edgar Allan Poe, Leo Tolstoy, Charles Dickens, Virginia Woolf, and Peter Ilich Tchaikovsky. More contemporary personalities with this problem include Whoopi Goldberg, Star Jones, Lisa Kudrow, Carly Simon, Loretta Lynn, Scotty Pippin, and Kareem Abdul-Jabbar.

Other global challenges including hunger, weather-related phenomena such as devastating hurricanes and earthquakes, military conflicts in many regions of the Middle East and Africa, disease control, education, financial instability in underdeveloped countries, widespread corruption within the global business community, migration, trade barriers, and access to water are putting pressures on the resources of both communities and the world as a whole. Domestic violence, also a widespread phenomenon, is so prevalent in the United States that its burden exceeds the toll of some epidemics caused by contagion and adversely affects 1.5 million individuals (mostly women) annually (Sorenson & Wiebe, 2004).

CULTURAL CONNECTION 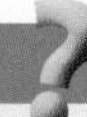

A patient's culture and meaning of pain can influence the management of chronic illness. Think of how different cultures express pain or discomfort and how these variations will affect the community health nurse's interventions.

Individuals with chronic illnesses whose lives are affected by these overarching issues may find fewer resources available to them to address their health problems and to provide preventive care aimed at increasing their lifespan and quality of life. It is increasingly important that community health nurses become involved in future planning for management of chronic illness care so they are able to advocate for those affected by changing local and global resource allocation. Age has long been recognized as a source of stigma in health care. The aged, chronically ill, or disabled are frequently unwelcome consumers in the current healthcare system, which has been designed around the episodic, acute care needs of middle-aged and younger persons. In many cases, caring for these individuals has been relegated to the least experienced, least educated, and, occasionally, least desirable segments of the healthcare community.

Ethnic and racial disparities in health constitute a persistent and formidable challenge to those in the United States with chronic illnesses and disability (see **Box 28-2**). Cardiovascular disease, in particular, is problematic in this regard. Despite the fact that it is the most frequent killer worldwide, this disease affects some groups more frequently than others. Rates of death from diseases of the heart are 30% higher among African Americans than among whites, and mortality resulting from stroke is 41% higher in African Americans (National Center for Chronic Disease Prevention and Health Promotion, 2010). It is well recognized that the proportion of African Americans who are hypertensive exceeds the proportions of other population groups with high blood pressure. In many cases, Type 2 diabetes disproportionately affects American Indians and Alaska Natives, who develop this disease 2.3 times more frequently than do whites. African Americans experience type 2 diabetes 1.6 times more frequently than whites, and Hispanic Americans are 1.5 times more likely to have diagnosed diabetes. HIV/AIDS disproportionately affects these groups, which account for 75% of both AIDS and new HIV infections among U.S. adults and 62% of all people living with HIV/AIDS in the United States. Rates of pediatric AIDS cases are similarly disproportionate in the United States, with such cases being composed of 82% minority individuals.

BOX 28-2 Ethnicity and Disability

Ethnicity plays an important role in quality of life for the disabled. According to the CDC (2011), reports of fair or poor health among adults with a disability by race and ethnicity were:

- Hispanic, 55.2%
- American Indian or Alaska Native, 50.5%
- Non-Hispanic Black or African American, 46.6%
- Non-Hispanic White, 36.9%
- Native Hawaiian or Other Pacific Islander, 36.5%
- Asian, 24.9%

We have learned a great deal about infectious disease epidemics globally during the past 2 centuries. The burden of chronic illness has been less well documented, because large numbers of those persons with acute diseases perished before their diseases became chronic. During the 19th century, immigration from Europe taxed sanitation and housing resources in many East Coast cities in the United States. With repeated epidemics, poor health conditions among established and relocated populations dwindled. Chronic conditions such as heart disease, diabetes, neurological problems, and blood disorders are identified in literature of that time. Because drugs and therapeutic regimens were scarce, overall survival rates for these diseases were poor in those eras, especially in vulnerable populations.

Major inroads into treatment, management, and prevention were made worldwide during the 20th century. Because of improved sanitation, widespread use of antibiotics and technology, rapid advances in research and communication, and comprehensive, nurse-driven health initiatives and education, the standard of living for many Americans has improved. However, these relatively recent developments have fostered trends of developing chronic illnesses that have become more prevalent in the 21st century in the United States. Aging baby boomers and their predicted healthcare needs are bringing these nursing specialty areas to the forefront.

An example of this trend can be seen with chronic renal failure. Until dialysis became available in the 1960s, renal failure was essentially untreatable and, therefore, fatal. Dialysis is now a common intervention for both acute and chronic phases of treatment. Additionally, organ transplantation is now considered a routine surgical procedure aimed at restoring renal function and improving the associated quality of life.

This consideration is especially important to community health nurses, because they are often involved with encouraging follow-up appointments and monitoring patients who experience uremic symptoms. Chronic renal insufficiency may present early in the disease trajectory with symptoms of sleep disturbance, muscle spasms/stiffness, excessive fatigue, and bone pain in addition to altered lab values (Pugh-Clarke, 2004). In this predialysis phase, patients often report that the intrusiveness of disease symptoms adversely affects their quality of life.

Another example of the development of a chronic condition from a formerly fatal condition is HIV/AIDS. Initially, few patients survived the opportunistic infections that manifested with disease progression. The discovery of multiple targeted therapies to suppress the virus and limit its impact on the immune system has changed HIV into a chronic illness that can be managed medically over years and even decades. Although it is still an extremely serious condition, HIV/AIDS is no longer synonymous with rapid progression, unmitigated suffering, and certain death (Mitchell & Linsk, 2004). Many infected individuals now survive for years with HIV and AIDS thanks to newly formulated medications and combination antiretroviral drug regimens. They are living highly productive and satisfying lives for many years. With effective prophylaxis and treatment, many are able to return to their jobs on a full-time basis and remain largely self-sufficient and autonomous. As a chronic, long-term illness, HIV/AIDS can affect patients, families, and communities in numerous and complex ways. Understanding the context in which those individuals are living with the condition will assist community health nurses to assess and intervene by supporting their initiation of medical treatment, suggesting coping strategies, and teaching and reinforcing understanding of the complex and challenging medical regimen.

Defining Disability and Chronic Illness

Disability is a permanent condition or constellation of related symptoms that result in impairment or diminished ability to do a job or live independently (see **Box 28-3**). According to the CDC (2014), those with disabilities face many barriers to good health. Studies show that individuals with disabilities are more likely than people without disabilities to experience having poorer overall health, having limited access to adequate health care, and engaging in risky health behaviors including smoking and physical inactivity. Those with disabilities are frequently more susceptible to preventable health problems that decrease their overall health and quality of life. Secondary conditions such as pain, fatigue, obesity, and depression may result from having a disabling condition. Health-related quality of life (HRQoL) is a multidimensional concept that includes domains related to physical, mental, emotional, and social functioning. It goes beyond direct measures of population health, life expectancy, and causes of death, and focuses on the impact health status has on quality of life. A related concept of HRQoL is wellbeing, which assesses the positive aspects of a person's life, such as positive emotions and life satisfaction. Public health efforts, from the individual to the national level, can affect the health and wellbeing of people with disabilities. These efforts must respond to known determinants of disability and health (CDC, 2012).

There are many social and physical factors that influence the health of people with disabilities. The following three areas for public health action have been identified,

BOX 28-3 WHO Definition of Disability

WHO, the United Nations' public health arm, published its new framework for disability and health in 2001 called the International Classification of Functioning, Disability and Health, known as the ICF. WHO's new definition of disability did the following:

- Established parity between "mental" and "physical" reasons for disability
- Mainstreamed the experience of disability and recognized it as a universal human experience
- Called for the identification of "facilitators" that not only eliminate barriers but enhance experience and performance

RESEARCH ALERT

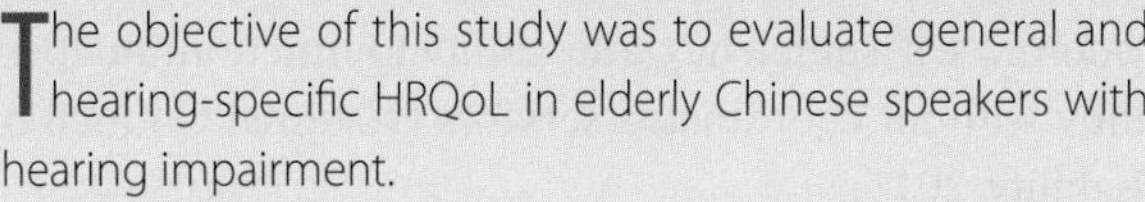

The objective of this study was to evaluate general and hearing-specific HRQoL in elderly Chinese speakers with hearing impairment.

Sixty-four Chinese speakers older than 65 years who did not use hearing aids were evaluated using Chinese versions

(continues)

RESEARCH ALERT (*continued*) 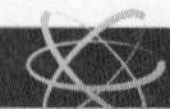

of the Short-Form 36 health survey (SF-36) and the Hearing Handicap Inventory for the Elderly (Screening Version) (HHIE-S). Results on the SF-36 were compared to norms obtained in a general elderly Chinese population. The relationships between HRQoL and degree of hearing impairment and between SF-36 and HHIE-S were evaluated.

Elderly Chinese speakers with hearing impairment rated six of the eight scales of the SF-36 poorer, compared to a general elderly Chinese population. When average hearing impairment in the better ear exceeded 40 dB HL, SF-36 ratings were poorer than for those with better hearing. Poorer better ear hearing was significantly related to poorer ratings on the vitality scale of the SF-36 and the three scales of the HHIE-S, after controlling for age, gender, and number of coexisting chronic health problems. Ratings on SF-36 and HHIE-S did not correlate.

Elderly Chinese who are hearing impaired experienced poorer general and hearing-specific HRQoL, and HRQoL was further reduced among those with greater hearing impairment.

Source: Wong, L. L., & Cheng, L. K. (2012). Quality of life in older Chinese-speaking adults with hearing impairment. *Disability & Rehabilitation, 34*(8), 655–664.

using the International Classification of Functioning, Disability, and Health (ICF) and the three WHO principles of action for addressing health determinants.

Disability is defined by the ADA as having a three-part meaning: An individual with a disability is a person who has a physical or **mental impairment** that (1) substantially limits one or more major life activities, (2) has a history or a record of such an impairment, or (3) is regarded by others as having such an impairment (U.S. Department of Justice, 2014). The ADA itself does not define what qualifies as a disabling condition. This rather broad definition is refined into several subareas. A **developmental disability** is defined as a severe, lifelong disability attributable to mental and/or **physical impairments** that manifest themselves before age 22 and are likely to continue indefinitely. Developmental disabilities result in substantial limitations in three or more of the following areas: self-care, comprehension and language skills (receptive and expressive language), learning, mobility, self-direction, and the capacity for independent living, economic self-sufficiency, and ability to function independently without coordinated services (National Council on Disability, 2011).

According to the WHO Family of International Classifications (WHO, 2014a), the following statements regarding health, disease, and classification are commonly used and understood in order to provide a baseline understanding of language and purpose enabling ease in communication of terms:

> The WHO constitution mandates the production of international classifications on health so that there is a consensual, meaningful and useful framework which governments, providers and consumers can use as a common language. Internationally endorsed classifications facilitate the storage, retrieval, analysis, and interpretation of data. They also permit the comparison of data within populations over time and between populations at the same point in time as well as the compilation of nationally consistent specifics based on data.

International Classification of Functioning, Disability, and Health (ICF)

The International Classification of Functioning, Disability, and Health, known more commonly as ICF, is a classification of health and health-related topics. These topics or domains are classified from body, individual, and societal perspectives by means of two lists: a list of body functions and structure (physiology and anatomy), and a list of topics of activity and sharing. Because an individual's functioning and disability occur within a context, the ICF also includes a list of environmental factors. The ICF is WHO's framework for measuring health and disability at both individual and population levels. The ICF was officially endorsed by all 191 WHO Member States in the 54th World Health Assembly in 2001. Unlike its predecessor, which was endorsed for field trial purposes only, the ICF was endorsed for use in Member States as the international standard to describe and measure health and disability.

The ICF situates the ideas of "health" and "disability" in a distinctive manner. It concedes that each individual may undergo a variance or change in health and may therefore confront some degree of disability. The manifestation of disability may affect many more than a minority population, rendering disability a frequently encountered phenomenon rather than the exception. By providing the commonly held idea of this experience of disability, the ICF acknowledges it as a collective human experience. Shifting the focus from reason to influence, it positions all health conditions on a uniform standpoint enabling comparison using a common metric—the ruler of health and disability. Additionally, ICF takes into account the social aspects of disability and does not see disability only as a "medical" or "biological" dysfunction. By including contextual factors, in which environmental factors are listed, ICF allows the impact of the environment on the person's functioning.

The disability prevalence rate increases with age. First, about one-fifth of the non-institutionalized population or 49.7 million people report disabilities. According to Iezonni & O'Day (2006), among those of working age, about 21.5 million or 13% have some type of disability. Seven percent of people ages 21–29 have a disability compared to 26% of people ages 60–64. These rates increase even more dramatically for the population over age 65: 30% of people ages 65–74 have a disability, and more than two-thirds (69%) of people over age 85 have some type of disability. Undoubtedly, the numbers of elderly will grow substantially in coming decades. Those who acquire significant physical disabilities in early life are living longer than formerly because of medical advancements. Healthy aging with a disability has become an important clinical consideration and research topic, as persons with such conditions as cerebral palsy, polio, and spina bifida increasingly live into their 7th decade and beyond (see **Table 28-1**).

TABLE 28-1 Examples of Disability, Etiology, Incidence, and Effects

Disability	Etiology	Incidence	Effects (Selected)
• Amputation	Trauma, bone cancer, diabetes	Not available	Impaired mobility
• Autism	Brain damage, abnormality in brain development, genetic predisposition	10/10,000 live births[1]	Impaired reciprocal social interaction, impaired communication and imaginative activity, markedly restricted repertoire of interests and activities
• Cerebral palsy	Perinatal anoxia, trauma, intraventricular hemorrhage, or stroke; trauma, meningitis in early childhood	1.4–2.4/1,000 births[1]	Difficulty with balance, coordination, and movement, hypertonicity; associated with sensory impairments, seizures, mental retardation
• Down syndrome	Genetic; extra chromosome 21	1/700–1/1,000 live births[1]	Mental retardation, hypotonia, physical characteristics, sensory impairments, decreased immunity, frequent respiratory infections and otitis media, increased incidence of leukemia, thyroid problems, early onset Alzheimer's-type dementia
• Duchenne's muscular dystrophy (MD)	Genetic, inherited as a sex-linked trait, affects males	1/3,500 males[1]	Increasing muscle weakness beginning with waddling gait and resulting in need for crutches or wheelchair; eventually heart and diaphragm are affected; usually causes death before adulthood
• Fetal alcohol syndrome (FAS)	Maternal alcohol ingestion resulting in prenatal exposure (leading known cause of mental retardation)	1–2/1,000 births[1]	Mental retardation, decreased height and weight, facial characteristics, behavior problems including hyperactivity and noncompliance
• Fragile X syndrome	Genetic; inherited as a sex-linked trait	1/1,500 males 1/500 females[1]	Mental retardation, hypotonia, physical characteristics, behavior problems such as self-stimulatory behavior, self-injurious -behavior, and aggression
• Hearing impairment	Otitis media (middle ear infections), congenital malformation, genetic, exposure to maternal virus or drug, meningitis, head trauma	1/1,000 infants born with severe to profound hearing loss[1]	Ranges from mild hearing impairment to deafness; developmental delay, language impairment, need for prenatal hearing aid, FM trainer, speech-language therapy, sign language

(*continues*)

TABLE 28-1 (*continued*)

Disability	Etiology	Incidence	Effects (Selected)
• Polio	Polio virus causes paralysis below part of spinal column damaged by virus	Eliminated since 1991 but 16,316 cases of paralytic polio occurred during the period 1951–1954[2]	Paralysis, complications related to immobility (decubiti, fractures), postpolio syndrome in mid to late adulthood causing increased severity of symptoms
• Spina bifida (myelomeningocele)	Multifactorial etiology; environmental causes including folic acid deficiency and genetic influences	60/100,000 births[1]	Paralysis below level of defect, impaired ambulation requiring crutches and walker or wheelchair, lack of bowel and bladder control, hydrocephalus requiring shunt, seizures, vision problems, mental retardation, complications related to immobility
• Spinal cord injury (SCI)	Trauma from diving accidents and motor vehicle accidents	250,000 individuals with SCI in the United States[3]	Paralysis, hypotonia and muscle wasting, incontinence, complications related to immobility and repeated catheterization; high-level injuries can also cause inability to breathe without assistance
• Traumatic brain injury (TBI)	Trauma from motor vehicle accidents, gunshots, child abuse	71–125/100,000 (22% of those died)[3]	Motor, communication, cognitive, sensory, and behavioral deficits
• Vision impairment	Prenatal exposure to viruses or bacteria, prematurity and oxygen treatment, eye trauma, chemical burns, diabetes, glaucoma, cataracts	1/3,000 children are blind[1]; vision impairment increases significantly in older adults	Ranges from poor sight to total blindness

1. Batshaw, M. L., Pellegrino, M. D., & Roizen, M. D. (2007). Children with disabilities (6th ed.). Baltimore, MD: Brookes Publishing Company.
2. Centers for Disease Control and Prevention. (2010).
3. Marino, M. J. (1999). CDC report shows prevalence of brain injury. *TBI Challenge, 3*(3).

Disabled individuals are generally unable to initiate or complete self-care activities alone because of physical impairments. To achieve independence or optimal levels of self-care, focused rehabilitative efforts are usually required. In some cases, rehabilitation is also useful in maintaining established progress in self-care activities. Likewise, rehabilitation is employed in conditions of disability associated with chronic health problems and degenerative diseases such as Parkinson's disease, amyotrophic lateral sclerosis, and multiple sclerosis (Hickey, 2003).

Understanding the Differences Between Disability and Chronic Illness

The terms *disability* and *disabled* are not used to diminish or label persons or groups for the purpose of undermining their individual rights or freedoms; rather, they are meant only to provide a context in which needs may be addressed from a position of specificity. An example of this notion may be found in professional literature discussing and describing assistive devices and equipment that are fabricated to meet specific needs and possess specific functions (Dewsbury, Clarke, Randall, Rouncefield, & Somerville, 2004).

Chronic illness differs from disability in that disability does not necessarily imply sickness or less-than-optimal health, whereas chronic illness is always related to a permanent decrease in health status that will not, in all likelihood, result in restoration of former or normal health status. Chronic illness is contrasted to disability in the following three examples: (1) type 1 diabetes results in chronic illness but not disability in every individual (Klang & Clyne, 1997); (2) a hip fracture may result in disability but not necessarily in chronic illness; and (3) a spinal cord injury may result in both conditions, because disability immediately develops as a consequence of spinal cord damage, and chronic illness may ensue if prolonged immobility causes development of decubitus ulcers, urinary tract infections, or muscle spasms unrelieved by medications. Disability resulting from spinal cord injury may, for example, cause numerous problems of chronic illness that relate to development of decubitus ulcers. Patients may require surgical interventions to enable healing. Because of inadequate sensory innervation, necessary position changes may be overlooked while individuals are in wheelchair-sitting positions.

Patients with chronic disability often define themselves in terms of their illness role and diagnosis. Definitions of this type may be limiting. When individuals with disabilities are viewed as striving toward higher level wellness, they may be supported by interacting with their environment in an integrated manner, thereby promoting their personhood and emphasizing their human qualities, instead of their disabilities (Davidhizar & Shearer, 1997).

NOTE THIS!

Stable, chronic conditions affect as much as 30% of the U.S. adult population.

RESEARCH ALERT

Many home health agencies are actively recruiting new home health nurses while trying to retain qualified home health nurses. According to a survey of home health administrators, 82% of them reported difficulty attracting nurses, and 63% reported difficulty retaining nurses. Due to rising healthcare costs and the desire of patients and families to receive care in their home environment, more and more health care is being provided outside the typical acute care setting. Because of the unique demands of the home healthcare setting, nurses must have a strong clinical background, usually with at least 1 year of acute care experience. Homecare nurses need a wide variety of clinical and technical skills to provide care safely in a patient's home. Nurses with a high degree of self-efficacy and varied clinical experience tend to be more successful and satisfied in homecare positions. Nurse autonomy and control over the practice environment are two factors attracting and retaining homecare nurses. Nurses go into community health nursing (CHN) because of the level of the independence and autonomy that this career allows, and because of the flexibility associated with the community setting.

Although healthcare delivery is moving away from institutions toward a variety of community settings, nursing education continues to concentrate on acute care settings, and most prelicensure bachelor of science in nursing (BSN) students do not perceive themselves as pursuing a career in community or public health nursing.

In one study, students' attitudes changed somewhat after they had a positive clinical experience in CHN, although CHN did not rank as the students' first choice for a career in nursing. This may have been due to the students' awareness that nurses are required to have at least 1 year of experience before being employed in CHN.

Source: Prestia, M. (2008). Nursing students' attitudes about home health nursing. *Home Healthcare Nurse, 28*(8), 496.

Needs of Those with Chronic Illness and Disability

Overall, people with disabilities have lower employment rates, lower annual earnings, lower educational attainment and achievement; lack adequate access to housing, transportation, technology, and health care; and are more likely to live in poverty. According to the U.S. Department of Labor's (2012) Bureau of Labor Statistics, disability employment statistics for January 2012 show that the percentage of people with disabilities participating in the labor force was (compared to 68.9% for people without disabilities). The unemployment rate of people with disabilities was 12.9%, compared to 8.7% for people without disabilities. The unemployment rate for people with disabilities has been steadily improving (it was 13.6% previously), but the number of unemployed was still disproportionately high in comparison to persons without disabilities. The number may be actually higher considering that many people with disabilities may have given up looking for work.

Because the incidence of disability increases with age, we can anticipate that the numbers of people with disabilities and chronic diseases will climb as the baby-boomer generation ages and as life expectancy increases with the further development and refinement of medical, surgical, and genetic technology. Quality of life for individuals with disabilities has not increased as rapidly as strides in technology; however, expectations of living a sustained, satisfying, and rewarding life have risen. Full inclusion in community living is an important dimension of a rewarding quality of life.

Community health nurses' knowledge of the healthcare needs of those with disabilities provide pivotal integration into community services and programs; employment; leisure and recreational activities; advocacy; accessible housing and transportation; current disability legislation; awareness, understanding, and use of technology for adaptive and mainstreamed activities; and a resource for the provision of care.

The community presents a myriad of challenges in the sometimes patchwork availability of resources and client care needs of those disabled moving within and among facilities and providers. The ADA has had limited impact on the ways health care is delivered for those with disabilities. Significant architectural and programmatic accessibility barriers still remain, and healthcare providers continue to lack awareness about steps they are required to take to ensure that patients with disabilities have access to appropriate, culturally competent care. Further, although many with disabilities have some type of health insurance, a significant number of individuals with chronic health conditions remain uninsured.

According to the CDC, the uninsured have a higher risk of death when compared to the privately insured, even after taking into account socioeconomics, health behaviors, and baseline health. In a 2009 study by Wilper and Woolhandler, nearly 45,000 excess deaths were linked annually to a lack of health coverage. The study found that deaths associated with lack of health insurance now exceed those caused by many common killers such as kidney disease. Of those lacking the ability to pay for their medications, nearly half of all uninsured, nonelderly adults report having a chronic condition, and almost half of these individuals report forgoing medical care or prescription drugs because of the cost or their lack of insurance. Nonelderly adults who lack health insurance include those with hypertension (14% uninsured), high cholesterol (11% uninsured), heart disease (13% uninsured), asthma (18% uninsured), diabetes (15% uninsured), and arthritis-related conditions (12% uninsured). Case/care management strategies may uncover funding and other resource inconsistencies necessitating critical thinking abilities and flexibilities. Knowledge and understanding are essential to successful navigation of community health nursing roles to enable crucial care. At the time of this writing, it is unclear how, if at all, the changes initiated by the ACA will impact this issue.

BOX 28-4 Janet Reno: A Public Experience with Parkinson's Disease

From 1993–2001, Janet Reno served as the Attorney General, the United States' top law enforcer, with the longest tenure in the history of the office. Since 1995, she has also lived with Parkinson's disease, with little self-acknowledgment of the affects it had on her demanding professional role as U.S. Attorney General. Reno made no effort to hide her tremors and continued to embrace her responsibility with the same vigor and tenacity. By being public with a disease that has in the past been hidden and restrictive, she moved forward for all persons who have such a chronic illness.

Caregivers for Individuals with Chronic Conditions

Because increasing numbers of those with chronic illness and disability remain in community-based care settings, including their homes, swelling numbers of caregivers—many of them unpaid family members—face a new role for which they are poorly prepared. In particular, caregivers for those with neurological impairments, including Parkinson's disease, multiple sclerosis, neuropathy, spinal cord diseases, amyotrophic lateral sclerosis, cerebrovascular disease, Alzheimer's disease, and chronic pain from arthritis, osteoporosis, or back problems, may experience problems with their own health associated with caregiving activities (Hilton & Henderson, 2003). Osteoporosis, in particular, is of great concern because the volume of cases is increasing at an astonishing pace; 30% of all women older than age 65 are estimated to have this painful and debilitating disease (U.S. Department of Health and Human Services [HHS], 2011). This condition of bone demineralization places those affected at increased risk for vertebral, pelvic, and hip fractures. For those who are family caregivers, osteoporosis adds a component of silent deterioration that may be aggravated by the lifting, turning, bending, stooping, and walking that are inherent in many caregiving activities.

RESEARCH ALERT

Chronically ill persons in communities may include those with chemical dependency, chronic mental illness, tuberculosis, and hepatitis C. Stable chronic conditions, affecting as much as 30% of the U.S. adult population, include cardiovascular disease, neurological diseases such as Alzheimer's disease, some slow-developing forms of cancer, emphysema, diabetes, fetal alcohol syndrome, learning disabilities, adjustment disorders, genetically linked diseases such as Down syndrome (trisomy 18 and 21), sickle cell disease, cystic fibrosis, Tay-Sachs disease, and schizophrenia. New medications are enabling individuals with these and other chronic diseases to live longer than ever before. Many chronically ill individuals remain in community settings and depend on others to render all or part of their physical and/or mental care. Despite our attention to the acute outbreak of SARS, the continuing threat of bioterrorism, and the effect of overseas wars, the most costly health problems in the United States are still the result of chronic diseases. We have come a long way, yet sadly, we also have not gone far. Attacking the problem of chronic illness in the United States presents us with a set of challenges that is complex and difficult to disentangle, especially when we focus on improving outcomes for populations. Chronic health problems provide ample opportunity to engage in primary, secondary, and tertiary preventive measures that use our nursing strengths.

Source: Abrams, S. E. (2003). Chronic illness: "Chronic" boredom. *Public Health Nursing, 20*(4), 250.

> Cancer didn't bring me to my knees, it brought me to my feet.
>
> —*Michael Douglas*

Care of individuals in the United States with the previously mentioned neurological diagnoses may include activities such as supervision, assistance with the execution of various tasks, and decision making about aspects of care (Lopes, Piementa, Kurita, & Oliveira, 2003). Caregivers for individuals with such diagnoses may feel the care they provide constitutes a burden. Because caregivers may have few or no resources to share the tasks and responsibility necessary to maintain or restore the chronically ill or disabled individual, and because caring activities may persist for an undetermined length of time, caregivers may experience fatigue, depression, emotional distress, sadness, loss of leisure activities, difficulties in their sexual activities, future planning, personal grooming, and disrupted family relationships.

Perhaps not unexpectedly, caregivers in Japan and in Brazil experience nearly identical issues while in the caregiving role, suggesting caregiver role strain is not unique to the U.S. population. Cultural differences may affect the perceived value of the caregiving role in which the individual is dependent upon a caregiver while sick, however. In the case of chronicity for an indeterminate interval, this caregiving role is recognized as essential in both Japan and Brazil. For those individuals experiencing chronic pain, caregivers may provide extensive psychological support aimed at promoting successful coping and restoring the locus of control for analgesic modalities and relaxation interventions. This type of care may be extremely taxing to caregivers because of the frequency of interventions required and because of the inherent discouragement that may accompany the recurrence of symptoms as the patient and the caregiver seek to establish order out of chaos (Bullington, Nordemar, Nordemar, & Sjöström-Flanagan, 2003).

The importance of family caregiver issues related to the challenging and difficult work of caring for an individual with chronic conditions cannot be overemphasized (Grey, Knaft, & McCorkle, 2006). Supports including respite care services and social workers are useful and important in providing long-term care. In caring for the caregivers, however, it is also important to recognize the nurse and his or her contributions to the therapeutic relationship (Hickey, 2003). Both conscious and unconscious responses of the community health nurse should be considered. Nurses may also experience caregiver burden if they go unrelieved in dealing with the consistent demands of care necessitated by individuals with disabilities and chronic illnesses. If possible, this problem should be anticipated and addressed by a "break" in the assignments of this population so the nurse is able to attend to his or her own self-care and spiritual renewal.

ETHICAL CONNECTION 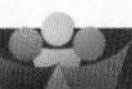

What are the ethical implications of a healthcare system that focuses on acute care interventions while the majority of patients in the system suffer from chronic and debilitating health issues?

Prevention Measures

Recent data indicate that increasing numbers of Americans believe their physical and mental HRQoL is deteriorating and that they are less able to engage in their usual activities (Zack, Moriarity, Stroup, Ford, & Mokdad, 2004). Given that disability and chronic illness contribute overwhelmingly to these factors, prevention and management are increasingly important to individuals and health agencies.

According to the CDC (2009), chronic health conditions affect both individuals and the larger society. U.S. healthcare costs are greatly affected by chronic illness. As a nation, more than 75% of our healthcare spending is on people with chronic conditions.

Vulnerable Populations

Some populations are more likely than others to develop chronic illnesses. Chronic illnesses affect various ethnic and racial groups, and some disease processes are gender preferential. Examples of this relate to all types of cancer. Cancer incidence rates for men are highest among blacks, followed by whites, Hispanics, Asian/Pacific Islanders, and American Indian/Alaska Natives. However, the cancer incidence rates for women are highest among whites, followed by blacks, Hispanics, Asian/Pacific Islanders, and American Indian/Alaska Natives. Cancer death rates for men are highest among blacks, followed by whites, Hispanics, American/Indians/Alaska Natives, and Asian/Pacific Islanders. Among women, the cancer death rates are highest among blacks, followed by whites,

American Indian/Alaska Natives, Hispanics, and Asian/Pacific Islanders. Cancer incidence rates and cancer death rates do not match according to gender and ethnicity. American Indian/Alaska Native men have the lowest incidence rates of cancer; however, Asian/Pacific Islander men have the lowest death rates. White women have the highest incidence rates of cancer; however, black women have the highest death rates. American Indian/Alaska Native women have the lowest incidence rates of cancer and the third highest death rates (U.S. Cancer Statistics Working Group, 2007). Population-specific vulnerability is especially important to consider when projecting needs for development of community resources.

ENVIRONMENTAL CONNECTION

For patients with asthma and allergies, any change in household products or household items, such as rugs and furniture, can result in a severe allergic reaction.

Because of their limited defense mechanisms, such as diminished or slowed reflexes, people with chronic illness are more susceptible to environmental sources of pollution. The destruction of the World Trade Center on September 11, 2001, created the largest acute environmental disaster that ever has befallen New York (Landrigan et al., 2004). In addition to experiencing severe posttraumatic stress disorder, those individuals with asthma and emphysema living in the area most closely affected by the buildings' collapse experienced exposure-related exacerbations of their diseases.

Disability

The composition of disability is intricate. It is embedded in societal values of mind–body functioning that separate mental and physical impairments (Imrie, 2004). According to Kaplan (2008), disability policy scholars identify four distinctive social and historical models of disability: a moral model that regards disability as the result of sin; a medical model that considers disability as a sickness or defect that must be cured; a rehabilitation model that regards disability as a deficiency that must be fixed; and the disability model under which the problem is defined as a dominating attitude toward the person with a disability by professionals and others.

WHO's ICF (2001; see also WHO, 2014b) employs performance-based contexts as a vehicle for delimiting disabilities based on individual attributes and societal values ascribed to limitations. WHO defines *disability* as any restriction or lack (resulting from an impairment) of ability to perform an activity in the manner or within the range considered normal for a human being. **Impairment** is defined as any loss or abnormality of psychological or anatomical structure or function; **handicap** is defined as a disadvantage for a given individual, resulting from an impairment or disability that limits or prevents the fulfillment of a role that is normal, depending on age, sex, and social and cultural factors, for that individual (WHO, 2001).

The original purpose of the ADA was to protect individuals from discrimination. Current thinking reflects a trend in public policy to regard disability as a functional status, not a list of physical impairments. Unfortunately, stigmatization and stereotyping accompany the delineation of disabled, so many choose not to identify themselves as disabled (Kaplan, 2008). Disability is viewed by some as social prejudice, and by others as a physical condition affecting life quality (Koch, 2001). The nature of disability may be linked to social variables such as class, ethnicity, gender, and geographical location (Morgan, 1996). According to Hurst (2000), disability may be construed as "something that happens to you, not something you have."

ETHICAL CONNECTION 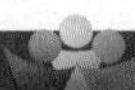

Chronic illness is not typically a focus of public health services in a community. This bias may result in persons with chronic illnesses having few resources for drug and medical expenses. Why do you think chronic illness has not typically been considered a public health "problem" until very recently?

HEALTHY PEOPLE 2020 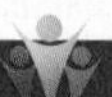

Objectives Related to Chronic Illness

Access to Health Services

- AHS-1 Increase the proportion of persons with health insurance
- AHS-5 Increase the proportion of persons who have a specific source of ongoing care

Arthritis, Osteoporosis, and Chronic Back Conditions

Arthritis

- AOCBC-1 Reduce the mean level of joint pain among adults with doctor-diagnosed arthritis
- AOCBC-2 Reduce the proportion of adults with doctor-diagnosed arthritis who experience a limitation in activity due to arthritis or joint symptoms

- AOCBC-3 Reduce the proportion of adults with doctor-diagnosed arthritis who find it "very difficult" to perform specific joint-related activities
- AOCBC-4 Reduce the proportion of adults with doctor-diagnosed arthritis who have difficulty performing two or more personal care activities, thereby preserving independence
- AOCBC-5 Reduce the proportion of adults with doctor-diagnosed arthritis who report serious psychological distress
- AOCBC-6 Reduce the impact of doctor-diagnosed arthritis on employment in the working-age population
- AOCBC-7 Increase the proportion of adults with doctor-diagnosed arthritis who receive healthcare provider counseling
- AOCBC-8 Increase the proportion of adults with doctor-diagnosed arthritis who have had effective, evidence-based arthritis education as an integral part of the management of their condition
- AOCBC-9 Increase the proportion of adults with chronic joint symptoms who have seen a healthcare provider for their symptoms

Osteoporosis

- AOCBC-10 Reduce the proportion of adults with osteoporosis
- AOCBC-11 Reduce hip fractures among older adults

Chronic Back Conditions

- AOCBC-12 Reduce activity limitation due to chronic back conditions.

Cancer

- C-13 Increase the proportion of cancer survivors who are living 5 years or longer after diagnosis
- C-14 Increase the mental and physical health-related quality of life of cancer survivors

Chronic Kidney Disease

- CKD-1 Reduce the proportion of the U.S. population with chronic kidney disease
- CKD-2 Increase the proportion of persons with chronic kidney disease (CKD) who know they have impaired renal function
- CKD-4 Increase the proportion of persons with diabetes and chronic kidney disease who receive recommended medical evaluation
- CKD-5 Increase the proportion of persons with diabetes and chronic kidney disease who receive recommended medical treatment with angiotensin-converting enzyme (ACE) inhibitors or angiotensin II receptor blockers (ARBs)
- CKD-6 Improve cardiovascular care in persons with chronic kidney disease
- CKD-7 Reduce the number of deaths among persons with chronic kidney disease
- CKD-8 Reduce the number of new cases of end-stage renal disease (ESRD)
- CKD-9 Reduce kidney failure due to diabetes
- CKD-10 Increase the proportion of chronic kidney disease patients receiving care from a nephrologist at least 12 months before the start of renal replacement therapy

Diabetes

- D-1 Reduce the annual number of new cases of diagnosed diabetes in the population
- D-4 Reduce the rate of lower extremity amputations in persons with diagnosed diabetes
- D-5 Improve glycemic control among persons with diabetes
- D-6 Improve lipid control among persons with diagnosed diabetes
- D-7 Increase the proportion of persons with diagnosed diabetes whose blood pressure is under control
- D-8 Increase the proportion of persons with diagnosed diabetes who have at least an annual dental examination
- D-9 Increase the proportion of adults with diabetes who have at least an annual foot examination
- D-10 Increase the proportion of adults with diabetes who have an annual dilated eye examination
- D-11 Increase the proportion of adults with diabetes who have a glycosylated hemoglobin measurement at least twice a year
- D-12 Increase the proportion of persons with diagnosed diabetes who obtain an annual urinary microalbumin measurement
- D-13 Increase the proportion of adults with diabetes who perform self–blood glucose monitoring at least once daily
- D-14 Increase the proportion of persons with diagnosed diabetes who receive formal diabetes education
- D-15 Increase the proportion of persons with diabetes whose condition has been diagnosed
- D-16 Increase prevention behaviors in persons at high risk for diabetes with prediabetes

Disability and Health

Systems and Policies

- DH-1 Increase the number of population-based data systems used to monitor *Healthy People 2020* objectives that include in their core a standardized set of questions that identify people with disabilities
- DH-2 Increase the number of tribes, states, and the District of Columbia that have public health surveillance and health promotion programs for people with disabilities and caregivers
- DH-3 Increase the proportion of U.S. master of public health (MPH) programs that offer graduate-level courses in disability and health

Barriers to Health Care

- DH-4 Reduce the proportion of people with disabilities who report delays in receiving primary and periodic preventive care due to specific barriers

(*continues*)

HEALTHY PEOPLE 2020 (continued) 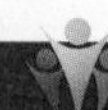

- DH-5 Increase the proportion of youth with special healthcare needs whose healthcare providers have discussed transition planning from pediatric to adult health care
- DH-6 Increase the proportion of people with epilepsy and uncontrolled seizures who receive appropriate medical care

Heart Disease and Stroke

- HDS-5 Reduce the proportion of persons in the population with hypertension
- HDS-6 Increase the proportion of adults who have had their blood cholesterol checked within the preceding 5 years
- HDS-7 Reduce the proportion of adults with high total blood cholesterol levels
- HDS-8 Reduce the mean total blood cholesterol levels among adults
- HDS-12 Increase the proportion of adults with hypertension whose blood pressure is under control
- HDS-22 Increase the proportion of adult heart attack survivors who are referred to a cardiac rehabilitation program at discharge
- HDS-23 Increase the proportion of adult stroke survivors who are referred to a stroke rehabilitation program at discharge

Hearing and Other Sensory Communication Disorders

Newborn Hearing Screening

- ENT-VSL-1 Increase the proportion of newborns who are screened for hearing loss by no later than age 1 month, have audiologic evaluation by age 3 months, and are enrolled in appropriate intervention services no later than age 6 months

Hearing

- ENT-VSL-3 Increase the proportion of persons with hearing impairments who have ever used a hearing aid or assistive listening devices or who have cochlear implants
- ENT-VSL-4 Increase the proportion of persons who have had a hearing examination on schedule
- ENT-VSL-5 Increase the number of persons who are referred by their primary care physician or other healthcare provider for hearing evaluation and treatment

Tinnitus (Ringing in the Ears or Head)

- ENT-VSL-9 Increase the proportion of adults bothered by tinnitus who have seen a doctor or other healthcare professional
- ENT-VSL-10 Increase the proportion of adults for whom tinnitus is a moderate to severe problem who have tried appropriate treatments

Balance and Dizziness

- ENT-VSL-11 Increase the proportion of adults with balance or dizziness problems in the past 12 months who have ever seen a healthcare provider about their balance or dizziness problems
- ENT-VSL-12 Increase the proportion of adults with moderate to severe balance or dizziness problems who have seen or been referred to a healthcare specialist for evaluation or treatment
- ENT-VSL-13 Increase the proportion of persons who have tried recommended methods for treating their balance or dizziness problems
- ENT-VSL-14 Reduce the proportion of adults with balance and dizziness problems who experienced negative or adverse outcomes in the past 12 months
- ENT-VSL-15 Reduce the proportion of adults with balance and dizziness problems who have fallen and been injured

Voice, Speech, and Language

- ENT-VSL-19 Increase the proportion of persons with communication disorders of voice, swallowing, speech, or language who have seen a speech-language pathologist (SLP) for evaluation or treatment
- ENT-VSL-20 Increase the proportion of persons with communication disorders of voice, swallowing, speech, or language who have participated in rehabilitation services
- ENT-VSL-21 Increase the proportion of young children with phonological disorders, language delay, or other developmental language problems who have participated in speech-language or other intervention services
- ENT-VSL-22 Increase the proportion of persons with communication disorders of voice, swallowing, speech, or language in the past 12 months whose personal or social functioning at home, school, or work improved after participation in speech-language therapy or other rehabilitative or intervention services

Internet Healthcare Resources for ENT-VSL

- ENT-VSL-23 Increase the proportion of persons with hearing loss and other sensory or communication disorders who have used Internet resources for healthcare information, guidance, or advice in the past 12 months

Medical Product Safety

- MPS-2 Increase the safe and effective treatment of pain
- MPS-5 Reduce emergency department (ED) visits for common, preventable adverse events from medications

Nutrition and Weight Status

- NWS-8 Increase the proportion of adults who are at a healthy weight
- NWS-9 Reduce the proportion of adults who are obese
- NWS-10 Reduce the proportion of children and adolescents who are considered obese
- NWS-11 Prevent inappropriate weight gain in youth and adults

Respiratory Diseases

Asthma

- RD-2 Reduce hospitalizations for asthma
- RD-3 Reduce ED visits for asthma

- RD-4 Reduce activity limitations among persons with current asthma
- RD-5 Reduce the proportion of persons with asthma who miss school or work days
- RD-6 Increase the proportion of persons with current asthma who receive formal patient education
- RD-7 Increase the proportion of persons with current asthma who receive appropriate asthma care according to National Asthma Education and Prevention Program (NAEPP) guidelines

Chronic Obstructive Pulmonary Disease

- RD-9 Reduce activity limitations among adults with chronic obstructive pulmonary disease (COPD)
- RD-10 Reduce deaths from COPD among adults
- RD-11 Reduce hospitalizations for COPD
- RD-12 Reduce ED visits for COPD
- RD-13 Increase the proportion of adults with abnormal lung function whose underlying obstructive disease has been diagnosed

Source: U.S. Department of Health and Human Services. (2014b). 2020 Topics and Objectives. Retrieved from http://www.healthypeople.gov/2020/topicsobjectives2020/default.aspx

As defined in 1956 by the Commission on Chronic Illness (cited in Strauss, 1975), impairments or deviations from normal have one or more of the following characteristics: (1) They are permanent; (2) they leave residual disability; (3) they are caused by nonreversible pathological alterations; (4) they require special training of the patient for rehabilitation; and (5) they may be expected to require a long period of supervision, observation, or care. In addition to chronic illness, multiple chronic conditions in the same person are frequently noted (Strauss, 1975). For example, diabetes may affect nerve tissue, causing damage to sensory nerve pathways, leading to diabetic-induced visual loss from retinal disease, and coexisting with hypertension.

Acute illness is defined as a disease (or process) with a sudden, dynamic onset with signs and symptoms related to the disease process itself, which either resolves shortly with complete recovery or results in death. Differences between acute and chronic illness are notable in terms of their treatment, duration, and perceived significance. Another important difference between acute and chronic illness relates to coping abilities taxed during severe and sustained illness.

Acute and chronic illnesses also occur together. Examples of this phenomenon include asthma and diabetes, in which acute manifestations emerge from chronic problems in regulating the diseases. One challenge presented by chronic illness is that of keeping patients motivated to achieve and maintain optimal levels of health. Supporting patients' efforts to learn to manage their chronic illness requires skill, creativity, and persistence to keep each patient's entire life pattern in focus.

Experiences of Populations with Chronic Illnesses and Disabilities

Chronic illness may assume many forms. Psychiatric and mental illness including dysthymia, major depression, and unipolar depression are typically considered more chronic than other forms of depression (Antai-Otong, 1995). Women's health was studied across the United States, and the results were reported in the *American Journal of Public Health* (Bromberger, Harlow, Kravitz, & Cordal, 2004). Data indicated that 22% of middle-aged women residing in the community reported clinically significant depressive symptoms. Furthermore, women who had previous depressive episodes were at increased risk for recurrences. Middle-aged women were examined for racial/ethnic differences in significant depressive symptoms. The researchers reported Hispanic and African American women had the highest risk of developing severe symptoms, and Chinese and Japanese women the lowest. Contributing factors included low socioeconomic status, financial strain, physical inactivity, low social support, stress, and poor physical health. Social support is of particular importance to individuals whose chronic illness waxes and wanes, such as is seen in depression.

RESEARCH ALERT

Although medical illness and physical disability are strongly associated with depression, the majority of older adults who experience medical illness or disability at any given time are not depressed. The aim of these analyses was to identify risk factors for new-onset depression in a sample of medically ill, disabled older adults.

The authors used data from a representative sample of homebound older adults who recently started receiving Medicare home healthcare services for medical or surgical problems (n = 539). The authors reported on the rate and baseline predictors of new-onset major or minor depression using the *Diagnostic and Statistical Manual of Mental Disorders, Fourth Edition* (*DSM-IV*) criteria and made assessments at 1-year follow up with the Structured Clinical Interview for *DSM-IV* Axis I Disorders. The analyses were conducted with a subsample of older adults (n = 268) who did not meet criteria for major or minor depression and were not on an antidepressant medication at the time of baseline interviews.

(continues)

RESEARCH ALERT (*continued*)

At 1-year follow up, 10% (28 out of 268) of patients met criteria for either major (3%; 9 out of 268) or minor depression (7%; 19 out of 268). In multivariate analyses, the authors found that worse self-rated health (odds ratio [OR] = 0.53, $p = 0.042$), more somatic depressive symptoms (OR = 1.19, $p = 0.015$), greater number of activities of daily living (ADL) limitations at baseline (OR = 1.63, $p = 0.014$), and greater decline in ADL functioning from baseline to 1 year (OR = 1.59, $p = 0.022$) were all independently associated with onset of depression.

These findings underscore the significant fluctuations in depression and disability in high-risk older adults and suggest that persistent and new-onset disability increase the risk of depression. They may also help in designing preventive strategies to promote the ongoing good mental health of these high-risk patients over time.

Source: Weinberger, M., Raue, P., Meyers, B., & Bruce, M. (2011). Predictors of new onset depression in medically ill disabled older adults at 1 year follow-up. White Plains, NY: Department of Psychiatry, Weill Cornell Medical College.

Paradox and Loss

In each chronic illness, disease forms a path through lives that is not always apparent at outset and may not be clearly understood. Wellness and optimal health are subjectively described by each person experiencing those conditions, and chronic illness is best described and experienced by those living the phenomenon. A seeming contradiction associated with chronic illness is that patients often present with minor or mysterious symptoms. An example of this paradox is described by a woman with chronic asthma:

> I didn't have a fever and my doctor said all my blood tests and x-rays were fine. At first my friends were sympathetic, but then they began asking whether I was really taking care of myself. Even my doctor seemed exasperated, and so I began to think I was crazy and had made all this up. Little did I know when this happened two years ago that I was heading for chronic asthma. My asthma finally got so bad that I had to stop teaching. (Wilson, 1992, p. 42)

Paradox is present in many chronic disease processes and contributes to feelings of loss, fear, and frustration. Johnson (1991) explains the paradoxical nature of myocardial infarction:

> The signs and symptoms of a heart attack often begin insidiously and escalate over a period of hours. Heart attacks have a paradoxical nature. Although potentially fatal, the early signs of a heart attack mimic minor and trivial complaints. Unless the heart attack is extensive, the early symptoms may be interpreted as indigestion, the flu, a pulled muscle, or food poisoning. The irony of delaying treatment is caused in part by the mixed messages given to the public. On the one hand, the signs and symptoms of heart attack are well publicized because it is assumed that people will … seek help early. On the other hand, people are reluctant to go to the hospital emergency room or "bother" their physicians with seemingly minor complaints. (p. 33)

Losses may be the first awareness of chronic disease processes "taking hold." Fear of loss sets in quickly and is accompanied by awareness and understanding of chronic disease processes (Schaefer, 1995). Losses associated with chronic illness may include fear, social status, self-concept, self-esteem, role, family support, recognition by the healthcare community, and loss of independence related to financial and personal issues. Losses may also relate to insufficiency of status or stigmatization by feelings of imperfection; by being different, some feel as though they fall short of cultural norms relating to identity (Scambler, 2004).

This perception of loss is especially important in hidden conditions in which no visual validation is apparent. The paradox of lived disability that presents with no outward signs may compel the individual to conceal the disabling condition in an effort to preserve social acceptance. Secondary gains may enhance the "invisible" sick role such as that seen in diabetes, in which marginal control of blood glucose may prompt individuals to abandon their careers. Children may experience paradox when their developmental tasks conflict with limitations imposed by their chronic illness. For example, a child with asthma may find his or her medication regimen leaves the child unprepared to engage in the rigorous activities of many of his or her peers unless medications are adjusted (Agius, 2003).

Uncertainty coupled with numerous losses makes chronic illness particularly devastating for patients who also face challenges of an evolving disease process. Those with chronic heart failure, for example, describe feelings of physical incapacity that adversely affect the whole life situation. Those with chronicity identify with feelings of fear, anxiety, fatigue, pain, grief, astonishment, anger, dependence, loss, and hopelessness. A diagnosis of heart failure is associated with high morbidity and mortality and is being increasingly identified in the aging population (Dosh, 2004). Despite well-recognized symptom manifestation of heart failure, onset of progressive changes heralds a downward spiral that results in mortality in 59% of men and 45% of women at 5 years. Losses associated with heart failure include uncertainty and lessened endurance, because symptoms may be silent yet contribute to overall fatigue related to an inability of the heart to deliver sufficient oxygenated blood to meet the needs of organs and tissues during rest or exercise.

Fatigue associated with ADLs may promote discouragement, depression, and contribute to social isolation.

Individuals with chronic kidney disease face some similar challenges in that the disease process unfolds in a predictable manner and is associated with significant mortality and morbidity. However, the disease differs from heart failure in several important ways. Most notably, early in the disease process, renal disease (which currently affects nearly 20 million Americans) involves nearly all body systems. The incidence and prevalence of renal failure doubled from the late 1990s to the early 2000s, and associated causal conditions of renal failure—including diabetes mellitus, hypertension, ischemia, increased susceptibility to infections, obstructions, toxins, and autoimmune and infiltrative diseases—have also been on the rise (Snively & Gutierrez, 2004). The prospects of additional numbers of aging individuals developing this disease, and the implications of such a trend, are staggering.

Disease progression is frequently discussed in terms of treatment response. However, actions to slow progression of the disease—maintaining glycemic control, in particular—can slow the progression of associated nephropathy and, therefore, enhance quality of life. Maintaining excellent glycemic control is a daily struggle for many with chronic renal disease. The renal diet is generally low in protein, and many patients find this and other stringent dietary restrictions burdensome to comply with and difficult to remember. Frequently, renal disease leads to malnutrition and hypoalbuminemia. These conditions may result in fatigue, decreased endurance, and poor stamina, all of which may worsen as the disease inevitably progresses. Community health nurses can play a major role in helping patients to understand the effects of their behaviors. Assistance with dietary planning to better suit the tastes and budgets of patients can have a great influence on compliance with dietary restrictions and improved outcomes for diabetes management.

In chronic hepatitis C, diagnostic testing sensitivity and specificity are as high as 99%, yet diagnosis remains elusive in those who are not screened or tested for previous exposure or current, active infection. Because the symptoms of fatigue and nausea are commonly seen in other chronic processes, carriers may not seek or receive appropriate treatment until symptoms of cirrhosis develop (Ward, Kugelmas, & Libsch, 2004). Although 3.2 million persons in the United States are estimated to have this condition, most remain undiagnosed. Highly successful treatment modalities exist and afford relief in 50% to 80% of all persons who receive medications for hepatitis C. Disease progression is of great concern, because cirrhosis is essentially irreversible and progression accelerates in the presence of increased age, male gender, and use of alcohol. Nurses can make a huge difference in hepatitis C outcomes by encouraging high-risk patients to be tested so that hepatitis C infection can be diagnosed early and treated before cirrhosis develops.

In the United States, back pain accounts for nearly 25% of all workers' compensation claims and is the most frequent type of claim filed (Strunin & Boden, 2004). The social and personal aspects of back pain are substantial and interfere with personal integrity and role functioning. The following statements reflect these concerns: "You feel a lot of times that you are half a person," "I don't think I'm as good as I was," and "It kind of made me feel like an invalid." Family responsibilities may have to be assumed by others if back pain persists and becomes chronic.

Because the etiology of back pain is often unclear and damage is obscure in many cases, persons with back pain may have no defined path to symptom relief or cure. They may visit a variety of healthcare providers seeking both validation and relief of their symptoms. "Individuals who experience bodily suffering but who fail to gain acceptance for this suffering find themselves with illness but without sickness and can be described as inhabiting a liminal space, being both well and sick, and being neither" (Dumit, 1998). This statement tacitly refers to the importance of the sick role in which individuals seek relief from particular duties in acknowledgment of their suffering for a stipulated period of time. In the **sick role** in Western society, the physician functions as a "gatekeeper" and is responsible for monitoring signs of disease, worsening of the condition, or improvement. The patient is expected to "act sick," cooperate with physicians and their designees, and be cared for until able to resume his or her productive place in society. Because of the nature of back pain and the current state of the science and its limited ability to provide relief, individuals may experience loss and burden related to the chronic pain experience. However, because the individual is increasingly responsible for his or her improvement and ultimate recovery, the person may be challenged to use support groups, alternative and complementary strategies, and coping behaviors including courage, empowerment, and partnership with the healthcare community to master this situation.

Losses and resulting sorrow may lead to development of **chronic sorrow** that develops from grief emerging from continual loss during the trajectory of an illness or disability. For example, persons with Parkinson's disease—a slowly developing, progressive neurological disorder—and their spouses often experience chronic sorrow. Losses triggering sorrow include loss of future plans, restrictions on social life, inability to travel, and decreased ability to participate in hobbies (Lindgren, 1996).

The meaning of chronic illness to individuals and to society varies widely. Individuals may undertake to control chronic physical or psychiatric illnesses using strict adherence to treatment regimens, or they may eschew traditional healthcare practices in favor of nontraditional methods. Control of healthcare behaviors, however, does not always relate to successful outcomes, and some chronic diseases remain difficult to manage with current therapy options.

Adjustment to losses becomes a recurrent theme in many chronic illnesses, but each loss may represent a singular and significant experience that must be grieved. Diagnosis of chronic illness may result in releases of powerful emotions, including denial, shock, depression, and suicidal ideation. Consider the following example of a woman with chronic illness:

> I wanted to go jump in front of a car, and I can remember one day staying home. I was just so depressed that my husband got very alarmed and took off a day of work to stay with me because he was concerned about what I might do. As I thought about jumping in front of a car, I thought it would be my luck just to be maimed. (Wolf, 1994, p. 372)

By trying to protect herself from facing the reality that something is wrong, this woman pretends not to be ill and hopes that people will not notice her intrusive symptoms (Wolf, 1994).

Suffering

The socialization process ensures that adults will be able to assume roles in society recognized as necessary for members of society and for continuation of society. Socialization in children and adolescents with chronic illness can also present problems. Adolescents with cancer, for example, believe that hopefulness is essential to their successful coping with the cancer experience (Hinds, 2004). Celiac disease and the ensuing dietary control essential for maintenance of health have many far-reaching effects on both the ill child and family. Children with asthma or bronchitis related to environmental sources experience interference with socialization and with developmental tasks. Children who spend more time outdoors and who engage in team sports in areas with excessive ozone levels associated with automobile exhaust have more respiratory symptoms, including increased respiratory rate, persistent mucus production, increased respiratory illness, and decreased endurance. Long-term consequences of these problems are being identified with increasing frequency in urban areas.

> We are healed of a suffering only by experiencing it in full.
>
> —*Marcel Proust, 1871–1922*

Not all chronic illnesses are physical in nature. For instance, abilities and determinations that are aspects of personality may also be compromised in cases of chronic mental illness. Additionally, mental illness carries a social stigma that is not commonly encountered with physical problems, such that supports that are readily available to some chronically ill persons are not universally available to individuals with mental illness. **Geriatric depression**—a frequently noted condition in elders with chronic illness—is associated with lower quality of life (Small et al., 1996). Geriatric depression has been found to respond well to treatment, when it is instituted. Specifically, medication provided relief to elders with depression as frequently as younger patients in a comparison group without chronic illness (Small et al., 1996).

Younger individuals also face stigma with chronic physical or mental illness. A woman with asthma shares the following story:

> I was really embarrassed so I was trying to pretend that I wasn't short of breath. So I'd get up and turn around for a minute so that they wouldn't see. When I finally caught my breath, I'd start lecturing again. . . . I hid the inhaler in my pocket and went to the ladies room; I always hid it from my employer and my teachers. (Wolf, 1994)

Another woman with ulcerative colitis recalls her feelings:

> I never wanted to be stigmatized as someone who has a chronic problem or who is labeled as a chronic disease-type person. I've known people who just call out sick. I've never wanted to be stigmatized as one who abused sick time in that way. (Wolf, 1994)

ETHICAL CONNECTION 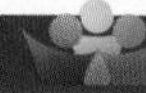

What do you think?

"Either he didn't take his medication or he's acting," said radio host Rush Limbaugh, on October 23, 2006, accusing actor Michael J. Fox, who has Parkinson's disease, of exaggerating his disease in democratic political ads. Fox, who supported democratic candidates nationwide in midterm elections through a series of political ads, was instrumental in moving the stem cell research debate into the public arena.

Did Limbaugh have the right to criticize Michael J. Fox for exercising his "freedom of speech"? What do you think of celebrities who advocate for scientific research simply based on their own personal experiences with disease? What are some of the influences, in addition to celebrity involvement, that contribute to changes in policies regarding people with disabilities and their future?

Power and Powerlessness

Power can be equated to individual possession of adequate resources enabling chronically ill people to be in control of their lives, or in substantial control of important aspects of their lives (Miller, 1992). Resources include perceptions of power that unfold with other inner attributes and coping strategies that emerge as a consequence of diminished health capacity and confronting of adversity (Miller, 1992).

Powerlessness is a nonadaptive coping mechanism resulting from loss of self, loss of self-esteem, loss of autonomy, and loss of hope. Chronic illness may result in additional losses without appropriate healthcare interventions that are sensitive to needs of individuals with ongoing challenges, uncertainty, and suffering for prolonged intervals. During illness, it is the fear of loss of the whole or a part of the body that is a focus of great psychological concern (Smith, 1974).

Survival of chronically ill individuals depends, in some measure, on individual ability and determination to endure aspects of suffering for long periods of time that must be endured if they cannot be altered or avoided. Community nurses may help to alleviate powerlessness by providing both physical and emotional support and by providing education related to self-care skills and the availability of community resources.

Caring for Persons with Long-Term Health Problems

Knowledge of patient perceptions of care is essential to community health nurses who plan, coordinate, manage, and evaluate community-based care. Maintaining an optimal quality of life becomes a paramount consideration when the future is uncertain and when limitations are both recognized and anticipated. Limitations and permanent disability can be daunting prospects to those who never considered themselves to be vulnerable to long-term health issues.

Facing devastating physical limitations may cause individuals to question their future and to wonder if they will be able to tolerate rigors of chronicity (Johnson, 1991). A challenging example is chronic pain resulting from development or deterioration of many conditions related to aging. Management of chronic pain is essential to avoid debilitating physical limitations. Another common problem is hypertension, which is a major risk factor for heart disease, stroke, and renal failure, among other serious conditions. Because this condition is "silent," many affected individuals do not seek care from their primary providers or adhere to necessary regimens once the condition has been diagnosed. Given that the risk of cardiovascular disease increases substantially in women after menopause, follow up with community health nurses is essential to optimal blood pressure management and will result in decreased mortality and morbidity, especially in women who are age 50 or older (Hirao-Try, 2003).

Nurses can be instrumental in facilitating adaptation to chronic disease processes and promote optimal health within a framework of disease-imposed limitations. Nurses can also support patient-generated activities that sustain endurance and alleviate suffering. Community-based nurses are in an optimal position to identify and promote adaptation to chronic disease processes resulting in diminished limitations.

MEDIA MOMENT 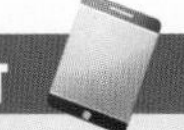

Persons with chronic health conditions are seldom portrayed on network television and in movies. Conversely, many advertisements for products and drugs to treat chronic illnesses appear on a daily basis. How would you explain this dichotomy?

Quality of Life in Disability and Chronic Illness

Acute phases of many chronic illnesses are managed in a hospital or nursing home by healthcare professionals, but the majority of ongoing care takes place in the home. Because the needs of chronically ill persons often outstrip the resources available to them, community health nurses must seek out solutions to care for chronically ill individuals in the most cost-effective manner using available resources of the extended family. This situation is especially relevant in older adult populations; increased longevity and aging of the baby boomers will result in not only a larger population of older adults, but also a higher prevalence of disability (Spillman, 2004). Medical interventions must be designed and implemented not only to prolong life, but also to promote health and independence.

APPLICATION TO PRACTICE 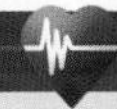

Osteoporosis

Mrs. A. was discharged to her home 3 weeks after having her right hip replaced. She was in a long-term care facility for 2 weeks after she was released from the hospital and was happy to be home again, among familiar surroundings. Mrs. A. had just passed her 77th birthday

(continues)

APPLICATION TO PRACTICE (*continued*)

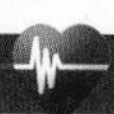

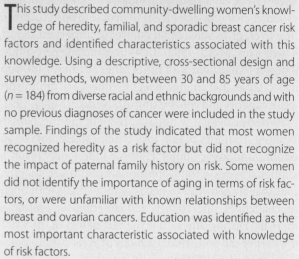

when she fell getting out of her bathtub at home. She managed to reach the telephone and called a neighbor, who came over and helped get Mrs. A. to the hospital in an ambulance. Although always ambulatory, Mrs. A. spent the next week recovering in bed from hip replacement surgery. She had physical therapy twice daily and ambulated with assistance in her room. She was surprised to learn from her physician that she had experienced a significant overall loss of bone.

Factors contributing to loss of bone density include small bones, smoking, low calcium intake, early menopause without estrogen replacement, amenorrhea, lack of exercise, excessive cola intake, and a familial history of osteoporosis. Other factors related to osteoporosis include chronic diseases, excessive alcohol consumption, and eating disorders (Dowd & Cavalieri, 1999).

After sustaining the fracture, suspicions that Mrs. A. had weakened and fragile bones were confirmed by bone densitometry that was arranged by her community health nurse. Medicare recently added bone mass measurements to its benefits for those fitting risk criteria, so Mrs. A.'s bone density scan was covered. Her osteoporosis could have been diagnosed much earlier if she had known the risks associated with its development. Her community health nurse explained symptoms and factors contributing to development of osteoporosis. Looking back, Mrs. A. recalled one symptom in particular: losing her height. She had been 5'5" and was now just over 5'1". The community health nurse also explained how to prevent falls and directed Mrs. A. to an equipment supply store, where she ordered a metal grab-bar for her bathtub, which would reduce the possibility of future falls while bathing. Now home, Mrs. A. continued the calcium and Vitamin D supplements and bisphosphonates therapy initiated in the hospital and planned to start a walking program at the senior center near her house. Her progress will be monitored for the next few weeks by her community health nurse.

Bone density is also important in those with chronic HIV. They are at increased risk for loss of bone density as a consequence of continued use of antiretrovirals.A baseline DXA scan should be performed initially and every 2–3 years based on the results. The community health nurse is well situated to initiate discussions with the client and physician about this important screening test. Alterations in bone strength predispose to fragility fractures, which are associated with increased morbidity and mortality in the HIV-negative population.

Source: Adapted from Dowd, R. & Cavalieri, J. (1999). Help your patient live with osteoporosis: Identifying risk, managing pain, overseeing treatment. *American Journal of Nursing, 99*(4), 55–60.

RESEARCH ALERT

This study described community-dwelling women's knowledge of heredity, familial, and sporadic breast cancer risk factors and identified characteristics associated with this knowledge. Using a descriptive, cross-sectional design and survey methods, women between 30 and 85 years of age ($n = 184$) from diverse racial and ethnic backgrounds and with no previous diagnoses of cancer were included in the study sample. Findings of the study indicated that most women recognized heredity as a risk factor but did not recognize the impact of paternal family history on risk. Some women did not identify the importance of aging in terms of risk factors, or were unfamiliar with known relationships between breast and ovarian cancers. Education was identified as the most important characteristic associated with knowledge of risk factors.

Interestingly, 49% of those surveyed in the study were college graduates. Despite this demographic, knowledge of breast cancer risk factors was incomplete. Implications for nursing relate to the need for women to receive education about the three types of breast cancer: hereditary, familial, and sporadic. Additionally, advanced practice nurses should provide individualized counseling to women seeking information about their risk factors.

Source: Katapodi, M. C., & Aouizerat, B. E. (2005). Do women in the community recognize heredity and sporadic breast cancer risk factors? *Oncology Nursing Forum, 32*(3), 617–623.

RESEARCH ALERT

This study sought to assess patterns of medical consultation, diagnosis, and medication use in representative samples of adults with migraine in England and the United States. Validated computer-assisted telephone interviews were conducted in the United Kingdom ($n = 4,007$) and the United States ($n = 4,376$). Individuals who reported six or more headaches per year meeting the criteria for migraine were interviewed.

Patients with migraine in the United Kingdom were more likely to have consulted a doctor for headache at least once in their lifetime (86% versus 69%, $p < 0.0001$), but also were more likely to have lapsed from medical care (37% versus 21%, $p < 0.001$). In the United States, patients with migraine who had consulted physicians made more office visits for headache and were more likely to see a specialist. In the United States but not in the United Kingdom, women with migraine were more likely than men to consult doctors for headache. Patients with migraine in the United Kingdom were more likely to receive a medical diagnosis of migraine (United

Kingdom, 67%; United States, 56%; $p < 0.05$). Patterns of medication use were similar in both countries, with most people treating the headaches with over-the-counter (OTC) medications. Substantial disability occurred in a high proportion of those who never consulted physicians (United Kingdom, 60%; United States, 68%), never received a correct medical diagnosis (United Kingdom, 64%; United States, 77%), and treated only with OTC medication (United Kingdom, 72%; United States, 70%).

Implications for community health nurses are that medically unrecognized migraine remains an important health problem both in the United States and the United Kingdom. Furthermore, there may be barriers to consultation for men in the United States that do not operate in the United Kingdom. While effective treatment exists for preventing and treating migraines, patterns of OTC treatment and lack of follow up exist in both countries, which indicates a need for greater emphasis on population-focused education.

Source: Lipton, R. B., Scher, A. I., Steiner, T. J., Bigal, M. E., Kolodner, K., Liberman, J. N., & Stewart, W. F. (2003). Patterns of health care utilization for migraine in England and in the United States. *Neurology, 60*(3), 441–448.

Many times, chronic illnesses are not immediately fatal but are disabling by virtue of their progression and side effects of social isolation and fatigue. Despite the nonfatal nature of some chronic diseases, they erode quality of life and diminish individual, family, and community resources. Part of the suffering that accompanies chronic health problems is increased by uncertainty, by remissions and exacerbations, by depleted or inadequate coping mechanisms, and by fatigue, which is a factor to consider while planning appropriate activities. The most predictable outcome of chronic illness is unpredictability (Schaefer, 1995). Patient autonomy characterizes the current era of health care, which is safeguarded by nursing (Miller, 1992). Patient quality of life is an appropriate consideration in chronic illness. Assessment of quality of life is directly related to the goals of nursing care, including promotion of health and restoration of maximal functioning of the patient.

These nursing goals become increasingly important when thinking about cancer as an acute event shifts to consideration of cancer as a chronic condition. Increasing numbers of adult cancer survivors have indicated to the healthcare community that, when it comes to treatment choice, quality of life is as important as overall therapeutic effect. Patients are concerned with the impact of cancer therapy on their daily lives. Chemotherapy-induced nausea and vomiting is one of the most devastating adverse effects of cancer treatment and adversely affects quality of life (Wickham, Goodin, & Lynch, 2004). Abandonment of chemotherapy owing to this problem is common. Improving control of this distressing side effect of cancer treatment greatly enhances the patient's ability to tolerate the full dose of chemotherapy. Serotonin-receptor antagonists, neurokinin, and steroids are part of current treatment protocols that accomplish this useful goal (Wickham et al., 2004). By mitigating side effects, chemotherapies are more easily tolerated; hence improved outcomes become possible.

Age alone is not the sole determinant of enhanced or diminished quality of life. The specific condition or disease process may adversely affect individuals differently at different points during their lives. Consider the chronic illness and disability associated with Parkinson's disease. Although related to age, Parkinson's disease also affects some persons who are younger (21–40 years) and may alter their quality of life because of the earlier onset of motor complications and disease progression (Jung, 2004). As expected, older adults with Parkinson's disease also face issues related to quality of life. They may encounter daily issues associated with disease onset and progression including tremor, bradykinesia, postural instability, cognitive changes, and depression (Whitney, 2004). Worsening symptoms that indicate deterioration, although more gradual than in younger adults, may adversely affect quality of life. Maintaining their usual activities, modifying their physical environment to enable maximal autonomy, accepting their limitations, and modifying the daily routine to make the most of their functional capabilities help preserve quality of life for individuals with this disease (Whitney, 2004).

Not surprisingly, racial and ethnic variations in household dynamics may produce differing perceptions of health-related issues including quality of life. Accordingly, because older African Americans are disproportionately more likely to acquire caregiving responsibilities for family members with chronic illness or disability, they may distinguish quality of life in different ways than whites with similar responsibilities.

The Chronic Care Model

In the United States, the federally funded National Institute on Disability and Rehabilitation Research (NIDRR), the most significant funder of disability research in our nation, has also participated in this historical evolution. According to the NIDRR Long Range Plan (2005–2009):

> The disability paradigm that undergirds NIDRR's research strategy for the future maintains that disability is a product of an interaction between characteristics

(e.g., conditions or impairments, functional status, or personal and social qualities) of the individual and characteristics of the natural, built, cultural, and social environments. The construct of disability is located on a continuum from enablement to disablement. Personal characteristics, as well as environmental ones, may be enabling or disabling.

Broadly defined, models are illustrative representations of the interrelations that exist within a system or process (*Mosby's Dictionary,* 2007). They are frequently used in nursing to explain phenomena and to make predictions about patients or outcomes. Prediction and control of outcomes are highly desirable when managing chronic illness and disability on a case-by-case basis and in contemplating future needs and settings. The model of chronic care discussed here was developed by E. H. Wagner and refined and further developed by a group supported by the Robert Wood Johnson Foundation (2010). The model was tested nationally and revised accordingly. Discussion of this model provides information about advancements in chronic care gleaned from research and numerous clinical applications and offers insights into innovative programs that have been identified by leading experts in the United States (ICIC, 2008).

The **chronic care model** identifies the essential elements of a healthcare system that promotes high-quality chronic disease care (see **Figure 28-1**). High-quality chronic disease care encompasses several interrelated elements, including the community, the health system, self-management support, delivery system design, decision support, and clinical information systems (ICIC, 2008). When informed patients interact with these elements and have access to providers with resources and expertise, the result is healthier patients, more satisfied providers, and cost savings.

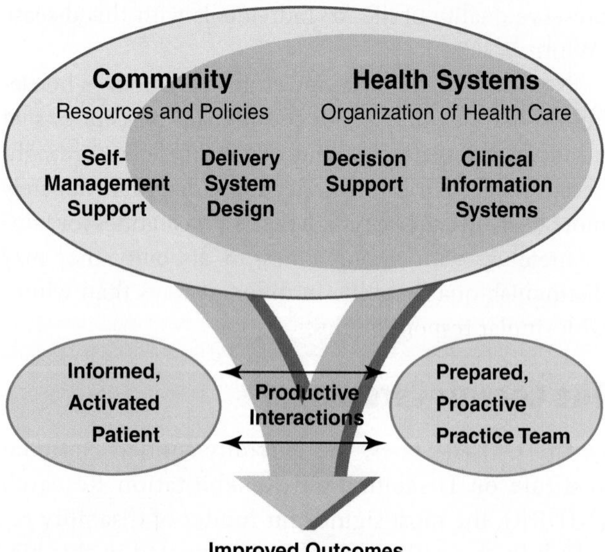

Figure 28-1 The Chronic Care Model.

Source: Chronic Care Model. Edward H. Wagner, MD, MPH, Chronic disease management: What will it take to improve care for chronic illness? *Effective Clinical Practice*, August/September 1998, Vol. 1, Figure 1. Used with permission.

According to this model (ICIC, 2008), community resources must be mobilized to meet the needs of patients and avoid costly duplication of services. Shared services such as mobile clinics or meals-on-wheels programs are examples of this idea. Self-help strategies may be promoted by partnering with national patient organizations such as the American Diabetes Association. Additionally, local and state health policies, insurance benefits, and civil rights for those with disabilities should be emphasized by patient advocates.

A culture, organization, and mechanisms that promote safe, high-quality treatment must be created if chronic illness care is to be improved. According to the ICIC (2008), care improvement goals must be clearly articulated by senior management and implemented through the use of incentives. Prevention of errors through reporting mechanisms and analysis of problem areas with corrective action must be incorporated into the working plans of system management. Communication should be facilitated and data sharing should be optimized as patients navigate across settings and providers.

The ICIC (2008) model emphasizes empowerment of patients to enable them to effectively manage their own health and health care. By acknowledging the central role of the patient in chronic illness care, self-management support strategies provided by the community health nurse and others lay the foundation for better disease control and desirable outcomes. By fostering a sense of responsibility for their individual health, patients and providers work collaboratively to prioritize goals, define problems, and monitor for progress throughout the process.

In the chronic care model, the delivery of effective and efficient clinical care and self-management support are essential. Because the current healthcare system is reactive and responds primarily to those who are ill, it provides few opportunities for keeping people healthy. The chronic care model emphasizes the importance of keeping in close communication with all patients to facilitate aftercare and proposes the implementation of **case management** or care management, depending on the complexity of each case. To facilitate efforts to reach this goal, tasks and responsibilities should be distributed among community-based health team members. The role of prevention is especially emphasized to enable optimal health for chronically ill individuals. Intensive management of those with complicated or multiple chronic processes is articulated. Finally, the model stresses the need for cultural sensitivity and health literacy in the health professionals who support those with chronic illnesses.

The model supports the use of evidenced-based care and consideration of patient preferences. Treatments should be based solely on explicit proven guidelines that are supported by clinical research. Providers must stay up to date on trends, and supportive specialists are considered an essential part of the treatment team that provides expert guidance. Changes to the treatment plan should result from the application of timely reminders, feedback, and standing orders. Finally, the performance of the practice team and care system should be monitored.

The model of chronic care has unique utility for community health nurses in that it can be applied to a broad, diverse cross-section of patients. Those who are permanently disabled *and* chronically ill, in particular, may identify strengths in the enduring nature of the evaluation component and note the ongoing advocacy built into the model. A further strength of this model is its ability to adapt to changing needs and changing characteristics of specific disease states as progression or improvement of symptoms develops. Finally, the use of functional and clinical outcomes ensures standard measures are applied to persons with disabilities and chronic, progressive diseases.

Stages of Adjusting to a New Form of Disability

Adjusting to a new form of disability follows four basic stages: shock, denial, anger/depression, and adjustment/acceptance. People progress through these stages at their own pace. **Shock** involves a state of both emotional and physical numbness that can last from a few hours to several days. **Denial** may last anywhere from 3 weeks to 2 months and is a defense mechanism that allows the implications of the new disability the person has experienced to be gradually introduced or taken in. Denial becomes an issue only when it interferes with the person's life, forms of treatment, or rehabilitation efforts. **Anger and depression** are reactions to loss and the person's change in social treatment and status. The person may experience a number of different emotions during this stage and grieve for the changes in body image, function, loss of future expectations, or former satisfaction based upon any function that has vanished.

The stage of **adjustment and acceptance** does not necessarily mean the person is happy about the disability now experienced, although it does allow for the relinquishment of any false hopes, as well as the successful adaptation of new roles based upon realistic potentials and limitations (Taormina-Weiss, 2012). At this stage, persons might benefit from interactions with others who experience forms of disabilities, which can help them become comfortable with who they have become.

Emotional aspects associated with a new form of disability may be a major factor in determining the person's outcome and the benefits related to rehabilitative efforts. Effective psychological intervention is beneficial when ensuring recovery from an injury resulting in a disability. Many people experience more than four stages of adjustment to a physical disability; in fact, people might experience as many as 12 stages that include shock, anxiety, bargaining, denial, mourning, depression, withdrawal, internalized anger, externalized aggression, acknowledgment, acceptance, and adjustment. As with all adjustment activities, times and tasks of each activity are individualized and variable.

People with Disabilities

According to Taormina-Weiss (2012), in every single way that matters, disability does not change a person. Instead, disability threatens concepts persons hold about who they are. People bring to their disability whatever mix of beliefs, attitudes, talents, charisma, fears, or social skills they have or have the capacity to develop. Who a person is impacts the ability to adjust to disability.

One of the common questions people with disabilities are asked by those who are not disabled is, "What can be done to help?" Perhaps the first thing someone can do is to understand that persons with disabilities are the same persons they were before experiencing their form of disability. It is important not to treat them differently simply because they have a form of disability. Do not expect them to be any weaker or stronger, and do not be surprised if they have found new qualities within themselves that have not surfaced before.

The experience of a form of disability forces the issue of "finding one's self." Some people take pride in the things they learn about themselves through the experience of a form of disability. They may appreciate the way disability helps to define their values (Taormina-Weiss, 2012). A number of psychological adjustments have little to do with the disability a person experiences; they are issues everyone encounters. It is important for people with disabilities to avoid making disability a scapegoat for issues that might have emerged nonetheless. For the majority of people with disabilities, disability does not define who they are; it is something they manage when it becomes necessary to do so.

The Experience of a New Disability

Most able-bodied individuals who have no or very few physical challenges envision the experience of disability as far more demanding and complicated than it is in reality. A person may have no concept of how someone functions with a wheelchair, for example, and it might seem that life for a person who uses a wheelchair is completely helpless, reliant, and complicated—yet the reality is very different. When a person suddenly experiences a form of disability due to an injury or a diagnosis of a form of degenerative disease, he or she brings prior notions of disabilities to it. It is not surprising that a number of people find themselves experiencing anger, depression, fear, anxiety, and a deep sense of loss during the early stages of their disability experience. Despite how well adjusted, emotionally strong, or mature a person may be, the experience of a new form of disability is an event that shakes many persons' basic beliefs about their life. A new form of disability also demands the individual draw upon his or her coping skills—possibly using skills the person may not have needed previously (Taormina-Weiss, 2012).

A person's experience with a new form of disability may be marked by fatigue, negative emotions, or a sense of powerlessness or confusion. It is important to remember that there is also the chance to experience confidence and hope as the person witnesses new abilities to cope with what is often a challenging situation. The majority of people who experience a new form of disability adjust in ways they never believed possible. With positive social support from family members, friends, and society at large, the vast majority of people who experience a new form of disability adapt and adjust.

Disability Diversity in Society

Those with disabilities are the nation's largest minority—the only minority group that any person can join at any time for any reason. For those who are able-bodied, there is about a 20% chance of becoming disabled at some point during the normally expected work life. Those with disabilities cross all racial, gender, educational, socioeconomic, and organizational lines. Discussion regarding diversity has often focused on gender and race. In contrast, limited attention has been given to people with disabilities as the world's largest minority group.

According to the Office of Diversity Employment, those companies that include people with disabilities in their diversity programs increase their competitive advantage. People with disabilities add to the variety of viewpoints needed to be successful and bring effective solutions to today's business challenges. The American economy is made stronger when all segments of the population are included in the workforce and in the customer base. The federal government realizes that opportunity for employment is an important way to give people with disabilities the means to provide for themselves, while lowering federal support costs. There are several unique programs, such as the Work Incentives Planning and Assistance (WIPA) program, the Plan to Achieve Self-Support (PASS), and the Ticket to Work, that have been set up to help people with disabilities succeed at work while maintaining their benefits. The disability employment benefits system can assist with housing, jobs, medical costs, and career security.

BOX 28-5 Diversity, Chronic Illness, and Disabilities

The concept of diversity encompasses acceptance and respect. It means understanding that each individual is unique, and recognizing our individual similarities and differences. These can be along the dimensions of race, ethnicity, gender, sexual orientation, socioeconomic status, age, physical abilities, or religious or political beliefs or other ideologies. The concept of diversity is best explored in a safe, positive, and nurturing environment. The concept of diversity embraces understanding and acceptance while moving beyond simple tolerance to comprehending differences and celebrating the rich dimensions of variety and multiplicity held within each individual (Disability World, 2012).

GLOBAL CONNECTION

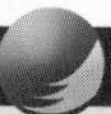

In addition to the immediate devastating effects of war, chronic disease and disabilities are long-term consequences that persist for decades in countries where conflicts occur. Conditions such as cancer from chemical warfare, stress-related illnesses, and injuries to the musculoskeletal system are just a few of the chronic, debilitating conditions that plague countries even after war ends.

GOT AN ALTERNATIVE?

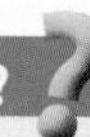

Persons with chronic illness are more likely to embrace nontraditional interventions than other patients. Why do you think this is true? What is the role of the community health nurse in educating persons with chronic illness related to complementary and alternative health choices?

Roles for Community Health Nurses

Community health nurses caring for individuals with chronic illness attempt to mitigate effects of chronic, disabling conditions for individuals and communities by functioning in many roles in established and nontraditional settings. Settings in which they work include free-standing clinics, homeless shelters, shopping malls, schools, apartments, hospitals, churches, rural settings, urban residences, and wherever healthcare needs occur.

Nurses identify risk factors associated with chronic diseases, and they anticipate complications arising from acute illnesses superimposed on chronicity. Further, nurses provide direction for modification of current health policy to reflect changing priorities and identify silent and underserved groups of chronically ill persons.

Community health nurses may intervene to facilitate use of adaptive coping mechanisms. Coping enhancement involves incorporation of social support—for example—which is believed to mediate and buffer effects of stressors associated with chronic illness. Another coping mechanism that may mitigate feelings of hopelessness and loss is spiritual support, which is also identified as a helpful mechanism of coping by chronically ill populations (Miller, 1992). Use of spiritual support may provide comfort and alleviate prolonged grieving.

Nurses function as change agents, advocates, professional caregivers, and role models. The role of prevention grows more important every year. Nursing interventions help delineate areas in which nurses have specialty knowledge and expertise. Some nursing interventions that have had limited applications in research may be explicated further in future clinical investigations, thereby providing additional support for practice.

Change Agent

As the number of NPs and family practice physicians entering primary care within the community multiply, community health nurses will have increasing opportunities to identify changing needs that require immediate attention. Long waiting periods to access primary care will be shortened, and turnaround times for maintenance care activities will decrease. Nurses will be an important source of support, facilitating better and faster follow-up care, and more in-depth prevention activities for all disabled and chronically ill persons.

Nurse Life-Care Planners are a relatively new addition to community-based health care. According to the American Association of Nurse Life Care Planners (AANLCP), nurse care planning is defined as the specialty practice in which the planner utilizes the nursing process in the collection and analysis of comprehensive client-specific data in the preparation of a dynamic document. Developed for individuals who have experienced an injury or have chronic healthcare issues, this document provides an organized, concise plan stipulating estimates for reasonable and necessary current and future healthcare needs with the associated costs and frequencies for goods and services. The plan may be updated as needed. Nurse life-care planners engage in a specialty nursing practice that encompasses many roles that directly and indirectly influence patient outcomes. In addition, the nurse life-care planner serving as a testifying expert provides testimony on the facts of nursing care needs, projecting reasonable and necessary future care needs and costs for the injured or chronically ill individual. Nurse life-care planner roles cross into testifying as expert witnesses, case management, medical-legal advisers, insurance, and private industries. They also may work with trust administrators, health workers' compensation insurance carriers, the federal government's national vaccine program, and private families to assist them with planning future healthcare needs for their loved ones, both young and old. They also develop medical cost projections.

> Every time I think that I'm getting old, and gradually going to the grave, something else happens.
>
> —*Lillian Carter, nurse and mother of President Jimmy Carter*

Advocate

Advocating for chronically ill patients may result in provision and expansion of services where they are either currently unavailable or are of limited availability. By increasing necessary services, additional supports and effective interventions may be identified in the future that capitalize on use of extended familial caregivers and community-based volunteers. Political activity associated with enabling increased access to health-promoting activities may be of increasing importance in the future, as populations of the chronically ill increase in the new millennium.

Professional Caregiver

An area of great need will be that of professional caregivers who assist chronically ill persons to cope over the long term. Coping with chronic illness may mean development of personal and societal resources as a means of enhancing quality of life and survival. Development of personal resources may include increasing coping abilities so as to endure painful or prolonged aspects of disease. Adjustment to losses associated with chronic diseases becomes essential. Adjustment entails coping with physical symptoms and uncertainty. Facilitating adjustment may include use of nursing interventions such as family integrity promotion, decision-making support, and mutual goal setting (Luckmann, 1997).

Role Models

Role-modeling behaviors of the community health nurse will include smoking cessation, weight control, and physical fitness to encourage preventive behaviors in the chronically ill. Health teaching will increase in importance, and nurses in community settings will be sought to initiate effective educational programs specifically designed to address the needs of the chronically ill population.

Interdisciplinary Roles and Responsibilities

As care providers, change agents, and advocates, community health nurses work as an integral part of interdisciplinary healthcare teams. Other team members include both paraprofessional and professional individuals. Some of these individuals will have no direct contact with, or knowledge of, the chronically ill patient. Others will have day-to-day contact with the patient and will depend on the community health nurse for essential information and opinions.

CULTURAL CONNECTION 

A patient's culture and meaning of pain can influence the management of chronic illness and disabilities. Think of how different cultures express pain or discomfort and how this will affect the public health nurse's interventions.

ENVIRONMENTAL CONNECTION

For patients with asthma and allergies, any change in new household products or household items, such as rugs and furniture, can result in a severe allergic reaction.

Use of the rehabilitation interdisciplinary model frequently adds to the team concept of care that has long been in place and effectively used by healthcare personnel (Hickey, 2003). Rehabilitative treatments of patients depend on the efforts of many healthcare specialists and demand that patients be actively engaged in their treatment protocols. Community health nurses will continue to have an active role in supporting rehabilitation efforts in chronically ill populations to optimize these patients' functional independence and self-reliance.

Financing Costs of Chronic Illness

By 2020, nearly 157 million Americans are expected to have at least one chronic condition (about 80 million will have multiple chronic illnesses). Direct medical costs for these conditions are expected to be more than $685 billion annually; adding in the indirect costs, it is estimated that the total cost of just seven chronic illnesses will top $4 trillion by 2023, accounting for more than 20% of total U.S. gross domestic product (GDP) (Fahey, 2008). Despite the encouraging impact of recent healthcare reforms, thousands of Americans and immigrants residing in the United States lack health insurance or have inadequate access to healthcare services.

Fees for health care are generally set by formulas put forth by federal and state governments (Hickey, 2003). Medicare, Medicaid, and third-party payers are involved in establishment of fee schedules and cost-management efforts that determine "who gets what" in terms of services. Both direct and indirect healthcare costs are considered when estimating the magnitude of chronic illness. Chronic illness costs society millions of dollars annually and results in massive productivity losses. Treatments for chronic illnesses are rising in cost as more people survive longer because of earlier and more accurate diagnostics. Cancer and heart disease are examples of these phenomena, with heart disease alone affecting an estimated 80 million people in the United States (CDC, 2008a).

Age and chronic illness are positively related. Persons older than age 65 represent a rapidly growing segment of the world's population. Elderly have the highest rates of hospitalizations and visits to physicians in the United States, even though they experience the lowest rates of acute illnesses (CDC, 2008a, 2008b). The cost of caring for such individuals is a substantial concern, as chronically ill elders may experience a long-term financial burden related to their needed care.

Funding initiatives for community-based supports vary. Some private funds are available through service organizations, religious, and secular groups. Public funds for community supports for home-based caregivers vary widely from region to region. Use and availability of supports affect the indirect costs of caring for chronically ill persons. Additional or indirect costs of caring for the chronically ill population include time lost from work in the case of home-based caregivers, resulting in lost productivity. The cost of hospitalizations secondary to exacerbations of symptoms and medications, supplies, and treatments are other indirect costs. For example, diabetic supplies can cost hundreds of dollars monthly; this cost is often offset, at least in part, by federal tax dollars. Prioritizing these issues has engendered fierce debate in political arenas, as rising healthcare costs and increasing numbers of chronically ill require new funding sources.

ETHICAL CONNECTION 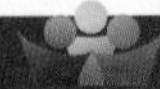

Chronic illness is not typically a focus of public health services in a community. This may result in persons with chronic illnesses having few resources for drug and medical expenses. Why do you think chronic illness has not typically been considered a public health "problem" until very recently?

President Obama placed comprehensive health reform at the top of his domestic policy agenda. The president signed into law the ACA, which provides many benefits for disabled persons who previously were unable to procure health insurance due to prior existing conditions. The ACA's provisions include the following:

- Discrimination on the basis of pre-existing condition is banned, as are caps on lifetime benefits.
- Starting in 2015, insurance companies are barred from discrimination on the basis of medical history or genetic information.
- Establishment of the Community Living Assistance Services and Supports (CLASS) program, a self-funded and voluntary long-term care insurance choice that would help people with disabilities remain in their homes, communities, and jobs through cash benefits to pay for community support services.
- Extension of the Money Follows the Person program, improving the Medicaid home-and-community-based services (HCBS) option.
- Establishment of the Community First Choice Option covering community-based attendant services and supports to help Medicaid beneficiaries with daily activities and health-related tasks.
- Establishment of standards for medical diagnostic equipment so people with disabilities can access vital preventive care.

Chronically ill individuals are particularly vulnerable to reforms in healthcare policy that decrease or eliminate essential services, including home-based nursing care, needed to improve and maintain their health status. These patients are often unable to effectively advocate for themselves, so they rely on healthcare professionals to secure needed services for them. If fragmentation of health care continues, the chronically ill population will experience increased difficulties in accessing adequate health care. According to the National Council on Disability (2013), many Medicaid enrollees with disabilities are difficult and costly to serve, primarily because of the wide-ranging needs within the target population; hence the importance of coordinating and synchronizing services and supports across multiple service-delivery systems. The fact that Medicaid recipients with disabilities frequently require healthcare services and long-term supports adds to the complexity of the service-delivery equation, because the latter services, historically, have been provided through networks that operate outside the healthcare delivery system.

The Future of Managed Care for People with Disabilities

Three factors are driving states to expand managed care enrollments: (1) the severe budget constraints under which most states presently operate and predictions that budget shortfalls will continue to plague states for at least the next few years, (2) the expansion of Medicaid roles in 2014 under the ACA, and (3) a growing consensus among health experts and government officials that high-cost Medicaid recipients—including frail seniors and people with disabilities and chronic diseases—can be served more effectively and at lower costs through managed care plans.

Viewed from a disability perspective, federal and state Medicaid officials see Medicaid as a key device for accomplishing all of the discussed delivery reforms, and state officials also hope to significantly improve the cost-effectiveness of health services provided to high-cost beneficiaries by enrolling more people with chronic illnesses and disabilities in Medicaid managed care programs. Moreover, a growing number of states see managed care as a more effective and less costly approach to (1) delivering behavioral health services to people with serious mental illnesses and substance use disorders; (2) providing long-term services and support to people with physical, sensory, and developmental disabilities; and (3) providing a coordinated array of health services and long-term supports to those with dual eligibilities.

All of the signs indicate that Medicaid services to beneficiaries with disabilities are on the edge of a major transformation, driven primarily by the introduction of managed care principles to the financing and delivery of such services. The changes inherent in a managed care approach pose both opportunities and challenges in providing services for people with disabilities, whether they are eligible for Medicaid services only or for both Medicare and Medicaid services.

Racial Disparities in Health Care in Chronic Illness and Disability

According to the Center to Reduce Cancer Health Disparities, an agency of the National Cancer Institute (2013), poor people are at greatest risk of being diagnosed and treated for cancer at late stages of disease. Death rates from lung cancer are four to five times higher in the least educated than in the most educated individuals. African American males have the highest incidence and mortality rates for colon, prostate, and lung cancers. Treatment delays encountered by minorities contribute to poorer outcomes in cancer treatment. Stokes et al. (2013) found African American patients with prostate cancer experienced longer time from diagnosis to treatment than Caucasian patients with prostate cancer. The authors further concluded that African American patients appear to experience disparities across all aspects of this disease process, and together these factors in receipt of care plausibly contribute to the observed differences in rates of recurrence and mortality among African American and Caucasian patients with prostate cancer.

Self-Determination: The Patient as Partner

Chronically ill patients frequently experience perceptions of life quality that are not shared by physicians. Elderly, chronically ill outpatients may perceive their lives to have acceptable quality, despite the physician's perceptions to the contrary. Research suggests patients' perceived emotional, socioeconomic, intellectual, and physical functioning affect their perceptions of quality of life (Wilson & Satterfield, 2007). Quality of care may directly affect quality of life. Those who experience adequate management of symptoms and undesirable side effects may rate their quality of life as acceptable or better. In cases characterized by uncontrolled relief from chronic symptoms that result in reduced or unbearable daily symptoms, quality of life will decrease markedly.

Sensitivity in Community-Based Caring

More than 50 million Americans are currently involved in assisting chronically ill or elderly persons with either personal or household management issues (National Family Caregivers Association, 2008). All ethnic, racial, and gender groups are involved in caring for chronically ill individuals. Community health nurses are in the unique position of entering private homes to render or assist in care provision. Each of these groups and each individual have issues and expectations that may present unique challenges to healthcare workers in provision of gender-, ethnic-, and racially sensitive care. Care rendered in ethnic- and culturally sensitive ways will enhance the nurse's efforts to individualize important interventions.

Gender-Specific Considerations

Overall, women live longer than men. In addition, women tend to rely more on daughters, sisters, mothers, and female friends than on male children or spouses when chronic illnesses occur. Men tend to rely on these same groups of caregivers but most often rely on female spouses. Consequently, there are many more women functioning as caregivers than men. For many reasons, including societal expectations, women tend to put the needs of others before their own needs. Many women, especially older women, may have difficulty articulating their needs and preferences in aspects of care, and need to be reassured, offered options, and consulted about all aspects of care as both patients and caregivers.

Chronically ill women may use a variety of coping strategies to handle the effects of their disease or illness. Effective coping strategies will underscore their desire to maintain normalcy to the greatest extent possible. Women with early-onset disability may strive to prevent secondary complications from developing (Goodwin & Compton, 2004). Consequently, many more women are invested in health promotion to improve their day-to-day experiences and to extend their life expectancy. An example of this idea is controlling the fatigue associated with cancer: Scheduled exercises may be carefully planned around levels of least fatigue in an effort to promote a sense of normalcy and encourage women to take control of their physical symptoms (Coon & Coleman, 2004). The role of motivation and engagement in rehabilitation makes a strong case for those with disability to achieve and maintain high-level wellness.

One issue of increasing concern is women's increasing mortality rate compared to men. An example of this problem is the rapidly rising rate of lung cancer from cigarette smoking in women. Nicotine addiction, in particular, has increased among women since the late 1980s and greatly hampers their ability to achieve high-level wellness. This particular form of addiction results from a distinct, routine, and harmful social behavior that reflects the changing role and status of women (Pampel, 2003). This disturbing trend has been documented in nine high-income industrialized nations—the United States, the United Kingdom, Ireland, Australia, Austria, Canada, Denmark, New Zealand, and Sweden. Not surprisingly, the United Kingdom and the United States have the highest rates of mortality from smoking and lung cancer in women (Pampel, 2003). Activities of the community health nurse should include leading by example, repeatedly encouraging patients to quit smoking, and discouraging women from starting smoking, with the knowledge that prevention is far easier to promote than cessation.

APPLICATION TO PRACTICE 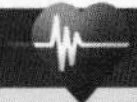

Arthritis

Rose is an 87-year-old woman who has been dependent on others for many years for her daily care. She is unable to ambulate and is in a wheelchair. She lives in a long-term care facility and experiences chronic pain from arthritis in nearly all her joints. She has been in arthritic pain for many years and has used different drugs at intervals, but she continues to experience severe pain that interrupts all other activities. Rose grimaces as she moves in her wheelchair, and speaks about her pain:

> The pain is always there. I would like to be without it just for a day, now and then. I've really forgotten how it is to just get up and do for yourself. I never wanted to have to ask other people to help me all the time, but lately, that's how it is. I'm so tired all the time. The pain keeps me awake, and when I fall asleep, if I try to turn over, it reminds me right away by waking me up! I have the pain all the time, more or less. I take some of the arthritis medicine for it, and it helps a good bit, but it always wears off, and then it feels like the pain comes back real strong. Either sittin' or standin' it bothers me, and I can't walk any distance at all. My niece comes to take me out some, but I don't always feel like going. 'Course, it's real nice to have her come, it's just that I can't go like I used to. We both miss getting out together, but then, at my age, I'm expecting to have pain. They all tell me you don't die from it, but it sure keeps you from doing like you want to.

Issues Community Health Nurses Encounter

Professional issues encountered in providing and managing community-based care for chronically ill individuals include understanding long- and short-term goals, patterns of disease progression, resource allocation, development of support systems, education, and home-based caregiver roles. In daily care, routines provide a framework and format for use of the nursing process. Continuous supervision by nurses is generally not needed by all chronically ill individuals, but ADLs may be supported by home-based caregivers. These caregivers, who are frequently relatives or close friends of the individual with chronic illness, provide valuable services that enable chronically ill persons to retain autonomy in their homes. Paraprofessional caregivers who work in the community and function with a great deal of autonomy include nurse aides, therapy assistants, and transport staff, all of whom facilitate ADLs, maximal independence, and travel within the community. The home setting is desirable for many chronically ill patients and supports self-identity and self-determination, whereas institutional settings may depersonalize and socially isolate some chronically ill individuals from familiar surroundings, personal belongings, and cherished supports. Institutional settings may be desirable in situations in which home-based caregiving is not realistic.

RESEARCH ALERT 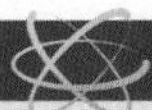

A qualitative study was undertaken to detect differences in the way caregivers in three ethnic groups (African American, Puerto Rican, and Caucasian) describe their reactions to caregiving. An ethnographic method was appropriately used to focus on scientific descriptions of cultural groups. The stratified, random sample consisted of 18 caregivers who were selected from a sample of 409 caregivers. All interviews were conducted in informants' homes, with one exception. Informed consent was ensured, and data were collected through use of CES-D and guided, unstructured conversations. The CES-D scale is a short self-report scale designed to measure depressive symptomatology in the general population. Data were analyzed using content analysis to discover themes and meanings expressed by caregivers.

Findings revealed differences in expression of burden, both by ethnicity and gender within ethnicity groups. Generally, caregiving was associated with negative feelings and situations. Almost all Caucasians described their situations negatively. African Americans described their situations as demanding and time-consuming. Puerto Rican caregivers reported that it was difficult to meet the demands of the care required. Several reported caregiving to be a rewarding and satisfying experience. These individuals had an extended network of support in which there were other people involved in the care and assistance of the disabled. Level of outside support was key in decreasing caregiver burden. The authors state that their findings can assist practitioners to better understand the cultural idiosyncrasies that are important in developing a culturally sensitive plan.

Source: Calderon, V., & Tennstedt, S. L. (1998). Ethnic differences in the expression of caregiver burden: Results of a qualitative study. *Journal of Gerontological Social Work, 30*(1–2), 159–178.

Supporting Community-Based Caregivers

In addition to provision and direction of care, another role of importance for community health nurses is providing support to home-based caregivers. Daily provision of care to chronically ill persons can be both challenging and rewarding for home-based caregivers, and support systems, both formal and informal, may be necessary for a positive experience. Their anticipation of needs and understanding of disease progression make nurses invaluable assets to home-based caregivers who may have unrealistic or unachievable goals. For example, home-based caregivers for persons with chronic obstructive pulmonary disease need to understand that perceived quality of life and use of coping mechanisms may contribute more to comfort and adaptation than does use of oxygen and medications (Herbert & Gregor, 1997).

Respite services are urgently needed by family caregivers who provide care to homebound elders with chronic illness and/or disability. Because of the nature of chronic illness and disability, home care may be provided for extended periods and may challenge the resources of the caregiver. Respite involves four elements: (1) purpose, (2) time, (3) activities, and (4) place; it may occur in the home or elsewhere (Lubkin & Larsen, 2013). In addition to home-based care, sites of respite care include senior centers, daycare centers, long-term care facilities, and group living facilities. Respite care has the unique purpose of relieving caregivers so as to provide them with time for themselves so they are able to resume their caregiving role. The community health nurse may underscore these efforts by devising flexible schedules and interventions to address the needs of both care recipient and caregiver.

Support groups have become popular since the late 1990s as a means of facilitating coping with illness and/or disability. They may offer concrete assistance with adjustment to illness and associated role changes in addition to providing a neutral "sounding board" and informational services. Larger cities tend to have more support groups for specific needs, but because the Internet has eliminated many communication barriers, numerous support groups may be accessed online. Group leaders are frequently health professionals who have expertise in topical areas related to disabilities identified by potential group members. Some groups may be particularly helpful to individuals who are returning home from a hospitalization or who are working through illness-related issues. By taking advantage of the link to an empathetic community, individuals may feel better connected to others with similar issues and will reintegrate more easily. For those who live in rural areas, an Internet group may be especially useful if social contacts are limited by distance.

In addition to the Internet, the postal service and the telephone are excellent tools to encourage connectedness and engagement. Handwritten letters may provide a continuing source of enjoyment to the recipient. Those with memory loss are often comforted and reassured by "hard-copy" or tangible reminders of others. Similarly, phone calls are frequently welcome reminders of social connections and common interests. Each of these modalities may provide indispensable links and social support that is instrumental in preventing social isolation and loneliness.

Nonnursing caregivers provide care and services for chronically ill individuals in numerous community and institutional settings. Familial caretakers most frequently include women in the roles of wife, mother, daughter, sibling, or grandparent. Often, these female caregivers have chronic or unmet health needs themselves, and must subordinate their own needs to render care to their relative on a continuing basis. Continuing care can be extremely demanding and exhausting, if the familial caregiver is unrelieved. Neglect of self may develop in these circumstances, and depression, decreased overall health, and exhaustion may follow.

It is important to anticipate caregiver burnout and to suggest alternatives to prevent it from developing. Community-based programs and resources have been developed in some areas to help familial caregivers to take care of themselves. Respite and episodic care of chronically ill programs enable these caregivers to receive physical and psychological support at periodic intervals, while nurses and other members of the healthcare team assume responsibility for care of the chronically ill individual. Both of these options are available through some Veterans Administration (VA) hospitals, nursing homes, public hospitals, and community health agencies. These services are available only to provide temporary relief to community-based, familial caregivers. If the burdens of giving full-time care exceed the abilities and resources of the familial or home-based caregiver over the long term, institutionalization becomes the primary source of care.

Issues encountered by familial caregivers include other family commitments, personal physical health, recreational needs, fear of using needed equipment, stress, loss of independence, role change, loss of privacy, decreased wellbeing, depression, negative feelings, physical strain, anxiety, anger, guilt, loss of self, and caregiver burnout. Effects of chronic illness on families are a major problem for some parental caregivers of children, who often attempt to cope with illness by adapting. Parental caregivers who lack professional help and support in care of their children may feel burdened and overwhelmed. These feelings may lead to development of abusive behaviors. Home-based caregivers of chronically ill children and adults may perpetrate abuse because of feelings of overwhelming frustration, social isolation, and powerlessness. Some family systems may have characteristics that promote abuse, including lack of family support, familial caregiver reluctance, overcrowding, isolation, family burdens, marital conflict, or differing opinions about institutionalization (Lubkin & Larsen, 2013).

In chronic illness, abuse may be obvious or covert. If neglect, self-neglect, exploitation, and coercion are not readily apparent, the community health nurse needs to be sensitive to suspected cases of abuse (Luckmann, 1997). Use of several familial caregivers may relieve the frustration and feelings of isolation that underlie abuse. Another important factor in diminishing burdens of familial caregiving is engagement in social interaction, fun, and recreation, which may enhance the caregiver's sense of wellbeing (Thompson, Futterman, Gallagher-Thompson, Rose, & Lovett, 1993). Caregiver burnout has been linked with lack of assistance in day-to-day activities and should be examined proactively to incorporate supports necessary to benefit both the familial or home-based caregiver and the patient.

BOX 28-6 Social Security Announces New Compassionate Allowances Conditions: Fast-Track Disability Process Will Now Include 200 Conditions

Michael J. Astrue, Commissioner of Social Security, today announced 35 additional Compassionate Allowances are in effect, bringing the total number of conditions in the expedited disability process to 200. Compassionate Allowances are a way to quickly identify diseases and other medical conditions that, by definition, meet Social Security's standards for disability benefits. The program fast-tracks disability decisions to ensure that Americans with the most serious disabilities receive their benefit decisions within days instead of months or years. These conditions primarily include certain cancers, adult brain disorders, and a number of rare disorders that affect children.

"We have achieved another milestone for the Compassionate Allowances program, reaching 200 conditions," Commissioner Astrue said. "Nearly 200,000 people with severe disabilities nationwide have been quickly approved, usually in less than 2 weeks, through the program since it began in October 2008."

By definition, these conditions are so severe that Social Security does not need to fully develop the applicant's work history to make a decision. As a result, Social Security eliminated this part of the application process for people who have a condition on the list.

Social Security has held seven public hearings and worked with experts to develop the list of conditions considered to be Compassionate Allowances. The hearings also have helped the agency identify ways to improve the disability process for applicants with conditions classified as Compassionate Allowances.

For more information on the Compassionate Allowances initiative, visit http://www.ssa.gov/pressoffice/pr//compassionateallowances200conditions-pr.html

New Compassionate Allowances Conditions

1. Adult non-Hodgkin's lymphoma
2. Adult-onset Huntington disease
3. Allan-Herndon-Dudley syndrome
4. Alveolar soft part sarcoma
5. Aplastic anemia
6. Beta thalassemia major
7. Bilateral optic atrophy—infantile
8. Caudal regression syndrome—Types III and IV
9. Child T-cell lymphoblastic lymphoma
10. Congenital lymphedema
11. DeSanctis cacchione syndrome
12. Dravet syndrome
13. Endometrial stromal sarcoma
14. Erdheim-Chester disease
15. Fatal familial insomnia
16. Fryns syndrome
17. Fulminant giant cell myocarditis
18. Hepatopulmonary syndrome
19. Hepatorenal syndrome
20. Jervell and Lange-Nielsen syndrome
21. Leiomyosarcoma
22. Malignant gastrointestinal stromal tumor
23. Malignant germ cell tumor
24. MECP 2 duplication syndrome
25. Menkes disease—classic or infantile onset form
26. NFU-1 mitochondrial disease
27. Non-ketotic hyperglycemia
28. Peritoneal mucinous carcinomatosis
29. Phelan-McDermid syndrome
30. Retinopathy of prematurity—Stage V
31. Roberts syndrome
32. Severe combined immunodeficiency—childhood
33. Sinonasal cancer
34. Transplant coronary artery vasculopathy
35. Usher syndrome—type

Palliative and Hospice Care

Hospice or palliative services provide care and support to terminally ill individuals and their families in the final stages of life, and support death with respect and dignity. For those with chronic illnesses, great comfort may be obtained by having hospice services provided within the home. This allows the familial caregiver to have a rest from caring activities and to have an opportunity to consider relevant quality-of-life issues. The role of community health nurses in hospice care varies but usually includes referral through the attending physician, facilitation of transfer of care of the chronically ill patient, and consultation as needed. Community-based hospice nurses may also provide education, coordination, and support services. Although palliative and hospice services had their roots in oncology, the principles underlying that field have been applied to care for those with other diseases such as HIV/AIDS. Since the advent of highly effective antiretroviral therapies, the disease trajectory of HIV/AIDS has been altered, such that it is not always predictable. Community health nurses may be involved in caring for HIV/AIDS patients who have an uncertain future and who may not fit in the traditional paradigm of palliative or hospice care (Cochrane, 2003).

Congregate housing is another option for care that maximizes resources while carefully considering quality of life. *Congregate housing* and *assisted living* are considered interchangeable terms. Those who qualify for this type of living arrangement characteristically have a stable chronic condition and require assistance with three or more functional ADLs. Bringing needed services into individuals' homes, whether private or congregate, is an effective way to reduce institutionalization in those with chronic conditions (Sheehan & Oakes, 2003). Congregate housing services typically include the following core services: three meals daily, housekeeping and laundry services, transportation, social programs, and 24-hour security. Additionally, nursing supervision is available 20 hours per week, and emergency services are always available. Community health nurses may be involved with planning and supervision of care in these dwellings, which emphasize autonomy.

THINK ABOUT THIS 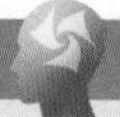

Sometimes I look at the sarcoidosis as a mean monkey on my back. In a way, I tried to mourn for the person who I was and figure out who I am now. I did as much research as I could and I took ownership of this illness, because if you don't take care of your body, where are you going to live?

—Karen Duffy

Institutionalization

Chronically ill persons who elect to receive institutional-based care are relatively few in number; however, they may be frail and require care that is not available in the community. The population requiring institutional provision of care, which currently includes fewer than 2 million individuals in the United States, is expected to increase rapidly over the next 40 years as baby boomers age and experience health problems.

Physical restraints actually increase injuries. Restraints also have the effect of reducing mobility, inhibiting communication, preventing individual reorientation, and restricting patterns of socialization within and outside of the facility. In facilities with decreased use of physical restraints, security and safety of residents may be enhanced by use of cameras, alarm systems, and staff surveillance. Unfortunately, falls and patient injuries continue to be a major problem encountered in institutional settings due to staffing levels and the age and physical condition of patients. Many are frail and require frequent assistance with all ADLs. Other problematic issues related to long-term care include loss of privacy, decreased choices in routines, diminished autonomy, and adverse relocation consequences.

Facility selection is an important decision, and community health nurses should support consultation of the chronically ill patient with family members who may assist in the process. The physical environment, accessibility, nurse-to-patient ratio, friendliness of the staff, availability of medical and support services, cost, and location will all be of concern to patients and families considering placement.

Both private and publicly funded facilities for long-term care of chronically ill patients exist. Long-term care facilities with religious affiliations are available in many geographic areas and may be Medicare certified for reimbursement purposes. Nonsectarian facilities are also available and may be affiliated with state or local governments. Both public and private institutions must adhere to standards of care that are put forth and monitored by local, state, and federal agencies. Areas subject to regulation in all long-term care facilities include resident rights; admission, transfer, and discharge rights; resident behavior and facility practice; administration; physical environment; infection control; quality of life; resident assessment; quality of care; nursing; rehabilitation; and medical services.

Nursing home selection may cause emotional distress to chronically ill individuals, who may have decreased coping skills and decreased endurance to withstand a major lifestyle change. Often, the community health nurse is aware of plans to move an individual to a nursing home. Elderly persons with chronic health problems may experience severe adjustment issues related to perceived and actual losses, feelings of powerlessness, and despair. Coping with these changes will require sensitive support and time to process changes. Rapid adjustment to lifestyle changes should not be expected.

Health Promotion in Chronic Illness and Disability

Health-promotion activities that focus on improving function across a spectrum of diagnoses and a range of age groups are effective in reducing secondary conditions experienced by, and outpatient physician visits made by, people with disabilities. Health-promotion strategies for persons with chronic illnesses and/or disability may be adapted from those activities already identified for the mainstream population. An example of this idea is maintenance of normal weight. Obesity—once stigmatized as an unfortunate and undesirable condition—has dramatically increased in frequency and now adversely affects American adults and children in record numbers. Considered the worst health problem in the United States, obesity affects those living in poverty much more frequently than the affluent (Colvin, 2004). Obesity is associated with a 50% to 100% increased risk of death from all causes. Persons with chronic conditions are at even greater risk for mortality and increased morbidity if they develop obesity.

Health-promotion strategies, including encouragement of a regular exercise program and patient education teaching healthy eating practices, will benefit both healthy and chronically ill populations. Those with disabilities also must strive to achieve or maintain normal weight. Those with mobility or endurance challenges will be adversely affected if they develop obesity, so prevention is a top priority with this population. Meal replacements may warrant consideration for those with difficulty in limiting portions, managing food preparation, or maintaining weight in a normal range (Noakes, Foster, Keogh, & Clifton, 2004).

Indeed, health-promotion activities for all groups are increasingly important. Preventing the development of secondary complications related to risk behaviors is essential. Complications are far more costly to treat than health-promoting behaviors are to adopt. This is surely the case for the chronically ill and disabled. Many persons with disability have no additional health problems and are well; these individuals may benefit substantially from health-promotion activities. Structural changes associated with normal aging may also be mitigated by health-promoting behaviors. With the projected growth in the number of aging individuals worldwide, health promotion must soon move to the top of the health agenda for all providers as resources are stretched to accommodate greater-than-ever-numbers. Complications associated with preventable cardiovascular disease alone consume astonishing quantities of resources that could be beneficially directed in numerous other ways. Historically, nurses have optimized all available resources to promote healing and health (Phillips, 2005). Because of their proximity to the patient base, community health nurses are ideally positioned to provide leadership in the area of health promotion for their disabled and chronically ill patients.

Community Living Needs of People Who Have Disabilities

Legislation has been passed to ensure that environments in which people with disabilities live and work follow the patterns of life and conditions that most people experience. Children and adults with disabilities have the right to live in homes and attend school or work within integrated settings with their peers without disabilities. For example, most adults live in settings of their choosing, with people of their choice, getting up and going to bed at "normal" times, eating three meals a day about 5 hours apart, going to work, and choosing their own recreational activities and friends. Social movements (e.g., "normalization" and now "inclusion") have urged the provision of opportunities and supports for individuals with disabilities to enable them to live and work in their communities (DiLeo, 2007; Wehman, 2006).

Similar to individualized family services plans and individualized education plans, which are discussed later in this chapter as plans of service for children, individual service plans of assistance and skill enhancement can be written for adolescents and adults to identify the supports needed to transition to work, further education, or other living arrangements. These plans are written with the individual with a disability and/or family members as the most important members of the team.

Person-centered planning is an approach whose goals are to reduce social isolation and segregation, establish friendships, increase opportunities to engage in preferred activities, develop competencies, and promote respect. Person-centered planning brings together the most important people in the life of a person, envisions a better life for the person, and discovers ways to achieve the vision. Participation is voluntary and the group is typically diverse, not consisting solely of service providers. The views of the family members, friends, and the focus person are foremost, instead of the professional authority hierarchy of a clinical team meeting, with an orientation toward the deficiencies of the individual. The process is guided by a facilitator who keeps the group focused on creating a lifestyle based on the aspirations of the focus person. The facilitator typically partners with a recorder or maps what people say on large sheets of paper, under categories such as history, preferences, dreams, and fears; these items then become the basis for developing a vision for the future. The group continues to meet periodically to reflect on successes and setbacks and adjusts strategies to accommodate changing circumstances and sometimes changing aspirations (Holburn, 2002).

Unfortunately, service plans are still being written that segregate individuals with disabilities. Segregated situations are often established under the premise that people need to "get ready" for living and working in the community. Work and living skills, however, are best learned in real jobs, homes, and communities. Program activities with self-contained groups of people with disabilities in perpetual preparation for the real world by traveling, recreating, working, and living together do not promote the uniqueness and value of each individual with a disability, nor do they prepare individuals for life in the community (DiLeo, 2007; Wehman, 2006).

Our society, with cultural values of productivity, skill, attractiveness, and affluence, still views people with disabilities as different in a negative way, perceived as incompetent or as children who never grew up, "funny looking," or even dangerous. The most powerful way to change negative societal attitudes is for individuals with disabilities to participate successfully in their communities, as skilled and productive workers and managers of their own homes (with the right supports). As neighbors, coworkers, and friends, people with disabilities demonstrate their adult needs for expression of personal accomplishment, responsibility, interdependence, privacy, and sexuality. The more opportunities for choice and the more competencies an individual possesses, the more self-esteem and status he or she will have in the community. Community health nurses who provide assistance should show care in interactions, choosing moments to teach and methods of support provision that are professionally appropriate and demonstrate personal respect. For example, the community health nurse should use minimal cues, gestures, and words (the less assistance the better, to counteract dependency), watching tone and volume, to promote the dignity of the individual and not convey an attitude of pity or assume a parental role.

The movement away from a focus on an individual's deficits to a focus on self-determination and inclusion has influenced decisions on which supports are needed for individuals to participate in their communities, assume valued social roles, and experience greater satisfaction and fulfillment. Supports are defined as resources and strategies that promote the interests and welfare of individuals and result in enhanced personal independence and productivity, greater participation in an interdependent society, increased community integration, and an improved quality of life. Types of supports should be tailored to individual needs and preferences and be provided in a flexible manner. Supports are more important to some individuals than to others. Systematic assessments of support needs should consider multiple factors and guide the development and revision of individual support plans. Assessment and planning should begin with identifying an individual's desirable life experiences and goals. After determining the intensity of support needs, an individual support plan should be developed that will be monitored for progress (Thompson et al., 2002).

Homes of Their Own

Historically, people with significant disabilities, particularly those with mental impairments, had two living options. Either the family could care for the individual at home indefinitely, with little, if any, public assistance, or the family could place the individual in a state residential facility. Current beliefs about the rights of people with disabilities support that (1) all children, including those with severe disabilities, have the right to live at home with their family; and (2) adults with disabilities have the right to the supports necessary to live in a home in the community, either alone or with another adult of their choosing.

Living options for people with disabilities are often presented on a continuum from large, segregated facilities at one end to group homes or homes of their own at the other. Such a continuum reinforces the past belief that large residential institutions or large group homes can be legitimate options as places to live. Most professionals believe that "the people who were most often viewed as needing to live in larger, specialized facilities, such as institutions and group homes, were often the very people who most benefited from the opportunities a smaller place offered" (Racino & Taylor, 1993, p. 36). When these smaller group homes are managed based on the same model of services as the large facilities, however, people with disabilities are still shortchanged. The pseudo-home can be highly routinized, "run" by service providers, and while "homelike" in atmosphere, not truly a home.

Living arrangements can vary from a home of one's own, a semi-independent or supported apartment (with staff available to assist), a home with one's family, a foster home, or a group home (Kirk, Gallagher, Anastasiow, & Coleman, 2006; Wehman, 2006). Regardless of the type of living arrangement a person wants, needs, and can reasonably afford, there should be opportunity for choice, ownership of personal property, and privacy. For example, the individual should choose the type of neighborhood, style of home, landscaping, furnishings, and decorations—all choices demonstrating the individual is a competent adult. Also, a person should own his or her possessions, make choices in how to spend his or her own money, and choose activities he or she wishes to participate in. If there is a roommate (by choice of the individual), arrangements should be made for privacy, such as providing personal space and securing private items.

Housing must be accessible for the individual with a disability. Contractors and builders may be unaware of modifications or regulations involving accessibility, and few accessible houses or apartments are available, particularly in rural areas. The community health nurse can educate community members and leaders regarding housing needs of adults with disabilities, which in many ways overlap the needs of older adults in the community: the need for safe, affordable, and accessible housing choices. Information related to accessibility is available through each state's Department of Rehabilitation Services or Office of Vocational Rehabilitation Services, along with ample information available on the Internet.

A person with a disability may require assistance in the home to carry out ADLs such as bathing, dressing, cooking, eating, and toileting (LaPlante, Harrington, & Kang, 2002). It is estimated that about 9 million individuals in the United States need personal assistance to carry out typical daily activities. Although most of these helpers are relatives (80%), in many cases the individual with a disability must hire a helper to come into the home (U.S. Census Bureau, 2006). A **personal care attendant** can be employed to assist with ADLs, transportation, pet care, and household chores and maintenance. Personal assistant services also include interpreting, mobility assistance, social support, medical assistance, reading, and recreation. Unfortunately, availability of attendants, coordinating agencies, and public funding options vary greatly from state to state.

GLOBAL CONNECTION 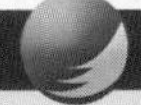

Disabling conditions throughout the world are often the result of war and conflict. When governments in other developing countries are unable to assume responsibility for the rehabilitation of the population's veterans and war victims, how do these people recover? How does this differ from U.S. policy related to veterans?

Families who may be caring for a child or adult with a significant disability 24 hours a day need the option of **respite care** to prevent caregiver burnout. Respite care provides another caregiver to assume the round-the-clock care of the family member with a disability, allowing the caretaker a vacation, a mental health break, time to recover from illness, or merely time to oneself. Because of the significant medical problems that individuals with severe disabilities may have, the respite provider (e.g., church, civic group, the Association for the Rights of Citizens with Developmental Disabilities) often will recruit nurses in the community to serve as respite caregivers. Respite may be provided in the patient's home, at a group home, in a private home, or at an organization's facility.

An Accessible Community

Accessibility to all that a community offers is critical if persons with disabilities are to participate to the fullest extent possible in community life. Many individuals with disabilities cannot afford to own customized vehicles to drive or may be physically or mentally unable to drive. Accessible public transportation is needed by many persons who are disabled so that they may work, recreate, worship, seek medical attention, socialize, and so on, as we all do on a daily basis. Inadequate transportation was cited as a problem by 30% of adults with disabilities in a 2000 Harris poll. Many areas are lacking adequate public transportation, particularly in rural areas of the country. By the year 2002, all public buses were required to be accessible. Facility accessibility is also necessary and required by the ADA. It is accomplished by accommodations such as curb cuts, ramps, large doorways with easily opened doors, elevators, and wide hallways. The community health nurse can educate community leaders about these needs for access and may become involved in advocating for individuals with disabilities or working with legislators for policy reform. Individuals who use wheelchairs for mobility are often frustrated with the inadequate involvement of people with disabilities in the development of facilities that comply with ADA accessibility requirements (Pierce, 2012). Ideally, a person who uses a wheelchair should serve on committees involved in designing buildings to ensure that they not only meet ADA requirements, but also are functional for those who use wheelchairs or who have other types of disabilities.

Meaningful Work

Work is highly valued in our society. Society often judges an individual's worth by his or her productivity; thus performing real work and paying taxes can enhance a person's dignity. The stigma associated with disability decreases when individuals are seen as productive and competent workers (Wehman, 2003). Work that includes regular coworker contact and shared common experience offers opportunities for development of personal relationships, arranged social activities after work hours, and a network of social support in the community that is often lacking in the life of individuals with developmental disabilities (Green & Schleien, 1991). The wages and fringe benefits earned at work can also offer increased financial security, greater independence and mobility in the community, control over life choices, and greater personal satisfaction (Wehman, 2003b).

Vocational options for individuals with mild to severe disabilities range from day treatment programs and sheltered workshops to supportive employment and competitive employment in community businesses. Each of the options represents less and less supervision and assistance for the individual with disabilities in a work setting. For many years, the only vocational option for individuals with mental retardation or developmental disabilities was training in segregated work settings (e.g., adult activity centers, sheltered workshops, nursing homes, and institutions). Maintaining an individual who can be productive on the Social Security disability rolls is not an efficient use of human resources or public funds. Individuals with developmental disabilities can and should work in competitive community employment settings (Revell, Kregel, Wehman, & Bond, 2000).

Competitive employment as a possibility for individuals with significant developmental disabilities has grown with the use of trained employment specialists, informed coworkers, mentors, technology supports, and legislation such as the ADA. Supported employment, with its focus on valuing the abilities of individuals with disabilities and their productivity in the workplace, has given these individuals an opportunity to be included in community business environments. The goal of supported employment is to help individuals with the most significant disabilities be successful in paid employment in the integrated work setting of their choice. Supported employment emphasizes the benefits of competitive employment for all involved. Community employment provides the individual with a disability with a real job plus the benefits and dignity that come with contribution. The employer gets a good worker and receives specialized support to train and maintain the individual. The family is able to see its family member in a competent role in the workplace. Taxpayers spend less money than they would to support the individual in a segregated program (Wehman, Revell, & Brooke, 2003; Wehman, Targett, & Cifi, 2006).

There are a number of factors that facilitate beginning or continuing employment for people with disabilities. According to the National Organization on Disability (2004), three major factors identified as helpful were assistance from vocational rehabilitation (23%); getting equipment or a device that they needed to do their work, talk with other workers, or get around at work (21%); and getting an interpreter or personal care attendant (7%). For those individuals with disabilities who did not work full-time, reasons given included the following: employers do not recognize they are capable of doing the job (42%); they lack skills, education, or training needed to get the job (33%); they need a personal assistant to help get to work or to do the job (32%); they risk losing benefits or insurance (31%); no work is available in the line of work respondent could do (29%); and special equipment or devices are needed to do the work, talk to or hear other workers, or get around at work (28%) (Toldrá & Santos, 2013). However, a recent study suggested that older adults in general, and older adults with disabilities in particular, face a greater level of workplace discrimination (Bjelland et al., 2010).

Many businesses have made changes in how they think and act about hiring individuals with disabilities since the signing of the ADA. Supervisors are indicating they are satisfied at the same or even a higher level compared to workers without disabilities regarding the performance of workers with disabilities in the areas of timeliness of arrival and departure, punctuality, attendance, and consistency in task. The business community appears to be increasingly embracing the employment of individuals with disabilities as a sound business strategy, investing in appropriate supports to ensure these employees' success. Businesses are changing their procedures for hiring new employees to better accommodate job applicants and new hires with disabilities. Written return-to-work policies for workers with disabilities are also becoming more popular. Accommodations for workers with disabilities (and without) are including job carving, job restructuring and schedule modifications, transitional work, telework, and use of assistive technology (Wehman, 2003a).

Innovations in natural supports, coworker training, and employer leadership within the business community have helped increase the capacity of service providers to include people with disabilities in the workforce. New methods of job development, modern marketing techniques, assistive technology, transition services from school to work, expansion of choice and self-determination, and person-centered planning have all contributed to the increase in integrated employment. Today segregated employment of activity centers and sheltered workshops are giving way to alternatives such as work crews and enclaves and now individual placements in community businesses, although these jobs are largely entry-level positions in the service industry (Lubkin & Larsen, 2013). Years of research have confirmed that individuals with disabilities who need long-term employment assistance fare better in supported employment than in sheltered workshops. To assist individuals with severe disabilities to succeed in employment, professionals must identify suitable opportunities within community businesses and develop the supports that those individuals need. Inclusive employment within the community is the right of all people, including those with significant disabilities (Wehman, Brooke, Green, Hewett, & Tipton, 2008).

GOT AN ALTERNATIVE?

Persons with chronic, disabling conditions often use complementary and alternative interventions. What is the role of the community health nurse as patients seek alternative treatments?

Relationships

All people experience sexual feelings, and individuals with disabilities are no exception. Sexual activity is one of the most controversial issues pertaining to the lives of individuals with disabilities, particularly mental retardation. Sexual development for individuals with mental retardation is for the most part similar to persons without mental retardation. Many professionals argue that individuals have the right to socially appropriate sexual expression. Others disagree and are concerned about outcomes, including unwanted advances (e.g., rape, incest) and sexually transmitted diseases. Appropriate sexual expression is more difficult for individuals with mental retardation who have higher levels of supervision and support. They may not have information about sexual development and functioning and typically have fewer socialization opportunities in which to practice appropriate behaviors, roles, and expectations (Beirne-Smith, Patton, & Kim, 2006).

Individuals with physical disabilities such as spinal cord injuries or cerebral palsy also may need education regarding sexuality. The community health nurse and other professionals assisting individuals with disabilities may have to set aside their own sexual values so as not to deny, limit, or inhibit an individual's interest in romance and sex. People with disabilities should receive sex education, sexual healthcare information, and opportunities for socializing, sexual expression, and intimacy.

Recreation

Participating in recreational activities is an important aspect of life for individuals with disabilities, just as it is for others in our society. Individuals with disabilities usually participate in sedentary leisure, commonly watching television or listening to the radio with family or possibly a few friends. This pattern of leisure does not help them maintain their health or fitness level. Without coordinated preventive health care for increasing fitness, secondary health conditions often result for individuals with disabilities, such as high blood pressure and high cholesterol levels, heart disease, diabetes, obesity, chronic skin problems, and hygiene-related issues. With inclusive community recreation programs for individuals with disabilities, not only will there be increased opportunity for improved health and fitness, but individuals also have increased opportunities for social contact—an additional critical variable for improved quality of life (Carter & Van Andel, 2002). Recreation may take the form of individual or team games, athletic programs in schools, college-sponsored recreational sports, employer-sponsored activities, church-sponsored activities, and family recreation. Specific activities include outdoor recreation (e.g., birding, hiking, bike riding, canoeing, softball) and indoor activities (e.g., ceramics, painting, aerobics, weight lifting, racquetball). Ideally, recreational activities in the community serve to promote physical health and conditioning, improve social skills, facilitate friendships, and develop specific skills. Although achieving a balance between work and leisure is important for everyone, it is especially critical for people with disabilities. Many individuals with disabilities who work do not have recreational outlets for evenings and weekends. Community recreation programs have been slow to accept responsibility for offering programming that includes people with disabilities:

> It is not enough merely to open programs to people with disabilities; the professionals in charge of the programs must go further and actively recruit and encourage the participation of people with disabilities and provide them with successful and ongoing mechanisms of support. (Schleien, Ray, & Green, 1997, p. 19)

Community recreational opportunities ranging from individual skill building to competitive international competition are becoming increasingly available to people with disabilities and are supported by recreational specialists and special equipment (e.g., modified bowling balls, walkers for ice skating, sit-skis for snow skiing). In addition to group participation in community-based opportunities for recreation, home-centered hobbies such as card games, board games, collections, and other leisure interests should be encouraged.

The camp movement for children with disabilities is on the rise. Currently there are hundreds of camps for children with diabetes, cancer, HIV/AIDS, multiple sclerosis, muscular dystrophy, cystic fibrosis, cerebral palsy, spina bifida, blindness, and hearing impairments. Camps may be sponsored on a national basis or supported by local chapters of national charitable organizations (Mayo, 2002). Children and youth with developmental disabilities usually attend separate recreation and leisure activities and need additional options to participate in community activities with other children and youth. With assistance and accommodation recommendations from knowledgeable personnel, all participants can benefit from inclusive recreation programs created by community recreation agencies, nonprofit sports organizations, schools, parks and recreation departments, universities, local governments, religious organizations, and private activity providers. Some children will need one-on-one assistance for safety or other very individualized accommodations to meet their unique learning or equipment needs and communication styles (Fennick & James, 2003).

Adults with disabilities may attend fewer social and cultural activities than adults without disabilities. Although they attend a place of worship almost as often as individuals without disabilities (54% as compared with 57%), their participation in other social events is typically less.

Transition from Education to Work and Living in the Community

Students with disabilities are now placed in regular education programs as much as possible because the best preparation for living and working in an integrated environment is to be taught in an inclusive school setting. Educational programming available to students with disabilities includes four major areas: (1) general education academic content, (2) basic academic skills and social skills, (3) learning strategies, and (4) vocational and life skills. A balance of these instructional areas should also address relevant adolescent issues such as biological changes and sexuality; social values and behavioral competence; identification of personal interests, talents, and areas of need; and a desire for emotional independence (Patton, Blackbourn, & Fad, 2004; Wehman, 2006).

Educational systems are expanding their roles in preparing students for transition to work and living in the community (Dolyniuk et al., 2002). Employers and employees of industries and businesses should be invited to address school systems about their workforce needs. Business connections and alliances offering students opportunities for work experiences and employment before graduation are having success. Many students with disabilities are staying employed upon graduation and are not remaining dependent on their families or the social service system.

To facilitate successful transition from the school environment to more independent living and work environments, key connections should be built with community businesses, community colleges, recreation centers, and adult supports for living. Appropriate planning focusing on student/family choice is also critical. Major options for students with disabilities include (1) employment (full-time or part-time, supported or non-supported), (2) further education (2- and 4-year colleges, technical schools, trade schools, adult education), (3) military service, (4) volunteer work, (5) "domestic engineering" (house husband/wife), or (6) absence of gainful employment or purposeful activity (Patton et al., 2004).

Transition planning is shifting the decision making to individuals with disabilities and their families. Students are now learning to make choices, be more self-determined, and be self-advocates assuming control and management responsibilities for their own lives. Professionals are shifting away from "curing" individuals with disabilities to supporting them for improved quality of life. Before students leave the school environment, they and their family members must learn how to access the supports (informal and unpaid or formal and paid) they need and want in the communities. Person-centered planning focuses on the desires of the individuals and their families and identifies the formal and informal supports the individuals will need to achieve their future dreams. A planning meeting focuses on the individual's abilities and preferences and identifies possible resources needed to provide desired assistance and support for adult living and work.

Rehabilitation

Rehabilitation is a term used for interventions aimed at restoring or optimizing functioning after an injury or significant medical problem. Rehabilitation nurses work to reduce the stigma associated with disabilities, restore maximum levels of independent functioning, advocate for optimal quality of life, help the individual and family adapt to an altered lifestyle, and improve the overall outcome for the individual with disabilities. Individuals having experienced spinal cord injuries or cerebrovascular accidents are examples of types of persons who would be involved in rehabilitation. Initially, after a significant injury, the individual with disabilities is involved in inpatient rehabilitation, which may use nursing, physical therapy (PT), occupational therapy (OT), speech language therapy, recreation therapy, music therapy, and counseling. Later, after discharge from the facility, the individual may receive home visits from a home health nurse and PT or

OT sessions at an outpatient rehabilitation facility. Both the length of the initial hospital stay and the number of outpatient rehabilitation visits permitted after discharge have been severely curtailed in recent years by insurance providers.

Medical Technology

Many individuals with disabilities require technology assistance, nonmedical or medical, immediately after an injury, during rehabilitation, and/or throughout their lives. **Medical assistive devices** assist or replace necessary body functions and are necessary to keep the individual alive or prevent further disability. Persons using medical technologies also typically require daily skilled nursing care. Medical technology is used to assist with respiration, nutrition, excretion, and surveillance of vital functions and oxygen levels.

Individuals with chronic respiratory failure may require oxygen supplementation by nasal cannula, face mask, oxygen tent or hood, or a tracheostomy. These individuals often may require chest physiotherapy and suctioning several times a day to clear pulmonary secretions. When assistance is needed to replace or augment the individual's own breathing, mechanical ventilation and tracheostomy are used. Training nurses in rehabilitation facilities about ventilators can expedite the discharge of ventilator-dependent individuals from the hospital acute care unit to rehabilitation facilities.

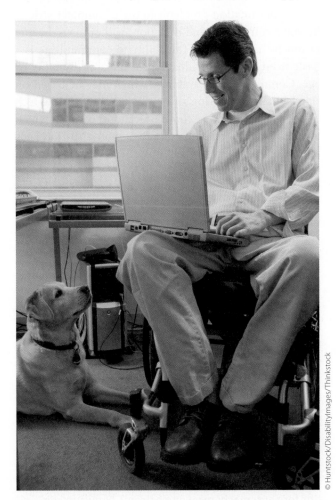

© Huntstock/DisabilityImages/Thinkstock

Faculty member with disability uses service dog to function more independently.

> There are two kinds of 'disabled' persons. Those who dwell on what they have lost and those who concentrate on what they have left.
>
> —*Thomas S. Szasz*

According to King (2012), patients requiring prolonged mechanical ventilation are rapidly increasing in number. Improved intensive care unit (ICU) care has resulted in many patients surviving acute respiratory failure to require prolonged mechanical ventilation during convalescence. Also, mechanical ventilation is increasingly used as a therapeutic option for patients with symptomatic chronic hypoventilation, with an increased effort to predict nocturnal hypoventilation to initiate ventilation earlier. There are continued efforts by ventilator manufacturers to improve home ventilators. These factors point to a likely increase in the number of patients receiving home mechanical ventilation in the United States. Unfortunately, there are no comprehensive databases or national registry of home ventilator patients—therefore the number of home ventilator patients is unknown.

King also states, "There are real challenges to providing mechanical ventilation in the home, which include caregiver training, adequacy of respiratory care, and reimbursement." Technology, expertise, and funding were now available to support ventilator-dependent patients outside of the hospital. The door was now open for many chronic ventilator patients, both children and adults, to live at home.

Why Is Home the Preferred Location for Long-Term Mechanical Ventilation?

Ideally, the preferred location for long-term mechanical ventilation is in the home, because costs are reduced (hospital costs $21,570, homecare costs $7,050, dollar savings per patient, per month $14,520 (Bach, Intola, Alba, & Holland, 2000). Quality of life is enhanced, and integration into the community is maximized (Marchese, Coco, & Coco, 2008). For the pediatric ventilator patient, the advantages of home ventilation also include being reunited with parents and family, which greatly enhances normal development and relationships. Home mechanical ventilation also reduces exposure to hospital-borne infections and frees hospital ICU beds for other acutely ill patients (Downes, Boroughs, Doughterty, & Parra, 2007).

Recent research suggests long-held beliefs about preterm children having dyscalculia from invasive ventilation may be incorrect. Dyscalculia is a lack of ability to perform math operations including addition, subtraction, multiplication and division. Jäkel found children in the study had no specific math deficits if their general IQ was factored in. However, they do have math difficulties that may go unrecognized if parents are not aware of their children's problems. Also, Jäkel found that schools lacked ways to deliver specific support to affected children (Jäkel, 2014). This is important for community health nurses to be aware of since these children may experience frustration and discouragement in math classes and lack the ability to express their problems.

Medical technology or equipment may be necessary to promote excretion of wastes. Indwelling urinary catheters may be used to empty the bladder and keep the individual dry. Two main problems with long-term indwelling catheters are frequent urinary tract infections, which can cause permanent kidney damage, and the bulkiness and unsightliness of the urine collection bag. Many persons with spina bifida (accompanied by paralysis below the level of the defect) or spinal cord injuries prefer to perform clean intermittent self-catheterization throughout the day, eliminating the need for the urine collection bag and indwelling catheter. An ostomy or opening in the abdominal wall may also be used, either to empty the bladder or to allow evacuation of the bowel contents through the abdominal wall. In the past, adults with kidney failure could receive hemodialysis at home, and now children with kidney failure can receive peritoneal dialysis at home and avoid hospitalization. Peritoneal dialysis, in which fluid is passed into the abdominal cavity via an abdominal catheter and allowed to drain back out, takes several hours to complete and may be needed up to 3 to 5 days per week (Batshaw, Pellegrino, & Roizen, 2007).

Another category of medical technology commonly used at home or in rehabilitation settings includes monitoring devices such as left ventricular assist devices, cardiorespiratory monitors, and pulse oximeters. Monitors are important for alerting caregivers to problems requiring prompt intervention, such as a kink in the oxygen tubing or an occluded airway, but the beeping and alarms of the monitors can unfortunately compete with the patient as the focus of the caregiver.

Nonmedical Assistive Technology

Nonmedical assistive technology is often a critical part of the continuum of services needed by a person with a disability. Areas in which assistive technology is helpful include employment tasks, ADLs, environmental control, communication, mobility, transportation, and recreation. Within each of these areas, technology can be either low tech (easy to make and inexpensive) or high tech (more difficult to make, often computerized or electronic, and expensive).

Technology for everyday living, or those adaptations and devices that will enable the individual to perform ADLs, are the first needs of consumers. Examples of technology to help with ADLs include "grabbers," adapted eating utensils, shower chairs, and Braille or large-print labels on appliances. Environmental control can be achieved through the use of switch extenders to place light switches within reach of a person in a wheelchair, adapters to convert lamps into "touch" lamps, or voice-controlled lights and heating/cooling. Voice recognition software is available that enables a person with vision, motor, or coordination problems to use a computer strictly by voice commands and dictation, without ever having to touch the keyboard. The ability to communicate is a basic need of all individuals, regardless of disability or age. Communication systems (which may be based on sign language, gesturing, or Braille) may require low-tech devices such as simple communication boards at which to point or gaze, or high-tech computers that "talk" for the person such as the Liberator. Telecommunication devices for the deaf (TDDs) allow individuals with severe hearing impairments to transmit and receive typed messages over the telephone. Text messaging and social media platforms such as Facebook and Twitter, accessed via computers, smart phones, tablets, and other mobile devices, have increased communication opportunities for persons with a wide range of disabilities. Mobility devices include the traditional walkers, canes, and crutches along with scooters and wheelchairs. Scooters and wheelchairs have become costly and highly technical pieces of equipment that are custom-made to fit the size, posture, and lifestyle of the person with a disability. In addition to manual wheelchairs, power wheelchairs with joystick control and tilt and recline options are available. For persons without upper-extremity control, sip and puff or breath-controlled power chairs are available. Specialized wheelchairs have also been developed for rough outdoor terrain and for specific sports such as wheelchair basketball, track, or rugby. Technological adaptations for vehicles include wheelchair lifts for vans, mechanical or electronic hand controls, and steering devices.

Ideally, evaluations for assistive technology devices should be conducted by appropriate individuals. Team members may include physical therapists, occupational therapists, and technology suppliers. Although many of the low-tech devices can be made or purchased for a moderate price, other pieces of technology such as computerized communication devices, specialized wheelchairs, and customized vans require significant financial resources.

Advances in technology are enhancing the possibilities for individuals with disabilities to communicate and move more effectively. With the advances in technology, service providers can plan solutions to everyday problems in social and personal spaces.

Adaptive/assistive devices have moved some individuals from dependence to independence but include sometimes costly equipment such as customized electric wheelchairs and electronic communication systems. Technology, both low and high tech, has made the difference for many people with disabilities between a life of dependency and limited options and an independent, productive life in which the person is included in all aspects of community life. According to Sprayberry (2014), a disabled person and an advocate for persons with muscular dystrophy, about 40 million people with disabilities currently live in the United States. Technology that would provide relief of the many problems and conditions imposed by various disorders is expensive and therefore unavailable to many disabled persons.

The Assistive Technology Act of 1998 was not reauthorized when it expired in 2010, and a substantial number of disabled individuals still lack assistive technology access. *Healthy People 2020* (HHS, 2014a) includes the following objective under the category of Disability and Health: "Reduce the proportion of people with disabilities who report barriers to obtaining the assistive devices, service animals, technology services, and accessible technologies that they need" (DH-10).

Assistance Animals

In addition to technological assistance, individuals with disabilities and chronic illnesses may benefit from animal assistance. Using pets to enhance health status dates back to the 18th and 19th centuries, when pets were used in Great Britain to give institutionalized people with mental retardation a sense of purpose and meaning. Caring for pets has been shown to help individuals improve mood, lower blood pressure, overcome physical limitations, and increase social skills (DeLaune & Ladner, 2006). A variety of animals can be used to provide companionship and give purpose to daily living (e.g., cats, dogs, rabbits, guinea pigs, birds, and miniature horses) or to assist individuals in daily activities (e.g., dogs, monkeys). Some animals are trained to detect changes in blood glucose, respiration, or other cues and to alert caregivers to assist children with disorders such as type 1 diabetes, epilepsy, and respiratory disorders in a potential crisis.

The most commonly used animal to assist patients with disabilities is the dog (Eames & Eames, 1997). Assistance dogs, although commonly thought to include only guide dogs for people who are blind, actually include several types of dogs serving a variety of purposes. Guide dogs are specially trained dogs who, when working, stay at their owner's side and provide behavioral cues about the environment. Examples would be warnings of steps, streets, or other obstacles in the path of movement. Hearing dogs, also specially trained, may be used by individuals with significant hearing impairments to cue the individual about meaningful sounds in the environment such as a doorbell, telephone, smoke detector, or an approaching person. Service dogs for persons with physical disabilities are especially useful to persons using wheelchairs. These dogs are trained to be helpful by picking up dropped objects (e.g., a pen, car keys, a wallet), carrying items in a dog backpack, and retrieving objects (e.g., a telephone) for the owner. For an individual who can walk short distances between a chair and a nearby bathroom, for instance, a large dog can help the person balance and provide stability for the short walk. A lesser-known type of assistance dog is the seizure detection dog. Certain dogs seem to have an innate ability to sense an impending seizure. Dogs with this ability can be trained to warn the owner that a seizure is about to begin, enabling the owner to position himself or herself in a safe position away from sharp and hard objects and to summon help. Once the seizure begins, if no one else is present, the dog is trained to bark to get help. Diabetes service dogs, similar to seizure detection dogs, detect hypoglycemia and sound an alert in much the same manner. All of the aforementioned types of assistance dogs require specialized training for both the dog and the prospective owner, funds to purchase the dog (often available through a civic organization), and owner commitment.

The ADA protects the rights of a person with a disability who uses an assistance dog to have full access to any public facility, including hospitals and outpatient rehabilitation facilities. The community health nurse may be involved in developing or revising a healthcare agency's policies regarding service animals to ensure that the facility is in compliance with ADA guidelines (Eames & Eames, 1997). Questions about access to places of public accommodation can be directed to the U.S. Department of Justice's ADA hotline (800-514-0301).

NOTE THIS!

Theresa Uchytil, as former Miss Iowa, was born without a left hand and adopted as her slogan for the 2000 Miss America contest: "Americans with disabilities, think ability."

Ethical Issues Related to Disabilities

A number of ethical issues exist in the disability field. Newborn screening for diseases such as phenylketonuria (PKU) is one area of question. Presently, in many states, newborn screening is conducted without parental consent. This screening detects several diseases, including PKU, which respond profoundly to early treatment. It is more economical for states to detect and treat a disease such as PKU early rather than provide lifelong support for an untreated child who will develop severe mental retardation. Does this law violate parents' rights to give informed consent? Would it be ethical to expand mandatory screening of newborns for other genetic diseases such as cystic fibrosis when the disease course will not be significantly improved by newborn diagnosis?

ETHICAL CONNECTION 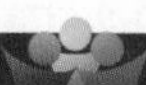

Recent disasters in the United States, including the September 11, 2001 terrorist attacks and Hurricane Katrina, exposed the lack of awareness of the need for plans to accommodate those persons with disabilities in all evacuation and disaster plans. For most of the people with disabilities who were affected by these two disasters, there were virtually no plans to manage the special needs of this vulnerable population. What can be done at the local, state, and national levels to provide safe, appropriate prevention and intervention in the workplace, homes, and communities for people with disabilities? What role does the community health nurse play in promoting disaster preparation for this vulnerable population?

Historically, another ethical debate centered on the relatively common occurrence of withholding lifesaving surgical treatment of newborns with obvious disabilities such as Down syndrome, hydrocephalus, or spina bifida. Although withholding treatment from infants with disabilities had been common, the 1982 birth of "Baby Doe" in Indiana brought this practice under public scrutiny. An infant was born with Down syndrome and tracheoesophageal fistula, a connection between the trachea and esophagus. Without corrective surgery, oral feedings would be routed into the baby's lungs via the fistula. Following the advice of their obstetrician, the parents refused to consent to the corrective surgery and the infant was not given food or water. A consulting pediatrician tried to stop the starvation of the infant, but the courts upheld the parents' decision and the infant died a number of days later. In response to the public outrage resulting from the death of this infant, the federal government enacted the "Baby Doe" ruling and notified all hospitals that such activity would be penalized. Since 1982, it has been unlawful to withhold treatment from a baby born with a disability; however, violation of this "Baby Doe" ruling carries minor penalties such as loss of federal dollars, rather than criminal or civil action.

Sexual and reproductive rights of individuals with disabilities have been another area of ethical debate. Not only have people with disabilities reported feeling violated by the personnel caring for them, but in individuals with mental retardation the person may not learn appropriate physical boundaries. In the past, programs for individuals with mental retardation separated males and females and punished sexual behavior such as masturbation. These methods are being questioned because they forbid individuals to express their autonomy through activities that are pleasurable and potentially harmless to others. Individuals with mental retardation or other mental disabilities should receive instruction in using judgment in choosing when and with whom to engage in sexual activity, in the use of birth control, and in the prevention of sexually transmitted diseases. Sterilization is considered in some cases in which the individual is unable to learn to use birth control, would be unable to competently raise a child, or would experience a serious health risk if pregnant. Sterilization should not be done, however, strictly for the convenience of family members, caretakers, schools, or institutions. If it is determined that sterilization is necessary, informed consent should be obtained from the individual to the fullest extent possible.

Informed consent means that the individual understands the risks and benefits of the procedure, is presented with alternatives, and is given the opportunity to express a choice. Acquiring informed consent from an individual with mental retardation can be time-consuming, requiring simplification of information and multiple meetings. Informed consent is a sensitive issue in the United States because of the eugenics policies of the 1920s and 1930s. These policies were in some cases a model for the eugenics programs in Nazi Germany and required compulsory, involuntary sterilization of individuals who were "feebleminded" or "mental defectives" in an effort to improve public health and the gene pool. A 1927 U.S. Supreme

Court ruling defending sterilization resulted in more than 60,000 persons with mental retardation being sterilized without their consent. Before sterilization is performed, the motives of those in favor of the procedure along with documented efforts to use a less restrictive alternative must be examined (Batshaw et al., 2007).

The Role of Community Health in Chronic Illness and Disability Care in the Future

According to Brown and Brown (2003), disability is a challenge of considerable magnitude throughout the world. These authors are concerned with the practice of disability therapy and research. They believe that in the future, we may face increasing numbers of challenges. Genetic, medical, and social advances are resulting in the detection of new disabilities. New health and social conditions such as HIV are emerging that present with new disabilities. People are increasingly living longer and with a scale of incapacity unknown in previous generations. Today, between 40 million and 50 million people in the United States report some kind of disability. That number will likely grow significantly over the next few decades as the baby boom generation enters late life, when the risk of disability is the highest. If one considers people who now have disabilities (at least one in seven Americans), people who are likely to develop disabilities in the future, and people who are or who will be affected by the disabilities of family members and others close to them, then disability affects today or will affect tomorrow the lives of most Americans. Clearly, disability is not a minority issue.

Surveillance in chronic disease may monitor the current epidemics of diabetes and obesity, the array of cardiovascular diseases, and smoking cessation. Cancer surveillance may be aimed at tracking prevention efforts, stage at diagnosis, and treatment effectiveness community-wide, not merely detailing occurrences. Surveillance is currently being used to monitor chronic disease development in communities with the highest acuity of smoking, diabetes, hypertension, hypercholesterolemia, depression, and obesity (Friedan, 2004).

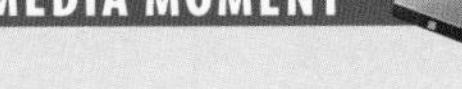

My Left Foot (1989)

Physical disability: The story of Christy Brown, who was born with cerebral palsy. He learned to paint and write with his only controllable limb, his left foot.

Brother's Keeper (1992)

Mental retardation: This documentary by Joe Berlinger and Bruce Sinofsky details the murder trial of Delbert Ward.

Scent of a Woman (1992)

Physical disability: A blind retired army officer hires a young man to be his guide as he seeks out a few final pleasures in life before his planned suicide.

Girl, Interrupted (1999)

Mental illness: Based on writer Susanna Kaysen's account of her 18-month stay at a mental hospital in the 1960s.

Prozac Nation (2001)

Mental illness and treatment issues: Based on a novel by Elizabeth Wurtzel, a young woman struggles with depression during her first year at Harvard.

A Beautiful Mind (2002)

Mental illness: After a brilliant but asocial mathematician accepts secret work in cryptography, his life takes a turn to the nightmarish as he develops paranoid schizophrenia.

I Am Sam (2002)

Mental retardation: A mentally retarded man fights for custody of his 7-year-old daughter, and in the process teaches his cold-hearted lawyer the value of love and family.

Murderball (2005)

Physical disability: A documentary film about quadriplegic athletes who play wheelchair rugby and the rivalries that precede the Paralympics.

The King's Speech (2010)

Developmental disability: This film is based on the true story of Britain's Prince Albert, who suffered from a severe speech impediment that was not addressed until he was on the verge of unexpectedly ascending to the throne as King George VI. The film chronicles his relationship with speech therapist Lionel Logue.

The Sessions (2012)

Physical disability: Based on a true story, the film recounts the relationship between a man paralyzed by polio and living in an iron lung and the sex surrogate he hires so that he can lose his virginity before he dies.

NOTE THIS!

Runner Marla Runyan became the first blind athlete in history to qualify for the 2000 U.S. Olympic team.

In communities in which this type of monitoring is ongoing, definitive, community-specific data are being generated to guide local action. Disease registries and those used to track local treatment progress and outcomes have great potential to improve chronic disease management.

Environmental interventions might be used to encourage and promote more active lifestyles and to eliminate architectural barriers. Preventive services may be placed at points of contact to encourage their use.

Clinical care efforts may lead to provision of smoking-cessation clinics and cancer screening areas as well as supplement local efforts in hypertension control, diabetes management, and cholesterol monitoring. These initiatives will extend local efforts aimed at achieving optimal control, not eliminating primary care sites. Use of public health efforts will require increased funding but will result in improved chronic disease prevention and control (Friedan, 2004).

Conclusion

Traditionally, community health nurses have cared for many chronically ill patients and patients with disabilities. By assessing the severity of the illness as well as the person's barriers, resources, self-efficacy, acceptance, current health-promoting behaviors, and current quality of life, the community health nurse will formulate a plan of care that will enable achievement of both long- and short-term wellness goals (Secrest, 2005). The current climate in healthcare services and distribution of healthcare resources make continued provision of care to chronically ill members of the community a challenge. As advocates and leaders in health care, community health nurses must ensure that appropriate and effective provision of services to chronically ill individuals expands by engaging in education, participating in political activity, and becoming involved in healthcare policy and research. Persons with disabilities are living longer and more productive lives than ever. Community health nurses are in settings where the opportunity to promote the health of persons, families, and populations with disabilities and chronic health issues are ample. Using knowledge gained from this chapter, community health nurses can assist these populations with preventing health problems and enhancing their ability to make informed health decisions.

HEALTHY ME 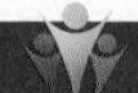

How can you prevent any acute health problems you might be experiencing in nursing school from becoming a chronic or disabling condition?

Critical Thinking Activities

1. Discuss power and powerlessness. What aspects of each are essential to consider in planning care for the chronically ill? Consider how the same chronic disease may affect perceptions of power and powerlessness differently in children and adults.
2. Think of an image that would help you forget about the unpleasant sensation of nausea. Describe an image that might help you to focus on positive thoughts about disease outcomes like gaining strength or taking control.
3. Analyze health teaching strategies that enhance retention of new material. Think of two specific techniques you can use to involve chronically ill children in prevention activities. Contrast these activities with those of an elderly adult. Develop a teaching plan that incorporates use of visual aids for each population.
4. How does having a disability or a chronic illness affect a person's self-concept?
5. Can a person with a disability ever be autonomous? Why or why not?
6. When community health nurses assist patients with disabilities in areas of health promotion, what are the most difficult challenges in regard to self-care and independence?
7. How can community health nurses promote positive self-regard for persons with disabilities and chronic conditions in the media? Give some examples of projects that could enhance the perception of "abilities" rather than disabilities for this vulnerable population group.

References

Agius, R. (2003). *Airborne environmental pollutants and asthma.* Retrieved from http://www.agius.com/hew/resource/asthma.htm

Antai-Otong, D. (1995). *Psychiatric nursing: Biological and behavioral concepts.* Philadelphia, PA: Saunders.

Batshaw, M. L., Pellegrino, M. D. and Roizen, M. D. (2007). *Children with disabilities* (6th ed). Baltimore, MD: Brookes Publishing Company.

Beirne-Smith, M., Patton, J. R., & Kim, S. H. (2006). *Mental retardation: An introduction to intellectual disabilities* (7th ed). Upper Saddle River, NJ: Pearson Merrill Prentice Hall.

Bjelland, M. J., Bruyère, S. M., von Schrader, S., Houtenville, A. J., Ruiz-Quintanilla, A., & Webber, D. A. (2010). Age and disability employment discrimination: Occupational rehabilitation implications. *Journal of Occupational Rehabilitation, 20*(4), 456–471.

Bromberger, J. T., Harlow, S. A., Kravitz, H. M., & Cordal, A. (2004). Racial/ethnic differences in the prevalence of depressive symptoms among middle-aged women: The study of women's health across the nation (SWAN). *American Journal of Public Health, 94*(8), 1378–1385.

Brown, I., & Brown, R. I. (2003). *Quality of life in disability: An approach for community practitioners.* London, England: Jessica Kingsley.

Bullington, J., Nordemar, R., Nordemar, K., & Sjöström-Flanagan, C. (2003). Meaning out of chaos: A way to understand chronic pain. *Scandinavian Journal of Caring Sciences, 17*(4), 325–331.

Carter, M.J., & Van Andel, G. (2002). *Therapeutic recreation: A practical approach* (4th ed.). Long Grove, IL: Waveland Press.

Centers for Disease Control and Prevention (CDC). (2008a). *Chronic disease overview.* Retrieved from http://www.cdc.gov/nccdphp/overview.htm

Centers for Disease Control and Prevention (CDC). (2008b). *Death rates by age and age-adjusted death rates for the 15 leading causes of death in 2005: United States, 1999–2005.* Retrieved from http://www.disastercenter.com/cdc/Leading%20Cause%20of%20Death%201999-2005.html

Centers for Disease Control and Prevention (CDC). (2009). The power of prevention. Chronic disease ... the public health challenge of the 21st century. Retrieved from http://www.cdc.gov/chronicdisease/pdf/2009-power-of-prevention.pdf

Centers for Disease Control and Prevention (CDC). (2011). Rationale for regular reporting on health disparities and inequalities-United States. *Morbidity and Mortality Weekly Report, 60*(1), 3–10.

Centers for Disease Control and Prevention (CDC). (2012). Prevalence of autism spectrum disorders—Autism and developmental disabilities monitoring network, 14 sites, United States, 2008. *Morbidity and Mortality Weekly Report, 61*(SS03), 1–19.

Centers for Disease Control and Prevention (CDC). (2014). *Chronic disease prevention and health promotion: Statistics and tracking.* Retrieved from http://www.cdc.gov/chronicdisease/stats/index.htm

Cochrane, J. (2003). The experience of uncertainty for individuals with HIV/AIDS and the palliative care paradigm. *International Journal of Palliative Nursing, 9*(9), 382–388.

Colvin, G. (2004). Get ready for a life and death battle over obesity. *Fortune, 150*(1), 64.

Coon, S. K., & Coleman, E. A. (2004). Keep moving: Patients with myeloma talk about exercise and fatigue. *Oncology Nursing Forum, 31*(6), 1127–1135.

Davidhizar, R., & Shearer, R. (1997). Helping the patient with disability achieve high-level wellness. *Rehabilitation Nursing, 22*(3), 131–134.

DeLaune, S. C., & Ladner, P. K. (2006). *Fundamentals of nursing: Standards of practice* (3rd ed.). Florence, KY: Cengage.

Dewsbury, G., Clarke, K., Randall, D., Rouncefield, M., & Somerville, I. (2004). The anti-social model of disability. *Disability and Society, 19*(2).

DiLeo, D. (2007). Raymond's room: Ending the segregation of citizens with disabilities. Training resource network, St. Augustine, FL.

Disability World. (2012). Retrieved from http://www.disability-world.org/

Dolyniuk, C., Kamens, M. W., Corman, H., DiNardo, P. O., Totaro, R. M., & Rockoff, J. C. (2002). Students with developmental disabilities go to college. *Focus on Autism and Other Developmental Disabilities, 17*(4), 236–242.

Dosh, S. A. (2004). Diagnosis of heart failure in adults. *American Family Physician, 70*(11), 2145–2152. Retrieved from http://www.aafp.org/afp/20041201/2145.html

Dowd, R., & Cavalieri, J. (1999). Help your patient live with osteoporosis: Identifying risk, managing pain, overseeing treatment. *American Journal of Nursing, 99*(4), 55–60.

Downes, J. J., Boroughs, D. S., Dougherty, J., & Parra, M. (2007). A statewide program for home care of children with chronic respiratory failure. *Caring, 26*(9), 16–18.

Dumit, J. (1998). Symptomatic, ill, and structurally damned: Notes on liminal creativity and social movements. Unpublished work.

Eames, E., & Eames, T. (1997). Interpreting legal mandates: Assistance dogs in medical facilities. *Nursing Management, 28*(6), 49–51.

Fahey, D. F. (2008.). *Cost and consequences of chronic disease management.* Presentation given April 30, 2008, at the University of Galway, Ireland. Retrieved from http://www.nuigalway.ie/cchsrd/documents/daniel_fahey__23.04.08.ppt

Fennick, E., & James, R. (2003). Community inclusion for children and youth with developmental disabilities. *Focus on Autism and Other Developmental Disabilities, 18*(1), 20–28.

Friedan, T. R. (2004). Asleep at the switch: Local public health and chronic disease. [Editorial]. *American Journal of Public Health, 94*(12), 2059–2061.

Gerber, L. (2012). Community health nursing: A partnership of care. *American Journal of Nursing, 112*(1), 19–20.

Goodwin, D. L., & Compton, S. G. (2004). Physical activity experiences of women aging with disabilities. *Adapted Physical Activity Quarterly, 21*(2), 122–138.

Green, F. P., & Schleien, S. J. (1991). Understanding friendship and recreation: A theoretical sampling. *Therapeutic Recreation Journal, 25*(4), 29–40.

Grey, M., Knaft, K., & McCorkle, R. (2006). A framework for the study of self and family management of chronic conditions. *Nursing Outlook, 54*, 278–286.

Herbert, R., & Gregor, S. (1997). Quality of life and coping strategies of patients with COPD. *Rehabilitation Nursing, 22*(4), 182–187.

Hickey, J. V. (2003). *The clinical practice of neurological and neurosurgical nursing.* Philadelphia, PA: Lippincott Williams & Wilkins.

Hilton, E. L., & Henderson, L. J. (2003). The nature, meanings, and dynamics of lived experiences of syringomyelia in a middle-aged man: A phenomenological case study. *SCI Nursing, 20*(1), 10–17.

Hinds, P. S. (2004). The hopes and wishes of adolescents with cancer and the nursing care that helps. *Oncology Nursing Forum, 31*(5), 927–944.

Hirao-Try, Y. (2003). Hypertension and women: Gender specific differences. *Clinical Excellence for Nurse Practitioners, 7*(1–2), 4–8.

Holburn, S. (2002). How science can evaluate and enhance person-centered planning. *Research & Practice for Persons with Severe Disabilities, 27*(4), 250–260.

Horrocks, S., Anderson, E., & Salisbury, C. (2002, April 6). Systematic review of whether nurse practitioners working in primary care can provide equivalent care to doctors. *British Medical Journal*, 324, 819.

Hurst, R. (2000). To revise or not to revise. *Disability and Society, 12*(3), 325–340.

Iezonni, L., & O'Day, B. (2006). *More than ramps: A guide to improving health care quality and access for people with disabilities.*

Improving Chronic Illness Care (ICIC). (2008). *The chronic care model elements: Delivery system design.* Retrieved from http://www.improvingchroniccare.org/index.php?p=The_Chronic_Care_Model&s=2

Imrie, R. (2004). Demystifying disability: A review of the International Classification of Functioning, Disability, and Health. *Sociology of Health and Illness, 26*(3), 287–305.

Jäkel, J. (2014). Preterm children do not have an increased risk for dyscalculia. *ScienceDaily: Ruhr Universitaet-Bochum.* Retrieved from http://www.sciencedaily.com/releases/2014/08/140801091120.htm

Jaffe, H. (2004). Whatever happened to the U.S. AIDS epidemic? *Science, 305*, 5688.

Johnson, J. (1991). Adjustment following a heart attack. In J. M. Morse & J. I. Johnson (Eds.), *The illness experience* (pp. 13–88). Newbury Park, CA: Sage.

Jung, S. K. (2004). A young onset Parkinson's patient: A case study. *Journal of Neuroscience Nursing, 36*(5), 273–277.

Kaplan, D. (2008). *The definition of disability.* The Center for an Accessible Society. Retrieved from http://www.accessiblesociety.org/topics/demographics-identity/dkaplanpaper.htm

King, A. C. (2012). Long-term home mechanical ventilation in the United States. *Respiratory Care, 57*(6), 921–932.

Kirk, S. A., Gallagher, J. J., Anastasiow, N. J., & Coleman, M. R. (2006). *Educating exceptional children* (11th ed.). Boston, MA: Houghton Mifflin.

Klang, B., & Clyne, N. (1997). Well-being and functional ability in uremic patients before and after having started dialysis treatment. *Scandinavian Journal of Caring Science, 11*(3), 159–166.

Klein, S. J., Cruz, H., O'Connell, D., Scully, M. A., & Birkhead, G. (2005). A public health approach to "prevention with positives": The New York State HIV/AIDS Service Delivery System. *Journal of Health Management Practice, 11*(1), 7–17.

Koch, T. (2001). Disability and difference: Balancing social and physical constructions. *Journal of Medical Ethics, 27*(6), 370–376.

Landrigan, P. J., Lioy, G., Thurston, G., Berkowitz, G., Chen, L. C., Chillrud, S. N., . . . Small, C. (2004). Health and environmental consequences of the World Trade Center disaster. *Environmental Health Perspectives, 112*(6), 731–739.

LaPlante, M. P., Harrington, C., & Kang, T. (2002). Estimating paid and unpaid hours of personal assistance services in activities of daily living provided to adults living at home. *Health Services Research, 37*(2), 397–415.

Lewis-Washington, C., & Holcomb, L. (2010). Empowering community health: An educational approach. *Journal of Community Health Nursing, 27*(4), 197–206.

Lindgren, C. L. (1996). Chronic sorrow in persons with Parkinson's disease and their spouses. *Scholarly Inquiry for Nursing Practice, 10*(4), 351–366.

Lopes, D., Piementa, C., Kurita, A., & Oliveira, A. C. (2003). Caregivers of patients with chronic pain: Responses to care. *International Journal of Nursing Terminologies and Classifications, 15*(1), 5–14.

Lubkin, I. M., & Larsen, P. D. (2013). *Chronic illness impact and interventions* (8th ed.) Burlington, MA: Jones & Bartlett Learning.

Luckmann, J. (1997). *Saunders manual of nursing care.* Philadelphia, PA: Saunders.

Marchese, S., Coco, D. L., & Coco, A. L. (2008). Outcome and attitudes toward home tracheostomy ventilation of consecutive patients: A 10-year experience. *Respiratory Medicine, 102*(3), 430–436.

Mayo, L. (1956). *Chronic illness.* Paper presented at the meeting of the Commission on Chronic Illness, Washington, DC.

Mayo, M. (2002). Camps for children with illnesses on the rise: Normalcy and fun help with coping and healing of disease and disabilities. *Camping Magazine, 75*(6), 20–24.

Meadows, P. (2009). Rationale for regular reporting on health disparities and inequalities—United States: Great challenges and great opportunities. *Morbidity and Mortality Weekly Report, 60*(1), 3–10.

Miller, J. F. (1992). *Coping with chronic illness: Overcoming powerlessness* (2nd ed.) Philadelphia, PA: F. A. Davis.

Mitchell, C., & Linsk, N. L. (2004). A multidimensional conceptual framework for understanding HIV/AIDS as a chronic long-term illness. *Social Work, 49*(3), 469–477.

Molyneux, D. H. (2004, July 24). Neglected diseases but unrecognized successes—challenges and opportunities for infectious disease control. *Lancet, 364.*

Morgan, M. (1996). The meaning of high blood pressure among Afro-Caribbean and white patients. In D. Kelleher & S. Hillier (Eds.), *Researching cultural differences in health.* London, England: Routledge.

Mosby. (2007). *Mosby's dictionary of medicine, nursing, and health professionals* (8th ed.). St. Louis, MO: Elsevier Health Sciences.

National Council on Disability. (2011). *Bullying and students with disabilities*. Retrieved from http://www.ncd.gov/publications/2011/March92011

National Council on Disability. (2013). *Medicaid, managed care, and people with disabilities*. Washington, DC: Author.

National Family Caregivers Association. (2008). About NFCA. Retrieved from http://www.thefamilycaregiver.org/about_nfca/

National Organization on Disability. (2004). 2004 N.O.D./Harris Survey documents trends impacting 54 million Americans.

Noakes, M., Foster, P., Keogh, J. B., & Clifton, P. M. (2004). Meal replacements as effective as weight-loss diets for treating obesity in adults with features of metabolic syndrome 1, 2. *Journal of Nutrition*, *134*(8), 1894–1899.

Pampel, F. (2003). Declining sex differences in mortality from lung cancer in high-income nations. *Demography*, *40*(1), 45–65.

Patton, J. R., Blackbourne, J. M., & Fad, K. (2004). *Exceptional individuals in focus* (7th ed.). Englewood-Cliffs, NJ: Prentice Hall.

Phillips, L. J. (2005). Analysis of the explanatory model of health promotion and quality of life in chronic disabling conditions. *Rehabilitation Nursing*, *30*(1), 18–24.

Pierce, L. (2012). Barriers to Access: Frustrations of People Who Use a Wheelchair for Full-Time Mobility. *Rehabilitation Nursing*, *23*(3), 120–125.

Pugh-Clarke, K. (2004). Quality of life and symptomatology in chronic renal insufficiency. *Nephrology Nursing Journal*, *31*(2).

Racino, J. A., & Taylor, S. J. (1993). People first: Approaches to housing and support. In J. A. Racino, P. Walker, S. O'Connor, & S. J. Taylor (Eds.), *Housing, support and community: Choices and strategies for adults with disabilities* (vol. 2, pp. 33–56). Baltimore, MD: Paul H. Brookes.

Revell, G., Kregel, J., Wehman, P., & Bond, G. (2000). Cost effectiveness of supported employment programs: What we need to do to improve outcomes. *Journal of Vocational Rehabilitation*, *14*, 173–178.

Robert Wood Johnson Foundation. *Chronic care: Making the case for ongoing care.* (2010). Princeton, NJ: Robert Wood Johnson Foundation, 16. Retrieved from http://www.rwjf.org/content/dam/farm/reports/reports/2010/rwjf54583

Scambler, G. (2004). Re-framing stigma: Felt and enacted stigma and challenges to the sociology of chronic and disabling conditions. *Social Theory and Health*, *2*, 29–46.

Schleien, S. J., Ray, M. T, and Green, F. P. (1997). *Community recreation and people with disabilities: Strategies for inclusion* (2nd ed). Baltimore, MD: Paul H. Brookes.

Schaefer, K. M. (1995). Women living in paradox: Loss and discovery in chronic illness. *Holistic Nursing Practice*, *9*(3), 63–74.

Secrest, J. (2005). Commentary. *Rehabilitation Nursing*, *30*(1), 24.

Sheehan, N. W., & Oakes, C. E. (2003). Bringing assisted living services into congregate housing: Residents' perspectives. *Gerontologist*, *43*(5), 766–770.

Small, G. W., Birkett, M., Meyers, B. S., Loran, L. M., Bystricky, A., & Nemeroff, C. B. (1996). Impact of physical illness on quality of life and antidepressant response in geriatric major depression. *Journal of the American Geriatric Society*, *44*(10), 1220–1225.

Smith, S. (1974). The psychology of illness. In V. A. Christopherson, P. P. Coulter, & M. O. Wolanin (Eds.), *Rehabilitation nursing*. New York, NY: McGraw-Hill.

Snively, C. S., & Gutierrez, C. (2004). Chronic kidney disease: Prevention and treatment of common complications. *American Family Physician*, *70*(10), 1921–1928.

Social Security announces new compassionate allowances conditions. Retrieved from http://www.ssa.gov/pressoffice/pr/compassionate-allowances200conditions-pr.html

Sorenson, S. B., & Wiebe, D. J. (2004). Weapons in the lives of battered women. *American Journal of Public Health*, *94*(8), 1412–1417.

Spillman, B. C. (2004). Changes in elderly disability rates and the implications for health care utilization and cost. *Milbank Quarterly*, *82*(1), 157–194.

Sprayberry, T. L. (2014). Applying current technology to positively change disability for tomorrow. Retrieved from http://www.huffingtonpost.com/trisha-lynn-sprayberry/applying-current-technolo_b_5438756.html

Stokes, W. A., Hendrix, L. H., Royce, T. J., Allen, I. M., Godley, P. A., Wang, A. Z., & Chen, R. C. (2013). Racial differences in time from prostate cancer diagnosis to treatment initiation: A population-based study. *Cancer,* 1.

Strauss, A. L. (1975). *Chronic illness and the quality of life*. St. Louis, MO: Mosby.

Strunin, L., & Boden, L. I. (2004). Family consequences of chronic back pain. *Social Science and Medicine*, *58*, 1385–1393.

Taormina-Weiss, W. (2012). Psychological and social aspects of disability. *Disability World.* Retrieved from http://www.disabled-world.com/disability/social-aspects.php accessed 8/26/2012

Thompson, B., Wickham, D., Wegner, J., Mulligan-Ault, M., Shanks, P., & Reinertson, B. (2002). *Handbook for the inclusion of young children with severe disabilities.* Lawrence, KS: Learner Managed Designs.

Thompson, E. H., Futterman, A. M., Gallagher-Thompson, D., Rose, J. M., & Lovett, S. B. (1993). Social support and caregiving burden in family caregivers of frail elders. *Journal of Gerontology: Social Sciences*, *48*(5), S245–S254.

Toldrá, R. C., & Santos, M. C. (2013). People with disabilities in the labor market: Facilitators and barriers. *Work*, *45*(4), 553–563.

U.S. Cancer Statistics Working Group. (2007). *United States cancer statistics: 2004 incidence and mortality.* Atlanta, GA: Department of Health and Human Service, Centers for Disease Control and Prevention, and National Cancer Institute.

U.S. Census Bureau (2006). American community survey: Disability characteristics.

U.S. Department of Health and Human Services (HHS). (2011). *Women's Health USA 2011*. Rockville, MD: Author.

U.S. Department of Health and Human Services (HHS). (2014b). 2020 topics and objectives. Retrieved from http://www.healthypeople.gov/2020/topicsobjectives2020/default.aspx

U.S. Department of Justice, Civil Rights Division. (2014). *Information and technical assistance on the ADA: Introduction to the ADA.* Retrieved from http://www.ada.gov/ada_intro.htm

U.S. Department of Labor. (2012). Employment rates for people with disabilities. Bureau of Labor Statistics.

Ward, R. P., Kugelmas, M., & Libsch, K. D. (2004). Management of hepatitis C: Evaluating suitability for drug therapy. *American Family Physician, 69*(6), 1429–1436.

Wehman, P. (2003a). Business collaboration with public sector. Journal of Vocational Rehabilitation, 19, 3–4.

Wehman, P. (2003b). Workplace inclusion: Persons with disabilities and coworkers working together. Journal of Vocational Rehabilitation, 18, 131–141.

Wehman, P. (2006). *Life beyond the classroom: Transition strategies for young people with disabilities* (4th ed.). Baltimore, MD: Brookes.

Wehman, P. H., Revell, W. G., & Brooke, V. (2003). Competetive employment: Has it become the "first choice" yet? *Journal of Disability Policy Studies, 14*(3), 163–173.

Wehman, P. H., Targett, P. S., & Cifi, D. X. (2006). Job coaches: A Workplace support. *American Journal of Physical Medicine and Rehabilitation, 85*(8), 704.

Wehman, P., Brooke, V., Green, H., Hewett, M., & Tipton, M. (2008). Public/private partnerships and employment of people with disabilities: Preliminary evidence from a pilot project. *Journal of Vocational Rehabilitation, 28*, 53–66.

Whitney, C. M. (2004). Maintaining the square: How older adults with Parkinson's disease sustain quality in their lives. *Journal of Gerontological Nursing, 30*(1), 28.

Wickham, R. S., Goodin, S., & Lynch, K. (2004). Demystifying CINV control in the complex aging patient: Assessing the complexities of the aging oncology pt. *Spotlight on Symposia, ONS News, 19*(9).

Wilper, A., & Woolhandler, S. (2009). Health insurance and mortality in U.S. adults. *American Journal of Public Health, 9*(9), 1542–1542.

Wilson, J. S. (1992). Our nation's walking wounded: The chronically ill. *Home Healthcare Nurse, 5*(5), 42–43.

Wilson, K. M., & Satterfield, D. W. (2007, July). Where are we to be in these times? The place of chronic disease prevention in community health promotion. *Preventing Chronic Disease* [serial online], *4*(3). Retrieved from http://www.cdc.gov/pcd/issues/2007/jul/07_0014.htm

Wolf, Z. R. (1994). Seeking harmony. Chronic physical illness. In P. Munhall (Ed.), *In women's experience.* New York, NY: National League for Nursing.

World Health Organization (WHO). (2001). *International classification of functioning, disability, and health.* Geneva, Switzerland: Author.

World Health Organization (WHO). (2010). *Pandemic (H1N1) 2009—update 103.* Retrieved from http://www.who.int/csr/don/2010_06_04/en/

World Health Organization (WHO). (2013). *WHO update on polio outbreak in Middle East.* Retrieved from http://www.who.int/mediacentre/news/statements/2013/polio-syria-20131113/en/

World Health Organization (WHO). (2014a). *The WHO family of international classifications.* Retrieved from http://www.who.int/classifications/en/

World Health Organization (WHO). (2014b). *List of official ICF updates.* Retrieved from http://www.who.int/classifications/icfupdates/en/

Zack, M. M., Moriarity, D. G., Stroup, D. F., Ford, E. S., & Mokdad, A. H. (2004, August). *Adult Americans health-related quality of life has recently gotten worse.* Retrieved from http//www.cdc.gov/nccdphp/press/trends.htm

Appendix: Appropriate Language for Communicating About Persons with Disabilities

Dr. Valerie Rachal

The community health nurse should use language that is current and endorsed by the disability community when speaking or writing about people with disabilities. The words we choose and the way we structure sentences can create a clear, positive view of persons with disabilities or a negative, discriminatory portrayal that reinforces common stereotypes. One of the best known guidelines is that of **people-first language**, with which the speaker puts the person first, not the disability. For example, the community health nurse should refer to "the child with mental retardation" or "a man with Down syndrome." One exception to the people-first language guideline is when speaking about deaf people. Many deaf people do not consider themselves disabled and prefer to be called a "deaf person" rather than a "person who is deaf" or a "person with a hearing impairment." When in doubt, the community health nurse should ask persons with disabilities how they wish to be described.

The community health nurse must avoid using language that characterizes the person with a disability as pitiable. Do not say "afflicted with," "crippled with," or "suffers from." Rather, say, "the person *has* a spinal cord injury" or speak about "the person *with* spina bifida." Words such as *crippled* or *deformed* are never acceptable. The word *handicapped*, which was once used to refer to a person with a disability, has been redefined. *Handicap* now refers to a functional limitation that varies based on the conditions in the environment of the individual. For example, although a person with a spinal cord injury has a disability, whether or not that individual has a handicap in a certain situation would depend on conditions such as lack of a ramp to a building entrance. Finally, emphasize abilities, not limitations.

UNIT 6

Health Across the Lifespan

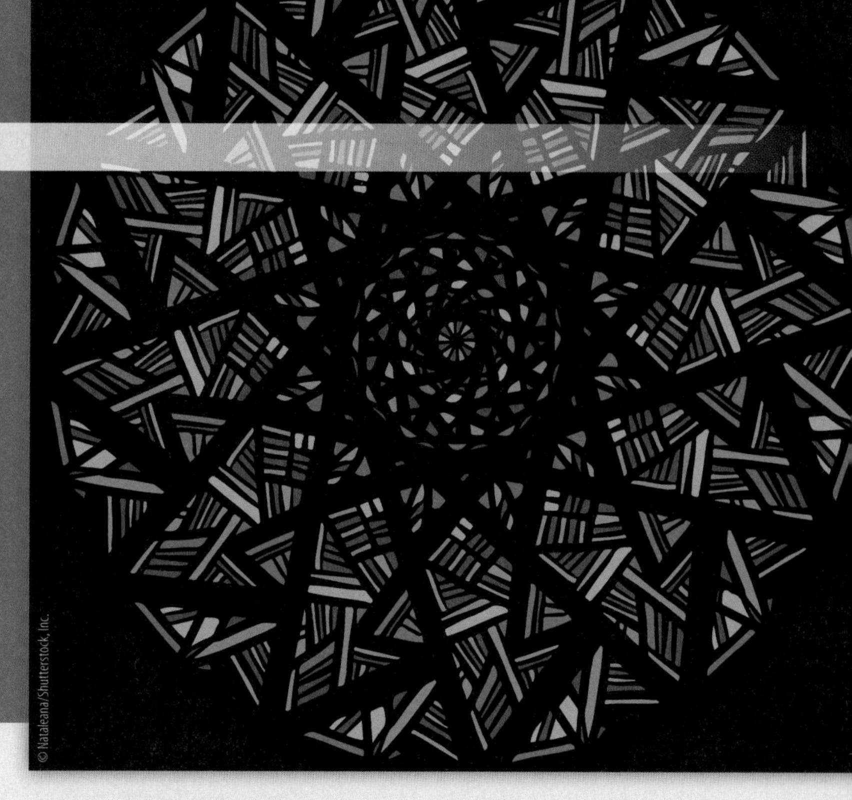

CHAPTER FOCUS

Definition of Family

Health Responsibilities of the Family

- Development of Members' Sense of Personal Identity and Self-Worth
- Emotional Support and Guidance During Lifecycle Transitions
- Socialization of Family Members to Value and Maintain Health
- Education About When and How to Use the Healthcare System
- Care Provision and Management for Chronically Ill, Disabled, and Aging Family Members

Theoretical Approaches to the Family

- Human Ecology Theory
- Family Systems Theory
- Family Development Theory

Family-Oriented Versus Family-Focused Nursing Role

A Conceptual Framework for Family Assessment

- Energy
- Consciousness
- Role Structure
- Decision-Making Processes
- Communication Patterns
- Values
- Family Boundaries

A Self-Efficacy Model of Nurse–Family Intervention

- Identification of Family Health Concerns and Needs
- Mutual Setting of Goals
- Delineation of Alternatives
- Implementation of the Plan
- Evaluation

QUESTIONS TO CONSIDER

After reading this chapter, you will know the answers to the following questions:

1. How is *family* defined?
2. What are the health responsibilities of the family?
3. What is the difference between family-oriented and family-focused nursing care?
4. What is an example of a conceptual framework for family assessment?
5. How is the self-efficacy model of family interventions used in promoting the health of families?

"If the family were a container, it would be a nest, an enduring nest, loosely woven, expansive and open.

If the family were a fruit, it would be an orange, a circle of sections, held together but separately—each segment distinct.

If the family were a boat, it would be a canoe that makes no progress unless everyone paddles.

If the family were a sport, it would be baseball: a long, slow, non-violent game that is never over until the last out.

If the family were a building, it would be an old, but solid structure that contains human history, and appeals to those who see the carved moldings under all the plaster, the wide plank floors under the linoleum, the possibilities . . ."

—Letty Cottin Pogrebin

CHAPTER 29

Foundations of Family Care

Ruth A. O'Brien and Karen Saucier Lundy

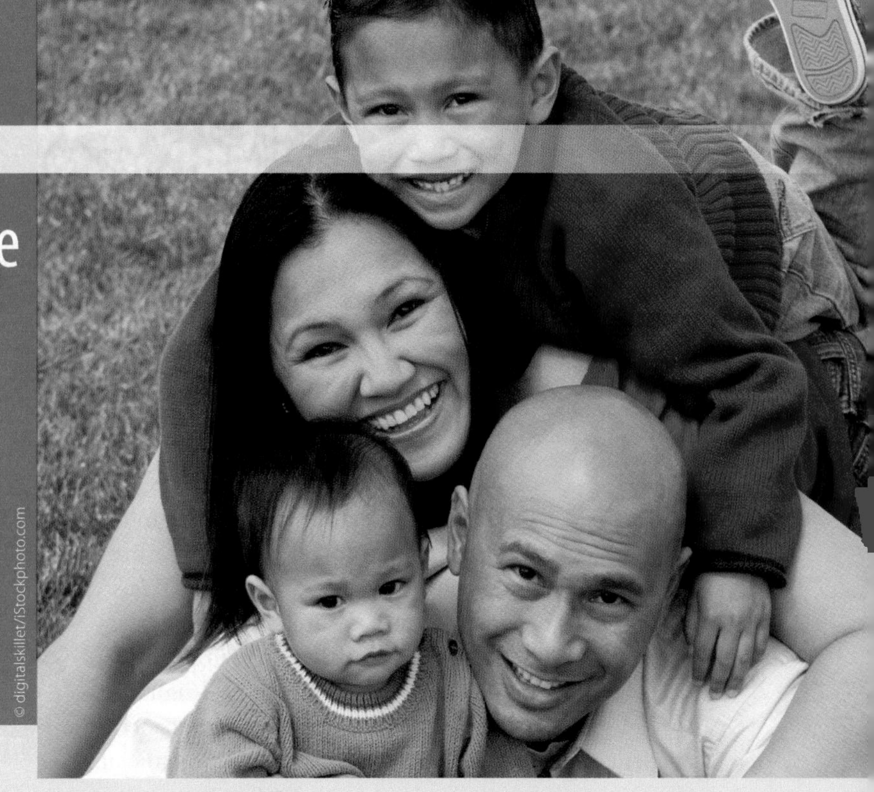

KEY TERMS

affect
beliefs
communication
contracting
environment
family
family developmental tasks
function
interdependence
meaning
negative feedback
nonsummativity
positive feedback
power
self-regulation
structure

> We all enter the world with fairly simple needs: to be protected, to be nurtured, to be loved unconditionally, and to belong.
>
> —*Louise Hart*

REFLECTIONS

As you reflect on this quotation and on the one accompanying the photo, think about your definition of family. Who do you consider your family? Does your definition include friends and non-blood-related members? How did your family of origin (the family of your childhood) affect your values about life, about health? As an adult, have your values about families changed or remained the same? As nurses, we often have "idealized" notions about family, which influence our care. Think about your own experiences as a child with your family as well as your present family as you read this chapter.

WHAT IS A FAMILY? Perhaps no other word in today's society would yield as many different responses from people who should know: After all, we have all been raised in some form of family. As the basic unit of society, the family has certainly undergone dramatic changes in the last few decades. Since World War II, through the civil rights and women's rights movements of the 1960s and the economic challenges of the latter part of the 20th century, to the national insecurity post–September 11, 2001, in this century, society has faced conflicting ideas about how and what to think about the institution we call "family." We all care about our own families, and most of us have definite ideas about how they have influenced our lives. In recent years, however, society has also moved to caring about the *idea* of family and the future of the family in the United States.

Family is not a precise or universally understood word: It has many different meanings and provokes strong reactions depending on the context in which it is used. To give us some idea of how family is used in different contexts, consider the following:

- When are you two going to settle down and raise a family? In this context, *family* means children.
- We refer to orphans as children "without a family."
- When abused children are removed from the custody of their father and mother, they are taken "from their family," so in this context, *family* means parents.
- The media often refer to the "single-parent family," but this usually means the parent is a "mother."
- When a question of care is involved (as in parenting courses, and class parents), "parent" means "mother."
- When a man is arrested for a horrible crime, neighbors often refer to their surprise because he had been a "real family man." Is a "family man" somehow distinct from other men? Is such a man less likely to commit a crime? Do you hear people refer to women as a "real family woman"?
- When a woman runs for office, she is often asked how she will manage as a "working mother." Yet, is that same question ever asked of a "working father"?

In this chapter, you will learn about how community health nurses can assist all families, whatever form they take, to live healthier lives. The family may be defined in many ways but, most importantly, *our family is who we think it is.*

NOTE THIS!

Denmark became the first country in the world to legalize same-sex marriage when it did so in 1989.

Definition of Family

Dramatic changes in family structure over the past few decades are highlighted in contrasting media images portrayed in popular television sitcoms, from *Ozzie and Harriet* and *Father Knows Best* in the 1950s to the 1960s and 1970s families portrayed in *The Brady Bunch* and *The Partridge Family*. The 1980s and 1990s brought *The Simpsons, The Cosby Show, The Golden Girls, Full House, Roseanne, Will & Grace, Married . . . With Children,* and *Everybody Loves Raymond* to showcase a great variety of family structures, ranging from traditional nuclear families to novel partnerships and some outright dysfunctional groupings. More recent offerings include *How I Met Your Mother, Parenthood,* and *Modern Family*. It is clear that at least since the 1980s, the popular image of the family as a nuclear two-parent unit raising their own children, with father as the breadwinner and mother as the homemaker, as portrayed in *Ozzie and Harriet* and *Father Knows Best,* and with minor alterations in *The Brady Bunch,* is no longer the dominant pattern in American society. Only one in five families in the 21st century comes close to this stereotype.

Single-parent, stepfamilies or blended families, dual-career families in which both parents work, married couples without children, cohabitating couples, and gay and lesbian families/marriages are more typical of the diverse family patterns today. Social, demographic, and economic

APPLICATION TO PRACTICE 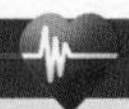

Joyce Williams, a school nurse at Sagebrush Elementary, reflected on her recent meeting with Mrs. Carson, the first-grade teacher for Kevin Johnson. Mrs. Carson had contacted her to discuss Kevin's increasing episodes of toileting accidents and inattention in class over the past 2 months. Mrs. Carson questioned whether Kevin's behavior was indicative of problems coping with his parents' divorce; she told Joyce that the 3rd-grade teacher who had Kevin's sister in class related that the children's father recently remarried and moved to another city about 50 miles away. According to Kevin's school file, Mrs. Johnson was a legal secretary for a large law firm downtown. Recognizing the strains that a single, working parent raising two children, 6 and 8 years old, might be experiencing, Joyce decided that she would call Mrs. Johnson to schedule a home visit to talk with her about the problems Kevin's teacher had reported. A home visit, rather than a conference at the school, would provide an opportunity for her to observe parent–child interaction and also to gain a better appreciation of how Mrs. Johnson is handling being a single parent and what other supports are available.

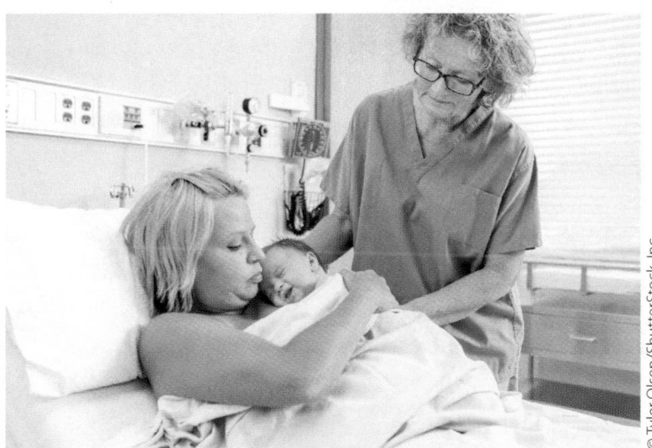

The single-mother family has increased in number during the past decade. These families are at special risks for poverty and a lack of health insurance.

factors have all contributed to the changing composition of the family. Close to 40% of all births in the United States are now to unmarried women (Kaiser Family Foundation, 2010). Contrary to common perceptions that teens are responsible for most of the out-of-wedlock births, rates of out-of-wedlock births are highest among single women in their 20s. Based on the trend toward a higher proportion of births to single women, coupled with the higher incidence of divorce, about half of all children today are expected to spend some part of their time in a single-parent home. Given that most people who divorce remarry, stepfamilies or blended families are fast becoming the norm in the 21st century. The number of dual-career families also has markedly increased, with almost three-fourths of married mothers with children reporting some paid employment. Furthermore, the continued growth of the older population will increase both the number of elderly couples and the number of frail elderly persons living alone who will require supportive services in an era when adult daughters hold jobs and are not as readily available as earlier generations to be family caregivers.

Heightened attention to demographic changes in the composition of the family since the 1960s has generated considerable debate among social scientists on whether the family is declining in importance in our society. In reflecting on the passion that often surrounds the debate, Cowan, Field, Hansen, Skolnick, and Swanson (1992) asserted, "Families mattered in the past; they continue to matter in the present; and they will matter still, in the uncertain years of our future" (p. 481). Valuing the family, however, should not be confused with valuing a particular family form. These authors urged that, rather than viewing demographic changes in the composition of the family unit as indicative of family decline, we need to reconsider traditional definitions of family that emphasize

RESEARCH ALERT 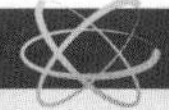

What makes a happy marriage? Lauer and Lauer (1992) interviewed 351 couples who had been married for 15 years or longer. Fifty-one of these couples were unhappy with their marriages but stayed together for the children, tradition, and other reasons. The other 300 "happy" couples all had the following in common:

- Think of their spouse as their best friend
- Like their spouse as a person
- Think of marriage as a long-term commitment
- Believe that marriage is sacred
- Agree with their spouse on goals
- Believe that their spouse has grown more interesting over the years
- Strongly want the relationship to succeed
- Laugh together

Source: Lauer, J., & Lauer, R. (1992). Marriages made to last. In J. M. Henslin (Ed.), *Marriage and family in a changing society* (4th ed., pp. 481–486). New York, NY: Free Press.

legal and biological ties between members and conceptualize how diverse types of families fulfill different functions to address the complexity of their health needs. As example of the changing concept of family in the United States, the Defense of Marriage Act (DOMA), enacted in 1996, prevented the federal government from recognizing same-sex marriages but was ruled unconstitutional by the U.S. Supreme Court on June 26, 2013, in United States v. Windsor. As of August 2014, 19 states and the District of Columbia have legalized same-sex marriage,

How should we define the family for community health nursing assessment and intervention? Although community health nursing's primary target of service is the community, work with the family as a population is one strategy that nurses may use to improve the health of communities. Thus, community health nurses need a broad conceptual perspective of the family that recognizes diverse compositions. **Family** in this chapter refers to two or more individuals who identify themselves as family and manifest some degree of interdependence in interactions with each other and their **environment** in meeting basic human needs for affection and meaning. Themes central to this definition are members' **interdependence** in meeting basic needs and members' **beliefs** that they are a family. This intentionally broad view of family encompasses the traditional two-parent nuclear family, single-parent families, stepfamilies or blended families, childless couples, and relationships that (in many states) are not built on legal or biological ties, such as gay or lesbian families.

Health Responsibilities of the Family

How well the family functions has a great impact on individual family members' wellbeing and health behaviors. Health professionals' encounters with the family are episodic, with the family assuming primary responsibility for the health care of its members. An assessment of family functioning in promoting and protecting its members' health requires a clear understanding of its responsibilities in this arena. Five major responsibilities of the family for members' health are presented in this section.

Development of Members' Sense of Personal Identity and Self-Worth

The family plays a significant role in the development of one's mental health (Hanson & Boyd, 1996; Loveland-Cherry, 1996). Family interactions may facilitate or impede members' access to (1) **affect**, the sense of loving and being loved; (2) **power**, the freedom to decide what one wants and the ability to obtain it; and (3) **meaning**, a sense of who and what one is. The functionally healthy family is one that maintains a balance between all members' access to affect, power, and meaning so that no member consistently and systematically is denied actualization of these basic human needs. Community health nurses often receive referrals to conduct a family assessment in situations in which parents have experienced difficulties in meeting the socioemotional needs of infants and young children, resulting in impaired attachment and inadequate weight gain associated with the syndrome referred to as *failure to thrive.* Early parent–infant attachment is critical to the development of trust and ability to form intimate relationships with others later in life. Parents who have difficulty forming appropriate attachments with their infants may have lacked appropriate role models as young children themselves. Such individuals often are suspicious of professionals, and much interpersonal skill and patience are needed to establish working relationships with them. By conveying warmth

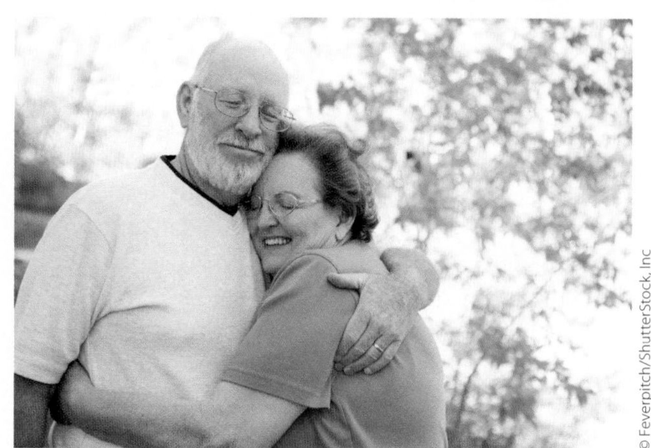

A strong and mutually respectful relationship between partners promotes healthy development in children and families.

CULTURAL CONNECTION

- Fewer than half of Hispanics and African Americans own homes, compared with 73.4% of whites in 2013 (U.S. Department of Commerce, 2014).
- The median net worth of African American and Hispanic households fell 60% to \$4,995 and \$7424, respectively, from 2005 to 2010; over the same period, the median net worth of white households dropped only 23% to \$110,729 (Luhby, 2012).

and caring, coupled with a nonjudgmental attitude, nurses can assist parents in learning how to meet the socioemotional needs of their children.

Emotional Support and Guidance During Lifecycle Transitions

As individuals grow and mature, they are expected to meet new performance expectations consistent with their current life stage. For example, a child is expected to learn to read when he or she goes to school. Should the child find reading difficult, school progress is slowed and the child's sense of personal worth is threatened. Support and guidance from the family are essential in helping individuals achieve their developmental tasks across the lifecycle (Duvall & Miller, 1985). In fact, the family as a whole is described as having responsibilities, goals, and developmental tasks that parallel the developmental tasks of individual family members. Thus, while children are expected to learn to read and develop other cognitive skills when they go to school, the family has the corresponding developmental task of encouraging children's educational achievement and learning to relate to the educational system in an effective manner.

Community health nurses have many opportunities to provide guidance to families undergoing lifecycle transitions. Prenatal and postpartum visits for new parents can offer health teaching to ease the transition to parenthood. Changes in family structure as a result of divorce and/or remarriage also present new developmental tasks for family members, such as single parenthood and the addition of stepparents into children's lives. As noted in the Application to Practice feature earlier in this chapter, Kevin Johnson's teacher, in making a referral to the school nurse, questioned whether his toileting accidents in school might be symptomatic of difficulty in coping with his parents' divorce and the subsequent move and remarriage of his father.

ETHICAL CONNECTION 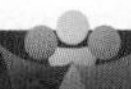

The poorest people in our country today, on the whole, are working every day. But they are earning wages so low that they cannot begin to function in the mainstream of the economic life of our nation.... We have thousands and thousands of people working on full-time jobs, with part-time incomes.

—Martin Luther King, Jr., January 1968

How different is today's society from what it was in 1968? Are the poorest families still "outside of the mainstream"?

Socialization of Family Members to Value and Maintain Health

Family members acquire values about health and learn personal health practices relative to nutrition, exercise, smoking, alcohol consumption, and hygiene through their family of origin and later transmit these values and beliefs to children as they become parents. Recognition that lifestyle factors are the single most important determinant of most of our chronic diseases has focused attention on the importance of the family's responsibility to teach its members how to maintain and preserve health (Antonovsky, 1987).

Healthy People 2020 (U.S. Department of Health and Human Services [HHS], 2012) offers a vision for preventing unnecessary death and disability and enhancing the quality of life for all Americans through the establishment of specific health promotion and disease prevention objectives. Many of the objectives focus on lifestyle risks that have their origin in health practices learned within the family context. In their interactions with families, nurses may assist members to assess health risks and to incorporate health promotion into their lifestyle (Duffy, 1988). Schools and the workplace also offer natural loci for helping children and adults to improve their health knowledge and develop attitudes that facilitate healthier behaviors.

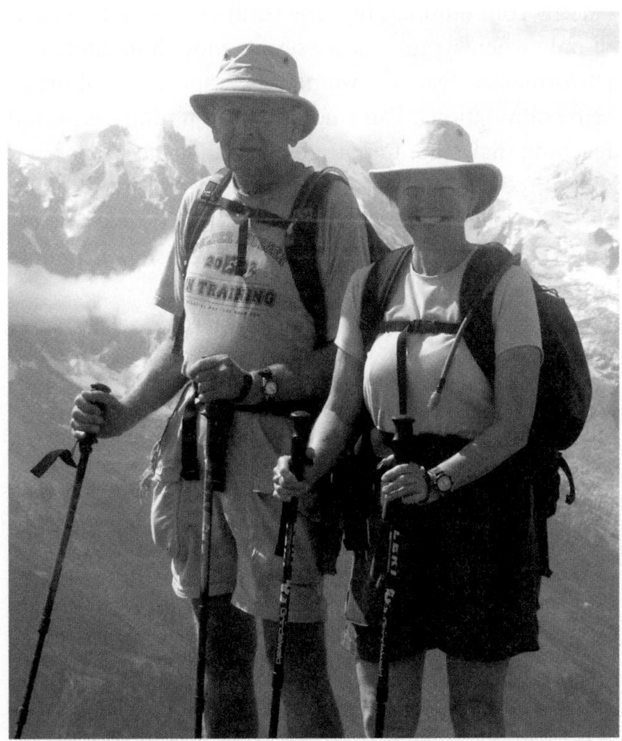

Elders today are more active. This couple climbs mountains throughout the world after retirement.

THINK ABOUT THIS 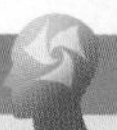

The 300 millionth American was born in 2006. A baby is born every 8 seconds in the United States.

Education About When and How to Use the Healthcare System

The family also serves as the basic referent for defining illness and what should be done about it (Doherty & Campbell, 1988). The process by which the ill person seeks information and advice from family, friends, neighbors, other nonprofessionals, and Internet-media sources has been labeled the "lay referral network." Whether a family member's symptoms should be treated with home remedies and over-the-counter medications or professional help should be sought is negotiated within the family based on interpretations of the seriousness of the symptoms, the possible cause, costs versus benefits of the action, and the impact that illness may have on the member's fulfillment of role responsibilities (Doherty, 1992). While *Healthy People 2020* has shifted national attention toward primary prevention by emphasizing health promotion and health protection activities, secondary prevention, which involves early detection and treatment of illness, is recognized as another important approach for fostering healthy communities. In some families, one is defined as ill only when symptoms are severe enough to affect role performance. Teaching women the importance of breast self-examinations, Pap smears, and mammograms and teaching males the importance of regular testicular and digital rectal examinations are examples of ways nurses can encourage family members to value the early detection of disease and to use the healthcare system in a more proactive way.

With recent national disasters, there has been a greater awareness of the need for disaster preparedness for families. Additionally, families need assistance in evaluating the quality of Internet-based health information.

Care Provision and Management for Chronically Ill, Disabled, and Aging Family Members

Families assume a major share of the responsibility for intergenerational support and assistance. Among older disabled persons who live in the community, more than 90% rely in part or entirely on family for care (Houser, Gibson, Redfoot, & AARP Public Policy Institute, 2010). Two distinct caregiving roles that may be assumed by the family are direct care provider and indirect care manager. The direct care provider actively assists family members with those activities and tasks that they are no longer able to perform independently. The indirect care manager identifies the needed services an impaired relative requires and manages their provision by others. Problems in meeting societal expectations of families for caring for disabled and aging members are emerging because the caregiving role previously filled by women has dramatically changed as a result of the increase in dual-career families. Women still account for the largest percentage of caregivers for these family members. Recognition of this fact has led to the rapid expansion of home health services and hospice programs to facilitate care of family members within their home environment.

Theoretical Approaches to the Family

Theory provides the practitioner with a systematic way of viewing a particular phenomenon. A variety of theoretical frameworks have been used to describe family interaction and behavior. No single theory is sufficiently broad enough to deal with the complex dynamics that undergird the family's competence to fulfill its health responsibilities. Thus, an integrated approach that blends family systems theory with family development and human ecology theory will be used here. This ecological systems perspective is particularly relevant to the discipline of nursing because it considers interrelationships between individuals within the family as well as between the family unit and the community over time.

Human Ecology Theory

Human ecology theory emphasizes the importance of social contexts as influences on human development. Bronfenbrenner (1986) notes that the parent–child relationship is enhanced as a context for development to the extent that the family's interrelationships with social networks, neighborhoods, communities, institutions, and cultures are supportive of its efforts to care for children. A similar perspective is presented by Hillary Rodham Clinton in her 1996 book *It Takes a Village: And Other Lessons Children Teach Us.* Thus, the extent to which work settings provide quality day care or flexible working hours can strongly influence the success of dual-career couples in fulfilling their childrearing functions. Similarly, adolescent parents are more likely to be able to continue to meet their own developmental needs for education when school policies support pregnant teens' remaining in school throughout the pregnancy and/or provide child care for teens returning to school after the baby's birth.

Another distinctive feature of human ecology theory is its recognition that the family is both influenced by and actively influences the larger social systems with which it interacts. This perspective of human ecology theory encourages us to look at interactions between the family and its multilevel environment as reciprocal rather than unidirectional processes. For example, although governmental policies often strongly influence the healthcare services available to a family, families can also shape policy. Parents concerned about pressures from health maintenance organizations (HMOs) and insurance companies, which often forced mothers and their newborns to be discharged within 24 hours of birth, joined professional and citizen lobby groups to help pass the Newborns' and Mothers' Health Protection Act in 1996. This bill requires insurers to cover a minimum stay of 48 hours for mothers and their newborns.

NOTE THIS!

Two-thirds of women work for pay during the same years that they are bearing and raising children.

Source: International Law Office. (1999). *Maternity protection at work.* Geneva, Switzerland: International Labor Office.

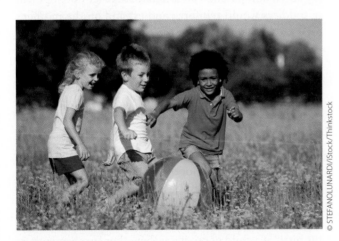

© STEFANOLUNARDI/iStock/Thinkstock

The socialization of children is one of the most important functions of the family.

Family Systems Theory

Although human ecology theory provides us with a conception of how interrelationships between the family and its social context influence the family's capacity to foster health, it does not address how internal processes within the family may facilitate or impede health. Family systems theory, however, does provide us with several key concepts to understand the role of internal family processes on health. First is the concept of **nonsummativity**, which states that the family as a whole is greater than the sum of its parts, such that a change in one family member affects all family members (Wright & Leahey, 1994). Because the whole is more than and different from the sum of its parts, the family's ability to fulfill its health responsibilities cannot be predicted from knowledge about an individual's behavior and health practices. Instead, the nurse must assess how family relationships and their social environments either impede or foster health (see the Research Alert).

RESEARCH ALERT 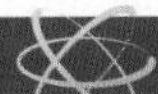

A study of 35 mothers with multiple sclerosis and their children found that both mothers and children perceived that mothers were less physically affectionate when mothers' symptoms of illness were exacerbated. Mothers, however, significantly underestimated the changes in their physical affection compared with children's perceptions. Qualitative data further revealed that affective issues were linked with tremendous fears of the children, particularly the younger children, as reflected in the following comments: "I cry when she's sick. Sometimes I think that she is going to die."

Source: Deatrick, J. A., Brennan, D., & Cameron, M. E. (1998). Mothers with multiple sclerosis and their children: Effects of fatigue and exacerbations on maternal support. *Nursing Research, 47*(4), 205–210.

For example, one cannot judge that an infant is developing adequate attachment without assessing the relationships between the parent and infant. Are bids of the infant to mother for attention when distressed responded to with soothing behaviors on the part of the mother? Healthfulness is reflected in the dyad's capacity to achieve patterns of interaction that are mutually rewarding (Robinson, Emde, & Korfmacher, 1997). Another example of the principle of nonsummativity is illustrated in the Application to Practice feature presented at the beginning of this chapter. Rather than simply viewing Kevin's toileting accidents and inattention as indicators only of a potential underlying physical health problem, the school nurse and the teacher recognize the importance of considering that Kevin's symptoms may reflect problems he is having in coping with changes in family relationships. Moreover, the school nurse chooses to follow up on the problem by scheduling a home visit to gather more data on how the mother is handling the transition to being a single parent.

Two other concepts important in understanding how the family operates as a system are structure and function. **Structure** refers to the organization of relationships among family members (i.e., roles), whereas **function** defines the purposes or goals of the family, such as activities necessary to ensure health and growth of its members (Walsh, 1982). Structure and function are interrelated in that the structure of a family influences how well it is able to fulfill its purposes or goals. Roles within a family must be integrated, much like the meshing of gears in a finely tuned engine, to facilitate attainment of common goals. Nurses working in the community often encounter families who are struggling with children's behavioral problems, because the parents cannot agree on what are reasonable bedtimes for young children or how to consistently set limits, and consequently each defines different expectations for the child. Although adults may learn to balance multiple role expectations (e.g., spouse, parent, worker, volunteer), young children need clarity in role expectations to begin to develop a sense of identity and self-worth (one of the family's five health responsibilities).

Finally, understanding the role that **self-regulation** processes play in how the family functions in meeting its health responsibilities is important for nurses working in the community. A balance between stability and change is needed for a family to effectively address the differing needs of its members over time (Klein & White, 1996). Self-regulation involves processing the internal and external feedback that a family receives regarding its behavior. Feedback can be positive or negative. **Positive feedback** moves the family toward change, whereas **negative feedback** tends to promote stability. In assessing a family, the nurse seeks to identify those behaviors that are detrimental to health and provides feedback in the form of health teaching. In the previous example in which parents are having difficulty in agreeing on limits for their children, teaching by the nurse about realistic expectations for the child's developmental age and the importance of consistency in parental discipline would be directed toward behavioral change. Conversely, when working with a mother who the nurse observes reads to her toddler, teaching about how parents can facilitate language development of toddlers would reinforce and expand on the mother's existing behaviors.

NOTE THIS!

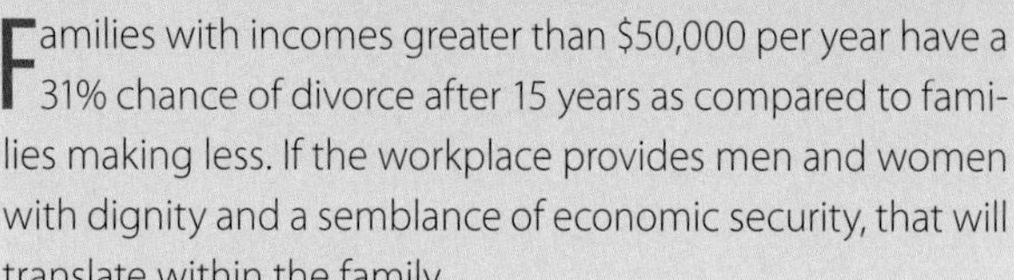
Families with incomes greater than $50,000 per year have a 31% chance of divorce after 15 years as compared to families making less. If the workplace provides men and women with dignity and a semblance of economic security, that will translate within the family.

Source: Blumer, R. (2006). *National marriage project.* New Brunswick, NJ: Rutgers, The State University of New Jersey.

MEDIA MOMENT

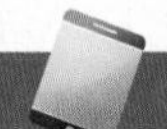

The Family in Movies

Nebraska (2013)

An aging alcoholic believes he's struck it rich after receiving a sweepstakes letter, and he ropes his son into helping him travel from Montana to Nebraska to collect his prize.

August, Osage County (2013)

Their father's death brings mean-spirited Violet Weston's daughters and sister back to her Oklahoma home for a dysfunctional family reunion.

Mother and Child (2010)

A middle-aged woman seeks the daughter she gave up for adoption 35 years ago, only to find that the daughter has recently died in childbirth—and that her long-lost granddaughter has been adopted by another local couple.

Rachel, Getting Married (2008)

Drug addict Kim is released from rehab to attend her sister Rachel's wedding, but old family troubles haunt the festivities.

The Long Walk Home (2002)

On a long walk, a man remembers the events that led to the death of his wife.

Family Development Theory

Family development theory highlights that change is an inherent aspect of family life. The family lifecycle is described in terms of developmental stages characterized by major family events—in particular, the addition and exiting of members (Carter & McGoldrick, 1989). The concept of **family developmental tasks** refers to growth responsibilities that must be achieved by a family during each stage of its lifecycle to successively meet the health and developmental needs of its members. For example, the birth of a child necessitates that other family members learn new role behaviors for protecting and fostering the health and development of the infant.

Variations in the family lifecycle and its developmental tasks are changing with the increasing diversity of family types. Although the single-parent family experiences the same lifecycle changes as the traditional two-parent nuclear family, the absence of the second parent to carry a share of the family tasks with respect to support, childrearing, companionship, and gender role-modeling for children may result in increased stressors for single parents. Divorce and possibly remarriage, with their losses and shifts in family membership, create new developmental tasks. For example, after divorce, spouses need to work through resolution of the attachment to one another while promoting ongoing parental contact between the ex-spouse and children (Carter & McGoldrick, 1989). With stepparent or blended families, crucial developmental tasks involve the restructuring of family boundaries and roles to allow for inclusion of new family members (stepparent and possibly stepchildren).

Bain (1978) has advanced a theory to predict the capacity of families to cope with lifecycle transitions that helps integrate human ecology and family systems with family development theory. According to his theory, families who are likely to have the least capacity to cope with lifecycle transitions, or who are at most risk, are (1) those who are experiencing a greater number of concurrent lifecycle changes involving (2) role transitions of great magnitude (e.g., blended families) and who (3) have a social support network that is small and nonsupportive and (4) live in a community that has few available services to assist them with the transitions confronting them.

Family-Oriented Versus Family-Focused Nursing Role

Nurses working in the community generally advocate a family approach in the delivery of services. In practice, a family approach has varied meanings. Many times, nursing interventions are directed toward the health concerns of referred individuals, with other family members being considered only as a support system for helping the individual cope with his or her health concerns. This family-oriented approach is most typical of nurses working in ambulatory care centers and home health agencies. For example, in working with a person with newly diagnosed diabetes, the nurse may assess the extent to which other family members understand and support the diabetic individual's need to modify dietary patterns to manage the disease effectively and prevent further complications.

The complexity of health issues confronting families may, at times, necessitate a more sophisticated holistic approach. With a family-focused approach, as contrasted with a family-oriented approach, the family as a whole is viewed as having specific health responsibilities, and the extent to which family processes support these functions is the nursing focus. Assessments of the family as a group are made and interventions are directed toward helping the family grow in its abilities to meet its health responsibilities.

A typical example often encountered by nurses working in public health departments is the family with a 13-year-old pregnant adolescent. From an ecological systems perspective, the adolescent's pregnancy necessitates role changes for all family members as the new baby is incorporated into the family. Hence, a family-focused approach is needed to help family members deal effectively with the lifecycle transitions triggered by the adolescent's pregnancy.

As nurses move into community settings, they need to be aware of the differences between a family-oriented and family-focused approach and select the one that is best suited to the needs of the healthcare situations they encounter. The mission of the healthcare delivery system in which the nurse works also may influence the choice of approach. For example, where the mission of the organization is disease control or rehabilitation, the family-oriented approach may be a better fit. Nurses working in organizations such as health departments, which have a population-focused perspective and emphasize health promotion and disease reduction, are likely to find more support for a family-focused approach.

MEDIA MOMENT 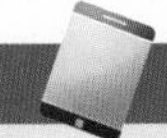

Ordinary People (1980)

Robert Redford made his Academy Award–winning directorial debut with this highly acclaimed, poignantly observant drama (based on the novel by Judith Guest) about a well-to-do family's painful adjustment to tragedy. Mary Tyler Moore and Donald Sutherland play a seemingly happy couple who lose the older of their two sons to a boating accident; Timothy Hutton plays the surviving teenage son, who blames himself for his brother's death and has attempted suicide to end his pain. The family lives in a meticulously kept home in an affluent Chicago suburb, never allowing themselves to speak openly of the grief that threatens to tear them apart. Only when the son begins to see a psychiatrist (Judd Hirsch) does the veneer of denial begin to crack. Superior performances and an Oscar-winning script by Alvin Sargent make this one of the most uncompromising dramas ever made about the psychology of dysfunctional families in grief.

A Conceptual Framework for Family Assessment

A conceptual framework provides direction to the collection, organization, and interpretation of data about the family's health situation. The conceptual framework for family assessment presented in this chapter builds on the perspective of the family as an ecological system and is designed to assist nurses in evaluating the extent to which a family is able to fulfill its health responsibilities (**Box 29-1**). The conclusion reached by conducting the assessment is an evaluation that the family is functioning more or less optimally in meeting

BOX 29-1 Family Health Responsibilities

- Promote mental health of family members by providing opportunities for each to achieve a satisfactory sense of personal identity and self-worth.
- Provide support and cognitive guidance for family members to achieve developmental tasks associated with lifecycle transitions.
- Socialize family members to adopt health practices that foster health and reduce risks for disease.
- Educate family members about when and how to use healthcare services when disruptions in health occur.
- Assist ill, disabled, and aging family members to meet their basic needs either through direct care provision or through helping them access community services.

its health responsibilities, as opposed to an evaluation regarding the health status of a particular family member.

To meet its health responsibilities, a family needs to be conscious of the health needs of its members at varying stages in the lifecycle and have sufficient energy to undertake the desired healthful behaviors (O'Brien, 1979; O'Brien & Robinson, 1984). At times, a family may have sufficient energy but lack the necessary awareness of members' needs to use its energy constructively to attain desired goals. The reverse also may be true. Thus, it is only when energy and consciousness interface and overlap that the family has the potential to effectively fulfill its health responsibilities (see **Figure 29-1**).

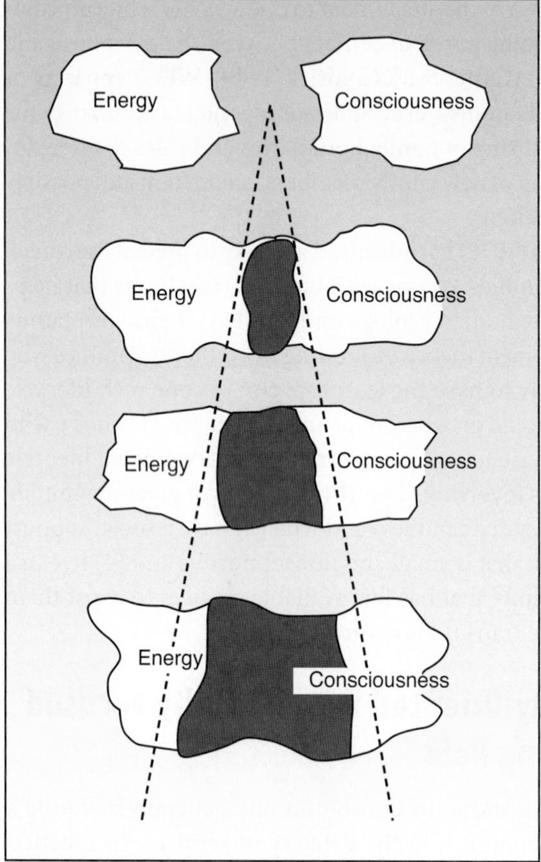

Figure 29-1 Expanding family health potential.

Source: "Expanding Family Health Potential" by O'Brien and Robinson, from *Directions in community health nursing*, edited by Judith Ann Sullivan, Blackwell Scientific Publications, 1984.

CULTURAL CONNECTION 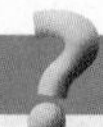

I am convinced that our American society will become more and more vulgarized and that it will be fragmentized into contending economic, racial, and religious pressure groups lacking in unity and common will, unless we can arrest the disintegration of the family and of community solidarity.

—Agnes E. Meyer, 1953

A more detailed discussion of these two core concepts as well as those family attributes and processes that may influence the level of energy and consciousness within a family system is presented here.

Energy

To teach family members good health practices, to use the professional care system to foster health maintenance, to provide members with supportive and effective relationships necessary for positive mental health, and to actively cope with lifecycle transitions all require the investment of energy (Newman, 1994; Rogers, 1983). A critical issue in family functioning is the regulation of energy flow to attain balance as opposed to imbalance—too much or too little energy (O'Brien & Robinson, 1984). When the energy flow within families is excessive, behavior is likely to be chaotic and ineffectual, resulting in crisis-oriented problem solving when members' needs or concerns become too great to ignore. The latter is often the case in families that lack clear boundaries and where extended kin, neighbors, and friends move in and out of the household at will. In contrast, when energy is low or depleted, family members' needs are likely to be unmet, as illustrated in the experience of a mother suffering from postpartum depression.

In addition to assessing the energy that the family has available to invest in meeting members' health needs, it is important to identify how it replenishes its energy. The potential sources of energy vary from family to family, from individual to individual. For some, the source may be religious beliefs, cultural traditions, shared time together, school or work activities, or social relationships with friends. The nature of the sources is unimportant, provided that the family acquires sufficient energy to meet the demands placed on it. With a family that manifests a low energy level, nursing intervention may take the form of helping the family identify new ways of acquiring energy.

Pertinent questions to consider in assessing a family's energy level include the following:

- How does the family acquire energy?
- What are its sources?
- Is there sufficient energy to meet the varying needs of its members? If not, where is the family's energy directed?
- Does the expenditure of energy in meeting family demands occur repeatedly at the expense of one particular family member?

GLOBAL CONNECTION 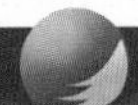

What difference does it make to the dead, the orphans, and the homeless whether the mad destruction is wrought under the name of totalitarianism or the holy name of liberty or democracy?

—Mahatma Gandhi

Consciousness

Consciousness is being aware of one's own feelings, needs, and actions as well as what is happening with others; in essence, it is the information that a system has available to effectively fulfill its functions (Newman, 1994). Growth and change within a family are directly linked to the family's level of consciousness, because it enables knowledge to be translated into goal-directed behavior. That is, the greater the consciousness, the more aware the family will be of its health responsibilities at any given stage of the lifecycle, and the more refined repertoire of choices generated for meeting those responsibilities (Newman, 1994; O'Brien & Robinson, 1984). A thoughtful assessment of the family's level of consciousness provides the foundation for planning health-promotion activities.

Another important aspect of the family's consciousness is the myths it creates about how it operates as a family (O'Brien & Robinson, 1984). For example, a family may describe relationships among members as close and intimate because all members spend a lot of time watching television together. Yet an observer might note that family

BOX 29-2 Keeping Your Drugs in the Home Safe and Your Teen Safer

The new trend in drug abuse among teens is no longer street drugs—they are easily found in every home in the United States.

The drugs of choice among teens are no longer street drugs like marijuana, cocaine, or LSD. While some teens still use these drugs, many more abuse drugs that don't carry the same stigma and are easier to get, but provide the same type of high—prescription and over-the-counter (OTC) drugs. Confused? Wondering how something that a doctor prescribes to patients can be so bad? Prescription and OTC drugs are very effective when people follow proper dosages and are supervised by a medical doctor. However, there is a new and disturbing trend parents need to know about.

Some teens are abusing prescription and OTC drugs, intentionally, to get high. And these drugs can be just as addictive as illegal drugs, like marijuana, cocaine, and LSD.[1]

This is not a problem to ignore, because you think prescription or OTC drugs are safe. They are only safe when used properly. When teens intentionally abuse these drugs to get high, it's not just a couple of pills or an extra swig of cough syrup. In some cases, teens are ingesting anywhere from a few pills to dozens or more a day, or drinking up to three to five bottles of cough syrup a day, or mixing them with alcohol.

Taking prescription drugs without a doctor's approval and supervision can be a dangerous—even deadly—decision. According to the Substance Abuse and Mental Health Services Administration (SAMHSA), almost half (48%) of all emergency department visits resulting from overdoses from an ingredient found in many cough syrups, dextromethorphan (DXM), were patients 12–20 years old.[2]

In addition, some teens in cities across the country get together and "party" with prescription and OTC drugs. "Pharming," as this alarming behavior is often referred to, describes grabbing a handful of prescription drugs and swallowing some or all of them, often with alcohol. Some of these young people are taking pills from the family medicine cabinet or ordering them online from illegal pharmacies (among other places) and giving them to their friends at school. What they don't realize is that ingesting a mix of known or unknown drugs, especially in high dosages, is always dangerous and sometimes fatal, especially with alcohol.

Parents can prevent drug abuse by setting clear expectations, communicating with their children early, knowing the signs and symptoms of abuse, and keeping all potentially abused prescription drugs locked in a safe place in the home.

Sources:

[1] SAMHSA, Office of Applied Studies, National Survey on Drug Use and Health, 2005.

[2] SAMHSA. Emergency Department Visits Involving Dextromethorphan, DAWN Report, Issue 32, 2006.

members hardly ever communicate with one another during the time spent in the same room. Quite obviously, family myths may at times impede addressing family members' needs, because the family is unable to recognize the need for behavioral change as a result of the belief that it is already behaving in the desired way. A useful assessment technique to begin to help family members become more aware of their own behavior is to engage them in reflective exercises. For example, in responding to a mother who complains that her son is "always misbehaving and won't listen" to her, the nurse might ask the mother to describe in detail a typical incident, including what her son was doing at the time and how she responded to his behavior. A common error that parents make in setting limits is to tell the child what not to do but offer no explanation for why the behavior is unacceptable.

Pertinent questions to consider in assessing a family's level of consciousness include the following:

- How aware and knowledgeable is the family of specific health and developmental needs of its members?
- Does it hold incorrect beliefs that are likely to lead to unsound health practices?
- Is its perception of how it functions congruent with reality?
- What are the sources that the family utilizes in acquiring knowledge?
- How do past family experiences influence its consciousness of health issues?
- Does it actively seek to expand its level of consciousness or does it respond only to crisis demands?

Role Structure

Roles define the goals and actions that are expected to characterize the occupant of a specific position such as mother or father (Hardy & Conway, 1988). Identification of the varying roles of family members provides the nurse with important information about the organization of relationships among family members, such as who is expected to do what and for whom. Flexibility of role definitions enables the family to deal more effectively with developmental transitions and situational crises resulting from illness or disability of one of its members (Boss, 1988).

Difficulty in the performance of one's role is defined as role insufficiency. A basic concept in role theory is that roles are reciprocal in that they are patterned to complement that of a role partner. Thus, the mothering role cannot be understood without looking at the corresponding role of the child at a particular developmental stage. Role behaviors expected of mothers of infants will differ from those expected of mothers whose children are in their adolescent years. When role insufficiency occurs, one or more family members' health and developmental needs are likely to be unmet.

In assessing family members' role performance, nurses need to be aware that role behaviors are learned according to the cultural values of the family. Collecting information about the family's customs and traditions is important for interpreting whether family members' roles are appropriate within their social context. For example, the maternal grandmother often assumes the mothering role for young children in African American single-parent families (Burton & deVries, 1995). Furthermore, it often is helpful to gather information about their early role models and to determine how these experiences have affected present role behaviors (Friedman, 1998). It is not uncommon for parents' expectations and behaviors toward children to be similar to those they experienced in their families of origin (see the Research Alert that follows).

Role overload leading to increased stress and reduced levels of wellness has been cited as an issue for single-parent families (Burden, 1986; Popenoe, 1995). The single parent must fulfill both mother and father roles, often in addition to the work role, whereas role ambiguity and conflict are often major sources of stress in stepparent and blended families as members attempt to define whether the stepparent should assume the role of parent or nonparent and how children of the respective parents should relate as siblings. A typical example of resulting role conflict is the stepfather who disciplines his wife's child for misbehavior and is confronted by his wife for "overstepping" the boundaries of his role as a stepfather. In addition, ongoing relationships with the biological parent and the addition of relationships with the kin of the stepparent further compound the clear definition of family roles (Carter & McGoldrick, 1989).

It is important for the nurse to carefully assess role strain and conflict occurring within the family because tension and conflict may negatively impact members' emotional wellbeing. Clarity of role expectations is crucial to helping family members develop a sense of personal identity and self-worth. Moreover, role strain and conflict, if left unresolved, may deplete the usable energy available for meeting the family's other health responsibilities, such as teaching members basic health practices to maintain health and ways to use healthcare services appropriately (Pratt, 1976, 1982).

Pertinent questions to consider in assessing a family's role structure include the following:

- Which roles do each of the family members fulfill? How competently do members perform their roles?

- How do past family experiences influence members' role performance?
- If role strain or conflict exists, what are the contributing factors?
- Is there flexibility in roles when needed?

GLOBAL CONNECTION 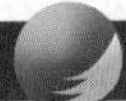

Globally, there were an estimated 33 million people living with HIV in 2007. The percentage of women worldwide among people living with HIV has remained stable at 50% for several years (UNAIDS, 2008).

RESEARCH ALERT 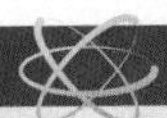

This literature review focuses on family identity formation within a social cultural context for families, couples, and women who are in committed Black-White interracial relationships that include biracial children. This review was limited to U.S. research studies completed between 1990 and 2002. The American racial lens represented the environmental context that this article seeks to capture. Family nurses who can assess and intervene in a culturally competent manner will be essential to promoting health and eliminating health disparities for these interracial families.

Source: Byrd, M., & Garwick, A. (2004). A feminist critique of research on interracial family identity: Implications for family health. *Journal of Family Nursing, 10*(3), 302–322.

Decision-Making Processes

Decision making is central to the fulfillment of family responsibilities in meeting members' health and developmental needs. It is a process that involves (1) recognizing the need for a decision, (2) identifying and weighing alternatives, and (3) selecting an alternative and facilitating its implementation. Central to effective decision making is the processing of information; the decision maker must be able to discriminate between what is important and what is not, between what is relevant and what is irrelevant, between actions that will achieve goals and those that will not.

The family's use of healthcare services often provides insight into their decision-making processes. Families often seek the advice of extended kin and friends about how to interpret untoward symptoms and whether they are sufficiently serious to warrant professional care. In some families, illness may be equated with inability to perform one's expected roles, resulting in a delay in seeking health care until symptoms are advanced. Studies have shown that poor health-related decision-making skills often reflect difficulty in decision making in other areas of family life. Conversely, parents who make general lifestyle decisions that are growth-oriented and motivated toward change are more likely to practice and encourage health-promotion behaviors for themselves and their children (Duffy, 1988).

MEDIA MOMENT 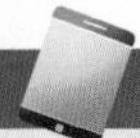

Love in the Driest Season: A Family Memoir (2004)

By Neely Tucker, New York, NY: Crown.

This memoir was written by Neely Tucker, a writer for the *Washington Post* and a white Mississippi native, married to a black woman, Vita, whom he met in Detroit. The book focuses on their journey to Zimbabwe with their intent to adopt Chipo, a baby black girl abandoned in a field of dry grass, one of thousands of children left orphaned by AIDS, civil war, and the Rwandan genocides. Tucker is an engaging writer who combines a lively style with the emotionally moving story of the couple driven to achieve what seems to be the impossible: adopt a Zimbabwe child in a country where foreign adoptions are prohibited. They encounter seemingly insurmountable obstacles from President Robert Mugabe's policies, which eventually even endanger their own lives. Their courage and commitment to adopt Chipo makes for a creative and engaging story about love and family, all set against the backdrop of the tense situation in Africa. Overall, this tale of the journey between two worlds offers many lessons about the power of love that truly can conquer all odds.

RESEARCH ALERT 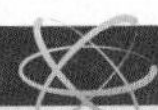

The ability of a nurse home visitation program for first-time mothers and their infants to effect changes in the quality of the caregiving environment was found to vary with household structure. Mothers who lived alone and those who lived with their husbands or boyfriends were able to create safer and more stimulating child-rearing environments than mothers who lived with grandmothers or with other adults. The investigators interpreted these findings as suggesting that when the mother is able to plan and take a course of action on her own, or in concert with someone over whom she is likely to exert some decision-making influence such as a husband or boyfriend, she is more able to implement changes in the home suggested by nurse home visitors.

Source: Cole, R., Kitzman, H., Olds, D., & Sidora, K. (1998). Family context as a moderator of program effects in prenatal and early childhood home visitation. *Journal of Community Psychology, 26*(1), 37–48.

Nursing assessment of the family's decision-making processes focuses on identifying strengths or limitations in the information-processing function as well as the generation of alternative solutions. Immediate closure through the selection of a single option without explicit ranking or elimination of alternatives is characteristic of dysfunctional families, whereas healthy, functioning families explore numerous options, and if one alternative does not work, the family backs off and tries another, instead of trying to just make one option work (O'Brien & Robinson, 1984; Walsh, 1982).

Of equal importance to note are those situations in which families arrive at no decision. Discussions finish inconclusively and are then decided by events, as with a couple who argues about which form of birth control to use until the wife discovers she is pregnant. Such an event is called *de facto decision making* in that things are allowed to happen without planning. De facto decision making is characteristic of multiproblem families, many of whose members feel powerless and/or lack the energy to actively manage their lives. It also may occur in healthy families dealing with highly stressful situations when members' abilities to process information are reduced (Friedman, 1998).

Observations about family decision-making processes also help clarify the family's power structure. Families tend to reach decisions either by consensus or by accommodation (Friedman, 1998). With consensus, a particular course of action is mutually agreed on by all concerned. With accommodation, some members assent to allow a decision to be reached. Accommodation occurs by use of compromising, bargaining, and coercion. Thus, by recognizing situations involving accommodation and who was identified with the decision reached, the nurse can identify the "power" brokers in the family. Identification of who has the power in family decision making is crucial for nurses working with families because interventions must be designed to include these family members (see the preceding Research Alert).

Pertinent questions to consider in assessing family decision making include the following:

- Who makes which decisions?
- Are there particular health needs or issues that are not recognized or addressed?
- Is the family able to discriminate between information that is relevant and information that is irrelevant to the decision?
- Are alternative solutions generated and weighed? Is the selected alternative implemented?
- Who holds the power in family decision making? To what extent do family decisions involve consensus or coercion?

Communication Patterns

Observation of a family's communication patterns yields valuable information about the meaning accorded to various family members as well as the clarity of interpersonal boundaries (Sieburg, 1985). **Communication** is a transactional process between two or more individuals in which feelings, needs, information, and opinions are shared. One of the most basic assessments regarding the family's communication patterns is the identification of who communicates what with whom. Individuals within the family may selectively disclose feelings, needs, and information to other members. Thus, communication patterns are linked to the family's level of consciousness. When individuals share their ideas and feelings freely and completely, they have a broad base of cues and provisional solutions on which to base their final actions. Problem solving is more effective in such families because members contribute to the solution of concern and are more likely to be committed to the decisions reached.

Still another important assessment is the identification of covert rules governing communication among family members. Satir (1983) defines rules as the "shoulds" and "should nots" of family life. For example, a family rule may be that only positive feelings should be expressed or that sex is not an appropriate topic of discussion. An illustration of the importance that family rules play in understanding communication exchanges among family members may be found in a spousal argument over the wife's allowing the couple's 10-year-old son to attend a movie with a group of friends. After much heated discussion, the husband acknowledges that he did not object to his son's having gone to the movies with his friends, but he felt his wife should have consulted him before giving the son permission. In reality, the argument between husband and wife stems from the husband's perception that his wife violated a family rule—namely, that decisions about the son's peer activities are joint parental decisions.

One fundamental principle of communication theory is that every exchange not only conveys information or content, but a definitional meaning of how one views self and others (Sieburg, 1985). In fact, the recognition accorded to the other is more crucial than the content. By attending to the recognition accorded to others, the nurse can gain an understanding of how communication shapes members' feelings of self-worth and self-efficacy. Confirming messages validate the intrinsic worth of the person and endorse the other's self-experience as unique and valuable. Confirmation is conveyed by direct verbal acknowledgment of the other's message, expanding or elaborating on its content, requesting clarification of what another has said—all behaviors reflective of active listening.

Child: "Mom, look—I tied my own sneakers."

Mother: "Let me see. Yes, you did do a fine job of tying your laces. You have worked very hard at learning to do that. I'm proud of you."

In contrast, disconfirming messages question the other's perception or validity of self-experience through such behaviors as looking away from the other when speaking, interrupting the other, turning to speak to a third person while the other is still talking, interjecting comments that are irrelevant, engaging in other activities while talking, exiting while another is talking, or remaining silent when a response is required or expected (Sieburg, 1985). Obviously, such behaviors leave the recipient with a feeling of powerlessness and, over time, result in lowered self-esteem.

Child: "Mom, look—I tied my own sneakers."

Mother: "Don't bother me now. Can't you see that I'm reading the newspaper?"

Another important principle of communication relates to the congruence between the verbal and nonverbal aspects of the exchange. Verbal language conveys the substance of the message, whereas nonverbal language transmits the more subtle nature of the intent of the message. The degree of congruence and balance between the verbal and nonverbal portions of an exchange define the degree of clarity of the message for the recipient. Given that much verbal conflict among family members often stems from faulty interpretation of nonverbal aspects of communication, it is particularly important to assess the extent to which family members are able to elicit feedback and validate messages to minimize misinterpretation of cues and faulty mind reading (Sieburg, 1985).

Communication patterns also are the most observable indicators of the clarity of interpersonal boundaries among family members. The use of "I" statements as opposed to "we" statements and the extent of mind reading and censorship (e.g., "You shouldn't say that," "You have no reason to feel angry") present in members'

RESEARCH ALERT 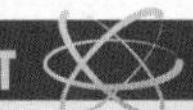

This qualitative study explored the experience of delayed parenthood for women who had children for the first time after the age of 30. Unstructured, conjoint interviews with both parents were conducted with couples. The findings suggested that older parents experience parenthood differently from younger parents concerning negotiation of childcare roles and career roles, greater interest and participation of the father in childbirth and childrearing, a general concern over career involvement among the mothers, and greater selectivity in terms of healthcare professionals. When women choose to become parents at a later age, their maturity, career status, and values about sharing of parenting responsibilities are significantly different from those of younger first-time mothers. As women age, especially for those who are childless, they tend to become more independent in their marriage roles and are more career oriented. Having a baby past the age of 30 presents somewhat different challenges to women whose lives are "already in progress." Mothers in the study consistently mentioned that the baby was "joining" a family, rather than the family adapting to the baby. This is a significant difference relative to younger women whose lives have not been well defined by work and other adult roles. The traditional norm for beginning parenthood has been changing since the 1970s. This change is clearly evidenced by the increasing number of adults who are delaying parenthood until age 30 or older. This situation appears to represent a significant change in the attitudes of some women and men toward traditional parenting roles. For example, while birth rates for younger women have decreased, the age at first birth for U.S. women aged 30 to 39 has increased steadily over the past several years.

First-time parenthood has long been recognized as one of the most important events in adult development and in the formation of the family. Changing demographic patterns of fertility have been the result of and catalyst for changes in parenting roles and statuses for men and women. With advanced reproductive technologies, women and men are facing new options regarding the decision to have children, including issues of timing, number of children, and even the method of conception. Although delayed childbearing has occurred in the past, the current trend should be of particular interest, not only because of the numbers involved, but also because the reasons for the delay may reflect general structural changes in society that may cause more and more people to delay parenthood. These reasons include changing attitudes toward marriage and family, changing parenting and gender role patterns, increasing levels of education for both men and women, greater employment opportunities for women in particular, and technological advances. These findings have implications for nurses and other caregivers who work with childbearing families, especially those involved in parent education, labor and delivery, prenatal health care, and newborn nurseries.

Source: Saucier, K. A. (1997). *The experience of having children late: A qualitative study about delayed parenthood.* Unpublished dissertation, University of Colorado, Boulder, CO.

THINK ABOUT THIS 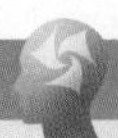

Words of Wisdom from Anne Morrow Lindbergh
A Good Relationship Has a Pattern Like a Dance

A good relationship has a pattern like a dance and is built on some of the same rules. The partners do not need to hold on tightly, because they move confidently in the same pattern, intricate but gay and swift and free, like a country dance of Mozart's. To touch heavily would be to arrest the pattern and freeze the movement, to check the endlessly changing beauty of its unfolding. There is no place here for the possessive clutch, the clinging arm, the heavy hand; only the barest touch in passing. Now arm in arm, now face to face, now back to back—it does not matter which. Because they know they are partners moving to the same rhythm, creating a pattern together, and being invisibly nourished by it.

Marriage is tough, because it is woven of all these various elements, the weak and the strong. "In love-ness" is fragile, for it is woven only with the gossamer threads of beauty. It seems to me absurd to talk about "happy" and "unhappy" marriages.

When the wedding march sounds the resolute approach, the clock no longer ticks, it tolls the hour. The figures in the aisle are no longer individuals, they symbolize the human race.

communications with one another provide important clues to the clarity of interpersonal boundaries and members' sense of separateness and personal autonomy (Sieburg, 1985). Clear and functional communication among family members is considered a cornerstone of the healthy family (Goldenberg & Goldenberg, 1996; Janosik & Green, 1992; Satir, 1983). It is foundational in enabling the family to fulfill its health responsibility in assisting members to develop a sense of personal identity and self-worth. Moreover, clarity and openness of communication among family members facilitates effective decision making when disruptions to health arise. Families whose members lack good communications skills also often have difficulty accessing community services to help with their needs.

Pertinent questions to consider in assessing a family's communication patterns include the following:

- Who talks to whom?
- Which feelings or issues are closed to discussion?
- Are members able to clearly state their needs and feelings?
- Is there congruence between verbal and nonverbal aspects of communication?
- How well do members listen when others are communicating?
- Do members elicit feedback and validation in communicating with one another?
- What are the predominant patterns of acknowledgment accorded various members?
- Is communication among members age appropriate?

Values

Knowledge of the value orientations of the family provides direction to understanding the why of family dynamics. A family's configuration of values ascribes meaning to certain health events and suggests ways to respond to them (Friedman, 1998). The identification of family values, however, is often compounded by the family's own lack of awareness of how it ascribes worth to people, events, and things. It is important to distinguish both the overt and covert values operative in family behavior.

A particularly important value orientation to assess is how the family views itself in relation to the environment. The family that feels it has little control over what happens does not take the initiative to seek out new ideas, information, or resources and apply them to the solution of family problems or to minimize health risks (Boss, 1988). Similarly, the time orientation of the family influences the extent to which it actively addresses lifecycle transitions and change. Families who emphasize past traditions may experience lifecycle transitions as more stressful (Carter & McGoldrick, 1989). Likewise, a predominant focus on the present is likely to minimize anticipatory planning and emphasize de facto decision making (Duffy, 1988). As noted in the discussion of family decision making, families who rely on de facto decision making are less likely to engage in health-promotion activities or use preventive health services.

Furthermore, there is a hierarchical nature to family values that influences the family's perceptions of risks and benefits of taking certain actions. The relative ranking of health in the family's hierarchy of values is important in determining the extent to which forces within the family tend to sustain or undermine healthcare behaviors. For example, the family who places a high value on home ownership may choose to forgo preventive health care if economic resources are limited. An accurate assessment of a family's value system should help tailor interventions to goals that are important to the family.

A family's values are a reflection of its subculture as well as of the community in which it resides. Obviously, the greater the degree of congruence between a family's subcultural values and the community's values, the more the community supports the family's identity. Incompatibility in values between the family and the community generates conflict that increases stress within the family as a whole or between varying members of the family who have assimilated the community's values in differing degrees. Such stress may deplete the energy available to meet health responsibilities and negatively affect members' self-esteem (Friedman, 1998; Pratt, 1982).

It is equally important to recognize that nurses often have their own personal and professional values that define how the "ideal family" should behave. Unless nurses are aware of their own values, interactions with families may become conflictual as they pursue interventions directed toward expectations they hold for the family that are incongruent with its own values and beliefs. Generally, nursing's code of ethics encourages respect for the family's autonomy to make its own choices involving health matters unless such choices are likely to result in serious harm for others, such as spread of communicable disease and physical or sexual abuse of children.

Given that values cannot be seen directly, Friedman (1998) advocates the use of a "compare and contrast" method to assist the nurse in identifying specific family values. The compare and contrast method involves using a list of central values of the dominant culture or the family's subcultural reference group to engage the family in a discussion of their own values. Through discussion with the family, the nurse seeks not only to identify values held by the family and their overall relative importance to one another, but also to identify value differences and clashes between family members.

Pertinent questions to consider in assessing a family's values include the following:

- What are the important values held by the family?
- To what extent do family values foster active coping and mastery of concerns?
- What is the family's orientation to the past, present, and future?
- What is the relative ranking of health in the family's hierarchy of values?
- Are there value conflicts evident within the family, between the family and the subculture/community, or between the family and the nurse?

Family Boundaries

Family boundaries serve to distinguish the family from the social contexts or environments with which it interacts. In essence, family boundaries serve as a conceptual filter controlling the degree of exchange that family members have with their environment (Klein & White, 1996). Having selectively permeable boundaries allows for family growth and change, because the use of resources outside the family is enhanced (see the Research Alert). The latter can contribute to family functioning by developing awareness of alternative courses of action (e.g., greater consciousness) and by increasing understanding of personal health practices and the value of self-directed action for promoting health (Pratt, 1982). Conversely, the amount of information a family can handle adequately is limited, and loose boundaries that result in an excess of information or conflicting information from the environment may amplify and create family disorganization (Walsh, 1982).

RESEARCH ALERT

This article presents guidelines for spiritual assessment and interventions explicitly for families, while considering each family member's unique spirituality. The category of spiritual interpretation to represent diagnosis is introduced. Case studies exemplify how to integrate the guideline and illustrate elements that may favor specific interpretations that would guide the interventions. As nurses continually strive to assist families with their health needs, they must also attend to their spiritual needs.

Source: Tanyi, R. (2006). Spirituality and family nursing: Spiritual assessment and interventions for families. *Journal of Advanced Nursing, 53*(3), 287–294.

MEDIA MOMENT

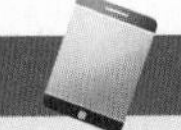

Prince of Tides (1991)

A troubled man from a dysfunctional family talks to his suicidal sister's psychiatrist about their family history and falls in love with her in the process.

The Squid and the Whale (2006)

Based on the true childhood experiences of Noah Baumbach and his brother, *The Squid and the Whale* tells the touching story of two young boys dealing with their parents' divorce in Brooklyn in the 1980s.

Orange County (2002)

A guidance counselor mistakenly sends out the wrong transcripts to Stanford University under the name of an overachieving high schooler. The student wants desperately to leave his dysfunctional family.

Garden State (2004)

A quietly troubled young man returns home for his mother's funeral after being estranged from his family for a decade.

Markedly restricted interchange with the environment creates a greater reliance on inner family resources. Relatively closed families may exhibit more energy, in the form of tension, than they can discharge in constructive ways. Studies repeatedly have noted that child abuse clusters in

APPLICATION TO PRACTICE

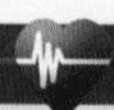

Family Lifecycle Transition: Teenage Pregnancy

Nancy, a 16-year-old unmarried Caucasian teen, lives in a housing project with her mother, her mother's current boyfriend, and two brothers—Jerome, 17 years old, and Derrick, 3 years old. She is 25 weeks pregnant. The pregnancy was unplanned; she was not using any form of contraception. Ronald, her 26-year-old boyfriend, is the father of the expectant child. Ronald has two previous children (ages 2 and 4 years) by another woman whom he rarely sees.

Nancy did not seek prenatal care until the beginning of her second trimester of pregnancy. To date, she has gained 13 pounds. Her health practices include the use of home remedies and self-comfort measures that she learned from her grandmother. She began smoking at age 13 and now smokes 1 to 2 packs of cigarettes per day. A frequent problem is urinary tract infections. Nancy told the clinic nurse who made the referral, "I can hardly get up in the morning to face the day now that I am pregnant. Sometimes life just doesn't seem worth it."

The two-bedroom apartment is too small for the five-person family; Nancy sleeps on a pull-out couch in the living room. She complains that she never has any privacy. The home is cluttered and in need of cleaning. Much cigarette smoke permeates the environment. Nancy says she feels unsafe in her neighborhood, where groups of males congregate outside the project complex; thus she stays indoors most of the day.

Nancy dropped out of school in the 9th grade to stay home and care for Derrick while her mother works. She states that she knows that she will not be able to get a very good job in the future without finishing high school and wishes she could find a way to continue her education. Her mother works long hours as a certified care assistant in a nursing home trying to support herself and her children. The mother's current boyfriend is looking for employment because he had to quit his job in construction as a result of a back injury from an automobile accident.

Nancy is ambivalent about her pregnancy. She reports that Ronald has become more distant as her pregnancy has progressed; she is concerned that he may not assume financial responsibility for the baby and that this will be a further strain on her mother. She expresses confidence about being able to take care of a baby, because she has had significant responsibility for her younger brother. The nurse observes that Nancy displays much warmth and patience in interactions with Derrick during the visit.

Nancy receives Medicaid and help from the Women, Infants and Children (WIC) program. Although she could not be specific as to how Ronald makes a living, she states, "He always seems to have plenty of money." He has given her some money to buy baby equipment and clothes.

1. What initial family diagnosis would you make?
2. What other information would you need to know to assist Nancy in promoting a healthy pregnancy?
3. Which community resources could you use to promote family health in this family?

families that are isolated from other families, neighbors, and society. In healthier isolated families, the members tend to believe that all or most of the needs of the members can be met within the family or the family's reference group (Sedgwick, 1981). Yet such exclusive reliance on internal resources may occur to the detriment of one or more family members in situations involving long-term chronic illness or disability, as evidenced by caregiver burden (Kramer & Kipnis, 1995; Smith, Tobin, & Fullmer, 1995).

Pertinent questions to consider in assessing family boundaries include the following:

- Are family boundaries overly rigid or overly loose?
- What ongoing relationships does the family maintain with extended kin, friends, or other social groups?
- Do interactions with its support network foster or impede the family's ability to cope with its health responsibilities?
- Is the family satisfied with its support network?
- Is the family willing and able to access community services?

Although the framework for family assessment presented in this chapter emphasizes critical areas of family functioning that have been found to contribute to the family's effectiveness in meeting its health responsibilities, one usually begins by obtaining basic identifying data about the family and its immediate environment: names and ages of family members, health history of each family member, racial/ethnic background, education, employment, income, health insurance, housing, characteristics of the immediate neighborhood, and availability of health and other basic services in the neighborhood (e.g., grocery stores, schools, churches, transportation). The purpose or reason for the nurse's contact with the family guides the initial information collected about pertinent areas of family functioning. For example, in making a home visit to the Johnson family (described in the Application to Practice at the beginning of this chapter) to follow up on Kevin's toileting accidents and inattention in school, the nurse might begin by asking Mrs. Johnson what she thinks may be contributing to the changes in Kevin's behavior.

Initial information shared by the family will help guide the nurse in determining what other data to collect. The data are synthesized to identify family strengths in meeting its health responsibilities and areas where the family could use help to cope more effectively. The latter serves as a guide for negotiating the nurse's continuing role and activities with the family.

A Self-Efficacy Model for Nurse–Family Intervention

Because the family's ability to effectively fulfill its health responsibilities requires self-direction and self-governance, the nurse–family intervention should facilitate the family's active participation in dealing with the health concerns or issues that it is experiencing. Indeed, the family's active participation in nurse–family interactions may be a significant variable in determining the effectiveness of nursing intervention (Kemp et al., 2006; O'Brien & Robinson, 1984).

The **contracting** process provides a means for enhancing family participation in its own health maintenance. Contracting is based on the belief that families have the potential for self-growth and the right to self-determination. It calls for an active participative and collaborative role for both family and nurse, because the goal is to build family self-efficacy in addressing its needs. The contracting process may be subdivided into five interlinking, sequenced phases (Sloan & Schommer, 1982). As with any relationship, the phases denote an ebb and flow of movement rather than discrete points at which something begins or ends. In the description that follows, each phase is discussed separately, although in reality they may overlap.

Identification of Family Health Concerns and Needs

This phase begins with the initial contact between the family and the nurse. Data, both subjective and objective, are gained about each other through observation and exchange of information. The use of a conceptual framework for assessing family functioning facilitates a clear identification of how the family is meeting its health responsibilities and any accompanying concerns (see the Appendix at the end of this chapter). The preferable outcome of this first phase is an agreement between the nurse and the family on the definition of the problems, needs, and concerns to be addressed in subsequent interactions. Two other outcomes are also possible: (1) referral to a more appropriate service or (2) termination because congruence between nurse and family does not exist and effective problem solving is not feasible (Williamson, 1981).

Mutual Setting of Goals

What does the family hope to accomplish? This is a crucial question, and one that is not asked often enough by nurses. By asking what the family hopes to gain from the intervention, the nurse assists the family to focus on its own goals and priorities. The nurse also can gain a sense of congruency between individual member and family goals, which are often a potential source of conflict (Lynch & Tiedje, 1991). In essence, this phase involves collaborative negotiations and democratic compromise rather than the nurse deciding what the goals will be. The nurse, however, expands the family's consciousness by sharing observations and knowledge that can facilitate the family's identification of goals.

The communication style used by the nurse can foster or hinder the family's acceptance of a suggested goal. For instance, saying, "Perhaps we need to work on ways to reduce the distress your son's behavior is causing" is likely to be met with a more favorable response than, "You need to work on improving your relationships with one another." The second approach will invariably raise the family's defenses, whereas the first fosters its willingness to allow the nurse to help them work toward a solution to their concern. Helping the family to set realistic, attainable goals is one of the nurse's key functions. Goals should be stated in a precise manner capable of being monitored, and a timeframe for their accomplishment should be specified. For example, "Mother will spend half an hour each evening in some planned activity with children" is a more measurable goal than "Mother will improve attention given to children." Even when specific goals are set, there may be lack of progress. The family's prioritizing of goals may conflict with the nurse's. The nurse may need to support the family's priorities to free its energy for other goal attainment. If the nurse cannot offer such support because of possible injury to a particular family member, the family needs to be informed of what action will be taken.

Delineation of Alternatives

Once the goals are established, the nurse and the family need to discuss how those goals can be attained. This process involves (1) the exploration and determination of the family's strengths and available resources, (2) the steps or actions needed to attain the goals, (3) the negotiation and division of responsibilities of the family and nurse for goal attainment, and (4) the establishment of a reasonable time limit for implementing the plan.

Emphasizing the existing family strengths reinforces the family's belief in its own ability to solve problems and meet goals. In working with a mother having difficulty with limit setting and discipline with a toddler, the nurse might begin by acknowledging the attempts the mother has made to solve the problem and emphasize how well she is managing other areas of child care. Such an approach fosters esteem and confidence in the mother and facilitates her acceptance of the nurse as a helping person. A temptation to be avoided is the offering of numerous suggestions about how to do something better or differently before recognizing and drawing out the family's estimation of its own resources and potential solutions. The nurse can then supplement the family's developing knowledge base by introducing family and/or community resources not identified for its consideration.

Equally important in the planning process are decisions on the sequence of activities and the time frame needed to achieve the goal. The nurse generally plays a supportive role in this process, encouraging the family to make specific and detailed plans that are likely to maximize goal attainment. Agreement on the nurse's role and ways to monitor progress are crucial outcomes of this phase.

Implementation of the Plan

The plan and division of responsibilities mutually agreed on are tried. The nurse plays particularly vital roles during this phase. First is the anticipation of problems or setbacks that may arise, followed by helping the family recognize and deal with them in as positive a way as possible. A series of minor setbacks can discourage and demoralize family members to the extent that the carefully negotiated plan may be prematurely abandoned. Frequent contacts for guidance and support during the implementation phase can help individual family members accomplish their tasks. Second, the nurse has an important role-modeling function in that nursing responsibilities are carried out as agreed, within the given time limit. If problems are encountered in fulfilling the agreed-on nursing activities, the nurse should communicate them openly to the family and seek help in making alternative plans.

Evaluation

Evaluation is an ongoing process throughout all phases of the nurse–family transaction as well as an end phase. Results may range from successful goal attainment to discovering that the selected solution is not acceptable to the family. The latter may happen when the family and nurse fail to identify the "real" problem, they select unrealistic solutions, or unforeseen outcomes occur. As in other phases, the family should be encouraged to participate equally by sharing feelings and concerns about its course and about the nurse's role in accomplishing outlined responsibilities. Emphasis on positive strides, although they may be small, can bolster the family's sense of self-efficacy.

The Long Walk

We have walked a long way—the old woman said.
I no longer know the way—
The trees are so tall—they all look the same.
Are we near to the end?
We are close—
You see—right there—the cleared meadow on the top of the next hill—we have just one more hill to climb.
We are very close to the end my dear—the old man said.
I am growing tired—is it much farther—she asked.
See my dear we are close. Just beyond the next hill
See how the trees part—just one more hill to climb.
Are you sure this is the way? We have walked for such a long time and climbed so many hills.
We are close now my dear—you can almost see the stream.
Listen we are very close—just behind that hill—see how the valley opens.
It's growing late—have we reached the end?
My legs are tired and I would like to rest.
See the top of the hill—see how the trees are black picture cuts—you can almost see it now.
Look where the sun is setting—home is just beyond that bend—we can hear the stream if we listen—my dear.
The shadows are growing long and I would like to rest.
Are we near home?
Just one more hill to climb—then we can rest.
It is growing so dark and my eyes are not so good—do you see the end of our journey?
This is our last hill to climb. We will soon rest—my dear.

—*Ann Thedford Lanier*

Crucial questions to consider in end-phase evaluation include the following:

- Was the goal(s) achieved?
- Was the selected solution(s) appropriate?
- Which factors facilitated or impeded goal attainment?
- Should the nurse–family relationship be terminated or should other goals and plans be developed?

The manner in which the nurse–family relationship is concluded is as vital as the way in which it is begun. The establishment of a plan for continuity of care, if needed, is crucial. Often, after a period of intensive nursing supervision, a plan for periodic reassessment of the situation is warranted. This is particularly applicable to families dealing with long-term chronic illness or disability. The family should know how to contact the nurse should unanticipated changes occur before the scheduled interval for reappraisal.

APPLICATION TO PRACTICE 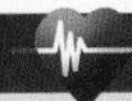

Application of Nurse–Family Intervention Model: Johnson Family

Mrs. Williams, the school nurse at Sagebrush Elementary, called Mrs. Johnson and scheduled a home visit for 5:30 p.m. She began the visit by clarifying for Mrs. Johnson the changes in Kevin's behavior that his teacher had noted in recent months and asked her if she had observed similar problems at home. Mrs. Johnson reported that Kevin had begun to have episodes of nighttime bedwetting and she felt he was more moody and, at times, quite argumentative with her when she would not let him "have his way." She stated that she had spoken with Kevin's pediatrician about the bedwetting, and he felt that Kevin was probably having trouble with the changes with his father. Kevin had no history of bedwetting or toileting accidents since about 3 years of age. The pediatrician encouraged her not to scold Kevin for his accidents and to try to give him a little more attention to help him deal with his separation from his father.

When asked what she thought of the pediatrician's advice, Mrs. Johnson acknowledged that she knew the divorce had been hard for the children. Their father's former job had made it possible for him to be home with them after school, and he had spent a lot of time with Kevin, helping him with schoolwork, games, and other activities. Since her ex-husband's remarriage, he had spent less time visiting with the children. She knew that Kevin missed his father's attention, but planning time to do all the things his dad had done was difficult for her along with working and managing the home. Moreover, she knew Kevin resented going to the "after-school program" because of her work hours. In fact, she sometimes had to ask her mother-in-law to pick up the children from the childcare center because she had to work late. Mrs. Johnson indicated that she didn't want to refuse her boss's request to work late because she was hoping to qualify for a promotion. One of the women she worked with was retiring in another 6 months, and her position as office manager would need to be filled. Although her mother-in-law was always willing to be helpful with caring for the children, she didn't like to ask too often. She felt that her in-laws might have some feelings that she contributed to the divorce because of her interest in "getting ahead in her career." Her own parents did not live nearby.

During the visit, Mrs. Williams observed that Mrs. Johnson often seemed impatient with Kevin, responding rather sharply to him when he came into the room where they were meeting to ask questions. She often redirected him to go to his sister for help. At one point, Mrs. Johnson even remarked to the nurse that she had difficulty coping with Kevin's many requests of her and that it hurt her when he made comments to her about how things were different "when Daddy lived here." When she set limits with him, he often remarked, "I want to go live with my Daddy."

Using Mrs. Johnson's descriptions of the problems she was facing in dealing with Kevin at the time of the divorce (Kevin's bedwetting and increased demands for her attention, his remark that "things were different when Daddy lived here"), her own observations about parent–child interactions, and Mrs. Johnson's hesitation to turn down requests for overtime work and to ask for too much help from in-laws, the nurse felt it appeared that the family was experiencing difficulty with new family developmental tasks resulting from the divorce and remarriage of the father, such as learning to be a single parent and promoting ongoing parental contact between the ex-spouse and children. In discussing with Mrs. Johnson ways that she thought the nurse might be helpful, they identified the goal as helping Mrs. Johnson to assist her children with the divorce and developed the following immediate plan:

- The nurse would set up a conference with the school psychologist for Mrs. Johnson to have some counseling about how to deal with Kevin's reaction to the divorce and his behavior.
- Mrs. Johnson would take her children to the neighborhood library on the weekend and borrow some children's books that deal with parental divorce. Together she and her children would read the books.
- Mrs. Johnson would try to spend half an hour each evening with her children in some planned activity that the children helped choose.
- The nurse would revisit in 2 weeks to follow up on Mrs. Johnson's meeting with the school psychologist and to assess how the children had responded to the books on parental divorce and their mother's efforts to plan some activity with them each evening.

I Planned It This Way

I planned it this way you know.
I planned it to happen at the very height of Spring.
I loved the Spring.
The time of rebirth, remember, this is a new beginning for me.
Bert loved the Spring too you know.
Remember our big garden?
Oh how I enjoyed our big garden, snapping the beans while sitting in the swing, Bert cooking pork chops on the grill, watermelon, ice cream …
Oh how I love my home and Bert, and my children, my family, my church, my community, all of you.
I liked to keep my house in order you know.
So I decided it was a good time for me to go home, back with Bert again,
At the very height of Spring.

—*Dr. Judith A. Barton, written about her mother-in-law after her death*

Judith A. Barton, PhD, RN

Conclusion

Understanding the family as a focal unit for nursing care will become more important in the future as healthcare delivery increasingly takes place in community settings. A family is two or more individuals who manifest some degree of interdependence in their interaction with each other and their environment in meeting basic needs for affection and meaning. The family lifecycle is described in terms of developmental stages corresponding to major family events—in particular, the addition and exiting of members.

Families who are likely to have the most difficulty coping with lifecycle transitions are those who experience a large number of concurrent lifecycle changes involving transitions of great magnitude; who have a small, nonsupportive social network; and who live in a community with few resources to assist them.

Health responsibilities of the family include (1) provision of opportunities for members to achieve a sense of personal identity and work, (2) emotional support and cognitive guidance for members experiencing lifecycle transitions, (3) education of members about how to maintain health and when and how to use professional services, (4) the socialization of members to value health and to accept personal responsibility for its maintenance, and (5) care provision for chronically ill, disabled, or aging family members. To fulfill its health responsibilities, the family needs sufficient energy and knowledge to invest in goal-directed behavior.

Nurses' work with families is facilitated through the use of a conceptual framework for collecting, organizing, and interpreting data about how the family is fulfilling its health responsibilities and issues and concerns they are experiencing. The self-efficacy model for nurse–family intervention involves a contracting process in which the nurse and family pursue mutually established goals.

AFFORDABLE CARE ACT (ACA)

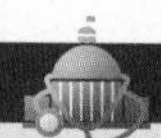

Children and young adults can stay on their parents' health insurance until the age of 26.

Coverage of services provided at freestanding birth centers is required.

Individuals are allowed to apply for and enroll in Medicaid, the Children's Health Insurance Program (CHIP), or the Exchange through a state-run website for families.

LEVELS OF PREVENTION

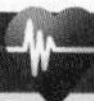

Primary: Educating parents about keeping prescription drugs safe in a home with children

Secondary: Assisting parents with locating resources for teens who are abusing prescription drugs at home

Tertiary: For the chronic drug user, providing guidance for the family in locating groups such as Al-Anon and other supportive resources in the community

HEALTHY ME

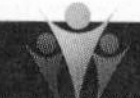

How does your family shape your ideas about health and illness? How did your family approach health education for their children?

Critical Thinking Activities

1. Reflect on your own experience in growing up in a family. Identify how your family met each of the five health responsibilities. How are your beliefs about health and ways to maintain your health similar to or different from those practiced in your family?
2. Using the Application to Practice on "Family Lifecycle Transition: Teenage Pregnancy," address the following questions:
   - What are some factors that may have led Nancy to become pregnant? As you answer this question, think about her life history.
   - What are the potential health threats to Nancy and her unborn baby, given her current health habits and living situation?
   - Using the framework for assessment presented in this chapter, how would you assess the family's current capacity to deal with this lifecycle transition given the information provided?
   - Which additional information would you want to gather?
   - Which ethical principles should guide your interactions with Nancy and her family?

References

Antonovsky, A. (1987). *Unraveling the mystery of health: How people manage stress and stay well.* San Francisco, CA: Jossey-Bass.

Bain, A. (1978). The capacity of families to cope with transition: A theoretical essay. *Human Relations, 8,* 675.

Boss, P. (1988). *Family stress management.* Newbury Park, CA: Sage.

Bronfenbrenner, U. (1986). Ecology of the family as a context for human development. Research perspectives. *Developmental Psychology, 22*(6), 723–742.

Burden, D. S. (1986). Single parents and the work setting: The impact of multiple job and homelife responsibilities. *Family Relations, 35*(1), 37–43.

Burton, L., & deVries, C. (1995). Challenges and rewards: African-American grandparents as surrogate parents. In L. M. Burton (Ed.), *Families and aging* (pp. 175–190). Amityville, NY: Baywood.

Carter, E. A., & McGoldrick, M. (Eds.). (1989). *The changing family life cycle: A framework for family therapists* (2nd ed.) New York, NY: Gardner Press.

Clinton, H. R. (1996). *It takes a village: And other lessons children teach us.* New York, NY: Touchstone Books.

Cole, R., Kitzman, H., Olds, D., & Sidora, K. (1998). Family context as a moderator of program effects in prenatal and early childhood home visitation. *Journal of Community Psychology, 26*(1), 37–48.

Cowan, P. A., Field, D., Hansen, D. A., Skolnick, A., & Swanson, G. E. (Eds.). (1992). *Family, self, and society: Toward a new agenda for family research.* Hillsdale, NJ: Lawrence Erlbaum.

Deatrick, J. A., Brennan, D., & Cameron, M. E. (1998). Mothers with multiple sclerosis and their children: Effects of fatigue and exacerbations on maternal support. *Nursing Research, 47*(4), 205–210.

Doherty, W. J. (1992). Linkages between family theories and primary health care. In R. Sawa (Ed.), *Family health care* (pp. 30–39). Newbury Park, CA: Sage.

Doherty, W. J., & Campbell, T. L. (1988). *Families and health.* Newbury Park, CA: Sage.

Duffy, M. E. (1988). Health promotion in the family: Current findings and directives for nursing research. *Journal of Advanced Nursing, 13,* 142–148.

Duvall, E. M., & Miller, B. L. (1985). *Marriage and family development* (6th ed.). New York, NY: Harper & Row.

Friedman, M. M. (1998). *Family nursing: Research, theory and practice* (4th ed.). Stamford, CT: Appleton & Lange.

Goldenberg, I., & Goldenberg, H. (1996). *Family therapy: An overview* (4th ed.). Monterey, CA: Brooks/Cole.

Hanson, S. M. H., & Boyd, S. T. (Eds.). (1996). *Family health nursing: Theory, practice and research.* Philadelphia, PA: F. A. Davis.

Hardy, M. E., & Conway, M. (1988). *Role theory: Perspectives for health professionals.* New York, NY: Appleton-Century-Crofts.

Houser, A., Gibson, M. J., Redfoot, D. L., & AARP Public Policy Institute. (2010). *Trends in family caregiving and paid home care for older people: Data from the National Long-Term Care Survey.* Retrieved from http://assets.aarp.org/rgcenter/ppi/ltc/2010-09-caregiving.pdf

Janosik, E. H., & Green, E. (1992). *Family life.* Boston, MA: Jones and Bartlett.

Kaiser Family Foundation. (2010). *Parents, media and public policy.* Menlo Park, CA: Author.

Kemp, L., Eisbacher, L., McIntyre, L., O'Sullivan, K., Taylor, J., Clark, T., & Harris, E. (2006). Working in partnership in the antenatal period: What do child and family health nurses do? *Contemporary Nurse: A Journal for the Australian Nursing Profession, 23*(2), 312–320.

Klein, D. M., & White, J. M. (1996). *Family theories: An introduction.* Thousand Oaks, CA: Sage.

Kramer, B. J., & Kipnis, S. (1995). Eldercare and work-role conflict: Toward an understanding of gender differences in caregiving burden. *The Gerontologist, 35*(3), 273–278.

Loveland-Cherry, C. (1996). Family health promotion and health protection. In P. J. Bomar (Ed.), *Nurses and family health promotion* (2nd ed., pp. 22–35). Philadelphia, PA: Saunders.

Luhby, T. (2012). Worsening wealth inequality by race. *CNN Money*. Retrieved from http://money.cnn.com/2012/06/21/news/economy/wealth-gap-race/

Lynch, I., & Tiedje, L. B. (1991). Working with multiproblem families: An intervention model for community health nurses. *Public Health Nursing, 8*(3), 147–153.

Newman, M. A. (1994). *Health as expanding consciousness* (2nd ed.). New York, NY: National League for Nursing Press.

O'Brien, R. A. (1979). *A conceptualization of family health. Clinical and scientific sessions.* Kansas City, MI: American Nurses Association.

O'Brien, R. A., & Robinson, A. G. (1984). Family as client. In J. A. Sullivan (Ed.), *Directions in community health nursing* (pp. 138–152). Boston, MA: Blackwell Scientific.

Popenoe, D. (1995). The American family crisis. *National Forum, 75*(3), 15–19.

Pratt, L. (1976). *Family structure and effective health behavior: The energized family.* Boston, MA: Houghton Mifflin.

Pratt, L. (1982). Family structure and health work: Coping in the context of social change. In H. I. McCubbin, A. E. Cauble, & J. M. Patterson (Eds.), *Family stress, coping, and social support* (pp. 73–89). Springfield, IL: Charles C Thomas.

Robinson, J. L., Emde, R. N., & Korfmacher, J. (1997). Integrating an emotional regulation perspective in a program of prenatal and early childhood home visitation. *Journal of Community Psychology, 25*(1), 59–75.

Rogers, M. E. (1983). Analysis and application of Rogers' theory of nursing. In J. W. Clements & F. B. Roberts (Eds.), *Family health: A theoretical approach to nursing care* (pp. 219–228). New York, NY: Wiley.

Satir, V. (1983). *Conjoint family therapy* (3rd ed.). Palo Alto, CA: Science and Behavior Books.

Sedgwick, R. (1981). *Family mental health: Theory and practice.* St. Louis, MO: Mosby.

Sieburg, E. (1985). *Family communication: An integrated systems approach.* New York, NY: Gardner Press.

Sloan, M. R., & Schommer, B. T. (1982). The process of contracting in community health nursing. In B. W. Spradley (Ed.), *Readings in community health nursing* (2nd ed., pp. 197–204). New York, NY: Little, Brown.

Smith, G. C., Tobin, S. S., & Fullmer, E. M. (1995). Elderly mothers caring at home for offspring with mental retardation: A model of permanency planning. *American Journal on Mental Retardation, 99*(5), 487–499.

UNAIDS, Joint United Nations Programme on HIV/AIDS. (2008). *UNAIDS 2008 report on the global AIDS epidemic.* Geneva, Switzerland: World Health Organization.

U.S. Department of Commerce. (2014). U.S. Census Bureau news. Retrieved from http://www.census.gov/housing/hvs/files/qtr413/q413press.pdf

U.S. Department of Health and Human Services (HHS). (2012). *Healthy people 2020.* Retrieved from http://www.healthypeople.gov/2020/default.aspx

Walsh, F. (Ed.). (1982). *Normal family processes.* New York, NY: Guilford Press.

Williamson, J. A. (1981). Mutual interaction: A model of nursing practice. *Nursing Outlook, 29*, 104.

Wright, L. M., & Leahey, M. (1994). *Nurses and families: A guide to family assessment and intervention* (2nd ed.). Philadelphia, PA: F. A. Davis.

Appendix: Family Assessment Guide

1. Family Composition and Identifying Data
    - Names, ages of family members
    - Address
    - Racial/ethnic background
    - Education/school attendance
    - Employment
    - Income
    - Health insurance
2. Environmental Data
    - Is housing adequate to meet the family's needs?
    - What are the characteristics of the immediate neighborhood and community?
    - What health and other basic services are available in the neighborhood? In the community?
    - What is the availability of public transportation?
    - How is the family prepared for disasters? How have they responded in the past?
3. Energy
    - What are the sources of energy for the family?
    - Is there sufficient energy to meet the varying health needs of its members? If not, where is the family's energy directed?
    - Does the expenditure of energy in meeting family demands occur repeatedly at the expense of one particular family member?
4. Consciousness
    - How aware and knowledgeable is the family of specific health and developmental needs of its members?
    - Does it hold incorrect beliefs that are likely to lead to unsound healthcare practices?
    - Is its perception of how it functions congruent with reality?
    - What are the sources that the family utilizes in acquiring knowledge?
    - Does the family actively seek to expand its level of consciousness or does it respond only to crisis demands?
    - How do past family experiences influence its consciousness about health issues?
5. Role Structure
    - Which roles do each of the family members fulfill?
    - How competently do members perform their roles?
    - How do past family experiences influence members' role performance?
    - If role strain or conflict exists, what are the contributing factors?
    - How are role conflicts resolved?
    - Is there flexibility in roles when needed?
6. Decision-Making Processes
    - Who makes which decisions?
    - Are there particular needs or issues that are not recognized or addressed?
    - Is the family able to discriminate between information that is relevant and information that is irrelevant to the decision?
    - Are alternative solutions generated and weighed?
    - Is the selected alternative implemented?
    - To what extent does family decision making involve consensus or coercion?
    - Does the mode of decision making affect its implementation?
    - Is the family satisfied with the results of its members' choices?
    - How does the family react to change?
7. Communication Patterns
    - Who talks to whom?
    - Which feelings or issues are closed to discussion?
    - Are members able to clearly state their needs and feelings?
    - Is there congruence between verbal and nonverbal aspects of communication?
    - How well do members listen when others are communicating?
    - Do members elicit feedback and validation in communicating with one another?
    - What are the predominant patterns of acknowledgment accorded varying members?
    - Is communication among members age appropriate?
8. Values
    - What are the important values held by the family?
    - To what extent do family values foster active coping and mastery of concerns?
    - What is the family's orientation to the past, present, and future?
    - What is the relative ranking of health in the family's hierarchy of values?
    - Are there value conflicts evident within the family, between the family and the subculture/community, or between the family and the nurse?
9. System Boundaries
    - Are family boundaries overly rigid or overly loose?
    - Which ongoing relationships does the family maintain with extended kin, friends, or other social groups?
    - To what degree do interactions with its support network foster or impede the family's abilities to cope with its health responsibilities?
    - Is the family satisfied with its support network?
    - To what extent is the family willing and able to access community services?

CHAPTER FOCUS

Thinking Differently About Family Health
- Thinking Upstream
- Thinking of a Bottom-Down Health System
- The Human Ecology Model: Thinking in Layers

Community-Based Services for Promoting Family Health
- Preventive Support Services for All Families
- Targeted Programs for More Vulnerable Families
- Families in Crisis

Characteristics of Successful Interventions: Creating Healthy Families and Communities
- Relationship-Focused Care
- Intensity and Timing of Interventions
- Nursing Skills and Strategies

Issues in Family Nursing Today

Values: A Challenge for the Future

QUESTIONS TO CONSIDER

After reading this chapter, you will know the answers to the following questions:

1. What is thinking upstream? What is its relevance to caring for families?
2. What are community-based services in the promotion of health for families?
3. What are characteristics of successful family interventions?
4. What is the nurse's role in relationship-focused care?
5. What are necessary nursing skills and strategies in promoting positive family interventions?
6. What are current issues in family nursing?
7. What are current nursing values?

Caring for families in health and illness is not new to nurses. Lillian Wald, Margaret Sanger, and Mary Breckenridge are a few of the nurses who helped establish a tradition of family care. Indeed, some count public health nurses as one of the unique contributions the United States has made to the cause of public health. Much has changed in the social and economic system since the days of Wald, Sanger, and Breckenridge. Each generation of nurses must reclaim this tradition of family care: keeping relevant wisdom of the past and learning new ways to help families in the ever-changing world in which we live.

CHAPTER 30

Caring for the Family in Health and Illness

Linda Beth Tiedje and
Karen Saucier Lundy

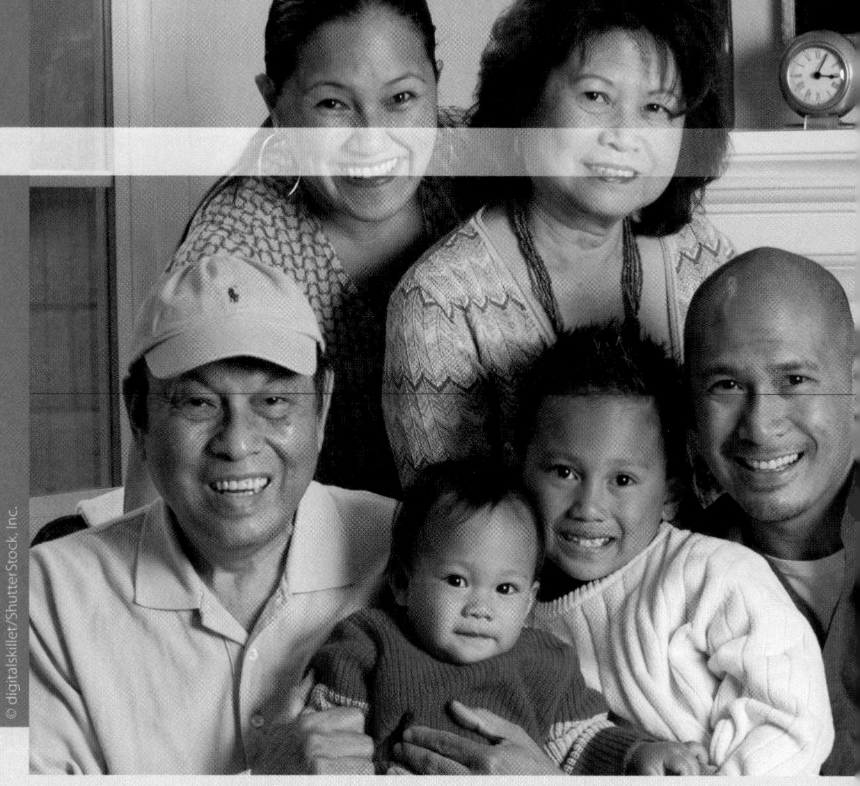

KEY TERMS

Ad Hoc Committee to Defend Health Care
bottom-down health system
caring
comprehensive community initiatives (CCIs)
courage
human ecology model
inclusion
intensity
intensive services
least possible contribution theory
nursing skills and strategies
preventive support services
reflective thinking
relationship-focused care
social responsibility
strength-based approach
targeted programs
think upstream
timing

> Call it a clan, call it a network, call it a tribe, call it a family: Whatever you call it, whoever you are, you need one.
>
> —Jane Howard

> In an ideal society, mothers and fathers would produce potty-trained, civilized, responsible new citizens while government and corporate leaders would provide a safe, healthy, economically just community.
>
> —Mary Kay Blakely

REFLECTIONS

Community health nurses most often come in contact with families who are experiencing illnesses or family dysfunctions. Think about how your own family has reacted to health and illness. Do your values about family health influence how you evaluate a family's health status? How does U.S. society assist or hinder families who are experiencing health risks?

WHAT IS FAMILY HEALTH, and what does it mean to care for the family in health and illness? Family health is a whole series of activities that are designed to promote health, to prevent disease and injury, to prevent premature death, and to create conditions in which we can all be safe and healthy (Levy, 1998). There are many examples of activities nurses do every day to promote family health:

- Supporting a family with a chronically ill child to find community resources and respite care
- Working with a family with a schizophrenic young adult to establish consistent drug therapy and vocational training
- Discussing eating patterns learned in families of origin when providing support and information for weight reduction
- Reflecting on family learned values as we attempt to understand others for whom health is not a priority
- Assessing whether other women in the family have breastfed in the process of helping a new mother initiate breastfeeding
- Working for the enforcement of laws that prohibit sales of tobacco to minors
- Being part of school curriculum committees to ensure a focus on social skills so that students learn skills such as sharing, listening to others, and working cooperatively in groups
- Teaching parenting competency skills in parent education classes
- Participating in community-based sex education committees
- Promoting awareness of the need for disaster preparedness, including terrorism
- Educating families about Internet use and abuse, and the importance of parental involvement

A more specific example of family nursing to prevent disease, injury, and premature death occurred in Hawaii. A group of emergency department (ED) nurses there noted the numbers of individual children who were coming to the ED as a result of drownings and near-drownings. Some of the children were resuscitated; others died. Over time the nurses collected data from families and found that none of the pools in which the children drowned had fences. Working with families, the fire department, and other community groups, they raised funds to help families fence their private pools, and the accidental drownings among children decreased. This is an example of a family-focused, community-targeted intervention that served to prevent disease and injury and premature death. Nurses in EDs each day save children in tertiary care settings; they can also move beyond this "downstream" approach, to thinking about how to work with families in *preventing* such accidents from occurring in the first place.

Thinking Differently About Family Health

As novice healthcare providers, we may view provision of health care to families as an "extra," a nonessential part of individually focused, technically oriented care. As we become more confident of our physical assessment, communication, and psychomotor skills, we learn that health care is more than the provision of individual-level physical care. Indeed, we begin to appreciate that factors at the level of the family, group, and society affect the health of individuals within them. Overall family health challenges us to think in new ways about influences on the family. Specifically, this new way of thinking challenges us to (1) **think upstream**, always asking, "What would have prevented this in the first place?" (Butterfield, 1991, 2002; McKinlay, 1979); (2) think of working with families in a **bottom-down health system** (Hancock, 1993) where homes and neighborhood meeting places are the basis of healthcare delivery, not hospitals; and (3) use the **human ecology model** (Bronfenbrenner, 1986) in thinking beyond what happens within individual families to factors outside families that influence family health.

Thinking Upstream

If we think of illness as people drowning in swiftly flowing water, thinking upstream means we have to think beyond rescuing people from the water and look upstream to see what is "pushing" the people into the dangerous water in the first place (McKinlay, 1979). Rescuing people is a "downstream endeavor." In health care, downstream endeavors are short-term, individually focused interventions such as lung transplants for two-pack-a-day smokers or treating myocardial infarctions instead of the sedentary, stressful lifestyles that lead to them. Upstream interventions focus on the social and physical environments in which families live. Upstream interventions focus on changing the behavioral, social, political, and environmental factors that lead to poor health, not waiting "downstream" for poor health to occur (Butterfield, 1991, 2002).

In the late 1990s and into the 21st century, school violence has erupted several times throughout the United States: Springfield, Oregon; Littleton, Colorado; Pearl, Mississippi; Paducah, Kentucky; Fayetteville, Tennessee; Jonesboro, Arkansas; the 2006 Amish school tragedy in Lancaster, Pennsylvania; and the horrific mass shooting of young children and their teachers at Sandy Hook Elementary School in Newtown, Connecticut in 2012. In the 14 months following the Sandy Hook shooting, 44 separate incidents of gun violence in educational settings were reported. At least 13 such incidents took place during the first 6 weeks of 2014—four of these in the span of just 8 days (Moms Demand Action/Mayors Against Illegal Guns, 2014). School violence has been an unpredictable and increasingly common phenomenon that has fueled a search for "answers." The answers and the causes, of course, are multifaceted. A steady diet of violent media, the availability of guns, increasing feelings of alienation and unchecked rage, lack of access to mental health services, racism, and poor communication within families are all implicated as causes. School violence is a complicated phenomenon with no easy answers. In the real world, downstream thinking (dealing with consequences of school violence) and upstream thinking (dealing with its prevention) are both required. To focus only on downstream thinking is a mistake. The other mistake often made is to focus blame on singular causes.

ENVIRONMENTAL CONNECTION

Family members with allergies can reduce allergens significantly by avoiding household products with added perfume, such as dryer sheets, carpet cleaner, and bathroom products.

President Bill Clinton, in a radio address to the nation (May 1, 1999), urged all citizens to focus on responsibility instead of blame. What responsibility could be taken by each citizen to help prevent such violence in the future? Thinking responsibly means thinking upstream about what would prevent such school violence in the first place. Consider these comments taken from a *USA Today* story the week of the Littleton, Colorado, shootings. Recall that in Littleton, the student gunmen targeted people of color and athletes:

- "I think one of our jobs as students is to include everybody; I would want to do that." Mario Francisco Penaiver, 18-year-old student from Puyallup, Washington.
- "These kids were not genetically programmed to be racist. They have been taught by the people around them." Stanley Wilson, 39, Montgomery, Alabama.
- "We, as a society, have to ask, 'What is the impact of a steady diet of violent media content on a growing child?'" Kathryn Montgomery, the Center for Media Education.
- Urging parents to take any guns in their homes to the police, Rosie O'Donnell, talk show host, said, "If you have a gun in the house, you are 43 times more likely to be a victim of gun violence."

The National Association of Attorneys General and the National School Boards Association have also published a manual with tips on preventing violence in schools, focusing on parents as a key in prevention. Some of the upstream thinking includes encouraging parents to participate and volunteer at school and encouraging students and teachers to talk about problems. The National School Safety Center also encourages parents to talk with their children about fears and feelings and to be part of their children's lives. Community health nurses, in the spirit of such upstream thinking, could start school-based parent groups. If parental involvement is one of the keys to prevention, parents need to know *how* to communicate, offer support, and open the dialogue. Community health nurse–led parent groups would be a preventive start. See the box for selected *Healthy People 2020* objectives focusing on families.

Thinking of a Bottom-Down Health System

Hancock (1993) suggests that instead of thinking of a healthcare delivery system based in tertiary or hospital-specialty-based care, we should focus on how to keep people healthy (see **Figure 30-1**). Such a system would be a health system, as opposed to the current illness-focused system. Most resources would then be prevention focused at the neighborhood and community levels. In a bottom-down health system, the services link people and families with others in support groups, neighborhood activities, parent training groups, early childhood education, and

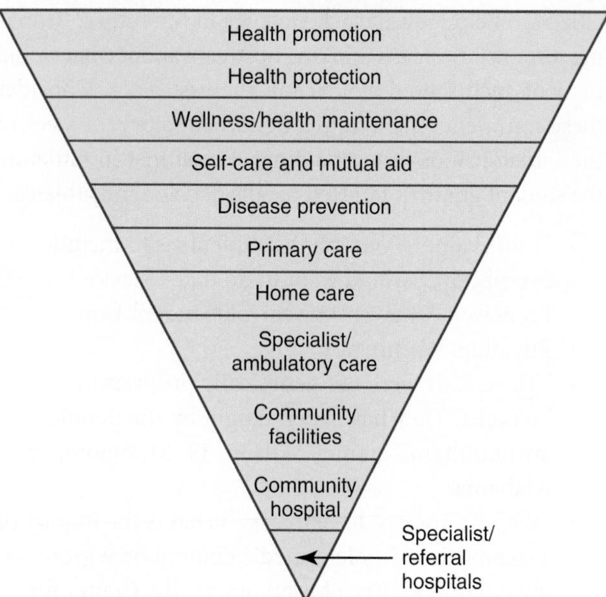

Figure 30-1 Bottom-down health system.

after-school recreation programs. Such services can be provided by primary care teams in the home and primary health centers based in schools and neighborhoods.

HEALTHY PEOPLE 2020 

Objectives Related to Families: Maternal, Infant, and Child Health

- MICH-20 Increase the proportion of infants who are put to sleep on their backs
- MICH-21 Increase the proportion of infants who are breastfed
- MICH-22 Increase the proportion of employers that have worksite lactation support programs

Nutrition and Overweight: Food Insecurity

- NWS-13 Reduce household food insecurity and in doing so reduce hunger

Older Adults: Long-Term Services and Supports

- OA-8 Reduce the proportion of noninstitutionalized older adults with disabilities who have an unmet need for long-term services and supports
- OA-9 Reduce the proportion of unpaid caregivers of older adults who report an unmet need for caregiver support services

Social Determinants of Health: Economic Stability

- SDOH-1 Proportion of children age 0–17 years living with at least one parent employed year round, full time
- SDOH-3 Proportion of persons living in poverty

Source: U.S. Department of Health and Human Services. (2012). *Healthy people 2020.* Retrieved from http://www.healthypeople.gov/2020/default.aspx

BOX 30-1 The Affordable Care Act (ACA) of 2010 and the Family

The ACA provided U.S. families more options and greater control over managing their health care by:

- Lowering healthcare costs through federal and state insurance exchanges.
- Expanding Medicaid to include more working families.
- Offering families more options for healthcare coverage that is more affordable, accessible, and secure
- Extending dependent coverage to the age of 26
- Providing preventive care for better healthcare outcomes
- Preventing denial of coverage for those who have preexisting conditions

The Human Ecology Model: Thinking in Layers

The family can be conceived of as an ecological system using general systems and human ecology theories. These theories focus on the external influences that affect families and their ability to function. These forces outside the family have a powerful influence on what goes on inside the family. Some of these systems outside the family are neighborhoods, institutions, the media, and government. The human ecology model (see **Figure 30-2**) shows how

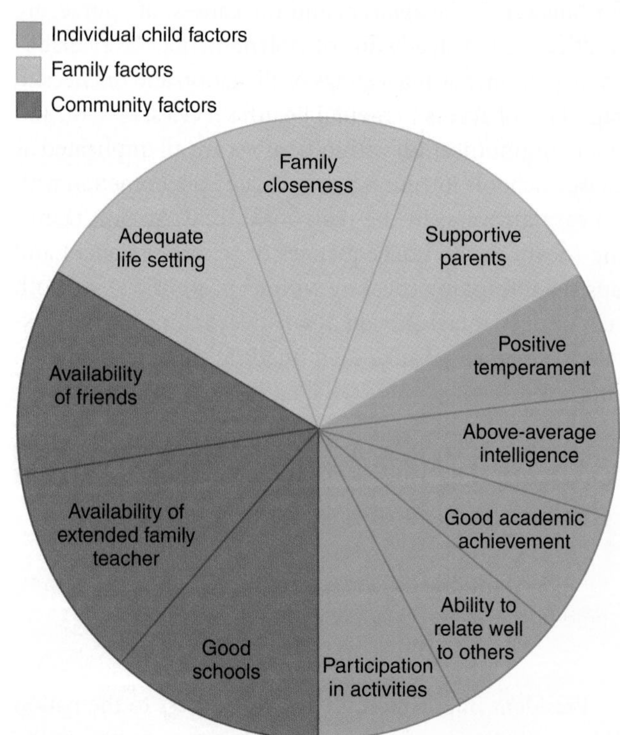

Figure 30-2 Factors that contribute to invulnerability or resistance of stress in children.

individual and family health are nested within and influenced by these macro-level forces, like Russian dolls stacked neatly one inside the other (Bronfenbrenner, 1986).

In this human ecology model, many factors inside and outside the family influence family health. Are community factors more important than family factors? Are individual factors more important than family factors? Are community factors more important than individual factors? Each of the three broad categories of factors—community, family, and individual—contributes about the same amount to making people within families—especially children—resilient and resistant to stress.

A bottom-down health system is based on the concept of social capital (Kawachi, Kennedy, Lochner, & Prothrow-Stith, 1997; Lomas, 1998) and the importance of increasing social cohesion in communities. Features of social capital in communities include "social organization such as networks, norms and trust that facilitate coordination and cooperation for mutual benefit" (Putnam, 1995, p. 66). This can be done by creating meeting places, sports leagues, clubs, and associations. Creating spaces in communities for people to come together allows for idea exchange and fosters trust. Building a community structure is the focus for health, not the individual (Minkler, 1998). Some experts now think that social capital is the most important determinant of our health (Lomas, 1998).

An example of building social cohesion in a community occurs in Grand Ledge, Michigan, each spring. On a spring weekend, several activities are planned to bring people of all ages together. Children gather to make May baskets to deliver to friends, and a May Pole dance is held at a city park. Other activities include a teddy bear tea, a quilt show, and a pie contest. Such community building is "for health" because it increases social contact. A vast group of studies has already linked social support networks to health outcomes (House, Landis, & Umberson, 1988). But more than that, research is emerging that supports the additional health benefits of cohesive, caring communities (Lomas, 1998).

RESEARCH ALERT 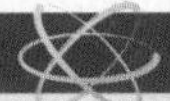

This meta review focused on recent research to identify implications for designing sustainable programs of psychosocial care for children and young people who are affected by disasters and terrorism. Recent research confirms previous knowledge that most children and young people are resilient, but also very vulnerable to the psychosocial effects of disasters. Most children are distressed in the immediate aftermath, until they recover a sense of safety from adults, predictable routines, and consistent support systems. Others may develop serious mental disorders, though posttraumatic mental disorders may not develop until weeks, months, or years later. Research instruments may be sensitive to cultural variability; simply translating measures into other languages is insufficient. International experience of different types of disasters and terrorist incidents suggests that the broad principles of good service design include integrating responses to the psychosocial needs of children and adolescents into general disaster preparedness and recovery plans, working with families rather than individual children to address their needs, identifying professionals who specialize in responding to disasters and are skilled in working with children prior to events, and focusing resources on increasing the capabilities of staff members of community facilities to recognize and respond to children's common reactions to trauma and to provide assistance.

Source: Williams, R., Alexander, D., Bolsover, D., & Bakke, F. (2008, July). Children, resilience and disasters: Recent evidence that should influence a model of psychosocial care. *Current Opinion in Psychiatry, 21*(4), 338–344.

Most traditional interventions focus mainly on individuals, occasionally on families, and less often on institutions and communities. For example, when a community health nurse makes a home visit to an adolescent mother, her baby, and her extended family, traditionally, the primary focus has been on individuals within that family, such as how much the baby weighs and health follow up for mother and baby. Bronfenbrenner (1986) would encourage us also to look at the family and community: Does the workplace or school have a designated place for women to privately breastfeed or pump milk? Do friends support the adolescent mother by providing child care from time to time? What encouragement is the mother receiving to return to school? Does the mother have a list of friends she can call when she needs to talk? What messages do the media (e.g., television, the Internet, magazines) provide to adolescent women? Do local churches provide quality drop-in child care? What are school policies regarding child care for adolescent parents? What are government programs for employment or educational support for teen parents? Does this adolescent mother have access to contraceptive services?

The human ecology model emphasizes, "the way we organize our society, the extent to which we encourage interaction among the citizenry, and the degree to which we trust and associate with each other in caring communities is probably the most important determinant of our health" (Lomas, 1998, p. 1181).

Community-Based Services for Promoting Family Health

Recall that in the introduction to this chapter one aspect of family health was to create conditions in which we can all be safe and healthy. "Every community must have a range of family-based programs, starting with **preventive support services** for all families, continuing through **targeted programs** for more vulnerable families, and ending with highly **intensive services** for families in crisis" (Children's Defense Fund, 1994, p. 4).

Preventive Support Services for All Families

In contrast to the United States, where programs are most commonly developed for "at-risk" groups with problems, in other parts of the world community-based social support for all families is part of a comprehensive program of health care. *All* families receive postpartum home visits after they leave the hospital, and health visitors continue to see *all* families of preschool children on a regular basis (Crockenberg, 1985; Heaman, Chalmers, Woodgate, & Brown, 2007; Kemp et al., 2006).

Another example of preventive support services for all families is a preterm birth prevention program begun in France, based on a communitywide public health approach. In contrast to approaches in the United States, which have unsuccessfully attempted to identify women at risk for preterm birth, in France all families, regardless of income, were targeted by a national media campaign. The purpose of the campaign was to make everyone more aware of symptoms of preterm labor. In addition, the effects of employment, such as long-term standing, were widely publicized as affecting preterm labor. This universal preterm birth prevention approach has become a successful national policy in France and has markedly reduced infant mortality there. France has been recognized as an international model in its efforts to focus on prevention of preterm births (Papiernik et al., 1986; World Health Organization, 2005).

Another example of preventive support services for all families is a widely disseminated program created by the Search Institute in Minneapolis. This program uses a **strength-based approach** and focuses on building assets broadly in all individuals, families, and communities (Hill, 2008; Laursen, 2000; Roehlkepartain, 1995). The assumptions include that all people and environments possess strengths that can be used toward improving their quality of life and that all environments, even the most bleak, contain resources.

ETHICAL CONNECTION 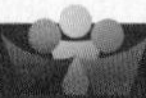

Parents often seek advice from community health nurses about the need for circumcision of infant boys. What are the ethical considerations for the nurse in assisting parents with such decisions?

APPLICATION TO PRACTICE 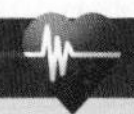

Key Concept: The Human Ecology Model

Think of an individual patient you have taken care of in the past. List family, neighborhood, community, media, and government factors that influence his or her health or illness. Then identify one prevention-targeted intervention that would help prevent disease and injury or promote health. For example, research has established connections between asthma and the exposure to environmental chemicals and passive smoke. In addition to treating asthma (tertiary care), a more prevention-oriented approach would examine family, neighborhood, community, media, and government factors that influence asthma and then develop interventions targeted at prevention of these factors. For instance:

- *Government*: Email legislators about air quality standards.
- *Media*: Use principles of marketing, public relations, and advertising to design a public service campaign working with the state health department, such as public service announcements or a website to increase awareness of asthma and who is affected. Use experts such as William DeJong and Jay Winsten, who wrote *The Media and the Message: Lessons Learned from Past Public Service Campaigns* (which provides guidelines and is available from the National Campaign to Prevent Teen Pregnancy, 2100 M Street NW, Suite 300, Washington, DC, 20037).
- *Community*: Petition local restaurants to provide no-smoking sections or to ban smoking indoors.
- *Neighborhood*: Plan neighborhood health fairs, with information about how to avoid use of tobacco.
- *Family*: Role-play with patients ways to persuade those they live with not to expose them to passive smoke.
- *Individual*: Encourage those with asthma to write about their stressful experiences. One study documented the positive effects of such a writing intervention for people with asthma (Smyth, Stone, Hurewitz, & Kaell, 1999).

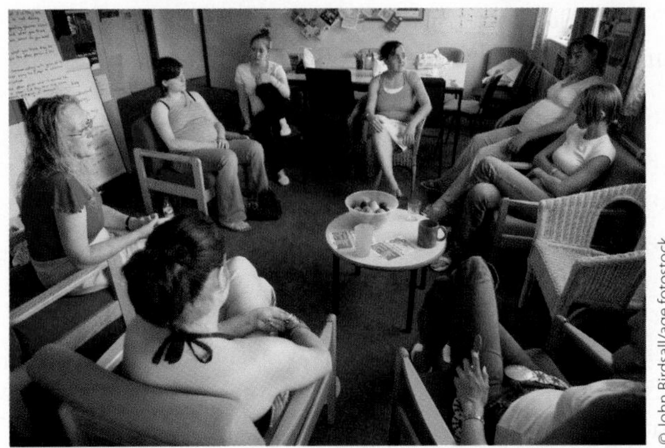

Nurses work to promote health with teen mothers through hands-on education and by including family members in interventions.

Targeted Programs for More Vulnerable Families

What does an "at-risk" family look like? Who is vulnerable? Some define vulnerable populations as groups who experience limited resources and have a consequent high risk for morbidity and premature mortality (Flaskerud & Winslow, 1998), such as families with a chronically ill child who do not have respite care. Families who are least likely to cope with lifecycle transitions are those defined to be most at risk, such as families with a history of abuse who are moving to a new city with a new baby. Vulnerable families might also have a small and nonsupportive social network or live in communities with few available services. All of these factors may make families at risk from time to time.

For example, during the 2005 Hurricane Katrina disaster, the most vulnerable families in New Orleans suffered the most, and not just from the storm itself. These families were unable to leave their homes because they lacked adequate transportation. When they did escape to expected safety in the New Orleans Convention Center and the Superdome, they found chaotic conditions there. Many died, and even more continue to face extreme health problems as a result of their ordeal.

Economic factors also help define risk in families, poverty being an especially potent factor. One-third of all children in the United States will live in poverty at some time before reaching adulthood. Surprisingly, fewer than 20% of poor families live in inner-city urban areas (Federman et al., 1996; Tandon, 2007). Individuals in these poor families are indeed vulnerable, facing multiple problems such as joblessness, substance use, crime, violence, and poor schools. These multiproblem families vary in size, composition, location, and the nature of problems they present (Lynch & Tiedje, 1991).

RESEARCH ALERT 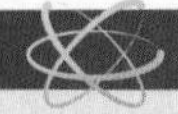

This article reviews family and conceptual research on the concept of family resilience. Family resilience is the successful coping of family members under adversity that enables them to flourish with warmth, support, and cohesion. An increasingly important realm of family nursing is to identify, enhance, and promote family resiliency. Prominent factors of resilient families include positive outlook, spirituality, family member accord, flexibility, family communication, financial management, family time, shared recreation, routines and rituals, and support networks. A family resilience orientation, based on the conviction that all families have inherent strengths and the potential for growth, provides the family nurse with an opportunity to facilitate family protective and recovery factors and to secure extrafamilial resources to help foster resilience.

Source: Black, K., & Lobo, M. (2008). A conceptual review of family resilience factors. *Journal of Family Nursing, 14*(1), 33–55.

APPLICATION TO PRACTICE 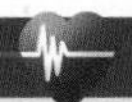

Strength-Based Approaches

At a prenatal clinic, a nurse approached a teenage mother and her boyfriend with their new baby who seemed thin for her age of 6 weeks. The father was holding the baby and burping her, vigorously pounding on her back. Overcoming her urge to negatively comment on the father's burping technique, the nurse asked how things were going. The family related that the baby had already had surgery for pyloric stenosis and had several repeat visits at child health clinic to check on her small head circumference. Later in a discussion with other families in the clinic waiting room, the father strongly voiced his opinion that babies needed lots of holding and "couldn't be spoiled." Reflecting back on this encounter, if the nurse had acted on her initial impulse to judge this teen couple and their childcare techniques, she would have missed the opportunity to see their real strengths: attentiveness at keeping healthcare appointments, shared care of the child, and knowing that the child needed holding and touch.

1. How could the nurse be most effective in working with this young family?
2. What might be a priority intervention for these parents?

Although not all poor families are multiproblem families, certain family qualities help define families as multiproblem. Women in multiproblem families often feel exploited and powerless in relationships with males. Men in these families, if present, often do not see themselves as responsible for taking care of children either physically or emotionally. Children in multiproblem families depend on proximal control and lack home orientation to school norms (Lynch & Tiedje, 1991; Tandon, 2007). These defining qualities are not intended as value judgments or descriptors for *each* family in this category. Multiproblem families have problems both within the family and between the family and the wider community. They often feel insecure and fearful in the wider community. Multiproblem families span both vulnerable and crisis family categories and are known for both the chronic problems that make them vulnerable and the crises they frequently experience. Comprehensive, community-based services targeting family economics, social support, and education are more successful with multiproblem families than services that focus narrowly on one type of problem at a time.

NOTE THIS!

Refugee Families

In 1999 in Kosovo, thousands of families were displaced, causing crisis and chaos. Once refugee camps were established to provide for basic needs, schools were set up to provide education and a unifying social support for the families. Finally, the United Nations trained preventive mental health workers to work with groups of children. Healthcare workers assisted the children in playing games, telling stories, and expressing their grief, because many of them were separated from parents. The components of these interventions are common to interventions for all families in crisis.

Families in Crisis

A family may be in crisis for several reasons. Families may run out of food. Home fires may leave a family without shelter. Families in which physical and emotional abuse occur are certainly families in crisis. Families displaced by war, terrorism, and natural disasters are also families in crisis. Regardless of the cause, interventions to help families in crisis share common components. First, their basic needs of food, clothing, and shelter must be provided for and their safety ensured. Next, both social and community support networks must be initiated or maintained. Finally, longer term mental health prevention programs must be referred to or established.

Characteristics of Successful Interventions: Creating Healthy Families and Communities

Launching and sustaining work with families are difficult. Successful nursing interventions with families contain several similar components: (1) **relationship-focused care**, (2) attention to **intensity** and **timing** of the interventions, and (3) particular **nursing skills and strategies**.

Relationship-Focused Care

The ability of sensitive nurses to develop ongoing, meaningful relationships with families makes a difference in the ultimate effectiveness of an intervention. Nursing is more than a series of tasks to be performed "on" families or information delivered to educate them. Through interactions with families, nurses weave a "tapestry of care" (Gordon, 1997). Interpersonal connections become the foundation for effectively influencing health behaviors and helping people take charge of their health and healing (Heaman et al., 2007; Kemp et al., 2006; Remen, 1996; Tanner, 1995; Zerwekh, 1997).

Intensity and Timing of Interventions

Programs with successful results offer opportunities for multiple contacts with families over a short time. Programs during the childbearing years are particularly useful because they furnish potential continuity over time and multiple contacts. Multiple contacts in and of themselves do not ensure success, however. Other factors, such as provider credibility, are also important for successful results.

School-based clubs and groups offer opportunities for multiple contacts over time. One such group, begun by a school nurse, targeted preadolescent girls, who during the second decade of life appear to be substantially more vulnerable than boys to environmental and psychological

RESEARCH ALERT 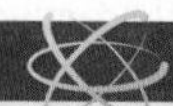

Several North American studies have found a connection between domestic violence and animal abuse. This article reports on the first Australian research to examine this connection. A group of 102 women recruited through 24 domestic violence services in the state of Victoria and a non–domestic violence comparison group (102 women) recruited from the community took part in the study. Significantly higher rates of partner pet abuse, partner threats of pet abuse, and pet abuse by other family members were found in the violent families compared with the non–domestic violence group. As hypothesized, children from the violent families were reported by their mothers to have witnessed and committed significantly more animal abuse than children from the nonviolent families. Logistic regression analyses revealed, for the group as a whole, that a woman whose partner had threatened the pets was five times more likely to belong to the intimate partner violence group.

Source: Volant, A., Johnson, J., Gullone, E., & Coleman, G. (2008). The relationship between domestic violence and animal abuse: An Australian study. *Journal of Interpersonal Violence, 23*(9), 1277–1295.

stressors (Pipher, 1994). A school nurse started a girls club with girls from the 4th grade. The girls met weekly over the noon hour at school, at first to talk. A softball team, field trips to sporting and cultural events, and a presentation on grooming and hygiene were soon club activities. Such a club, building assets such as self-esteem and communication skills, is health promoting and helps prevent adolescent pregnancy. Positive, asset-building activities with preadolescent girls are prime examples of intensive interventions.

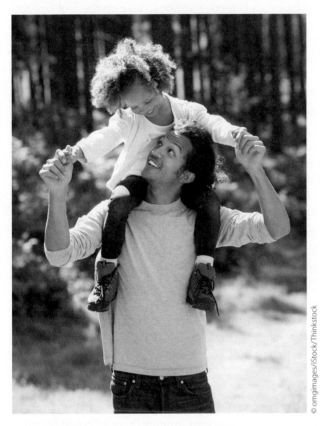

The family provides the framework for learning from parents and siblings about health risks and health behavior.

Nursing Skills and Strategies

Nurses delivering interventions to families must have skills specific to the intervention delivered. Five skills are particularly important: communicating, problem solving, listening, connecting, and evaluating.

Communicating

In addition to the skills nurses need to communicate, communication is a core issue in families and communities. Community health nurses can facilitate communication and also teach particular communication skills to people in families and groups. The following program example is one way nurses may provide parents with practical advice about ways of communicating with their children. The content area is human sexuality.

In New York, Jo Leonard and Marcia Siegel (1998) implemented a workshop for mothers and daughters called "Mother–Daughter Workshop: Getting Your Period." Offering the class to girls ages 9 to 13, no class was bigger than eight mother–daughter pairs. The class was based on the premise that parents are the first and most important sexuality educators and that family support and guidance have a significant effect on sexual activity. The class provided opportunities for parents and children to practice communicating about sexuality. It also provided opportunities to ask questions about sexuality in a neutral atmosphere. The class is a prime example of a strategy nurses may use to enhance family communication.

APPLICATION TO PRACTICE 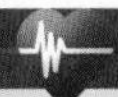

Establishing Trust for Relationship-Focused Care

At the request of a children's clinic, a nurse made a home visit because clinic personnel were concerned that a 6-month-old child had not been brought in for cast changes. The cast was the result of treatment for congenital foot deformities. At the first home visit, the mother was guarded and uncommunicative and admitted the nurse to her home with obvious reluctance. The dominant feature in the dark, cluttered room was a slate pool table. The nurse, sensing that so costly an item in all probability was highly prized, shared that observation with the mother. The nurse then admired the pool table, noting its many features. The mother responded immediately. She explained at length about how much it meant to the family to have it, how friends and neighbors gathered to use it, and its contribution to her life. She then angrily described the previous nurse who had scolded her for spending money foolishly instead of using her resources to better meet the needs of her children. She was grateful to the current nurse for being a more understanding person and immediately switched the conversation to questions she had about her children. She then proceeded to plan with the nurse how she could arrange for necessary clinic follow up for the 6-month-old, thanked the nurse for all her help, and asked when she would return.

Source: Lynch, I., & Tiedje, L. B. (1991). Working with multiproblem families: An intervention model for community health nurses. *Public Health Nursing, 8*(3), 147–153.

> Most people learn how to avoid emotional hijackings from the time they are infants. If they have supportive and caring adults around them, they pick up the social cues that enable them to develop self-discipline and empathy.
>
> —Hillary Rodham Clinton, 1996, in *It Takes a Village*

In addition to intensity, most family interventions require time and living through difficulties. Family interventions do not provide immediate answers; it takes time for families to experiment with new ideas and strategies. It also takes time for families to come to their own solutions.

For example, there is a growing number of community-based programs for couples who present for domestic violence counseling and want to be treated jointly (Dawe & Harnett, 2007; Johannson & Tutty, 1998; LaTaillade, Epstein, & Werlinich, 2006). Although controversial, in cases of domestic abuse, the conjoint treatment of couples is increasing because unless both men and women are treated, the cycle of abuse repeats even when a relationship with a particular abusive partner ends. Conjoint treatment requires patience and time. Most conjoint groups last 12 weeks and are preceded by gender-specific (all-men or all-women groups), 24-week treatment groups. The conjoint groups are often held in community centers, schools, or YWCAs and emphasize alternatives to domestic violence. Cessation of physical violence between the partners is a condition for group membership.

MEDIA MOMENT 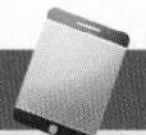

Bradshaw On: The Family: A New Way of Creating Solid Self-Esteem (1996)

By John Bradshaw, Deerfield Beach, Florida: Health Communications, Inc.

John Bradshaw is a well-recognized speaker and author on the family and addiction, recovery, and spirituality. This book is based on his 1984 television series. Bradshaw contends that the patriarchal model of childrearing is outdated and calls for a more democratic model of family relations. The book provides insights into the evolution of parenting and family relations and suggests how to create healthier families.

GLOBAL CONNECTION 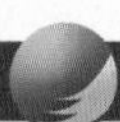

Families in many parts of the world are given paid leave after a child's birth. In many Scandinavian countries, women or men can take as much as 6 months paid leave to stay with their newborn baby.

MEDIA MOMENT 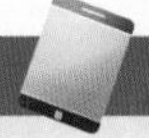

Life as a House (2001)

Faced with a diagnosis of terminal cancer, George (Kevin Kline) decides to construct a beautiful new house on his land overlooking the Pacific Ocean, while at the same time trying to connect with his estranged son (Hayden Christensen). Kristin Scott Thomas and Mary Steenburgen co-star in a drama that speaks eloquent volumes about the fragility—and resilience—of the human condition within the family.

Problem Solving

Problem solving is a skill that must be done with—and not for—families and communities. Nurses may have "rescue fantasies" as helpers, wanting to take on the problem and tell others what to do. Coming to terms with who owns the problem leads to mutual goal setting and gives patients the power of solving their own problems.

For example, a nurse in a prenatal clinic was discussing the importance of finishing high school with a pregnant mother who had dropped out of school. The pregnant woman was accompanied by her mother, who also was a high school dropout. As the nurse talked with both women, it was obvious that the grandmother was proud of her longstanding job as a hotel maid. She also believed high school had been unnecessary for her achievement. For the nurse to assume an authoritarian, directive role in this situation and insist on high school completion would have been unproductive. Instead, talking with the mother and daughter about education, jobs, and life success over the course of the pregnancy helped the nurse better understand the mother–daughter perspective. The mutual problem solving that evolved enabled the daughter to "own the problem" of high school completion and take the necessary steps for it to happen.

Listening

Nurses have vast amounts of health information to share with families and communities in an effort to improve health outcomes. Often, our first impulse is to give advice and information. Sometimes, especially in response to particular patient questions, advice is appropriate. However, we have entered an era in which health information is no longer a commodity exclusively owned by health systems. Many individuals, families, and communities can access health information from many sources. Self-care and wellness reflect a growing awareness that maintaining and enhancing health is a shared enterprise between providers and consumers. In such a shared enterprise, listening becomes a more vital skill. What does the patient already know? Which experiences has the patient already had? Listening through storytelling has recently been reclaimed as a powerful educational and therapeutic tool (Banks-Wallace, 1998). When a nurse truly listens to patients' or families' stories, he or she can more fully understand where they are coming from. Storytelling can reveal the way patients and families think about health issues, as well as gaps in their understanding. The use of storytelling as an educational tool also has been expanded to include groups of patients within prenatal and other clinical settings (Banks-Wallace, 1999; Carter, 2008; Nelson, McClintock, Perez-Ferguson, Shawver, & Thompson, 2008).

Connecting

Caring for families in health and illness requires the ability to connect with other agencies and programs, to coordinate and reinforce interventions. Being assertive, phoning other providers, planning family meetings—all these actions require skill and a definite lack of shyness! Nurses often know the many other agencies involved with a family and initiate care conferences to coordinate services. Long before case managers were popular, community health nurses were coordinating services for individuals and families. It is nurses who often are the best patient advocates, articulating family needs for and with families.

During the late 1980s and the early 1990s, an approach emerged to facilitate connecting: **comprehensive community initiatives (CCIs)**. Instead of focusing on one type of problem at a time, CCIs focus on creating systems of comprehensive services (e.g., health care, social services, education, housing) through a variety of programs and community building to better the lives of urban poor families (Stagner & Duran, 1997). The overall purpose is to provide neighborhood conditions in which families can succeed. CCIs share certain attributes such as emphasizing participation and providing a variety of services with their predecessors: settlement houses (early 1900s), neighborhood programs (1930s), war on poverty programs (1960s), and community action agencies (1970s).

Evaluating

Outcomes of what community health nurses do are important. To measure outcomes, evidence-based practice guidelines are especially critical. In addition to evaluating interventions with individuals and families, nurses are often asked to serve on evaluation teams to review the impact of community planning or intervention efforts. Traditional evaluation methods include pretesting and post-testing, interviews, surveys, record review, and focus groups (Minkler, 1998). A new approach that expands on some of these traditional methods is called *empowerment evaluation*. It is used as a tool for both evaluation and community building (Fetterman, Kaftarian, & Wandersman, 1996).

Empowerment evaluation was used in the evaluation of a human immunodeficiency virus (HIV) prevention community planning effort funded by the Centers for Disease Control and Prevention and consists of four steps. The first step in the empowerment evaluation process is taking stock. This involves a review of documents (e.g., budgets, reports, organizational charts) and interviews and focus groups with community participants to uncover background experiences. The purpose of this step is to reveal a common history and broad shared experience. In the second step, setting goals, the evaluator helps community group members identify where they want to go and the kind of evaluation they want to create. Note that the evaluation process is not a preconceived idea of the evaluator.

The third step, developing strategies, is often difficult. Uneasy group dynamics and underfunding often create hassles and obstacles as communities struggle to decide on particular strategies to meet high expectations. In the example of the HIV prevention planning, one team encountered many difficulties when generating strategies. In an effort to overcome these difficulties, participants were asked to name the biggest hassle of community planning and to identify what they particularly appreciated in each of the other participants. The written responses were then organized into hassles, uplifts, and ways of changing course. These responses were circulated and then discussed at a community meeting. This helped the participants move beyond the difficulties to the work they needed to do: developing strategies.

The fourth and final step of empowering evaluation is documenting the process—that is, keeping a written record of what occurred and why, in a way accessible to all participants. The usefulness of this step was apparent in the HIV prevention planning process when the planning group, after nearly a year, faced some difficult decisions. Planning group members were on a 3-day retreat and faced a vote about how to proceed. Behind-the-scenes maneuvering, miscommunication, and longstanding alliances left the planners angry and divided. The empowering evaluation team found some data collected after an ice breaker exercise early in the planning process when participants had been asked to share their personal mottoes and messages for the world. One of the messages was from a group member who had died of acquired immune deficiency syndrome (AIDS) just a few months before. Stunned, the group was reminded of their collective vision, and they were then able to vote in a more unified spirit. This use of data is a prime example of how documenting the process can be used to empower communities in evaluation efforts (Roe, Berenstein, Goette, & Roe, 1996).

The five nursing skills and strategies of communicating, problem solving, listening, connecting, and evaluating are a necessary foundation for community health nurses as they seek to provide services to individuals, families, and communities. These skills are necessary but not sufficient in a healthcare system where changes are massive, swift, and without precedent. Therefore, in the next section, issues in family nursing resulting from large-scale integrated healthcare enterprises, managed care plans, intense market competition, and a pervasive concern for operational efficiency and cost reduction are discussed.

Issues in Family Nursing Today

The healthcare climate in which we practice may constrain what we want to do with families and communities. For example, many states have community programs in which nursing visits are reimbursed in a fragmented way for childbearing families: maternal support services for mothers; infant support services for children; Women, Infants, and Children (WIC) for nutrition; and family planning services for contraception. The "family" sees many healthcare providers, with little concern for coordination of services. As nurses, we may find ourselves in situations we have not created and without much power. It is difficult—but not impossible—to provide family-centered care in an environment that reimburses for individual services and that is not designed for time with families. The nation's estimated 2.7 million nurses make up the clinical backbone of the care delivery system (Bureau of Labor Statistics, 2012). Nurses are uniquely suited in this emerging healthcare system. We have the exact skills the healthcare delivery system needs: communicating, problem solving, listening, connecting, and evaluating.

Nursing reinvented itself in the past when social changes demanded it. Before the Great Depression, most nurses worked in private duty. As the depression grew worse, nurses moved into hospitals and were employed at a salary. We can reinvent ourselves again, as we have done before (Salmon, 1999). How do we accomplish this reinvention?

One strategy is based on the **least possible contribution theory** (Weisman, 1981). A little can go a long way, and the least possible contribution is the one with the best chance of making a difference, however small. Making one small, seemingly insignificant contribution furnishes a foundation on which one can continue to add other contributions until something surprising but substantial results. Of course, least possible contribution does not mean doing as little as possible. Least possible contribution means doing something that the nurse is really good at and something that is only a little bit beyond the ordinary (Weisman, 1981).

GOT AN ALTERNATIVE?

Gentle massage for infants has been linked to improvements with sleep and food intolerance.

RESEARCH ALERT 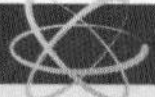

A caring inquiry grounded in the hermeneutic–phenomenological philosophical perspectives was conducted to uncover the family experience of living with childhood chronic illness. The purpose of this study was to describe and interpret the family's experience and to sensitize healthcare professionals about this experience. The presence of a child with chronic illness in a family is a unique, yet not uncommon experience. Chronic illness is both a personal misfortune and a sign of progress. No longer solely terminal, but still not thoroughly curable, these illnesses become illnesses to live with.

Data were generated from audiotaped interviews, photographs taken by the families, the artwork of the children, and the researcher's journaling. Eight family interviews and 32 individual interviews were the source of text for analysis. Data analysis was guided by a caring inquiry combining the hermeneutic–phenomenological approaches of van Manen and Ray and other philosophers.

The analysis included several levels of reflection. The first level of reflection revealed the descriptions and themes of the families. The families' metaphor of "traveling a different road" also emerged. In the second level of reflection, literature and poetry were used to illuminate the experiences of these families, and the themes were linguistically transformed into the seven meta-themes of the experience: "embodiment of illness: being in tune"; "temporal changes: living with uncertainty"; "relationships: creating a caring community"; "interacting with our environment: being aware"; "endowing the illness with meaning: understanding the illness"; "confronting death, affirming life: living with dying"; and "a spiritual transcendence: faith, hope, and love." Through deeper reflection, the unity of meaning, "a way of life: a new beginning each day," was revealed as metaphor. A theory of coming to understand the meaning of chronic illness, "a way of life: a new beginning each day" integrates the themes, meta-themes, and family metaphor. This research makes a strong plea for transforming healthcare delivery for children with chronic illnesses from a medically based, categorical, illness structure to an experiential, holistic, family-centered process. Implications for healthcare professionals in practice, education, healthcare policy development, and research are described.

Source: Hagedorn, M. I. E. (1993). *A way of life: A new beginning each day: The family's lived experience of childhood chronic illness.* Doctoral dissertation, University of Colorado Health Sciences Center.

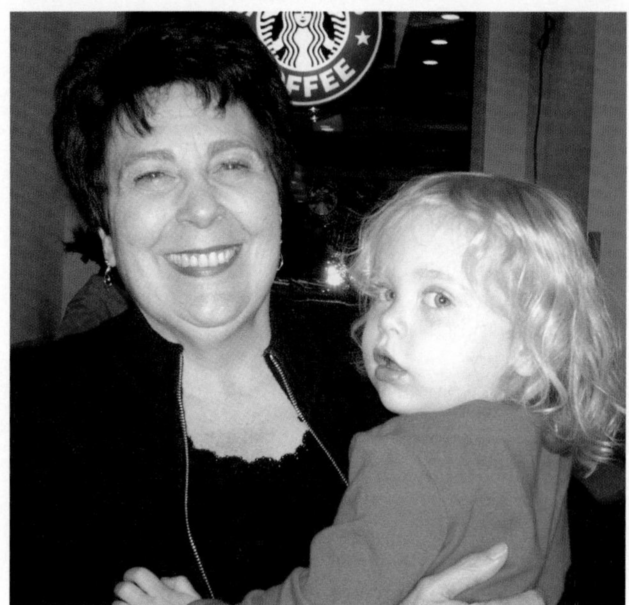

Children form a healthy self-identity through positive and caring relationships in the family.

An example of the least possible contribution theory in action occurred in 1997 when a group of Massachusetts healthcare providers created the **Ad Hoc Committee to Defend Health Care**. Together these physicians and nurses worked to reestablish caregiving from those who were trying to make health care a business driven by the bottom line. This committee has become a national movement against "a corporate-driven health care system" (Shindul-Rothschild, 1998). The committee's agenda was based on the following legislative initiatives: (1) Give the public information so that they can make informed choices, (2) assure patients that they will be cared for by registered nurses, and (3) extend whistle-blower protection to all healthcare workers so that they are not put in the position of choosing between a job and advocacy for patients. Only through such group efforts can the healthcare delivery scale be tilted back toward care instead of profits. Human and capital resources can then be put back into direct patient care instead of where the true inefficiencies lie in the delivery system—in the huge administrative overhead.

Values: A Challenge for the Future

The value of inclusion rather than exclusion and the embracing of diversity as a means of enriching the social fabric remain two of our greatest challenges in community health. Perhaps the Hurricane Katrina national disaster and our perceived vulnerability to acts of terrorism have made these challenges to the U.S. public more essential to our wellbeing as a nation. To deliver relationship-focused care to families, nurses must get emotionally free to focus on the family without judgment or bias. As nurses we may perceive people's situations differently because of our own value systems, which are created by our own experiences. We live in a heterogeneous society, a society with many different kinds of people and families. There are recent immigrant families from all over the world, as well as families whose ancestors came from Northern Europe, England, Eastern and Southern Europe, and Scandinavia. We must not simply assess minorities for cultural norms, customs, and rituals; the majority culture also has cultural norms, customs, and rituals that must be owned. To ignore cultural assessment of everyone is to imply that the majority culture is the "norm" and is beyond assessing.

The structure of families is also increasingly diverse: single parent, two parent, gay or lesbian parent, and so on. Therefore, healthcare providers often find themselves relating to families that are different from the ones they grew up in either in culture or in structure. It is common when confronting such differences to feel strange or uncomfortable. Sometimes, healthcare providers react by thinking of ways all people and families are alike, such as that we all have similar needs (e.g., food, clothing, shelter) and we all need love and affection. As healthcare providers, we also need to preserve the differences in people and families. That is more difficult. At times, we may just want everyone to be like us.

To better meet the values challenges of a diverse culture, three activities are outlined in this section. The first is a self-assessment quiz in **Box 30-2** to increase value and community awareness. The second is a critical thinking exercise in **Box 30-3** about providing support for families when there are scarce resources. Decisions about such family support ultimately involve values. The third activity is to recall how core nursing values may help us meet the challenges of a diverse society.

In the area of values, looking where we have come from may help us in where we are going. Nursing may provide guidance to meeting the values challenges in providing care to families and communities in a diverse culture. Salmon (1999) reminds us that there are five core values in nursing: **caring**, **courage**, **inclusion**, **reflective thinking**, and **social responsibility**. The value of caring is what has allowed us to move from the "doing for" approach to the current focus on enabling and empowering. The second value of courage needs to be shared and taught with exemplars and living models. We need to share and call attention to the daily courageous acts of nurses, particularly as they care for diverse groups. The third nursing value of inclusion seems most appropriate for the values challenge of working with diverse groups. But have we as

BOX 30-2 Self-Assessment Quiz for Providers Working with Families and Communities

In the spirit of thinking of similarities and differences in people, this self-assessment is intended as a means for you as a provider to become more aware of your values. In addition, questions 4 to 9 are intended to assess your awareness of your community, because community cohesion and the degree to which you associate with others in creating caring communities will be important to your success as a community health nurse.

1. Do you respect others' beliefs?
2. Do you believe that life is good and positive?
3. What is your ethnic/cultural heritage? List some norms/customs/rituals.
4. When was the last time you took public transportation?
5. Have you given blood recently?
6. Have you ever served on a jury?
7. How many of your neighbors do you know by name?
8. When was the last time you went to a free public event or amusement like a museum or the zoo?
9. When was the last time you checked a book out of the local library?
10. Do you do volunteer work in your community?

Source: Questions 1 to 3 are based on Benson, 1996; questions 4 to 10 are based on a community quotient quiz adapted by the *Utne Reader* (Cordes & Walljasper, 1997).

nurses, so long marginalized and excluded, learned our lessons so well that we in turn oppress others? Consider Salmon on this point:

> I wonder what we teach our students about inclusion. Do they understand that our health care system serves only some people, and that more than 40 million others have no real access to care? ... Does our science teach students to care only for those who are part of the system? ... Or do we convey the value that nursing's job is not complete until all receive the care they need? (p. 23).

The fourth nursing core value is that of reflective thinking, not easy to come by in our fast-paced lives. However, as community health nurses, we must become more than just technicians: "We must also educate people who are equipped intellectually to deal with the meaning of what they do and who they are in the context of humanity" (Salmon, 1999, p. 24). Reflection is needed as we deal with the issues of value conflicts in a complex and diverse society.

Finally, the last core value—the linchpin for all the others—is social responsibility. Florence Nightingale's vision of nursing's responsibility to the common good was based on social responsibility. She saw a society like ours in which certain groups were marginalized and in poor health because of unjust systems, and "Her response was to engage nursing in addressing these injustices" (Salmon, 1999, p. 25). Nursing is only as good as what it does for all the people. Do we, like Lillian Wald, have a firm grasp of the way in which society functions to impact the health of individuals? Our sense of social responsibility will help us meet the challenges of values conflicts in a diverse culture.

BOX 30-3 Value Checkpoint: Critical Thinking

The issue of who is responsible for children affects not only how we as healthcare providers care for families, but also how resources get allocated in our society. People from widely different points of view can agree that valuing families is important in our society. What is harder is agreeing on how much the family needs to be supported by social institutions, including churches, schools, community agencies, and government.

The conservative view is that families should be self-reliant and self-sufficient, not relying on community and government support. The liberal view is that "parents are and should be the most important people in their children's lives. But that doesn't mean they can or should raise their children without any help" (Children's Defense Fund, 1994). Liberals maintain that many forms of assistance are needed to maintain strong families, including sufficient family income and access to health care, child care, and adequate housing.

Think for a moment about your attitudes and beliefs regarding family support. How much family support is needed? What kind of support is needed? Should government ensure basic health care for all families, including children and parents? How does increasing the supply of affordable housing promote health in families? What is the best environment for families if we want to create families who are self-reliant, self-sufficient, and responsible? At what point does the conservative model threaten the overall health of the community? At what point does the liberal model threaten self-reliance in families?

MEDIA MOMENT

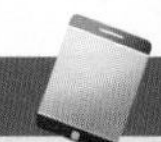

Kramer vs. Kramer (1979)

Winner of five Academy Awards, including Best Picture, Actor, and Screenplay, *Kramer vs. Kramer* remains one of the most powerful dramas ever made about divorce and child custody issues. Adapted from the novel by Avery Corman, the film chronicles the failure of a marriage and the tumultuous shift of parental roles within the family. Joanna Kramer (Meryl Streep) suddenly informs her husband Ted (Dustin Hoffman) that she is leaving him, just as his advertising career is advancing and demanding most of his waking hours. Ted's self-centeredness and Joanna's search for her own identity interplay with the 7-year-old son's future (Justin Henry). The son now finds himself living with a workaholic father he barely knows. Balancing his domestic challenge with professional deadlines, Ted is further pressured when his wife files for custody of their son. The drama of the legal battle for the child's custody explores complex issues related to gender, parenting, and legal accountability.

Terms of Endearment (1983)

Terms of Endearment was adapted from Larry McMurtry's novel and won five Academy Awards, including the Best Adapted Screenplay, Best Picture, Best Actress (Shirley MacLaine), Best Director (James Brooks), and Best Supporting Actor (Jack Nicholson). The cast includes Debra Winger, John Lithgow, Jeff Daniels, and Danny DeVito. The story focuses on a mother, Aurora Greenway (Shirley MacLaine), and her daughter, Emma (Debra Winger), and explores how their relationship develops over the years, from the day that their husband/father dies. Aurora disapproves of Emma's marriage to Flap Horton (Jeff Daniels), a college professor. Emma has three children with Flap, even as his infidelity continues throughout their marriage. .

The event that ties everyone together is Emma's cancer diagnosis. One of the film's most dramatic scenes occurs when Aurora confronts the nurses at the nurses' station, demanding that her daughter's pain medication be given early. The nurses appear more concerned with protocol and schedules than with relieving her daughter's pain; Aurora's shouting match with the nurses is perhaps the most memorable in the movie. After Emma's death, it becomes apparent that Flap is not the one who should be raising the children; Aurora takes the two boys and Emma's best friend raises the girl. The ending reveals the complexities of how families function in good times and in bad times. Many critics consider the film one of the best of the last century, with outstanding performances and a touching and dramatic analysis of family.

THINK ABOUT THIS

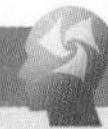

Parents who are stressed or disturbed will have more difficulty in meeting their children's needs. Parents who have little support—from friends, relatives, neighbors, or the community—are more likely to be overburdened by the demands of their babies and to be unable to respond to them adequately. Parents who experience severe poverty or economic insecurity, who cannot satisfy their own basic needs, are likely to have difficulty in responding to their children's needs.

—Sheila B. Kamerman

MEDIA MOMENT

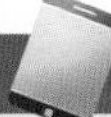

Merry Christmas 1953: A Story About Family

Ann Thedford Lanier

> It is amazing how quickly the years go by. I can still feel the sun on my face that day, smell the turkey cooking in the kitchen, hear the sounds of the children playing, and sense the joy of being home.
>
> I also remember that within a few minutes of this photo a neighbor child shot out our picture window with his new 22 rifle as a Christmas gift and mortally wounded our dog "Mutt." Daddy, in anger and frustration, slapped Lynda so hard that her Christmas watch flew off her arm and was broken. I ran away to hide in the playhouse next door. In my rush to get away, I fell down with my new skates and ripped the knee of my only pair of jeans. My two brothers, Howard and David, got into a fistfight—blackened each other's eyes and bloodied each other's noses. Mother screamed at all of us for being such heathens on "this Day of Our Lord's Birth." She then locked herself in her bedroom and cried. The only member of the family that got away unharmed was "Felix" the cat. Well, so much for happy childhood memories.

What are you thinking as you read this account of one family's holiday? What are ways that the community health nurse could assist this family in making positive changes in family functioning and managing conflict in a healthier way?

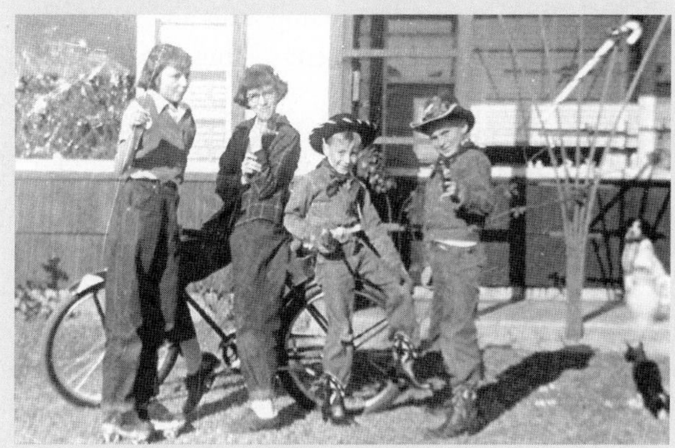

Highly intensive services	Targeted services	Preventive support
↓	↓	↓
Families in crisis	Vulnerable families	All families
↓	↓	↓
Safe houses; foster care	Multiproblem families	Parental/support

Figure 30-3 Continuum of services.

Conclusion

Community health nurses must not only care for individuals and families, but also create caring and cohesive communities. Key concepts highlighted in this chapter, which serve as a foundation for community-based family nursing, include the following:

- Family health is a series of activities designed to promote health, to prevent disease and injury, to prevent premature death, and to create conditions in which we all can be safe and healthy.
- Family health challenges us to think in new, broader ways. Thinking differently about family health means (1) thinking upstream about prevention, (2) thinking of a bottom-down health system focused on increasing cohesion in communities and providing services at the neighborhood level, and (3) thinking in layers in terms of the human ecology model about the many external influences on family health.
- There are three general strategies for promoting family health: preventive services for all families, targeted programs for more vulnerable families, and intensive services for families in crisis.
- There are three characteristics of all successful interventions with families embedded in neighborhoods and larger social systems. Successful interventions involve (1) relationship-focused care, (2) attention to intensity and timing of interventions, and (3) the use of the nursing skills and strategies of communicating, problem solving, listening, connecting, and evaluating.
- The issues in family nursing today are varied and complex. Most important are the constraints of the healthcare delivery system.
- There are many challenges facing community health nurses as they build and organize communities for health. A special challenge is the value conflicts that result when we work with diverse families and communities.
- Salmon's five core values of nursing are proposed as ways to meet the value conflicts of diversity. The five core values are caring, courage, inclusion, reflective thinking, and social responsibility.

Toys

Color washed from years,
At awkward angles,
Tension springs still wound
Grandchildren—children no longer

Waiting to be touched—once again
To dance—march—beat the drum—play the music

Alone in the lower drawer
They wait
Company kept with
Orange green photographs of—
What summer day—what winter night?

—Ann Thedford Lanier, PhD

HEALTHY ME

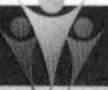

What were your family's values about health and illness? How have these values influenced you during nursing school?

LEVELS OF PREVENTION

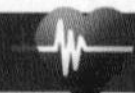

Primary: Teaching expectant parents about anticipated changes in the family with a new baby

Secondary: Leading a recovery group for spouses who have lost their partners to sudden death

Tertiary: Assisting school staff and parents with selecting appropriate and safe sporting equipment for children with special needs and disabilities

Critical Thinking Activities

1. As a community health nurse you have been assigned to a community action committee to design a parent support group for parents of teens in your local high school. The purpose of the group is to teach communication, conflict resolution, and problem-solving skills and to provide a forum for social support for parents. A major emphasis will be on practicing skills. Explore the following questions and give rationales for your decisions:
   - Would you have a group for parents only, for parents and teens, or separate groups for parents and teens?
   - Which resources would you use to teach communication, conflict resolution, and problem-solving skills? Remember that a major emphasis of the groups is to practice these skills.
   - The teaching of social skills to children is important, especially children who feel alienated and left out. In her book, *Why Doesn't Anybody Like Me?: A Guide to Raising Socially Confident Kids,* Hara Estroff Marano (1998) gives several suggestions to parents. How would you incorporate some of these suggestions into your parent group? Which activities would you use to make the suggestions come alive?
   - How many weeks will the group meet, when (e.g., evening, weekend), and for how long (e.g., 1 hour, 2 hours)?
   - Who would you have lead the groups? Which experts in your community would you utilize to help you if you were chosen to lead the groups?
2. Explore the factors contributing to the gap in mortality between the rich and the poor. Especially look at factors other than health behaviors. Explain how some of the other factors suggested by the research might contribute to increased mortality in the poor. How might these factors affect physical health? What are interventions that would address the following other factors?
   - Lack of social relationships and social supports

     Intervention:
   - Personality factors such as a lost sense of mastery, optimism, sense of control, and self-esteem

     Intervention:
   - Factors such as heightened level of anger and hostility

     Intervention:
   - Chronic and acute stress in jobs and at home as a result of lack of resources

     Intervention:
   - The stress of racism and classicism and other stress related to the unequal distribution of power and resources

     Intervention:
   - Differences in exposure to occupational and environmental health hazards (poor people tend to have more exposure to these hazards, such as lead)

     Intervention:
   - Differences in access to health care

     Intervention:
3. Think of a family you are currently working with. Name one skill that each family member possesses that is a strength. Does the documentation system used in your nursing agency, hospital, or community clinic have a place for listing strengths of individuals and families?
4. Most conjoint domestic abuse after-treatment groups are co-led by a man and a woman. Leaders should have experience in counseling, group work, and family violence. Assume you are co-leading a conjoint after-treatment group.
   - Which safety considerations would you have for the formerly abused women in the group?
   - Which skills would be particularly important for couples to practice in the group?
   - Which built-in strategies would you use to monitor current physical abuse in these relationships?
   - Which kind of system would you have in place for crisis intervention if abuse developed between sessions?

5. Explain why someone in a family or community would respond differently to a problem than you do. Discuss the following questions with the family/community to enhance their problem solving (adapted from Schorr, 1997).
   - What do you think is the problem?
   - What do you think you should do?
   - What would help?
   - What have you done in the past when this happened? Did it work?
   - What are your options?
   - Who might help you?

References

Banks-Wallace, J. (1998). Emancipatory potential of storytelling in a group. *Image: The Journal of Nursing Scholarship, 30*(1), 17–21.

Banks-Wallace, J. (1999). Storytelling as a tool for providing holistic care to women. *American Journal of Maternal/Child Nursing, 24*(1), 20–24.

Benson, H. (1996). *Timeless healing. The power and biology of belief.* New York, NY: Simon & Schuster.

Bronfenbrenner, U. (1986). Ecology of the family as a context for human development. Research perspectives. *Developmental Psychology, 22*(6), 723–742.

Bureau of Labor Statistics. (2012). *Occupational outlook handbook: Registered nurses.* Retrieved from http://www.bls.gov/ooh/healthcare/registered-nurses.htm

Butterfield, P. G. (1991). Thinking upstream: Nurturing a conceptual understanding of the societal context of health behavior. In K. A. Saucier (Ed.), *Perspectives in family and community health* (pp. 66–71). St. Louis, MO: Mosby.

Butterfield, P. G. (2002). Upstream reflections on environmental health: An abbreviated history and framework for action. *Advances in Nursing Science, 25*(1), 32–50.

Carter, B. (2008). "Good" and "bad" stories: Decisive moments, "Shock and awe," and being moral. *Journal of Clinical Nursing, 17*(8), 1063–1070.

Children's Defense Fund. (1994). *Helping children by strengthening families: A look at family support programs.* Washington, DC: Author.

Clinton, H. R. (1996). *It takes a village: And other lessons children teach us* (p. 65). New York, NY: Touchstone Books.

Cordes, H., & Walljasper, J. (Eds.). (1997). *Goodlife: Mastering the art of everyday living.* Minneapolis, MN: Utne Reader.

Crockenberg, S. B. (1985). Professional support and care of infants by adolescent mothers in England and the United States. *Journal of Pediatric Psychology, 10*, 413–428.

Dawe, S., & Harnett, P. (2007). Reducing potential for child abuse among methadone-maintained parents: Results from a randomized controlled trial. *Journal of Substance Abuse Treatment, 32*(4), 381–390.

Federman, M., Garner, T. I., Short, K., Cutter, W. N., 4th, Kiely, J., Levine, D., ... McMillen, M. (1996). What does it mean to be poor in America? *Monthly Labor Review, 119*(5), 3–17.

Fetterman, D. M., Kaftarian, S. J., & Wandersman, A. (Eds.). (1996). *Empowerment evaluation: Knowledge and tools for self-assessment and accountability.* Thousand Oaks, CA: Sage.

Flaskerud, J. H., & Winslow, B. J. (1998). Conceptualizing vulnerable populations: Health-related research. *Nursing Research, 47*(2), 69–78.

Gordon, S. (1997). *Life support: Three nurses on the front lines.* Boston, MA: Little, Brown.

Hancock, T. (1993). Re-designing healthcare from the bottom down. In *Healthier communities action kit* (vol. 2). San Francisco, CA: Healthcare Forum.

Heaman, M., Chalmers, K., Woodgate, R., & Brown, J. (2007). Relationship work in an early childhood home visiting program. *Journal of Pediatric Nursing, 22*(4), 319–330.

Hill, K. (2008). A strengths-based framework for social policy: Barriers and possibilities. *Journal of Policy Practice, 7*(2/3), 106–121.

House, J. S., Landis, K. R., & Umberson, D. (1988). Social relationships and health. *Science, 241*(4865), 540–545.

Johannson, M. A., & Tutty, L. M. (1998). An evaluation of after-treatment couples' groups for wife abuse. *Family Relations, 47*(1), 27–35.

Kawachi, I., Kennedy, B. P., Lochner, K., & Prothrow-Stith, D. (1997). Social capital, income inequality, and mortality. *American Journal of Public Health, 87*(9), 1491–1498.

Kemp, L., Eisbacher, L., McIntyre, L., O'Sullivan, K., Taylor, J., Clark, T., & Harris, E. (2006). Working in partnership in the antenatal period: What do child and family health nurses do? *Contemporary Nurse: A Journal for the Australian Nursing Profession, 23*(2), 312–320.

LaTaillade, J., Epstein, N., & Werlinich, C. (2006). Conjoint treatment of intimate partner violence: A cognitive behavioral approach. *Journal of Cognitive Psychotherapy, 20*(4), 393–410.

Laursen, E. (2000). Strength-based practice with children in trouble. *Reclaiming Children and Youth, 9*(2), 70–75.

Leonard, J., & Siegel, M. (1998). Mother and daughter workshops. *Childbirth Instructor Magazine,* March/April, 34–35.

Levy, B. S. (1998). Creating the future of public health: Values, vision, and leadership. *American Journal of Public Health, 88*(2), 188–192.

Lomas, J. (1998). Social capital and health: Implications for public health and epidemiology. *Social Science and Medicine, 47*(9), 1181–1188.

Lynch, I., & Tiedje, L. B. (1991). Working with multiproblem families: An intervention model for community health nurses. *Public Health Nursing, 8*(3), 147–153.

Marano, H. E. (1998). *Why doesn't anybody like me?: A guide to raising socially confident kids.* New York, NY: William Morrow.

McKinlay, J. B. (1979). A case for refocusing upstream: The political economy of illness. In E. G. Jaco (Ed.), *Patients, physicians, and illness* (3rd ed., pp. 9–25). New York, NY: Free Press.

Minkler, M. (Ed.). (1998). *Community organizing & community building for health.* New Brunswick, NJ: Rutgers University Press.

Moms Demand Action/Mayors Against Illegal Guns. (2014). Analysis of school shootings. Retrieved from https://s3.amazonaws.com/s3.mayorsagainstillegalguns.org/images/SchoolShootingsReport.pdf

Nelson, A., McClintock, C., Perez-Ferguson, A., Shawver, M., & Thompson, G. (2008). Storytelling narratives: Social bonding as key for youth at risk. *Child & Youth Care Forum, 37*(3), 127–137.

Papiernik, E., Bouyer, J., Yaffe, K., Winisdorffer, G., Collin, D., & Dreyfus, J. (1986). Women's acceptance of a preterm birth prevention program. *American Journal of Obstetrics and Gynecology, 155*, 939–946.

Pipher, M. (1994). *Reviving Ophelia: Saving the selves of adolescent girls.* New York, NY: Ballantine.

Putnam, R. D. (1995). Bowling alone. American's declining social capital. *Journal of Democracy, 6*, 65–78.

Remen, R. N. (1996). *Kitchen table wisdom.* New York, NY: Riverhead Books.

Roe, K. M., Berenstein, C., Goette, C., & Roe, K. (1996). Community building through empowering evaluation. In M. Winkler (Ed.), *Community organizing & community building for health* (pp. 308–322). New Brunswick, NJ: Rutgers University Press.

Roehlkepartain, J. L. (1995). *Building assets together.* Minneapolis, MN: Search Institute.

Salmon, M. E. (1999). Thoughts on nursing: Where it has been and where it is going. *Nursing and Health Care Perspectives, 20*(1), 20–25.

Schorr, L. B. (1997). *Common purpose: Strengthening families and neighborhoods to rebuild America.* New York, NY: Anchor Books.

Shindul-Rothschild, J. (1998). Nurses week tribute: A nursing call to action. *American Journal of Nursing, 98*(5), 36.

Smyth, J., Stone, A. A., Hurewitz, A., & Kaell, A. (1999). Effects of writing about stressful experiences on symptom reduction in patients with asthma or rheumatoid arthritis. *Journal of the American Medical Association, 281*(14), 1304–1309.

Stagner, M. W., & Duran, M. A. (1997). Comprehensive community initiatives: Principles, practice, and lessons learned. In R. E. Behrman (Ed.), *The future of children: Children and poverty* (pp. 44–68). Los Altos, CA: Center for the Future of Children.

Tandon, D. (2007). Promotion of service integration among home visiting programs and community coalitions working with low-income, pregnant, and parenting women. *Health Promotion Practice, 8*(1), 79–87.

Tanner, C. A. (1995). Living in the midst of a paradigm shift. *Journal of Nursing Education, 34*(2), 51–52.

U.S. Department of Health and Human Services. (2012). *Healthy people 2020.* Retrieved from http://www.healthypeople.gov/2020/default.aspx

Weisman, A. D. (1981). Understanding the cancer patient: The syndrome of caregiver's plight. *Psychiatry, 44*, 161–168.

World Health Organization (WHO). (2005). *The world health report 2005—Make every mother and child count.* Retrieved from http://www.who.int/whr/2005/en/

Zerwekh, J. V. (1997). Making the connection during home visits: Narratives of expert nurses. *International Journal for Human Caring, I*(1), 25–29.

CHAPTER FOCUS

Profile of Women's Health
- Education
- Employment
- Poverty
- Marital Status/Family Configuration
- Reproductive Health and Risks
- Patterns of Health and Illness

Health Issues, Health Promotion, and Health Prevention Across the Lifespan
- Adolescence (12 to 18 Years Old)
- Young Adulthood (19 to 35 Years Old)
- Perimenopausal/Menopausal (36 to 55 Years Old)
- Mature (55 and Older)

Specific Disease Conditions of Women Throughout the Lifespan
- Cancer
- Osteoporosis

Diversity and Women's Health
- Cultural Influences
- Sexual Orientation
- Women and Aging
- Global Issues and Women's Health

Special Issues Affecting Women's Health
- Violence
- Homelessness
- Incarceration
- Poverty
- Workplace Health

Toward the Future
- Women's Ways of Knowing
- Feminism
- Empowerment
- Healthcare Policy

QUESTIONS TO CONSIDER

After reading this chapter, you will know the answers to the following questions:

1. How are demographic variables related to women's health status?
2. As women age, which specific health concerns and issues are most prevalent?
3. What are special health concerns of lesbians, women of color, and elder women?
4. What are the special ethical issues related to health that concern women?
5. Which populations of women are more vulnerable to health risks?
6. How can nurses provide preventive-based care to the diverse population of women in the promotion of health?
7. What are sources of empowerment for women related to improved health?
8. Which future issues will likely influence the health of women?

CHAPTER 31

Women's Health

Karen Saucier Lundy and
Norma G. Cuellar

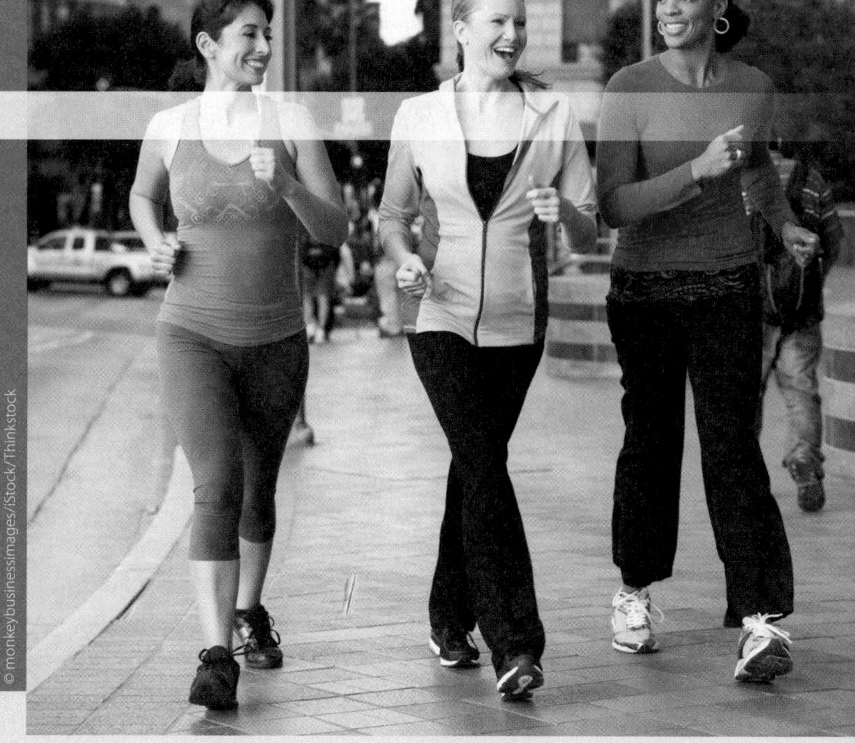

KEY TERMS

caregivers
Commission on the Status of Women
constructed knowledge
empowerment
feminism
feminization of poverty
heterosexism
homophobia
hormone replacement therapy (HRT)
mammography
perimenopausal period
procedural knowledge
United Nations Platform for Action for Women
urinary incontinence
World Conference on Women

> A woman's health is her capital.
>
> —Harriet Beecher Stowe

> Women do two-thirds of the world's work. Yet they earn only one-tenth of the world's income and own less than 1% of the world's property. They are among the poorest of the world's poor.
>
> —Barber B. Conable

> Women never have a half-hour in all their lives (excepting before or after anybody is up in the house) that they can call their own, without fear of offending or of hurting someone. Why do people sit up so late, or, more rarely, get up so early? Not because the day is not long enough, but because they have 'no time in the day to themselves.'
>
> —Florence Nightingale, 1852

REFLECTIONS

When you reflect on these women's quotes, how are women different from men in their caring for themselves as well as caring for others? What are the health risks that women have as compared to men? Has the feminist movement affected the way society values women? Is the feminist movement still relevant today, especially for young women?

Women now live an average of 30 years longer than they did 100 years ago. A woman born in 1900 was expected to live 49 years; today's baby girls can expect a lifespan of 80 years. Significant changes and increased opportunities in the lives of American women have broadened the focus of women's health to include physiological, emotional, social, cultural, and economic wellbeing. Women, as the primary caregivers of families, are key to achieving the goal of healthy communities. However, women face significant barriers in gaining access to health care and in caring for themselves, even as they care for others. Often, inadequate education, gender bias in the healthcare system, and low socioeconomic status prevent women from assuming the responsibilities for their own health and wellbeing. As consumers of health services, women must be involved in the development of health policy to achieve parity in availability and access to healthcare resources for women. Community health nurses play key roles in collaborating with women to achieve the national goal of health care for all. This chapter provides information about the context of women's health and describes how community health nurses can assist women of all ages to meet health needs.

For much of the 20th century, women's health focused almost exclusively on reproductive functions such as menstruation, childbearing, and menopause. In 1990, a landmark report by the General Accounting Office (GAO) revealed shocking gaps in research on women's health issues. During the 20th century, women had been left out of most research on cancer, heart disease, and interventions, such as the development of new technology and medications. Such inequities resulted in women's health lagging considerably behind in advances known to benefit men.

In the 1990s, the federal government mobilized the greatest effort ever to improve women's health through research and services. We now have better and safer **mammography** and breast cancer treatment, have more effective ways to prevent and treat osteoporosis, and know more about alternatives for women during the **perimenopausal period**. As the lives of women have been extended, chronic diseases and disability have taken the place of acute illness and childbirth as leading causes of death. Women are living longer lives, challenging community health nurses to help women improve the quality of these added years.

Profile of Women's Health

The U.S. Census Bureau (2012) reports a ratio at birth of 105 males to 100 females; the median age for females in the United States is currently 38.5 years. In most countries, women typically have longer lifespans than men and consequently make up 52% of the world's population. In the United States, the average lifespan for a woman is 79.9 years, compared with 74.4 years for men. Because males are more likely to die at any given age, the proportion of females to males increases over the lifespan (U.S. Census Bureau, 2012). The difference in the life expectancy of men and women in the United States has narrowed over the years, and the difference of 5.2 years in 2013 was the smallest difference ever recorded, and is below the average for most other Organization for Economic Cooperation and Development (OECD; 2013) nations. Among persons 65 years and older, women make up 58% of this age group. By the age of 85, women outnumber men about 2.5 to 1. For community health nurses, many gerontological health issues in the future will be those involving elder women. With a decline in mortality in certain diseases for men (e.g., cardiovascular disease) and an increase in the number of women who have assumed many lifestyle behaviors and health habits previously characteristic of men (e.g., cigarette smoking, alcohol use, stress associated with full-time work in the labor force, and added challenges of maintaining traditional gender roles, such as housekeeping and family care as well as head of household responsibilities), the differences in lifespans for women and men are expected to converge even more in the future.

Education

Education is positively correlated with health status for both men and women. While women in the United States have high literacy rates (equal to those of men), almost 1 billion adults around the world cannot read,

CULTURAL CONNECTION 

Research has consistently found that mothers who create a "culture of weight fixation" are more likely to have daughters with eating disorders than are less self-conscious moms. The media influence daughters, but daughters more often tend to model their mothers' behaviors, such as noticing what they eat, how they talk about their bodies, how often they weigh themselves, and especially whether they have "self-loathing" attitudes. Self-contempt passes from generation to generation as a cultural trait; for daughters to accept their bodies, mothers need to accept their own as only a part of their self-worth. With self-awareness, the culture can become more balanced and healthy for both mothers and daughters throughout their lives.

GOT AN ALTERNATIVE? 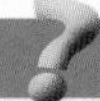

Medicinal herbs often used by women include the following:

- Black cohosh—used for treating hot flashes as symptoms of menopause
- Chaste tree berry (*Vitex agnus-castus*)—for premenstrual syndrome (PMS)
- Cranberry (*Vaccinium macrocarpon*)—for prevention of urinary tract infections
- Dong quai (*Angelica sinensis*)—for general female wellness, irregular periods, fatigue
- Flaxseed (*Linum usitatissimum*)—for cardiovascular health and fiber supplement
- Feverfew (*Tanacetum parthenium*)—for treatment of symptoms of migraine headache
- Turmeric (*Curcuma longa*)—as an anti-inflammatory and antioxidant
- Green tea (*Camellia sinensis*)—for cancer prevention
- Ginger (*Zingiber officinale*)—for nausea and vomiting, especially during pregnancy

Before advising patients about the use of any herbs, nurses should conduct a thorough literature review of current research on specific herbs, contraindications, and recommendations for specific use. The National Center for Complementary and Alternative Medicine (NCCAM), a division of the U.S. National Institutes of Health (NIH), is the best resource for clinical trial data on herbs and other complementary therapies. NCCAM can be accessed online at http://nccam.nih.gov/.

Source: Parch, L. (2006). The nine best herbs for women. *Natural Health, 36*(8), 74–79.

and two-thirds of those are women (U.S. Department of Education, 2007). In the past, the predominant roles professional women chose were in education, nursing, library science, and social work. However, since the late 1980s, more women have entered professions traditionally dominated by men, such as engineering, theology, medicine, law, and dentistry. A continuing concern is that ethnic minority women have been slow to enter these major areas of study. An emerging trend, according to the U.S. Census Bureau (2013a), is an overall significant increase in college enrollment among African Americans and Hispanics since 1970. Such a trend holds promise for increasing the number of all women and women of color pursuing advanced specialty degrees as these cohorts move through the educational ranks.

Employment

More women are in the U.S. workforce than ever before, and they are entering the workforce at increasingly earlier ages. As compared to 1960, when one of every three workers in the United States was female, half of all workers today are women. However, increased opportunities in the workforce are creating more challenges and risks for their families, such as child and elder caregiving issues. The job market remains male dominated, with average annual salaries differing by gender. Recent data indicate that women earn 77% of the average man's salary in the United States (Johnson, 2012). This ratio varies considerably throughout the world, according to educational levels and chosen professions. A contributing factor to the significant gender differences in salary relates to women choosing lower paying jobs by career preparation: Half of the pay difference in salaries for women is attributed to this factor alone. Other factors include caring for family and children during peak earning years.

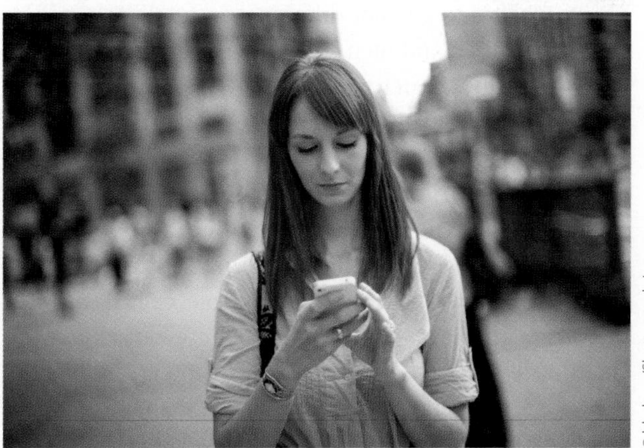

Technology has improved our lives dramatically, especially "anywhere" instant communication and availability. The use of cellular phones in automobiles, as a result, has also added stress and risk for many women as they have extended their multitasking to travel time.

NOTE THIS!

In the United States, women live on average 5.2 years longer than men.

Traditional female occupations generally pay less than comparable men's jobs and have fewer healthcare and retirement benefits. Sixty-five percent of women are in the workforce as librarians, teachers, social workers, and nurses with lower mean salaries than members of other professions. Working women continue to assume responsibility for child care, housework, and elder care. More than 50% of women with an infant are in the workforce, up 35.3% since 1978. The percentage of new mothers who work tends to increase with both age and education. Men are more likely to be employed in higher level management positions, with jobs that offer health benefits, medical leave, and insurance. Women continue to face the "glass ceiling" in regard to career advancement to managerial positions. The "glass ceiling" refers to the barriers that keep women from reaching the executive suite in their chosen professions. Women tend to be outside the

> pipeline to success, choosing limited upward mobility options, such as public relations and human resource positions. Men tend to be in more upwardly mobile marketing and sales positions. Women often do not have mentors in higher positions and are often stuck in the "mommy track," limiting their overnight travel and night/weekend work. (Clarke, 2000)

This translates to a major difference in total life earnings between women and men.

Universally, greater prestige is given to male work activities, regardless of what they are. For example, when most infants were delivered by midwives in the 19th and early 20th centuries, the job had low prestige and an associated small salary. When men took over the job of "birthing babies" as medicine specialized in obstetrics and gynecology, the prestige of the role rose along with the salary. This is but one example of how the value of the "nature" of work changes according to the gender of the worker and societal values. Thus, it is not about the work itself that promotes privilege and salary, but rather the gender of the worker.

Women with limited health benefits and lower salaries tend to have limited healthcare options. As a consequence, they may not seek out health care when needed and are less likely to practice preventive health care.

Poverty

Women often earn less than men working in comparable jobs. One result of this disparity is a greater proportion of women in poverty; women account for two-thirds of all poor adults. This statistic is greatly influenced by culture and race, with the largest increases in poverty occurring among African American and Hispanic women. Women in poverty are usually 18 to 24 years old, live in the South, and reside outside central cities. Women and children make up a majority of the homeless population in the United States. Many factors contribute to poverty, including the gender wage gap, single mothers as heads of households, teenage birth rates, lack of adequate child care, and lack of enforcement of child support payments. Of all the countries in the industrialized world, the United States is the only country without a system that provides subsidized child care for working parents.

ENVIRONMENTAL CONNECTION

Consider the following possible environmental threats affecting women:

- Household chemicals (e.g., insect spray, plant food)
- Inhalants (e.g., hair products, powders)
- Hair dyes and coloring agents
- Nail polish and polish removers

How do these environmental hazards specifically pose a threat to women's health and reproduction?

Single-earner families headed by women are more than twice as likely to be impoverished as families where the single earner is male, and five times more likely to be living below the poverty line than dual-earner families (U.S. Census Bureau, 2013b). All of these risk factors of poverty as related to women have been referred to as the **feminization of poverty** (Albelda & Tilly, 1997; Dujan & Withorn, 1996).

Marital Status/Family Configuration

Women's roles in marriage and the family are in a state of transition and have been since the 1960s. The traditional role of the unemployed mother working in the home has become a small minority. Only 6% of households have a male working full-time supporting a full-time homemaker with children in the home—and yet the image of the traditional family (stay-at-home mom, working dad) persists as the norm. We see evidence of this in the media, such as in commercials where housekeeping advertisements target women and business advertisements target men. The necessary goal of any family, however defined, is to maintain the safety, wellbeing, and health of the family. More than half of adult women in the United States are single, with their number having increased 50% since 1970.

Racial differences in lifestyles can affect attitudes and beliefs about health. African Americans, as compared with Caucasians, are more often single or married with no spouse present or living with extended families. More Caucasians are divorced or widowed, and they tend to have fewer children than do African Americans and Hispanics. Families maintained by women with no husband present are more likely to be poor. Among those men who are present in their families, African American and Hispanic men tend to spend more time with their family tasks than do Caucasian men.

Women, on top of their everyday family obligations, continue to care for older family members: More than one in 10 women care for a sick or aging relative. Meeting these multiple obligations is demanding and leaves many women concerned about the challenge of meeting all their family and work commitments as well as managing their own health. An overwhelming majority of women are responsible for the vast majority of routine healthcare decisions and responsibilities for their families. For example:

- Eight in 10 women are responsible for choosing their children's healthcare provider.
- Forty-eight percent of working mothers have no alternative but to miss work if a child gets sick; 47% of these women lack paid time off benefits and therefore lose income when they do so.
- Fifty-seven percent of mothers are primarily responsible for decisions about their children's health insurance.
- One in 8 women cares for a sick or aging relative; in nearly two-thirds of these cases, these women are primary caregivers for the sick individual and manage the majority of daily needs, including doing housework, providing transportation, making various financial decisions, and managing health care, medication administration, and basic care such as assisting with bathing and dressing.
- Fifty-one percent of women who are caring for others have a chronic health condition of their own; of those who don't, 28% consider their own health to be only "fair" or "poor." Forty-one percent of those caring for a sick relative are also caring for children under 18. Approximately 19% assist their relative for more than 40 hours per week, while 21% state that providing care strains family finances (Kaiser Family Foundation, 2011).

ETHICAL CONNECTION 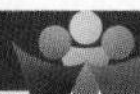

Dana Reeve lost her battle with lung cancer at age 44 on March 6, 2006, just 17 months after the death of her husband Christopher Reeve. Dana, a nonsmoker, often said, "I learned a long time ago life just isn't fair . . . you just forge ahead."

Lung cancer accounts for the most cancer deaths among women and yet often goes unrecognized as the "top killer" that it is. Smokers used to account for 95% of all lung cancer cases. Today, however, as many as 15% of lung cancer patients are nonsmokers; of those, about 60% are women. Breast cancer kills about 35,000 women each year in the United States, while lung cancer kills about twice that many—70,000 women per year. Research is unclear about the exact reasons for this trend but some factors have emerged as possible epidemiological factors: genetics, estrogen, and the increase in environmental toxins (e.g., radon gas, secondhand smoke, pollution). To further emphasize the political significance of public perception of cancer risks, between 2008 and 2010 the National Cancer Institute (NCI) spent $1.8 billion on research for breast cancer while spending $776 million on lung cancer—even though lung cancer kills more people each year than the next three most common cancers (breast cancer, colon cancer, and pancreatic cancer) *combined* (American Cancer Society [ACS], 2014). The research inputs from NCI, the Centers for Disease Control and Prevention (CDC), and the Department of Defense amounted to $17,835 per breast cancer death, but only $1,378 per lung cancer death (Ganti, 2013).

Part of the problem is the perception that lung cancer is a "self-inflicted" disease of smokers. What are the ethical implications of this view?

For more information, go to http://www.lung.org.

Reproductive Health and Risks

Women are uniquely at risk during pregnancy and childbirth, including the risks of induced and spontaneous abortions. Even in the 21st century, women continue to die during childbirth, with pulmonary embolism being the leading cause of death in pregnant women. However, thanks to partnerships between community health nurses and the healthcare system, maternal mortality has been dramatically reduced through prenatal care, education related to maternal risk factors, blood transfusions, anesthesia, and antibiotics. Racial discrepancies persist in the number of maternal deaths, with women of color having a threefold greater incidence of death during pregnancy than Caucasian women (CDC, 2013a). Contributing factors include late or no prenatal care, poor nutrition, and substandard living conditions. Concurrent infant death rates are also disproportionate among races, with twice

RESEARCH ALERT

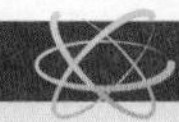

That's What Makes Me Care: Empowering Women as Community Health Workers to Promote Personal and Public Health

Susan Mayfield-Johnson, PhD, MPH, CHES
Director, Education and Training
Center for Sustainable Health Outreach
University of Southern Mississippi
Hattiesburg, Mississippi

Because the cost of health care is continuing to rise and resources are not, innovative solutions must be employed to mobilize our largely untapped but most valuable resource, the people in our community and neighborhoods. The lack of coordination between various health service delivery agencies and programs has often led to duplication of efforts and widening gaps in meeting community needs. Community health advisors (CHAs) have emerged as a viable solution to bridge the gap between health service delivery systems and the community. As trusted community members, community health advisors are able to integrate health information about prevention of disease and the health system into the community's culture, language, and value systems, and as a result, they reduce cultural, linguistic, social, and financial barriers to health care. They can increase access to care and facilitate appropriate use of health resources by providing outreach and cultural linkages between communities and health systems. Community health advisors are often described as natural helpers or individuals to whom people naturally turn to for advice, emotional support, and tangible aid.

Because community health advisors are members of the communities they serve, they are agents of change within these communities. However, little research exists that described how these women as change agents experience growth themselves in the empowerment process. The purpose of this phenomenological study was to examine and describe the empowerment change processes of CHAs utilizing photovoice, an innovative method that incorporates documentary photography within a group setting, and separately through reflective in-depth interviews. Using photos and narratives as primary research methods, the women who served as CHAs in this study gave voice to an often overlooked resource in the improvement of vulnerable populations in the promotion of the public's health.

Photovoice is an innovative participatory tool based on health-promotion principles and the theoretical literature on education for critical consciousness, feminist theory, and a community-based approach to documentary photography (Wang, 2003). Photovoice was chosen because it provided a means for participants to narrate their perceptions and experiences through an emic perspective. Instead of placing cameras into the hands of professional photographers or researchers who are often in control of photo data generation, the photovoice method puts cameras into the hands of the individuals whose lives are daily affected and the focus of the study. The goal of photovoice is to use people's photographic documentation of their everyday lives as an educational tool to record and reflect their needs, promote dialogue, encourage action, and inform policy. Photovoice has three main goals: (1) enable people to record and reflect their community's strengths and concerns through taking photographs; (2) promote critical dialogue and knowledge about important personal and community issues through discussion of their photographs; and (3) to reach policymakers (Wang, 1999; Wang & Burris, 1994). It is a participatory process that integrates empowerment education, feminist theory, and documentary photography. After the photovoice sessions, semi-structured, in-depth reflective interviews were also chosen to complement the study design.

In this study, 31 female African American community health advisors in a cancer control and prevention program in Mississippi and Alabama participated in four photovoice focus groups, and 15 additional women participated in reflective interviews. Analysis of the data in the sample revealed the following:

1. The experiences of a CHA profoundly affect her desire to help her community. The typical CHA came from a large family with little to low income and expressed a desire to make a difference in the community.
2. Most CHAs are either the eldest child, eldest female child, or had a position of authority and/or caregiving in the family structure.
3. Most CHAs are older women who have experienced significant hardship and struggle in their lives. They have lived through major social and political movements in history, and the significant struggle to obtain equality has left a lasting impression in their philosophy and activities.
4. CHAs expressed dismay at the apathy and destructiveness of African Americans related to other African Americans. CHAs in the research study believed that they have a duty to their families, communities, and the African American race to change the health disparities and oppression that exist in predominantly African American communities.
5. History, culture, and family are intertwined layers that define who they are and where they come from. These layers cannot be severed in describing their experience. While the remnants of slavery still exist, progress is evident.
6. Spirituality and faith are essential components for service in the community. Their role was often described as "a calling."

7. Participation in a community health worker program served two purposes: individual change in knowledge, attitudes, and beliefs and application of efficacy in practice.
8. CHAs feel that they have made a difference in their communities. They see the changes in their communities.
9. CHAs described their role in the community as a leader, educator, caregiver, mentor, and servant. They credit these roles to the leadership development and skill building characteristics of the program.
10. CHAs draw on other women for support. The social networking function of a CHA group was expressed by the participants as essential to professional growth and development.

One CHA in Alabama described her perception of race and class in the African American community in this way:

> So we had a class system, just because you're Black doesn't mean class doesn't exist. You can have class system between light color Blacks and dark color Blacks, you have it between poor Blacks and better-off Blacks, you know, so you had the class system. And in that point, considering my dad's job status, we were the poorer Blacks and the darker color Blacks.
>
> —54-year-old mother of three, who lost her daughter to cancer

Another CHA in Mississippi describes her personal growth and empowerment in the following narrative account:

> I had a pair of black pumps and I had had them for I don't know, three or four years but anyway they were all ran over and the heel was crooked on them. You know, my mama told me that when I got ready to graduate she said, "Why don't you go and get you a new pair of shoes?" I said, "No." So every event that I had to attend when I went to school, I wore those shoes ... I'm gonna wear these shoes and even after I graduate, I kept those shoes until they really dry rotted. And the reason why I kept those shoes, is because I didn't want to forget where I came from so everyday I looked in that closet and I saw those shoes and I remembered the struggle that I had to be where I came from. But now I look back and I see that I had to go through that to get to where I am now. And I thank God and He let me go through that. Because the people that I work with now, the abused women, the low self-esteem women, I can related to those women because I been through that. And I think that's what makes me care.
>
> 51-year-old mother of three, sister to a lung and liver cancer survivor

Implications of the Study

Describing what it means to be a CHA gives important recognition and value to the role of change agents in the community. Discovering how the empowerment change process takes place in CHAs is crucial for public health professionals in their efforts to promote community health. Community health education research can be designed to enhance individual and population-focused learning by understanding the needs of the people within the framework and culture of the community. Allowing the emergence of a theoretical framework shaped by the perspectives of community health advisors will enable members of the community to collaborate with researchers and practitioners in designing effective interventions in their communities. Involving CHAs in developing and implementing interventions that are socially and culturally appropriate to their learning needs has the potential to result in changes in the paradigm of public health promotion, specifically related to health education. These implications for change go beyond how programs are developed and administered by examining empowerment, social action, and community capacity. Inclusive and consistent program design and methodology can then form the basis for true community participatory research.

Sources: Mayfield-Johnson, S. (2007). Her story through photovoice and reflective interviews: Describing changes in empowerment among community health advisors as research partners in Mississippi and Alabama. *Dissertation Abstracts International: The Humanities and Social Sciences, 68*(06), UMI No. 3268458; Wang, C. (1999). Photovoice: A participatory action research strategy applied to women's health. *Journal of Women's Health, 8*, 185–192; Wang, C. C. (2003). Using photovoice as a participatory assessment and issue selection tool: A case study with the homeless in Ann Arbor. In M. Minkler & N. Wallerstein (Eds.), *Community-based participator research for health* (pp. 179–186). San Francisco, CA: Jossey-Bass; Wang, C., & Burris, M. A. (1994). Empowerment through photo novella: Portraits of participation. *Health Education Quarterly, 21*, 171–186.

the number of infants of color dying as Caucasian infants during the first year of life.

Trends in U.S. birth rates have major implications for the growth of the population and the evolution of health care. Fertility rates continue to drop, with an overall decline in birth rates in the United States (U.S. Census Bureau, 2013b). The number of births is expected to decline further as the majority of baby boomers have aged past their childbearing years. More women are delaying childbearing or choosing to remain childless. Birth rates vary by age and ethnicity, with the number of births for unmarried women declining in all age groups.

Women are beginning prenatal care earlier and seeking it out in greater numbers, although this tendency varies, with women of color and those in poverty seeking prenatal care later or not at all. Twice as many African American women deliver low-birth-weight babies compared with Caucasian women (CDC, 2013a). Parenting classes, health care for children, quality daycare facilities, and flexible employment opportunities for working mothers are not consistently available to women in the United States; the health and wellbeing of working families has not been a national funding priority. By contrast, many countries throughout the world have established policies that ensure protection and support of mothers, infants, and families and can serve as role models for such positive family investments.

Madam Chairperson

Must I wear my skirts longer than most
So I can put my feet upon my desk
And smoke
And learn to drink
Jack Daniels?
"Just because you were born deformed
doesn't mean you can't
stand up just as straight
and be heard just as far
as those born with a
talie-wacker!"
I believe gentlemen, I will
Smoke that cigar
And a brandy sounds
Quite nice
I think I'll stay

—*Ann Thedford Lanier*

RESEARCH ALERT 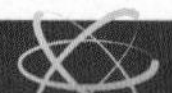

Rap music videos as a media genre have long concerned the public owing to their graphic depiction of violence and sexual exploitation of women. Little research has examined the effect of rap music videos on adolescent behavior. This study sought to determine whether exposure to rap music videos at baseline could predict the occurrence of health-risk behaviors and sexually transmitted diseases (STDs) among African American adolescent females over a 12-month follow-up period.

The study followed 522 single African American females ages 14 and 18 who had been sexually active in the previous 6 months. Level of exposure to rap music videos—the predictor variable—was determined by asking the subjects to estimate the number of hours they viewed rap music videos during an average day. This was multiplied by the number of days in the week that rap music videos were viewed. Music video viewing characteristics assessed included which primary type of rap music videos was viewed (gangsta, bass, or hip-hop), with whom they viewed rap music videos, and where the videos were viewed. Covariates included age, employment status, involvement in extracurricular activities and religious events, family composition, public assistance, parental monitoring, and group assignment to HIV intervention. Health-risk behaviors assessed included teacher violence, fighting in school, arrest, alcohol or drug use, multiple sex partners, condom use, and STD infection over the 12-month period.

Greater exposure to rap music videos was associated with unemployment and less parental monitoring. Greater exposure was also independently associated with a broad spectrum of health outcomes. Compared with adolescents who had less exposure to rap music videos, adolescents who had greater exposure to such videos were 3 times more likely to have hit a teacher, more than 2.4 times as likely to have been arrested, 2 times as likely to have had multiple sexual partners, and more than 1.5 times as likely to have acquired a new STD, used drugs, and used alcohol over the 12-month follow-up period. Although this was one of the first studies to empirically show that greater exposure to rap music videos at baseline was prospectively associated with the occurrence of health-risk behaviors and having lab-confirmed new STDs 1 year later, the authors were careful to note that it is difficult to determine whether the relationship between exposure to rap music videos and adolescent health status was causal.

Social cognitive theory was used to explain the findings. Modeling occurs more readily when the modeled behavior is salient, simple, and prevalent and when it has functional value. Thus, exposure to rap music videos—and specifically gangsta rap, which is explicit about sex and violence and rarely shows the potential long-term adverse effects of risky behaviors—may influence adolescents modeling these unhealthy practices. Moreover, African American females desiring greater independence may rebel against parental medical restrictions and engage in risky behaviors. Implications for community health nurses are that education efforts should focus on these high-risk groups in determining risky behaviors and mediating factors.

Source: Wingood, G., DiClemente, R. J., Bernhardt, J. M., Harrington, K., Davies, S.L., Robillard, A., & Hook, E. W., 3rd. (2003). A prospective study of exposure to rap music videos and African American female adolescents' health. *American Journal of Public Health, 93*(3), 437–440.

Patterns of Health and Illness

Women are generally healthier and live longer than men, yet women miss more sick days from work, visit physicians more often than men, and are more likely to take on what sociologists refer to as the "sick role." Differences are often explained in terms of the way men and women are socialized to health and illness. Roughly 35% of women have a chronic condition that requires ongoing medical attention, and more than half (51%) take at least one prescription drug on a regular basis. Not surprisingly, this rate increases with age: 63% of women ages 45–64 take prescription medications, with 23% of these taking at least six medications regularly (Kaiser Family Foundation, 2011). The prevalence of certain chronic conditions has been increasing earlier in women's lives, too. Between 2001 and 2011, significant changes included the rise in diabetes from 5% to 9% of non-elderly women, anxiety and depression rose from 21% to 26%, and obesity rates increased from 11% to 16%. The three major chronic conditions women experience are arthritis, hypertension, and high cholesterol, all of which increase with age. However, it is striking that among women with incomes below 200% of the poverty level, two additional chronic conditions—asthma and obesity—are equally prevalent to high cholesterol, while incidence of arthritis and hypertension are 4% higher in this group than in women with incomes above 200% poverty level (Kaiser Family Foundation, 2011).

The leading causes of death in women are heart disease, cancer, and stroke, with differences in mortality observed by age and across racial groups. The leading causes of death in women older than age 65 are heart disease, cancer, cerebrovascular accident (CVA), pneumonia, and influenza. These diseases can be attributed to lifestyle, environmental, and social factors and are often preventable. Alcohol and drug use and abuse, unprotected sex, cigarette smoking, lack of exercise, obesity, and environmental threats are all associated with the leading causes of death in women.

Women's health needs are reflected in their provider choices as they age. Nearly all elderly women (95%) age 65 and older have regular health providers, compared to 77% of women ages 18 to 44 and 90% of women ages 45 to 64. Predictably, as women age, they are also less likely to visit a women's healthcare specialist on a regular basis. Only 5% of women 44 and older consider these women's healthcare specialists among their regular providers, compared to 14% of women in their reproductive years, and more than one in five (21%) reported being unable to see a specialist when they felt such care was needed. Of concern to health professionals, there have been declines in mammogram and Pap smear rates in both younger and middle-age women. While the changes are modest, these findings cause concern, because they reverse gains in previous years as women became more aware of the value of these early detection screening tests in improving the outcomes of breast and reproductive cancer. Mammography rates reported by women ages 40 to 64 dropped from 73% to 69%; Pap testing rates for women ages 18 to 64 fell from 81% to 70%. Possible reasons for these declining rates include media attention about the accuracy of mammography in detecting early-stage breast cancer. Further, the guidance on mammography for women ages 40 to 49 can be ambiguous, with major breast cancer organizations and researchers in disagreement over the recommendations for this age group. There have also been changes in recommendations for timing of Pap smears, which are now based on risk and presence of other health conditions, rather than uniform guidelines based on age. While these changes were intended to improve the targeting of screening programs and reduce the costs of unnecessary testing, they could be creating some confusion among women and their healthcare providers (Kaiser Family Foundation, 2011).

> **NOTE THIS!**
>
> For all persons who live to be 100 years of age, there will be five women for every two men.

Women may delay seeking care when sick because of family and work obligations, may not take symptoms of pain seriously, and may not pursue health care for themselves while focusing on the care of others. In addition, physicians may minimize women's complaints and delay necessary diagnostic tests, which results in a greater chance for a poor health outcome. One study examined the differences in women's survival rates from open-heart coronary bypass surgery as compared to men. The researchers found a significant survival rate difference between men and women. Women were almost twice as likely to die (at 4.6%) as men (2.6%) following the exact same open-heart surgical procedure. Factors identified by the researchers as explaining the difference are related to women's cardiac symptoms being different from those experienced by men, with healthcare providers taking women's complaints less seriously than men's. Physicians were 10 times more likely to order stress tests and scans with the first symptom for men, but they waited longer until women had clear-cut symptoms before ordering these diagnostics and doing surgery. By operating on a patient with more severe and late-manifested cardiac damage, the mortality goes up (Bell et al., 1995). All of these factors may contribute to women entering the healthcare system at a high acuity level with a greater chance of either dying or requiring more expensive and advanced medical and health interventions.

Mental health is an often overlooked but critical aspect of women's health care. One out of every four women (23%) reports that she has been diagnosed with depression or anxiety, more than twice the rate for men (11%). Even among senior women, who have lower rates of depression than young women do, these mental health issues affect 16% (Kaiser Family Foundation, 2011).

Health coverage, public or private, continues to be a major concern for women and is highly correlated with health and illness patterns in women throughout the lifespan. Nearly one in six women younger than age 65 is uninsured (17%). Women who are Latina, low income, single, and young are particularly at risk for being uninsured. Uninsured women are least likely to have visited a healthcare provider even once a year (67%), compared to women with either private insurance (90%) or public insurance—Medicaid (88%) and Medicare (93%) (*Kaiser Family Foundation*, 2011). Clearly, when women cannot afford insurance, pay for drugs, or qualify for public insurance, their health suffers. Compared to women with insurance, uninsured women consistently report lower rates of preventive screening tests for many conditions, including breast cancer, cervical cancer, hypertension, high cholesterol, and osteoporosis. Even insured women face barriers when seeking and accessing health care: One in 6 women with private coverage and one-

RESEARCH ALERT 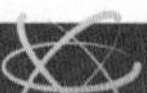

Skin cancer has historically been a condition of the elderly. Yet, it is now becoming common in women younger than age 30 at alarming rates due to the popularity and availability of tanning salons. Despite increasing awareness of skin cancer, particularly melanoma, and growing popularity of "spray tan" products, use of tanning beds is still significant among certain subpopulations, particularly among young adult and adolescent females. Many are obsessed with having a year-round tan, often thought of as a "healthy" and celebrity-type look. Of concern is the fact that among those who use tanning beds, more than half (57%) of females and 40% of males report using tanning beds frequently (more than 10 uses per 12 months).

Evidence of this growing public health problem can be seen in the prevalence of skin cancer among the young. The rate of new melanoma cases, the most lethal form of skin cancer, has doubled in the United States since 1975 for women ages 15 to 29. The World Health Organization (WHO, 2002) estimates that as many as 60,000 deaths worldwide are caused each year by excessive ultraviolet (UV) exposure and urges youth (especially those younger than age 18) to stay away from indoor tanning.

The "tanning business" is a profitable $5 billion per year quest for the year-round tan. This easy access to instant, year-round tans may be contributing to a frightening spike in skin cancer of the young. Consequences of this practice may include skin wrinkles, skin melanoma, cataracts, and premature aging. In addition, melanoma in dark-skinned people is more likely to be fatal: African Americans and Hispanics are at greater risks for late detection and death. Musician and reggae innovator Bob Marley, of Jamaica, died of melanoma.

Why do teen girls and others ignore the warnings about tanning salons and skin cancer? The popularity of this rotisserie style of tanning is related to the celebrity image of a year-round tan, especially among girls who are cheerleaders, majorettes, and aspiring models and actors. Many do it with their mothers, who often accompany them for tanning. Researchers have even posed the idea that tanning can be addictive. Tanning through either artificial light or natural light may produce endorphins and feeling of relaxation, and, therefore, withdrawal symptoms may be experienced when tanning is not available.

There is also a historical association between tanning and health. The myth that a tan is a sign of good health is not supported by research, even though sunshine is associated with vitamin D production, which is vital for good bone health. Vitamin D has been added to milk for decades, but we need only a few minutes on face and arms in winter to meet our need for vitamin D. Any change in skin color is a sign of UV damage. Even two sunburns by the age of 20 raise a person's lifetime risk of cancer significantly.

What are possible solutions? Restrictions and oversight by health departments have been slow to materialize. Only five states, and some local jurisdictions such as the cities of Chicago and Washington, DC, prohibit children under 18 from using tanning salons; 33 others place restrictions upon their use by minors, but often these restrictions may be easily circumvented. Campaigns and policy enactments are needed, much as occurred with successful antismoking campaigns, pushing laws to limit access, and raising taxes on tanning salons. Mass-media campaigns featuring celebrities who discourage tanning salons for teens would be wise as well.

Community health nurses should teach individuals about UV risk and tanning salons and promote the use of sunscreen on a daily basis, not just when tanning. Early detection of skin cancer, such as irregularly shaped moles and changes in existing skin lesions (e.g., oozing moles), should be emphasized in all contact with teenagers. Schools can be an excellent forum to warn teens about indoor tanning and encourage the use of sunless lotions.

Sources: Centers for Disease Control and Prevention. (2012a). Use of indoor tanning devices by adults—United States, 2010. *Morbidity and Mortality Weekly Report, 61*(18), 323–326; National Conference of State Legislatures (NCSL). (2014). *Indoor tanning restrictions for minors—a state-by-state comparison.* Retrieved from http://www.ncsl.org/research/health/indoor-tanning-restrictions.aspx; World Health Organization. (2004). *Ultraviolet radiation: Global solar UV index.* Retrieved from http://www.who.int/mediacentre/factsheets/fs271/en

third of women with Medicaid report that they postponed or went without needed health services in the past year because they could not afford it. Women are more likely (56%) than men (42%) to use prescription medicine on a regular basis and are more likely to report difficulties affording their medications. One in five women (20%) reports not filling at least one prescription, compared to 14% of men. Approximately 41% of uninsured women fail to fill prescriptions because of the drugs' costs. Related to these cost barriers, one in seven women reports skipping or taking lower doses of prescribed medication to make them last longer (*Kaiser Family Foundation,* 2011).

> Be who you are and say what you feel, because those who mind don't matter and those who matter don't mind.
>
> —*Dr. Seuss*

African American women are at elevated risk for certain health problems, and these risks increase with age. For example, African American women have arthritis and diabetes at significantly higher rates than do white women.

Health Issues, Health Promotion, and Health Prevention Across the Lifespan

Community health nurses, because of their unique relationship with clients and their awareness of community problems and resources, occupy a pivotal role in influencing women's beliefs and practices for health promotion and illness prevention. Community health nurses, as educators of women about health issues, incorporate the health-promotion and disease-prevention aims of *Healthy People 2020* to accomplish the primary goal of identifying and implementing behavioral and social interventions that are effective in motivating women to use preventive health services across the lifespan.

Adolescence (12 to 18 Years Old)

Today's teenage females in the United States face many health and social issues that their mothers and grandmothers could never have imagined. The present generation of teens is more likely to have an abundance of "screen" time, including tablets, computers, and smartphones, enabling a variety of ways to be "plugged in" to the Internet and to communicate with others. Opportunities are unlimited in the use of these media in influencing healthy behaviors, as these forms of communication are often more effective in reaching teens than in traditional clinic settings. Teens are more likely than adults to seek health information on the Internet, for example, due to the anonymity it provides. Community health nurses can play an important role in promoting the health of adolescent females through teaching, counseling, and role modeling, and can gainfully employ these various new technologies for sharing health information.

Community health nurses need to establish trusting relationships with adolescents, thereby gaining their confidence. This is a most challenging task, as parents of teens can relate to. As nurses, we must be able to ask the tough questions that might reveal alcohol and other drug abuse, high-risk sexual activity, or emotional distress. Community health nurses working with adolescents face challenges in communication, peer influences, and the stigma of teens being seen in local health clinics or settings that offer reproductive health resources. Effective programs that have a positive impact on the health of adolescents are often specifically targeted to teens in schools, night clinics, and malls, as well as through celebrity and teen role model spokespersons.

Young women in adolescence have many issues to deal with, including puberty, menarche, body image, eat-

TABLE 31-1 Births and Percentage of Births of Women by Age and Race, 2012

Age Group	Total Births	Non-Hispanic White	Non-Hispanic Black	American Indian	Asian or Pacific Islander	Hispanic
10–14	3,672	24%	34%	2%	2%	38%
15–19	305,388	39%	23%	2%	2%	34%
20–24	916,811	48%	21%	2%	3%	26%
25–34	2,137,316	58%	12%	1%	8%	21%
35–44	581,897	55%	11%	<1%	11%	21%
45–54	7,757	54%	13%	<1%	12%	16%

Source: Data from Martin, J. A., Hamilton, B. E., Osterman, M. J. K., Curtin, S. C., & Mathews, T. J. (2013). Births: Final data for 2012. *National Vital Statistics Reports, 62*(9), 1–87. Retrieved from http://www.cdc.gov/nchs/data/nvsr/nvsr62/nvsr62_09.pdf

ing disorders, and sexual issues, including sexual identity, contraception decisions, and STDs. Attitudes about these issues are influenced by the media, peers, society, and family relationships. *Healthy People 2020* objectives should guide the direction of educational efforts targeting this age group. School-based health programs for health promotion, exercise and fitness, sex education, and prevention of drug use should address social concerns related to teenage girls. Because the greatest number of new smokers are adolescent females, primary lung cancer prevention must start at the elementary school level, with aggressive counseling programs to decrease the number of new smokers among young girls. Successful programs with teen girls and the prevention of smoking initiation have focused on assertiveness training and decision-making models of accountability.

Parents should be included in these targeted interventions, as one media campaign advises: "Parents: The Anti Drug." Research supports this advice, with studies linking consistent attention by parents to drug prevention in their everyday conversations and decreased risks of their children engaging in drug experimentation (including smoking) and use.

While illegal drug use has decreased in past years, over-the-counter (OTC) and prescription drug abuse have continued to increase at alarming rates. Parents should remain constantly vigilant about the availability or misuse potential of their own prescribed drugs, especially those with high risk for abuse, such as narcotics, antihistamines, antidepressant drugs, and cough and cold preparations. They should also monitor online purchases via credit card on a monthly basis, checking out any suspicious charges. Drugs sold over the Internet are often charged on credit cards as innocent miscellaneous product or service sales. Nurses should be also vigilant about including this information when counseling teens, their parents, and educators who are in frequent contact with members of this age group.

The Youth Risk Behavior Surveillance System, which exists under the auspices of the CDC, monitors health-risk behaviors among youth and young adults on an annual basis. These health-risk behaviors contribute to unintentional and intentional injuries, tobacco use, alcohol and other illegal and prescription drug use, sexual behaviors, dietary behaviors, and physical activity, and should guide the community health nurse in planning interventions directed toward the female adolescent. Nurses should check the CDC website (http://www.cdc.gov) on a regular basis for current research and trends related to this age group, as well as review suggestions for applying the information in community settings. Schools, churches, and recreational groups all provide the community health nurse with opportunities to influence health decisions through education and media campaigns (CDC, 2008).

Adolescents' misconception that they are "immortal" sometimes leads to risk-taking behaviors that make them more susceptible to injury and death. During the past few years, females have been gaining on males as greater numbers engage in risk taking traditionally associated with males. Increases in automobile accidents, often in conjunction with cell phone use, and aggressive acts toward both males and other females have increased significantly. These trends are most likely to continue as gender roles move toward less rigid stereotypical expressions and the boundaries of appropriate behavior as distinguished by gender continue to blur. Female adolescents face potential threats to health such as substance abuse, pregnancy, acne, menstrual disorders, eating disorders, and STDs. Every year, nearly one-fourth of all new human immunodeficiency virus (HIV) infections, one-fourth of new STD infections, and hundreds

HEALTHY PEOPLE 2020 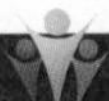

Objectives Related to Women's Health

Arthritis, Osteoporosis, and Chronic Back Conditions: Osteoporosis

- AOCBC-11.1 Reduce hip fractures among females age 65 years and older

Blood Disorders and Blood Safety

- BDBS-14 Increase the proportion of providers who refer women with symptoms suggestive of inherited bleeding disorders for diagnosis and treatment
- BDBS-15 Increase the proportion of females with von Willebrand disease (vWD) who are timely and accurately diagnosed

Cancer

- C-2 Reduce the lung cancer death rate
- C-3 Reduce the female breast cancer death rate
- C-4 Reduce the death rate from cancer of the uterine cervix
- C-10 Reduce invasive uterine cervical cancer
- C-11 Reduce late-stage female breast cancer
- C-15 Increase the proportion of women who receive a cervical cancer screening based on the most recent guidelines
- C-17 Increase the proportion of women who receive a breast cancer screening based on the most recent guidelines
- C-18.1 Increase the proportion of women who were counseled by their providers about mammograms
- C-18.2 Increase the proportion of women who were counseled by their providers about Pap tests

Family Planning

- FP-1 Increase the proportion of pregnancies that are intended
- FP-2 Reduce the proportion of females experiencing pregnancy despite use of a reversible contraceptive method
- FP-3 Increase the proportion of publicly funded family planning clinics that offer the full range of FDA-approved methods of contraception, including emergency contraception, onsite
- FP-4 Increase the proportion of health insurance plans that cover contraceptive supplies and services
- FP-5 Reduce the proportion of pregnancies conceived within 18 months of a previous birth
- FP-6 Increase the proportion of females at risk of unintended pregnancy or their partners who used contraception at most recent sexual intercourse
- FP-7.1 Increase the proportion of sexually experienced females age 15 to 44 years who received reproductive health services in the past 12 months
- FP-8 Reduce pregnancies among adolescent females
- FP-9.1 Increase the proportion of female adolescents age 15 to 17 years who have never had sexual intercourse
- FP-9.3 Increase the proportion of female adolescents age 15 years and under who have never had sexual intercourse
- FP-10.1 Increase the proportion of sexually active females age 15 to 19 years who use a condom at first intercourse
- FP-10.3 Increase the proportion of sexually active females age 15 to 19 years who use a condom at last intercourse
- FP-11.1 Increase the proportion of sexually active females age 15 to 19 years who use a condom and hormonal or intrauterine contraception at first intercourse
- FP-11.3 Increase the proportion of sexually active females age 15 to 19 years who use a condom and hormonal or intrauterine contraception at last intercourse
- FP-12.1 Increase the proportion of female adolescents who received formal instruction on abstinence before they were 18 years old
- FP-12.3 Increase the proportion of female adolescents who received formal instruction on birth control methods before they were 18 years old
- FP-12.5 Increase the proportion of female adolescents who received formal instruction on HIV/AIDS prevention before they were 18 years old
- FP-12.7 Increase the proportion of female adolescents who received formal instruction on sexually transmitted diseases before they were 18 years old
- FP-13.1 Increase the proportion of female adolescents who talked to a parent or guardian about abstinence before they were 18 years old
- FP-13.3 Increase the proportion of female adolescents who talked to a parent or guardian about birth control methods before they were 18 years old
- FP-13.5 Increase the proportion of female adolescents who talked to a parent or guardian about HIV/AIDS prevention before they were 18 years old
- FP-13.7 Increase the proportion of female adolescents who talked to a parent or guardian about sexually transmitted diseases before they were 18 years old
- FP-14 Increase the number of states that set the income eligibility level for Medicaid-covered family planning services to at least the same level used to determine eligibility for Medicaid-covered, pregnancy-related care
- FP-15 Increase the proportion of females in need of publicly supported contraceptive services and supplies who receive those services and supplies

HIV

- HIV-14.3 Increase the proportion of pregnant women who have been tested for HIV in the past 12 months.
- HIV-17.1 Increase the proportion of sexually active unmarried females age 15 to 44 years who use condoms

(*continues*)

HEALTHY PEOPLE 2020 (*continued*)

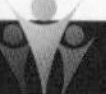

Injury and Violence Prevention: Violence and Abuse Prevention

- IVP-39 Reduce violence by current or former intimate partners
- IVP-40 Reduce sexual violence

Lesbian, Gay, Bisexual, and Transgender Health

- LGBT-1 (Developmental) Increase the number of population-based data systems used to monitor *Healthy People 2020* objectives that include in their core a standardized set of questions that identify lesbian, gay, bisexual, and transgender (LGBT) populations

Maternal, Infant, and Child Health

Maternal Death and Illness

- MICH-5 Reduce the rate of maternal mortality
- MICH-6 Reduce maternal illness and complications due to pregnancy (complications during hospitalized labor and delivery)
- MICH-7 Reduce cesarean births among low-risk (full-term, singleton, and vertex presentation) women

Pregnancy Health and Behaviors

- MICH-10 Increase the proportion of pregnant women who receive early and adequate prenatal care
- MICH-11 Increase abstinence from alcohol, cigarettes, and illicit drugs among pregnant women
- MICH-12 Increase the proportion of pregnant women who attend a series of prepared childbirth classes
- MICH-13 Increase the proportion of mothers who achieve a recommended weight gain during their pregnancies
- MICH-16 Increase the proportion of women delivering a live birth who received preconception care services and practiced key recommended preconception health behaviors
- MICH-17 Reduce the proportion of persons age 18 to 44 years who have impaired fecundity (i.e., a physical barrier preventing pregnancy or carrying a pregnancy to term)

Postpartum Health and Behavior

- MICH-18 Reduce postpartum relapse of smoking among women who quit smoking during pregnancy
- MICH-19 Increase the proportion of women giving birth who attend a postpartum care visit with a health worker

Nutrition and Weight Status: Iron Deficiency Anemia

- NWS-21 Reduce iron deficiency among young children and females of childbearing age
- NWS-22 Reduce iron deficiency among pregnant females

Sexually Transmitted Diseases: STD Complications Affecting Females

- STD-1.1 Reduce the proportion of females age 15 to 24 years with *Chlamydia trachomatis* infections attending family planning clinics
- STD-1.2 Reduce the proportion of females age 24 years and under with *Chlamydia trachomatis* infections enrolled in a National Job Training Program
- STD-2 Reduce *Chlamydia* rates among females age 15 to 44 years
- STD-3 Increase the proportion of sexually active females age 24 years and under enrolled in Medicaid plans who are screened for genital *Chlamydia* infections during the measurement year
- STD-4 Increase the proportion of sexually active females age 24 years and under enrolled in commercial health insurance plans who are screened for genital *Chlamydia* infections during the measurement year
- STD-5 Reduce the proportion of females age 15 to 44 years who have ever required treatment for pelvic inflammatory disease (PID)
- STD-6.1 Reduce gonorrhea rates among females age 15 to 44 years
- STD-7.1 Reduce domestic transmission of primary and secondary syphilis among females
- STD-9 Reduce the proportion of females with human papillomavirus (HPV) infection

Source: U.S. Department of Health and Human Services (HHS). (2012). *Healthy People 2020: Topics and Objectives*. Retrieved from http://www.healthypeople.gov/2020/topicsobjectives2020/default.aspx

of thousands of unintended pregnancies occur among U.S. teenagers.

The community health nurse can be a pivotal force in promoting the health of adolescents through health assessment, risk analysis, screening, anticipatory guidance, health teaching, and counseling with both adolescents and parents. The most common healthcare requests of adolescent females are related to pregnancy, sexual choices, and pregnancy prevention. As part of any visit with a teen female, the nurse should conduct a health screening assessment, including last missed menstrual period; contraception, if any, being used; living arrangements; financial status; and significant sex partners. This provides the nurse with opportunities to determine the teen's concerns about the initiation of a sexual relationship, the risks involved with such initiation, and concerns arising from the teen's own moral and ethical feelings about sex and attachment.

Young females are having sex at younger ages and approaching the percentage of teen boys who begin hav-

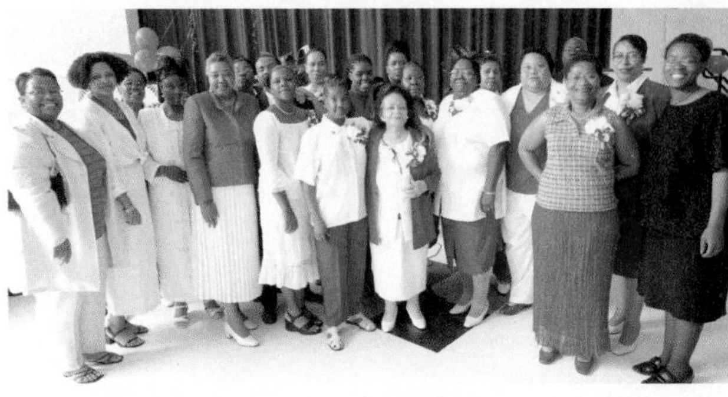

Women who are involved in their communities, such as this community lay advisor group, are very effective in promoting health among specific populations, such as elder African American women.

ing sex as early as 15. Teen girls are at risk for acquaintance rape during high school, and this problem only escalates in the college years. The frequent use of the "date rape" drug Rohypnol ("roofies") placed in drinks exposes girls who overuse alcohol in social settings to an even greater risk of sexual assault and rape. Because of the effects of Rohypnol, girls have little to no memory of the sexual assault or the person involved, which lessens the likelihood of the rape being reported. The nurse should offer suggestions about how to avoid this ever-increasing problem, as teen girls' alcohol use has increased significantly in the past 5 years, leaving them even more vulnerable to date and acquaintance rape.

If an adolescent is pregnant, anticipatory guidance is needed. This includes referral to a local prenatal health clinic or health department, encouragement of open communication regarding the pregnancy with family members or the significant other, and referral to the local department of human services for Medicaid enrollment if necessary. Health teaching must include the effects of alcohol and drugs on the fetus, the potential side effects of x-rays on the fetus, nutrition, and Women, Infants, and Children (WIC) nutrition program enrollment. The counseling services of the nurse should include a meeting with the adolescent and parent to inform them of the pregnancy.

For sexually active adolescents who are not pregnant, the nurse should encourage enrollment in a family planning clinic for contraceptives and STD education, and take the time to discuss sexual values and concerns that are often difficult for the teen to talk about with friends or family. Instead of asking, "Do you have any other concerns?", the nurse can often open up the discussion with, "Many young women your age have concerns and questions about intimacy and decisions about sex. I know that it is very hard to talk about these things with our friends and family. Do you have any questions or concerns that we might need to talk about?"

MEDIA MOMENT

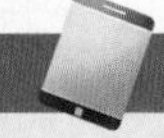

Songs About Women and Women's Issues

"Independence Day," Martina McBride
"I Am Woman," Helen Reddy
"Goodbye Earl," The Dixie Chicks
"Eleanor Rigby," The Beatles
"Hey Hey Cinderella," Suzy Bogguss
"Stand by Your Man," Tammy Wynette
"It Wasn't God Who Made Honky Tonk Angels," Kitty Wells
"The Pill," Loretta Lynn

Young Adulthood (19 to 35 Years Old)

Two main concerns of women in this age group include making career choices and establishing relationships that may lead to marriage and pregnancy. Since the 1990s, women in increasing numbers have been delaying marriage and children, which has led to an increase in infertility rates for women in their 30s and 40s. Community health nurses can address health-promotion interventions in the context of these two life tasks. Nurses need to be knowledgeable about the various resources that are available in the community to assist women in this age range with such decisions. The nurse can be an effective model/mentor for young women in this developmental stage and should be able to address such concerns as fertility counseling, parenting skills, contraception options, domestic violence, and occupational health issues. Women in young adulthood face concerns such as STDs, contraceptive choices, safety, intentional and unintentional injury, stress management, alcohol and drug abuse, unhealthy dietary behaviors and relationships, physical activity, and role stress and strain. As women marry and establish families, they face issues such as learning to balance work and children, sexual harassment in the workplace, and establishing habits of self-care. The community health nurse must be cognizant of the problems of this age group and skillful in locating and accessing the resources available to intervene with this age group in setting lifelong healthy patterns.

Violent deaths, homicide, suicide, and accidents (particularly motor vehicle accidents) are responsible for the majority of deaths in this age group. For young adults and college students, as for adolescents, violent death or injury, alcohol and substance abuse, unwanted pregnancies, and STDs are major health threats. Females in this age group may find themselves more vulnerable to "date rape," especially in college, where the use of alcohol and binge drinking have increased (see **Box 31-1**). Most health problems in this stage are related to lifestyle behaviors and can

TABLE 31-2 Recommended Healthcare Calendar

Test or Procedure	Who Needs It?	How Often?
• General physical exam (including blood pressure and lifestyle counseling)	Everyone	Every year
• Pelvic examination	Everyone	Every year
• Dental examination	Everyone	Every year
• Eye examination	Everyone	Every year
• Breast examination	Everyone	Every year
• Breast self-examination (BSE)	Everyone	Every month
• Skin cancer check	Everyone	Every 3 years
• Rectal examination	Everyone	Every year
• Pap smear	Everyone	Every year
• Blood cholesterol	Everyone	Every 3 years (if first test was normal); as recommended by health professional if level is elevated
• Mammogram	Everyone	Every 1 to 2 years between ages 40 and 50 and once a year after age 50
• Tests for STDs	Anyone who is sexually active	Every 6–12 months if multiple partners, otherwise as recommended by health professional
• Electrocardiogram	Anyone with two or more of the following: risk factors for heart disease: family history, smoking, high cholesterol, diabetes, high blood pressure	Every 3 to 5 years
• Sigmoidoscopy	Anyone over 50	Every 3 years
• Fecal occult–blood test	Everyone	Every year
• Tuberculin skin test	Anyone who is at increased risk	Every year or as recommended by health professional
• Tetanus booster	Everyone	Every 10 years
• Diphtheria booster	Everyone	Every 10 years
• Human Papillomavirus vaccination	Girls, ages 11–26	Once

Sources: Data from Centers for Disease Control and Prevention (CDC). (2012b). *HPV Vaccine recommendations*. Retrieved from http://www.cdc.gov/STD/hpv/STDFact-HPV-vaccine-hcp.htm#vaccrec.

alter individuals' chances for a healthy life in the future. Weight concerns and eating problems are often reported as concerns for young women. Media images and social influences may pressure young women desiring to be thin into abusive habits, such as purging, vomiting, laxative and diuretic abuse, and poor nutrition. Young women should be aware of interventions to delay onset of osteoporosis, including increasing calcium intake and weight-bearing exercises to promote bone density and decreasing cola intake, which decreases reabsorption of calcium. Ingesting excessive soft drinks is associated in research studies with decreasing bone mass, and many members of this age group consume soft drinks on a daily basis as a habit started during the teen years. Diet sodas have been found to be associated with a greater risk for obesity, despite the traditional belief their use reduces calorie intake. The use of diet sodas apparently keeps the need for and consequent consumption of foods and drinks that are high in sugar higher than in those who do not drink excessive diet sodas.

BOX 31-1 Acquaintance Rape: A New Name for an Old Crime?

Acquaintance rape occurs when a friend or former acquaintance sexually molests a woman. While this act of violence was more likely to have occurred in the past, studies of young women—especially those in college—have indicated a wider incidence than previously thought. In one study, 24% of women reported that they had sex at least once when they "did not want to" (Felton, Gumm, & Pittenger, 2001). A majority of women in the study reported unwanted sexual advances, particularly when drugs and alcohol were involved. Because this crime occurs with acquaintances and can occur under the influence of "date rape" drugs, few report the incidents. A woman is often reluctant to report the incident because she knows the person and was with him voluntarily, at least to some degree. Women often define rape erroneously as occurring only with strangers. Many times, women have no memory of the incident or the identity of the man or men involved.

Young women must be educated while still in middle and high school about the additional risk of sexual assault while under the influence of alcohol and drugs and told to avoid drinking any liquid from an opened bottle or cup at any time during social gatherings. Having a "buddy system," similar to the one used in scuba diving and other risky sports, can also reduce the risk of unwanted sexual assault during college and young adulthood.

MEDIA MOMENT 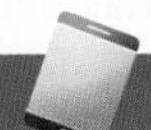

***Half the Sky* (2012)**

A documentary based on the book of the same title by the Pulitzer-winning team of *New York Times* journalists Nicholas Kristof and Sheryl WuDunn, who argue that a more aggressive stance opposing the oppression of women worldwide is the paramount humanitarian issue of the modern era. Both book and documentary look at a wide range of issues affecting women's status, health, and wellbeing, from economic inequities to sex trafficking to gender violence.

The community health nurse can play a vital role in educating this group regarding behaviors that will positively affect their lifestyles. The proper use of condoms to help prevent STDs and the availability and variety of contraceptive choices to prevent unwanted pregnancy must be discussed with the young adult. Many young adults continue to erroneously believe that the use of oral contraceptives eliminates the need for condom use. Nurses must be vigilant about reminding young women of the continued STD risks even with the use of alternative birth control methods; using a condom every time is a good practice for all young women who have multiple sex partners. Addressing these concerns and seeking mutual solutions together can accomplish the ultimate goal of improved health and risk reduction with young women in this age group.

Perimenopausal/Menopausal (36 to 55 Years Old)

A comprehensive assessment of women in this age group should include the changes of life that a woman goes through, including physiological, psychological, and emotional changes. The community health nurse must assess the woman's knowledge regarding the changes in her body, including her beliefs about menopause and the implications for her health. The nurse must be aware of complementary therapies women may choose for their health care and should remain open-minded about what is acceptable for their clients. Cardiovascular disease, cancer, and osteoporosis are the three major diseases that occur during the perimenopausal/menopausal period of a woman's life. The community health nurse must address health priorities with this age group of women, including:

- Benefits and risks of **hormone replacement therapy (HRT)**
- Early signs and symptoms of cardiovascular disease
- Benefits of monitoring and controlling cholesterol and blood pressure levels
- Maintaining bone strength and density
- Maintaining healthy weight
- Exercising regularly
- Benefits of regular mammograms and Pap smears
- Maintaining meaningful sexual relations with a partner
- Maintaining healthy eating habits and adjusting to nutritional needs as they age

As women delay childbearing and then resort to advanced reproductive technology, more women may be having their first child during this late reproductive stage. Women may also be caring for their own parents during this time while building careers, putting even greater time and energy demands on themselves.

During this period of a woman's life, the ovaries begin to slow down and eventually cease production of estrogen. Because of this decrease in estrogen, women may experience symptoms such as hot flashes, vaginal dryness, or night sweats. All perimenopausal women should be counseled about the benefits and risks of HRT. HRT has been associated with greater risks for certain groups of women, and research continues to help nurses better inform all women about their choices during menopause. With declining estrogen levels, bone density decreases dramatically

RESEARCH ALERT

Artificial insemination by donor (AID) is an option being selected by increasing numbers of single women who desire parenthood. Although AID has been reported to have positive outcomes for couples, there is a paucity of research about the experience of single women who choose this alternative, perhaps, because of cultural and social prohibitions. Thus, nurses who provide health care with this "emerging family" have little knowledge available related to the unique needs of these patients.

This case study can be utilized by nurses as more women choose alternative ways of becoming mothers. In this case, a 38-year-old single female, well established in her career, delivered her first child, a son, from artificial insemination. The baby is now 3 months old. The nursing theory of Man-Living-Health provided the framework to elicit, organize, and analyze nursing care. Research questions were derived from the principles of this theory and focused on three areas: the processes of structuring and giving meaning in situations, developing and changing relationships, and transcending or actualizing one's dreams and future goals. A fourth question focused specifically on the subject's perceptions of her health care and health needs. The researcher conducted an unstructured, tape-recorded interview to collect data.

Themes emerging from data analysis suggested that valuing independence, making choices related to directing health decisions, and assuming self-responsibility for outcomes of decisions were associated with the decision to have insemination. A period of relationship flux appeared to occur as the woman took on the maternal role. While there were some dramatic positive effects on the new mother's perspectives about her quality of like experience, themes of vulnerability and aloneness were also predominant.

Implications to promote optimal health and effective maternal role transition were identified, especially directed toward fostering the woman's sense of security and community. The need for the nurse to initiate immediate and anticipatory guidance was viewed as critical because the mother's intense feelings of self-responsibility could conflict with the desire to ask for support and guidance. Because the new mother was acutely aware of potential censure from others, a critical element of effective nursing care was the nurse's examination of his or her own moral/ethical values about insemination. Because of the growing numbers of women who are choosing to have children through AID, there is a significant need for further research to validate health needs in this population.

Source: Frank, D. (1987). *The health experience of a single woman having a child through artificial insemination by donor (AID).* Presented at the 8th Annual Research Symposium, Gamma Zeta Chapter, Sigma Theta Tau, University of North Carolina, Greensboro.

during and after menopause, resulting in greater risks for fractures and other complications. As estrogen levels drop, a decrease in high-density lipoprotein (HDL) cholesterol and an increase in low-density lipoprotein (LDL) cholesterol increase the risk of cardiovascular problems, such as myocardial infarction and CVA. Women may react differently to these menopausal physiological changes in the body, and nurses should consider individual risk factors, tolerance of symptoms, and comfort as women face a myriad of choices and options available to them during this period of change.

CULTURAL CONNECTION

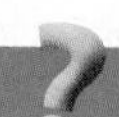

We black women must forgive black men for not protecting us against slavery, racism, white men, our confusion, their doubts. And black men must forgive black women for our own sometimes dubious choices, divided loyalties, and lack of belief in their possibilities. Only when our sons and our daughters know that forgiveness is real, existent, and that those who love them practice it, can they form bonds as men and women that really can save and change our community.

—*Marita Golden*

During this time, a woman may reexamine her life, which may result in a new self-identity. Women must explore what aging means to them and go through an acceptance of what their life has been and what it may still become. Sexuality of women also changes during this time. Our society, with its focus on youth and sexuality, rarely acknowledges the sexuality of women as they age. Health professionals more often than not exclude sexuality in their assessment of women in the postmenopausal years. Most women continue to have healthy sex drives and, when this consideration is included as an integral part of health assessment and care, maintain their interest in sexuality as they age. Research indicates that for many women, the post-reproductive years become better sexually once children and family obligations are less demanding. Many women view this time as the best years of their lives: Children are grown, careers are more stable, career changes are possible, and acceptance of self-identity is well established. For women who have devoted their younger years to childrearing, they may be returning to school, reentering the career market, or making career changes.

Mature (55 and Older)

As more women are reaching the mature stage of the lifecycle, the community health nurse must realize that a shift of health emphasis from infectious and acute diseases to chronic diseases occurs in this age group. Because of the chronic nature of diseases in this age group, the historical definition of health (absence of disease) is less applicable. Rather, the emphasis should be placed on functional health, independence, and autonomy. Health promotion should be aimed at preserving the mature woman's ability to function at the highest spectrum of wellness. Health-promoting activities to enhance wellness are listed in **Box 31-2**. Career choices and lifestyle changes, such as dating after divorce or death of a spouse, bring both challenges and opportunities as women move into this new phase of their lives. Most women find the freedom of this period in their lives very exciting, as it is often filled with choices and opportunities not possible or considered when younger.

Mature women deal with many healthcare issues as they age. Many of the issues and health conditions discussed in the previous section on menopausal women apply here as well. However, as women live longer, their chronic conditions may increase in severity. Depression, dementia, and **urinary incontinence** are some of the illnesses that occur later in life. Arthritis, osteoporosis, hypertension, and cardiovascular disease (CVD) continue to be health concerns for women in this age group (Fogel & Woods, 1995; Kaiser Family Foundation, 2011).

Community health nurses often must deal with depression in mature women. Many may have outlived their spouses and are dealing with the loss daily. This depression often goes untreated. Many medications may also contribute to the depression. If dementia is present, safety considerations in the surrounding environment become essential. Urinary incontinence is seen as much as four to seven times as often in women as in men (Nitti, 2001). Nurses must also be aware of medications that may cause urinary retention or urinary incontinence, possibly leading to urinary tract infections.

BOX 31-2 Health-Promotion Activities for the Mature Woman

- Health screenings
- Blood pressure, early cancer detection, hearing and vision screenings
- Health education
- Stress reduction, nutrition, general health, smoking cessation, classes about seasonal health issues such as hypothermia, heart-related illness, colds/flu
- Immunizations
- Influenza shots
- Safety
- Safe driving courses, self-protection measures
- Exercise
- Walking, aerobics, water aerobics, weight lifting, weight-bearing exercise

GLOBAL CONNECTION 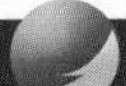

The idea of female genital mutilation/circumcision (FGM/C) is so horrifying that it is difficult to comprehend how the practice became so widespread globally. It is common in 29 countries located primarily in central and south-Saharan Africa and the Middle East as well as (to a lesser extent) in Pakistan, Afghanistan, Malaysia, India, and Indonesia. It is sometimes encountered among immigrants from these cultures living in Western countries, although in the United States, performing FGM/C on anyone under 18 is illegal and subject to prosecution if identified. While it is a practice primarily encountered in Islamic countries, it is not a religious ritual related to Islam, Office of Women's Health [OWH], 2012). Some 100–140 million women and girls have been subjected to FGM/C, usually before reaching puberty. In Egypt, an estimated 90% of girls undergo the procedure between the ages of 5 and 14, but in Yemen more than three-quarters of the procedures are done on infants younger than 2 weeks of age (OWH, 2012). The most common victim of this practice is 4 to 8 years of age, and the procedure is done without anesthesia. Complications include shock, excessive bleeding, and chronic urinary tract infections.

In female circumcision, the clitoris (and often the labia) is removed, with only a small opening left for urination. The cut is opened wider when the woman is married (often by her husband) and for childbirth. After birth, the opening is once again sutured shut.

Why is this practice done? Factors associated with female circumcision include ensuring the woman is a virgin from birth to marriage, removing pleasure from sex to ensure faithfulness in the marriage, and enhancing "cleanliness." A common myth is that this act enhances the fertility of the woman, but the World Health Organization identifies no health benefits, in contrast to multiple short- and long-term harms (WHO). Mothers often support the practice because it makes a girl "more marriageable" (Boyle, Songora, & Foss, 2001).

There is hope on the horizon, as the horror of female circumcision has become more widely known outside of these countries. Women across the globe have condemned the practice and led political action to stop it. Significant advances in eliminating this practice include the West African Regional Fatwa of 2010, in which 34 religious leaders from 10 Islamic countries, including Sudan and Egypt, denounced the practice

(continues)

GLOBAL CONNECTION (*continued*) 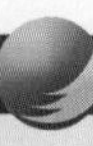

(UNFPA-UNICEF, 2011) and national legislation passed in Kenya and Guinea-Bissau outlawing FGM/C (UNFPA-UNICEF, 2011), bringing the total number of African countries that explicitly forbid it to 16, with a 17th country, Sudan, outlawing the most severe practices but not other, less invasive forms. Other indicators of progress include the following:

- Nearly 2,744 communities publicly declared their abandonment of FGM/C.
- Across 15 countries, 141 cases violating national laws against FGM/C were prosecuted in court.
- Nearly 19,584 community education sessions took place.
- More than 3,485 newspaper articles and TV and radio programs discussed the benefits of ending the practice.
- Nearly 300 health facilities included FGM/C prevention in their antenatal and neonatal care.
- Nearly 4,107 religious leaders taught their followers that FGM/C is not sanctioned by Islam.
- Nearly 1,000 religious edicts were issued in support of the abandonment of the practice.

Do you think that the United States should intervene in other countries' cultural practices? Are there legitimate reasons to do so?

Source: UNFPA-UNICEF, 2011.

Specific Disease Conditions of Women Throughout the Lifespan

Cardiovascular disease (CVD) is the largest single cause of mortality among women, accounting for 25% of all deaths among females in the United States. The most effective strategies for CVD reduction target the primary prevention level. In reality, almost all women are at risk for CVD; consequently, women and their healthcare providers should consider the use of guidelines as part of routine visits and preventive health education. The public health impact of CVD in women is not solely related to mortality, as advances in science and medicine now allow many women to survive heart disease. Modifiable risk factors for such disease include cigarette smoking, hypertension, hypercholesterolemia, and physical inactivity, with less direct but still important risk factors being obesity, diabetes, stress, and menopause. The American Heart Association publishes guidelines for preventing CVD in women, which are updated annually based on current research about risk factors and CVD in women. The guidelines provide research-based health information that should be used by women and their healthcare providers to reduce CVD risks throughout a woman's lifetime.

NOTE THIS!

- Cardiovascular disease affects more than one in three women in the United States and is the cause of death for nearly 400,000 women each year.
- The number of deaths due to cardiovascular disease in women has outstripped the number in men each year since 1984.
- Almost two-thirds (64%) of women who die suddenly from heart disease have no prior symptoms.

The typical warning signs of heart attack in women are not the same as those in men. Chest pain is number one in men; the most common warning signs in women include unusual fatigue, sleep disturbances, and shortness of breath. Women are more likely to describe chest pain that is sharp, burning and more frequently have pain in the neck, jaw, throat, abdomen, or back.

Source: American Heart Association. (2013). *Cardiovascular disease: Women's No. 1 health threat*. Retrieved from http://www.heart.org/idc/groups/heart-public/@wcm/@adv/documents/downloadable/ucm_302256.pdf; Centers for Disease Control and Prevention (CDC). (2013b). Women and heart disease fact sheet. Retrieved from http://www.cdc.gov/dhdsp/data_statistics/fact_sheets/fs_women_heart.htm

Community health nurses need to first become aware of the modifiable risk factors and then develop a cardiovascular health plan with an emphasis on prevention. When a woman seeks health care, either for herself or for a family member, the community health nurse should seize the opportunity to emphasize heart health. The relationship between estrogen and CVD, along with cardiac risk factors, must be discussed and assessed. The use of medications in the home should be reinforced by client teaching, including when to take prescribed nitroglycerin and when to seek medical attention for chest pains. By empowering women with knowledge, nurses can help women employ appropriate prevention strategies in their lives and seek health care early should CVD become a health problem. By following preventive measures regarding heart health, women can improve their chances for living longer and enjoying a better quality of life.

Cancer

Cancer is the second leading cause of death in women in the United States. Lung cancer has surpassed breast cancer as the leading cause of cancer deaths in women. The most common types of cancer in women are lung, breast, colorectal, ovarian, and pancreatic. Tobacco is the single most toxic carcinogenic substance responsible for the occurrence of lung cancer and has been linked to cancers of the mouth, pharynx, larynx, esophagus, pancreas, uterine cervix, kidney, and bladder. For this reason, smoking cessation programs for women who smoke need to be readily accessible.

Breast cancer is the second leading cause of cancer death in women overall and is the leading cause of cancer deaths in women age 50 to 54. It is imperative that community health nurses educate women about breast self-examination, the signs and symptoms of breast cancer, and the need for age-appropriate mammography (American Cancer Society, 2008). If symptoms are detected, women must be educated that seeking health care is critical in the reduction of morbidity and mortality risks associated with breast cancer. When breast cancer is detected in the early stages (localized), the 5-year survival rate for women is more than 94%.

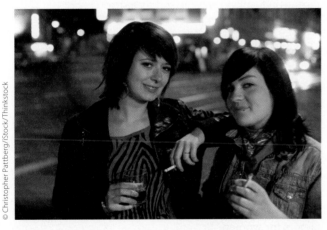

Women in high stress careers may be at greater risk for substance abuse although educated and better informed than previous years as to the problems associated with alcohol and smoking behaviors.

When a woman is receiving chemotherapy for cancer, the nurse should be aware of the side effects of this treatment and know what can be done in the home to decrease or alleviate symptoms of discomfort (e.g., nausea, vomiting, pain). Nurses must also be aware of local resources to ensure that women have prompt access to care as soon as a definite cancer diagnosis has been obtained, along with support groups and referral agencies for cancer victims. (See **Box 31-3**.) Reach to Recovery is the American Cancer Association's peer support program, which provides women with both individual and group support in the promotion of recovery from breast cancer.

Osteoporosis

Bone mass peaks at the end of the growth period, usually around age 17. Some small gains in bone mass occur up to age 30; this is then followed by a progressive loss of bone mass. Osteoporosis is largely a disease affecting women, with 80% of females suffering from this preventable disorder. Osteoporosis is a major public health problem in the United States. Vertebral fractures generally occur in women 55 years and older and result in back pain, height loss and kyphosis, anterior rib pain, negatively changed body image, difficulty in fitting clothes, a protuberant abdomen, and abdominal discomfort (as a result of reduced lumbar vertebral height). Hip fractures occur twice as often in women older than 75 than in men and are associated with excess mortality of 5% to 20% as a result of preoperative and postoperative complications, such as deep vein thrombosis, pulmonary embolism, and pneumonia.

RESEARCH ALERT

This descriptive research study examined the effectiveness of exercise as an aid for smoking cessation in women. The sample was composed of 281 healthy but sedentary female smokers between the ages of 18 and 65 who had smoked routinely for at least 1 year. The subjects were followed in a 12-week smoking cessation program. Of the 134 women who exercised three times per week, 19.4% gave up smoking for at least 2 months after their program ended, compared with 10.2% of the 147 nonexercisers. Three months later, 16.4% of the exercisers were still not smoking, compared with 8.2% of the nonexercisers. One year after the study, the difference was 11.9% and 5.4%, respectively. The study provides evidence that vigorous exercise leads to improved rates of continuous abstinence from smoking in women.

Source: Marcus, B., & Albrecht, A. (1999). The efficacy of exercise as an aid for smoking cessation in women. *Archives of Internal Medicine, 159*(11), 1229–1235.

RESEARCH ALERT 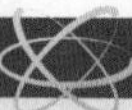

The American Heart Association's "Effectiveness-Based Guidelines for the Prevention of Cardiovascular Disease Women—2011 Update" emphasize the following points:

- Make lifestyle changes to help manage blood pressure, including weight control, increased physical activity, alcohol moderation, sodium restriction, and an emphasis on eating fresh fruits, vegetables, and low-fat dairy products.
- Cease all tobacco use through counseling, nicotine replacement, or other forms of smoking cessation therapy.
- Recommend physical activity for women who need to lose weight or who want to sustain weight loss, including a minimum of 60 to 90 minutes of moderate-intensity activity (e.g., brisk walking) on most, and preferably all, days of the week.
- Reduce saturated fats intake to less than 7% of calories, if possible.
- Consume oily fish at least twice weekly, for omega-3 fatty acid intake; use a capsule supplement of 850 to 1,000 mg of eicosapentaenoic acid (EPA) and docosahexaenoic acid (DHA) in women with heart disease, and 2 to 4 g for women with high cholesterol or high triglycerides.
- Hormone replacement therapy and selective estrogen-receptor modulators (SERMs) are not recommended to prevent heart disease in women.
- Antioxidant supplements (such as vitamin E, vitamin C, and beta-carotene) should not be used for primary or secondary prevention of CVD.
- Folic acid should not be used to prevent CVD.
- Routine low-dose aspirin therapy is not recommended in women over 65 years of age, but low-dose aspirin may be used if benefit in myocardial infarction (MI) or ischemic stroke prevention outweighs risks of gastrointestinal (GI) bleeding or hemorrhagic stroke.
- The upper dosage of aspirin for high-risk women is up to 325 mg per day.
- Reduce LDL cholesterol to less than 70 mg/dL in very high-risk women with heart disease, which may require a combination of cholesterol-lowering drugs.

These guidelines are published by the American Heart Association and written by an expert panel of cardiovascular specialists and researchers, and are updated based on new research findings and designed for use by women to reduce their cardiovascular risks. Emphasis in the latest version of the guidelines is on the *lifetime* risk of women for CVD, and as such they include a new paradigm for risk assessment based on risk factors and family history. Women and health professionals focusing on the prevention of CVD should use the guidelines over the lifespan.

The new guidelines include expanded recommendations on lifestyle factors, such as physical activity, nutrition, and smoking cessation, as well as more in-depth recommendations on drug treatments for blood pressure and cholesterol control.

Source: Mosca, L., Benjamin, E. J., Berra, K., Bezanson, J. L., Dolor, R. J., Lloyd-Jones, D. M, ... Wenger, N. K. (2011). Effectiveness-based guidelines for cardiovascular disease prevention in women—2011 update: A guideline from the American Heart Association. *Circulation, 123*, 1243–1262.

BOX 31-3 Cancer Support Groups

American Cancer Society
800-227-2345
http://www.cancer.org/treatment/supportprogramsservices/index

Candlelighters Childhood Cancer Family Alliance
713-270-4700
https://www.candle.org/

National Breast Cancer Foundation
http://www.nationalbreastcancer.org/

National Coalition for Cancer Survivorship
877-NCCS-YES |
http://www.canceradvocacy.org/

SHARE: Self-Help for Women with Breast or Ovarian Cancer
http://www.sharecancersupport.org/share-new/
844-ASK-SHARE

The community nurse must be aware of lifestyle changes that can help prevent osteoporosis, including calcium intake, weight control, and weight-bearing exercise, as well as HRT used to treat osteoporosis. Nurses can apply the osteoporosis profile (**Table 31-3**) to identify risk factors for women.

Diversity and Women's Health

Cultural Influences

Gender roles are greatly influenced by culture and affect where, when, and how women seek health information and advice. The impact of culture on women is imperative for the community health nurse to understand. An awareness of family dominance patterns is essential when teaching clients and communicating with family members about the specific health issues affecting women. Although many cultures are still largely patriarchal, matriarchal influences are also important. Acceptable

TABLE 31-3 Osteoporosis Risk-Factor Profile for Women

- 65 years or older
- Family history of osteoporosis
- Caucasian or Asian
- Postmenopausal, especially premature
- History of a traumatic fracture
- Loss of 1 inch or more in height
- Slender build
- Estrogen deficiency/menopause
- Sedentary lifestyle
- Low calcium intake
- Low serum vitamin D
- Failure to achieve peak bone mass
- Cigarette smoking
- High alcohol consumption
- Weight below normal
- Steroid use

BOX 31-4 Questions for Assessing Cultural Communication Patterns

1. Is the individual willing to share thoughts, feelings, and ideas?
2. What does touching mean in the culture? Is touching certain body parts appropriate?
3. What does silence mean in the culture? A loud voice?
4. Which spatial and distancing characteristics when communicating are observed for family members versus strangers?
5. What kind of eye contact is used (avoidance; changes among family, friends, strangers, or socioeconomic groups)? Is it a sign of respect or insult?
6. Which facial expressions are used? Do individuals smile a lot, show emotions?
7. How are people greeted?

Source: Adapted from Purnell, L., & Paulanka, B. (1998). *Transcultural health care: A culturally competent approach.* Philadelphia, PA: F. A. Davis.

ways of communicating and touching should be assessed by community health nurses and included in any interventions for the client. In some cultures, women may not speak unless they are given permission to do so by a spouse or father. In other cultures, the elder female in the household may speak for the entire family. Men and women interact with each other according to their cultural values. Community health nurses should always remain sensitive to a woman's cultural influences in the promotion of healthy interventions (Lipson, Dibble, & Minarik, 1996; Purnell & Paulanka, 1998). Guidelines for a cultural communication assessment appear in **Box 31-4**.

Sexual Orientation

As lesbianism has become more widely accepted, its effects on families and health care should be acknowledged by the community health nurse. Family structures are no longer made up only of the typical married couple with children. Gay and lesbian couples are more open in today's society and may live with other persons, including communal communities where responsibilities are shared, based on their common beliefs. Many lesbian women choose to adopt children or conceive a child through artificial insemination or heterosexual intercourse. Women whose sexual orientation is lesbian or bisexual still face discrimination and insensitivity in the healthcare system, where heterosexuality is still considered the norm. Healthcare providers may continue to employ narrow definitions of families and partners and often exhibit prejudice by ignoring the specific healthcare considerations of this population.

Lesbian women are more likely to neglect their own healthcare needs and avoid examinations by healthcare providers because of the stigma and humiliation that often accompany the disclosure of being a lesbian. They are more likely to reveal their identity to nurses and other healthcare providers who are open and nonjudgmental (Stevens, Tatum, & White, 1996). Lesbians are at low risk for vaginal infections, STDs, and HIV. In contrast, they are at higher risk for breast and uterine cancer than their heterosexual cohorts (Brandenburg, Matthews, Johnson, & Hughes, 2007; Dibble, Eliason, DeJoseph, & Chinn, 2008; Rosser, 1995). They also are more likely to experience stress and depression because of social isolation. Substance abuse has been reported in 30% of lesbian women, compared with 7% of the general female population (Roberts, 2006). **Heterosexism** and **homophobia** contribute to prejudice, fear, and continued discrimination against lesbians, which in turn place these women at higher risks for health problems.

The community health nurse should learn to communicate without bias with women of all sexual orientations. Lesbians are often insulted when healthcare workers assume they are heterosexual and ask gender-specific questions, such as, "What form of birth control do you use?" Alternative questions should be phrased in the form of open-ended, nongender statements such as,

"Tell me about your sexual activity." The nurse should encourage lesbian women to have regular pelvic examinations and to avoid unprotected oral sex by using latex barriers (Zeidenstein, 1990). Mental health counseling and support networks are also options for dealing with troublesome psychosocial issues, such an addiction and depression.

Women and Aging

The elderly population will more than double by the year 2050, with the oldest old—those older than 85—the most rapidly growing segment in the United States (U.S. Census Bureau, 2010). The majority of this population will be female; these women are much more likely to be widowed, live alone, and live in poverty. Women belonging to racial and ethnic groups are in "quadruple jeopardy" because they are elderly, minority, female, and poor. Elderly women are also at greater risk than their younger counterparts for depression related to loneliness and isolating health conditions.

Differences have been identified regarding why women are living longer, including differences related to gender, exposure to environmental hazards, health habits, personality styles, and reactions to illness. Men have traditionally held jobs that expose them to more hazardous environmental factors, such as asbestos and carcinogens. Women have traditionally smoked less and managed stress better. These differences are expected to narrow in the future as a result of changes in our society, equal rights for women, and greater participation of women in the workforce.

Because women generally outlive men, more women live alone or live in long-term care facilities. Women currently outnumber elderly men by six to five from age 65

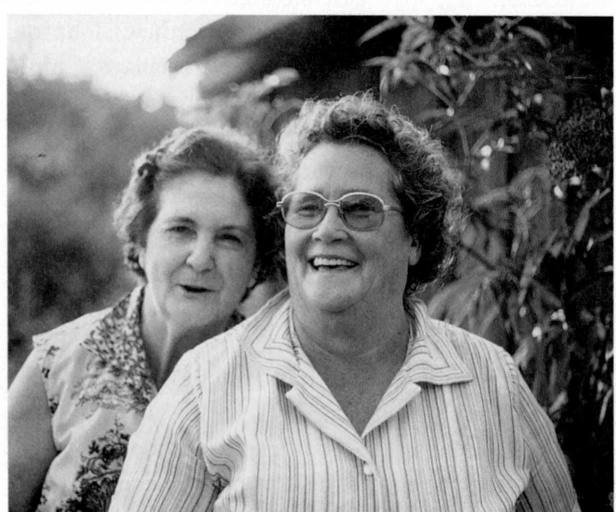

As women age, friendships become more important in promoting a sense of wellbeing.

MEDIA MOMENT

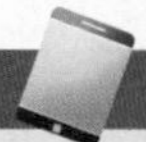

The Turning Point (1977)

This movie is about the friendship between two professional ballerinas who chose different paths. One becomes a world-renowned ballerina, while the other chooses homemaking and raising children. Their often conflicted relationship surfaces when the daughter of the stay-at-home mom wins a role as a prima ballerina in the friend's dance company.

Extremities (1986)

Farrah Fawcett plays one of several roommates who face a rapist in their home. After an attempted rape, the women tie him up and torture him, which sets off a soul-wrenching ethical conflict among the women. This is the first movie of its kind—where the woman is not the victim, the man becomes the trapped and vulnerable rapist.

Steel Magnolias (1989)

The story follows older Southern women in a small town in Louisiana, where the daughter of one of the women has developed diabetes but decides to have a baby even with the risks. It is a story about the power of women's friendships.

Thelma and Louise (1991)

This is the classic women's freedom, take-to-the-highway movie. Thelma and Louise take off on a vacation road trip to escape their unsatisfactory relationships with their spouses and end up facing rape, committing murder, and engaging in crime. Ultimately, they are cornered by police and must make a choice whether to give up their freedom or drive into the unknown.

Like Water for Chocolate (1992)

A Mexican-produced movie, which combines food and passion effectively in a mystical setting where one daughter has exceptional powers regarding male and female interactions. This is a must-see film about the value of love and family.

Monster's Ball (2001)

A poor, black widow becomes romantically involved with the white prison warden who oversaw her husband's execution. The film explores themes of racism, family, and honesty in intimate relationships.

Vera Drake (2004)

A working-class woman in 1950s London is revealed as a back-room abortionist when one of her patients nearly dies.

The Help (2011)

Based on the best-selling book, this movie tells the story of the relationship between a white girl and her Southern family's black maids during the civil rights era.

> Freedom is what you do with what's been done to you.
>
> —*Jean-Paul Sartre*

to 69, and by five to two at ages older than 85 (U.S. Census Bureau, 2010). More families are opting to care for their elderly parents at home; however, women (especially Caucasian women) continue to make up a larger percentage in nursing homes, with 50% childless or having outlived their own children. The financial consequences for elderly women are of major concern. Elderly women often have saved little, because many grew up in a male-dominated era in which women did not manage their finances. The few resources that these women have must last for a longer period. Additionally, older women may have limited Social Security benefits owing to their lack of participation in the workforce. With rising healthcare costs, many elderly women rely on Medicare and Medicaid resources with fewer Social Security benefits of their own, due to limited contributions during their lifetime.

Elderly women often report they are disappointed with health care and their treatment by healthcare personnel. As the women age, they report that physicians often dismiss their complaints as compared with their male cohorts. An example of this phenomenon is often seen in women with cardiac conditions. Until recently, women have been largely ignored in cardiovascular research and have not had the benefits of the same interventions as men, such as early intervention and cardiac rehabilitation. Many elderly women report feeling disrespected and mistreated by their healthcare providers. Discrimination based on race and sexual orientation is also a concern. Elderly lesbian women are often discounted in healthcare practices, with their significant other being eliminated from major healthcare decisions. Elderly women may not have been socialized to deal with finances, and this lack of knowledge may place them at significant risk. Rural elderly women may also be disadvantaged because of the greater risks associated with their often low educational and socioeconomic status.

Community health nurses must acknowledge the diverse needs of elderly women. Health promotion should be encouraged, including sleeping, exercising, weight control, and diet. Nurses in the community should work with elderly women, listening to their needs and problems, and promoting autonomy as they age. The cultural prejudices against the elderly in the United States influence how women perceive themselves as they age, how they care for themselves, how they relate to healthcare providers, and ultimately how healthy they remain in their later years of life.

Global Issues and Women's Health

The **Commission on the Status of Women** was one of the first bodies established by the United Nations (UN) Economic and Social Council to monitor the situation of women and promote their rights in all societies around the world. The UN's fourth **World Conference on Women** was held in Beijing, China, in 1995. Ethical issues related to women were explored, and universal standards regarding equality between women and men were set. Women's concerns should be brought to the forefront with issues related to human rights. Mutilation of female body parts, prostitution for survival, and female child slavery are all considered culturally acceptable in some countries. Women must participate in the political arena and in decision making related to legislation to fully address these ethical concerns. Women should also have a role in the development of their countries, including in the realms of policy, employment, education, the economy, and the environment.

Discussion of the need for a fifth conference has been underway for a number of years, and the UN's Secretary-General and President jointly proposed in 2012 that such a conference be held in 2015; however, to date the UN has not announced specific plans for a fifth conference.

The Death of a Soft Snowflake

My friend Babs always reminded me of a soft snowflake,
From her outward appearance to her inner core.

Her outward appearance was a soft one—her perpetual sweet smile, her blond hair, her radiant light complexioned skin, her preference for pastels.

Her inner core a caring one—for family, friends, and strangers;

Never an unkind thought or word towards anyone.

It is hard to say what will be missed the most about my friend Babs,

She was a wonderful loving daughter, wife, and mother; She was a true friend;

She was a tireless community worker.

The qualities that I will probably miss the most about my friend Babs will be her smiling face, and her authenticity.

It was almost unnerving to be in the company of someone as authentic as Babs—could she be real?

But it was genuine—the softness, the caring, the tenderness.

My heart is broken over the loss of my friend Babs.

My heart is also broken for her family;

I know she had to be a sparkling light in their lives—a sparkling soft snowflake.

(continues)

(continued)

Our prayer for this family is for strength to go on without her, for thankfulness for having had Babs in their lives.

Please dear Lord, take care of Babs—our sparkling soft snowflake.

—Judith A. Barton, PhD, RN

Three of Us

Three of us
Talk among the simmering pots
And bubbling ham
Of gifts and debts
And years behind—ahead
Of pimples and diaper rash
And falling out of love
Of bombs and war
And Mary Kay
The pots boil over and we rush about
Finding ways to save the family dinner.

—Ann Thedford Lanier

Special Issues Affecting Women's Health

Violence

Violence against women takes many forms, including physical and verbal assault, sexual assault, and homicide. Age has been identified as the most significant trait that puts women at risk for a violent attack: Younger women are more likely to be victims of abuse. The health consequences of violence against women are vast, including physical, psychological, and social effects. Societal consequences are more subtle, but are nonetheless damaging to women's sense of security and safety. More than 1.3 million physical or sexual assaults are committed by current or former partners each year in the United Sates. One in four women reports having been harmed by an intimate partner during her lifetime (Wiebe, 2003). On a personal level, violence touches one in four families and is responsible for more than one in three female murder victims (Tjaden & Thoennes, 2000). To put this in perspective, acts of violence in the United States kill as many women every 5 years as the total number of U.S. citizens killed in the Vietnam War. Violence is the single largest cause of injury to women in the United States—it is more common than automobile accidents and muggings combined. While evidence from research during the 1990s and early 2000s reveals that one in four women will experience violence at some point in her life, healthcare providers rarely assess women as potential victims of violence, even when symptoms of abuse present as the primary complaint (Scholle et al., 2003).

While abuse in a marriage or relationship is commonly assumed to involve men abusing women, sociologists for many years have found that men and women are about equally likely to attack each other. An important distinction that should be of concern to nurses, however, is that 85% of the injured parties are women (Goetting, 2001). A primary reason for this discrepancy is that men are generally larger and stronger than women, putting women at a physical disadvantage in the relationship. Men are much more likely to use not only their strength, but also firearms, which leaves women more vulnerable to severe and often life-threatening injuries (Strauss, 1992).

Violence directed toward women is related to the sexist structure of our society. Because men are socialized with norms that encourage aggressive behavior and the use of violence, men who abuse often feel it is their right to control women. When the inevitable frustrations of life occur within a relationship—and sometimes as a result of events outside the couple's lives—male abusers may turn violent toward their partners. Equality between the sexes in the United

GLOBAL CONNECTION 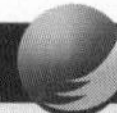

In 2012, a woman's life expectancy at birth in the United States was 81 years, as compared to 86 years in Japan, 77 years in Saudi Arabia, 68 years in India, 65 years in Haiti, and 46 years in Botswana.

Source: World Bank. (2014). *World development indicator data: Life expectancy at birth, female (years).* Retrieved from http://data.worldbank.org/indicator/SP.DYN.LE00.FE.IN

I Planned It This Way

I planned it this way, you know.
I planned it to happen at the very height of Spring.
I loved the Spring.
The time of rebirth, remember, this is a new beginning for me.

Bert loved the Spring too, you know.
Remember our big garden?
Oh how I enjoyed our big garden, snapping the beans while sitting in the swing, Bert cooking pork chops on the grill, watermelon, ice cream …
Oh how I love my home and Bert, and my children, my family, my church, my community, all of you.

I liked to keep my house in order, you know.
So I decided it was a good time for me to go home, back with Bert again,
At the very height of Spring.

—Judith A. Barton, PhD, RN

States has certainly become more valued than in previous generations, yet we have made less progress in socializing males to handle frustration and disagreements without resorting to aggressive and violent behavior (Strauss, 1992).

The poem "I Planned It This Way" is about an elderly woman's death. How do you interpret this poem's meaning concerning gender roles and culture?

NOTE THIS!

The National Resource Center on Homelessness and Mental Illness provides technical assistance and information about services and housing for the homeless and mentally ill population. It is sponsored by the Center for Mental Health Services, Substance Abuse and Mental Health Services Administration, and can be found at http://homeless.samhsa.gov/.

GOT AN ALTERNATIVE?

Naomi Judd, country music singer and registered nurse, contracted hepatitis when she was a nurse in an intensive care unit (ICU). She has approached this chronic illness with a combination of traditional treatments and complementary interventions by seeking out consultation with Dr. Deepak Chopra, a leading researcher in mind–body healing.

> Most of what they teach us in nursing school is like a mental enema. Let's separate the wheat from the chaff and start emphasizing nutrition, music, humor, altruism, support system, faith, and an open belief system. We need to be freed of the useless, time-consuming, soul-draining stuff. When you combine psychology and spirituality, healing takes place. This is the mind–body connection. The mind controls the body and our bodies want to heal us. My motto these days is "Slow down, simplify, and be kind."
>
> Your belief becomes your biology. For instance, if you're having a bad day and all of a sudden you realize that you're holding the winning lottery ticket, everything just completely changes. Unfortunately, data shows that 3 months later, you return to your prior emotional state. So the mind is the body's control tower, and it tells the body what hormones, neuropeptides and neurochemicals to secrete. The brain is like a drug store.

Naomi Judd is the author of the book *Naomi's Breakthrough Guide: 20 Choices to Transform Your Life* (Simon and Schuster, 2004).

Sources: Siegler, B. (2004). Love built a bridge. *Better Nutrition, 66*, 10; Lee, M. (1994). Naomi Judd: One of country music's brightest stars is also a nurse living with a chronic illness. *American Journal of Nursing*, March, 40–45.

NOTE THIS!

Emergency contraception (EC) is often misconstrued by the public and health professionals alike. EC, which is commonly referred to as the "morning after pill," is a form of backup birth control that can be taken up to a few days after intercourse and still prevent pregnancy. It was approved by the Food and Drug Administration (FDA) in 1999 for distribution by prescription, in 2006 for nonprescription behind-the counter availability for women 18 years of age and older, and since that time it has been made available to 15 year olds who can show proof of age, and President Obama has worked to make EC available to all ages. EC supporters believe that this contraceptive has enormous potential to reduce the rate of unintended pregnancies.

EC consists of a series of pills or a single pill containing progestin, the same hormone found in daily oral contraceptives. It is not intended for use as a regular contraceptive method, but rather as a backup in the event of unprotected sex or contraceptive failure. EC does not affect an established pregnancy, nor is it a medical abortion drug like mifepristone (RU-486). Plan B, the most widely used form of EC, is a one- or two-dose regimen that must be taken within days of unprotected sex to be effective.

EC prevents pregnancy by inhibiting or delaying ovulation or by preventing implantation of a fertilized egg in the uterus. It reduces the likelihood of pregnancy by 81% to 90% when taken within 72 hours of intercourse (the earlier it is taken, the higher the effectiveness). There are no known serious side effects of EC, though approximately 23% of women report nausea and vomiting. Researchers estimate that widespread use of EC could potentially prevent as many as half of the approximately 3 million unintended pregnancies that occur annually in the United States and as many as 700,000 pregnancies that now result in abortion.

Source: *Women's health policy facts*. (2005). Henry J. Kaiser Family Foundation.

A common question asked about women in abusive relationships is "Why do women stay in abusive relationships?" Researchers have studied such issues for many years and have found some common characteristics of women who stay and those who leave a violent relationship. Goetting (2001) studied women who had left their abusive partners and provides insights into why other women stay. She found the following common characteristics among the women who had left an abusive relationship: The women had a positive self-concept and believed that they could "do better," broke with traditional values about staying in a relationship "for better or worse," found adequate finances, and had supportive friends and family who provided a social network that helped them "rescue" themselves. Conversely, the women who remained in abusive relationships did not have good self-worth, believed in the duty of staying with a relationship at any cost, did not believe they could make it financially, and lacked a supportive network. These findings are not all equally important in explaining why women stay or leave a destructive relationship, and they do not apply to all women. However, community health nurses should be aware of the possible barriers and solutions to assisting women who are victims of abuse. This includes assisting these women in improving their abilities to care for themselves, financially and emotionally, and affirming their right to living in a safe and healthy relationship. Safe houses for women and families can provide job and financial counseling, as well as a supportive network for helping them envision a new life outside of the abusive relationship. Nurses should not consider the sexual orientation of the woman as either greater or lesser risk for abuse.

Community health nurses should be aware of "red flag" identifiers associated with domestic violence, such as women who (1) often have bruises on the limbs, torso, and face; (2) come to the clinic with vague symptoms of illness, such as pain in lower abdomen, chronic diarrhea, or pain of undetermined origin; (3) have trouble making eye contact; (4) have controlling partners; and (5) consistently wear sunglasses indoors. Because of the significant number of women at risk for abuse, community health nurses should assess every woman's relationship as part of their routine health assessments, regardless of the individual's sexual orientation. The stigma and fear associated with relationship abuse keep most women from expressing or admitting any information about this very serious "invisible" health problem in our society.

Community health nurses should be aware of local resources that can be accessed to assist women who find themselves in an abusive situation. National crisis lines such as the Domestic Violence Crisis Line and the Sexual Assault Crisis Line are accessible nationwide, and safe houses are available in most cities throughout the United States.

ETHICAL CONNECTION

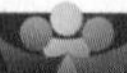

Stand by Your Man—But Keep a Gun Just in Case

As women have become more unwilling to tolerate abusive relationships and risky social situations, one of the more controversial outcomes has been the increase in the number of women who buy and use firearms. Current or former partners commit more than 1.5 million physical or sexual assaults against women each year in the United States. An intimate partner has harmed an estimated one in four women during their lifetime (Tjaden & Thoennes, 2000). Most of these women do not press charges against the accused or even report repeated attacks and harassment to proper authorities. Emergency room healthcare professionals are often faced with obvious physical and sexual abuse of women presenting for treatment, only to have the woman refuse to report her abuser's name or contact authorities. For women who do report such abuse, the legal system often puts her "on trial," and convictions—especially of present or former partners—are difficult to obtain.

In their study, Sorenson and Wiebe (2004) found that the common weapons used against and by women during a violent incident with a partner were words, hands/feet, household objects (e.g., telephones, pots, pans, dishes, ashtrays), kitchen knives, hammers, screwdrivers, and belts. A majority of the women had had a door slammed against their bodies or limbs and had been slammed against a door or wall.

Approximately one-third of the women interviewed had a firearm in the home. Previous research has linked firearm ownership with a greater potential for abuse in the family. The proportion of homes with a firearm in which abuse occurs is about 20% higher than in the general population (Lund, 2002; Smith & Martos, 2002). In two-thirds of these households, the partner eventually used the gun against the woman, usually threatening to shoot or kill her. The women in the Sorenson and Wiebe (2004) study expressed the need for partner/spousal notification regarding gun purchases by partners and stated that a personal firearm in the home creates greater risk for harm to them.

Implications for nurses include the assessment of household presence of firearms and experiences of women at risk for abuse concerning other forms of violence. The presence of firearms in the home poses an especially dangerous threat to women, given the lethality of guns. Firearms can also be used to intimidate or threaten a woman into doing something or allowing something to be done to her. Although physical harm may not result, emotional abuse occurs just the same. Further research in this area should go beyond gunshot wounds to the role of firearms in the home used to harass, abuse, and intimidate women.

"Goodbye Earl"

In 2001, the Dixie Chicks released a song about a subject rarely broached in country music: spousal abuse. "Goodbye Earl" asked an age-old question about violent relationships:

What does an abused wife (Mary Ann) do with a mean, unrepentant, and drunk partner (Earl) after all legal options have failed? The song, which was banned by many radio stations as being too controversial, presented an equally violent solution: Earl had to die, and the wife's best friend became her enthusiastic partner. In the song, Earl physically abused Mary Ann from the beginning of their marriage. When she reported his attacks, nothing changed: "He walked right through that restraining order and put her in intensive care." The two friends plotted the only permanent solution to Mary Ann's plight—they poisoned Earl's black-eyed peas, put him in the back of the car trunk, dumped his body, and reported him as a "missing person, that no one missed at all." The two get away with the murder and live happily ever after selling home-grown fruit at a roadside stand.

A similar country song that won numerous awards, "Independence Day" by Martina McBride, is about a young girl's account of her mother burning down their house after abuse from her alcoholic father. Both her mother and father are killed in the blaze. The song reflects an association with "freedom" and eliminating the problem through her mother's death. Again, lyrics reflect the community "looking the other way" even though the abuse was a widely known occurrence.

Women make up the fastest growing demographic group in the United States who buy handguns. This fact has caught the attention of both pro- and anti-gun advocacy groups, because women have traditionally avoided the purchase or use of firearms. For a man to die at the hand of a woman (or women) has rarely been the subject of songs in any musical genre, whereas having men kill their "cheating" women is common in songs. One such example is Jimi Hendrix's song "Hey Joe," about a woman who is shot because of her philandering ways, and the folk song about "Pretty Polly," who also does not make it to the end of the song alive.

1. What are the ethical implications of a popular song, such as "Goodbye Earl," when violence is presented as a solution to spousal abuse?
2. Can songs change the way we think about social problems, such as abuse?
3. Do you think such a song should be banned from the public, why or why not?

Homelessness

Homelessness is a growing problem in all urban and rural regions of the United States. Women and children continue to make up the fastest growing segment of the homeless and, as such, are among the most vulnerable in this already hazardous environment. For women, many factors can lead to homelessness, including divorce, poverty, eroding work opportunities, decline in public assistance, domestic violence, substance abuse, and mental illness. Substance abuse often accompanies homelessness and increases the risk of homeless women engaging in prostitution and experiencing other health-related conditions such as HIV, STDs, tuberculosis, and malnutrition.

The community health nurse can assist homeless women and families through primary, secondary, and tertiary prevention interventions at individual, community, and national levels. The community health nurse may be a first-line defense for the homeless woman and her family. Maintaining a long-term relationship with this vulnerable group is perhaps the most challenging among all populations. Establishing trust is difficult because of sporadic and infrequent contact with these families, so the nurse must be creative and take immediate steps to provide safe and acceptable care at the time of contact. Knowledge about community resources is vital; the nurse can act as an advocate to assist the client through the "red tape" of the bureaucratic process.

RESEARCH ALERT 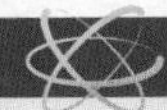

Women's increasing alcohol consumption has come under intense scrutiny from the British press. The coverage overall presents women who drink as problematic. Although feminist researchers have examined media constructions of gender, and although men's drinking has been the subject of critical analyses, there appears to be little feminist work on women's drinking per se. This is a significant omission, because gender representations related to eating, drinking, or sex tend to draw on conventional ideals of femininity and, as such, invite feminist deconstruction. It is also necessary for feminists working in this area to examine critically scientific thinking on women's drinking, as media constructions and everyday understandings will inevitably be distilled from mainstream psychological knowledge.

Source: Day, K., Gough, B., & McFadden, M. (2004). Warning! Alcohol can seriously damage your feminine health. *Feminist Media Studies, 4*(2), 165–183.

Working with the community to prevent homelessness through policy changes should also be a priority for nurses who work with this vulnerable and often forgotten population. Nurses must work in the community by challenging government officials to examine the homeless problem and soliciting concerned citizens to develop shelters and programs for homeless individuals and families.

Incarceration

Since the 1980s, due to the decline in economic conditions and the crackdown on drugs and crime, the number of women in U.S. prisons has increased nearly 650%, with more than 1 million women incarcerated as of 2010 (The Sentencing Project, 2012). The typical conviction of an incarcerated women is for property crimes—for example, check forgery and illegal credit card use. The increase in the female population in jails and prisons more recently is attributed to drug possession and abuse, often as a result of partner involvement. Women are increasingly more likely to be arrested for drug crimes, even though they may have been simply residing with a drug user or distributor. Single mothers account for 90% of women inmates. Poverty, age, race, and lack of education are primary risk factors for women in prison.

The majority of incarcerated women have a dependency on drugs and/or alcohol and have incomes at or below the poverty level. Given these lifestyle patterns, health care has often been neglected before incarceration. Many of these women have a host of chronic medical problems, such as tuberculosis, HIV, and other STDs. Historically, prison systems have not had enough resources to provide sufficient or appropriate health care for women.

Community health nurses need to be politically active and act as advocates for this hidden population of vulnerable women. The community health nurse should assume the role of client advocate in regard to child care and visitation while incarcerated. Parenting and childcare classes should be made available to the inmates. Programs that provide occupational training and that promote self-esteem and assertiveness have been linked with better outcomes for women who are released from prison.

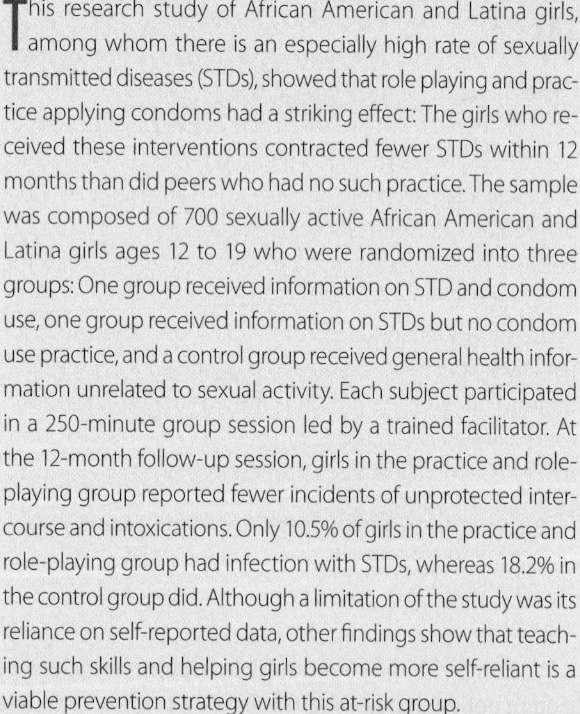

RESEARCH ALERT

This research study of African American and Latina girls, among whom there is an especially high rate of sexually transmitted diseases (STDs), showed that role playing and practice applying condoms had a striking effect: The girls who received these interventions contracted fewer STDs within 12 months than did peers who had no such practice. The sample was composed of 700 sexually active African American and Latina girls ages 12 to 19 who were randomized into three groups: One group received information on STD and condom use, one group received information on STDs but no condom use practice, and a control group received general health information unrelated to sexual activity. Each subject participated in a 250-minute group session led by a trained facilitator. At the 12-month follow-up session, girls in the practice and role-playing group reported fewer incidents of unprotected intercourse and intoxications. Only 10.5% of girls in the practice and role-playing group had infection with STDs, whereas 18.2% in the control group did. Although a limitation of the study was its reliance on self-reported data, other findings show that teaching such skills and helping girls become more self-reliant is a viable prevention strategy with this at-risk group.

Source: Jemmott, J. B., Jemmott, L. S., Braverman, P. K., & Fong, G. T. (2005). HIV/STD risk reduction interventions for African American and Latino adolescent girls at an adolescent medicine clinic: A randomized controlled trial. *Archives of Pediatrics & Adolescent Medicine, 159*(5), 440–449.

The Unplanned Gift

I hold my breath
My head up high
Now I breathe deep and smooth,
Straighten my shoulders

I hear your voice
"Don't let them see you blink."

God I wish I could remember
What happened?
When I heard your voice
The first time?

Were you really there
Standing beside me?
Or was I so frightened
I conjured your spirit?

And your voice comes to me now
"Do what you have to do
and don't look back."

A wealth of wisdom in such simple phrases.
A wealth of strength when I have needed it.
There are times when such down-home guidance
Comes in handy,
There are times when I must stand and be a man.
What thing for a mother to teach
A Southern daughter!

—Ann Thedford Lanier

Poverty

Poverty dramatically affects women's health. Women who are poor, sick, uninsured, or members of a racial minority are at particularly high risk for experiencing barriers in affording and accessing appropriate preventive care. Poor women have limited access to health care and preventive healthcare services, which results in delay of diagnosis of disease and injury, and consequently leads to shorter lifespans. For women in poverty, healthcare problems often exacerbate other existing challenges in their lives. Half of poor women and 38% of near-poor women (100–199% of poverty) report that they have delayed or did not get needed healthcare because of the cost.

Medicaid serves the poorest and sickest populations of women in the United States. Almost one in four women on Medicaid (23%) reports being turned away by a physician or healthcare provider who was not taking new patients or did not accept Medicaid (Kaiser Family Foundation, 2011).

Factors unique to women in regard to poverty include the following:

- Women are usually responsible for children, and many are single parents with no extended support.
- Women are not traditionally socialized to assume the breadwinner role and usually accept lower paying jobs, often leading to a choice between public assistance and inadequate child care while they work.
- Health care is an expendable luxury when placed alongside child care, food, and lodging.
- Jobs women take may not have healthcare benefits comparable to the benefits associated with men's jobs.

Community health nurses need to be knowledgeable about local resources if they are to assist women who are poor to gain access to appropriate health care. Church-based programs and other community resources can provide community health nurses with excellent opportunities to identify this vulnerable population and to provide much-needed health interventions. Some local resources that are available in most areas include religious groups, county and state health departments, federal health clinics, United Way support, Medicaid, and the Social Security Administration.

Workplace Health

Women represent approximately half of the current workforce in the United States. Many factors have contributed to the increasing number of women in the workforce, including economic necessity, fewer children, changes in women's attitudes toward work, and changes in society. Women face a variety of concerns in the workplace, including reproductive risks, job stress, role conflict, sexual harassment, discrimination, and salary inequality.

Women account for the largest percentage of healthcare workers in the United States. Major occupational hazards for healthcare workers include biological, chemical, environmental, physical, and psychosocial hazards. All of these factors may influence a woman's physical and emotional/mental health at work, in the family, and in her community. The community health nurse in the occupational setting should address sensitive issues for women, including effects of cancer, reproductive problems (e.g., menstrual disorders, reduced fertility, genetic damage, spontaneous abortion, stillbirths), back problems, carpal tunnel syndrome, and sexual harassment issues (Fogel & Woods, 1995).

RESEARCH ALERT 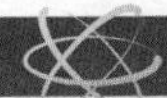

Eighty-nine percent of female veterans who served in the Vietnam War were nurses. Agent Orange, a toxin used in Vietnam to clear out dense vegetation and crops, is well known for its serious adverse health effects and role in cancer and Hodgkin's disease in men. Virtually no research had been conducted on the women who were exposed to Agent Orange. Dr. Linda Schwartz has studied this "forgotten population" and found that they are at great risk for increased cancer rates and miscarriages. Agent Orange was used to keep down weeds around the camps, and the empty containers were often used to store supplies and as barbecue grills. Nurses handled the containers and were exposed to the toxin as well. The outcome of this study has been to influence policy in the Veterans Administration to compensate women for these damages.

Source: Trossman, S. (1999, May/June). RN explores Agent Orange's lasting effects on women vets. *American Nurse, 24.*

Occupations known to place women at a greater risk for health problems should be considered by nurses in the community when assessing personal health. Even though many factors affect health in the workplace, very little research has been conducted with regard to women and work. Instead, most research has been conducted with male workers, resulting in gender-biased findings. This bias has led to designs and practices in the work environment that may compromise the working woman's health and safety. Community health nurses must act as advocates for women in the workplace by promoting research specific to female workers and educating women about gender-specific risks associated with work.

Toward the Future

Women's Ways of Knowing

Women must play a major role in their acquisition of knowledge to make informed health decisions. Historically, most women have not been as well educated as men in basic or health sciences. The way in which women have been educated directly influences their health knowledge. Poorly educated women may participate in the healthcare system in silence—afraid to ask questions, feeling inadequate, with minimal knowledge of their own health care. They may accept answers without question. They may not

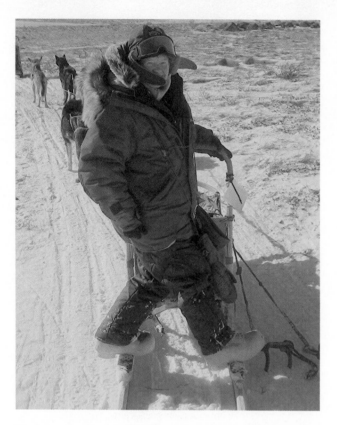

Women who remain active after retirement are generally healthier than more sedentary counterparts. This woman at 65 is on a five-day dog-sledding excursion in Alaska.

be able to understand the complex healthcare system or understand why they are expected to change from old patterns. Some distrust anyone of authority and reject science and medicine, relying on tradition or family influence.

As women become better educated through college, life, and work experiences they learn **procedural knowledge**, including critical thinking and logical reasoning skills. Some women acquire **constructed knowledge** and are able to synthesize knowledge from many areas. The logic of women's ways of knowing is related to a degree to the lack of formal education for many women's programs (Rosser, 1995). Education can play a key role in eliminating the subservient way women react to the healthcare industry. Community health nurses play a critical role in the education of women throughout the lifespan.

> For us who nurse, our nursing is a thing, which unless we are making progress every year, every month, every week, take my word for it, we are going back.
>
> —*Florence Nightingale, Graduation address, St. Thomas School of Nursing, 1872*

Feminism

The politics of women's healthcare issues have long been priorities of the feminist movement. Traditionally, few women have been invited to attend or participate in legislative forums related to women's health. Women have often been absent in the establishment of research priorities related to their health until recently. **Feminism** and the promotion of women's rights in society today are closely associated with the promotion of a national women's health agenda.

Feminist theory deals with gender by race and class, along with individuals, groups, and communities. There are many feminist theories, including liberal feminism, Marxist feminism, socialist feminism, African American feminism, lesbian separatist feminism, conservative feminism, existential feminism, psychoanalytic feminism, and radical feminism. Women's issues focus on economics, health care, and violence toward women. The correlation between the feminist movement and the political arena and the impact on women's health is obvious. Women must continue in their quest for a voice in healthcare policy and the implementation of policies that affect women (Rosser, 1995). Community health nurses can promote the feminist agenda through public policy activism and service on boards where women's health issues are concerned.

MEDIA MOMENT

Gail Sheehy wrote the landmark book *Passages* in 1974 about the stages of continuing development of adulthood. More than 30 years later, as she reflected on the changes in women's lives:

> The incredible shrinking traditional family with a stay-at-home mom and breadwinner dad is down to only one-tenth of all American households. More and more contemporary women are choosing to remain single or to raise a child on their own. This dramatic demographic shift is driven only in part by women's desire for independence; their male contemporaries also have more choices, including prolonged bachelorhood or dual-income, childfree cohabitation.

Source: Sheehy, G. (2004). Passages redux. *More*, July/August, 62–65.

> I myself have never been able to find out precisely what feminism is: I only know that people call me a feminist whenever I express sentiments that differentiate me from a door mat.
>
> —*Rebecca West, 1913*

Empowerment

Empowerment is based on the assumption that all people are created equal. Each person has the opportunity to recognize one's assets and develop from them on a professional, physical, spiritual, and emotional level. Recognizing and respecting the fact that all people have assets supports humility and dismisses the threat that others are better or more deserving. People feel powerful in themselves when they feel secure and safe. Community health nurses can be the "mirror" that reflects the woman's steps toward recognizing her own special assets. By affirming and reinforcing a woman's ability to recognize these assets, women can gain confidence to move forward in the search for security, wellbeing, and improved self-esteem.

One of the most empowering events for women was the formation of the **United Nations Platforms for Action for Women** with the purpose of challenging governments to raise the status of women. Global conferences are held on a regular basis and focus on the identification of commonly held beliefs about women's rights to health care, global healthcare needs of women and children, and proposed solutions for these identified problems. Some recent strategic objectives for women's health are listed in **Box 31-5**. A specific action plan was developed for achievement of each of the four objectives.

Healthcare Policy

Policymakers in health care have historically ignored women's issues when developing healthcare policy. However, many policies were established in the last decade of the 20th century that influence the health promotion and wellbeing of women.

The Women's Health Equity Act of 1990 identified the inequality of research into women's health issues and required that women and underrepresented racial and ethnic groups be included in research. At the same time, the National Institutes of Health established the Office of Research on Women's Health, based on the concept that women's research must expand from its traditional focus on women's reproductive systems to include all body systems and behavioral factors that influence women's health care. Recommendations for priority research for women included health promotion and wellness, elimination of barriers to healthcare services, prevention of illness, health education, and recognition of differences among women. **Box 31-6** identifies areas of research needed for women across the lifespan.

BOX 31-5 Strategic Objectives of the World Conference on Women

- Increase women's access throughout the lifespan to appropriate, affordable, and quality health care; information; and related services
- Strengthen preventive programs that promote women's health
- Undertake gender-sensitive initiatives that address sexually transmitted diseases, HIV/AIDS, and sexual and reproductive health issues
- Increase resources and monitor follow up for women's health

DAY IN THE LIFE

Retired schoolteacher Margie E. Richard became a local hero when she took on Shell petrochemical plants in her small community of Norco, Louisiana, upriver from New Orleans. Shell was the main employer in the community, which surrounded the African American community, and was illegally venting toxic chemicals from its plant. Richard convinced the petroleum giant to clean up its act and pay each homeowner in a four-block area surrounding the plant a minimum of $80,000 to buy a house elsewhere—an offer all homeowners accepted. She set up a webcam to show the venting of chemicals, installed her own atmospheric monitors, and even traveled to Shell headquarters in the Netherlands to invite company executives to "take a whiff" of Norco's air for themselves. The end result—Shell agreed to invest more than $20 million in emission reduction and relocation, which was a historic victory for the "fence-line communities" living with energy industries.

Richard became the first African American to win the Goldman Environmental Prize in 2004.

Source: AARP Magazine, January/February 2006. "Margie Richard: Pollution Fighter."

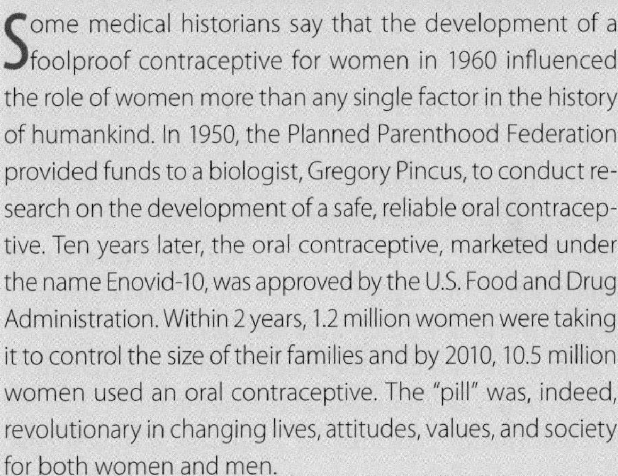

NOTE THIS!

Some medical historians say that the development of a foolproof contraceptive for women in 1960 influenced the role of women more than any single factor in the history of humankind. In 1950, the Planned Parenthood Federation provided funds to a biologist, Gregory Pincus, to conduct research on the development of a safe, reliable oral contraceptive. Ten years later, the oral contraceptive, marketed under the name Enovid-10, was approved by the U.S. Food and Drug Administration. Within 2 years, 1.2 million women were taking it to control the size of their families and by 2010, 10.5 million women used an oral contraceptive. The "pill" was, indeed, revolutionary in changing lives, attitudes, values, and society for both women and men.

BOX 31-6 Research Areas for Women Across the Lifespan

- *Adolescence*: Prevention of accidents, suicide prevention, HIV, sexuality, alcohol, tobacco, diet and exercise
- *Young adult/college*: Low-birth-weight babies, pregnancies dangerously complicated by hypertension, ectopic pregnancies resulting in death, infertility, sexually transmitted diseases, cancer prevention (breast), safety (alcohol/drugs), health education, contraception, eating disorders, discomforts of pregnancy, obesity, HIV, family planning
- *Midlife*: Disease prevention (cancer, hypertension, stroke, heart disease), health promotion, health education, strengths of single-parent head of household, multiple role adaptation, obesity, influence of diet on osteoporosis, domestic violence, early detection of cancer, arthritis, pain
- *Perimenopausal*: Heart disease, health promotion, health education, impact of diet on osteoporosis, domestic violence, urinary incontinence, hormone replacement therapy, dietary influence on breast cancer, calcium and vitamin D supplements
- *Mature*: Coping with chronic illnesses and disability, urinary incontinence, depression, institutionalization, respite care, social and economic contributions to health status, older women and health policy, racial/cultural influences on health care, caregivers, cost-effectiveness of health care to elder women

The Family Medical Leave Act of 1993 allows for 12 weeks of unpaid leave time from work for family or medical reasons. Employees are guaranteed the same job, pay, and benefits when they return to work after a leave. Because women are the primary family **caregivers** in the United States, this legislation was considered a major victory for working women with families.

Although women are the dominant caregivers in our society, policy development at the national level has been slow to formally recognize the "second shift" that so many women work when caring for sick family members. Caring for family members has long been an expectation of women. In addition to working outside the home, women are required to care for children, spouses, and aging parents. Women often must give up their employment to care for family members, with loss of wages, employee benefits—health and retirement—and social support. Many women who lack health insurance may not have adequate resources for health care. Owing to the extra stresses of caregiving, women may end up divorced, with the additional loss of security from the employee benefits of their spouses (e.g., health insurance). With the passage of the ACA in 2010, women now have expanded insurance options, free wellness screenings, and other age-appropriate testing at no cost.

RESEARCH ALERT 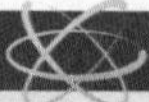

This research examined mental health and birth outcomes among women exposed to Hurricane Katrina. Data were collected prospectively from a cohort of 301 women from New Orleans, Louisiana. Pregnant women were interviewed about their experiences during the hurricane, and whether they had experienced symptoms of posttraumatic stress disorder (PTSD) or depression. High hurricane exposure was defined as having three or more of the eight severe hurricane experiences, such as feeling that one's life was in danger, walking through floodwaters, or having a loved one die. Study results found that the frequency of low birth weight was higher in women with high hurricane exposure (14.0%) than women without high hurricane exposure (4.7%), with an adjusted odds ratio (aOR) of 3.3; 95% confidence interval (CI): 1.13–9.89; $p < 0.01$. The frequency of preterm birth was higher in women with high hurricane exposure (14.0%) than in women without high hurricane exposure (6.3%), with aOR of 2.3; 95% CI: 0.82–6.38; $p > 0.05$. Rather than a general exposure to disaster, exposure to specific severe disaster events and the intensity of the disaster experience may be better predictors of poor pregnancy outcomes. To prevent poor pregnancy outcomes during and after disasters, future disaster preparedness may need to include the planning of earlier evacuation of pregnant women to minimize their exposure to severe disaster events.

Source: Xiong, X., Harville, E., Mattison, D., Elkind-Hirsch, K., Pridjian, G., & Buekens, P. (2008). Exposure to Hurricane Katrina, post-traumatic stress disorder and birth outcomes. *The American Journal of the Medical Sciences, 336*(2), 111–115.

Healthcare policy for female caregivers should be promoted as a critical social need that benefits not only women but also society as a whole. Examples of policy issues related to unpaid caregiver responsibilities of women in their families include reimbursement and respite services. Changes in healthcare policy that relate to the challenges of female caregivers will serve to improve the quality of women's lives and the lives of their families and communities. These critical policy issues are not just about women, but affect the health of the entire nation.

Health behaviors of women are affected by the availability of healthcare resources and are influenced by education and income. Women get health insurance either through employment or marriage. Well-educated women are more likely to practice positive health-promotion activities such as healthy eating, exercising, not smoking, and drinking less alcohol (Fogel & Woods, 1995). Poverty and lack of education have a negative influence on health, however, often leading to stress, depression, and poor health-promotion habits. Usually, poor women wait until an acute episode to seek health care. Many may rely on home remedies or alternative interventions for health care. Inadequate healthcare access for women, especially the most vulnerable, results in needless personal suffering and economic losses for society.

Despite the reality that women are the major caregivers for families in the United States, they play a small role in public decision making regarding healthcare issues. Women have traditionally remained outside the circle of influence in the national political arena. This trend is changing, however, as more women become better educated and assume roles with greater power in their professional lives. More women are being elected to public office, as evidenced by the outcome of the 2006 elections when Representative Nancy Pelosi of California became the first woman in history to serve as Speaker of the House of Representatives. Women in the United States are entitled to equal health care, and community health nurses are in a position to lead the way toward a healthier future for all women.

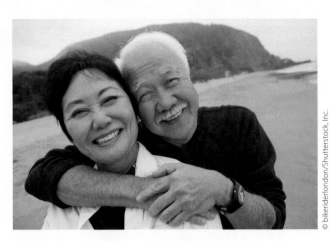

Healthy relationships are characterized by open communication, a sense of humor, and truly liking one's mate.

APPLICATION TO PRACTICE 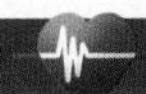

Frances Benton is a 68-year-old widow who has recently been referred to your community health clinic by Rachel Jackson, a concerned neighbor. According to Ms. Jackson, Mrs. Benton's husband died about 8 months ago. Mr. Benton had been Mrs. Benton's caretaker. The couple did not have children, and there are no close relatives. Mrs. Benton had fallen and sustained a hip fracture approximately 1 year ago, and she recently cracked a vertebra. She has begun to have lapses of memory and has lost her way home from the grocery store. Two days ago, Mrs. Benton was out in the yard with only her slip on, which was definitely out of character, according to Ms. Jackson. The landlord stopped by several times to collect the rent but could not get Mrs. Benton to understand that she had not paid it in 3 months. He had spoken with Ms. Jackson and was planning to evict Mrs. Benton.

1. What are your nursing diagnoses in this situation?
2. Which secondary and tertiary preventive measures might be appropriate in working with Mrs. Benton?
3. Which community resources could you collaborate with to address the health risks for Mrs. Benton?

Conclusion

Community health nurses are invaluable in assisting women with healthcare needs in the community. They should be knowledgeable regarding the various health concerns that women face, such as violence, homelessness, incarceration, poverty, and health conditions such as osteoporosis and cancer, and they must be able to define these women's needs. Community health nurses should be aware of the local resources that are available and be skilled in linking these resources with clients and their communities. Finally, they should be able to evaluate the process, fill in the gaps, and provide continuity of care for the individual client and the community as a whole.

AFFORDABLE CARE ACT (ACA) 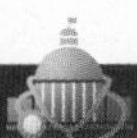

ACA Preventive Health Services for Women

Most health plans must cover additional preventive health services for women, ensuring a comprehensive set of preventive services like breast cancer screenings to meet women's unique healthcare needs. These preventive services are critical to keeping women healthy. For example, breast cancer is the most common cancer affecting women and the second leading cause of cancer death for women in the United States, after lung cancer. But when breast cancer is caught early and treated, survival rates can be near 100%.

The Affordable Care Act also protects women's access to quality health care. No one can be denied health insurance coverage because of a preexisting health condition, such as breast cancer, pregnancy, depression, or being a victim of domestic violence. And there are no more annual and lifetime dollar limits on coverage.

(continues)

AFFORDABLE CARE ACT (ACA) (*continued*)

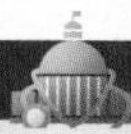

Today, health plans in the ACA Marketplace offer a comprehensive package of 10 essential health benefits (EHB), including maternity care. An estimated 8.7 million American women currently purchasing individual insurance will gain coverage for maternity services, and most women will no longer need a referral from a primary care provider to obtain obstetrical or gynecological services.

Cost has also been a significant barrier to care for many women. For low-income women, that situation is much worse: More than half of women who make $11,490 per year or less spend at least $1,149 a year on care. But through the Marketplace 6 out of 10 uninsured individuals can get coverage for $100 or less.

Comprehensive Coverage for Women's Preventive Care

All ACA Marketplace health plans and many other plans must cover the following list of preventive services for women without charging a copayment or coinsurance (This is true even if the yearly deductible has NOT been met. This applies only when these services are delivered by an in-network provider.):

- Anemia screening on a routine basis for pregnant women
- Breast cancer genetic test counseling (for the BRCA gene) for women at higher risk for breast cancer
- Breast cancer mammography screenings every 1 to 2 years for women over 40
- Breast cancer chemoprevention counseling for women at higher risk
- Breastfeeding comprehensive support and counseling from trained providers and access to breastfeeding supplies for pregnant and nursing women
- Cervical cancer screening for sexually active women
- Chlamydia infection screening for younger women and other women at higher risk
- Contraception: FDA-approved contraceptive methods, sterilization procedures, and patient education and counseling, as prescribed by a healthcare provider for women with reproductive capacity (not including abortifacient drugs); this does not apply to health plans sponsored by certain exempt "religious employers"
- Domestic and interpersonal violence screening and counseling for all women
- Folic acid supplements for women who may become pregnant
- Gestational diabetes screening for women 24 to 28 weeks pregnant and those at high risk of developing gestational diabetes
- Gonorrhea screening for all women at higher risk
- Hepatitis B screening for pregnant women at their first prenatal visit
- HIV screening and counseling for sexually active women
- Human papillomavirus (HPV) DNA test every 3 years for women with normal cytology results who are 30 or older
- Osteoporosis screening for women over age 60, depending on risk factors
- Rh incompatibility screening for all pregnant women and follow-up testing for women at higher risk
- Sexually transmitted infections counseling for sexually active women
- Syphilis screening for all pregnant women or other women at increased risk
- Tobacco use screening and interventions for all women, and expanded counseling for pregnant tobacco users
- Urinary tract or other infection screening for pregnant women
- Well-woman visits to get recommended services for women under 65

For specifics on additional mandatory coverage under the ACA, refer to https://www.healthcare.gov

LEVELS OF PREVENTION

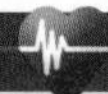

Primary: Presenting a community talk on the preventive services required by ACA for women

Secondary: Screening for hypertension in a women's church group

Tertiary: Assisting a woman after a mastectomy for breast cancer with range of motion exercises

Critical Thinking Activities

1. You are a rural community health nurse working on a mobile van visiting a large migrant community at a local farm. Selena King, a 16-year-old Hispanic female, comes into the van to have her blood pressure checked because she has been feeling tired and nauseated lately and is having difficulty working in the fields. She is also complaining of a coin-shaped rash on her arms, palms, and trunk. In completing your history, you find that she has not had any medical care since she was 8, when she had her appendix removed in Florida. Her blood pressure is 100/68 mmHg.

Selena cannot remember when her last menstrual period was, but she thinks it was 2 months ago. She is sexually active and uses condoms occasionally. She lives with her mother, four sisters, two brothers, and her father (who has forbidden her to see her boyfriend, Juan) in a travel trailer that they pull from town to town.

- What are your nursing diagnoses in this situation?
- How would you address the two dimensions of secondary prevention (diagnosis and treatment) of pregnancy and secondary syphilis?
- Which secondary and tertiary preventive measures might be appropriate in working with Selena?
- Which resources could you as a community nurse tap to assist Selena?

2. Mrs. Wise, a 67-year-old woman, is being discharged from the hospital after having surgery to repair a broken hip and bilateral wrist fractures. She will have bilateral casts for 8 weeks. Mrs. Wise is a widow and has two sons who live within 2 miles of her. She lives alone. Her daughters-in-law will be the main caretakers. Both daughters-in-law work outside the home, neither has had any medical training, and both are afraid of assuming the health care of their mother-in-law. Mrs. Wise is reluctant to move in with her sons and would rather return to her small townhouse. The discharge diagnosis includes hip and wrist repair as a result of osteoporosis, diabetes, hypertension, and obesity.
   - What are your nursing diagnoses in this situation?
   - How would you address considerations of competence, time management, and supervision in planning the care of Mrs. Wise?
   - Which resources could you as a community nurse use to assist this family in caring for Mrs. Wise and at the same time address Mrs. Wise's concerns regarding her independence?
3. Empowerment of women may well be seen in a depiction of the Hindu goddess Sarasvati (sa-RAS-vah-tee). The goddess of knowledge, she is credited with the creation of the fruits of civilization, arts, and music. Her color and brightness represent the powerful, pure light of education, which destroys the darkness of ignorance. Sarasvati is depicted with four arms, showing that her power extends in all directions. In one of her hands, she holds a book (representing learning) and in another a strand of beads (representing spiritual knowledge). In the other hands, she holds and plays the vina, an Indian lute, representing the art of music (Waldherr, 1996).
   - How does this depiction reflect our society's view of women in the United States today?
   - Is education encouraged in women?
   - What is spirituality, and how is it seen in our society? How is it seen in Sarasvati?
   - What does music represent to Sarasvati or to the women of many other cultures and diversities?
   - What is the darkness of ignorance?

HEALTHY ME 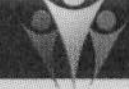

Do you set health goals for yourself? How do women differ from men in their experiences in and frequency of use of the healthcare system? Women, especially nurses, tend to care for others before caring for themselves. Do you?

References

Albelda, R., & Tilly, C. (1997). *Glass ceilings and bottomless pits: Women's work, women's poverty.* Cambridge, MA: South End Press.

American Cancer Society. (2008). *All about breast cancer.* Retrieved from http://www.cancer.org/docroot/CRI/CRI_2x.asp?sitearea=&dt=5

American Cancer Society. (2014). *Cancer facts and figures 2014.* Retrieved from http://www.cancer.org/research/cancerfactsstatistics/cancerfactsfigures2014/index

American Heart Association. (2013). *Cardiovascular disease: Women's No. 1 health threat.* Retrieved from http://www.heart.org/idc/groups/heart-public/@wcm/@adv/documents/downloadable/ucm_302256.pdf

Bell, M. R., Grill, G. E., Garrett, K. N., Berger, P., Gersh, B. J., & Holmes D. R. Jr. (1995). Long-term outcome of women compared with men after successful coronary angioplasty. *Circulation, 91*, 2876–2881.

Boyle, E. H., Songora, F., & Foss, G. (2001). International discourse and local politics: Anti-female-genital-cutting laws in Egypt, Tanzania and the United States. *Social Problems, 48*(4), 524–544.

Brandenburg, D., Matthews, A., Johnson, T., & Hughes, T. (2007). Breast cancer risk and screening: A comparison of lesbian and heterosexual women. *Women & Health, 45*(4), 109–130.

Centers for Disease Control and Prevention (CDC). (2008). Youth risk behavior surveillance—United States, 2007. *Morbidity and Mortality Weekly Report, 57*(SS-4), 1–136.

Centers for Disease Control and Prevention (CDC). (2012a). Use of indoor tanning devices by adults—United States, 2010. *Morbidity and Mortality Weekly Report, 61*(18), 323–326.

Centers for Disease Control and Prevention (CDC). (2012b). *HPV vaccine recommendations.* Retrieved from http://www.cdc.gov/STD/hpv/STDFact-HPV-vaccine-hcp.htm#vaccrec

Centers for Disease Control and Prevention (CDC). (2013a). *Pregnancy mortality surveillance system.* Retrieved from http://www.cdc.gov/reproductivehealth/maternalinfanthealth/pmss.html

Centers for Disease Control and Prevention (CDC). (2013b). Women and heart disease fact sheet. Retrieved from http://www.cdc.gov/dhdsp/data_statistics/fact_sheets/fs_women_heart.htm

Clarke, R. D. (2000). Has the glass ceiling really been shattered? *Black Enterprise, 30*(7), 145–158.

Dibble, S., Eliason, M., DeJoseph, J., & Chinn, P. (2008). Sexual issues in special populations: Lesbian and gay individuals. *Seminars in Oncology Nursing, 24*(2), 127–130.

Dujan, D., & Withorn, A. (1996). *For crying out loud: Women's poverty in the United States.* Cambridge, MA: Southend Press.

Felton, L. A., Gumm, A., & Pittenger, D. J. (2001). The recipients of unwanted sexual encounters among college students. *College Student Journal, 35*(1), 135–143.

Fogel, C., & Woods, N. (1995). *Women's health care: A comprehensive handbook.* Thousand Oaks, CA: Sage.

Ganti, A. K. (2013). Will funding for lung cancer ever improve? *ASCO Post, 4*(14). Retrieved from http://www.ascopost.com/issues/september-1,-2013/will-funding-for-lung-cancer-ever-improve.aspx

Goetting, A. (2001). *Getting out: Life stories of women who left abusive men.* New York, NY: Columbia University Press.

Johnson, D. S. (2012). *Webinar on 2011 income, poverty, and health insurance estimates from the current population survey.* Retrieved from http://www.census.gov/newsroom/releases/pdf/20120912_ip_remarks_johnson.pdf

Kaiser Family Foundation. (2011). *Women's health care chartbook: Key findings from the Kaiser Women's Health Survey.* Retrieved from http://kff.org/womens-health-policy/report/womens-health-care-chartbook-key-findings-from/

Lipson, J., Dibble, S., & Minarik, P. (1996). *Culture and nursing care: A pocket guide.* San Francisco, CA: UCSF Nursing Press.

Lund, L. E. (2002). *Incidence of non-fatal intimate partner violence against women in California, 1998–1999* (Report No. 4). Sacramento, CA: California Department of Health Services, Epidemiology for Prevention and Injury Control Branch.

Martin, J. A., Hamilton, B. E., Osterman, M. J. K., Curtin, S. C., & Mathews, T. J. (2013). Births: Final data for 2012. *National Vital Statistics Reports, 62*(9), 1–87. Retrieved from http://www.cdc.gov/nchs/data/nvsr/nvsr62/nvsr62_09.pdf

Mosca, L., Benjamin, E. J., Berra, K., Bezanson, J. L., Dolor, R. J., Lloyd-Jones, D. M, … Wenger, N. (2011). Effectiveness-based guidelines for cardiovascular disease prevention in women—2011 update: A guideline from the American Heart Association. *Circulation, 123*, 1243–1262.

National Conference of State Legislatures (NCSL). (2014). *Indoor tanning restrictions for minors—A state-by-state comparison.* Retrieved from http://www.ncsl.org/research/health/indoor-tanning-restrictions.aspx

Nitti, V. W. (2001). The prevalence of urinary incontinence. *Reviews in Urology, 3*(Suppl 1), S2–S6.

Office of Women's Health (OWS). (2012). *Female genital cutting fact sheet.* Retrieved from https://www.womenshealth.gov/publications/our-publications/fact-sheet/female-genital-cutting.html

Organization for Economic Cooperation and Development (OECD). (2013). *Health at a glance—OECD indicators.* Retrieved from http://www.oecd.org/els/health-systems/health-at-a-glance.htm

Purnell, L., & Paulanka, B. (1998). *Transcultural health care: A culturally competent approach.* Philadelphia, PA: F. A. Davis.

Roberts, S. (2006). Healthcare recommendations for lesbian women. *Journal of Obstetric, Gynecologic, & Neonatal Nursing, 35*(5), 583–591.

Rosser, S. (1995). *Women's health—missing from U.S. medicine.* Bloomington, IN: Indiana University Press.

Scholle, S. H., Buranosky, R., Hanusa, B. H., Ranieri, L., Dowd, K., & Valappil, B. (2003). Routine screening for intimate partner violence in an obstetrics and gynecology clinic. *American Journal of Public Health, 93*(7), 1070–1073.

Smith, R. W., & Martos, L. (2002). *Attitudes towards and experience with guns: A state level perspective.* Chicago, IL: National Opinion Research Center.

Sorenson, S. B., & Wiebe, D. J. (2004). Weapons in the lives of battered women. *American Journal of Public Health, 94*(8), 1412–1417.

Stevens, P., Tatum, N., & White, J. (1996). Optimal care for lesbian patients. *Patient Care, 30*(5), 121–134.

Strauss, M. A. (1992). Explaining family violence. In J. M. Henslin (Ed.), *Marriage and family in a changing society* (4th ed., pp. 344–356). New York, NY: Free Press.

The Sentencing Project. (2012). Fact sheet: Incarcerated women. Retrieved from http://www.sentencingproject.org/doc/publications/cc_Incarcerated_Women_Factsheet_Sep24sp.pdf

Tjaden, P., & Thoennes, N. (2000). *Full report of the prevalence, incidence and consequences of violence against women* (Publication NCJ 183781). Washington, DC: U.S. Department of Justice, Office of Justice Program, National Institute of Justice.

UNFPA-UNICEF (2013). Joint programme on female mutilation/cutting: Accelerating change, 2008-2012. New York, NY: Author.

U.S. Census Bureau. (2010). *Statistical abstract of the United States: The national data book.* Retrieved from https://www.census.gov/prod/2010pubs/p25-1138.pdf

U.S. Census Bureau. (2012). *The next four decades: The older population in the United States: 2010–2050.* Retrieved from http://www.census.gov/compendia/statab/

U.S. Census Bureau. (2013a). *Educational attainment in the United States: 2013—Detailed tables.* Retrieved from http://www.census.gov/hhes/socdemo/education/data/cps/2013/tables.html

U.S. Census Bureau. (2013b). Births: Preliminary data for 2012. *National Vital Statistics Reports, 62*(3). Retrieved from http://www.cdc.gov/nchs/products/nvsr.htm#vol63

U.S. Department of Education. (2007). *Secretary Spelling's remarks at UNESCO General Conference Plenary Debate in Paris, France.* Retrieved from http://www.ed.gov/news/speeches/2007/10/10182007.html

U.S. Department of Health and Human Services (HHS). (2012). *Healthy People 2020: Topics and Objectives.* Retrieved from http://www.healthypeople.gov/2020/topicsobjectives2020/default.aspx

Waldherr, K. (1996). *The book of goddesses.* Hillsboro, OR: Beyond Words.

Wiebe, J. (2003). Firearms in the home as a risk factor for homicide and suicide: A national case-control study. *Annals of Emergency Medicine, 4,* 771–782.

World Bank. (2014). *World development indicator data: Life expectancy at birth, female (years).* Retrieved from http://data.worldbank.org/indicator/SP.DYN.LE00.FE.IN

World Health Organization. (2002). *Ultraviolet radiation: Global solar UV index.* Retrieved from http://www.who.int/mediacentre/factsheets/fs271/en/

Zeidenstein, L. (1990). Gynecological and childbearing needs of lesbians. *Journal of Nurse Midwifery, 35,* 10–18.

CHAPTER FOCUS

Men's Health
- Genetic Factors
- Sociocultural and Ethnic Factors
- Environmental Factors
- Behavioral Factors
- *Healthy People 2020*

Healthcare System Utilization
- Ambulatory Care
- Hospital Care
- Preventive Care

Specific Male Health Issues
- Prostate Cancer
- Testicular Cancer
- Erectile Dysfunction
- Cardiovascular Disease

Selected At-Risk Populations
- Men with HIV/AIDS
- Homosexual Men and Families

Community Health Nursing Roles
- Patient Advocate
- Educator
- Facilitator

Men's Health Research Issues

QUESTIONS TO CONSIDER

After reading this chapter, you will know the answers to the following questions:

1. What are some of the major factors affecting men's health?
2. How are risk factors for illness or injury different for men compared with women?
3. How does the threat of testicular and prostate cancer affect the lives of young and middle-aged men?
4. What is the nurse's role in the treatment of erectile dysfunction?
5. What are some roles for the community health nurse in the promotion of men's health?

Nurses on the gridiron: Undergraduate nursing students who were on the 2007 Case Western Reserve University Spartans football team. Case Western Reserve University's 2007 season was its best record in history. One of the nursing student football players was quoted as saying, "It was a great experience to be part of the record-setting team. Teammates gave me a hard time on the days I had to wear my clinical uniform. I would walk in with my scrubs on and they would joke—but all in good fun."

CHAPTER 32

Men's Health

Sharyn Janes, Karen Saucier Lundy, and Joseph Farmer

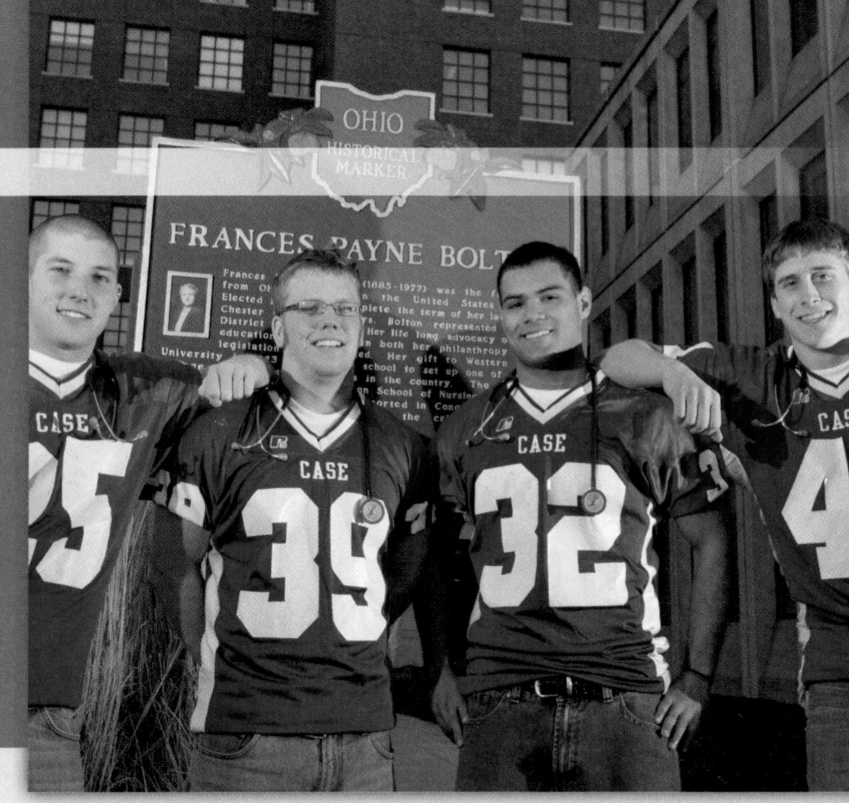

KEY TERMS

erectile dysfunction (ED) and treatment
fertility
gender differences
health status
homosexuality
socialization process
stress
violence

REFLECTIONS

Historically, most research studies have been based on male subjects. In many Western cultures, years of a predominantly male workforce have resulted in healthcare systems and policies being established by men. Despite this dominance of men in healthcare systems, women still have longer life expectancies than men.

It has been said that the most dangerous substance on earth is testosterone. What do you think and why? How do biology, gender, and culture affect the health of men?

Gender matters. Men and women have different death rates from the same diseases. Most men have shorter lifespans than women, particularly among minorities. What are your stereotypes of men and how they differ from women? How do these images affect nursing care? This chapter explores the specific threats to men's health based on physiological, social, and cultural differences.

AS A NURSING STUDENT, you have most likely had a course in women's health. What you most likely have *not* had is a specific course on men's health. The male gender has been neglected as the "other half" of the human population. Especially today, men are most likely to be in need of health care. When you hold clinics in community-based settings, it is unlikely that you will have seen many men in waiting rooms where primary health and prevention health services were provided. Whether through media campaigns or in focused efforts by health professionals, few health efforts have been directed toward men. Poor men and men of color are even more at risk in a society that rewards wealth and career success, particularly for men. Men typically die earlier than women, have fewer contacts with the healthcare system as compared to women, and have the highest risks for most diseases such as heart disease and cancer, and for accidents, including those associated with violent behavior. More than women, many men focus more intensely on work and providing for their families on a daily basis, and do not see health as a priority.

This chapter focuses on men's health, the risks that men face, and the role of the community health nurse in making the wellbeing of men a priority.

Men's Health

Women live longer than men. Men are many times more likely to die of lung cancer, motor vehicle accidents, cirrhosis of the liver, heart disease, and acquired immune deficiency syndrome (AIDS) than women. Suicide rates are three times higher for men. **Gender differences** in health are caused by genetic, sociocultural, environmental, and behavioral factors (Harrisson, Chin, & Ficarotto, 1992).

Genetic Factors

Genetic factors related to gender influence a man's physiological and psychological wellbeing. According to the genetic approach, some gender differences are natural in origin. They are driven by instinctual, hormonal, structural, or neurological characteristics of the male gender (Blekhman et al., 2008; Galdas, Cheater, & Marshall, 2005; Sabo & Gordon, 1995). For example, gender differences in ischemic heart disease mortality may be a result of the protective effects of female sex hormones and men's tendency to accumulate fat in the upper abdomen (Courtenay, 2000b; Fackelmann, 1998; Waldron, 1995). Higher levels of testosterone contribute to men's predisposition to **violence**. Some of the other physiological differences between men and women include the following (Tanne, 1997):

- Men's brain cells die faster than women's as they age.
- There are structural differences between men and women in the mitral valve, which separates the left atrium of the heart from the left ventricle.
- Women's hearts beat more rapidly than men's hearts.
- Men have weaker immune systems than women.
- Men and women often react differently to medications, therapies, and diagnostics.

RESEARCH ALERT

Rooted in a qualitative research project with 70 stay-at-home fathers in Canada, this paper explores the ways that work and family interact for fathers who "trade cash for care." While fathers are at home, they also remain connected to traditionally masculine sources of identity such as paid work and they take on unpaid masculine self-provisioning work at home and community work that builds on traditional male interests. They thus carve out complex sets of relations between home, paid and unpaid work, community work, and their own sense of masculinity. Narratives from stay-at-home fathers speak volumes about the ways in which the long shadow of hegemonic masculinity hangs over them while also pointing to hints of resistance and change as fathers begin to critique concepts of "male time" and market capitalism approaches to work and care. The research concludes by pointing to several theoretical contributions to research on fatherhood and masculinities as well as to policy implications that arise from this study on the social valuing of unpaid work."

Source: Doucet, A. (2004) "It's almost like I have a job, but I don't get paid": Fathers at home reconfiguring work, care, and masculinity. *Fathering: A Journal of Theory, Research, & Practice about Men as Fathers*, 2(3), 277–304.

Sociocultural and Ethnic Factors

In many cultures, particularly Western cultures, the male **socialization process** has emphasized traits such as the following (Torres, 1998):

- Assertiveness
- Preoccupation with achievement and success (individualism, status, aggression, toughness, and winning)
- Restricted emotionality and affectionate behavior
- Concerns about power and control
- Fear and bias related to **homosexuality**

As a result, most males tend to conform to these stereotyped gender expectations and behaviors, leading to definite health consequences. Some men may experience and endure more trauma because of their belief that taking physical risks is a sign of masculinity. Boys are socialized into competitive games at an early age and learn to endure physical punishment as part of having fun or as a prerequisite to becoming a man (Charles & Walters, 2008; Courtenay, 2000b; Stillion, 1995; Williams, 2008). From Little League on, a boy is told to "act like a man" (or given negative messaging when chided that he "throws like a girl"). Hence, to admit to having pain or some other health problem may be seen as a reflection of weakness. This male denial factor is pervasive and not related to occupation, age, race, or socioeconomic status. High death rates from coronary heart disease for men in the United States may be due in part to these stereotyped gender expectations, which increase the risk of the disease (Charles & Walters, 2008; Glassner, 1992; Harrisson et al., 1992; Men's Health Network, 2008; Pease, 1997).

THINK ABOUT THIS 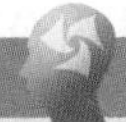

President Bill Clinton and Heart Surgery: Did He Ignore the Early Warnings of a Pending Heart Attack?

President Bill Clinton was hospitalized in 2004 and had successful coronary bypass surgery immediately. He had complained of shortness of breath and chest pain, and drove himself to the hospital.

Physicians were alarmed enough to insist that Clinton, 58, undergo bypass surgery with minimal delay at Manhattan's New York–Presbyterian Hospital.

In a call from the hospital to CNN's *Larry King Live*, Clinton said, "I guess I'm a little scared, but not much. I'm looking forward to it. I want to get back; I want to see what it's like to run five miles again.

"My blockage is so substantial, I think if I don't do this, there's virtually a 100% chance that I'll have a heart attack," he said.

Clinton's health scare took most of the nation by surprise for a man who had been declared in good health after years of intensive annual physicals in his White House years and afterward.

The former president, though he has labored against a tendency toward overweight, has been particularly fit over the years after the presidency. He has lifted weights and uses an elliptical trainer and has lost weight using a modified version of the South Beach Diet. However, he told CNN that he had regained 10 pounds during a tour promoting his memoir, *My Life*.

Clinton has a family history of heart disease and a history of eating fast-food meals. "Some of this is genetic, and I may have done some damage in those years when I was too careless about what I ate," the former president said.

Clinton has described himself as a child as "fat, uncool, and hardly popular with the girls." His grandmother was 5 feet tall and 180 pounds, and one of her main goals in life was to get people to eat. "When I was little, it was generally believed that a fat baby was a healthy baby."

Heart bypass surgeries are performed when one or more of the arteries feeding the heart are blocked or choked off by buildups of fatty plaque—of which high cholesterol levels are the leading cause. The chest pains that brought Clinton into the hospital appear to have developed abruptly, but the root causes of the problem are likely to be several years old: During his last physical before he left the White House, Clinton had a total cholesterol count of 233 and a "bad" cholesterol count of 177. Clinton acknowledged he needed "to keep my cholesterol down, keep my blood pressure down." The American Heart Association recommends that total cholesterol should be below 200.

Men often ignore the early signs of heart failure. President Clinton admitted that he had experienced a few symptoms in the past, but he thought it was reflux. This is a common misconception about heart disease because of the overlap of the symptoms. The two conditions are very different, even with similar symptoms. Men who experience symptoms of reflux should have a complete workup to rule out heart disease.

Sources: Harris, J. F., & Vedantam, S. (September 4, 2004). *Washington Post*, p. A01; A look at heart disease. (September 11, 2004). *CNN House Call with Dr. Sanjay Gupta*.

The lack of healthy emotional channels for men contributes to higher risks among men for suicide, heart disease, accidents, and violence. The traditional male socialization process has historically emphasized restricted emotionality and affectionate behavior. This traditional male gender role is inconsistent with the provision and receipt of social support, particularly emotional support that includes expressiveness and disclosure. Such characteristics may have adverse health consequences (Galdas et al., 2005). The lack of expressiveness becomes especially significant in the way men deal with **stress** and depression. Most men tend not to cry and try to keep emotions hidden (Vogel, Heimerdinger-Edwards, Hammer, & Hubbard, 2011; Williams, 2008). They are far less likely to seek psychological counseling than are women. Along with other cultural messages that men need to be strong, powerful, and independent, men are taught not to react to physical, psychological, or spiritual pain. Some men are unwilling to seek health care simply because they fear the risk of appearing "unmanly" or the exposure of their sense of vulnerability (Charles & Walters, 2008; Harrisson et al., 1992; Will, 1998).

ENVIRONMENTAL CONNECTION

Men are more vulnerable to accidents due to their risk-taking behavior. How does the environment in which we live affect the choices we make about health? For example, in rural areas, four-wheeler accidents occur almost exclusively among men. Compared to their female counterparts, teenage boys in the United States remain at higher risk for death from automobile accidents and acts of violence, most notably in urban environments. How does the environment affect these outcomes?

The sociocultural differences between men and women must be considered when planning and developing intervention and prevention programs. Strategies that target the general population may not consider the diversity of expectations and behaviors of men. Although some publicly funded programs may attempt to target as many people as possible, programs with more specifically focused segments or populations may be more effective with men. The nurse must consider the vast number of socialization possibilities that exist within male societies (Isenhart & Silvermith, 1994). This gender difference in regard to socialization also extends to nursing. The media image of a nurse as female has often been cited in research as a deterrent in the recruitment of males to nursing. Health interventions directed toward men may be more effective when men are separated from women, divided into age-specific groups, or grouped into a larger audience. For example, instead of a smoking cessation program for all people, with an emphasis on the long-term effects of smoking, a program targeting men ages 15 to 25, with an emphasis on the sex appeal of nonsmokers, may be more effective.

Environmental Factors

Physical and occupational environments affect the **health status** of men. More men are employed than women, and male-dominated occupations such as mining, construction, and farming are often more hazardous. Accidents on the job are a major contributor to higher death rates among men. In addition, men in these types of occupations are more likely to be exposed to carcinogens and other toxins that are associated with higher rates of pneumoconiosis (black lung), asbestosis, leukemia, and cancer of the bladder. Men's greater exposure to occupational hazards accounts for about 5% to 10% of the gender difference in mortality (Hudak & Hagan, 2002; Miniclier, 2002; Parker, 2002; Roman & Carroll, 2003; Waldron, 1995).

The high number of men in high-risk employment settings may be advantageous to community health nurses, who can use these environments to introduce men to health care. Prevention and screening programs in the workplace can be effective interventions for men who would not seek health care in traditional settings. Recent West Virginia coal mining accidents have exposed the public to the often invisible, yet hazardous work of men. Fire fighters, especially those involved in the September 11, 2001 terrorist attacks, have suffered extraordinary health consequences (Delsohn, 1996; Hauser & Sokol, 2008; Poppius, Virkkunen, Hakama, & Tenkanen, 2008).

Behavioral Factors

Unlike genetic factors, behaviors such as diet, tobacco use, alcohol consumption, illicit drug use, lack of physical exercise, physical and sexual risk taking, and suicide and violence are controllable and subject to human influence and intervention. Individuals can make wiser choices such as wearing seatbelts; exercising and eating right; not using tobacco, drugs, or alcohol, or at least not driving while under the influence of alcohol or drugs; not bungee jumping; or not committing acts of violence against themselves or others (Courtenay, 2000c; Harrisson et al., 1992; Steenbergh, Whelan, Meyers, Klesges, & DeBon, 2008). Partly as a result of the cultural expectations of society and the gender socialization process, men's behavior is consistently less healthy than that of women. As a result, behavior is the cause of the largest differences in mortality between men and women (Courtenay, 2000a; Galdas et al., 2005; Stillion, 1995; Stoltenberg, Batien, & Birgenheir, 2008).

Data in the United States indicate that men's diets have had higher ratios of saturated to polyunsaturated fat, which contribute to higher ischemic heart disease mortality among men (Power & Schulkin, 2008). More males than females smoke cigarettes and drink heavily. Men's smoking habits account for as much as 90% of gender differences in cancer mortality and roughly one-third of gender differences in ischemic heart disease mortality. Similarly, men's drinking contributes to higher mortality in liver disease, accidents, suicide, and homicide (Courtenay, 2000a; Galdas et al., 2005; Stoltenberg et al., 2008; Waldron, 1995).

Diet

Obesity and consumption of fatty foods increase the risk of cardiovascular disease, which is a major killer for men. Men consume a large amount of fatty foods and are less likely than women to change their eating habits, even though more than 33% of men meet the definition of obesity (a body mass index of 27.8 kg/m^2). Researchers suggest that low-fat diet programs for men should target worksite and peer-group organizations and include meal modifications with all family members (Coakley, Rimm, Colditz, Kawachi, & Willett, 1998; Nguyen, Otis, & Potvin, 1996; Power & Schulkin, 2008).

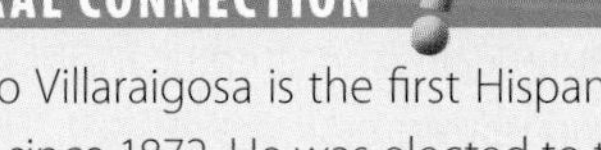

Antonio Villaraigosa is the first Hispanic mayor of Los Angeles since 1872. He was elected to the office on May 17, 2005.

Born Antonio Villar in the Boyle Heights neighborhood of Los Angeles' east side of Mexican American parentage, Villaraigosa had a troubled childhood. He added his wife's surname, Raigosa, after he married Corina Raigosa and, combining their names, changed his name from Villar to Villaraigosa.

Although he dropped out of high school, Villaraigosa received an honorary degree from Theodore Roosevelt High School. He was a gang member but eventually shook off that lifestyle and went on to attend East Los Angeles College and the University of California at Los Angeles (UCLA). While at UCLA, he was active in MEChA, a student-based civil rights organization. He obtained his degree in history, and then attended the People's College of Law, an unaccredited law school. After failing the bar four times, he moved on to labor.

As early as 15 years old, Villaraigosa had been volunteering with the farm workers movement. He has been active in labor, the American Civil Liberties Union, and the American Federation of Government Employees. He has also campaigned for smaller school districts, sought more funding for the homeless, and is an advocate for the environment.

Los Angeles is the second largest city in the United States, with a population of 3.7 million. The city is plagued by school violence, racial and ethnic tensions, and poverty. Approximately 40% of the people in Los Angeles are foreign born, according to the U.S. Census. Nearly half of the population is Hispanic, 11% is black, and 11% is Asian.

The Academy Award–winning *Crash,* which was released in 2005, is about the brutal ethnic and racial tensions in Los Angeles.

Tobacco

Gender differences in smoking prevalence have been decreasing for decades, but still more males than females smoke cigarettes. Smoking is positively correlated with men's higher mortality from bronchitis, emphysema, and asthma.

Men, especially rural men, are more likely to use smokeless (chewing) tobacco. Despite the general declining trends in the use of cigarettes, there has not been a concomitant decline in the use of smokeless tobacco. Smokeless tobacco use is associated with higher risks of cardiovascular disease and cancers of the oral cavity, as well as gum recession and nicotine addiction. Heavy marketing efforts by tobacco companies toward rural men might explain the slight increase in the use of smokeless tobacco (Dutta & Boyd, 2007; Hede, 2007; Nelson, Tomar, Mowery, & Siegel, 1996).

Alcohol and Drug Use

Alcohol abuse is well known for its devastating effects on physical and emotional health. More men drink than women, and men are five times more likely to drink heavily. Higher numbers of male drinkers contribute to males' higher mortality, related to chronic liver disease, cirrhosis of the liver, accidents, and homicide. In addition, male drivers have substantially higher risk of fatal motor vehicle accidents because they are more likely to have high blood alcohol levels when driving and are also more likely to exhibit riskier driving behaviors (Gefou-Madianou, 1992; Gough & Edwards, 1998;

Poppius et al., 2008; Stoltenberg et al., 2008; Thornton, 2004; Waldron, 1995).

Alcohol use must be taken into consideration in developing strategies to prevent the transmission of sexually transmitted diseases (STDs), including human immunodeficiency virus (HIV), because alcohol consumption is related to risky sexual behavior. A number of studies have suggested that people who drink more heavily are more likely to have multiple partners, and among young men, consistent use of condoms decreases at higher levels of alcohol use (Graves, 1995; Isenhart & Silversmith, 1994). It is estimated that two-thirds of all alcoholics are men, more than 80% of those who have serious drug addictions are men, more than 80% of those who die of drug abuse are men, and 90% of those arrested for alcohol or drug abuse are men (Thornton, 2004).

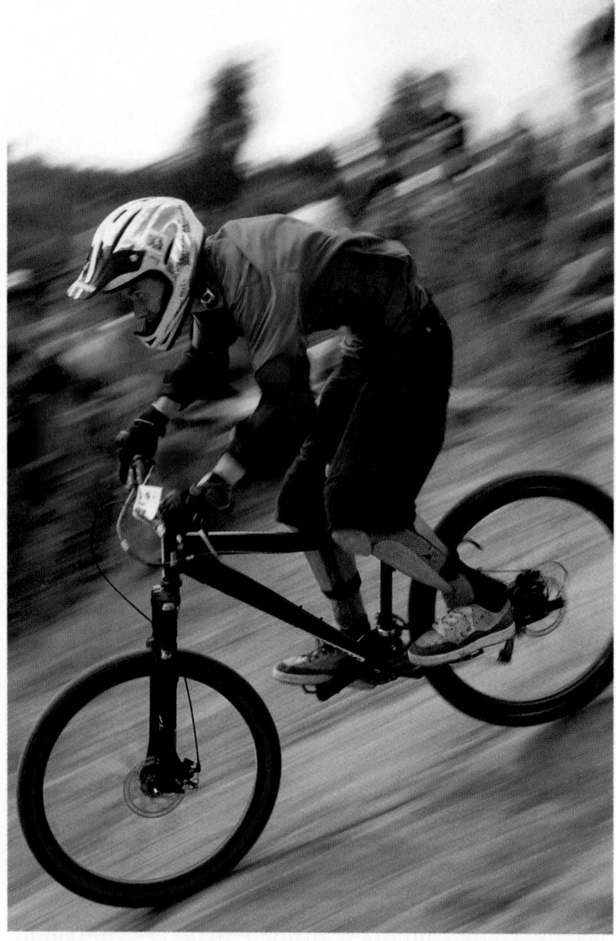

Young males are likely to be involved in risk-taking behavior. However, risk can be decreased through the use of protective gear.

Suicide and Violence

Deaths by suicide and violence are a predominantly male phenomenon. The suicide rate among males is 4 times that of females in all age groups (American Foundation for Suicide Prevention, 2014), but in specific age groups, the rate is even higher: Between the ages of 20 and 24, for example, men are six times more likely to commit suicide than women, and over the age of 85, men are more than 11 times more likely to kill themselves than women (Men's Health Network, 2008). Suicide rates for specific groups of men, such as veterans, divorced men, and homosexual teenagers, are even higher. Researchers argue that men's higher suicide rates are due to men's greater frequency of substance abuse, subjection to more stress, lack of emotional channels, and use of more violent, lethal means of taking their lives in comparison with women (Femquist, 2001; Williams, 2008; Yip et al., 2012).

The world of men is much more violent than that of women. White men are three times more likely to die in a homicide than white women; and African American men are five times more likely to die in a homicide than black women (Black & Breiding, 2008; Centers for Disease Control and Prevention [CDC], 2012). The persons at greatest risk for violence victimization, as well as becoming the perpetrators of violence, are young males who are members of underrepresented ethnic groups and live in poor urban communities. These young men risk injury to themselves, disrupted personal lives, damaging criminal records, extended imprisonment, and in some cases, capital punishment.

RESEARCH ALERT

In this study, risk factors for college male sexual aggression that were both theoretically and empirically based were tested using multivariate regression analyses. These risk factors included substance abuse patterns, pornography consumption, negative gender-based attitudes, and child sexual abuse experiences. Regression analyses indicated that some gender attitudes, pornography use, and alcohol abuse were significant predictors of perpetration of sexual violence. Although a number of men were sexually abused as children, this risk factor did not predict sexual aggression as an adult. Many men reported alcohol-related sexual coercion and held many rape-supportive attitudes and beliefs. These practices by college men contribute to the pro-rape cultures found on many campuses. Strategies are needed to identify and intervene with high-risk men to prevent sexual victimization of women in college.

Source: Carr, J., & VanDeusen, K. M. (2004). Risk factors for male sexual aggression on college campuses. *Journal of Family Violence, 19*(5), 279–290.

HEALTHY PEOPLE 2020 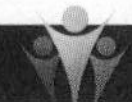

Objectives Related to Men's Health

Cancer

- C-2 Reduce the lung cancer death rate.
- C-7 Reduce the prostate cancer death rate.
- C-19 Increase the proportion of men who have discussed the advantages and disadvantages of the prostate-specific antigen (PSA) test to screen for prostate cancer with their healthcare provider.

Family Planning

- FP-7.2 Increase the proportion of sexually experienced males age 15 to 44 years who received reproductive health services.
- FP-9.2 Increase the proportion of male adolescents age 15 to 17 years who have never had sexual intercourse.
- FP-9.4 Increase the proportion of male adolescents age 15 years and under who have never had sexual intercourse.
- FP-10.2 Increase the proportion of sexually active males age 15 to 19 years who use a condom at first intercourse.
- FP-10.4 Increase the proportion of sexually active males age 15 to 19 years who used a condom at last intercourse.
- FP-11.2 Increase the proportion of sexually active males age 15 to 19 years who use a condom and hormonal or intrauterine contraception at first intercourse.
- FP-11.4 Increase the proportion of sexually active males age 15 to 19 years who used a condom and hormonal or intrauterine contraception at last intercourse.
- FP-12.2 Increase the proportion of male adolescents who received formal instruction on abstinence before they were 18 years old.
- FP-12.4 Increase the proportion of male adolescents who received formal instruction on birth control methods before they were 18 years old.
- FP-12.6 Increase the proportion of male adolescents who received formal instruction on HIV/AIDS prevention before they were 18 years old.
- FP-12.8 Increase the proportion of male adolescents who received formal instruction on sexually transmitted diseases before they were 18 years old.
- FP-13.2 Increase the proportion of male adolescents who talked to a parent or guardian about abstinence before they were 18 years old.
- FP-13.4 Increase the proportion of male adolescents who talked to a parent or guardian about birth control methods before they were 18 years old.
- FP-13.6 Increase the proportion of male adolescents who talked to a parent or guardian about HIV/AIDS prevention before they were 18 years old.
- FP-13.8 Increase the proportion of male adolescents who talked to a parent or guardian about sexually transmitted diseases before they were 18 years old.

Heart Disease and Stroke

- HDS-1 Increase overall cardiovascular health in the U.S. population.
- HDS-2 Reduce coronary heart disease deaths.
- HDS-3 Reduce stroke deaths.
- HDS-15.2 Increase aspirin use as recommended among men age 45 to 79 years with no history of cardiovascular disease.

HIV/AIDS

- HIV-6 Reduce new AIDS cases among adolescents and adult men who have sex with men (MSM).
- HIV-14.2 Increase the proportion of MSM who have been tested for HIV in the past 12 months.
- HIV-17.2 Increase the proportion of sexually active unmarried males age 15 to 44 years who use condoms.
- HIV-18 Reduce the proportion of MSM who reported unprotected anal sex in the past 12 months.

Injury and Violence Prevention

Unintentional Injury Prevention

- IPV-13 Reduce motor vehicle crash-related deaths.
- IPV-21 Increase the number of states and the District of Columbia with laws requiring bicycle helmets for bicycle riders.
- IPV-22 Increase the proportion of motorcycle operators and passengers using helmets.

Violence and Abuse Prevention

- IPV-29 Reduce homicides.
- IPV-30 Reduce firearm-related deaths.
- IPV-31 Reduce firearm-related injuries.
- IPV-34 Reduce physical fighting among adolescents.
- IPV-36 Reduce weapon carrying by adolescents on school property.
- IPV-39 Reduce violence by current or former intimate partners.
- IPV-40 Reduce sexual violence.

Mental Health and Mental Disorders

Mental Health Status Improvement

- MHMD-1 Reduce the suicide rate.
- MHMD-9 Increase the proportion of adults with mental health disorders who receive treatment.
- MHMD-10 Increase the proportion of persons with co-occurring substance abuse and mental disorders who receive treatment for both disorders.
- MHMD-12 Increase the proportion of homeless adults with mental health problems who receive mental health services.

Occupational Safety and Health

- OSH-1 Reduce deaths from work-related injuries.
- OSH-2 Reduce nonfatal work-related injuries.
- OSH-3 Reduce the rate of injury and illness cases involving days away from work due to overexertion or repetitive motion.

(*continues*)

HEALTHY PEOPLE 2020 (*continued*) 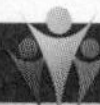

- OSH-7 Reduce the proportion of persons who have elevated blood lead concentrations from work exposures.
- OSH-10 Reduce new cases of work-related, noise-induced hearing loss.

Substance Abuse

Adverse Consequences of Substance Use and Abuse

- SA-6 Increase the number of states with mandatory ignition interlock laws for first and repeat impaired driving offenders in the United States.
- SA-12 Reduce drug-induced deaths.
- SA-16 Reduce average annual alcohol consumption.
- SA-18 Reduce steroid use among adolescents.
- SA-19 Reduce the past-year nonmedical use of prescription drugs.

Tobacco Use

Tobacco Use in Population Groups

- TU-1 Reduce tobacco use by adults.
- TU-2 Reduce tobacco use by adolescents.

Source: U.S. Department of Health and Human Services. (2013). *Healthy People 2020: Topics and Objectives.* Retrieved from http://www.healthypeople.gov/2020/TopicsObjectives2020/default.aspx

Much of the violent actions of men are directed at women. In the United States, female murder victims are most often (63%, likely an underestimate) killed by their husbands, boyfriends, other male family members, or close male friends (Carr & VanDeusen, 2004; National Center for Health Statistics, 2002; New York State Office for the Prevention of Domestic Violence, 2011). Violence against women will not cease until greater emphasis is put on prevention, treatment, and rehabilitation programs for the men who perform the violent acts. The nursing literature that addresses the issue of working with men who batter women and children is almost nonexistent, yet nurses who work in hospitals and community settings deal with the results of domestic violence every day. Because nurses are on the front line, they are in the best position to intervene in ways that are sensitive to both the perpetrators and the victims of family violence. Nurses working in settings such as schools, churches, and worksites can conduct education programs to promote awareness of the potential for and prevention of family violence (Carr & VanDeusen, 2004; Goldstein, Chesir-Teran, & McFaul, 2008; Rynerson & Fishel, 1998).

Healthy People 2020

The purpose of *Healthy People 2020* is to improve the health of Americans with specific objectives in many health-related areas. Although men are not specifically listed as a targeted group, several objectives do focus on specific subpopulations of males. Selected objectives are listed in the *Healthy People 2020* box.

THINK ABOUT THIS 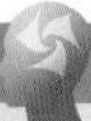

Men are more likely to speed, drive aggressively, fail to wear seat belts, and drive drunk (Thornton, 2004).

RESEARCH ALERT 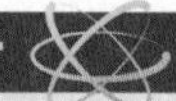

Osteoporosis: Not Just a Woman's Disease—2 Million American Men Have Osteoporosis, and Another 12 Million Are at Risk

Osteoporosis ... isn't that a woman's disease? While it is true that more women than men have been diagnosed with osteoporosis, men have no "immunity" to osteoporosis. Some of the factors that contribute to the gender differences in bone density are:

1. Men usually have larger bones than women do.
2. The life expectancy for men in the United States is shorter than that of women. One of the factors in the development of osteoporosis is age-related loss of bone density. Women live long enough to be diagnosed with osteoporosis.
3. Bone density is affected by estrogen and testosterone. Decreases in estrogen usually occur in the late 4th or early 5th decade of life for women, while testosterone decreases in the 5th or 6th decade. Another variable that affects women is surgical menopause; many women in the United States have lost the bone-protective effects of estrogen earlier than age 50. There are very few medical indications for male castration, so men do not suffer from surgical andropause!

The bad news for men is:

Even though there are fewer cases of osteoporosis in men, and fewer osteoporotic fractures in men, the chances of dying from an osteoporotic fracture are higher for a man than for a woman! Men, such as the Pope and former President Ronald Reagan, suffered from osteoporosis-related complications, which contributed to their deaths.

The good news for men is:

1. Even at the same bone mineral density level, men generally do not fracture at the same rate as women.
2. Effective treatments are available.

Risk factors for men include:

1. Alcohol use of more than two drinks per day
2. Use of corticosteroids for diseases such as asthma, Addison's disease, and Crohn's Disease
3. Advanced age (70 years or more)
4. Use of anticonvulsants (such as Dilantin)
5. Use of thyroid supplements (such as Synthroid)

Recommendations for slowing progress in osteoporosis, according to the National Osteoporosis Foundation (2008), include:

- Adults age 50 and older should consume 1,200 mg of calcium per day.
- Adults age 50 and older should consume 800–1,000 IU of vitamin D_3 per day.
- Fortified dairy products are among the best food sources of calcium and vitamin D.
- For those concerned with fat and cholesterol counts, reducing fat content does not adversely affect calcium and vitamin D content of dairy products.
- Exposure of the forearms to sunlight for 15 minutes three or four times a week is recommended to stimulate the production of vitamin D.
- In addition to calcium and vitamin D intake, weight-bearing exercise is known to be protective for bones. Walking for 20 minutes three to four times a week will help maintain bone mass.

—Dr. Cynthia Luther, ANP
Assistant Professor
The University of Southern Mississippi
School of Nursing

Source: National Osteoporosis Foundation. (2008). *Clinician's guide to prevention and treatment of osteoporosis*. Washington, DC: Author.

Healthcare System Utilization

Patterns of healthcare utilization by men are cited as an important contributor to the inferior health status of men. One-third of American men do not have a checkup every year. Men visit doctors 25% less often than women. At the same time, men account for the majority of the patients admitted to emergency departments (Courtenay, 2000a, 2000b). Men tend to have fewer contacts with the healthcare system, perhaps as a result of psychological and sociological factors such as a reluctance to admit that they need assistance. This situation is exacerbated by the fact that the U.S. healthcare system tends to focus on health from an illness perspective, with relatively little attention paid to prevention. As a result, unlike women who have annual gynecological examinations that include screening for other conditions, men are less likely to enter the healthcare system for a physical examination on a routine basis. Moreover, although men come in contact with many healthcare professionals in a wide variety of settings, they have no specialist to whom they can go for their specific care needs. Men have to be attended by generalists, such as family practitioners, or by other specialists such as urologists who also see women. There is a growing national movement to create men's health as a medical and nursing specialty, a long overlooked but necessary change in improving the health of men (Pinkhasov et al., 2010; Treadwell & Ro, 2003).

Strategies to improve men's utilization of preventive health care must target all ages. Men must establish a committed relationship with preventive health care as early as possible. For men to use preventive health care, programs that present health prevention as masculine and strengthening must be developed and implemented. The required school physical before participation in extracurricular activities may be used in the resocialization of men for the active and lifelong usage of preventive health care.

Ambulatory Care

Men have significantly lower rates of visits to ambulatory care settings, such as physician offices and outpatient services, than women, but the visit rates to hospital emergency departments do not differ by gender. By age 75, men have approximately half of the contacts with healthcare providers compared to women. This discrepancy persists even when the contribution of pregnancy and birth control–related issues is not counted in women's contacts. The patterns in provider contacts indicate that, for all ages, the difference between men and women has been increasing. Although the total number of healthcare provider contacts is lower for men, men are seen more frequently than women for chronic diseases, such as heart and lung disease, which are more prevalent among men (Galdas et al., 2005; Harrisson et al., 1992; Pattison, 1998).

Hospital Care

Hospitalization rates and length of stays in hospitals vary by gender. Hospital discharge rates, the numbers used to determine usage, from short-stay hospitals are higher for women than for men (Galdas et al., 2005; Harrisson et al.,

1992; Pattison, 1998). When gynecological disorders in women and reproductive disorders in men are excluded, rates of hospitalization for men are about the same as for women. The lower rate of discharge and longer hospital stays may be due to the fact that when men are hospitalized their conditions are more severe.

Preventive Care

Men and women differ in their ability to seek preventive care for the early diagnosis of healthcare problems. Unlike women, who seek routine reproductive health screening, most men do not have routine checkups that would detect health problems at an early stage. Men are more likely to have examinations at the insistence of their employers, and they do not perceive that they need a regular source of care. More often than women, men perceive their health as very good or excellent and therefore may not think that they need to be involved in health-promotion activities (Clark, 1999; Galdas et al., 2005; Harrisson et al., 1992). Women are more likely than men to exhibit stronger health-promotion behaviors in terms of blood pressure checks, dental flossing, diet, smoking, drinking, physical activity, weight, and hours of sleep. Men tend to view exercise as sufficient to compensate for unhealthy behaviors such as poor diets. As a result, men are at greater risk for several of the top killers such as heart disease, cancer, suicide, accidents, and violence. Because most of these killers are preventable, changes in eating habits, workplace environments, and educational strategies are needed to improve preventive care for men (Pattison, 1998).

Specific Male Health Issues

Prostate Cancer

The American Cancer Society lists prostate cancer as the second leading cause of cancer death in American men after lung cancer. Prostate cancer is most common in men older than 40, and the risk increases with each decade thereafter. Most often, prostate cancer is asymptomatic until the disease has progressed. Symptoms that may indicate prostate disease include the following (Wigle, Turner et al., 2008).

- Difficulty or pain with urination
- Painful ejaculation
- Blood in urine or semen

Although prostate cancer is the second leading cause of cancer deaths in American men, how many prostate cancer prevention and awareness campaigns have you seen? Can the same be said for breast cancer? Consider the financial appropriations and expenditures for cancer in the United States detailed in **Table 32-1**.

TABLE 32-1 Breast Versus Prostate Cancer Expenditures

	Breast	Prostate
National Institutes of Health research (FY 2013)	$657 million	$286 million
Department of Defense research (FY 2013)	$120 million	$80 million
National Cancer Institute funds (2008):		
Per person diagnosed	$2,596	$1,318
Per death	$13,452	$11,298

Sources: National Institutes of Health (NIH). (2014). Research portfolio online reporting tools: Estimates of funding for research, condition, and disease categories (RCDC). Retrieved from http://report.nih.gov/categorical_spending.aspx; Parker-Pope, T. (2008). Cancer funding: Does it add up? *The New York Times* (blog). Retrieved from http://well.blogs.nytimes.com/2008/03/06/cancer-funding-does-it-add-up

NOTE THIS!

Several high-profile men came forward in the 1990s to talk about their experiences with prostate cancer in an effort to remove the embarrassment surrounding the disease. As a result of the openness of men like former U.S. Senator and presidential candidate Bob Dole, professional golfer Arnold Palmer, and retired General H. Norman Schwarzkopf, many books and journal articles appeared and support groups surfaced all over the country.

Information about the necessity of digital rectal examinations beginning at age 40 for all men, with possible earlier intervention for those with signs and symptoms of problems or a positive family history, must be included and incorporated into health fairs and promotions. Up-to-date information related to prostate-specific antigen (PSA) blood testing that is used in conjunction with the digital rectal examination for certain subsets of men should also be provided. In 1986, the U.S. Food and Drug Administration (FDA) approved the PSA test for prostate cancer screening, and for many years it was used routinely for all males; however, current guidelines from the American Urological Association (AUA) state that routine PSA testing be used only where the benefit outweighs the risk of potential harms related to false-positive findings. In men under 40 and men under 55 without known risk factors (e.g., family history or African American race), routine PSA testing is generally not recommended (AUA, 2013). This position is not without controversy, as many physicians believe that the subsequent fall in prostate cancer

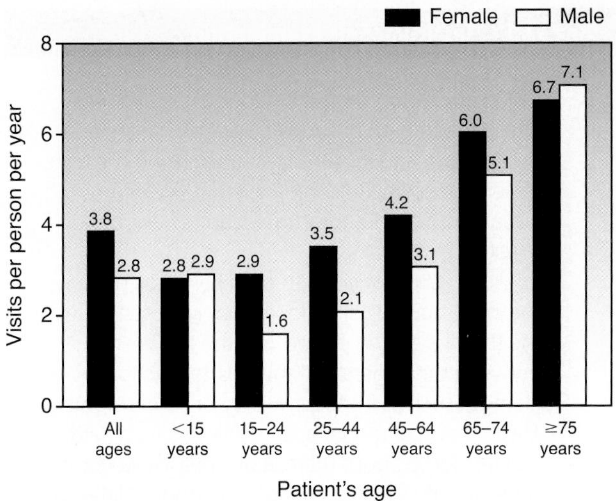

Figure 32-1 Annual rate of ambulatory care visits by patient's age and gender.

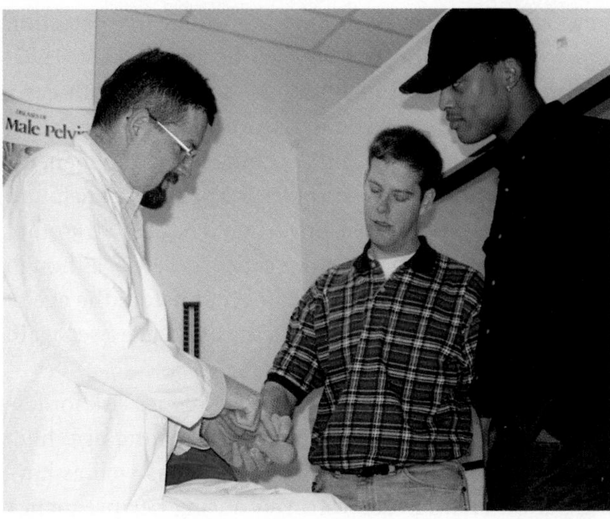

Chapter author Joseph Farmer uses a model to teach young men how to do a testicular self-examination.

mortality rates can be attributed to early diagnosis stemming from PSA testing (Courtenay, 2001; Feuer & Merrill, 1999). Current thinking holds that individualized decision making, rather than a "one-size-fits-all" approach, balances the need for early detection with a desire to avoid overly aggressive screening (McNaughton-Collins & Barry, 2011).

DAY IN THE LIFE

Lance Armstrong, testicular cancer survivor

Lance Armstrong is a father, cancer survivor, advocate, and philanthropist. In 1996, at age 25, Lance found himself struggling for his life against testicular cancer that had spread to his brain, lungs, and abdomen. Lance aggressively educated himself about his diagnosis and treatment. Even as he battled against overwhelming odds, he made the decision to declare himself a cancer survivor rather than a victim. During his personal battle with cancer, Lance recognized the lack of resources available to those facing this disease. In an effort to help fellow survivors and their families, Lance created a foundation with the express purpose of helping others manage life through and beyond a cancer diagnosis.

In the years since, the organization Lance founded—now the LIVESTRONG Foundation—has served millions of people affected by cancer through direct support services that fill critical financial, emotional, physical, and practical gaps in care for them and their loved ones. The Foundation has raised more than $500 million to serve cancer survivors, advocated on behalf of cancer patients in major policy debates, and fought the stigma many cancer survivors throughout the world face.

Source: http://www.livestrong.org

The importance of the procedure and information regarding signs, symptoms, and the screening process should be emphasized in promotions. Nurses should also include written information for distribution because some men are ill at ease discussing the procedure and testing in public.

The community health nurse can also organize targeted prostate-specific screenings, during which the men have the digital rectal examination and PSA blood tests on site. In a study that explored the relationship between attitudes toward digital rectal examinations and prostate screening among African American men, the results revealed that fear of the procedure did not prevent men from participating in the screening (Gelfand, Parzuchowski, Cort, & Powell, 1995; Treadwell & Ro, 2003).

Testicular Cancer

Testicular cancer accounts for only 1% of all cancers in men. However, testicular cancer is the most common form of cancer in men between the ages of 20 and 34 (Anderson, 2002). It is the second most common cancer for men between the ages of 35 and 39 and the third most common for men between the ages of 15 and 19. This type of cancer is 4.5 times more common among Caucasian men than African American men, with rates for Hispanics/Latinos, Native Americans, and Asians falling somewhere in between.

Epidemiological data show an increase in the incidence of testicular cancer since the 1970s (Clore, 1993; Koshti-Richman, 1996). As recent as the early 1980s, testicular cancer was fatal for 8 out of 10 patients (Brock et al., 1993; Walbrecker, 1995). Today, because of advances in chemotherapy and improved surgical techniques, testicular cancer is one of the most curable forms of cancer. Testicular cancer has a nearly 100% cure rate with early detection and treatment (Brakey, 1994; Clore, 1993; Peate, 1997; Walbrecker, 1995). This optimistic prognosis with early intervention makes testicular self-examination (TSE) a critical component of health teaching for young men, especially because most cases of testicular cancer are found by the patients themselves. Boys should begin TSE around age 13 and make it a lifelong practice, because, although testicular cancer is most likely to occur before the age of 40, it can occur at any age. In fact, the incidence rises again after the age of 70.

The characteristics that put men at higher risk for testicular cancer include Caucasian race, young age, high socioeconomic status, or family history, as well as having a mother who took estrogen during her pregnancy (Bertuccio et al., 2007; Brakey, 1994; Cheung et al., 2007; Feldman, Bosl, Sheinfeld, & Motzer, 2008; Kinkade, 1999; Wigle, Turner, Gomes, & Parent, 2008). Males with undescended testicles or late descending testicles (after age 6) have a 3 to 17 times higher than average risk for developing testicular cancer. In recent years, there have also been suggestions that use of endogenous steroids as performance-enhancing drugs may promote testicular and prostate cancer (Pinto et al., 2010). Despite this information, the health education literature suggests that most of the men who are most susceptible to testicular cancer are unaware of the signs and symptoms of the disease and how to detect them (Cook, 2000; Rovito, Gordon, Bass, & Ducette, 2011). Research has indicated that although information has been readily available to young women regarding breast self-examination (BSE) and the importance of regular Pap smears, the information related to TSE has not been as widely communicated.

> "I wouldn't be half the person I am today if I hadn't gone through cancer. People ask me the biggest blessing in my life. My boys and my wife are my top priority, but cancer was the biggest character builder I could've ever gone through."
>
> —*Josh Bidwell, former Green Bay Packers punter and testicular cancer survivor (Clemmons, 2008)*

Nurses are in the best position to provide young men with the information to learn the self-examination techniques needed for early detection and cure (Peate, 1997; Walbrecker, 1995). TSE education and screening programs can be set up in high schools and presented simultaneously with BSE and screening programs. Models can be used for practicing self-examination with lifelike lumps and abnormalities to teach young men what they should be looking for. Testicular examination and TSE education should be part of every routine physical examination for adolescent and young adult males. Instructions for self-examination of the testicles are given in **Box 32-1**.

Box 32-1 Testicular Self-Examination

- Self-examination should be done once a month after a warm bath or shower because heat relaxes the scrotum and loosens the skin, making the testes easier to examine.
- Visually inspect the scrotum for any swelling or changes in color.
- Examine each testicle with both hands by placing the index and middle fingers under the testicle with the thumbs placed on top. Roll the testicle gently between the fingers and thumbs, feeling for any changes such as lumps, swelling, or painful spots.
- The first sign of testicular cancer is usually a hard, painless lump about the size of a pea. However, if there are any kinds of changes or abnormalities, immediately notify your healthcare provider, because only he or she can make a positive diagnosis.

Sources: Adapted from Henkel, J. (1996, January/February). Testicular cancer: Survival high with early treatment. *FDA Consumer*. Retrieved from http://www.menweb.org/fdatesti.htm; Testicular cancer—What to look for. (1999, May 1). *American Family Physician, 59*(9), 2549–2550; Walbrecker, J. (1995, January). Start talking about testicular cancer. *RN*, pp. 34–35.

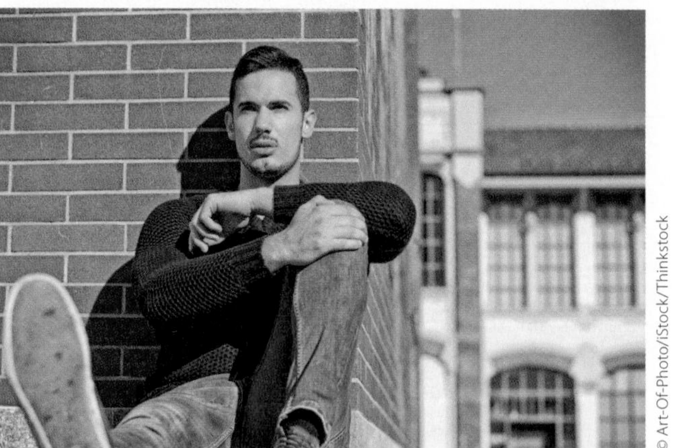

Young men are less likely than young women to practice preventive health care.

The only way a positive diagnosis of testicular cancer can be made is through surgical removal (orchiectomy) of the affected testicle for direct examination. Because testicular cancer occurs most often in men of reproductive age, **fertility** is a major concern. Although sperm count may be lowered, a unilateral orchiectomy usually does not affect sexual function or fertility (Brakey, 1994; Henkel, 1996; Walbrecker, 1995). However, abnormalities in the remaining testicle or the effects of radiation and chemotherapy may have adverse effects on sexual function and fertility (Brakey, 1994), although studies have shown that many men recover fertility within 2 to 3 years after chemotherapy (Bertuccio et al., 2007; Blekhman et al., 2008; Feldman et al., 2008; Henkel, 1996; Paduch, 2006; Pettersson, Richiardi, Nordenskjold, Kaijser, & Akre, 2007).

Erectile Dysfunction

Many sexual topics are now discussed openly, but **erectile dysfunction** (ED) is still a subject that causes fear and anxiety for many men and women. Although a significant amount of scientific data are available about erectile dysfunction (also called *impotence*), large segments of the public, including healthcare professionals, are still uninformed, or even worse, misinformed. A lack of accurate information, in addition to reluctance on the part of many healthcare providers to deal openly with sexual issues, has left many patients without a source of help for their sexual concerns. Improving both public and professional knowledge and attaining a comfort level in talking about erectile dysfunction will provide both men and their sexual partners with an avenue for obtaining needed information and effective treatment.

THINK ABOUT THIS 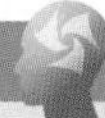

The Peyton family is football royalty. Archie Manning, the father, was a legendary quarterback at the University of Mississippi and with the New Orleans Saints. His middle son Peyton, an All Pro with the Indianapolis Colts and later quarterback for the Broncos, is one of the most popular and respected players in the game. Youngest son Eli led the New York Giants to victory in the 2008 and 2012 Super Bowls.

Cooper Manning the first son born to Archie and Olivia Manning in 1974. In the beginning, he was the most gifted athlete among Archie's sons—smart, witty, and fearless. His problems began in his sophomore year at Ole Miss, when he began dropping balls and experiencing numbness on his right side. He was eventually diagnosed at Baylor Medical center as having spinal stenosis, a congenital disorder. In 1993, Cooper underwent surgery on his spine and had to learn to walk again. He is now a stock trader for an energy investment company, but cannot do any kind of risky sports. He is married and has a daughter.

Source: Bradley, J. E. (November 10, 2003). The other brother. *Sports Illustrated,* 79–86.

ETHICAL CONNECTION 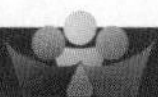

Should healthcare providers address men differently than women in their assessments of behaviors, such as the number of sex partners, risky behavior, and rate of seeking primary health care? Women go to healthcare providers much more frequently than men do; they also take more prescription medications over a lifetime than men do. How would this information affect your care of men as patients?

What Is Erectile Dysfunction?

Erectile dysfunction is the inability to achieve or maintain a penile erection sufficient for sexual intercourse. Approximately 18 million American men suffer from erectile dysfunction, and the incidence increases with age. Approximately 5% of men experience erectile dysfunction by the age of 40, increasing to between 15% and 25% by the age of 65 (National Kidney and Urologic Disease Information Clearinghouse, 2012). Sex researchers Masters and Johnson discovered that although sexual activity slows down with advancing age, it does not end. Most men and women between the ages of 50 and 60 are still interested in remaining sexually active.

Causes

Most cases of erectile dysfunction have a physical cause such as disease, injury, or drug side effects. Diabetes mellitus, kidney disease, multiple sclerosis, atherosclerosis, chronic alcoholism, hypertension, and vascular disease account for approximately 70% of all cases of erectile dysfunction. Of men with diabetes mellitus, 35% to 50% experience erectile dysfunction (Herbert et al., 2008; National Kidney and Urologic Diseases Information Clearinghouse, 2012). Various kinds of surgeries are also associated with increased incidence of erectile dysfunction. The most common are surgeries that can cause injury to nerves and arteries near the penis. These include surgeries for prostate, colon, rectal, and bladder cancers. Any type of vascular surgery can increase a man's risk for erectile dysfunction. Many common medications list erectile dysfunction as a side effect, including drugs used to treat hypertension, antihistamines, antidepressants, sedatives, tranquilizers, appetite suppressants, and pain medications. Smoking has also been shown to have an adverse effect on erectile function by increasing the effects of other risk factors such as vascular disease or hypertension. Vasectomy, however, has not been associated with increased risk for erectile dysfunction (Herbert et al., 2008).

In 10% to 20% of cases of erectile dysfunction, the cause is deemed to be psychological. Factors such as stress, anxiety, guilt, depression, low self-esteem, and fear of sexual failure can cause erectile dysfunction without the presence of any physical problems or can be secondary reactions to underlying physical causes (Herbert et al., 2008). Important facts that should be emphasized when counseling a man and his sexual partner about erectile dysfunction include the following:

- Most men experience erectile dysfunction related to stress or alcohol at some time in their lives.
- Past sexual practices, including masturbation, do not cause erectile dysfunction.
- Physical disorders can directly affect sexual functioning.
- An occasional problem with erectile dysfunction does not mean a chronic problem will develop.
- A man can sabotage his ability to have an erection by worrying about it.

RESEARCH ALERT

We have neglected a significant part of the population most in need of health care. We have been blind to the fact that when we visited clinics and worked with communities to address their health needs, there were few men in the waiting rooms of the clinics where primary health and prevention services were being provided. Virtually no health efforts were directed toward men. Poor men had become invisible and their health needs neglected. Poor men and men of color live with tremendous emotional and physical pain, are demeaned and devalued in a system that rewards wealth and values some people over others, and die early. Poor men are less likely to have health insurance, less likely to seek needed health service, and less likely to receive adequate care when they do. Even among the poor, some men are less than equal.

Those men of African descent demonstrate the great peril that poor men have to face (Treadwell & Ro, 2003). Life expectancy for African American men is 7.1 years shorter than that for men overall. African American men are 30% more likely to die from cardiovascular disease compared with non-Hispanic white men (Office of Minority Health, 2012). Death rates for HIV/AIDS are nearly five times higher for African American men than for white men (CDC, 2013a).

Society has no system in place to support the health and health-seeking behaviors of men who work at lower wage levels or who are unable to work because of poor education, absence of jobs, mismatch in skills, or other reasons. Men are so concerned about their daily survival—that is, caring for their families and having a good job—that they do not make health a priority. Working conditions of low-income men are frequently hazardous, and policies designed to protect these workers are often grossly inadequate. Most often, low-paid and low-skilled workers are not offered health insurance coverage through work. With the passing of the Affordable Care Act in 2010, men without insurance may purchase it at a reduced rate and coverage includes free preventive health based on age-appropriate interventions. Low-income men who are childless are excluded from publicly funded insurance programs (Barstow & Bergman, 2003; Hudak & Hagan, 2002; Miniclier, 2002; Parker, 2002; Roman & Carroll, 2003).

Sadly, the penal system is the only place where men have the right to health care, under the U.S. Constitution's protection against "cruel and unusual punishment." There are currently more than 1.5 million inmates in federal and state prisons, plus an additional 750,000 in local jails, and more than 637,000 are released during each year. Some 93% of U.S. inmates are male and 58% are people of color (Bureau of Justice Statistics, 2013).

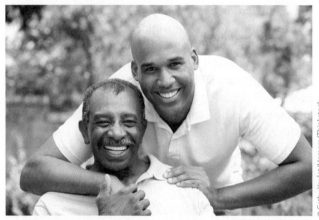

Men with at least two close relatives with prostate cancer have a very high risk of developing the disease before the age of 70. Men with a family history of prostate cancer should have PSA screening and prostate examinations between the ages of 50 and 70.

Treatment

Treatment varies according to the severity and cause of the dysfunction. Healthcare providers start with the least invasive treatment and progress to more invasive treatments until erectile dysfunction is corrected. Reducing the dosage or eliminating drugs that may be causing erectile dysfunction is the first step. Psychotherapy and behavior modifications are next. Vacuum devices, oral drugs, drugs injected into the urethra, and finally surgically implanted penile devices or vascular surgery are offered as treatment if the problem persists (National Kidney and Urologic Disease Information Clearinghouse, 2012).

In 1998, a new "wonder drug" called *sildenafil citrate* (commonly known by its trade name, Viagra) was approved by the FDA. Viagra is taken 1 hour before sexual intercourse and works by boosting the effects of nitric oxide, a chemical produced by the body to relax smooth muscle in the penis and allow increased blood flow during sexual stimulation. This drug does not trigger automatic erection as other drugs used to treat erectile dysfunction do, but rather just allows the man to respond to sexual stimulation (National Kidney and Urologic Disease Information Clearinghouse, 2012). The drug is very successful in treating many forms of erectile dysfunction, although some fear the drug may be overused by middle-aged and older men who may not actually suffer from erectile dysfunction but just want to "boost" their sex lives.

THINK ABOUT THIS 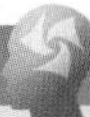

Men experience notable midlife physical changes. After age 40, testosterone decreases; muscle mass loss, cognition problems, and osteoporosis risk increase. Lower testosterone levels are known to increase a man's prostate cancer risk.

RESEARCH ALERT 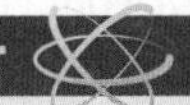

Socialization of men into the masculine role influences their health-related beliefs, attitudes, perceptions, and risk-taking behavior. Yet, traditionally men's health has been primarily defined in terms suggesting that biological factors, such as hormones, are the main determinants of morbidity and mortality. Men's health must be viewed within the broader context of family health. Across the population, the main differences in mortality and morbidity are related to variations in exposure to risk factors. Men stress the importance of being fit, strong, energetic, physically active, and in control, whereas women stress not being ill and not needing to see a doctor. Men see their body as a machine and view exercise as more important than nutrition and rest, whereas women place more emphasis on nutrition, rest, and relaxation and less emphasis on exercise.

Men are not encouraged to express their feelings, such as pain and other symptoms of illness. Instead, men often mask their feelings by engaging in aggressive and risk-taking behaviors, which can expose them to illness, injury, or death.

STD incidence is higher in men, especially among the 25- to 34-year-old age group, because men in this age cohort tend to have more sexual partners than women of the corresponding age do.

Male infertility appears to be on the increase, possibly due to environmental factors and chemicals that increase risk of testicular disease and affect sperm production.

What can nurses do to correct this imbalance? Here are some practical steps:

- Establish men's health-awareness-raising groups, and involve women in seeking a solution to the problem.
- Educate nurses and others on risk-reduction strategies, and help men ventilate their feelings in a healthy way.
- Teach men testicular self-examination.
- Organize campaigns to increase men's contact with health services.
- Identify and focus interventions on high-risk groups such as young men; poor men; men of color; single, divorced, and widowed men with chronic disease; and men who abuse substances.
- Promote safer sex practices.
- Promote regular screening for rectal, prostate, and other cancers.

Source: Lloyd, R. (1996). Men's health review. Men's Health Forum, London Royal College of Nursing.

Role of the Community Health Nurse

The most important things the community health nurse can do for men with erectile dysfunction are to provide accurate and easily understandable information and to encourage the man and his sex partner to talk openly and comfortably about the problem. Including the man's sex partner in the discussion acknowledges his or her importance in the relationship. The partner may also have questions, doubts, and insecurities that need to be addressed. Many persons whose partners are impotent blame themselves for the problem. The partner may also feel hurt and angry because the male has withdrawn physically and emotionally. Understanding that he or she is not to blame can go a long way in enabling the partner to support the diagnosis and treatment. It is important for nurses to be sensitive to the needs of patients whose values or sexual orientation may be different from their own. Whatever the relationship of the partners, all couples should be treated with dignity and respect.

Cardiovascular Disease

Cardiovascular disease is the single greatest cause of death in men. Approximately one in three male deaths is related to cardiovascular disease. Similarly, more than one-third of men dying between the ages of 45 and 65 die of a heart attack. Cardiovascular disease is caused by the accumulation of fatty deposits within the artery wall that causes stiffness and reduced blood flow. When the brain interprets reduced blood flow as low blood pressure, it sends a signal to the heart to compensate. The heart works faster with less rest and increases the pressure on each contraction. Although there are many explanations for higher cardiovascular disease rates among men than women, research points to two major factors:

1. Men's diets have higher ratios of saturated to polyunsaturated fat, which contributes to cardiovascular disease (Power & Schulkin, 2008).
2. Men's sociocultural environments lead to higher levels of stress, which contributes to cardiovascular disease (Hall, 2007; Williams, 2008).

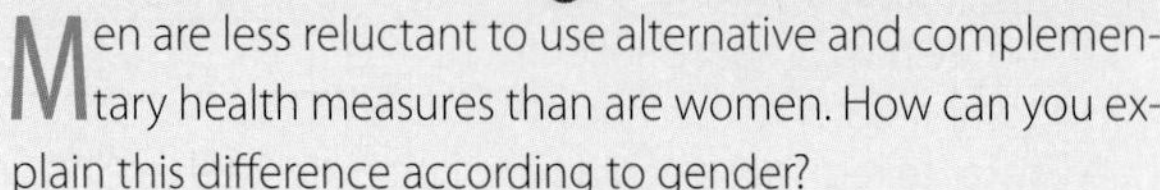

Men are less reluctant to use alternative and complementary health measures than are women. How can you explain this difference according to gender?

Cardiovascular disease and hypertension can often be prevented by changes in behavior, including stopping smoking, increasing activity, and improving diet. Community health nurses can design educational programs that target men to promote behavior changes that reduce the risk of cardiovascular disease (Barnett et al., 2001; Gregory, Blanck, Gillespie, Maynard, & Serdula, 2008; Woloshin, Schwartz, & Welch, 2008). These recommendations may include the following:

- Losing weight
- Reducing salt intake
- Smoking cessation
- Eating foods rich in natural sources of fiber and antioxidant vitamins
- Exercising
- Relaxing

In addition, consumption of moderate amounts of alcohol and sexual activity are associated with reduced risks of cardiovascular disease.

Selected At-Risk Populations

Men with HIV/AIDS

According to the CDC, by 1994 HIV/AIDS had become a leading cause of death in the United States for men between the ages of 25 and 44. With the introduction of new medications in recent years, HIV/AIDS-related death rates have steadily declined, but the incidence of new HIV/AIDS cases continues to rise. HIV/AIDS has historically been viewed in the United States as a disease targeting a specific population—homosexual men. Although the initial cases in the United States, Canada, Australia, and Western Europe were found among this population, this was not the case for the rest of the world. After three decades of the pandemic, many still view HIV/AIDS as something that will not affect them (Stoltenberg et al., 2008). As a result of this apathy, the safer sexual practices adopted in the homosexual communities have not been applied as readily in heterosexual communities. High-risk behaviors, such as alcohol and drug use and unprotected sex with numerous partners, continue to put heterosexual men at risk (Williams, 2008). Heterosexual transmission rates continue to escalate, especially in the African American and Hispanic communities as well as in urban poor populations regardless of race (CDC, 2013b).

The introduction of new medications has reduced the number of HIV/AIDS-related deaths, which means persons with HIV/AIDS are living longer. HIV/AIDS, when appropriately treated, is now considered more of a chronic illness. What does this mean to younger men? An entire generation of sexually active men has never known of a world without HIV or AIDS. To some, this may be interpreted as, "Why bother to protect myself, because I can always take the medications." Some are applying safer sexual practices haphazardly, thus allowing the introduction of drug-resistant strains of HIV into their bodies. To others, especially an alarming number of young homosexual men, the principle of "I'd rather die young and beautiful" applies. Intervention and prevention programs must address these issues and concerns. The community health nurse's best option would include the education of young men who would act as role models for their peers.

RESEARCH ALERT

This research study explored young men's perceptions of and participation in hip hop culture—urban social and artistic expressions, such as clothing style, breakdancing, graffiti, and rap music—and how contextual factors of the hip hop scene may be associated with their condom use, condom-use self-efficacy, and sense of community. A cross-sectional survey design was conducted of 95 African American and Latino men age 15 to 25 years as part of a 4-year ethnographic study in New York City. Results indicated that differences in young men's perceptions of and levels of affiliation with hip hop culture were not statistically associated with differences in their sense of community or condom-use self-efficacy. Frequency of participation in the hip hop nightclub scene was the strongest factor negatively associated with condom use. The researchers concluded that popular discourses on young men's health risks often blame youths' cultures such as the hip hop culture for increased risk practices but do not critically examine how risk emerges in urban young men's lives and what aspects of youths' culture can be protective. Further research needs to focus on contextual factors of risk such as the role of hip hop nightlife on increased HIV risk.

Source: Muñoz-Laboy, M., Castellanos, D., Haliburton, C., Del Aguila, E., Weinstein, H., & Parker, R. (2008). Condom use and hip hop culture: The case of urban young men in New York City. *American Journal of Public Health, 98*(6), 1081–1085.

APPLICATION TO PRACTICE

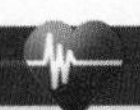

You are a nurse working in a community clinic. One of your patients is Rick Fernandez, a 34-year-old married man who complains about fever and swollen glands. Fearing the possibility of HIV/AIDS, you ask Rick the typical textbook questions to assess his HIV/AIDS risk behaviors: You ask if he uses intravenous drugs, if he has had any blood transfusions, if he has sex with men, and if he is homosexual. He responds with a no to all questions. Based on his replies, you do not pursue HIV/AIDS testing. When he comes back a few months later with complaints of recurrent skin lesions, you again ask about his HIV/AIDS risk behaviors and receive the same answers as before. Rick insists that he is a happily married man in a monogamous relationship and does not use any sort of drugs. Rick seems offended by your questions. You approach the physician and ask if he has considered testing Rick for HIV/AIDS. The physician has assessed the risk behaviors and concluded that Rick does not have any of the risk factors associated with HIV/AIDS. When Rick returns to the clinic for a third visit, you are more assertive and convince Rick to have an HIV test. The test comes back positive. Rick reveals to the HIV/AIDS counselor that he had been imprisoned a while back and that his only potential exposure to HIV/AIDS might have been through another inmate who raped him.

1. What is your reaction to Rick's situation?
2. Do you feel that your personal beliefs and values influenced your reaction?
3. Why do you think Rick did not disclose the key information earlier?
4. What could you have done to obtain the accurate information?
5. What specific questions could you have asked Rick to obtain this information?

What does the increase in HIV/AIDS cases within the African American and Hispanic communities mean to the community health nurse? Intervention and prevention programs need to specifically target these communities. The church is an institution generally accepted as having a powerful influence within both of these communities. By securing the commitment from religious leaders and their congregations, the community health nurse can create positive change from within the system. Developing role models and implementing prevention programs that include members of the community results in much more effective outcomes.

For example, the community health nurse working within a community often develops a relationship with community members. Once a trusting relationship has been established, the nurse can approach some of the unofficial leaders within the community to enlist their support and discuss strategies and objectives to decrease the epidemic of infection affecting the population. This needs to be done in a nonjudgmental manner, in which the nurse details the problems and possible solutions without passing blame or creating fear. By enlisting the members' support in the initial stages, the nurse can formulate plans and develop goals that are perceived as important to the community, thus securing support for the intervention.

Homosexual Men and Families

The special needs of homosexual men include more than just HIV/AIDS education. Homosexual men and their families exist in virtually every community, regardless of how restrictive or liberal the community proclaims to be. However, societal stigmatization of homosexuality forces many to remain "in the closet." Homosexual myths and stereotypes abound, particularly in cultures that value male dominance or masculinity. Homosexual men and their sexual practices run the entire spectrum, just as in the heterosexual community. Also, homosexual men may be married or have children, live alone or with a partner. Individuals define who makes up their family group, not nurses or official definitions.

MEDIA MOMENT

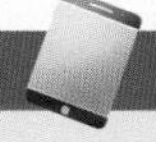

Age Proofing—My Way

David Cartwright

What does a man do when the "medical system" takes over his life? Go on a bicycle trip across the country!

Why would a man over the age of 60 ride a bicycle half way across the country? I have no idea; I had never done anything like this before. Maybe we ride because we're mad—we want to do the wild thing. For men of a certain age, it is called the *Ulysses Factor.*

How else can one explain chafing your backside, battling heat and thirst, living with numbness in your feet and hands—and being literally scared to death at the mercy of those on four wheels who claim to "share" the road with you. There is certainly no money in it for most of us, in this boot camp approach to wellbeing. In this complex world, I can barely manage myself. The simple life of an adventure cyclist is a wonderful tonic. It's a fine thing, to do—a kind of age proofing. I get outdoors. It keeps me in good physical shape. For me, it helps me keep

(continues)

MEDIA MOMENT (*continued*)

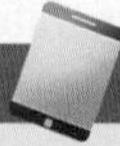

a good mental attitude and have the time to reflect on the meaning of life.

I am no romantic cycling bum but I talked myself into this last long trip. I kept it a secret. Why? Because there is always somebody who will find something wrong with what you are doing or about to do.

The germ of the idea began when I saw myself as a growing victim of the medical system, mentally, physically, and emotionally—undergoing surgeries, popping pills, and receiving reassurance with recommendations for more treatments—in short I was rapidly becoming a crock. Somehow I had to break the chains and regain control. I did it by hopping on a bicycle, laden with tent and sleeping bag, waving goodbye to my loved ones—for a test of my survival skills. For a nonthinker, I even did some planning—such as how far, best routes, what to take, when to go, and whom to avoid. And I just did it.

1,700 miles later, I am back to my old life, back to work. But I am ready to do it again. The best thing about my trip was the hospitality I found on my trip and the people I met. I'm a new man now with an extraordinary sense of freedom and energy, looking forward to the weekends for those short rides and forever planning the next really long one. You know the one that keeps me age-proofed.

Although there is little research on violence between male homosexuals, early reports indicate that abusive behavior in these relationships is significant (Harrison & Beck, 2002). The experience of both verbal and physical abuse among homosexual men appears to differ little from intimate partner violence rates reported for heterosexual women (Blosnich & Bossarte, 2009; Stephenson, Sato, & Finneran, 2013).

The community health nurse's role in interactions with any group of men is inclusion instead of exclusion. Nurses should ask questions in such a manner that the man does not feel obligated to give an answer he believes the nurse expects. When using such items as risk assessments, questions should be phrased in a general manner. For example, the nurse should ask about "the number of sexual partners" instead of "the number of female sex partners." Nurses should maintain a nonjudgmental tone and manner throughout all interactions. Just as in any interaction, including the entire family whenever possible is recommended. By developing a trusting and honest relationship, the nurse can be instrumental in generating assistance and implementing change of unsafe or risky behaviors (Kaufman & Gregory, 2007).

MEDIA MOMENT

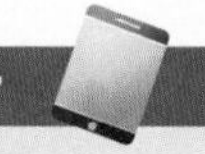

My Life (1993)

Bob (Michael Keaton) and Gail (Nicole Kidman) Jones are expecting their first child, but Bob has been diagnosed with kidney cancer, which may take his life before his child is born. Heartbroken at the prospect of not ever getting to know his child, he decides to make a video about himself and his life so that his child will know him.

TABLE 32-2 Life Expectancy at Birth

	2011*	1970**	1950**	1920**
Classification	**Life Expectancy**			
Population	78.7	70.8	68.2	54.1
All females	81.1	74.7	71.1	54.6
All males	76.3	67.1	65.6	53.6
White females	81.3	75.6	72.2	55.6
Black females	78.2	68.3	62.9***	45.2***
White males	76.6	68.0	66.5	54.4
Black males	72.1	60.0	59.1***	45.5***

*Data from Hoyert, D. L. & Xu, J. (2012). Deaths: Preliminary data for 2011. *National Vital Statistics Reports, 61*(6), 1–52.

**Anderson, R. N. (2001). United States life tables, 1998. *National Vital Statistics Reports, 48*(18), 33–34.

***Prior to 1970, data for the black population are not available; data shown prior to 1970 are for the nonwhite population.

Community Health Nursing Roles

The community health nurse assumes a wide range of duties and responsibilities while providing health care to men. A typical week could include hundreds of miles traveled, diverse teaching methods and strategies, and numerous new encounters. Community health nursing roles may include patient advocate, educator, and facilitator.

Patient Advocate

As a patient advocate, the role of the community health nurse includes interfacing with healthcare providers and healthcare agencies to support the best care for the patient. For instance, a nurse realizes that a recently diagnosed HIV-positive man has been prescribed zidovudine (AZT) alone, rather than the more effective cocktail combination medications and latest research-based interventions. A proper assessment must be made to determine whether alternative medications should be prescribed. With the permission of the patient, the nurse can contact the appropriate healthcare provider and discuss the patient's options with a nonthreatening and nonjudgmental stance to allow for future interactions. Any new information must be shared with the patient.

Educator

The role of a health educator for men can often be challenging. Education can occur in any setting from the stockyards to the corporate boardroom. Safety issues, violence, diet, sexual relationships, stress, and physical exercise are examples of topics that may be addressed. The community health nurse must customize education efforts to the specific needs of the patient population. The first step involves a correct assessment of the educational needs of the individuals. The nurse determines the level of the learners to ensure that the level of the educational program is neither too low nor too high for the specific group. Providing educational programs for men in their own environments requires versatility, flexibility, and consideration of cultural issues.

Facilitator

The community health nurse as facilitator brings various people and groups together to talk about issues and needs. The most significant facilitator role involves helping people and groups with different views to reach a compromise so that they can find a common ground to solve problems and bring about positive changes to alleviate a specific community health issue. For instance, a community health nurse, as the facilitator, may initiate positive change through programs with specific targeted groups such as adolescent boys. This can be accomplished by teaching safer sexual practices to prevent STDs and teenage pregnancies by bringing together parents, school administrators, politicians, healthcare providers, and teens.

Men's Health Research Issues

Despite the advances in medical technology and research, men continue to live an average of 5 years less than women. Although most medical research was historically based on men, men's health issues no longer dominate the research agenda because of recent federal mandates. Research on men's health must focus on the areas where prevention, early detection, and treatment efforts will significantly improve the quality of life of men across the lifespan. Men's health should be considered a specialty, including clinics and programs especially designed for men.

In addition, research studies must be more inclusive and utilize subjects that represent the diversity within the male population. Studies need to report findings based not only on middle-aged, middle class, Caucasian males, but also on other males representing various ethnic and socioeconomic groups.

Historically, most research studies have been based on male subjects. In many Western cultures, years of a predominantly male workforce have resulted in healthcare systems and policies being established by men. Despite this dominance of men in healthcare systems, women still have longer life expectancies than men.

NOTE THIS!

Men who smoke a pack of cigarettes or more per day are nearly 40% more likely to have erectile dysfunction compared to nonsmokers.

Conclusion

Men's health care is not easily defined as a single issue with a limited focus or target population. Although men constitute half the population, their needs and health system utilization vary greatly from those of women. Men's health has failed to be recognized as a specialty, and the declining health of men in the United States may be a result of this lack of specialization. Issues faced by men must be addressed to improve their overall health and decrease the variance in life expectancy between men and women.

The community health nurse can be instrumental in securing access to and promoting the utilization of health care by men. Health promotion and screening programs can be implemented with specifically targeted groups of men. The community health nurse also assumes the roles of patient advocate, educator, and facilitator to secure the most advantageous outcomes for the improvement of men's health.

AFFORDABLE CARE ACT

Good News

Like many Americans, men have much to gain from the Affordable Care Act. The healthcare law includes a variety of benefits that can help men of all ages lead longer and healthier lives. Under the Affordable Care Act, many young men can benefit by being able to stay on their parent's health insurance until they turn 26 years old. For insured middle-aged and older men, the Affordable Care Act requires most private insurance plans to cover—without a copay or deductible—preventive services such as screenings for blood pressure, cholesterol,[1] colorectal cancer,[2] depression, HIV,[3] obesity,[4] and type 2 diabetes.[5] Again, these preventive services are at no cost for many consumers who have insurance.[6]

Preventive Health Services for Adults

Most ACA health plans must cover a set of preventive services such as shots and screening tests at no cost to the patient. This includes ACA Marketplace private insurance plans.

Free Preventive Services

All Marketplace plans and many other plans must cover the following list of preventive services without charging you a copayment or coinsurance (This is true even if you haven't met your yearly deductible. This applies only when these services are delivered by a network provider.):

- Abdominal aortic aneurysm one-time screening for men of specified ages who have ever smoked
- Alcohol misuse screening and counseling
- Aspirin use to prevent cardiovascular disease for men and women of certain ages
- Blood pressure screening for all adults
- Cholesterol screening for adults of certain ages or at higher risk
- Colorectal cancer screening for adults over 50
- Depression screening for adults
- Diabetes (type 2) screening for adults with high blood pressure
- Diet counseling for adults at higher risk for chronic disease
- HIV screening for everyone ages 15 to 65, and other ages at increased risk
- Immunization vaccines for adults—doses, recommended ages, and recommended populations vary:
    - Hepatitis A
    - Hepatitis B
    - Herpes zoster
    - Human papillomavirus
    - Influenza (flu shot)
    - Measles, mumps, rubella
    - Meningococcal
    - Pneumococcal
    - Tetanus, diphtheria, pertussis
    - Varicella
- Obesity screening and counseling for all adults
- Sexually Transmitted Infection (STI) prevention counseling for adults at higher risk
- Syphilis screening for all adults at higher risk
- Tobacco Use screening for all adults and cessation interventions for tobacco users

Please visit http://www.healthcare.gov to learn more about the Affordable Care Act and your healthcare coverage options in your state.

[1] Cholesterol screening for adults of certain ages or at higher risk.
[2] Colorectal cancer screening for adults over 50.
[3] HIV screening for adults at higher risk.
[4] Obesity screening and counseling for all adults.
[5] Type 2 diabetes screenings for adults with high blood pressure.
[6] Check with your insurance provider to find out if these and other preventive services are included in your plan.

LEVELS OF PREVENTION

Primary: Presenting a community talk on the preventive services required by the Affordable Care Act for men

Secondary: Screening for hypertension in a men's prayer group at a local church

Tertiary: Assisting a man after prostate surgery with mobility issues

Critical Thinking Activities

1. Smoking is a behavior issue that plays an important role in the reduction of the length and quality of life of men. As a community health nurse, which programs would you develop to improve this situation? Which groups would you specifically target? How would you most effectively implement your plans?
2. Based on the information provided regarding men's utilization of preventive health care, what would be the most effective intervention(s) to ensure participation? Where should the intervention(s) be implemented? How would the intervention(s) be modified to address differences in age, religion, education, or socioeconomic status?

HEALTHY ME

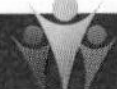

Do you set health goals for yourself? How do men differ from women in their experiences in and frequency of use of the healthcare system?

References

American Foundation for Suicide Prevention. (2014). *Facts and figures: Suicide deaths*. Retrieved from http://www.afsp.org/understanding-suicide/facts-and-figures

American Urological Association (AUA). (2013). *Early detection of prostate cancer: AUA guideline*. Retrieved from http://www.auanet.org/education/guidelines/prostate-cancer-detection.cfm

Anderson, R. N. (2002). Deaths: Leading causes for 2000. *National Vital Statistics Report 2002, 50*(16), 1–85.

Barnett, E., Casper, M. L., Halverson, J. A., et al. (2001, June). *Men and heart disease: An atlas of racial and ethnic disparities in mortality*. Morgantown, WV: West Virginia University, Office for Social Environment and Health Research.

Barstow, D., & Bergman, L. (2003). At a tax foundry, an indifference to life. *New York Times*, January 8, p. A1.

Bertuccio, P., Malvezzi, M., Chatenoud, L., Bosetti, C., Negri, E., Levi, F., & La Vecchia, C. (2007). Testicular cancer mortality in the Americas, 1980–2003. *Cancer (0008543X), 109*(4), 776–779.

Black, M., & Breiding, M. (2008). Adverse health conditions and health risk behaviors associated with intimate partner violence—United States, 2005. *Journal of the American Medical Association, 300*(6), 646–649

Blekhman, R., Man, O., Herrmann, L., Boyko, A., Indap, A., Kosiol, C., … Przeworski, M. (2008). Natural selection on genes that underlie human disease susceptibility. *Current Biology, 18*(12), 883–889.

Blosnich, J. R., & Bossarte, R. M. (2009). Comparisons of intimate partner violence among partners in same-sex and opposite-sex relationships in the United States. *American Journal of Public Health, 99*(12), 2182–2184.

Brakey, M. R. (1994, September). Myths and facts … About testicular cancer. *Nursing, 24*.

Brock, D., Fox, S., Gosling, G., Haney, L., Kneebone, P., Nagy, C., & Qualitza, B. (1993). Testicular cancer. *Seminars in Oncology Nursing, 9*(4), 224–236.

Bureau of Justice Statistics. (2013). Total U.S. correctional population declined in 2012 for fourth year (press release). Retrieved from http://www.bjs.gov/content/pub/press/cpus12pr.cfm

Carr, J., & VanDeusen, K. M. (2004). Risk factors for male sexual aggression on college campuses. *Journal of Family Violence, 19*(5), 279–290.

Centers for Disease Control and Prevention (CDC). (2012). Surveillance for violent deaths—National Violent Death Reporting System, 16 states, 2009. *Morbidity and Mortality Weekly Report, 61*(ss06), 1–43.

Centers for Disease Control and Prevention (CDC). (2013a). QuickStats: Human immunodeficiency virus (HIV) disease death rates among men aged 25–54 years, by race and age group —National Vital Statistics System, United States, 2000–2010. *Morbidity and Mortality Weekly Report, 62*(03), 58.

Centers for Disease Control and Prevention (CDC). (2013b). HIV infection among heterosexuals at increased risk—United States, 2010. *Morbidity and Mortality Weekly Report, 62*(10), 183–188.

Charles, N., & Walters, V. (2008). "Men are leavers alone and women are worriers": Gender differences in discourses of health. *Health, Risk & Society, 10*(2), 117–132.

Cheung, W., Demers, A., Hossain, D., Owen, T., Ahmed, S., & Czaykowski, P. (2007). Appropriateness of testicular cancer management: A population-based cohort study. *The Canadian Journal of Urology, 14*(3), 3542–3550.

Clark, M. J. (1999). *Nursing in the community* (3rd ed.). Stamford, CT: Appleton & Lange.

Clemmons, A. K. (2008). Bucs punter had cancer scare as rookie. *ESPN Page2*. Retrieved from http://sports.espn.go.com/espn/page2/story?page=clemmons/081205&sportCat=nfl

Clore, E. R. (1993). A guide for the testicular self-examination. *Journal of Pediatric Health Care, 7*(6), 264–268.

Coakley, E. H., Rimm, E. B., Colditz, G., Kawachi, I., & Willet, W. (1998). Predictors of weight change in men: Results from the Health Professionals Follow-Up Study. *International Journal of Obesity, 22*, 89–96.

Cook, N. (2000). Testicular cancer: Testicular self-examination and screening. *British Journal of Nursing, 9*(6), 338–343.

Courtenay, W. H. (2000a). Behavioral factors associated with disease, injury, and death among men: Evidence and implications for prevention. *Journal of Men's Studies, 9*(1), 81–142.

Courtenay, W. H. (2000b). Constructions of masculinity and their influence on men's well-being: A theory of gender and health. *Social Sciences Medicine, 50*(10), 1385–1401.

Courtenay, W. H. (2000c). Engendering health: A social constructionist examination of men's health beliefs and behaviors. *Psychology of Men & Masculinity, 1*(1).

Courtenay, W. H. (2001). Men's health: Ethnicity matters. *Social Work Today, 1*(8), 20–22.

Delsohn, S. (1996). *The fire inside: Firefighters talk about their lives.* New York, NY: HarperCollins.

Dutta, M., & Boyd, J. (2007). Turning smoking man images around: Portrayals of smoking in men's magazines as a blueprint for smoking cessation campaigns. *Health Communication, 22*(3), 253–263.

Fackelmann, K. (1998). An enzymatic sex difference. *Science News, 153*(13), 204.

Feldman, D., Bosl, G., Sheinfeld, J., & Motzer, R. (2008). Medical treatment of advanced testicular cancer. *Journal of the American Medical Association, 299*(6), 672–684.

Femquist, R. M. (2001). Education, race/ethnicity, age, sex, and suicide: Individual-level data in the United States. *Current Research in Social Psychology, 3*, 277–290.

Feuer, E. J., & Merrill, R. M. (1999). Cancer surveillance series: Interpreting trends in prostate cancer—Part II: Cause of death misclassification and the recent rise and fall in prostate cancer mortality. *Journal of the National Cancer Institute, 91*(12), 1025–1032.

Galdas, P. M., Cheater, F., & Marshall, P. (2005). Men and health help-seeking behaviour: Literature review. *Journal of Advanced Nursing, 49*(6), 616–623.

Gefou-Madianou, D. (Ed.). (1992). *Alcohol, gender, and culture.* London & New York: Routledge.

Gelfand, D. E., Parzuchowski, J., Cort, M., & Powell, I. (1995). Digital rectal examinations and prostate cancer screening: Attitudes of African American men. *Oncology Nursing Forum, 22*, 1253–1255.

Glassner, B. (1992). Men and muscles. In M. Kimmel & M. Messner (Eds.), *Men's lives* (2nd ed.). New York/Toronto: Macmillan/Maxwell.

Goldstein, S., Chesir-Teran, D., & McFaul, A. (2008). Profiles and correlates of relational aggression in young adults' romantic relationships. *Journal of Youth & Adolescence, 37*(3), 251–265.

Gough, B., & Edwards, G. (1998). The beer talking: Four lads, a carry out and the reproduction of masculinities. *Sociological Review, 46*(3), 409–435.

Graves, K. L. (1995). Risky sexual behavior and alcohol use among young adults: Results from a national survey. *American Journal of Health Promotion, 10*(1), 27–36.

Gregory, C., Blanck, H., Gillespie, C., Maynard, L., & Serdula, M. (2008). Perceived health risk of excess body weight among overweight and obese men and women: Differences by sex. *Preventive Medicine, 47*(1), 46–52.

Hall, R. (2007). Racism as health risk for African-American males: Correlations between hypertension and skin color. *Journal of African American Studies, 11*(3/4), 204–213.

Harrison, P. M., & Beck, A. J. (2002). *Prisoners in 2001.* Washington, DC: U.S. Department of Justice, Bureau of Justice Statistics.

Harrisson, J., Chin, J., & Ficarotto, T. (1992). Warning: Masculinity may be dangerous to your health. In M. Kimmel & M. Messner (Eds.), *Men's lives* (2nd ed.). New York/Toronto: Macmillan/Maxwell.

Hauser, R., & Sokol, R. (2008). Science linking environmental contaminant exposures with fertility and reproductive health impacts in the adult male. *Fertility & Sterility, 89*(2), e59–e65.

Hede, K. (2007). Lung cancer may be different for men and women, but researchers ponder what to do. *Journal of the National Cancer Institute, 99*(24), 1830–1832.

Henkel, J. (1996, January/February). Testicular cancer: Survival high with early treatment. *FDA Consumer.* Retrieved from http://www.menweb.org/fdatesti.htm

Herbert, K., Lopez, B., Castellano, J., Palacio, A., Tamari, L., & Arcemen, L. (2008). The prevalence of erectile dysfunction in heart failure patients by race and ethnicity. *International Journal of Impotence Research, 20*(5), 507–511.

Hudak, S., & Hagan, J. F. (2002). Asbestos: The lethal legacy, families of workers blame deaths on plants' use of asbestos. *Plain Dealer* (Cleveland, OH), November 4, p. A1.

Isenhart, C. E., & Silversmith, D. J. (1994). The influence of the traditional male role on alcohol abuse and the therapeutic process. *Journal of Men's Studies, 3*(2), 127–135.

Kaufman, K., & Gregory, W. (2007). Discriminators of complementary and alternative medicine provider use among men with HIV/AIDS. *American Journal of Health Behavior, 31*(6), 591–601.

Kinkade, S. (1999, May 1). Testicular cancer. *American Family Physician, 59*(9), 2539–2544.

Koshti-Richman, A. (1996). The role of nurses in promoting testicular self-examination. *Nursing Times, 92*(33), 40–41.

McNaughton-Collins, M. F., & Barry, M. J. (2011). One man at a time—resolving the PSA controversy. *New England Journal of Medicine, 365*, 1951–1953.

Men's Health Network. (2008). *Men's health network.* Retrieved from http://www.menshealthnetwork.org

Miniclier, K. (2002). Coal miners dig for pay, perks: Workers at Rangeley site brush aside issue of danger. *Denver Post,* August 25, p. B01.

National Center for Health Statistics. (2002). *Health, United States, 2002, with chartbook on trends in the health of Americans.* Hyattsville, MD: Department of Health and Human Services.

National Institutes of Health (NIH). (2014). Research portfolio online reporting tools: Estimates of funding for research, condition, and disease categories (RCDC). Retrieved from http://report.nih.gov/categorical_spending.aspx

National Kidney and Urologic Disease Information Clearinghouse. (2012). *Erectile dysfunction.* Retrieved from http://kidney.niddk.nih.gov/kudiseases/pubs/ED/

Nelson, D. E., Tomar, S. L., Mowery, P., & Siegel, P. Z. (1996). Trends in smokeless tobacco use among men in four states, 1988 through 1993. *American Journal of Public Health, 86*(9), 1300–1303.

New York State Office for the Prevention of Domestic Violence. (2011). *National data on intimate partner violence.* Retrieved from http://www.opdv.ny.gov/statistics/nationaldvdata/

Nguyen, M. N., Otis, J., & Potvin, L. (1996). Determinants of intention to adopt a low-fat diet in men 30 to 60 years old: Implications for heart health promotion. *American Journal of Health Promotion, 10*(3), 201–207.

Office of Minority Health. (2012). *Heart disease and African Americans.* Retrieved from http://minorityhealth.hhs.gov/templates/content.aspx

Paduch, D. (2006). Testicular cancer and male infertility. *Current Opinion in Urology, 16*(6), 419–427.

Parker, D. (2002). Hazardous job workers learn to live with fear. *Corpus Christi Caller-Times,* August 11, p. H1.

Parker-Pope, T. (2008). Cancer funding: Does it add up? *The New York Times* (blog). Retrieved from http://well.blogs.nytimes.com/2008/03/06/cancer-funding-does-it-add-up/

Pattison, A. (1998). *The M factor: Men and their health.* East Roseville, NSW: Simon & Schuster.

Pease, B. (1997). Masculinity and health: The emotional and physical costs of dominance. In B. Pease (Ed.), *Men and sexual politics: Towards a profeminist practice.* Adelaide: Dulwich Centre Publications.

Peate, I. (1997). Clinical. Testicular cancer. The importance of effective health education. *British Journal of Nursing, 6*(6), 311–316.

Pettersson, A., Richiardi, L., Nordenskjold, A., Kaijser, M., & Akre, O. (2007). Age at surgery for undescended testis and risk of testicular cancer. *New England Journal of Medicine, 356*(18), 1835–1841.

Pinkhasov, R. M., Wong, J., Kashanian, J., Lee, M., Samadi, D. B., Pinkhasov, M. M., & Shabsigh, R. (2010). Are men shortchanged on health? Perspective on health care utilization and health risk behavior in men and women in the United States. *International Journal of Clinical Practice, 64*(4), 475–487.

Pinto, F., Sacco, E., Volpe, A., Gardi, M., Totaro, A., Calarco, A., … Bassi, P. F. (2010). Doping and urologic tumors [Italian]. *Urologia, 77*(2), 92–99.

Poppius, E., Virkkunen, H., Hakama, M., & Tenkanen, L. (2008). The sense of coherence and risk of injuries: Role of alcohol consumption and occupation. *Journal of Epidemiology & Community Health, 62*(1), 35–41.

Power, M., & Schulkin, J. (2008). Sex differences in fat storage, fat metabolism, and the health risks from obesity: Possible evolutionary origins. *The British Journal of Nutrition, 99*(5), 931–940.

Roman, S., & Carroll, S. (2003). Migrant farmworkers live their lives in shadows. *Sarasota Herald-Tribune,* January 16, p. A1.

Rovito, M. J., Gordon, T. F., Bass, S. B., & Ducette, J. (2011). Perceptions of testicular cancer and testicular self-examination among college men: A report on intention, vulnerability, and promotional material preferences. *American Journal of Men's Health, 5*(6), 500–507.

Rynerson, B. C., & Fishel, A. H. (1998). Expressions of men who batter: Implications for nursing. *Journal of the American Psychiatric Nurses Association, 4*(2), 41–47.

Sabo, D., & Gordon, D. F. (1995). Rethinking men's health and illness. In D. Sabo & D. F. Gordon (Eds.), *Men's health and illness: Gender, power, and the body* (p. 21). London: Sage.

Steenbergh, T., Whelan, J., Meyers, A., Klesges, R., & DeBon, M. (2008). Gambling and health risk-taking behavior in a military sample. *Military Medicine, 173*(5), 452–459.

Stephenson, R., Sato, K. N., & Finneran, C. (2013). Dyadic, partner, and social network influences on intimate partner violence among male-male couples. *Western Journal of Emergency Medicine, 14*(4), 316–323.

Stillion, J. (1995). Premature death among males. In D. Sabo & D. F. Gordon (Eds.), *Men's health and illness: Gender, power, and the body* (pp. 47–67). London, England: Sage.

Stoltenberg, S., Batien, B., & Birgenheir, D. (2008). Does gender moderate associations among impulsivity and health-risk behaviors? *Addictive Behaviors, 33*(2), 252–265.

Tanne, J. H. (1997). Medicine's new motto: One sex does not fit all. *American Health For Women, 16*(5), 54–58.

Testicular cancer—What to look for. (1999, May 1). *American Family Physician, 59*(9), 2549–2550.

Thornton, J. (2004). Driving while male. *Men's Health, 19*(7), 96–99.

Torres, J. B. (1998). Masculinity and gender roles among Puerto Rican men: Machismo on the US mainland. *American Journal of Orthopsychiatry, 68*(1), 16–26.

Treadwell, H. M., & Ro, M. (2003). Poverty, race, and the invisible men. *American Journal of Public Health, 93*(5), 705–707.

U.S. Department of Health and Human Services. (2013). *Healthy People 2020: Topics and objectives.* Retrieved from http://www.healthypeople.gov/2020/TopicsObjectives2020/default.aspx

Vogel, D. L., Heimerdinger-Edwards, S. R., Hammer, J. H., & Hubbard, A. (2011). "Boys don't cry": Examination of the links between endorsement of masculine norms, self-stigma, and help-seeking attitudes for men from diverse backgrounds. *Journal of Counseling Psychology, 58*(3), 368–382.

Walbrecker, J. (1995, January). Start talking about testicular cancer. *RN,* pp. 34–35.

Waldron, I. (1995). Contributions of changing gender differences in behavior and social roles to changing gender differences in mortality. In D. Sabo & D. F. Gordon (Eds.), *Men's health and illness: Gender, power, and the body* (pp. 22–35). London, England: Sage.

Wigle, D., Turner, M., Gomes, J., & Parent, M. (2008). Role of hormonal and other factors in human prostate cancer. *Journal of Toxicology & Environmental Health: Part B, 11*(3/4), 242–259.

Will, H. (1998). Better to die than cry? A longitudinal and constructionist study of masculinity and the health risk behavior of young American men. Doctoral dissertation, University of California at Berkeley. *Dissertation Abstracts International, 59*(08A), (publication number AAT 9902042).

Williams, D. (2008). The health of men: Structured inequalities and opportunities. *American Journal of Public Health, 98,* S150–S157.

Woloshin, S., Schwartz, L., & Welch, H. (2008). The risk of death by age, sex, and smoking status in the United States: Putting health risks in context. *Journal of the National Cancer Institute, 100*(12), 845–853.

Yip, P. S., Caine, E., Yousuf, S., Chang, S. S., Wu, K. C., & Chen, Y. Y. (2012). Means restriction for suicide prevention. *Lancet, 379*(9834), 2393–2399.

CHAPTER FOCUS

Improving Children's Health: Working with Families
- Preventing Maternal and Infant Mortality and Morbidity
- Immunizing Children
- Preventing Childhood and Youth Injuries and Violence
- Promoting Child and Youth Mental and Spiritual Health

Selected Nursing Interventions
- Transition from Hospital to Home and Community for High-Risk Children and Youth
- Weaving Spirituality into Nursing Interventions
- School-Based Programs
- Home-Based Programs

Improving Child and Youth Health: Systems of Care

Ecology of Child and Youth Health: Contexts for Growth and Development
- Poverty
- Neighborhood Contexts
- Parents' Work Context
- Childcare Context
- Public Policy Context

QUESTIONS TO CONSIDER

After reading this chapter, you will know the answers to the following questions:

1. What is the significance of the infant mortality rate in the assessment of a community's health?
2. What are three common health problems of children?
3. How is chronic disease manifested in children?
4. How are risk-taking behaviors of adolescents related to health?
5. What are common behavioral problems that have health consequences during adolescence?
6. What is the scope of maltreatment of children in the United States?
7. What is the ecology of child health?
8. What delivery-of-care issues exist in relation to child health?
9. How does the role of the community health nurse in child and youth health differ from the acute care setting?

"There are two lasting bequests we can give our children. One is roots. The other is wings."

—Hodding Carter, Jr.

CHAPTER 33

Child and Adolescent Health

Angela Blackburn and Harriet Kitzman

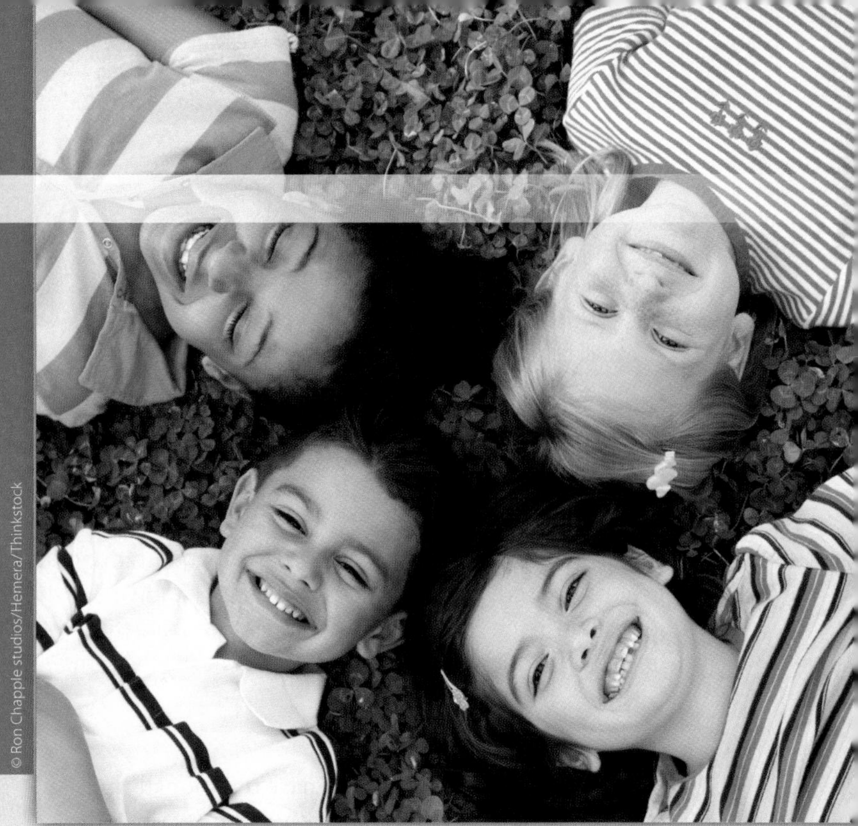

KEY TERMS

Children's Defense Fund
externalizing behavior
Individuals with Disabilities Education Act (IDEA)
multisystemic therapy model
Nurse–Family Partnership
recidivism
system of care
Temporary Assistance for Needy Families (TANF)

REFLECTIONS

Ring-a-round o'roses
A pocket full of posies,
A-tishoo! A-tishoo!
We all fall down.

Old English children's rhyme that dates back to the Great Plagues refers to the "rosy rash"; "posies" of herbs were kept in pockets as protection from the disease, and sneezing was often a final, fatal symptom with resulting death and "falling down."

—*The Oxford Dictionary of Nursery Rhymes*

You have most likely heard this children's rhyme throughout your childhood. Until the last century, children were at greatest risk of dying from infectious diseases. How have the changes in antibiotics and vaccines affected children's health care in the 20th and 21st centuries? What are the vulnerabilities of children today as compared to those in "Ring Around the Rosies"? Are there some that are still the same?

COMMUNITY HEALTH nurses have traditionally had a strong focus on children's health. In the early 20th century, nurses from settlement houses taught immigrant families how to care for their children. In the 21st century, community nurses are involved in many programs addressing children's health, from giving immunizations, to helping communities identify unmet needs, to finding ways to improve the health of mothers and infants as members of local child fatality review (CFR) teams.

It makes sense for a society to be child centered. In European nations, where the "aging" of the population is even more marked than in the United States, it is national policy to provide extra resources to families with newborns and young children. For example, the French government provides paid pregnancy and infancy leaves for mothers, stipends for each additional child, and free preschools. As a result, France has some of the best health outcomes in the world, including a longer life expectancy and a lower infant mortality rate than the United States and most post-industrialized nations.

To some degree, focusing on children's health is self-serving for adults: Children are the wage earners of the future. But children's health is more important to a thriving nation than just having new young workers to pay taxes. If children are not healthy in the broadest sense—physically healthy, but also well educated, mentally healthy, competent citizens—then a nation lacks future leaders, scientists, and parents capable of continuously renewing human capital.

Community nurses use all of the themes presented in this text, but especially upstream programming, family, environmental health, and systems of care, to plan and carry out effective child health programs. In many states, public health nursing is changing from providing direct services, such as well-child clinics, to assessing community needs and resources, developing policies to improve population health, and ensuring the quality and accessibility of health services. This change in roles from direct care to population-based care offers nurses an opportunity to lead the community in providing comprehensive, excellent services addressing children's physical, mental, spiritual, and social health.

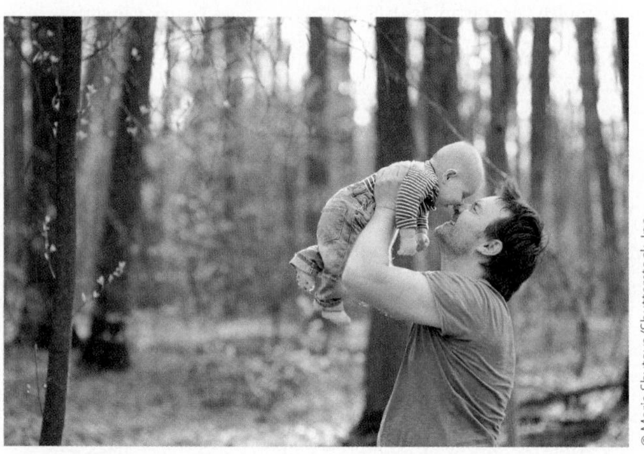

Father's involvement with babies is a critical part of healthy development.

The chapter has three sections. The first section addresses progress in improving children's health at the individual and family levels. The *Healthy People 2020* goals for children and family health focus on salient, preventable children's diseases and causes of death, especially those that unfairly affect children of certain social classes, races, or ethnicities. Stories of successful nursing interventions—many of them related to the 2020 goals for children—confirm the promise of upstream or preventive measures. These stories bring to life how nursing research and practice in the community or in the transition from hospital to home address common childhood illnesses.

The second section of this chapter addresses systems of care for children—not only the healthcare system, but also systems of justice, welfare, education, and public housing. Surprisingly, the serious violent crime offending rate was 6 crimes per 1,000 juveniles ages 12–17, with a total of 154,000 such crimes involving juveniles. This was similar to the rate in 2010, but it was substantially lower than the 1993 peak rate of 52 crimes per 1,000 juveniles ages 12–17 (Federal Bureau of Investigation, 2012; Federal Interagency Forum on Child and Family Statistics [FIFCFS], 2013). Knowledge of systems of care helps community health nurses find resources and coordinate care

Finally, the third section considers the contexts or settings other than the family that make a difference in children's health. The home and the family context are most important to children, but nurses must attend to the health consequences of other contexts. The air children breathe, their parents' workplaces, neighborhoods, and public policy all affect children's health and development.

Improving Children's Health: Working with Families

Community health nurses must always see the child both as an individual and as a member of a family. Our society tries to balance the right of the family to make decisions for children against older children's rights for self-determination and against society's responsibility to keep children safe. Ideally, families will understand and meet their children's needs on their own. Unfortunately, during 2011, data from all 50 states plus the District of Columbia indicate that there were 676,569 victims (unique count) of child abuse and neglect in the United States. The unique count of child victims counts a child only once regardless of the number of times he or she was found to be a victim during the reporting year, so the actual incidence of child abuse is considerably higher, because many children are subject to repeated abuse. The 2011 unique victim rate was 9.1 victims per 1,000 children in the population ages 0–17 years (U.S. Department of Health and Human Services [HHS], 2013b). Younger children are more frequently victims of maltreatment than are older children. In 2011, there were 23 substantiated child maltreatment reports per 1,000 children under age 1, compared with 13 reports for children ages 1–3, 11 for children ages 4–7, 8 for children ages 8–11, 8 for children ages 12–15, and 5 for adolescents ages 16–18 (HHS, 2012, 2013b).

According to data from the National Child Abuse and Neglect Data System (NCANDS) cited in Child Maltreatment (HHS, 2013), 49 states reported a total of 1,640 fatalities. Based on these data, 2.2 per 100,000 children in the population died from abuse. This translates into 4.7% decrease from 2008 when 1,720 children died of abuse and neglect. While the national estimate and rate are lower for 2012 than 2008, both the number and rate of child abuse and neglect have increased since 2010 (HHS, 2013b). NCANDS defines "child fatality" as the death of a child caused by an injury resulting from abuse or neglect or where abuse or neglect was a contributing factor (HHS, 2013b).

Economic stress on families, such as occurs in single-parent and low-income families, increases the risk of abuse or neglect of children.

HEALTHY PEOPLE 2020 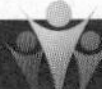

Objectives Related to Children

Adolescent Health

- AH-1 Increase the proportion of adolescents who have had a wellness checkup in the past 12 months
- AH-2 Increase the proportion of adolescents who participate in extracurricular and/or out-of-school activities
- AH-3 Increase the proportion of adolescents who are connected to a parent or other positive adult caregiver
- AH-5.2 Increase the proportion of students who are served under the Individuals with Disabilities Education Act who graduate high school with a diploma
- AH-5.6 Decrease school absenteeism among adolescents due to illness or injury
- AH-6 Increase the proportion of schools with a school breakfast program
- AH-7 Reduce the proportion of adolescents who have been offered, sold, or given an illegal drug on school property
- AH-9 Increase the proportion of middle and high schools that prohibit harassment based on a student's sexual orientation or gender identity
- AH-10 Reduce the proportion of public schools with a serious violent incident
- AH-11 Reduce adolescent and young adult perpetration of, and victimization by, crimes

Early and Middle Childhood

- EMC-1 Increase the proportion of children who are ready for school in all five domains of healthy development: physical development, social-emotional

(continues)

HEALTHY PEOPLE 2020 (*continued*)

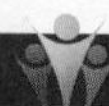

development, approaches to learning, language, and cognitive development

- EMC-2 Increase the proportion of parents who use positive parenting and communicate with their doctors or other healthcare professionals about positive parenting
  - EMC-2.1 Increase the proportion of parents who report a close relationship with their child
  - EMC-2.2 Increase the proportion of parents who use positive communication with their child
  - EMC-2.3 Increase the proportion of parents who read to their young child
  - EMC-2.4 Increase the proportion of parents who receive information from their doctors or other healthcare professionals when they have a concern about their children's learning, development, or behavior
  - EMC-2.5 Increase the proportion of parents with children under the age of 3 years whose doctors or other healthcare professionals talk with them about positive parenting practices
- EMC-3 Reduce the proportion of children who have poor quality of sleep
- EMC-4 Increase the proportion of elementary, middle, and senior high schools that require school health education

Maternal, Infant, and Child Health

- MICH-1 Reduce the rate of fetal and infant deaths
- MICH-2 Reduce the 1-year mortality rate for infants with Down syndrome
- MICH-3 Reduce the rate of child deaths
- MICH-4.1 Reduce the rate of deaths among adolescents age 10 to 14 years
- MICH-4.2 Reduce the rate of deaths among adolescents age 15 to 19 years

Immunizations and Infectious Disease

- IID-1 Reduce, eliminate, or maintain elimination of cases of vaccine-preventable diseases
- IID-4.1 Reduce new invasive pneumococcal infections among children under age 5 years
- IID-4.3 Reduce invasive antibiotic-resistant pneumococcal infections among children under age 5 years
- IID-5 Reduce the number of courses of antibiotics for ear infections for young children
- IID-7 Achieve and maintain effective vaccination coverage levels for universally recommended vaccines among young children
- IID-8 Increase the percentage of children age 19 to 35 months who receive the recommended doses of DTaP, polio, MMR, Hib, hepatitis B, varicella, and pneumococcal conjugate vaccine (PCV)
- IID-9 Decrease the percentage of children in the United States who receive 0 doses of recommended vaccines by age 19 to 35 months
- IID-10 Maintain vaccination coverage levels for children in kindergarten
- IID-11 Increase routine vaccination coverage levels for adolescents
- IID-17 Increase the percentage of providers who have had vaccination coverage levels among children in their practice population measured within the past year

Mental Health and Mental Disorders

- MHMD-2 Reduce suicide attempts by adolescents
- MHMD-3 Reduce the proportion of adolescents who engage in disordered eating behaviors in an attempt to control their weight
- MHMD-4.1 Reduce the proportion of adolescents age 12 to 17 years who experience major depressive episodes (MDEs)
- MHMD-6 Increase the proportion of children with mental health problems who receive treatment
- MHMD-7 Increase the proportion of juvenile residential facilities that screen admissions for mental health problems

Nutrition and Weight Status

- NWS-1 Increase the number of states with nutrition standards for foods and beverages provided to preschool-aged children in child care
- NWS-2 Increase the proportion of schools that offer nutritious foods and beverages outside of school meals
- NWS-5.2 Increase the proportion of primary care physicians who regularly assess body mass index (BMI) for age and sex of their child or adolescent patients
- NWS-6.3 Increase the proportion of physician visits made by all child or adult patients that include counseling about nutrition or diet
- NWS-10 Reduce the proportion of children and adolescents who are considered obese
- NWS-11 Prevent inappropriate weight gain in youth and adults
- NWS-12 Eliminate very low food security among children
- NWS-14 Increase the contribution of fruits to the diets of the population age 2 years and older
- NWS-15 Increase the variety and contribution of vegetables to the diets of the population age 2 years and older
- NWS-16 Increase the contribution of whole grains to the diets of the population age 2 years and older
- NWS-17 Reduce consumption of calories from solid fats and added sugars in the population age 2 years and older
- NWS-18 Reduce consumption of saturated fat in the population age 2 years and older
- NWS-19 Reduce consumption of sodium in the population age 2 years and older
- NWS-20 Increase consumption of calcium in the population age 2 years and older
- NWS-21 Reduce iron deficiency among young children and females of childbearing age

Source: HealthyPeople.gov

When families need support in meeting a child's health and development needs, the nurse's approach to the family is important. Nurses should spend the time needed to create a partnership with the family using a warm, nonjudgmental approach. When families feel threatened and defensive, use your nursing knowledge and experience of adult health to open doors. Remember that by showing interest and concern for parents, nurses can "get in the door" to address the child's needs.

As a result of our sometimes contradictory values—family privacy and children's safety, for example—the United States has more violence against children than any developed country. Two of the nursing interventions discussed later in the chapter—nurse home visits and nurse-run parenting clinics—show promise in helping parents decrease harsh parenting and foster their children's safety, growth, and development.

Preventing Maternal and Infant Mortality and Morbidity

The infant mortality rate decreased by 11.6% between 2000 and 2010, from 6.9 infant deaths per 1,000 live births to 6.1 (HHS, 2013a). There is still work to do, particularly in decreasing health disparities among children of different ethnic and socioeconomic groups. Some health researchers believe that disparities such as the difference in infant mortality between blacks and other groups suggest a need for more social justice in access to basic resources—better access for minorities to good jobs and education, not just more health care.

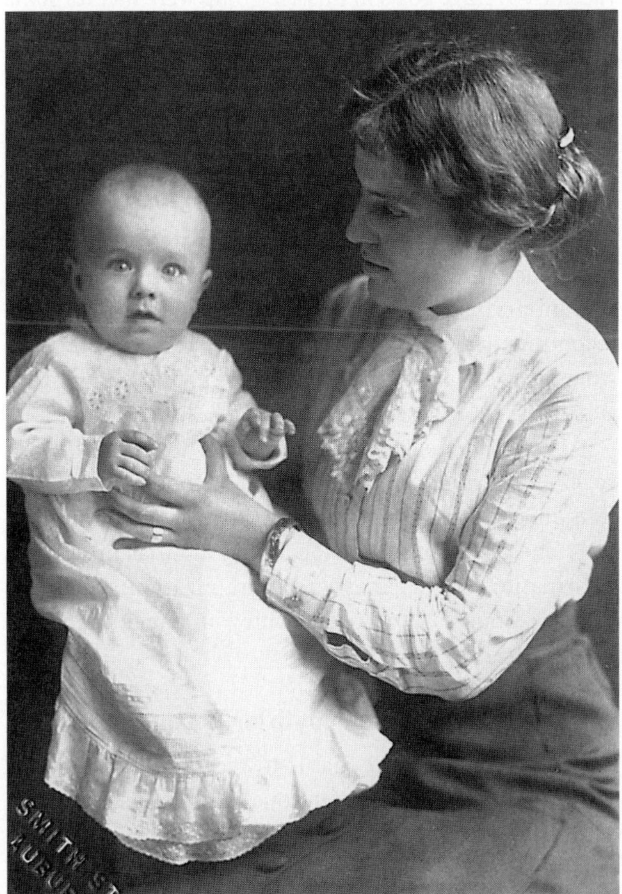

Mothers and babies during the first half of the twentieth century were at a greater risk for dying from acute infection.

Discrepancies in health outcomes between racial or ethnic groups within the United States, and between the United States and other countries, led to a government task force setting *Healthy People 2020* objectives. There are differences between race/ethnicities in infants' and pregnant women's mortality; for example, black infants are nearly twice as likely to die as white infants (Matthews & MacDorman, 2013). Few women die during childbirth, but black women are more than three times as likely to die as white women (CDC, 2014).

CULTURAL CONNECTION

Youths who identify themselves with the "Goth" culture may be more at risk for suicide attempts and self-mutilation than those in the general population of adolescents. Research is not clear on whether participation in the Goth culture leads to self-destructive behavior or whether adolescents with more suicidal tendencies gravitate toward the Goth culture. Goth culture is defined as "a dark and sinister aesthetic, with aficionados conspicuous by the range of distinctive clothing and makeup and tastes in music." A British study found that self-identification with a Goth subculture was associated with a 14-fold increase in the risk for self-harming behavior and a 16-fold increase in the risk for suicide attempts as compared with non-Goth youth. These findings held true even after adjusting for other known predictive factors, such as being female, having divorced or separated parents, smoking, drug use, and depression. Goth identification remained the single strongest predictor of self-harm and suicide attempt.

Source: Young, R. (2006, April 13). Prevalence of deliberate self-harm and attempted suicide within contemporary Goth youth subculture: A longitudinal cohort study. *British Medical Journal*, 10. doi: 1136/bmj.38790.495544.7C

Nurses have traditionally been strong advocates of social justice. You can learn more about these issues by doing community participatory research about local causes of disparities in child health outcomes. For more background information on racial and ethnic health disparities, start at the Maternal and Child Health Library (http://www.mchlibrary.info), which has several "knowledge paths," including one on racial and ethnic disparities in health.

Immunizing Children

Another *Healthy People 2020* goal focuses on childhood immunizations. Vaccines are the true "miracle drugs." Before the polio vaccine became available in 1955, summers were a time of terror for parents. A child's neck ache could turn into paralyzing polio overnight. In addition to preventing suffering, childhood immunizations save billions of dollars in health-related and other expenditures.

Vaccines are among the most cost-effective clinical preventive services and are a core component of any preventive services package. Childhood immunization programs provide a very high return on investment. For example, for each birth cohort vaccinated with the routine immunization schedule (this includes DTap, Td, Hib, Polio, MMR, Hep B, and varicella vaccines), society:

- Saves 33,000 lives
- Prevents 14 million cases of disease
- Reduces direct healthcare costs by $9.9 billion
- Saves $33.4 billion in indirect costs

Despite progress, approximately 300 children in the United States die each year from vaccine-preventable diseases. Communities with pockets of unvaccinated and undervaccinated populations are at increased risk for outbreaks of vaccine-preventable diseases. In 2008, imported measles resulted in 140 reported cases—nearly a three-fold increase over the previous year. The emergence of new or replacement strains of vaccine-preventable disease can result in a significant increase in serious illnesses and death (HHS, 2013a).

In 2011, about 78% of children ages 19–35 months had received the recommended combined six-vaccine series. Children living in families with incomes below the poverty level had lower rates of coverage (75%), compared with children in families with incomes at or above the poverty level (79%).

Since 2006, vaccination coverage with routinely recommended vaccines among U.S. adolescents ages 13–17 has increased, but coverage with vaccines recommended at 11 or 12 years of age remains low, especially for human papillomavirus (HPV) vaccine. In the United States each year, there are about 17,000 women and 9,000 men affected by HPV-related cancers. Many of these cancers are preventable with vaccinations in both women and men. The HPV vaccination is recommended for preteen girls and boys at age 11 or 12 years. There are two vaccines available, distributed under the trade names Cervarix and Gardasil. Only one of these, Gardasil, has been tested and licensed for use in males (Centers for Disease Control and Prevention [CDC], 2013a; Dunne et al., 2011)

In 2011, vaccination coverage among U.S. adolescents ages 13–17 for one dose (or more) of tetanus, diphtheria, acellular pertussis (Tdap) vaccine was 78%; one dose (or more) of meningococcal conjugate (MenACWY) vaccine was 71%; and one dose (or more) of HPV vaccine among females was 53%.

Haemophilus influenzae type B (Hib) is a serious bacterial infection that is particularly significant in very young children. Before the introduction of the Hib vaccine, *H. influenzae* was the leading cause of bacterial meningitis among children younger than 5 years of age in the United States, with roughly 20,000 children younger than 5 years of age developing severe infections and about 1,000 deaths annually. More than half of these children were younger than 1 year. In the years since use of Hib vaccine became routine, this has changed dramatically; in 2010, fewer than 50 cases of Hib-related disease (bacteremia, meningitis, epiglottitis, pneumonia, and cellulitis) occurred annually in children younger than 5 years old (CDC, 2013b).

At its 2014 progress report, the *Healthy People 2020* goal of 80% vaccine coverage for all recommended doses in children ages 19–35 months had not been met; it stood at 68.5% in 2011. However, this represents a significant improvement in just 2 years, given that data from 2009 indicated less than half (44.3%) of children had received all recommended vaccines (HHS, 2014), and it is likely that still more progress has been made toward the goal in the interim. Moreover, vaccine coverage goals in this age group were met for *some* vaccines: Hib, hepatitis B, measles–mumps–rubella (MMR), polio, and varicella. The 2020 goals have not been met for DTaP, pneumococcal conjugate vaccine (PCV), hepatitis A, and rotavirus (CDC, 2013b).

Despite these vaccine success stories, we cannot let our guard down. For example, more than 48,000 cases of whooping cough (pertussis) were reported in 2012, the most since 1955. Vaccination is the most effective way to prevent pertussis in your patients. Pertussis vaccines are recommended across the lifespan, including for pregnant women. The main focus is on protecting infants, who are at greatest risk for serious illness, including death.

Tips for increasing immunization levels and other vaccine information can be found at the website of the Immunization Action Coalition (http://www.immunize.org). The CDC (http://www.cdc.gov) also has up-to-date information on vaccines and immunization schedules, clinical resources, tools to use with your patients, and national outbreak trends.

Preventing Childhood and Youth Injuries and Violence

A *Healthy People 2020* goal is to reduce the number of children dying from unintentional injuries and violence. After age 1, the most common cause of child death is injury. While rates of childhood injuries have decreased over the last decade, injury is still a leading cause of death from infancy to adolescence.

Dying due to a motor vehicle accident is the number one cause of all such injury deaths. Safety restraints appropriate to the age and size of the child can save lives, but the family must make their use a habit at all times.

ETHICAL CONNECTION 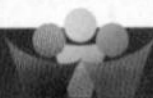

Parents who practice certain religions may choose not to immunize their children and instead homeschool them to avoid the school-mandated schedule of required immunizations. How do you feel about this practice? How does it affect public health in the community?

The racial and gender disparities in child deaths send a compelling message that we must act to prevent violent deaths. Black adolescents and young men are nearly twice as likely to die as their peers of other races. As we will discuss later in this chapter, school and neighborhood violence pose a mental and physical health threat to all children.

The CDC (2012) reported that childhood unintentional injuries are the leading cause of death among children ages 1 to 19 years, representing nearly 40% of all deaths in this age group. Each year, an estimated 8.7 million children and teens from birth to age 19 are treated in emergency departments (EDs) for unintentional injuries, and more than 9,000 die as a result of their injuries—one every hour. Common causes of fatal and nonfatal unintentional childhood injuries include: drowning, falls, fires or burns, poisoning, suffocation, and transportation-related injuries. Injuries claim the lives of 25 children every day (CDC, 2012).

Every hour, nearly 150 children between ages 0 and 19 are treated in emergency departments for injuries sustained in motor vehicle accidents. More children ages 5 to 19 die from crash-related injuries than from any other type of injury. One CDC study found that, in one year, more than 618,000 children ages 0–12 rode in vehicles without the use of a child safety seat or booster seat or a seat belt at least some of the time (Greenspan, Dellinger, & Chen, 2010). But many of these deaths can be prevented. Placing children in age- and size-appropriate car seats and booster seats reduces serious and fatal injuries by more than half (U.S. Department of Transportation, National Highway Traffic Safety Administration, 2012).

Youth suicide is a major, preventable public health problem. The CDC (2013c) reported that teen suicide is the third leading cause of death, behind accidents and homicide, of people ages 15 to 24. An equally disturbing statistic reported by the CDC is that suicide is the fourth leading cause of death for children between the ages of 10 and 14. Lesbian, gay, bisexual, and transgendered (LGBT) youth were significantly more likely to attempt suicide compared with heterosexuals (21.5% versus 4.2%) (Hatzenbuehler, 2011).

Studies have shown that connectedness is an important factor for suicide. Strong, positive relationships with others (individuals, families, community organizations) can be protective against suicidal thoughts and behaviors, lower levels of isolation, increase a sense of belonging, strengthen identity and personal worth, and provide access to communities of support. However, research also warns that youth's connectedness to negative peer groups may increase their risk for suicidal behavior (CDC, 2014; Hatzenbuehler, 2011).

Community health nurses are in a position to address factors that place children and youth at risk for, or protect them from, engaging in suicidal behavior by taking a population approach to the problem (suicide awareness with a focus on the individual, peers, family, and community), providing primary prevention that assists parents and youth in building positive relationships and fostering connectedness, incorporating evidence-based interventions in the plan of care, and using a multidisciplinary perspective to address the youths' complex health concerns (CDC, 2013c).

Underage drinking is an often overlooked public health problem in the United States (Lewis & Hession, 2012). The Center on Alcohol Marketing and Youth (CAMY, 2010) reported that every day in the United States, 4,750 young people younger than 16 years have their first drink of alcohol. Alcohol proves to have detrimental effects on the physiological, psychological, and sociological aspects of developing young children. Young people who start drinking before the age of 15 years are 4 times more likely to become alcohol dependent, 7 times more likely to be in a motor vehicle accident because of drinking, and 11 times more likely to be in a physical fight after drinking (CAMY, 2010).

Promoting Child and Youth Mental and Spiritual Health

The 2020 goal for improved mental health for children is as important as the goals for improving children's physical health. Surveys estimate that 13–20% of children living in the United States (up to one out of five children) experience mental health problems in a given year, but fewer than half of those children receive treatment for the problem. Mental health problems that are not treated in childhood do not just go away; many tend to linger or even flare up and become more serious in adulthood. Mental health problems such as depression are among the most costly health problem for adults, due to loss of wages as well as the cost of care (CDC, 2013d).

Clearly, there is a lot of work to be done to protect and improve children's physical and mental health. In this work it is important to see the child in an ecological framework. Children's physical and mental health are affected by factors at many levels: biological, family, neighborhood, and national health policy. The book *From Neurons to Neighborhoods*, published by National Academies (Shonkoff & Phillips, 2000), supports this ecological view of child development. This book told parents and professionals that young children need early emotional responsiveness and spoken language from their parents as well as protection from neighborhood violence. The third section of this chapter more specifically addresses the ecological factors that affect children's health and development.

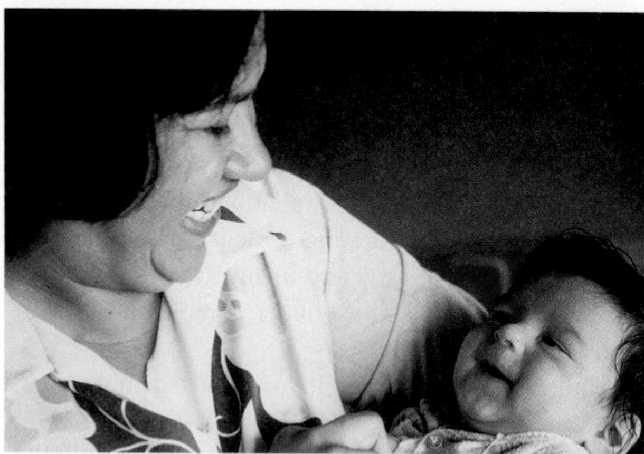

The health of an infant is greatly influenced by the ability of the mother to meet the infant's security needs.

> We have not all had the good fortune to be ladies. We have not all been generals, or poets, or statesmen; but when the toast works down to the babies, we stand on common ground.
>
> —*Mark Twain*

> Children begin by loving their parents; as they grow older they judge them; sometimes they forgive them.
>
> —*Oscar Wilde*

Selected Nursing Interventions

The excitement of being a community health nurse is best communicated by learning about real nurses who have created and carried out programs addressing common child health problems at various ages and in various community settings. Two examples of interventions specifically focused on mental health and child development are presented here. However, nurses also address mental health and development when intervening with children with any physical illness, such as asthma or cancer.

Transition from Hospital to Home and Community for High-Risk Children and Youth

The transition from hospital to home is an opportunity for community health nurses to improve children's health. Children are rarely hospitalized, but when they are, the nurse must prevent long-term physical or mental health effects from the trauma of illness and being in strange surroundings. Two nurses have had important impacts on this transition. Dorothy Brooten and colleagues (1986) asked why healthy, but low-birth-weight infants were being kept in the hospital so long. She and her colleagues then designed a research study that answered this question and changed the protocols for keeping low-birth-weight children in the hospital. In their work, these researchers found that, as long as the infant had no serious complications, parents with support and instruction from advanced practice nurses could provide care at home at less cost and less distress for the infant and the parents.

Another nurse, Bernadette Melynk, identified the need to support, educate, and involve parents of sick children in their children's care. In her evaluation of Creating Opportunities for Parent Empowerment (COPE), Melynk and her colleagues (2004) found that when parents of low-birth-weight infants or children needing intensive hospital care for other reasons received preventive educational–behavioral support from specially trained nurses, fewer child adjustment problems (such as posttraumatic stress disorder) occurred when children went home.

Nursing interventions for chronically and acutely ill children also address the transition from hospital to home. Cancer is a serious chronic illness that kills more children than any cause other than injuries. Pamela Hinds and colleagues (2001) at St. Jude Children's Research Hospital in Memphis value improving the quality of life for children, even when they have incurable cancer. In addition to inquiring into ways to support nurses who work with very sick and dying children, these nurses developed guidelines to involve adolescents and their parents in making decisions about their care. These nurses concluded that adolescent patients want to know about their treatment and are able and willing to help make decisions. The research team published guidelines to help nurses in the hospital or the community give the best quality of care from diagnosis to end-of-life decision making (Hinds et al., 2001). Since 2012, hospitals are responsible for the cost of 30-day readmissions that are deemed avoidable (Centers for Medicare & Medicaid Services [CMS], 2014). Models to improve the quality of care as clients transition from one care setting to another are evolving, and a body of evidence suggesting best practices is being formulated (Agency for Healthcare Research and Quality [AHRQ], 2007).

Weaving Spirituality into Nursing Interventions

Nursing interventions are an excellent place to address children and spirituality. Hinds and colleagues (2001) found that both parents and children identified "religious beliefs" as "belief in a god and the certainty of life after death" as important factors in making an end-of-life decision. The 31 factors considered by physicians in making end-of-life decisions addressed staff recommendations, family preferences, therapeutic options, and the family and child's comfort and preferences, but not spiritual issues. This indicates that caregivers may often not help children and their parents explore and integrate their spiritual beliefs into the care plan.

NOTE THIS!

Melanoma—the most serious and potentially deadly form of skin cancer—was until recently almost unheard of in children. From 1973 through 2009, rates of pediatric melanoma increased by an average of 2% per year (Wong, Harris, Rodriguez-Galindo, & Johnson, 2013). Recent studies have also reported increases in England, Sweden, and Australia. Although the reasons for the increase are uncertain, many researchers speculate that depletion of the ozone layer might be allowing children to be exposed to more of the sun's damaging ultraviolet radiation. Other factors may be excessive sun exposure and blistering sunburns in early childhood and use of tanning beds. The rate of melanoma has more than doubled among adults as well.

Melanoma is often missed in children, not only because of its rarity but also because of its very different appearance than in adults. Melanoma in children comprises lighter-colored lesions that have well-defined borders. Also, unlike adults, most children presenting with melanoma have no family history of the disease.

GOT AN ALTERNATIVE?

Yoga and tai chi can be effectively used as stress-relieving exercises as well as flexibility-enhancing interventions for children.

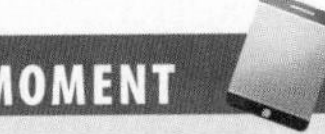

MEDIA MOMENT

Born into Brothels (2004)

This Academy Award–winning documentary is a study of several unforgettable children who live in Calcutta's red-light district, where their mothers work as prostitutes. Zana Briski, a photographer documenting life in the brothels, decides to teach these children photography. They are fascinated with the camera. As they begin to record their world, the children come to a recognition of their own worth and talents.

Children, like adults, see themselves as part of a narrative or a story with meaning. While considering the child's developmental stage and respecting religious and cultural beliefs, the nurse can help the child tell his or her own story and find meaning not just in the stress of illness or violence, but also in the joy of living. By asking a few questions appropriate for the child's developmental age, the nurse can explore the child's preconceived ideas about illness or death, fears, fantasies, and concerns about separation, isolation, or death. Simple questions that might work with children or adults are: "What is most important to you?", "What do you think is happening to you?", "What brings you joy?", and "What scares you?"

School-Based Programs

Community health nurses are in contact with children and can see important trends in children's health even before they become newsworthy. For example, nurses in schools and community clinics knew that children's asthma and obesity were serious problems long before official statistics confirmed the fact.

In the United States, asthma is a major cause of morbidity in children ages 0–17. Nearly one in 10 children (10%) have asthma, and 59% of these children miss at least 1 day of school each year—the average days lost per child is 4—because of their asthma (American Academy of Allergy, Asthma & Immunology [AAAAI], 2014). Although medications and therapeutic regimens to control the disease have improved, asthma continues to have devastating effects on the lives of large numbers of children and their families. The prevalence and severity of the disease are greater in African American children living in poverty and in crowded conditions (FIFCFS, 2013). In 2011:

- About 10% of children were reported to currently have asthma, including children with active asthma symptoms and those whose asthma was well controlled.
- Approximately 5% of all children had one or more asthma attacks in the previous 12 months. These children have ongoing asthma symptoms that could put them at risk for poorer health outcomes, including hospitalizations and death.
- About three out of five children who currently have asthma have ongoing asthma symptoms.
- About 16% of black, non-Hispanic children were reported to currently have asthma, compared with 8% of white, non-Hispanic and 10% of Hispanic children. Disparities exist within the Hispanic population such that 25% of Puerto Rican children were reported to currently have asthma, compared with 8% of children of Mexican origin.

- From 2001 to 2011, there was an increasing trend in the percentage of children reported to currently have asthma. Between 1980 and 1995, childhood asthma more than doubled (from about 4% in 1980 to approximately 8% in 1995). Methods for measurement of childhood asthma changed in 1997, so earlier data cannot be compared to data from 1997–2011.

Viral respiratory infections and exposure to specific allergens, such as cigarette and other smoke, dust mites, molds, cockroaches, and pet dander, often provoke this disease. Nurses and nurse researchers working in schools have developed and implemented asthma education programs in schools that increase adherence to prescribed medical regimens and reduce exposure to allergens (Engelke, Swanson, & Guttu, 2013; Toole, 2013; Yoos et al., 1997).

These programs have had varying degrees of success in helping families change their lifestyles. One of the explanations for limited adherence to asthma-prevention regimens is that the disease produces intermittent symptoms. It is often difficult for families to maintain regular day-to-day prevention practices during times when the child is well.

Prevention of childhood obesity is one of the *Healthy People* 2020 priorities. Childhood obesity has more than doubled in children (from 7% to 18%) and tripled in adolescents (from 5% to 18%) since the 1980s, causing an epidemic and public healthcare crisis (Ogden, Carroll, Kit, & Flegal, 2012). The consequences of youth obesity include risk factors for cardiovascular disease, pre-diabetes, diabetes, bone and joint problems, sleep apnea, and social and psychological problems such as stigmatization and poor self-esteem (Chen, Kim, Houtrow, & Newacheck, 2010). There are racial and ethnic disparities in these percentages, with black and Hispanic children twice as likely to be overweight as white children (Taveras, Gillman, Kleinman, Rich-Edwards, & Rifas-Shiman, 2013).

Children and adolescents with developmental disabilities such as autism spectrum disorder (ASD) may be particularly vulnerable to obesity due to the behavioral, physical, and psychological complications related to their condition (Strahan & Elder, 2013).

Waters and colleagues (2011) found strong evidence to support beneficial effects of child obesity prevention programs on body mass index, particularly for programs targeted at children ages 6 to 12 years. As a result, they found the following to be promising policies and strategies:

- School curriculum that includes healthy eating, physical activity, and positive body image
- Increased sessions for physical activity and the development of fundamental movement skills throughout the school week
- Improvements to nutritional quality of the food supply in schools
- Environments and cultural practices that support children eating healthier foods and being active throughout each day
- Support for teachers and other staff to implement health-promotion strategies and activities (e.g., professional development, capacity-building activities)
- Parent support and home activities that encourage children to be more active, eat more nutritious foods, and spend less time doing screen-based activities

However, study and evaluation designs need to be strengthened, and reporting should be extended to capture process and implementation factors, outcomes in relation to measures of equity, longer term outcomes, potential harms, and costs. Childhood obesity prevention research must now move toward identifying how effective intervention components can be embedded within health, education, and care systems and achieve long-term, sustainable impacts.

GLOBAL CONNECTION

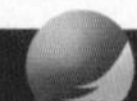

Teenagers in the United States weigh more than their counterparts in most other industrialized countries, and fast-food availability and consumption are most likely the leading cause. According to a study of 15-year-olds in 15 developed nations, 15% of U.S. girls and nearly 14% of U.S. boys are classified as obese. The next highest numbers (5.5% of girls and almost 11% of boys) come from Greece. By comparison, only 4% of French girls and not quite 3% of French boys were obese. (Lissau et al., 2004). In another study, one-third of U.S. children ages 4 to 19 were found to eat at least one fast-food meal daily and take in 187 calories more a day than those who don't, for an average gain of about 6 extra pounds per year (Bowman, Gortmaker, Ebbeling, Pereira, & Ludwig, 2004).

Sources: Lissau, I., Overpeck, M. D., Ruan, W. J., Due, P., Holstein, B. E., & Hediger, M. L. (2004). Body mass index and overweight in adolescents in 13 European countries, Israel and the United States. *Archives of Pediatric and Adolescent Medicine, 158*(1), 27–33;. Bowman, S. A., Gortmaker, S. L., Ebbeling, C. B., Pereira, M. A., & Ludwig, D. S. (2004). Effects of fast-food consumption on energy intake and diet quality among children in a national household survey. *Pediatrics, 113*(1), 112–118.

The American Public Health Association (APHA) has developed an action plan to address the goal of preventing childhood obesity. **Table 33-1** outlines its recommendations.

A mental health program designed by a creative community health nurse, Carolyn Webster-Stratton (2014),

TABLE 33-1 APHA Action Plan: Childhood Obesity

Goal 1: Increase daily physical activity among children and adolescents.
Goal 2: Reduce the amount of time kids spend on television, video games, and the Internet.
Goal 3: Decrease the consumption of energy-dense, high-sugar/high-fat foods such as soda, ice cream, junk food, and fast food.
Goal 4: Increase the consumption of nutritious foods such as fruits, vegetables, whole grains, and skim milk.
Goal 5: Create social, monetary, and policy-driven incentives that reinforce long-term environmental and behavioral change.

Source: American Public Health Association. (2014). Tackling childhood obesity: Vision and guiding principles. Retrieved from http://www.apha.org/programs/resources/obesity/tacklingobesity.htm

focuses on elementary-school-age children with behavior problems that could escalate into antisocial behavior or crime if not addressed. This work is very important because as many as one out of four high-risk children may already exhibit aggressive, disruptive behavior in preschool. Furthermore, if these children are not helped to learn more positive behaviors, they are at high risk of adopting criminally delinquent behavior and/or dropping out of school. (Le Blanc, Swisher, Vitaro, & Tremblay, 2007).

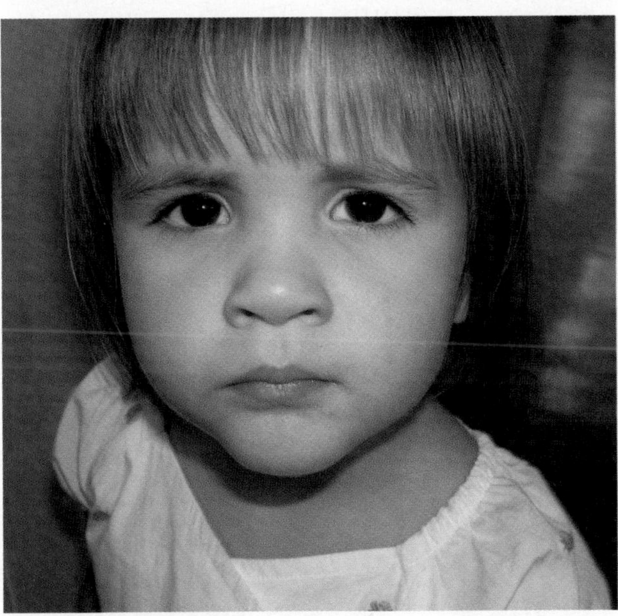

Children are one-third of our population and all of our future.

Her work with children, teachers, and parents earned Webster-Stratton a prestigious Research Scientist Award from the National Institute of Mental Health. In a nurse-run parenting clinic and in schools, nurses help parents and teachers understand how to change from negative to positive teaching and parenting strategies (Webster-Stratton & Reid, 2014). It is counterintuitive to most adults, but praising children when you "catch" them behaving well works better than focusing on punishing misbehavior. Children are also taught to recognize and express their emotions, to solve problems without fighting, and to apologize and pay compliments to other children. Learning new positive social skills helps suppress children's misbehavior.

Home-Based Programs

The **Nurse–Family Partnership** (NFP) links low-income families with nurses who visit in the home from pregnancy until the baby is 2 years of age. These visits focus on the mother's health and life choices as well as her knowledge of child development and other needs. They not only prevent child abuse and neglect, but also improve the child's health and development. Studies (Olds & Kitzman, 1993; Olds, Kitzman, Knudtson, Anson, Smith, & Cole, 2014) have demonstrated that NFP reduced preventable death among both low-income mothers and their first-born children living in disadvantaged, urban neighborhoods. More importantly, even after the visits stop, both mothers and children make wiser, healthier choices that save money in welfare and other costs. The NFP is based on three decades of randomized controlled trials, with consistent and enduring effects on maternal and child health (Olds et al., 2013). You can learn more about this program at the website of the NFP (http://www.nursefamilypartnership.org/) or from special reports on the program on the website of the Robert Wood Johnson Foundation (http://www.rwjf.org/en/research-publications/find-rwjf-research/2013/11/improving-the-nurse-family-partnership-in-community-practice.html).

These kinds of programs involving community health nurses, ranging from helping tiny newborn babies move safely from the hospital to the home to visiting new mothers at home, highlight the importance of systems of care. In addition to forming partnerships with families, nurses in these programs must collaborate with many other community agencies to provide holistic care. Children and their families also need resources from the justice, welfare, housing, and political systems. The next section of the chapter addresses these systems of care and explores how they affect children and offer opportunities for nursing leadership.

Improving Child and Youth Health: Systems of Care

Community health nurses must often intervene at the system level to ensure that children receive needed and effective education, housing, economic assistance, and spiritual

BOX 33-1 Challenging Question for Students

Compare the action plan and explanation of the causes of obesity in children cited by the APHA with the areas addressed by nurse researcher Margaret Grey and colleagues (2004). Why would Grey include measures of spirituality in her school health program to decrease obesity in minority youth? What does it mean to be holistic in addressing obesity in children? How is a child's spirituality different at different ages, and how would that affect your treatment plan for an obese child?

The following are additional resources on children's spirituality:

Catlin, E. A., Guillemin, J. H., Thiel, M. M., Hammond, S., Wang, M. L., & O'Donnell, J. (2001). Spiritual and religious components of patient care in the neonatal intensive care unit: Sacred themes in a secular setting. *Journal of Perinatology, 21*, 426–430.

Smith, J., & McSherry, W. (2004). Spirituality and child development: A concept analysis. *Journal of Advanced Nursing, 45*(3), 307–315.

Lawson, K. E. (Ed). (2012). *Understanding children's spirituality: Theology, research and practice.* Eugene, OR: Cascade Books.

guidance as well as health care. The term **system of care** was coined to describe comprehensive mental health care for disabled children. This section first addresses the system of mental health care for children. The term *system of care* is used generically to address healthcare, justice, education, welfare, spiritual/religious, and public housing systems.

The mental health system of care aims to bring together many agencies and service providers into a coordinated network to meet the "multiple and changing needs of children and adolescents [and their families] with severe emotional disturbances" (Stroul & Friedman, 1986, p. xx). The visionary system of care has core values that are also important to community health nurses. The values shared by systems of care and community nurses are:

- Being child centered and family focused
- Being community based so that children can live at home
- Being culturally competent about racial, ethnic, and cultural differences among families
- Providing individualized services that build on the strengths of families
- Providing integrated, coordinated, effective, and efficient services
- Identifying and treating problems early (Cook & Kilmer, 2004)

These values are important but hard to achieve.

One of the oldest mental health systems is the system of services for children with disabilities funded by the **Individuals with Disabilities Education Act (IDEA)**. The Early Intervention program is part of IDEA. Early Intervention grants to each state are used for comprehensive statewide programs to work with children (and their families) from birth to age 2 with disabilities or slowed development. The expectation is that, by providing early intervention measures such as physical therapy and developmental child care, children will be less likely to have permanent disabilities with the attendant extra human and financial costs. This system of screening, diagnosis, and treatment for infants and young children is run by different agencies in different states. You can find out which government agencies have grants at the website of the Early Childhood Technical Assistance Center (http://ectacenter.org/).

IDEA is more than just early intervention. Public law No. 94-142 (Education for All Handicapped Children, now known as Individuals with Disabilities Act [IDEA]) was first passed in 1975 and was most recently reauthorized by Congress in 2004. IDEA covers children with disabilities ranging from Down syndrome to attention deficit hyperactivity disorder (ADHD) from birth to age 18. The public school system is responsible for providing educational and assistive services to children from age 3 to age 18. Parents, sometimes the child, and school representatives meet to set goals for the child and to agree on which special resources the school must provide to ensure that the child has the best chance of meeting his or her educational and developmental goals.

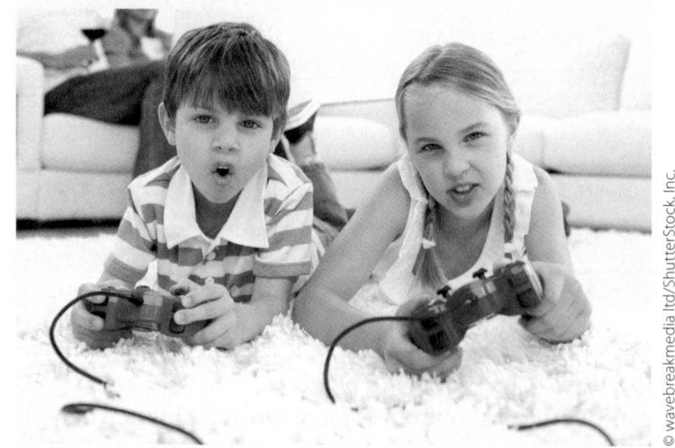

Video games, on television and portable devices and via computers, should be carefully monitored by parents for violent and inappropriate content as well as setting time limits on their use.

In most states, mental health systems of care focus on children already diagnosed with serious mental health problems such as emotional disturbance. Except for early

NOTE THIS!

Children's illnesses—the top four causes of missed school are:

1. Colds
2. Gastroenteritis ("stomach flu")
3. Conjunctivitis ("pink eye")
4. Strep throat

Source: The Mayo Foundation for Medical Education and Research, August 8, 2005.

NOTE THIS!

The Children's Health Insurance Program (CHIP) was approved in 1997 by the U.S. government to cover uninsured children whose families earn too much to qualify for Medicaid. More than a dozen states have expanded the program, which also insures nearly 8 million children and families (CMS, 2014).

identification of children with developmental delays, the concept of "upstream programming" is rare in the mental health system. There are two main reasons that mental health care is usually remediation-based rather than preventive care: Mental health care is stigmatized and poorly funded.

For many persons, there is a negative stigma connected with seeking mental health care. Depression, obsessive thoughts, and oppositional behavior are often considered personal weaknesses rather than illnesses that can be treated with medications or counseling. Consequently, parents may not want to get care for their mental health problems even when those problems also harm family relationships. Perhaps because of this stigma, policymakers do not believe that mental health care should be funded on an equal basis with physical health care.

The CDC (2013d) reports that in any given year, 13–20% (one of five) of U.S. children ages 3 to 17 years need mental health care for serious problems. Fewer than 10% of the children needing mental health services get them within 3 months of recommendation, and fewer than half of those diagnosed with a serious emotional disorder ever get treatment from an appropriate mental health clinician (Behrens, Lear, & Price, 2013). This problem is equally shared by children of all races and ethnicities. In fact, children on Medicaid public insurance are *more* likely than privately insured children to receive developmental and mental health screening (Kataoka et al., 2002).

Evaluations of the impact of creating a formal interagency system of care for severely emotionally disturbed children have yielded mixed results. The children served by these systems have significant functional impairment at home and school. They have diagnoses of one or more of the following: ADHD, oppositional defiant disorder, conduct disorder, and/or depression (often bipolar). The families of these children often have economic, social, mental, and legal problems. Many agencies, and informal helpers such as churches and neighbors, must work together to help these families and children. While there was variation across community sites where systems of care were funded and put in place, overall the outcomes were no better for children provided with services from a formal system of care (Cook & Kilmer, 2004) compared to children with usual community care.

The explanation for the lack of improved outcomes in these funded interagency systems of care for severely emotionally disturbed children and their families is unclear. Traditionally, community agencies have had their own unique cultures and are accustomed to working alone. It takes skilled leadership to create long-term collaboration among agencies.

There may be more hope in single agencies using multiple therapists to address all the problems of these children and families. In the **multisystemic therapy model** (Henggeler, 2003), one agency works intensively with families and connects them with other community resources. This model has improved children's school performance, kept more children living at home, decreased substance abuse, and improved families' functioning.

There may be a take-home lesson from these efforts for community health nurses trying to create coordinated, integrated systems of care for children. Groups of agencies and informal helpers can learn to work together by solving specific, immediate problems of a real family in crisis. Trying to reform a system by convening meetings to address abstract needs of generic families may not lead to efficient collaboration among agencies. In other words, community systems seem to learn to work together using inductive, bottom-up processes rather than top-down, deductive processes.

It is an easy transition from talking about children in the mental health system for children to talking about other systems of care and children. Mental health is an important factor in the justice, school, healthcare, welfare, and public housing systems:

- Most of the children in the justice system have mental health problems.
- School systems are the largest providers of mental health services for children.
- Mental health problems increase the cost of care for physical health problems.
- Medicaid public insurance for poor children covers more mental health services than most private insurance.

- Public housing systems provide housing specifically for homeless mentally ill persons because it is nearly impossible for them to get well without safe housing.

When systems of care work well for children, they are efficient, comprehensive, and just. Unfortunately, systems, like individuals, can get "stuck" and fail to adopt the best practices or to meet new and growing needs of those who depend on them. For example, starting in 1970 the justice system began punishing juvenile offenders with rough scare tactics and "adult punishment for adult crimes." More juvenile offenders who are sent to boot camps or to adult jails end up being chronic criminals than those who receive more developmentally appropriate support and guidance (Muscar, 2008). It is hard to know the exact number of children arrested or the percentage of crimes attributed to juveniles. The juvenile justice system in the United States is actually 51 separate systems in each state and the District of Columbia. One report estimates that more than 100,000 youths are incarcerated on any given day. Juvenile arrests have been declining since the 1980s, whereas adult arrests have continued to increase. However, four times as many youths are stopped, interrogated, and searched than are actually arrested. Minority youth, particularly black males, are stopped and arrested at higher rates than other youth. More than half of all incarcerated youth have a severe mental disorder such as conduct disorder, depression, ADHD, learning disability, posttraumatic stress disorder, or developmental disability. Such disorders contribute to risky or violent behaviors leading to arrest. There is little or no treatment for mental disorders in the juvenile system; indeed, the harsh conditions found there often exacerbate these disorders.

Intensive treatment of mental disorders and problem behaviors aimed at the child and the family can divert the child from incarceration and prevent further criminal behaviors. Harsh, punitive treatment, which occurs when a child is forced to move to the adult justice system for serious crimes, usually increases **recidivism** or chances of rearrest and results in more jail time.

Community health nurses may feel helpless to change this situation or even to continue contact with youthful patients who happen to be arrested and incarcerated. Mental Health America provides descriptions of programs aimed at children involved with the juvenile justice system. It also provides descriptions of programs that do not work. Sharing knowledge of best practices in juvenile justice with parents and politicians is a first step to changing the juvenile justice system where you practice.

NOTE THIS!

Children raised with pets are less allergic. In one study, children who were raised in households with two or more dogs or cats in infancy were about half as likely to develop common allergies as children who had no pets in the home. Research found that the group exposed to animals had fewer positive skin tests to both indoor allergens (e.g., pet dander, dust mites) and outdoor allergens (e.g., ragweed, grass). The children exposed to cats and dogs were almost half as likely to have hyperresponsive and easily irritated airways—a risk factor for asthma. Researchers propose that the difference may lie in endotoxins, the breakdown products of bacteria found in the animals' mouth. These endotoxins are thought to force the body's immune system into developing a response pattern that is less likely to lead to allergic reactions.

Source: Ownby, D. R., Johnson, C. C., & Peterson, E. L. (2002). Exposure to dogs and cats in the first year of life and risk of allergic sensitization at 6 to 7 years of age. *Journal of the American Medical Association, 288*(8), 963–972.

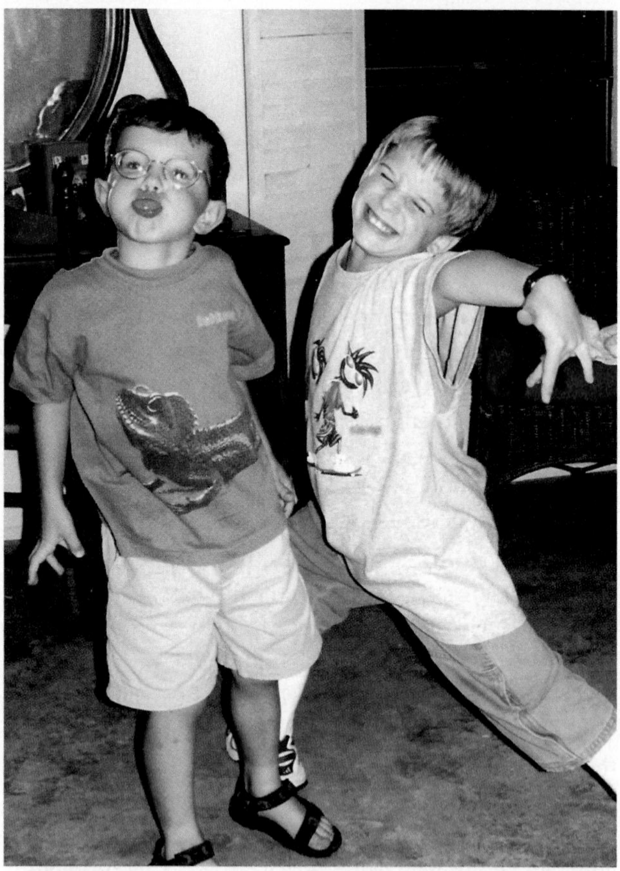

> You are worried about seeing him spending his early years in doing nothing. What! Is it nothing to be happy? Nothing to skip, play, and run around all day long? Never in his life will he be so busy again.
>
> —*Jean Jacques Rousseau, 1762*

Antique Doll

Hair set with sugar
Face painted
Brittle she waits

Patient in the dark room
Petals are lost
From the wedding bouquet

Children are grown
More children are on the way
The house fills with sound

For a brief span
Time will pass more rapidly.

—*Ann Thedford Lanier*

School systems usually have their own health component. Even without designated health programs, schools are so central to children's healthy growth and development that the community health nurse must collaborate with this system. The "health" program at a school can vary from a secretary handing out Band-Aids to a comprehensive program with the following standards set by the CDC:

- Community based
- Integrated within and supportive of the educational system
- Managed by a qualified nursing leader who is integrated into the school administrative structure as part of the management team
- Advised by a school and community group, including parents and students
- Based on accepted standards, regulations, and statutes
- Supported by a health service management information system
- Offering a range of prevention and treatment services, including tobacco control
- Implemented by sufficient numbers of qualified school nurses and support personnel during the entire school day
- Culturally competent and linguistically relevant
- Coordinated with the eight components of a comprehensive school health program, as defined by the CDC: health education, health services, social and physical environment, physical education, guidance and support services, food service, school and worksite health promotion, and integrated school and community health promotion
- Linked with community primary care, mental health and dental health providers, local youth and family serving agencies, local and state public health and emergency providers, and public insurance outreach programs
- Making maximum use of available public and nonpublic funds (e.g., Municipal Medicaid, grants, insurance reimbursement, business partnerships, Foundation Budget, Community Benefits Program)
- Evaluated regularly to determine its effectiveness and efficiency

RESEARCH ALERT 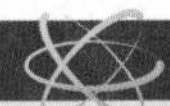

This study looked at the protective effectiveness of speed bumps in reducing child pedestrian injuries in residential neighborhoods. A matched case-control study design was conducted over a 5-year period among children seen in a pediatric emergency department after being struck by an automobile. A multivariate conditional logistic regression analysis showed that speed bumps were associated with lower odds of children being injured within their neighborhood and being struck in front of their home. Children living within a block of a speed bump had significantly lower odds of being struck. Living within a block of a speed bump was associated with a roughly twofold reduction in the odds of injury within one's neighborhood. This protective effect was even more pronounced among the subset of children who were injured on the block immediately in front of their house.

Source: Tester, J. M., Rutherford, G. W., Wald, Z., & Rutherford, M. W. (2004). A matched case-control study evaluating the effectiveness of speed humps in reducing child pedestrian injuries. *American Journal of Public Health, 94*(4), 646–649.

School clinics are becoming more common. They were first implemented in high schools, but can now be found in middle and elementary schools. While children must have their parents' permission to receive care from a school clinic, these clinics increase access to health care and improve school attendance and school performance. Evaluations of school clinics show that they can decrease emergency room use (Key, Washington, & Hulsey, 2002), improve immunization coverage, promote responsive sexuality, and identify serious untreated health problems ranging from asthma to heart disease.

Unfortunately, community health nurses seldom work in or with the school systems unless they are school employees. Providing a continuing nursing education program or collaborating on a school health fair is a great way to break the ice and start working together. If you can collaborate with the school system, you will have access to all but the youngest children in your community. There are wonderful opportunities for health promotion and health education with school children.

The community nurse focusing on child health should remember that almost all divisions of the healthcare system are potential partners in promoting health and preventing disease in children. Home health agencies have child patients with diagnoses ranging from cancer to cerebral palsy. Occasionally children must be placed in nursing homes when their families can no longer care for them at home. To care for children in the transition from hospital to home, the community nurse must have contacts with local hospitals to receive referrals when children are discharged.

The last two systems of care addressed here are essential resources for low-income children and their families. There resources are not thought of as health resources, but a child cannot be healthy and develop well if the family has no money for food and other essentials or if the family does not have a safe place to live. The human services or welfare department has traditionally provided financial assistance to poor families. The U.S. Department of Housing and Urban Development (HUD) oversees most of the publicly owned housing in the United States and has a program that discounts the amount of rent paid in private housing.

In 1996, drastic changes were made in a cash-payment program formerly called Aid to Families with Dependent Children (AFDC). In addition to changing its name to **Temporary Assistance for Needy Families (TANF)**, the program was redesigned to provide only short-term cash assistance while adults in the family were getting education and/or job placement help so that they would support themselves. There are many requirements for families receiving cash assistance. Adults must be looking for work, in school, or in some other worthy endeavor such as job training or volunteering to keep getting assistance. Furthermore, adults must immediately report changes of address and income or risk losing their cash grant or even being prosecuted.

At the same time that AFDC was abolished, Medicaid health insurance was separated from the cash grant system. While the federal government provides part of the money to pay for Medicaid insurance, each state must also fund a portion of this publicly funded insurance. Two-thirds of the Medicaid-insured population are poor children and their families; the other third are low-income elderly or disabled adults. Medicaid is one of the largest expenses of state governments and is frequently seen as a place to cut benefits. As a community health nurse interested in children, you should know that the one-third of patients who are elderly or disabled adults account for two-thirds of the costs incurred by Medicaid programs. One of the largest costs of Medicaid is elderly people who use this insurance to pay for care in nursing homes. Compared to the cost of nursing home care, children's health care is inexpensive.

Safe housing is very important to a child's health and development. HUD agencies provide safe public housing and other services in almost every city in the country. Just as for people receiving cash assistance, there are also many rules for families living in public housing. Families must keep the apartment clean and agree to regular inspections. Families can be evicted if they allow anyone who has been convicted of dealing illegal drugs to live with them in public housing. While these rules may seem harsh, the resources are so important to family survival that adults can usually understand and follow the rules. Furthermore, there was a time when public housing projects were considered the most unsafe place to life; these harsh rules help make the needed housing option safer. The community health nurse should learn about agencies providing cash grants and housing and understand their regulations to help in providing referrals to families who need these services.

Captured

I saw you this morning
  holding your oldest son

Love can be captured—only the color will change

Locked inside the plastic case
  of paper and chemicals

Miniature hands grasping

He smiles up at you—mouth open for your breast.

—*Ann Thedford Lanier*

Ecology of Child and Youth Health: Contexts for Growth and Development

The first section of this chapter addressed the family context and the need for community nurses to work as partners with families to improve children's health and development. Other, larger contexts also affect children's growth and development. The neighborhood, work, and public policy contexts form the child's ecology (see Bronfenbrenner, 1979, for a discussion of the theory of human ecology) and are of particular interest for children.

Poverty

Living in the context of poverty places children at risk for poor health and developmental outcomes (Wagmiller, Kuang, Aber, Lennon, & Alberti, 2006). Kids Count, a project of the Annie E. Casey Foundation, estimates that 23% of children in the United States live in families whose income is below the federal poverty line. Nearly half of these children live in extreme poverty, which means the family of four has an annual income of less than $11,641 per year

THINK ABOUT THIS 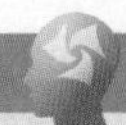

Each year, an average of 37 children die from heat-related causes after being left in a car by a parent. In many cases, this is an inadvertent act, but some parents intentionally left the child in the car, either because they didn't want to disturb a sleeping child or because they were only planning to be away a short time. In either case, the parent lacked awareness of how fast a car might heat up to dangerously high temperatures. Experiments using a common model of car (Honda Civic) in a popular color (silver) showed that in just 10 minutes, a car parked in the sun at mid-morning (~10:30 a.m.) had the potential to go from a comfortable 70°F temperature to 84°F. This increased temperature is uncomfortable for an older child, and dangerous for an infant or toddler. Twenty minutes more, and the car's ambient temperature rises to over 100°F, which is actively harmful to even school-age children and adolescents. At 1 hour, the once-comfortable car becomes a 122°F oven—a death trap for children inside. And if the car is already hot to begin with—say, 90°F, as it might be on a July day (even when outdoor temperatures are slightly cooler), the temperature reaches the danger point even faster. A car that starts out at 90° will heat to over 100° in under 10 minutes.

Source: Grundstein, A., Dowd, J., & Meentemeyer, V. (2010). Quantifying the heat-related hazard for children in motor vehicles. *Bulletin of the American Meteorological Society, 91,* 1183–1191.

(Kids Count Data Center, 2012). The risks of being poor increase with single parenthood, low educational attainment, part-time employment, or low wages. The educational level of parents is a strong predictor of family income.

Effects of Poverty on Children's Physical Health

There is evidence that family poverty and neighborhood physical and socioeconomic conditions affect a child's health status.

Low-birth-weight and prematurity are highly correlated with poor health status in the infancy period. Sequelae of both these conditions (neurological damage or poor respiratory function, for example) or their treatment (retinopathy of prematurity from high concentrations of administered oxygen) may be long lasting. There are two mechanisms of low birth weight—fetal growth restriction and preterm delivery; both are more common in low-income families and neighborhoods (Pless, 1994). Chronic stress, particularly in relation to food insecurity and poor coping skills, was identified as being significantly related to the likelihood of bearing a low-birth-weight infant (Borders, Grobman, Amsden, & Holl, 2007). Predisposing factors for fetal growth retardation include pregnancy in an adolescent or unsupported mother; intrauterine exposure to drugs, nicotine, or alcohol; intrauterine infection; maternal ill health; maternal short stature or underweight; multiple births; and fetal anomalies. Preterm deliveries are related to vaginal infections, which are in turn related to the number of sexual partners.

The chances of a child's thriving if born preterm or with low birth weight are strongly related to the socioeconomic status of the family. Factors that appear to explain why children are born at low birth weight and are more likely to die in infancy in impoverished neighborhoods include public and substandard market housing, high crime rates, single-parent and female-headed families, and high male unemployment (Anthony, Vu, & Austin, 2008). These neighborhood conditions have direct effects on the child, but also indirectly affect the child's chance of thriving by shaping the home environment (Cohen & Reutter, 2007; Klebanov, Brooks-Gunn, Chase-Lansdale, & Gordon, 1997).

Respiratory illnesses are the most common illnesses for which children seek medical care and are hospitalized. They are still important causes of death. The number of respiratory illnesses appears to be constant at six to eight episodes per child per year throughout the world (Durani, Friedman, & Attia, 2008). Children living in poverty are more likely to have severe viral or bacterial infections that progress to the lower respiratory tract and cause pneumonia, bronchitis, bronchiolitis, or croup. The following factors are related to the severity of respiratory infections:

- Air pollution, both outdoor and indoor (Bateson & Schwartz, 2008)
- Crowding, particularly with many young children in a home (Collins, Kasap, & Holland, 1971)
- Malnutrition (Harsten, Prellner, & Heldrup, 1990)
- Daycare attendance (Harsten et al., 1990)

Maternal stress, perhaps by increasing the child's stress and causing related declines in immunity, increases the risk of a child's having respiratory infections (Graham, Ryan, & Douglas, 1990).

Gastroenteritis is yet another common physical illness that is more prevalent and more serious when children live in poverty and when sanitation is poor. In the United States, 10% of preventable postneonatal infant deaths are attributable to diarrhea and occur primarily in the most disadvantaged groups (Pless, 1994).

It would be expected from discussions of the increased severity of illness that the likelihood of sequelae of low birth weight and prematurity for children in poverty would have lower average reported health status. Children have better access to health care since implementation of Medicaid in 1965, but when health status is controlled, poor children still make far fewer visits to physicians and are less likely to have a personal physician than nonpoor children (Coiro, Zill, & Bloom, 1994).

Cognitive Skills in the Context of Poverty

Family and neighborhood conditions also have important influences on children's ability to take in and process information. The effects can be subtle or devastating. The presence of both biological risks and poor environmental conditions can be disastrous. Physical illness, which is more common in poor families and neighborhoods, causes a child to miss school or perform poorly when present. The combination of physical illness, stress, and living in communities where most adults are poorly educated and lack the energy, vision, and skills to spend time helping children learn can place the young child at higher risk of school failure.

RESEARCH ALERT 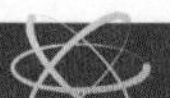

A study of mothers' neonatal intensive care unit (NICU) experiences identified three core narratives: enchantment, disenchantment, and re-enchantment stories. Enchantment stories were the stories mothers told about their hopes, dreams, and ideals for their first pregnancy, birth, and baby. Disenchantment stories were stories that mothers told when things didn't go as planned and babies required care in the NICU. Re-enchantment stories were told by mothers about their attempts to create normalcy in the chaos of the NICU. The research makes a case that through narrative understanding, care providers can maintain a better balance between the highly technological nature of the NICU and also achieve therapeutic relationships with patients. The study also explored a second level of reflection that revealed descriptions of five narrative features and transcendent themes.

Source: Blackburn, A. C. (2009). *Stories, ethics and the interpretation of meaning: Bearing witness to mothers' stories of their neonatal intensive care unit experience.* Ann Arbor, MI: ProQuest, UMI Dissertation Publishing.

MEDIA MOMENT 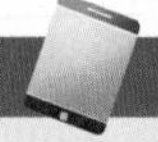

The Secret Life of Bees

By Sue Monk Kidd (2003), Penguin Publishers, New York

In Sue Monk Kidd's *The Secret Life of Bees*, 14-year-old Lily Owen, neglected by her father and isolated on their Georgia peach farm, spends hours imagining a blissful infancy when she was loved and nurtured by her mother, Deborah, whom she barely remembers. This coming of age story set in the turmoil of the early 1960s takes the reader on a journey with Lily and her beloved nanny, Rosaleen, to the colorful world of the Black Madonna. The search for a mother, and the need to mother oneself, are themes of this critically acclaimed bestseller. The women who take Lily and Rosaleen into their homes and hearts teach her about love, life, and beekeeping, all metaphors for healing and growing up.

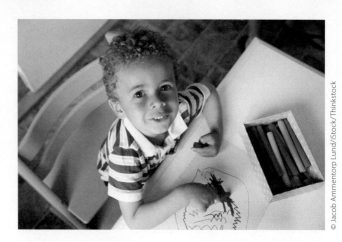

As children grow, they need a stimulating environment for optimal development.

We have long known that children raised in poverty are at a disadvantage at school entry (National Scientific Council on the Developing Child (2005/2014). While some claim this inequality is a result of poor genetic endowment, others fault the lack of cognitive and sensory stimulation—and research is beginning to support the latter position (National Scientific Council on the Developing Child, 2014).

Early intervention programs such as Head Start have not only shown immediate improvements in terms of children's elementary school math and reading capabilities, but long-term effects in terms of outcomes such as high school graduation, years of education completed, earnings, and reduced crime and teen pregnancy (Radner & Shonkoff, 2012; Yoshikawa et al., 2013). Continuing services into the elementary school grades, however, does appear to reinforce and prolong the effects (Shonkoff & Fisher, 2013).

Poverty and poor neighborhoods are also the major risk factors for childhood injuries. Poor children are more than twice as likely to die from trauma as nonpoor children, and they are five times more likely to die from fires and burns (Nersesian, Petit, & Shaper, 1985; Rodgers & Payne, 2007). Poor housing, violence, high traffic volume, and lack of smoke detectors in poor neighborhoods put children at very high risk of injury.

While children are able to report their own emotional disorders, they are less able to report **externalizing behavior** such as disrupting others, negative, hostile, and defiant behaviors (Liu, 2004). Externalizing behaviors have an early onset, and without treatment or a change in environment can lead to patterns of escalating hostility between the child and adults. Children who have externalizing behaviors often have poor self-esteem and problems with personal and work relationships, and these behavior problems are important predispositions to later juvenile delinquency, adult crime and violence (Liu, 2004).

THINK ABOUT THIS 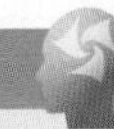

Children and Terrorism

Parents, teachers, and caregivers were challenged with how to communicate with children and adolescents about the cataclysmic events surrounding the terrorist attacks on September 11, 2001. As nurses, it is important that we take a leadership role in raising awareness of how children may understand, interpret, and respond to related and persistent fears and concerns of these events. Although being honest with our children and reassuring them about their safety is important, it is critical to provide information that is developmentally appropriate. By providing information that is appropriate to the age and circumstances of the child, stress and fear can be reduced and children can better understand the chaotic events facing our nation in terms of terrorism and war. This interaction can also lay the foundation for future communication should additional terrorist attacks or acts of war occur.

Source: Adapted from DeRanieri, J. T., Clements, P. T., Clark, K., Kuhn, D. W., & Manno, M. S. (2004). War, terrorism and children. *Journal of School Nursing, 20*(2), 69–72.

Risk factors for externalizing behaviors are multifactorial (biological, psychological, protective factors, interaction between biology and psychological). Chaotic and unpredictable environments can contribute to poor self-regulation behaviors and impulse control. Identifying early risk factors is an important first step in preventing juvenile delinquency, adult crime, and violence. There is sufficient evidence to suggest that capacities for executive function skills can be improved through focused early intervention programs and education programs. (Center on the Developing Child, 2011; Liu, 2004; 2011).

This review provides evidence that family poverty and various correlates of being poor, such as young maternal age, crowding, low birth weight, malnutrition, parental stress, and dysfunctional adult relationships, are important predictors of poor outcomes in physical health, cognitive performance, and emotional or behavioral problems (Holzer, Schanzenbach, Duncan, & Ludwig, 2008). The family environment is very important to a child's health and development. There is also evidence that neighborhoods

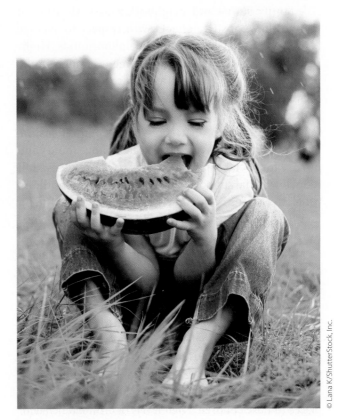

Female children learn early healthy habits, which can promote their wellbeing as adults.

have direct and indirect effects on health and development (Guthrie, 2007; Prentice, 2007).

Environmental Hazards in the Poverty Context

Pollutants such as tobacco smoke or nitrous oxide in the air we breathe inside and outside the home increase the risk for impaired lung growth, middle ear infection, respiratory infections, asthma attacks, and even cancer. Community health nurses can provide information to parents about the risks of secondhand smoke to children and can support parents as they try to stop smoking.

In addition to the toxins in the air, toxic chemicals such as lead, diazinon, and mercury are found in common household objects and substances. Young children are most at risk for harm from exposure to toxins. Children who eat large amounts of flaking old paint containing lead can get sick, and even be left intellectually disabled. Children crawling in grass that has been sprayed with insecticides may absorb the insecticide through their skin.

Neighborhood Contexts

Protective factors in families and neighborhoods are more important than risk factors for important outcomes such as developmental test scores. That is, low-risk family status and neighborhoods with affluent families have positive effects with respect to average family risk and average income neighborhoods. High-risk scores for a family and few affluent families in the neighborhood do not further decrease child developmental test scores. Family protective or risk status has been measured by proxies for human capital (e.g., maternal education, maternal verbal comprehension, maternal age, employment of head of household) and proxies for social capital measures (e.g., child-to-adult ratio, low social support network score). Neighborhood protective status is based on the percentage of affluent families; risk status is based on the percentage of families below the poverty line.

When neighborhood risk factors rise above a threshold level, they become important. Neighborhoods with extreme impoverishment and a high childcare burden (high child-to-adult ratio, high population turnover, and many female-headed households) tend to have high rates of child abuse and neglect (Anthony et al., 2008; Cancian, Slack, & Yang, 2010; Rodgers & Payne, 2007). Furthermore, residents in these neighborhoods perceive that neighborhoods with crime, drugs, and violence are poor places to raise children. High levels of criminal behavior and physical evidence of poverty and neglect, such as broken windows, abandoned cars, and weeds, may either elicit or be markers for fear and hopelessness.

Research suggests that neighborhood effects on child development start after family effects, but exist as early as age 3. For a population of low-birth-weight infants, Klebanov, Brooks-Gunn, McCarton, and McCormick (1998) concluded that there are significant nonlinear effects of family risk factors, such as maternal education, employment of head of household, and child-to-adult ratio, on child developmental test scores as early as age 1. Family poverty became significant at age 2. Neighborhood income showed significant nonlinear effects at age 3. Thus, living in poverty during early childhood appears to be more harmful than the same duration of living in poverty in later childhood (Anthony et al., 2008; Rodgers & Payne, 2007).

Neighborhood poverty, family risk status, and family poverty effects have been shown to be mediated by the quality of the home environment—primarily by learning opportunities within the home, such as appropriate toys, books, pets, and interaction with male and female caregivers (Klebanov et al., 1998). Other possible mediators of the effect of neighborhood poverty and its sequelae (e.g., violence, isolation, and lack of basic services) are the mother's depression or lack of self-efficacy. These mediators have not been extensively studied but will be considered in this research.

Perhaps the clearest statement from research is the vulnerability of black children, particularly black males. Black children are more concentrated in poor neighborhoods than white or Hispanic children (Massey & Kanaiaupuni, 1993). Male joblessness is significantly related to black children's, but not white children's, internalizing and externalizing problems (Chase-Lansdale, 1997).

The detrimental effects of long-term exposure to neighborhood risks are clear in African American male adolescents. Spencer (1977) concluded from his research on African American adolescents living in high- and low-risk neighborhoods in Atlanta that African American "boys require more protection from adverse circumstances in the most extreme neighborhood conditions" (p. 217).

Parents' Work Context

The family friendliness of the workplace affects children's health and development indirectly. If parents cannot take leave to care for a sick child without the fear of losing their job, the child suffers.

Childcare Context

A dramatic increase in the number of women with children who work occurred in the last part of the 20th century. Nearly three out of four U.S. mothers work. Even among mothers with very young children, nearly two out of three are employed outside the home. Unmarried mothers are more likely than married mothers to work (Bureau of Labor Statistics, 2013). While most children of working mothers are still cared for by other family members, more children than ever are now in site-based child care.

It is difficult for parents to balance work, time with children, caring for the home, and adult social life. The stress and resultant anxiety of feeling that, as a parent, you are not spending enough time with your child can contribute to depression and fatigue. Parents can feel better about their work if they are sure that their child is in a safe, developmentally rich childcare setting. Unfortunately, there are not enough government-funded childcare programs such as Head Start and Early Head Start. Furthermore, government subsidies to working parents needing child care are limited. Parents often must take whatever child care they can afford. While childcare providers want to provide good care, that is expensive, and childcare care workers are typically paid little more than minimum wage.

Public Policy Context

One of the challenges for community health nurses focusing on children's health and development is the lack of a public policy system focused on children's rights and needs. Why should children have their own policy system? Because it works. For example, elderly persons in the United States have a network of public agencies called Area Agencies on Aging in every medium-size or larger city to advocate for their rights.

Nothing like this exists for children. The state of California and certain cities have attempted to establish and fund formal agencies to plan and implement a well thought-out set of programs to ensure that children grow and develop into productive and happy citizens. One of the most powerful policy advocates for U.S. children is the **Children's Defense Fund**, a nonprofit agency. See its website for news on children's policy issues (http://www.childrensdefense.org).

Another public policy dilemma for children is that children don't vote, and low-income parents struggling to work and care for their children often don't vote either. These parents are the last to know when Medicaid insurance or child care for the working poor is cut to balance the budget.

As a community health nurse, you can find out which agencies in your town advocate for children and their families. Encourage families you work with as a nurse to tell their political representatives how public programs help their children. Encourage people to vote.

Conclusion

Nurses working in the community have a unique opportunity to provide individualized services to families in their homes and community. Nurses observe parents struggling to do the best for their children, often in the face of tremendous adversity. Nurses then have unique perspectives and information from their work with children and families. Consequently, community nurses are critical members of community efforts to plan services for children and families.

AFFORDABLE CARE ACT (ACA) 

Preventive Health Services for Children

Most ACA health plans must cover a set of preventive health services for children at no cost when delivered by an in-network provider. This includes ACA Marketplace and Medicaid coverage.

Children and young adults under the age of 26 can now be covered under their parents' health insurance. As of 2010, all new health insurance plans are required to include recommended preventive service and immunizations to which no deductible and copayments apply. One of the required areas for coverage includes preventive services recommended for infants, children, and adolescents by the U.S. Health Resources and Services Administration's Bright Futures project. In addition to immunizations and other screening services, these include behavioral and developmental assessments; irons and fluoride supplements; and screening for autism, vision impairment, lipid disorders, tuberculosis, and diabetes. Under the ACA, all insurance marketplace plans and many other plans must cover the following list of preventive services without charging a copayment or coinsurance. This is true even if the yearly deductible has not been met. This applies only when these services are delivered by a network provider.

Coverage for Children's Preventive Health Services

All Marketplace health plans and many other plans must cover the following list of preventive services for children without charging you a copayment or coinsurance (This is true even if you haven't met your yearly deductible.):

- Autism screening for children at 18 and 24 months
- Behavioral assessments for children at the following ages: 0 to 11 months, 1 to 4 years, 5 to 10 years, 11 to 14 years, 15 to 17 years
- Blood pressure screening for children at the following ages: 0 to 11 months, 1 to 4 years, 5 to 10 years, 11 to 14 years, 15 to 17 years
- Cervical dysplasia screening for sexually active females
- Depression screening for adolescents
- Developmental screening for children under age 3
- Dyslipidemia screening for children at higher risk of lipid disorders at the following ages: 1 to 4 years, 5 to 10 years, 11 to 14 years, 15 to 17 years
- Fluoride chemoprevention supplements for children without fluoride in their water source
- Gonorrhea preventive medication for the eyes of all newborns
- Hearing screening for all newborns
- Height, weight, and body mass index measurements for children at the following ages: 0 to 11 months, 1 to 4 years, 5 to 10 years, 11 to 14 years, 15 to 17 years
- Hematocrit or hemoglobin screening for children
- Hemoglobinopathies or sickle cell screening for newborns
- HIV screening for adolescents at higher risk
- Hypothyroidism screening for newborns

(continues)

AFFORDABLE CARE ACT (ACA) (*continued*)

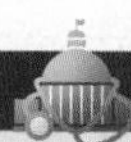

- Immunization vaccines for children from birth to age 18; doses, recommended ages, and recommended populations vary:
  - Diphtheria, tetanus, pertussis
  - Haemophilus influenzae type b
  - Hepatitis A
  - Hepatitis B
  - Human papillomavirus
  - Inactivated poliovirus
  - Influenza (flu shot)
  - Measles, mumps, rubella
  - Meningococcal
  - Pneumococcal
  - Rotavirus
  - Varicella
- Iron supplements for children ages 6 to 12 months at risk for anemia
- Lead screening for children at risk of exposure
- Medical history for all children throughout development at the following ages: 0 to 11 months, 1 to 4 years, 5 to 10 years, 11 to 14 years, 15 to 17 years
- Obesity screening and counseling
- Oral health risk assessment for young children ages: 0 to 11 months, 1 to 4 years, 5 to 10 years
- Phenylketonuria (PKU) screening for this genetic disorder in newborns
- Sexually transmitted infection (STI) prevention counseling and screening for adolescents at higher risk
- Tuberculin testing for children at higher risk of tuberculosis at the following ages: 0 to 11 months, 1 to 4 years, 5 to 10 years, 11 to 14 years, 15 to 17 years
- Vision screening for all children.

Source: U.S. Centers for Medicare & Medicaid Services. (2014). Preventive health services for children. Retrieved from https://www.healthcare.gov/what-are-my-preventive-care-benefits/children

APPLICATION TO PRACTICE

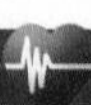

Ben is a 16-year-old, Hispanic male with severe asthma. Originally diagnosed at 6 months of age, Ben's asthma has escalated in severity over the past 3 years. He has experienced multiple emergency department visits and hospitalizations, often requiring intensive care.

Ben's parents are divorced. He lives with his father but often spends time at his mother's home or at his maternal grandmother's residence. Ben has experienced many school absences throughout this academic year as a result of the persistent nature of his symptoms and frequent need for hospitalization. He thinks his grades are suffering because of his absences. Ben's usual asthma triggers include dust, cigarette smoke, upper respiratory infection, and weather change.

Ben is currently being discharged after a 3-day hospitalization for an asthma exacerbation. One week before admission, Ben began to experience nasal congestion and cough. On the day of admission, he developed labored breathing and wheezing despite increased use of his albuterol inhaler. In the emergency department, Ben did not respond to continuous albuterol nebulizer treatments and was transferred to the pediatric intensive care unit. His condition gradually improved with supportive medical therapy. Because of Ben's anxiety associated with his asthma attacks, the psychiatry service was consulted and relaxation therapy was initiated.

At the time of discharge Ben was feeling well, with peak-flow readings of 560 before and after albuterol treatments.

Chest examination at discharge revealed an occasional expiratory wheeze but was otherwise clear to auscultation. His discharge medications included the following: prednisone 30 mg/day orally; fluticasone (Flovent) twice daily; nedocromil (Tilade) metered-dose inhaler (MDI) 2 puffs twice daily; albuterol MDI 2 puffs every 6 hours, increasing to 2 puffs every 4 hours for cough or wheeze. A community health nursing referral was initiated.

1. What lifestyle changes might you recommend to Ben and his family for avoiding his asthma triggers? Be sensitive to his family situation and needs and consider cultural influences.
2. Education about asthma and its management is an essential part of your care. Develop a teaching plan for Ben and his family including learning objectives, content, and appropriate teaching strategies.
3. His father is very concerned about Ben's absences from school and the work that he has missed. Which options might you consider for approaching this problem? How might you work with school personnel to help Ben remain in school?
4. Community-based, comprehensive service programs are needed to provide the full continuum of required services to asthmatic children and their families. Describe the role of the community health nurse in advocating for and developing such services. Which resources are available in your community?

LEVELS OF PREVENTION 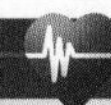

Primary: Teaching a program about using safe toys for new parents

Secondary: Screening for lead poisoning in toddlers

Tertiary: Teaching family about recognizing signs and symptoms of complications from diabetes in their newly diagnosed child

HEALTHY ME 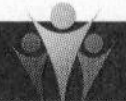

As a child, how did your parents or caregivers provide for your health care? How does this affect your role as a nursing student when working with children?

Critical Thinking Activities

1. Is it necessary for prospective parents to be prepared for pregnancy and parenthood?
2. The United Nations Convention on the Rights of the Child suggests that a woman planning on becoming pregnant should be in a state of optimal health. She should schedule a pre-conception health examination (including a review of nutritional status); have a plan for regular prenatal care with early detection and treatment of complication and have a plan for managing day-to-day demands during pregnancy; be free from infections and chemical agents that may affect the sperm, ovum, and fetus; be emotionally, psychologically, and economically committed to being a parent and be socially connected with a supportive network and living in a community that values the rights of children.
   - Are these suggested conditions feasible?
   - What are the social implications of these recommendations?
   - Do these recommendations conflict with the rights of individuals as they have been operationalized?
   - What is the role of the community health nurse in education and advocacy regarding the bases for these recommended conditions?
   - What role should nurses play when working with families who do not meet these conditions?

References

Agency for Healthcare Research and Quality (AHRQ). (2007). *Highlights of AQRH children's health care quality findings*. Retrieved from http://www.ahrq.gov/research/findings/factsheets/children/child-qfindings/index.html

American Academy of Allergy, Asthma & Immunology (AAAAI). (2014). *Asthma statistics*. Retrieved from http://www.aaaai.org/about-the-aaaai/newsroom/asthma-statistics.aspx

Anthony, E., Vu, C., & Austin, M. (2008). TANF child-only cases: Identifying the characteristics and needs of children living in low-income families. *Journal of Children & Poverty, 14*(1), 1–20.

Bateson, T. E., & Schwartz, J. (2008). Children's response to air pollutants. *Journal of Toxicology and Environmental Health, 71*(3), 238–243.

Behrens, D., Lear, J. G., & Price, O. A. (2013). Improving access to children's mental health care: Lessons from a study of eleven states. Retrieved from http://healthinschools.org/School-Based-Mental-Health/Eleven-State-Report.aspx

Blackburn, A. C. (2009). *Stories, ethics and the interpretation of meaning: Bearing witness to mothers' stories of their neonatal intensive care unit experience*. Ann Arbor, MI: ProQuest, UMI Dissertation Publishing.

Borders, A. E. B., Grobman, W. A., Amsden, L. B., & Holl, J. L. (2007). Chronic stress and low birth weight neonates in a low-income population of women. *Obstetrics & Gynecology, 109*(2, part 1), 331–338.

Bronfenbrenner, U. (1979). *The ecology of human development: Experiments by nature and design*. Cambridge, MA: Harvard University Press.

Brooten, D., Kumar, S., Brown, L. P., Butts, P., Finkler, S. A., Bakewell-Sachs, S., ... Delivoria-Papadopoulos, M. (1986). A randomized clinical trial of early hospital discharge and home follow-up of very-low-birthweight infants. *New England Journal of Medicine, 315*(15), 934–939.

Bureau of Labor Statistics, U.S. Department of Labor, *The Editor's Desk*. (2013). Happy Mother's Day from BLS: Working mothers in 2012. Retrieved from http://www.bls.gov/opub/ted/2013/ted_20130510.htm

Cancian, M., Slack, K. S., & Yang, M. Y. (2010). The effect of family income on risk of child maltreatment (Institute for Research on Poverty Discussion Paper No. 1385-10). Retrieved from http://www.irp.wisc.edu/publications/dps/pdfs/dp138510.pdf

Center on the Developing Child at Harvard University. (2011). *Building the Brain's "Air Traffic Control" System: How Early Experiences Shape the Development of Executive Function: Working Paper No. 11*. Retrieved from www.developingchild.harvard.edu

Center on the Developing Child at Harvard University. (2012). *The Science of Neglect: The Persistent Absence of Responsive Care Disrupts the Developing Brain: Working Paper 12*. www.developingchild.harvard.edu

Centers for Disease Control and Prevention (CDC). (2012). National action plan for child injury prevention. Retrieved from http://www.cdc.gov/safechild/pdf/National_Action_Plan_for_Child_Injury_Prevention.pdf

Centers for Disease Control and Prevention (CDC). (2013a). HPV. Retrieved from http://www.cdc.gov/vaccines/vpd-vac/hpv/downloads/dis-HPV-color-office.pdf

Centers for Disease Control and Prevention (CDC). (2013b). National, state, and local area vaccination coverage among children aged 19-35 months—United States, 2012. *Morbidity and Mortality Weekly Report*, *62*(36), 733–740. Retrieved from http://www.cdc.gov/mmwr/preview/mmwrhtml/mm6236a1.htm

Centers for Disease Control and Prevention (CDC). (2013c). *Suicide prevention: A public health issue.* Retrieved from http://www.cdc.gov/violenceprevention/pdf/asap_suicide_issue2-a.pdf

Centers for Disease Control and Prevention (CDC). (2013d). Mental health surveillance among children—United States, 2005–2011. *Morbidity and Mortality Weekly Report*, *2*(Suppl 2), 1–35.

Centers for Disease Control and Prevention (CDC). (2014). National Center for Chronic Disease Prevention and Health Promotion, Division of adolescent and school health. *Lesbian, Gay, Bisexual and Transgender Health.* Retrieved from http://www.cdc.gov/lgbthealth/youth.htm

Centers for Disease Control and Prevention (CDC). *Pregnancy Mortality Surveillance System.* Retrieved from http://www.cdc.gov/reproductivehealth/MaternalInfantHealth/PMSS.html

Centers for Medicare & Medicaid Services (CMS). (2014). *Readmissions reduction program.* Retrieved from http://www.cms.gov/Medicare/Medicare-Fee-for-Service-Payment/AcuteInpatientPPS/Readmissions-Reduction-Program.html

Chase-Lansdale, P. L. (1997). Neighborhood and family influences on the intellectual and behavioral competence of preschool and early school-age children. In G. J. Duncan, J. Brooks-Gunn, & J. L. Aber (Eds.), *Neighborhood poverty* (vol. *1*). New York, NY: Russell Sage Foundation.

Chen, A. Y., Kim, S. E., Houtrow, A. J., & Newacheck, P. W. (2010). Prevalence of obesity among children with chronic conditions. *Obesity*, *18*(1), 210–213. Retrieved from http://onlinelibrary.wiley.com/doi/10.1038/oby.2009.185/pdf

Cohen, B., & Reutter, L. (2007). Development of the role of public health nurses in addressing child and family poverty: A framework for action. *Journal of Advanced Nursing*, *60*(1), 96–107.

Coiro, M. J., Zill, N., & Bloom, B. (1994). Health of our nation's children. *Vital Health Statistics*, *10*, 191.

Colley, J. R. T., & Reid, D. D. (1970). Urban and social origins of childhood bronchitis in England and Wales. *British Medical Journal*, *2*, 213–217.

Collins, J. J., Kasap, H. S., & Holland, W. W. (1971). Environmental factors in child mortality in England and Wales. *American Journal of Epidemiology*, *93*, 10–22.

Cook, J. R., & Kilmer, R. P. (2004). Evaluating systems of care: Missing links in children's mental health research. *Journal of Community Psychology*, *32*(6), 655–674.

Dunne, E. F., Markowitz, L. E., Chesson, H., Curtis, C. R., Saraiya, M., Gee, J., & Unger, E. R. (2011). Recommendations on the use of quadrivalent human papillomavirus vaccine in males. Advisory Committee on Immunization Practices (ACIP), 2011. *Morbidity and Mortality Weekly Report*, *60*(50), 1705–1708.

Durani, Y., Friedman, M. J., & Attia, M. W. (2008). Clinical predictors of respiratory syncytial virus infection in children. *Pediatrics International*, *50*(3), 352–356.

Engelke, M. K., Swanson, M., & Guttu, M. (2013). Process and outcomes of school nurse case management for students with asthma. *The Journal of School Nursing*, *30*(3), 195–205.

Federal Bureau of Investigation (FBI). (2012). *Uniform crime report: Crime in the United States, 2012.* Retrieved from http://www.fbi.gov/about-us/cjis/ucr/crime-in-the-u.s/2012/crime-in-the-u.s.-2012

Federal Interagency Forum on Child and Family Statistics (FIFCFS). (2013). *America's Children: Key National Indicators of Well-Being, 2013.* Washington, DC: U.S. Government Printing Office. Retrieved from http://www.childstats.gov/pdf/ac2013/ac_13.pdf

Graham, N. M. J., Ryan, P., & Douglas, R. M. (1990). Acute respiratory illness in Adelaide children. II: The relationship of maternal stress, social supports and family functioning. *International Journal of Epidemiology*, *19*(4), 937–940.

Greenspan, A. I., Dellinger, A. M., & Chen, J. (2010). Restraint use and seating position among children less than 13 years of age: Is it still a problem? *Journal of Safety Research*, *41*, 183–185.

Grey, M., Berry, D., Davidson, M., Galasso, P., Gustafson, E., & Melkus, G. (2004). Preliminary testing of a program to prevent type 2 diabetes among high-risk youth. *Journal of School Health*, *74*(81), 10–15.

Grundstein, A., Dowd, J., & Meentemeyer, V. (2010). Quantifying the heat-related hazard for children in motor vehicles. *Bulletin of the American Meteorological Society*, *91*, 1183–1191.

Guthrie, B. (2007). An inconvenient truth. *Journal for Specialists in Pediatric Nursing*, 213–214.

Harsten, G., Prellner, K., & Heldrup, J. (1990). Acute respiratory tract infections in children: A three year follow-up from birth. *Acta Paediatrica Scandinavia*, *79*, 402–409.

Hatzenbuehler, M. L. (2011). The social environment and suicide attempts in lesbian, gay, and bisexual youth. *Pediatrics*, *127*(5), 896–903. Retrieved from http://pediatrics.aappublications.org/content/127/5/896.full.pdf+html

Henggeler, S. (2003). Advantages and disadvantages of multisystemic therapy and other evidence-based practices for treating juvenile offenders. *Journal of Forensic Psychology Practice*, *3*(4), 53–59.

Hinds, P. S., Oakes, L., Furman, W., Quargnenti, A., Olson, M. S., Foppiano, P., & Srivastava, D. K. (2001). End-of-life decision making by adolescents, parents, and healthcare providers in pediatric oncology: Research to evidence-based practice guidelines. *Cancer Nursing*, *24*(2), 122–134.

Holzer, H., Schanzenbach, D., Duncan, G., & Ludwig, J. (2008). The economic costs of childhood poverty in the United States. *Journal of Children & Poverty, 14*(1), 41–61.

Hoyert, D. L., & Xu, J. (2012). Deaths: Preliminary data for 2011. *National Vital Statistics Reports, 61*(6), 1–52. Retrieved from http://www.cdc.gov/nchs/data/nvsr/nvsr61/nvsr61_06.pdf

Kataoka, S. H., Stein, B. D., Jaycox, L. H., Wong, M., Escudero, P., Tu, W., ... Fink, A. (2002). A school-based mental health program for traumatized Latino immigrant children. *Journal of the American Academy of Child and Adolescent Psychiatry, 42*(3), 311–319.

Key, J. D., Washington, E. C., & Hulsey, T. C. (2002). Reduced emergency department utilization associated with school-based clinic enrollment. *Journal of Adolescent Health, 30*(4), 273–278.

Kids Count Data Center. (2012). Retrieved from datacenter.kidscount.org

Klebanov, P. K., Brooks-Gunn, J., Chase-Lansdale, P. L., & Gordon, R. A. (1997). Are neighborhood effects on young children mediated by features of the home environment? In J. Brooks-Gunn, G. J. Duncan, & J. L. Aber (Eds.), *Neighborhood poverty: Context and consequences for children* (vol. I, pp. 119–145). New York, NY: Russell Sage.

Klebanov, P. K., Brooks-Gunn, J., McCarton, C., & McCormick, M. C. (1998). The contribution of neighborhood and family income to developmental test scores over the first three years of life. *Child Development, 69*(5), 1420–1436.

Le Blanc, L., Swisher, R., Vitaro, F., Suppl Tremblay, R. E. (2007). school social climate and teachers' perceptions of classroom behavior problems: A ten-year longitudinal and multilevel study. *Social Psychology of Education, 10*(4), 429–442.

Lewis, T., & Hession, C. (2012). Alcohol use: From childhood through adolescence. *Journal of Pediatric Nursing, 27*, e50–e58.

Liu, J. (2004). Childhood externalizing behavior: Theory and implications. *Journal of Child Adolescent Psychiatric Nursing, 17*(3), 93–103.

Liu, J. (2011). Early health risk factors for violence: Conceptualization, review of the evidence, and implications. *Aggression and Violent Behavior, 16*(1), 63–73.

Massey, D. S., & Kanaiaupuni, S. M. (1993). Public housing and the concentration of poverty. *Social Science Quarterly, 74*(1), 109–122.

Matthews, T. J., & MacDorman, M. F. (2013). Infant mortality statistics from the 2010 period linked birth/infant death data set. *National Vital Statistics Report, 62*(8), 1–26.

Melnyk, B. M., Alert-Gillis, L., Feinstein, N. F., Crean, H. F., Johnson, J., Fairbanks, E., ... Corbo-Richert, B. (2004). Creating opportunities for parent empowerment: Program effects on the mental health/coping outcomes of critically ill young children and their mothers. *Pediatrics, 113*(6), 597–607.

Muscar, J. (2008). Advocating the end of juvenile boot camps: Why the military model does not belong in the juvenile justice system. *UC Davis Journal of Juvenile Law and Policy, 12*(1), 2–50.

National Scientific Council on the Developing Child. (2005/2014). *Excessive Stress Disrupts the Architecture of the Developing Brain: Working Paper 3*. Updated Edition. Retrieved from www.developingchild.harvard.edu

Nersesian, W. S., Petit, M. R., & Shaper, R. (1985). Childhood death and poverty: A study of all childhood deaths in Maine, 1976 to 1980. *Pediatrics, 75*, 41–50.

Ogden, C. L., Carroll, M. D., Kit, B. K., & Flegal, K. M. (2012). Prevalence of obesity and trends in body mass index among US children and adolescents, 1999–2010. *Journal of the American Medical Association, 307*(5), 483–490.

Olds, D. L., & Kitzman, H. (1993). Review of research on home visiting for pregnant women and parents of young children. *Future of Children, 3*(Winter), 53–92.

Olds, D. L., Kitzman, H., Knudtson, M. D., Anson, E., Smith, J.A., & Cole,. R. (2014). Effect of Home Visiting by Nurses on Maternal and Child Mortality: Results of a 2-Decade Follow-up of a Randomized Clinical Trial. *JAMA Pediatrics, 168*(9):800–806. doi:10.1001/jamapediatrics.2014.472

Olds, D., Donelan-McCall, N., O'Brien, R., MacMillan, H., Jack, S., Jenkins, T., ... Beeber, L. (2013). Improving the nurse-family partnership in community practice. *Pediatrics, 132*(Suppl), S110–S117. Retrieved from http://pediatrics.aappublications.org/content/132/Supplement_2/S110.full.html

Press, I. B. (1994). *The epidemiology of childhood disorders*. New York, NY: Oxford University Press.

Prentice, S. (2007). Less access, worse quality. *Journal of Children & Poverty, 13*(1), 57–73.

Radner, J. M., & Shonkoff, J. P. (2012). Mobilizing science to reduce intergenerational poverty. In N. O. Andrews & D. J. Erickson (Eds.), *Investing in what works for America's communities* (pp. 338–350). San Francisco , CA: Federal Reserve Bank of San Francisco and Low Income Investment Fund.

Rodgers, Jr., H., & Payne, L. (2007). Child poverty in the American states: The impact of welfare reform economics, and demographics. *Policy Studies Journal, 35*(1), 1–21.

Shonkoff, J. P., & Fisher, P. A. (2013). Rethinking evidence-based practice and two-generation programs to create the future of early childhood policy. *Development and Psychopathology, 25*(4, part 2), 1635–1653.

Shonkoff, J. P., & Phillips, J. A. (Eds.). (2000). *From neurons to neighborhoods: The science of early childhood development*. Washington, DC: National Academies Press.

Spencer, M. E. (1977). History and sociology: An analysis & Weber's The city. *Sociology, 11*(3), 507–525.

Strahan, B. E., & Elder, J. H. (2013). Obesity in adolescents with autism spectrum disorders. *Research in Autism Spectrum Disorders, 7*, 1497–1500.

Stroul, B. A., & Friedman, R. M. (1986). *A system of care for children and youth with severe emotional disturbances* (rev. ed.). Washington, DC: Georgetown University Child Development Center, CASSP Technical Assistance Center.

The Center on Alcohol Marketing and Youth (CAMY). (2010). Youth exposure to alcohol advertising on television: 2001 to 2009. Washington, DC: The Center on Alcohol Marketing and Youth.

Toole, K. P. (2013). Helping children gain asthma control: Bundled school-based interventions. *Pediatric Nursing, 39*(3), 115–124.

Taveras, E. M., Gillman, M. W., Kleinman, K. P., Rich-Edwards, J. W., & Rifas-Shiman, S. L. (2013). Reducing racial/ethnic disparities in childhood obesity: The role of early life risk factors. *Journal of the American Medical Associates Pediatrics, 167*(8), 731–738. Retrieved from http://archpedi.jamanetwork.com/article.aspx?articleid=1692336

U.S. Department of Health and Human Services (HHS). (2013a). *Healthy People 2020: Immunization and infectious diseases overview*. Retrieved from http://www.healthypeople.gov/2020/topicsobjectives2020/overview.aspx?topicid=23

U.S. Department of Health and Human Services (HHS). (2013a). *Healthy People 2020: Maternal, infant, and child health*. Retrieved from http://healthypeople.gov/2020/LHI/micHealth.aspx?tab=data

U.S. Department of Health and Human Services (HHS). (2013b). *Child maltreatment 2012*. Retrieved from http://www.acf.hhs.gov/sites/default/files/cb/cm2012.pdf#page=16.

U.S. Department of Health and Human Services (HHS). (2013c). *Child abuse and neglect fatalities 2011: Statistics and interventions*. Retrieved from https://www.childwelfare.gov/pubs/factsheets/fatality.pdf

U.S. Department of Health and Human Services (HHS). (2014). *Healthy People 2020 leading health indicators: Progress update*. Retrieved from http://www.healthypeople.gov/2020/LHI/LHI-ProgressReport-ExecSum.pdf

U.S. Department of Transportation, National Highway Traffic Safety Administration (NHTSA). (2012). Traffic Safety Facts 2010: Children. Washington (DC): NHTSA.

Wagmiller, R. L., Kuang, L., Aber, J. L., Lennon, M. C., & Alberti, P. M. (2006). The dynamics of economic disadvantage and children's life chances. *American Sociological Review 71*(5), 847–866.

Waters, E., de Silva-Sanigorski, A., Burford, B. J., Brown, T., Campbell, K. J., Gao, Y., ... Summerbell, C. D. (2011). Interventions for preventing obesity in children. *Cochrane Database of Systematic Reviews, 12*(CD001871). doi: 10.1002/14651858.CD001871.pub3.

Webster-Stratton, C., Jamila, R. M., & Stoolmiller, M. (2004). Preventing conduct problems and improving school readiness: Evaluation of the Incredible Years teacher and child training programs in high-risk schools. *Journal of Child Psychology and Psychiatry and Applied Health Disciplines 59*(5), 471–488.

Webster-Stratton, C., & Reid, J. (2014). Parent, teacher and child interventions: Tailoring the incredible years for young children with ADHD. In J. K. Ghuman & H. S. Ghuman (Eds.), *ADHD in Preschool Children: Assessment and Treatment*. New York, NY: Oxford University Press.

Wong, J. R., Harris, J. K., Rodriquez-Galindo, C., & Johnson, K. (2013). Incidence of childhood and adolescent melanoma in the United States: 1973–2009. *Pediatrics, 131*(5), 846–854.

Yoos, H. L., McMullen, A., Bezek, S., Hondorf, C., Berry, S., Herendeen, N., ... Schwartzberg, M. L. (1997). An asthma management program for urban minority children. *Journal of Pediatric Health Care, 11*, 66–74.

Yoshikawa, H., Weiland, C., Brooks-Gunn, J., Burchinal, M. R., Espinosa, L. M., Gormley, W. T., ... Zaslow, M. J. (2013). *Investing in our future: The evidence base on preschool education*. Retrieved from http://fcd-us.org/sites/default/files/Evidence%20Base%20on%20Preschool%20Education%20FINAL.pdf

CHAPTER FOCUS

Aging
- Aging Terminology
- Aging and Health

Nursing of Elders
- Older Adults in the Community
- Older Adults in the Family
- Older Adults as Individuals

Preventive Health Care
- Sensory Integrity
- Nutrition and Sleep
- Elimination
- Mobility and Communication
- Cognition and Affect
- Employment and Retirement
- Thermal Regulation and Skin Integrity
- Comfort and Spirituality

Special Older Adult Health Issues
- Immunizations
- Medications
- Chemical Addictions
- Ethical Dilemmas

QUESTIONS TO CONSIDER

After reading this chapter, you will know the answers to the following questions:

1. What are the various meanings of *aging*?
2. What are the major health concerns of the aging population?
3. How are ideas and misconceptions about aging related to the care of older adults?
4. What are the major preventive health issues of the older adults?
5. What are specific intervention strategies for the community health nurse in promoting the health of older adults?
6. What are special health considerations that the community health nurse should be aware of in caring for older adults?
7. Which ethical issues are involved when working with older adults?

Community health nurses in the 21st century face the challenge of caring for an unprecedented number of people in the "older adult" age category. The first post–World War II baby boomers reached 65 in 2011, and 10,000 Americans will turn 65 each day for the next 20 years! The last of the baby boomers will turn 65 in 2030; by then, one in five people will be 65 or older. By 2050, it is anticipated that the number of Americans age 65 and older will more than double the number in this age category in 2010. The people who comprise this population are diverse- in terms of health status, culture, and expectations. Two-thirds of older Americans have multiple chronic illnesses and require more healthcare services than any other age group.

CHAPTER 34

Older Adults

Virginia Lee Cora and Cindy Luther

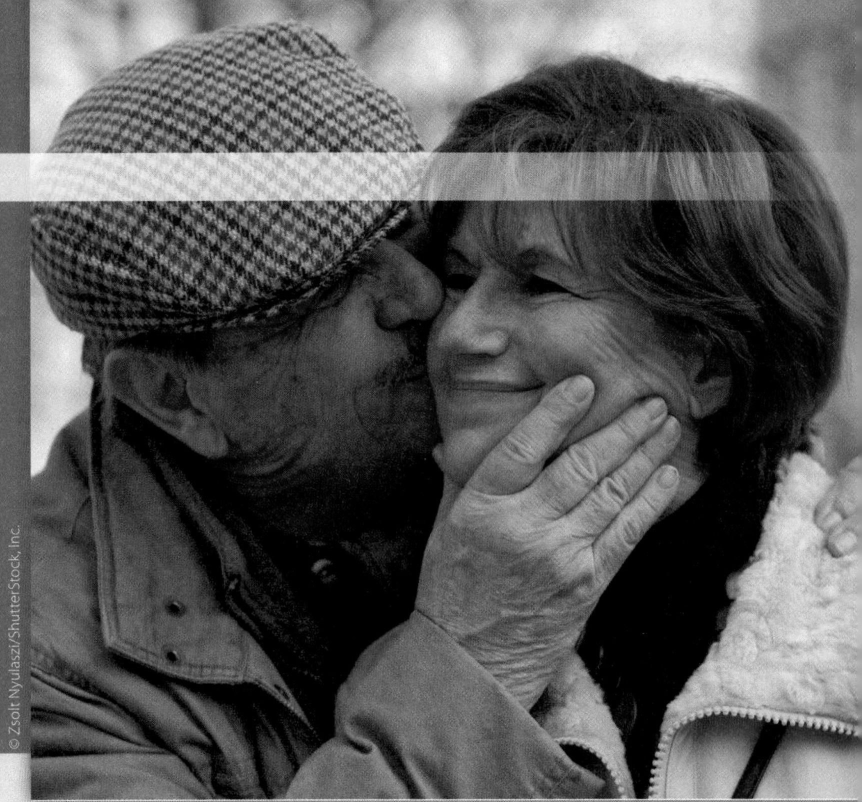

KEY TERMS

activity of daily living (ADL)
advance directives
age
ageism
aging
Alzheimer's disease
cohort
confusion
delirium
dementia
depression
elder abuse (maltreatment)
elder neglect
geriatrics
gerontology
instrumental activity of daily living (IADL)
life expectancy
life review
lifespan
longevity
mild cognitive impairment
osteoporosis
PLISSIT model
polypharmacy
presbycusis
presbyopia
respite care
senescence

> Just remember, once you're over the hill, you pick up speed.
>
> —Charles Schultz

> You can't help getting older.
> But you don't have to get old.
>
> —George Burns

REFLECTIONS

When we are younger, it was almost impossible to imagine what it was like to grow old, lose some of our physical strength, and face sensory limitations and the reality of our own mortality. What is your idea of growing old? How do you see yourself at age 65? At age 85? Are you comfortable with older people? What is your experience living or working with people older than yourself?

IN CARING FOR OLDER ADULTS, nurses cannot look to the past for direction because never have so many people lived to age 65 and older. Traditionally, all persons who survived childhood and adolescence were grouped together as "adults." Only in the last generation have healthcare providers begun to realize that older adults represent a unique population with healthcare needs requiring specialized knowledge and skills. Old ways of thinking about aging and models of caring for older adult populations are outdated. Promoting functional capacity, mobility, independence, dignity, and self-care are fundamental goals of care of older adults.

In the past, most of society's investments in health care have focused on child and adult healthcare issues. Health care for older adults has had greater emphasis on institution-based, disease-focused strategies, and little attention has been paid to preventive, holistic, care and "aging-in-place." Yet, home- and community-based alternatives are becoming the norm for older adults, and nurses provide the leadership to promote independence and the highest possible quality of life for older adults and their families. Addressing these evolving views of aging and health from the perspective of community health nursing is the focus of this chapter on older adults and their families. With the passage of the Patient Protection and Affordable Care Act (ACA), more older adults will be living outside of traditional institutions than ever before, as care changes to one that is home and community based.

Aging

Older adults differ from young and middle-aged adults in many ways. Persons 80 years old are not the same as persons 20 or 50 years old. **Aging** is the sum of all the changes that normally occur in a person with the passage of time; it begins at conception and ends at death. Aging is a natural, lifelong, and total process that varies among individuals and within various domains and organ systems of each individual. Aging is *universal*—it occurs at different rates and degrees; *progressive*—it interferes with lifestyle; *decremental*—it has a general gradual decline; and *intrinsic*—it is unmodifiable, as opposed to *extrinsic* (modifiable by lifestyle changes) (Blazer & Steffens, 2009).

Nurses have opportunities to influence the health status of older adults by identifying genetic predispositions in family health histories, using data from screening tests, and teaching lifestyle changes to alter risk factors and ensure safety. For example, if the patient's family history includes heart disease in both parents and a sibling, total cholesterol levels greater than 200, and low-density lipoprotein (LDL) levels greater than 100, the nurse might encourage dietary modifications and exercise; the primary care provider (physician, practitioner, or physician's assistant) might prescribe pharmacological therapies.

Aging Terminology

Age is the length of time a person has existed. **Lifespan** is the maximum potential for survival of a particular species. The maximum duration of existence for a human being currently is believed to be 115 to 120 years.

Life expectancy ("expected life") is the average observed years of life of a species from birth to death or at any stated age. American males born in 2010 have an estimated life expectancy of 76 years, an increase of 5 years from 20 years previously. A man reaching age 65 in 2010 can expect to live, on average, until age 82, while women turning age 65 in 2010 can expect to live, on average, to age 85. Approximately one of four of those 65-year-olds will live past the age of 90, and one of 10 will live past age 95 (National Center for Health Statistics [NCHS], 2013).

In his memoir, *An Hour Before Daylight*, former U.S. President Jimmy Carter (2001) recalled the type of nursing his mother practiced:

> Since we lived several miles from town among neighbors who were very poor and whose best transportation, if any, was a mule and wagon, my mother cared for many of them almost as a doctor, often providing both diagnosis and treatment. There may have been other nurses who did this, but I never heard of it. Mama was a special person, who refused to acknowledge most racial distinctions and spent many hours with our black neighbors. She never charged them anything for her help, but they would usually bring her what they could afford—a shoat, some chickens, a few dozen eggs, or perhaps blackberries or chestnuts.

> I'm not afraid of growing old, because I am. That's just a fact of life. I'm not out to 'arrest' life, the way some people do. I'm living with it. That's a part of your journey, that's part of who you are. You carry it with you.
>
> *—Robert Redford, actor, reflection on turning 60 years of age*

The life expectancy during the Stone Age was 15 years; in the time of Hippocrates (460–377 B.C.), it was about 18 years; in the time of George Washington (1732–1799), it was 30 years; in the time of Florence Nightingale (1820–1910), it was 50 years. The "graying of America" refers to the longer life expectancy of the U.S. population.

Longevity ("long life") usually is the expected length of an individual's life, based on the lives of their immediate family members. **Senescence** ("grown old") is the last stage of a lifelong process of aging. In the United States, old age, or senescence, was designated by the 1935 Social Security Act as being over age 67.

Cohort is a group of people who share a particular age, historical moment, or geographical area (i.e., born between 1900 and 1920, in the Depression era, during the baby boom, or in an urban ghetto). Cohorts of people who share experiences of a certain place or period tend to develop similar attitudes and values (e.g., the frugality seen in many elders who survived the Great Depression and awareness of personal rights of baby boomers).

Older adults usually are persons age 65 years or older. They often are referred to as *pre-old* at ages 55 to 64 years, *young-old* or "almost-old" at ages 65 to 74 years, *middle-old* or "already-old" at ages 75 to 84 years, *old-old* or "very-old" at ages 85 and over, and *elite-old*—the centenarians 100 years and older (Ebersole, Hess, Touhy, & Jett, 2005).

Geriatrics (*geras*, "old age"; *iatros*, "physician") is the branch of health science concerned with the diseases and problems of old age. **Gerontology** (*geron*, "old man"; *logos*, "word") is the study of old age and aging.

Aging and Health

With this country's many advantages, most Americans are able to live long enough to grow old. As community health nurses, we must examine our own attitudes and values about aging and older people to gain holistic, realistic views and provide age-appropriate care for this population.

Aging does not equal health. The changes associated with normal aging are differentiated from the changes associated with health problems. For example, a 65-year-old may be confined to bed with end-stage rheumatoid arthritis, while an 85-year-old may run a marathon (26.2 miles).

Aging is a comprehensive process. It is not only an accumulation of biological changes, but also a complex series of psychosocial, socioeconomic, and spiritual changes that influence and are influenced by the individuals, their families, communities, and society. Any changes that affect one domain simultaneously affect all other domains.

Old age is a time of continued growth, development, and fulfillment (i.e., achieving self-actualization or ego integrity). This culmination of the life cycle is a balance of both gains and losses in the processes of change. As with other transitional periods of life, old age is a time of holding on and letting go.

The older adult population is heterogeneous and diverse. Human beings tend to be more homogeneous (similar) at birth and become quite heterogeneous (different) in old age. As with other age or ethnic groups, the nurse must avoid simplistic generalizations and neither romanticize older adults nor stigmatize them. Rather, we must balance their positive aspects with their negatives to accept them as they are with specific health problems countered by many real strengths.

Older adults are tough. Very few elders are frail; a great majority are hardy, vigorous, and active through the very end of their lives. They are not *victims* of aging processes, but rather *survivors* of life's experiences as part of family systems within their environment.

Nursing of Elders

The "age wave" of baby boomers began arriving throughout the first decade of the 21st century. Society needs well-educated and experienced nurses to meet the challenge of providing care to this ever-increasing, complex segment of the population. In providing holistic care, community health nurses consider older adults within the context of their community, their family, and their individual selves. Recent disasters in the United States, such as Hurricane Katrina, demonstrate the need of society to recognize the specific needs of older adults as compared to the younger population. In New Orleans, Hurricane Katrina caused unprecedented damage to property and demands for mass evacuation of an entire city. Disaster plans had not included the special issues related to the older adult population, such as mobility, driving ability, awareness of disaster risk, and specific health needs. As a result, many older adults remained in their homes or long-term care facilities, had limited ability to evacuate to safe shelters, and made up a large percentage of those who died. This is but one example of society's failure to address the complexities and unique risks of this vulnerable population.

Older Adults in the Community

The status and roles of older people in the community are influenced by the values placed on aging by society. In some cultures, elders and their collective wisdom are held in very high esteem; in other cultures, old age exemplifies loss of productivity, loss of status, and stigmatization. **Ageism** is the systematic stereotyping of and discrimination against people because they are old (Butler, 2003). Learned at an early age, these prejudices may surface in younger people's negative beliefs about older people as well as in the older persons' beliefs about themselves. These views can influence the outcomes of health care. For example, older adults may be viewed as too old for surgical procedures, even though most tolerate surgery well. A person with a dementing illness may have needs for pain relief or comfort measures that are overlooked. Nurses and caregivers can unintentionally contribute to dependency and declines in function by using "elderspeak" (terms of endearment) or "doing for" older adults what they could do for themselves, given assistance and time. Nurses need to be aware of ageism in themselves and others, and confront it as they would racism or sexism through education about the realities of old age, both positive and negative.

Demography of Elders

The aging population is growing by both absolute and relative numbers (U.S. Census Bureau, 2010). The old-old (age 85 and older) are the fastest growing segment of the population, having increased in number by more than 1 million between 2000 and 2010, representing a growth rate of almost 30% (by way of comparison, the population of persons 65–85 years old grew by only 12.6%). The oldest old are projected to reach 8.7 million by 2030, representing an increase of nearly 50% from 2010.

Older women have long outnumbered older men, and the skewed gender ratio increases by age: in the 2010 census, women made up 54% of those 65–74, 58% of those 75–84, and 67% of those 85 and older. However, the gap is decreasing: projections for 2030 and 2050 anticipate that the gap will narrow significantly in all age groups, although the oldest old will remain over 60% female (U.S. Census Bureau, 2010). Most older men (74.5%) are married, and most older women (55.5%) are not (U.S. Census Bureau, 2012).

The older adult population in the United States also is becoming more racially, ethnically, and culturally diverse. Older adults of various cultural groups may have different responses to health problems, modifiable risk factors, and health-promotion activities such as education. Community health nurses need to determine the distributions and values of elderly populations within their area and figure out how these cultural differences affect health care. For example, older family members may be immigrants to the United States. They may not understand or speak English; they may not be literate in any language. These individuals may delay seeking health care because of fear of the system.

The distribution of the elderly population is biased 4:1 rural over urban settings. Rural elders are the oldest old, are poorer, and have more chronic illnesses, compounded by greater problems with access, transportation, and inadequate healthcare facilities.

Economically, the median annual income of older adult men and women is $25,877 and $15,282, respectively. Only 8.9% are below the poverty line, but 27% are near poor. Women account for 74% of poor elders; blacks account for 24% of these poor. The major source of income for older adults is the federal Social Security program; more than half have pensions, and 19% have private pensions. Eight percent are on public assistance, 6% receive food stamps, and 12% have Medicaid.

As many as 50% to 80% of older adults have inadequate *functional health literacy*—that is, they are unable to read prescription bottle labels, comprehend health literature and appointment slips, complete health insurance forms, follow diagnostic test instructions, and perform other reading comprehension tasks (Williams et al., 1995).

Because of their economic status, disabilities, or social needs, many elders resort to a wide variety of living arrangements, including senior housing units, home sharing, home equity conversion, group homes, "granny flats," and others. Although only 4.5% of U.S. elders age 65 live in nursing homes, at age 85 years 18.2% live in these facilities, with more women and Caucasians than men or other ethnic groups being part of this population (U.S. Census Bureau, 2012). A growing variety of alternative housing arrangements and number of facilities for frail and/older adults with dementing illnesses are emerging. These newer services include adult daycare centers, personal care homes, assisted-living facilities, and dementia care units.

With regard to healthcare access, the older adult population accounts for 36% of U.S. healthcare expenditures. Although only 12% of the total U.S. population, older adults account for approximately 39% of patients in hospitals, 69% of home health patients, and 88% of nursing home residents (Centers for Disease Control and Prevention [CDC], 2011, 2013a). For the older adult population, *Healthy People 2020* goals are to maintain their health and functional independence and compress morbidity and dependence into the shortest possible time. The 10 leading health indicators (i.e., physical activity, overweight and obesity, tobacco use, substance abuse, responsible sexual behavior, mental health, injury and violence, environmental quality, immunization, and access to health care) all have implications for older adults. Community health nurses can help address the need for more health education and programs for older adults. For example, only 30% of elders participate in moderate physical activity (e.g., walking, gardening) and less than 10% in vigorous physical activity.

Walk with Me

Long ago I was a young man
I had children and friends
Remember?
Moments I recall slip away.
Brown and gray
  Orange and green still life
Between paper and plastic
Memories
  child, wife, mother
Fade
Remember for me.

—*Ann Thedford Lanier*

HEALTHY PEOPLE 2020 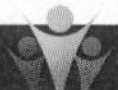

- OA-1 Increase the proportion of older adults who use the Welcome to Medicare benefit
- OA-2 Increase the proportion of older adults who are up to date on a core set of clinical preventive services
- OA-3 Increase the proportion of older adults with one or more chronic health conditions who report confidence in managing their conditions
- OA-4 Increase the proportion of older adults who receive Diabetes Self-Management Benefits
- OA-5 Reduce the proportion of older adults who have moderate to severe functional limitations
- OA-6 Increase the proportion of older adults with reduced physical or cognitive function who engage in light, moderate, or vigorous leisure-time physical activities
- OA-7 Increase the proportion of the healthcare workforce with geriatric certification

Long-Term Services and Supports

- OA-8 Reduce the proportion of noninstitutionalized older adults with disabilities who have an unmet need for long-term services and supports
- OA-9 Reduce the proportion of unpaid caregivers of older adults who report an unmet need for caregiver support services
- OA-10 Reduce the rate of pressure ulcer–related hospitalizations among older adults
- OA-11 Reduce the rate of emergency department (ED) visits due to falls among older adults
- OA-12 Increase the number of states, the District of Columbia, and tribes that collect and make publicly available information on the characteristics of victims, perpetrators, and cases of elder abuse, neglect, and exploitation

Objectives Related to Older Adults

Selected objectives for older adults are summarized in the *Healthy People 2020* box. Some programs and organizations concerned with improving the living situations and health of older persons are identified in **Box 34-1**.

Older Adults in the Family

As the basic social unit mediating between the individual person and the whole of society, the family is the focus of intervention for older adults in the community. A family is "a social system of multiple, interdependent generations of persons who identify each other as being related by birth, marriage, adoption, or mutual consent, as being committed to one another over time, and as having common properties, rights, and responsibilities" (Cora, 1985). By helping families maintain positive attitudes toward aging, nurses can assist older adults to enjoy their longevity and life experiences. Elders then give their families one final gift: a positive model of old age.

Aging Families

Aging families are assessed according to their structure, functions, or development, or as systems that encompass all of these attributes. No matter the setting, older adults should be approached as members of multigenerational families.

Even when older adults live alone, their families influence their needs, behaviors, and health care. When assessing older adults' families, nurses may need to develop brief genograms of immediate, distant, or extended family members to understand their beliefs and values and explain their behaviors. Nurses may need to help contact these family members to establish support systems for older adults with frailty or dementing illnesses or to create surrogate families to assist with health care.

Family Caregivers

As part of the intergenerational family life process, family members accept responsibility in times of crisis. More than 42.1 million family caregivers provide ongoing daily assistance to an older adult fam-

BOX 34-1 Federal Programs

- Social Security Act of 1935: Social Security Administration (SSA); Old Age, Survivors, and Disability Insurance (OASDI); Social Security (SS); Supplemental Security Income (SSI).
- Older Americans Act (OAA) of 1965: Administered by the U.S. Department of Health and Human Services' (HHS) Administration on Aging (AoA), it provides state and area agencies on aging with multipurpose senior centers (social, recreational, educational, and nutritional services for senior citizens), senior employment and volunteer programs (ACTION: Foster Grandparents, RSVP, Senior Companions), senior nutrition programs, health education and prevention activities, senior transportation services, and in-home health care. Call the National Institute on Aging Information Center (800-222-2225) or Eldercare Locator (800-677-1116) for more information.
- Research on Aging Act of 1974: Created the National Institute on Aging (NIA) within the National Institutes of Health; publishes a resource guide for older Americans (*Age Pages*).
- Centers for Medicare and Medicaid Services (CMS): Administers Medicare and Medicaid insurance programs.
- Department of Agriculture: Offers food and nutrition programs, including food stamps.
- Department of Veterans Affairs: Provides services and benefits to veterans.
- Department of Housing and Urban Development: Provides low-cost public housing for elders.
- Department of Treasury, Internal Revenue Service (IRS): Offers assistance with income tax problems and filing.
- Department of Interior: Provides access to federal park system; Gold Age Passports (free), Golden Eagle Passports (low-cost).

National Private and Voluntary Nonprofit Organizations

- National Council on Aging (NCOA): Established in 1950 as a national resource for information, consultation; sponsors publications, special programs, advocacy activities, research, training, Health Promotion Institute.
- American Association of Retired Persons (AARP): largest nonprofit, nonpartisan membership organization in the world; purpose is to enhance quality of life for older persons; promote independence, dignity, and purpose for older persons; provide leadership in determining the role of older persons in society; and improve the image of aging; members are 50 or older; provides *Modern Maturity* magazine and *AARP Bulletin* for news; and driver safety program, tax assistance, health insurance, mail-order drugs, information.
- Andrus Foundation on gerontological research.
- American Society on Aging (ASA): Enhances knowledge and skills of those working with older adults and their families.
- Gerontological Society of America (GSA): A multidisciplinary professional and scientific organization for those working in the field of gerontology.
- American Geriatrics Society
- Alzheimer's Association
- Geriatric Advanced Practice Nurses Association (GAPNA)
- Gray Panthers: Founded by Maggie Kuhn (1905–1995) who said, "Speak your mind. Even if your voice shakes, well-aimed slingshots can topple giants. . . . The best age to be is the age you are." An intergenerational activist group dedicated to social change.

ily member, and 61.6 million—one-fifth of the total U.S. population—provide at least temporary care (AARP, 2011). The average age of caregivers is 46 years. These individuals often represent the "sandwich generation"—adults who may be raising children and caring for older adults at the same time, often while working outside the home. However, persons 65 years and older comprise 12% of caregivers. More than 2.4 million grandparents also are raising 4.5 million grandchildren—20% of them without assistance from either parent (AARP, 2011). More than 73% of the caregivers are female; two-thirds are working.

Most caregivers provide assistance with at least one **instrumental activity of daily living (IADL)**, about one-half assist with one **activity of daily living (ADL)**, and one-third help with at least three ADLs. Most view caregiving as having some impact on family life, leisure time, work life, and personal finances. They also see caregiving as an overall positive experience (AARP, 2011).

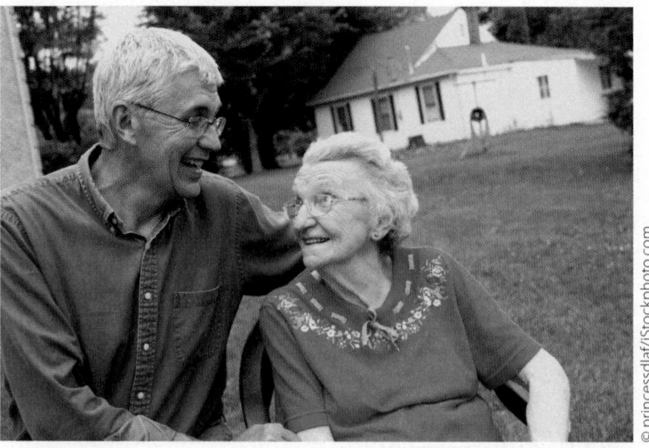

More women than men survive, and the very old are often cared for by their older children.

Community health nurses need to assess caregivers for their *competence* (i.e., caregiving knowledge, skills, confidence, and objectivity), *burden* (number of hours of caregiving per day/week, nature of tasks to be completed), and *burnout* (psychological stress related to nature of illness and necessary care and support system). Because many caregivers are older adults themselves, their own health issues needs to be addressed, especially if they are too frail to give care. When problems are identified, caregivers may need to expand their support systems through family, friends, or community agencies (e.g., home health social services, area agencies on aging, religious groups). Caregivers may need assistance to manage financial and legal concerns, or they may benefit from participation in caregiver groups for their educational and social support. Those who are caregivers to people with dementing illnesses, such as Alzheimer's disease, may benefit from support groups and resources, such as "hotline" services, offered by the Alzheimer's Association.

Respite care provides family members with temporary relief of caregiving responsibilities. The availability of these services varies widely in rural and urban areas and across different regions of the country. Respite may be offered in the home by other family members, religious organizations, or federal or state programs; alternatively, this service may be offered in institutional settings by adult daycare centers, assisted-living facilities, or nursing homes. Social workers may be helpful in locating respite services in various communities, or the community health nurse may need to help create opportunities for respite for overburdened caregivers.

Elder Abuse, Exploitation, and Neglect

With most caregiving for older adults occurring in homes, community health nurses must be aware of the potential for abusive, dysfunctional family relationships. More than 1 million elderly women are victims of abuse each year. They often fail to report maltreatment because of shame, fear of retaliation, or previous unsatisfactory experiences with police, district attorneys, or social workers who may have lacked sensitivity to the concerns and needs of older people. As a form of domestic violence, **elder abuse** or **maltreatment** is defined by the CDC (2014) as "any abuse and neglect of persons age 60 or older by a caregiver or another person in a relationship involving an expectation of trust." This fairly broad definition encompasses not only physical and sexual abuse and neglect, but also financial malfeasance, isolation, abandonment, intimidation, and emotional abuse, all of which have been identified as additional means by which older adults may be mistreated by family members, caregivers, or acquaintances. **Elder neglect** refers to older adults who are either living alone and not able to provide for themselves the services that are necessary to maintain physical and mental health or are not receiving necessary services from responsible caretakers (O'Malley, 1987). Types of elder maltreatment are described in **Table 34-1**.

TABLE 34-1 Types of Elder Maltreatment

Types	Behaviors of Abusers and/or Elders
Abuse	
Physical or sexual	Slapping, pushing, restraining, molesting
Psychological	Threats, intimidation
Exploitative	Misappropriation of funds or property
Medical	Withholding necessary medications, treatments, or assistive devices
Neglect	
Passive	Unintentional lack of caregiving because of lack of knowledge and/or skills
Active	Abandonment or intentional failure to provide caregiving
Self-neglect	Intentional or unintentional lack of attention to self-care

Maltreatment occurs with 5% to 10% of elders, typically by family members. The most frequently abused, exploited, and neglected elders are those who are frail, confused, and dependent with functional disabilities; are older than 70 years of age, female, and of minority status; and have poor social networks. The abuse often is invisible—it is repeated, not reported. Adult protective service laws require mandatory or voluntary reporting of suspected abuse or neglect in all states. Also, older adults can be abusive to their family members and caregivers. Sensitivity to these dysfunctional family relationships is essential for community health nurses.

Nurses who encounter older adults in the community have opportunities to assist with both primary and secondary prevention of elder maltreatment. The goals of primary prevention are to support caregivers and reduce the potential for abuse. The goals of secondary prevention are early case finding of abusive situations and crisis intervention, referrals, and follow up with elders and family caregivers. Techniques for interventions in the maltreatment of elders are summarized in **Box 34-2**.

Older Adults as Individuals

The goals of health care for individual older adults are to maximize independence and to minimize dependence. For nurses working directly with older adults in the community, the focus of intervention is on health promotion and primary prevention to maintain autonomy of the older

BOX 34-2 Techniques for Intervention in the Maltreatment of Elders

Primary Prevention

- Be aware of the risk factors for potentially abusive situations—in both elders and caregivers (e.g., frailty, confusion, dependence, functional disabilities, age 70+ years, female, minority status, poor social networks).
- Provide anticipatory guidance to help families plan for future needs of frail and/or demented elders.
- Broaden support systems for families with dependent elders by involving other family and friends in caregiving activities.
- Teach families stress management techniques and provide information about caregiving and local resources (e.g., caregiver classes, support groups, respite and day care, financial aid, counseling).

Secondary Prevention

- Observe for physical injuries (e.g., bruises, lacerations, burns, fractures, pressure sores, malnutrition, poor hygiene, dehydration, recurring injuries) and/or psychological damage (e.g., unusual fears, caregiver not letting elder be alone with providers).
- Ask direct questions while alone with the older adult: "Has anyone tried to hurt you or make you do things you didn't want to do?"
- Do a complete physical examination, including the skin, head, neck, breasts, abdomen, genitals, and rectum.
- Document findings with the person's own words, detailed descriptions, and, if possible, photographs of injuries.
- Assess the severity and frequency of the abuse and the safety of the elder. Report findings to adult protective services. If potentially lethal, make immediate referrals (call the police).
- Provide follow up with the elder and family, because many abusive situations are repetitive.

adults as members of family systems with their environment. Emphasis is on the individuals' abilities (i.e., what can be built upon) rather than disabilities (i.e., what's been lost). Functional ability depends on individual characteristics and the setting/environment. The healthcare provider's role is to enhance coping ability by careful clinical assessment and management of remediable problems and by facilitating changes in the environment to maximize function in the face of those problems that remain (Kane, Ouslander, & Abrass, 2003).

NOTE THIS!

Elders Have Their Own Dreams

John Glenn, Oseola McCarty, and Lillian Carter are well known public figures who pursued their dreams throughout their lives. Each took different paths toward realizing their dreams as they grew older.

John Glenn took his first ride in space in 1962, becoming the first man to orbit the earth. Thirty-six years later, he became the oldest person in space when at the age of 77 he returned as part of the crew of the *Discovery*. When Glenn went into space in 1962 as a young man, the thought of sending a 77-year-old into orbit seemed unthinkable; today it is not only possible but expected. Glenn states, "Just because we grow older, doesn't mean we give up our dreams."

Ms. Oseola McCarty never set out to get attention. McCarty, a tiny 87-year-old woman, washed clothes all her life. She lived a simple life, never married, and never had children, yet amazingly she was able to amass a small fortune of $250,000. When she donated $150,000 to the University of Southern Mississippi (USM) to fund scholarships for African American students, she was surprised at the reaction. Her generosity so touched people the world over that she became a cultural heroine. She shared the spotlight with Oprah Winfrey and Jesse Jackson and received the Presidential Citizen's Medal from President Bill Clinton. She simply said, "If you can help somebody, help them." She had dreamed of a future in nursing but was forced to drop out of school in the 6th grade. The University of Southern Mississippi College of Nursing made her an honorary graduate of its nursing program in 1996. Because of Miss McCartney's generosity, Ted Turner was inspired to give $1 billion to the United Nations.

Lillian Carter, mother of President Jimmy Carter, was a retired RN at the age of 68 when she joined the Peace Corps and served as a nurse in Bombay, India, for 2 years.

Older adults usually exhibit multiple health problems with complex interactions. As a consequence, healthcare interventions often require multidisciplinary approaches. Nurses work in collaboration with primary care providers (e.g., physicians, nurse practitioners, physician assistants), therapists (e.g., physical, occupational, and speech therapists), pharmacists, dietitians, social workers, psychologists, and many others. Health care for these elders must consider the issues of access, quality, and cost.

In the community, providers of health care become integral to the older adult's environment. Nurses may be viewed as friendly visitors or surrogate family members rather than as healthcare providers. Nurses must be aware of factors that foster dependency, including their own attitudes and behaviors. The aversion to risk of healthcare providers, families, and the elders themselves can bias thinking toward conservative interventions without a full consideration of quality-of-life issues (Kane et al., 2003). For example, fear of falling in an elder may lead to a suggestion of using a wheelchair, which promotes further deconditioning, rather than emphasizing walking to strengthen muscles and improve balance and gait. Nurses can help keep older adults as active and healthy as possible, encourage their independence, and support their health decisions.

Chronic Illness

The cost of surviving the acute illnesses and injuries of young and middle age is the chronic illnesses of old age. Approximately two of three older adults have multiple chronic conditions. Common conditions include diabetes, arthritis, asthma, chronic respiratory disease, heart disease, hypertension, depression, chronic kidney disease, and Alzheimer's disease. People who have multiple chronic diseases often see multiple specialists and are at risk for conflicting medical advice, duplicative tests, and adverse drug effects (CDC, 2013b).

With the focus of nursing for health promotion being on self-care, a universal prescription for patients of every age, including older adults, is reduction of health risks. In the United States, ample evidence shows that we are living better as well as longer. The disability rate, although high for older adults, has been falling steadily since the early 1980s. All of this improvement is most likely the result of the improved treatment of disease and the accelerated study of aging. A growing body of knowledge confirms that chronic illness and disability are not inevitable consequences of aging, as previously believed, but result from unhealthy lifestyle choices, such as smoking, obesity, sedentary lifestyle, or poor adaptation to stress. The way we age is often more dependent on how we live than who our parents are.

NOTE THIS!

President George W. Bush turned 60 in 2006. He was in good company among the baby-boomer generation that, many have said, changed the world. Among those who turned 60 in 2006: Bill Clinton, Cher, Dolly Parton, Donald Trump, Reggie Jackson, and Jimmy Buffett. Bush was among the first wave of the 78 million strong baby boomers to enter their senior years. Upon turning 60, Bush remarked that, while he considered 60 practically "ancient" when he was younger, he has been inspired by changing circumstances and has adjusted his perspective: "It's all in your mind. It's not that old, it really isn't."

Assessment of Older Adults

Nurses in community health emphasize wellness with the goal of maintaining optimal function—physically, mentally, socially, and spiritually—so as to be as independent as possible for as long as possible. The four primary domains of geriatric assessment are functional ability, physical health, mental health, and socioenvironmental factors.

Functional Assessment As a measure of physical and mental abilities to manage ADLs and IADLs, functional assessment is an important parameter for determining an older adult's potential for self-care at home (see Appendix B). In addition to self-reports by the older adult and family member(s), the ability to perform the ADLs needs to be observed by the nurse by having the individual perform as many of these activities as possible (e.g., putting on a button-front shirt, getting on the toilet, picking up a penny). Individuals' risk for falls is assessed by checking balance and gait (see Appendix C).

Physical Assessment In the physical assessment of older adults, emphasis is placed on those areas that most directly affect functional ability (i.e., vision, hearing, strength). The health history for older adults must include frequent inquiries about exercise, nutrition, medications, substance use (tobacco, alcohol, caffeine), incontinence, memory, depression, social activities, and isolation. In addition to the usual height, weight, and vital signs, blood pressures need to be checked sitting, lying, and standing for orthostatic hypotension. Along with the usual adult physical examination, vision and hearing, mouth, skin, breasts (women), prostate (men), and feet need to be checked regularly. Nurses should be aware that the normal values for diagnostic laboratory tests and other physical findings may differ between younger and older adults. For example, uric acid and alkaline phosphatase increase slightly with age; erythrocyte sedimentation rate (ESR) and C-reactive protein increase significantly with age.

Mental Assessment The assessment of mental health in older adults focuses primarily on memory and mood. The Folstein, Folstein, and McHugh (1975) Mini-Mental State Examination is an 11-item instrument designed to screen five areas of cognitive functioning: orientation, registration, attention and calculation, recall, and language and praxis. Scores may be adjusted for educational and visual deficits, but generally a score of 24 to 30 indicates no cognitive impairment, 18 to 23 is mild impairment, and 0 to 17 is severe impairment (see Appendix D). The Clock Drawing Test, a performance test of freehand clock drawing, measures constructional skills and visual–spatial abilities, usually with scoring on a 10-point system.

TABLE 34-2 Recommended Primary and Secondary Disease Prevention for People Age 65 and Older

Preventive Strategy	Frequency
U.S. Preventive Services Task Force (USPSTF) or CDC[a] Recommendations for Primary Prevention	
Bone mineral density (BMD) (women)	At least once after age 65
Blood pressure (BP) screening	Yearly
Diabetes mellitus (DM) screening	Every 3 years in people with BP > 135/80 mmHg
Exercise, vitamin D supplementation	Adults age 65 or older at increased risk of falls
Herpes zoster immunization	Once after age 60 in immunocompetent people[b]
Influenza immunization	Yearly
Lipid disorder screening	Every 5 years, more often in coronary artery disease (CAD), DM, peripheral artery disease (PAD), prior stroke
Obesity (height and weight)	Yearly
Pneumonia immunization	Once at age 65[c]
Smoking cessation	At every office visit
Tetanus immunization	Every 10 years
USPSTF[a] Recommendations for Secondary Prevention	
Abdominal aortic aneurysm (AAA) ultrasonography	Once between age 65 and 75 in men who have ever smoked
Alcohol abuse screening	Unspecified but should be done periodically
Depression screening	Yearly
Fecal occult blood test (FOBT)/sigmoidoscopy/colonoscopy	Yearly/every 5 years/every 10 years from age 50 to age 75[d]
Mammography[e]	Every 2 years in women age 50–74
Other[f] Recommendations for Primary Prevention	
Aspirin (ASA) to prevent myocardial infarction (MI)[g]	Daily
BMD (men)	At least once after age 70
Calcium (1200 mg) and vitamin D (≥ 800 IU) to prevent osteoporosis	Daily
Measurement of serum C-reactive protein	At least once in people with one CAD risk factor
Omega-3 fatty acids to prevent MI, stroke	At least twice weekly
Multivitamin	1–2 times per day
Other[f] Recommendations for Secondary Prevention	
Skin examination	Yearly
Cognitive impairment screening	Yearly
Electron-beam CT	At least once in people at intermediate risk (5–20% over 10 years) of a coronary event
Glaucoma screening	Yearly
Hearing impairment screening	Yearly

(continues)

TABLE 34-2 Recommended Primary and Secondary Disease Prevention for People Age 65 and Older *(continued)*

Preventive Strategy	Frequency
Inquiry about falls	Yearly
Thyroid-stimulation hormone (TSH) in women	Yearly
Visual impairment screening	Yearly

The USPSTF recommends against screening for:

- Asymptomatic bacteriuria with urinalysis (UA)
- Bladder cancer with hematuria detection, bladder tumor antigen measurement, NMP22 urinary enzyme immunoassay, or urine cytology
- CAD with ECG, exercise treadmill test, or electron-beam CT in people with few or no CAD risk factors
- Carotid artery stenosis with duplex ultrasonography
- Cervical cancer in women age 65 or older who have had adequate prior screening or who have had a hysterectomy for benign disease
- Colon cancer with FOBT/sigmoidoscopy/colonoscopy in people 85 years old or older. Screening may be modestly beneficial in people 76–85 years old with long life expectancy and no or few comorbidities.
- Chronic obstructive pulmonary disease (COPD) with spirometry
- Ovarian cancer with transvaginal ultrasonography or CA-125 measurement
- PAD with measurement of ankle-brachial index (ABI)
- Pancreatic cancer with ultrasonography or serologic markers
- Prostate cancer with prostate-specific antigen (PSA) and/or digital rectal examination

Cancer Screening and Medical Decision Making

- Many decisions about whether or not to perform preventive activities are based on the estimated life expectancy of the patient.
- Most cancer screening tests do not realize a survival benefit for the patient until after 5 years from the time of the test. Cancer screening should be discouraged or very carefully considered in patients with 5 or fewer years of estimated life expectancy.

[a] See http://www.ahrq.gov/clinic/uspstfix.htm and http://www.cdc.gov/vaccines/schedules/hcp/adult.html.

[b] May vaccinate patients 1 year after zoster infection; patients on chronic acyclovir, famciclovir, or valacyclovir treatment should discontinue the medication 24 hours before zoster vaccination and resume the medication 14 days after vaccination.

[c] Consider repeating pneumococcal vaccine every 6–7 years.

[d] Do not repeat colorectal cancer screening (by any method) for 10 years after a high-quality colonoscopy is negative in average-risk individuals.

[e] Mammograms to age 70 are almost universally recommended; many organizations recommend that mammography should be continued in women over 70 who have a reasonable life expectancy.

[f] Not endorsed by USPSTF/CDC for all older adults, but recommended in selected patients or by other professional organizations.

[g] Use with caution in adults 80 years old or older.

Source: Reuben, D. B., Herr, K. A., Pacala, J. T., Pollock, B. G., Potter, J. F., & Semla, T. P. (2013). *Geriatrics at your fingertips* (15th ed.). New York, NY: American Geriatrics Society.

The 30-item Yesavage and Brink (1983) Geriatric Depression Scale is used to screen for depression in elders with intact cognition or only mild cognitive impairment (MCI) (see Appendix E). The 15-item short form is used for initial screening and, if depression is indicated by missing 5 or more items, the remaining 15 items are administered. Depression is suspected if the elder misses 11 or more items on the full instrument. Elders with significant mental/emotional impairments are referred to their primary care provider for further evaluation and treatment.

MEDIA MOMENT

Driving Miss Daisy **(1989)**

This four-time Academy Award–winning story about a strong-willed Southern matron, Daisy Werthan (Jessica Tandy), and her elderly chauffeur, Hoke (Morgan Freeman), is based on Alfred Uhry's Pulitzer Prize–winning play. It is a contest of wills as the pair learn that for two people so different, they have much in common. The bumpy road they travel ultimately leads to the friendship of a lifetime.

Socioenvironmental Assessment Socioenvironmental factors are assessed to identify family and living situations, social support systems, financial status, and environmental hazards. A home and community safety checklist may be administered on the initial visit and periodically thereafter to monitor for the hazards contributing to accidents, falls, and injuries (see Appendix F).

NOTE THIS!

Clinical Pearls for the Community Health Nurse (Virginia Lee Cora)

- *Ten pennies make one dime.* Loss of independence in elders may be the result of many subtle changes accumulated over time rather than sudden, dramatic events. Look for multiple simple interventions (the pennies) to support existing strengths and maximize function (the dime). For example, correcting poor vision, losing a few pounds of excess weight, and strengthening deconditioned extremities through a walking program may enable elders threatened with impending relocation to become more mobile and remain in their own homes living independently.
- *Never ask an elder's age.* Rather than ask elders their ages, ask when they were born to identify their cohort. This fact provides rich information about the physical, psychological, and social factors that have influenced elders' lives. For example, to know a man is 97 in 2014 identifies him as old-old; to know he was born in 1917 places him at the end of the Great Depression and prior to World War II during his early adulthood while trying to establish work and family roles.
- *Listen to be heard.* Community health nurses usually are younger than their elderly patients. There is a tendency for nurses to "preach" about health care and for elders to "turn off" these young "know-it-alls." After all, elders are the survivors of many hardships in their life experience (not victims). If you are talking more than 50% of the time, you are not listening. To avoid this common pitfall, each nurse needs to center the self; ask clarifying questions and then listen to the elder's answers; reinforce the positive and support the elder's control, and then listen to the elder's concerns; verify understandings and then listen to the elder's responses; reinforce outcomes and enable maximum autonomy, and, yes, *listen* to the elder!
- *To hydrate elders, encourage them to drink fluids in small, frequent amounts.* Offer a 4- to 6-ounce juice glass every 1 to 2 hours; or provide a 1-pint, covered plastic mug to be sipped frequently between breakfast and lunch, refilled, and consumed again between lunch and supper; or a half-gallon plastic carton of water kept in the refrigerator and drunk throughout the day. Avoid fluids after the evening meal to reduce nocturia.
- *Be realistic about weight management goals for elders.* Rather than using ideal body weight (IBW), ask about the usual body weight (UBW) at about age 30 to 50 to establish more individualized goals for gaining or losing weight.
- *For health teaching with elders, remember the four S's:* Start Small and Stay Simple. Take more time, break content into smaller units, present one idea at a time, be concrete (not abstract), increase repetitions (three to seven times), and use more than one modality (visual, verbal, and written).
- *Be aware of bowel function.* Any time an elder presents with anorexia, nausea and vomiting, constipation, abdominal pain, loose stool, fecal incontinence, urinary retention or incontinence, confusion, delirium, fever, dysrhythmia, or tachypnea, inquire about the last bowel movement and check for a fecal impaction.
- *Teach elders to use it or lose it.* "The right amount of exercise in old age is 'more than yesterday.' If you don't do it today, you can't do it tomorrow."

AFFORDABLE CARE ACT (ACA) 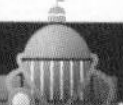

With the passage of ACA, Medicare beneficiaries have increased access to preventive healthcare benefits, including a Welcome to Medicare preventive visit and an Annual Wellness Visit. The ACA increased access to preventive services, including preventive visits for review of medications, family and personal history, identification of risk factors, and coverage for screening tests, immunizations, and self-management education. (http://www.medicare.gov/coverage/preventive-and screening)

A community assessment can be completed as described elsewhere in this text.

Interpreting Assessment Data In analyzing the findings of geriatric assessments, nurses must remember that the effects of normal aging are continuously being redefined. The presentation of signs and symptoms of illnesses in older adults may be atypical. They may under- or over-report symptoms of illnesses or have multiple, nonspecific complaints that require explication. Older adults may have a decreased tolerance for stress, yet have difficulty communicating their health needs.

Preventive Health Care

In providing preventive health care for older adults in the community, nurses can use 16 verbs (eight verb sets) that represent basic functions. These eight verb sets are easily understood by older adults and their families and provide a framework for a functional approach to this section on preventive health care.

How well does the elder:

- See and hear?
- Eat and sleep?
- Eliminate bladder and bowel?
- Walk and talk?

- Think and feel?
- Work and play?
- Heat/cool and touch/feel?
- Hurt and believe?

Sensory Integrity

The older adult depends on accurate perception of environmental information from all the senses to maintain independence. Interventions to maximize perception are essential for success in living alone or with families. In addition to regular assessment of vision and hearing, the community health nurse needs to be aware of the potential for sensory overload or sensory isolation in elders.

Vision

Normal aging is associated with increasing impairment of vision, most commonly a progressive farsightedness called **presbyopia**. In addition, four major ocular diseases frequently are seen in persons older than age 75: cataracts, macular degeneration, glaucoma, and diabetic retinopathy (Kane et al., 2003). Approximately 92% of adults older than age 65 wear eyeglasses; however, the vision of only 65% of those older than 85 is corrected well enough to be able to recognize a friend across the street or read newsprint. Yellowing of the lens reduces color clarity so that reds, oranges, and yellows are seen more clearly than greens, blues, and purples. Decreased lens elasticity and pupil size (miosis) decrease accommodation and contribute to central ("tunnel") vision and night blindness. Diminished lacrimation may cause xerophthalmia ("dry eyes"). Loss of skin elasticity may result in entropion (inversion) or ectropion (eversion) of the eyelids, both of which are associated with conjunctivitis and blindness.

Visual acuity should be assessed annually. Individuals with scores greater than 20/40 should be referred to an ophthalmologist. Correction typically involves magnification with bifocal glasses.

Hearing

Because of its implications for social interactions and safety, hearing is an essential component of sensory integrity. Hearing impairment is the most common sensory problem experienced by older adults: It occurs in 25–30% of people older than 60, especially males. It is the most poorly recognized and undercorrected sensory deficit. Only 25% of those who might benefit from a hearing aid actually use one (Cobb, Duthie, & Murphy, 2002). The most common impairment of aging is **presbycusis**, a gradual, progressive bilateral sensorineural hearing loss of predominately higher frequencies and impairment of speech discrimination (especially the consonants *f*, *s*, *th*, *h*, and *sh*). Hearing sensitivity may be assessed with the simple whisper test: whisper random numbers about 12 inches from each ear while covering the opposite ear. Older adults with hearing deficits require referral to an audiologist for amplification with a hearing aid or an assistive listening device.

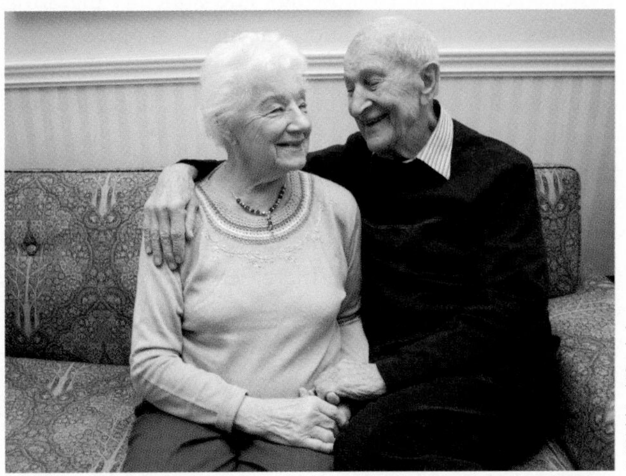

Healthy elders often find assisted living facilities provide them with privacy, modified and accessible compact living quarters, and supervision of health issues by registered nurses on site.

Because of the increased viscosity of cerumen and coarseness of hairs lining the auditory canal, another common problem found in older adults is cerumen impaction. A simple intervention is to soften the earwax daily for 3 or 4 days with an over-the-counter (OTC) cerumenolytic agent and then irrigate with warm water until the wax is removed (see the package instructions). Refer the older adult to a primary care provider if the impaction is not resolved.

Nutrition and Sleep

In every culture, food and meals have great social significance in addition to nutritional value. Changes in appetite and weight may be the first indicators of altered health status. A balance of activity and rest are important for feelings of wellbeing. Therefore, "eat and sleep" are functions to be assessed thoroughly and often in older adults.

Nutrition

Of community-dwelling elders, 15% to 50% are believed to have poor nutrition or be malnourished. Factors often associated with malnutrition in community-dwelling older adults include physical illness, medications, lack of hydration, social isolation, oral health problems, limited mobility, lack of transportation, poor vision, limited income, dementia, depression, and alcoholism.

The nutritional needs of adults change significantly with advanced age. For example, calorie requirements progressively decrease because of decreases in physical activity and metabolic rate. There is a decrease in the acuity and differentiation of taste and smell, which contributes to anorexia and malnutrition. With loss of salty and sweet tastes, foods taste more bitter and sour. Less volume and acidity of salivation contribute to xerostomia (dry mouth), dysphagia (difficult swallowing), and difficulty digesting starches. Loss of gingiva and wearing down of teeth contribute to gingivitis, loss of teeth, edentulism, ill-fitting dentures, and potentially mouth ulcers. Thinning of the esophageal wall and relaxation of the cardiac sphincter contribute to early satiety and dyspepsia, as do less mucin, decreased gastric juices, and slower peristalsis in the stomach. Thinning of the intestinal wall and slower peristalsis in the colon contribute to increased flatulence, polyps, and diverticula.

Changes in weight may be early indicators of health problems in older adults (e.g., depression, dementia, congestive heart failure, diabetes). Height and weight need to be measured to calculate the body mass index (BMI; 24 to 29 is ideal in older adults) during the initial assessment of the nutritional status. Then, on *every visit*, the weight is rechecked.

MEDIA MOMENT

What's Happening to Grandpa? (2004)

by Maria Shriver, New York, NY: Little, Brown

This book for children facing the challenge of having a grandparent with Alzheimer's disease helps children understand not only the disease, but also ways they can communicate and maintain a relationship with their grandparents. Shriver presents the relationship between a young girl and her grandfather. The book discusses the questions the granddaughter has about the changes produced by Alzheimer's disease, and ways, such as photos and scrapbooks, to stay connected throughout the progression of the disease. Resources for families facing this situation are also included.

The community health nurse can begin the nutritional assessment with a 3-day diet recall and calorie count. Consider *financial* (fixed income, buying habits), *physical* (transportation, limited mobility, poor vision), and *personal barriers* (food preparation, preferences, eating problems, medications). Oral assessment includes checking for ill-fitting dentures, lost teeth, periodontal disease, and the last dental visit. Home health nurses' assessments may include an inspection of refrigerator and pantry contents; the combined effects of sensory impairments, limited access to foods, and frugality often lead to consumption of foods that are unhealthy.

THINK ABOUT THIS

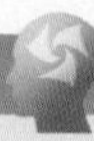

More baby boomers and middle-age Americans are getting motorcycles as the baby boomer generation continues to defy previous trends of "aging gracefully." Unfortunately, aging adults often buy more powerful machines than their aging and out-of-practice bodies can handle. From 2003 to 2012, the annual number of motorcycle fatalities among those age 65 and older in the United States increased by 201% (males increased by 194% and females increased by 333%), according to the National Highway Traffic Safety Administration.

Source: National Highway Traffic Safety Administration, 2014.

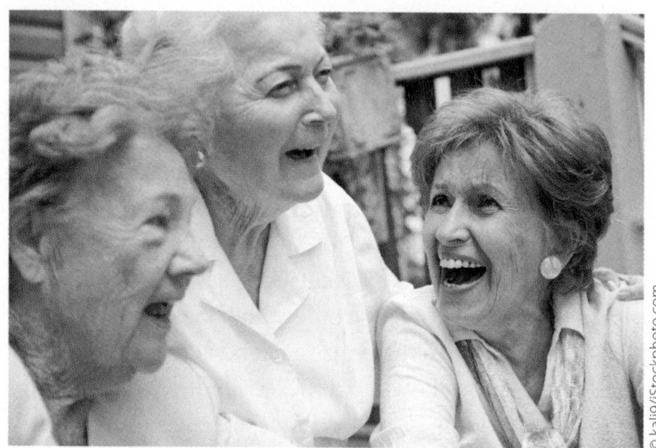

Elders are living longer than in generations past and are healthier than their predecessors.

Nutritional services might start with shopping assistance, which can be provided by family, friends, religious groups, senior centers, and local homemaker services. Grocery stores may offer senior parking and electric shopping carts. Community services include aggregate meal sites in senior centers, Meals on Wheels, area agencies on aging, and county extension services.

For older adults with limited income, stretching money to purchase both food and medications can be a challenge. They may buy easy-to-prepare "empty-calorie" foods rather than foods for a balanced diet. The nurse can suggest a variety of foods that will not break the budget: dried legumes, beans, whole cereal grains, poultry, fish, dried fortified milk, less expensive cuts of meat, low-fat cheeses, yogurt, and powdered instant breakfast mixes.

The goals for nutrition are to assist older adults to plan and provide a well-balanced diet with a variety of foods from each food group and to maintain a desirable weight. The goal of weight management is to help older adults approach an ideal body weight (IBW) for their age, sex, and body frame. As individuals age, they may involuntarily gain or lose weight and may need to stabilize their weight; or they may have a long history of being seriously overweight or underweight and now are experiencing health problems.

Underweight

For elders who are malnourished or underweight (BMI less than 20 or more than 10% *below* IBW), the goal is to increase the calorie intake, including taking a daily multivitamin with mineral supplementation. Loss of smell affects taste and enjoyment; loss of appetite may be from loneliness and depression.

Overweight

For elders who are obese or overweight (BMI greater than 29 or more than 20% *above* IBW), the weight management goals are to decrease calories and increase activity levels. Diets to promote weight loss generally limit intake to 1,500 to 1,800 calories per day (including a daily multivitamin with mineral supplementation) with adjustments for age, sex, and body frame. The lifestyle adjustments required for weight loss are difficult to accomplish and maintain at any age, and no less so with older adults. In addition to reducing amounts or eliminating certain types of foods, individuals must incorporate exercise into daily routines to achieve their goals. They are especially prone to fads and gimmicks rather than adjustment of lifelong eating and exercise patterns. Appetite suppressants are to be avoided; they may have serious side effects in older adults.

To assist with weight loss, many nutritionally sound, holistic commercial weight-loss programs (e.g., Weight Watchers) are available. Public television may offer low-impact exercise programs, such as chair aerobics. Community and religious groups also may offer weight-loss and exercise programs, or the nurse can facilitate the formation of a neighborhood weight-loss group. Whatever the approach, overweight older adults often need weight-loss programs that are relatively inexpensive, easily accessible, and socially supportive. Obese persons on weight-loss diets also need to be weighed weekly.

Hydration

Often overlooked as part of nutrition, adequate hydration is a key factor to prevent dehydration, soften stools, increase salivation and expectoration, maintain skin and renal function, and aid in absorption of medications and high-fiber foods. Older adults usually require at least 1.5 quarts (1,500 mL) of fluids per day, especially water. For diabetic or overweight elders or those who dislike the taste of water, sugar-free flavors added to water (e.g., Crystal Light, Sugar-Free Kool-Aid) can be encouraged.

Like infants, elders are particularly vulnerable to variations in fluid volume (overhydration or underhydration) because of their decreased cardiovascular and renal reserves. Signs of dehydration include weight loss; concentrated urine and decreased output; elevated temperature; sunken eyeballs; dry, parched, coated tongue; poor skin turgor; and dry mucous membranes. Depending on thirst for the intake of fluids is unreliable in older adults. A weight loss of 2% to 4% is considered mild dehydration, 5% to 9% is moderate dehydration, and 10% or more is severe (potentially lethal) dehydration. These individuals require immediate referral to their primary care provider for careful rehydration.

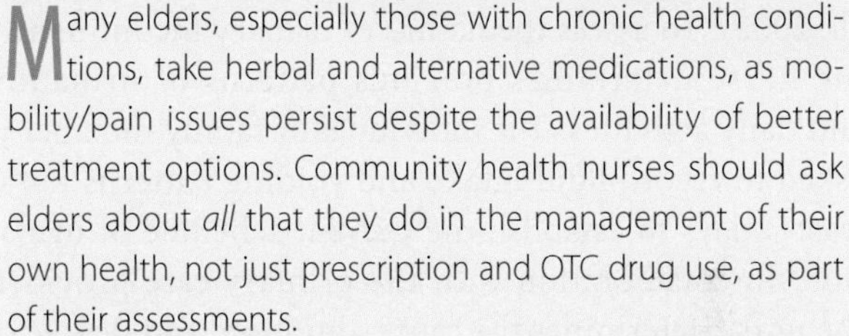

GOT AN ALTERNATIVE?

Many elders, especially those with chronic health conditions, take herbal and alternative medications, as mobility/pain issues persist despite the availability of better treatment options. Community health nurses should ask elders about *all* that they do in the management of their own health, not just prescription and OTC drug use, as part of their assessments.

Sleep

Adequate periods of sleep and rest are essential for the restoration of energy. Older persons commonly experience changes in sleep patterns and sleep structure. These changes can result in initial insomnia (disturbances and difficulty falling asleep), interim insomnia (frequent awakenings), and terminal insomnia (earlier morning awakenings), or hypersomnolence (excessive sleep).

Community health nurses can prevent or intervene in many of these problems by thorough assessments of patterns of activity and rest. Consider the nature of the sleep problem by determining its onset and duration (i.e., acute, transient, chronic [more than 3 weeks]). A sleep history can be obtained by having the individual keep a "sleep log" for several days and nights. The log is analyzed for patterns of wakefulness and sleep: total sleep time, total time in bed, nap times, and night problems and day problems that interfere with sleep. The nurse inquires about changes in behavior or performance and evaluates use of caffeine (e.g., coffee, tea, cola), xanthine (e.g., chocolate), nicotine, alcohol, and medications that interfere with sleep (prescription and OTC drugs). Health problems that may interfere with sleep are considered (e.g., arthritis, heart failure, chronic obstructive pulmonary disease [COPD], gastroesophageal reflux disease [GERD], diabetes, anxiety, depression, dementia, nocturnal myoclonus, sleep apnea). The nurse teaches the elder and family good sleep hygiene.

Elimination

Problems with elimination can have devastating consequences for older adults. Fear of "accidents" may contribute to social withdrawal and isolation. Inability to control the bladder and bowels are major precipitants to institutionalization. Therefore, nurses must take every opportunity to maintain elimination patterns in older adults.

Urinary Elimination

Although aging alone does not cause urinary incontinence, several age-related changes can contribute to its development (e.g., childbirth, menopause, prostate surgery, stroke). Urinary incontinence is the involuntary loss of urine severe enough to have social or hygienic consequences. It is prevalent in 15% to 30% of community-dwelling men and women, respectively (Cobb et al., 2002). To assess the nature of urinary incontinence, the nurse determines previous patterns of urination and daily activities. The individual or family member is asked to record fluid intake and voiding patterns for at least 3 days to establish the current schedule of urination. In collaboration with the primary care provider, the nurse determines the cause, duration, and degree of incontinence.

Factors commonly associated with this problem include medications, caffeine, and fecal impactions. With frail or confused elders, it is especially helpful to observe toileting activities (e.g., walking, dressing, transfers, hygiene). When establishing realistic goals for urinary incontinence, the nurse considers the level of cooperation anticipated from the patient and family for bladder rehabilitation activities (e.g., total continence, daytime continence with night-time padding).

Treatments for urinary incontinence include pelvic muscle rehabilitation (Kegel exercises, biofeedback, vaginal weight training, pelvic floor electrical stimulation), behavioral therapies (bladder training, toileting assistance), pharmacotherapy, and surgical interventions.

Fecal Elimination

Bowel elimination has significant implications for the older adult's comfort and quality of life. Common problems include diarrhea, constipation, and fecal incontinence.

Diarrhea For diarrhea in older adults, the criterion is the volume of stool per day, rather than the number or consistency of stools, which may be altered with changes in food or fluid intake but still be within normal limits. Diarrhea can be infectious or noninfectious and is a significant cause of morbidity and mortality among those elders who are frail and more susceptible to fluid and electrolyte imbalances. This condition is prevented by scrupulous food preparation and storage, frequent handwashing, and avoidance of fecal contamination and polypharmacy. Initial assessments include onset, volume, number, consistency of stools; duration (acute versus chronic); the presence of bright red blood (hematochezia) or black, tarry stool (melena); the presence of other symptoms (e.g., abdominal cramping or distention, lassitude, thirst, nausea, vomiting, fever, malaise); diet; and medications. The nurse evaluates the elder's general appearance, vital signs, and weight and performs an abdominal exam for pain or tenderness.

Although common diarrhea often is treated in the home, any condition lasting more than 24 hours in older adults should be referred to the primary care provider for evaluation and possible rehydration.

Constipation For elders, the most common bowel problem is constipation, a difficulty in passing stools or incomplete or infrequent passage of stools (usually less than three per week). The usual causes of small, hard, or infrequent stools are poor bowel habits, including a lack of dietary fiber, poor fluid intake, inadequate exercise, psychological factors, and medications, often with inappropriate use of laxatives. Common complications are fecal impaction and fecal incontinence.

MEDIA MOMENT 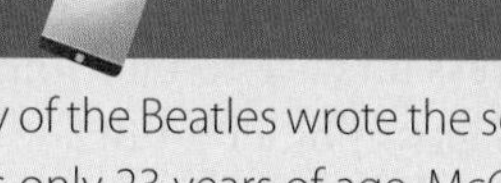

Sir Paul McCartney of the Beatles wrote the song "When I'm 64" when he was only 23 years of age. McCartney turned 64 years old in 2006. Of this event, he said, "I still believe that 'all you need is love.'"

To assess the nature of constipation, the nurse must determine previous patterns of bowel habits and daily activities. The older adult is asked to record food and fluid intake (noting dietary fiber and water) and bowel movements (frequency, timing, difficulty) for at least 3 days. The person's general physical and mental condition is evaluated and, if frail or confused, the level of function for toileting activities (e.g., walking, dressing, transfers, hygiene) is observed. The nurse considers possible associated factors (e.g., medications, fecal impactions, illnesses) and makes a referral to the primary care provider, if indicated. When setting goals for bowel elimination, the nurse considers the level of cooperation anticipated for the elder and family with bowel rehabilitation activities. By working with older adults, their caregivers, and primary care providers, community health nurses often can prevent and intervene with a bowel rehabilitation including a high-fiber diet, adequate fluids, daily exercise, and reduction of reliance on stimulant laxatives. Monitor activities daily and evaluate them at least weekly until a bowel pattern is established. Check for constipation, use of the toilet for defecation, fecal impaction, skin integrity, and self concept. If relapses occur, restart the program with suppositories for 3 days. Encourage the person frequently, praise successes, reinforce teaching frequently, and do not permit discouragement when accidents occur. Reconditioning of the bowel may require several weeks to overcome years of poor bowel habits, but with patience and persistence, it usually is successful.

Mobility and Communication

The ability to move about the environment is crucial for independent living. The ability to communicate thoughts and feelings to others is also essential for wellbeing. Therefore, nurses must take an active role in maintenance of an elder's ability to "walk and talk" while striving to remain in the community.

Mobility

Adequate mobility is critical for elders to maintain their functional independence. Even brief periods of immobility can lead to rapid deconditioning and loss of flexibility and strength in older adults, increasing the risk of falls and injury. Conversely, daily physical activity helps the individual to prevent diseases (e.g., osteoporosis, arterial/venous insufficiency, gastrointestinal stasis, coronary heart disease, obesity, stroke, depression, anxiety); improve sleep, mobility, strength, flexibility, and mood; increase life expectancy; and improve quality of life. Community health nurses can encourage elders to exercise individually, with families, or in groups.

Impaired mobility usually involves multiple factors, including an initial physical deficit (e.g., a fractured hip or degenerative joint disease), compounded by a sedentary lifestyle, deconditioning, inadequate daily exercise patterns, sensory impairment (i.e., vision and hearing), confusion, inappropriate medications, improper assistive devices, and/or environmental hazards. To assess mobility in older adults, the nurse determines the person's previous types and levels of exercise and daily activity patterns, any history of activity-related injuries and falls, and possible associated factors influencing mobility (e.g., medications, confusion, illnesses). The nurse evaluates the individual's general physical and mental condition, food and fluid intake, environmental safety, and availability of assistive devices, and observes the individual's level of function for physical activities (e.g., posture, gait, balance, strength, endurance). When establishing a program for exercise or physical rehabilitation, the nurse considers the level of cooperation anticipated from the elder and family for physical activities and addresses both the physical deficits and any contributing factors.

Falls

Accidents are the fifth leading cause of death among elders, and falls account for two-thirds of these deaths. Seventy percent of fall injuries occur in persons older than 75 years of age; 50% of those hospitalized for such an injury do not survive for 1 year. Fear of falling further inhibits many elders from performing activities that would prevent falls and contributes to functional decline, depression, helplessness, and social isolation. Falls may be caused by environmental hazards, deconditioning, sensory deficits, and impaired central processing. The best prevention for falls is a combination of rehabilitative, environmental, and behavioral strategies. For example, correcting vision, using assistive devices, installing bathroom grab bars, and implementing a progressive exercise program that emphasizes conditioning of the lower extremities all help reduce the occurrence of falls.

Osteoporosis

A multifactorial disease of increased skeletal fragility, **osteoporosis** increases risk of fractures. Postmenopausal women usually are affected initially, but men are also subject to this type of bone loss. The vertebral bodies, proximal femur, and distal radius are common fracture sites in older adults. In collaboration with primary care providers, community health nurses can assist with preventive strategies for osteoporosis (**Box 34-3**).

> Wrinkles should merely indicate where smiles have been.
>
> —*Mark Twain*

BOX 34-3 Prevention of Osteoporosis in Elders

- Establish a daily exercise program.
- Encourage dietary intake of calcium (1,200 to 1,500 mg/day) with dairy products (milk, cheese, yogurt) and/or calcium supplementation .
- Encourage dietary intake of vitamin D (> 800 IU/day) and/or supplementation, and, with the primary care provider, consider pharmacological therapies, including selective estrogen receptor modulators, (SERMS), antiresorptives, or anabolic agents.
- On sunny days, sit outside for 1 to 2 hours (avoiding 11 a.m. to 2 p.m.) to enhance vitamin D intake.

Communication

Other than development of slower speech, verbal communication usually is unaffected by aging. The most common causes of language disorders in older adults are strokes and dementia resulting in some form of aphasia.

Cognition and Affect

Because people are sentient beings, attention, memory, and emotion are integrally intertwined with personal identity, environmental adaptation, and quality of life. Changes in cognitive abilities may be stereotyped as "senility" and either minimized or maximized by elders and family members. Altered mood and emotional responses may further confound the situation. Impaired cognition and affect may exhaust family resources and precipitate relocation from the home to a long-term care facility. Therefore, nurses can assist older adults to remain independent in their own environments by being sensitive to changes in how they "think and feel."

> The old believe everything.
> The middle-aged suspect everything.
> The young know everything.
>
> —*Oscar Wilde*

Cognition

Cognitive functioning changes very little with normal aging. Intelligence is unchanged and, with the wisdom gathered from life experience, problem solving often is improved. Memory involves pattern recognition and is both declarative (factual, "what") and procedural (process, "how"). With diminished attention and immediate recall, older adults may have some declarative memory loss (forgetfulness), but their procedural memory usually is not affected by the aging process. Learning, which depends on memory, also is undisturbed, although it proceeds more slowly. Performance may be slower, but it is more precise. **Confusion** is a common problem in elders and may result from alterations in sensory or central processing. The most common causes of confusion are delirium, dementia, and depression.

Delirium Acute confusional state (**delirium**) is a physiological state that usually is reversible and is characterized as an altered level of consciousness and disorganized thinking (incoherent speech, repetitive speech, and behavior), with a rapid onset and fluctuating course, often worse at night. Delirium has an underlying medical cause (e.g., pneumonia, urinary tract infection, fecal impaction, septicemia). Prevention involves adequate oxygenation, hydration, nutrition, elimination, sensory stimulation, exercise, and avoidance of certain medications.

Dementia **Mild cognitive impairment** (MCI) is the mild, gradual deterioration in memory performance, speed of cognitive processing, and executive functions that may accompany normal aging but does not interfere with activities or relationships. Older adults with MCI may have *subjective* memory complaints and *objective* memory impairments, yet may be within the normal range or in early stages of dementia.

Dementia is a syndrome of progressive decline that relentlessly erodes intellectual abilities, causing cognitive function deterioration and leading to impairment in social and occupational functioning (Agency for Health Care Policy and Research, 1996, p. 1). Dementia occurs in 5% of persons aged 65; the rate doubles every 5 years after age 65, until dementia affects almost 50% of persons age 85 or older. This cognitive impairment is irreversible, has an insidious onset, and is relatively stable over time, though it leads to progressive amnesia (loss of memory), aphasia (loss of language), agnosia (loss of object recognition), apraxia (loss of motor function), and loss of executive function (abstract thinking and complex behavior). **Alzheimer's disease** is a cortical degeneration that accounts for 80% of dementia.

Most older adults with mild or moderate dementia live at home and are cared for by family members. Community health nurses can assist with early case finding and referral to a primary care provider or specialist (geriatrician, neuropsychologist, or psychiatrist). Cognitive functioning is screened in community settings with mental status exams, which test orientation, memory, attention, language, and praxis.

The basic principles for working with elders who have cognitive deficits are to *simplify the environment, provide a structure* for daily activities, *minimize changes* in that structure, and, when changes are necessary, *prepare for changes* well in advance. The goals of cognitive behavioral programs are to help individuals maintain their highest level of function, enable them to continue living at home, and offer support to caregivers. These programs are based on strengths, areas of deficit, and realistic goals for their living situations. Strategies for the management of dementia are summarized in **Box 34-4**.

Realizing the impact of the "age wave" and the potential for a higher percentage of the U.S. population to have Alzheimer's dementia, the U.S. Department of Health and Human Services acknowledges Alzheimer's disease as a major public health issue. In 2011, President Barack Obama signed the National Alzheimer's Project Act

BOX 34-4 Strategies for Management of Dementia in Elders

- *Structure time and place.* Use daily and weekly schedules that provide consistency, predictability, and repetition. Structure and simplify activities of daily living, family activities, specific tasks, and the environment to maximize ability in conjunction with less clutter, complexity, and hurry. For example, activities may be done in the same order and at the same times and places each day (e.g., arise at 7:00, breakfast at 7:30); certain activities take place on certain days of the week every week (e.g., bathe on Tuesday and Saturday, laundry on Monday).
- *Anticipate change.* Known events, such as holidays and family gatherings, may be anticipated several weeks in advance by mentioning every day the names of people who will be involved and using photos, stories, or other aids to familiarize the elder with the anticipated situation. Persons with cognitive deficits can learn, but the key is repetition.
- *Modify the environment.* Reorganize the elder's living situation to compensate for sensory and functional impairments. Use memory aids (e.g., clocks, calendars, simple written cues) for orientation and identification of items and places. Keep the environment as simple and uncluttered as possible. Avoid situations that stress intellectual capabilities. For those with early dementia, newspapers, television, telephone calls, and email may be helpful. For those with severe dementia, security devices and electronic monitoring may be indicated. Recommend identification jewelry, photo ID, and current photos; suggest MedicAlert or the Alzheimer's Association Safe Return Program (800-272-3900).
- *Manage problem behavior.* Analyze each behavioral problem in three parts:

  A: Antecedents (what happens before to trigger or cause the behavior)

  B: Behavior (which specific actions can be seen and described)

  C: Consequences (what happens after or because of the behavior)

  Develop a plan to either avoid or prevent problem behaviors by changing either the antecedents or the consequences of the behavior. Avoid catastrophic reactions by minimizing the common antecedents (too much too fast, fatigue).
- *Support the caregiver.* Because persons with dementia may not be able to change as a result of their illness, the caregivers have to be the ones to change. Altering problem behaviors is not easy and not every attempt will be successful. If the plan isn't working, look at the situation again and try another approach. Be flexible and willing to try new approaches as the person changes over time. Reward successes, no matter how small. Remember to laugh.
- *Provide information and referral*: Encourage family members to contact the Alzheimer's Association (800-272-3900), Alzheimer's Disease Education and Referral (ADEAR) Center, area agency on aging, community mental health centers, and/or Internet support groups.
- *Community-based care*: adult day centers, home health agencies.
- *Caregiver burden*: caregivers support groups, respite care.
- *Long-term care*: personal care/assisted living homes, skilled care nursing homes.

(NAPA) into law. The CDC established the Healthy Brain Initiative in 2005, which included development of a coordinated approach to Alzheimer's disease, and it is developing a second road map for state and national partnerships.

Depression The most common disturbance of mood experienced by elders is **depression**. Its prevalence varies by setting: 5% to 20% in community-dwelling elders, 25% in hospitalized elders, and 40% in nursing home residents (Cobb et al., 2002). Its presentation may differ from younger populations, with somatic complaints being more likely than emotional statements about guilt, anger, or depressed mood in elders. The etiology may be situational—resulting from finances, disability, bereavement, loneliness, or social isolation—or biochemical—resulting from physical illnesses, pain, or medications.

The assessment of depression in elders requires information from the elder and family members. New physical complaints or exacerbations of previous pain, gastrointestinal symptoms, cardiovascular symptoms, preoccupation with poor health or physical limitations, diminished interest in pleasurable activities (anhedonia), sleep disturbances, fatigue, poor concentration, memory loss, and expressions of negativism should be noted. The Geriatric Depression Scale (see Appendix E) is administered to screen for depression, and the individual is referred to the primary care provider as indicated by assessments. In collaboration with the primary care provider, the nurse checks for physical problems and medications that cause depression. Interventions for depression in community-dwelling elders are summarized in **Box 34-5**.

Suicide Among Elders Given the high prevalence of depression among elders, it is not surprising that they have the highest suicide rate among any demographic group. Suicides among elders are characterized more by physical illnesses and functional losses than by the problems with employment, finances, and family relations that are more

BOX 34-5 Strategies for Management of Depression in Elders

- Offer unconditional, positive regard for the changes of aging and altered function.
- Emphasize with the person and family that depression is manageable and reversible; offer hope.
- Encourage the person to maintain control over self and the situation by offering choices for decision making.
- Assist the individual to identify the positives of the situation and opportunities for gains as well as losses.
- In collaboration with the primary care provider, encourage the use of medications, psychotherapy, and exercise to treat the depression.

BOX 34-6 Strategies for Prevention of Suicide in Older Adults at Risk

- Reduce immediate danger by removing hazardous articles.
- Refer any potentially suicidal elder promptly to his or her primary care provider (same day). Provide a constant companion (family, friend) en route.
- Extract a promise from the person not to attempt suicide before the agreed intervention (e.g., clinic visit, your next visit).
- Mobilize resources by restoring a sense of control in the person's life, reconnecting the elder with significant others, and developing life lines of support systems and community resources.
- Follow up with regular calls and maintenance of support systems.

frequently encountered among younger adults who attempt suicide. Suicides are more often completed by men (60%); suicides are more often attempted by women (75%). The methods include guns, hanging, drug overdose, and cutting or slashing. Threats are real, and first attempts usually are successful. More insidious suicide activities among elders include refusal to eat, take medications, or follow simple safety procedures and overuse of alcohol and drugs.

Nurses should consider the potential for suicide in any elders who are depressed or exhibit negativism and hopelessness. Older adults often fear loneliness, abandonment, loss of control, and pain, but not always death. Incidence of suicide is higher among elders who are white, male, Protestant, or widowed; they often live alone, have financial problems, have a history of alcoholism, and have poor health, especially a recent diagnosis of terminal illness. The nurse must not hesitate to inquire about suicidal fantasies and ideation. If these thoughts are present, ask directly about plans, method, and means. Behavioral clues such as putting personal affairs in order, giving away possessions, making wills and funeral arrangements, self-neglect, erratic behavior, suspiciousness, hoarding pills or neglecting to refill prescriptions, and personality changes must be addressed. Community health nurses have unique opportunities for suicide prevention through early case finding and enrichment of resources and support systems (**Box 34-6**).

Affect

Self-concept evolves from what persons think and feel about themselves, what they think and feel about others, and what they think and feel others think and feel about them (Satir, 1964). Assurance of personal worth is based on feeling valued, useful, and competent. Old age is accompanied by many epoch events—retirement, altered health, relocation of home, deaths of family and friends, and finally one's own transition from life to death. With the frequent, multiple losses associated with old age, older adults may experience feelings of powerlessness, hopelessness, and spiritual distress. These feelings may result in the anxiety, fear, and anger of depression.

Employment and Retirement

With a life expectancy of 20 or more years at age 65, transition from work into retirement—which is a 20th-century phenomenon—is the major normative event of the second half of life. Issues to be considered in retirement planning include financial security; role restructuring; location; new or part-time careers; educational, recreational, and leisure activities; and relationships with family and friends. Many older adults enjoy volunteering with community agencies or through programs such as the Foster Grandparents or Retired Senior Volunteer Program (RSVP) through the local area agency on aging. Others pursue lifelong learning by way of community education programs through schools (including high school equivalency programs), colleges, and universities, and elder hostel programs throughout the world. Travel about the country or abroad may be an option.

For those who are able to redefine themselves with meaningful activities, the latter stages of life can be times for achieving ego integrity (Erikson, 1963) and self-actualization (Maslow, 1968) through lifelong learning and creativity. For those who are unable to make these transitions, old age may become a time of loneliness, hopelessness, and boredom. Quality of life rather than quantity of life becomes the issue. Mastery of the past is the basis for adaptation to the present and hope for the future. Family, friends, and faith are integral to self-concept and spirituality.

Nurses can help alert elders to the characteristics and normality of aging and employ the **life review** process to find purpose in life (Ebersole et al., 2005). For frail and/or demented elders, special programs (e.g., the Eden Alternative) are needed to combat the plagues of loneliness, boredom, and helplessness in nursing homes by using companionship, variety, and helpfulness. The integration of resident animals, abundant plants, children, and community activities into this environment makes it a more human habitat. For example, a nursing home may adopt suitable dogs and cats from animal shelters, sponsor a scout troop, offer its meeting rooms for local gardener groups, and provide summer day camps for children.

Sexuality

Aging does not end the need for love and belongingness. Older adults in any community setting need social interaction with their peers. Their sexual expressions may take a variety of forms, including touching, holding, kissing, fondling, petting, and intercourse, and may be heterosexual or homosexual. For older adults living with children or in institutions, nurses may need to facilitate their needs for privacy and intimacy. For those with no spouse or partner, masturbation or fantasy may be alternatives. As with any age group, sexually active elders are at risk for sexually transmitted diseases (STDs), including human immunodeficiency virus (HIV) infection and acquired immunodeficiency syndrome (AIDS).

The **PLISSIT model** (Permission, Limited Information, Specific Suggestions, Intensive Therapy) is helpful to assess and intervene in sexual problems with elders (Annon, 1976). For example, nurses can support the sexuality of elders indirectly by saying gently that romance does not end at a certain age and wonder if the person has any questions or concerns in this area (e.g., getting permission to discuss sexuality). If men indicate a problem, the nurse can ask more directly, but tactfully, if they are having problems with erections or intercourse; if women indicate a problem, the nurse can ask about lubrication; both can be asked about satisfaction and what they want to do about their intimacy needs. The nurse can provide limited information and make specific suggestions for simple problems (e.g., mild analgesia and alternative positions for painful joints), and then make referrals to a primary care provider for intensive therapy as indicated.

MEDIA MOMENT

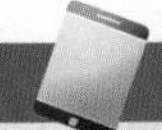

"100 Years," Five for Fighting (John Ondrasik, 2004)

The song "100 Years" by Five for Fighting shot to the top of the worldwide charts in 2004. Listen to the entire song and describe the meaning of the stages of life in the lyrics.

THINK ABOUT THIS

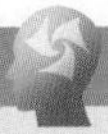

The endlessly youthful baby-boomer generation turned 60 in 2005 and they are *not* in their rocking chairs!

The baby-boomer generation that couldn't "get no satisfaction" are now senior citizens. Kathleen Casey has the distinction of being the first baby born in the baby-boomer generation at 12:01 a.m. on January 1, 1946. She was the first of 76 million Americans brought into the world between 1946 and 1964 when, in a sharp reversal of a steady century of decline, the national birth rate skyrocketed, creating a massive demographic upheaval. This generation is showing no signs of slowing down or changing the lifestyles that changed the world more than 40 years ago. For example, 40 years after the Rolling Stones hit the top of the charts with "I Can't Get No Satisfaction," the Stones launched their 2005 world tour at Boston's Fenway Park. The band continues to be among the top five grossing concert groups in the United States. This generation has gained unprecedented affluence—no matter how much they have, they can't ever seem to get enough or do enough. Here are just a few well-known Americans who are in their 50s and 60s:

Dolly Parton (born in 1946)

Former President Bill Clinton (1946)

Former President George W. Bush (1946)

Katie Couric (1957)

Samuel L. Jackson (1948)

Oprah Winfrey (1954)

Bill Gates (1955)

Bruce Springsteen (1949)

Cher (1946)

Jimmy Buffett (1946)

Reggie Jackson (1946)

Meryl Streep (1949)

Antonio Banderas (1950)

Angela Merkel (1954)

Yo-Yo Ma (1955)

Neil deGrasse Tyson (1958)

Angela Bassett (1958)

President Barack Obama (1961)

George Clooney (1961)

Brad Pitt (1963)

Safety and Security

As an aspect of work and play, safety for elders is concerned with accidental injuries in the home and community, especially from falls, fires, and motor vehicle accidents (see **Box 34-7**). Older adults with generalized weakness, slow reaction time, unstable gait, visual changes, hearing loss, and on multiple medications are at greater risk for accidents and crime. Unfortunately, their vulnerability makes them frequent targets of purse snatchings, pickpocketing, fraud, theft, vandalism, and harassment. Community health nurses need to assess home safety to eliminate hazards (see Appendix F).

Thermal Regulation and Skin Integrity

With less efficient thermal regulation, elders are at higher risk for health problems during temperature extremes. As the largest organ of the body, the skin of elderly people undergoes many age-related changes, and it is subject to serious complications. Nurses are at the forefront of preventive health care for the functions of both "heat/cool" and "touch/feel."

Thermal Regulation

Internal body temperature is a balance of cellular metabolism, muscle activity, and heat loss by radiation, convection, and evaporation through the skin (Ebersole et al., 2005). The ability to feel heat and cold is impaired in elders, and their return to core body temperature in response to heating or cooling takes twice as long as in their youth. Drugs such as sedative-hypnotics, phenothiazines, and alcohol may further impair thermoregulatory mechanisms (Cobb et al., 2002). Fear of costly utility bills may inhibit their use of air conditioning or heating systems during extreme temperatures. These factors place community-dwelling elders at high risk for hypothermia and hyperthermia during very hot and cold weather.

Community health nurses can help prevent life-threatening emergencies and death by encouraging elders and families to check homes for insulation and caulking to maintain heat and cool. Assistance with fuel costs, which is available in most states, also may be needed. Nurses can help establish "buddy" systems among family, friends, and neighbors to make daily checks on elders during weather extremes. A low threshold of suspicion should be used for referrals of at-risk elders to primary care providers or emergency care centers for thermal regulatory problems.

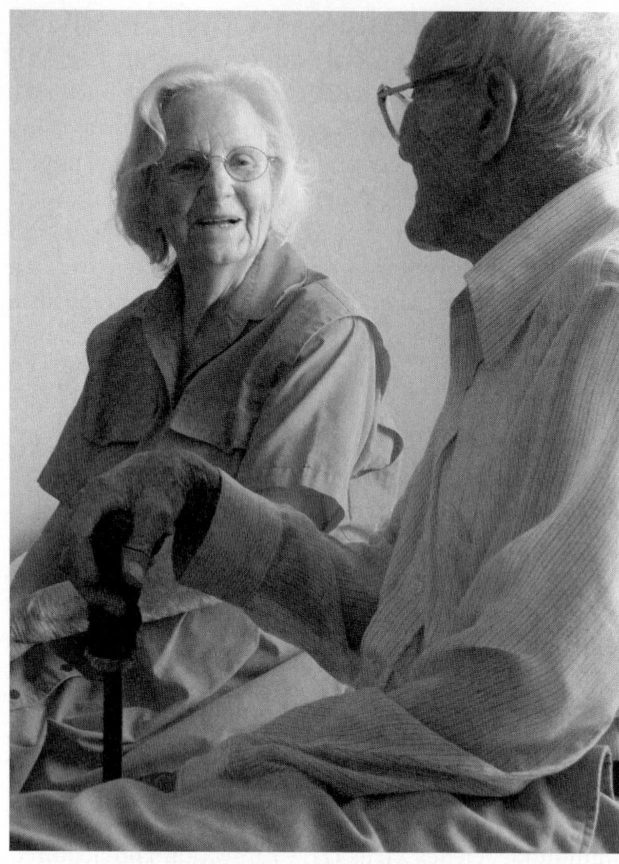

Although as a culture we often associate romance, dating, and marriage with youth, elders can continue to have healthy, loving, and passionate relationships throughout the lifespan. This couple dated for two years and married at the age of 90, after being widowed for several years.

BOX 34-7 Safety Precautions for Elders

- Check to see that stairs are well lighted, are free of clutter, and have nonskid surface and handrails.
- Check bathrooms for handrails, nonslip adhesive surfaces in tubs/showers, and nonslip flooring.
- Provide rooms with adequate, nonglare lighting; eliminate clutter and throw rugs, casters on chairs, dangling cords, and waxed floors.
- Avoid sedation with narcotics and sedatives.
- Use carbon monoxide and smoke detectors.
- Encourage defensive driving; suggest the local AARP mature/defensive driving program.
- Provide for easy access to the local emergency system, including telephone numbers. If the individual is frail and/or homebound, suggest "Friendly Caller" or lifeline services.
- Recommend identification jewelry (i.e., bracelet or necklace) and have current photo identification readily available.
- When accidents occur, investigate as to specific information on location, time, and environmental factors, and intervene to prevent their recurrence.

Hypothermia Elders produce less heat per kilogram of body weight. They usually have decreased muscle mass and subcutaneous fat, reduced muscle activity, and less efficient shivering. The vasoconstriction response of their skin arterioles to cooling is diminished, so heat within the body is not conserved. Elders are also less able to discriminate temperature differences and may have delayed perception of being cold. These age-related changes contribute to an increased risk of hypothermia in elders when indoor temperatures are below 65°F. Symptoms of hypothermia include a body temperature of 95°F (96°F rectal) or less, cold to touch, absent shivering and piloerection, slow capillary refill, pallor or cyanosis, bradypnea, arrhythmia and bradycardia, hypotension, slurred speech, and lethargy. Treatment requires slow warming and may require hospitalization for metabolic imbalances if cooling is prolonged or extreme. See **Box 34-8** for techniques to prevent hypothermia.

Hyperthermia The vasodilatation response of the arterioles to heating is diminished in elders, such that heat is not delivered to the skin for dissipation. As a consequence, a greater threshold temperature is needed to initiate perspiration, and less sweat is produced in response to heating. Older adults also are less sensitive to thirst. Individuals with cardiovascular and peripheral vascular diseases, diabetes, and infections, and those taking certain medications (e.g., anticholinergics, antihistamines, diuretics, beta blockers, antidepressants, antiparkinsonian drugs), are at risk for hyperthermia.

The three types of hyperthermic emergencies are heat syncope, heat exhaustion, and heat stroke. Symptoms include increased body temperature (especially 105°F and higher), flushed skin, tachypnea, headache, weakness, and seizures. Suggested techniques to prevent hyperthermia in older adults are listed in Box 34-8.

BOX 34-8 Techniques to Improve Thermal Regulation in Elders

Prevention of Hypothermia

- Drink adequate warm fluids and eat hot, calorie-rich foods.
- Warm hands and feet; cover them with warm blankets. Warm the room to 68° to 70°F when elders are inactive, and use electric blankets at night.
- During the day, wear head coverings; warm, layered clothing; and socks and shoes. Use leg warmers on arms and legs. At night, wear a bed cap and leg and foot warmers.
- Encourage indoor physical activity.
- Avoid alcohol and drugs that lower regulatory mechanisms.

Prevention of Hyperthermia

- During heat extremes, drink 2,000 to 3,000 mL of cool fluids per day, if tolerated.
- Avoid exertion, especially during the heat of the day, between 10 a.m. and 4 p.m.
- Alternate periods of heat exposure with cooling; stay in air conditioning or use fans when possible.
- Avoid alcohol and drugs that inhibit thermal regulation.

Skin Integrity

As a result of increased elasticity, decreased surface acidity, dryness of the epidermis (xerosis), thinning of the dermis, and loss of subcutaneous fat, skin integrity is an ever-present potential problem in elders. Nurses need to inspect the skin during any clinical encounter or procedure to check for the many skin disorders of elders (e.g., pruritus [itching], urticaria, intertrigo, seborrheic dermatitis and keratosis, rosacea, psoriasis). Several skin cancers are common in elders (e.g., actinic keratoses [precancerous], basal-cell and squamous-cell carcinomas, and melanomas). The nurse should check skin lesions for the ABCDEs of skin cancers: *a*symmetry, irregular *b*orders, multiple *c*olors, *d*iameter greater than 1 cm, and *e*volving (changing in size, shape, color, elevation, or another trait, or exhibiting new symptoms such as bleeding, itching, or crusting). Suspicious findings should be reported promptly to the primary care provider. Lacerations (especially skin tears), abrasions, and pressure ulcers also are common in elders.

Maintenance of skin integrity can be accomplished by limiting bathing (i.e., two to three times per week in warm weather, once or twice per week in cold weather), liberally using emollients, and avoiding prolonged direct sun exposure (i.e., wearing protective clothing or sunscreens). Bath oils are to be avoided because they may exacerbate skin problems and increase the risk of falls.

Pressure Ulcers Maintenance of skin integrity and prevention of pressure ulcers require an ever-present vigilance of older adults, family caregivers, and nurses in the community. As with other age groups, skin problems are prevented with adequate nutrition and avoidance of pressure, friction, shear, and moisture. Individuals most at risk are immobile, incontinent, malnourished, frail, or confused. With elders who are confined to bed or wheelchairs, the most common sites of pressure ulcers are the ischium (24%), sacrum (23%), trochanters (15%), and malleolus (7%). Community health nurses can help prevent these painful, costly, and life-threatening complications by being systematic, comprehensive, and routine about skin care. Two instruments often used for assessment of risk factors are the Braden Scale, for predicting pressure sore risk, and the Norton Risk Assessment Scale.

Comfort and Spirituality

Older adults may not complain of discomfort or pain, healthcare providers may treat it inadequately, and poorly managed pain may aggravate other health problems. Given the many age-related health and lifestyle changes experienced by elders, an intact spiritual belief system is essential. "Hurt" and "believe" conclude this functional approach to preventive health care.

MEDIA MOMENT 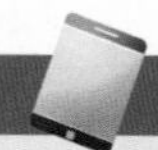

***Tuesdays with Morrie: An Old Man, a Young Man, and Life's Greatest Lessons* (1997)**

by Mitch Albom, New York, NY: Doubleday

This book details the relationship between a former student and his professor, Morrie, as the professor battles Lou Gehrig's disease (amyotrophic lateral sclerosis). A nonfiction bestseller, this book is an outstanding story about life, death, and the meaning of it all.

Spirituality

With the experiences of aging and changes in health status, many older adults and families are faced with the need to discover a continuing purpose in the elder's life, find new meanings in their existence, and prepare for their transcendence from life to death. As they approach the end of their lives, elders may contemplate their movement from the concrete reality of their physical existence toward more abstract, metaphorical conceptualizations of their oneness with God, a divine being, or a higher power. Spirituality—the essence of the soul—may be integral to elders' beliefs, hope, energy, creativity, acceptance of life and death, and transcendence (Ebersole et al., 2005).

As with other age groups, nurses assess the spiritual health of elders by inquiring discretely about their spiritual perspectives and religious commitments. Observations include their ability to discover continuing meaning and purpose in life, give and receive love, have hope, be creative, and share humor. The goals of spiritual care are to preserve the elders' unique beliefs and values and support their religious practices. Nurses may need to help older adults make contact with religious advisors (e.g., minister, priest, rabbi, shaman) and use religious articles (e.g., Bible, Koran, crucifix, medals, prayer shawls, incense). They may need to have privacy for prayer and meditation or may want to sing hymns, read or write poetry, or offer other forms of self-expression. Older adults may ask the nurse to share in these practices, as is appropriate for the situation. However the older adults express their spirituality, it is important that nurses recognize these needs and assist with their being met.

Comfort

Altered proprioception is more common in elders, who typically have increased light touch and pain thresholds. Maintaining comfort and managing pain—both acute and chronic—are essential to keep older adults mobile and fully involved in their daily activities. Community health nurses need to assess comfort levels frequently using standard pain scales for persistent problems. Gentle massage, warm (*not* hot) baths, and fragrances are just a few of the techniques that may be helpful for common discomforts. Use of analgesics, including those that are available without prescription (acetaminophen and nonsteroidal anti-inflammatory drugs), must be discussed with the primary care provider because of increased risks of organ damage and gastrointestinal bleeding.

MEDIA MOMENT 

Don't miss these movies about aging:

On Golden Pond

Driving Miss Daisy

The Notebook

Hanging Up

Songs about aging include:

"Old Man," Neil Young

"100 Years," Five for Fighting

"Living Years," Mike and the Mechanics

"When I'm 64," The Beatles

"Eleanor Rigby," The Beatles

Special Older Adults Health Issues

Community health nurses must consider special aspects of health care in elderly populations. Comprehensive health care for elders includes immunizations, medication review, chemical abuse, and ethical dilemmas.

Immunizations

Taken together, pneumonia and influenza are a leading cause of death in the United States. Older adults with chronic illnesses are at the highest risk for these respiratory illnesses. In the older adult population, immunizations usually are limited to four vaccines: influenza, pneumococcal, tetanus/diphtheria, and the zoster vaccine for shingles (Herpes zoster) (CDC, 2008). For older adults who travel to foreign countries, other immunizations may be indicated.

Medications

Elderly individuals purchase 40% of all prescription drugs (most commonly cardiovascular, anti-infective, antipsychotic, antidepressant, and diuretic agents) and 40% of OTC medicines (mostly analgesics, laxatives, and antacids). An average of five prescription drugs and three OTC drugs are taken by 90% of elders (U.S. Food and Drug Administration, 2003). Because aging changes affect the absorption, distribution, metabolism, and elimination of pharmacological agents, older adults are more vulnerable to drug interactions, adverse reactions, and toxicities.

Polypharmacy (use of many drugs simultaneously) is a multifactorial problem that results from a "pill-oriented" society, older adults' beliefs about health care and their various acute and chronic health problems, the prescribing practices of primary care providers, and the use of multiple primary and specialty providers. Problems of adherence to drug regimens occur with 25% to 50% of medications, including underuse, overuse, and misuse; many of these errors contribute to unnecessary hospitalizations (Ebersole et al., 2005). Because of the expense of drugs, older adults may not fill prescriptions or may discontinue medications or decrease dosages and/or frequencies to stretch their medicines.

Community health nurses must be attentive for errors of omission (e.g., unfilled prescriptions, skipped doses, discontinuing medicines) and errors of commission (e.g., self-medication by increasing or decreasing dosages, changing times, using another person's drugs, taking OTC drugs). Nursing interventions for drug therapies are summarized in **Box 34-9**.

Chemical Addictions

Among elders, chemical addictions include all of the psychoactive chemicals used by younger populations, with alcohol being the substance that is most frequently abused. Alcoholism is estimated to affect 10% to 15% of community-dwelling older adults. Given their decreased tolerance to alcohol, combined with normal aging changes and use of multiple prescription and OTC drugs, older adults are at higher risk for falls, accidents, and burns.

BOX 34-9 Strategies to Improve Medication Use by Elders

- Obtain a medication history and consider the ability of elders to manage their medications, including financial status (purchase), environmental situation (storage), educational level (literacy), cognitive status (memory), visual acuity (reading labels), functional status (opening containers), and drug allergies.
- Remind elders to bring their medicines to each clinic visit; do a drug review ("brown-bag check") for correct medications, dosages, instructions, refills, and drug knowledge.
- Check medications frequently during home visits, including storage arrangements and the disposition of old medications.
- In collaboration with primary care providers, simplify drug regimens and eliminate all unnecessary drugs, both prescribed and OTC. Use once- or twice-daily dosing whenever possible.
- Teach individuals and family members about all their medications and prepare a written schedule, including each drug name and strength, size/color, purpose, frequency with specific times or days (e.g., 8 a.m. and 4 p.m. instead of "twice daily"; Monday, Wednesday, Friday instead of "every other day"), and important side effects.
- Encourage elders and family members to purchase all medications through the same pharmacy to check for drug allergies and interactions.
- Encourage elders to take medications at the same time and place every day with 4 to 6 ounces of water. Use memory aids to assist with adherence to drug regimens (e.g., written lists, medication calendars, pill boxes).
- Store all medicines together in a safe dry place, in their original containers, and out of the reach of small children. Some medications require refrigeration.
- Remind older adults to take a sufficient supply of all medicines when traveling away from home.
- If elders have memory problems, functional impairments, or complicated drug regimens, suggest the use of medication boxes prefilled by the caregiver either daily or weekly.
- If elders have arthritic problems, suggest easy-opening containers; if they have visual problems, use large print for labels; and if they have swallowing problems, use liquid forms. Caution against crushing tablets or emptying capsules into food or fluid before checking with a pharmacist.
- Monitor elders continually for efficacy and side effects of medications. Use the Abnormal Involuntary Movement Scale (AIMS) to monitor drugs (especially antipsychotics) with extrapyramidal side effects such as tremors, akinesia, akathisia, and rigidity (tardive dyskinesia).

Nurses in the community can help identify these individuals by noting changes in behavior (e.g., anxiety, memory loss, depression, blackouts, confusion), health status (e.g., weight loss), hygiene, falls, and injuries. Older adults can be screened with the TWEACK test (Cobb et al., 2002):

Tolerance	How many drinks before you feel the effects of alcohol?
Worry	Have you ever felt worried by criticism of your drinking?
Eye opener	Have you ever taken a morning "eye opener"?
Amnesia	Are there times after drinking when you can't remember what you did?
Cut down	Have you ever felt the need to cut down on drinking?
Drin**k**ing	How many drinks before you fall asleep or pass out?

Those persons and families found to have alcohol problems may be referred to their primary care providers, community mental health centers, Alcoholics Anonymous, or other local agencies for chemical abuse. Because denial of alcohol abuse is so prevalent and the necessary lifestyle changes are so difficult to maintain, recovery often is a long, irregular process. Nurses need to persist in their support, referral, and follow up for these individuals and their families.

Other substances abused by older adults include nicotine, caffeine, prescription and OTC drugs, illicit street drugs, and food. Assessments and interventions for these chemicals are similar to those for younger populations.

Ethical Dilemmas

Because community health nurses become so involved with older people in their own environment, they often encounter ethical dilemmas and end-of-life issues. All too often, there is no simple, easy, "right" answer to these complex situations.Usually the choice is between two or more "bad" options. Beware of simple solutions, which usually ignore the complex nature of dilemmas. For example, when a frail, demented elder is anorexic, losing weight, and at risk for complications, one option is to insert an enteral feeding tube. That measure may improve nutrition, but it may also prolong the person's suffering and dying and may be against his or her wishes for end-of-life care.

In American society, critical values in most ethical dilemmas are concerned with autonomy (freedom of choice), nonmaleficence or beneficence (do no harm/do good), and distributive justice (use of resources). Because older adults consume large amounts of healthcare resources, ethical conflicts occur around the quantity of life (adding years to life) versus quality of life (adding life to years). For many individuals,, the finality of death must be weighed against dependence, pain, abandonment, and loneliness. Clarification of beliefs and values of the individual, the family, and the healthcare providers may offer insights into these differing perspectives and facilitate satisfactory resolution of these conflicts.

Advance directives can help clarify elders' desire for healthcare interventions in the event of life-threatening situations. Nurses can encourage families to discuss end-of-life issues (e.g., cardiopulmonary resuscitation, hospitalization, antibiotics, intravenous and enteral feedings) while older adults are relatively young, healthy, and competent to express their wishes. The older adult can complete a durable power of attorney for health care in accordance with state statutes to assist family members and healthcare providers in implementing these wishes. In elders, intellectual competence for informed consent can be determined with the Folstein Mini-Mental State Examination (see Appendix D).

For elders who have no advance directives and are very frail or demented, the occurrence of end-of-life issues frequently can be anticipated. Nurses can take the initiative to approach families with these decisions *early*, encourage them to talk with extended family members as appropriate, and consider what the elders would prefer if they were able to express their wishes. Criteria for decision making are to be considered (e.g., reversibility or irreversibility of the condition), communicated with the primary care provider, and decisions documented appropriately. If elders are able to participate in these decisions, the nurse should encourage them to do so. Supporting the spiritual integrity of all concerned helps sort out the issues and maintain positive attitudes and behaviors.

ETHICAL CONNECTION 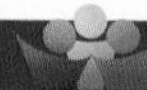

The number of older female drivers will increase dramatically as baby boomers continue to work past 65 years of age. Currently, 75% of women older than 55 have a driver's license, but 90% of women younger than 55 drive. As the percentage of the population older than age 65 rises sharply after 2010, a key question will be how many continue to work and, therefore, commute in their cars.

Retired people have traditionally been very careful about staying off interstate highways, taking back roads, and not driving after dark. Those who are still working may not have that choice, which leads to a safety question that remains to be answered.

What are the ethical implications for nursing, the healthcare system, and society?

Source: Pisarski, A. (October 16, 2006). *Commuting in America III*. Transportation Research Board, National Research Council.

An Old Woman Lives in My Mother's House

An old woman lives in my mother's house;
she sits alone and watches TV.
An old woman lives where my mother once did,
in the house Daddy built in '53.

An old woman wears my mother's clothes
though they don't fit; they hang on her back.
The old woman shuffles in Mother's shoes
when we go for a walk at the walking track.

An old woman cries in my mother's bed,
cries for the things she thinks someone took.
The old woman stops and scratches her head
And looks for her keys or her puzzle book.

The old woman says no one ever comes
to visit, though we go every day.
My mother would not complain like that
but the old woman took my mother away.

The old woman wants my mother's checks,
screams that she has no money at all.
My sister patiently pays the bills,
takes the old woman to shop at the mall.

They buy more yarn for my mother to knit,
to make afghans for little ones' toes.
The old woman bundles the skeins in bags
and hides it away where only she knows.

The old woman screams when I clean her house;
I shut the door and change the bed.
Sometimes I cry when she throws me out,
though I know it's not Mother's anger I dread.

My brothers help out whenever they can.
The old woman swears they never come.
We write in a book, keep a daily log,
for Mother to read, should she ever come home.

—Brenda Finnegan

This poem was written by the author about her experiences with her mother, who has Alzheimer's disease.

RESEARCH ALERT 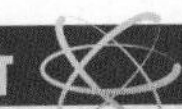

This article presents information on a Great Britain National Health Service (NHS) report titled "Prescriptions Dispensed in the Community 1997–2007," which revealed that polypharmacy is on the rise in older people in England. It also says that people over age 60 are prescribed twice as many drugs as they were 10 years ago. The report further says that older people receive more prescription items per head than any other group, 42.4 items on average compared with 9.5 items for those ages 16–59.

Source: Birmingham, K. (2008). Older people take twice as many drugs. *Nursing Older People, 20*(7), 4–4.

Conclusion

With the "graying of America," older adults have become an integral concern in the delivery of community health care. These older adults were socialized in a reactive healthcare system that focused on illness. Until recently, they have not been especially proactive or focused on wellness or prevention. Community health nurses in the 21st century can help older adults by promoting the three A's: awareness, assessment, and advocacy. Nurses can help older adults practice health promotion and primary disease prevention through good nutrition, regular exercise, family and community involvement, stress management, anticipatory guidance, and safety checks. Secondary prevention requires self-monitoring activities (e.g., breast or testicular self-examinations), periodic screening, regular physical and oral health exams, and adherence to therapeutic regimens. By working collaboratively with primary care providers, nurses can improve the health and quality of life of older adults—and help them celebrate the joy of aging.

HEALTHY ME 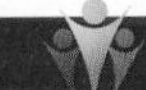

Spend time with an older adult who is in your family or circle of friends. Ask them what kind of health advice they would give to someone your age, as their younger 'self'.

LEVELS OF PREVENTION 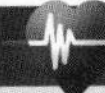

Primary: Teaching a class for older adults about household safety

Secondary: Instructions for home health patients regarding medication noncompliance

Tertiary: Leading an exercise class for older adults with osteoarthritis

Critical Thinking Activities

1. After reading the following excerpt, what are some ways that community health nurses can help "reconnect" elders with other patients in the healthcare delivery system? Identify settings where health-promotion interventions might be created to meet this need.

On the need to reconnect with elders:

> A great deal of America's social sickness comes from age segregation. … We segregate the old for many reasons: prejudice, ignorance, and a lack of good alternatives. … If we aren't around dying people, we don't have to think about dying … and, the more involved we are with the old, the more pain we feel at their suffering. … The old often save the young. And the young save the old. … If 10 people ages 2 to 80 are grouped together, they will fall into a natural hierarchy that nurtures and teaches them all … the incredible calculus of old age—that as more is taken, there is more love for what remains.

Source: Pipher, M. (1999, March 19–21). The new generation gap: For the nation's health, we need to reconnect young and old. *USA Weekend*, p. 12.

2. Using photographs, assist an elderly patient with visualizing independence in his or her life today. How can photographs throughout our lives assist in maximizing our ability to care for ourselves and promote our autonomy? Think of times in your own life when you were dependent and had limitations. What kinds of images helped improve your confidence in becoming self-sufficient again?

AFFORDABLE CARE ACT

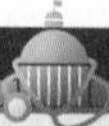

With the passage of the Patient Protection and Affordable Care Act (ACA) of 2010, more older adults will be living outside of traditional institutions than ever before, as care changes to one that is home and community based. What implications does this have for nursing education?

References

Agency for Health Care Policy and Research (AHCPR). (1996). *Recognition and treatment of Alzheimer's disease and related dementias*. Rockville, MD: U.S. Government Printing Office.

American Association of Retired Persons (AARP). (2011). *Valuing the invaluable: 2011 update. The growing contributions and cost of family caregiving*. Retrieved from http://assets.aarp.org/rgcenter/ppi/ltc/i51-caregiving.pdf

Annon, J. (1976, January). The PLISSIT model: A proposed conceptual scheme for behavioral treatment of sexual problems. *Journal of Sex Education and Therapy*, pp. 18–20.

Blazer, D. G., & Steffens, D. C. (2009). *The American Psychiatric Publishing textbook of geriatric psychology* (4th ed.). Arlington, VA: American Psychiatric Publishing.

Burnside, I. (1988). *Nursing and the aged: A self-care approach* (2nd ed.). New York, NY: McGraw-Hill.

Butler, R. (2003). *Why survive? Being old in America*. Baltimore, MD: Johns Hopkins University Press.

Carter, J. (2001). *An hour before daylight*. New York, NY: Simon & Schuster.

Centers for Disease Control and Prevention (CDC). (2008). *National immunization project: Adult immunization schedule*. Retrieved from http://www.cdc.gov/vaccines/schedules/hcp/adult.html

Centers for Disease Control and Prevention (CDC). (2011). Home health care and discharged hospice care patients: United States, 2000 and 2007. *National Health Statistics Reports, 38*, 1–28.

Centers for Disease Control and Prevention (CDC). (2013a). FastStats: Nursing Home Care. Retrieved from http://www.cdc.gov/nchs/data/nnhsd/Estimates/nnhs/Estimates_PaymentSource_Tables.pdf

Centers for Disease Control and Prevention (CDC). (2013b). *The State of Aging & Health in America, 2013*. Retrieved from http://www.cdc.gov/features/agingandhealth/state_of_aging_and_health_in_america_2013.pdf

Centers for Disease Control and Prevention (CDC). (2014). Elder Abuse: Definitions. Retrieved from http://www.cdc.gov/violenceprevention/elderabuse/definitions.html

Cobb, E., Duthie, E., & Murphy, J. (Eds.). (2002). *Geriatrics review syllabus: A core curriculum in geriatric medicine* (5th ed.). Malden, MA: Blackwell Publishing for the American Geriatrics Society.

Cora, V. L. (1985). *Family life process of intergenerational families with functionally dependent elders*. Dissertation. University of Alabama at Birmingham.

Ebersole, P., Hess, P., Touhy, T., & Jett, K. (2005). *Gerontological nursing and healthy aging*. St. Louis, MO: Mosby.

Erikson, E. (1963). *Childhood and society*. New York, NY: Norton.

Folstein, M., Folstein, S., & McHugh, P. (1975). Mini-mental state: A practical method for grading the cognitive state of patients for the clinician. *Journal of Psychiatric Research, 12*, 189–198.

Kane, R., Ouslander, J., & Abrass, I. (2003). *Essentials of clinical geriatrics* (5th ed.). New York, NY: McGraw-Hill.

Maslow, A. (1968). *Toward a psychology of being* (2nd ed.). Princeton, NJ: Van Nostrand.

National Center for Health Statistics (NCHS), Centers for Disease Control and Prevention. (2013). *Health, United States*, U.S. Public Health Service, DHHS Publication No. 2013–1232. Retrieved from http://www.cdc.gov/nchs/data/hus/hus12.pdf#018

O'Malley, R. (1987). *Inadequate care of the elderly: A health care perspective on abuse and neglect*. New York, NY: Springer.

Satir, V. (1964). *Conjunct family therapy: A guide to theory and technique*. Palo Alto, CA: Science & Behavioral Books.

U.S. Census Bureau. (2010). *The next four decades: The older population of the United States, 2010 to 2050*. Retrieved from https://www.census.gov/prod/2010pubs/p25-1138.pdf

U.S. Census Bureau. (2012). *Statistical abstract of the United States*. Retrieved from https://www.census.gov/compendia/statab/

U.S. Food and Drug Administration. (2003). Medications and older people. *FDA Consumer*. Retrieved from http://www.fda.gov/fdac/features/1997/697_old.html

Williams, M., Parker, R., Baker, D., Parikh, N. S., Pitkin, K., Coates, W. C., & Nurss, J. R. (1995). Inadequate functional health literacy among patients at two public hospitals. *Journal of the American Medical Association, 274*, 1677–1720.

Yesavage, J., & Brink, T. (1983). Development and validation of a geriatric depression screening scale: A preliminary report. *Journal of Psychiatric Research, 17*, 37–49.

APPENDIX A

Selected Theories of Aging

Biological Theories

Molecular Theories

- Gene: selected genes become active in later life, causing the organism to fail to survive
- Error, error catastrophe
    - Somatic mutation
    - Transcription
- Programmed senescence
    - Run-out-of-program

System-Level Theories

- Neuroendocrine control (pacemakers)
- Immunologic/autoimmune

Cellular Theories

- Free radicals, antioxidants
- Cross-link/connective tissue
- Clinker
- Wear-and-tear

Sociological Theories

- Disengagement (Cummings & Henry, 1961)
- Activity (Lemon, 1972)
- Continuity (Havighurst, 1963)
- Age stratification
- Person–environment fit
- Sociological aging: life course, life transitions, status and role changes, social supports

Psychological Theories

- Maslow's hierarchy of human needs
- Jung's individualism
- Course of human life
- Erikson's eight stages of life: Sense of ego integrity versus sense of despair
- Peck: ego differentiation versus work-role preoccupation; body transcendence versus body preoccupation; ego transcendence versus ego preoccupation
- Feil: resolution of the past versus vegetation
- Butler's life review
- Levinson's seasons of life
- Lowenthal's life transitions
- Havighurst's developmental tasks: establishing satisfactory living arrangements, adjusting to retirement and reduced income, adjusting to decreasing physical strength and health, establishing an explicit affiliation with one's age group

APPENDIX B

Activities of Daily Living and Instrumental Activities of Daily Living

	Independent	Assisted	Dependent
• Bathing	0	1	2
• Dressing	0	1	2
• Toileting	0	1	2
• Transfer	0	1	2
• Continence	0	1	2
• Feeding	0	1	2
• Telephoning	0	1	2
• Shopping	0	1	2
• Transporting	0	1	2
• Medicating	0	1	2
• Handling money	0	1	2
• Preparing food	0	1	2
• Housekeeping	0	1	2
• Laundry	0	1	2

ADL Score (0–12) ____		**IADL Score (0–16)____**		**Total Score (0–28)____**	
0	Independent	0	Independent	0	Independent
1–6	Assisted	1–8	Assisted	1–14	Assisted
7–12	Dependent	7–16	Dependent	15–28	Dependent

APPENDIX C

Tinetti Fall Assessment Scale

Balance	(Seated in Hard, Armless Chair)	Scoring
· **Sitting balance**	Leans or slides in chair	5 0
	Steady, safe	5 1______
· **Arises**	Unable without help	5 0
	Able, uses arms to help	5 1
	Able without using arms	5 2______
· **Attempts to rise**	Unable without help	5 0
	Able, requires 1 attempt	5 1
	Able to rise, 1 attempt	5 2______
· **Immediate standing**	Balance (first 5 seconds)	
	Unsteady (staggers, moves feet, trunk sway)	5 0
	Steady but uses walker or other support	5 1
	Narrow stance without other support	5 2______
· **Standing balance**	Unsteady	5 0
	Steady but wide stance and uses other support	5 1
	Narrow stance without support	5 2______
· **Nudged**	Begins to fall	5 0
	Staggers, grabs, catches self	5 1
	Steady	5 2______
· **Eyes closed**	Unsteady	5 0
	Steady	5 1______
· **Turning 360°**	Discontinuous steps	5 0
	Continuous steps	5 1
	Unsteady (grabs, staggers)	5 0
	Steady	5 1______
· **Sitting down**	Unsafe (misjudged distance, falls into chair)	5 0
	Uses arms or not a smooth motion	5 1
	Safe, smooth motion	5 2______
· **Balance Score:**		____**/16**

Gait:	(Stands, walks about 10 feet at usual pace, then back at rapid, but safe pace with aids)	Scoring
· **Initiation of gate**	Any hesitancy or multiple attempts to start	5 0
	No hesitancy	5 1_____
· **Step length and height**		
Right swing foot	Does not pass left stance foot with step	5 0
	Passes left stance foot	5 1
	Right foot does not clear floor completely	5 0
	Right foot completely clears floor	5 1
Left swing foot	Does not pass right stance foot with step	5 0
	Passes right stance foot	5 1
	Left foot doesn't clear floor completely	5 0
	Left foot completely clears floor	5 1
· **Step symmetry**	Right and left step length not equal (estimate)	5 0
	Right and left step appear equal	5 1_____
· **Step continuity**	Stopping or discontinuity between steps	5 0
	Steps appear continuous	5 1_____
· **Path**	Marked deviation	5 0
	Mild/moderate deviation or uses walking aid	5 1
	Straight without walking aid	5 2_____
· **Trunk**	Marked sway or uses walking aid	5 0
	No sway but flexion of knees or back or spread arms out while walking	5 1
	No sway, no flexion, no use of arms, and no use of walking aid	5 2_____
· **Walking time**	Heels apart	5 0
	Heels almost touching while walking	5 1_____
· **Gait Score:**		**___/12**
· **Balance 1 Gait Score:**		**Score ___/28**
· **Key to Risk for Falls:**	**Score**	
Low	25–28	
Moderate	19–24	
High	0–18	

APPENDIX D

Folstein Mini-Mental State Exam

Highest school grade completed ______

Maximum	Score	Orientation
5	______	What is the (year), (season), (date), (day), (month)?
5	______	Where are we: (state, (city), (county), (facility), (floor)?
		Attention and Calculation
5	______	Serial 7s. One point for each correct. Stop after five answers. 93 86 79 72 65.
		Alternatively, spell "world" backward: D L R O W
		Recall
3	______	Ask for three objects repeated above. Give 1 point for each correct answer.
		Language and Praxis
2	______	Name a pencil and a watch.
1	______	Repeat the following phrase: "No ifs, ands, or buts."
		Registration
3	______	Name three objects: 1 second to say each; ask person all three objects after they are said.
		Give 1 point for each correct answer. Then repeat objects until all three are learned. Count trials and record: ______
3	______	Follow a three-stage command: "Take this paper in your right hand, fold it in half, and put it on the table."
1	______	Read and obey the following command:
		CLOSE YOUR EYES
1	______	Write a sentence:
1	______	Copy this design:
—	______	
30		
Key to FMMSE Scores:		
No cognitive impairment	24–30	
Mild cognitive impairment	18–23	
Severe cognitive impairment	0–17	

Source: Folstein, Folstein, & McHugh, 1975.

APPENDIX E

Geriatric Depression Scale

Mood Scale		
1. ARE YOU BASICALLY SATISFIED WITH YOUR LIFE?	yes	NO
2. HAVE YOU DROPPED MANY OF YOUR ACTIVITIES AND INTERESTS?	YES	no
3. DO YOU FEEL THAT YOUR LIFE IS EMPTY?	YES	no
4. DO YOU OFTEN GET BORED?	YES	no
5. Are you hopeful about the future?	yes	NO
6. Are you bothered by thoughts that you just can't get out of your head?	YES	no
7. ARE YOU IN GOOD SPIRITS MOST OF THE TIME?	yes	NO
8. ARE YOU AFRAID THAT SOMETHING BAD IS GOING TO HAPPEN TO YOU?	YES	no
9. DO YOU FEEL HAPPY MOST OF THE TIME?	yes	NO
10. DO YOU OFTEN FEEL HELPLESS?	YES	no
11. Do you often get restless and fidgety?	YES	no
12. Do you prefer to stay home at night rather than go out and do new things?	YES	no
13. Do you frequently worry about the future?	YES	no
14. DO YOU FEEL THAT YOU HAVE MORE PROBLEMS WITH MEMORY THAN MOST?	YES	no
15. DO YOU THINK IT IS WONDERFUL TO BE ALIVE NOW?	yes	NO
16. Do you often feel downhearted and blue?	YES	no
17. DO YOU FEEL PRETTY WORTHLESS THE WAY YOU ARE NOW?	YES	no
18. Do you worry a lot about the past?	YES	no
19. Do you find life very exciting?	yes	NO
20. Is it hard for you to get started on new projects?	YES	no
21. DO YOU FEEL FULL OF ENERGY?	yes	NO
22. DO YOU FEEL THAT YOUR SITUATION IS HOPELESS?	YES	no
23. DO YOU THINK THAT MOST PERSONS YOUR AGE ARE BETTER OFF THAN YOU ARE?	YES	no
24. Do you frequently get upset over little things?	YES	no
25. Do you frequently feel like crying?	YES	no
26. Do you have trouble concentrating?	YES	no
27. Do you enjoy getting up in the morning?	yes	NO
28. Do you prefer to avoid social gatherings?	YES	no

29. Is it easy for you to make decisions?	yes	NO
30. Is your mind as clear as it used to be?	yes	NO
Score	Circled capitalized answers	______
	Crossed-out lowercase answers	______
	Total	15 or 30
Key to Scoring	**GDS**	
No depression	0–4 capitalized on 15-item screen	
Mild depression	5–10 capitalized on 30-item scale	
Severe depression	11–30 capitalized on 30-item scale	

Directions for Scoring: This scale is intended to be administered orally to the elderly person in a quiet, private setting. Circle the capitalized *answer* if the elder answers the question with the capitalized response. Draw a line through the lowercase *answer* if the elder answers with the lowercase response.

Score 1 point for each circled capitalized answer.

Score 0 for each lowercase answer.

For screening purposes, use the 15 short-form *questions*, which are capitalized. If the elder scores more than 5 points, administer the full 30-item scale.

Interpretation: A score of 5 or more capitalized responses on the 15-item screen is suggestive of depression and indicates the need to administer the full scale. A score of 0–10 is normal range; a score of 11 or more capitalized responses on the 30-item scale is positive for depression.

According to Yesavage and Brink (1983), a cut-off score of 11 has a sensitivity of 84% and a specificity of 95%. A cut-off score of 14 has a sensitivity of 80% and a specificity of 100%.

Source: Yesavage & Brink, 1983.

APPENDIX F

Home Safety Checklist

Home Interior

- Floors: clean, clutter-free, rugs anchored and in good repair (no throw rugs), surface smooth and nonskid wax
- Electrical appliances: cords in good repair and out of traffic lanes
- Lighting: adequate non-glare lighting; stairs illuminated; night lights where needed
- Temperature: range 70–75°F; adequate heating, cooling, and ventilation; insulation; fireplace/heaters with protective screens
- Furniture: sturdy, good repair
- Stairs: sturdy railings; nonskid steps; uncluttered
- Organization: uncluttered, navigable traffic lanes

Communication

- Lock/unlock door; reach light switches
- Emergency telephone numbers posted, legible (fire, ambulance, doctor, family)
- If no telephone, life line, neighbor, "buddy," or other means to summon help
- Smoke alarms available with working batteries

Kitchen

- Food: adequate supply, fresh
- Stove: free of grease and flammables, baking soda or fire extinguisher
- Refrigerator: cooling effectively, food available and fresh
- Sink: draining properly, hot (check temperature) and cold water; dishes washed
- Cleaning supplies: stored separately and clearly marked
- Garbage: taken out; regular pick-up
- Ladder or step stool: sturdy with handle

Bathroom

- Handrails for tub and toilet
- Skid-proof mats for tub and/or shower
- Nonskid rug on floor
- Electrical outlets safe distance from tub

Medications

- Stored safely; current; disposal of old medicines
- Current list with times, dosage, description, purpose

Outside

- Walks, driveways, and stairs: smooth surfaces in good repair (no raised or uneven places); edges painted or clearly visible; handrails secure
- Doors and windows: panes and screens in good repair
- Fire escape or alternate exit from house

Source: Adapted from Burnside, 1988.

APPENDIX G

Baccalaureate Competencies for Geriatric Nursing Care/Care of Older Adults (2010)

1. Incorporate professional attitudes, values, and expectations about physical and mental aging in the provision of patient-centered care for older adults and their families.
2. Assess barriers for older adults in receiving, understanding, and giving of information.
3. Use valid and reliable assessment tools to guide nursing practice for older adults.
4. Assess the living environment as it relates to functional, physical, cognitive, psychological, and social needs of older adults.
5. Intervene to assist older adults and their support network to achieve personal goals based on the analysis of the living environment and availability of community resources.
6. Identify actual or potential mistreatment (physical, mental, or financial abuse, and/or self-neglect) in older adults and refer appropriately.
7. Implement strategies and use online guidelines to prevent and/or identify and manage geriatric syndromes.
8. Recognize and respect the variations of care, the increased complexity, and the increased use of healthcare resources inherent in caring for older adults.
9. Recognize the complex interaction of acute and chronic comorbid physical and mental conditions and associated treatments common to older adults.
10. Compare models of care that promote safe, quality physical and mental health care for older adults such as PACE, NICHE, Guided Care, Culture Change, and Transitional Care Models.
11. Facilitate ethical, noncoercive decision making by older adults and/or families/caregivers for maintaining everyday living, receiving treatment, initiating advance directives, and implementing end-of-life care.
12. Promote adherence to the evidence-based practice of providing restraint-free care (both physical and chemical restraints).
13. Integrate leadership and communication techniques that foster discussion and reflection on the extent to which diversity (among nurses, nurse assistive personnel, therapists, physicians, and patients) has the potential to impact the care of older adults.
14. Facilitate safe and effective transitions across levels of care, including acute, community-based, and long-term care (e.g., home, assisted living, hospice, nursing homes) for older adults and their families.
15. Plan patient-centered care with consideration for mental and physical health and wellbeing of informal and formal caregivers of older adults.
16. Advocate for timely and appropriate palliative and hospice care for older adults with physical and cognitive impairments.
17. Implement and monitor strategies to prevent risk and promote quality and safety (e.g., falls, medication mismanagement, pressure ulcers) in the nursing care of older adults with physical and cognitive needs.
18. Utilize resources/programs to promote functional, physical, and mental wellness in older adults.
19. Integrate relevant theories and concepts included in a liberal education into the delivery of patient-centered care for older adults.

UNIT 7

Diversity in Community Health Nursing Roles

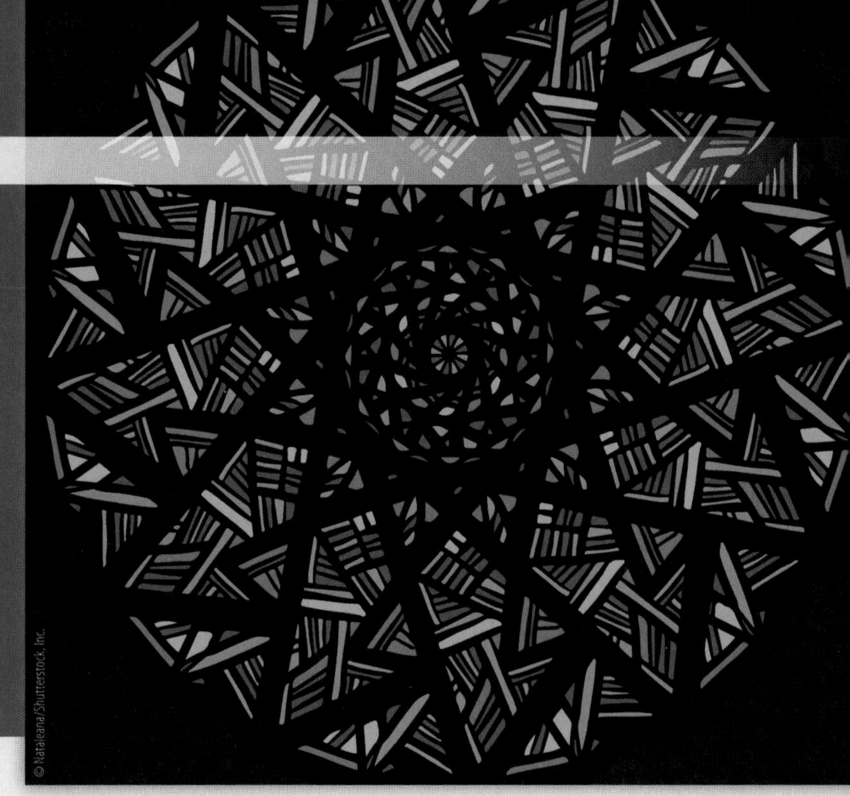

CHAPTER FOCUS

History of Public Health Nursing
- Early Healthcare Reform
- The Later Years

Public Health Nursing Philosophy
- Institute of Medicine Study
- Conceptual Basis for Public Health Nursing Practice
- Definition and Development of Public Health Nursing

Challenges and Issues for Public Health Nursing in the 21st Century
- Impact of the Nursing Shortage on Public Health Nursing
- Further Development of Public Health Nursing Models and Competencies
- National Public Health Performance Standards
- Other Challenges for Public Health Nursing

QUESTIONS TO CONSIDER

After reading this chapter, you will know the answers to the following questions:

1. What were the early public health reform efforts?
2. Who were the early public health nursing leaders?
3. What were the primary contributions of public health nurses during the early part of the 20th century?
4. What are characteristics of nursing from the 1960s through the 1980s?
5. What is the role and focus of public health nursing practice?
6. What is the significance of the Institute of Medicine's report of 1988?
7. How are conceptual models used in public health nursing?
8. What is the Construct for Public Health Nursing, and what is its usefulness in present public health nursing practice?
9. What is meant by *essential public health services*?
10. What is the future of public health nursing in the 21st century?

When Florence Nightingale founded modern nursing, the relationship between the environment and the health of the individual was a cornerstone. Nightingale's text *Notes on Nursing* described the nurse's role in altering the patient's immediate environment through ventilation and heating, cleanliness of housing, modification of noise, provision of light, and proper preparation and availability of food. These factors were found by Nightingale to be of importance to the health and wellbeing of individuals and, therefore, relevant to nursing intervention. The public health nurse role emerged from these early links between health and the environmental conditions under which we live.

CHAPTER 35

Public Health Nursing: Pioneers of Healthcare Reform

Kaye W. Bender and Marla E. Salmon

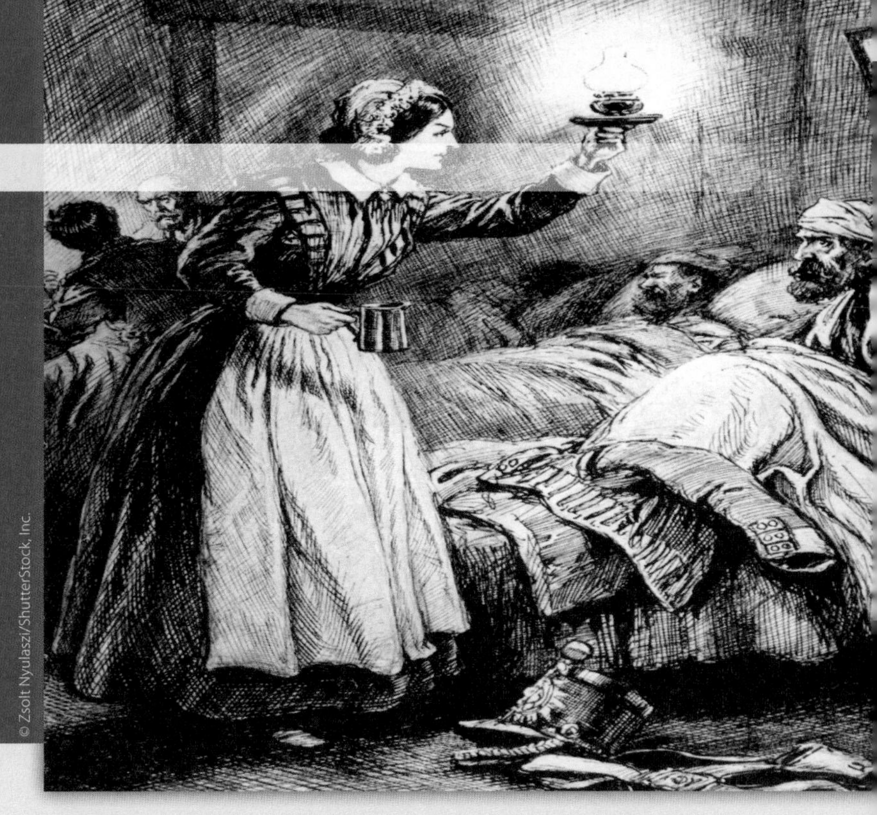

KEY TERMS

Commonwealth Fund
conceptual model
Construct for Public Health Nursing: A Framework for the Future
Hospital and Reconstruction Act of 1946
Institute of Medicine
Medicare
Milbank Report
Mary D. Osborne
Salk vaccine
Social Security Act of 1935
Lillian Wald

> Home Health bringing requires different, but not lower, qualifications and more varied. They require tact and judgment unlimited to prevent the work being regarded as interference and becoming unpopular. They require initiative and real belief in Sanitation and that Life and Death may lie in a grain of dust or drop of water or other such minutiae which are not minutiae but Goliaths and the Health Missioner must be Davids and slay them.
>
> —Florence Nightingale, 1891

> Over broken asphalt, over dirty mattresses and heaps of refuse we went … there were two rooms and a family of seven not only lived here but shared their quarters with boarders … I felt ashamed of being a part of society that permitted such conditions to exist… . What I had seen had shown me where my path lay.
>
> —Lillian Wald, 1893; Wald coined the phrase "public health nursing" and organized the first public health agency, the Henry Street Settlement in New York City

REFLECTIONS

As you reflect on these quotations, what comes to mind when you think of "public health"? The term *public health* in the past century has been associated with government programs, such as immunizations and blood tests for marriage licenses. What do you think of when you hear "public health nurse"?

History of Public Health Nursing

There have been public health problems in the United States since colonization, but it was not until after the Civil War that concerted efforts were made to improve morbidity and mortality and to control infectious diseases. Poverty, unsanitary living conditions, rampant spread of communicable diseases, natural disasters such as floods, malnutrition, and lack of health care were contributing factors to morbidity and mortality. Public health nursing pioneers emerged as public health efforts began, the most notable being **Lillian Wald**, who is recognized as the leader of public health nursing in the United States. Wald was the first to use the term *public health nurse* to describe visiting nurses who provided direct care to the sick in their homes. These nurses also taught basic hygiene, sanitation, care of children, and proper care and preparation of food. Public health nurses proved versatile: Their skills seemed endless, with a mission to prevent disease, promote health, and to provide care. Their communities truly became their workplace as they became involved in health concerns associated with access to health care, labor movements, maternal and child health, reproductive health, mental health, prison reform, and school health.

Early Healthcare Reform

Organized public health efforts were initiated across the United States in the late 1800s and early 1900s. This early healthcare reform movement was aimed at improving the health status of all citizens. Leading causes of death were tuberculosis, pneumonia and influenza, diarrhea, malaria, heart and cerebrovascular diseases, and infectious diseases in early infancy; complicating factors were the deplorable living conditions and malnutrition of many citizens. Most notable among the early public health nursing activities were services to river travelers in the South and seaports along the nation's coasts and preventive health services to immigrants in large Eastern Seaboard cities.

Many of the early efforts to establish public health nursing occurred as a result of collaborative agreements between municipalities and the American Red Cross. It was not uncommon for public health nurses to be assigned to posts in geographical areas other than the ones in which they lived at the time of their employment. One such early pioneer was **Mary D. Osborne**, who came to a rural Southern state to work toward the improvement of infant mortality. Her philosophy of public health nursing is reflected in her writings, in which she described qualities she deemed essential for public health nurses of the time: "nurses chosen for public health needed vision, a great desire to do community work, the ability to work up resources at hand, the adaptability to meet situations as they arose, and most of all infinite patience with people they serve" (Mississippi Department of Archives, 1920–1980); these qualities are as essential today for public health nurses as they were in Osborne's time. Osborne received national and international recognition in 1929 for her work in forging a strong network of public health nurses and for their accomplishments in lowering maternal and infant mortality through improved midwifery practice.

ENVIRONMENTAL CONNECTION

How Can Climate Change Harm the Public's Health?

The climate is changing and these changes impact the nation's health. The ebb and flow of disease are linked to climate. For example, warmer temperatures are often associated with increases in diseases such as West Nile virus. Scientists estimate that the changes in our climate are associated with increasing rather than decreasing risks of disease. Climate change may cause extreme weather events and changes in environmental conditions, leading to increases in disease and death. Populations already at increased risk from death and disease, such as communities of color, the elderly, young children, and the poor, will bear the burden of disease and death from climate change. The existing conditions that already cause worse health among these populations—lack of clean air and water and unhealthy living conditions—will be exacerbated by the adverse effects of climate change. These communities are not only at increased risk for disease, but they are also the least able to prepare, respond, and recover from effects of climate change.

Source: American Public Health Association. (2008). *Climate change is a public health issue*. Washington, DC: Author.

The Great Depression is remembered today as one of the most dramatic times in U.S. history, and most states felt the difficult economic effects of the early 1930s.

Public health and public health nursing struggled through this era; however, federal initiatives through Roosevelt's New Deal programs and private entities such as the **Commonwealth Fund** provided funding to expand public health nursing services. The hope was to place one public health nurse in each county in many of the states. Immunization efforts against smallpox, diphtheria, and typhoid were among the special initiatives with the expanded public health nursing workforce. New initiatives were integrated with previously established activities centered around communicable diseases, perinatal and infant care and midwifery supervision, and tuberculosis control. Their place of service delivery was literally all places in their community, as public health nurses made home visits, initiated school visits, and often set up clinic sites in rural churches or under shade trees.

The public health nurse was equipped with a large brown leather bag to carry essential items such as needles, syringes, a Sterno stove, and matches to set up clinic sites. A black nursing bag was added to provide a mechanism for carrying needed items for home visits. To get where they needed to be, the nurses might travel down muddy paths by riding a mule, borrowing a horse and buggy, or walking lengthy distances. Sometimes a boat might be the mode of transportation. An automobile was a luxury item and a prized possession when available.

CULTURAL CONNECTION

Motorcyclists often believe that they alone should decide if they will wear a helmet. In states where helmets are mandatory for all ages, how do you address the concerns of autonomy for the motorcyclist and the protection of the public's health?

Early Health Outcomes

The dramatic results of this healthcare movement are noted in mortality and morbidity statistics from 1926 to 1936, with reductions in typhoid fever, diphtheria, pulmonary tuberculosis, pellagra, puerperal septicemia, and eclampsia. One state health official gave much credit to public health nursing by noting that the public health nursing service had come to be recognized as a vital part of an efficient public health administration.

Syphilis had been recognized for several years as a major source of morbidity and mortality. Several boards of health participated with the United States Public Health Service (USPHS) in major studies in the 1930s and 1940s to develop means to conquer the disease. Public health nurses were recognized by the USPHS project director as the chief means to find cases, access medical care for treatment, provide education, find contacts, and follow up on lapsed cases.

Despite interferences of World War II, public health nurses continued to receive education in prevention and treatment of disease processes, including tuberculosis, vaccine-preventable diseases, maternal and child health, and syphilis. Remarkable advances in medical prevention and diagnostic and treatment measures such as the introduction of penicillin were changing public health service delivery and opening new challenges for public health nurses. After World War II, social and economic changes in the states (e.g., improved housing and transportation, movement from farms to towns, expansion of industry) also brought challenges for public health nursing. A public health nurse was employed to institute industrial nursing, which would focus on disease prevention, improvements of hazardous work conditions, promotion of personal health (including nutrition), and first aid.

The country had experienced cyclic polio epidemics since 1934, but disaster struck with the most virulent and widespread epidemic in 1951–1952. Public health nurses made home visits to assist in rehabilitative measures for persons affected with this crippling disease. Regional orthopedic clinics were manned by public health nurses to support access to medical care and set up patient treatment plans. With the availability of the injectable **Salk vaccine** in 1955, public health nurses set up mass immunization sites, while using needles and syringes that required sterilization between each use. These efforts prevented the occurrence of any further polio epidemics.

Healthcare reform was again under way as federal funds were made available through the **Hospital and Reconstruction Act of 1946**. The increased availability of local hospitals resulted in more physician-attended births, another significant contribution to lower maternal and infant mortality rates. A dilemma resulted, however, as newly constructed hospitals, expanding industry, and public health were competing for the short supply of nurses in the country. Concerns such as the turnover of nursing personnel, the below-average ratio of public health nurse to population, inadequate salaries, and increased responsibilities caused by a shortage of medical directors in county health departments were prevalent. During this era, public health nursing services shifted significantly from the community to the clinic, rendering the large brown bag used to set up outlying clinics extinct. A shift from family health to more technical, disease-oriented services occurred as a result of limited medical coverage and increased demands for nursing services.

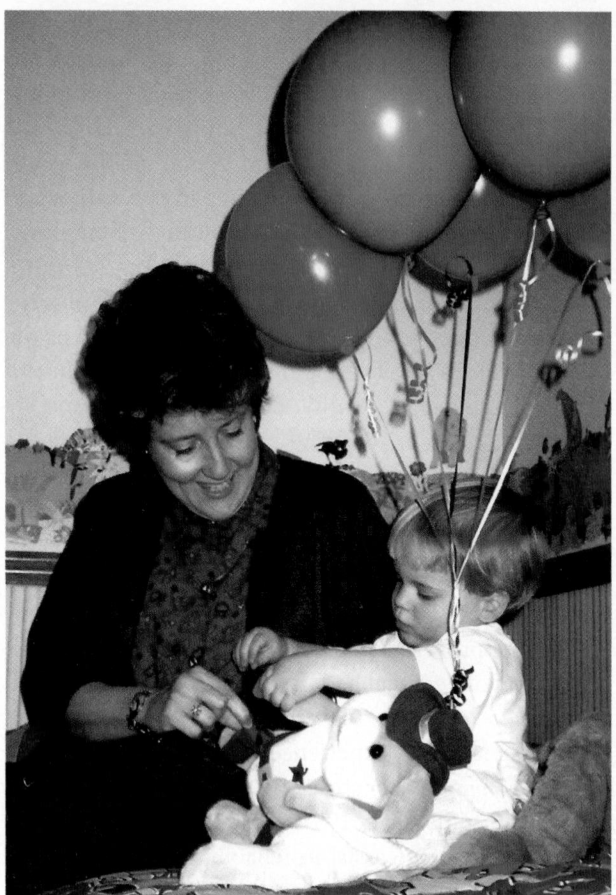

Dr. Kaye W. Bender, chapter author, on a well child home visit for the public health department.

The individual states, along with the rest of the nation, were flourishing economically as the 1960s began. Tuberculosis and several other infectious diseases were no longer the leading causes of death. Typhoid fever, diphtheria, malaria, smallpox, and pellagra had been leading causes of death in 1930–1931; by 1959–1960, only a few deaths were reported from these diseases. Heart disease, circulatory diseases, cancer, accidents, and diabetes were reported as the leading causes of death.

Changes in morbidity and mortality required evaluation by public health and, consequently, new strategies and public health programs were needed to continue the public health mission. Public health nursing established chronic illness objectives to identify cases and treat diabetic and hypertensive patients. Nursing interventions included referrals to local physicians to initiate treatment plans, nutrition and general health education, administration of medication, and teaching administration of insulin. In addition, new vaccines to prevent measles and rubella were integrated into routine immunization standards.

Tuberculosis, although no longer a leading cause of death, remained a public morbidity threat. Medications and treatment modalities had greatly advanced, however. Recognizing the value of early detection of persons susceptible to tuberculosis and providing prophylactic treatment, public health nurses accepted the challenge of a major initiative by boards of health to eradicate tuberculosis. Public health nurses identified contacts to active cases and others determined to be infected, coordinated medical evaluations, initiated plans of care for further diagnostic measures, and administered isonicotinylhydrazine (INH) medication.

Landmark federal legislation in 1965 transformed health care with an amendment to the **Social Security Act of 1935**, establishing **Medicare**, a health insurance plan for people 65 years and older and for those with long-term disabilities. Many boards of health supported expanded efforts to meet the federal conditions of participation and, over a 4- to 5-year period, implemented certified home health services. Educational opportunities provided public health nurses with knowledge and skills to provide skilled rehabilitative nursing care to persons who were essentially confined to their homes. Public health nurses had been providing home nursing services on a limited basis since the 1920s, but this would be the first reimbursement established for direct nursing services.

Another new federal initiative for public health nursing by the mid-1960s was family planning. The objective was aimed at lowering maternal and infant mortality rates and improving the general health of women and children, primary interests of public health nurses since the 1920s. With the development of oral contraceptives and the sexual revolution of the 1960s, public health nurses promoted family planning, taught contraception methods, and were key in identifying women at higher risk for such services.

The quantity and variance of public health nursing activities continued to increase. The number of public health nursing visits increased in the areas of communicable disease, maternal and child health, school health, tuberculosis control, sexually transmitted disease, home health, mental health, accident prevention, and chronic disease. Particularly in the Southern states, the work of public health nurses in all health programs was perhaps the greatest force in delivering health services to all citizens.

The Later Years

Social and political unrest begun in the 1960s continued into the 1970s, and simultaneously the nation was faced with inflation. Travel budgets were cut; public health nursing activities were again evaluated and were relocated from the field to the clinic setting. Continued vigilance in protecting the public's health was in order, and public health nursing rose to the occasion. Increased teen pregnancy rates, a higher incidence of premature births in poorer women, and frequent pregnancies were the focus for public health nursing interventions. More intense family planning initiatives and high-risk tracking systems were implemented to reduce unintended pregnancies and ensure quality, continuous care. In addition, public health nurses supported program implementations to improve nutrition to mothers and children and newborn screening with follow up for select genetic diseases.

Public health was confronted in the 1970s with increasing demands for services and a limited availability of physicians. Federal funds were made available to provide education to expand the scope of nursing in primary care. Many nurse practice acts were revised by legislation to allow for the expanded role of public health nurses. Boards of health, recognizing the value of this level of practitioner in public health, selected public health nurses to return to school with primary areas of study in maternal and child health. This proved to be an added advantage as nurses returned to more patient- and family-centered care, which had been the traditional philosophy of public health nursing.

Public health nurses since the 1980s have continued to provide an array of public health services to the general public, to medically underserved populations, and to culturally diverse populations. Their workplace remains the same, as they provide services in individual homes, schools, industry, jails and prisons, and the county health departments; and their mission, to prevent disease and to promote health, remains constant. With today's national and state focus on healthcare reform, public health nurses are positioned to assist communities and the individuals within to bridge the transitions of health care. Their versatile skills include assessing the health status of communities, translating and interpreting among healthcare disciplines, promoting and teaching health, delivering primary community-based health care, and sustaining measures to control communicable disease (Cohen & Reutter, 2007; Gebbie & Turnock, 2006).

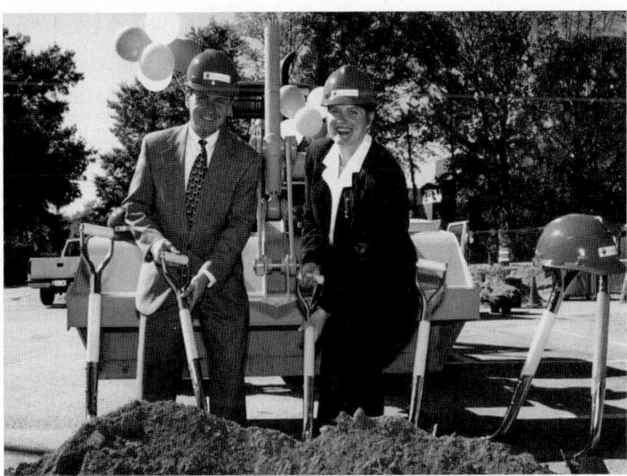

At the groundbreaking for the Nell Hodgson Woodruff School of Nursing of Emory University's new building, James Curran, MD, MPH, dean of the Rollins School of Public Health, and Marla Salmon, ScD, RN, FAAN, dean of the School of Nursing and chapter author, broke ground together. Drs. Curran and Salmon hold joint faculty appointments in each other's schools, concrete evidence of a collaboration and partnership between the two schools.

Public Health Nursing Philosophy

Fundamental to the philosophy of public health nursing are holistic beliefs about humanity, health, and nursing.

Public health nursing practice is a systematic process that accomplishes the following:

1. The health and healthcare needs of a population are assessed to identify subpopulations, families, and individuals who would benefit from health promotion or who are at increased risk of illness, injury, disability, or premature death.
2. A plan for intervention is developed with the community to meet identified needs that take into account available resources and the range of activities that contribute to health and the prevention of illness, disability, and premature death.
3. A plan is implemented effectively, efficiently, and equitably.
4. Evaluations are conducted to determine the extent to which the interventions have an effect on the health status of individuals and the population.
5. The results of the process are used to influence and direct the current delivery of care, deployment of health resources, and the development of local, regional, state, and national health policy and research to promote health and prevent disease.

This systematic process is based on and is consistent with (1) community strengths, needs, and expectations; (2) current scientific knowledge; (3) available resources; (4) accepted criteria and standards of nursing practice; (5) agency purpose, philosophy, and objectives; and (6) the participation, cooperation, and understanding of the population. Other services and organizations in the community are considered, and planning is coordinated to maximize the effective use of resources and enhance outcomes. The philosophy of public health nursing is based on the belief that patients (individuals, families, groups, or communities) have the right to quality health care that is available, accessible, and acceptable and that will include them in the planning of their health care (American Public Health Association [APHA], 1996; Easley & Allen, 2008; Gebbie & Turnock, 2006).

Institute of Medicine Study

Recognizing that organized public health efforts had been vital to ensuring the health of the nation, the **Institute of Medicine** (IOM) completed a 2-year study of the future of public health in 1988. During that 2-year period, the committee members interviewed an array of public health workers, policymakers, members of the general public, and public health academicians. The study's final recommendations have become a cornerstone for guiding public health's organizational development. Those recommendations included a description of the mission of public health.

> It is mere childishness to tell us that it is not important to know what houses people live in ... the connection between health and the dwellings of the population is one of the most important that exists.
>
> —*Florence Nightingale, 1861*

History reveals that healthcare reform is a continuous process, not a new phenomenon. The elements currently influencing healthcare reform are both old and new—tremendous technology advances, explosive and diverse population growth, political changes, an array of extreme social problems, escalating healthcare costs, access to care, financing for acute care rather than preventive health, and the need to encourage individual responsibility for health (Abrams, 2007; Kulbok & Reed, 2006; Polivka et al., 2008).

THINK ABOUT THIS

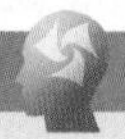

Can this really be true? Public health efforts are the reason we are living longer!

Public health's prevention efforts are responsible for 25 years of the nearly 30-year improvement in life expectancy at birth in the United States since 1900. Only 3.7 years can be attributed to medical treatment, and clinical preventive services (such as immunizations and screening tests) account for 1.5 years. The remaining 25 years have resulted primarily from prevention efforts in the form of social policies, community actions, and personal decisions. Examples that have added years to our lifespans are infectious disease control, improved nutrition to targeted populations (women and children), clean drinking water, environmental risk reduction, prenatal care, contraception use, and self-risk reduction and education (Turnock, 1997). And yet today, less than 3% of the federal budget is allotted to preventive health services.

What do you think? Are we putting our money on the right horse?

Source: Turnock, B. J. (1997). *Public health: What it is and how it works*. Gaithersburg, MD: Aspen.

GOT AN ALTERNATIVE?

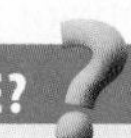

Public health nurses, perhaps more than other specialties, are confronted with "folk remedies" used by their patients. Because of the bond that exists between nurse and patient influenced by long-term contact, the public health nurse is often aware of what the patient and her family uses outside of traditional medical interventions. These items may include folk remedies such as medicinal herbal preparations, beliefs about childbearing and menstruation, and use of meditation and prayer. How can the public health nurse promote the health of patients, and prevent potential risks, considering his or her unique position with families?

The resulting mission statement said succinctly what public health nurses had been practicing for many years. With the goal of improving the health of the public as a whole, public health nurses systematically provide nursing interventions at both individual and community levels. These interventions vary with the changing health status of the citizens of the country. In the early years when living conditions and crowded housing created opportunities for diseases to spread, public health nurses provided assessment, treatment, and education on tuberculosis, sexually transmitted diseases, and general personal hygiene. In later years, as lifestyles and personal health habit choices became more significant to the causes of morbidity and mortality, public health nurses added education about the prevention of tobacco use, exercise benefits, and domestic violence to their menu of interventions (Cohen & Reutter, 2007; Gebbie & Turnock, 2006).

The role of ensuring that the public remains as healthy as possible is shared between government and the private sector. The Institute of Medicine (1988) described government's role in ensuring the public's health as follows:

- *Assessment*: Public health agencies systematically collect, analyze, and publish information on the health status of the community.

- *Policy development*: Public health agencies promote the use of scientific knowledge as the basis for formulating public policy about health.
- *Assurance*: Public health agencies assure that services that are needed to ensure the health of the public are in place and are of high quality.

Several levels of responsibility were attached to these roles. Local, state, and federal governments were all challenged with their respective responsibilities in ensuring the health of the public. Special linkages to environmental health, mental health, and the care of the indigent were also described in the study.

Public health nurses have the potential to develop roles in all of the areas described in the IOM report. Although the most commonly defined role of the public health nurse has been that of providing services to control communicable diseases, there are numerous other roles for public health nurses. Since the beginning of the 21st century, public health nurses have been working in epidemiology, policy development, administration, specialized research areas, and nurse-managed projects aimed at improving the health of special populations.

Conceptual Basis for Public Health Nursing Practice

The new millennium has brought forth countless predictions about the nature of tomorrow's healthcare delivery system. These scenarios range from visions of health care being delivered through primarily technological means as part of the many services provided by one of a few large health-related corporations to more humanistic portrayals of high-touch, community-based programs that reflect the unique nature of where people live and work. What is common to almost all scenarios is that they seem to ignore two very important factors: the changing social context worldwide and the ongoing role of government in the protection and assurance of the health of the public.

Clearly, it is difficult to predict what the world will be like over the next two to three decades; however, there are some crucial themes that will undoubtedly play major roles in shaping the health of all people. The first of these is globalization and the resulting interconnectedness of all people. Through increasingly interlaced economies, markets, and the media, it is now virtually impossible to remain unaffected by what is happening in other countries and cultures. In addition, travel, migration, and the forced movement of masses of people by political and natural disasters have mixed peoples together in ways never before seen. Communities based on shared culture and history are disappearing rapidly. The global disruption of people and communities, coupled with the rise in religious fundamentalism and nationalism worldwide, promises a highly unstable and challenging future for the health of all people.

Global changes of the magnitude described here place heavy burdens on individuals, communities, and governments. The United States is not immune to these changes and is already struggling to address these at all levels. Rising violence of all types and growing gang membership; increasing diversity in language, culture, and race; and growing separation between the rich and the poor are challenging every social institution and community. In the face of these enormous challenges, it is difficult to imagine any healthcare system without considering how governments at all levels will work to ensure that the health of the public is protected.

GLOBAL CONNECTION 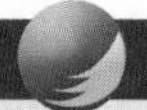

Public health nurses in many countries are responsible for geographical areas, such as city blocks or rural areas defined by miles. They care for all families in their "district" and are considered generalists.

It is in the context of ensuring the health of the public that the future of public health nursing will emerge. We will now look at those key themes that are critical to the creation of the future roles of public health nurses and propose the application of a fundamental **conceptual model** in the development of future public health nursing interventions.

When one examines health systems scenarios for the 21st century, there is an implicit assumption that the system of health care will be deeply embedded in the marketplace and governed by the principles of competition and a market economy. Often accompanying this assumption is the belief that the market has the ability in and of itself to deal with the problems of access and quality that plague our system. There is a view that the more troubling issues of equity and social justice—who receives care and in what ways—will be solved by letting the market do its work. As noted financier George Soros (1997) has observed, there are inherent dangers in this optimistic view of relying heavily on the marketplace to address these crucial issues. Our economy has as its fundamental purposes the creation of goods, services, and profit, based on willingness and ability to pay. Unfortunately, when health services become a commodity, not everyone can afford them or pay for them.

The reality that large sectors of the U.S. population are denied access to reasonable health care is not in the best interest of these individuals, nor does it work to the benefit of the overall public. The failure or inability of the marketplace to address public health needs—whether in provision of health care, protection of the environment, or containing and preventing disease and injury—is where much of public health's future lies (O'Fallon, 2006). It is comforting to know that this mandate of acting in the overall interest of the public has been in existence for well over a century. The historic **Milbank Report** on Higher Education for Public Health offered a timeless definition of public health:

> Public health is the effort organized by society to protect, promote, and restore the people's health. The programs, services, and institutions involved emphasize the prevention of disease and the health needs of the population as a whole. Public health activities change with changing technology and social values, but the goals remain the same: to reduce the amount of disease, premature death, and the disease-produced discomfort and disability. (Milbank Memorial Fund Commission, 1976, p. 3)

The history of public health nursing clearly illustrates both the changing nature and timelessness of ensuring the health of the people. For more than 100 years, public health nurses have filled multiple roles and created an endless variety of strategies, interventions, and programs to fulfill their mission. It is in both the constancy of the mission and the flexibility of its means that public health nursing will find its future (Chaudry, 2008; Salmon, 1993).

What this means in practical terms is that public health nursing needs to clearly understand the effects of the changing society on health and the forces that are at work either enhancing or eroding the health of the people. To do so, public health nurses need an overall operating framework that encompasses public health values, health determinants, practice priorities, types of interventions, and an understanding of the interplay of these at all levels. The model presented in this chapter is **Construct for Public Health Nursing: A Framework for the Future** (White, 1982). (See **Figure 35-1**.)

In 1982, the Construct for Public Health Nursing first appeared in *Nursing Outlook*. The purpose of the construct was to provide a systematic model through which public health nursing could be understood and practiced. Since

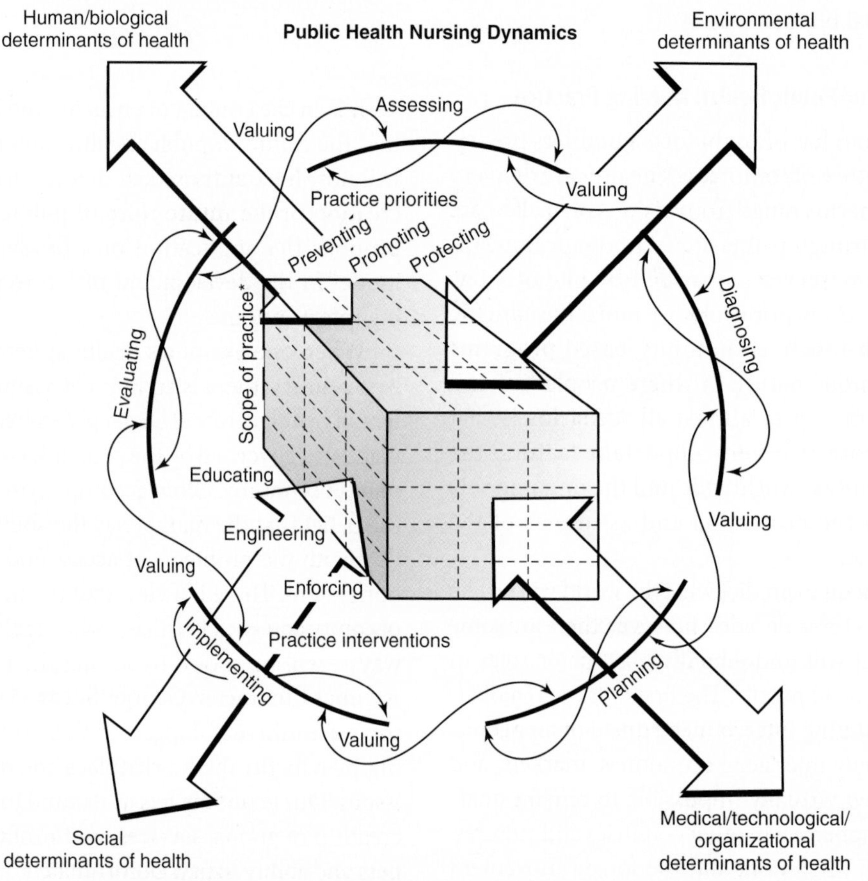

Figure 35-1 Construct for Public Health Nursing Model.

Source: From *Nursing Outlook*, Nov-Dec 1982, "Construct for Public Health Nursing Model" by Maria Salmon White, pages 30 and 527. Copyright Elsevier, 1982. Used by permission.

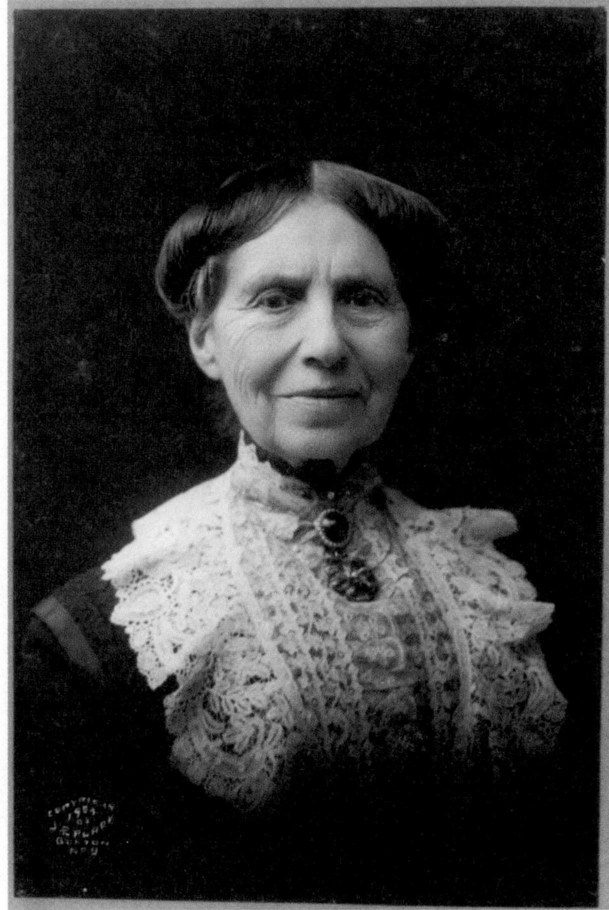

Clara Barton founded the American Red Cross by convincing Congress to ratify the Treaty of Geneva and was the driving force behind the creation of the Army Nurse Corps.

that time, the model has been incorporated into education and practice through its adoption in curricula, incorporation in a variety of texts and articles, and extensive use in the creation of public health nursing programs at a variety of levels.

THINK ABOUT THIS

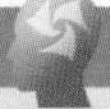

Florence Nightingale referred to public health nurses as District Nurses, because they were responsible for districts or geographical areas in their responsibilities of caregiving in the community. She held fast that District Nurses must have 1 year of experience in hospital nursing (which is still a widely held belief today for community health nurses) and additional formal training as a District Nurse. The additional training included patient teaching, the care of houses, preventive care, and hygiene education. Nightingale (December 16, 1896) believed that District Nurses would be "a great civilizer of the poor, training as well as nursing them out of ill health into good health, out of drink into self control, but all without preaching, without patronizing—as friends, in sympathy."

This model is particularly useful as public health nursing grapples with understanding and shaping the health of the public in the 21st century. The model itself is built on the premise that the fundamental difference between public health nursing and all other nursing rests in its commitment to the health of the public. This notion of the public good is understood to be the ethical base for public health nursing practice and the consequences of fundamentally social and political processes. As a result, the model depicts a practice that is based on explicit valuing of the public good and a "form follows function" approach to actual interventions. The values of public health nursing are interlaced in the circular depiction of the public health nursing process: assessing, diagnosing, planning, implementing, and evaluating. In other words, each of those actions is based on the primacy of the public's health and good.

This notion of valuing the public's good does not sit easy with most health professionals, whose ethics are grounded in advocacy for individual patients. It is for this reason that the explicit delineation of public health values is critical to the successful future practice of public health nursing. Most of our healthcare system has been built on the notion of serving individuals; very little consideration has been given to the impact on the wellbeing of the public.

In the model, the health of the public is seen as being impacted by four determinants of health: social, human/biological, environmental, and medical/technological/organizational. The first three are fairly well understood—it is the fourth that continues to be less a part of most practitioners' concept of health determinants. Another way of describing these determinants is that they are *made up* of the technology, organization, and policies relating to healthcare delivery. It is the content and organization of health care itself. This determinant has shown itself to be an extremely important point of consideration during this period of "healthcare reform," which has focused entirely on this factor.

In understanding the determinants of health and their dynamics, public health nursing has the knowledge on which to target interventions. In other words, public health nursing practice is fundamentally focused on influencing determinants of health as the primary mechanism for enhancing and protecting the health of people.

The practice of public health nursing that is described in the model has three priorities: prevention, protection, and health promotion. Understood as somewhat overlapping concepts, each is given its own prominence because of the importance of considering all three in actual practice. These priorities serve to focus the ways in which public health nurses interface with health determinants. The message in all three of these priorities is that early intervention is always most desirable, with prevention being the primary goal.

When one considers the mandate of ensuring the health of the public, the nature of health determinants, and the utilitarian notion that the form of public health nursing is sharpened to fulfill its function, it becomes apparent that public health nursing practice can occur in a variety of contexts at many levels. The magnitude of public health nursing practice possibilities is depicted through a scope of practice that extends from the individual at one end to the world at another. Along this continuum sit families, groups, communities, populations, and geopolitical entities, such as towns, counties, states, and countries. This enormous scope of practice provides tremendous latitude and opportunity; it also presents great challenges to the field. The successful practice of public health nursing requires practitioners with a variety of knowledge and skills. The foundations of these skills are found in the core content of both nursing and public health.

The Construct for Public Health Nursing describes three categories of interventions: education, engineering, and enforcement. These general classifications are consistent with the notion that their content is shaped by the priorities for practice, the determinants of health to be targeted, and their "location" on the scope of practice. An educational intervention that is aimed at prevention of lead poisoning, for example, is quite different at an individual level than one aimed at a family, group, community, or legislators. So also would be engineering strategies, which would be designed to alter the environment in a manner that protects people. Some of these strategies might focus on retrofitting plumbing at a community level or working on a house-to-house basis to reduce the presence of lead-based paint. Engineering strategies also include those of a societal nature—changing the social environment to prevent exposures. Consider, for example, preventing crime through changing social factors in a community—increasing employment, developing neighborhood watch strategies, encouraging community policing, and so on. Last, enforcement strategies are aimed at putting into place mechanisms for "compelling" behavior that results in better health. Laws that require motorcycle helmets are one such example. Enforcement strategies can also be used on an individual level, such as individually observed therapy for high-risk patients with drug-resistant tuberculosis.

The underlying theme throughout this model is that actions are guided by commitment, context, clear priorities, public health values, flexibility, and the melding of nursing and public health knowledge and skills. This means that public health nursing is really a practice that is shaped by intent, not by convention. The intent, of course, is serving the public's health.

Definition and Development of Public Health Nursing

There are four organizations that work together to develop policy and practice-related guidelines for public health nursing. Those organizations, collectively called the *QUAD Council of Public Health Nursing Organizations,* include the American Nurses Association (ANA) Council on Nursing Practice and Economics; the Public Health Nursing Section

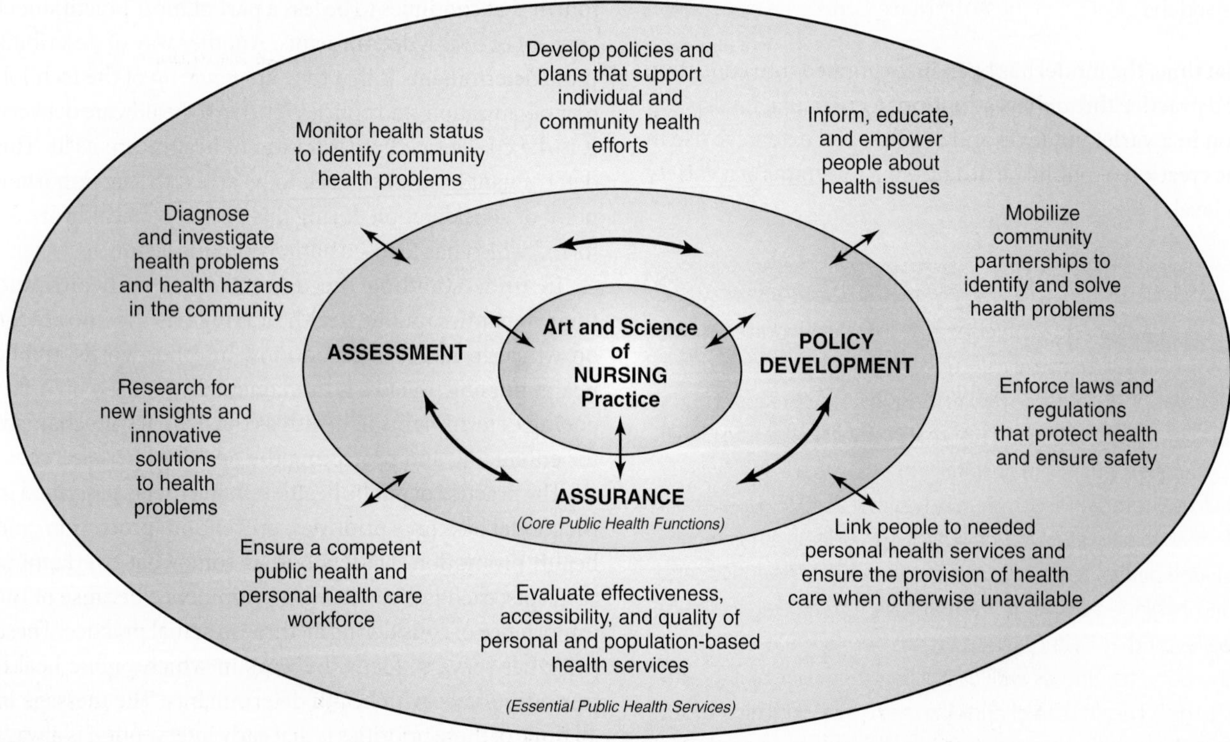

Figure 35-2 ASTDN Public Health Nursing Practice Model: Essential Public Health Services and Public Health Nursing, 1999.

of the American Public Health Association (PHN-APHA); the Association of Public Health Nurses (APHN); and the Association of Community Health Nurse Educators. (ACHNE). In the 1990s, these four organizations came together to develop descriptions of the scope of practice for public health nursing that are reflective of the diversity of the roles across the country. One key element in the work of these groups is the fundamental understanding that what it takes to maintain the health of the public differs across lifespans, across cultures, and across state and territorial boundaries. The process of public health nursing, however, combines the knowledge base of both public health and nursing to guide the intervention.

Challenges and Issues for Public Health Nursing in the 21st Century

Impact of the Nursing Shortage on Public Health Nursing

Numerous nursing organizations and healthcare agencies have documented the existing nursing shortage throughout the United States. This shortage is predicted to continue and become more acute by the year 2030, with a projected deficit of nearly 1 million registered nurses (RNs) compared to positions needing to be filled; some regions of the United States, such as southern and western states, will face more acute shortages than others

TABLE 35-1 Association of State and Territorial Directors of Nursing Public Health Nursing Practice Model: Essential Public Health Services and Public Health Nursing

Essential Service	Public Health Nursing Activity	Example
Monitor health status	Community assessment	A public health nurse asked a civic group and local health providers to participate in a study of major risk factors for disability in their community. As a result, the community developed a walking trail and wrote a federal grant for a health center.
Diagnose health hazards	Disease case identification	Public health nurses provided tuberculosis skin testing to a plant's workers. As a result, two cases of tuberculosis were identified early and contacts were placed on preventive therapy.
Inform and educate public	Community education	Public health nurses provided classes to a local community group on prevention of disease transmission in daycare centers.
Mobilize community partnerships	Community organization	A public health nurse called a community meeting to discuss accident prevention. As a result of several meetings, the community raised funds for streetlights.
Develop policies	Advocate for funding	Public health nurses organized efforts to secure funding for a school nurse in a community with high teen pregnancy rates, high school dropout rates, and increased drug use among the teen population.
Enforce health regulations	Implementation of health regulations	After hearing a complaint from a member of the public about finding needles and syringes in a public garbage area behind a medical clinic, the public health nurse assessed the complainant for potential blood and body fluid exposure testing and contacted the appropriate authorities to work with the local clinic to develop proper disposal policies.
Link people to services	Provision of health services	In an undeserved area, public health nurses provide prenatal care to women and then refer them to a nearby physician for delivery.
Ensure competency	Participation in organized educational sessions	Public health nurses attend a workshop on a new treatment for HIV-infected individuals.
Evaluate effectiveness	Participation in research	Public health nurses collaborate with a local university on a study to determine the effectiveness of a new home visiting program for preterm babies.
Research for new ideas	Implementation of new strategies	Public health nurses test a new health education model for reducing youth tobacco use.

(Juraschek, Zhang, Ranganathan, & Lin, 2012). Much of the information from the nursing profession on this shortage has focused on the institutional setting and associated working conditions. However, the shortage is affecting all areas of nursing practice.

The impact of a shortage on public health nursing differs in a number of respects from that in other settings. For example, job vacancy rates are not an adequate indicator of the shortage in public health nursing, because vacant positions are generally eliminated to cover local or state budget deficits or RN positions are converted to other types of positions. While other professionals in public health perform excellent jobs of connecting these individuals with community resources, they are not able to integrate the clinical status of the patient with their social needs—namely, the skill set of nurses. A better indicator of the shortage in public health nursing is the decreasing number of qualified applicants for vacant positions (resulting in agencies hiring people who are not qualified to do the job and trying to provide on-the-job training, or leaving positions open longer and, therefore, increasing the risk for elimination or transition to a position that does not require an RN). If the essential contributions that nursing can make to the health of a community are to continue, it is critical to have a public health nursing workforce that is educationally prepared at the baccalaureate or higher degree level with a strong knowledge base and skills in public health nursing. The ANA, the APHA, and the National Association of County & City Health Officials have passed policy statements reflecting their concern about a potential national shortage of public health nurses.

Further Development of Public Health Nursing Models and Competencies

The Council on Linkages between Academia and Public Health Practice (COL) developed a set of core competencies for public health professionals based on the Ten Essential Public Health Services framework in 2004. Recognizing the need for this work to become relevant for the specific specialty of public health nursing, the QUAD Council of Public Health Nursing Organizations (2004) initiated a national dialogue to explore nursing-specific applications of the public health core competencies. In 2000, the QUAD Council began work on developing a set of national public health nursing (PHN) competencies, culminating with the release of its ground-breaking document, "QUAD Council Public Health Nursing Competencies," which was published in 2004 in *Public Health Nursing*. Through this collaborative effort, the generalist level in public health nursing would reflect preparation at the baccalaureate level, public health practice would be population focused, and one of the unique contributions of public health nurses would be the ability to apply these principles at individual and family levels within the context of population-focused practice.

By placing public health nursing in this context, many of the competency statements indicate a level of awareness, knowledge, and proficiency at the individual and family levels. QUAD Council (2004) Public Health Nursing Competencies include the following domains:

- Domain 1: Analytic Skills
- Domain 2: Policy Development/Program Planning Skills
- Domain 3: Communication Skills
- Domain 4: Cultural Competency Skills and Cultural Dimensions of Practice Skills
- Domain 5: Community Dimensions of Practice Skills
- Domain 6: Basic Public Health Sciences Skills
- Domain 7: Financial Planning and Management Skills
- Domain 8: Leadership and Systems Thinking Skills

The Minnesota Department of Health, Center for Public Health Nursing, has developed a Public Health Interventions wheel to guide public health nursing practice based on the Ten Essential Public Health Services and related competencies. The Minnesota Model builds on a novice-to-expert population-focused nursing framework. A strong partnership between governmental public health and nursing education has encouraged incorporation of the model into public health nursing education as well.

National Public Health Performance Standards

A consortium of national public health organizations, under the leadership of the Centers for Disease Control and Prevention (CDC, 1998), recognized the need for a national set of performance standards for public health systems. Utilizing the Ten Essential Public Health Services as a framework, the National Public Health Performance Standards (NPHPS) provide guidance to state and local health departments on self-assessment of system performance.

In many public health jurisdictions, public health nurses working on public health system quality improvement initiatives have embraced NPHPS standards. The most significant difference in the application of the standards and a more familiar model of health facility regulatory standards lies in the definition of the public health system. The NPHPS employ a broad definition of public health system partners (Bender, 2007).

Other Challenges for Public Health Nursing

During the first years of the new millennium, public health nurses were confronted with new technology, the reemergence of "old" infectious diseases, bioterrorist threats to the public's health, and a larger population of people at risk. The United States is faced with the growing problem of a "too little, too late" attitude about protecting the public's health through preventive measures. The healthcare system continues to focus on personal health care and expensive disease interventions, while public health resources for preventive health services decline. The value of prevention has long been recognized in economic as well as humanistic terms. Yet in the United States, only about 3% of the gross national product (GNP) is spent on preventive health services (APHA, 2012). Access to care continues to challenge our patient populations, requiring even more skills on the part of the public health nurse in the maze of managed care.

Public health nursing is destined to play a vital part in the evolution of the healthcare system in the 21st century. There are three major areas that will affect these changes: personal responsibility in health promotion and disease prevention, international health, and biological and chemical terrorism (Jakeway, LaRosa, Cary, & Schoenfisch, 2008). If the nation and the states are to adequately address the escalating costs of health care, the individual must be a key factor in the design of a new system of care. To this end, public health nurses are the best equipped to deal with these changes.

RESEARCH ALERT

Collaboration with community partners and developing linkages with key stakeholders is included in the QUAD Council's Public Health Nursing Competencies and is an important aspect of the development of community health. Maltby's article describes a community–campus partnership between a school of nursing and the community that also included social work, physical therapy, and medical students. A shared learning experience was structured through the presentation of health fairs in collaboration with community agencies. An evaluation of the process, relationships, and outcomes of the health fairs demonstrated that the students attained beginning competencies in all public health nursing competency domains of the QUAD Council's Public Health Nursing Competencies.

Source: Maltby, H. (2006). Use of health fairs to develop public health nursing competencies. *Public Health Nursing, 23*(2), 183–189.

Adequate attention to the health and related socioeconomic problems in this country will require community-level interest and intervention. The public health nurse will be called on once again to mobilize communities to meet the needs of their citizens for the improvement of society as a whole. In empowering the community to act, the public health nurse will be challenged to develop a greater understanding of the significant effect that culture has on the individual's response to health promotion, intervention, and education. The explosive population growth and the resultant migration of families will result in a variety of cultures to be served, even in rural communities.

The greatest number of elderly ever seen in this country will emerge as the typical patient as the baby boomers reach retirement age. This phenomenon will occur as the workforce is getting smaller and more diversified, thereby creating a need to evaluate the role of the public health nurse. Health promotion and disease prevention activities will be primary among the services offered by the public health nurse. The created healthcare system will place greater emphasis on what public health nurses have known all along—that prevention is more cost-effective than technological intervention.

This millennium should be an exciting one for public health nurses. The challenges will be great, but the opportunity to practice traditional public health nursing will also be more available than it has been since its inception.

As public health nurses consider the future for their practice, a number of questions will surface over and over again. The framework provided by the Construct for Public Health Nursing is useful in helping public health nurses address these, given the rapidity and magnitude of changes that we are encountering.

As clinical services seem to be moving out of health departments, what will public health nurses' role be in the future? Clinical services should be understood as a strategy for providing needed services when they are otherwise not available. These services need to be seen as a way of ensuring health, not an end unto themselves. Public health nurses offer a tremendous breadth and depth of skills that are important to almost *any* public health intervention. When public health and public health nursing are understood through the frameworks of core functions and models like the Construct for Public Health Nursing, future roles are envisioned based on their utility, not their history.

Is it possible to be a public health nurse in a managed care setting? There is no question that the skills that public health nurses bring to managed care are extremely useful and needed, but the important distinction is the purposes for which these skills are used. The organizational values of public health and the mandate of ensuring the health of the public reside in the public sector; it is that sector alone that has this responsibility. Public health nurses can and do practice in a variety of settings, some of which focus on the health of populations. Their practice may be one of community health, but it lacks the essential public nature of public health.

Should public health nurses practice in the private sector? Having public health nurses practicing in the private sector benefits everyone. The skills certainly benefit patients, and the overall values and commitments help pave the way for networking and partnerships between the public and private sectors. It is important for these individual nurses to understand that there are some critical differences between the public and private sectors in their values, priorities, and "bottom lines."

What are the biggest challenges that public health nursing currently faces? Perhaps the most significant challenge facing public health nursing and public health in general is finding ways to address the broader issues of equity and social justice that are currently so much a part of the health "equation." As long as there are such huge inequities—disparities between the "haves" and "have nots"—the major health problems that we see today will only continue.

Public health nurses must now consider the public health threat of terrorism and how best to prepare communities for human-generated disasters, such as the September 11, 2001 terrorist attacks; bioterrorism, such as anthrax and smallpox; and devastating natural disasters, such as Hurricane Katrina. As a society, we have learned that being healthy and well prepared can strengthen the entire country, in contrast to the unprecedented public health breakdown that occurred during Hurricane Katrina. Public health nurses must view their practice in global terms, going beyond the narrow boundaries of personal health services, if they are to truly enhance the health of all people.

APPLICATION TO PRACTICE

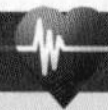

Case Presentation: Staphylococcus *Food Poisoning in a University Cafeteria*

Stephanie is a 19-year-old white female who is a sophomore at a local university. She lives on campus in one of the dormitories. After dinner one evening, she became ill with nausea, vomiting, diarrhea, and abdominal cramps. Five other women who live in Stephanie's building became ill that same evening with similar symptoms. When others in the dorm became aware of the symptoms, most of the women thought that there was a gastrointestinal virus that was making the women ill. None of these six women became ill enough to seek medical attention.

That same evening Mary, a 20-year-old African American female who lives on campus in another dormitory, also became ill with nausea, vomiting, and severe abdominal cramps. Mary was not able to get the vomiting under control, so her roommate brought her to the local hospital emergency department. Mary was hospitalized and placed on replacement intravenous fluids and medication for nausea and diarrhea.

The hospital, which serves the university town, is relatively small, and the staff soon became aware that nine individuals—all students from the university—had been admitted with the same symptoms within a period of approximately 6 hours that evening. The hospital staff notified the campus clinic physician. He verified that he had treated eight students that same evening for nausea, vomiting, and abdominal cramps. He notified the local county health department that he suspected a food-borne illness outbreak. The public health nurses organized the follow up of the problem, utilizing the core functions of public health and the definition of public health nursing.

1. Discuss the activities that the public health nurse might conduct in this follow up.
2. Identify the core functions and essential services that are described in this case.

MEDIA MOMENT

And the Band Played On (1987) (Book)

Acclaimed book by Randy Shilts: As the first major book on AIDS, *San Francisco Chronicle* reporter Randy Shilts chronicled the making of one of the most devastating epidemics of the 20th century. Shilts researched and reported the book exhaustively, chronicling almost day-by-day the first 5 years of AIDS. His work is critical of the medical and scientific communities' initial response, as well as the indifference of the mass media and country at large.

And the Band Played On (1993) (Film)

This film stars Matthew Modine as a doctor with the CDC at the time when the first reports of a disease plaguing the gay community were heard. Modine's character and his colleagues embark on an investigation that resembles a compelling detective story as they try to track the source of the disease and discover a cure. Their efforts are thwarted by an ambivalent government and a turf war between French physicians and a celebrated American researcher (Alan Alda) who seems to place his own glory above the dead and the dying. The cast includes Richard Gere, Glenne Headly, Anjelica Huston, Steve Martin, Ian McKellen, Saul Rubinek, and Lily Tomlin. The movie effectively captures Shilts' book on film and marks the early struggles in this monumental epic, and the politics that all too effectively wiped out these victims of this devastating epidemic.

Conclusion

Shakespeare's *The Tempest* contains a sage observation: "The past is prologue. The future is yours and mine to dispatch." So it is with public health nursing. Our history is our prologue, our foundation. Our future is what we create within the framework of what we value, what we understand, what we know, and what we can do. When one considers the work of Lillian Wald, which included her own "hands-on" reaching out to destitute individuals and families and helping create the League of Nations and the United States Children's Bureau, it is clear that our foundation can provide us with the inspiration and wisdom that we need to move forward. There are no promises for public health nursing in the 21st century. There is only the ironic assurance that within the significant challenges that will confront societies around the world will be opportunities for public health nurses. The ways in which we define ourselves and our practice will either limit or enable our abilities to take hold of these opportunities. In the final analysis, public health nursing in the future will be what we make it.

HEALTHY ME 

Have you used the services of the local health department? What was your experience like?

LEVELS OF PREVENTION 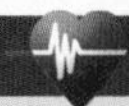

Primary Providing in-service to a group of discharge nurses at an acute care center about the use of public health services

Secondary Conducting an epidemiological investigation in a school setting after two cases of tuberculosis were found

Tertiary Assisting with after-disaster care with the public health needs of a community, such as shelter management

Critical Thinking Activities

1. What are the advantages of public health nurses working in the private health sector?
2. Compare the role of the public health nurse of today with that of public health nurses at the beginning of the 20th century. What are the challenges common to both roles?
3. Using the three priorities of prevention, protection, and health promotion identified by Dr. Salmon in her model Construct for Public Health Nursing, give examples from your own practice in community health nursing that illustrate these three priorities.

References

Abrams, S. (2007). For the good of a common discipline. *Public Health Nursing, 24*(3), 293–297.

American Public Health Association (APHA). (1996, March). *The definition and role of public health nursing. A statement of the Public Health Nursing Section.* Washington, DC: Author.

American Public Health Association (APHA). (2012). *The prevention and public health fund: A critical investment in our nation's physical and fiscal health.* Retrieved from http://www.apha.org/NR/rdonlyres/8FA13774-AA47-43F2-838B-1B0757D111C6/0/APHA_PrevFundBrief_June2012.pdf

Bender, K. (2007). Recommendations from the exploring accreditation for state and local health departments: Do we have the political will? *Public Health Nursing, 24*(5), 465–471.

Centers for Disease Control and Prevention (CDC). (1998). *National public health performance standards.* Atlanta, GA: Author.

Chaudry, R. (2008). The precautionary principle, public health, and public health nursing. *Public Health Nursing, 25*(3), 261–268.

Cohen, B., & Reutter, L. (2007, October). Development of the role of public health nurses in addressing child and family poverty: A framework for action. *Journal of Advanced Nursing, 60*(1), 96–107.

Council on Linkages between Academia and Public Health Practice (COL). (2001). *Core competencies for public health practice.* Washington, DC: Author.

Easley, C., & Allen, C. (2008). A critical intersection: Human rights, public health nursing, and nursing ethics. *Advances in Nursing Science, 30*(4), 367–382.

Gebbie, K. M., & Turnock, B. J. (2006). The public health workforce, 2006: New challenges. *Health Affairs, 25*(4), 923–933.

Institute of Medicine (IOM). (1988). *The future of public health.* Washington, DC: National Academies Press.

Jakeway, C., LaRosa, G., Cary, A., & Schoenfisch, S. (2008). The role of public health nurses in emergency preparedness and response: A position paper of the Association of State and Territorial Directors of Nursing. *Public Health Nursing, 25*(4), 353–361.

Juraschek, S. P., Zhang, X., Ranganathan, V., & Lin, V. W. (2012). United States registered nurse workforce report card and shortage forecast. *American Journal of Medical Quality, 27*(3), 241–249.

Kulbok, P., & Reed, J. (2006, March). PHN Competencies. *Public Health Nursing, 23*(2), 97, 98.

Milbank Memorial Fund Commission. (1976). *Higher education for public health: A report*. New York, NY: Prodist.

Mississippi Department of Archives. (1920–1980). *Correspondence, memoranda, and reports* (Mississippi Department of Health, Record Group 51, Public Health Nursing Division, Vol. 36). Jackson, MS: Author.

O'Fallon, L. (2006). Fostering the relationship between environmental health and nursing. *Public Health Nursing, 23*(5), 377–380.

Polivka, B., Stanley, S., Gordon, D., Taulbee, K., Kieffer, G., & McCorkle, S. (2008). Public health nursing competencies for public health surge events. *Public Health Nursing, 25*(2), 159–165.

QUAD Council of Public Health Nursing Organizations. (2004). Public health nursing competencies. *Public Health Nursing, 21*(5), 443–452.

Salmon, M. E. (1993). Public health nursing: The opportunity of a lifetime. *American Journal of Public Health, 83*(1), 674–675.

Soros, G. (1997). The capitalist threat. *The Atlantic Monthly, 279*(2), 45–58.

White, M. S. (1982, November–December). Construct for public health nursing. *Nursing Outlook, 30*, 527.

CHAPTER FOCUS

Home Health Nursing
Standards of Home Health Nursing

The Medicare Era

Types of Home Health Agencies
Home Health Documentation

Financing and Payment Systems for Home Health Services
Medicare
Medicaid
Private Insurance

Quality Assurance and Public Accountability
Regulation and Licensure
Quality Assurance in Home Health
Accreditation

Managed Care and Home Health

Interdisciplinary Team Approach in Home Health

Role of Family Caregivers in Home Health

Legal and Ethical Issues in Home Health
Home Care Bill of Rights
Advance Medical Directives

Information and Technology in Home Health
Communication and Data Management
Delivery of Care

Hospice Care in the Home
Quality Assurance and Hospice
Hospice Care for Children
Disaster and Home Health and Hospice: Incident Command System
Holistic Care

The Future of Health Care in the Home

QUESTIONS TO CONSIDER

After reading this chapter, you will know the answers to the following questions:

1. Which factors have contributed to the increased growth in home health care in the past 30 years?
2. What is a typical home health patient like in terms of diagnosis and age?
3. What are common reimbursement sources for home health services?
4. How does home health nursing differ from nursing that takes place in other healthcare settings?
5. How are technologies being used in home care?
6. What is hospice, and how does it differ from home health?
7. What is the future of home care nursing?

CHAPTER 36

Home Health and Hospice Nursing

Karen Saucier Lundy and
Ilene Purvis Bloxsom

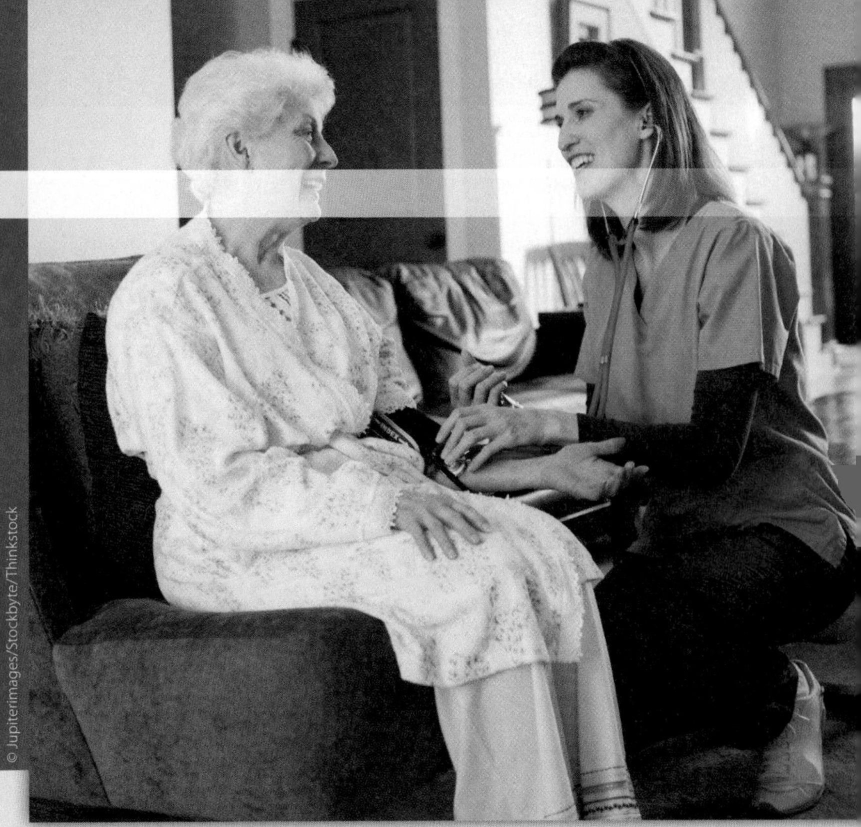

KEY TERMS

conditions of participation (CoP)
fee-for-service rate
home health care
home healthcare nurses
home healthcare nursing
hospice
informal caregivers
palliative care
plan of care (POC)
skilled nursing visits (SNVs)

> No matter how dreary and gray our homes are, we people of flesh and blood would rather live there than in any other country, be it ever so beautiful. There is no place like home.
>
> *The Wizard of Oz* —L. Frank Baum

> My view you know is that the ultimate destination is the nursing of the sick in their own home. I look to the abolition of all hospitals ... but no use to talk about the year 2000.
>
> —Florence Nightingale, 1867

REFLECTIONS

The home was the earliest setting for nursing care. Why do you think Florence Nightingale believed that care should ideally return to the home? How does home health differ now from Nightingale's era? It is often said that almost anything that can be done in the hospital, can be done in the home today. How do you feel about being a nurse in someone's home? How is this different from the secure environment of the hospital or healthcare facility?

HOME HEALTH CARE was established in the latter part of the nineteenth century, as nursing schools began graduating more and better-trained professional nurses. Influencing this movement to home care was the explosion of scientific knowledge about microorganism transmission and communicable disease and the accompanying advancement in technology.

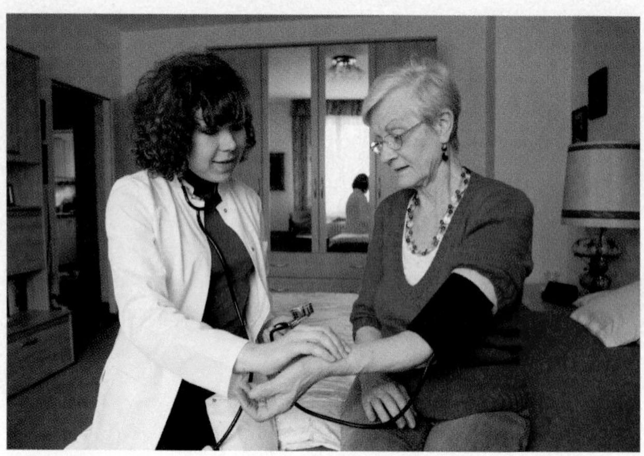

A home health nurse conducts a physical assessment.

Home Health Nursing

Home health care refers to the delivery of health services in the home setting for purposes of restoring or maintaining the health of individuals and families. The purpose of home health care is to provide the support, treatment, and information that caregivers and patients need to successfully manage their healthcare needs at home. The home health nurse's role is that of facilitator of home independence through patient education, patient advocacy, and case management. Managed care and technological advances and research have all contributed to the movement from the hospital to the home as a diverse and dynamic service delivery setting for care (National Association for Home Care & Hospice [NAHC], 2008; Rice, 2005). Providing homecare services to the millions who require health care, **home healthcare nursing** is the choice for many community health nurses who are attracted by the autonomy, flexibility, and challenge of caring for persons in their own homes. Home healthcare nursing involves the same primary preventive focus with home health patients and the secondary and tertiary prevention foci on the care of individuals in collaboration with the family and caregivers. **Home healthcare nurses** provide care to a broad spectrum of ages and clinical diagnoses (Duke & Street, 2003; Rice, 2005).

Home-based health care has been one of the most rapidly growing areas in the healthcare sector in the United States and other Western countries since the 1990s. Market forces and the development of government policies and mandates, especially with the passage of the Patient Protection and Affordable Care Act (ACA) of 2010, to control cost increases in the health sector have driven health care from acute care facilities to the home (American Academy of Nursing [AAN], 2010). Trends that have influenced the move to home health care include economic pressure to reduce the escalating cost of healthcare systems, the movement of healthcare delivery away from acute care into the community, the rapid growth of managed care systems, and the increasing percentage of older people in populations. Home healthcare nursing presents a challenge to nurses who must incorporate new technology, increasing patient acuity, and complex patient and family needs into their practice. Home care serves a number of functions for acute, continuing, preventive, and palliative care; each of these functions necessitates a different care provider mix, level of care, and need for health management in the home (Brennan, 2012; Congdon & Magilvy, 1998). Some examples of the types of activities of home health nurses include:

- *Acute care*: facilitates early discharge, reduces admission or readmission to hospitals and other more costly facilities, such as long-term care.
- *Continuing care or long-term care*: allows individuals to remain in their current home environment in the community as long as possible.
- *Preventive care*: prevents occurrence of injuries, illnesses, chronic conditions, and their resulting disabilities.
- *Palliative care*: offers total care to a person and supports caregiver(s) to improve the person's quality of life for life-threatening and terminal conditions.

Home health care is holistic and focused on the individual patient, integrating family, caregivers, and

BOX 36-1 Summary Description of Patients in Sample Home Health Daily Nursing Schedule

On each skilled nursing visit:

1. Wash hands.
2. Set up equipment, including laptop computer.
3. Obtain complete assessment with review of systems. DOCUMENT.
4. Contact physician with assessment results, if indicated. DOCUMENT.
5. Ask the patient or caregiver to recall previous instruction, making corrections if needed. DOCUMENT.
6. Wash hands. Perform procedures; wash hands. Note response to care. DOCUMENT.
7. Instruct patient/caregiver from plan of care. Note response to instruction. Review as needed. DOCUMENT.
8. Schedule next visit with the patient/caregiver.
9. Clean equipment; wash hands.

Ms. Lottie AAA. Hx: 74 y/o with a longstanding history of osteoarthritis, using a walker for mobility in her small rural home. She has a recent diagnosis of type 2 DM. The physician has requested daily SNVs to instruct her in blood glucose monitoring, diabetic diet, and medication regimen after the initiation of an oral hypoglycemic agent. She lives alone but receives assistance from her many children and grandchildren in the community.

Mr. Ali BBB. Hx: 81 y/o with CHF for several years and is particularly forgetful since the death of his wife last year. His physician has requested SNVs because he has had two recent hospitalizations with exacerbations of his disease. Although he lives alone, his daughter drops by each morning at 9:00 to offer help. The nursing visit is set so that instruction can be given to both.

Mr. Carlo CCC. Hx: 26 y/o with paraplegia and development of a stage II sacral ulcer. He has a roommate who helps with shopping and some ADLs. He previously spent most of his day in the wheelchair but has begun to take rest periods midmorning, midafternoon, and early evening. He is pleased with the air cushion for his wheelchair and the gel overlay for his bed.

Ms. Helaria DDD. Hx: 78 y/o with recent onset of idiopathic HTN. She lives with her elderly husband and a very active dog, Maggie. Her children have hired a caregiver for ADLs and housekeeping. The physician has ordered BP assessments 2–3 times per week for 3 weeks to assess the effects of her new medication, quinapril HCl. Systolic pressure at 160 or greater and diastolic pressure at 94 or greater are to be reported. One dosage adjustment has been made, and she has been normotensive on the last two visits. Visit times are varied to give the physician an across-the-day view.

Mr. Paul EEE. Hx: 34 y/o with congenital lower extremity malformation, type 1 DM, and open wounds on both lower limbs. He helps his elderly father with financial matters and record keeping. The patient meticulously records his wound progress and emails any concerns to the nurse and physician. He provides wound care to the areas he can reach, and the nurse performs care to the area outside his reach. He is well educated about his health conditions. He depends on home health aides for most of his personal care. A supervised home health aide visit is planned.

Abbreviations: ADLs, activities of daily living; BP, blood pressure; CHF, congestive heart failure; DM, diabetes mellitus; HTN, hypertension; Hx, history; SNVs, skilled nursing visits; y/o, years old.

Source: Contributed by Jim Jones, RN, BEd, Case Manager Home Health Nurse, South Mississippi Home Health, Hattiesburg, Mississippi.

environmental and community resources to promote optimal health for the patient confined to the home. **Boxes 36-1** and **36-2** describe the typical home health nurse's day and patient load.

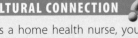

CULTURAL CONNECTION 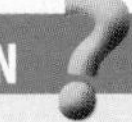

As a home health nurse, you will experience many different cultural practices from your own. When entering the home of a person of the Muslim faith, it is customary to remove one's shoes at the door. Compare this to the hospital setting and our attempts to be sensitive to our patients' cultural values. Would you be likely to remove your shoes in the hospital when entering the room of a patient with similar values as above? Why or why not?

Almost any care that can now be provided in the hospital can also take place in the home, which has created numerous practice opportunities for home health nurses to improve the health of the population in a more convenient and cost-effective manner. Homecare services are provided to persons with acute care needs, long-term health conditions, permanent disabilities, or terminal illnesses.

Home health care is that component of the continuum of comprehensive health care whereby health services are provided to individuals and families in their places of residence for the purpose of promoting, maintaining, or restoring health, or of maximizing the level of independence while minimizing the effects of disability and illness, including terminal illness. The appropriate services to meet the needs of the individual patient and family are planned, coordinated, and made available by providers organized for

BOX 36-2 Sample Home Health Daily Nursing Schedule*

- 7:00 Get ready for the day: Check laptop and ensure that the nightly transfer of schedule and patient information completed successfully. [The laptop stores the vital scheduling information and the patients' electronic medical record and crucial teaching tools to assist the clinician in carrying out the specific plan of care or care path for the patient.] If so, unplug and pack up the laptop for the day. If the transfer did not complete successfully, this message will be present on the laptop and the process must be attempted again. If problems continue, contact the helpdesk at the office for assistance.
- Call office, check overnight voicemail for any last-minute messages.
  [Night on-call nurses may have taken calls that require a schedule change, such as notification that a patient has entered the hospital for care.]
- Organize patient visits by priority.
  [Some patients require a timed visit due to needed lab studies or the presence of a caregiver to receive instruction.]
- Check nursing bag and automobile to see that all needed supplies are available for assessment and procedures.
- 7:30 Turn on pager and cell phone; grab the lunch cooler. You need to travel about 30 minutes to the outlying community to see your first two patients.
- 8:00 Arrive at Ms. Lottie AAA's home. Ms. AAA is now testing her blood glucose with minimal prompting. You praise her for her performance and correct entry of the WNL results. Together, you review her meal plans for the day, and discuss some of your suggestions. You give her instruction on signs and symptoms of hyperglycemia/hypoglycemia with handouts of this in pictorial and text form. You remind her to fast for tomorrow's visit. The visit has lasted an hour and you will travel back toward town to see your next patient.
- 9:15 Arrive at Mr. Ali BBB's home. His daughter greets you at the door with his daily wt. record and the information that he has gained 3 pounds overnight. He is SOB, resp. 34, pulse is 100, BP is 150/92 mm Hg, temp. 98.3 °F. His 14:00 dose of furosemide is in the MediPlanner for the past 2 days. Ausc. of his lung fields, posterior, indicate fine crackles in the lower lobes bilaterally, and the mid lobe on the right. You contact his physician contact, and administer furosemide IV as ordered. The patient admits to forgetting medications that don't come at mealtimes. You give instructions to move the 14:00 dose to noon, and his daughter will call after lunch as a reminder on medications. You then reiterate signs and symptoms that require contact with the nurse/physician. Now vital signs indicate resp. at 26, pulse 92, and BP 132/84. He has voided twice. Arrangements are made to return later in the afternoon for reassessment. You call the office to move an afternoon visit to tomorrow, and your other patient is notified. You have spent an hour and 15 minutes here, and now you travel back into town for your remaining patients.
- 10:50 Arrive at Mr. Carlo CCC's home. You arrive at his home 15 minutes after the scheduled time with sincere apologies. You remove his old dressing, and gently clean the wound with NS. The 0.5-cm measurement reveals that healing is rapidly occurring. You apply skin preps to the intact skin, place a hydrocolloid dressing, and secure the edges with tape. You continue discharge planning because the wound is nearly healed. You provide a review of pressure-relief measures and discuss self-inspection using a mirror. The patient is eager to return to a more regular routine, and you encourage his plans. His roommate offers coffee, which you graciously decline. Your 40-minute visit is ended with traveling a short distance to the next patient.
- 11:40 Arrive at Ms. Helaria DDD's home. Maggie, an energetic poodle, has loudly announced your arrival, and she meets you at the door before the bell is rung. You are led to the bedroom for her positional BP checks, but extracting Maggie from the patient's lap is a problem. This accomplished, you find her sitting BP is 138/82, standing BP is 128/80, and supine BP is 144/88. She denies headache, dizziness, back pain, fatigue, dry mouth, or GI upset. She is still unclear about taking the medication because she feels "just fine." You repeat the silent threat of HTN, and the need to take her medication as ordered. She agrees and promises to call if any side effects are noted. At 12:10 you are ready to travel toward the next patient, with a pull-over for lunch.
- 12:15 After your fruit and cheese, you check your voicemail for any messages that may affect your afternoon travel.
- 12:50 Arrive at Mr. Paul EEE's home. The door is open when you arrive, and he calls out to "come on back." The aide has arrived just before you and is performing his routine care. You check the aide worksheet and note that the POC isn't being followed. You provide the needed supervision and document your findings. Before care can begin, a trip back to the car is needed to bring in sterile syringes. You observe Mr. EEE's wound self-care and note the wound characteristics. You irrigate the distal wound with ½ H_2O_2/½ NS using an 18-gauge blunt needle. Then you rinse the wound with NS, pack it with NS-moistened gauze packing, cover with gauze sponges, and wrap with roll gauze. Last you apply tape to secure the dressing. Your cell phone rings and requires a brief call to one of the patients with medication instruction. Your visit, with interruptions, has lasted an hour and 10 minutes.
- 14:15 Arrive at Mr. Ali BBB's home. He reports voiding several times since you left. You note that there is no apparent SOB, resp. is 22, pulse is 80, BP is 132/82, and temp. is 98.8 °F. His lungs have only faint, scattered crackles in the bases. You give instruction again

regarding which high-potassium foods to include in his diet. He has several bananas on hand and eats one while you talk. You then call his daughter at her home and remind her to call the agency if signs and symptoms indicate a fluid increase. This visit is over after 30 minutes, and you leave to return to the office.

- 15:05 Arrive at the office. Attend scheduled in-service training and competency testing at office. Submit notes, verbal order, and check voicemail for tomorrow's assignments and schedule. Load supplies, and return any calls. Make a note in your daily planner about the in-service on laptop use in the home for next Wednesday. Check the on-call schedule and leave a report for the night nurse should Mr. BBB call with continuing problems.
- 15:30 GO HOME. (Your own!) Plug laptop into phone jack and electrical outlet to recharge and be available for the automated data transfer set to occur during the night.

Abbreviations: Ausc., auscultation; BP, blood pressure; GI, gastrointestinal; H_2O_2, hydrogen peroxide; HTN, hypertension; IV, intravenous; NS, normal saline; POC, plan of care; resp., respirations; SOB, shortness of breath; temp., temperature; WNL, within normal limits; wt., weight.

*Refer to Box 36-1 for a summary description of each patient.

Source: Contributed by Jim Jones, RN, BEd, Case Manager Home Health Nurse, South Mississippi Home Health, Hattiesburg, Mississippi.

the delivery of home care through the use of employed staff, contractual arrangements, or a combination of the two patterns (Brennan, 2012; Rice, 2005; Shick & Balinsky, 2006).

ENVIRONMENTAL CONNECTION

A home visit provides the community health nurse with ample opportunities for assessing environmental risks. When you enter a patient's home for the first time, what kinds of things do you notice first? How does this differ from a visit to a friend's house?

NOTE THIS!

What are ADLs (Activities of Daily Living)?

ADLs refer to activities that reflect the patient's capacity for self-care.

OASIS requires the assessment of seven ADLs:

- Grooming
- Dressing the upper and lower body
- Bathing
- Toileting
- Transferring
- Ambulation/locomotion
- Feeding or eating

ETHICAL CONNECTION

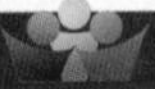

During a home visit to an elderly patient, you notice several empty liquor bottles in the trash and on the kitchen table. The patient's husband is a recovering alcoholic and their 22-year-old grandson is living with them while attending college. Would you respond to this observation? What ethical issues exist in the home setting, using this example, as compared to the hospital environment?

Changes in the healthcare system, healthcare reform as a result of the ACA, and advances in technology and information are challenging nurses to redefine the terms *home* and *care* (Affordable Care Act is Still the Law, 2012; Franz, 1997). Clarke and Cody (1994) have challenged nurses to rethink the central concepts of nursing: person, environment, health, and nursing. In the home, boundaries between nurse and family as caregivers become blurred, with each party providing essential care to the patient. The home has long been considered the private domain of the family—but it is increasingly becoming the "employment setting" for the home health nurse, where nurse and patient needs intersect. In the hospital, there are often dramatic changes from illness to health; in the community home setting, the changes are often subtle as a chronic disease state emerges as the dominant mode of health and illness. In the home setting, the autonomy of the family and patient is vital, and maintaining it requires a collaborative effort between caregivers and health providers.

Standards of Home Health Nursing

The American Nurses Association (ANA) endorses and continues to update the Standards of Home Health Nursing as the basis for home health nursing practice. These standards, similar to other nursing practice standards, use the nursing process and identify two levels of nursing practice—the generalist and the specialist—to detail the role and function of the home health nurse. Generalist roles include direct care provider, educator, resource manager, collaborator, and supervisor of ancillary personnel. The nurse as specialist has a master's degree and serves as consultant, administrator, researcher, and clinical specialist. The nurse in the specialist role may develop and evaluate agency policy, perform staff development, and be responsible for organizing and managing interdisciplinary staffing services.

The nurse in home health nursing must have excellent critical thinking and decision-making skills. In the home health setting, the nurse practices autonomously and without the support of a traditional peer group. In addition, giving care in the home of the patient necessitates a sensitivity for the patient's environment and culture to a much greater degree than does delivering care in other practice settings (Ward-Griffin & McKeever, 2000). Current advances in technology and pharmacology have also resulted in the need for the home care nurse to be increasingly more competent in infusion therapies, complex wound therapies, and advanced computer technologies.

The Medicare Era

Following the establishment of the Medicare program in 1965, significant growth and change throughout the U.S. healthcare system created a broad spectrum of health services for the elderly population (Davitt & Choi, 2008). Medicare made homecare services, primarily **skilled nursing visits (SNVs)** and curative or restorative therapy, available for all persons older than 65. These services were extended to the disabled population in 1973, and hospice services were added in 1983. **Hospice** services provide **palliative care** and supportive social, emotional, and spiritual services to the terminally ill and their families (NAHC, 2008). Medicare is the largest single payer of healthcare services in the home.

RESEARCH ALERT

Hospice nurses know that all their patients will die. There are several potential benefits of including rituals and healing practices into the hospice care setting for staff. Evidence suggests that not only does it provide an outlet for hospice workers to express their grief and reflect on their work in an accepting environment; it also provides closure for their patient's passing and has also been shown to decrease the risk of burnout and compassion fatigue. This article discusses the important aspects of grief rituals and provides an illustrative example of one such ritual.

Source: Running, A., Tolle, L., & Girard, D. (2008). Ritual: The final expression of care. *International Journal of Nursing Practice, 14*(4), 303–307.

> I have the highest respect for them, especially for the nurses, aides and therapists, who devote their lives to caring for people with disabilities, the infirm and dying Americans. There are few more noble professions.
>
> —*President Barack Obama*

Certainly, one of the primary benefits of health care in the home is that it is significantly less expensive than in the hospital. Home health care can reduce per-patient expenditures, as well as reduce the number, length, and frequency of hospitalization episodes.

More than half the patients who receive home health care are older than 65, and the amount of home health they use tends to increase with age. Approximately 40% of these patients have one or more functional limitations. The most common single diagnostic category for home health services is for diabetes. Diseases and conditions associated with the circulatory system are next, including hypertension and heart failure. These diagnoses are followed in frequency by chronic ulcers of the skin and osteoarthritis. The services provided by home healthcare nurses focus on assisting the patient to reach or maintain an optimal state of health, independence, and comfort in their home setting.

The persons who most need home health care require assistance in ADLs (NAHC, 2008; National Institute on Disability and Rehabilitation Research, 1996). **Informal caregivers**, such as family members, friends, and others who provide services on an unpaid basis, provide the bulk of home care with guidance and support from home health professionals.

The provision of care in the patient's place of residence contributes to the unique nature of this part of the healthcare delivery system. Home care represents a cost-effective and satisfying means of meeting the patient's healthcare needs (Rice, 2005; Shamansky, 1988). Many factors have contributed significantly to the growth of the homecare industry in recent years, including the aging of the U.S. population, advances in technology, shorter inpatient hospital stays, and the increasing availability of outpatient services (Curtin, 2008; Davitt & Choi, 2008). According to Maraldo (1989), "Home care is most suited to become the centerpiece of a new healthcare delivery system, because survey after survey demonstrates that consumers prefer home care to other types of care" (p. 303).

Many complex therapies previously administered only in hospital intensive care units are now safe and available in the home setting. For example, intravenous (IV) therapy has now become common in the home setting, infusing antibiotics, chemotherapy, analgesics, total parenteral nutrition (TPN), and blood products (Sheldon & Bender, 1994). Pediatric hospitalizations have dropped significantly, by 46% since the 1980s, as more procedures and treatments have been done on an outpatient basis and in the home. Pediatric postoperative recovery often occurs in the home (Curtin, 2008; Dougherty, 1998). The ability to provide sophisticated pain control and other comfort measures to the terminally ill, along with an increased understanding and recognition of the importance of preserving dignity in the dying process, have contributed to the growth of hospice services. Often, with the provision of an intermittent skilled service along with the assistance of the home health aide for personal care and exercise therapy, the patient is able to remain in the comforts of his or her own home rather than requiring institutional care (Davitt & Choi, 2008; Milone-Nuzzo, 1998).

RESEARCH ALERT

This qualitative study of 38 hospice patients examines how people answered questions about what mattered the most to them or was of ultimate concern in their lives at the time of the interviews. Responses participants gave when asked what they found most troubling and of ultimate concern at the time of the interviews are reported here. While this sample of hospice recipients reported that dependence, religious or spiritual matters, incapacitation, and money were matters of concern, the largest response category by far was concern for others.

Source: Pevey, C. (2008). Death, god, flesh, and other: Hospice recipients reflect on what matters. *Illness, Crisis & Loss, 16*(3), 203–226.

Types of Home Health Agencies

Home health agency structures vary depending on the type of organization and their corporate structure (Shick & Balinsky, 2006). These differences affect the entity's obligations to local, state, and federal law and regulations. The structure also determines the agency's tax obligation. Agencies are classified as official, nonprofit, proprietary, and institution based. **Box 36-3** describes the various classifications of agencies.

Official agencies are publicly funded units in state or local health departments that are supported by taxes. These agencies provide home health services through legislative statutes. Home health services when offered through official agencies may be provided by community health nurses who also function in various other roles, such as in health promotion and communicable disease prevention. Medicare, Medicaid, and private insurance companies all reimburse for home health services, though the reimbursement formulas used are often complex. Because of the proliferation of private agencies and a reevaluation of the priorities for public health for disease prevention, most public health services that provide home health are located in underserved and isolated areas.

Nonprofit home health agencies are made up of voluntary agencies and private, nonprofit agencies. Voluntary agencies are supported by charities such as United Way or private endowments. The earliest Visiting Nurse Associations are examples of voluntary agencies. This type of agency is privately owned and exempt from federal income tax. Such agencies do not receive any state or local tax revenues. Certain nonprofit hospitals may also have home health agencies as part of their community services. These types of agencies are usually governed by boards of directors composed of representatives from the community from which they serve. With the increase in the number of for-profit private agencies in the United States, the number of these agencies has declined in recent years. With voluntary agencies, service is provided based on the patient's need for home health rather than on his or her ability to pay.

Proprietary agencies include private, profit-making agencies and profit-making hospitals. These agencies receive the largest percentage of their revenue through third-party payers. Because of a trend toward a highly competitive, managed care market, many proprietary agencies are now part of national healthcare organizational chains managed through corporate headquarters. Another trend is the development of alliances among home

BOX 36-3 Home Health Agency Classifications

- *Public/governmental agency*: A public or governmental agency is an agency operated by a state or local government. Examples are state-operated health departments and county hospitals.
- *Nonprofit agency*: A private, nongovernmental agency exempt from federal income tax. These agencies are often supported, in part, by private contributions or other philanthropic sources, such as foundations. Examples include Visiting Nurse Associations and Easter Seal Societies, as well as nonprofit hospitals.
- *Proprietary agency*: A private, profit-making agency or profit-making hospital.
- *Institution-based agency*: An institution-based agency can be propriety, nonprofit, official, or voluntary and operates within the organizational structure of a hospital or health maintenance organization (HMO). The nature of the home health agency will be dictated by the type of hospital structure.

Source: Home Health Agency (HHA). (1998). *Med-Manual 2180. Citations and description, state operations manual* (CMS Publication No. 7). Washington, DC: U.S. Government Printing Office.

healthcare agencies and other agencies that become contracting partners in networks. Proprietary agencies make up approximately 40% of all Medicare-certified agencies.

Institution-based agencies emerged in the 1970s as hospitals began putting a greater emphasis on continuity of care. As the high cost of hospitalization and movement toward diagnosis-related groups (DRGs) led to earlier discharges, hospitals developed their own home health agencies, with their inpatient population serving as the major source of referrals to home health. Under such a structure, patients have the advantage of staying within the same system and enjoy greater ease of movement between and among services. These agencies are second only to proprietary agencies in total number of Medicare-certified agencies in the United States, accounting for approximately 30% of these agencies.

MEDIA MOMENT

The House on Henry Street (1915)

By Lillian Wald, New York, NY: Holt, Rinehart and Winston

Lillian Wald, who coined the term *public health nursing* and founded the historic Henry Street Settlement in New York City in 1893 for home visiting, is truly a larger than life figure in the field of home health. One of the most influential and respected social reformers of the 20th century, Henry Street Settlement founder Lillian Wald was a tireless and accomplished humanitarian. Born into a life of privilege, Wald came to Manhattan to attend the New York Hospital School of Nursing at age 22. In 1893, Wald founded the Henry Street Settlement and began teaching health and hygiene to immigrant women on the impoverished Lower East Side.

This book, written by Wald, is a fascinating look at her background, passion for delivering quality professional nursing care in the home, and the art and science of providing nursing care in the home. In 1915, at the peak of her career, Wald published the history of Henry Street and her work in *The House on Henry Street.* Dedicated to "the comrades who have built the house," the book became a classic for generations of nursing, sociology, and social welfare students. The settlement's services continued to grow; in 1915 alone 100 nurses cared for more than 26,575 patients and made more than 227,000 home visits.

One day, while teaching, a little girl approached Wald and asked her to attend to her sick mother. The child led her through the tenements, "over broken roadways ... between tall, reeking houses ... across a court where open and unscreened closets were promiscuously used by men and women, up into a rear tenement, by slimy steps ... and finally into the sickroom" where Wald attended to the child's mother. Her encounter with the young girl's family prompted Wald to dedicate her life's work to the tenement community. Wald wrote, "That morning's experience was a baptism of fire. Deserted were the laboratory and academic work of college. I never returned to them ... I rejoiced that I had training in the care of the sick that in itself would give me an organic relationship to the neighborhood in which this awakening had come." With funding from philanthropists and friends, Wald and Mary Brewster, her friend and colleague, established the Visiting Nurses Service in 1893. By January 1894, the two had visited more than 125 families and offered advice to many more. Wald wrote of one of her home visits in a poor, immigrant neighborhood

> Over broken asphalt, over dirty mattresses and heaps of refuse we went ... There were two rooms and a family of seven not only lived here but shared their quarters with boarders ... [I felt] ashamed of being a part of society that permitted such conditions to exist ... What I had seen had shown me where my path lay.

Wald provided leadership to the settlement until 1930. During that time, she established herself as a national leader of social reform, and as an international crusader for human rights. Wald pioneered public health nursing by placing nurses in public schools and with corporations, and by helping found the National Organization for Public Health Nursing and Columbia University's School of Nursing.

For more information on the Henry Street Settlement that still serves patients in New York City today go to: http://www.henrystreet.org

Home Health Documentation

Because of the reimbursement policies of the Medicare program, accurate and appropriate documentation by the home health nurse is critical to ensure current and future reimbursement of the agency and maintenance of certification of the agency. Documentation activities affect home health to a much greater degree than care delivered in perhaps any other setting (Rice, 2005). Documentation requirements are defined in the Medicare conditions of participation. These documentation requirements have a direct impact on reimbursement for the home health agency. Put simply, the documentation requirements for home health care are among the most stringent seen in any healthcare settings. Each professional note of documentation must demonstrate a skilled level of care and must be inclusive of all care rendered. The professional nurse is responsible for documenting the supervision of the licensed practice nurse (LPN) and the home health aide. As Lovejoy (1997) states, "Because visits and supplies translate to costs, nurses enter the frontline of margin producing responsibility when moving from hospital or other settings to home care" (p. 12). See **Figure 36-1**.

NOTE THIS!

How is home health paid for?

- Medicare
- Medicaid
- Private insurance
- Out-of-pocket expenses paid by patient
- OASIS sources of payment for home care

(M0150) Current Payment Sources for Home Care: (Mark all that apply.)

☐ 0 - None; no charge for current services
☐ 1 - Medicare (traditional fee-for-service)
☐ 2 - Medicare (HMO/managed care/Advantage plan)
☐ 3 - Medicaid (traditional fee-for-service)
☐ 4 - Medicaid (HMO/managed care)
☐ 5 - Workers' compensation
☐ 6 - Title programs (e.g., Title III, V, or XX)
☐ 7 - Other government (e.g., TriCare, VA, etc.)
☐ 8 - Private insurance
☐ 9 - Private HMO/managed care
☐ 10 - Self-pay
☐ 11 - Other (specify)
☐ UK - Unknown

Source: http://www.cms.gov/Medicare/Quality-Initiatives-Patient-Assessment-Instruments/HomeHealthQualityInits/HHQIOASISDataSet.html

ETHICAL CONNECTION 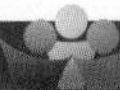

A nurse on a home visit is offered a bouquet of flowers from the patient's garden in honor of the nurse's birthday. How would you respond to this situation? Is it always appropriate to refuse gifts from a patient? Why or why not?

Financing and Payment Systems for Home Health Services

Medicare

The U.S. federal government, through the Centers for Medicare & Medicaid Services (CMS), contracts with regional insurance companies or fiscal intermediaries to provide reimbursement for homecare services. To qualify for Medicare benefits for their patient population, home health agencies must follow the federal regulatory requirements called **conditions of participation (CoP)**. The CoP for home health agencies and hospice services define the requirements that an agency must meet to participate in the Medicare program. They are detailed and prescriptive. Requirements related to organizational structure, patients' rights, and the covered disciplines, which include skilled nursing, physical therapy, speech therapy, occupational therapy, home health aides, and medical social services, are all specified in the CoP. The CoP also address the specific skilled services that each of these disciplines can provide, training requirements for aides, and other requirements that the agency must abide by to become an approved provider of Medicare home care or hospice services. The standards set forth in the CoP not only stipulate what agencies must do to qualify for Medicare, but also form the basis for evaluation of the quality of the services provided. Each agency must incorporate these requirements in its policies and procedures. The home health agency must follow these policies and procedures with absolute compliance to the regulations to ensure Medicare reimbursement of visits.

Medicare Payment for an Episode of Care

Under the current Medicare program, home health services are paid for either on a fee-for-service basis, or on an episode-of-care basis. The Medicare program defines an episode of care as being 60 days in length. Payment for the

BOX 36-4 Disease State Management Concepts

Coordination of Primary and Specialty Care

1. Referrals are coordinated from one provider to another.
2. Patients are treated by the most appropriate caregiver in the most appropriate setting.

Practice Guidelines

1. The optimal approach to patient care is established.
2. Providers are educated to follow the established practice guidelines given the patients' individual needs.
3. Patient care and cost-effective treatment are enhanced.
4. Patients achieve optimal outcomes.

Patient Education and Empowerment

1. Patients are educated in appropriate self-care.
2. Health awareness is increased, and complications are decreased.

Preventive Care and Wellness

1. Individuals at risk for a given disease are targeted.
2. Individuals are taught wellness and prevention strategies.
3. Future complications and costs are minimized.

(M2100) Types and Sources of Assistance: Determine the level of caregiver ability and willingness to provide assistance for the following activities, if assistance is needed. (Check only *one* box in each row.)

Type of Assistance	No assistance needed in this area	Caregiver(s) currently provide assistance	Caregiver(s) need training/ supportive services to provide assistance	Caregiver(s) *not likely* to provide assistance	Unclear if caregiver(s) will provide assistance	Assistance needed, but no caregiver(s) available
a. **ADL assistance** (e.g., transfer/ ambulation, bathing, dressing, toileting, eating/feeding)	0	1	2	3	4	5
b. **IADL assistance** (e.g., meals, housekeeping, laundry, telephone, shopping, finances)	0	1	2	3	4	5
c. **Medication administration** (e.g., oral, inhaled, or injectable)	0	1	2	3	4	5
d. **Medical procedures/ treatments** (e.g., changing wound dressing)	0	1	2	3	4	5
e. **Management of Equipment** (includes oxygen, IV/infusion equipment, enteral/parenteral nutrition, ventilator therapy equipment or supplies)	0	1	2	3	4	5
f. **Supervision and safety** (e.g., due to cognitive impairment)	0	1	2	3	4	5
g. **Advocacy or facilitation** of patient's participation in appropriate medical care (includes transportation to or from appointments)	0	1	2	3	4	5

BOX 36-5 Key Words to Use in Documentation of Care

Unstable	Does not comprehend
Deteriorating	New problem
Change in	Leaving
Improving	Remaining at
Taught	Deterioration in
Assessed	Complains of
Instructed	Needs assistance with
Observed	Unable to perform
Evaluated	Specific limitations
Comprehends	Remains

Source: Courtesy of North Mississippi Medical Center Home Health and Hospice.

60-day episode of care is determined by the results of the Outcome and Assessment Information Set (OASIS)—an assessment data set that groups patients into payment episodes for reimbursement purposes. This data set, which is used to determine patient outcomes of care, is completed at specific time points throughout the patient's course of home health care. A number of circumstances might result in the payment rate for the episode being prorated for the agency—for example, if the patient required four or fewer visits in a 60-day episode (Schneider, Barkauskas, & Keenan, 2008).

As previously discussed, documentation requirements and recordkeeping standards must be adhered to strictly and are primary responsibilities of the home healthcare nurse. The completion of these tasks is required to ensure coverage for the care rendered. The visit and progress notes completed by the direct care staff are essential to justifying the need for the services rendered. Each visit made by the agency must be considered "reasonable and necessary" to the plan of treatment established by the physician for Medicare to consider the service to be covered. The fiscal intermediaries for Medicare are responsible for reviewing a portion of the agency's clinical documentation on an ongoing basis. This scrutiny is intended to ascertain that the services provided by the agency were appropriately ordered by the physician, were reasonable and necessary, and met the qualifying and coverage criteria for payment.

Agencies are responsible for filing detailed cost reports. These cost reports identify expenditures made by the agency in providing direct care to the patient, including the number of complete and prorated episodes of care, the number of visits made per discipline, the number of Medicare patients, and indirect care such as administration and other overhead expenses. This cost report is used to determine the future rate setting and payment levels for the Medicare home health services.

The CoP require that the patient meet several qualifying criteria to receive covered services by Medicare. These qualifying criteria for home health services are that the patient (1) be under the care of a physician, (2) be essentially confined to the home, and (3) require skilled services of a registered nurse, physical therapist, or speech pathologist on an intermittent basis. **Box 36-6** lists some general questions that can guide the nurse in the documentation of homebound status.

The physician must certify that the patient is essentially homebound and establish an individual **plan of care (POC)** for the patient. The POC is established by the physician in collaboration with the home health team and must be updated as changes occur in the patient's condition, or at least every 60 days. The nurse plays a key role in establishing the POC for both home care and hospice, in collaboration with the physician and with other health team members. The POC is based on the patient's health history and a current comprehensive assessment of the patient's physical, psychological, social, and spiritual needs inclusive of the OASIS data set. The nurse's knowledge of the resources available in the community is very important to establish the plan that will optimally meet the patient's needs (Cho, 2005).

BOX 36-6 General Questions to Guide the Nurse in Documentation of Homebound Status

- How often does the patient leave home for social reasons?
- How long does he or she stay gone?
- How taxing or difficult is it for the patient to leave home?
- What kind of assistive devices are used when the patient leaves home?

Source: Courtesy of North Mississippi Medical Center Home Health and Hospice.

GOT AN ALTERNATIVE?

On a home health visit, a nurse discovers that his patient is using numerous over-the-counter vitamins and herbal supplements not previously identified by the home health agency admission nurse on a previous visit. The patient states, "I told the first nurse who came here that I was taking these but did not want my doctor to know so to please not write them down in my record." How should the nurse respond to the patient and to the other agency nurse about these unidentified vitamins and supplements?

Medicaid

Medicaid is authorized by Title XIX of the Social Security Act and provides health services to low-income persons. As a source of reimbursement for home health services, Medicaid is federally aided but state operated and state administered. Each state determines program eligibility, benefits covered, and the rates of payment for providers in that state.

Clinical guidelines for Medicaid reimbursement basically follow those of the Medicare program. Medicaid covers home health services, including skilled and unskilled services. If a patient qualifies for both Medicare and Medicaid, Medicare is generally the primary reimbursement source.

Private Insurance

For a growing number of home health patients, private insurance offered by a third-party payer in the private sector provides reimbursement for home healthcare services. Three major types of organizations provide this type of reimbursement: indemnity insurance companies that pay a percentage of billed charges, nonprofit Blue Cross and Blue Shield, and HMOs. As more managed care networks emerge as reimbursement mechanisms, HMOs are growing in number and scope in comprehensive healthcare services. The services provided in the private sector vary by payer, but most often the documentation and clinical guidelines follow Medicare standards for reimbursement (Cochran & Brennan, 1998; Shick & Balinsky, 2006).

GLOBAL CONNECTION 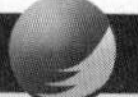

Home health in the United States is often very different from home visiting programs in other countries. Do an Internet search on home health services in France or Canada and identify the differences in purpose, funding, and utilization of home health services as compared to the United States.

RESEARCH ALERT 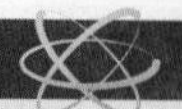

Patients with heart failure represent a common patient population in home health care, yet little is known about their outcomes. Patients with heart failure, regardless of site of care, experience substantial numbers of rehospitalizations in the United States. Home health care is a common post-acute care service for patients with heart failure. The study used a retrospective design and employed a large administrative database from 2003—the Outcome and Assessment Information Set, which is required for all U.S. Medicare and Medicaid patients receiving home health care. There were 145,191 patients with a primary diagnosis of heart failure represented in the data set. The outcomes of interest were the trajectory of care (point of entry and discharge from home health care), hospitalization, length of stay, and change in functional status. Almost three-quarters (73.9%) of patients entered home health care following a hospital stay. Nearly two-thirds (64%) remained at home at discharge from home health care. Approximately 15% of patients are hospitalized during the home healthcare episode, most often for symptoms consistent with exacerbation of the heart failure, if a reason could be identified. The average length of stay in home health care was 44 days. There was only a small improvement in functional status: 0.50 points for activities of daily living and 0.57 points for instrumental activities of daily living. Similar small improvement occurred in depressive symptoms, 0.68. There may be room for improvement in these outcomes with more recent evidence that suggests strategies for reducing hospitalization and improving patient functional status abilities. Yet, the chronic progressive nature of heart failure may also provide a limiting factor in the outcomes that can be attained.

Source: Madigan, E. A. (2008). People with heart failure and home health care resource use and outcomes. *Journal of Clinical Nursing*, 17(7B), 253–259.

Quality Assurance and Public Accountability

Regulation and Licensure

In addition to Medicare requirements, most states require that home health and hospice agencies be licensed to operate within their state. Agencies operating in states that require licensure must abide by the state's minimum standards for licensure, in addition to the regulations included in the CoP. The CMS, under the direction of the U.S. Department of Health and Human Services (HHS), contracts with state licensing and certification authorities to provide survey and audit services for the purposes of certifying homecare agencies to participate in the Medicare program. Surveys are performed at regular intervals, and at least every 3 years to ensure compliance with state licensure requirements and continued certification to participate in the Medicare and Medicaid programs. These surveys may be conducted more often for new providers or providers that had deficiencies on their previous evaluations. These surveys involve record reviews, staff and patient interviews, and home visits. The purpose of the survey process is to ascertain that all regulations are being met in providing homecare services to the Medicare and Medicaid beneficiaries. State authorities are responsible for responding to and investigating any complaints lodged against the agency and initiating any action indicated through the appropriate regulatory body.

Quality Assurance in Home Health

In 2000, as part of a broad quality improvement (QI) initiative, the federal government began requiring that every Medicare-certified home health agency complete and submit health assessment information for their patients. The instrument/data collection tool used to collect and report performance data by home health agencies is called the Outcome and Assessment Information Set (OASIS). Since fall 2003, CMS has posted on www.medicare.gov a subset of OASIS–based quality performance information showing how well home health agencies assist their patients in regaining or maintaining their ability to function. Measures of how well people can get along in their homes performing ADLs form a core of the measures, but these are supplemented with questions about physical status and use-of-service measures (hospitalization and emergent care).

OASIS is a group of data items developed, tested, and refined over the past decade. The OASIS items were designed for the purpose of enabling the rigorous and systematic measurement of patient home healthcare outcomes, with appropriate adjustment for patient risk factors affecting those outcomes. Outcomes have been defined in many ways, but those derived from OASIS items have a very specific definition: they measure changes in a patient's health status between two or more time points.

In 2004 and 2005, a private, nonprofit organization, the National Quality Forum (NQF), convened technical experts representing varying perspectives to review quality measures for home health care. Following a long review and consensus development process, the group endorsed measures for use in public reporting. The 2005 measures (all collected via the OASIS data set) are:

- Improvement in ambulation/locomotion
- Improvement in bathing
- Improvement in transferring
- Improvement in management of oral medication
- Improvement in pain interfering with activity
- Acute care hospitalization
- Emergent care
- Discharge to community
- Improvement in dyspnea (shortness of breath)
- Improvement in urinary incontinence

NQF had previously endorsed additional measures, and two of those related to wounds were added to Home Health Compare in December 2007. A variety of additional measures were added in 2009 (NQF, 2009).

Another part of the HHS/CMS quality initiative includes Quality Improvement Organizations (QIOs). QIOs exist in each state and are private organizations that contract with CMS to help improve the quality of care provided to Medicare patients. In addition to assisting beneficiaries with complaints about the quality of care they receive, physicians and other healthcare experts work with home health agencies to encourage the adoption, use, and monitoring of best practices and quality measures. These best practice measures will assist agencies in adapting to process measures in testing for future OASIS revisions.

While the current home health assessment and reporting tool, OASIS, will remain in use in the foreseeable future, several new priorities have emerged and are expected to be part of planning for the future, including Pay for Performance which ties a portion of reimbursement to delivery of care. The generalist nurse will always be involved in the QI process, whether data collecting, planning, implementing, evaluating, or being the performance improvement (PI) project quality manager. QI is a continuous process tool used to assist in the goal of delivering excellent patient care (CMS, 2012; Schneider et al., 2008).

Monitoring systems have been established that require agencies to report certain quality indicator data to CMS for the Home Health Quality Initiative. These quality indicator data are linked to payment, thus being a critical influence in the home health nurse's documentation and reporting of care. Agency submission of quality data was mandated beginning in 2007, with financial penalties for failure to submit (CMS, 2007; Davitt & Choi, 2008). The focus is on providing consumers with information on the practice effectiveness of home health agencies. In addition, some analysts have recommended incorporating Medicare–agency risk sharing in relation to profit–loss margins and/or tying agency payment to outcome indicators.

The Home Health Compare website is one of the central features of the Home Health Quality Initiative (http://www.medicare.gov/homehealthcompare). The Home Health Quality Initiative is part of an ongoing HHS effort that also focuses on improving the quality of care in nursing homes and hospitals. Public reporting is also intended to stimulate and support providers and clinicians to improve the quality of care provided. Home Health Compare is one of a number of search tools and other valuable information available at the public Medicare website, http://www.medicare.gov/. Consumers can search for Medicare-certified home health agencies by selecting a state and entering a county or zip code.

Once agencies are located in the search, consumers can view data on 11 quality measures that provide information about how well the home health agency provides care for some of their patients. This information should assist the healthcare consumer to make an informed decision when choosing a home health agency.

RESEARCH ALERT

Applying Roy's Adaptation Model, the purposes of this study were to explore hospice support of family caregivers in their decision to provide care at home and the relationships between hospice support, coping, and spiritual wellbeing. Data were collected in home visits of 21 recently bereaved family caregivers of hospice patients. Instruments included a demographic questionnaire, a Hospice Social Support questionnaire, the Jalowiec Coping Scale, the Spiritual Well-Being (SWB) Scale, and a postbereavement interview. Hospice workers were frequently identified as providing significant emotional support, making the caregiver feel highly cared for, respected, and supported. Subjects scored moderately high on the SWB Scale and reported low use of coping strategies. A significant negative correlation was found between reported use of coping strategies and hospice support. Hospice family caregivers rated this support highly as a major factor in making and sustaining the homecare decision.

Source: Hunt Raleigh, E., Robinson, J., Marold, K., & Jamison, M. (2006). Family caregiver perception of hospice support. *Journal of Hospice & Palliative Nursing, 8*(1), 25–33.

APPLICATION TO PRACTICE

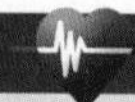

Mrs. Mae Thompson is a 68-year-old woman. Her referral diagnosis is congestive heart failure. Mrs. Thompson was discharged from Baxterville General Hospital after a 5-day stay. She lives with her 75-year-old sister in a two-bedroom house in a small rural community.

Upon arrival at the home, the health nurse finds Mrs. Thompson lying in bed. Her sister is watching television in the living room. During the visit, Mrs. Thompson relates the history of her illness. About a month ago, she noticed swelling in her feet and legs and extreme shortness of breath while picking tomatoes from her garden. She had to rest after picking only a small bucket of tomatoes. She also noticed that she had to stop midway between the house and the mailbox to catch her breath. Mrs. Thompson recalled that she had to use two or more pillows to breathe easy enough to sleep. She began awakening during the night with shortness of breath and had to sit up in the bedside chair to "get her breath back again" before going back to sleep. She also reported getting up several times a night to urinate, which was a change in her usual habits. She grew increasingly more concerned about herself when she became so fatigued that she neglected her garden crops.

The nurse, when conducting a medication review, found that Mrs. Thompson had been taking digoxin following a myocardial infarction 9 months earlier. Immediately before the present symptoms began, Mrs. Thompson had discontinued taking the digoxin, because, "I felt fine and didn't think I needed it anymore."

Mrs. Thompson's present medications are as follows: digoxin 0.25 mg/day, furosemide (Lasix) 40 mg/day, and KCl 20% tsp per day in juice. She reports that she is taking the "heart pill" but has stopped the "fluid pill," because it makes her have to urinate frequently and getting up makes her dizzy. She took the "other liquid" for about 2 days but has since quit taking it, "because it makes the juice taste funny." Since her discharge from the hospital, Mrs. Thompson has required assistance with self-care and is using a wheelchair for most ambulation. She spends much of her day in bed, because, "I feel so weak, I can't stand for very long." Her physician told her to "cut down on her salt," and she was given a diet sheet in the hospital, which she misplaced before reading it. She has a return appointment to see her physician in 2 weeks.

Mrs. Thompson's breakfast today consisted of two fried eggs, two pork sausage patties, two slices of toast with butter and jelly, and two cups of regular coffee. She is complaining of shortness of breath and is expressing frustration that "I will never be able to grow my own vegetables again." Her legs are extremely swollen with 3+ pitting edema; they are cool to the touch. Mrs. Thompson does not have socks on. She reports that she is concerned about her sister's "back problems" and that she fears relying on her too much for care such as bathing and ambulating. Her vital signs are as follows: blood pressure, 140/90 mmHg; pulse, 54 beats/min; and respiratory rate, 24 breaths/min.

1. Based on the preceding information, is Mrs. Thompson homebound?
2. Identify two nursing goals for Mrs. Thompson.
3. What action would you take regarding Mrs. Thompson's physical findings?
4. Identify one nursing goal related to Mrs. Thompson's caregiver.
5. What further information would you need about Mrs. Thompson?

Accreditation

Accreditation of agencies is another aspect of quality assurance (QA). Unlike state licensure, however, it is not required for Medicare or Medicaid participation. Accreditation is a demonstration of a commitment to providing a high standard of excellence in the delivery of care. Some third-party payers, such as managed care networks or insurance companies, may require accreditation. To meet the stringent standards of accreditation, an agency must demonstrate a team effort from all involved in the delivery of care (Lovejoy, 1997).

Three nationally recognized organizations provide voluntary accreditation for home health agencies: the Joint Commission's Home Care Accreditation Program (JCHCA); the Community Health Accreditation Program, (CHAP), a subsidiary of the National League for Nursing; (NLN); and the National Home Caring Council.

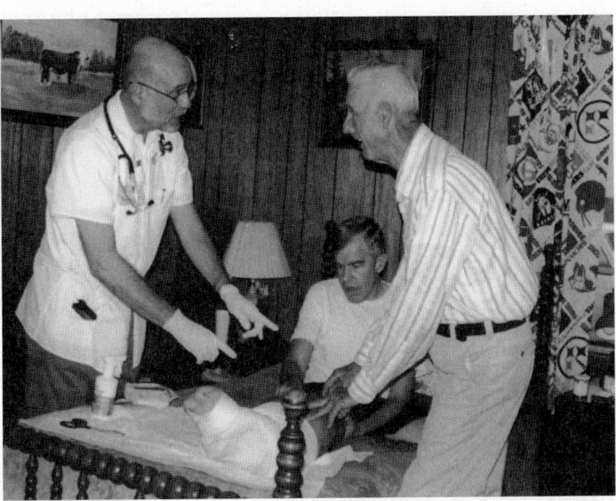

Home health nurses work with the family caregiver to implement the plan of care.

Managed Care and Home Health

Managed care became the primary pattern of organizational reimbursement in the United States in the first decade of the 21st century. As a result, most persons in the United States with private health insurance are in some type of managed care arrangement or network. A majority of states are in some form of Medicaid managed care program. Managed care will influence nursing practice as agencies respond to strong incentives to lower costs. As has been discussed, nursing interventions and their effectiveness will be measured against patient outcomes and patient satisfaction with care (Lin, Kane, Mehr, Madsen, & Petroski, 2006). Home health nurses will continue to focus on the family as caregiver, with a greater emphasis on teaching the family/caregiver more effective ways of caring for the patient. With increasing responsibilities resting with the caregiver, more efficient use of the nurse's time can occur resulting in shorter illness episodes. All home health nurses must be effective case managers to ensure that the highest quality care is delivered in the shortest time possible (Duke & Street, 2003; Peters & Eigsti, 1991).

Managed care plans generally reimburse home health agencies based on a fee-for-service or capitated rate methodology. A **fee-for-service rate** is generally based on a per-visit or hourly rate for each discipline. A capitated rate is generally awarded based on a population or group of "lives" for which the agency is paid a "per member per month" rate. Reimbursement of this nature requires that the agency make an estimation of the anticipated needs of the population to determine if the arrangement is financially feasible (McKnight, 2006; Spector, Cohen, & Pesis-Katz, 2004).

As the focus in managed care shifts to outcomes of care, research linking outcomes to care delivery has resulted in Medicare's OASIS: Standardized Outcome and Assessment Information Set for Home Health Care. Shaughnessy (1996) developed the OASIS instrument as a data set with the following categories of items: demographics and patient history, living arrangements, supportive assistance, body systems, activities of daily living/instrumental activities of daily living (ADLs/IADLs), medications, equipment management, and emergent care. Data are collected for a patient upon admission to the home health agency, at a specified time during care, and upon discharge of home health services. OASIS is used to measure outcomes of care based on the home health interventions provided. The instrument is mandated by Medicare and is the condition of participation for certified home health agencies. These data are being used by the CMS to provide information about the population of Medicare and Medicaid patients receiving home health care and their clinical outcomes.

DAY IN THE LIFE

You have to be prepared for anything in home health. Home health nurses use the nursing process just like other nurses; one difference is that they begin the assessment when they pull into the driveway or yard. The nurse may see a 2-month-old for an evaluation for failure to thrive at 8:00 a.m., a 10-year-old for post-appendectomy nonhealing surgical wound care at 9:30 a.m., and a 101-year-old for catheter care at 10:45 a.m. I believe that more than any other nursing care, the art and science of nursing must hold hands in home health. You must know how to administer a high-powered antibiotic IV, know the science, and possess the skill it calls for to do it properly.

(continues)

DAY IN THE LIFE (*continued*)

And at the same time, the home health nurse must use the art of caring when a patient hammers a nail into his wall for you to hang that IV on when the medical equipment company fails to deliver the IV pole on time. The true art is to use the patient's nail and tell him how important he is in the delivery of his care.

—Ilene Purvis Bloxsom, RN, BSN, MSHA, home health nurse

Interdisciplinary Team Approach in Home Health

Collaboration is mandatory in home health nursing. In fact, Medicare requires an interdisciplinary team approach for agencies to be Medicare certified. A collaborative approach is clearly evident in the definitions and standards of home health nursing. Collaboration is necessary to ensure the continuity of care as the patient moves from hospital to home. *Discharge* has traditionally referred to the patient's exit from the hospital to the home; in today's fluid healthcare system, patients are transitioned in and out of different realms of agency service, necessitating complex professional referrals. To be in legal compliance with federal regulatory statutes, the physician must certify the plan of treatment for the patient. In most instances, it becomes the responsibility of other team members to evaluate the patient's status and response to treatment and then, with the physician, modify the plan of treatment accordingly.

The nurse serves as manager or coordinator of care for this interdisciplinary team effort. To function in this role, the nurse must have a clear understanding of the roles of the other team members and a working knowledge of community resources. Traditionally, the roles and functions of the homecare nurse have been that of direct care provider, educator, and case manager or coordinator of care. Direct care activities or skills include assessments, performing procedures and treatments, and patient and family teaching. Indirect care includes ancillary personnel supervision, referrals, consultation, and team conferences. The nurse assesses and identifies the problems and needs. Referrals to other disciplines and community agencies may be needed, and this care is coordinated by the nurse under the direction of the physician. For example, if a nurse identifies a home health patient who is having financial difficulty owing to out-of-pocket deductibles for necessary equipment, a referral to a social worker would be appropriate (Boxer & Meadows, 2008).

Within an interdisciplinary model, the unit of care should be the family/caregivers, and nursing care is designed and provided within the context of the community in which the patient lives. The homecare nurse cares for patients across the lifespan with multiple medical diagnoses and responses to illness. Health promotion and disease prevention are the focus of care. The nurse develops a POC under the direction of a physician with the assistance of a multidisciplinary team, which becomes the home healthcare team and may include social workers, therapists, chaplains, nutritionists, and others as appropriate. The patient also participates in developing his or her POC, and evaluating, along with the team, the outcomes of care. The nurse and team members plan their visit schedule around patient preferences, other discipline visits, physician appointments, and geographic areas (Milton, 2005).

Appropriate planning by all disciplines before the visit is essential. This includes laboratory work or any supplies needed, along with the activities of the visit that center on the goals set for the patient in the previously established POC. Some agencies have care maps or critical paths that define the day-to-day activities and outcomes to be met during each visit; others use goals established on admission and modify them as appropriate. Detailed descriptions of

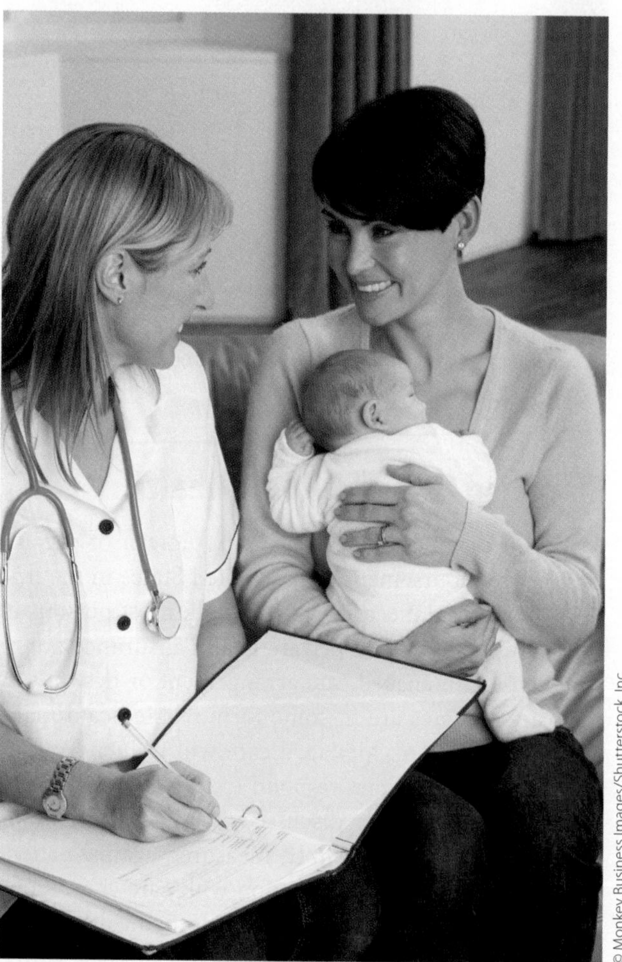

Home health nurses see a variety of patients with diverse healthcare needs.

member roles of the home healthcare interdisciplinary team are provided in **Box 36-7**.

BOX 36-7 Members of the Home Healthcare Interdisciplinary Team

- *Home health nurse* is the traditional provider of care in the home. Home health nurses provide skilled nursing services and coordinate care within the interdisciplinary team.
- *Physician* refers patients for homecare services and approves the plan of care.
- *Home health aides* provide personal care that includes activities such as bathing, shaving, and skin and nail care. The home health aide also performs basic tasks that include things such as emptying urinary drainage bags, taking vital signs, assisting with ambulation and performing exercises assigned, and light homemaking activities such as preparing a meal, changing linens, cleaning, and laundry.
- *Physical therapists* provide evaluation of the patient's rehabilitation needs and potential, which may include areas such as range of motion, strength, balance and coordination, gait analysis, muscle tone, pain, endurance, equipment needs, and home safety. The physical therapist then develops and implements the treatment plan that includes teaching the patient and family the home therapy regime and establishing a maintenance therapy program.
- *Speech therapists* provide services related to the evaluation of rehabilitation needs and potential in patients with speech and language disorders and swallowing disorders. The speech therapist develops and implements a restorative treatment program involving the patient and family.
- *Occupational therapists* focus on evaluation and treatment of the patient's upper extremities by assisting to restore muscle strength and mobility for functional skills. The program established is designed to restore physical function and sensory-integrative function or develop compensatory techniques. Vocational and prevocational assessment and training, and design and fitting of orthotic and self-help devices, are also provided by the occupational therapist.
- *Medical social workers* provide assessment of the social and emotional factors related to the patient's illness and plan of treatment. This includes assessment of the relationship of the patient's medical/nursing requirements to the home situation, financial resources, and community resources. The Medical social worker may provide counseling for the patient related to areas such as depression, addictions, reaction/adjustment to illness, and strengthening family support systems. Counseling for the patient's family may be necessary to treat the patient's illness/injury in resolving family problems that are obstructing or preventing the patient's treatment.

Role of Family Caregivers in Home Health

As community health nurses have long been aware, home health nurses contribute less to the wellbeing of a home health patient than the more significant influence of family caregivers. Informal caregiving provided by family caregivers is an integral part of our healthcare system (Bradley, 2003; Milton, 2005). Among people 45 and older, approximately two out of five report some experience with long-term care in their families. As the population ages, the demand for informal family caregivers will escalate over the coming decades. Home health patients would be unable to stay in their homes even to be the recipient of home health nursing care were it not for the family members and other caregivers who dedicate themselves to their care.

Community health nurses have traditionally been family oriented when conducting home visits. One need only look at our legacy of Lillian Wald and the Henry Street nurses to see the foundation of family-oriented care. Only when the family becomes recognized as the unit of service within the context of the larger community can significant, long-lasting change occur.

With the ever-present influence of Medicare and other funding sources, however, today's nurses often focus their care efforts on providing only those services that are reimbursable in the home setting. The individual ill patient has steadily become the focus in home care, with the family and other caregivers fading to a contextual backdrop (Bradley, 2003; Davitt & Choi, 2008; Kenyon et al., 1990).

NOTE THIS!

Who Are the Caregivers?

The 2004 caregiving in the United States survey, sponsored by the National Alliance for Caregiving and AARP, documented the prevalence of caregiving in the United States. The study found that more than one in five U.S. households (an estimated 44.4 million caregivers over age 18) are informal caregivers for a person older than age 18. This report also showed that 62% of caregivers are married and/or living with a partner, and nearly two-thirds (61%) are women. The typical caregiver is a 46-year-old woman with at least some college experience who provides more than 20 hours of care each week to her mother.

Source: National Alliance for Caregiving and AARP. (2004). *Caregiving in the U.S.* Retrieved from http://www.caregiving.org/data04final-report.pdf

The family caregivers of home health patients often have unmet health needs, and the role of caregiver is associated with high stress and increased illness when compared with similar populations. This role, which is often unpaid, is associated with isolation and selfless dedication to the health of the home health patient (Levine, 1999). Quite often, the caregiver is the only other adult in the home and, as such, has little choice about being the one responsible for the household and ill patient. Many studies report that family caregivers tend to be female and themselves in late adulthood (see Bradley, 2003; Bull, 1990; Kiecolt-Glaser et al., 1987; Pruchno & Potashnik, 1989).

The community health nurse must strive to consider these caregivers in the assessment of the environment and resources, because if the family caregiver has unmet health needs, eventually his or her caretaking abilities will be affected. Zelwesky and Deitrick (1987) go so far as to state, "Accurate needs assessment of the patient and his or her family may prevent family burn-out, extend care-giving abilities, conserve family resources, and delay or prevent institutionalization" (p. 77). In her 1996 study, Bradley contends that, although prevention activities are not covered by Medicare in home health,

> We depend on the family caregiver to provide needed care to many of our patients. If the caregivers become ill, their caregiving ability decreases. The likelihood of our losing the original home health patient to nursing home care or hospitalization increases when we do not promote the family caregiver's health. (p. 287)

Thus, although a financial gain might be apparent in the short term, there may be significant long-term financial benefits in caring for the ones who care for our patients day in and day out.

The home health nurse must assess the role of the family caregiver in the context of how well the patient functions in the home environment (Bradley, 2003). Supporting the caregiver may mean little more than listening carefully to his or her needs regarding personal health status and providing suggestions for health promotion and time management apart from the patient. Support groups for caregivers can also provide valuable resources that ultimately strengthen the care provided to the patient. The home health nurse has many opportunities to praise the caregiver and remind him or her of the need to pay attention to self for the sake of the patient. Daycare programs and respite care can provide needed breaks for the family caregiver and should be encouraged by the home health nurse. As the need for informal caregiving increases in the future, home health nurses will need to become more involved in the promotion of local, state, and national healthcare policy development related to the support of family caregivers as a healthcare resource.

Legal and Ethical Issues in Home Health

Home health nurses are confronted with legal and ethical issues related to nursing practice daily. Complex family situations create daily dilemmas for the home health nurse, such as questions regarding caretaking abilities of the family caregivers, financial constraints, and respect for autonomous decision making with the vulnerable patient. In the home, nurses are often caring for patients over a long period, as compared with the acute care setting; as a result, they face boundary issues related to self-responsibility for care (Gremmen, 1999; Liaschenko, 1997; Sorrell, 2012).

One source of ethical dilemma in health care is in providing necessary nursing care for identified patient needs when financial coverage is no longer available. Agency policy may include options for temporary services or the nurse may assist the patient and family in making alternative plans for care. Patients' noncompliance with treatment plans is an ongoing challenge, and ethical issues related to use of resources can be sources of significant ethical conflict. Reporting abusive, neglectful, and unsafe conditions, care, or practices may often be necessary as a legal and ethical mandatory practice.

Knowing a patient's rights and responsibilities, as well as the rights and limitations of the home healthcare nurse, is a critical component of home healthcare nursing practice (Gremmen, 1999). Referral to social work, support groups, and appropriate agencies is often the appropriate response (Sorrell, 2012).

RESEARCH ALERT

The aim of this research study was to explore and interpret the diverse subject of positions or roles that nurses construct when caring for patients in their own homes. Ten interviews were analyzed and interpreted using discourse analysis. The findings show that these nurses working in home care constructed two positions: "guest" and "professional." They had to make a choice between these positions because it was impossible to be both at the same time. An ethic of care and an ethic of justice were present in these positions, both of which create diverse ethical appeals, that is, implicit demands to perform according to a guest or to a professional norm.

Source: Öresland, S., Määttä, S., Norberg, A., Winther Jörgensen, M., & Lützén, K. (2008). Nurses as guests or professionals in home health care. *Nursing Ethics, 15*(3), 371–383.

Lovejoy (1997) recommends the creation of agency support groups for home health nurses and other professionals. A support group can provide needed discussion and conflict resolution in the environment of shared

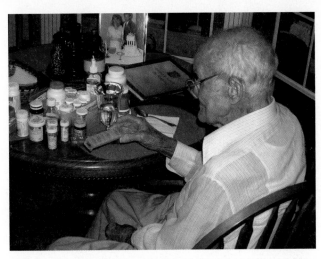

Home health nurses see a variety of patients with diverse healthcare needs.

experiences with others. Lovejoy (1997) makes the following recommendations in the creation of an efficient support group in home health:

- A clinical nurse specialist should facilitate and coordinate the support group. This clinical nurse specialist should have experience in leading support groups and ideally should have experience in the field as a home health staff nurse.
- Support group meetings should not be mandatory. Nurses should be encouraged to attend meetings but never required to attend.
- Support groups should include a mix of new and experienced nurses. All other health professionals should be encouraged to be a part of the group as well.

The support group should be sponsored by the agency, be a part of the formal organizational structure, and have rules and bylaws as appropriate. If the group is informal, minimal rules should relate to frequency of meetings, commitment of members, confidentiality issues, and termination of membership.

An effective support group should help make members feel better about themselves and their abilities and more at ease in the complex home environment. One unexpected benefit of the support group in home health agencies is that members often are able to see coworkers in a new light and learn to trust them as resources. Home care is often a lonely profession, because nurses do not have the benefit of working closely with colleagues on a daily basis. The support group, along with modern telecommunication strategies, can bridge the isolation of "nursing on the road" (Lovejoy, 1997).

Home Care Bill of Rights

Medicare-certified agencies are required to provide home health patients with a written bill of rights before the initiation of service. Each home health patient is required to be informed of his or her right for healthcare treatment, and this education must be documented in the patient's permanent record. To assist home health provider agencies with this requirement, the NAHC (2014) has developed a model home care bill of rights. This document provides the patient with details of what can be expected from homecare agencies in the delivery of their care. Agencies often use a modified form of the NAHC bill of rights.

Advance Medical Directives

Home health nurses must also be involved in the requirements for informed decision making as specified in the home care bill of rights related to treatment options and refusal when the patient is unable to make decisions and communicate those decisions to the healthcare provider (NAHC, 2014). An advance medical directive is a document that describes patient intent and wishes regarding various types of medical treatment in selected situations (Pevey, 2008). Medical directives were developed in the early part of the 1990s in response to increased technology in the treatment of acute and chronic illnesses and the increased awareness by the consumer population of the need to make informed decisions regarding treatment options and the refusal of medical interventions.

APPLICATION TO PRACTICE 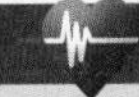

With the recent public health concerns related to increased rates of community-acquired methicillin-resistant *Staphylococcus aureus* (CA-MRSA), infection control in the home setting is even more critical than before. Home visits should be made in sequence based on vulnerability of the patient and risk to other patients. The home health nurse should prioritize his or her visit schedule to go from the least infectious patient to the one with greatest risk for infection or existing infection. Using these guidelines, the following visits would be conducted in this order: blood pressure check for patient on new hypertensive medication, diabetic instruction for newly diagnosed patient, pediatric wound care post-appendectomy patient, and HIV patient with MRSA wound.

Two types of advance medical directives are distinguished: living wills and healthcare proxies. Either type of directive specifically addresses the patient's desire for health care or refusal in the event of becoming incapacitated and unable to make decisions. The living will documents a patient's decision to decline life-prolonging interventions if that patient becomes terminally ill. A healthcare proxy, also known as durable power of attorney, specifies the name of a person who will make healthcare decisions if the patient becomes incapacitated and cannot make them.

The patient maintains the right to change any of these documents at any time. Each state differs in terms of its laws and regulations related to the implementation of advance directives, and the home health nurse must remain informed about such statutes.

Information and Technology in Home Health

Communication and Data Management

Home healthcare nurses depend on the use of information technology in clinical practice. There is continued demand for and improvement in the information systems available for use in the home. Technology is changing the way patient care is being delivered in all settings. As health care becomes more mobile, remote points of access within a safe and secure infrastructure will become the norm (Lind, Karlsson, & Fridlund, 2007; Seibert et al., 2008). Computerized records and care planning tools, such as critical pathways, are helping the homecare nurses achieve greater time and patient management. Many home health nurses now practice almost exclusively from home and use laptop computers to document visits. Although working from home does not allow for the camaraderie of team communication that occurs in other settings, it does provide many nurses with more work flexibility (Neal, 1997). Along with tools to manage this information, many healthcare organizations have decision-support systems that would benefit the management of patient care in the home by issuing reminders, offering a menu of options, or linking the nurse to important educational tools and information needed (Pare, Sicotte, St. Jules, & Gauthier, 2006).

As improvements in health networks continue, the nurse will be able to access test results from the laboratory and information from other providers involved in the coordination of care in the home. Electronic commerce may replace traditional home health methods of communicating with partners in health care, especially as disease management programs continue to grow (Doolittle, Whitten, McCartney, Cook, & Nazir, 2005).

Security programs within the organization should protect the confidentiality of individually identifiable healthcare information. This includes training, security audits, and policies regarding access to different types of information (Lind et al., 2007; Pare et al., 2006).

Healthcare information systems of the 21st century should guide QI efforts, improve the coordination of care, advance evidence-based healthcare practice, and support continued research (Monsen et al., 2006). Because the healthcare industry is so fragmented, it will be important to work toward data sharing as is common now in so many nonhealth industries (Doolittle et al., 2005; Waters, 2007). Although all healthcare organizations collect information, it is uncommon for this information to be brought together in a way that can shed light on how variations in the process of care affect outcomes. Information on the experiences and perspectives of patients and the healthcare team can now be collected with available computer systems. The home health nurse also works with patients as they research their health online, assisting them in evaluating the vast amount of information as to quality and application. Information on healthcare outcomes is becoming standard practice in most homecare settings (President's Advisory Commission on Consumer Protection and Quality in the Health Care Industry, 1998; Waters, 2007).

Delivery of Care

Homecare nursing must redefine the assessment parameters that are critical to be performed in person and those that can be done through technology such as telenursing. Nurses must also redefine "touch." Do we touch a patient physically, as in palpation, or do we also use the term generically, in that we can touch a patient with a few therapeutic words over the phone, television, or computer (Franz, 1997; Waters, 2007)? The homecare nurse can now deliver care and information through a lens, a screen, or a telephone into the home. Home telenursing can never fully replace in-person home health care, of course. Nevertheless, the appropriate mix of in-person and electronic visitation, along with the appropriate level of providers to accomplish both, will provide better and more holistic care for the home patient and family. Telenursing technology can assist the homecare nurse in managing the POC remotely to capture vital signs and in teaching patients and their families self-care management.

Laptop-based medical management systems have been used in the home setting for monitoring wound care and linking the home health nurses to physician consultation. This allows the physician consultants to view patient wounds from a live video image. The traditional method in the home requires the nurse to take Polaroid photographs of wounds and forward them to the physician for review. Using the telemedicine system, visiting nurses dial the physician and forward the image in real time; decisions regarding treatment protocols are then exchanged between the providers and the patient (Kincade, 1997; Seibert et al., 2008; Waters, 2007).

As home telemedicine and telenursing systems mature, they will evolve so that physical therapy can be administered, nutrition counseling conducted, and occupational therapy supervised. As computer ownership and use in the home become as common as television use, email can be used to communicate with patients and patients can report directly to healthcare providers. Successful programs have used email to remind patients about medication dosing and educational information for postsurgery patients on a daily basis (Jerant, 1999). Patient access to the Internet is becoming more common. Such systems allow nurse's aides to conduct physical home visits and be supervised by nurses at an agency or at home. The homecare industry now uses these technologies to track patient outcomes, reduce service redundancy, and supplement care provided by visiting nurses and other disciplines.

RESEARCH ALERT

A telemedicine approach was used to facilitate follow up and training of patients prescribed continuous positive airway pressure (CPAP) therapy for obstructive sleep apnea (OSA). In two back-to-back studies, researchers examined whether telemedical follow up was effective in and acceptable to patients. In the first study, the researchers enrolled 50 OSA patients who came to the sleep center for a CPAP follow-up visit. Patients were given a teleconsultation with a physician, after which they were asked to answer an anonymous questionnaire to obtain their opinions about the teleconsultation. In the second study, which was a randomized controlled trial, 40 OSA patients scheduled for CPAP training were included, with 20 receiving the usual face-to-face training and 20 who received the training via videoconference. After the session, all patients were blindly evaluated on what they learned about OSA and mask placement. More than 95% (49/50) of the interviewed patients in the first study were satisfied with the teleconsultation, and 66% (33/50) of them answered that the teleconsultation could replace 50–100% of their CPAP follow-up visits. In the second study, patients who received the CPAP training via videoconference demonstrated the same knowledge about OSA and CPAP therapy as the face-to-face group (mean 93.6% of correct answers vs. mean 92.1%; $p = 0.935$). Performance on practical skills (mask and headgear placement, leak avoidance) was also similar between the two groups. These results support the use of this telemedicine-based approach as a valuable strategy for patients' CPAP training and clinical follow up.

Source: Isetta, V., León, C., Torres, M., Embid, C., Roca, J., Navajas, D., … Montserrat, J. M. (2014). Telemedicine-based approach for obstructive sleep apnea management: Building evidence. *Interactive Journal of Medical Research, 3*(1), e6. doi: 10.2196/ijmr.3060

Hospice Care in the Home

Hospice services for the terminally ill became covered expenses under Medicare in 1983. Hospice nursing provides palliative nursing care for terminally ill patients and their families, with an emphasis on physical, psychosocial, emotional, and spiritual needs. Palliative care is comfort-oriented care and refers to interventions that alleviate or lessen the severity of disease or illness without curing it. The goal of the hospice program for home care is to improve the quality of life for people who are no longer able to benefit from curative interventions, with an emphasis on treating the symptoms of the disease to promote comfort. The word "hospice" comes from Latin *hospitium*, meaning "guesthouse." Hospice is holistic in nature and views dying as a normal part of living. Through hospice care in the home, the patient can live in dignity and comfort in the context of home and family. Hospice care is primarily provided at home, although facilities also exist that provide these services in an inpatient setting while still offering support for families in a homelike environment. Patients in long-term care facilities can also receive hospice services, with the facility being considered by Medicare as the place of residence of the patient (Acorn, 2008; Brooks, 1997). Medicare may pay for bereavement counseling for as long as a year after the loved one's death.

Many HMOs and insurance companies also cover hospice services for their patients, and the majority of states now offer hospice coverage under their Medicaid programs. Although each hospice service has individual policies concerning payment for care, a common principle of hospice care is to offer services based on need rather than the ability to pay. For this reason, hospice services may often rely more than other home health services on grants and voluntary donations (Forcina Hill, 2008).

Quality Assurance and Hospice

QA/PI/outcome-based quality improvement (OBQI) and QI have been a priority focus in the home healthcare arena for many years. Hospice care was thought to have an anticipated outcome of inevitability, and hospice agencies were not required to develop the types of lengthy quality PI plans and programs mandatory for the home health agency. However, in 2005, CMS published proposed CoP for hospices that included a new requirement that hospices develop, implement, and maintain an effective, data-driven quality assessment and PI (QAPI) program. These QA plans may look at such activities as patient place of death, patient pain medication status, and bowel status to determine how the agency might improve the care of the patient.

Beyond the Grave

Rattling tin piano
Voices crying softly,
Through sun flecked
Tabernacle roof.
We stand,
Singing of life beyond
That open grave.
Beyond early summer jam,
Beyond racing through her
Fall dry cornfield,
Beyond rocking to sleep,
Feet drag softly,
Beyond the smell of lilac talc,
Starch, snuff, Ponds Soap,
Beyond the Christmas lights,
Story of magic
Beyond
Just beyond
The better life.

—Ann Thedford Lanier

Do not go gentle into that good night. Old age should burn and rage at close of day; Rage, rage against the dying of the light.

—Dylan Thomas

RESEARCH ALERT

Three out of every four hospice patients (74.1%) died in a private residence, nursing home, or other residential facility versus acute-care hospital settings in 2006. This exceeds the rate seen in the general population, in which about 50% die in acute-care hospitals.

While the majority of patient care is provided in the place the patient calls home, 19.6% of hospices also operate a dedicated inpatient unit or facility. Most of these facilities (87.1%) are either freestanding or located within a hospital and provide a mix of acute and residential care. These facilities are typically found in larger agencies with an average daily census greater than 200 patients. Only 8.8% of hospice patients died in a hospital setting that was not managed by the hospice organization.

Source: Brown University Center for Gerontology and Health Care Research. (2004). *Facts on dying: Policy relevant data on care at the end of lie.* Retrieved from http://www.chcr.brown.edu/dying

Another facet of Quality is the proposed Hospice Experience of Care Survey.

Overview: The Hospice Experience of Care Survey is intended to gather information on the experiences of hospice patients and their caregivers with hospice services. Current trends are toward increased use of hospice services in the United States. More than a million American are receiving hospice services annually. The Hospice Experience of Care Survey will be national in scope and will require standardized survey administration protocols. The questionnaire is currently under development.

About the survey: The Hospice Experience of Care Survey will sample the primary caregivers of deceased hospice patients. Administration of the survey will occur several months after the death. The survey encompasses the following key topics: starting hospice care; the patients' hospice care (including controlling pain, help with difficulty breathing, help with constipation, and help with anxiety or sadness); special medical equipment; the caregivers' own experience with hospice; and overall rating of hospice care. We anticipate that there will be three approved modes of administration: mail only, telephone only, and mixed (mail followed by telephone).

Public reporting and policy relevance: The proposed rule published in the *Federal Register* (78FR48234) may be used by CMS to determine payments for hospice. The importance of patient satisfaction and quality in payment of services is fairly new to the healthcare industry. The role of the nurse in maintaining clear, concise documentation for quality measures and providing excellent, compassionate bedside care may determine the viability of the hospice agency.

For hospice services, the physician must certify that the patient has a life expectancy that would normally be expected to be 6 months or less and is seeking palliative treatment only. Hospice patients must be recertified every 60 days.

Patients and family are encouraged to be involved in all decisions about caregiving and medical interventions. Admission to a hospice should not be viewed as a failure of other therapies. Rather, a more holistic approach would suggest that previous treatments had become inappropriate and referral to a hospice as movement into another model of more appropriate therapy for terminal care (Hospice Foundation of America, 2008).

The nurse has traditionally cared for the dying and the bereaved, whether on the battlefield or in the trauma unit or in the home—so how is hospice different? Hospice emerged as an organized movement in England with the founding of the first hospice at St. Christopher in London in 1950 by Dr. Dame Cicely Saunders. The hospice movement was strongly influenced by the research of Dr. Elisabeth Kübler-Ross, who conceptualized death as the final stage of growth as contrasted with the prevailing fear of death and the dying process as failure on the part of the medical system (Kübler-Ross, 1969, 1975). Since the 1980s, with the prolongation of life, advanced technology, and a growing recognition that dying and terminally ill patients require a special kind of care, hospice as a community health nursing specialty has grown. Thousands of persons with life-limiting diseases have relied on hospice services for comfort, dignity, and compassion at the end of life.

Medicare hospice care for the terminally ill in the home generally costs significantly less than care for patients in the standard Medicare program. Reasons for this difference include less technology used in the care of the patient and family and friends who provide most of the daily care at home. Although hospice care does not provide 24-hour-a-day care in the home, hospice staff members are usually on call 24 hours a day. Volunteers make up an integral part of hospice care and are required to be a part of Medicare-certified hospice service. Inpatient respite care is available for the family, which provides family caregivers with periodic relief. A written POC is also required.

> Hospice does not speed up or slow down the dying process. It does not prolong life and it does not hasten death.
>
> —*National Hospice Foundation*

NOTE THIS!

In 2011, an estimated 1.651 million patients received services from hospice.

Source: National Hospice and Palliative Care Organization. (2012). NHPCO Facts and Figures: Hospice Care in America. Retrieved from http://www.nhpco.org/sites/default/files/public/Statistics_Research/2012_Facts_Figures.pdf

NOTE THIS!

Home Health Care During and After a Disaster

On August 30, 2005, displaced residents of New Orleans first learned that the levees of their city had been overtopped and then breached by the storm surge from Hurricane Katrina. New Orleans would soon be 80% flooded. Within a month, Hurricane Rita arrived in New Orleans, making cleanup and recovery an even more difficult process. This article discusses the preparation and follow up that was still going on in 2007 and the role of healthcare providers, particularly homecare providers, in the aftermath of Hurricanes Katrina and Rita.

Source: Weeber, S. (2007). Home health care after Hurricanes Katrina and Rita: A report from the field. *Home Health Care Management & Practice, 19*(2), 104–111.

Medicare mandates that four core services be provided directly by the hospice: nursing, medical care, social work, and counseling (Wilson, 1993). Services provided by hospice are as follows:

- Nursing service on an intermittent basis
- Physician services
- Drugs for pain relief
- Physical, occupational, and speech therapy
- Home health aides
- Medical supplies
- Spiritual and pastoral services
- Continuous care during a crisis
- Bereavement services for the family, up to a year following death

Hospice provides coordinated services for the family of the patient with a terminal illness. Hospice, as a specialized kind of home health care, is designed to provide comfort and support to patients and families in the final stages of terminal illness. Goals center on providing care in which patients can spend their last days with dignity, at home or in a homelike setting, surrounded by family members and loved ones. Comfort involves physical and spiritual comfort and emotional support of the patient, family, and caregivers (Acorn, 2008; Reese & Brown, 1997). See **Box 36-8** for a sample agency hospice philosophy.

Hospice Care for Children

Although hospice services have traditionally been associated with adults, recognition has grown among healthcare professionals that children with terminal illnesses can also benefit from hospice care. The epidemic of children with acquired immune deficiency syndrome (AIDS) has prompted the development of pediatric hospice services for children with life-limiting illnesses

BOX 36-8 Hospice Philosophy: One Agency's Commitment

Hospice affirms life. Hospice exists to provide support and care for persons in the last phases of incurable disease so that they might live as fully and comfortably as possible. Hospice recognizes dying as a normal process, whether or not resulting from a disease. Hospice exists in the hope and belief that, through appropriate care and the promotion of a caring community sensitive to their needs, patients and families may be free to attain a degree of mental and spiritual preparation for death that is satisfactory to them.

Source: Courtesy of North Mississippi Medical Center Home Health and Hospice.

(Oleske & Czarniecki, 1999). The first hospice home for children, The Helen House, was established in 1982 in the United Kingdom.

Palliative care for children with terminal diseases, such as cancer, can ensure the child's comfort through the course of his or her illness. Oleske and Czarniecki (1999) advocate that children with life-limiting illnesses, regardless of diagnosis, socioeconomic status, or geographic location, should receive a continuum of palliative care and have access to hospice services that enhance life and ease the burden of dying. They contend that "children should know, in an age appropriate way, that death is near but that it will not be painful, not faced alone, but rather in the company of those they love" (Oleske & Czarniecki, 1999, p. 1291). Opportunities for hospice nursing with children will most likely increase in the future.

Disaster and Home Health and Hospice: Incident Command System

The Incident Command System (ICS) was developed in California after the devastation of out-of-control wildfires. ICS is a disaster plan that is interdisciplinary in scope and response. The ICS mandates that hospitals, home health, hospices, cities, counties, and states have incorporated this system into their emergency preparedness plans. Home health and hospice agencies incorporate an Emergency Disaster Plan into their POC for each individual patient along with teaching the patients the plan. Upon admission the Home health nurses assign a disaster priority code to the patient who requires skilled intervention and the care must be provided such as ventilator care and management. A lesser priority code may be assigned for those patients with a skilled need that may be safely visited in 24 to 48 hours.; a lesser priority code number for a patient means that the nurse may miss a visit. In addition, nurses develop evacuation plans for and with their home health patients. They also have to have an emergency/disaster plan for the home health and hospice office, based on the ICS mandates.

Holistic Care

Nurses who work in hospice care have specialized training in grief and bereavement management. Although spiritual care has been a major component of nursing practice since its inception, nurses are often uncomfortable with spiritual components related to death (Brant, 1998). Hospice nurses must be especially comfortable in their skills related to the spiritual needs of their patients. Holistic nursing care for the hospice patient means assessing for suffering in the spiritual realm, because the total person is incomplete without such consideration (Running et al., 2008). Providing spiritual care does not mean that hospice nurses must hold the same beliefs of those for whom they care. Hospice nurses who provide palliative care approach patients with a nonjudgmental, listening ear. Nurses provide spiritual care by assisting patients in their final days in their search for meaning of past, present, and future events. Patients attempt to make sense of their life experiences, and nurses, in the holistic tradition, must be involved in this healing aspect of this last stage of life (Acorn, 2008; Reese & Brown, 1997).

CMS has added a CoP that on a federal level has major implications for the advanced nurse practitioner. See **Box 36-9**.

BOX 36-9 Advanced Practice Nursing and Home Health and Hospice Care

Interpretive Guidelines §418.64(b)(2)

- If state law permits registered nurses (RNs) to see, treat, and write orders for patients, then RNs may provide services to beneficiaries receiving hospice care. If an RN, including a nurse practitioner, advanced practice nurse, or other advanced practice nurse, is permitted by state law and regulation to see, treat, and write orders, then the RN may perform this function while providing nursing services for hospice patients. Hospices are free to use the services of all types of advanced practice nurses within their respective scopes of practice to enhance the nursing care furnished to their patients. Services provided by a nurse practitioner (NP) who is not the patient's attending physician are included under nursing care.

Source: CMS State Operations Manual Hospice.

Nurses as team members in hospice care are often the ones with the prolonged, close contact with patients and family members and, as such, can provide comprehensive information about the wellbeing of the family and caregivers to the physician and other members of the hospice team (Goldstein, et al. 2004).

Ethical issues include special considerations for hospice workers. Working with families during a family member's imminent death brings challenges related to professional boundaries, family responsibilities, and complex decisions about care (Hunt, 1991). The threat of legalized suicide is of concern to all nurses but is an especially significant issue in the field of hospice nursing. Legalized suicide and euthanasia practices threaten the natural cycle of dying and the final stage of growth. Providing appropriate, holistic, and comforting end-of-life care, as larger numbers of the baby boomer generation age, will continue to emerge as critical professional issues for home health nurses who specialize in hospice care (Ekman Ladd, Pasquerella, & Smith, 2008; Tilden, Tolle, Drach, & Perrin, 2004).

Other future issues for hospice nursing care include the expansion of community-based residential hospice care facilities, which include respite care, home care, acute inpatient care, and expanded bereavement counseling for families (Pevey, 2008). With the growing number of elders, adults with AIDS, and children with prolonged terminal illnesses, hospice services will be challenged to provide myriad home- and community-based services for families caring for the terminally ill. Humane care for the dying strains families who are already overburdened with dual-career demands and child care. Such facilities can provide nurse-managed, holistic care for the terminally ill in a non-institutional, natural environment more conducive to the promotion of health in the final stage of life (Brännström, Brulin, Norberg, Boman, & Strandberg, 2005; Doolittle et al., 2005; Wilson, 1993).

Life Goes On

I felt like a rainbow covered with dirt in this room.
I couldn't bear seeing
my uncle and aunt washed
with sad feelings.
My grandpa's hand had no life to it.
Though life went on and the
trees kept swaying.
I wondered what would life
be like without his hand to
cross my hair.
My rainbow just did not shine that day.
The wind took over everything.
I love the wind.
It changed everything in that room.
It made me feel like a hundred
butterflies had flown from his
chest.
His stuck together lips and
hard breathing harmed me.
I couldn't stand there.
Water was pulled from my eyes.
Our hands parted and I
kissed him and walked into
reality.

—Alexandra Zacharias, age 10, on the occasion of the death of her grandfather

Source: The Educational Forum, 55(3), Spring 1991.

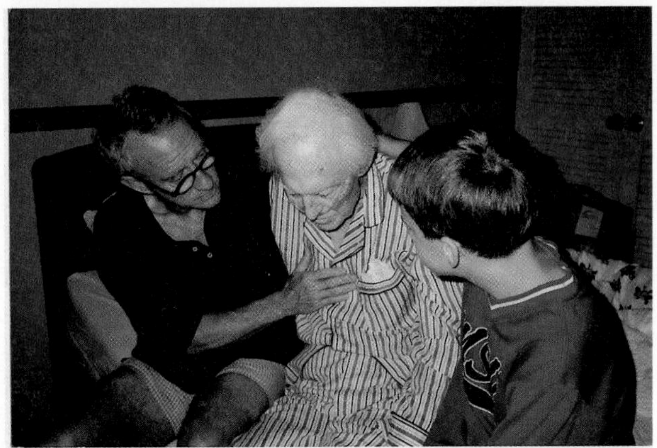

Hospice provides patients with the comfort and support of their families in the home as they face terminal illness.

RESEARCH ALERT

When hospice care in the United States was established in the 1970s, cancer patients made up the largest percentage of hospice admissions. Today, cancer diagnoses account for less than half of all hospice admissions (37.7%). Currently, less than 25% of U.S. deaths are now caused by cancer, with the majority of deaths due to other terminal diseases. The top four noncancer primary diagnoses for patients admitted to hospice in 2011 were debility unspecified (13.9%), dementia (12.5%), heart disease (11.4%), and lung disease (8.5%).

Source: National Hospice and Palliative Care Organization. (2012). NHPCO Facts and Figures: Hospice Care in America. Retrieved from http://www.nhpco.org/sites/default/files/public/Statistics_Research/2012_Facts_Figures.pdf

The Future of Health Care in the Home

As the home health industry continues to evolve, the homecare nurse will require advanced clinical skills in community health nursing and an understanding of data management and information technology systems. Knowledge of case management concepts to reach positive clinical and financial outcomes by using resources more effectively will be required. Case managers within home care will have clinical nursing expertise and a sense of measuring nursing impact on specific patient populations, such as individuals with heart disease or cancer. These case managers will be increasingly required in home health nursing practice to possess problem-solving and decision-making skills that require negotiation and a strong sense of patient collaboration. Principles of managed care and practicing in coalitions are important skills for all healthcare workers, but especially for those who work in the home health field.

The opportunities for professional growth in home care nursing are endless. The quest to provide patients and their caregivers with the best of home care continues to be a challenge given the myriad changes in health care today. Growth in information systems and advances in decision-making technology are offering business solutions to home health care. These advances enhance the practice of homecare nursing by offering additional resources to manage patient care to achieve quantifiable positive health outcomes (Hartung, 2005; Hawks, 2012).

Advanced practice nurses and nurse specialists will become required roles on the interdisciplinary team that offer direction, education, and support (Hartung, 2005; Rice, 2005). As advanced practice nurses assume service privileges in acute care facilities, it is expected that they will eventually demand the ability to discharge patients to home health. Home health nurses not only will be increasingly accountable for patient outcomes but will also be called on to use business skills, such as cost–benefit analysis, to objectively support the total cost of care. The planning for care based on expected outcomes and participating in policy-making decisions that involve nursing practice will be an expectation of all staff home health nurses (Blaha, 1997; Boxer & Meadows, 2008; Duke & Street, 2003).

> One's suffering disappears when one lets oneself go, when one yields—even to sadness.
>
> —*Antoine de Saint-Exupery*

> Who looks outside, dreams.
>
> Who looks inside, awakens.
>
> —*Carl Jung*

BOX 36-10 Thoughts on Being a Home Health Nurse—from the Field

- "Probably the best part of the job is being on your own and being able to spend quality time with patients who really believe you can help them."
- "There have been so many good memories and experiences—all of my patients are very special, they are like family. I really get to know them, their families, their fears, and their dreams. Home health is very rewarding."
- "After working for many years in intensive care, I had grown weary of less and less time getting to know my patients as I was getting better and better at managing the machines that really cared for them. In home health, each day I am doing exactly what I went into nursing for—helping people feel better, using the skills I have worked so hard to develop."
- "One of the more memorable home visits was the time the patient's pigs got out of the pen and the physical therapist and I had to chase the pigs before we could attend to the patient's needs."

Conclusion

In a managed care environment where the most efficient and effective delivery setting is chosen, nurses will find the home setting a likely practice environment. Community health nursing will continue to include the home as a viable and attractive setting for practice in sickness and in health, especially with the passage of the ACA. See **Box 36-10** for some nurses' thoughts about being home health nurses.

RESEARCH ALERT 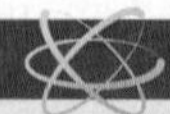

This study reported that hospice care may prolong the lives of some terminally ill patients. Among the patient populations studied, the mean survival was 29 days longer for hospice patients than for nonhospice patients. In other words, patients who chose hospice care lived an average of 1 month longer than similar patients who did not choose hospice care. Researchers selected 4,493 terminally ill patients with either congestive heart failure (CHF) or cancer of the breast, colon, lung, pancreas, or prostate. They then analyzed the difference in survival periods between those who received hospice care and those who did not. Longer lengths of survival were found in four of the six disease categories studied. The largest difference in survival between the hospice and nonhospice cohorts was observed in CHF patients where the mean survival period jumped from 321 days to 402 days. The mean survival period was also significantly longer for the hospice patients with lung cancer (39 days) and pancreatic cancer (21 days), while marginally significant for colon cancer (33 days).

Source: Connor, S. R., Pyenson, B., Fitch, K., Spence, C., & Iwasaki, K. (2007). Comparing hospice and nonhospice patient survival among patients who die within a three-year window. *Journal of Pain Symptom Management, 33*(3), 238–246.

AFFORDABLE CARE ACT

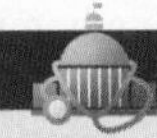

The ACA provides funding to states, tribes, and territories to develop and implement one or more evidence-based maternal, infant, and early childhood visitation model(s).

HEALTHY ME

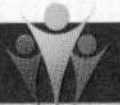

Have you ever given thought to where you would prefer to be cared for during illness or injury? Why might you choose a hospital over your own home, assuming all services could be provided equally? What are the challenges of being cared for in the home versus those in the hospital and vice versa?

LEVELS OF PREVENTION

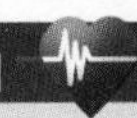

Primary: Making a home visit to a first-time new mother with a healthy newborn to assist with the challenges of a new baby and provide education concerning raising a healthy newborn

Secondary: Making a home visit to a child who has been discharged from the hospital after a fractured arm suffered during a soccer game

Tertiary: Following up care for a teenaged male who has been hospitalized due to unmanaged chronic asthma

Critical Thinking Activities

1. Home health care is one of the fastest growing nursing roles in health care today. Managed care has created incentives for hospitals to limit acute-care episodes and patient admissions. Patients continue to be discharged earlier than ever after surgery, childbirth, and acute episodes of chronic diseases. More and more "high-tech" health care can be replicated in the home, such as chemotherapy, intravenous therapy, and assisted ventilation. Given that this trend is likely to continue as all health agencies struggle to contain costs, consider the following opinions about home health nursing. Respond to each statement and document your agreement or disagreement with the opinion.
   - Home health nursing is more accurately described as "hospital care at home."
   - Home health nursing is a new, emerging specialty in preventive acute care and is not really a community health role or a hospital role.
   - Home health nurses are generalists who can provide health-promotion services to well patients, such as newly discharged mothers and babies, as well as newly discharged post–heart transplant patients with complex intravenous immunosuppressive drug therapy.

References

Acorn, M. (2008). In-home palliative care increased patient satisfaction and reduced use and costs of medical services. *Evidence-Based Nursing, 11*(1), 22.

Affordable Care Act is still the law. (2012). *American Nurse, 44*(4), 1–13.

American Academy of Nursing (AAN). (2010). *Implementing health care reform: Issues for nursing*. Washington, DC: Author.

Blaha, A. (1997). The current and future national voice for home healthcare nursing. *Home Healthcare Nurse, 15*(12), 873.

Boxer, M., & Meadows, B. (2008). Improving care transition from hospital to home health care through collaboration: The referral process between hospital and home health agency. *Remington Report, 16*(2), 32–34.

Bradley, P. J. (1996). Home healthcare nurses should regain their family focus. *Home Healthcare Nurse, 14*(4), 281–288.

Bradley, P. J. (2003). Family caregiver assessment: Essential for effective home health care. *Journal of Gerontological Nursing, 29*(2), 29–36.

Brant, J. (1998). The art of palliative care: Living with hope, dying with dignity. *Oncology Nursing Forum, 25*(6), 995–1004.

Brännström, M., Brulin, C., Norberg, A., Boman, K., & Strandberg, G. (2005). Being a palliative nurse for persons with severe congestive heart failure in advanced home care. *European Journal of Cardiovascular Nursing, 4*, 314–323.

Brennan, A. M. (2012). The paradigm shift. *Nursing Clinics of North America, 47*(4), 455–462.

Brooks, S. (1997). Of hope and hospice. *Contemporary Longterm Care, 20*(7), 56–61.

Buerhaus, P. I., DesRoches, C., Applebaum, S., Hess, R., Norman, L. D., & Donelan, K. (2012). Are nurses ready for health care reform? A decade of survey research. *Nursing Economic$, 30*(6), 318–330.

Bull, M. J. (1990). Factors influencing family caregiver burden and health. *Western Journal of Nursing Research, 12*, 758–776.

Centers for Medicare & Medicaid Services (CMS). (2007). Home health prospective payment system refinement and rate update for calendar year 2008: Final rule. *Federal Register, 72*(167), 49762–49810.

Centers for Medicare & Medicaid Services (CMS). (2008). *Medicare announces new proposed rule to improve hospice care.* Baltimore, MD: Author.

Centers for Medicare & Medicaid Services (CMS). (2012). *Outcomes and Assessment Information Set (OASIS).* Retrieved from http://www.cms.hhs.gov/oasis

Cho, S. (2005). Older people's willingness to use home care nursing services. *Journal of Advanced Nursing, 51*(2), 166–173.

Clarke, P., & Cody, W. (1994). Nursing theory-based practice in the home and community: The crux of professional nursing education. *Advances in Nursing Science, 17*, 41–53.

Cochran, M., & Brennan, S. (1998). Home healthcare nursing in the managed care environment: Part I. *Home Healthcare Nurse, 16*(4), 214–219.

Congdon, J., & Magilvy, J. (1998). Home health care: Supporting vitality for rural elders. *Journal of Long Term Home Health Care, 17*(4), 9–17.

Curtin, M. (2008). News from CCMC. Home health care: An integral part of the continuum. *Care Management, 14*(1), 6.

Davitt, J., & Choi, S. (2008). Tracing the history of Medicare home health care: The impact of policy on benefit use. *Journal of Sociology & Social Welfare, 35*(1), 247–276.

Doolittle, G., Whitten, P., McCartney, M., Cook, D., & Nazir, N. (2005). An empirical chart analysis of the suitability of telemedicine for hospice visits. *Telemedicine Journal & E-Health, 11*(1), 90–97.

Dougherty, G. (1998). When should a child be in the hospital? A. Frederick North, Jr, M.D. Revisited. *Pediatrics, 101*(1), 19–25.

Duke, M., & Street, A. (2003). Hospital in the home: Constructions of the nursing role—A literature review. *Journal of Clinical Nursing, 12*, 852–859.

Ekman Ladd, R., Pasquerella, I., & Smith, S. (2008). What to do when the end is near: Ethical issues in home health care nursing. *Public Health Nursing, 17*, 103–110.

Forcina Hill, J. (2008). Factors associated with hospice use after referral. *Journal of Hospice & Palliative Nursing, 10*(4), 240–252.

Franz, A. (1997). Prognosis: Home care nursing. *Home Healthcare Nurse, 15*(12), 876–877.

Goldstein, N., Concator, J., Fried, T., Kasl, S., Johnson-Hurzeler, R., & Bradley, F. (2004). Factors associated with caregiver burden among caregivers of terminally ill patients with cancer. *Palliative Care, 20*(1), 38–43.

Gremmen, I. (1999). Visiting nurses' situated ethics: Beyond "care versus justice". *Nursing Ethics, 6*, 515–527.

Hartung, S. (2005). Choosing home health as a specialty and successfully transitioning into practice. *Home Health Care Management and Practice, 17*(5), 370–387.

Hawks, J. (2012). The Affordable Care Act: Emphasis on population health. *Urologic Nursing, 32*(5), 233–234.

Hospice Foundation of America. (2008). What is hospice? Retrieved from http://hospicefoundation.org

Hunt, M. (1991). Being friendly and informal: Reflected in nurses' terminally ill patients' and relatives' conversations at home. *Journal of Advanced Nursing, 16*, 929–938.

Jerant, A. (1999). Home telemedicine: Merging the old and new ways. *American Family Physician, 60*(4), 1096–1098.

Jerant, A. F., Schlachta, L., Epperly, T. D., & Barnes-Camp, J. (1998). Back to the future: The telemedicine house call. *Family Practice Management, 5*, 18–22, 25–26, 28.

Kenyon, V., Smith, E., Hefty, L. V., Bell, M. L., McNeil, J., & Maraus, T. (1990). Clinical competencies for public health nursing. *Public Health Nursing, 7*, 33–39.

Kiecolt-Glaser, J. K., Glaser, R., Shuttleworth, E. C., Dyer, C. S., Ogrocki, B. S., & Speicher, C. E. (1987). Chronic stress and immunity in family care givers of Alzheimer's disease victims. *Psychosomatic Medicine, 49*, 523–535.

Kincade, K. (1997). Growing home-care business benefits from telemedicine TLC. *Telemedicine*, p. 4.

Kübler-Ross, E. (1969). *On death and dying: What the dying have to teach doctors, nurses, clergy and their own families.* New York, NY: Macmillan.

Kübler-Ross, E. (1975). *Death: The final stage of growth.* New York, NY: Simon & Schuster.

Levine, C. (1999). Home sweet hospital: The nature and limits of private responsibilities for home health care. *Journal of Aging and Health Care, 11*(2), 341–360.

Liaschenko, J. (1997). Ethics and the geography of the nurse-patient relationship: Spatial vulnerabilities and gendered space. *Scholarly Inquiry Nursing Practice, 11*, 45–49.

Lin, W., Kane, R. L., Mehr, D. R., Madsen, R. W., & Petroski, G. F. (2006). Changes in the use of postacute care during the initial Medicare payment reforms. *Health Services Research, 41*(4), 1338–1356.

Lind, L., Karlsson, D., & Fridlund, B. (2007). Digital pens and pain diaries in palliative home health care: Professional caregivers' experiences. *Medical Informatics & the Internet in Medicine, 32*(4), 287–296.

Lovejoy, D. (1997). *Making the transition to home health nursing.* New York, NY: Springer.

Maraldo, P. (1989). Home care should be the heart of a nursing sponsored national health plan. *Nursing and Health Care, 10*(6), 301–306.

McKnight, R. (2006). Home care reimbursement, long-term utilization, and health outcomes. *Journal of Public Economics, 90*(1), 293–323.

Milone-Nuzzo, P. (1998). Beyond venipuncture as the qualifying service for Medicare: Seeing the forest for the trees. *Home Healthcare Nurse, 16*(3), 177–183.

Milton, C. L. (2005). The metaphor of nurse as guest with ethical implications for nursing and healthcare. *Nursing Science Quarterly, 18*, 301–303.

Monsen, K., Fitzsimmons, L., Lescenski, B., Lytton, A., Schwichtenberg, L., & Martin, K. (2006). A public health nursing informatics date-and-practice quality project. *CIN: Computers, Informatics, Nursing, 24*(3), 152–158.

National Association for Home Care & Hospice (NAHC). (2008). *Basic statistics about home care*. Washington, DC: Author.

National Association for Home Care & Hospice (NAHC). (2014). Rights as a patient. Retrieved from http://www.nahc.org/what-are-my-rights-as-a-patient/

National Institute on Disability and Rehabilitation Research and Training Center. (1996). *U.S. Department of Education disability statistics abstract* (Number 17). San Francisco, CA: University of California, San Francisco.

National Quality Forum (NQF). (2009). *National Voluntary Consensus Standards for Home Health Care—Additional Performance Measures 2008: A Consensus Report*. Washington, DC: NQF. Retrieved from http://www.qualityforum.org/Publications/2010/10/National_Voluntary_Consensus_Standards_for_Home_Health_Care_%E2%80%94_Additional_Performance_Measures_2008.aspx

Neal, L. (1997). Current clinical practice of home care nursing. *Home Healthcare Nurse, 15*(12), 881–882.

Oleske, J., & Czarniecki, L. (1999). Continuum of palliative care: Lessons from caring for children infected with HIV-1. *Lancet, 354*(9186), 1287–1291.

Pare, G., Sicotte, C., St. Jules, D., & Gauthier, R. (2006). Cost minimization analysis of a telehome care program for patients with chronic obstructive pulmonary disease. *Telemedicine Journal and e-health, 12*(2), 114–121.

Peters, D., & Eigsti, D. (1991). Utilizing outcomes in home care. *Caring, 10*, 44–51.

Pevey, C. (2008). Death, God, flesh, and other: Hospice recipients reflect on what matters. *Illness, Crisis & Loss, 16*(3), 203–226.

The President's Advisory Commission on Consumer Protection and Quality in the Health Care Industry. (1998). *Quality first: Better health care for all Americans*. Washington, DC: U.S. Government Printing Office.

Pruchno, R. A., & Potashnik, S. L. (1989). Caregiving spouses: Physical and mental health in perspective. *Journal of the American Geriatric Society, 37*, 697–705.

Reese, D., & Brown, D. (1997). Psychosocial and spiritual care in hospice: Differences between nursing, social work, and clergy. *Hospice Journal, 12*(1), 29.

Rice, R. (1996). *Home health nursing: Concepts and application* (2nd ed.). St. Louis , MO: Mosby.

Rice, R. (2005). *Home care nursing practice: Concepts and application*. St. Louis, MO: Mosby.

Running, A., Tolle, L., & Girard, D. (2008). Ritual: The final expression of care. *International Journal of Nursing Practice, 14*(4), 303–307.

Schneider, J., Barkauskas, V., & Keenan, G. (2008). Evaluating home health care nursing outcomes with OASIS and NOC. *Journal of Nursing Scholarship, 40*(1), 76–82.

Seibert, P., Whitmore, T., Patterson, C., Parker, P., Otto, C., Basom, J., . . . Zimmerman, C. G. (2008). Telemedicine facilitates CHF home health care for those with systolic dysfunction. *International Journal of Telemedicine and Applications, Article ID 235031*, 7 pages.

Shamansky, S. (1988, June). Providing home care services in a for-profit environment. *Nursing Clinics of North America, 23*(2), 387–398.

Shaughnessy, P. W. (June 14, 1996). Using outcomes to build a continuous quality improvement program for home care. Presented at the 11th National Nursing Symposium on Home Health Care, University of Michigan School of Nursing, Ann Arbor, MI.

Sheldon, P., & Bender, M. (1994). High-technology in home care. *Nursing Clinics of North America, 29*(3), 508–519.

Shick, R., & Balinsky, W. (2006). Home health care services: Management and effectiveness in changing times. *Journal of Health and Human Services Administration, 28*(3), 423–462.

Sorrell, J. (2012). Ethics: The Patient Protection and Affordable Care Act: Ethical perspectives in 21st century health care. *OJIN: The Online Journal of Issues in Nursing, 18*(1). doi: 10.3912/OJIN.Vol18No02EthCol01

Spector, W. D., Cohen, J. W., & Pesis-Katz, I. (2004). Home care before and after the Balanced Budget Act of 1997: Shifts in financing and services. *The Gerontologist, 44*(4), 39–47.

Tilden, V., Tolle, S., Drach, L., & Perrin, N. (2004). Out-of-hospital death: Advance care planning, decedent symptoms, and caregiver burden. *American Geriatric Society, 52*, 532–559.

Ward-Griffin, C., & McKeever, P. (2000). Relationships between nurses and family caregivers: Partners in care? *Advances in Nursing Science, 22*(3), 89–103.

Waters, R. (2007). Technology. Measuring quality: An important tool in ensuring top notch home health care. *Caring, 26*(8), 54.

Weeber, S. (2007). Home health care after Hurricanes Katrina and Rita: A report from the field. *Home Health Care Management & Practice, 19*(2), 104–111.

Wilson, S. (1993). Hospice and Medicare benefits: Overview, issues, and implications. *Journal of Holistic Nursing, 11*(4), 356–368.

Zelwesky, M. G., & Deitrick, E. P. (1987). Rx for caregivers: Respite care. *Journal of Community Health Nursing, 4*, 77–84.

CHAPTER FOCUS

History of School Health Nursing
- Origins
- Evolution of School Nursing
- Federal Mandates in School Health

The Education System and the School Nurse

Education and Credentials of the School Nurse
- Continuing Professional Education of the School Nurse

Role Definition of the School Nurse
- Provider of Health Care
- Communicator
- Planner and Coordinator of Student Health Care
- Teacher
- Investigator
- Role Within the Profession

Healthy People 2020
- At-Risk Populations
- Nurse as Team Member

School Health Nursing Practice
- Health-Related Services
- Case Finding
- Practice Issues in School Health

Legal Issues in School Nursing
- Documentation
- Supervision and Accountability
- Funding Issues in School Health
- Delegation

Community Issues in School Health
- School–Health Linkages
- Collaboration
- Resources

Innovations
- School-Based Clinics and Primary Health Care
- Increased Role of the Media in School Health
- Technology

QUESTIONS TO CONSIDER

After reading this chapter, you will know the answers to the following questions:

1. What is school nursing?
2. Which services are typically offered as school health services?
3. Who was the first school nurse in the United States?
4. What role did Lillian Wald play in the development of school nursing?
5. What is a school nurse practitioner?
6. What are the major federal programs that relate to school health?
7. What is the relationship between educational goals and school nurse goals?
8. What are educational requirements of the school nurse?
9. Which kinds of health issues do school nurses deal with?
10. Which kinds of roles do school nurses play?
11. What are current practice issues in school nursing?
12. What are community issues related to school health?
13. What is a school-based clinic?

CHAPTER 37

School Health Nursing

Frances Martin and Karen Saucier Lundy

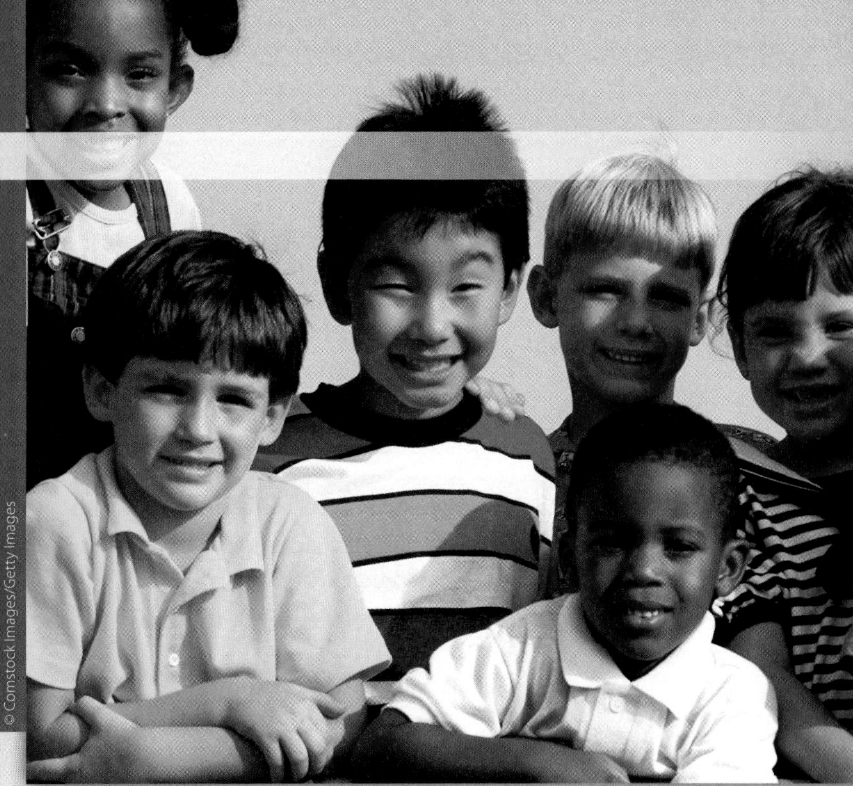

KEY TERMS

delegation
health-related services
inclusion ("mainstreaming")
individualized educational plan (IEP)
individualized family service plan (IFSP)
individualized health plan (IHP)
medically fragile children
school-based clinic
school-based services
school health services
school nursing
unlicensed assistive personnel

REFLECTIONS

All of us have experienced an educational system of some type, even home schooling. How was your school experience? Was elementary school different than high school? Did you experience unhealthy conditions in your school that threatened your safety or health? Did you develop health habits during your high school years that still influence you as a nursing student?

Do you see college health as a school health setting? Why or why not?

NOTE THIS!

A survey of 1,546 school districts with an identifiable school health program showed that in only 60% of these was "nursing" listed as the major field of the person in charge of school nursing.

EFFECTIVE SCHOOL NURSES are "bilingual"; they speak "education" and "health" (Costante, 1996). **School nursing** is a specialized practice of professional nursing that advances the wellbeing, academic success and lifelong achievement, and health of students. To that end, school nurses facilitate positive student responses to normal development; promote health and safety including a healthy environment; intervene with actual and potential health problems; provide case management services; and actively collaborate with others to build student and family capacity for adaptation, self-management, self advocacy, and learning (National Association of School Nurses [NASN], 2010).

Since 1975, Congress has required that students with disabilities receive an education in the "least restrictive environment." Data since 1988 suggest that U.S. schools have found regular education classrooms to be the "least restrictive environment" for increasing numbers of students with disabilities. In the 2010–2011 school year, 95% of students 6–21 years old with disabilities were served in regular schools (U.S. Department of Education, 2013). Depending on the nature of the disability, students may spend some (40% or less) or most (80% or more) of their time in special education classrooms with teachers and staff trained to manage the child's specific needs. Notably, the children categorized as having orthopedic impairments or "other health impairments"—including chronic illnesses such as heart conditions, tuberculosis, rheumatic fever, nephritis, asthma, sickle cell anemia, hemophilia, epilepsy, lead poisoning, leukemia, or diabetes—generally spend a significant amount of time outside general class despite the fact that their disease conditions do not inherently impair their ability to learn, as is the case with most of the other categories.

Schools by themselves cannot, and should not be expected to, address the nation's most serious health and social problems. Families, healthcare workers, the media, religious organizations, community organizations that serve youth, and young people themselves also must be systematically involved (Schwartz & Laughlin, 2008). There is a natural relationship between schools and child health care (Concepcion, Murphy, & Canham, 2007). Since 1992, the Centers for Disease Control and Prevention (CDC) has provided funding for Coordinated School Health Programs (CSHPs) as a means for reducing chronic disease risk factors. The CDC (2014) supported CSHPs in 22 states and one tribal government in 2013.

Today's children are different in many ways from those of the last generation. There are children today who may have been exposed in utero to cocaine and opiates; studies are under way to evaluate these effects (Messinger et al., 2004). Almost all children entering school will have had experience with a computer. A 2001 study of participants in a Head Start program with 122 preschool children enrolled in a rural county showed that 53% had a computer at home; more than a decade later, the U.S. Census Bureau (2012) provides statistics that 82% of children 3 years of age and older have Internet access in the home. The expansion of cellular telephone networks and especially the wide availability of Internet-ready smart phones has helped to increase access of even lower income families to the Internet; moreover, the vast majority of public school systems have incorporated technology into their teaching resources (Gray & Lewis, 2009). Children who have access to a computer perform better on measures of school readiness and cognitive development, controlling for children's developmental stage and family socioeconomic status (Li & Atkins, 2004).

Terrorism and war worries have become a part of our society (Laraque et al., 2004). Television coverage of news from war zones, for example, has created a climate of anxiety new to this country (van der Molen, 2004). How can school nurses make a difference for children growing up with these problems today? There is a short-term answer, and there is a long-term answer. In the short term, school nurses will need to grasp the impact that values and certain relevant societal problems have on education's goals. The school nurse shows evidence of understanding these issues by promoting physical, mental, and environmental health in the school. In this way, children may obtain and maintain appropriate learning experiences.

In the long term, there is a need to emphasize prevention of chronic diseases while the child is still in childhood. Among adults older than 25 years, 62.9% of all deaths result from two causes: cardiovascular disease and cancer (CDC, 2008). The majority of risk behaviors associated with these two causes of death are initiated during adolescence. Research has shown that chronic disease is often the outcome of modifiable lifestyle choices.

In the United States, more than 6 million adults work in school-related activities. The school setting is the workplace for more than 20% of the U.S. population (children and adults). Fifty-three million young people attend 129,000 public and private schools for about 6 hours of classroom time each day, for as many as 13 of the most formative years of their lives (Snyder & Hoffman, 2002).

APPLICATION TO PRACTICE

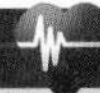

A Day in the Life of a School Nurse

Pleasantville Elementary School, early September: The school nurse, Ms. Davis, RN, plans to do the 1st-grade vision screening today, but first she will see the children who are waiting outside her clinic office door. First in line is Jason. Jason's mother wants him to be "checked out for chickenpox." Jason's cousin, Tommy, a 2nd-grader, now has chickenpox.

The school secretary knocks on the door. She has Mrs. Perez, who is visibly upset, and her three children with her. "We have a problem," says the secretary. "These children, ages 8, 6, and 5 years old, have not had any shots since their birth in Mexico. School policy will not allow me to register them. I told the mother that you could help them."

In the hallway sits 8-year-old Shelly Strong. Mr. Bullen, her teacher, is concerned because Shelly says she has asthma and needs a "breathing treatment." This is Mr. Bullen's first year to teach school. He is not sure what Shelly is talking about and says that he never has seen a breathing machine like the one Shelly brought to school in her backpack today.

Out in the hall, 9-year-old Steven (who is taking Ritalin for ADHD) and Hiram (who has a physical disability and uses crutches) are yelling and shoving each other. Both 9-year-olds have a history of poor anger control. Mr. Bullen assists Ms. Davis in breaking up the fist fight. Their teacher, Mrs. Adams, has become very frustrated with their behavior.

Ms. Davis seems to be in control of the situation. She has learned to be flexible with her schedule and to prioritize her nursing duties. Ms. Davis assesses Shelly's respiratory condition. Shelly has the signed papers from her mother and the physician giving permission for the inhalation treatment. The school nurse documents her condition and begins Shelly's treatment. She also records the time of treatment and the amount of albuterol as prescribed by her physician. She calls Mrs. Strong, Shelly's mother, at work and sets up an appointment for that afternoon to discuss Shelly's emergency care plan for future asthma attacks. Ms. Davis informs Mr. Bullen of the meeting and requests his presence. She makes a note to schedule a staff in-service on asthma: its signs, symptoms, medications, and treatments.

Ms. Davis assesses Jason for chickenpox and finds him presently free of eruptions. She sends him back to class with an excuse, then records the office visit in a nurse's note for the day. She schedules herself to check Jason in 1 week, because he has been exposed to herpes zoster and has not had chickenpox.

Ms. Davis has not forgotten about the Perez family. She discusses the immunization schedule with the mother. She teaches her about the diseases covered by the immunizations, reviews their medical records and a brief medical history for each child, and then prepares the correct immunizations for each one. Ms. Davis administers the immunizations and discusses possible side effects with the mother. Ms. Davis gives the mother and the school secretary the proper paperwork for the children to be registered in school that day.

Mrs. Perez speaks mostly Spanish. Ms. Davis has been taking Spanish night classes at a local college to communicate with the growing Spanish population in her area. Mrs. Perez requests information on applying for Medicaid. Ms. Davis sets up an appointment with the Medicaid office for Mrs. Perez to discuss this and draws a map for the mother. Ms. Davis asks if she can visit with her and the children at home to assess for other needs. The mother agrees.

Shelly's treatment has been completed. Ms. Davis assesses her respiratory condition and allows her to return to Mr. Bullen's class. Ms. Davis then schedules an appointment with Mrs. Adams (Steven's and Hiram's teacher). She wants to share some resource materials on behavior management that are now available. Also, she wants to discuss Steven's medication dosage and classroom behavior. Ms. Davis then makes a referral to the school psychologist regarding the repeat incident between the two boys. She schedules time on her calendar for classroom education regarding children with disabilities in grades K–6. By 10:00 a.m. she is ready to begin calling on her first class for vision screening.

More than 95% of youth ages 5 to 17 years are enrolled in school. Many of these children come to school with learning disabilities. The high school completion rate has remained relatively steady, growing to 72.5% in 2001 (National Center for Education Statistics [NCES], 2003) and then increasing substantially to 78.2% in 2009–2010 (NCES, 2013), the highest rate since 77.1% being attained in 1968–1969.

High-risk behaviors can lead to substantial morbidity and social problems among young people in the 9th to 12th grades. Over the past two decades, the percentage of children and adolescents who are overweight has doubled. The increase in type 2 diabetes may be one of the first consequences of this epidemic of obesity among young people. Statistics and trends show that "a choice is at hand: invest now in children's physical and emotional health to create tomorrow's healthy citizens, or pay ten-fold down the road" (National Council of State Boards of Nursing [NCSBN], 1990).

There have been encouraging statistics showing improvement in certain health indicators. The percentage of children immunized before the age of 3 was up from 67% in 1999 to 77% in 2006 (Federal Interagency Forum on Child and Family Statistics, 2008). Data from 2001 showed that the average percentage of children younger than age 18 years who were below poverty in urban areas was 15.8%, down from 21% in 1994. The percentage range differed by geographic area (The Annie E. Casey Foundation, 2008).

Mental health needs continue to require more attention than there are resources to meet them. The school nurse may become involved when a teacher suspects child abuse or neglect. For calendar year 2002, an estimated 1.8 million referrals alleging child abuse or neglect were accepted by state and local child protective services (CPS) agencies for investigation or assessment. The referrals included more than 3 million children; of those children, approximately 896,000 were victims of child abuse or neglect, with neglect being present in 60% of the cases reported. In 2002, there were 1,400 fatalities (Child Welfare Information Gateway, 2008).

Abuse and other mental health challenges involve more than just the child; they involve families, too. Home visits are the best strategy for assessing the child's living conditions more accurately.

The National Longitudinal Study of Adolescent Health (NLSAH—a congressionally mandated study of 90,000 teenagers across the United States) highlighted the importance of a child feeling "connected" to the school for greater success (Resnick et al., 1997). Continued data collection by Blum (2004) has contradicted the widely held assumptions of the predictive value of race, income, and family structure on an adolescent's choice of participating in unhealthy behaviors: "Failure in school, too much unstructured time, and poor family relationships were shown to be three to eight times more likely to predict the kinds of risk behaviors studied" (Resnick et al., 1997).

Immigration numbers have increased in the United States. Unlike previous immigrants, who often came from countries where education was valued, immigrant children today tend to come from countries where survival has taken precedence over education. The language barriers they experience have implications for health access, learning, and socialization. The percentage of children who are linguistically isolated ranged from 23.1% in Texas to 7% in Colorado (The Annie E. Casey Foundation, 2008). Members of this group are also at risk for poor physical and mental health, as well as challenges to their learning ability.

Many children currently in schools do not constitute an at-risk population but still can be healthier with school nurse interventions. Rates of "lifestyle-related" diseases such as diabetes, hypertension, obesity, cardiovascular disease, and cancer have risen dramatically, even among children. School nurses are in a strategic position to help address these issues. Currently, however, only limited school resources have been devoted to prioritized areas, such as meeting the needs of medically fragile students with severe asthma, diabetes, behavioral problems requiring medications, seizures, and human immunodeficiency virus (HIV)/acquired immune deficiency syndrome (AIDS), as well as students dependent on medical devices for life and health (Schwartz & Laughlin, 2008).

CULTURAL CONNECTION

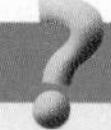

The Columbine High School shootings apparently resulted from a complex series of events where the two shooters had experienced perceived harassment (according to their online journals). How can school nurses mediate and introduce positive primary health intervention strategies to reduce harassment in an increasingly more diverse school population?

ENVIRONMENTAL CONNECTION

How do the cultural and physical environments of a school affect both health and learning? Compare an urban high school to a rural high school.

Nurses provide a variety of health services at schools. These services include assessing, promoting, and maintaining the health of staff and students. One school nurse, for example, arranged for her three schools to have a contest among staff and teachers at each school. Each school worked from January to May, striving to have the lowest cholesterol levels, the most normal blood pressures, the greatest numbers of average body mass index (BMI), and the most normal glucose levels. Health problems identified through this contest required referral to primary healthcare providers in the community. Health promotion in school staff has improved productivity, decreased absenteeism, and reduced health insurance costs (Schwartz & Laughlin, 2008).

Prevention and control of communicable diseases, management of chronic medical conditions, and emergency care for illness or injury can be well managed by school nurses. School health services that include mental, emotional, and social components contribute not only to the wellbeing of the individual student, but also to the school environment. School nurses are in a key position to foster better health, thereby handling concerns about promoting safe and sanitary school environments. The health curriculum also provides educational opportunities. Counseling needs are many and varied, and at times may require family involvement. If a school-based clinic (SBC) is available, follow up may be expedited.

Initially, school health services had limited meaning for many educational administrators; they viewed the scope of school health as compliance with regulatory laws regarding immunizations, and monitoring health screening results. Boyer (1991), and many others since, have supported the findings that a direct link exists between health and academic performance.

The Secretaries of the U.S. Department of Education and the U.S. Department of Health and Human Services (HHS) formally recognized the importance of school health to a community's health in a joint statement supporting comprehensive school health programs. School nurses, therefore, work under two entities: education and health; school nurses provide services in these two worlds. The joint document issued by these agencies supported school-based centers as a means of facilitating access to health care.

School health services may consist of basic health, expanded health, or comprehensive health services. School nurses provide episodic or emergency care, monitor health status through screenings, identify health problems that adversely affect students' progress, administer medications, and assist students with medical devices such as tracheostomies, urinary catheters, and orthopedic devices (Passarelli, 1996). They supervise medical care that has been delegated to nonprofessionals, develop programs and evaluate outcomes, and monitor family outreach as part of their expected practice. In addition, school nurses often participate in health education to staff and students. In 1998, Congress encouraged the CDC to promote CSHPs.

BOX 37-1 Selected Federal Mandates Related to School Health

1973	Section 504, Rehabilitation Act
1975	Education for all Handicapped Children Act (PL 94-142)
1978	Health Education Act (PL 95-561)
1979	Office of Comprehensive School Health
1988	Office of School Health (Health, Education, and Welfare)
1990	Birth to Twenty-One legislation (PL 99-457)
1991	IDEA (Individuals with Disabilities Education Act)
2001	No Child Left Behind federal mandates
2004	CDC Healthy Schools Initiative
2010	Patient Protection and Affordable Care Act (ACA)

At the local school district level, the principal may choose which health service model to implement. Funding often dictates the extent of services chosen for implementation. According to the Secretary of Education:

> Some schools have been run as centralized, bureaucratic, monopolies with little accountability and few standards of measurement. . . . When budgets are tight, and funds needed elsewhere, many of these schools are fiscally plundered by their state or local politicians. . . . As a result, millions of students have suffered from bureaucratic imprisonment and poorly delivered services. ("Paige," 2004)

History of School Health Nursing

Origins

School nursing grew out of a need identified by a school official in England around 1891. Without immunizations or antibiotics, children were losing school time to "minor ailments and infectious troubles" (Oda, 1981). A lack of parental support for education was pervasive; poorer families often used children as breadwinners or as babysitters for younger siblings. A school official and a nurse were concerned that some children's education was being hampered by absenteeism due to poor health, so the school official asked the nurse to visit the children at home. This was the beginning of school health nursing.

Around the same time (1902) in the United States, Lillian Wald became concerned about the education and general welfare of tenement children in New York. In particular, the health and education status of tenement children excluded from school due to illness or disabilities distressed Wald. At Wald's suggestion, Lina Rogers Struthers, the first school nurse in America, was hired by the Board of Education. Her task was to treat children in the school, if possible, or visit homes to monitor environmental conditions in need of attention (Pollitt, 1994).

Wald worked out of her home, known as the Henry Street Settlement. Wald's lifetime efforts brought nurses into the New York schools. Even though she was a nurse, she addressed social problems such as child labor. She established the first neighborhood playgrounds, centers, youth clubs, vocational classes, and foster homes. With remarkable foresight, Wald was the forerunner of comprehensive school health services: special education classes began with her development of the first ungraded classrooms for "defectives," or children with disabilities.

Evolution of School Nursing

During the first half of the 20th century, school nurses were seen as the people at school who made sure immunizations were up to date, who identified communicable diseases, who did vision and hearing screening, and who helped students in wheelchairs. Lina Rogers Struthers is considered the first school nurse in the United States, serving with Lillian Wald at the Henry Street Settlement in New York City during the early part of the 20th century. Miss Wald placed Lina Rogers Struthers in four NYC schools on October 1, 1902. New York City became the first city in the world to publicly fund school nursing services (Wold, 2001). Often, parents or support staff viewed their role at school as "Band-Aid" nurses, taking care of minor emergencies occurring at school. When mainstreaming began, the school nurse trained the teachers if a child needed medical attention (children with asthma, hearing impairments, or domestic abuse situations).

Drs. Loretta Ford and Henry Silver proposed the vision for the nurse practitioner movement in the early 1960s, in collaboration with nursing and medicine programs at the University of Colorado. A new role, school nurse practitioner, evolved along with the rest of the nurse practitioner movement. An impetus for the school nurse practitioner movement was the obvious need to improve children's access to health care, and to prepare practitioners who could focus on the needs of children and adolescents.

In 1969, the School Nurse Practitioner (SNP) program was first implemented. Under this model, the school nurse practitioner provided primary care in schools. This practice was funded through partnerships with managed care models and third-party reimbursements to SBCs. There was also the possibility of patient-generated revenue at such clinics (Urbinati, Steele, Harter, & Harrell, 1996).

In the 1970s, changes in funding and in public expectations of the government's role in health care reduced school health services to episodic and uncoordinated situational care. Parents and educators disagreed about how to teach sensitive and value-laden materials. To some parents, school health services became synonymous with sex education—a controversial position, to say the least. Schools began to decline as centers for providing primary care to children and the community. As increasing numbers of disabled and technology-dependent children were integrated into regular classrooms, the focus of school nursing changed to one of increased responsibility for training teachers and staff in how to meet the needs of these children. The school nurse provided in-service and one-on-one education for school personnel as needed.

Landmark research conducted during the 1980s by Judith Igoe and colleagues in Colorado (Igoe, 1990, 2002; Igoe & Giordano, 1992) highlighted the great potential for impacting the health and academic experiences of school children when adequately prepared nurses are present in the schools. Their federally funded research addressed issues such as shifting student health needs, volatile societal expectations, unpredictable legislation, and the need for reliable sources of funding. These authors even suggested a new paradigm for delivering services: the **school-based clinic**. Patient outcomes in school nursing were measured in educational terms such as school attendance and test scores, rather than as changes in morbidity. This work gave a broader context for school health nursing, which was now seen as relevant both within and outside the school setting (Gustafson, 2005).

Federal Mandates in School Health

In 1973, Section 504 of the Rehabilitation Act required that schools provide "free and appropriate education" for children with disabilities. Included in Section 504 were mandates for specially designed classroom instruction, and additional services such as specialized transportation. The school nurse became a necessary part of "special education" at schools attended by **medically fragile children** with chronic disorders such as cerebral palsy, seizure disorders, mental retardation, and emotional or behavioral problems.

In 1975, Public Law (PL) 94-142 (the Education for All Handicapped Children Act) broadened the definition of "free and appropriate education" by bringing children with various disabilities into regular classrooms. Called **inclusion** (or **mainstreaming**), this legislation-mandated movement focused on appropriate in-class support to students with various educational risks or disabilities, for the maximum time possible during each school day. The nurse's role was to train staff and teachers in the care of children with spina bifida, asthma, attention deficit hyperactivity disorder (ADHD), and other medical conditions on an individual basis.

Congress passed the Health Education Act (PL 95-561) in 1978. This act proposed that comprehensive school health services be delivered in the least restrictive environments for handicapped children, in settings outside the home. Subsequent state court cases gave legal weight to allowing severely disabled students to enter public schools in record numbers.

The Office of Comprehensive School Health (OCSH) was established in 1979 to extend school health services to include preschool children (Head Start) and expand coverage to include school nutrition. Two years later, the OCSH was abolished. In 1983, school health services were placed with the U.S. Public Health Service, Department of Maternal–Child Health. Funding was not sufficient to meet the increased demands brought about by funding of school health nursing on that department's budget, so funding for school health services was divided between multiple agencies.

In 1988, Congress authorized the establishment of the Office of School Health in the Department of Education. School health services would no longer be funded from health-related departments. Since 1988, as many as 300 federal agencies related to child health, school health, mental health, and environmental health have taken an interest in school children and adolescents. These agencies include the CDC, the Health Resources and Services Administration (HRSA; within the HHS), the Department of Agriculture, and agencies that focus on physical fitness and environmental issues.

The initial legislation passed in 1975 (PL 94-142) was modified through the passage of the Individuals with Disabilities Act (IDEA) in 1991. This legislation (PL 99-457) mandated school health services for specific conditions, starting from birth and continuing to age 21 years. Thirteen conditions included in the 1991 IDEA legislation were amended to 12, as follows: autism, deaf-blindness, emotional disturbance, hearing impairments, mental retardation, multiple disabilities, orthopedic impairments, other health impairments (chronic diseases such as asthma, epilepsy, or diabetes), specific learning disabilities, speech or language impairments, traumatic brain injury, and visual impairments (NASN, 2004a). However, IDEA is still funded at 17% of full funding (NASN, 2004b).

In 1965, the Elementary and Secondary Education Act (EASA) was enacted to provide guidance and funds to K–12 schools. Since then, Title 1 of EASA has provided trillions of dollars in financial assistance to schools educating low-income students. Half of all public schools in the United States currently receive funds under Title 1.

Funding and coordination of services are major issues for school nurses and other health professionals providing care to school children. The CDC's Healthy Schools Initiative forms the basis for coordination of agencies serving schools. An increasing number of states are availing themselves of CDC funding for these programs (CDC, Division of Adolescent School Health, 2004).

The most sweeping federal education legislative changes in decades were enacted into law in 2001. The No Child Left Behind (NCLB) legislation is the most recent reauthorization of EASA; it addresses all areas of K–12 education. NCLB seeks to address educational equity on the basis of educational *opportunity*, rather than on equalized *funding* for schools.

MEDIA MOMENT 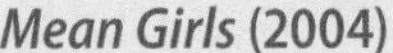

Mean Girls (2004)

This film centers on the daughter of world-trekking zoologists, Cady Heron, who had never known what "high school" truly meant. She lived her first 15 years in the African jungle, home-schooled living life with only her parents and the animals of the wilderness, knowing all of the rules of survival. However, when she moves out of Africa, she had to learn the rules of high school, a jungle in itself. She instantly makes friends with Damian and Janis, who, in the terms of the high school, are in the "out crowd" but are kind and interesting. Soon Cady meets the Plastics, three crude, beautiful, popular girls: Regina, the unofficial leader; Gretchen, Regina's full-time follower; and Karen, "one of the dumbest people you will ever meet." They immediately let Cady into their group, but Cady, wanting to keep her first friends, is unsure about the situation. Damian and Janis convince Cady to keep her relationship with the Plastics, as a sort of social experiment so that they can learn their "dark secrets." However, events become complicated when Cady falls for Regina's ex-boyfriend, Aaron. This leads to members of each group of friends plotting against each other, and as Cady spends more time with the Plastics, she becomes more and more like them. Eventually, a teacher and the school principal decide to intervene in the girls' feud.

Under NCLB, schools must make "annual yearly progress" (AYP) reports as a basis for funding. Without documented progress, distribution of federal monies is adversely affected, or parents are entitled to change their child's school.

This legislation has implications for schools that serve students with disabilities. There is a group of children, referred to as "gap kids" in the past, to whom the term "significant cognitive impairment" is applied. These children might have language barriers, be homeless, have parents in the military and have moved frequently, or have significant disabilities. Despite their unique challenges, the federal mandate of "no child left behind" still applies to this population. Initially, the definition of "significant cognitive impairment" could affect the AYP data on which school funding was based. Waivers are available to schools that provide adequate documentation.

The Education System and the School Nurse

Educators and school administrators measure school success, in large part, by first whether a student successfully completes each school year, and then whether each completes the K–12 curriculum. Costante (1996) claimed, "Health-related activities that affect daily class attendance are perhaps the hallmark of school nursing services" (p. 5). Teachers find that students who are not distracted by unmet health needs in themselves or their classmates are more motivated and attentive in class. Decreased vision or hearing, emotional distress, or adolescent pregnancy, by contrast, can affect the educational experience.

Having qualified nurses in schools has been shown to decrease student absenteeism (Allen, 2003). Absenteeism affects funding; it is, therefore, an important indicator for school administrators. Absenteeism is often an indication of family problems, neglect or abuse, or lack of resources and medical access. These issues might not be addressed without the assistance of a school nurse.

For many years, principals of each school district considered the school nurse as their employee (Zimmerman, Wagoner, & Kelly, 1996). Meeting health service needs in the educational setting poses a dilemma—not because the needs are questioned or the benefits disputed, but rather because the responsibilities and priorities for service are poorly funded.

School administrators have many constituents. They often operate in a more politicized arena than most nurses do, and they know that health issues can be surrounded by conflicting values. Administrators face societal mores that vary greatly within each individual school, in terms of cultural, religious, and even language differences. As one principal stated, "If I make even one parent unhappy, it may cost me my job."

Since "mainstreaming" came to schools in 1975, school resources have been stretched to cover the special health needs of disabled or chronically ill students. Services to just one child with disabilities in Alabama ran as high as $30,000 per year in 1999, compared with $15,000 budgeted per year to educate a nondisabled child. Efforts to cut their budgets have often forced schools to cut nursing positions and replace them with health aides.

ETHICAL CONNECTION 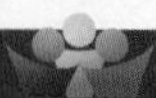

Colleges and universities in the United States are increasingly taking a more cautious approach to students who demonstrate suicidal tendencies and severe depressive symptoms. Faced with the threat of liability suits from parents when students kill themselves on campus, schools are taking more of an aggressive approach with students they believe are a risk to themselves and to the morale and mental health of those around them. With suicide ranking as the number two cause of death for college students (claiming 1,100 lives each year), college mental health officials defend their concerns about how to address the problem.

As the number of students with mental health issues who enter college each year grows, who should bear the responsibility for their safety? Will this trend toward identifying at-risk students affect their likelihood of seeking treatment for depression in student health services if this may eventually lead to their dismissal? How can nurses in school health settings serve as advocates for students while complying with university policies?

A CSHP has eight components. The CSHP is meant to provide a way for schools to become facilities where many agencies can cooperate and address the health needs of school children and staff. The CDC supported CSHPs in 22 states in 2013 (see **Figure 37-1**).

Education and Credentials of the School Nurse

The broad scope of knowledge expected of school nurses requires a minimum of a baccalaureate degree in nursing. Passarelli (1994) proposed that academic institutions design graduate-level and practitioner programs that correspond to the broad scope of school nursing. One NASN strategic goal was "to pursue and advocate for greater access to undergraduate, graduate, and practitioner programs by influencing higher education to provide appropriate professional content to a larger school nursing enrollment" (NASN, 2004a, p. 9). Both the NASN and the American Nurses Association (ANA) take the position that "school nursing requires advanced skills that include the ability to practice independently, supervise others, and delegate care in a community, rather than a hospital or clinic setting" (ANA & NASN, 2011).

In recent years, the family nurse practitioner (FNP) specialty has thrived, while the school nurse practitioner focus has become too restrictive, particularly in light of

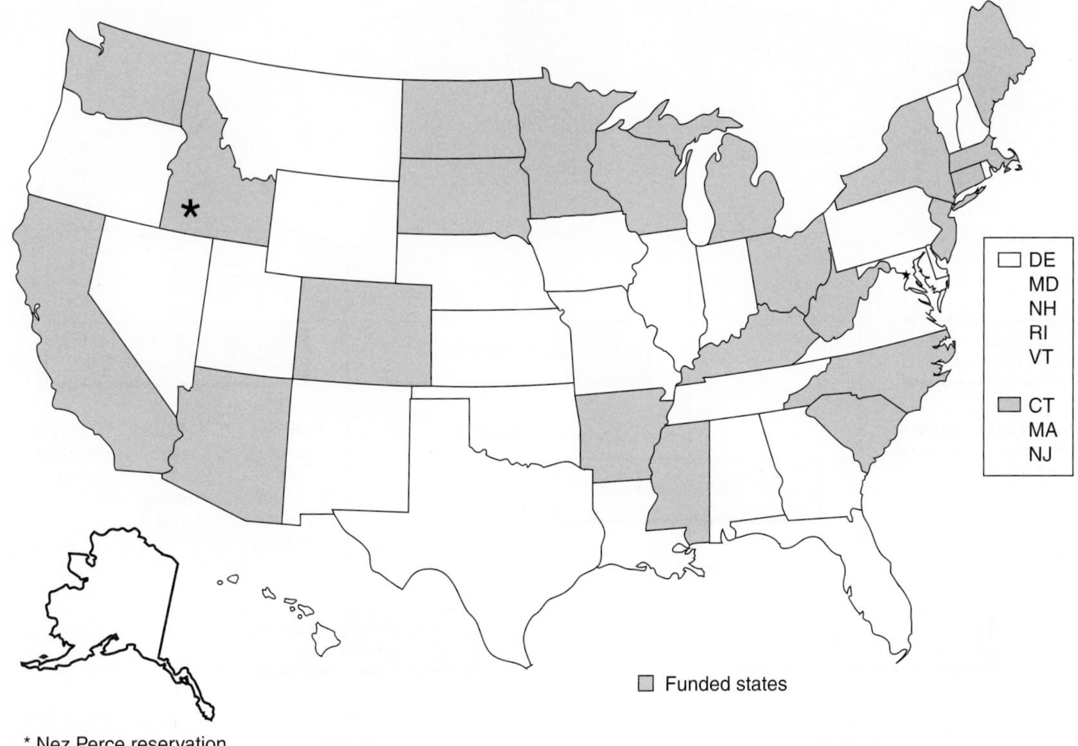

Figure 37-1 CDC Funding for Coordinated School Health Programs, Fiscal Year 2008.

Reproduced from Centers for Disease Control and Prevention (2002). Division of Adolescent School Health. Healthy Youth. At-lanta, GA: CDC. http://www.cdc.gov/HealthyYouth/about/healthyyouth.htm#map

higher education funding issues. FNP programs include content related to child and adolescent health, which makes FNPs educationally prepared to provide appropriate care in the school setting, particularly in SBCs.

Continuing Professional Education of the School Nurse

Continuing professional education is crucial, particularly given that school nurses often practice alone. Updates on clinical skills, pharmacology, and evidence-based research help maintain clinical competence. Topics related to management, supervision, and **delegation** have specific relevance to administrative expectations of the school nurse. The networking and collegiality of continuing professional education meetings may also help prevent the burnout that characterizes the careers of many otherwise motivated nurses.

Increased access to current information via the Internet has provided greater opportunities for school nurses to research a current need or to continue professional education. Nurses may negotiate for the use of staff development days to continue their own professional development. In addition, NASN offers an annual update program for school nurses. Journals addressing child health and illness, mental health, family health, and educational theory have increased in number.

Many school districts continue to require their school nurses to hold a valid school nurse certificate if they are to remain on the teacher's salary schedule. Every state requires that school nurses have an active nursing license to practice. State departments of education generally require school nurse certification as Education Specialists 1. School nurse specialists are educationally prepared to evaluate and care for children at risk and for medically fragile children. School nurses also support the educational goals of health promotion to students, staff, and (sometimes) families.

An increasing number of institutions of higher education are offering courses that meet these requirements for continuing professional education. Generally, school nurse certification requires 12 semester hours of coursework. Course offerings include courses on management of school nurse practice, educational psychology, physical assessment of the school-aged child, and nursing care of the child with developmental disabilities.

Role Definition of the School Nurse

"School nursing is at once the best and least understood form of practice on the part of the lay public and nursing professionals," wrote Oda in 1979. This is still largely

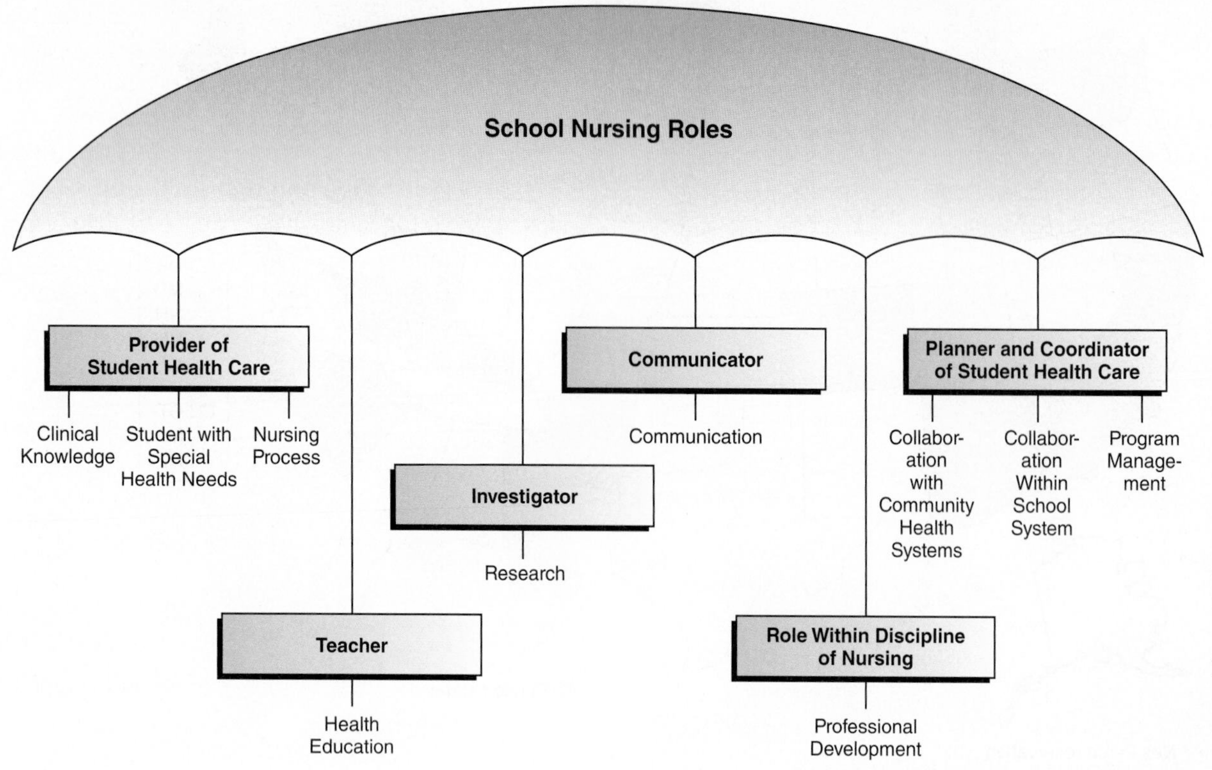

Figure 37-2 School nursing roles.

true. The dual-focused role is ripe for role ambiguity. Igoe (1990) coined the term "boundary-dwellers" to describe school nurses. Frequently school nurses must decide between two competing priorities: health and education. What may be prudent healthwise may be disruptive of education, because screening takes class time.

The school nurse role is often defined for nurses by others, such as school administrators, who do not clearly understand the nursing role (see **Figure 37-2**). The NASN has addressed this role ambiguity through its position statement on the "Education, Licensure and Certification of School Nurses" (NASN, 2012). The position statement can assist school nurses in translating their role to school administrators and others. School health services may consist of basic health, expanded health, or comprehensive health services (**Table 37-1**).

Provider of Health Care

Assessment of healthy children and recognition of the potential for health problems in children and adolescents are main preventive focuses for the school nurse. Minor emergencies and illnesses come up on a daily basis. Technology-dependent or chronically ill children also require competent nursing care. Nursing interventions may range from education and screening, to providing direct care to students with disabilities. Nurses can provide health services for school staff. Educational

TABLE 37-1 Examples of Selected Health Services Provided in Schools

Type of Service
Administration of first aid
Administration of medication
Screens (height/weight, sensory)
Abuse evaluation/follow up
Emotional/behaviors
Monitoring of vital signs
Cleaning/changing of dressings
Health component of IEP
Case management
Nutritional counseling
Mental health counseling
Cardiovascular screenings
Complex nursing to at-risk students
Employee wellness
Fitness screenings
Urinary catheterizations
Health risk appraisals

personnel often have chronic, stable medical conditions. School nurses are concerned for the health of the bus driver and the cafeteria worker as well as the health of teachers and students.

Familiarity with theory can guide decision making by the school nurse. Besides nursing theory, such theories include change theory, developmental theory, management theory, role theory, and systems theory. School nurses, like all other nurses, use the nursing process as the framework for all assessment, diagnosis, planning, intervention, and evaluation activities.

Communicator

The following parent's story illustrates the importance of communication with parents:

> I was adamant that our daughter would have at least one setting where she was treated as a "typical" kid. Because she has spina bifida, we see a lot of specialists. I wanted her child care program to be a place where we could escape the disability focus. So when the program director asked me to sign an information request form so she could get a copy of Karen's records, I refused. I wanted the child care staff to treat Karen just like all the other children.
>
> A few months later, Karen's teacher again asked if I would be willing to share information from the Individualized Family Service Plan (IFSP). She explained that it would help her develop better lesson plans if she knew more about what Karen could do, and the skills we were working on. It was the first time I realized that Karen's special needs could be incorporated into the games and activities that happened in her school day. A little reluctant, I gave my permission.
>
> Now, I wish that at the very beginning, the director had explained why it was important for them to have the IFSP and other information. You can't blame a parent for wanting to protect their child's (and their own) privacy. I remember being offended when asked to release Karen's records, and I am sure other parents feel that way. ("Notes from Home," 1997, p. 7)

Health, welfare, and social services for students are often complex, fragmented, or even unavailable. Good written and verbal communication skills are needed for the school nurse to work efficiently with the learners (students), teachers, parents, and the medical community.

School nurses who can identify problems and recommend solutions in terms that evoke policy responses are desperately needed. To date, this fourth component of school health (policy development) is lagging behind the other three. Communicating the problems and the positive contributions that school nurses make to the school's mission is an important part of nursing activities, often directly affecting funding for school nurse positions.

Student health has been shown to have "peace dividends" (intangible, but real, rewards), but cost containment is a byword of current policy activities. A long-term investment in health makes sense—but immediate needs with potential for quick success may receive greater attention from policymakers. Unless the school nurse's voice is heard loud and clear, policies may not reflect school health as a priority.

Many school nurses provide health education inside and outside the classroom, with individuals, with groups, and with families. Good communication skills help get important messages across to the children, school staff, and the community.

Planner and Coordinator of Student Health Care

Case management is a demanding component of school health services. Children with complex health problems may require home visits and referrals to medical services or resource agencies such as the health department. One individual responsible to coordinate this activity is the school nurse.

The school nurse must be self-motivated, organized, and flexible, while performing multiple activities. Many times, the school nurse is assessing rapidly changing situations, planning with teachers for addressing behavioral and emotional problems, evaluating the student and sometimes the family, or coordinating care with a physician. School nurses must also be ready to deal with unforeseen events (e.g., emergencies) in the midst of everything else.

Monitoring school health through recordkeeping and tracking is a part of coordinating services. The area of sexual health is often an area of discomfort in terms of documentation.

Teacher

School nurses serve as teachers to students, to school staff, to parents, and to community agencies. Staff consultation regarding individual students is a major component of the school nurse activity (Anderson, 1994). Teachers and staff are open to assistance with behavioral problems, conflict resolution, and student performance in general. School nurses may also be asked to provide training on how to render first aid or handle emergency situations (e.g., injuries, fighting).

Students with disabilities and their parents may need individualized education provided by the school nurse. However, it is not only the chronically ill or at-risk stu-

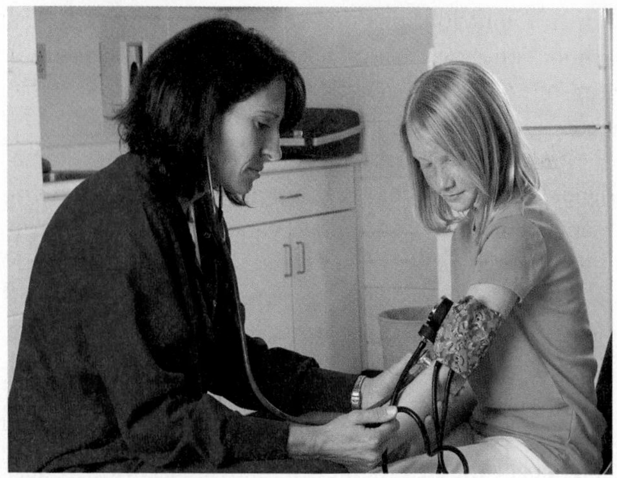

School nurse seeing student in office.

dents who need the teaching role of the nurse; all students benefit by receiving specific health-related information about nutrition, maintaining a safe environment, and proper rest and exercise.

Investigator

Currently, there are very few meaningful data on school health nursing services. In the past, outcome parameters have included (1) number of teen pregnancies, (2) degree of substance abuse, (3) school attendance, and (4) dropout rates.

School nurses collect data from health records, home visits, and teacher conferences. These data have been used to demonstrate improved school performance in a child receiving glasses following a vision screening, for example.

School nurses may note an increased number of obese children during a weight screening. The school nurse may recommend, and then implement, a weight-management intervention for such an aggregate group, often in conjunction with nutrition and physical fitness school personnel.

MEDIA MOMENT 

American History X (1998)

Derek Vinyard (Edward Norton) returns from prison to find his younger brother, Danny (Edward Furlong), caught in the same web of racism and hatred that landed him in prison. After Derek's father, a police officer, is killed in the line of duty by a minority, Derek's view of mankind is altered. While in prison, he discovers that there is good and bad in every race. The task before him now is to convince Danny of his new-found enlightenment.

School health records maintained by school nurses were used by Swanson and Leonard (1994) to provide (with 85% accuracy) an estimate of actual dropout rates. Students who dropped out of school used school health services less than those who did not drop out and who received follow up on identified health problems. Capturing the cost–benefit data of health services validates the benefits of having qualified nurses to provide such services. Studies that demonstrate the need for programs, or the impact of school nurses on absenteeism, for example, speak to educational leaders.

Utilization of the school as a research site is on the rise (Puskar, Weaver, & DeBlassio, 1994). A national survey to identify nursing interventions used in school settings (Cavendish, Lunney, Luise, & Richardson, 1999) found that there were 60 core interventions with school children. These interventions covered a wide range of nursing diagnoses. Their research supports the need for consistent language to document school nurse activities.

Role Within the Profession

The school nurse is a member of a profession now seriously committed to looking at school health. The ANA has established a Nursing Center for School Health, in collaboration with the National Nursing Coalition for School Health. In 1990, more than 50 organizations participated to form the National Consortium for Health Science Education (NCHSE), which was formed to bridge the health and education fields (Passarelli, 1994), conduct research, and develop policy to promote the education of children. Even in systems employing more than one nurse, school nurses often work alone. Remaining an active member of the profession is important for the professional development of school nurses.

Healthy People 2020

Although no single plan of action can be applied to all schools, a body of problems common to school-aged and adolescent youth has been identified in *Healthy People 2020*. Indicators include physical activity, overweight and obesity, tobacco use, substance abuse, responsible sexual behavior, mental health, injury and violence, environmental quality, immunization, and access to health care (HHS, 2004). Health risk behaviors have been measured by the CDC's Youth Risk Behavior Surveillance System (YRBSS) since 1991, and the survey's results provide data related to the national goals. See **Table 37-2**.

Of deaths in persons ages 10–24 in the United States, 70.8% result from only four causes: motor vehicle crashes, other unintentional injuries, homicide, and suicide. Encouraging data trends from 1991 to 2011 from the YRBSS

TABLE 37-2 Indicators from the Youth Risk Behavior Surveillance System for Students in Grades 9–12, 1991–2011

Indicator	1991 (%)	2003 (%)	2011 (%)
Never or rarely wore seatbelts	25.9	18.2	7.7
Rode with driver who had been drinking alcohol	39.9	30.2	24.1
Drove after drinking alcohol	16.7	12.1	8.2
Carried a weapon	26.1	17.1	16.6
Plan to attempt suicide	18.6	16.5	12.8
Cigarette smoking	70.1	58.4	44.7
Smokeless tobacco	—	6.7	7.7
Ever used alcohol	81.6	74.9	70.8
Ever used marijuana	31.3	40.2	39.9
Ever used cocaine	5.9	8.7	6.8
Sexual activity with more than four partners	18.7	14.2	15.3
Used condoms	46.2	63	60.2
Drank or used drugs before sex	21.6	25.4	22.1
Not eaten fruits or vegetables (ate less than five per day)	—	6.1	4.8

HEALTHY PEOPLE 2020 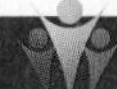

Objectives Related to School Health

Adolescent Health

- AH-5 Increase educational achievement of adolescents and young adults
- AH-6 Increase the proportion of schools with a school breakfast program
- AH-7 Reduce the proportion of adolescents who have been offered, sold, or given an illegal drug on school property
- AH-8 Increase the proportion of adolescents whose parents consider them to be safe at school
- AH-9 Increase the proportion of middle and high schools that prohibit harassment based on a student's sexual orientation or gender identity
- AH-10 Reduce the proportion of public schools with a serious violent incident

Disability and Health

- DH-9 Reduce the proportion of people with disabilities who encounter barriers to participating in home, school, work, or community activities
- DH-14 Increase the proportion of children and youth with disabilities who spend at least 80% of their time in regular education programs

Early and Middle Childhood

- EMC-4 Increase the proportion of elementary, middle, and senior high schools that require school health education

Educational and Community-Based Programs

- ECBP-1 Increase the proportion of preschool Early Head Start and Head Start programs that provide health education to prevent health problems in the following areas: unintentional injury; violence; tobacco use and addiction; alcohol or other drug use; unhealthy dietary patterns; and inadequate physical activity, dental health, and safety
- ECBP-2 Increase the proportion of middle, junior high, and senior high schools that provide comprehensive school health education to prevent health problems in the following areas: violence, suicide, tobacco use and addiction, alcohol and other drug use, unintended pregnancy, HIV/AIDS and STD infection, unhealthy dietary patterns, inadequate physical activity, and environmental health
- ECBP-3 Increase the proportion of elementary, middle, and senior high schools that have health education goals or objectives that address the knowledge and skills articulated in the National Health Education Standards (high school, middle, and elementary)
- ECBP-4 Increase the proportion of elementary, middle, and senior high schools that provide school health education to promote personal health and wellness in the following areas: handwashing or hand hygiene, oral health, growth and development, sun safety and skin cancer prevention, benefits of rest and sleep, ways to prevent vision and hearing loss, and the importance of health screenings and checkups

(continues)

HEALTHY PEOPLE 2020 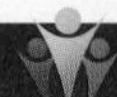 *(continued)*

- ECBP-5 Increase the proportion of elementary, middle, and senior high schools that have a full-time registered school nurse-to-student ratio of at least 1:750

Injury and Violence Prevention

- IVP-27 Increase the proportion of public and private schools that require use of appropriate head, face, eye, and mouth protection for students participating in school-sponsored physical activities

Violence and Abuse Prevention

- IVP-34 Reduce physical fighting among adolescents
- IVP-35 Reduce bullying among adolescents
- IVP-36 Reduce weapon carrying by adolescents on school property

Physical Activity and Fitness

Physical Activity in Children and Adolescents

- PA-3 Increase the proportion of adolescents who meet current federal physical activity guidelines for aerobic physical activity and for muscle-strengthening activity
- PA-4 Increase the proportion of the nation's public and private schools that require daily physical education for all students
- PA-5 Increase the proportion of adolescents who participate in daily school physical education
- PA-6 Increase regularly scheduled elementary school recess in the United States
- PA-7 Increase the proportion of school districts that require or recommend elementary school recess for an appropriate period of time
- PA-8 Increase the proportion of children and adolescents who do not exceed recommended limits for screen time

Tobacco Use

Exposure to Secondhand Smoke

- TU-15 Increase smoke-free and tobacco-free environments in schools, including all school facilities, property, vehicles, and school events

Source: HHS, 2000.

show significant decreases in the percentage of students who never or rarely wore their seatbelts, a decreased percentage of students who rode with a driver who had been drinking alcohol, and fewer students driving after drinking alcohol.

The percentage of students who carried a weapon also decreased significantly from 1991 to 2011. Fewer youths also reported a plan to attempt suicide in 2011 than in 1991. From 1991 to 2011, there was also a significant decrease both in the use of cigarettes, and in use of smokeless tobacco by 9th to 12th graders. The percentage of students who reported ever using alcohol also significantly decreased from 1991 to 2011. Trends from 1991 to 2011 show a decrease in the percentage of students who reported having sexual activity with four or more partners. There was also an increase in the number reporting use of a condom during sexual intercourse.

Health education is one strategy for meeting the *Healthy People 2020* goals. However, coordinated health education is not the norm. Some risk behaviors have worsened, despite educational efforts. Despite the fact that since 1991 selected risk behaviors monitored by the YRBSS have shown some decreases among high school students nationwide, the risk for chronic health problems might actually have increased including the rise in student obesity, sedentary lifestyle, nutritional inadequacy related to the inclusion of fruits and vegetables in their diet, and the increasing use of high-sugar energy drinks.

While there have been improvements in certain behaviors over time, far too many high school students continue to engage in health risk behaviors, such as:

- Failing to wear seatbelts
- Texting/talking on phone while driving
- Smoking cigarettes or consuming tobacco products
- Abusing alcohol and prescription drugs
- Using marijuana
- Engaging in risky sexual behavior

At-Risk Populations

Students at risk, such as technologically dependent children, may experience stigma from other children in the classroom because of their disability. Helping the child with socialization and addressing mental health needs are relevant school nurse roles.

Poverty may influence a child's ability to learn because parents lack the resources or the education to teach the child. When their problems are compounded with a chronic illness, these children constitute an at-risk population. Because of advancing medical technologies that have allowed tiny premature infants or children born with fetal alcohol syndrome and chromosomal abnormalities to survive, increasing numbers of medically fragile children now attend public schools across the country.

Blum (2004) found that:

> how young people do in school and what they do with their free time are the most important determinants for

> every risky behavior studied—regardless of whether they were rich or poor; white, black or Hispanic; or come from one- or two-parent families. (p. 12)

Blum makes the following recommendations on the basis of findings from the most recent NLSAH study on healthy adolescents:

> Policies must move away from the notion that youngsters' behavior choices are predetermined by their race, economic status, or family background—factors they cannot change. Efforts need to focus instead on the strong influences in children's lives that cut across demographic frameworks—the quality of involvement with friends, family, and school. (p. 15)

Peer pressure has a significant impact on youth behaviors. The data show that when teenagers band together on prevention issues such as not drinking and driving, lifestyles are modified much more successfully than with a course on driving sober (Blum, 2004).

Nurse as Team Member

A model of nursing services proposed by the School Nurse Organization of Minnesota (SNOM) captures the complexity of school nursing. Nursing services to children from birth to 21 years include case management, health assessment, disease-prevention activities, nursing care, policy development, and health promotion. In addition to this load, many school nurses collaborate with managed care organizations or private providers and with public health agencies.

Roles are fluid. Collaboration is the key to building an effective team. Schools operate under three levels of rules and regulations, as well as under parental and business community expectations (*Bridging the Gap*, 1992). Educators often feel they are "under siege" just to educate.

The entire school community is the school nurse's patient. School nurses work with families, with access health services, and with the environment in which learning activities occur. The health of the greater community is important to school nurses. Issues of concern to school nurses are similar to those of public health nurses. Bachman (1995) claims, "as the school nurse role expands to accommodate the multiple needs of a diverse patient population, a wide variety of collaborative practitioners is essential to the school setting" (p. 22).

School Health Nursing Practice

Health problems exist in every school, but the nature of these health problems varies. The NLSAH elucidated geographic, economic, and gender differences among the 20,000 teens and families surveyed (Blum & Rinehart, 1997).

The scope of clinical knowledge required ranges from wellness, to developmental delays, to other special needs of children and families. Screening for communicable diseases (e.g., lice, fever) and for developmental disorders (e.g., impairments in vision, hearing, emotional health, and scoliosis) is a large component of school nursing practice. Immunization surveillance is another important duty. Great strides have been made regarding immunization in the United States; however, healthcare providers should maintain a high index of suspicion regarding communicable diseases, especially in those persons who have traveled abroad recently.

The cost of providing one-on-one care is more than the hourly cost of the care provider. In addition to actually caring for patients, school nurses spend many hours coordinating care; developing, implementing, and monitoring individual health plans; determining the qualifications of care providers; and delegating procedures and training designated personnel. Being able to provide one-on-one care also takes time from other staff for training on how to be prepared to provide services in the absence of the care provider, or to help the care provider in an emergency. Each of these elements is an essential part of continuous nursing care and must be considered in planning. Districts will need added resources to provide such comprehensive school health services.

RESEARCH ALERT 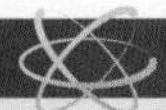

Teenage pregnancy outcomes remain an increasing concern in the United States. Education and support of pregnant teens are critical factors that may determine good or poor pregnancy outcomes. Poor outcomes may include low birth weight, developmental delays, and poor academic performance. Although the number of teenagers experiencing pregnancy and parenting has declined in the United States, school-based health clinics can be used to provide support and guidance designed to avoid the negative outcomes associated with teenage pregnancy and parenting. By having school-based health clinics, nurse practitioners and school nurses can provide much-needed services to pregnant and parenting teens. These services should include educational support, counseling, and community resources. This inquiry provides a metasynthesis of the literature and reviews, examines, and summarizes the literature relating to the effect of school-based clinics on teenage pregnancy and parenting outcomes.

Source: Strunk, J. A. (2008). The effect of school-based health clinics on teenage pregnancy and parenting outcomes: An integrated literature review. *Journal of School Nursing, 24*(1), 13–20.

It is, therefore, difficult to prescribe one specific set of health promotion guidelines for all school districts in the United States. Exercise, fitness activities, and good nutrition clearly affect physical and mental health in children and adolescents.

Health-Related Services

Health-related services is a term used to describe services that meet the distinct needs of medically fragile students: The child with tracheostomy equipment needs extra physical space, as will a child in a wheelchair. Other children may require medication administration for asthma, seizures, diabetes mellitus, ADHD, hemophilia, or other chronic illnesses such as HIV. Children using inhalers and oxygen may be common in regular classrooms.

At times, children in schools may need technology (e.g., catheters, respirators, gastrostomies) for survival. School personnel may be asked to perform tasks such as suctioning children with tracheostomies, providing parenteral nutrition in gastrostomies, and performing catheterization. Medication administration and emergency measures are often required as well.

An **individualized educational plan (IEP)** is written for at-risk students in regular classrooms. The IEP is an educational plan tailored to each child's unique needs to assist each child in meeting educational needs. IEPs may be written for a variety of children whether they are exceptionally bright or at risk.

Individualized health plans (IHPs) are plans of care used in the educational setting to identify, communicate, and document an individual student's healthcare needs. IHPs are the health-related component of the IEP. IHPs are based on the nursing process and are required by law to be written by a health team (Grabeel, 1996). Each child's IHP contains medical data, as well as plans for medication administration and emergency care (e.g., bee stings or anaphylaxis). Emergency care plans for IHPs must be written by a nurse. Emergency care plans anticipate injuries on the school grounds, exacerbation of chronic disease, and needed resources for health care.

The IHP is equivalent to the nursing care plan but is often implemented by nonnurses. The IHP is used along with the IEP to plan educational goals and activities.

For the medically fragile child, a multidisciplinary team writes an IHP. The school nurse is part of this team, which may consist of administrator, teachers, a local physician, social worker, speech pathologist, nutritionist, occupational/physical therapists, and parents.

The composition of the team is determined by district administration. An educational coordinator is responsible for the child's assessment, training, and monitoring. Input from parents or guardians is critical for optimal educational placement.

Case Finding

Early intervention programs to identify children from birth to 3 years of age who have disabilities may utilize schools to conduct screening. Input from primary physicians becomes part of the **individualized family service plan (IFSP)**. The IFSP is designed to assist in fostering the optimal development of children with disabilities from birth to 3 years of age.

All school personnel assist with identification of children and youth at risk for physical, emotional, or educational problems. The school nurse has a health perspective that can supplement the observations of teachers and staff, but teachers play a crucial role in assessing student health needs. Observations of children in the hallway, in the lunchroom, or on the playground provide teachers and school nurses with tips on physical, nutritional, or emotional needs.

Planned screening by the school nurse for developmental progress or vision, hearing, and dental screening are also important components in case finding. Review of attendance records is another form of case finding. Students who miss more than 10 days of school may need a home visit and/or family assessment, because high-risk families sometimes are unable to manage the tasks of getting their students off to school.

When a physician identifies a special need, referral to the school system may be less efficient. Hospital discharge planning may not include consideration of school needs. It may take months between the time a need is identified, the school is notified, and the child is actually enrolled in the school. This is particularly true for children experiencing the life changes that occur from a motor vehicle accident or other major traumatic event. A school nurse is a key contact for healthcare providers in the community.

Collaboration with the community healthcare providers requires case management, which begins with identifying the child's healthcare needs. The school nurse has all parents complete an emergency information card that includes the name of the child's healthcare provider (if any), and where the parent can usually be found during the day. If a student needs referral to a healthcare provider, parental permission is required to discuss the case with the provider.

Good documentation of the reason for referral and requests for feedback improves coordination of care with key contacts in the medical community. Some school nurses produce a newsletter with the goal of keeping community resource persons informed about school health.

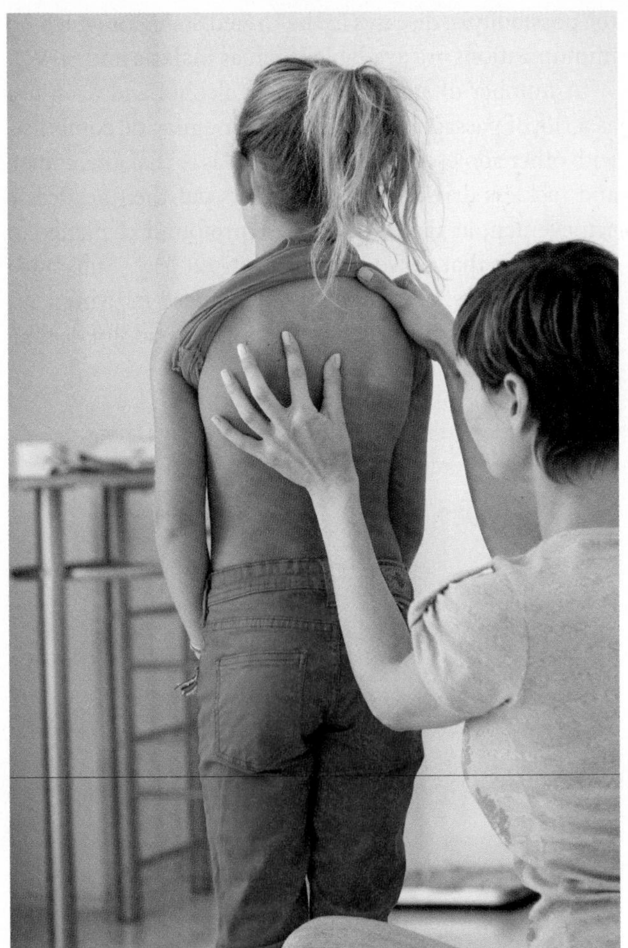

© BSIP SA/Alamy

A school nurse conducts a scoliosis screening for a girls basketball team at a local middle school.

All school personnel should assist with the identification of children and youth at risk for physical, emotional, and educational problems. Community issues such as war fears, violence and suffering in television news and other media, implications of terrorism, and sexual orientation issues may all affect the mental health of many school children. Teachers play a crucial role in identifying student health needs, but the school nurse has a health perspective that can supplement the observations of teachers and staff.

Many schools have delegated routine mandated school screenings (such as vision and hearing) to interdisciplinary teams for case finding and follow up. As mentioned earlier, review of attendance records is another form of case finding.

Practice Issues in School Health

Funding of school health care is a major practice issue. Many physical morbidities (such as childhood diseases and malnutrition) have steadily decreased as a result of immunizations and other screening programs (such as Early and Periodic Screening, Diagnostic, and Treatment [EPSDT]). However, many uninsured children with chronic diseases such as diabetes, asthma, recurrent otitis media, and poor vision (which are significant enough to affect functioning at school) are less likely to receive appropriate medical attention. Eye exams and eyeglasses, for example, may not be a priority for a low-income family.

The State Children's Health Insurance Program (SCHIP) offers health insurance to children 18 years and younger. This insurance covers children who are not eligible for Medicaid funding. Despite concerns that having insurance would lead families to abuse the healthcare system, the contrary has been found to be true (Lave, 1998). The school nurse is in a unique position of helping families enroll their children in this program. Each state has specific coverage.

In 1997, Congress passed legislation that allows states to provide health insurance to more children of working families. These programs build on the Medicaid program that started covering children and adults in the mid-1960s. For little or no cost, this insurance pays for physician and nurse practitioner visits, prescription medicines, hospitalizations, and much more. Most states also cover the cost of dental care, eye care, and medical equipment.

The changing structure of school health services is another practice issue. Other morbidities have taken center stage, as very tiny infants now survive into childhood, and the severely injured child may attend school despite the disabilities. In utero exposure to cocaine, marijuana, and alcohol is on the rise (Messinger et al., 2004). Health-risk behaviors of youth in alternative schools, those in the legal system, and those with no permanent home challenge the school health system (Kubik, Lytle, & Fulkerson, 2004). Sexual orientation has also emerged as a health issue (Frankowski, 2004).

There is a need to train leaders for school health programs. Expanding technology, changing disease trajectories, and increased accountability for patient outcomes contribute to the need for visionary innovations in school health services. School nurses work with a highly diverse population of well children and staff, as well as chronically ill children.

There are insufficient numbers of school nurses to cover all these needs. The nursing shortage has implications here, too. In fact, a membership survey of school nurses by NASN (Johnson, 2002) found that almost half of respondents were older than age 50. In 2000, the average

GLOBAL CONNECTION 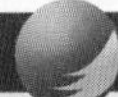

Select a country outside the United States and examine the differences in the school environment that influence the health of students. Compare a variety of factors, such as mental health services, violence, and sexually transmitted infections (STIs).

elementary school teacher earned $13,600 more than the average registered nurse. The number of school children younger than age 18 in the United States is expected to grow from 72.6 million to 77.2 million between 2000 and 2020. School nurses are clearly necessary in the educational system, as they have a central role in implementation of school health services.

Funding needs depend on a multitude of variables and cannot be assumed to be equal across regions. Common variables are socioeconomic status of the region, numbers of special needs students, the complexity of families and diversity of cultures, the number of sites being served by each nurse, and the distance between schools. However, nurse funding may not be based on student or program needs. A critical need in school health is to find sustainable funding.

Typical sources of funding for school-based health programs serving indigent children (IDEA Book, 1996) are federal grants (usually Public Health Service Act section 329, 330, or 340); state block grants, especially for maternal–child health; local government funds; grants from national or local foundations or local hospitals; and Medicaid reimbursement (primarily EPSDT).

According to the Secretary of Education, the United States spent more than half a trillion dollars on K–12 education in 2003 ("Paige," 2004). The NCLB Act has added new requirements for testing, which are expensive. Services that are not mandated by law, as is the case with some nursing services, may be cut disproportionately, regardless of their benefit to students.

Our awareness of the complex environmental impact on human health has grown exponentially in recent decades. Exposures to lead and to secondhand smoking are more damaging to growing children than they are to adults. Exposure may occur in the school setting (to cockroach parts, mold, ultraviolet light, and dust mites) or at home. The school nurse is also concerned about exposures that occur outside of the school setting. For example, one asthmatic student was riding the bus home when another student sprayed a perfume to which the asthmatic child was very allergic. The bus turned around and returned to the school to call for emergency assistance. Fortunately for the child, a clinic was located right across the street. Emergency inhalation treatment and parenteral medication assisted the needy student. It took the ambulance more than 45 minutes to reach this rural school. School policies are needed to address such emergencies (Reilly, 2002).

New infectious diseases, such as West Nile virus infection and severe acute respiratory syndrome (SARS), require school nurses to maintain vigilance and monitor the CDC's recommendations via the publication *Morbidity and Mortality Weekly Report.* Increased global travel raises the possibility of diseases in the United States for which no immunizations are available (such as malaria and HIV).

A number of students may see alcohol and drug use as a rite of passage. In fact, alcohol use may be combined with other adolescent behaviors such as sexual intercourse and reckless driving. These students put their academic achievement at risk and can be a profound challenge to the schools that serve them (NASN, 2004c). Substance use may also reflect problems experienced in living with alcohol or drugs at home, or as coping methods for dealing with depression and anxiety.

MEDIA MOMENT 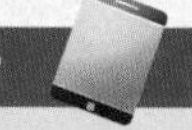

***Heathers* (1989)**

Veronica mingles with Heather Chandler, Heather Duke, and Heather McNamara so that she can be as popular as them, even though she hates them. Veronica hates them enough to wish they were dead, though she would never want to be their cause of death. When she starts dating J.D., however, she finds herself involved in the murders of most of her enemies, whose deaths are covered up as suicides.

Legal Issues in School Nursing

All nurses practice under their state's nurse practice act. Many legal and ethical considerations arise daily. Nurses are taught the importance of documentation, but in the school setting the perspective differs. Because of the lack of sufficient numbers of nurses to cover certain school health needs, delegation of tasks such as medication administration, and documentation of that care, may fall to unlicensed personnel (such as the school secretary). State nurse practice acts have clear guidelines related to delegation. Accountability in one's practice can place a tremendous burden on many school nurses. Although many school districts carry liability insurance on school nurses, school nurses should carry their own liability insurance as well.

Parental consent is required to provide health services to children. These services include health screening for psychological or learning disabilities, medication administration, immunization, medical treatment such as catheterization, and education on human sexuality. School districts must establish health policies that follow state and federal guidelines, especially for dealing with medical emergencies when a parent is not available or consent is urgently needed.

Legal issues sometimes clash with ethical issues, such as when a child's guardian has "do not resuscitate" (DNR) orders on file. In one case, when cardiopulmonary resuscitation was administered to such a child, responsible personnel were charged with assault.

APPLICATION TO PRACTICE

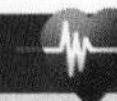

Blog Entry

Age: 18

Location: Colorado

Gender: Female

Date: 07 May 2014

Time: 13:01:43

I first got prescribed Paxil when I was 17. At that point in my life I was going through major depression and really bad anxiety attacks. I missed the first week of my senior year in high school because of my anxiety. When my mom decided to take me to the doctor, I had asked the doctor about Paxil since I had seen the advertisements on TV. He went ahead and wrote me the prescription, and I was put on therapy. I wasn't sure what to expect, but all I wanted was to feel like a normal person again.

I continued taking Paxil for a couple of months but when my insurance was up, I had no choice but to get off completely. I had no side effects at that point but my mom insisted that I get back on Paxil just to help me while I was still in school. I've been on it now for the past year and a half.

I've tried getting off Paxil, but it is so hard to do. I began experiencing extreme dizziness, shaking, nausea—any other bad feeling you can think of, I had. I'm not really all that sure what to do anymore. I still continue taking Paxil, but every other day. Even though it is every other day, I know I am addicted to this drug. As I try to shorten my dosage, it gets more and more difficult to go through each day at work and my first year at college.

My boyfriend tries so hard to help me but he's not sure how. I tell him how maybe I should see a doctor, but since he sees the side effects, he thinks they'll just try to give me another so-called wonder drug. So I guess I'm left to handle this alone and on my own. I can't believe my own doctor couldn't tell me the side effects of this drug that has now ruined my life and future.

How would you as a school nurse respond to this anonymous blog? Think of ways technology can expand the role of the school nurse beyond the physical school building.

GOT AN ALTERNATIVE?

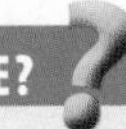

Teens are often a targeted population for "quick fix," alternative diet products, including herbal products and bodybuilding enhancements. How can the school nurse educate students to make healthy, informed choices about these marketing campaigns?

In schools, medicolegal aspects of care, such as confidentiality, may receive different emphasis than in the traditional nursing arena. Student confidentiality and parental consent are viewed differently; the school acts *in loco parentis* (that is, in the place of the parent). Sexuality, STIs, mental health, and substance abuse are recurring confidentiality issues among school children in traditional care settings.

Because of these differences, medicolegal aspects of medication administration, child abuse and neglect, documentation, and relevant licensure for care providers often challenge the school nurse. Many times these instances are managed by delegation, but the school nurse may ultimately be held responsible for the outcome. An example is medication administration to a child with ADHD. When no nurse is present at the school, but the time for the dose has come, a school staff member may be called on to "produce" the medication from a safe place, while the student is responsible for actually picking up the pill or pouring the liquid and swallowing it.

The federal Health Insurance Portability and Accountability Act (HIPAA) regulations cover personally identifiable health information. Initially (2000), it was applied only to healthcare providers, health plans, and health clearinghouses. Schools were exempt from HIPAA rules, because schools were covered under the Family Educational Rights and Privacy Act (FERPA) of 1974. Later, however, the federal government mandated confidentiality for health information held by schools.

NASN (2004a) is tracking changes in the law as they apply to schools. Confidentiality of information may be breached all too easily, as in a lunchroom conversation between teachers. Nevertheless, confidentiality of medical records is critical to parents and to administrators. FERPA gives parents the right to review and appeal records about their child, and it prohibits the release of student records without authorization.

Advance directives such as DNR orders raise serious ethical concerns for parents or guardians of a medically fragile child, as well as for teachers and other school personnel (Grant, Cureton, & Yahiro, 1998). Although any group of school nurses could list many other ethical concerns in school nursing, discussion of these issues is just beginning to take place on a broader scale (Proctor, 1998). Examples of ethical dilemmas include the following:

- The right of the school to exclude a child with chronic head lice, versus the need of the child to return to class for social and educational reasons

- The right of a school district to cut staff, including caregivers for severely disabled students, versus the child's right to safe, adequate, and competent care
- The refusal of a school district to implement DNR orders for a medically fragile child, versus the right of parents as guardians to forgo extraordinary procedures to prolong life

Documentation

Documentation is the only way to prove in a court of law that the nursing care was actually administered and that the standard of care was met. Malpractice suits against school nurses are rare; however, the increasing complexity of care and greater public expectations of healthcare accountability may increase the nurse's legal exposure if adequate documentation is lacking.

School health records also provide a way for the school nurse to communicate with families, students, multidisciplinary teams, emergency personnel, and other healthcare providers. Data can be used to identify student health problems, evaluate programs, provide quality assurance, and allow for continuity of care should the student move to another school district.

Student health records include documents such as immunization records, screening records, progress notes, physician orders, physical examination records, medication and treatment logs, IHPs, emergency healthcare plans, third-party medical records, consent forms, Medicaid and other insurance billing forms, and flow charts (NASN, 2004b). These may be in paper format. If so, these paper records should be kept in locked files. Records may also be stored via a number of electronic technologies, such as telephone databases, fax, email, and personal digital assistants (PDAs).

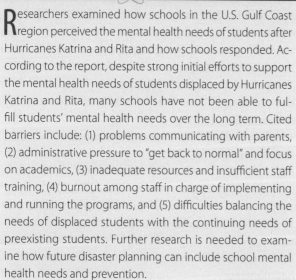

RESEARCH ALERT

Researchers examined how schools in the U.S. Gulf Coast region perceived the mental health needs of students after Hurricanes Katrina and Rita and how schools responded. According to the report, despite strong initial efforts to support the mental health needs of students displaced by Hurricanes Katrina and Rita, many schools have not been able to fulfill students' mental health needs over the long term. Cited barriers include: (1) problems communicating with parents, (2) administrative pressure to "get back to normal" and focus on academics, (3) inadequate resources and insufficient staff training, (4) burnout among staff in charge of implementing and running the programs, and (5) difficulties balancing the needs of displaced students with the continuing needs of preexisting students. Further research is needed to examine how future disaster planning can include school mental health needs and prevention.

Source: Jaycox, L. H., Tanielian, T. L., Sharma, P., Morse, L., Clum, G., & Stein, B. D. (2007). Schools' mental health responses after Hurricanes Katrina and Rita. *Psychiatric Services, 58*(10), 1339–1343.

Supervision and Accountability

Who is the school nurse's supervisor? Questions related to appropriate supervision of school nurse activities may arise almost daily. Some school nurses practice alone in their school settings and are accountable to school administration. Others work out of school health units in public health departments. The nurse must be clear on which decisions regarding health care rest with the school administration and which rest with the state's nurse practice laws.

Accountability involves meeting deadlines and following through with commitments, as well as providing competent nursing care. Being accountable involves risk. School nurses should request and welcome performance evaluations from peers.

An unlicensed assistive person (sometimes called a para-professional or a health aide) is an individual who is trained to function as an assistant to the licensed registered nurse in the provision of patient care activities as delegated by the registered nurse (NCSBN, 1990). These individuals have had specific training by the nurse related to tasks delegated to them—tasks such as catheterization, suctioning, or gastrostomy feedings.

Funding Issues in School Health

Parents become strong advocates for increased school health programs when they appreciate the valuable services provided by their school nurse (Brandt, 2002). There must be adequate pay to keep nurses and other providers in the workplace where they are needed. Funds from grants and contracts often do not suffice to meet financial realities, and they are not reliably renewed or increased over time (Igoe, 2002).

Creative fee structures have been used to fund school health care, including managed care (Igoe & Giordano, 1992) and business and school partnerships (Lever, Stephan, Axelrod, & Weist, 2004). SNOM (1995) has assisted local school districts to access federal funds for immunizations, Mantoux testing, and for EPSDT. Some states have designated money from tobacco settlements to fund school nurses. School nurses now have an increased number of partners and agencies to which they can appeal for support and innovation in school health nursing.

Business involvement in school health services has been used to fund CSHPs. A hospital on the Mississippi Gulf Coast helped set up six school-based, nurse-run clin-

THINK ABOUT THIS

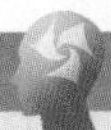

About one in five 9th graders reports having had oral sex. The teenagers (average age 14.5 years) say oral sex is less risky, more common, and more acceptable for their age group than intercourse. To study this issue, researchers surveyed 580 ethnically diverse 9th-graders in two California public high schools. Gender was not a factor, as girls and boys reported similar opinions and experiences. "I think the stereotypes don't exist as much anymore," reflected the study's lead author, Bonnie Halpern-Felsher, associate professor of pediatrics at University of California–San Francisco. "Girls and boys both see oral sex as not being a big deal." Teens often view oral sex as less risky, especially in regard to STIs and pregnancy.

While we know less about the risks of oral sex among heterosexuals, parents and school nurses should still inform teens about the potential risks for contracting STIs during oral sex. Further, there is the potential damage to the teen's relationships and self-esteem, which should also be discussed by healthcare providers and parents. While adults are focusing on avoiding sexual intercourse, teens are finding other ways to practice what they perceive as "safe sex" and parents are often "clueless" about these common and accepted practices among their children.

Source: Halpern-Felsher, B. L., Cornell, J. L., Kropp, R. Y., & Tschann, J. M. (2005). Adolescents and oral sex: Perceptions, attitudes, and behavior. *Journal of Adolescent Health, 36*(2), 443–456.

ics to provide health services (Clemen, 1997). The "Cities in Schools" model is an example of a program developed by city governments to connect appropriate human services with youth at risk for dropping out of school.

Ensuring security and privacy of data is critical. Computers have streamlined record keeping, but may also convey information inadvertently if a file is left open. Information transmitted electronically is particularly subject to confidentiality regulations (HIPAA-FERPA).

Traditional health agencies view school nursing as being largely unregulated, whereas primary care sites are typically heavily regulated. The totally different types of documentation further highlight differences from primary care.

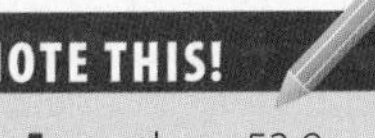

NOTE THIS!

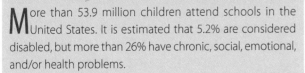

More than 53.9 million children attend schools in the United States. It is estimated that 5.2% are considered disabled, but more than 26% have chronic, social, emotional, and/or health problems.

Source: Van Cleave, J., Gortmaker, S. L., & Perrin, J. M. (2010). Dynamics of obesity and chronic health conditions among children and youth. *Journal of the American Medical Association, 303*(7), 623–630.

Delegation

Delegation is a legal issue. The ANA defines delegation as the transfer of responsibility for the performance of an activity from one individual to another, while retaining accountability for the outcome.

NASN recommends that the school nurse-to-pupil ratio be 1:750. Many school district administrators, not having this ratio of school nurses to students, may assign or delegate health-related activities to teachers, teachers' assistants, secretaries, or others. Such staff members are called **unlicensed assistive personnel** ("working with, or in the absence of, the school nurse"). A principal is not legally licensed to delegate such activities as medical treatments or use of assistive devices. A key duty of the school nurse, therefore, is to train persons to whom activities such as notification of a parent when the child is ill or injured may be delegated. Before agreeing to accept responsibility for these staff members' actions, the school nurse should be familiar with state and federal regulations regarding delegation.

A curriculum for basic training of school paraprofessionals is available from the School Health Resources Service's Project ASSIST. Other training aids related to appropriate medication administration or specific medical procedures are available from NASN and from state nurses' associations. Training also makes sure the paraprofessional is aware of school policies related to issues such as student self-administration of medication (e.g., an albuterol inhaler).

One example from business is the support provided by the American Cancer Society. In the 1990s, the American Cancer Society realized that eliminating cancer in the United States required more than delivery of cancer-prevention materials (Seffrin, 2004). Representatives went to the schools and listened to their needs. They heard about the need for community involvement, for collaboration with materials and curricula that addressed "their" area (cancer). They accepted the agenda for comprehensive school health education, viewing the full educational and school health picture. The American Cancer Society then moved from delivery of cancer-prevention materials to facilitating the expertise inherent in every community. Their mission became to create the strongest health environment for all school children.

Other community-based voluntary agencies are now beginning to creatively advocate for funding of school health care, as they strive to improve the health of children, and the adults these children will become.

The NCES (2003) has developed indicators for school crime and safety, which cover such topics as victimization, fights, bullying, disorder, teacher injury, weapons, and student perception of school safety, among others.

In 2011, students ages 12–18 were victims of nearly 1.25 million nonfatal crimes of violence or theft at school—a decrease of about 37.5% from 2001 (NCES, 2012). The majority (52%) of all school victimizations were property crimes such as theft or burglary. Bullying remains a problem, although there has been increased awareness and public campaigns against it. Reports on the extent of the issue vary in their estimates, with the CDC (2012) reporting that 20.1% of students in grades 9–12 experienced bullying on school property in 2011, while NCES (2012) reported for the same year that bullying was experienced by 28% of students ages 12–18—a similar, though not identical, cohort. With respect to cyberbullying, which is treated separately from in-person or in-school bullying, the CDC (2012) found 16% of students had experienced it, in contrast to the NCES's (2012) figure of 9%.

Children and adults have recently endured catastrophic events, which have resulted in death and injury to children and loved ones. Many children know little about the terrorist attacks on September 11, 2001 and the subsequent wars in Iraq and Afghanistan, but they experience the after-effects of these events in terms of heightened vigilance and security at airports and public events. Some may be aware of incidents such as the Boston Marathon bombing of 2013, in which an 8-year-old boy was killed and other children and adults were maimed. Many children are aware, in particular, of the increasing frequency of school shootings, particularly after the high-profile attack in Newtown, Connecticut that targeted the youngest children at the Sandy Hook Elementary School. All such factors have created a need to remain "on alert," which contributes to great anxiety (Webb, 2004). Children respond differently from adults, who are at the same time processing their own reactions. Since the September 11, 2001 attacks, researchers have identified more children with posttraumatic stress disorder symptoms than at any time in history (Hoven, Mandrell, & Duarte, 2003). There has been far less scientific research about children's exposure to the news than there has been to exposure to other entertainment media, but one study of children's responses to various types of disasters (natural or manmade) showed that three interventions are useful: (1) immediate crisis counseling after the incident, particularly for those directly impacted; (2) early intervention to promote a positive recovery environment; and (3) managing interactions with law enforcement and/or rescue workers so that the child's environment returns to a sense of safety and routine as quickly as possible (Reifels et al., 2013).

Disaster preparedness is an important part of the school health program. Disasters can occur within the school walls or beyond. Both types of disasters can impact the schools. In recent years, our country has experienced unprecedented disasters, from Hurricane Katrina to 9/11 and bioterrorism. Nurses in schools have special responsibilities and skills to act as first responders in mass casualty emergencies. They are in ideal positions to prepare school populations in disaster planning and preparedness. Schools are often utilized as shelters in disasters. The NASN (2005) contend in their position paper *School Nurse Role in Bioterrorism Emergency Preparedness and Response* that well-prepared nurses within the school environment have significant potential for minimizing the effects of disasters in school settings and, subsequently, in the community at large.

Community Issues in School Health

School–Health Linkages

School-based services are services delivered on the school grounds. School-linked services, by comparison, may be

ETHICAL CONNECTION 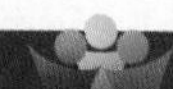

How can school nurses involve parents of children with obesity in the school setting?

Although the national health crisis of childhood obesity is a well-documented problem, few, if any, clinical interventions have had success in curbing its growth. In fact, childhood obesity, along with its associated morbidities, continues to climb even in the face of increased awareness. Research shows that factors contributing to obesity are almost entirely modifiable on some level. Furthermore, specific behavior changes have been shown to result in positive outcomes, yet these changes have not been widely implemented by practitioners, families, or individuals. The transtheoretical model of health behavior change offers insight into assessing individuals and targeting interventions for behavior change. This article focuses on guiding school nurses to assess parents of school-age children at risk for obesity for readiness for health behavior change, then choosing parent-focused interventions based on their stage of readiness for change.

Review this research article and identify ways in which school nurses can involve parents in addressing the epidemic of childhood obesity. Are there ethical issues involved in the sensitive issue of assessing parents' risk for obesity? How would you approach this with school administrators and parent–teacher groups?

Source: Howard, K. R. (2007). Childhood overweight: Parental perceptions and readiness for change. *Journal of School Nursing, 23*(2), 73–79.

delivered across the street or across town, but are initiated by school personnel. The definition of which services are "eligible" as school-linked services varies greatly from state to state.

Parental involvement and community linkages are crucial for success in each local school–health linkage. Unless the community is involved in planning and supporting the services, one single component of the program, such as pregnancy prevention education, can derail an entire health education program.

An example of a school–health linkage is the SBC. This type of clinic offers primary care to students, their families and siblings, and school personnel. SBC have been shown to be effective primary care providers of

DAY IN THE LIFE

From School Nurse to a Career in Politics

Marge Whaley, BSN, RN, MEd

My career in school nursing started at Howe High School in Indianapolis in 1963. I was all of 22 years old and newly married. There were 2,500 students enrolled and for the first 2 years, I taught health classes two periods a day. I think that is when I learned to love being in the classroom.

I had the opportunity to start a school nurse program in Pasco County, Florida, in 1977. We first hired five nurses for our 25 schools. Therefore, everyone was stretched pretty thin. We did have the advantage of having a health assistant at each school, so someone else took care of the daily "boo boos."

From the beginning, Pasco nurses were in the classroom. At first, it was simple lessons on cleanliness and nutrition. We soon advanced to STDs and birth control. Every year, when I interviewed for new positions, as we grew in numbers, I would ask each applicant to bring a lesson plan for a class they might offer. This usually surprised the applicants—this was not part of their perceived school nurse role. In addition, the new nurses mainly wanted to start an IV or dress a wound the first few months until they grew more comfortable in the education setting.

Each new nurse also had to learn how to make a good presentation in front of students. Other nurses were their mentors after they had attended my orientation class. I demanded they be as effective as any other teacher in the school was, so our classes on health would be requested.

As we grew, the needs of our students grew. The number of children on ADHD meds had tripled in the last 15 years. The number of profoundly mentally retarded children and those with severe developmental disabilities continued to grow as well. Our first student with acute health issues had a brain stem tumor, was 8 years old, fed through a stomach tube, and was blind and deaf. I was privileged to witness the dramatic improvement in conditions for a 7-year-old with a rare syndrome, who was at home with no services, incontinent, and fed mostly baby food. At the end of 1 year, he was in a standing box, toilet trained, and feeding himself. It was almost a miracle for his family and for us as well.

Today our nurses are still in the classroom, counseling girls about birth control and helping them manage pregnancies, referring kids with ruptured eardrums and creeping eruption, and dealing with the ever-present head lice in the student population. However, there are also children with catheters, heart monitors, nebulizers, communication boards, and more. Parents expect many of these children to be mainstreamed into the student population, so it takes a great deal of support from nurses to help their nervous teachers cope with these challenges in their classrooms. However, our school nurses continue to take time for classroom presentations as well.

I believe we have one of the best models for school nurses anywhere in Pasco County because our nurses do not use their professional skills taking care of tummy aches and putting on Band-Aids. A trained school paraprofessional—a health assistant—should do that, always under the guidance of the school nurse. This frees the school nurses to do population-focused care, such as screenings, referrals, and follow up for acutely ill students, helping teachers with mainstreamed students, counseling, and health education. I have *always* thought the nurse who must see every child who walks through the door with a minor health complaint is an inappropriate use of school nurses.

After several years of coordinating school health service, I decided to run for the county school board. I ran my first campaign in 1992 and have been a member for 14 years, serving as chair of the board three different times. Campaigning was terrible and foreign for me as a nurse—I hated asking people for money. What I learned after my first three elections where I had opposition is that most people pay almost no attention to the school board elections. We rank right above mosquito control in voters' concerns. Of course, when their child has a problem in the school system, they suddenly become much more interested.

I had a huge learning curve in my first term as a school board member; I thought, since I had been in the district for 17 years as a school nurse, I would be well prepared about school management and politics. Wow, was I ever surprised when I was the one at the orientation workshops asking the

(*continues*)

DAY IN THE LIFE *(continued)*

most questions. For instance, when I found out that giving the bus drivers a 50-cent raise would cost over $800,000 dollars, I was stunned. Because I know our health program is so good, I found my priorities focused on reading competency of our students in the district. Every child must learn to read or else nothing else matters. However, once a nurse, always a nurse, so I continue to keep my eye on the health of our student population.

As a school board member, I visit schools every month, staying the entire day. One of the joys of doing that is being asked to do a brief lesson in someone's classroom, often about health. So when asked if nurses should be involved in politics, I answer, "Haven't we always been?"

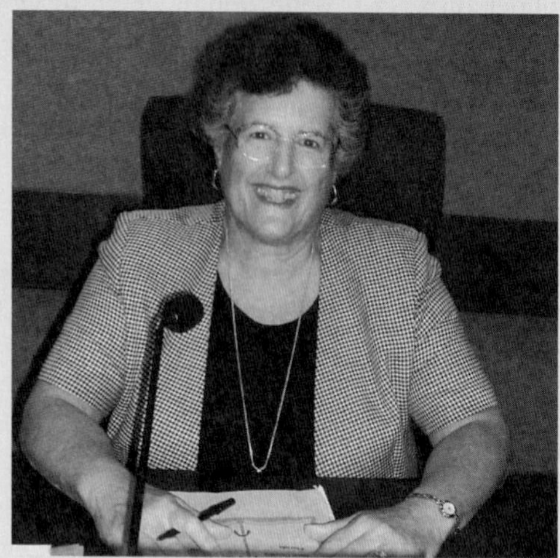

Marge Whaley served as a board member of the Pasco County School Board until 2008 and is retired as school nurse coordinator of the Pasco County, Florida, school system.

services to school children and youth, families, and their communities (Igoe & Giordano, 1992).

Collaboration

The trend toward delivery of health care in a community setting amounts to a paradigm shift for providers and consumers alike. Service through collaboration will become the norm, not the exception. There is the need for collaboration as a strategy for fostering healthy children. Parents, teachers, healthcare providers, mental health services, social workers, and physical fitness and nutrition agencies all have vested interest in the health of children.

Interdisciplinary practice is a term used in academia, but seldom do students practice with other disciplines before graduation. Thus, after graduation, interdisciplinary practice is seldom implemented. It will increasingly be required. Education majors, particularly those going into educational administration, may welcome interdisciplinary practice with schools of nursing preparing school nurses. Partnerships are no longer a wonderful idea, but an idea whose time has definitely come.

Resources

The School Health Resource Services (SHRS), from the Office of School Health, University of Colorado Health Sciences Center, provides a school health reference collection. Timely updates, linkages with programs already in operation in schools and communities across the United States, "starter kits" for specific topics in school health, information links with other projects, and bibliographic services for drawing together educational and health databases are available.

Innovations

Expanding technology, changing disease trajectories, and increased accountability for patient outcomes provide impetus for visionary innovations for school health services. The SBC movement began in the late 1960s in West Dallas. Staffed with nurse practitioners, part-time physicians, and social workers, the SBC in this town provided primary care. Funding was separate from the education budget and came from both private and public funds (Urbinati et al., 1996). The SBC movement has since grown and gained widespread acceptance as a means to address access to care.

Policymakers report that system-related factors may exacerbate poor health utilization. Examples of these factors include inaccessible hours of operation, inadequate number of health providers, and lack of continuity of care. SBCs have helped overcome these obstacles. Nevertheless, young people needing medical care may find lack of transportation, lack of information, and lack of money to be formidable barriers to care.

School-Based Clinics and Primary Health Care

SBCs have grown sevenfold in number, from 200 in the United States in 1990 to nearly 2,000 in 2014 (Button & Rienzo, 2002; HRSA, 2014). More than $200 million was earmarked in the 2010 Patient Protection and Affordable Care Act (ACA) for capital improvements and expansion of services at many of these clinics. One teacher explained the benefit to children and their families of the SBC:

> A lot of our kids are here without shots, without the appropriate care that they need because their parents can't reach the services—they don't have transportation or the motivation of getting up and going across town. Whereas at the school, the teachers can make sure the kids get the services. If health care providers can't get the kids to the health centers, then bring the health centers to the kids. (IDEA Book, 1996, p. 4)

A study of teenagers who used health clinics based in elementary and secondary schools found that they were nearly twice as likely to graduate from high school as those who didn't (Button & Rienzo, 2002); a follow-up study determined that even low to moderate use of SBCs made a difference (Kerns et al., 2011). Thus, SBCs are getting credit for keeping children in school, as well as decreasing parental absenteeism from work caused by the need to take a child to a doctor.

State funding for SBCs has increased dramatically, from $17 million in 1992 to $61.9 million in 2000, and the federal funds provided by the ACA have increased their capacity still more. With the downturn of the economy in the United States, these clinics are more important now than ever, in that they offer everything from physical examinations and mental health services to immunizations and reproductive counseling.

At present, there are insufficient numbers of educationally prepared (bachelor of science in nursing nurses, much less nurse practitioners, to meet the demands for staffing in SBCs. If these clinics were set up to provide care for only 5% of the 129,000 public schools, for example, it would create an immediate demand for 6,000 more nurse practitioners.

Some school nurses have expressed concerns that SBC staff will take on all of the school nurse's responsibilities, leading to confusion among students and staff about who does what. At one site, such concerns led to a grievance (IDEA Book, 1996, p. 49).

SBC nurses are covered by the health center's liability insurance and, therefore, are legally permitted to provide more services than school nurses can. Many school nurses are worried about their own liability, as discussed earlier.

Nurse practitioners who are knowledgeable about chronic illness in children and about educational requirements for children have a valuable role at SBCs. School nurse practitioners do not replace school nurses, however.

SBCs are portable in some geographic locations. For some communities, mobile clinics, like the bookmobiles of old, provide accessible health care. In rural states, physicians and nurse practitioners may schedule travel to provide predictable in-school opportunities for check-ups and immunizations.

Increased Role of the Media in School Health

Print and digital media represent an untapped source for developing school–health linkages and for advertising for school nurses. The media are always looking for news to disseminate: Nurses should step up and speak out! Coverage of successful programs like the CDC's "A Closer Look," updates on regional meetings, family training activities, and information from newsletters can be disseminated to the print media.

Television can also be very effective in portraying health providers at work (as in the show *Grey's Anatomy*). Updates on regional meetings and family training activities could make for very exciting programming on local newscasts.

School nurses must keep up to date on events occurring in their community and globally. These events are publicized through the news media. Events associated with war, violence against strangers, kidnappings (especially those involving children), natural disasters, and sexual assaults or well-touted murders show up all too frequently in news media outlets. The school nurse can take positive action by volunteering to participate in community efforts, educating both adults and children on coping strategies, or making referrals to mental health services. Experts at New York University's Child Study Center have also encouraged journalists to consider the way in which they cover tragic or traumatic events and how that perspective might affect children.

Technology

Information technology has become critical to group work, data management, and research. E-mail is often the quickest way to cover thousands of miles. Smith, Cureton, Hooper, and Deamer (1998) found that school nurses consistently express a need for more access to computers as a means for record keeping, information updating, and communication. Examples of computerized resources include Healthmaster's HealthOffice products (see http://www.healthmaster.com/) that can handle the networking needs of large districts and SNAP Health Center (http://www.promedsoftware.com/). Particularly with the emphasis on electronic health records (EHRs) written into the ACA, pressure to manage students' health records via technology is likely to increase; however, there are also widely available online resources to help nurses and school systems navigate the options (e.g., blogs like HealthITBuzz, which is available at http://www.healthit.gov/buzz-blog/ and run by the HHS, to help inform healthcare providers about technological changes).

Telemedicine is another innovative networking concept. Many rural health centers have gained access to large medical centers through this technology. Network-based linkages with students at the school may give an attending provider a diagnosis, a plan of care, and educational opportunities for the patient and family.

Increased telecommunication facilities are an innovation for education and for practice. PDAs, cell/smart phones, and paging equipment expedite the sharing and retrieving of information; they may even make the process much more satisfying. School nurses can be valuable resources to both students and teachers in using and evaluating web-based health information.

Conclusion

This chapter has highlighted the unique niche of school nursing found within the greater nursing profession.

LEVELS OF PREVENTION 

Primary: Teaching students about healthy nutritional habits

Secondary: Serving as an advocate for reducing the availability of soft drinks and unhealthy snacks in the school setting

Tertiary: Working with children experiencing obesity to plan increased physical activity and healthy eating

AFFORDABLE CARE ACT (ACA) 

The ACA authorizes a grant program for the operation of School-Based Health Clinics, which will provide comprehensive and accessible preventive and primary healthcare services to medically underserved children and families.

School districts face overwhelming constraints and competing demands. They need the invaluable assistance of school nurses to meet their agendas of improving student educational outcomes.

Significant factors that influence public and private schools as well as school nursing include the following:

- Societal and cultural contexts of school nursing
- Federal mandates
- Educational preparation of school nurses and FNPs
- At-risk children in school
- Legal–ethical considerations
- Violence and terrorism
- School-based health centers for primary care
- Increased role of the media
- Technology

A paradigm shift is required for both providers and the public if school nursing is to continue to provide basic nursing care. Nursing is not just part of the acute care setting; it is a critical element for the community. Formative use of media and far-reaching technologies may be better utilized to catch the attention of the government and the public. All nurses can contribute to enhancing the image of school nursing.

Critical Thinking Activities

1. Juan, a 10-year-old boy, has spina bifida and hydrocephalus. As a result, he has limited bowel function, wears a brace for severe curvature of the spine, and uses a wheelchair for mobility. In addition, Juan has only one kidney and wears a urine collection bag under his clothing. This appliance requires frequent emptying during the school day. He takes several medications to prevent infection and promote waste elimination. Juan lives in a single-parent family with his mother and two brothers. His extended family of aunts, uncles, and cousins is 200 miles away in another state. As a community health nurse, discuss four health outcomes that you and his family would plan for Juan's care. Give the rationale for each one.
2. Danielle, a 15-year-old student, recently learned that she is 3 months pregnant. When she informed her mother, Danielle was "thrown out" of the house and is now staying with her 28-year-old boyfriend. Danielle has been absent from school four times in the last 2 weeks. Select nursing interventions at the primary, secondary, and tertiary levels for Danielle. Include holistic interventions.

HEALTHY ME 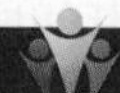

How has nursing school affected your health? What are ways that you as a nursing student can reduce and manage the stress of school? What resources should your school of nursing provide to assist you in the reduction of stress-related, damaging health risks?

References

Allen, G. (2003). The impact of elementary school nurses on student attendance. *Journal of School Nursing, 19*(4), 225–231.

American Nurses Association (ANA), & National Association of School Nurses (NASN). (2011). *School nursing: Scope and standards of practice* (2nd ed.). Silver Spring, MD: Nursebooks.org

Anderson, J. (1994). The changing role of school nurses: One state's experience. *Journal of School Nursing, 10*(3), 22–26.

The Annie E. Casey Foundation. (2008). *Create a report.* Retrieved from http://www.kidscount.org/datacenter

Bachman, B. (1995). A university's response to a need for school nurse education. *Journal of School Nursing, 11*(3), 20–23.

Blum, R. (2004). Success in school, healthy relationships can offset risky teen behavior. *NASP Communique, 30*(3), 12–14.

Blum, R., & Rinehart, P. (1997). *Reducing the risk: Connections that make a difference in the lives of youth.* Minneapolis, MN: Division of General Pediatrics and Adolescent Health, University of Minnesota.

Boyer, E. (1991). *Ready to learn: A mandate for the nation.* Princeton, NJ: Princeton University Press.

Brandt, C. (2002). Enhancing school nurse visibility. *Journal of School Nursing, 18*(1), 5–10.

Bridging the gap: Education primer for health professionals. (1992). National Health/Education Consortium.

Button, J., & Rienzo, B. (2002). *The politics of youth, sex, and health care in American schools.* Philadelphia, PA: Haworth Press.

Cavendish, R., Lunney, M., Luise, B., & Richardson, K. (1999). National survey to identify the nursing interventions used in school settings. *Journal of School Nursing, 15*(2), 14–21.

Centers for Disease Control and Prevention (CDC), Division of Adolescent School Health (HealthyYouth). (2004). *About us.* Atlanta, GA: Author.

Centers for Disease Control and Prevention (CDC). (2008). *School health guidelines and strategies.* Atlanta, GA: Author.

Centers for Disease Control and Prevention (CDC). (2014). *Adolescent and school health.* Retrieved from http://www.cdc.gov/HealthyYouth/CSHP

Child Welfare Information Gateway. (2008). *National clearinghouse on child abuse and neglect information.* Retrieved from http://www.childwelfare.gov

Clemen, P. (1997). Status of school health services in Mississippi: Executive summary. *HPER Journal, 14*(2), 19–21.

Concepcion, M., Murphy, S., & Canham, D. (2007). School nurses' perceptions of family-centered services: Commitment and challenges. *Journal of School Nursing, 24*(1), 315–321.

Costante, C. (1996). Supporting student success: School nurses make a difference. *Journal of School Nursing, 12*(3), 4–6.

Federal Interagency Forum on Child and Family Statistics. (2008). *America's children in brief: Key national indicators of well-being, 2008.* Retrieved from http://www.childstats.gov/americaschildren/glance.asp

Frankowski, B. (2004). Sexual orientation and adolescents. *Pediatrics, 113*(6), 1827–1832.

Grabeel, J. (1996). Nursing practice management: IHPs revisited. *Journal of School Nursing, 12*(4), 28–29.

Grant, L., Cureton, V., & Yahiro, M. (1998). Advance directives and do not resuscitate orders: Nurses' knowledge and the level of practice in school settings. *Journal of School Nursing, 14*(2), 4–13.

Gray, L., & Lewis, L. (2009). *Educational Technology in Public School Districts: Fall 2008* (NCES 2010–003). Washington, DC: National Center for Education Statistics, Institute of Education Sciences, U.S. Department of Education.

Gustafson, E. M. (2005). History and overview of school-based centers in the U.S. *Nursing Clinics of North America, 40*(4), 595–606.

Halpern-Felsher, B. L., Cornell, J. L., Kropp, R. Y., & Tschann, J. M. (2005). Adolescents and oral sex: Perceptions, attitudes, and behavior. *Journal of Adolescent Health, 36*(2), 443–456.

Health Resources and Services Administration (HRSA). (2014). *School-based health centers.* Retrieved from http://www.hrsa.gov/ourstories/schoolhealthcenters/

Hoven, C., Mandrell, D., & Duarte, C. (2003). Mental health of New York City public school children after 9/11: An epidemiologic investigation. In S. Coates, J. Rosenthal, & D. Schecter (Eds.), *September 11: Trauma and human bonds (pp. 46-54).* Hillsdale, NJ: Analytic Press.

IDEA Book. (1996). *Linking community health centers with school serving low-income children.* Washington, DC: Health Resources and Services Administration.

Igoe, J. (1990). School nursing and school health. In J. Natapoff & R. Wieczoirek (Eds.), *Maternal-child policy: A nursing perspective* (pp. 153–188). New York, NY: Springer.

Igoe, J. (2002). School nursing today: A search for new cheese. *Journal of School Nursing, 16*(5), 9–15.

Igoe, J., & Giordano, B. (1992). *Expanding school health services to serve families in the 21st century.* Washington, DC: American Nurses Publishing.

Jaycox, L. H., Tanielian, T. L., Sharma, P., Morse, L., Clum, G., & Stein, B. D. (2007). School's mental health responses after Hurricanes Katrina and Rita. *Psychiatric Services, 58*(10), 1339–1343.

Johnson, M. (2002). Choosing where we're going by knowing where we are: Results of the 2002 membership survey. *NASN Newsletter, 17*(6), 18–19.

Kerns, S. E. U., Pullman, M. D., Walker, S. C., Lyon, A. R., Cosgrove, T. J., & Bruns, E. J. (2011). Adolescent use of school-based health centers and high school dropout. *Archives of Pediatric and Adolescent Medicine, 165*(7), 617–623.

Kubik, M., Lytle, L., & Fulkerson, J. (2004). Physical activity, dietary practices, and other health behaviors of at-risk youth attending alternative high schools. *Journal of School Health, 74*(4), 119–124.

Laraque, D., Boscarino, J., Fleischman, A., Fleischman, A., Casalino, M., Hu, Y. Y., ... Chemtob, C. (2004). Reactions and needs of tristate area pediatricians after the events of September 11th: Implication for children's mental health services. *Pediatrics, 113*(5), 1357–1366.

Lave, J. (1998). Impact of a children's health insurance program on newly enrolled children. *Journal of the American Medical Association, 279*(22), 1820–1825.

Lever, N., Stephan, S., Axelrod, J., & Weist, M. (2004). Fee-for-service revenue for school mental health through a partnership with outpatient mental health centers. *Journal of School Health, 74*(3), 91.

Li, X., & Atkins, M. (2004). Early childhood computer experience and cognitive and motor development. *Pediatrics, 113*(6), 1715–1722.

Messinger, D., Bauer, C., Das, A., Seifer, R., Lester, B. M., Lagasse, L. L.,... Poole, W. K. (2004). The Maternal Lifestyle Study: Cognitive, motor and behavioral outcomes in cocaine-exposed and opiate-exposed infants through three years of age. *Pediatrics, 113*(6), 1677–1685.

National Association of School Nurses (NASN). (2004a). *Issue Brief: School health records.* North Branch, MN: Sunrise River Press.

National Association of School Nurses (NASN). (2004b). *Issue brief: State children's insurance program.* North Branch, MN: Sunrise River Press.

National Association of School Nurses (NASN). (2004c). *Privacy standards for school health records: Issue brief.* http://www.nasn.org

National Association of School Nurses (NASN). (2005). *School nurse role in bioterrorism emergency preparedness and response position paper.* Retrieved from http://www.nasn.org/Default.aspx?tabid=205

National Association of School Nurses (NASN). (2010). *Definition of school nursing.* North Branch, MN: Sunrise River Press. Retrieved from https://www.nasn.org/RoleCareer

National Association of School Nurses (NASN). (2012). *Position statement: Education, licensure, and certification of school nurses.* Scarborough, ME, & Castle Rock, CO: Author.

National Center for Education Statistics (NCES). (2003). *Indicators of school crime and safety.* Retrieved from http://nces.ed.gov/pubs2004/2004004.pdf

National Center for Education Statistics (NCES). (2012). *Indicators of school crime and safety: 2012.* Retrieved from http://nces.ed.gov/programs/crimeindicators/crimeindicators2012/key.asp

National Center for Education Statistics (NCES). (2013). *Public school graduates and dropouts from the common core of data: School year 2009–10.* Retrieved from http://nces.ed.gov/pubs2013/2013309rev.pdf

National Council of State Boards of Nursing (NCSBN). (1990). *Delegation: Concepts and decision-making process.* Chicago, IL: Author.

Notes from home: Parents want to know why. (1997). *Child Care Plus, 7*(2).

Oda, D. (1979). School nursing: Current observations and future projections. *Journal of School Health, 49*, 437–439.

Oda, D. (1981). A viewpoint on school nursing. *American Journal of Nursing, 9*, 674–678.

Paige links business and education. (2004, June 28). Retrieved from http://www.ed.gov/news/speeches/2004/06/06282004.htm

Passarelli, C. (1994). School nursing: Trends for the future. *Journal of School Nursing, 10*(2), 10–21.

Passarelli, C. (1996). School nursing services: Exploring national issues and priorities. *Journal of School Nursing, 12*(3), 24–36.

Pollitt, P. (1994). Lina Rogers Struthers: The first school nurse. *Journal of School Nursing, 10*(1), 34–36.

Proctor, S. (1998). School nurses and ethical dilemmas: Are schools short on ethics? *Journal of School Nursing, 14*(2), 3.

Puskar, K., Weaver, P., & DeBlassio, K. (1994). Nursing research in a school setting. *Journal of School Nursing, 10*(4), 8–14.

Reifels, L., Pietrantoni, L., Prati, G., Kim, Y., Kilpatrick, D. G., Dyb, G., ... O'Donnell, M. (2013). Lessons learned about psychosocial responses to disaster and mass trauma: An international perspective. *European Journal of Psychotraumatology, 4*, 10.3402/ejpt.v4i0.22897. Retrieved from http://www.ncbi.nlm.nih.gov/pmc/articles/PMC3873118/

Reilly, D. (2002). *Managing asthma triggers keeping students healthy: Air quality issues.* Castle Rock, CO: National Association of School Nurses.

Resnick, M., Bearman, P., Blum, R. W., Bauman, K. E., Harris, K. M., ... Udry, J. R. (1997). Protecting adolescents from harm: Findings from the National Longitudinal Study on Adolescent Health. *Journal of the American Medical Association, 278*(10), 823–832.

School Nurse Organization of Minnesota (SNOM). (1995). *Role for school nursing: A vision statement.* Ad Hoc Taskforce on Health Care Reform.

Schwartz, M., & Laughlin, A. (2008). Partnering with schools: A win-win experience. *Journal of Nursing Education, 47*(6), 279–282.

Seffrin, J. (2004). A changing view of schools. *Journal of School Health, 74*(3), 75.

Smith, C., Cureton, V., Hooper, C., & Deamer, P. (1998). A survey of computer technology utilization on school nursing. *Journal of School Nursing, 14*(2), 27–34.

Snyder, T., & Hoffman, C. (Eds.). (2002). *Digest of education statistics, 2001.* National Center for Education Statistics (Pub. # 2002130), Table 2.

Swanson, N., & Leonard, B. (1994). Identifying potential dropouts through school health records. *Journal of School Nursing, 10*(2), 22–26, 46.

Urbinati, D., Steele, P., Harter, B., & Harrell, D. (1996). The evolution of the school nurse practitioner: Past, present and future. *Journal of School Nursing, 12*(2), 609.

U.S. Census Bureau. (2012). *Computer and Internet Access in the United States: 2012.* Retrieved from https://www.census.gov/hhes/computer/publications/2012.html

U.S. Department of Education, National Center for Education Statistics. (2013). *Fast Facts: Students with disabilities, inclusion of.* Retrieved from https://nces.ed.gov/fastfacts/display.asp?id=59

U.S. Department of Health and Human Services (HHS). (2010). *Healthy people 2020: Conference edition.* Washington, DC: U.S. Government Printing Office.

Van Cleave, J., Gortmaker, S. L., & Perrin, J. M. (2010). Dynamics of obesity and chronic health conditions among children and youth. *Journal of the American Medical Association, 303*(7), 623–630.

van der Molen, J. (2004, June). Violence and suffering in television news: Toward a broader conception of harmful television content for children. *Pediatrics, 113*(6), 1771–1775.

Webb, N. (2004). *Mass trauma and violence: Helping families and children cope.* New York, NY: Guilford Press.

Wold, S. J. (2001). School health services: History and trends. In N. Schwab & M. Gelfman (Eds.), *Legal issues in school health services* (pp. 8–9). North Branch, MN: Sunrise River Press.

Zimmerman, B., Wagoner, E., & Kelly, L. (1996). A study of role ambiguity and role strain among school nurses. *Journal of School Nursing, 12*(4), 12–18.

Websites

- The Annie E. Casey Foundation. "Kids Count." Statistical information is available at this website: http://www.aecf.org/
- The American School Health Association: http://www.ashaweb.org
- *Morbidity and Mortality Weekly Report* facts from the Youth Risk Behavior Survey: http://www.cdc.gov/HealthyYouth/
- Facts and figures related to chronic diseases: http://www.cdc.gov/chronicdisease/index.htm
- Fact sheets addressing issues such as staffing, HIV/AIDS policies, school-based health centers, and screening requirements: http://www.cdc.gov/HealthyYouth/shpps/index.htm
- Updated statistics compiled by U.S. government on comprehensive health issues of children: http://www.childstats.gov/
- Federal legislative initiatives in education: http://www.ed.gov/
- Useful for searching the many websites linked with health and education from the federal level: http://www.usa.gov/
- Information related to food allergies, pharmacologic information when concerns over foods exist, and nutrition and strength training games: http://www.foodsafeschools.org/
- U.S. Department of Health and Human Services website offering information and advice regarding management of electronic health records: http://www.healthit.gov/
- National Association of School Nurses: http://www.nasn.org/
- National Association of School Psychologists: http://www.nasponline.org/
- National Longitudinal Study of Adolescent Health: http://www.cpc.unc.edu/projects/addhealth
- Updated briefs on many topics and concerns in school nursing: http://www.schoolnurse.com/med_info/

CHAPTER FOCUS

History of Occupational Health Nursing
Definition
Work and Workplace Hazards
Allergic and Irritant Dermatitis
Asthma and Chronic Obstructive Pulmonary Disease
Fertility and Pregnancy Abnormalities
Hearing Loss
Infectious Diseases
Low Back Disorders
Musculoskeletal Disorders of the Upper Extremities
Traumatic Injuries
Work/Workplace Change
Occupational Health Nursing Practice
Scope of Practice
Occupational Health Nursing Roles
Governmental Influence
Professionalism in Occupational Health Nursing
Education and Certification
Nurse-Managed Models in Occupational Health
Future Expansions
Environmental Health
Migrant Health
Health Promotion in the Workplace

QUESTIONS TO CONSIDER

After reading this chapter, you will know the answers to the following questions:

1. What is occupational health nursing, and how does it relate to community health?
2. Why has the practice of occupational health nursing changed so dramatically over time?
3. What are the work and workplace hazards that result in illness, injury, and loss of life to the worker?
4. How have these hazards changed over the years, and what is the role of the occupational health nurse in dealing with work-related illness and injuries?
5. What are the major laws governing occupational safety and health, and how have they affected workers and the role of the occupational health nurse?
6. What are the five models for worksite primary healthcare management in occupational health care?
7. How can the goal to provide quality, accessible, and cost-effective care be reached?
8. What is the critical link between occupational health nursing and environmental health?
9. Why will occupational health nurses need additional competencies in environmental health in the coming years and what competencies will be needed?

CHAPTER 38

Occupational Health Nursing

Bonnie Rogers

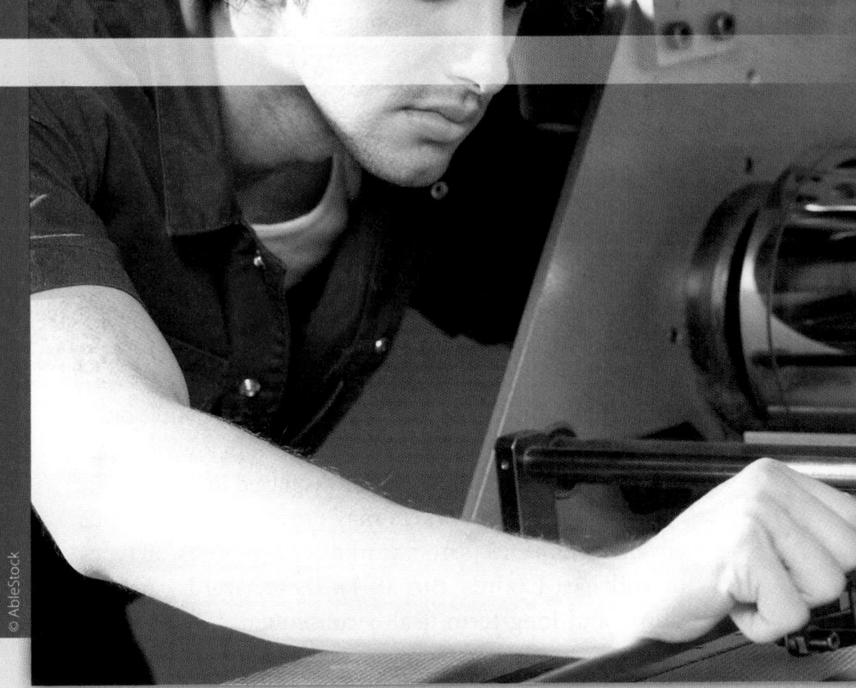

© AbleStock

KEY TERMS

- American Association of Occupational Health Nurses
- ergonomics
- National Institute for Occupational Safety and Health (NIOSH)
- occupational asthma
- occupational health nurse case manager
- occupational health nurse clinician
- occupational health nurse consultant
- occupational health nurse coordinator
- occupational health nurse corporate director
- occupational health nurse educator
- occupational health nurse health-promotion specialist
- occupational health nurse manager
- occupational health nurse practitioner
- occupational health nurse researcher
- occupational health nursing
- Occupational Safety and Health (OSH) Act of 1970
- worker/workplace assessment and surveillance

> It is not wealth, nor splendor, but tranquility and occupation which gives happiness.
>
> —Thomas Jefferson

> It is for us to pray not for tasks equal to our powers, but for powers equal to our tasks, to go forward with a great desire forever beating at the door of our hearts as we travel toward our distant goal.
>
> —Helen Keller

REFLECTIONS

Work gives meaning to our lives, yet also involves health risks according to what we do, how we react to our work, and under what conditions we work. What does "doing work" mean to you? Are you ever able to stop being a nursing student when you are "not at work"? How does this affect your health on a daily basis?

WORK IS GENERALLY considered one of life's worthwhile and exciting experiences. Most adults spend approximately one-fourth to one-third of their time at work, which becomes an integral part of their life. Work can be viewed as a source of strength, helping people build lives and communities. Americans work in a wide range of industries and jobs, which are displayed in **Table 38-1**.

Although most workers may never face any serious adverse health effects from workplace exposures, all types of work have hazards (**Box 38-1**). These hazards can have short- and long-term health consequences, and every effort must be made to prevent and control work-related illness and injury. Thus, the necessity to provide occupational health and safety services to prevent and manage occupational health illness and injuries is paramount in this mission. This chapter provides an overview of the practice of occupational health nursing, with emphasis on the scope of practice. Examples of work-related illnesses and injuries and a discussion of governmental and professional influences are also provided.

BOX 38-1 Categories of Work-Related Hazards

- *Biological/infectious hazards*: infectious/biological agents, such as bacteria, viruses, fungi, or parasites, that may be transmitted via contact with infected patients or contaminated body secretions/fluids to other individuals
- *Chemical hazards*: various forms of chemicals, including medications, solutions, gases, vapors, aerosols, and particulate matter, that are potentially toxic or irritating to the body system
- *Enviromechanical hazards*: factors encountered in the work environment that cause or potentiate accidents, injuries, strain, or discomfort (e.g., unsafe/inadequate equipment or lifting devices, slippery floors, workstation deficiencies)
- *Physical hazards*: agents within the work environment, such as radiation, electricity, extreme temperatures, and noise, that can cause tissue trauma
- *Psychosocial hazards*: factors and situations encountered or associated with one's job or work environment that create or potentiate stress, emotional strain, and/or interpersonal problems

Source: Rogers, B. (2003). *Occupational health nursing: Concepts and practice.* Philadelphia, PA: Saunders.

History of Occupational Health Nursing

Occupational health nursing, then called *industrial nursing*, began in the latter half of the 19th century in Norwich, England, when Phillipa Flowerday was hired by the J. & J. Coleman Company in 1878. Her work in the mustard company was primarily to work in the dispensary and provide homecare services to employees and their families (Godfrey, 1978). Although the company provided acute and tertiary care services for employees, the belief was that preventive care was better than cure in terms of healthy and quality living. Nurses were soon employed by other companies to provide healthcare services for employees who became ill and injured at work as well as health education services related to sanitation and hygiene, particularly given the high rates of tuberculosis (TB) at the time (Slaney, 1984).

In the United States, industrial or occupational health nursing, as it is now called, began in the late 19th century. In 1888, it is reported that a group of Pennsylvania coal mining companies hired Betty Moulder, a graduate of Philadelphia Blockley Hospital School of Nursing, to provide nursing care for ill and injured workers and their families (American Association of Industrial

TABLE 38-1 Labor Force by Job (2008)

Occupational Category	Number of Workers (in millions)
Management, business, financial	15.8
Professional & related	31.0
Service occupations	29.6
Sales	15.9
Office/administrative support	24.1
Farming, fishing, forestry	1.0
Construction/extraction	7.8
Installation, maintenance, & repair	5.8
Production	10.1
Transportation & materials moving	9.8

Source: Data from Lacey, T. A., & Wright, B. (2009). *Bureau of Labor Statistics: Occupational employment projections to 2018*. Retrieved from http://www.bls.gov/opub/mlr/2009/11/art5full.pdf

Nurses [AAIN], 1976; McGrath, 1945; Wright, 1919). However, little more is known about her or the services she provided. In 1895, Ada Mayo Stewart, who is often credited as being the first industrial nurse, was hired by the Vermont Marble Company. She had previously worked as a district nurse in several cities. During her tenure, she visited sick employees in their homes, provided emergency care, taught healthy living habits, taught mothers about child care, and gave speeches on health and hygiene to school children. In this era, there was much ethnic diversity, and Ada Stewart incorporated cultural customs and methods of caring for the sick and their families into her practice. She was later joined by a second nurse, her sister Harriet, who provided health care to employees in the west and central sections of the state (Felton, 1985; Rogers, 2003).

In the early 1900s, industrial health services proliferated rapidly across the country as it became apparent that nursing care related to worksite health issues could have a positive impact on productivity, could decrease illness and injury, and could reduce absenteeism. Working conditions in many factories were harsh and unrelenting, as the industrial ethic often placed the importance of profit above human rights. This type of ethic was not supported by the public, and the advent of worker's compensation (discussed later) came to being.

In 1913, the first organized effort in U.S. industrial nursing began in New England with the establishment of the first industrial nurse registry and the formation of the New England Industrial Nurses' Association in 1918. In 1917, Boston University's College of Business Administration offered the first specialty education course for industrial nurses that focused on industrial health issues and economics. This was followed in the 1920s by several colleges and universities offering short courses in industrial hygiene in which industrial nurses participated (Godfrey, 1978). The advent of World War II in the 1940s supported industrial growth and the concomitant demand for nursing services, with a reported 4,000 nurses employed in industrial health (Brown, 1981). With a viable group of nurses in need of professional support, the AAIN was created in 1942, with Catherine Dempsey as the first president. The purposes of AAIN were to improve industrial nursing practice, provide education, and increase interdisciplinary work (AAIN, 1976).

In the 1960s and 1970s, occupational health and safety became a public issue, with particular concern focused on mining accidents, cave-ins, and black lung disease, as well as the need for professional education and hiring in several disciplines. As a result, several laws were enacted to protect the health and safety of workers (e.g., Federal Coal Mine Health and Safety Act of 1969, Toxic Substances Control Act of 1976). The **Occupational Safety and Health (OSH) Act of 1970** was the first comprehensive law promulgated to ensure safe and healthful working conditions.

As the occupational health nurse's scope of practice broadened considerably, AAIN changed its name to the **American Association of Occupational Health Nurses** in 1977, with a current membership of approximately 13,000 occupational health nurses. The 1980s brought more role expansion into health promotion, management, policy development, research, and entrepreneurism. Several standards were promulgated to protect workers from unwarranted exposures (e.g., Hazard Communication Standard, 1983), and in 1988 the Occupational Safety and Health Administration (OSHA) hired the first occupational health nurse consultant to provide technical assistance in standards development, field consultation, and occupational health nursing expertise. In 1993, the Office of Occupational Health Nursing was established within the agency.

In 1990, American Association of Occupational Health Nurses (AAOHN) published its first occupational health nursing research priorities, updated in 1999, which provide the direction for occupational health nursing research (**Box 38-2**) (Rogers, Agnew, & Pompeii, 2000).

BOX 38-2 Research Priorities in Occupational Health Nursing

1. Effectiveness of primary healthcare delivery at the worksite
2. Effectiveness of health-promotion nursing intervention strategies
3. Methods for handling complex ethical issues related to occupational health
4. Strategies that minimize work-related adverse health outcomes (e.g., respiratory disease)
5. Health effects resulting from chemical exposures in the workplace
6. Occupational hazards of healthcare workers (e.g., latex allergy, blood-borne pathogens)
7. Factors that influence worker rehabilitation and return to work
8. Effectiveness of ergonomic strategies to reduce worker injury and illness
9. Effectiveness of case management approaches in occupational illness/injury
10. Evaluation of critical pathways to effectively improve worker health and safety and to enhance maximum recovery and safe return to work
11. Effects of shift work on worker health and safety
12. Strategies for increasing compliance with or motivating workers to use personal protective equipment

CULTURAL CONNECTION

Some workers, such as Orthodox Jews and Seventh Day Adventists, consider Saturday to be the Sabbath and a holy day. How would you be culturally sensitive to a patient who refuses to seek emergency treatment or use needed electricity for a health condition on the Sabbath?

The priorities will be used to target grant funding by AAOHN for occupational health nursing research. In 1996, the first National Occupational Research Agenda (NORA) was developed, spearheaded by the **National Institute for Occupational Safety and Health (NIOSH)** in partnership with more than 500 groups and individuals. NORA has identified 21 research priorities for occupational health and safety for which its funding is targeted. NORA priorities (NIOSH, 2006) are listed in **Box 38-3**.

MEDIA MOMENT

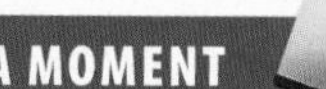

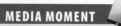

***Roger and Me* (1989)**

Roger and Me is a documentary directed and narrated by Michael Moore. When his hometown of Flint, Michigan, is devastated by a plant closure initiated by U.S. corporate giant General Motors, Moore attempts to interview GM Chairman Roger B. Smith, the elusive Roger of the film's title. The film is loosely structured around Moore's odyssey to track down the corporate titan for an interview. Throughout the movie, Moore encounters the disenfranchised poor and the unemployed. What results is a devastating look at the victims of downsizing in the midst of the 1980s economic boom. The documentary asks a simple question: What is corporate America's responsibility to the country's citizens?

BOX 38-3 National Occupational Research Agenda Priority Research Areas

Category	Areas
Disease and injury	Allergic and irritant dermatitis
	Asthma and chronic obstructive pulmonary disease
	Fertility and pregnancy abnormalities
	Hearing loss
	Infectious diseases
	Low back disorders
	Musculoskeletal disorders of upper extremities
	Traumatic injuries
Work environment	Indoor environment and workforce
	Mixed exposures
	Emerging technologies
	Organization of work
	Special populations at risk
Research tools and approaches	Cancer research methods
	Control technology and personal protective equipment
	Surveillance research methods
	Exposure assessment methods
	Risk assessment methods research
	Intervention effectiveness research
	Health services research
	Social and economic consequences of workplace illness and injury

Source: National Institute for Occupational Safety and Health. (2006). *The team document: Ten years of leadership advancing the National Occupation Research Agenda*. Washington, DC: Author.

Definition

In today's work environment, the delivery and management of occupational health services and programs are provided primarily by occupational and environmental health nurses. Collaboration with and referral to related occupational health and safety disciplines to resolve occupational health problems are essential to the practice. By definition, occupational and environmental health nursing is the specialty practice that focuses on the promotion, prevention, and restoration of health within the context of a safe and healthy environment. It includes the prevention of adverse health effects from occupational and environmental hazards. It provides for and delivers occupational and environmental health and safety services to workers, worker populations, and community groups. Occupational and environmental health nursing is an autonomous specialty, and nurses make independent nursing judgments in providing healthcare services (AAOHN, 2004).

Work and Workplace Hazards

Workers are exposed to many workplace hazards that result in illness and injury. There are about 155 million workers in the United States (Bureau of Labor Statistics [BLS], 2014). Each day, an average of 12 individuals die from work-related diseases or injuries on the job—a figure that is at its lowest level since 1970 (OSHA, 2012). Every 12 seconds, a worker is injured; more than 30% of these injuries result in lost time at work, with 8 days being the average time lost (BLS, 2013a). **Table 38-2** shows the highest work-related injuries by specific industry. Occupational injuries alone cost billions of dollars yearly in lost wages and productivity, administrative expenses, health care, and other costs. This figure does not include the cost of occupational illnesses.

TABLE 38-2 Nonfatal Occupational Injury Incidence Rates in the United States by Industry, Private Sector

	Work-Related Nonfatal Injuries (per 100 full-time workers)
Nursing and personal care facilities	13.6
Justice, public order/public safety	10.4
Construction (local government)	10.2
Hospitals	9.2
Air transportation	7.4
Couriers/Messengers	7.1
Beverage/tobacco manufacturing	6.5
Wood product manufacturing	6.5

Each of these 8 industries (ranked by occupational injury rate) reported more than 10,000 injuries in 2012. Air transportation reported the highest rate in the group (13.6 per 100 workers) followed by nursing and personal care facilities (13.0 per 100 workers). Together these 8 industry sectors accounted for about 1.4 million nonfatal injuries, or 29% of the 4.9 million total.

Source: Data from Bureau of Labor Statistics. (2013b). *Nonfatal occupational injuries and illnesses requiring days away from work, 2012.* Retrieved from http://www.bls.gov/news.release/pdf/osh2.pdf.

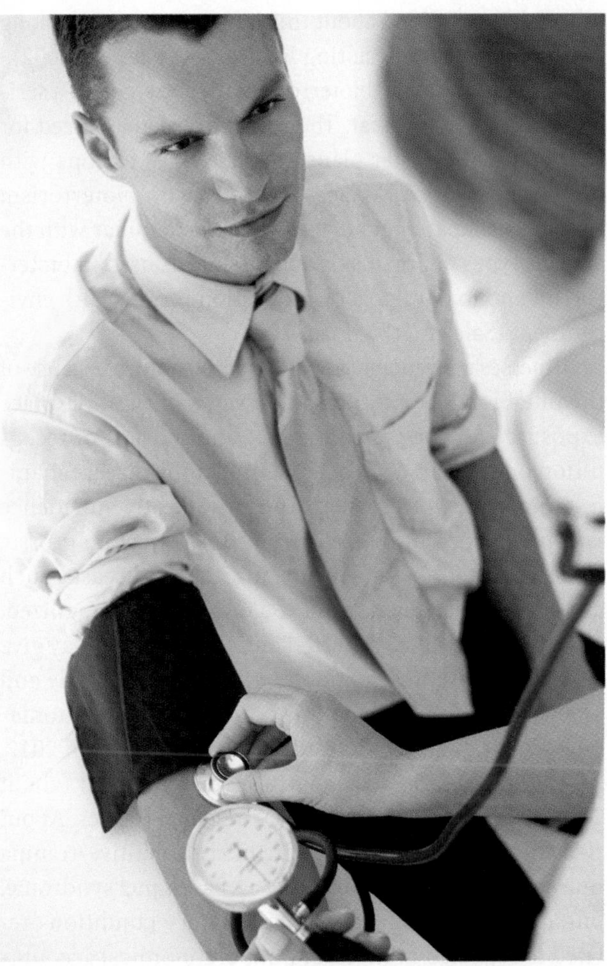

An occupational nurse conducts an assessment in the office setting.

Reports of injuries among nursing home workers and other personal caregivers have increased, with back injuries accounting for more than 40% of these reports. Construction workers have the highest injury rate in private industry, while trucking and warehousing have the highest injury rates in the service sector. Mining injuries, while declining, remain high. The January 2006 mining disaster at the Sago Mine in West Virginia, in which an explosion took the lives of 12 miners, is a grim reminder of the hazards of this occupation. Nearly half of the farm injuries in the United States result in permanent, disabling conditions; back injuries account for more than 40% of these injuries.

Vision and hearing problems due to exposure to noise and chemical exposure are also on the rise. Because of the long latency period between exposure and some of the long-term effects, such as cancer and asbestosis, adequate numbers are not available to account for all industrial hazards contributing to these chronic, and often fatal, diseases. Workers in nuclear power plants have been especially concerned about this issue because of the long period of exposure resulting in diseases (Landels, 2002).

In today's climate, bioterrorism has emerged as a serious occupational threat. There is an immediate need for occupational disaster plans and strategies to cope with bioterrorism in workplaces. Dealing with bioterrorism requires occupational nurses to become familiar with the various types of organisms and chemicals used in bioterrorism and to develop a plan of action for the work environment (Salazar & Kelman, 2002).

Illnesses are much more difficult to capture because of the often long latency period between initial workplace exposure and disease occurrence and the lack of recognition on the part of the clinician that the disease manifestations are work related. Thus, the relative incidence and prevalence of occupational illness may be grossly underreported. What this means is that diseases such as skin disorders, which may be more easily recognized, are more likely to be reported and treated. This may give a misleading representation of both the magnitude and severity of work-related illness. Of the 3 million nonfatal occupational injuries and illnesses reported in 2012, 2.8 million (94.8%) were injuries. The remainder (about 200,000 cases or 5.2%) were work-related illnesses. About two-thirds of these illnesses are likely repetitive-trauma musculoskeletal disorders (e.g., carpal tunnel syndrome, bursitis, or other chronic inflammatory conditions related to repeated motions or poor ergonomics) accounting for nearly 34% of lost workdays (OSHA, 2014). The sections that follow examine the eight groups of occupational diseases/injuries as targeted in the NORA priorities (NIOSH, 2006).

Allergic and Irritant Dermatitis

In the workplace, the skin is an important route of exposure to chemicals and other contaminants. According to the BLS, occupational skin diseases—mostly in the form of allergic and irritant (contact) dermatitis—are the second most common type of occupational disease. From 1983 to 1994, the rate of occupational skin diseases increased from 64 to 81 cases per 100,000 workers. Moreover, occupational skin diseases are believed to be severely underreported, such that the true rate of new cases may be many-fold higher than documented.

NOTE THIS!

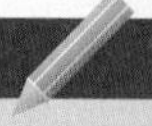

Back injuries are the most prevalent and most costly injury in the occupation of nursing.

THINK ABOUT THIS

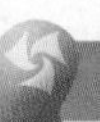

Irritant contact dermatitis is the most common occupational skin disease, usually resulting from toxic reactions to chemical irritants such as solvents and cutting fluids. Allergic dermatitis is estimated to constitute approximately 20% to 24% of all contact dermatitis; it is caused by a wide variety of substances such as latex and some pesticides that trigger an allergic (delayed hypersensitivity) reaction. Contact urticaria (hives occurring soon after an allergen or irritant contacts the skin) is considered here also because it may evolve into contact dermatitis. A number of substances may cause both irritant and allergic dermatitis as well as contact urticaria. For example, latex, which has been reported to cause skin disorders in as many as 10% of exposed healthcare workers, most commonly causes irritant dermatitis; however, it also results in allergic contact dermatitis and, least commonly, contact urticaria.

Because the prognosis of occupational irritant and allergic dermatitis is poor, prevention is imperative. Patients with occupational contact dermatitis often develop chronic skin disease. With thousands of potentially harmful chemicals being introduced into the workplace each year and with the threat of rapidly emerging skin diseases such as latex allergy, interventions need to be developed to reduce irritant and allergic contact dermatitis.

Asthma and Chronic Obstructive Pulmonary Disease

Asthma and chronic obstructive pulmonary disease (COPD—primarily chronic bronchitis and emphysema) are diseases of the lung airways. More than 20 million U.S. workers are potentially exposed to occupational agents capable of causing these diseases, including nearly 9 million workers occupationally exposed to known sensitizers such as toluene diisocyanate (TDI), a major ingredient in polyurethane manufacture, and irritants, such as ammonia, used in the manufacture of dyes, chemicals, plastics, and explosives (Levy & Wegman, 2000). Occupational asthma is now the most common occupational respiratory disease diagnosis among patients examined in occupational medicine clinics (Tarlo et al., 2008).

The Centers for Disease Control and Prevention (CDC; 2012) reports that asthma currently affects more than 18.7 million adults and 7 million children in the United States and is increasing in prevalence. In 2011, asthma and COPD caused more than 138,000 deaths in the United States, making airway diseases the third leading cause of death overall. Mortality from asthma and COPD is increasing annually, as is overall incidence of both disorders. **Occupational asthma** (asthma caused by exposures in the workplace) is estimated at 15–23% of new diagnoses in adults (American Lung Association [ALA], 2010; Kallstrom, 2008). In addition to those who develop occupational asthma as a result of workplace exposure to sensitizers or irritants, many workers are unaware that preexisting asthma may be worsened by the work environment. Each year, the number of asthma cases is increasing, and major new problem areas are emerging (Tarlo et al., 2008). For example, as a result of increased use of protective gloves, due to the introduction of universal precautions and the OSHA regulations on blood-borne pathogens (BBPs), latex allergies have become a major problem for healthcare workers. A significant number of these workers (8–12%, according to OSHA) have developed latex-related asthma.

MEDIA MOMENT 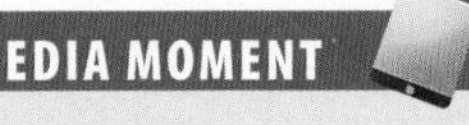

Antz **(1998)**

In an anthill with millions of inhabitants, Z 4195 is a worker ant. Feeling insignificant in a conformity-based system, he accidentally meets beautiful Princess Bala, who has a similar problem on the other end of the social scale. To meet her again, Z switches sides with his soldier friend Weaver—only to become a hero in the course of events. By doing so, he unwittingly upsets the sinister plans of ambitious General Mandible (Bala's fiancé, by the way), who wants to divide the ant society into a superior, strong race (soldiers) and an inferior, to-be-eliminated race (workers). Z and Bala, both unaware of the dangerous situation, try to leave the oppressive system by heading for Insectopia, a place where food paves the streets.

Morbidity from occupational asthma is preventable. Early diagnosis holds substantial promise for effective intervention. Complete resolution of symptoms and pulmonary function abnormalities is most likely when an affected individual's exposure is terminated early in the course of the illness, so early diagnosis holds substantial promise for effective intervention and reduces employer costs.

The relationship of COPD to workplace exposures is also well documented in studies of several occupational agents (e.g., coal dust, grain dust, cotton dust). Investigations of the health consequences of particulate exposure in the general environment, where exposures are at a far lower level than in the workplace, also suggest that COPD resulting from generally dusty conditions may be an important cause of preventable disease and death. Those with lung disease from other causes are especially vulnerable to occupational respiratory hazards. Although cigarettes remain the primary cause of pulmonary diseases in the United States, many occupational and environmental exposures, both by themselves and in combination with smoking, are known to cause COPD. One estimate of the proportion of COPD attributable to occupational exposure in the general population is 15% (Boschetto et al., 2006).

Fertility and Pregnancy Abnormalities

Disorders of reproduction include birth defects, developmental disorders, spontaneous abortion, low birth weight, preterm birth, and various other disorders affecting offspring; they also include reduced fertility, impotence, and menstrual disorders. Infertility is currently estimated to affect more than 2 million American couples. One in 12 couples finds themselves unable to conceive after 1 year of unprotected intercourse. Although numerous occupational exposures have been demonstrated to impair fertility (e.g., lead, some pesticides, solvents), the overall contribution of occupational exposures to male and female infertility is unknown (Paul, 1997). Moreover, observed global trends in men's decreasing sperm counts have increased concerns about the role of chemicals encountered at work and in the environment at large (Winker & Rüdiger, 2006).

Birth defects are the leading cause of infant mortality in the United States, accounting for 20% of infant deaths (more than 8,000) each year. Every year, approximately 120,000 babies are born in the United States with a major birth defect—about 3 per 100 live births. Neural tube defects, which include spina bifida and anencephaly, affect 3,000 pregnancies each year. Of all children in the United States, 14% have some type of developmental disability. The major developmental disabilities of mental retardation, cerebral palsy, hearing impairment, and vision impairment affect approximately 2% of all school-age children.

Most birth defects and developmental disabilities are of unknown cause. The overall contribution of workplace exposures to reproductive disorders and congenital abnormalities is also not known. Although some specific reproductive hazards have been identified in humans, most of the more than 1,000 workplace chemicals that have shown abnormal reproductive effects in animals have not been studied in humans. In addition, most of the 4 million other chemical mixtures in commercial use remain untested. Substances and activities that upset the normal hormonal activity of the reproductive system (e.g., shift work or pesticides that possess estrogenic activity) also need evaluation.

Similarly, the effects of physical factors such as prolonged standing, reaching or lifting, or the interactive effects of workplace stressors and exposures on pregnancy and fertility have not been rigorously investigated.

Although the total number of workers potentially exposed to reproductive hazards is difficult to estimate, three-fourths of employed women and an even greater proportion of employed men are of reproductive age. More than half of U.S. children are born to working mothers. The vast number of workers of reproductive age together with the substantial number of workplace chemical, physical, and biological agents suggest that a considerable number of workers are potentially at risk for adverse reproductive outcomes.

Although the causes of reproductive disorders and adverse pregnancy outcomes are poorly defined, lost productivity and deep suffering by affected individuals and families are evident. The contribution that may be made by occupational factors is largely unexplored, because the reproductive health of workers has only recently emerged as a serious focus of scientific investigation. Identifying reproductive hazards in the workplace has the potential for significantly reducing the multibillion-dollar costs and alleviating the personal suffering associated with disorders of reproduction.

ENVIRONMENTAL CONNECTION

Workers who are employed in highway construction may face a new health threat: silicosis from concrete destruction. Given the more than 163,000 miles of rural and urban roads, which also include the aging interstate system, more workers are involved in this type of occupation. Silicosis is a disabling, nonreversible, and sometimes fatal lung disease caused by inhaling dust containing extremely fine particles of crystalline silica. Crystalline silica is found in materials such as concrete, masonry, and rock. Working with these materials can produce airborne respirable dust, causing lung damage. Unfortunately, silicosis is a disease with a long latency period and usually takes 20 or more years to develop. Other diseases associated with the inhalation of crystalline silica are COPD, connective tissue disease, renal disease, and lung cancer.

While the dangers of silica exposure and silicosis have been well established as risks in the mining, iron, and steel manufacturing industries, the danger to construction workers is less clear. Highway workers seldom use protective face gear, so this problem will be a continuing threat for highway workers. Some states have begun surveillance of silicosis cases, but the issue is not yet a national priority at this time.

Source: Valiante, D. J., Schill, D. P., Rosenman, K. D., & Socie, E. (2004). Highway repair: A new silicosis threat. *American Journal of Public Health, 94*(5), 876–880.

GOT AN ALTERNATIVE?

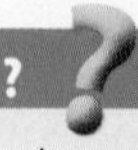

Musicians and other artists often develop health problems because of repetitive movements, poor technique, and poor posture due to the unique nature of their chosen professions. Damage can result from repetitive stress and overuse—that is, practicing the same movements repeatedly or increasing the workload prior to a concert or exhibit.

Dr. Kenneth Brandt founded the Performing Arts Medicine Program at Indiana University Medical Center in the early 1980s. Along with athletic trainers and occupational therapists and other specialists, he assists artists by developing exercises for them and offering pain management. Additionally, Dr. Brandt treats artists with diverse health problems, such as opera singers with throat problems, brass players with dental problems, and guitarists with rheumatism. Patients are treated with a holistic approach, including yoga, stress management, and other complementary therapies.

Source: Performing Arts Medicine Program, Indiana University School of Medicine.

RESEARCH ALERT

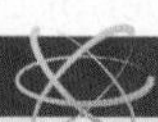

This study examined the effects of smoking, quitting, and time since quitting on absences from work. To do so, the researchers used data from the nationally representative Tobacco Use Supplements of the 1992–1993, 1995–1996, and 1998–1999 Current Population Surveys. The study included full-time workers ages 18–64 years, yielding a sample size of 383,778 workers. A binary indicator of absence due to sickness in the lost week was analyzed as a function of smoking status, including time since quitting for former smokers. Extensive demographic variables were included as controls in all models.

In initial comparisons between current and former smokers, smoking increased absences, but quitting did not reduce them. However, when length of time since quitting was examined, it was discovered that those who quit within the last year, and especially within the last 3 months, had a much greater probability of absences than did current smokers. As the time since quitting increased, absences returned to a rate somewhere between that of never smokers and current smokers. Interactions between health and smoking status significantly improved the fit of the model. Smokers who quit reduced their absences over time but increased their absences immediately after quitting. The benefits from smoking cessation appear to emerge over the long term rather than in the short term regarding work absenteeism.

Source: Sindelar, J. L., Duchovny, N., Falba, T. A., & Busch, S. H. (2005). If smoking increases absences, does quitting reduce them? *Tobacco Control, 14*(2), 99–106.

Hearing Loss

Occupational hearing loss is the most common occupational disease in the United States. It is so common that it is often accepted as a normal consequence of employment. More than 30 million workers are exposed to hazardous noise, and an additional 9 million are at risk from other ototraumatic agents. Occupational hearing loss knows no boundaries with respect to industries. Any worker, young or old, male or female, risks hearing loss when exposed to ototraumatic agents. Once the loss is acquired, it is irreversible.

Although noise-induced occupational hearing loss is the most common occupational disease and is the second most commonly self-reported occupational illness or injury, it has not been possible to create a sense of urgency about this problem. Efforts to prevent occupational hearing loss have been hindered because the problem is insidious and occurs without pain or obvious physical abnormalities in affected workers.

Problems created by occupational hearing loss include (1) reduced quality of life because of social isolation and unrelenting tinnitus (ringing in the ears); (2) impaired communication with family members, the public, and coworkers; (3) diminished ability to monitor the work environment (e.g., warning signals, equipment sounds); (4) lost productivity and increased accidents resulting from impaired communication and isolation; and (5) expenses for workers' compensation and hearing aids.

Infectious Diseases

Infections acquired in the work setting are diverse, with many different modes of transmission. Of particular concern are infectious diseases transmitted by humans (e.g., from patient to worker, from worker to worker) in a variety of work settings. BBPs and airborne pathogens represent a significant class of exposures for the 6 million U.S. healthcare workers. Occupational transmission of BBPs (including hepatitis B and C viruses and the human immunodeficiency virus [HIV]) occurs primarily by means of needlestick injuries but also through exposures to the eyes or mucous membranes. The risk of hepatitis B virus infection following a single needlestick injury with a contaminated needle varies from 2% to more than 40%, depending on the antigen status of the source individual. Similarly, the risk of hepatitis C virus transmission depends on the status of the source and ranges from 3.3% to 10%. Before widespread use of hepatitis B virus vaccine, approximately 8,700 acute cases of hepatitis B virus infection were reported among healthcare workers each year. Although the incidence of occupational hepatitis C virus infection among these workers is unknown, antibody to hepatitis C virus (evidence of previous infection) is found in 1% of hospital-based healthcare workers.

THINK ABOUT THIS

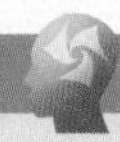

The kind of work we do provides important clues about our health. For example, taxi drivers have an increased prevalence of knee pain, which increases with drive time. Knee pain increases when taxi drivers have constant driving time of greater than 6 hours and can lead to work-related knee joint disorders. Which preventive measures can be taken to reduce the long-term disability risk among taxi cab drivers based on this research?

Source: Chen, J. C., Dennerlein, J. T., Shih, T. S., Chen, C. J., Cheng, Y., Chang, W. P., ... Christiani, D. C. (2004). Knee pain and driving duration: A secondary analysis of the Taxi Drivers' Health Study. *American Journal of Public Health, 94*(4), 575–578.

ETHICAL CONNECTION

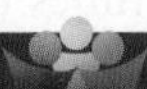

The number of uninsured Americans during 2010 was more than 49.9 million, and 29 million lacked enough insurance to cover all their medical bills (Schoen, Doty, Robertson, & Collins, 2011); this number is expected to fall as the provisions of the Patient Protection and Affordable Care Act (ACA) enable more uninsured persons and families to obtain coverage, but there will still be millions without coverage (Levy, 2014; Schoen et al., 2011). The recent sweeping changes to the healthcare coverage market are still ongoing as of this writing; the full impacts of health insurance reform efforts have yet to be assessed, as political jockeying around the topic continues.

Transmission of TB within healthcare settings, especially multidrug-resistant TB, has re-emerged as a major public health problem. Since 1989, outbreaks of this type of TB have been reported in U.S. hospitals. In addition, among workers of healthcare, social service, and corrections facilities who work with populations at increased risk of TB, hundreds have experienced tuberculin skin test conversions. Reliable data are lacking on the extent of possible work-related TB transmission among other groups of workers at risk for exposure. Some cases of influenza and other communicable respiratory infections are surely the result of exposure to infected persons at work. These are not generally considered occupational diseases, and the proportion acquired at work from coworkers, customers, patients, and the general public is unknown. The cost of lost work time and decreased productivity is likely to be substantial.

Low Back Disorders

Low back pain is one of the oldest and most common occupational health problems reported. Approximately 80% of workers will experience low back pain sometime during their active working life, and 11% of Americans report reduced functional ability. In 2012, back disorders occurred at a rate of 16 per 10,000 workers and accounted for 159,880 nonfatal occupational injuries and illnesses involving days away from work in the United States (BLS, 2013b). The economic costs of low back disorders are staggering. In 2005, the number of workdays lost per year due to back pain was calculated at approximately 149 million, costing the U.S. economy anywhere from $20 to $50 billion annually; at least two-thirds of these lost workdays stem from occupational injuries (Nguyen & Randolph, 2007).

As many as 30% of American workers are employed in jobs that routinely require them to perform activities that may increase their risk of developing low back disorders. For example, female nursing aides and licensed practical nurses were about 2.5 times more likely to experience a work-related low back disorder than all other female workers. Male construction laborers, carpenters, and truck and tractor operators were nearly two times more likely to experience a low back disorder than all other male workers.

MEDIA MOMENT

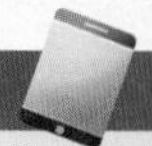

Nickel and Dimed: On (Not) Getting By in America (2001)

By Barbara Ehrenreich, New York, NY: Metropolitan Books.

Ehrenreich left behind her middle-class life as a journalist to live as a member of the working class. In 1999 and 2000, she worked as a waitress in Key West, Florida; as a cleaning woman and a nursing home aide in Portland, Maine; and in a Wal-Mart in Minneapolis. During the application process, she endured routine drug tests and "personality tests"; once on the job, she dealt with constant surveillance and punishing scoldings about minor infractions. She learned how to survive from her coworkers, some of whom slept in their cars, and many of whom suffered from job-related back problems and arthritis. Ehrenreich's income barely covered her month's expenses, even when she worked two jobs. This book is a must-read for exposing the working world for many women in the service industry today.

RESEARCH ALERT

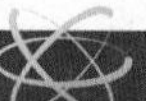

The Sago mining disaster on January 2, 2006, in Sago, West Virginia, claimed 12 men's lives. The mining accident occurred at the beginning of the first shift after the mine had closed for the New Year's holiday weekend. An examination conducted by a mine fireboss at 5:50 a.m. cleared the mine for use. Two carts of miners were making their way into the mine to begin work. The first group entered the mine approximately 8 to 10 minutes before the second.

The explosion occurred at approximately 6:30 a.m. and was heard and felt by many people outside the mine. The 13 trapped men were located about 2 miles inside the mine at approximately 280 feet below ground. Forty-one hours after the incident began, 12 of the miners were found dead in the early morning hours of January 4. One miner, Randal L. McCloy, Jr., was found alive, but in critical condition.

Hearings conducted during 2006 tentatively named the following as contributing causes of the explosion and fatalities:

- Sparks from restarting machinery after holiday.
- Use of "Omega blocks," a dense foam product, to seal the mine, rather than the required concrete blocks. The deputy director of the West Virginia Office of Miners' Health, Safety and Training told the state board of that group, "The seals, made with foam, could withhold pressures of five pounds per square inch."
- A lightning strike and seismic activity. Weatherbug, a Germantown, Maryland–headquartered weather tracking system reported on January 6, 2006, "The evidence suggests that the lightning strike could have caused the explosion due to the correlation between the timing and location of the lightning strike and seismic activity."
- Carbon monoxide levels. The levels in the area where the miners were found were in the range of 300–400 ppm when the rescue team arrived. This is near the safe threshold level to support life for 15 minutes. Carbon monoxide poisoning was the likely cause of the miners' deaths.

In 2005, the federal Mine Safety and Health Administration (MSHA) had cited the Sago mine 208 times for violating regulations, up from 68 citations in 2004. Of those, 96 violations were considered significant and substantial. Additionally, West Virginia's Office of Miners' Health, Safety and Training had issued 144 citations to the mine over that year, up from 74 in the previous year.

Some of those citations were for violations that could have been factors in the accident, such as failure to control methane and coal-dust accumulation and failure to properly shore up shafts against collapse. Former MSHA official Davitt McAteer also suggested that restarting operations after a holiday weekend may have caused sparks to ignite an excess buildup of methane gas and coal dust; he also noted that the mine had deficiencies in emergency planning. At least four natural gas wells were in close proximity to the mine. One appeared to be adjacent to the sealed area where the explosion was believed to have occurred.

Source: Mine Safety and Health Administration. (2006, March 9). Emergency mine evacuation. *Federal Register*, pp. 12252–12271.

The diagnosis of low back pain is primarily made by history and physical examination. The possibility of work-related origin must be explored in detail. Occupational factors often associated with the occurrence of low back pain include heavy physical work, static work postures, frequent bending and twisting, lifting, pushing and pulling, repetitive work, and vibrations.

In general, individuals with low back pain recover from an acute episode in a few days to a few weeks, requiring little treatment. Modifying work activities or work restriction may be needed in the short term. However, if indicated, employees with this problem may need to be placed in new jobs, even though this is not usual.

Prevention of work-related low back pain is key and involves several measures. These measures include a work process that is ergonomically sound, optimal work levels, good work organization to reduce repetitive loading and fatigue, and training and education of workers, managers, healthcare providers, and union representatives about disease etiology and control and prevention strategies.

Despite the overwhelming statistics on the magnitude of the problem, more complete information is needed to assess how changes implemented to reduce the physical demands of jobs will affect workplace safety and productivity in the future. A tremendous opportunity exists for prevention efforts to reduce the prevalence and costs of low back disorders.

Musculoskeletal Disorders of the Upper Extremities

Musculoskeletal disorders of the neck and upper extremities from work factors affect employees in every type of workplace and include such diverse workers as food processors, automobile and electronics assemblers, carpenters, office data-entry workers, grocery store cashiers, and garment workers. The highest rates of these disorders occur in the industries with a substantial amount of repetitive, forceful work. Musculoskeletal disorders affect the soft tissues of the neck, shoulder, elbow, hand, wrist, and fingers. These include the nerves (e.g., carpal tunnel syndrome), tendons (e.g., tenosynovitis, peritendinitis, epicondylitis), and muscles (e.g., tension neck syndrome). The costs associated with these disorders are high, including workers' compensation costs and indirect costs (hiring, training, overtime, and administrative costs) incurred annually for these musculoskeletal disorders. The most commonly reported musculoskeletal disorders of the upper extremities affect the hand–wrist region. Carpal tunnel syndrome, the most widely recognized condition, required the longest recuperation period of all conditions resulting in lost workdays.

Traumatic Injuries

Fatal Occupational Injuries

In 2012, 4,383 workers died as a result of work-related injuries (BLS, 2013c). The leading causes of occupational injury fatalities were transportation-related fatal injuries, aircraft incidents, violence (by persons and animals), falls/slips/trips, and equipment. Fatal work injuries in construction and extraction occupations rose for the second year in a row to 838. However, fatal work injuries in transportation and material moving; protective service; management; and farming, fishing, and forestry occupations, as well as military personnel declined.

Nonfatal Occupational Injuries

In 2012, more than 900,000 workers sustained job-related injuries that resulted in lost work time, medical treatment other than first aid, loss of consciousness, restriction of work or motion, or transfer to another job. The leading causes of nonfatal occupational injuries involving time away from work in 2012 were sprains, strains, and tears (BLS, 2013a). Industries experiencing the largest number of serious nonfatal injuries include seven occupations with rates greater than 375 cases per 10,000 full-time workers: transit and intercity bus drivers; police and sheriff department patrol officers; correctional officers and jailers; firefighters; nursing assistants; laborers and freight, stock, and material movers; and emergency medical technicians and paramedics. By way of comparison, the overall private sector rate was 102 cases per 10,000 workers.

Clearly, work-related injuries and fatalities result from multiple causes, affect different segments of the working population, and occur in myriad occupational and industrial settings. The total cost of work-related injuries and fatalities to industry and to society at large has not been fully recognized, but it is estimated to be greater than $121 billion annually.

Work/Workplace Change

The U.S. workplace is rapidly changing and becoming more diverse. Jobs in our economy continue to shift from manufacturing to services, with the service sector now employing 70% of all workers. Major changes are also occurring in the way work is organized. Longer hours, compressed workweeks, shift work, reduced job security, and part-time and temporary work are realities of the modern workplace. New chemicals, materials, processes, and equipment (e.g., latex gloves in health care, fermentation processes in biotechnology) are developed and marketed at an ever-accelerating pace.

Although much has been accomplished in controlling work-related illness and injury and reducing workplace fatalities, more needs to be done to ensure that worksites are safe and healthy for America's workforce (U.S. Department of Health and Human Services [HHS], 2011). *Healthy People 2020* outlines objectives related to reducing work-related risk and injury, improving worker health, supporting research, and increasing efforts in training and education of occupational health and safety professionals (see the *Healthy People 2020* box for selected objectives).

MEDIA MOMENT 

***Working Girl* (1988)**

This witty, romantic look at life in the corporate jungle stars Melanie Griffith as Tess McGill, an ambitious secretary with a unique approach for climbing the ladder to success. When her classy but villainous boss (Sigourney Weaver) breaks a leg while skiing, Tess simply takes over her office, her apartment, and even her wardrobe. She then creates a deal with a handsome investment banker (Harrison Ford) that will either take her straight to the top or finish her off for good.

HEALTHY PEOPLE 2020 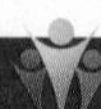

Objectives Related to Occupational Safety and Health

- OSH-1 Reduce deaths from work-related injuries
  OSH-1.1 Reduce deaths from work-related injuries in all industries
  - OSH-1.2 Reduce deaths from work-related injuries in mining
  - OSH-1.3 Reduce deaths from work-related injuries in construction
  - OSH-1.4 Reduce deaths from work-related injuries in transportation and warehousing
  - OSH-1.5 Reduce deaths from work-related injuries in agriculture, forestry, fishing, and hunting
- OSH-2 Reduce nonfatal work-related injuries
  - OSH-2.1 Reduce work-related injuries in private-sector industries resulting in medical treatment, lost time from work, or restricted work activity, as reported by employers
  - OSH-2.2 Reduce work-related injuries treated in emergency departments (EDs)
  - OSH-2.3 Reduce work-related injuries among adolescent workers age 15 to 19 years
- OSH-3 Reduce the rate of injury and illness cases involving days away from work due to overexertion or repetitive motion
- OSH-4 Reduce pneumoconiosis deaths
- OSH-5 Reduce deaths from work-related homicides
- OSH-6 Reduce work-related assaults
- OSH-7 Reduce the proportion of persons who have elevated blood lead concentrations from work exposures
- OSH-8 Reduce occupational skin diseases or disorders among full-time workers
- OSH-9 Increase the proportion of employees who have access to workplace programs that prevent or reduce employee stress
- OSH-10 Reduce new cases of work-related, noise-induced hearing loss

Source: Healthy People 2020. (2011). Leading health indicators: Development and framework. Retrieved from http://www.healthypeople. gov/2020/LHI/development.aspx

NOTE THIS!

With 1,247 fatalities, workers in transportation and materials moving industries suffered more workplace deaths in 2012 than any other profession.

Source: Bureau of Labor Statistics. (2014). Revisions to the 2012 census of fatal occupational injuries (CFOI) counts. Retrieved from http://www.bls.gov/iif/oshwc/cfoi/cfoi_revised12.pdf

Occupational Health Nursing Practice

The practice of occupational and environmental health nursing has changed dramatically over time, with increasing emphasis on autonomous decision making, independent practice, prevention and health promotion, analytical and investigative skills, management, and policy development (Rogers, 2003). This evolution is a result of the need to better deal with issues of changing workforce hazards, necessity for cost containment, and increased efforts to promote health and productivity at work.

This specialty practice has always been closely linked to public health nursing, which provides the practice underpinnings from a synthesis of the public health and nursing sciences directed at population health improvement (Rogers, 2003). Thus, familiarity with the definition of public health nursing is also important. The American Public Health Association (APHA), Public Health Nursing Section (2013) defines public health nursing practice as a systematic process by which:

1. The health and healthcare needs of a population are assessed in order to identify subpopulations, families, and individuals who would benefit from health promotion or who are at risk of illness, injury, disability, or premature death.
2. A plan for intervention is developed with the community to meet identified needs that takes into account available resources; the range of activities

that contribute to health; and the prevention of illness, injury, disability, and premature death.

3. The plan is implemented effectively, efficiently, and equitably.
4. Evaluations are conducted to determine the extent to which the interventions have an impact on the health status of individuals and the population.
5. The results of the process are used to influence and direct delivery of care, deployment of health resources, and the development of local, regional, state, and national health policy and research to promote health and prevent disease.

Occupational and environmental health nursing practice is guided by the *Standards of Occupational and Environmental Health Nursing Practice* (AAOHN, 2004), which are developed and published by the AAOHN. The professional standards provide the framework for evaluating the practice and a mechanism through which accountability with the public is maintained. AAOHN (2003) also has a *Code of Ethics* for occupational health nurses, which acts as a guide for the professional occupational health nurse to maintain and pursue professionally ethical behavior in providing occupational health services.

NOTE THIS!

Women are more likely to be murdered at work than to die in a traffic accident.

To apply practice skills, occupational health nursing practice requires more specific knowledge in fields nurses have some understanding of, including business and management, legal-regulatory fields, and behavioral sciences. In addition, it is essential that nurses be knowledgeable about the occupational health sciences, including industrial hygiene, toxicology, safety, and ergonomics (Rogers, 2003). A brief description of each of these occupational health science areas is provided next.

By definition, industrial hygiene includes the anticipation, recognition, evaluation, and control of occupational hazards, arising in or from the workplace, which may cause sickness, impaired health and wellbeing or significant discomfort, and inefficiency among workers or community citizens. This is done through identifying and quantifying exposures, through sampling techniques, and through implementation and evaluation of control strategies to mitigate exposures.

Toxicology is the study of harmful effects of chemicals on biological systems. In the occupational setting, toxicology is primarily concerned with evaluating human health effects posed by workplace chemical exposures, including dusts, gases, fumes, mists, and vapors. This involves the recognition of routes of exposure, the relativity of these exposures to acute and latent health effects such as burns or cancer, and dose–response relationships.

Safety in the workplace is everyone's responsibility, and safety is concerned with the design and implementation of strategies to prevent and control workplace exposures that result in injury or death.

The term **ergonomics** is derived from two Greek words *ergos,* meaning "work," and *nomos,* meaning "laws"; thus, the laws of work. The National Safety Council defines ergonomics as the science of designing the job and the workplace to fit the worker without undue stress. Within the framework of these definitions, the goal remains the same—that is, to match job demands and requirements to the abilities and capabilities of the worker (Sluchak, 1992). However, note that ergonomics is concerned with matching work and job design to fit the capabilities of most people by adapting the product to fit the user rather than vice versa.

Scope of Practice

The scope of occupational health nursing practice is broad and dynamic and includes the following areas (Rogers, 2003).

Worker/workplace assessment and surveillance focus on identification of potential worker health problems and determination of worker health status. This is accomplished through knowledge of worker jobs and their demands, work processes and related hazards, and working conditions and exposures. Expert occupational health history taking is essential, as are appropriate assessments that help match the job to the worker. In addition to general health information, the history must include an examination of all previous jobs and exposures that may indicate potential interactions (e.g., smoking, antineoplastic agent exposure). An example of an occupational health history form is shown in **Box 38-4**.

In addition, preplacement examinations to evaluate health status related to the work and gather baseline data, periodic examinations to determine any adverse work-related health effects, return-to-work evaluations to make certain the employee is fit for duty, screenings to detect health problems, and surveillance activities to monitor health status are needed.

The workplace also needs to be assessed and monitored to identify potential unhealthy working conditions. A collaborative walkthrough assessment provides for observation of the workforce doing the work, observation of the work processes for each specific job, and observation of the working conditions and work milieu. **Box 38-5** provides elements in the conduct of a worksite assessment.

BOX 38-4 Occupational and Environmental Health History Form

Work History

1. List your current and past longest-held jobs, including the military.

Company	Dates employed	Job title	Known exposures
____________	____________	____________	____________
____________	____________	____________	____________
____________	____________	____________	____________
____________	____________	____________	____________
____________	____________	____________	____________

2. Do you work full-time? No ___ Yes ___ How many hours per week? ___
3. Do you work part-time? No ___ Yes ___ How many hours per week? ___
4. Please describe any health problems or injuries that you have experienced in connection with your present or last jobs:
5. Have you ever had to change jobs due to health problems or injuries? If so, have any of your coworkers experienced similar problems?
6. In what type of business do you work currently?
7. Describe your work:
8. Have you had any current or past exposure (through breathing or touching) to any of the following?

___ acids ___ carbon ___ dichlorobenzene ___ manganese ___ pesticides ___ toluene

___ alcohols ___ tetrachloride ___ ethylene dibromide ___ mercury ___ phenol ___ TDI or MDI

___ alkalis ___ chlorinated naphthalenes ___ ethylene dichloride ___ methylene ___ phosgene ___ trichloroethylene

___ ammonia ___ fiberglass ___ chloride ___ radiation ___ trinitrotoluene

___ arsenic ___ chloroform ___ halothane ___ nickel ___ rock dust ___ vibration

___ asbestos ___ chloropurine ___ heat (severe) ___ noise (loud) ___ silica powder ___ vinyl chloride

___ benzene ___ chromates ___ isocyanates ___ PBBs ___ solvents ___ welding fumes

___ beryllium ___ coal dust ___ ketones ___ PCBs ___ styrene ___ x-rays

___ cadmium ___ cold (severe) ___ lead ___ perchloroethylene ___ talc

9. Did you receive any safety training about these agents?
10. Are you involved in any work processes, such as grinding, welding, soldering, or polishing, that create dust or fumes?
11. Did you use any of the following personal protective equipment when exposed?

___ respirator ___ gloves ___ earplugs or muffs ___ safety shoes

___ shield ___ sleeves ___ glasses or goggles ___ boots

___ welding mask ___ coveralls

12. Is your work environment generally clean? Describe:
13. What ventilation systems are used in your workspace?
14. Do the ventilation systems seem to work? Are you aware of any chemical odors in your environment?
15. Where do you eat, smoke, and take your breaks when you are on the job?
16. Do you use a uniform or have clothing that you wear to work only?
17. How is this laundered?
18. How often do you wash your hands at work, and how do you wash them?
19. Do you shower before leaving the worksite?
20. Do you have any physical symptoms associated with work?
21. Are other workers similarly affected?
22. Do you have any home exposures (e.g., pesticides, household cleaners), hobbies, or community exposures (e.g., live near waste site, landfill)? Please describe:

BOX 38-5 Elements of a Worksite Assessment

- The work, work processes, and related hazards, products, exposures
- Work environment (e.g., cleanliness, clutter, ventilation, noise, temperature, lighting, safety signs, wash disposal mechanisms)
- Worker population characteristics
- Staffing and personnel
- Corporate culture and philosophy
- Written policies/procedures for occupational health care
- Safety committee (frequency, interdisciplinary, measurements, recommendations)
- Occupational health and safety programs/services and types of occupational health visits
- Types and expenditures for medical/workers' compensation claims
- Most common illnesses/injuries
- Health-promotion/education programs
- Regulatory compliance with OSHA standards

THINK ABOUT THIS 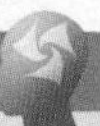

> That the birds of worry and care fly over your head, this you cannot help. But that they build nests in your hair, this you can prevent.
>
> —*Chinese Proverb*

Nurses who care for seriously ill patients can experience various stressors because of personal, interpersonal, healthcare system, and professional variables. We are caregivers who often fail to "care for ourselves"! In the nursing profession, the following stressors can affect our health:

- Personal variables: perfectionism and overinvolvement with patients, compassion fatigues, burnout
- Interpersonal variables: patient and family stressors, such as how the family is responding to the patient's illness; identification with the family and the nurse's own personal family situation
- Healthcare system variables: heavy workloads, scheduling conflicts, compromised time with family; physician–nurse conflicts
- Professional variables: moral and ethical dilemmas between nurse and family such as prolonging life and suffering, adverse effects of treatments, professional liability

Potential consequences of burnout and stress include the following problems:

- Eating disorders
- Gastrointestinal disturbances
- Somatic complaints: headaches, fatigue, insomnia
- Memory disturbances
- Hopelessness
- Depression
- Increased isolation
- Impaired judgment and reasoning
- Self-doubt
- Anger
- Low self-esteem
- Lack of meaning in profession
- Substance abuse
- Detachment from patients and colleagues

HEALTHY ME 

At the end of each day (or night!) ask yourself, "Which areas in my life are unhealthy and what have I done today to keep myself balanced and well?" Keep a journal and write *something* each day in response to this question.

- Physical health: eat well, exercise, rest, use relaxation techniques, do yoga, participate in support groups.
- Emotional health: use meditation; listen to quiet music after work on the drive home; play; speak with colleagues and friends about concerns; read fiction and watch funny movies; connect with friends outside of nursing; take long, hot baths.
- Mental health: set priorities, say *no*, let go of the day and the conflict, keep your mind open to possibilities, and find new hobbies that do not involve nursing.
- Intuitional health: Meditation and relaxation can balance your sense of inner peace, harmony, and wholeness. Be still at least once a day, create your own "sacred space," and learn to "self-comfort" no matter what the setting. Take a walk every day, rain or shine. Think about one good thing that you gave of yourself at work that day.

Contemplative Exercise

Find your sacred place and be still. Focus on the rhythm of your breathing and then read each of the following statements:

- May I offer my care and presence unconditionally, knowing that I may be met with gratitude, indifference, anger, or anguish.
- May I offer love, knowing that I cannot control the course of life's suffering and death.
- May I remain in ease and let go of my expectations.
- May I view my own suffering with compassion as I do the suffering of others.
- May I be aware that my suffering does not limit my good heart.
- May I forgive myself for things left undone.
- May I forgive those who have hurt me.
- May those whom I have hurt forgive me.
- May all beings and I live and die in peace.

Sources: Halifax, J. (2000). Art of Dying III. Open Center and Tibet House, New York City. As cited on p. 54 in Sherman, D. W. (2004). Nurses' stress and burnout. *American Journal of Nursing, 104*(5), 48–56.

The occupational health nurse should be knowledgeable about all work/work processes, the total work environment, and workforce characteristics so that hazards and potential interventions can be adequately identified. In addition, knowledge of the corporate culture and mission related to occupational health and safety, as well as policies, staffing, and programmatic initiatives, will provide a sense about the relative importance of occupational health and safety at the worksite. The occupational health nurse will also want to know the most common illnesses and injuries at the worksite so that appropriate healthcare interventions can be made. These data will also provide information for problem solving, research, and determination of cost-effective healthcare delivery strategies.

During assessment and surveillance activities, preventive and corrective strategies such as engineering, work practice, administrative, and personal protective controls can be discussed as approaches to reduce risk and minimize health problems. Occupational health nurses critically analyze each job task to detect task situations that place employees at risk. They also note work-related risk factors, such as bending or twisting, that may compromise the worker. The occupational health nurse is usually the first person to receive a complaint and must be prepared to recognize potential exposures and initiate exposure monitoring usually performed by an industrial hygienist.

RESEARCH ALERT

A 1999 research study examined associations between workers' reported exposure to occupational hazards and their risk for alcohol use. The sample was drawn from the National Health Interview Survey (NHIS) and included 15,907 working adults. *Occupational hazard exposures* were defined as chemical or biological substances, physical hazards, injury risk, and mental stress. *At-risk drinking* was defined as binge drinking and driving while drinking. Of the workers in the sample, 60% reported exposure to one or more occupational hazards, 31% of the sample reported binge drinking, and 15% drove after drinking too much. In a multivariate analysis that controlled for background of the subjects, workers who reported occupational hazard exposure were 1.2 to 1.4 times more likely to engage in binge drinking than workers without exposures. Similar results were found for drinking and driving and occupational exposure. All multivariate statistical analyses were statistically significant. Findings suggest that workers who perceive themselves as being at risk for occupational hazards are at greater risk for binge drinking and driving after drinking. Occupational nurses can lead workplace initiatives to reduce occupational risk exposures and, at the same time, reduce risks for workers at risk for alcohol consumption.

Source: Conrad, K. M., Furner, S. E., & Qian, Y. (1999). Occupational hazard exposure and at risk drinking. *American Association of Occupational Health Nurses Journal, 47*(1), 9–16.

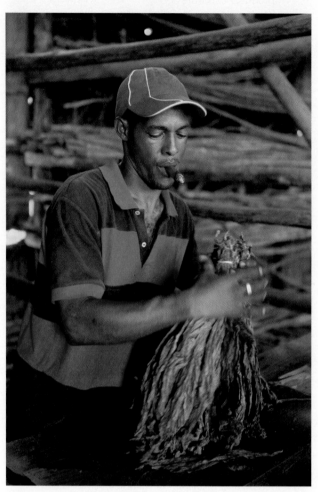

Man working in a cigar factory.

Occupational health and primary care for both occupational and nonoccupational illness and injury is provided in most worksites by the occupational health nurse within the context of a collaborative, multidisciplinary approach. Direct care is provided for emergency or urgent illness and injury (e.g., burns, head injuries), work-related acute illness and injury (e.g., back strain), minor health problems (e.g., headaches, lacerations), healthcare monitoring (e.g., high blood pressure), and preventive health care (e.g., immunizations, breast cancer screening). Also included here are mandatory or special programs such as hearing conservation, travel health, or drug and alcohol testing.

Case management is an integral component of occupational healthcare management involving conditions that may be occupational in origin (e.g., from an exposure) or nonoccupational in origin (e.g., cardiovascular disease).

Coordination and management of cost-effective, quality healthcare services from the onset of illness or injury to the return to work or optimal recovery are key. Early intervention and evaluation of outcomes, including cost savings, are essential components that provide for immediate problem identification and engage the worker in care planning from the beginning of the illness/injury to recovery. Early intervention helps prevent fragmented and delayed care by engaging appropriate healthcare providers at the beginning of care rather than later after complications may have developed. Case management requires knowledge of all factors that have an impact on worker health, including financial, spiritual, and cultural issues, and intense follow up.

MEDIA MOMENT

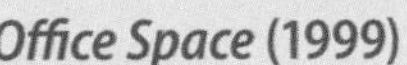

Office Space (1999)

Peter Gibbons just can't seem to catch a break. His girlfriend is cheating on him, he has an obnoxious neighbor, and he's completely miserable in his job as a small cog in a soulless company called Initech. Then he visits a hypnotherapist, who dies just after putting Peter into a state of complete bliss. Free of worrying about making a living, he no longer feels the need to keep his job, just as the company is going through a massive downsizing. His new, carefree attitude only makes him more valuable in the company's eyes, and his friends Michael and Samir are fired instead. Together, they scheme to plant a virus inside Initech's computer system that will pull money into their own bank account.

Health promotion/health protection activities are directed toward enhancing health and increasing the level of wellbeing toward optimal health. Activities are implemented at individual, group, and population levels through educational, behavioral, and environmental levels. Health protection is best described as preventive health behaviors designed to guard or defend an individual or group against specific illness or injury. Health protection is best achieved through a total range of prevention efforts incorporating primary, secondary, and tertiary prevention strategies. Primary, secondary, and tertiary prevention strategies, such as improved personal protective equipment, screening and surveillance activities, and return-to-work or cardiac rehabilitation programs, are used to reduce risks and restore health. Implementing a concept of health that is integrated into the business structure will be key to a healthy environment. This means that health and safety must be a priority in terms of program planning and resource allocation.

Counseling is provided about health with regard to prevention and management of occupational illness and injury, work-related stress, productivity issues, family, conflicts, finances, personal issues, interorganizational relationships, and other areas. Knowing risk factors about employees such as recurrent absenteeism, substance abuse, social withdrawal, or changes in mood or appearance is critical for successful interventions, including referrals. The occupational health nurse is in the best position to provide counseling services to the worker because he or she is the healthcare provider most available to the employee. Some issues may interfere with the worker's ability to work or perform the job, and the employee will probably benefit from some form of intervention, such as listening, supporting, or referral.

The occupational health nurse should have specific counseling knowledge and skills such as problem recognition; building a supportive, trusting, and confidential relationship; crisis intervention approaches; and knowledge about community resources for referral to effectively assist the employee and in some cases the family.

Management and administration, including the development of health policy, is a major role that focuses on ensuring effective occupational health and safety programs and services. Defining a corporate culture that is supportive of a healthy work environment is necessary for an effective occupational health and safety program. Increasingly, the occupational health nurse is assuming a major role in the management and administration of the occupational health unit and in policymaking decisions to ensure effective occupational health and safety programs and services for workers. At the unit level, the occupational health nurse manager is responsible for the overall operational management of the occupational health service, including program planning, organization, staffing, budget development and management, service coordination, and evaluation. Strategic or long-range planning shapes the future of the company and is key to the long-term success and growth of the occupational health program. When engaged in the strategic planning process, the occupational health nurse can use valuable expertise to set forth new ideas and positions and engage in policy development about furthering the occupational health and safety program within the context of the business mission. Understanding the business mission, the needs of the organization, and resource consumption variables is vital to a successful program. Keeping the workforce healthy and productive within the context of the cost containment is a major objective.

Community orientation emphasizes the development of partnerships and collaboration in the delivery of workplace health care. If used, services provided by voluntary or governmental agencies, such as parenting programs, cardiac or drug rehabilitation services, or home health care, can be cost beneficial to both the employee and employer. The occupational health nurse can help the industry create a health partnership with the community by working together on programs. Providing or sponsoring health fairs for workers, their families, and the community is another example of successful partnerships. Use of community programs and development of referral networks will aid the occupational health and safety program.

RESEARCH ALERT

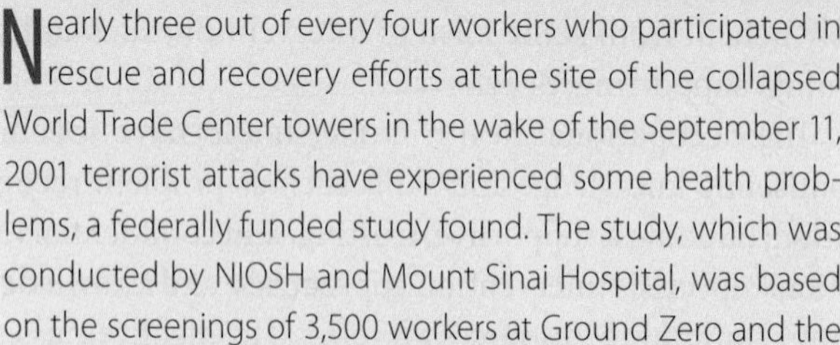

Nearly three out of every four workers who participated in rescue and recovery efforts at the site of the collapsed World Trade Center towers in the wake of the September 11, 2001 terrorist attacks have experienced some health problems, a federally funded study found. The study, which was conducted by NIOSH and Mount Sinai Hospital, was based on the screenings of 3,500 workers at Ground Zero and the Staten Island landfill, where tons of debris were trucked after the attacks. The preliminary results, based on 250 of the first screenings, suggest lingering health issues for a majority of the workers, and a delayed diagnosis for many.

"Seventy-three percent of the sample had ear, nose, and throat symptoms, or abnormal ear, nose, and throat physical exam findings, or both," said Dr. Robin Herbert, codirector of the screening program. Herbert said 57% of those tested had lung problems and 20% had symptoms of posttraumatic stress disorder.

An estimated 35,000 workers—who responded from all across the country after the worst terrorist attacks on U.S. soil—were exposed to concrete dust that may have contained asbestos, lead, fiberglass, and other particles released when the twin towers collapsed after being hit by two hijacked aircraft.

Source: Herbert, R., Moline, J., Skloot, G., Metzger, K., Baron, S., Luft, B., ... Levin, S. M. (2006). The World Trade Center disaster and the health of workers: Five-year assessment of a unique medical screening program. *Environmental Health Perspectives, 114*(12), 1853–1858.

NOTE THIS!

Since the war in Iraq began, the number of veterans returning home with limb amputations has increased dramatically. Prosthetic science has exploded, with NASA-tested titanium and carbon fiber that is strong and light enough for artificial limb replacement being developed. Today's artificial limb for an above-the-knee amputee will typically weigh 5 pounds; in previous years, it was twice as heavy. This makes it easier for an amputee to move. In addition, today's prosthesis contains a microprocessor that enhances life-like movement. These microprocessors anticipate what the person is doing, thereby helping the amputee prepare to absorb the impact as he or she is about to plant the foot on the ground.

Unfortunately, such progress has always come in an era of global conflict. The injuries in World War II inspired products that meshed wood and rubber, as well as the "soft heel," which featured a more flexible toe for the amputee. In the wake of the Vietnam War, prostheses bent and bounced in such a way that energy was returned to the amputee much like a spring on a diving board.

Today's veterans—both men and women—expect to live full lives, including returning to their previous careers and sports. With recent advances in the field of prosthetics, this expectation is becoming more often a reality.

Research and trend analysis is necessary to improve and foster the health and wellbeing of the worker and workforce, to improve working conditions by eliminating or minimizing hazards, and to build a body of occupational health nursing knowledge. Research and practice go hand in hand with the mission to improve and foster the health and wellbeing of the worker and workforce and to improve working conditions by eliminating or minimizing potential or actual hazards. For example, understanding the effects of toxic exposures, designing strategies to prevent work-related accident/injuries or illnesses, evaluating the cost-effectiveness of health interventions, and understanding human behavior and motivation related to health-promotion activities are important occupational health nursing investigations. Occupational health nursing research is essential in both preventive health management and control of workplace hazards.

Legal-ethical monitoring is paramount to ensure a safe and healthful work environment consistent with the OSH Act, related standards, and nurse practice acts. The occupational health nurse must be aware of occupational health and safety statutes and recommend programs and strategies to comply with mandated requirements. The nurse also should work to influence or help develop legislation such as confidentiality of employee health records protection or legislation specific to worker/workplace health protection.

Ethical issues abound in the work environment, and the occupational health nurse is faced with many challenges in ethical decision making. Issues related to confidentiality of employee health records, hazardous exposures, truth telling, inappropriate screening of employees, discrimination, and professional incompetence or illegal practice are but a few of these ethical challenges. As mentioned earlier, the AAOHN (2003) *Code of Ethics* will help guide practice and acts as a framework for implementation of values related to occupational health and safety. The nurse is obligated to always act in the best interest of the worker and provide effective leadership skills in ethical health care. In this role, the occupational health nurse not only brings a special expertise to occupational health dilemmas but also structures the issues so that sound and deliberate decisions are made using a reasoned approach.

Occupational Health Nursing Roles

Occupational health nursing roles have expanded enormously (Rogers & Cox, 1998) to match the increased scope of practice. The AAOHN describes the varied roles of occupational health nurses (see **Figure 38-1**).

The **occupational health nurse clinician** provides direct care for both occupational and nonoccupational illness and injuries using established protocols; performs health assessments, screenings, surveillance, and counseling; and conducts workplace walkthroughs/assessments and exposure follow up.

The **occupational health nurse case manager** coordinates healthcare services for the employee from the onset of injury or illness to a safe return to work or an optimal alternative. Quality outcome-focused care is delivered in a cost-effective manner.

The **occupational health nurse coordinator** functions as the single occupational health nurse for a company responsible for the occupational and environmental health and safety services. The occupational health nurse coordinator conducts needs assessments of the patient population and worksite and develops programs designed to address these needs. Evaluation is a component of the process.

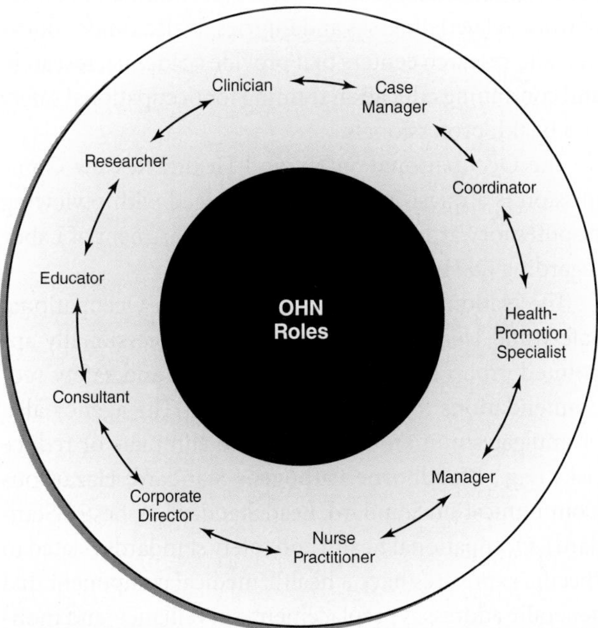

Figure 38-1 Occupational health nursing roles.

The **occupational health nurse health-promotion specialist** has primary responsibility for the overall management of the health-promotion program. This includes the development of a comprehensive program that meets the needs of the workforce population within the context of supporting organizational business objectives for a healthy workforce and work environment. These initiatives might include exercise, nutrition, or smoking-cessation programs.

The **occupational health nurse manager** is responsible for setting occupational health unit policy and directing, administering, and evaluating an occupational and environmental health and safety service. This includes the operational management of the occupational health unit, financial management consistent with organizational goals and objectives, and quality improvement of occupational health services.

The **occupational health nurse practitioner** uses independent and collaborative critical judgments in conducting health assessments, making differential diagnoses, promoting optimal health, and providing pharmacological and nonpharmacological treatments in the direct management of acute and chronic illness and injuries within the scope of state regulations. Services may range from preplacement physical examinations to comprehensive primary care for employees and their families.

The **occupational health nurse corporate director** functions as a policymaker at the corporate level and develops and directs the overall occupational and environmental health and safety programs in consultation with other health and safety specialists and corporate management. This individual also evaluates quantitative outcomes of occupational and environmental health and safety programs using cost–benefit analysis, engages in strategic planning and trend analysis in occupational and environmental health, and provides vision for the direction of the occupational health and safety program.

The **occupational health nurse consultant** provides advice for developing occupational and environmental health and safety services and for structuring the delivery of services, including managed care and case management. In addition, this individual consults about specific services such as hazard analysis, disability management review, hearing conservation, regulatory programming, and health promotion.

The **occupational health nurse educator** plans curricula appropriate to various levels of educational preparation and has responsibilities for occupational and environmental health nursing curricula and clinical experiences in college or university academic education, continuing professional education, or unit staff development programs. Evaluation is a continuous process.

The **occupational health nurse researcher** develops researchable questions, designs studies, conducts research, writes grants, and disseminates research findings to improve practice and build knowledge in the discipline.

These roles are multi-integrated, meaning that occupational health nurses often act in many capacities at the same time.

Within the knowledge context for role implementation, occupational health nurses must have a lifelong knowledge base in the public health and occupational health sciences (e.g., epidemiology, toxicology, industrial hygiene, safety/ergonomics), environmental health, business and economics, social and behavioral sciences, and legal and ethical parameters of practice. To implement the roles effectively, occupational health nurses must work within an interdisciplinary framework with other health disciplines, typically the industrial hygienist, safety specialist, and occupational medicine physician. These fields are briefly described in **Box 38-6**.

Governmental Influence

Although occupational health nursing practice is governed by state nurse practice acts, other federal and state laws affect these nurses' practice as well. The major law governing occupational safety and health is the OSH Act of 1970. This law was enacted to "assure so far as possible every man and woman in the Nation safe and healthful working conditions and to preserve our human resources." The act is administered by OSHA within the U.S. Department of Labor (although states may administer their own programs with OSHA approval) to do the following:

- Encourage employers and employees to reduce workplace hazards and to implement new or improve existing safety and health programs
- Provide for research in occupational safety and health to develop innovative ways of dealing with occupational safety and health problems
- Establish separate but dependent responsibilities and rights for employers and employees for the achievement of better safety and health conditions
- Maintain a reporting and recordkeeping system to monitor job-related illnesses and injuries
- Establish training programs to increase the number and competence of occupational safety and health personnel
- Develop mandatory job safety and health standards and enforce them effectively
- Provide for the development, analysis, evaluation, and approval of state occupational safety and health programs

Within the legislation for the OSH Act, several bodies were created to help carry out the mandates of the act. OSHA is the agency responsible to set and enforce the rules and regulations of the act and standards the agency develops. NIOSH conducts research and training and makes recommendations for the prevention and control of work-related illnesses and injuries. It also funds education and research centers that provide academic, research, and continuing education training for occupational safety and health professionals.

The Occupational Safety and Health Review Commission is a quasi-judicial body charged with reviewing disputes forwarded to it by the U.S. Department of Labor regarding OSHA inspections.

The National Advisory Committee on Occupational Safety and Health is a consumer and professionally appointed group that makes occupational and safety recommendations to OSHA and NIOSH. The agency also promulgates numerous standards to eliminate or reduce risks (e.g., Bloodborne Pathogens Standard, Hazardous Communication Standard, Lead Standard, Asbestos Standard). Occupational health and safety standards related to specific exposures have a health/medical component that generally addresses preplacement, surveillance, and monitoring activities. In most companies, the occupational

BOX 38-6 Interdisciplinary Fields of Practice Specific to Occupational Health Nursing

Occupational Medicine

The assessment, maintenance, restoration, and improvement of the health of the worker through the principles of preventive medicine, and promotion of worker health and productivity

Industrial Hygiene

The science devoted to the anticipation, recognition, evaluation, and control of environmental factors and stresses associated with work and work operations

Safety

The design and implementation of strategies aimed at preventing and controlling workplace exposures that result in unnecessary injuries and death

Ergonomics

The study of humans at work and the evaluation of the stresses that occur in the work environment and the ability of people to cope with these stresses so that the job demands are matched with human capabilities

health nurse manages implementation of these standards to ensure that employees are monitored appropriately for any adverse work-related health effects.

For example, the Bloodborne Pathogens Standard (29 CFR 1910.1030), established by OSHA in 1992, was designed to eliminate or minimize blood and body fluid exposure. The standard requires the employer to develop and implement an exposure control plan as follows:

- It must be written and accessible to employees.
- Documentation of exposure determination must be included.
- A method for implementing the exposure control plan, including methods of compliance, employee education and training, description of the hepatitis B vaccination program and postexposure follow-up procedures, and recordkeeping and communication procedures, must be provided.
- A procedure must be established for evaluating exposure incidents.

The occupational health nurse assists management in developing an effective program consistent with the standard's elements. Occupational health nurses also serve as consultants to assist in establishing methods of compliance, such as engineering and work practice controls.

The occupational health nurse is usually the person responsible for the development and implementation of the hepatitis B vaccination program and postexposure follow up. The standard requires that the hepatitis B vaccine be offered, at no expense, to all exposed employees. If the employee chooses not to accept the offer of the hepatitis B vaccination, he or she must sign a mandatory declination statement. The postexposure evaluation and follow up are critical to employee safety and health; therefore, the most important component of effective postexposure evaluation is the method for reporting exposures. Exposures must be reported and acted upon immediately. Counseling the employee about the risk of infection, importance of early testing to determine whether transmission has occurred, and recommendations for postexposure prophylaxis and prevention of transmission of disease are essential and should occur over several sessions.

Employee education and training are also provided by the occupational health nurse. Information about the hazards of BBPs and methods to prevent transmission to workers may be introduced at employee orientation. These programs are an ideal time to introduce the method for and importance of appropriate reporting of exposures. The occupational health nurse plays an active role in partnering with OSHA and the employer to reduce morbidity and mortality associated with exposures to BBPs, such as hepatitis B and HIV. Occupational health nurses participate in all aspects of compliance with the BBP Standard, beginning with development and implementation of an exposure control plan and ending with maintaining the health and training records for the appropriate number of years.

Within the OSH Act, the general duty clause states that employers are required to furnish all employees with "employment and a place of employment which are free from recognized hazards that are causing or likely to cause death or serious physical harm." If a specific hazard is not covered by a standard, the general duty clause can be invoked. OSHA also provides consultative services to identify and correct hazards, provide technical assistance, and provide education and training for health and safety personnel. Occupational health nurses must be fully cognizant of all occupational health and safety laws, standards, and the regulatory implications in the workplace.

In addition, the OSH Act requires most employers with 11 or more employees to prepare and maintain records of work-related illnesses and injuries. There are detailed rules and regulations regarding what constitutes a recordable event and how these events are to be recorded. In most instances in which there is an occupational health nurse, he or she is usually delegated this responsibility. Data are recorded in logs that are analyzed in aggregate form (by OSHA and the BLS) to identify companies with high-risk illnesses and injuries that may need enforcement and consultation efforts.

In addition to the OSH Act, examples of other pertinent laws affecting health and safety at the worksite include the following:

- Americans with Disabilities Act of 1990 (ADA): This act is intended to prevent discrimination against persons with disabilities. Under Title I of the act, persons with disabilities are entitled to equal employment opportunities without regard to their disability. Health assessments can be performed only after an offer of employment has been made, and applicants can be evaluated only in terms of their ability to perform essential job functions. In some situations, reasonable accommodations must be made by the employer for the disabled person to perform the work. The occupational health nurse may be actively involved in developing and implementing the company's ADA policy. This is done through the appropriate conduct of health examinations, review of job functions to determine job suitability, and recommendations for job accommodations.

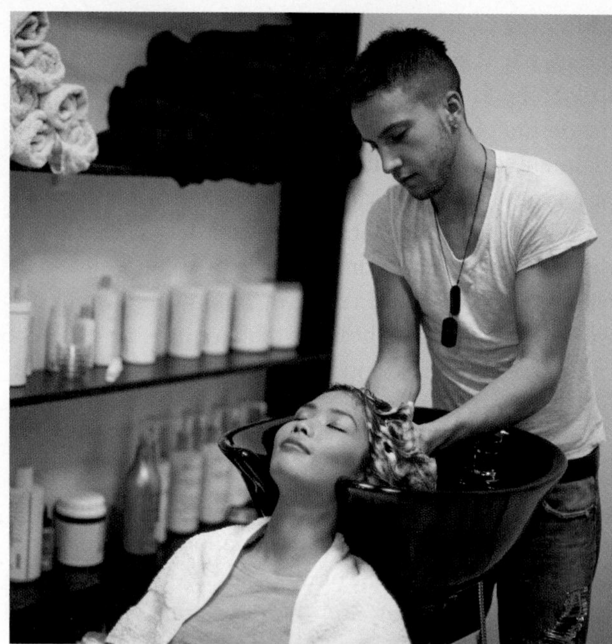

Hairdressers are exposed to hazardous chemicals, such as hair dye, bleach, and other skin and pulmonary irritants on a daily basis. Contact dermatitis and pulmonary problems are among the most common work-related health conditions that require preventive health care, such as well-ventilated mixing areas and the use of disposable gloves. They are also at risk for knee and back injuries.

- Family Medical Leave Act: This act requires employers with 50 or more employees to provide a maximum of 12 weeks unpaid job-related leave in a 12-month period to eligible employees. The occupational health nurse has the responsibility to educate eligible employees about what constitutes an eligible leave of absence and counsel the employee regarding health issues.
- Worker's Compensation: The worker's compensation system in each state and the District of Columbia is designed to cover monetary loss as a result of work-related injuries, including salary; medical, hospital, or funeral expenses; and dependent support in case of occupational death. In turn, there is no employer negligence or fault, safeguarding the employer from legal action. Federal civilian employees are covered by federal statutes.

The occupational health nurse often manages worker compensation claims, ensuring that injured workers are medically treated and managed. In addition, the occupational health nurse monitors the employee's return to work, cautioning against reinjury, but getting the employee back to functional work in a reasonable period.

Professionalism in Occupational Health Nursing

The professional society in occupational health nursing is AAOHN. AAOHN does the following:

- Promotes the health and safety of workers
- Defines the scope of practice and sets the standards of occupational health nursing practice
- Develops the *Code of Ethics* for occupational health nurses with interpretive statements
- Promotes and provides continuing education in the specialty
- Advances the profession through supporting research
- Responds to and influences public policy issues related to occupational health and safety

Its official journal is *Workplace Health & Safety: Promoting Environments Conducive to Well-Being and Productivity* (formerly *AAOHN Journal*).

Education and Certification

One must be a registered nurse to gain entry into professional occupational health nursing practice. Most companies prefer to hire occupational nurses with previous experience in occupational health, public health, or emergency care. As stated earlier, specialty academic education in occupational health and safety is generally offered at the graduate level (master's and doctoral) through NIOSH-funded Occupational Safety and Health Education and Research Centers (**Table 38-3**).

GLOBAL CONNECTION 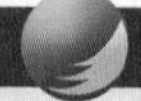

Many hospitals and other healthcare organizations recruit nurses from developing countries to work in U.S. healthcare facilities. What about the healthcare needs of these nurses' native countries? Should we be "poaching" these healthcare professionals from countries that have greater health needs than the United States simply because we are able to provide higher salaries? What do you think?

These centers provide academic, research, continuing education, and outreach programs. Grants support training and education of occupational health and safety professionals, including occupational health nurses, industrial hygienists, physicians, and safety specialists. In addition, a nurse practitioner option in occupational health is offered. Doctoral-level education prepares nurses as scientists in occupational health and safety research.

TABLE 38-3 National Institute for Occupational Safety and Health Education and Research Centers

Deep South Center for Occupational Health and Safety 1530 3rd Avenue South Birmingham, AL 35294 Phone: (205) 934-7178 http://www.soph.uab.edu/dsc/academicprogram
Northern California Education and Research Center 50 University Hall, MC #7360 Berkeley, CA 94720-7360 Phone: (510) 642-8365 http://coeh.berkeley.edu/
Southern California Education and Research Center 650 Charles E. Young South Drive Los Angeles, CA 90095 Phone: (310) 206-2304 http://www.ph.ucla.edu/erc/ced.php
University of Cincinnati Education and Research Center 231 Albert Sabin Way Cincinnati, OH 45267 Phone: (800) 207-9399 http://eh.uc.edu/erc/
Harvard Education and Research Center 677 Huntington Avenue Boston, MA 02115 Phone: (617) 432-2100 https://ecpe.sph.harvard.edu
Illinois Education and Research Center 2121 West Taylor Street Chicago, IL 60612 Phone: (312) 996-6904 http://www.uic.edu/sph/erc/
Johns Hopkins Education and Resource Center School of Hygiene and Public Health 615 North Wolfe Street Baltimore, MD 21205 Phone: (301) 955-0423 http://www.jhsph.edu/research/centers-and-institutes/johns-hopkins-education-and-research-center-for-occupational-safety-and-health/ce/index.html
Michigan Education and Research Center 1205 Beal Avenue Ann Arbor, MI 48109 Phone: (734) 936-0148 http://cohse.umich.edu/
Midwest Center for Occupational Health and Safety 2221 University Avenue SE Minneapolis, MN 55414 Phone: (612) 626-4515 http://www.mcohs.umn.edu/
New York/New Jersey Education and Resource Center 683 Hoes Lane West Piscataway, NJ 08854 Phone: (732) 235-9450 http://ophp.umdnj.edu/Office_of_Public_Health_Practice/Office_of_Public_Health_Practice.html
North Carolina Occupational Safety and Health Education and Research Center 1700 Martin Luther King, Jr. Blvd. Chapel Hill, NC 27516 Phone: (919) 962-2101 http://osherc.sph.unc.edu/
Southwest Center for Occupational and Environmental Health 1200 Herman Pressler Houston, TX 77030 Phone: (713) 500-9238 https://sph.uth.edu/research/centers/swcoeh/
Rocky Mountain Center for Occupational and Environmental Health 391 Chipeta Way Salt Lake City, UT 84108 Phone: (801) 581-7909 http://medicine.utah.edu/rmcoeh/
Northwest Center for Occupational Health and Safety 4225 Roosevelt Way NE Seattle, WA 98105 Phone: (206) 543-1069 http://depts.washington.edu/nwcohs/

(continues)

Mountain and Plains Education and Research Center
13001 E. 17th Place, B119
Aurora, CO 80045
Phone: (303) 724-4409
http://www.ucdenver.edu/academics/colleges/PublicHealth/research/centers/maperc/training/Pages/aboutmaperc.aspx

Sunshine Education and Research Center
13201 Bruce B. Downs Boulevard
Tampa, FL 33612
Phone: (813) 974-6624
http://health.usf.edu/publichealth/erc/index.htm

Central Appalachian Regional Education and Research Center University of Kentucky
111 Washington Ave, Suite 209
Lexington, KY 40536
Phone: (859) 218-2235
http://www.mc.uky.edu/erc/

Heartland Center for Occupational Health and Safety
2420 Old Farmstead Road
Iowa City, IA 52242
Phone: (319) 335-4684
http://www.public-health.uiowa.edu/Heartland/

Source: Educational Resource Centers for Occupational Safety and Health. (2014). ERC Locator. Retrieved from http://niosh-erc.org/courses/locator.shtml

Certification in occupational health nursing is conducted by the American Board of Occupational Health Nursing. Certification is met through educational qualifications, experience, continuing education, and examination.

As the occupational health nurse professionally progresses, the use of technology, in addition to print materials, may be the preferred approach to seek state-of-the-art information.

Nurse-Managed Models in Occupational Health

In 1993, an initiative of the American Nurses Association and the AAOHN about cost-effective healthcare services resulted in the publication *Innovations at the Worksite* (Burgel, 1993), which is still in use today. This document addresses five models of worksite primary health care managed and delivered by occupational health nurses as cost-effective healthcare providers. These models apply principles of health promotion and risk reduction through continuing integration of these strategies into practice. The goal is to provide quality, accessible, and cost-effective care. Following are brief descriptions of each model.

Model 1: One-Nurse Unit, On Site

This model may be the best choice for companies with limited resources, few workplace hazards, or a small workforce. The nurse acts as the in-house expert on health-related issues and develops a network of quality, community-based referrals for services not provided in house.

Model 2: Multiple Nurses, On-Site

This model is ideal for medium to large employers. Essential services are offered on site in a nurse-managed care center. The focus is on primary care and work-related illnesses and injuries.

Model 3: Consortium Model—Company Coalitions

This model is designed for groups of small employers to provide services in a centralized, nurse-managed, free-standing clinic. Essential services are provided on site during expanded hours of service, with a local hospital providing services during off hours through a preferred provider arrangement.

Model 4: Large Employers with Outreach to Small Employers

This model is best for a large employer with on-site services (as in model 2) that provides services to neighboring small employers through a contractual arrangement.

Model 5: Occupational Health Nurse Consultant

This model focuses on providing services by an occupational health nurse acting as consultant to small employers in geographically scattered locations. The occupational health nurse consultant is on site at each employer location on a periodic basis, providing some direct services and coordinating other services through a local hospital and nearby specialty providers.

In all of these models, a basic set of services is provided (e.g., direct care, health surveillance, regulatory compliance, case management, health promotion), either directly or by contracted arrangements. However, depending on the model, services may be modified to reflect the need.

Future Expansions

Environmental Health

More than ever before, the importance of integrating environmental health into occupational and environmental health nursing practice is well recognized. Environmental health can be defined as the interaction between individual and environmental agents that may affect health states. The workplace is included, because this is the place in which many of the most significant hazards occur. Environmental health has been a concept central to general nursing practice since its beginning. The nursing profession has long recognized that health is affected by many variables and has engaged a holistic approach to nursing care. Florence Nightingale viewed the environment as a fundamental aspect of nursing practice, and her interventions focused on modifying the environment as a primary means of promoting health. She cited five essential points in securing the health of individuals: pure air, pure water, efficient drainage, cleanliness, and light (Nightingale, 1869). Nightingale believed that the nurse was responsible for identifying any conditions that could affect the health of individuals and populations, such as ventilation, noise, heat, cold, and cleanliness, and for developing ways to alter the environment so that health and healing could flourish. Environmental health is a natural extension of occupational health nurses to identify environmental health hazards, explore their interaction, and work with members of the interdisciplinary team—management, workers, and communities—to reduce environmental and occupational health risks (Rogers & Cox, 1998).

The Institute of Medicine issued a report describing the importance of this integration and citing the important link between occupational health nursing and environmental health, which is supported by the professional organization AAOHN. Occupational health nurses therefore need additional competencies in environmental health, including the following:

- Understanding the interaction of environmental agents, such as lead and waste products, with human systems, and related signs and symptoms of disease
- Developing prevention, protection, and control strategies for environmental health problems, such as indoor air pollution, and using environmental health resources, including information from the Agency for Toxic Substances and Disease Registry
- Discussing ethical implications of environmental health exposures such as right to know about community toxic spills
- Influencing regulatory controls such as community residential exposures in environmental health as appropriate

APPLICATION TO PRACTICE 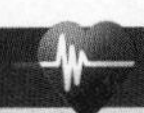

Polluted indoor air has become increasingly recognized as a potential public health problem. As an occupational health nurse, you have been asked to assess a small company with 75 workers who manufacture plant food. The workers have complained of headache, eye and throat irritations, and fatigue. Upon assessment, you find the company housed in a 30-year-old building with inconsistent maintenance. The ventilation system is old and has had cooling problems. The workers complain of inconsistent heating and cooling and "stuffiness." You find a greater-than-expected incidence of asthma, worker sick days, and headaches requiring neurologist care.

1. What are some likely contributing factors to worker illness?
2. What should the nurse suggest that the owner do next in determining the contributing causes to the worker health problems?
3. What role could the occupational health nurse play in the prevention of future problems in this work environment?

Migrant Health

According to the National Center for Farmworker Health (2008), the migrant population is diverse, and its composition varies from region to region. However, it is estimated that 85% of all migrant workers are minorities, of whom most are Hispanic (including Mexican Americans as well as Mexicans, Puerto Ricans, Cubans, and workers from Central and South America). The migrant population also includes African Americans, Jamaicans, Haitians, Laotians, Thais, and other racial and ethnic minorities.

Migrant and seasonal farmworkers hand-pick apples or peaches, harvest asparagus or chilies, stake up tomatoes, dig potatoes or beets, or work in packing plants. Hand labor is especially vital to the production of the blemish-free fruits and vegetables that U.S. consumers demand. The fruit, vegetable, and horticultural industries, in particular, rely on the labor of migrant and seasonal farmworkers. More than 85% of the fruits and vegetables produced in this country are hand harvested and/or cultivated. Although many people believe that fruit and vegetable production is declining in this country, in reality, domestic production has steadily increased in recent years.

Farm labor is seasonal and intensive. Planting, thinning, and harvesting are not year-round activities. However, they are crucial to crop production, and the timeframe in which they must occur is determined by the seasons and the weather. Failure to perform any of these activities at the appropriate time can result in a lost crop. The urgency to accomplish tasks according to nature's timetable compels farmworkers to work in the fields in all seasons and in all weather conditions, including extreme heat, extreme cold, rain, intense sun, and dampness.

Farmworkers' work hours accommodate the crops, not vice versa. Their work often requires stoop labor, working with the soil, climbing, carrying heavy loads, and having direct contact with plants. The plants and the soil are often treated with pesticides and chemical fertilizers. Some plants, such as tobacco and strawberries, exude chemicals that are toxic to humans or that can cause severe allergic reactions such as contact dermatitis. The Environmental Protection Agency (EPA) estimates that at least 300,000 farmworkers experience acute pesticide poisoning each year. Anecdotal reports from clinicians indicate that many cases of pesticide poisoning are unreported because patients do not seek treatment or are misdiagnosed because the symptoms of pesticide poisoning can resemble those of viral infection.

Many of the health problems found in the general population, particularly among minorities and the poor, also affect migrant farmworkers. The hardships of life as a farmworker result in unique challenges to the health of these workers and their families.

Some health concerns are clearly attributable to the occupational hazards of farm work. Dermatitis and respiratory problems caused by natural fungi, dusts, and pesticides are common. Lack of safe drinking water contributes to dehydration and heat stroke. Other health conditions such as TB, diabetes, cancer, hypertension, depression, and HIV, which require careful monitoring and frequent treatment, pose a special problem for farmworkers who must move frequently.

GOT AN ALTERNATIVE?

As an occupational health nurse in a high-tech environment, you might assess that many workers are stressed on the assembly line due to repetitive and boring work. Which kinds of complementary and alternative health interventions could you recommend to these workers that would not affect their work but would increase their relaxation?

Migrant and seasonal workers are a group of workers who could greatly benefit from occupational and environmental health nursing services. This can be done by providing direct-care clinic services, educating workers about occupational health and safety hazards, and initiating workplace/community outreach. The occupational and environmental health nurse can have a major impact on health promotion and protection in this vulnerable population of workers.

Health Promotion in the Workplace

In 2003, the HHS launched an initiative called Steps to a Healthier United States, now called the Healthy Communities Program, which was aimed at promoting healthier behaviors, actions, and programs in the context of both personal and social responsibility. As part of this effort NIOSH introduced Steps to a Healthier U.S. Workforce, now called the NIOSH WorkLife Initiative, which focuses on personal and workplace risk factors (CDC, 2013). The vision of this initiative is to integrate occupational safety and health protection with health-promotion activities into a coordinated system that addresses both workplace and worker health. Given that Americans spend an average of 8–12 hours per day at work, the workplace is an ideal locus for developing a healthier U.S. workforce. This initiative strongly supports the view that all illness and injury should be prevented when possible, controlled when necessary, and treated where appropriate. It emphasizes (1) preventing work-related illness, injury, and disability, and (2) promoting healthy living and lifestyles to reduce and prevent chronic disease. Health-promotion programs have traditionally focused on the individual's personal and lifestyle risk factors, such as lack of physical activity, poor nutrition, and tobacco use, whereas workplace safety and health programs have focused on workplace risks such as chemicals, noise, and other unsafe working conditions. The WorkLife Initiative creates an opportunity for the occupational and safety community and the health-promotion community to develop and implement workplace illness and injury programs collaboratively that prevent workplace illness and injury, promote health, and optimize the health of the U.S. workforce and workplace.

Many occupational and environmental health nurses are already engaged in developing and implementing health-promotion and health protection programs in the workplace. These efforts represent a wonderful opportunity to engage workers and employers in a significant movement to improve the health of America's workforce.

NOTE THIS!

Labor Day Holiday: Why Do We Celebrate It?

Labor Day is usually celebrated with barbecues and picnics and is associated with the beginning of school. We rarely remember that Labor Day was created as a way for us to remember the tremendous labor struggles to improve worker conditions in the United States. In the 19th century, workers often worked 16-hour days, 6 and 7 days a week. Children were commonly used as a labor resource. Injuries were common, thousands of workers died, "caught in the grinding machinery of our growing industries" (Rosner & Markowitz, 1999, p. 1319).

In the labor market of today, despite improvements, workers continue to die in the workplace, while many more are injured, sometimes for life. We should remember all workers, past and present, on Labor Day. Rosner and Markowitz (1999) encourage us to remember the "historical toll in lives and limbs that workers have paid to provide us with our modern prosperity ... the continuing toil is far too high and that workers who died and continue to die in order to produce our wealth" (p. 1320). They deserve to be remembered and honored on Labor Day.

> With employee health costs soaring to more than $1 trillion annually, the presence of an occupational health nurse (OHN) in a work environment can not only guarantee healthy, safe conditions for workers, but also can save employers the costs of illness- and injury-related absenteeism and disability claims.
>
> —*Richard Kowalski, Board President, American Association of Occupational Health Nurses*

Conclusion

Occupational health nursing is a specialty that provides nursing care to worker populations, creating and sustaining healthy and safe work environments. The specialty practice has grown enormously, encompassing expanded roles as independent practitioners, consultants, and policymakers. Expansion to focus on issues external to traditional workplace settings, including environmental health and migrant health, will be a significant and far-reaching opportunity. Prevention and health promotion are the cornerstones of care in occupational health nursing within an interdisciplinary framework. Research is critical in identifying work-related health issues and testing interventions to mitigate the risk. The specialty focus supports a healthy, productive workforce with not only a quality of work life but also a quality of life.

AFFORDABLE CARE ACT 

The Affordable Care Act creates new incentives and builds on existing wellness program policies to promote employer wellness programs and encourage opportunities to support healthier workplaces.

LEVELS OF PREVENTION 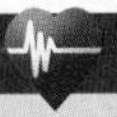

Primary: Conduct a workplace 'walk through' to identify any worker health risks in the work environment

Secondary: Provide a workshop for person's with carpal tunnel syndrome to enhance healing and return to work

Tertiary: Participate in rehab intervention education for workers after cardiovascular surgery

Critical Thinking Activities

1. The next time you go to a fast-food restaurant, observe the potential for occupational hazards in the workers who serve your food. Are there prevention strategies that could prevent those hazards?
2. Ask one of the staff members at your nursing school about workplace hazards in the office. Ask him or her to describe what the most prevalent injury or illness associated with his or her work is. What could be done to prevent this risk?
3. Investigate your nurses association's position on workplace violence in health care. How can nurses protect themselves from this occupational hazard?

References

American Association of Industrial Nurses (AAIN). (1976). *The nurse in industry.* New York, NY: Author.

American Association of Occupational Health Nurses (AAOHN). (2003). *Code of ethics.* Atlanta, GA: Author.

American Association of Occupational Health Nurses (AAOHN). (2004). *Standards of occupational health nursing practice.* Atlanta, GA: Author.

American Lung Association. (2010). *State of lung disease in diverse communities 2010: Occupational lung disease.* Retrieved from http://www.lung.org/assets/documents/publications/solddc-chapters/occupational.pdf

American Public Health Association. (2013). *The definition and role of public health nursing. A statement of the public health nursing section.* Washington, DC: Author.

Boschetto, P., Quintavalle, S., Miotto, D., Lo Cascio, N., Zeni, E., & Mapp, C. E. (2006). Chronic obstructive pulmonary disease (COPD) and occupational exposures. *Journal of Occupational Medicine and Toxicology, 1*(11). Retrieved from http://www.ncbi.nlm.nih.gov/pmc/articles/PMC1513231/

Brown, M. L. (1981). *Occupational health nursing.* Philadelphia, PA: Springer.

Bureau of Labor Statistics. (2013a). *Injuries, illnesses and fatalities: Latest numbers.* Washington, DC: U.S. Department of Labor. Retrieved from http://www.bls.gov/iif/

Bureau of Labor Statistics. (2013b). *Nonfatal occupational injuries and illnesses requiring days away from work, 2012.* Retrieved from http://www.bls.gov/news.release/pdf/osh2.pdf

Bureau of Labor Statistics. (2013c). *Census of fatal injuries summary, 2012.* Retrieved from http://www.bls.gov/news.release/cfoi.nr0.htm

Bureau of Labor Statistics. (2014). Revisions to the 2012 census of fatal occupational injuries (CFOI) counts. Retrieved from http://www.bls.gov/iif/oshwc/cfoi/cfoi_revised12.pdf

Burgel, B. (1993). *Innovations at the worksite: Delivery of nurse-managed primary care services.* Washington, DC: American Nurses Association.

Centers for Disease Control and Prevention (CDC). (2012). *Asthma's impact on the nation: Fact sheet.* Retrieved from http://www.cdc.gov/asthma/impacts_nation/asthmafactsheet.pdf

Centers for Disease Control and Prevention (CDC). (2013). *History of total worker health.* Retrieved from http://www.cdc.gov/niosh/twh/history.html

U.S. Department of Health and Human Services (HHS). (2011). *Healthy people 2020.*

Felton, J. (1985). The genesis of American occupational health nursing: Part I. *Occupational Health Nursing, 33,* 615–621.

Godfrey, H. (1978, November 30). One hundred years of industrial nursing. *Nursing Times,* 1966–1969.

Kallstrom, T. (2008). Focus on allergies & asthma. *AARC Times, 32*(5), 18–19.

Lacey, T. A., & Wright, B. (2009). *Bureau of Labor Statistics: Occupational employment projections to 2018.* Retrieved from http://www.bls.gov/opub/mlr/2009/11/art5full.pdf

Landels, M. (2002). Day in the life: An occupational health nurse at a nuclear power station. *Nursing Times, 98*(12), 65.

Levy, B., & Wegman, D. (2000). *Occupational health: Recognizing and preventing work-related disease.* Boston, MA: Little, Brown.

Levy, J. (2014). U.S. uninsured rate drops so far in first quarter of 2014. Gallup Well-Being Index. Retrieved from http://www.gallup.com/poll/167393/uninsured-rate-drops-far-first-quarter-2014.aspx

McGrath, B. J. (1945). Fifty years of industrial nursing. *Public Health Nurse, 37,* 119–124.

National Center for Farmworker Health. (2008). Migrant and farmworker demographics factsheet. Retrieved from http://www.ncfh.org/docs/fs=Migrant%20Demographics.pdf

National Institute for Occupational Safety and Health (NIOSH). (2006). *The team document: Ten years of leadership advancing the National Occupation Research Agenda* (Publication no. 2006-121). Washington, DC: U.S. Government Printing Office.

Nguyen, T. H., & Randolph, D. C. (2007). Nonspecific low back pain and return to work. *American Family Physician, 76*(10), 1497–1502.

Nightingale, F. (1869). *Notes on nursing: What it is and what it is not.* New York, NY: Dover Press.

Occupational Health and Safety Administration (OSHA). (2012). *Commonly used statistics.* Retrieved from https://www.osha.gov/oshstats/commonstats.html

Occupational Health and Safety Administration (OSHA). (2014). *2014: Prevention of work-related musculoskeletal disorders.* Retrieved from https://www.osha.gov/pls/oshaweb/owadisp.show_document?p_table=UNIFIED_AGENDA&p_id=4481

Paul, M. (1997). Occupational reproductive hazards. *Lancet, 349*(9062), 1385–1388.

Rogers, B. (2003). *Occupational health nursing: Concepts and practice.* Philadelphia, PA: Saunders.

Rogers, B., Agnew, J., & Pompeii, L. (2000). Occupational health nursing research priorities. *AAOHN Journal, 48*(1), 9–16.

Rogers, B., & Cox, A. (1998). Expanding horizons: Integrating environmental health in occupational health nursing. *AAOHN Journal, 46,* 9–13.

Rosner, D., & Markowitz, W. (1999). Labor Day and the war on workers. *American Journal of Public Health, 89*(9), 1319–1321.

Salazar, M., & Kelman, B. (2002). Planning for biological disasters: Occupational nurses as first responders. *AAOHN Journal, 50*(4), 174–181.

Schoen, C., Doty, M. M., Robertson, R. H., & Collins, S. R. (2011). Affordable Care Act reforms could reduce the number of uninsured US adults by 70 percent. *Health Affairs, 30*(9), 1762–1771.

Slaney, B. (1984). *The development of occupational health nursing.* Philadelphia, PA: Saunders.

Sluchak, T. J. (1992). Ergonomics: Origins, focus, and implementation considerations. *AAOHN Journal, 40*(3), 105–112, 147–149.

Tarlo, S., Balmes, J., Balkissoon, R., Beach, J., Beckett, W., Bernstein, D., ... Heitzer, J. (2008). Diagnosis and management of work-related asthma. *CHEST, 134,* 1S–41S.

Winker, R., & Rüdiger, H. (2006). Reproductive toxicology in occupational settings: An update. *International Archives of Occupational & Environmental Health, 79*(1), 1–10.

Wright, F. S. (1919). *Industrial nursing.* New York, NY: Macmillan.

Index

Note: Page numbers followed by *f*, *t*, and *b* refer to figures, tables, and boxes, respectively.

B

C

D

I

N

Q

T

U